D0448883

High Alert header highlights drugs that pose the greatest risk if administered improperly

...and other special dosages included throughout

cefibuten
ceftizoxime
ceftriaxone
See cephalosporins—3rd generation

cefuroxime
See cephalosporins—2nd generation

⚠ HIGH ALERT

celecoxib (Rx)
(cel-eh-cox'ib)
Celebrex
Func. class.: Nonsteroidal antiinflammatory, antirheumatic
Chem. class.: COX-2 inhibitor
Pregnancy category C (1st/2nd trimesters), D (3rd trimester)

Do not confuse:
CeleBREX/Celexa/Cerebra/Cerebyx

ACTION: Inhibits prostaglandin synthesis by selectively inhibiting cyclooxygenase 2 (COX-2), an enzyme needed for biosynthesis

Therapeutic outcome: Decreased pain, inflammation

USES: Acute, chronic rheumatoid arthritis, osteoarthritis, acute pain, primary dysmenorrhea, ankylosing spondylitis, juvenile rheumatoid arthritis (JRA)

Unlabeled uses: Colorectal adenoma prophylaxis

CONTRAINDICATIONS:
Pregnancy **D** (3rd trimester), hypersensitivity to salicylates, iodides, other NSAIDs, sulfonamides

BLACK BOX WARNING: CABG

Precautions: Pregnancy **C** (1st/2nd trimester), breastfeeding, children <18 yr, geriatric, renal/hepatic disease, hypertension, severe dehydration, bleeding, GI, cardiac disorders, PVD, asthma

BLACK BOX WARNING: GI bleeding/perforation, peptic ulcer disease, MI, stroke

DOSAGE AND ROUTES
Do not exceed recommended dose, deaths have occurred

Acute pain/primary dysmenorrhea
Adult: PO 400 mg initially, then 200 mg if needed on first day, then 200 mg bid on subsequent days, if needed; start with ½ dose in poor CYP2C9 metabolizers
Geriatric: PO use lowest possible dose

Osteoarthritis
Adult: PO 200 mg/day as a single dose or 100 mg bid; start with ½ dose in poor CYP2C9 metabolizers

Rheumatoid arthritis
Adult: PO 100-200 mg bid; start with ½ dose in poor CYP2C9 metabolizers

Ankylosing spondylitis
Adult: PO 200 mg daily or in divided dose (bid); start with ½ dose in poor CYP2C9 metabolizers

Juvenile rheumatoid arthritis (JRA)
Adolescent and child ≥2 yr (>25 kg): PO 100 mg bid; start with ½ dose in poor CYP2C9 metabolizers
Child ≥2 yr (10-25 kg): PO 50 mg bid; start with ½ dose in poor CYP2C9 metabolizers

Colorectal adenoma prophylaxis (unlabeled)
Adult: PO 400 mg bid × 6 mo

Hepatic dose
(Child-Pugh class II)
Adult: PO reduce dose by 50%

Available forms: Caps 50, 100, 200, 400 mg

Implementation
• Do not break, crush, chew, or dissolve caps; caps may be opened and mixed with applesauce, ingest immediately with water
• Administer with food or milk to decrease gastric symptoms
• Do not increase dose

ADVERSE EFFECTS
CNS: *Fatigue, anxiety, depression, nervousness, paresthesia,* dizziness, insomnia
CV: **Stroke, MI, tachycardia, CHF,** angina, palpitations, dysrhythmias, hypertension, fluid retention
EENT: Tinnitus, hearing loss, blurred vision, glaucoma, cataract, conjunctivitis, eye pain
GI: *Nausea, anorexia, vomiting, constipation, dry mouth,* diverticulitis, gastritis, gastro-

Subheadings indicate various administration routes

Common and life-threatening adverse effects grouped by body system

Adverse effects: *italics* = common; **bold** = life-threatening

Mosby's
DRUG GUIDE
for
NURSING
STUDENTS

TENTH EDITION

Linda Skidmore-Roth, RN, MSN, NP

Consultant
Littleton, Colorado

Formerly, Nursing Faculty
New Mexico State University
Las Cruces, New Mexico;
El Paso Community College
El Paso, Texas

ELSEVIER

ELSEVIER
MOSBY

3251 Riverport Lane
St. Louis, Missouri 63043

MOSBY'S DRUG GUIDE FOR NURSING STUDENTS,
TENTH EDITION

ISBN: 978-0-323-08643-1

Notices

Knowledge and best practice in this field are constantly changing. As new research and experience
broaden our understanding, changes in research methods, professional practices, or medical treatment may become necessary.

Practitioners and researchers must always rely on their own experience and knowledge in evaluating
and using any information, methods, compounds, or experiments described herein. In using such information or methods they should be mindful of their own safety and the safety of others, including
parties for whom they have a professional responsibility.

With respect to any drug or pharmaceutical products identified, readers are advised to check the
most current information provided (i) on procedures featured or (ii) by the manufacturer of each
product to be administered, to verify the recommended dose or formula, the method and duration of
administration, and contraindications. It is the responsibility of practitioners, relying on their own experience and knowledge of their patients, to make diagnoses, to determine dosages and the best treatment for each individual patient, and to take all appropriate safety precautions.

To the fullest extent of the law, neither the Publisher nor the authors, contributors, or editors, assume
any liability for any injury and/or damage to persons or property as a matter of products liability, neg-
ligence or otherwise, or from any use or operation of any methods, products, instructions, or ideas
contained in the material herein.

ISBN: 978-0-323-08643-1

Director, eContent Solutions: Robin Carter
Content Development Specialist: Shephali Graf
Content Coordinator: Kevin Korinek

Publishing Services Manager: Pat Joiner-Myers
Project Manager: Stephen Bancroft
Senior Book Designer: Amy Buxton

Printed in the United States of America

Last digit is the print number: 9 8 7 6 5 4 3 2 1

Working together to grow
libraries in developing countries

www.elsevier.com | www.bookaid.org | www.sabre.org

ELSEVIER   BOOK AID International   Sabre Foundation

Consultants

Timothy Loren Brenner, PharmD, BCOP
Clinical Pharmacy Specialist
UPMC Cancer Centers
Pittsburgh, Pennsylvania

Claudia Chiesa, PhD, RPh
Staff Pharmacist
Catalina Pharmacy Mangement Services
Tucson, Arizona

David S. Chun, PharmD
Richmond Heights, Missouri

Shelley Fess, MS, RN, AOCN, CRNI
Assistant Professor of Nursing
Monroe Community College
Rochester, New York

Amanda Gross, RPh
Clinical Pharmacist
University of Colorado Hospital
Aurora, Colorado

Nicholas B. Hampton, PharmD
Clinical Decision Support Pharmacist
BJC HealthCare
St. Louis, Missouri

Joshua J. Neumiller, PharmD, CDE, CGP, FASCP
Assistant Professor
Washington State University
Spokane, Washington

Christopher T. Owens, PharmD, BCPS
Associate Professor and Chair
Department of Pharmacy Practice
Idaho State University College of Pharmacy
Pocatello, Idaho

Adam B. Pesaturo, PharmD, BCPS
Critical Care Pharmacist
Department of Pharmacy Services
Baystate Medical Center
Springfield, Massachusetts

Randolph E. Regal, PharmD, RPh, BS
Clinical Associate Professor
Adult Internal Medicine
University of Michigan Hospitals and College of
  Pharmacy
Ann Arbor, Michigan

Sheila Seed, PharmD, MPh, RPh
Associate Professor of Pharmacy Practice
Massachusetts College of Pharmacy and Health
  Sciences–Worcester/Manchester
Worcester, Massachusetts

Travis E. Sonnett, PharmD, FASCP
Clinical Assistant Professor
Washington State University
Spokane, Washington

Patricia Ann Talbert, RN, AAS
Horticulturist, Aromatherapist, Herbalist
Baxter Regional Medical Center
Mountain Home, Arkansas

Shamin Tejani, PharmD
Clinical Pharmacist
Adelante Healthcare
Phoenix, Arizona

Kristin A. Tuiskula, PharmD, RPh
Assistant Professor
Massachusetts College of Pharmacy and Health
  Sciences
Worcester, Massachusetts

Kristine C. Willett, PharmD
Associate Professor
Massachusetts College of Pharmacy and Health
  Sciences
Manchester, New Hampshire

Preface

Mosby's Drug Guide for Nursing Students, tenth edition, is the most in-depth handbook available for nursing students! Since its first publication in 1996, more than 100 U.S. and Canadian pharmacists and consultants have reviewed the book's content closely. Today, *Mosby's Drug Guide for Nursing Students* is more up-to-date than ever—with features that make it easy to find critical information fast!

NEW FEATURES
- A new four-color design spotlights critical safety-related information.
- Over 20 recent FDA-approved drugs for 2013 located throughout the book and in Appendix A.
- The latest NANDA nursing diagnoses.

NEW FACTS
This edition features thousands of new drug facts, including:
- New drugs and new dosage information
- Newly researched adverse effects
- New Black Box Warnings
- The latest precautions, interactions, and contraindications
- IV therapy updates
- Revised nursing considerations
- Updated patient/family education guidelines
- Updates on key new drug research

ORGANIZATION
This handbook is organized into four main sections:
- Individual drug monographs (in alphabetical order by generic name)
- Drug Categories
- Appendixes
- Illustrated mechanisms and sites of action

The guiding principle behind this book is to provide fast, easy access to drug information and nursing considerations. Every detail—from the cover, binding, and paper to the typeface, four-color design, and appendixes—has been carefully chosen with the user in mind. Here's what you'll find in each section of the handbook:

Individual Drug Monographs
This book includes monographs for more than 4000 generic and trade medications—those most commonly administered by students. Common trade names are given for all drugs regularly used in the United States and Canada, with drugs available only in Canada identified by a maple leaf icon (✤).

Each monograph provides the following information, whenever possible, for safe, effective administration of each drug:

High-alert status: Identifies drugs with the most potential to cause harm to patients if administered incorrectly.

"Tall Man" lettering: Uses the capitalization of distinguishing letters to avoid medication errors and is required by the FDA for drug manufacturers.

Pronunciation: Helps the nurse master complex generic names.

Rx, OTC: Identifies prescription or over-the-counter drugs.

Functional and chemical classifications: Helps the nurse recognize similarities and differences among drugs in the same functional but different chemical classes.

Pregnancy category: FDA pregnancy categories A, B, C, D, and X are noted at the beginning of each monograph, as well as under Precautions or Contraindications depending on FDA category. Appendix D provides a detailed explanation of each category.

Do not confuse: Presents drug names that might easily be confused within each appropriate monograph.

Action: Describes pharmacologic properties concisely.

Therapeutic outcome: Details all possible results of medication use.

Uses: Lists the conditions the drug is used to treat.

Unlabeled uses: Describes drug uses that may be encountered in practice but are not yet FDA approved.

Dosages and routes: Lists all available and approved dosages and routes for adult, pediatric, and geriatric patients.

Available forms: Includes tablets, capsules, extended release, injectables (IV, IM, SUBCUT), solutions, creams, ointments, lotions, gels, shampoos, elixirs, suspensions, suppositories, sprays, aerosols, and lozenges.

Adverse effects: Groups these reactions by alphabetical body system, with common side effects *italicized* and life-threatening reactions in **bold, red type** for emphasis.

Contraindications: Lists conditions under which the drug absolutely should not be given, including FDA pregnancy safety categories D and X.

Precautions: Lists conditions that require special consideration when the drug is prescribed, including FDA pregnancy safety categories A, B, and C.

Black Box Warnings: Identifies FDA warnings that highlight serious and life-threatening adverse effects.

Pharmacokinetics/pharmacodynamics: Features a quick-reference chart of concise facts of pharmacokinetics (absorption, distribution, metabolism, excretion, half-life) and pharmacodynamics (onset, peak, duration).

Interactions: Lists confirmed drug, food, herb, and lab test interactions.

Nursing considerations: Identifies key nursing considerations for each step of the nursing process: Assessment, Nursing Diagnoses, Implementation, Patient/Family Education, and Evaluation, including positive therapeutic outcomes. Instructions for giving drugs by various routes (e.g., IV, PO, IM, SUBCUT, topically, rectally) appear under Implementation, with route subheadings in bold.

Compatibilities: Lists syringe, Y-site, and additive compatibilities and incompatibilities. If no compatibilities are listed for a drug, the necessary compatibility testing has not been done and that compatibility information is unknown. To ensure safety, assume that the drug may not be mixed with other drugs unless specifically stated.

Nursing Alert icon ⚠ : Highlights situations in which the patient could potentially be at risk.

Treatment of overdose: Lists drugs and treatments for overdoses where appropriate.

Drug Categories

The Drug Categories section, following the individual drug monographs, provides general information about the various functional classes to promote learning about the similarities and differences among drugs in the same functional class. It summarizes action, uses, adverse effects, contraindications, precautions, pharmacokinetics, interactions, and nursing considerations for each functional class.

Appendixes

Selected new drugs: Includes comprehensive information on 25 key drugs approved by the FDA during the last 12 months.

Ophthalmic, nasal, topical, and otic products: Provides essential information for 140 ophthalmic, nasal, topical, and otic products commonly used today, grouped by chemical drug class.

Vaccines and toxoids: Features an easy-to-use table with generic and trade names, uses, dosages and routes, and contraindications for 39 key vaccines and toxoids.

Abbreviations and pregnancy categories: Lists abbreviations alphabetically with their meanings and explains the five FDA pregnancy categories.

Immunization schedule: Recommended childhood and adolescent immunization schedules.

Standard Precautions: Precautions used in the care of all patients regardless of their diagnosis or disease.

Illustrated mechanisms and sites of action: These 13 detailed, full-color illustrations are added to help enhance the understanding of the mechanism or site of action for the following drugs and drug classes:
- Anticholinergic bronchodilators
- Antidepressants
- Antidiabetic agents
- Antifungal agents
- Antiinfective agents
- Antiretroviral agents
- Benzodiazepines
- Diuretics
- Laxatives
- Narcotic agonist-antagonist analgesics
- Narcotic analgesics
- Phenytoin
- Sympatholytics

Photo atlas of drug administration: This practical resource for students and practitioners lists standard precautions and provides more than 20 full-color illustrations depicting the physical landmarks and administration techniques used for IV, IM, SUBCUT, and ID drug delivery.

The following sources were consulted in the preparation of this edition:

Blumenthal M: *The Complete German Commission E Monographs: Therapeutic Guide to Herbal Medicines,* Austin, 1998, American Botanical Council.

Brunton L, Lazo J, Parker K: *Goodman and Gilman's The Pharmacological Basis of Therapeutics,* ed 11, New York, 2006, McGraw-Hill.

Clinical Pharmacology [database online], Tampa, 2010, Gold Standard, Inc. http://www.clinicalpharmacology.com. Updated March 2010.

Gahart BL, Nazareno AR: *Intravenous Medications,* ed 29, St. Louis, 2013, Mosby.

McKenry LM, Tessier E, Hogan MA: *Mosby's Pharmacology in Nursing,* ed 22, St. Louis, 2006, Mosby.

Acknowledgments

I am indebted to the nursing and pharmacology consultants who reviewed the manuscript and pages and thank them for their criticism and encouragement. I would also like to thank Robin Carter and Shephali Graf, my editors, whose active encouragement and enthusiasm have made this book better than it might otherwise have been. I am likewise grateful to Pat Joiner-Myers, Stephen Bancroft, and Graphic World Inc. for the coordination of the production process and assistance with the development of the new edition.

Linda Skidmore-Roth

Acknowledgments

Contents

abacavir (Rx)

(aba-ka'veer)
Ziagen
Func. class.: Antiretroviral
Chem. class.: Nucleoside reverse transcriptase inhibitor (NRTI)
Pregnancy category C

ACTION: A synthetic nucleoside analog with inhibitory action against HIV; inhibits replication of HIV by incorporating into cellular DNA by viral reverse transcriptase, thereby terminating the cellular DNA chain

Therapeutic outcome: Decreased symptoms of HIV

USES: In combination with other antiretroviral agents for HIV-1 infection (not to be used with lamivudine or tenofovir)

CONTRAINDICATIONS:

> **BLACK BOX WARNING:** Hypersensitivity, moderate to severe hepatic disease

Precautions: Pregnancy **C,** breastfeeding, child <3 mo, granulocyte count <1000/mm^3 or Hgb <9.5 g/dl, severe renal disease, impaired hepatic function, HLA B5701

> **BLACK BOX WARNING:** Lactic acidosis

DOSAGE AND ROUTES
Adults and adolescents ≥16 hr: PO 300 mg bid or 600 mg daily with other antiretrovirals
Adolescents <16 yr and children ≥3 mo: PO 8 mg/kg bid, max 300 mg bid with other antiretrovirals

Hepatic dose
Adult: (Child-Pugh 5-6) PO oral/sol 200 mg bid

Available forms: Tabs 300 mg; oral sol 20 mg/ml

Implementation
PO route
• Give on empty stomach, q12hr around the clock
• Give in combination with other antiretrovirals with or without food
• Store in cool environment; protect from light; do not freeze

ADVERSE EFFECTS
CNS: *Fever, headache, malaise, insomnia,* paresthesia
GI: *Nausea, vomiting, diarrhea, anorexia, cramps, abdominal pain, increased AST, ALT,* **hepatotoxicity, hepatomegaly with steatosis**
HEMA: Granulocytopenia, anemia, lymphopenia
INTEG: Rash, urticaria, hypersensitivity reactions
META: Lactic acidosis
MISC: Increased CPK, **fatal hypersensitivity reactions**
RESP: Dyspnea

Pharmacokinetics

Absorption	Rapid/extensive (PO)
Distribution	50% plasma protein binding, extravascular space, then erythrocytes
Metabolism	To inactive metabolite
Excretion	Kidneys, feces
Half-life	1^1/$_2$-2 hr

Pharmacodynamics
Unknown

INTERACTIONS
Individual drugs
Do not coadminister with abacavir-containing products
Alcohol: increased abacavir levels; do not use with alcohol
Ribavirin: possible lactic acidosis
Methadone: decreased levels of methadone
Tipranavir: decreased abacavir levels

Drug/lab test
Increased: glucose, triglycerides, GGT

NURSING CONSIDERATIONS
Assessment
• Assess for symptoms of HIV and possible infection, increased temp
• **Assess for lactic acidosis** (elevated lactate levels, increased liver function tests) and severe hepatomegaly with steatosis; discontinue treatment and do not restart

> **BLACK BOX WARNING:** Assess for fatal hypersensitivity reactions: fever, rash, nausea, vomiting, fatigue, cough, dyspnea, diarrhea, abdominal discomfort; treatment should be discontinued and not restarted

⚠ Assess for pancreatitis: abdominal pain, nausea, vomiting, elevated liver enzymes; product should be discontinued because condition can be fatal
• Monitor CBC, differential, platelet count qmo; withhold product if WBC is <4000/mm^3 or platelet count is <75,000/mm^3; notify prescriber of results; monitor viral load and CD4 counts during treatment
• Monitor renal function studies; BUN, serum uric acid, urine CCr before, during therapy; these may be elevated throughout treatment
• Monitor temp q4hr; may indicate beginning of infection

BLACK BOX WARNING: Monitor liver function tests before, during therapy (bilirubin, AST, ALT, amylase, alkaline phosphatase, creatine phosphokinase, creatinine prn or qmo)

Nursing diagnoses
• Infection, risk for (uses)
• Injury, risk for (adverse reactions)
• Knowledge, deficient (teaching)

Patient/family education
• Advise patient to report signs of infection: increased temp, sore throat, flulike symptoms; to avoid crowds and those with known infections
• Instruct patient to report signs of anemia: fatigue, headache, faintness, shortness of breath, irritability
• Advise patient to report bleeding; avoid use of razors or commercial mouthwash
• Inform patient that product is not a cure but will control symptoms
• Inform patient that major toxicities may necessitate discontinuing product
• Instruct patient to use contraception during treatment
• Caution patient to avoid OTC products or other medications without approval of prescriber
• Caution patient not to have any sexual contact without use of a condom; needles should not be shared; blood from infected individual should not come in contact with another's mucous membranes
• Give Medication Guide and Warning Card; discuss points on guide
• Advise patient to notify prescriber if skin rash, fever, cough, shortness of breath, GI symptoms occur; advise all health care providers that allergic reactions have occurred with this product

Evaluation
Positive therapeutic outcome
• Increased CD4 count
• Decreased viral load

abatacept (Rx)
(ab-a-ta'sept)
Orencia
Func. class.: Antirheumatic agent (disease modifying); biologic response modifier
Pregnancy category C

ACTION: A selective costimulation modulator, inhibits production of T-lymphocytes, inhibits tumor necrosis factor (TNF-α), interferon-γ, interleukin-2, which are involved in immune and inflammatory reactions

Therapeutic outcome: Decreased pain, inflammation in joints

USES: Polyarticular juvenile rheumatoid arthritis; acute chronic rheumatoid arthritis that has not responded to other disease-modifying agents; may use in combination with DMARDs; do not use with TNF antagonists (adalimumab, etanercept, infliximab) or anakinra

CONTRAINDICATIONS: Hypersensitivity, TB, viral hepatitis

Precautions: Pregnancy C, breastfeeding, children, geriatric, recurrent infections, COPD

DOSAGE AND ROUTES
Rheumatoid arthritis
Adult: SUBCUT 125 mg within a day after single IV loading dose, then 125 mg weekly, weekly subcut may be initiated without IV loading dose for those unable to receive an infusion; give at 2, 4 wk after first infusion, then q4wk
Adult >100 kg: IV INF 1 g over 30 min; give at 2, 4 wk after first infusion, then q4wk
Adult 60-100 kg: IV INF 750 mg over 30 min; give at 2, 4 wk after first infusion, then q4wk
Adult <60 kg: IV INF 500 mg over 30 min; give at 2, 4 wk after first infusion, then q4wk

Juvenile rheumatoid arthritis (JRA)/juvenile idiopathic arthritis (JIA)
Child/adolescent ≥6 yr >100 kg: IV 1000 mg over 30 min q2wk × 2 doses, then INF 1000 mg over 30 min q4wk starting at wk 8
Child/adolescent >6 yr >75 kg: IV INF 750 mg over 30 min q2wk × 2 doses, then 750 mg over 30 min q4wk starting at wk 8

Child/adolescent ≥6 yr <75 kg: IV INF 10 mg/kg over 30 min q2wk × 2 doses, then 10 mg/kg q4wk starting at wk 8

Available forms: Lyophilized powder, single-use vials 250 mg, sol for injection 125 mg/ml

Implementation
Intermittent IV infusion route
• To **reconstitute,** remove plastic flip top from vial and wipe the top with alcohol wipe; insert syringe needle into vial and direct stream of sterile water for inj on the wall of vial; rotate vial until mixed; vent with needle to rid foam after reconstitution 25 mg/ml; **further dilute** in 100 ml from a 100 ml NS infusion bag/bottle; withdraw the needed volume (2 vials remove 20 ml; 3 vials remove 30 ml, 4 vials remove 40 ml); slowly add the reconstituted Orencia sol from each vial into the infusion bag/bottle using the same disposable syringe supplied; mix gently, discard unused portions of vials; do not use if particulate is present or if discolored; **give** over 30 min; use non–protein binding filter (0.2-1.2 mcg)
• Do not admix with other sol or medications
• Store in refrigerator; do not use expired vials; protect from light

Subcut route
• Use prefilled syringe for subcut only, do not use for IV, only those trained should use this system; allow syringe to warm to room temperature (30-60 min) do not speed up warming process; the amount of liquid should be between the two lines on the barrel, do not use the syringe if there is more or less liquid; use front of thigh, outer area of the upper arm, or abdomen except 2-inch area around the navel, do not inject into tender, bruised area
• Gently pinch skin and hold firmly, insert needle at 45-degree angle, inject full amount in 125 mg syringe, rotate injection sites

ADVERSE EFFECTS
CNS: Headache, asthenia, dizziness
CV: *Hypertension, hypotension*
GI: Abdominal pain, dyspepsia, nausea
INTEG: Rash, *inj site reaction,* flushing, urticaria, pruritus
RESP: *Pharyngitis, cough, URI,* non-URI, *rhinitis,* wheezing
SYST: Anaphylaxis, malignancies, angioedema, serious infections

Pharmacokinetics
Absorption	Unknown
Distribution	Unknown
Metabolism	Increased clearance in obesity (subcut)
Excretion	Unknown
Half-life	Terminal 14.3 days, subcut 85 days, steady state 60 days

Pharmacodynamics
Unknown

INTERACTIONS
Individual drugs
Anakinra: do not use
Atropine, scopolamine, halothane: avoid concurrent use

Drug classifications
Corticosteroids, immunosuppressives: avoid concurrent use
TNF antagonists (adalimumab, etanercept, infliximab): do not use
Vaccines: do not give concurrently; immunizations should be brought up to date before treatment

NURSING CONSIDERATIONS
Assessment
• **RA:** Assess for pain, stiffness, ROM, swelling of joints during treatment
• Assess for latent/active TB before beginning treatment
• Assess for inj site pain, swelling
• Monitor patient's overall health on each visit; product should not be given with active infections
• **Infection:** sinusitis, urinary tract infection, influenza, bronchitis, serious infections have occurred

Nursing diagnoses
• Knowledge, deficient (teaching)
• Pain, chronic (uses)

Patient/family education
• Teach patient that product must be continued for prescribed time to be effective
• Advise patient to use caution when driving; dizziness may occur
• Advise patient not to have vaccinations while taking this product
• Discuss with patient information included in packaging

Adverse effects: *italics* = common; **bold** = life-threatening

Evaluation
Positive therapeutic outcome
• Decreased inflammation, pain in joints; decreased erythrocyte sedimentation rate (ESR)

---

abiraterone
Zytiga
(a-bir-a'ter-one)
Func. class.: Androgen inhibitor
Pregnancy category X

ACTION: Converted to abiraterone, which inhibits CYP17, the enzyme required for androgen biosynthesis; androgen-sensitive prostate cancer responds to treatment that decreases androgens

Therapeutic outcome: Decreases spread of malignancy

USES: Metastatic castration-resistant prostate cancer in combination with prednisone in patients who have received prior chemotherapy containing docetaxel

CONTRAINDICATIONS:
Pregnancy (X), women, children

Precautions:
Adrenal insufficiency, cardiac disease, MI, heart failure, hepatic disease, hypertension, hypokalemia, infection, surgery, ventricular dysrhythmia

DOSAGE AND ROUTES
Adult Males: PO 1000 mg q day with predniSONE 5 mg bid

Hepatic dose
Adult Males: (Child-Pugh B, 7-9) **PO** 250 mg q day with predniSONE; (Child-Pugh C, >10) do not use
Available forms: Tab 250 mg

Implementation
PO route
• Give whole, on empty stomach two hrs before or 1 hr after meals with full glass of water
• Women who are pregnant or may become pregnant should not touch tabs without gloves
• Storage of tabs at room temperature

ADVERSE EFFECTS
CV: Angina, **dysrhythmia exacerbation, atrial flutter/fibrillation/tachycardia, AV block,** chest pain, edema, **heart failure, MI,** hypertension, **QT prolongation, sinus**

tachycardia, supraventricular tachycardia, ventricular tachycardia
ENDO: Hot flashes
GI: Diarrhea, dyspepsia
GU: Increased urinary frequency, nocturia, urinary tract infection
META: Adrenocortical insufficiency, hyperbilirubinemia, hypertriglyceridemia, hypokalemia, hypophosphatemia
MS: Arthralgia, myalgia
RESP: Cough, upper respiratory infection
SYST: Infection

Pharmacokinetics

Absorption	Food increases effect; give on empty stomach; increased effect in hepatic disease
Distribution	99% protein binding
Metabolism	Converted to abiraterone (active metabolite)
Excretion	88% (feces), 5% (urine)
Half-life	Mean terminal half-life 7-17 hr

Pharmacodynamics

Onset	Unknown
Peak	Unknown
Duration	Unknown

INTERACTIONS
Drug classifications
CYP3A4 inhibitors (clarithromycin, atazanavir, nefazodone, saquinavir, telithromycin, ritonavir, indinavir, nelfinavir, voriconazole, ketoconazole, itraconazole); CYP3A4 inducers (carbamazepine, phenytoin, rifampin, rifabutin, rifapentine, phenobarbital): avoid use with this product
CYP2D6 substrate (dextromethorphan, thioridazine): increased action of these products; dose of these products should be reduced

NURSING CONSIDERATIONS
Assessment
• Monitor prostate specific antigen (PSA), serum potassium
• Monitor liver function tests (AST/ALT) baseline and every 2 wk for 3 mo and monthly thereafter in those with no known hepatic disease; interrupt treatment in patients without known hepatic disease at baseline who develop ALT/AST >5 times ULN or total bilirubin >3 times ULN; in baseline moderate hepatic disease, measure ALT, AST, and bilirubin before the start of treatment, every week for the first month,

every 2 weeks for the following 2 months, and monthly thereafter; if elevations in ALT and/or AST >5 times ULN or total bilirubin >3 times ULN occur in patients with baseline moderate hepatic impairment, discontinue and do NOT restart. Measure serum total bilirubin, AST, and ALT if hepatotoxicity is suspected. Elevations of AST, ALT, bilirubin from baseline should prompt more frequent monitoring.
• Monitor musculoskeletal pain, joint swelling, discomfort: Arthritis, arthralgia, joint swelling, and joint stiffness, some severe. Muscle discomfort that included muscle spasms, musculoskeletal pain, myalgia, musculoskeletal discomfort, and musculoskeletal stiffness may be relieved with analgesics
• Assess for signs and symptoms of adrenocorticoid insufficiency; monthly for hypertension, hypokalemia, and fluid retention
• Monitor ECG for QT prolongation, ejection fraction in those with cardiac disease, small increases in the QTc interval such as <10 ms have occurred; monitor for arrhythmia exacerbation such as sinus tachycardia, atrial fibrillation, supraventricular tachycardia (SVT), atrial tachycardia, ventricular tachycardia, atrial flutter, bradycardia, AV block complete, conduction disorder, and bradyarrhythmia

Patient/family education
• That women must not come in contact with tabs, wear gloves if product needs to be handled, pregnancy (X)
• To report chest pain, swelling of joints, burning/pain when urinating

acarbose (Rx)
(a-kar'bose)
Precose
Func. class.: Oral antidiabetic
Chem. class.: α-Glucosidase inhibitor
Pregnancy category B

Do not confuse:
Precose/PreCare

ACTION: Delays the digestion/absorption of ingested carbohydrates by inhibiting α-glucosidase, results in a smaller rise in blood glucose after meals; does not increase insulin production

Therapeutic outcome: Decreased blood glucose levels in diabetes mellitus

USES: Type 2 diabetes mellitus, alone or in combination with a sulfonylurea, metformin

CONTRAINDICATIONS:
Hypersensitivity, breastfeeding, diabetic ketoacidosis, cirrhosis, inflammatory bowel disease, ileus, colonic ulceration, partial intestinal obstruction, chronic intestinal disease, serum creatinine >2 mg/dl

Precautions: Pregnancy **B**, children, renal/hepatic disease

DOSAGE AND ROUTES
Initial dose
Adult >60 kg: PO 25 mg tid with first bite of meal

Maintenance dose
Adult: PO May be increased to 50-100 mg tid; dosage adjustment at 4-8 wk intervals
Adult <60 kg: PO Max 50 mg tid

Available forms: Tabs 25, 50, 100 mg

Implementation
• Give tid with first bite of each meal
• Provide storage in tight container in cool environment

ADVERSE EFFECTS
GI: *Abdominal pain, diarrhea, flatulence, increased serum transaminase level*

Pharmacokinetics
Absorption	Poor systemic
Distribution	Unknown
Metabolism	GI tract
Excretion	Kidneys as intact drug
Half-life	Elimination 2 hr

Pharmacodynamics
Onset	Unknown
Peak	1 hr
Duration	Unknown

INTERACTIONS
Individual drugs
Acetaminophen: increased toxicity combined with alcohol
Digoxin: decreased acarbose effect
Phenytoin: increased hypoglycemia
Baclofen, cycloSPORINE, tacrolimus, isoniazid: increased hyperglycemia

Drug classifications
Androgens, quinolones: increased or decreased glycemic control
Corticosteroids, diuretics, estrogens, oral contraceptives, phenothiazines, progestins, sympathomimetics: digestive enzymes, intestinal

---

absorbents, thiazide diuretics, loop diuretics, corticosteroids, protease inhibitors, atypical antipsychotics, carbonic anhydrase inhibitors: increased hyperglycemia, decreased effect of acarbose

MAOIs, salicylates, fibric acid derivatives, bile acid sequestrants, ACE inhibitors, angiotensin II receptor antagonists, β-blockers, sulfonylureas, insulins: increased hypoglycemia

Drug/herb
Chromium, garlic, horse chestnut: increased hypoglycemia

Drug/lab test
Increased: ALT, AST, bilirubin
Decreased: calcium, vit B_6, Hgb , Hct

NURSING CONSIDERATIONS

Assessment
• Assess for hypoglycemia (weakness, hunger, dizziness, tremors, anxiety, tachycardia, sweating), hyperglycemia; even though this product does not cause hypoglycemia, if on a sulfonylurea or insulin, hypoglycemia may be additive; if hypoglycemia occurs, treat with glucose or if severe, **IV** dextrose or IM glucagon
• Monitor 1 hr postprandial glucose for establishing effectiveness, then glycosylated Hgb q3mo
• Monitor AST, ALT q3mo × 1 yr, and periodically thereafter, if elevated dose, may need to be reduced or discontinued; obtain glycosylated Hgb periodically
• Assess for stress, surgery, or other trauma that may require change in dose

Nursing diagnoses
• Knowledge, deficient (teaching)
• Noncompliance (teaching)
• Nutrition, impaired: less than body requirements, imbalanced (adverse reactions)
• Nutrition, impaired: more than body requirements, imbalanced (uses)

Patient/family education
• Teach patient the symptoms of hypoglycemia, hyperglycemia, and what to do about each
• Instruct that medication must be taken as prescribed; explain consequences of discontinuing the medication abruptly; that insulin may need to be used during stress such as trauma, surgery, fever
• Tell patient to avoid OTC medications, herbal products unless approved by prescriber
• Teach patient that diabetes is a lifelong illness; product will not cure condition; that diet and exercise regimen must be followed

• Instruct patient to carry/wear emergency ID as diabetic
• Teach not to breastfeed
• Inform that GI side effects may occur

Evaluation
Positive therapeutic outcome
• Improved signs, symptoms of diabetes mellitus (decreased polyuria, polydipsia, polyphagia; clear sensorium, absence of dizziness, stable gait)

acebutolol (Rx)
(a-se-byoo' toe-lole)
Apo-Acebutolol ✤, **Gen-Acebutolol** ✤, **Nu-Acebutolol** ✤, **Sectral**
Func. class.: Antihypertensive
Chem. class.: Selective $β_1$-blocker; group II antidysrhythmic (II)
Pregnancy category B

ACTION: Competitively blocks stimulation of β-adrenergic receptors within vascular smooth muscle (decreases rate of SA node discharge, increases recovery time), slows conduction of AV node resulting in decreased heart rate (negative chronotropic effect), which decreases O_2 consumption in myocardium because of $β_1$-receptor antagonism; also decreases renin-aldosterone-angiotensin system at high doses, inhibits $β_2$-receptors in bronchial system (high doses)

Therapeutic outcome: Decreased B/P, heart rate, AV conduction; control of dysrhythmias

USES: Mild to moderate hypertension, management of PVCs

CONTRAINDICATIONS:
Hypersensitivity to this agent or β-blockers; cardiogenic shock, heart block (2nd or 3rd degree), sinus bradycardia, CHF, cardiac failure

Precautions: Pregnancy **B,** breastfeeding, children, major surgery, diabetes mellitus, renal/hepatic/thyroid disease, COPD, asthma, well-compensated heart failure, peripheral vascular disease, abrupt discontinuation, myasthenia gravis, vasospastic angina

DOSAGE AND ROUTES

Hypertension
Adult: PO 400 mg daily or in 2 divided doses; may be increased to desired response; maintenance 200-1200 mg daily in 2 divided doses
Geriatric: PO Max 800 mg daily

Ventricular dysrhythmia
Adult: PO 200 mg bid, may increase gradually; usual range 600-1200 mg daily; should be tapered over 2 wk before discontinuing
Geriatric: PO Max 800 mg daily

Renal dose
Adult: PO CCr 25-49 ml/min, reduce dose by 50%; if CCr <25 ml/min, reduce dose by 75%

Available forms: Caps 200, 400 mg; tabs 100, 200, 400 mg ❦

Implementation
PO route
• Given before meals, at bedtime; tablet may be crushed or swallowed whole; give with food to prevent GI upset; reduced dose in renal dysfunction; check pulse before giving, hold dose and notify prescriber if pulse is <60 bpm
• Store protected from light, moisture; place in cool environment

ADVERSE EFFECTS

CNS: *Insomnia, fatigue, dizziness, mental changes,* memory loss, hallucinations, depression, lethargy, drowsiness, strange dreams, catatonia, headache
CV: Profound hypotension, bradycardia, CHF, cold extremities, postural hypotension, **2nd- or 3rd-degree heart block,** edema
EENT: Sore throat; dry, burning eyes
ENDO: Increased hyper/hypoglycemic response to insulin
GI: *Nausea, diarrhea,* vomiting, **mesenteric arterial thrombosis, ischemic colitis,** flatulence
GU: *Impotence,* decreased libido, dysuria, nocturia, polyuria
HEMA: Agranulocytosis, thrombocytopenia, purpura
INTEG: Rash, flushing, pruritus, sweating, alopecia, dry skin
MISC: Facial swelling, weight gain, decreased exercise tolerance
MS: Joint pain, cramping
RESP: Bronchospasm, dyspnea, wheezing, cough

Pharmacokinetics

Absorption	Well absorbed, rapid, significant first-pass effect
Distribution	Crosses placenta, enters breast milk (small amounts), minimal CNS; protein binding 26%
Metabolism	Liver to diacetolol
Excretion	Urine
Half-life	8-13 hr diacetolol, 3-4 hr acebutolol

Pharmacodynamics

	PO
Onset	1-1½ hr
Peak	2.5-3.5 hr
Duration	12-24 hr

INTERACTIONS

Individual drugs
Calcium, cholestyramine, colestipol: decreased antihypertensive effect
Amiodarone, cimetidine, cloNIDine, diltiazem, haloperidol, hydrALAZINE, methyldopa, prazosin, respirine, verapamil: bradycardia, increased hypotension
Insulin: increased hypoglycemia

Drug classifications
Anticholinergics, calcium channel blockers, cardiac glycosides, diuretics, MAOIs: increased hypotension, bradycardia
Other antihypertensives, NSAIDs: decreased antihypertensive effect
Sulfonylureas: attenuated effects
Theophyllines, β_2-agonists: decreased bronchodilatation
Thyroid hormones: decreased thyroid hormone effect

Drug/herb
Ephedra: decreased antihypertensive effect
Hawthorn: increased acebutolol effect

Drug/lab test
Positive: antinuclear antibodies titer
Increased: serum lipoprotein levels, BUN, potassium, triglyceride, uric acid, LDH, AST, ALT, blood glucose, alkaline phosphatase

NURSING CONSIDERATIONS

Assessment
• Monitor B/P during beginning treatment, periodically thereafter; pulse q4hr; note rate, rhythm, quality; apical/radial pulse before ad-

ministration; notify prescriber of any significant changes (pulse <50 bpm)
• Check for baselines in renal, liver function tests before therapy begins
• Assess for edema in feet, legs daily, monitor I&O, daily weight; check for jugular vein distention, crackles bilaterally, dyspnea (CHF)
• Monitor skin turgor, dryness of mucous membranes for hydration status, especially geriatric

Nursing diagnoses
• Cardiac output, decreased (side effects)
• Injury, risk for (side effects)
• Knowledge, deficient (teaching)
• Noncompliance (teaching)

Patient/family education
⚠ Teach patient not to discontinue product abruptly, severe cardiac reactions may occur, taper over 2 wk; may cause precipitate angina if stopped abruptly
• Advise patient that product may mask signs of hypoglycemia or alter blood glucose levels
• Teach patient not to use OTC products containing α-adrenergic stimulants (such as nasal decongestants, cold preparations); to avoid alcohol, smoking; to limit sodium intake as prescribed
• Teach patient how to take pulse and B/P at home, advise when to notify prescriber
• Instruct patient to comply with weight control, dietary adjustments, modified exercise program
• Tell patient to carry/wear emergency ID to identify product(s) that patient is taking, allergies; tell patient that product controls symptoms but does not cure
• Caution patient to avoid hazardous activities if dizziness or drowsiness is present; that product may cause sensitivity to cold
• Teach patient to report symptoms of CHF: difficult breathing, especially on exertion or when lying down, night cough, swelling of extremities or bradycardia, dizziness, confusion, depression, fever
• Teach patient to take product as prescribed, not to double or skip doses; take any missed doses as soon as remembered if several hours until next dose
• Advise patient to continue with required lifestyle changes (exercise, diet, weight loss, stress reduction)

Evaluation
Positive therapeutic outcome
• Decreased B/P in hypertension (after 1-2 wk)
• Absence of dysrhythmias

TREATMENT OF OVERDOSE:
Lavage, **IV** atropine for bradycardia, **IV** theophylline for bronchospasm, digoxin, O_2, diuretic for cardiac failure, hemodialysis, glucagon for hypoglycemia, **IV** diazepam (or phenytoin) for seizures, calcium chloride, vasopressors

acetaminophen (OTC)
(a-seat-a-mee′noe-fen)
Acephen, Aceta, Aminofen, Apacet, APAP, Apo-Acetaminophen ✿, Apra, Children's Feverall, Equaline Children's Pain Relief, Equaline Infant's Pain Relief, Exdol ✿, Genapap, Good Sense Acetaminophen, Good Sense Children's Pain Relief, Infantaire, Leader Children's Pain Reliever, Mapap, Maranox, Meda, Neopap, Ofirmen, Oraphen-PD, Q-Pap, Q-Pap Children's, Redutemp, Ridenol, Silapap, Tapanol, Tempra, T-Painol, Tylenol, Uni-Ace, Walgreen's Acetaminophen, Walgreen's Non-Aspirin, XS Pain Reliever
Func. class.: Nonopioid analgesic
Chem. class.: Nonsalicylate, paraaminophenol derivative
Pregnancy category B

ACTION:
May block pain impulses peripherally that occur in response to inhibition of prostaglandin synthesis; does not possess antiinflammatory properties; antipyretic action results from inhibition of prostaglandins in the CNS (hypothalamic heat-regulating center)

Therapeutic outcome: Decreased pain, fever

USES:
Mild to moderate pain or fever; arthralgia, dental pain, dysmenorrhea, headache, myalgia, osteoarthritis

CONTRAINDICATIONS:
Hypersensitivity

Precautions: Pregnancy **B; C (IV)** breastfeeding, geriatric, anemia, renal/hepatic disease, chronic alcoholism

DOSAGE AND ROUTES
Adult and child >12 yr: PO/RECT 325-650 mg q4-6hr prn, max 4 g/day; weight ≥50 kg IV 1000 mg q6hr or 650 mg q4hr prn, max single

dose 1000 mg, minimum dosing interval 4 hr; weight <50 kg IV 15 mg/kg/dose q6hr or 12.5 mg/kg/dose q4hr, max single dose 15 mg/kg minimum dosing interval 4 hr, max 75 mg/kg/day from all sources

Child ≥2 yr and <50 kg: IV 15 mg/kg/dose q6hr or 12.5 mg/kg/dose q4hr, max single dose 15 mg/kg, minimum dosing interval 4 hr, max 75 mg/kg/day from all sources

Child 1-12 yr: PO 10-15 mg/kg q4-6hr, max 5 doses/24 hr; RECT 10-20 mg/kg/dose q4-6hr

Neonates: RECT 10-15 mg/kg/dose q6-8hr

Available forms: Rectal supp 80, 120, 325, 650 mg; chewable tabs 80, 160 mg; caps 500 mg; elix 120, 160, 325 mg/5 ml; tabs 160, 325, 500, 650 mg; sol for injection 1000 mg/100 ml; disintegrating tab 80, 160 mg; oral drops 80 mg/10.8 ml; liquid 500 mg/5 ml, 80 mg/ml

Implementation
PO route
• Administer to patient crushed or whole; chewable tabs may be chewed; do not crush or chew EXT REL product
• Give with food or milk to decrease gastric symptoms; give 30 min before or 2 hr after meals; absorption may be slowed
• Shake susp well; check all product concentrations carefully

Intermittent IV infusion route
• No further dilution needed, do not add other medications to vial or infusion device
• For doses equal to single vial, a vented IV set may be used to deliver directly from vial; for doses less than a single vial, withdraw dose and place in an empty sterile syringe, plastic IV container, or glass bottle, infuse over 15 mins
• Discard unused portion, once seal is broken or vial penetrated or transferred to another container, give within 6 hr

ADVERSE EFFECTS
CNS: Stimulation, *drowsiness*
GI: Nausea, vomiting, abdominal pain; **hepatotoxicity, hepatic seizure (overdose), GI bleeding**
GU: Renal failure (high, prolonged doses)
HEMA: Leukopenia, neutropenia, hemolytic anemia (long-term use), thrombocytopenia, pancytopenia
INTEG: Rash, urticaria
SYST: Hypersensitivity
TOXICITY: Cyanosis, anemia, neutropenia, jaundice, pancytopenia, CNS stimulation, delirium followed by vascular collapse, seizures, coma, death

Pharmacokinetics
Absorption	Well absorbed (PO), variable (RECT)
Distribution	Widely distributed; crosses placenta in low concentrations
Metabolism	Liver 85%-95%; metabolites are toxic at high levels
Excretion	Kidneys—metabolites, breast milk
Half-life	3-4 hr

Pharmacodynamics
	PO	RECT
Onset	1/2-1 hr	1/2-1 hr
Peak	1-3 hr	1-3 hr
Duration	3-4 hr	3-4 hr

INTERACTIONS
Individual drugs
Alcohol, carbamazepine, diflunisal, imatinib, isoniazid, lamotrigine, rifabutin, rifampin, zidovudine: increased hepatotoxicity
Colestipol, cholestyramine: decreased absorption of acetaminophen
Warfarin: hypoprothrombinemia; long-term use, high doses of acetaminophen

Drug classifications
Barbiturates, hydantoins: decreased effect; increased hepatotoxicity
NSAIDs, salicylates: increased renal adverse reactions

Drug/herb
St. John's wort: decreased acetaminophen effect
Echinacea: increased hepatotoxicity (rare)

Drug/lab test
Interference: Chemstrip G, Dextrostix, Visidex II, 5-HIAA

NURSING CONSIDERATIONS
Assessment
• Monitor liver function studies: AST, ALT, bilirubin, creatinine before therapy if long-term therapy is anticipated; may cause hepatic toxicity at doses >4 g/day with chronic use
• Monitor renal function studies: BUN, urine creatinine, occult blood; albumin indicates nephritis
• Monitor blood studies: CBC, PT if patient is on long-term therapy
• Check I&O ratio; decreasing output may indicate renal failure (long-term therapy)

Adverse effects: *italics* = common; **bold** = life-threatening

- Assess for fever and pain: type of pain, location, intensity, duration, temp, diaphoresis
- **Assess for chronic poisoning:** rapid, weak pulse; dyspnea; cold, clammy extremities; report immediately to prescriber
- **Assess hepatotoxicity:** dark urine, clay-colored stools, yellowing of skin and sclera; itching, abdominal pain, fever, diarrhea if patient is on long-term therapy
- **Assess allergic reactions:** if rash, urticaria occur, product may have to be discontinued

Nursing diagnoses
- Injury, risk for (side effects)
- Knowledge, deficient (teaching)
- Mobility, impaired physical (uses)
- Pain, acute (uses)
- Pain, chronic (uses)

Patient/family education
⚠ **Teach patient not to exceed recommended dosage; acute poisoning with liver damage may result; acute toxicity includes symptoms of nausea, vomiting, and abdominal pain; prescriber should be notified immediately**
- Inform patient that toxicity may occur when used with other combination products
- Advise patient not to use with alcohol or herbals without prescriber approval
- Teach patient to recognize signs of chronic overdose: bleeding, bruising, malaise, fever, sore throat
- Inform patient that urine may become dark brown as a result of phenacetin (metabolite of acetaminophen)
- Tell patient to notify prescriber for pain or fever lasting more than 3 days

Evaluation
Positive therapeutic outcome
- Decreased pain, use pain scoring
- Decreased fever

TREATMENT OF OVERDOSE:
Product level q4hr, gastric lavage, activated charcoal; administer oral acetylcysteine to prevent hepatic damage (*see acetylcysteine monograph,* p. 13)

acetaZOLAMIDE (Rx)
(a-set-a-zole'-a-mide)
Apo-Acetazolamide ✣, Diamox Sequels
Func. class.: Diuretic carbonic anhydrase inhibitor; antiglaucoma agent, antiepileptic
Chem. class.: Sulfonamide derivative
Pregnancy category C

Do not confuse:
acetaZOLAMIDE/acetoHEXAMIDE,
Diamox/Dobutrex/Trimox

ACTION: Decreases the aqueous humor in the eye, which lowers intraocular pressure by the inhibition of carbonic anhydrase; also inhibits carbonic anhydrase activity in proximal renal tubules to decrease reabsorption of water, sodium, potassium, bicarbonate; decreases carbonic anhydrase in CNS, increasing seizure threshold; prevents uric acid or cysteine buildup in the renal system by the decrease in pH, causing increased urine volume and alkaline urine

Therapeutic outcome: Decreased intraocular pressure; control of seizures; prevention and treatment of acute mountain sickness; prevention of uric acid/cysteine renal stones; decreased edema in lung tissue and peripherally; decreased B/P

USES: Open-angle glaucoma, angle closure glaucoma (preoperatively if surgery delayed), seizures (petit mal, grand mal, mixed, absence), edema in CHF, product-induced edema, acute altitude sickness

CONTRAINDICATIONS:
Hypersensitivity to sulfonamides, severe renal/hepatic disease, electrolyte imbalances (hyponatremia, hypokalemia), hyperchloremic acidosis, Addison's disease, long-term use in closed-angle glaucoma, adrenalcortical insufficiency

Precautions: Pregnancy **C**, breastfeeding, hypercalciuria, COPD, respiratory acidosis, pulmonary obstruction/emphysema

DOSAGE AND ROUTES
Angle closure glaucoma
Adult: PO/**IV** 250 mg q4hr or 250 mg bid, to be used for short-term therapy

Open-angle glaucoma
Adult: PO/IV 250 mg/day in divided doses for amounts over 250 mg or 500 mg **SR** bid, max 1 g/day

Edema in CHF
Adult: PO/IV 250-375 mg/day or 5 mg/kg in AM, give for 2 days, then 1-2 days drug-free
Child: PO/IV 5 mg/kg/day or 150 mg/m^2 in AM

Seizures
Adult: PO/IV 8-30 mg/kg/day in 1-4 divided doses, usual range 375-1000 mg/day; EXT REL not recommended in seizures
Child: PO/IV 8-30 mg/kg/day in divided doses tid or qid, or 300-900 mg/m^2/day, not to exceed 1 g/day

Altitude sickness
Adult: PO 250 mg q6-12hr; EXT REL 500 mg q12-24hr, start therapy 24-48 hr prior to ascent and $\geq$48 hr after arrival at high altitude
Geriatric: PO 250 mg bid; use lowest effective dose

Renal dose
Adult: PO/IV CCr 10-50 ml/min, give dose q12hr; CCr <10 ml/min, avoid use

Available forms: Tabs 125, 250 mg; ext rel caps 500 mg; inj 500 mg

Implementation
• Give in AM to avoid interference with sleep
• Administer fluids 2-3 L/day to prevent renal calculi, unless contraindicated
• Potassium replacement if potassium level is <3.0 ml/dl

PO route
• Do not crush or chew ext rel caps; caps may be opened and sprinkled on food
• Give with food; if nausea occurs, crush tabs and mix with sweet substance to counteract bitter taste

IV route
• Do not use solution that is yellow or has a precipitate or crystals
• **Dilute** 500 mg of product/5 ml or more sterile water for inj; use within 24 hr, **give** at 100-500 mg/min

IV, direct route
• Give over 1 min or more

Intermittent IV infusion route
• May be added to NS, D$_5$W, D$_{10}$W, 0.45% NaCl; **give** over 15-30 min

Additive compatibilities: Cimetidine, ranitidine

Additive incompatibilities: Multivitamins

ADVERSE EFFECTS
CNS: Drowsiness, paresthesia, anxiety, depression, headache, dizziness, confusion, stimulation, fatigue, **seizures**
EENT: Myopia, tinnitus
ENDO: Hyperglycemia
GI: Nausea, vomiting, anorexia, diarrhea, melena, weight loss, **hepatic insufficiency, cholestatic jaundice, fulminant hepatic necrosis,** taste alterations, **bleeding**
GU: Frequency, polyuria, **uremia,** glucosuria, hematuria, dysuria, crystalluria, renal calculi
HEMA: Aplastic anemia, hemolytic anemia, leukopenia, thrombocytopenia purpura, pancytopenia
INTEG: Rash, pruritus, urticaria, fever, **Stevens-Johnson syndrome,** photosensitivity, flushing, toxic epidermal necrolysis
META: *Hypokalemia, hyperchloremic acidosis,* hyponatremia, sulfonamide-like reactions, metabolic acidosis

Pharmacokinetics

Absorption	GI tract—65% if fasting, 75% with food; **IV**—complete
Distribution	Crosses placenta; widely distributed
Metabolism	None
Excretion	Kidneys, unchanged (80% within 24 hr); breast milk
Half-life	2^1/$_2$-5^1/$_2$ hr

Pharmacodynamics

	PO	PO–ext rel	IV
Onset	1^1/$_2$ hr	2 hr	2 min
Peak	8-12 hr	3-6 hr	15 min
Duration	8-12 hr	18-24 hr	4-5 hr

INTERACTIONS

Individual drugs
Amphotericin B, corticotropin, ACTH: increased hypokalemia
Arsenic trioxide, levomethadyl: increased cardiac toxicity if hypokalemia develops
CarBAMazepine, ethotoin: increased osteomalacia
CycloSPORINE: increased toxicity
Diflunisal: increased side effects
Lithium: increased excretion of lithium
Methenamine: decreased acetaZOLAMIDE effect
Primidone: decreased primidone level
Topiramate: increased renal stone formation, heat stroke, avoid concurrent use

Adverse effects: *italics* = common; **bold** = life-threatening

Drug classifications

Amphetamines: increased action

Anticholinergics, folic acid antagonists: increased action of each product

Cardiac glycosides: increased cardiac toxicity if hypokalemia develops

Corticosteroids: increased hypokalemia

Flecainide, memantine, phenytoin, procainamide, quiNIDine, mecamylamine, mexiletine: increased effect of each product

Salicylates: increased toxicity

Drug/lab test

Increased: glucose, bilirubin, calcium, uric acid

Decreased: thyroid iodine uptake

False positive: urinary protein, 17-hydroxysteroids

NURSING CONSIDERATIONS

Assessment

• Assess patient for tinnitus, hearing loss, ear pain; periodic testing of hearing is needed when high doses of this product are given by **IV** route

• **Assess for seizures:** type, location, duration; provide seizure precautions

• Assess fluid volume status: I&O ratio and record, count or weigh diapers as appropriate, distended neck veins, crackles in lung, color, quality, and specific gravity of urine, skin turgor, adequacy of pulses, moist mucous membranes, bilateral lung sounds, peripheral pitting edema; dehydration symptoms of decreasing output, thirst, hypotension, dry mouth, and mucous membranes should be reported

• Monitor electrolytes: potassium, sodium, calcium, magnesium; also include BUN, blood pH, ABGs, uric acid, CBC, blood glucose

• Assess B/P before and during therapy with patient lying, standing, and sitting as appropriate; orthostatic hypotension can occur rapidly

• Monitor blood, urine glucose in diabetic patients; glucose levels may be increased

• Assess for eye pain, change in vision when using product for intraocular pressure

• Assess neurologic status when using product for seizures

• **Assess for decreased symptoms of acute mountain sickness:** headache, nausea, vomiting, dizziness, fatigue, drowsiness, shortness of breath, insomnia

• Assess for cross-sensitivity between other sulfonamides and this product

Nursing diagnoses

• Fluid volume, deficient (side effects)

• Fluid volume, excess (uses)

• Knowledge, deficient (teaching)

• Sensory perception, disturbed (uses)

Patient/family education

• Teach patient to take the medication early in the day to prevent nocturia

• Instruct patient to take with food or milk if GI symptoms of nausea and anorexia occur

• Teach patient to maintain a record of weight on a weekly basis and notify prescriber of weight loss of >5 lb

• Caution patient that this product causes a loss of potassium, so food rich in potassium should be added to the diet; refer to a dietitian for assistance in planning

• Advise patient to wear protective clothing and sunscreen in the sun to prevent photosensitivity

• Teach patient not to use alcohol or any OTC medications without prescriber's approval; serious product reactions may occur

• Emphasize the need to contact prescriber immediately if muscle cramps, weakness, nausea, dizziness, or numbness, rapid weight changes, change in stools, rash, sore throat, bleeding/bruising, Stevens-Johnson syndrome, toxic epidermal necrolysis (red rash that spreads, blistering) occur

• Teach patient to take own B/P and pulse and record

• Teach patient to continue taking medication even if feeling better; this product controls symptoms but does not cure the condition

• Teach patient to see ophthalmologist periodically; glaucoma is a slow process

• Advise patient to increase fluids to 2-3 L/day if not contraindicated

Evaluation

Positive therapeutic outcome

• Decreased intraocular pressure (glaucoma)

• Decreased edema in feet, legs, sacral area daily (CHF)

• Decreased frequency of seizures

• Prevention of altitude sickness

TREATMENT OF OVERDOSE:

Lavage if taken orally, monitor electrolytes, administer dextrose in saline, monitor hydration, CV, renal status

acetylcholine ophthalmic

See Appendix B

⚠ Nurse Alert

acetylcysteine (Rx)

(a-se-teel-sis′tay-een)

Acetadote, Mucomyst ✖

Func. class.: Mucolytic; antidote—acetaminophen

Chem. class.: Amino acid L-cysteine

Pregnancy category B

ACTION: Decreases viscosity of secretions in respiratory tract by breaking disulfide links of mucoproteins; serves as a substrate of glutathione, which is necessary to inactivate toxic metabolites in acetaminophen overdose

Therapeutic outcome: Decreased hepatotoxicity from acetaminophen overdose (PO); decreased viscosity of mucus in respiratory disorders (inh)

USES: Acetaminophen toxicity, bronchitis, cystic fibrosis, COPD, atelectasis

CONTRAINDICATIONS: Hypersensitivity, increased intracranial pressure, status asthmaticus

Precautions: Pregnancy **B**, breastfeeding, hypothyroidism, Addison's disease, CNS depression, brain tumor, asthma, renal/hepatic disease, COPD, psychosis, alcoholism, seizure disorders, bronchospasms, asthma, anaphylactoid reactions, fluid restriction, weight <40 kg

DOSAGE AND ROUTES

Mucolytic

Adult and child: Instill 1-20 ml (10%-20% sol) q6-8hr prn, or 3-5 ml (20% sol) or 6-10 ml (10% sol) tid or qid; nebulization (face, mask, mouthpiece, tracheostomy) 1-10 ml of a 20% sol or 2-20 ml of a 10% sol q2-6hr; nebulization (tent, croupette) may require large dose, up to 300 ml/treatment

Acetaminophen toxicity

Adult and child: PO 140 mg/kg, then 70 mg/kg q4hr × 17 doses to total 1330 mg/kg; **IV** loading dose 150 mg/kg over 60 min (dilution 150 mg/kg in 200 ml of D₅); maintenance dose 1:50 mg/kg over 4 hr (dilution 50 mg/kg in 500 ml D₅); maintenance dose 2:100 mg/kg over 16 hr (dilution 100 mg/kg in 1000 ml D₅)

Available forms: Oral sol 10%, 20%; inj 20% (200 mg/ml)

Implementation

• Give decreased dosage to geriatric patients; their metabolism may be slowed; give gum, hard candy, frequent rinsing of mouth for dryness of oral cavity

• Use only if suction machine is available

PO route (Antidotal use)

• Lavage, then give within 24 hr; dilute 10% or 20% sol to a 5% sol with diet soda; may use water if giving via gastric tube; dilution of 10% sol 1:1, 20% sol 1:3; use within 1 hr

Direct intratracheal INSTILL

• Use ½-1 hr before meals for better absorption, to decrease nausea; only after patient clears airway by deep breathing, coughing

• Give by syringe 2-3 doses of 1-2 ml of 10%-20% sol up to q1hr; 20% sol diluted with NS or water for injection; may give 10% sol undiluted

• Store in refrigerator: use within 96 hr of opening

• Provide assistance with inhaled dose: bronchodilator if bronchospasm occurs; wash face and rinse mouth after use to remove sticky feeling

• Use decreased dose in geriatric, metabolism may be slowed

• Use mechanical suction if cough insufficient to remove excess bronchial secretions

IV route

21-hr regimen:

• Loading dose: **dilute** 150 mg/kg in 200 ml D₅W; maintenance dose no. 1 **dilute** 50 mg/kg in 500 ml D₅W; maintenance dose no. 2 **dilute** 100 mg/kg in 1000 ml D₅W

• **Give** loading over 15 min; **give** maintenance dose no. 1 over 4 hr; **give** maintenance dose no. 2 over 16 hr; **give** sequentially without time between doses

Incompatibilities: Rubber, metals, stability with other products unknown

ADVERSE EFFECTS

CNS: Chills, *dizziness, drowsiness,* fever, headache

CV: Flushing, hypotension, tachycardia

EENT: *Rhinorrhea,* tooth damage

GI: Anorexia, constipation, diarrhea, **hepatotoxicity,** *nausea,* stomatitis, vomiting

INTEG: Clamminess, fever, pruritus, rash, urticaria

MISC: Anaphylaxis, angioedema

RESP: Bronchospasm, burning, chest tightness, cough, **hemoptysis**

Pharmacokinetics

Absorption	Extensive (PO), locally (inh)
Distribution	Protein binding 83%
Metabolism	Liver
Excretion	Kidneys
Half-life	5.6 hr (adult), 11 hr (newborn)

Pharmacodynamics

	PO	Inh
Onset	Unknown	5-10 min
Peak	1-2 hr (antidote)	10 min
Duration	Up to 4 hr (antidote)	1 hr

INTERACTIONS

Individual drugs
Iron, copper, nickel, rubber: do not use with acetylcysteine

Drug classifications
Nitrates: increased effect

NURSING CONSIDERATIONS

Assessment
Mucolytic use
• **Assess cough:** type, frequency, character, including sputum
• **Assess characteristics, rate, rhythm of respirations,** increased dyspnea, sputum; discontinue if bronchospasm occurs; ABGs for increased CO_2 retention in asthma patients
• Monitor VS, cardiac status including checking for dysrhythmias, increased rate, palpitations
Antidotal use
• Assess liver function tests, acetaminophen levels, PT, glucose, electrolytes, BUN, creatinine; inform prescriber if dose is vomited or vomiting is persistent; provide adequate hydration; decrease dosage in hepatic encephalopathy
• Assess for nausea, vomiting, rash; notify prescriber if these occur

Nursing diagnoses
• Airway clearance, ineffective (uses) (mucolytic)
• Gas exchange, impaired (uses) (mucolytic)
• Injury, risk for (uses) (antidote)
• Knowledge, deficient (teaching)
• Poisoning, risk for (uses) (antidote)

Patient/family education
Mucolytic use
• Tell patient to avoid driving or other hazardous activities until patient is stabilized on this medication; avoid alcohol, other CNS depressants; will enhance sedating properties of this product
• Teach patient that unpleasant odor will decrease after repeated use; that discoloration of solution after bottle is opened does not impair its effectiveness; avoid smoking, smoke-filled rooms, perfume, dust, environmental pollutants, cleaners
• Teach patient to report vomiting, as dose may need to be repeated

Evaluation
Positive therapeutic outcome
• Absence of purulent secretions when coughing (mucolytic use)
• Clear lung sounds bilaterally (mucolytic use)
• Absence of hepatic damage (acetaminophen toxicity)
• Decreasing blood toxicology (acetaminophen toxicity)

---

acyclovir (Rx)
(ay-sye'kloe-veer)
Apo-Acyclovir ✦, Gen-Acyclovir ✦, Nu-Acyclovir ✦, ratio-Acyclovir ✦, Zovirax
Func. class.: Antiviral
Chem. class.: Acyclic purine nucleoside analog
Pregnancy category B

ACTION: Interferes with DNA synthesis by conversion to acyclovir triphosphate, causing decreased viral replication

Therapeutic outcome: Decreased amount and time of healing of lesions

USES: Mucocutaneous herpes simplex virus, herpes genitalis (HSV-1, HSV-2), varicella infections, herpes zoster, herpes simplex encephalitis

CONTRAINDICATIONS: Hypersensitivity to this product or valacyclovir

Precautions: Pregnancy **B**, breastfeeding, renal/hepatic disease, electrolyte imbalance, dehydration, neurologic disease; hypersensitivity to famciclovir, ganciclovir, penciclovir, valganciclovir

DOSAGE AND ROUTES

Renal dose
Adult and child: PO/IV CCr >50 ml/min 100% dose q8hr; CCr 25-50 ml/min 100% dose q12hr; CCr 10-24 ml/min 100% dose q24hr; CCr 0-10 ml/min 50% of dose q24hr

Herpes simplex
Adult: PO 400 mg 3 ×/day for 5 days or 200 mg 5 ×/day × 5 days
Adult and child >12 yr (use ideal weight in obesity): IV INF 5 mg/kg over 1 hr q8hr × 5 days
Infant >3 mo/child <12 yr: IV INF 250 mg/m² or 30 mg/kg/day divided q8hr over 1 hr × 5 days

Genital herpes
Adult: PO 200 mg q4hr (5 times a day while awake) × 5 days to 6 mo depending on whether initial, recurrent, or chronic; IV 5 mg/kg q8hr × 5 days

Herpes simplex encephalitis
Adult: IV 10 mg/kg over 1 hr q8hr × 10 days
Child 3 mo-12 yr: IV 20 mg/kg q8hr × 10 days
Child birth-3 mo: IV 10 mg/kg q8hr × 10 days

Herpes zoster (shingles): immuno-compromised patients
Adult and adolescent: PO 800 mg q4hr 5 times/day × 7-10 days; IV 10 mg/kg q8hr × 7 days
Child ≥12 yr: IV 10 mg/kg q8hr × 7 days
Infant and child <12 yr: IV 20 mg/kg q8hr × 7-10 days

Herpes zoster (shingles): immuno-competent patient
Adult: PO 800 mg q4hr 5 times/day × 7-10 days; start within 48-72 hr of rash onset

Varicella (chickenpox): immuno-competent patient
Adult, adolescent, and child >40 kg: PO 800 mg 4 times/day × 5 days
Child ≥2 yr and ≤40 kg: PO 20 mg/kg (max 800 mg) PO 4 times per day × 5 days

Mucosal/cutaneous herpes simplex infections in immunosuppressed patients
Adult and child >12 yr: IV 5 mg/kg q8hr × 7 days
Infant >3 mo/child <12 yr: IV 10 mg/kg q8hr × 7 days

Available forms: Caps 200 mg; tabs 400, 800 mg; powder for inj 500, 1000 mg; sol for inj 50 mg/ml; oral susp 200 mg/5 ml

Implementation
PO route
• Do not break, crush, or chew caps
• Give with food to lessen GI symptoms; may give without regard to meals with 8 oz of water
• Store at room temperature in dry place
• May be taken orally before infection occurs or when itching or pain occurs, usually before eruptions
• Must be taken at equal intervals around the clock
• Shake susp before use

IV route
• Provide increased fluids to 3 L/day to decrease crystalluria, most critical during first 2 hr after IV infusion
Intermittent IV infusion route
• Reconstitute with 10 ml sterile water for injection/500 mg of product (50 mg/ml); shake; **further dilute** in 50-125 ml compatible sol, use within 12 hr; **give** over at least 1 hr (constant rate) by infusion pump to prevent nephrotoxicity; do not reconstitute with sol containing benzyl alcohol or parabens; check infusion site for redness, pain, induration; rotate sites
• Lower dosage in acute or chronic renal failure
• Store at room temp for up to 12 hr after reconstitution; if refrigerated, sol may show a precipitate that clears at room temperature; yellow discoloration does not affect potency

Y-site compatibilities: Alemtazumab, allopurinol, amikacin, aminophylline, amphotericin B cholesteryl, amphotericin B liposome, ampicillin, anidulafungin, argatroban, atracurium, bivalirudin, buprenorphine, busulfan, butorphanol, calcium chloride/gluconate, CARBOplatin, ceFAZolin, cefonicid, cefoperazone, cefotaxime, cefoxitin, ceftazidime, ceftizoxime, cefTRIAXone, cefuroxime, cephapirin, chloramphenicol, chlolesteryl sulfate compex, cimetidine, clindamycin, dexamethasone sodium phosphate, dimenhyDRINATE, DOXOrubicin, doxycycline, erythromycin, famotidine, filgrastim, fluconazole, gentamicin, granisetron, heparin, hydrocortisone sodium succinate, HYDROmorphone, imipenemcilastatin, LORazepam, magnesium sulfate, melphalan, methylPREDNISolone sodium succinate, metoclopramide, metroNIDAZOLE, multivitamin, nafcillin, oxacillin, paclitaxel, penicillin G potassium, PENTobarbital, perphenazine, piperacillin, potassium chloride, propofol, ranitidine,

Adverse effects: *italics* = common; **bold** = life-threatening

remifentanil, sodium bicarbonate, teniposide, theophylline, thiotepa, ticarcillin, tobramycin, trimethoprim-sulfamethoxazole, vancomycin, vasopressin, voriconazole, zidovudine

Y-site incompatibilities: DOBUTamine, DOPamine, ondansetron, verapamil

ADVERSE EFFECTS

CNS: Tremors, confusion, lethargy, hallucinations, **seizures,** *dizziness, headache,* encephalopathic changes
EENT: Gingival hyperplasia
GI: Nausea, vomiting, diarrhea, increased ALT, AST, abdominal pain, glossitis, colitis
GU: Oliguria, proteinuria, hematuria, vaginitis, moniliasis, **glomerulonephritis, acute renal failure,** changes in menses, polydipsia
HEMA: Thrombotic thrombocytopenia purpura, hemolytic uremic syndrome (immunocompromised patient)
INTEG: Rash, urticaria, pruritus, pain or phlebitis at **IV** site, unusual sweating, alopecia, **Stevens-Johnson syndrome**
MS: Joint pain, leg pain, muscle cramps

Pharmacokinetics

Absorption	Minimal (PO)
Distribution	Widely distributed, crosses placenta; CSF concentration 50% plasma; protein binding 9%-33%
Metabolism	Liver, minimal
Excretion	Kidneys, 95% unchanged
Half-life	2.0-3.5 hr, increased in renal disease

Pharmacodynamics

	PO	IV
Onset	Unknown	Rapid
Peak	$1^{1}/_{2}$-$2^{1}/_{2}$ hr	Infusion's end
Duration	Unknown	Unknown

INTERACTIONS

Individual drugs

Aminoglycosides: increased nephrotoxicity
Entecavir, pemetrexed, tenofovir: increased concentration of each product
Mycophenolate, probenecid: increased neurotoxicity, nephrotoxicity
Valproic acid: decreased action of valproic acid
Zidovudine, IT methotrexate: increased CNS side effects
Zoster vaccine: avoid concurrent use

Drug classifications

Hydantoins: decreased actions of hydantoins

NURSING CONSIDERATIONS

Assessment

• **Monitor for signs of infection,** type of lesions, area of body covered, purulent drainage
• Check I&O ratio; report hematuria, oliguria, fatigue, weakness; may indicate nephrotoxicity; check for protein in urine during treatment
• **Toxicity:** monitor any patient with compromised renal system, since product is excreted slowly in poor renal system function; toxicity may occur rapidly
• Monitor liver studies: AST, ALT
• Monitor blood studies: WBC, RBC, Hct, Hgb, bleeding time; blood dyscrasias may occur; product should be discontinued
• Monitor renal studies: urinalysis, protein, BUN, creatinine, CCr; increased BUN, creatinine indicates renal failure and **nephrotoxicity**
• Obtain C&S before product therapy; product may be taken as soon as culture is taken; repeat C&S after treatment; determine the presence of other sexually transmitted diseases
• Monitor bowel pattern before, during treatment; if severe abdominal pain with bleeding occurs, product should be discontinued
• Assess allergies before treatment, reaction of each medication; place allergies on chart in bright red letters; allergic reaction: burning, stinging, swelling, redness, rash, vulvitis, pruritus
• Assess neurologic status in herpes encephalitis

Nursing diagnoses

• Infection, risk for (uses)
• Knowledge, deficient (teaching)

Patient/family education
PO route
• Teach patient that product may be taken orally before infection occurs or when itching or pain occur, usually before eruptions; that partners need to be told that patient has herpes; they can become infected, so condoms must be worn to prevent reinfections
⚠ **Tell patient to report sore throat, fever, fatigue; may indicate superinfection; that product must be taken at equal intervals around the clock to maintain blood levels for duration of therapy**
• Tell patient to notify prescriber of side effects: bruising, bleeding, fatigue, malaise; may indicate blood dyscrasias

- Tell patient to seek dental care during treatment to prevent gingival hyperplasia
- Teach female patients with genital herpes to have regular Pap smears to prevent undetected cervical cancer

Evaluation
Positive therapeutic outcome
- Absence of itching, painful lesions
- Crusting and healed lesions

TREATMENT OF OVERDOSE:
Discontinue product, hemodialysis, resuscitate if needed

---

acyclovir topical
See Appendix B

adalimumab (Rx)
(add-a-lim'yu-mab)
Humira
Func. class.: Antirheumatic agent (disease modifying), immunomodulator, anti-TNF
Pregnancy category B

Do not confuse:
Humira/Humalin/Humalog

ACTION: A form of human IgG1 monoclonal antibody specific for human tumor necrosis factor (TNF); elevated levels of TNF are found in patients with rheumatoid arthritis

Therapeutic outcome: Decreased pain, inflammation in joints, better ROM

USES: Reduction in signs and symptoms and inhibiting progression of structural damage in patients with moderate to severe active rheumatoid arthritis in patients ≥18 years of age who have not responded to other disease-modifying agents, JRA, psoriatic arthritis, Crohn's disease, moderate-severe plaque psoriasis, ankylosing spondylitis

CONTRAINDICATIONS:
Hypersensitivity

Precautions: Pregnancy **B**, breastfeeding, children, geriatric, CNS demyelinating disease, lymphoma, latent TB, CHF, hepatitis B carriers, manitol hypersensitivity, latex allergy, neoplastic disease

> **BLACK BOX WARNING:** Active infections, risk of lymphomas/leukemias, TB

DOSAGE AND ROUTES
Rheumatoid arthritis, ankylosing spondylitis, psoriatic arthritis
Adult: SUBCUT 40 mg every other wk or every week if not combined with methotrexate

Juvenile rheumatoid arthritis (JRA)
Child ≥4 yr/adolescent ≥30 kg: SUBCUT 40 mg every other wk
Child ≥4 yr/adolescent ≥15 kg to <30 kg: SUBCUT 20 mg every other wk
Child ≥4 yr/adolescent <15 kg: SUBCUT 24 mg/m^2 BSA (up to 40 mg total) every other wk, then 20 mg every other wk

Crohn's disease
Adult: SUBCUT 160 mg given as 4 inj on day 1, or 2 inj on days 1 and 2, then 80 mg at wk 2 and 40 mg every other wk, starting at wk 4

Plaque psoriasis
Adult: SUBCUT 80 mg baseline as 2 inj, then 40 mg every other week starting 1 wk after initial dose × 16 wk

Available forms: Inj 40 mg/0.8 ml; 20 mg/0.4 ml (pediatric)

Implementation
SUBCUT route
- Do not admix with other sol or medications, do not use filter, protect from light

ADVERSE EFFECTS
CNS: Headache
CV: Hypertension
EENT: Sinusitis
GI: Abdominal pain, nausea, hepatic damage
HEMA: Leukopenia, pancytopenia, aplastic anemia, agranulocytopenia
INTEG: Rash, *inj site reaction*
MISC: Flulike symptoms, UTI, hypertension, back pain, lupuslike syndrome, risk of cancer, antibody development to this drug, **risk of infection (TB, invasive fungal infections, other opportunistic infections); may be fatal, Stevens-Johnson syndrome**
RESP: *URI,* **pulmonary fibrosis**

Pharmacokinetics

Absorption	Unknown
Distribution	Unknown
Metabolism	Unknown
Excretion	Unknown
Half-life	Terminal 2 wk

Pharmacodynamics
Unknown

Adverse effects: *italics* = common; **bold** = life-threatening

INTERACTIONS

Individual drugs
Anakinra: do not use together
Rilonacept: increase serious infections

Drug classifications
Vaccines: do not give concurrently; immunization should be brought up to date before treatment
Other TNF blockers: increased serious infections

NURSING CONSIDERATIONS

Assessment
• Rheumatoid arthritis: assess for pain, stiffness, ROM, swelling of joints during treatment
• Check for inj site pain, swelling, redness; usually occur after 2 inj (4-5 days) use cold compress to relieve pain/swelling

> **BLACK BOX WARNING:** Check for infections, fever, flulike symptoms, dyspnea, change in urination, redness/swelling around wounds, stop treatment if present, some serious infections, including sepsis, may occur; patients with active infections should not be started on this product

• Assess for latent TB prior to therapy; treat before starting this product
• Assess for anaphylaxis, latex allergic; stop therapy if lupuslike syndrome develops
• Assess for blood dyscrasias: CBC, differential periodically

> **BLACK BOX WARNING:** Assess for neoplastic disease (lymphomas/leukemia)

Nursing diagnoses
• Activity intolerance, risk for (uses)
• Knowledge, deficient (teaching)
• Mobility, impaired physical (uses)
• Pain, chronic (uses)

Patient/family education
• Teach patient about self-administration if appropriate: inj should be made in thigh, abdomen, upper arm; rotate sites at least 1 inch from old site; do not inject in areas that are bruised, red, hard
• Advise patient that if medication is not taken when due, inject next dose as soon as remembered and inject next dose as scheduled
• Advise patient not to take any live-virus vaccines during treatment
• Instruct patient to report signs of infection, allergic reactions, lupuslike syndrome

Evaluation
Positive therapeutic outcome
• Decreased inflammation, pain in joints, decreased joint destruction

---

adefovir (Rx)
(add-ee-foh′veer)
Hepsera
Func. class.: Antiviral
Pregnancy category C

ACTION: Inhibits hepatitis B virus DNA polymerase by competing with natural substrates and by causing DNA termination after its incorporation into viral DNA; causes viral DNA death

Therapeutic outcome: Improving liver function tests, lessening symptoms of chronic hepatitis B

USES: Chronic hepatitis B

CONTRAINDICATIONS:
Hypersensitivity

Precautions: Pregnancy **C**, breastfeeding, children, geriatric, dialysis, females, labor, obesity, organ transplant

> **BLACK BOX WARNING:** Severe renal disease, impaired hepatic disease, lactic acidosis, HIV

DOSAGE AND ROUTES
Adult/adolescent: PO 10 mg daily, optimal duration unknown

Renal dose
Adult: PO CCr ≥50 ml/min 10 mg q24hr; CCr 30-49 ml/min 10 mg q48hr; CCr 10-29 ml/min 10 mg q72hr; hemodialysis 10 mg q7 days following dialysis

Available forms: Tabs 10 mg

Implementation
• Give by mouth without regard to food
• Store in cool environment; protect from light

ADVERSE EFFECTS
CNS: *Headache*
GI: *Dyspepsia*, abdominal pain, nausea, vomiting, diarrhea, hepatomegaly, flatulence, **pancreatitis**
GU: Hematuria, glycosuria, **nephrotoxicity, Fanconi syndrome, renal failure**
MISC: Fever, rash, weight loss, cough

⚠ Nurse Alert

Pharmacokinetics

Absorption	Rapidly from GI tract
Distribution	Unknown
Metabolism	Unknown
Excretion	Kidneys 45%
Half-life	7.48 hr

Pharmacodynamics

Onset	Unknown
Peak	$1^3/_4$ hr
Duration	Unknown

INTERACTIONS

Individual drugs
Amiloride, cimetidine, cycloSPORINE, digoxin, dofetilide, efavirenz, emtricitabine, memantine, metformin, midodrine, morphine, pemetrexed, procainamide, quiNIDine, quinine, ranitidine, tacrolimus, tenofovir, triamterene, trospium, vancomycin: increased serum concentrations, toxicity

Drug classifications
Benzodiazepines, nucleoside analogs (experimental), NSAIDs, sulfonamides: increased serum concentrations, toxicity

> **BLACK BOX WARNING:** NNRTIs, NRTIs, antiretroviral protease-inhibitors, aminoglycosides

Drug/lab test
Increased: ALT, AST, amylase, creatine kinase

NURSING CONSIDERATIONS

Assessment

> **BLACK BOX WARNING:** Assess for **nephrotoxicity:** increasing CCr, BUN

• Assess for HIV before beginning treatment because HIV resistance may occur in chronic hepatitis B patients

> **BLACK BOX WARNING:** Assess for **lactic acidosis,** severe hepatomegaly with stenosis

• Assess geriatric patients more carefully; may develop renal, cardiac symptoms more rapidly

> **BLACK BOX WARNING:** Assess for exacerbations of **hepatitis** after discontinuing treatment, monitor liver function tests, hepatitis B serology

Nursing diagnoses
• Infection, risk for (uses)
• Knowledge, deficient (teaching)

Patient/family education
• Advise patient that optimal duration of treatment is unknown, that drug is not a cure; transmission may still occur
• Advise patient to avoid use with other medications unless approved by prescriber
• Advise patient to notify prescriber of decreased urinary output
• Avoid breastfeeding

Evaluation
Positive therapeutic outcome
• Decreased symptoms of chronic hepatitis B, improving liver function tests

> **⚠ HIGH ALERT**
>
> ## adenosine (Rx)
> (ah-den′oh-seen)
> **Adenocard, Adenoscan**
> *Func. class.:* Antidysrhythmic—miscellaneous
> *Chem. class.:* Endogenous nucleoside
> **Pregnancy category C**

Do not confuse:
Adenocard/adenosine phosphate

ACTION: Slows conduction through AV node, can interrupt reentry pathways through AV node, and can restore normal sinus rhythm in patients with paroxysmal supraventricular tachycardia (PSVT)

Therapeutic outcome: Normal sinus rhythm in patients diagnosed with SVT or diagnosis of perfusion defect

USES: PSVT, as a diagnostic aid to assess myocardial perfusion defects in CAD; Wolff-Parkinson-White (WPW) syndrome

CONTRAINDICATIONS:
Hypersensitivity, 2nd- or 3rd-degree heart block, AV block, sick sinus syndrome, atrial flutter, atrial fibrillation, ventricular tachycardia, bronchospastic lung disease, symptomatic bradycardia, bundle branch block, heart transplant, unstable angina

Precautions: Pregnancy C, breastfeeding, children, geriatric, asthma

DOSAGE AND ROUTES

Antidysrhythmic
Adult and child >50 kg: IV BOL 6 mg; if conversion to normal sinus rhythm does not oc-

---

cur within 1-2 min, give 12 mg by rapid **IV** BOL; may repeat 12 mg dose again in 1-2 min
Infant and child <50 kg: IV BOL 0.05 mg/kg; if not effective, increase dose by 0.05-0.1 mg/kg q2min to a max of 0.3 mg/kg/dose
Neonate: IV BOL: 0.05 mg/kg by rapid **IV** BOL, may increase by 0.05 mg/kg q2min, max 0.3 mg/kg/dose

Diagnostic use
Adult: IV 140 mcg/kg/min × 6 min

Wolff-Parkinson-White (WPW)
Adult/adolescent/child ≥50 kg: IV BOL 6 mg by rapid inf, follow with saline flush; then **IV** BOL 12 mg if needed

Available forms: Adenocard: Inj 3 mg/ml in prefilled syringes; Adenocard: 3 mg/ml in vials

Implementation
IV, direct (bolus) route
• Give **IV** BOL undiluted; give 6 mg or less by rapid inj; if using an **IV** line, use port near insertion site, flush with 0.9% NaCl (20 ml), then elevate arm
Intermittent infusion route (diagnostic testing)
• Give 30-ml vial undiluted via peripheral vein at a rate of 140 mcg/kg/min over 6 min for a total dose of 0.84 mg/kg, inject thallium 201 as close to venous access as possible after 3 min of infusion

Solution compatibilities: D₅LR, D₅W, LR, 0.9% NaCl
• Store at room temperature; sol should be clear; discard unused product

ADVERSE EFFECTS
CNS: Light-headedness, dizziness, arm tingling, numbness, apprehension, blurred vision, headache
CV: Chest pain/pressure, **atrial tachydysrhythmias,** sweating, palpitations, hypotension, *facial flushing,* **AV block, cardiac arrest, ventricular dysrhythmias**
GI: *Nausea,* metallic taste, throat tightness, groin pressure
RESP: *Dyspnea, chest pressure,* hyperventilation, **bronchospasm (asthmatics)**

Pharmacokinetics	
Absorption	Complete bioavailability
Distribution	Erythrocytes, cardiovascular endothelium
Metabolism	Liver, converted to inosine and adenosine monophosphate
Excretion	Kidneys
Half-life	10 sec

Pharmacodynamics	
Onset	Rapid
Peak	Unknown
Duration	1-2 min

INTERACTIONS
Individual drugs
Caffeine, theophylline: decreased effects of adenosine
CarBAMazepine: increased heart block
Digoxin, verapamil: increased ventricular fibrillation
Dipyridamole: increased effects of adenosine
Smoking: increased tachycardia

Drug/herb
Ginger: increased effect
Green tea, guarana: decreased effect

NURSING CONSIDERATIONS
Assessment
• Monitor I&O ratio, electrolytes (potassium, sodium, chloride)
• **Assess cardiopulmonary status:** pulse, respiration, ECG intervals (PR, QRS, QT); check for transient dysrhythmias (PVCs, PACs, sinus tachycardia, AV block)
• Assess respiratory status: rate, rhythm, lung fields for crackles, watch for respiratory depression; bilateral crackles may occur in CHF patient; if increased respiration, increased pulse occurs, product should be discontinued
• Assess CNS effects: dizziness, confusion, paresthesias; product should be discontinued

Nursing diagnoses
• Cardiac output, decreased (uses)
• Gas exchange, impaired (adverse reactions)
• Knowledge, deficient (teaching)

Patient/family education
• Tell patient to report facial flushing, dizziness, sweating, palpitations, chest pain
• Instruct patient to rise from sitting or standing slowly to prevent orthostatic hypotension

Evaluation
Positive therapeutic outcome
- Normal sinus rhythm
- Diagnosis of perfusion defect

albumin, human 5%/25% (Rx)
(al-byoo'min)
Albuked, Albuminar, Albutein, Buminate, Plasbumin, Flexbumin
Func. class.: Blood derivative—plasma volume expander
Chem. class.: Placental human plasma
Pregnancy category C

ACTION: Exerts colloidal oncotic pressure, which expands volume of circulating blood by pulling fluid from extravascular to intravascular spaces, and maintains cardiac output

Therapeutic outcome: Increased B/P, decreased edema, increased serum albumin levels, increased plasma protein

USES: Restores plasma volume in burns, hyperbilirubinemia, shock, hypoproteinemia, prevention of cerebral edema, cardiopulmonary bypass procedures, ARDS, hemorrhage; also replacement in nephrotic syndrome

CONTRAINDICATIONS:
Hypersensitivity, CHF, severe anemia, renal insufficiency, pulmonary edema

Precautions: Pregnancy **C,** decreased salt intake, decreased cardiac reserve, lack of albumin deficiency, renal/hepatic disease, chronic anemia

DOSAGE AND ROUTES
Burns
Adult: **IV** dose to maintain plasma albumin at 3-4 mg/dl

Shock
Adult: **IV** Rapidly give 5% sol; when close to normal, infuse at ≤2-4 ml/min; 25% sol ≤1 ml/min
Child: 0.5-1 g/kg/dose, 5% sol, may repeat as needed; max 6 g/kg/day

Nephrotic syndrome
Adult: **IV** 100-200 mg of 25% and loop diuretic × 7-10 days

Hypoproteinemia
Adult: **IV** 25 g, may repeat in 15-30 min, or 50-75 g of 25% albumin infused at ≤2 ml/min
Child/infant: **IV** 0.5-1 g/kg/dose over 2-4 hr, may repeat q1-2days

Hyperbilirubinemia/erythroblastosis fetalis
Infant: **IV** 1 g/kg 1-2 hr before transfusion

Available forms: Inj 50, 250 mg/ml (5%, 25%)

Implementation
IV route
- Check type of albumin; some are stored at room temperature, some need to be refrigerated; use only amber-colored sol without precipitate; solution should be clear, use within 4 hr of opening
- Give **IV** slowly to prevent fluid overload; 5% sol may be given undiluted; 25% sol may be given diluted (D_5W, 0.9% NaCl) or undiluted; give over 4 hr, use infusion pump
- Provide adequate hydration before, during administration; whole blood may need to be given to prevent anemia; monitor hydration during treatment
- 5% sol may be used in hypovolemic/intravascular depletion
- 25% sol may be used in sodium/fluid restriction

Y-site compatibilities: Diltiazem

Solution compatibilities: LR, NaCl, Ringer's, D_5W, $D_{10}W$, $D_2\frac{1}{2}W$, dextrose/saline, dextran$_6$ D_5, dextran$_6$ NaCl 0.9%, dextrose/Ringer's, dextrose/LR

ADVERSE EFFECTS
CNS: Fever, chills, flushing, headache
CV: Fluid overload, hypotension, erratic pulse, tachycardia
GI: Nausea, vomiting, increased salivation
INTEG: Rash, urticaria
RESP: Altered respirations, **pulmonary edema**

Pharmacokinetics	
Absorption	Complete bioavailability
Distribution	Intravascular spaces
Metabolism	Liver
Excretion	Unknown
Half-life	Terminal, 21 days

Pharmacodynamics

Onset	15-30 min
Peak	Unknown
Duration	Unknown

INTERACTIONS

Drug/lab test
Increased: alkaline phosphatase
Decreased: Hct, Hgb
False increase: alk phos

NURSING CONSIDERATIONS

Assessment
• Monitor blood studies: Hct, Hgb; if serum protein declines, dyspnea, hypoxemia can result; check for decreasing B/P, erratic pulse, respiration

⚠ Monitor CVP: pulmonary wedge pressure will increase if overload occurs; I&O ratio: urinary output may decrease; CVP reading: distended neck veins indicate circulatory overload; shortness of breath, anxiety, insomnia, expiratory crackles, frothy blood-tinged sputum, cough, cyanosis indicate pulmonary overload

• Assess for allergy: fever, rash, itching, chills, flushing, urticaria, nausea, vomiting, hypotension; requires discontinuation of infusion, use of new lot if therapy reinstituted; premedicate with diphenhydrAMINE

Nursing diagnoses
• Fluid volume, deficit (uses)
• Fluid volume, excess (adverse reactions)
• Injury, risk for (uses)
• Knowledge, deficient (teaching)

Patient/family education
• Explain use, reason for albumin; provide information on what to report to prescriber (hypersensitivity, fluid overload)

Evaluation
Positive therapeutic outcome
• Increased B/P, decreased edema (shock, burns)
• Increased serum albumin levels
• Increased plasma protein (hypoproteinemia)

albuterol (Rx)
(al-byoo′ter-ole)
AccuNeb, Gen-Salbutamol ✤, Novo-Salmol ✤, Proair HFA, Proventil, Proventil HFA, Relion, Ventolin HFA, Vospire ER
Func. class.: Bronchodilator
Chem. class.: Adrenergic β_2-agonist, sympathomimetic, bronchodilator
Pregnancy category C

Do not confuse:
albuterol/atenolol, **Proventil**/ Prinivil, **Salbutamol**/salmeterol, **Ventolin**/Vantin

ACTION: Causes bronchodilatation by action on β_2 (pulmonary) receptors by increasing levels of cyclic AMP, which relaxes smooth muscle; produces bronchodilatation; CNS, cardiac stimulation, increased diuresis, and increased gastric acid secretion; longer acting than isoproterenol

Therapeutic outcome: Increased ability to breathe because of bronchodilatation

USES: Prevention of exercise-induced asthma, acute bronchospasm, bronchitis, emphysema, bronchiectasis, reversible airway obstruction

Unlabeled uses: Hyperkalemia in dialysis patients

CONTRAINDICATIONS:
Hypersensitivity to sympathomimetics, tachydys-rhythmias, severe cardiac disease, heart block

Precautions: Pregnancy **C**, breastfeeding, exercise-induced bronchospasm (aerosol) in children <12 yr, cardiac/renal disease, hyperthyroidism, diabetes mellitus, hypertension, prostatic hypertrophy, closed-angle glaucoma, seizures, hypoglycemia

DOSAGE AND ROUTES

Bronchospasm
Adult and child ≥4 yr: INH (metered dose inhaler) 2 puffs q4-6hr prn

Other respiratory conditions
Adult and child ≥12 yr: INH (metered dose inhaler) 1 puff q4-6hr; PO 2-4 mg tid-qid, max 32 mg/day, depending on formulation; NEB/IPPB 2.5 mg tid-qid
Geriatric: PO 2 mg tid-qid, may increase gradually to 8 mg tid-qid

Child 2-12 yr: INH (metered dose inhaler) 0.1 mg/kg tid (max 2.5 mg tid-qid); NEB/IPPB 0.1-0.15 mg/kg/dose tid-qid or 1.25 mg tid-qid for child 10-15 kg or 2.5 mg tid-qid >15 kg

Available forms: Aerosol 90 mcg/actuation; tabs 2, 4 mg; oral syr 2 mg/5 ml; ext rel 4, 8 mg; inh sol 0.5, 0.83, 1, 2, 5 mg/ml; powder for inh (Ventodisk) 200, 400 mcg; inh caps 200 mcg; 100 mcg/spray, 80 inh/canister, 200 inh/canister

Implementation
PO route
- Do not break, crush, or chew ext rel tabs
- Give PO with meals to decrease gastric irritation; oral sol for children (no alcohol, sugar)
- In geriatric patients, a spacing device is advised

Aerosol route
- Give after shaking metered dose inhaler; have patient exhale and place mouthpiece in mouth, inhale slowly while depressing inhaler, hold breath, remove inhaler, exhale slowly; allow at least 1 min between inhalations; avoid using near flames or source of heat
- Track number of inhalations used and discard when labeled inhalations have been used
- Store in light-resistant container; do not expose to temperatures >86° F (30° C)

Nebulizer/IPPB route
- **Dilute** 5 mg/ml sol/2.5 ml 0.9% NaCl for inhalation; other solutions do not require dilution for nebulizer O_2 flow or compressed air 6-10 L/min

ADVERSE EFFECTS
CNS: *Tremors, anxiety,* insomnia, headache, dizziness, stimulation, *restlessness,* hallucinations, flushing, irritability
CV: *Palpitations, tachycardia, hypertension,* angina, hypotension, dysrhythmias
EENT: Dry nose, irritation of nose and throat
GI: *Heartburn, nausea, vomiting*
MISC: Flushing, sweating, anorexia, bad taste/smell changes, hypokalemia
MS: Muscle cramps
RESP: Cough, wheezing, dyspnea, **bronchospasm,** dry throat

Pharmacokinetics

Absorption	Well absorbed (PO)
Distribution	Unknown
Metabolism	Liver extensively, tissues
Excretion	Unknown, breast milk
Half-life	3-4 hr

Pharmacodynamics

	PO	PO–ext rel	INH
Onset	$\frac{1}{2}$ hr	$\frac{1}{2}$ hr	5-15 min
Peak	$2\frac{1}{2}$ hr	2-3 hr	1-$1\frac{1}{2}$ hr
Duration	4-6 hr	12 hr	4-6 hr

INTERACTIONS
Individual drugs
Atomoxetine, selegiline: increased CV effects

Drug classifications
Adrenergics: increased action of albuterol; do not use together
β-Adrenergic blockers: block therapeutic effect
Bronchodilators (aerosol): increased action of bronchodilator
Diuretics (potassium-losing): increased ECG changes/hypokalemia
MAOIs, tricyclics: increased chance of hypertensive crisis; do not use together
Oxytocics: severe hypotension; do not use together
Theophylline: toxicity

Drug/herb
Black tea, green tea, kola nut, guarana, yerba maté: increased stimulation

Drug/food
Caffeine products, chocolate: increased stimulation

NURSING CONSIDERATIONS
Assessment
- Assess respiratory function: vital capacity, forced expiratory volume, ABGs, lung sounds; heart rate, rhythm; B/P, sputum (baseline and during therapy)
- Determine that patient has not received theophylline therapy before giving dose, to prevent additive effect; client's ability to self-medicate
- Monitor for evidence of allergic reactions; paradoxic bronchospasm; withhold dose; notify prescriber if bronchospasm occurs

Nursing diagnoses
- Airway clearance, ineffective (uses)
- Gas exchange, impaired (uses)
- Knowledge, deficient (teaching)

Patient/family education
- Tell patient not to use OTC medications before consulting prescriber; excess stimulation may occur; instruct patient to use this medication before other medications and allow at least 5 min between each to prevent overstimulation; to limit caffeine products such as chocolate, coffee, tea, and cola

Adverse effects: *italics* = common; **bold** = life-threatening

• Teach patient to use inhaler; review package insert with patient; to avoid getting aerosol in eyes or blurring may result; to wash inhaler in warm water and dry daily; to rinse mouth after using; to avoid smoking, smoke-filled rooms, persons with respiratory infections

⚠ **Teach patient that if paradoxic broncho-spasm occurs to stop product immediately and notify prescriber**

• Instruct patient on administration of dose, not to use more than prescribed; serious side effects may occur; if taking PO regularly and dose is missed, take when remembered; space other doses on new time schedule; do not double doses

• In geriatric patients, a spacing device is advised

Evaluation

Positive therapeutic outcome

• Absence of dyspnea and wheezing after 1 hr
• Improved airway exchange
• Improved ABGs

TREATMENT OF OVERDOSE:

Administer a β_1-adrenergic blocker, **IV** fluids

⚠ HIGH ALERT

aldesleukin, IL-2 (Rx)

(al-dess-loo'kin)

Proleukin

Func. class.: Antineoplastics—miscellaneous

Chem. class.: Interleukin-2, human recombinant, cytokine

Pregnancy category C

Do not confuse:

aldesleukin/oprelvekin,
Proleukin/Oprelvekin/ Prokine

ACTION: Enhancement of lymphocyte mitogenesis and stimulation of IL-2–dependent cell lines; enhancement of lymphocyte cytotoxicity; induction of killer cell activity; induction of interferon-γ production; results in activation of cellular immunity and cytokines and inhibition of tumor growth

Therapeutic outcome: Prevention of rapid growth of malignant cells

USES: Metastatic renal cell carcinoma in adults, melanoma (metastatic)

Unlabeled uses: Acute myelogenous leukemia (AML), cutaneous T-cell lymphoma (CTCL), HIV, Hansen's disease (leprosy), mycosis fungoides, non-Hodgkin's lymphoma

CONTRAINDICATIONS:

Hypersensitivity, abnormal thallium stress test or pulmonary function tests, organ allografts, angina, cardiac tamponade, MI, GI bleeding/perforation, psychosis, renal failure, pulmonary insufficiency, seizures, ventricular tachycardia

> **BLACK BOX WARNING:** Cardiac/pulmonary disease, coma

Precautions: Pregnancy **C**, breastfeeding, children, CNS metastases, bacterial infections, renal/hepatic disease, anemia, thrombocytopenia, scleroderma, vasculitis

> **BLACK BOX WARNING:** Capillary leak syndrome, infection

DOSAGE AND ROUTES

Renal cell cancer, malignant melanoma

Adult: **IV** INF 600,000 international units/kg (without LAK cells) over 15 min q8hr × 14 doses; off 9 days; repeat schedule for another 14 doses, for a maximum of 28 doses/course

Available forms: Powder for inj 22 million international units/vial

Implementation

Intermittent IV infusion route

• Premedicate with an antipyretic, H_2 blocker, antiemetics, antibiotic; use meperidine; DOPamine for hypotension, IV fluids

• Give by intermittent **IV** INF after diluting 22 million international units (1.3 mg)/1.2 ml sterile (1.1 mg/ml) water for inj at side of vial and swirl, do not shake; dilute dose with 50 ml D_5W and give over 15 min; use plastic bag; do not use an in-line filter; give through Y-tube or 3-way stopcock

• Give DOPamine 1-5 kg/min before onset of hypotension; decreased dose preserves kidney output

Continuous IV infusion route

• Dilute appropriate reconstituted IV solution in a sufficient amount of D_5W inj containing 0.1% albumin human to 5-60 mcg/ml

• Do not use in-line filter

• Give hydrocortisone, dexamethasone, or sodium bicarbonate (1 mEq/1 ml) for extravasation, apply ice compresses

---

• Store any diluted product in refrigerator; do not freeze; administer within 48 hr; bring to room temperature before infusing; discard unused portion

Y-site compatibilities: Amikacin, **IV** fat emulsion, gentamicin, morphine, piperacillin, potassium chloride, ticarcillin, tobramycin, TPN #145, amphotericin B, calcium gluconate, diphenhydrAMINE, DOPamine, fluconazole, foscarnet, heparin, magnesium sulfate, metoclopramide, ondansetron, ranitidine, trimethoprim/sulfamethoxazole

ADVERSE EFFECTS

CNS: Mental status changes, dizziness, sensory dysfunction, syncope, motor dysfunction, fever, chills, headache, impaired memory, depression, sleep disturbances, hallucinations, rigors, neuropathy

CV: Hypotension, sinus tachycardia, dysrhythmias, bradycardia, PVCs, PACs, myocardial ischemia, **myocardial infarction, cardiac arrest,** capillary leak syndrome, **CVA**

EENT: Reversible visual changes

GI: Nausea, vomiting, *diarrhea*, stomatitis, anorexia, GI bleeding, dyspepsia, constipation, **intestinal perforation/ileus,** jaundice, ascites

GU: Oliguria/anuria, proteinuria, hematuria, dysuria, **renal failure**

HEMA: *Anemia*, **thrombocytopenia, leukopenia, coagulation disorders, leukocytosis, eosinophilia**

INTEG: Pruritus, *erythema*, *rash*, dry skin, **exfoliative dermatitis,** purpura, petechiae, urticaria

MS: Arthralgia, myalgia

RESP: Pulmonary congestion, dyspnea, **pulmonary edema, respiratory failure,** tachypnea, pleural effusion, wheezing, **apnea**

SYST: Infection

Pharmacokinetics

Absorption	Complete bioavailability
Distribution	Rapid extracellular, intravascular
Metabolism	Kidneys (convoluted tubules)
Excretion	Kidneys
Half-life	85 min

Pharmacodynamics

Onset	4 wk
Peak	Unknown
Duration	≤12 mo

INTERACTIONS

Individual drugs
Indomethacin, methotrexate, asparaginase, DOXOrubicin: increased toxicity

Drug classifications
Aminoglycosides: increased toxicity
Antihypertensives: increased hypotension
Cytotoxic chemotherapy: increased toxicity
Glucocorticosteroids: decreased tumor effectiveness
Live-virus vaccines: decreased immune response; do not use concurrently
Psychotropics: unpredictable reactions

Drug/lab test
Increased: bilirubin, BUN, serum creatinine, transaminase, alkaline phosphatase, hypomagnesemia, acidosis hypocalcemia, hypophosphatemia, hypokalemia, hyperuricemia, hypoalbuminemia, hypoproteinemia, hyponatremia, hyperkalemia, alkalosis (toxic effect of product)

NURSING CONSIDERATIONS

Assessment
• Monitor CBC, differential, platelet count weekly; withhold product if WBC is <2000/mm^3 or platelet count is <75,000/mm^3; notify prescriber of these results; transfusion of RBCs, platelets may be required

> **BLACK BOX WARNING:** Identify capillary leak syndrome (CLS), including a drop in mean arterial pressure (2-12 hr after initiating therapy); hypotension and hypoperfusion will occur; if B/P <90 mm Hg, monitor ECG, CVP in cardiac patients

• Monitor renal function studies: BUN, serum uric acid, urine CCr, electrolytes before, during therapy; I&O ratio; report fall in urine output to <30 ml/hr
• Monitor temp q4hr; fever may indicate beginning infection
• Check liver function tests before, during therapy: bilirubin, AST, ALT, alkaline phosphatase, LDH prn or monthly
• Monitor ECG; watch for ST-T wave changes, low QRS and T, possible dysrhythmias (sinus tachycardia, PVCs)

> **BLACK BOX WARNING:** Monitor baselines in pulmonary function; document FEV >2 L or ≥75% before therapy; check daily VS, pulse oximetry, dyspnea, crackles, ABGs, watch for respiratory failure, intubate if necessary

- Obtain stress thallium study before therapy; document normal ejection fraction, unimpaired wall motion
- Assess for bleeding: hematuria, guaiac, bruising or petechiae, mucosa, or orifices
- Assess for GI symptoms: frequency of stools, cramping
- Assess for acidosis, signs of dehydration: rapid respirations, poor skin turgor, decreased urine output, dry skin, restlessness, weakness
- Assess for cardiac status: B/P, pulse, character, rhythm, rate, ABGs, ECG
- Assess for infection: sore throat; antibiotics may be prescribed prophylactically

Nursing diagnoses
- Body image, disturbed (adverse reactions)
- Infection, risk for (adverse reactions)
- Injury, risk for (adverse reactions)
- Knowledge, deficient (teaching)

Patient/family education
- Teach patient to avoid use of products containing aspirin or ibuprofen, razors, commercial mouthwash because bleeding may occur; to report symptoms of bleeding, hematuria, tarry stools
- Tell patient to report signs of anemia: fatigue, headache, irritability, faintness, shortness of breath
- Tell patient to report any changes in breathing or coughing even several months after treatment
- Advise patient that contraception will be necessary during treatment; teratogenesis may occur
- Teach patient to report signs/symptoms of infection: fever, chills, sore throat; patient should avoid crowds or persons with known infections
- Advise patient to avoid alcohol, NSAIDs, salicylates; GI bleeding may occur
- Advise patient that visual problems may occur but are reversible

Evaluation
Positive therapeutic outcome
- Decreased spread of malignancy

alemtuzumab (Rx)
(al-em-tuz'uh-mab)
Campath
Func. class.: Antineoplastic—miscellaneous
Chem. class.: Monoclonal antibody
Pregnancy category C

ACTION: Composed of recombinant DNA-derived humanized monoclonal antibody (campath-1H), binds to CD52 antigen that is present on surface of B and T lymphocytes, causes lysis of leukemic cells

Therapeutic outcome: Decreased number of white blood cells

USES: B-cell chronic lymphocytic leukemia that has been treated with alkylating agents and that has failed fludarabine therapy

CONTRAINDICATIONS:
Hypersensitivity

Precautions: Pregnancy **C**, breastfeeding, children

> **BLACK BOX WARNING:** Infusion-related reactions, bone marrow suppression, fungal/viral infection, active systemic infection, immunodeficiency

DOSAGE AND ROUTES
Adult: **IV** 3 mg over 2 hr daily; when tolerated, increase to 10 mg; when 10 mg tolerated, increase to 30 mg daily; maintenance is 30 mg/day 3 ×/wk on alternate days for 12 wk; titration usually takes 3-7 days; max single dose 30 mg; max weekly dose 90 mg

Dosage adjustments for neutropenia/thrombocytopenia
Adult: **IV** ANC ≤250/mol; platelets ≤25,000: 1st time hold dose; 2nd time hold dose; then resume at 10 mg; if delay longer than 7 days, start at 3 mg; 3rd time, stop completely; ANC 500/mol, platelets 50,000 if delay ≥7 days start at 3 mg and increase as tolerated

Available forms: Sol for inj 30 mg/ml

Implementation
IV route
- Do not give **IV** push or bolus
- Withdraw amount needed; do not shake ampule; use 5 mcm filter prior to dilution, check for particulate matter and discoloration; inject into 100 ml sterile 0.9% NaCl or D₅W, invert to mix, do not add other products or infuse in same **IV** tubing
- Do not shake ampule

> **BLACK BOX WARNING:** Give diphenhydrA-MINE 50 mg and acetaminophen 650 mg ¹/₂ hr prior to inf; give hydrocortisone 200 mg to decrease severe inf reactions; give trimethoprim-sulfamethoxazole DS bid 3×/wk and famciclovir 250 mg bid; continue for 2 mo or until CD4+ ≥200 cells/mm3, whichever is later

• Store reconstituted sol for ≤8 hr at room temperature, do not freeze; protect from light

ADVERSE EFFECTS

CNS: *Dizziness,* insomnia, depression, headache, tremor, somnolence, fatigue, drowsiness, weakness, anxiety
CV: *Hypo/hypertension, tachycardia, edema, chest pain, supraventricular tachycardia,* **CHF**
GI: *Anorexia, diarrhea,* constipation, *nausea, stomatitis, vomiting, abdominal pain, dyspepsia*
HEMA: Anemia, neutropenia, thrombocytopenia, pancytopenia, purpura, epistaxis
INTEG: *Rash,* local reaction, pruritus
MISC: Rigors, fever, *infusion reactions,* **sepsis, risk for fatal infection**
MS: Back pain
RESP: Cough, pneumonia, rhinitis, **bronchospasm,** dyspnea, pharyngitis

Pharmacokinetics

Absorption	Unknown
Distribution	Unknown; steady state 6 wk
Metabolism	Unknown
Excretion	Unknown
Half-life	12 days

Pharmacodynamics

Unknown

INTERACTIONS

Individual drugs

Radiation: increased bone marrow depression

Drug classifications

Live-virus vaccines: decreased antibody reaction
Other neoplastics: increased bone marrow depression

Drug/lab test

Diagnostic tests using antibodies

NURSING CONSIDERATIONS

Assessment

• Assess CBC, platelets qwk or more often if myelosuppression occurs; assess CD4+ after therapy until recovery of >200 cells/mcL

BLACK BOX WARNING: Assess for symptoms of infection; chills, fever, headache, may be masked by product fever; do not administer product if infection is present

• Assess CNS reaction: LOC, mental status, dizziness, confusion

• Assess cardiac status: lung sounds; ECG before and during treatment, especially in those with cardiac disease

BLACK BOX WARNING: Assess for bone marrow depression: bruising, bleeding, blood in stools, urine, sputum, emesis

Nursing diagnoses

• Body image, disturbed (adverse reactions)
• Infection, risk for (adverse reactions)
• Injury, risk for (adverse reactions)
• Knowledge, deficient (teaching)
• Nutrition, impaired: less than body requirements, imbalanced (side effects)

Patient/family education

• Instruct patient to take acetaminophen for fever
• Advise patient to avoid hazardous tasks, since confusion, dizziness may occur
• Instruct patient to report signs of infection: sore throat, fever, diarrhea, vomiting

Evaluation

Positive therapeutic outcome
• Decreased production of malignant lymphocytes

---

alendronate (Rx)

(al-en'droe-nate)
Apo-Alendronate ✦, CO Alendronate, Fosamax, Gen-Alendronate ✦, Novo-Alendronate ✦, PMS-Alendronate
Func. class.: Bone-resorption inhibitor
Chem. class.: Bisphosphonate
Pregnancy category C

Do not confuse:
Fosamax/Flomax

ACTION: Decreases rate of bone resorption and may directly block dissolution of hydroxyapatite crystals of bone; inhibits osteoclast activity

Therapeutic outcome: Decreased symptoms of osteoporosis, Paget's disease

USES: Treatment and prevention of osteoporosis in postmenopausal women, treatment of osteoporosis in men, Paget's disease, treatment of corticosteroid-induced osteoporosis in postmenopausal women not receiving estrogen, or in men who are continuing corticosteroid treatment with low bone mass

---

Adverse effects: *italics* = common; **bold** = life-threatening

CONTRAINDICATIONS:

Hypersensitivity to bisphosphonates, delayed esophageal emptying, inability to sit or stand for 30 min, hypocalcemia

Precautions: Pregnancy **C**, breastfeeding, children, CCr <35 ml/min, esophageal disease, increased esophageal cancer risk, ulcers, gastritis, poor dental health

DOSAGE AND ROUTES

Osteoporosis in postmenopausal women
Adult and geriatric: PO 10 mg daily or 70 mg qwk

Osteoporosis in men
Adult: PO 10 mg/day or 70 mg qwk

Paget's disease
Adult and geriatric: PO 40 mg daily × 6 mo, consider retreatment for relapse

Prevention of osteoporosis
Adult (postmenopausal females): PO 5 mg daily or 35 mg qwk

Corticosteroid-induced osteoporosis in postmenopausal women (not receiving estrogen)
Adult: PO 10 mg daily

Corticosteroid-induced osteoporosis in men or premenopausal women (not receiving estrogen)
Adult: PO 5 mg daily

Renal dose
Adult: PO CCr ≤35 ml/min, not recommended

Available forms: Tabs 5, 10, 35, 40, 70 mg; oral sol 70 mg/75 ml

Implementation
- Give PO for 6 mo to be effective in Paget's disease; take with 8 oz of water 30 min before 1st food, beverage, or medication of the day
- Patient to remain upright for 30 min after dose to prevent esophageal irritation
- Store in cool environment out of direct sunlight

Tablet:
- Do not lie down for ≥30 min after dose, do not take at bedtime

Liquid:
- Use oral syringe or calibrated device; give in AM with ≥2 oz of water ≥30 min before food, beverage, or medication

ADVERSE EFFECTS

CNS: Headache
CV: Atrial fibrillation
GI: Abdominal pain, constipation, nausea, vomiting, esophageal ulceration, acid reflux, dyspepsia, **esophageal perforation,** diarrhea, **esophageal cancer**
META: Hypophosphatemia, hypocalcemia
MS: Bone pain, osteonecrosis of the jaw, bone fractures
SYST: Angioedema, Stevens-Johnson syndrome, toxic epidermal necrolysis

Pharmacokinetics

Absorption	Bioavailability 60%
Distribution	Mainly to bones; protein binding 78%
Metabolism	Unknown
Excretion	Via kidneys after bound to bone
Half-life	>10 yrs

Pharmacodynamics

Unknown

INTERACTIONS

Drug classifications
Aminoglycosides, antacids, calcium supplements: decreased absorption
H_2 blockers, proton pump inhibitors (PPIs), gastric mucosal agents, NSAIDs, salicylates: adverse GI reactions

Drug/food
Caffeine, food, orange juice: decreased product absorption

NURSING CONSIDERATIONS

Assessment
⚠ **Assess for serious reactions: angioedema, Stevens-Johnson syndrome, toxic epidermal necrolysis, atrial fibrillation**
- Assess dental status, regular dental exams should be done; dental extractions (cover with antiinfectives) prior to procedure
- Hormonal status if a woman, prior to treatment
- Assess for **osteoporosis:** bone density testing
- For **Paget's disease:** increased skull size, bone pain, headache
- Monitor renal studies and electrolytes (calcium, potassium, magnesium, phosphorous) BUN/creatinine
- Assess for **hypercalcemia:** paresthesia, twitching, laryngospasm, Chvostek's, Trousseau's signs

---

⚠ Nurse Alert

• Monitor alkaline phosphatase; level of 2 ×
upper limit of normal is indicated for Paget's
disease

Nursing diagnoses
• Injury, risk for (uses)
• Knowledge, deficient (teaching)

Patient/family education
• Teach patient to remain upright for 30 min
after dose to prevent esophageal irritation; if
dose is missed, skip dose, do not double doses
or take later in day
• Teach patient to take in AM, only before food,
other meds, to take with 6-8 oz of water (not
mineral water)
• Teach patient to take calcium, vit D if instructed by provider
• Teach patient to use weight-bearing exercise
to increase bone density
• Teach patient to let provider know if pregnancy is planned or suspected or if nursing
• Advise to maintain good oral hygiene

Evaluation
Positive therapeutic outcome
• Increased bone mass, absence of fractures

---

alfuzosin (Rx)
(al-fyoo′zoe-sin)
Apo-Alfuzosin ✦, Uroxatral
Func. class.: Urinary tract, antispasmodic,
α_1-agonist
Chem. class.: Quinazolone
Pregnancy category B

ACTION: Binds preferentially to α_{1A}-
adrenoceptor subtype located mainly in the
prostate, relaxing smooth muscles

Therapeutic outcome: Resolution of
symptoms of benign prostatic hyperplasia

USES: Symptoms of benign prostatic
hyperplasia

CONTRAINDICATIONS:
Hypersensitivity, moderate to severe hepatic
impairment, not indicated for use in women
or children, breastfeeding (but not used in
women)

Precautions: Pregnancy **B**, geriatric, coronary artery disease, coronary insufficiency, mild
hepatic disease, mild/moderate/severe renal
disease, history of QT prolongation or coadministration with medications known to prolong QT
interval, torsades de pointes, syncope, surgery,
prostate cancer, orthostatic hypotension, ocular
surgery, CAD, dysrhythmias, angina

DOSAGE AND ROUTES
Adult: PO EXT REL 10 mg daily, taken after
same meal each day

Available forms: EXT REL tabs 10 mg

Implementation
• Swallow tabs whole; do not break, crush, or
chew tabs
• Store in tight container in cool environment

ADVERSE EFFECTS
CNS: *Dizziness, headache,* fatigue, flushing
CV: Postural hypotension (dizziness, light-
headedness, fainting) within a few hours of
administration, chest pain, tachycardia, angina
GI: Nausea, abdominal pain, dyspepsia, consti-
pation, diarrhea, liver injury, jaundice
GU: Impotence, priapism
INTEG: Rash, urticaria, **angioedema,**
pruritus
MISC: Body pain in general, xerostomia,
rhinitis
RESP: Upper respiratory tract infection,
pharyngitis, bronchitis, sinusitis

Pharmacokinetics

Absorption	Unknown
Distribution	Moderately protein bound (82%-90%)
Metabolism	Liver (by CYP3A4 enzyme)
Excretion	Urine
Half-life	10 hr

Pharmacodynamics
Unknown

INTERACTIONS
Individual drugs
Alcohol: possible increased effects of alfuzosin
Doxazosin, itraconazole, ketoconazole,
prazosin, ritonavir, terazosin: do not take
concurrently

Drug classifications
b-Blockers, nitrates, phosphodiesterase 5
inhibitors: increased hypotension
CYP3A4 inhibitors (ketoconazole, itraconazole,
ritonavir): do not take concurrently

NURSING CONSIDERATIONS
Assessment
• Assess for prostatic hyperplasia: change in
urinary patterns, baseline and throughout treatment

Adverse effects: *italics* = common; **bold** = life-threatening

• Monitor CBC with differential and liver function tests; B/P and heart rate; QT prolongation
• Monitor BUN, uric acid, urodynamic studies (urinary flow rates, residual volume)
• Monitor I&O ratios, weight daily, edema; report weight gain or edema

Nursing diagnoses
• Urinary elimination, impaired (uses)
• Knowledge, deficient (teaching)

Patient/family education
• Advise not to drive or operate machinery for 4 hr after first dose or after dosage increase

Evaluation
Positive therapeutic outcome
• Decreased symptoms of benign prostatic hyperplasia

aliskiren (Rx)
(a-lis'kir-en)
Tekturna
Func. class.: Antihypertensive
Chem. class.: Direct renin inhibitor
Pregnancy category
C (1st trimester)
D (2nd/3rd trimesters)

ACTION: Renin inhibitor that acts on the renin-angiotensin system (RAS)

Therapeutic outcome: Decrease in B/P

USES: Hypertension, alone or in combination with other antihypertensives

CONTRAINDICATIONS:
Hypersensitivity

> **BLACK BOX WARNING:** Pregnancy **D** (2nd/3rd trimester)

Precautions: Pregnancy **C** (1st trimester), breastfeeding, children, geriatric, angioedema, aortic/renal artery stenosis, cirrhosis, CAD, dialysis, hyper/hypokalemia, hyponatremia, hypotension, hypovolemia, renal/hepatic disease, surgery, diabetes, seizures

DOSAGE AND ROUTES
Adult: PO 150 mg/day, may increase to 300 mg/day if needed, max 300 mg/day

Available forms: Tabs 150, 300 mg

Implementation
• PO; do not use with a high-fat meal
• Give daily with a full glass of water, titrate up to achieve correct dose

• Do not discontinue abruptly; correct electrolyte/volume depletion prior to treatment
• Store in tight container at room temperature

ADVERSE EFFECTS
CNS: Headache, dizziness
CV: Orthostatic hypotension, hypotension
GI: Diarrhea
GU: Renal stones, increased uric acid
INTEG: Rash
META: Hyperkalemia
MISC: Angioedema, cough

Pharmacokinetics	
Absorption	Poor, bioavailability 2.3%
Distribution	Steady state 7-8 days
Metabolism	Unknown
Excretion	91% unchanged in the feces
Half-life	Unknown

Pharmacodynamics	
Onset	Unknown
Peak	1-3 hr
Duration	Unknown

INTERACTIONS
Individual drugs
Atorvastatin, cycloSPORINE, itraconazole, ketoconazole: increased aliskiren levels, concurrent use is not recommended
Warfarin: decreased levels of warfarin

Drug classifications
ACE inhibitors, angiotensin receptor antagonists, potassium-sparing diuretics, potassium supplements: increased potassium levels
Diuretics, other antihypertensives: increased hypotension

Drug/food
High-fat meal: decreased absorption

Drug/lab test
Increased: uric acid, CPK, BUN, serum creatinine, potassium
Decreased: Hct, Hgb

NURSING CONSIDERATIONS
Assessment
• Monitor renal tests: uric acid, serum creatinine, BUN may be increased; hyperkalemia may occur
• Assess for allergic reactions: angioedema may occur
• Monitor daily dependent edema in feet, legs; weight, B/P, orthostatic hypotension, if there is a significant drop in B/P, place in supine position, give **IV** 0.9% NaCl

Nursing diagnoses
- Cardiac output, decreased (uses)
- Knowledge, deficient (teaching)
- Noncompliance (teaching)

Patient/family education
- Teach patient the importance of complying with dosage schedule even if feeling better
- Instruct patient to notify if pregnancy is planned or suspected; if pregnant, product needs to be discontinued
- Teach patient how to take B/P and normal reading for age-group
- Advise patient that if dose is missed, take as soon as possible; if it is almost time for the next dose, take only that dose; do not double dose
- Instruct patient not to use OTC products, including herbs, supplements unless approved by prescriber
- Advise patient to report to prescriber immediately: dizziness, faintness, chest pain, palpitations, uneven or rapid heart beat, headache, severe diarrhea, swelling of tongue or lips, trouble breathing, difficulty swallowing, tightening of the throat
- Caution patient not to operate machinery or perform hazardous tasks if dizziness occurs
- Advise patient to avoid faintness; do not get up or stand up rapidly

BLACK BOX WARNING: Advise patient to notify prescriber if pregnancy is planned or suspected; if pregnant, product should be discontinued (pregnancy **D** 2nd/3rd trimester)

Evaluation
Positive therapeutic outcome
- Decrease in B/P

allopurinol (Rx)
(al-oh-pure′i-nole)
Aloprim, Apo-Allopurinol ✦, Zyloprim
Func. class.: Antigout drug, antihyperuricemic
Chem. class.: Xanthine enzyme inhibitor
Pregnancy category C

Do not confuse:
allopurinol/apresoline, **Zyloprim**/Zovirax

ACTION: Inhibits the enzyme xanthine oxidase, reducing uric acid synthesis

Therapeutic outcome: Decreasing serum uric acid levels, decreasing joint pain

USES: Chronic gout, hyperuricemia associated with malignancies, recurrent calcium oxalate calculi, uric acid calculi

CONTRAINDICATIONS:
Hypersensitivity

Precautions: Pregnancy **C**, breastfeeding, children, renal/hepatic disease

DOSAGE AND ROUTES
Increased uric acid levels in malignancies
Adult: PO 600-800 mg/day in divided doses, for 2-3 days; start up to 1-2 days prior to chemotherapy; **IV** INF 200-400 mg/m²/day, max 600 mg/day 24-48 hr prior to chemotherapy, may be divided at 6-, 8-, 12-hr intervals
Child 6-10 yr: PO 300 mg/day, adjust dose after 48 hr
Child <6 yr: PO 150 mg/day, adjust dose after 48 hr
Child: IV INF 200 mg/m²/day, initially as a single dose or divided q6-12hr

Gout (mild)
Adult: PO 100 mg/day, increase qwk based on uric acid levels, max 800 mg/day, maintenance dose 100-200 mg bid-tid

Gout (moderate-severe)
Adult: PO 400-600 mg/day in a single dose or divided bid-tid, max 800 mg/day, doses >300 mg should be given in divided doses

Recurrent calculi
Adult: PO 200-300 mg/day in a single dose or divided bid-tid, max 300 mg/dose, 800 mg/day

Uric acid nephropathy prevention
Adult and child >10 yr: PO 600-800 mg daily × 2-3 days

Renal dose
Adult: PO/IV CCr 81-100 ml/min 300 mg/day; CCr 61-80 ml/min 250 mg/day; CCr 41-60 ml/min 200 mg/day; CCr 21-40 ml/min 150 mg/day; CCr 10-20 ml/min 100-200 mg/day; CCr 3-9 ml/min 100 mg/day or 100 mg every other day; CCr <3 ml/min 100 mg q24hr or longer or 100 mg every third day

Available forms: Tabs, scored, 100, 300 mg; powder for inj 500 mg/vial

Implementation
PO route
- Give with meals to prevent GI symptoms; crush and mix with food or fluids for patients with swallowing difficulties

- Increase fluid intake to 2 L/day
- Give a few days before antineoplastic therapy if using for hyperuricemia associated with malignancy

Intermittent IV infusion route
- Reconstitute 30-ml vial with 25 ml of sterile water for inj; dilute to desired conc (≤6 mg/ml) with 0.9% NaCl for inj or D₅ for inj, begin inf within 10 hr

IV compatibilities: Acyclovir, aminophylline, amphotericin B lipid complex, anidulafungin, argatroban, atenolol, aztreonam, bivalirudin, bleomycin, bumetanide, buprenorphine, butorphanol, calcium gluconate, CARBOplatin, caspofungin, ceFAZolin, cefoperazone, cefotetan, ceftazidime, ceftizoxime, cefTRIAXone, cefuroxime, CISplatin, cyclophosphamide, DACTINomycin, DAUNOrubicin liposome, dexamethasone, dexmedetomidine, docetaxel, DOXOrubicin liposomal, enalaprilat, etoposide, famotidine, fenoldopam, filgrastim, fluconazole, fludarabine, fluorouracil, furosemide, gallium, ganciclovir, gatifloxacin, gemcitabine, gemtuzumab, granisetron, heparin, hydrocortisone phosphate, hydrocortisone succinate, HYDROmorphone, ifosfamide, linezolid, LORazepam, mannitol, mesna, methotrexate, metroNIDAZOLE, milrinone, mitoxantrone, morphine, nesiritide, octreotide, oxytocin, paclitaxel, pamidronate, pantoprazole, pemetrexed, piperacillin, piperacillin-tazobactam, plicamycin, potassium chloride, ranitidine, sodium, sulfamethoxazole-trimethoprim, teniposide, thiotepa, ticarcillin, ticarcillin clavulanate, tigecycline, tirofiban, vancomycin, vasopressin, vinBLAStine, vinCRIStine, voriconazole, zidovudine, zoledronic acid

ADVERSE EFFECTS
CNS: *Headache,* drowsiness, neuritis, paresthesia
EENT: Retinopathy, cataracts, epistaxis
GI: *Nausea, vomiting, anorexia, malaise,* metallic taste, cramps, peptic ulcer, diarrhea, stomatitis
HEMA: Agranulocytosis, thrombocytopenia, aplastic anemia, pancytopenia, leukopenia, bone marrow suppression, eosinophilia
INTEG: Fever, chills, dermatitis, pruritus, purpura, erythema, ecchymosis, alopecia, rash, **Stevens-Johnson syndrome**
MISC: Myopathy, arthralgia, hepatomegaly, **cholestatic jaundice, renal failure, exfoliative dermatitis**

Pharmacokinetics
Absorption	80%
Distribution	Widely distributed
Metabolism	Liver to oxypurinol
Excretion	Kidneys
Half-life	1-2 hr

Pharmacodynamics
	PO	IV
Onset	Unknown	Unknown
Peak	1½ hr	Up to 30 min
Duration	Unknown	Unknown

INTERACTIONS
Individual drugs
Ammonium chloride, potassium/sodium phosphate, vit C: increased kidney stone formation
Ampicillin, amoxicillin: increased risk of rash
Azathioprine: increased bone marrow depression
Mercaptopurine: increased bone marrow depression
Rasburicase: increased xanthine nephropathy, calculi
Theophylline: increased action of theophylline

Drug classifications
ACE inhibitors: increased hypersensitivity
Anticoagulants (oral): increased action of oral anticoagulants
Antidiabetics (oral): increased action of antidiabetics
Antineoplastics: increased bone marrow suppression
Diuretics (thiazide): increased hypersensitivity

NURSING CONSIDERATIONS
Assessment
- Assess for **pain** including location, characteristics, onset/duration, frequency, quality, intensity or severity of pain, precipitating factors; **gout:** joint pain, swelling, may use with NSAIDs for acute gouty attacks
- Monitor uric acid levels q2wk; normal uric acid levels are 6 mg/dl or less; check I&O ratio; increase fluids to 2 L/day to prevent stone formation, toxicity
- Monitor CBC, AST, BUN, creatinine before starting treatment, monthly; check blood glucose in diabetic patients receiving oral antidiabetic agents

Nursing diagnoses
- Knowledge, deficient (teaching)

- Nutrition, impaired: more than body requirements, imbalanced (uses)

Patient/family education
- Tell patient to increase fluid intake to 2 L/day; to avoid taking large doses of vit C; kidney stone formation may occur; to maintain a diet enhancing urine alkalinity (e.g., milk, other dairy products); if taking for calcium oxalate stones, reduce dairy products, refined sugar, sodium, meat
- Tell patient to report skin rash, stomatitis, malaise, fever, aching; product should be discontinued
- Advise patient to avoid hazardous activities if drowsiness or dizziness occurs; response may take several days to determine
- Tell patient to avoid alcohol, caffeine; these substances increase uric acid levels and decrease allopurinol levels
- Teach patient to report side effects and adverse reactions to prescriber, including rash, itching, nausea, vomiting

Evaluation
Positive therapeutic outcome
- Decreased pain in joints
- Decreased stone formation in kidney
- Decreased uric acid level to 6 mg/dl

---

almotriptan (Rx)
(al-moh-trip′tan)
Axert
Func. class.: Antimigraine agent
Chem. class.: 5-HT₁ receptor agonist, triptan

Pregnancy category C

ACTION: Binds selectively to the vascular 5-HT$_{1B/1D/1F}$ receptor subtype, exerts antimigraine effect; causes vasoconstriction in cranial arteries

Therapeutic outcome: Absence of migraines

USES: Acute treatment of migraine with or without aura (Adults/adolescents/children ≥12 yr)

CONTRAINDICATIONS:
Hypersensitivity, acute MI, angina, CV disease, CAD, stroke, vasospastic angina, ischemic heart disease or risk for, peripheral vascular syndrome; uncontrolled hypertension, basilar or hemiplegic migraine

Precautions: Pregnancy **C**, breastfeeding, children <18 yr, geriatric, postmenopausal women, men >40 yr, risk factors for coronary artery disease, MI, hypercholesterolemia, obesity, diabetes, impaired renal/hepatic function, sulfonamide hypersensitivity, cardiac dysrhythmias, Raynaud's disease, tobacco smoking, Wolff-Parkinson-White syndrome

DOSAGE AND ROUTES
Adult/adolescent/child ≥12 yr: PO 6.25-12.5 mg, may repeat dose after 2 hr; max 2 doses/24 hr, 25 mg/day, or 4 treatment cycles within any 30-day period

Renal/hepatic dose (CCr 10-30 ml/hr)
Adult: PO 6.25 mg initially, max 12.5 mg

Available forms: Tabs 6.25, 12.5 mg

Implementation
- Swallow tabs whole; do not break, crush, or chew tabs
- Provide quiet, calm environment with decreased stimulation from noise, bright light, excessive talking

ADVERSE EFFECTS
CNS: *Tingling, hot sensation, burning, feeling of pressure, tightness, numbness, dizziness, sedation,* headache, anxiety, fatigue, cold sensation, **seizures**
CV: *Flushing,* palpitations, tachycardia, **coronary artery vasospasm, MI, ventricular fibrillation, ventricular tachycardia**
EENT: Throat, mouth, nasal discomfort; vision changes
GI: Nausea, xerostomia
INTEG: Sweating
MS: *Weakness, neck stiffness,* myalgia
RESP: Chest tightness, pressure

Pharmacokinetics
Absorption	Well absorbed (~70%)
Distribution	35% protein bound
Metabolism	Liver (metabolite); metabolized by MAO-A, CYP2D6, CYP3A4
Excretion	Urine, feces
Half-life	3-4 hr

Pharmacodynamics
Onset	Unknown
Peak	1-3 hr
Duration	3-4 hr

INTERACTIONS
Individual drugs
Ergot: increased vasospastic effects, avoid concurrent use

Erythromycin, itraconazole, ketoconazole, ritonavir: increased plasma concentration of almotriptan

Drug classifications
5-HT$_1$ agonists, ergot derivatives: increased vasospastic effects, avoid concurrent use

CYP2D6 inhibitors: increased almotriptan effect; do not use together

MAOIs: increased almotriptan effect; do not use together

SSRIs, SNRIs, serotonin-receptor agonists, sibutramine: increased serotinin syndrome

Drug/herb
Feverfew: avoid use

St. John's wort: increased serotonin syndrome

NURSING CONSIDERATIONS
Assessment
• Assess B/P, signs/symptoms of coronary vasospasms
• Assess for tingling, hot sensation, burning, feeling of pressure, numbness, flushing
• Assess for stress level, activity, recreation, coping mechanisms
• Assess neurologic status: LOC, blurring vision, nausea, vomiting, tingling in extremities preceding headache
• Assess for ingestion of **tyramine-containing foods** (pickled products, beer, wine, aged cheese), food additives, preservatives, colorings, artificial sweeteners, chocolate, caffeine, which may precipitate these types of headaches
• Assess for **migraine:** pain, location, aura, duration, intensity, nausea, vomiting
• Assess for **serotonin syndrome:** occurs in those taking SSRIs, SNRIs; agitation, confusion, hallucinations, diaphoresis, hypertension, diarrhea, fever, tremor

Nursing diagnoses
• Knowledge, deficient (teaching)
• Pain, acute (uses)

Patient/family education
• Instruct patient to use contraception while taking product, notify prescriber if pregnancy is planned or suspected, avoid breastfeeding
• Advise patient to have dark, quiet environment available
• Inform patient that product does not prevent or reduce number of migraine attacks

• Advise patient to report chest pain, drowsiness, dizziness, tingling, flushing

Evaluation
Positive therapeutic outcome
• Decrease in severity of migraine

TREATMENT OF OVERDOSE:
Gastric lavage followed by activated charcoal; clinical and ECG monitoring for ≥ 20 hr after overdose

ALPRAZolam (Rx)
(al-pray'zoe-lam)
Gen-Alprazolam ✦, **Niravam, Xanax, Xanax XR**
Func. class.: Antianxiety/sedative/hypnotic
Chem. class.: Benzodiazepine, short/intermediate acting
Pregnancy category D
Controlled substance schedule IV

Do not confuse:
ALPRAZolam/LORazepam,
Xanax/Lanoxin/Tylox/Zantac

ACTION: Depresses subcortical levels of CNS, including limbic system, reticular formation

Therapeutic outcome: Decreased anxiety

USES: Anxiety, panic disorders with or without agoraphobia, anxiety with depressive symptoms

Unlabeled uses: Premenstrual dysphoric disorder, insomnia, PMS, alcohol withdrawal syndrome

CONTRAINDICATIONS:
Pregnancy **D,** breastfeeding, hypersensitivity to benzodiazepines, closed-angle glaucoma, psychosis, addiction

Precautions: Geriatric, debilitated, hepatic disease, obesity, severe pulmonary disease

DOSAGE AND ROUTES
Anxiety disorder
Adult: PO 0.25-0.5 mg tid, may increase q3-4days if needed, max 4 mg/day in divided doses
Geriatric: PO 0.125-0.25 mg bid; increase by 0.125 mg prn

Panic disorder
Adult: PO 0.5 mg tid, may increase up to 1 mg/day q3-4days, max 10 mg/day; EXT REL TABS (Xanax XR) give daily in AM 0.5-1 mg initially, maintenance 3-6 mg daily

Premenstrual dysphoric disorder (unlabeled)
Adult: PO 0.25 mg bid-qid, starting on day 16-18 of menses cycle, taper over 2-3 days when menses occurs, max 4 mg/day

Hepatic dose
Reduce dose

Insomnia (unlabeled)
Adult: PO 0.25-0.5 mg at bedtime

Available forms: Tabs 0.25, 0.5, 1, 2 mg; ext rel tabs (Xanax XR) 0.5, 1, 2, 3 mg; orally disintegrating tabs 0.25, 0.5, 1, 2 mg; oral sol, 1 mg/ml

Implementation
• Give with food or milk for GI symptoms; high-fat meal decreases absorption; tab may be crushed, if patient is unable to swallow medication whole, and mixed with foods or fluids; may divide total daily dose into more times/day, if anxiety occurs between doses
• Give sugarless gum, hard candy, frequent sips of water for dry mouth
• Discontinue, decrease by 0.5 mg q3days
• Place orally disintegrating tabs on tongue to dissolve and swallow
• Give ext rel tab in AM

ADVERSE EFFECTS
CNS: *Dizziness, drowsiness,* confusion, headache, anxiety, tremors, stimulation, fatigue, depression, insomnia, hallucinations, memory impairment, poor coordination
CV: *Orthostatic hypotension,* **ECG changes, tachycardia,** hypotension
EENT: *Blurred vision,* tinnitus, mydriasis
GI: Constipation, dry mouth, nausea, vomiting, anorexia, diarrhea, weight gain/loss, increased appetite
GU: Decreased libido
INTEG: Rash, dermatitis, itching, angioedema

Pharmacokinetics

Absorption	Slow, complete
Distribution	Widely distributed; crosses placenta; crosses blood-brain barrier, protein binding 80%
Metabolism	Liver, to active metabolites
Excretion	Kidneys, breast milk
Half-life	12-15 hr

Pharmacodynamics

	PO	Oral Disintegrating
Onset	1 hr	
Peak	1-2 hr	1.5-2 hr
Duration	4-6 hr, therapeutic response 2-3 days	

INTERACTIONS
Individual drugs
Alcohol: increased CNS depression
Cigarette smoking: decreased drug level
Levodopa: decreased action of levodopa
Rifampin: decreased action of ALPRAZolam

Drug classifications
Anticonvulsants, antihistamines, opioids, sedatives/hypnotics: increased CNS depression
CYP3A4 inducers (barbiturates): decreased action of ALPRAZolam
CYP3A4 inhibitors (cimetidine, disulfiram, erythromycin, fluoxetine, isoniazid, itraconazole, ketoconazole, metoprolol, propoxyphene, propranolol, valproic acid): increased action of ALPRAZolam
Xanthines: decreased sedation

Drug/herb
Chamomile, kava, melatonin, St. John's wort, valerian: increased CNS depression

Drug/food
Grapefruit juice: increased product level

Drug/lab test
Increased: ALT, AST, alkaline phosphatase

NURSING CONSIDERATIONS
Assessment
⚠ **Assess mental status: mood, sensorium, anxiety, affect, sleeping pattern, drowsiness, dizziness, especially geriatric; physical dependency, withdrawal symptoms: anxiety, panic attacks, agitation, seizures, headache, nausea, vomiting, muscle pain,**

weakness; suicidal tendencies; withdrawal seizures may occur after rapid decrease in dose or abrupt discontinuation; short duration of action makes it the product of choice in the geriatric

• Monitor B/P (with patient lying, standing), pulse; if systolic B/P drops 20 mm Hg, hold product, notify prescriber

• Monitor blood studies: CBC during long-term therapy; blood dyscrasias have occurred rarely; decreased hematocrit, neutropenia may occur

• Monitor hepatic studies: AST, ALT, bilirubin, creatinine LDH, alkaline phosphatase, if on long-term treatment

• Monitor I&O; indicate renal dysfunction if on long-term treatment

Nursing diagnoses
• Anxiety (uses)
• Injury, risk for (adverse reactions)
• Knowledge, deficient (teaching)

Patient/family education
• Tell patient that product may be taken with food or fluids and tabs may be crushed or swallowed whole

• Tell patient not to use for everyday stress or longer than 4 mo unless directed by prescriber; not to take more than prescribed amount; may be habit forming; not to double doses or skip doses; memory impairment is a sign of long-term use

• Tell patient to avoid OTC preparations unless approved by prescriber; alcohol and CNS depressants increase CNS depression

• Tell patient to avoid driving, activities that require alertness, since drowsiness may occur; to avoid alcohol ingestion or other psychotropic medications; to rise slowly, or fainting may occur, especially geriatric; that drowsiness may worsen at beginning of treatment

• Tell patient not to discontinue medication abruptly after long-term use; withdrawal symptoms include vomiting, cramping, tremors, seizures

Evaluation
Positive therapeutic outcome
• Decreased anxiety, restlessness, sleeplessness (short-term treatment only)

TREATMENT OF OVERDOSE:
Lavage, VS, supportive care, flumazenil

⚠ HIGH ALERT

alteplase (tissue plasminogen activator, t-PA) (Rx)
(al-ti-plaze')
Activase, Cathflo
Func. class.: Thrombolytic enzyme
Chem. class.: Tissue plasminogen activator (TPA)
Pregnancy category C

Do not confuse:
alteplase/Altace

ACTION: Produces fibrin conversion of plasminogen to plasmin; able to bind to fibrin, convert plasminogen in thrombus to plasmin, which leads to local fibrinolysis, limited systemic proteolysis

Therapeutic outcome: Lysis of thrombi in MI, pulmonary emboli (life threatening)

USES: Lysis of obstructing thrombi associated with acute MI; conditions requiring thrombolysis (e.g., PE, unclotting arteriovenous shunts, acute ischemic CVA); central venous catheter occlusion (Cathflo)

Unlabeled uses: Arterial thromboembolism, deep vein thrombosis (DVT), occlusion prophylaxis, percutaneous coronary intervention (PCI)

CONTRAINDICATIONS:
Active internal bleeding, recent CVA, severe uncontrolled hypertension, intracranial/intraspinal surgery/trauma (within 3 mo), aneurysm, brain tumor, platelets <100,000 mm³, bleeding diathesis including INR >1.7 or PT >15 sec, arteriovenous malformation, subarachnoid hemorrhage, intracranial hemorrhage, uncontrolled hypertension, seizure at onset of stroke

Precautions: Pregnancy **C**, breastfeeding, children, geriatric, neurologic deficits, mitral stenosis, recent GI/GU bleeding, diabetic retinopathy, subacute bacterial endocarditis, arrhythmias, diabetic hemorrhage retinopathy, CVA, recent major surgery, hypertension, acute pericarditis, hemostatic defects, significant hepatic disease, septic thrombophlebitis, occluded AV cannula at seriously infected site

---

DOSAGE AND ROUTES

Pulmonary embolism
Adult: IV 100 mg over 2 hr, then heparin

Acute ischemic stroke
Adult: IV 0.9 mg/kg, max 90 mg; give as INF over 1 hr, give 10% of dose **IV** BOL over 1st min

Myocardial infarction (standard infusion)
Adult >65 kg: IV a total of 100 mg, given over 3 hr; 6-10 given **IV** BOL over 1-2 min, then the remaining 50-54 mg over the remainder of the hr, during 2nd, 3rd hr 20 mg is given by cont **IV** INF (20 mg/hr)

Adult <65 kg: IV 1.25 mg/kg over 3 hr; 60% in first 1 hr (10% as a bolus), remaining 40% over next 2 hr

Myocardial infarction (accelerated infusion)
Adult >67 kg: 100 mg total dose: give 15 mg **IV** BOL, then 50 mg over 30 min, then 35 mg over 60 min

Adult <67 kg: 15 mg **IV** BOL: then 0.75 mg/kg over 30 min (max 50 mg); 0.5 mg/kg over the next 60 min (max 35 mg)

Occlusion prophylaxis (unlabeled)
Adult ≥30 kg: Max 2 mg in 2 ml; may use up to 2 doses (120 min apart)

Available forms: Powder for inj 50 mg (29 million international units/vial), 100 mg (58 million international units/vial), lyophilized powder for injection 2 mg

Implementation
Intermittent IV infusion route
• Give after reconstituting with provided diluent; add appropriate amount of sterile water for inj (no preservatives); 20-mg vial/20 ml or 50-mg vial/50 ml (1 mg/ml); mix by slow inversion or dilute with 0.9% NaCl, D$_5$W to a concentration of 0.5 mg/ml further dilution; 1.5 to <0.5 mg/ml may result in precipitation of product; use 18-G needle; flush line with 0.9% NaCl after administration; use reconstituted **IV** sol within 8 hr or discard, within 6 hr of coronary occlusion for best results

⚠ **Do not use 150 mg or more total dose; intracranial bleeding may occur**
• Give heparin therapy after thrombolytic therapy is discontinued and when thrombin time, ACT, and APTT <2 times control (about 3-4 hr), treatment can be initiated before coagulation study results, infusion should be discontinued if pretreatment is INR >1.7, PT >15 sec, or an elevated APPT is identified

• Avoid invasive procedures, inj, rect temp; apply pressure for 30 sec to minor bleeding sites; 30 min to sites of atrial puncture, followed by pressure dressing; inform prescriber if this does not attain hemostasis; apply pressure dressing
• **Cathflo Activase:** reconstitute by using 2.2 ml of sterile water provided and injecting in vial, direct flow into powder (1 mg/ml), foam will disappear after standing, swirl, do not shake, sol will be pale yellow or clear, use sol within 8 hr, instill 2 ml of reconstituted sol into occluded catheter, try to aspirate after ½ hr, if unable to remove allow 2 hrs; a second dose may be used; aspirate 5 ml of blood to remove clot and product; irrigate with normal saline
• Store powder at room temperature or refrigerate; protect from excessive light

Y-site compatibilities: Eptifibatide, lidocaine, metoprolol, propranolol

Y-site incompatibilities: DOBUTamine, DOPamine, heparin, nitroglycerin

ADVERSE EFFECTS
CV: *Sinus bradycardia, ventricular tachycardia, accelerated idioventricular rhythm, bradycardia, recurrent ischemic stroke, cholesterol microembolization,* hypotension
EENT: Orolingual angioedema
INTEG: *Urticaria, rash*
SYST: **GI, GU, intracranial, retroperitoneal bleeding,** *surface bleeding,* **anaphylaxis,** fever

Pharmacokinetics
Absorption	Complete
Distribution	Unknown
Metabolism	>80% liver
Excretion	Kidneys
Half-life	35 min

Pharmacodynamics
Onset	Immediate
Peak	30-45 min
Duration	4 hr

INTERACTIONS
Individual drugs
Abciximab, clopidogrel, dipyridamole, eptifibatide, plicamycin, ticlopidine, tirofiban, valproic acid: increased bleeding
ACE inhibitors: increased orolingual angioedema
Nitroglycerin: decreased effect

Drug classifications
Anticoagulants (oral), cephalosporins (some), NSAIDs, salicylates: increased bleeding

Drug/herb
Feverfew, garlic, ginger, ginkgo, ginseng, green tea: increased risk of bleeding

Drug/lab test
Increased: PT, APTT, TT

NURSING CONSIDERATIONS

Assessment
• Treatment is not recommended in patient with acute ischemic stroke >3 hr after symptom onset, with minor neurologic deficit, or with rapidly improving symptoms
• Monitor VS q15min, B/P, pulse, respirations (including peripheral), neurologic signs, temp at least q4hr; temp >104° F (40° C) indicates internal bleeding; monitor rhythm closely; ventricular dysrhythmias may occur with hyperfusion; monitor heart, breath sounds, neurologic status, and peripheral pulses, those with severe neurologic deficit (NIHSS >22) at presentation (increased risk of hemorrhage)
⚠ **Assess for bleeding during first hr of treatment and 24 hr after procedure: hematuria, hematemesis, bleeding from mucous membranes, epistaxis, ecchymosis, puncture sites; guaiac all body fluids and stools; obtain blood studies (Hct, platelets, PTT, PT, TT, APTT) before starting therapy; PT or APTT must be <2 times control before starting therapy; TT or PT q3-4hr during treatment; obtain CPK-MB to identify product effectiveness**
• Assess **hypersensitivity:** fever, rash, facial swelling, dyspnea, itching, chills; mild reaction may be treated with antihistamines; report to prescriber
• **Pulmonary embolism:** monitor pulse, B/P, ABGs, rate/rhythm of respirations
• **Occlusion:** have patient exhale then hold breath when connecting/disconnecting syringe to prevent air embolism
• **Cholesterol embolism:** assess for purple toe syndrome, acute renal failure, gangrenous digits, hypertension, livedo reticularis, pancreatitis, MI, cerebral infarction, spinal cord infarction, retinal artery occlusion, bowel infarction, rhabdomyolysis
• **Myocardial infarction:** monitor ECG; on monitor, watch for segment changes, changes in rhythm: sinus bradycardia, ventricular tachycardia, accelerated idioventricular rhythm may occur due to reperfusion, cardiac enzymes, radionuclide myocardial scanning/coronary angiography
• **Pulmonary embolism:** monitor pulse, B/P, ABGs, rate/rhythm of respirations; symptoms include dyspnea, tachypnea, chest pain, cough, hemoptysis
• **Occlusion:** have patient exhale then hold breath when connecting/disconnecting syringe to prevent air embolism

Nursing diagnoses
• Injury, risk for (adverse reactions)
• Pain, chronic (uses)
• Tissue perfusion, ineffective cardiac (uses)

Patient/family education
• Teach patient reason for alteplase, signs and symptoms of bleeding, allergic reactions, when to notify prescriber

Evaluation
Positive therapeutic outcome
• Lysis of pulmonary thrombi
• Adequate hemodynamic state
• Absence of congestive heart failure

aluminum hydroxide (OTC)
Func. class.: Antacid, hypophosphatemic, antiulcer
Chem. class.: Aluminum product, phosphate binder
Pregnancy category C

ACTION: Neutralizes gastric acidity, binds phosphates in GI tract; these phosphates are excreted

Therapeutic outcome: Decreased acidity, healing of ulcers; decreased phosphate levels in chronic renal failure

USES: Antacid, adjunct in peptic, gastric, duodenal ulcers; hyperphosphatemia in chronic renal failure; reflux esophagitis, hyperacidity, heartburn, stress ulcer prevention in critically ill, GERD

Unlabeled uses: GI bleeding

CONTRAINDICATIONS: Hypersensitivity to this product or aluminum products

Precautions: Pregnancy C, breastfeeding, geriatric, fluid restriction, decreased GI motility, GI obstruction, dehydration, renal disease, sodium-restricted diets

DOSAGE AND ROUTES

Antacid
Adult: SUSP PO 600 mg 1 hr after meals, at bedtime; max 6 times/day

Hyperphosphatemia
Adult: PO 300-600 mg tid
Child: PO 50-150 mg/kg/day in 4-6 divided doses

GI bleeding (unlabeled)
Infant: PO 2-5 ml/dose q1-2hr
Child: PO 5-15 ml/dose q1-2hr

Available forms: SUSP 320 mg/5 ml, 600 mg/5 ml

Implementation
• 2 tsp (10 ml) neutralizes 20 mEq of acid
PO route
• Give laxatives or stool softeners if constipation occurs, especially geriatric
• Give after shaking suspension; follow with water to facilitate passage
• Tab may be chewed if patient is unable to swallow, drink 8 oz of water after chewing; or by nasogastric tube if patient unable to swallow
• Give with 8 oz of water for hyperphosphatemia unless contraindicated
• Give 1 hr before or after other medications to prevent poor absorption
• Give 15 ml 30 min after meals and at bedtime (esophagitis)
NG tube route
• May be given as prescribed q1-2hr and given by gastric tube after diluting with water (peptic ulcer)

ADVERSE EFFECTS

GI: *Constipation,* anorexia, **obstruction,** fecal impaction
META: *Hypophosphatemia,* hypercalciuria

Pharmacokinetics

Absorption	Not usually absorbed
Distribution	Widely distributed if absorbed; crosses placenta
Metabolism	Unknown
Excretion	Feces, kidneys (small amounts), breast milk
Half-life	Unknown

Pharmacodynamics

Onset	20-40 min
Peak	$^1/_2$ hr
Duration	1-3 hr

INTERACTIONS

Individual drugs
Allopurinol, amprenavir, delavirdine, digoxin, gabapentin, gatifloxacin, isoniazid, ketoconazole, penicillamine, phenytoin, quinidine, ticlopidine: decreased effect of each of these drugs

Drug classifications
Anticholinergics, cephalosporins, corticosteroids, H_2 antagonists, iron salts, phenothiazines, quinolones, tetracyclines, thyroid hormones: decreased effect of each of these drug classifications

Drug/food
High-protein meal: decreased product effect

NURSING CONSIDERATIONS

Assessment
• Assess pain symptoms: location, duration, intensity, alleviating/precipitating factors
• Monitor phosphate levels, since product is bound in GI system; urinary pH, calcium, electrolytes; hypophosphatemia: anorexia, weakness, fatigue, bone pain, hyperreflexia
• Monitor constipation; increase bulk in diet if needed

Nursing diagnoses
• Constipation, risk for (adverse reactions)
• Knowledge, deficient (teaching)
• Pain, chronic (uses)

Patient/family education
• Instruct patient to increase fluids to 2000 ml/day unless contraindicated
• Instruct patient to avoid phosphate-containing foods (most dairy products, eggs, fruits, carbonated beverages) during product therapy; to add cheese, corn, pasta, plums, prunes, lentils after product (hyperphosphatemia)
• Instruct patient not to use for prolonged periods if serum phosphate is low or if on a low-sodium diet; CHF patients should check for sodium content and use sodium-reduced products
• Instruct patient that stools may appear white or speckled; constipation may result; to report black tarry stools, which indicate gastric bleeding
• Instruct patient to check with prescriber after 2 wk of self-prescribed antacid use; may be used for 4-6 wk after symptoms subside or as prescribed
• Instruct patient to separate other medications by 2 hr

Evaluation
Positive therapeutic outcome
- Absence of pain, decreased acidity
- Increased pH of gastric secretions
- Decreased phosphate levels

alvimopan (Rx)
(al-vi′moe-pan)
Entereg
Func. class.: Functional GI disorder agent
Chem. class.: Peripheral μ-opioid receptor antagonist
Pregnancy category B

ACTION: Acts within the GI tract, antagonizes opioid-induced GI dysfunction

Therapeutic outcome: Resolution of ileus

USES: Ileus, postoperative

CONTRAINDICATIONS:
Hypersensitivity

BLACK BOX WARNING: No more than 15 doses

Precautions: Pregnancy **B**, breastfeeding, renal/hepatic disease, children, GI obstruction, MI, complete GI obstruction surgery

DOSAGE AND ROUTES
Ileus, postoperative
Adult: PO 12 mg given $1/2$-5 hr before surgery, then 12 mg bid beginning the day after surgery, max 7 days (15 doses)

Available forms: Caps 12 mg

Implementation
- Use in hospital only; therapeutic doses of opiates should not be used for >7 consecutive days
- Must register in EASE program
- Do not give >15 doses (short-term hospital only)
- Give without regard to food
- Store at room temperature

ADVERSE EFFECTS
CV: MI
GI: Dyspepsia, flatulence, constipation
GU: Urinary retention
MISC: Anemia, hypokalemia
MS: Back pain

Pharmacokinetics

Absorption	High-fat meal decreases absorption
Distribution	Protein binding 80%-94%
Metabolism	Unknown
Excretion	Kidneys (35%)
Half-life	Terminal 10-18 hr

Pharmacodynamics
Unknown

INTERACTIONS
Individual drugs
Amiodarone, bepridil, cycloSPORINE, diltiazem, itraconazole, quinidine, quinine, spironolactone, verapamil: increased alvimopan effect
Methylnaltrexone: duplicate therapy

Drug classifications
Opiate agonists: increased GI adverse reactions; do not give if opiate agonists were taken for ≥7 days
Opiate antagonists: duplicate therapy

NURSING CONSIDERATIONS
Assessment
- Monitor Hgb, Hct, serum potassium

Nursing diagnoses
- Knowledge, deficient (teaching)

Patient/family education
- Instruct the patient in the reason for the product

Evaluation
Positive therapeutic outcome
- Resolution of ileus

amantadine (Rx)
(a-man′ta-deen)
Gen-Amantadine ✤
Func. class.: Antiviral, antiparkinsonian agent
Chem. class.: Tricyclic amine
Pregnancy category C

Do not confuse:
amantadine/ranitidine/rimantidine

ACTION: Prevents uncoating of nucleic acid in viral cell, preventing penetration of virus to host; causes release of dopamine from neurons

Therapeutic outcome: Resolution of infection, lessening of parkinsonism symptoms

USES: Prophylaxis or treatment of influenza type A, extrapyramidal reactions, parkinsonism, Parkinson's disease

Unlabeled uses: Neuroleptic malignant syndrome, MS-associated fatigue

CONTRAINDICATIONS:
Breastfeeding, child <1 yr, hypersensitivity, eczematic rash

Precautions: Pregnancy **C**, geriatric, epilepsy, CHF, orthostatic hypotension, psychiatric disorders, renal/hepatic disease, peripheral edema

DOSAGE AND ROUTES
Influenza type A
Adult and child >9 yr: PO 200 mg/day in single dose or divided bid
Geriatric: PO no more than 100 mg/day
Child 9-12 yr: PO 100 mg bid
Child 1-8 yr: PO 4.4-8.8 mg/kg/day divided bid-tid, max 150 mg/day

Extrapyramidal reaction/parkinsonism
Adult: PO 100 mg bid, up to 400 mg/day in EPS; give for 1 wk, then 100 mg prn up to 400 mg in parkinsonism

Renal dose
Adult: PO CCr 30-50 ml/min 200 mg first day, then 100 mg/day; CCr 15-29 ml/min 100 mg first day, then 100 mg on alternate days; CCr 15 ml/min reduce dose and interval to 200 mg q7days

MS-associated fatigue (unlabeled)
Adult: PO 200 mg daily or 100 mg bid

Neuroleptic malignant syndrome (unlabeled)
Adult: PO 100 mg bid × 3 wk

Available forms: Caps 100 mg; oral sol 50 mg/5 ml, tab 100 mg

Implementation
• **Prophylaxis:** give before exposure to influenza; continue for 10 days after contact; **treatment:** initiate within 24-48 hr after onset of symptoms, continue for 24-48 hr after symptoms disappear
• Give at least 4 hr before bedtime to prevent insomnia
• Give after meals for better absorption, to decrease GI symptoms
• Give in divided doses to prevent CNS disturbances: headache, dizziness, fatigue, drowsiness
• Store in tight, dry container
• Caps may be opened and mixed with food

ADVERSE EFFECTS
CNS: *Headache, dizziness,* drowsiness, fatigue, *anxiety,* psychosis, *depression, hallucinations,* tremors, **seizures,** confusion, *insomnia*
CV: *Orthostatic hypotension,* **CHF**
EENT: Blurred vision
GI: *Nausea, vomiting,* constipation, dry mouth, anorexia
GU: *Frequency, retention*
HEMA: **Leukopenia, agranulocytosis**
INTEG: Photosensitivity, dermatitis, livedo reticularis

Pharmacokinetics
Absorption	Unknown
Distribution	Crosses placenta
Metabolism	Not metabolized
Excretion	Urine unchanged (90%), breast milk
Half-life	11-15 hr

Pharmacodynamics
Onset	48 hr
Peak	2-4 hr
Duration	Unknown

INTERACTIONS
Individual drugs
Atropine: increased anticholinergic response
Intranasal influenzae vaccine: decreased effect of vaccine; avoid use 2 wk before or 48 hr after amantadine
Metoclopramide: decreased amantadine effect
Triamterene, hydrochlorothiazide: decreased excretion of amantadine

Drug classifications
Anticholinergics (other): increased anticholinergic response
CNS stimulants: increased CNS stimulation
Phenothiazines: decreased amantadine effect

Drug/lab test
Increase: BUN, creatinine, alk phos, CK, LDH, bilirubin, AST, ALT, GGT

NURSING CONSIDERATIONS
Assessment
• Monitor I&O ratio; report frequency, hesitancy; serum BUN, creatinine baseline

- Assess **CHF**, confusion, mottling of skin
- Assess bowel pattern before, during treatment
- Assess skin eruptions, photosensitivity after administration of product
- Assess respiratory status: rate, character, wheezing, tightness in chest
- Assess allergies before initiation of treatment, reaction of each medication
- Assess signs of infection
- Assess hematologic status for leukopenia, agranulocytosis
- Assess for **livedo reticularis:** mottling of the skin, usually red, edema, itching in lower extremities
- Assess for **Parkinson's disease:** gait, tremors, akinesia, rigidity
- Assess for **toxicity:** confusion, behavioral changes, hypotension, seizures

Nursing diagnoses
- Infection, risk for (uses)
- Knowledge, deficient (teaching)

Patient/family education
- Advise patient to change body position slowly to prevent orthostatic hypotension
- Teach about aspects of product therapy: need to report dyspnea, weight gain, dizziness, poor concentration, dysuria, behavioral changes
- Advise patient to avoid hazardous activities if dizziness, blurred vision occurs
- Advise patient to take product exactly as prescribed; parkinsonian crisis may occur if product is discontinued abruptly; do not double dose; if a dose is missed, do not take within 4 hr of next dose
- Teach to avoid alcohol; do not breastfeed

Evaluation
Positive therapeutic outcome
- Absence of fever, malaise, cough, dyspnea in infection; tremors, shuffling gait in Parkinson's disease

TREATMENT OF OVERDOSE:
Withdraw product, maintain airway, administer EPINEPHrine, aminophylline, O$_2$, **IV** corticosteroids, physostigmine

ambrisentan (Rx)
(am-bri-sen'tan)
Letairis
Func. class.: Antihypertensive
Chem. class.: Vasodilator/endothelin receptor antagonist
Pregnancy category X

ACTION: Endothelin-1 receptor antagonist; endothelin-1 is vasoconstrictor

Therapeutic outcome: Decreased shortness of breath, dizziness

USES: Pulmonary arterial hypertension, alone or in combination with other antihypertensives

CONTRAINDICATIONS:
Breastfeeding, hypersensitivity

BLACK BOX WARNING: Pregnancy **X**

Precautions: Children, women, geriatric, hepatitis, anemia, heart failure, jaundice, peripheral edema, hepatic disease

DOSAGE AND ROUTES
Adult: PO 5 mg/day; may increase to 10 mg if needed

Hepatic dose
Adult: Discontinue if AST/ALT >5 or if elevations are accompanied by bilirubin >2 ULN or other signs of liver dysfunction

Available forms: Tabs 5, 10 mg

Implementation
- Do not break, crush, or chew tabs
- Give daily with a full glass of water without regard to food
- Do not discontinue abruptly
- Only those facilities enrolled in the LEAP program may administer this product
- Store in tight container at room temperature

ADVERSE EFFECTS
CNS: Headache, fever, flushing, fatigue
CV: Orthostatic hypotension, hypotension, peripheral edema, palpitations
EENT: Sinusitis, rhinitis
GI: Abdominal pain, constipation, anorexia, **hepatotoxicity**
GU: Decreased sperm counts
HEMA: Anemia
INTEG: Rash, **angioedema**

RESP: Pharyngitis, dyspnea, **pulmonary edema, venoocclusive disease (VOD)**

Pharmacokinetics

Absorption	Rapid
Distribution	Protein binding 99%
Metabolism	By CYP3A4, CYP2C19
Excretion	Unknown
Half-life	Terminal 15 hr, effective half-life 9 hr

Pharmacodynamics

Onset	Unknown
Peak	2 hr
Duration	Unknown

INTERACTIONS

Individual drugs

Cimetidine, clopidogrel, efavirenz, felbamate, fluoxetine, modafinil, oxcarbazepine, ticlopidine: possibly increased ambrisentan

Mefloquine, nicardipine, propafenone, quiNIDine, ranolazine, tacrolimus, testosterone: decreased ambrisentan absorption

Drug classifications

Antihypertensives (other), diuretics, MAOIs: increased hypotension

Barbiturates: need for ambrisentan dosage change

CYP3A4 inhibitors (amprenavir, aprepitant, atazanavir, clarithromycin, conivaptan, cyclo-SPORINE, dalfopristin, danazol, darunavir, erythromycin, estradiol, imatinib, itraconazole, ketoconazole, nefazodone, nelfinavir, propoxyphene, quinupristin, ritonavir, RU-486, saquinavir, tamoxifen, telithromycin, troleandomycin, zafirlukast), CYP2C19/CYP3A4 (chloramphenicol, delavirdine, fluconazole, fluvoxamine, isoniazid, voriconazole): increased ambrisentan

CYP3A4 inducers (carBAMazepine, PHENobarbitol, phenytoin, rifampin): decreased ambrisentan

Drug/herb

Ephedra (ma huang), St. John's wort: need for ambrisentan dosage change

Drug/food

Grapefruit products: avoid use

Drug/lab test

Decreased: Hct, Hgb
Increased: LFTs

NURSING CONSIDERATIONS

Assessment

• Assess pulmonary status: improvement in breathing, ability to exercise; pulmonary edema that may indicate venoocclusive disease
• Monitor blood studies: CBC with differential; Hct, Hgb may be decreased
• Monitor liver function tests: AST, ALT, blirubin

> **BLACK BOX WARNING:** Assess pregnancy status before giving this product; pregnancy category **X**

Nursing diagnoses

• Activity intolerance, risk for (uses)
• Breathing pattern, ineffective (uses)
• Knowledge, deficient (teaching)

Patient/family education

• Teach patient the importance of complying with dosage schedule even if feeling better
• Advise patient that if a dose is missed, take as soon as possible; if it is almost time for the next dose, take only that dose; do not double dose
• Instruct patient not to use OTC products, including herbs, supplements unless approved by prescriber
• Advise patient to report to prescriber immediately: dizziness, faintness, chest pain, palpitations, uneven or rapid heart rate, headache
• Caution patient not to operate machinery or perform hazardous tasks if dizziness occurs
• Advise patient to avoid faintness; do not get up or stand up rapidly

> **BLACK BOX WARNING:** To notify if pregnancy is planned or suspected; if pregnant, product will need to be discontinued, pregnancy test done monthly, to use two contraception methods while taking this product

• To report hepatic dysfunction: nausea/vomiting, anorexia, fatigue, jaundice, right upper quadrant abdominal pain, itching, fever, malaise

Evaluation

Positive therapeutic outcome
• Decrease in B/P
• Decreased shortness of breath

amifostine (Rx)

(a-mi-foss'teen)
Ethyol
Func. class.: Cytoprotective agent for
CISplatin/radiation
Pregnancy category C

ACTION: Binds and detoxifies damaging metabolites of cisplatin, alkylating agents, DNA-reactive agents, and ionizing radiation by converting this product by alkaline phosphatase in tissue to an active free thiol compound

Therapeutic outcome: Decreased toxic reaction from cisplatin

USES: Used to reduce renal toxicity when CISplatin is given in ovarian cancer; reduces xerostomia (dry mouth) in radiation therapy for head, neck cancer

Unlabeled uses: To prevent or reduce cisplatin-induced neurotoxicity, cyclophosphamide-induced granulocytopenia; prevent or reduce toxicity of radiation therapy; reduce toxicity of paclitaxel, myelodysplastic syndrome (MDS)

CONTRAINDICATIONS:

Breastfeeding, hypersensitivity to mannitol, aminothiol; hypotension, dehydration

Precautions: Pregnancy **C**, children, geriatric, CV disease, hypocalcemia, MI radiation therapy, stroke, dehydration, hypotension, chemotherapy, exfoliative dermatitis

DOSAGE AND ROUTES

Reduction of renal damage with CISplatin

Adult: **IV** 910 mg/m² daily, within ½ hr before chemotherapy; give over 15 min; may reduce dose to 740 mg/m² if higher dose is poorly tolerated

Xerostomia prophylaxis

Adult: **IV** 200 mg/m² daily over 3 min as INF 15-30 min before radiation therapy

Bone marrow suppression prophylaxis, nephrotoxicity prophylaxis, neurotoxicity prophylaxis (unlabeled)

Adult: **IV** 100-340 mg/m²/day over 15 min prior to each dose of chemotherapy/radiation

Myelodysplastic syndrome (MDS) (unlabeled)

Adult: **IV** 100 mg/m² 3 ×/wk, max 300 mg/m² 3 ×/wk

Available forms: Powder for inj lyophilized 500 mg/vial

Implementation

Intermittent IV infusion route

• Give by **IV** intermittent inf after reconstituting 500 mg/9.5 ml of sterile 0.9% NaCl, further dilute with 0.9% NaCl to a concentration of 5-40 mg/ml, give at a rate over 15 min within ½ hr of chemotherapy
• Patient to be in supine position during infusion

Y-site compatibilities: Amikacin, aminophylline, amphotericin B liposome, ampicillin, ampicillin-sulbactam, aztreonam, bivalirudin, bleomycin, bumetanide, buprenorphine, butorphanol, calcium gluconate, CARBOplatin, carmustine, caspofungin, ceFAZolin, cefotaxime, cefotetan, cefoxitin, ceftazidime, ceftizoxime, cefTRIAXone, cefuroxime, cimetidine, ciprofloxacin, clindamycin, cyclophosphamide, cytarabine, dacarbazine, DACTINomycin, DAPTOmycin, DAUNOrubicin, dexamethasone, dexmedetomidine, diltiazem, diphenhydrA-MINE, DOBUTamine, docetaxel, DOPamine, DOXOrubicin, doxycycline, droperidol, enalaprilat, epirubicin, ertapenem, etoposide, famotidine, fenoldopam, floxuridine, fluconazole, fludarabine, fluorouracil, furosemide, gallium, gentamicin, granisetron, haloperidol, heparin, hydrocortisone, HYDROmorphone, IDArubicin, ifosfamide, imipenem-cilastatin, leucovorin, levofloxacin, linezolid, LORazepam, magnesium sulfate, mannitol, mechlorethamine, meperidine, mesna, methotrexate, methylPRED-NISolone, metoclopramide, metroNIDAZOLE, mezlocillin, milrinone, mitomycin, morphine, nalbuphine, nesiritide, netilmicin, octreotide, ondansetron, oxaliplatin, paclitaxel, palonosetron, pantoprazole, pemetrexed, piperacillin, plicamycin, potassium chloride, promethazine, ranitidine, sodium bicarbonate, streptozocin, tacrolimus, teniposide, thiotepa, ticarcillin, ticarcillin/clavulanate, tigecycline, tirofiban, tobramycin, trastuzumab, trimethoprim-sulfamethoxazole, trimetrexate, vancomycin, vinBLAStine, vinCRIStine, voriconazole, zidovudine

Additive incompatibilities: Do not mix with other products or solutions

ADVERSE EFFECTS

CNS: Dizziness, somnolence, loss of consciousness, **seizures**
CV: Hypotension
EENT: Sneezing
GI: Nausea, vomiting, hiccups, diarrhea
INTEG: Flushing, feeling of warmth
MISC: Hypocalcemia, rash, chills, **anaphylaxis, toxic epidermal necrolysis, toxicoderma, Stevens-Johnson syndrome, exfoliative dermatitis, erythema multiforme**

Pharmacokinetics

Absorption	Complete
Distribution	Unknown
Metabolism	To free thiol compound
Excretion	Unknown
Half-life	5-8 min

Pharmacodynamics

Unknown

INTERACTIONS

Drug classfications
Antihypertensives: increased hypotension

Drug/lab
Decrease: calcium

NURSING CONSIDERATIONS

Assessment
• Assess for **xerostomia:** mouth lesion, dry mouth during therapy
• Assess fluid status before administration; administer antiemetic before administration to prevent severe nausea and vomiting; also, dexamethasone 20 mg **IV** and a serotonin antagonist such as ondansetron, dolasetron, or granisetron
• Monitor calcium levels before, during treatment; may cause hypocalcemia; calcium supplements may be given for hypocalcemia
• Monitor blood pressure before and q5min during infusion; antihypertensive should be discontinued 24 hr prior to infusion; if severe hypotension occurs, give **IV** 0.9% NaCl to expand fluid volume, place in modified Trendelenburg position
• **Anaphylaxis:** Assess for rash, pruritus, wheezing, laryngeal edema, discontinue; give antihistamines, EPINEPHrine depending on severity; reactions may be delayed, if severe, product should be permanently discontinued; other serious skin disorders (Stevens-Johnson syndrome, toxic epidermal necrolysis, *Toxicoderma*, erythema multiforme, exfoliative dermatitis)

Nursing diagnoses
• Injury, risk for (uses)
• Knowledge, deficient (teaching)

Patient/family education
• Teach reason for medication and expected results
• Teach that side effects may cause severe nausea, vomiting, decreased B/P, chills, dizziness, somnolence, hiccups, sneezing

Evaluation
Positive therapeutic outcome
• Absence of renal damage

---

amikacin (Rx)
(am-i-kay′sin)
Amikin
Func. class.: Antibiotic
Chem. class.: Aminoglycoside
Pregnancy category D

Do not confuse:
Amikin/Amicar, amikacin/anakinra

ACTION: Interferes with protein synthesis in bacterial cell by binding to ribosomal subunit, which causes misreading of genetic code; inaccurate peptide sequence forms in protein chain, causing bacterial death

Therapeutic outcome: Bactericidal effects for the following organisms: *Pseudomonas aeruginosa, Escherichia coli, Enterobacter, Acinetobacter, Providencia, Citrobacter, Staphylococcus, Serratia, Proteus*

USES: Severe systemic infections of CNS, respiratory, GI, urinary tract, bone, skin, soft tissues caused by *Staphylococcus aureus (MSSA), Pseudomonas aeruginosa, Escherichia coli, Enterobacter, Acinetobacter, Providencia, Citrobacter, Serratia, Proteus, Klebsiella pneumoniae*

Unlabeled uses: *Mycobacterium avium* complex (intrathecal or intraventricular) in combination; aerosolization, actinomycotic mycetoma

CONTRAINDICATIONS:
Pregnancy **D,** mild to moderate infections, hypersensitivity to aminoglycosides, sulfites

Precautions: Neonates, breastfeeding, geriatric, myasthenia gravis, Parkinson's disease

---

BLACK BOX WARNING: Hearing impairment, renal/neuromuscular disease

DOSAGE AND ROUTES

Severe systemic infections

Adult and child: IV INF 10-15 mg/kg/day in 2-3 divided doses q8-12hr in 100-200 ml D₅W over 30-60 min, not to exceed 1.5 g; use for 7-10 days; decreased dosages are needed in poor renal function as determined by blood levels, renal function studies; **pulse dosing** (once-daily dosing) may be used with some infections; IM 10-15 mg/kg/day in divided doses q8-12hr; daily or extended internal dosing as an alternative dosing regimen

Infant: IV/IM 10 mg/kg initially, then 7.5 mg/kg q12hr

Neonate: IM/IV 10 mg/kg initially, then 7.5 mg/kg q12hr

Premature neonate: IV 10 mg/kg initially, then 7.5 mg/kg q8-12hr

Severe urinary tract infections

Adult: IM 10-15 mg/kg/day divided q8-12hr

Hemodialysis

Adult: IM/IV 7.5 mg/kg followed by 5 mg/kg 3 ×/wk after each dialysis session (for TIW dialysis)

Mycobacterium avian complex (unlabeled)

Adult and adolescent: IV 7.5-15 mg/kg divided q12-24hr as part of a multiple-drug regimen

Child: IV 15-30 mg/kg/day divided q12-24hr as part of a multiple-drug regimen, max 1.5 g/day

Renal dose

Adult: IV/IM CCr 40-59 ml/min 15 mg/kg IV q36hr; CCr 20-39 ml/min 15 mg/kg IV q48hr; <20 ml/min adjust based on serum concentrations and MIC

Available forms: Inj IM, IV 50, 250 mg/ml

Implementation

IM route

• Give deeply in large muscle mass, rotate inj sites

Intermittent IV INF route

• **Dilute** 500 mg of product/100-200 ml of **IV** D₅W, 0.9% NaCl and **give** over ¹/₂-1 hr; dilute insufficient volume to allow inf over 1-2 hr (infants); **flush** after administration with D₅W or 0.9% NaCl; solution is clear or pale yellow; discard if precipitate or dark color develops
• In children, amount of fluid depends on ordered dose; in infants infuse over 1-2 hr

• Give in evenly spaced doses to maintain blood level

Y-site compatibilities: Acyclovir, aldesleukin, alfentanil, amifostine, aminophylline, amiodarone, amsacrine, anidulafungin, ascorbic acid, atracurium, atropine, aztreonam, benztropine, bivalirudin, bumetanide, buprenorphine, butorphanol, calcium chloride/gluconate, CARBOplatin, caspofungin, ceFAZolin, cefepime, cefonicid, cefotaxime, cefotetan, cefoxitin, ceftazidime, ceftizoxime, cefTRIAXone, cefuroxime, chloramphenicol, chlorproMAZINE, cimetidine, cisatracurium, CISplatin, clindamycin, codeine, cyanocobalamin, cyclophosphamide, cycloSPORINE, cytarabine, DACTINomycin, DAPTOmycin, dexamethasone, dexmedetomidine, digoxin, diltiazem, diphenhydrAMINE, DOBUTamine, docetaxel, DOPamine, doripenem, doxacurium, DOXOrubicin, doxycycline, enalaprilat, ePHEDrine, EPINEPHrine, epirubicin, epoetin alfa, eptifibatide, ertapenem, erythromycin, esmolol, etoposide, famotidine, fentaNYL, filgrastim, fluconazole, fludarabine, fluorouracil, foscarnet, furosemide, gemcitabine, gentamicin, glycopyrrolate, granisetron, hydrocortisone, HYDROmorphone, IDArubicin, ifosfamide, IL-2, imipenem-cilastatin, isoproterenol, ketorolac, labetalol, levofloxacin, lidocaine, linezolid, LORazepam, magnesium sulfate, mannitol, mechlorethamine, melphalan, meperidine, metaraminol, methotrexate, methoxamine, methyldopate, methylPREDNISolone, metoclopramide, metoprolol, metroNIDAZOLE, midazolam, milrinone, mitoxantrone, morphine, multivitamins, nafcillin, nalbuphine, naloxone, niCARdipine, nitroglycerin, nitroprusside, norepinephrine, octreotide, ondansetron, oxaliplatin, oxytocin, paclitaxel, palonosetron, pantoprazole, papaverine, pemetrexed, penicillin G, pentazocine, perphenazine, PHENobarbital, phenylephrine, phytonadione, piperacillin-tazobactam, potassium chloride, procainamide, prochlorperazine, promethazine, propranolol, protamine, pyridoxine, quinupristin-dalfopristin, ranitidine, remifentanil, riTUXimab, rocuronium, sargramostim, sodium acetate, sodium bicarbonate, succinylcholine, SUFentanil, tacrolimus, teniposide, theophylline, thiamine, thiotepa, ticarcillin/clavulanate, tigecycline, tirofiban, tobramycin, tolazoline, trimetaphan, urokinase, vancomycin, vasopressin, vecuronium, verapamil, vinCRIStine, vinorelbine, voriconazole, warfarin, zidovudine

ADVERSE EFFECTS

CNS: Confusion, depression, numbness, tremors, **seizures**, muscle twitching, **neurotoxicity,**

dizziness, vertigo, tinnitus, **neuromuscular blockade with respiratory paralysis**
CV: Hypotension or hypertension, palpitations
EENT: Ototoxicity, deafness, visual disturbances
GI: *Nausea, vomiting, anorexia,* increased ALT, AST, bilirubin, hepatomegaly, **hepatic necrosis,** splenomegaly
GU: Oliguria, hematuria, renal damage, azotemia, renal failure, nephrotoxicity
HEMA: Agranulocytosis, thrombocytopenia, leukopenia, eosinophilia, anemia
INTEG: *Rash,* burning, urticaria, dermatitis, alopecia

Pharmacokinetics

Absorption	Well absorbed (IM), completely absorbed (IV)
Distribution	Widely distributed in extracellular fluids, poor in CSF; crosses placenta
Metabolism	Minimal; liver
Excretion	Mostly unchanged (79%) in kidneys, removed by hemodialysis
Half-life	2-3 hr, prolonged up to 7 hr in infants; increased in renal disease

Pharmacodynamics

	IM	IV
Onset	Rapid	Rapid
Peak	15-30 min	1-2 hr
Duration	Unknown	Unknown

INTERACTIONS

Individual drugs
Acyclovir, amphotericin B, cidofovir, cycloSPORINE, vancomycin: nephrotoxicity
DimenhyDRINATE, ethacrynic acid: increased masking of ototoxicity

Drug classifications
Anesthetics, nondepolarizing neuromuscular blockers: increased neuromuscular blockade, respiratory depression
Cephalosporins: inactivation of amikacin, nephrotoxicity
NSAIDs: increased serum trough and peak

Drug/lab test
Increased: BUN, ALT, AST, bilirubin, LDH, alkaline phosphatase, creatinine
Decreased: calcium, sodium, potassium, magnesium

NURSING CONSIDERATIONS

Assessment
• Assess patient for previous sensitivity reaction
• Assess patient for signs and symptoms of infection, including characteristics of wounds, sputum, urine, stool, WBC >10,000/mm^3, earache, temp; obtain baseline information before and during treatment
• Obtain C&S tests before beginning product therapy to identify if correct treatment has been initiated
• Assess for allergic reactions: rash, urticaria, pruritus

> **BLACK BOX WARNING:** Assess renal impairment by securing urine for CCr, BUN, serum creatinine; lower dosage should be given in renal impairment; nephrotoxicity may be reversible if product is stopped at first sign

• Notify prescriber of increased BUN and creatinine, urine CCr <80 ml/min; urinalysis daily for protein, cells, casts
• Monitor blood studies: AST, ALT, CBC, Hct, bilirubin, LDH, alkaline phosphatase; Coombs' test monthly if patient is on long-term therapy
• Monitor electrolytes: potassium, sodium, chloride, magnesium monthly if patient is on long-term therapy
• Assess bowel pattern daily; if severe diarrhea occurs, product should be discontinued
• Monitor for bleeding: ecchymosis, bleeding gums, hematuria, stool guaiac daily if on long-term therapy
• Assess for **overgrowth of infection:** perineal itching, fever, malaise, redness, pain, swelling, drainage, rash, diarrhea, change in cough, sputum
• Obtain weight before treatment; calculation of dosage is usually based on ideal body weight but may be calculated on actual body weight
• Monitor VS during infusion, watch for hypotension, change in pulse
• Assess **IV** site for thrombophlebitis including pain, redness, swelling q30min; change site if needed; apply warm compresses to discontinued site
• Obtain serum peak, drawn 30-60 min after **IV** infusion or 60 min after IM injection; trough level drawn just before next dose; 20-30 mcg/ml, trough 4-8 mcg/ml, blood level should be 2-4 times bacteriostatic level
• Urine pH if product is used for UTI; urine should be kept alkaline

> **BLACK BOX WARNING:** Deafness by audiometric testing, ringing, roaring in ears, vertigo; assess hearing before, during, after treatment

- **Dehydration:** high specific gravity, decrease in skin turgor, dry mucous membranes, dark urine
- **Vestibular dysfunction:** nausea, vomiting, dizziness, headache; product should be discontinued if severe

Nursing diagnoses
- Diarrhea (side effects)
- Infection, risk for (uses)
- Injury, risk for (side effects)
- Knowledge, deficient (teaching)

Patient/family education
- Teach patient to report sore throat, bruising, bleeding, joint pain; may indicate blood dyscrasias (rare)
- Advise patient to contact prescriber if vaginal itching, loose foul-smelling stools, furry tongue occur; may indicate superinfection
- Advise patient to report hypersensitivity: rash, itching, trouble breathing, facial edema and notify prescriber

Evaluation
Positive therapeutic outcome
- Absence of signs/symptoms of infection: WBC <10,000/mm³, temp WNL; absence of red draining wounds; absence of earache
- Reported improvement in symptoms of infection

TREATMENT OF OVERDOSE:
Withdraw product; administer epinephrine, O_2, hemodialysis, exchange transfusion in the newborn; monitor serum levels of product; may give ticarcillin or carbenicillin

---

amiloride (Rx)
(a-mill'oh-ride)
Apo-Amiloride ✦, Midamor
Func. class.: Potassium-sparing diuretic
Chem. class.: Pyrazine
Pregnancy category B

Do not confuse:
amiloride/amlodipine

ACTION: Inhibits sodium, potassium ATPase in the distal tubule, cortical collecting duct resulting in inhibition of sodium reabsorption and decreasing potassium secretion

Therapeutic outcome: Diuretic and antihypertensive effect while retaining potassium

USES: Edema in CHF in combination with other diuretics; for hypertension, adjunct with other diuretics to maintain potassium; polyuria due to lithium administration

Unlabeled uses: Ascites

CONTRAINDICATIONS:
Anuria, hypersensitivity, impaired renal function, diabetic neuropathy

> **BLACK BOX WARNING:** Hyperkalemia

Precautions: Pregnancy **B**, breastfeeding, children, geriatric, dehydration, diabetes, acidosis, respiratory hyponatremia

DOSAGE AND ROUTES
Adult: PO 5-10 mg daily in 1-2 divided doses; may be increased to 10-20 mg daily if needed

Renal dose
Adult: PO CCr 10-50 ml/min reduce dose by 50%; however, avoid if possible, CCr <10 ml/min contraindicated

Ascites (unlabeled)
Adult: PO 10 mg/day, max 40 mg

Available forms: Tabs 5 mg

Implementation
- Give in AM to avoid interference with sleep
- With food; if nausea occurs, absorption may be increased

ADVERSE EFFECTS
CNS: *Headache,* dizziness, fatigue, weakness, paresthesias, tremor, depression, anxiety, encephalopathy
CV: Orthostatic hypotension, dysrhythmias, angina
EENT: Blurred vision, increased intraocular pressure
ELECT: **Hyperkalemia,** dehydration, hyponatremia, hypochloremia
GI: *Nausea, diarrhea,* dry mouth, *vomiting, anorexia,* cramps, constipation, abdominal pain, jaundice
GU: *Polyuria,* dysuria, frequency, impotence
HEMA: Aplastic anemia, **neutropenia**
INTEG: *Rash, pruritus,* alopecia, urticaria
MS: *Cramps*
RESP: Cough, dyspnea, shortness of breath

Pharmacokinetics

Absorption	Variable (10%-15%)
Distribution	Widely distributed
Metabolism	Unchanged in urine (50%), in feces (40%)
Excretion	Renal; breast milk
Half-life	6-9 hr

Pharmacodynamics

Onset	2 hr
Peak	6-10 hr
Duration	24 hr

INTERACTIONS

Individual drugs

> **BLACK BOX WARNING:** CycloSPORINE, tacrolimus: increased hyperkalemia

Lithium: increased lithium toxicity

Drug classifications

> **BLACK BOX WARNING:** ACE inhibitors, diuretics (potassium-sparing), potassium products, salt substitutes: increased hyperkalemia

Antihypertensives: increased action
NSAIDs: decreased effectiveness of amiloride

Drug/herb
Hawthorn, horse chestnut: increased amiloride effect

Drug/food
Potassium foods: increased hyperkalemia

Drug/lab test
Interference: GTT

NURSING CONSIDERATIONS

Assessment
• Monitor for **hyperkalemia:** *MS:* fatigue, muscle weakness; *CARDIAC:* dysrhythmias, hypotension; *NEURO:* paresthesias, confusion; *RESP:* dyspnea
• Monitor for **hypokalemia:** weakness, polyuria, polydipsia, fatigue, ECG ∪ wave
• Assess fluid volume status: I&O ratios and record weight, distended red veins, crackles in lung, color, quality, and specific gravity of urine, skin turgor, adequacy of pulses, moist mucous membranes, bilateral lung sounds, peripheral pitting edema; dehydration symptoms of decreasing output, thirst, hypotension, dry mouth and mucous membranes should be reported
• Monitor electrolytes: potassium, sodium, calcium, magnesium; also include BUN, ABGs, uric acid, CBC, blood glucose
• Assess B/P before, during therapy with patient lying, standing, and sitting as appropriate; orthostatic hypotension can occur rapidly

Nursing diagnoses
• Fluid volume, deficient (side effects)
• Fluid volume, excess (uses)
• Knowledge, deficient (teaching)

Patient/family education
• Teach patient to take medication early in the day to prevent nocturia
• Instruct patient to take with food or milk if GI symptoms of nausea and anorexia occur
• Teach patient to maintain a weekly record of weight and notify prescriber of weight loss >5 lb
• Caution patient that this product causes an increase in potassium levels, so foods high in potassium should be avoided; refer to dietitian for assistance, planning
• Caution patient not to exercise in hot weather or stand for prolonged periods since orthostatic hypotension is enhanced
• Teach patient not to use alcohol or any OTC medications without prescriber's approval; serious product reactions may occur
• Emphasize the need to contact prescriber immediately if muscle cramps, weakness, nausea, dizziness, or numbness occurs
• Teach patient to take own B/P and pulse and record
• Advise patient that dizziness and confusion may occur; avoid driving or other hazardous activities if alertness is decreased
• Teach patient to continue taking medication even if feeling better; this product controls symptoms but does not cure the condition
• Advise patient with hypertension to continue other medical treatment (exercise, weight loss, relaxation techniques, cessation of smoking)

Evaluation
Positive therapeutic outcome
• Prevention of hypokalemia (diuretic use)
• Decreased edema
• Decreased B/P
• Increased diuresis

TREATMENT OF OVERDOSE:
Lavage if taken orally; monitor electrolytes; administer **IV** fluids; monitor hydration, CV, renal status

amino acid (Rx)

(a-mee'noe)
**Injection: FreAmine, HepatAmine
Solution: Aminess, Aminosyn, Branch
Amin, FreAmine III, NephrAmine,
Novamine, ProcalAmine, Ren Amin,
Travasol, Troph Amine**
Func. class.: Caloric agent
Chem. class.: Nitrogen product
Pregnancy category C

ACTION: Needed for anabolism to maintain structure; decreases catabolism, promotes healing

Therapeutic outcome: Positive nitrogen balance, decreased catabolism

USES: Hepatic encephalopathy, cirrhosis, hepatitis, nutritional support in cancer, burn, or solid organ transplant patients; to prevent nitrogen loss when adequate nutrition by mouth, gastric, or duodenal tube cannot be used; intestinal obstruction, short bowel syndrome, severe malabsorption

CONTRAINDICATIONS:

Hypersensitivity, severe electrolyte imbalances, anuria, severe liver damage, maple syrup urine disease, PKU, azotemia, genetic disease of amino acid metabolism

Precautions: Pregnancy **C**, children, renal disease, diabetes mellitus, CHF, breastfeeding, sulfite sensitivity

DOSAGE AND ROUTES

Amino acid injection
Adult: **IV** 80-120 g/day; 500 ml of amino acids/500 ml D_{50} given over 24 hr

Amino acid solution
Adult: **IV** 1-1.5 g/kg/day titrated to patient's needs
Child: **IV** 2-3 g/kg/day titrated to patient's needs

Available forms: Inj; many strengths, types

Implementation
Continuous IV route
• Give up to 40% protein and dextrose (up to 12.5%) via peripheral vein; stronger solutions require central **IV** administration; TPN only mixed with dextrose to promote protein synthesis
• Use immediately after mixing in pharmacy under strict aseptic technique using laminar flowhood; use infusion pump, in-line filter (0.22 μm) unless mixed with fat emulsion and dextrose (3 in 1)
⚠ **Use careful monitoring technique; do not speed up infusion; pulmonary edema, glucose overload will result**
• Storage depends on type of solution; consult manufacturer
• Change dressing and **IV** tubing to prevent infection q24-48hr or q5-7days if transparent dressing is used

ADVERSE EFFECTS

CNS: *Dizziness, headache,* confusion, **loss of consciousness**
CV: Hypertension, **CHF, pulmonary edema**
ENDO: *Hyperglycemia, rebound hypoglycemia, electrolyte imbalances, hyperosmolar syndrome, hyperosmolar hyperglycemic nonketotic syndrome,* alkalosis, acidosis, hypophosphatemia, hyperammonemia, dehydration, hypocalcemia
GI: Nausea, vomiting, liver fat deposits, abdominal pain, jaundice
GU: Glycosuria, osmotic diuresis
INTEG: Chills, flushing, warm feeling, rash, urticaria, extravasation necrosis, phlebitis at inj site

Pharmacokinetics
Absorption	Complete bioavailability
Distribution	Widely distributed
Metabolism	Anabolism
Excretion	Kidney to urea nitrogen
Half-life	Unknown

Pharmacodynamics
Unknown

INTERACTIONS

Drug classifications
Tetracycline: decreased protein-sparing effects (inj only)

NURSING CONSIDERATIONS

Assessment
• Monitor electrolytes (potassium, sodium, calcium, chloride, magnesium), blood glucose, ammonia, phosphate, ketones; renal, liver function studies: BUN, creatinine, ALT, AST, bilirubin; urine glucose q6hr using Chemstrips, which are not affected by infusion substances; if BUN increases over 15%, therapy may need to be discontinued

⚠ Nurse Alert

• Check inj site for extravasation: redness along vein, edema at site, necrosis, pain; for a hard, tender area
• Monitor respiratory function q4hr: auscultate lung fields bilaterally for crackles; monitor respirations for quality, rate, rhythm that indicates fluid overload
• Monitor temp q4hr for increased fever, indicating infection; if infection is suspected, infusion is discontinued and tubing, bottle, catheter tip cultured; blood catheter may be obtained
⚠ Monitor for impending hepatic coma: **asterixis, confusion, fetor, lethargy**
• **Hyperammonemia:** nausea, vomiting, malaise, tremors, anorexia, seizures; increased ammonia, ketone levels may occur

Nursing diagnoses
• Infection, risk for (adverse reactions)
• Injury, risk for (uses, adverse reactions)
• Knowledge, deficient (teaching)
• Nutrition, impaired: less than body requirements, imbalanced (uses)

Patient/family education
• Teach reason for use of amino acids as part of nutrition (TPN)
• Instruct patient to report at once to prescriber if chills, sweating are experienced

Evaluation
Positive therapeutic outcome
• Weight gain
• Decreased jaundice in liver disorders
• Increased LOC

---

aminophylline (theophylline ethylenediamine) (Rx)
(am-in-off′i-lin)
Phyllocontin ♣
Func. class.: Bronchodilator, spasmolytic
Chem. class.: Xanthine, ethylenediamine
Pregnancy category C

ACTION: Exact mechanism unknown; relaxes smooth muscle of respiratory system by blocking phosphodiesterase, which increases cyclic AMP; increased cyclic AMP alters intracellular calcium ion movements; produces bronchodilatation, increased pulmonary blood flow, relaxation of respiratory tract

Therapeutic outcome: Increased ability to breathe

USES: Apnea in infancy for respiratory/myocardial stimulation, bronchial asthma, bronchospasm associated with chronic bronchitis, emphysema

Unlabeled uses: Methotrexate toxicity, sleep apnea, status asthmaticus

CONTRAINDICATIONS:
Hypersensitivity to xanthines, tachydysrhythmias

Precautions: Pregnancy **C,** breastfeeding, children, geriatric, CHF, cor pulmonale, hepatic disease, diabetes mellitus, hyperthyroidism, hypertension, seizure disorder, irritation of the rectum or lower colon, alcoholism, active peptic ulcer disease

DOSAGE AND ROUTES
Adult: PO 6 mg/kg, then 3 mg/kg q6hr × 2 doses, then 3 mg/kg q8hr maintenance, max 900 mg/day or 13 mg/kg; PO in CHF 6 mg/kg, then 2 mg/kg q8hr × 2 doses, then 1-2 mg/kg q12hr maintenance; **IV** 4.7 mg/kg, then 0.55 mg/kg/hr × 12 hr, then 0.36 mg/kg/hr maintenance; **IV** in CHF 4.7 mg/kg, then 0.39 mg/kg/hr × 12 hr; then 0.08-0.16 mg/kg/hr maintenance
Geriatric and in cor pulmonale: PO 6 mg/kg, then 2 mg/kg q6hr × 2 doses, then 2 mg/kg q8hr maintenance; **IV** 4.7 mg/kg, then 0.47 mg/kg/hr × 12 hr, then 0.24 mg/kg/hr maintenance
Child 9-16 yr: PO 6 mg/kg, then 3 mg/kg q4hr × 3 doses, then 3 mg/kg q6hr maintenance, max 18 mg/kg/day 12-16 yr, or 20 mg/kg/day 9-12 yr; **IV** 4.7 mg/kg, then 0.79 mg/kg/hr × 12 hr, then 0.63 mg/kg/hr maintenance
Child 6 mo-9 yr: PO 4 mg/kg q4hr × 3 doses, then 4 mg/kg q6hr maintenance, max 24 mg/kg/day; **IV** 4.7 mg/kg, then 0.95 mg/kg/hr × 12 hr, then 0.79 mg/kg/hr maintenance
Infants 6-52 wk: Dose (0.2 × age in wk) ÷ 5 × kg = 24 hr dose in mg
Neonates up to 40 wk premature postconception age: PO/IV 1 mg/kg q12hr
Neonates at birth or 40 wk postconception age: PO/IV >8 wk postnatal 1-3 mg/kg q6hr; 4-8 wk postnatal 1-2 mg/kg q8hr; up to 4 wk postnatal 1-2 mg/kg q12hr

Hepatic disease
Adult: PO 6 mg/kg, then 2 mg/kg q8hr × 2 doses, then 1-2 mg/kg q12hr maintenance; **IV** 4.7 mg/kg, then 0.39 mg/kg/hr × 12 hr, then 0.08-0.16 mg/kg/hr maintenance

Available forms: Inj 250 mg/10 ml, 500 mg/20 ml, 100 mg/100 ml in 0.45% NaCl; 200 mg/100 ml in 0.45% NaCl; rectal supp 250 mg, 500 mg; oral liq 105 mg/5 ml; tabs 100, 200 mg; cont rel tabs 225, 350 mg

---

Adverse effects: *italics* = common; **bold** = life-threatening

Implementation
- Give around the clock to maintain blood (theophylline) levels
- If switching from **IV** to PO, give controlled-release dose at time **IV** infusion is discontinued; if giving tab (immediate release), discontinue **IV** and wait >4 hr
- If GI upset occurs, take with 8 oz of water or food
- Increase fluids to 2 L/day

PO route
- Do not break, crush, or chew enteric-coated or cont rel tabs
- Avoid giving with food

Continuous IV Infusion route
- May be diluted for **IV** inf in 100-200 ml in D_5W, $D_{10}W$, $D_{20}W$, 0.9% NaCl, 0.45% NaCl, LR
- Give loading dose over $1/2$ hr, max rate of inf 25 mg/min, use infusion pump; after loading dose, give by cont inf
- Avoid IM inj; pain and tissue damage may occur
- Only clear sol; flush **IV** line before dose; store diluted sol for 24 hr if refrigerated

Syringe compatibilities: Heparin, metoclopramide, pentobarbital, thiopental

Y-site compatibilities: Allopurinol, amifostine, amphotericin B sulfate complex, inamrinone, aztreonam, ceftazidime, cimetidine, cladribine, DOXOrubicin liposome, enalaprilat, esmolol, famotidine, filgrastim, fluconazole, fludarabine, foscarnet, gallium, granisetron, heparin sodium with hydrocortisone sodium succinate, labetalol, melphalan, meropenem, netilmicin, paclitaxel, pancuronium, piperacillin/tazobactam, potassium chloride, propofol, ranitidine, remifentanil, sargramostim, tacrolimus, teniposide, thiotepa, tolazoline, vecuronium

Y-site incompatibilities: DOBUTamine, hydrALAZINE, ondansetron

ADVERSE EFFECTS
CNS: Anxiety, restlessness, insomnia, *dizziness,* **seizures,** headache, light-headedness, muscle twitching, tremors
CV: *Palpitations, sinus tachycardia,* hypotension, flushing, **dysrhythmias,** edema
GI: *Nausea, vomiting,* diarrhea, dyspepsia, anal irritation (suppositories), epigastric pain, reflux, anorexia
GU: Urinary frequency, SIADH
INTEG: Flushing, urticaria
MISC: Hyperglycemia
RESP: Tachypnea, increased respiratory rate

Pharmacokinetics
Absorption	Well absorbed (PO), slow (PO–EXT REL), erratic (RECT)
Distribution	Widely distributed; crosses placenta
Metabolism	Liver to caffeine
Excretion	Kidneys
Half-life	3-12 hr, increased in renal disease, CHF, geriatric patients, smokers

Pharmacodynamics
	PO	PO–EXT REL	IV
Onset	15-60 min	Unknown	Immediate
Peak	1-2 hr	4-7 hr	Infusion's end
Duration	6-8 hr	8-12 hr	6-8 hr

INTERACTIONS
Individual drugs
Allopurinol (high doses), cimetidine, clarithromycin, disulfiram, erythromycin, fluvoxamine, interferon, mexiletine: decreased metabolism, increased toxicity of aminophylline
CarBAMazepine, isoniazid: increased or decreased aminophylline levels
Halothane: increased risk of dysrhythmias
Ketoconazole, phenytoin, rifampin: decreased aminophylline effect
Lithium: decreased effect of lithium
Smoking: increased metabolism, decreased effect

Drug classifications
Barbiturates, β-adrenergic blockers: decreased effect of aminophylline
Benzodiazepines, β-blockers (nonselective), corticosteroids, diuretics (loop), fluoroquinolones, influenza vaccines, oral contraceptives: increased aminophylline levels
Corticosteroids, influenza vaccines: increased aminophylline toxicity
Diuretics (loop): may increase or decrease aminophylline levels
Dose-dependent reversal of neuromuscular blockade
Fluoroquinolones: decreased metabolism, increased toxicity
Sympathomimetics: increased CNS, CV adverse reactions
Tetracyclines: increased adverse reactions

Drug/herb
Cola tree, ginseng, guarana, horsetail, Siberian ginseng, tea (black, green), yerba maté: increased effects

St. John's wort: decreased effects

Drug/food
High-carbohydrate, low-protein diet: decreased elimination

Low-carbohydrate, high-protein diet, charcoal-broiled beef: increased elimination

Xanthines: increased effect

Drug/lab test
Increased: plasma free fatty acids

NURSING CONSIDERATIONS

Assessment
• Monitor theophylline blood levels (therapeutic level is 10-20 mcg/ml); toxicity may occur with small increase above 20 mcg/ml, especially geriatric; determine whether theophylline was given recently (24 hr); check for toxicity: nausea, vomiting, anxiety, restlessness, insomnia, tachycardia, dysrhythmias, seizures; notify prescriber immediately

• Monitor I&O; diuresis will occur; dehydration may result in geriatric or children in whom diuresis is great

• Monitor liver function tests: periodically, lower doses may be required in those with moderate to severe hepatic disease

• Monitor respiratory rate, rhythm, depth; auscultate lung fields bilaterally, pulmonary function tests; notify prescriber of abnormalities; check ECG for tachycardia, PVCs, PACs in patients with cardiac problems

• Monitor allergic reactions: rash, urticaria; if these occur, product should be discontinued, prescriber notified

Nursing diagnoses
• Activity intolerance, risk for (uses)
• Airway clearance, ineffective (uses)
• Injury, risk for (uses, adverse reactions)
• Knowledge, deficient (teaching)

Patient/family education
• Teach patient to take doses as prescribed, not to skip dose; to check OTC medications, current prescription medications for ephedrine, which will increase CNS stimulation; advise patient not to drink alcohol or caffeine products (tea, coffee, chocolate, colas), which will increase action

• Teach patient to avoid hazardous activities; dizziness may occur

• Teach patient if GI upset occurs, to take product with 8 oz of water or food; absorption may be decreased

• Teach patient to remain in bed 15-20 min after rect supp is inserted to prevent removal

• Instruct patient to avoid smoking because it increases metabolism; decreases blood levels and terminal half-life; dosage may need to be increased

• Teach patient to obtain blood levels of product every few months to prevent toxicity; not to change brands, since effect may not be the same

• Teach patient to increase fluids to 2 L/day to decrease viscosity of secretions

• Advise patient to report **toxicity:** nausea, vomiting, anxiety, insomnia, rapid pulse, seizures, flushing, headache, diarrhea

Evaluation
Positive therapeutic outcome
• Decreased dyspnea
• Respiratory stimulation in infants
• Clear lung fields bilaterally

⚠ HIGH ALERT

amiodarone (Rx)
(a-mee-oh′da-rone)
Apo-Amiodarone ✦, Cordarone, Gen-Amiodarone ✦, Nexterone, Novo-Amiodarone ✦, Pacerone, PMS-Amiodarone ✦, ratio-Amiodarone ✦, Sandoz Amiodarone
Func. class.: Antidysrhythmic (Class III)
Chem. class.: Iodinated benzofuran derivative
Pregnancy category D

Do not confuse:
amiodarone/inamrinone, **Cordarone**/Inocor

ACTION: Prolongs action potential duration and effective refractory period, noncompetitive α- and β-adrenergic inhibition; increases PR and QT intervals, decreases sinus rate, decreases peripheral vascular resistance

Therapeutic outcome: Decreased amount and severity of ventricular dysrhythmias

USES: Hemodynamically unstable ventricular tachycardia, supraventricular tachycardia, ventricular fibrillation not controlled by 1st-line agents

CONTRAINDICATIONS:
Pregnancy **D**, breastfeeding, neonates, infants, severe sinus node dysfunction, hypersensitivity, cardiogenic shock

---

> **BLACK BOX WARNING:** 2nd-3rd degree AV
> block, bradycardia

Precautions: Goiter, Hashimoto's thyroiditis,
electrolyte imbalances, CHF, severe respiratory
disease, children

> **BLACK BOX WARNING:** Cardiac arrhythmias,
> pneumonitis, pulmonary fibrosis, severe
> hepatic disease

DOSAGE AND ROUTES
Ventricular dysrhythmias
Adult: PO loading dose 800-1600 mg/day for
1-3 wk; then 600-800 mg/day × 1 mo; maintenance 400 mg/day; IV loading dose (first rapid)
150 mg over the first 10 min then slow 360 mg
over the next 6 hr; maintenance 540 mg given
over the remaining 18 hr, decrease rate of the
slow infusion to 0.5 mg/min
Child (unlabeled): PO loading dose 10-15 mg/
kg/day in 1-2 divided doses for 4-14 days then
5 mg/kg/day
Child and infant: IV/INTRAOSSEOUS during
CPR 5 mg/kg as a bolus (PALS guidelines)
Perfusion tachycardia: IV 5 mg/kg loading
dose given over 20-60 min

Supraventricular tachycardia
Adult: PO 600-800 mg/day × 7 days or until
desired response, then 400 mg/day × 21 days,
then 200-400 mg/day maintenance
Child: PO 10 mg/kg/day (800 mg/1.72 m²/day)
× 10 days or until desired response, then 5 mg/
kg/day (400 mg/1.72 m²/day) × 21-28 days,
then 2.5 mg/kg/day (200 mg/1.72 m²/day) (not
recommended in children)

Available forms: Tabs 100, 200, 400 mg;
inj 50 mg/ml

Implementation
Start with patient hospitalized and monitored
PO route
• Give reduced dosage slowly with ECG moni-
toring only
• Loading dose with food to decrease nausea

IV, direct route
• **Peripheral:** max 2 mg/ml for longer than 1
hr; preferred through central venous line with
in-line filter; concentration >2 ml should be
given by central line
• **Cardiac arrest:** give 300 mg bol; may repeat
150 mg after 3-5 min
Intermittent IV INF route
• **Rapid loading:** add 3 ml (150 mg), 100 ml
D₅W (1.5 mg/ml), give over 10 min

• **Slow loading:** add 18 ml (900 mg), 500 ml
D₅W (1.8 mg/ml), give over next 6 hr
Continuous IV infusion route
• After 24 hr, dilute 50 ml to 1-6 mg/ml, give
1-6 mg/ml at 1 mg/ml for the first 6 hr, then 0.5
mg/min

Y-site compatibilities: Amikacin, bretylium, clindamycin, DOBUTamine, DOPamine,
doxycycline, erythromycin, esmolol, gentamicin,
insulin (regular), isoproterenol, labetalol, lidocaine, metaraminol, metronidazole, midazolam,
morphine, nitroglycerin, norepinephrine,
penicillin G potassium, phentolamine, phenylephrine, potassium chloride, procainamide,
tobramycin, vancomycin

Solution compatibilities: D₅W, 0.9%
NaCl

ADVERSE EFFECTS
CNS: *Headache, dizziness,* involuntary move-
ment, tremors, peripheral neuropathy, malaise,
fatigue, ataxia, paresthesias, insomnia
CV: *Hypotension,* **bradycardia, sinus arrest,
CHF, dysrhythmias, SA node dysfunction,
AV block,** increased defibrillation energy
requirement
EENT: Blurred vision, halos, photophobia,
corneal microdeposits, dry eyes
ENDO: Hyper/hypothyroidism
GI: Nausea, vomiting, diarrhea, abdominal
pain, anorexia, constipation, **hepatotoxicity**
GU: Epididymitis, ED
INTEG: Rash, photosensitivity, blue-gray
skin discoloration, alopecia, spontaneous ecchy-
mosis, **toxic epidermal necrolysis,** urticaria,
pancreatitis, phlebitis (IV)
MISC: Flushing, abnormal taste or smell,
edema, abnormal salivation, coagulation
abnormalities
MS: Weakness, pain in extremities
RESP: Pulmonary fibrosis/toxicity, pulmonary inflammation, **ARDS, gasping syndrome
in neonates**

Pharmacokinetics

Absorption	Slow, variable (PO) up to 65%
Distribution	Body tissues; crosses placenta
Metabolism	Liver
Excretion	Bile, kidney (minimal)
Half-life	15-100 days

	PO
Onset	1-3 wk
Peak	Unknown
Duration	Up to months

Pharmacodynamics

INTERACTIONS

Individual drugs
CycloSPORINE, dextromethorphan, digoxin, disopyramide, flecainide, methotrexate, phenytoin, procainamide, quinidine, theophylline: increased blood levels, increased toxicity
Warfarin: increased bleeding

Drug classifications
Azoles, fluoroquinolones, macrolides: increased QT prolongation
β-Adrenergic blockers, calcium channel blockers: increased bradycardia
Class I antidysrhythmics: increased levels
HMG-CoA reductase inhibitors: increased myopathy
Protease inhibitors: increased amiodarone concentrations, possible serious dysrhythmias

Drug/herb
St. John's wort: decreased amiodarone effect

Drug/food
Grapefruit juice: toxicity

Drug/lab test
Increased: T_4, ALT, AST, GGT, alk phos, cholesterol, lipids, PT, INR
Decrease: T_3

NURSING CONSIDERATIONS

Assessment
• Monitor I&O ratio; monitor electrolytes: potassium, sodium, chloride
• Monitor chest x-ray, thyroid function tests
• Monitor liver function studies: AST, ALT, bilirubin, alkaline phosphatase

> **BLACK BOX WARNING:** Monitor ECG continuously to determine product effectiveness; measure PR, QRS, QT intervals; check for PVCs, other dysrhythmias; monitor B/P continuously for hypo/hypertension; check for rebound hypertension after 1-2 hr

• Monitor for dehydration or hypovolemia
• Assess for CNS symptoms: confusion, psychosis, numbness, depression, involuntary movements; if these occur, product should be discontinued

• Assess for hypothyroidism: lethargy, dizziness, constipation, enlarged thyroid gland, edema of extremities, cool, pale skin
• Monitor hyperthyroidism: restlessness, tachycardia, eyelid puffiness, weight loss, frequent urination, menstrual irregularities, dyspnea, warm, moist skin

> **BLACK BOX WARNING:** Assess for pulmonary toxicity including ARDS, pulmonary fibrosis: dyspnea, fatigue, cough, fever, chest pain; product should be discontinued if these occur

• Monitor cardiac rate, respiration: rate, rhythm, character, chest pain, ventricular tachycardia, supraventricular tachycardia or fibrillation
• Assess sight and vision before treatment and throughout therapy; microdeposits on the cornea may cause blurred vision, halos, and photophobia

Nursing diagnoses
• Cardiac output, decreased (uses)
• Gas exchange, impaired (adverse reactions)
• Knowledge, deficient (teaching)

Patient/family education
• Instruct patient to report side effects immediately to prescriber
• Instruct patient that skin discoloration is usually reversible, but skin may turn bluish on neck, face, arms when used for long periods
• Advise patient that dark glasses may be needed for photophobia
• Instruct patient to use sunscreen and protective clothing to prevent burning associated with photosensitivity
• Instruct patient to take medication as prescribed, not to double doses
• Instruct patient to complete follow-up appointment with health care provider including pulmonary function studies, chest x-ray, ophthalmic examinations

Evaluation
Positive therapeutic outcome
• Decreased ventricular tachycardia
• Decreased supraventricular tachycardia or fibrillation

TREATMENT OF OVERDOSE:
Administer O_2, artificial ventilation, ECG, DOPamine for circulatory depression, diazepam or thiopental for seizures, isoproterenol

amitriptyline (Rx)
(a-mee-trip′ti-leen)
Apo-Amitriptyline ✿
Func. class.: Antidepressant—tricyclic
Chem. class.: Tertiary amine
Pregnancy category C

Do not confuse:
amitriptyline/nortriptyline/aminophylline

ACTION: Blocks reuptake of norepinephrine, serotonin into nerve endings that increase action of norepinephrine, serotonin in nerve cells

USES: Major depression

Unlabeled uses: Neuropathic pain, prevention of cluster/migraine headaches, fibromyalgia

Therapeutic outcome: Decreased symptoms of depression after 2-3 wk

CONTRAINDICATIONS:
Hypersensitivity to tricyclics, recovery phase of MI

Precautions: Pregnancy C, breastfeeding, geriatric, seizure disorders, prostatic hypertrophy, schizophrenia, psychosis, severe depression, increased intraocular pressure, closed-angle glaucoma, urinary retention, cardiac disease, renal/hepatic disease, hyperthyroidism, electroshock therapy, elective surgery

> **BLACK BOX WARNING:** Child <12 yr, suicidal patients

DOSAGE AND ROUTES
Depression
Adult/adolescent: PO 25-75 mg/day as a single dose at bedtime or in divided doses; may increase to 200 mg/day, max 300 mg/day (hospitalized)
Geriatric: PO 10-25 mg at bedtime; may be increased to 150 mg/day

Cluster/migraine headaches (unlabeled)
Adult: PO 100-300 mg/day

Pain (unlabeled)
Adult: PO 75-300 mg/day

Fibromyalgia/insomnia (unlabeled)
Adult: PO 10-50 mg nightly

Available forms: Tabs 10, 25, 50, 75, 100, 150 mg

Implementation
• Give with food or milk for GI symptoms
• Crush if patient is unable to swallow medication whole
• Give dose at bedtime if oversedation occurs during day; may take entire dose at bedtime; geriatric may not tolerate once/day dosing
• Store at room temperature; do not freeze

ADVERSE EFFECTS
CNS: *Dizziness, drowsiness,* confusion, headache, anxiety, tremors, stimulation, weakness, insomnia, nightmares, EPS (geriatric), increased psychiatric symptoms, **seizures, suicidal thoughts**
CV: *Orthostatic hypotension,* **ECG changes, tachycardia, hypertension,** palpitations, dysrhythmias
EENT: *Blurred vision,* tinnitus, mydriasis, ophthalmoplegia
GI: *Constipation, dry mouth,* weight gain, nausea, vomiting, **paralytic ileus,** increased appetite, cramps, epigastric distress, jaundice, **hepatitis,** stomatitis
GU: *Urinary retention*
HEMA: **Agranulocytosis, thrombocytopenia, eosinophilia, leukopenia, aplastic anemia**
INTEG: Rash, urticaria, sweating, pruritus, photosensitivity

Pharmacokinetics

Absorption	Well absorbed
Distribution	Widely distributed; crosses placenta
Metabolism	Liver, extensively
Excretion	Kidneys, breast milk
Half-life	10-46 hr

Pharmacodynamics

	PO
Onset	45 min
Peak	2-12 hr
Duration	Unknown

INTERACTIONS
Individual drugs
Alcohol: increased CNS depression
Amiodarone, procainamide, quiNIDine: increased QT prolongation
CarBAMazepine: increased amitriptyline levels, increased toxicity

Cimetidine, fluoxetine: increased levels, increased toxicity

CloNIDine: decreased effects

Guanethidine: decreased effects

Drug classifications

Antidepressants, antidysrhythmics (class IC), phenothiazines: increased amitriptyline levels, toxicity

Antidysrhythmics (class IA, III), tricyclic antidepressants: increased QT prolongation

Antithyroid agents: increased risk of agranulocytosis

Barbiturates, benzodiazepines, CNS depressants, opioids, sedative/hypnotics, sympathomimetics (direct acting): increased CNS effects

MAOIs: hypertensive crisis, seizures, hyperpyretic crisis

Oral contraceptives: increased effects, toxicity

Sympathomimetics (indirect acting): decreased effects

Drug/herb

Chamomile, hops, kava, lavender, valerian: increased CNS depression

SAM-e, St. John's wort, yohimbe: serotonin syndrome

Drug/lab test

Increased: serum bilirubin, blood glucose, alkaline phosphatase, LFTs

Decreased: WBCs, platelets, granulocytes

NURSING CONSIDERATIONS

Assessment

• Monitor B/P (with patient lying, standing), pulse q4hr; if systolic B/P drops 20 mm Hg, hold product, notify prescriber; take VS q4hr in patients with cardiovascular disease

• Monitor blood studies: CBC, leukocytes, differential, cardiac enzymes if patient is receiving long-term therapy

• Monitor hepatic studies: AST, ALT, bilirubin

• Check weight weekly; appetite may increase with product

• Assess ECG for flattening of T wave, bundle branch block, AV block, prolongation of QTc interval, dysrhythmias in cardiac patients

• Assess for EPS primarily in geriatric: rigidity, dystonia, akathisia

• Assess mental status: mood, sensorium, affect, suicidal tendencies; increase in psychiatric symptoms: depression, panic

• Monitor urinary retention, constipation; constipation is more likely to occur in children or geriatric

• Assess for **withdrawal symptoms:** headache, nausea, vomiting, muscle pain, weakness; do not usually occur unless product was discontinued abruptly

• Identify alcohol consumption; if alcohol is consumed, hold dose until morning

• Assess for sexual dysfunction: erectile dysfunction, decreased libido; usually resolves after discontinuing product

Nursing diagnoses

• Coping, ineffective (uses)
• Injury, risk for (side effects)
• Knowledge, deficient (teaching)
• Noncompliance (teaching)

Patient/family education

• Teach patient that therapeutic effects may take 2-3 wk

• Instruct patient to use caution in driving or other activities requiring alertness because of drowsiness, dizziness, blurred vision; to avoid rising quickly from sitting to standing, especially geriatric; management of anticholinergic effects

• Advise patient to avoid alcohol ingestion, other CNS depressants; overheating

• Teach patient not to discontinue medication quickly after long-term use; may cause nausea, headache, malaise

• Advise patient to wear sunscreen or large hat, since photosensitivity occurs; hyperthermia can occur

• Teach patient to increase fluids, bulk in diet if constipation, urinary retention occur, especially geriatric

• Teach patient to use gum, hard sugarless candy, or frequent sips of water for dry mouth

• Instruct patient to use contraception during treatment

Evaluation

Positive therapeutic outcome

• Decreased depression
• Absence of suicidal thoughts

TREATMENT OF OVERDOSE:

ECG monitoring, lavage, administer anticonvulsant, sodium bicarbonate

amLODIPine (Rx)

(am-loe'di-peen)

Norvasc

Func. class.: Antianginal, calcium channel blocker, antihypertensive

Chem. class.: Dihydropyridine

Pregnancy category C

Do not confuse:

amLODIPine/amiloride,
Norvasc/Navane/Norvir/Nascor

ACTION: Inhibits calcium ion influx across cell membrane during cardiac depolarization; produces relaxation of coronary vascular smooth muscle and peripheral vascular smooth muscle; dilates coronary vascular arteries; increases myocardial oxygen delivery in patients with vasospastic angina

Therapeutic outcome: Decreased angina pectoris, dysrhythmias, B/P

USES: Chronic stable angina pectoris, hypertension, variant angina (Prinzmetal's angina); may coadminister with other antihypertensives, antianginals

CONTRAINDICATIONS:

Hypersensitivity to this product, severe aortic stenosis, severe obstructive CAD

> **BLACK BOX WARNING:** Hypersensitivity to dihydropyridine

Precautions: Pregnancy C, breastfeeding, children, geriatric, CHF, hypotension, hepatic injury

DOSAGE AND ROUTES

Coronary artery disease

Adult: PO 5-10 mg daily

Geriatric: PO 5 mg daily, may increase; max 10 mg/day

Hypertension

Adult: PO 5 mg daily initially, max 10 mg/day

Geriatric: PO 2.5 mg/day; may increase to 5 mg/day, max 10 mg/day

Hepatic dose

Adult: PO 2.5 mg/day, may increase to 10 mg/day (antihypertensive); 5 mg/day, may increase to 10 mg/day (antianginal)

Available forms: Tabs 2.5, 5, 10 mg

Implementation

• Give once a day, without regard to meals

ADVERSE EFFECTS

CNS: Headache, fatigue, dizziness, asthenia, anxiety, depression, insomnia, paresthesia, somnolence

CV: Peripheral edema, bradycardia, hypotension, palpitations, syncope, chest pain

GI: Nausea, vomiting, diarrhea, gastric upset, constipation, flatulence, anorexia, gingival hyperplasia, dyspepsia, dysphagia

GU: Nocturia, polyuria, sexual difficulties

INTEG: Rash, pruritus, urticaria, alopecia

MISC: Flushing, muscle cramps, cough, weight gain, tinnitus, epistaxis

Pharmacokinetics

Absorption	Well absorbed up to 90%
Distribution	Crosses placenta, protein binding 93%
Metabolism	Liver, extensively by CYP3A4
Excretion	Kidneys to metabolites (90%)
Half-life	30-50 hr; increased in geriatric, hepatic disease

Pharmacodynamics

Onset	Unknown
Peak	6-10 hr
Duration	24 hr

INTERACTIONS

Individual drugs

Alcohol, fentaNYL, quiNIDine: increased hypotension

Diltiazem: increased amLODIPine level

Lithium: increased neurotoxicity

Drug classifications

Antihypertensives, nitrates: increased hypotension

NSAIDs: decreased antihypertensive effect

Drug/food

Grapefruit juice: increased hypotension

NURSING CONSIDERATIONS

Assessment

• Assess fluid volume status: I&O ratio and record, weight; CHF: distended red veins, crackles in lung; color, quality, and specific gravity of urine, skin turgor, adequacy of pulses, moist mucous membranes, bilateral lung sounds, peripheral pitting edema; dehydration symptoms of decreasing output, thirst, hypotension, dry

mouth and mucous membranes should be reported
• Assess for angina: intensity, location, duration of pain
• Monitor B/P and pulse; if B/P drops, call prescriber
• Monitor ALT, AST, bilirubin daily; if these are elevated, hepatotoxicity is suspected
• Monitor platelet count: if <150,000/mm³, product is usually discontinued and another product started
• Monitor cardiac status: B/P, pulse, respiration, ECG

Nursing diagnoses
• Cardiac output, decreased (uses)
• Knowledge, deficient (teaching)

Patient/family education
• Advise patient to avoid hazardous activities until stabilized on product, dizziness is no longer a problem
• Instruct patient to avoid alcohol and OTC products unless directed by prescriber
• Advise patient to comply in all areas of medical regimen: diet, exercise, stress reduction, smoking cessation, product therapy; to notify prescriber of irregular heartbeat, shortness of breath, swelling of feet, face, and hands, severe dizziness, constipation, nausea, hypotension
• Teach patient to use as directed even if feeling better; may be taken with other cardiovascular products (nitrates, β-blockers)
• Advise to avoid large amounts of grapefruit juice or alcohol

Evaluation
Positive therapeutic outcome
• Decreased anginal pain
• Decreased B/P
• Increased exercise tolerance

TREATMENT OF OVERDOSE:
Defibrillation, β-agonists, **IV** calcium inotropic agents, diuretics, atropine for AV block, vasopressor for hypotension

---

amoxicillin (Rx)
(a-mox-i-sill′in)
Gen-Amoxicillin ❦, Moxatag
Func. class.: Antiinfective, antiulcer
Chem. class.: Aminopenicillin
Pregnancy category B

Do not confuse:
amoxicillin/amoxapine/Amoxil,
Trimen/Diamox/Tylox, **Wymox**/Tylox

ACTION: Interferes with cell wall replication of susceptible organisms by binding to the bacterial cell wall; the cell wall, rendered osmotically unstable, swells and bursts from osmotic pressure; bactericidal, lysis mediated by bacterial cell wall autolysis

Therapeutic outcome: Bactericidal effects for the following organisms: effective for gram-positive cocci *(Staphylococcus aureus, Streptococcus pyogenes, Streptococcus faecalis, Streptococcus pneumoniae)*, gram-negative cocci *(Neisseria gonorrhoeae, Neisseria meningitidis)*, gram-negative bacilli *(Haemophilus influenzae, Proteus mirabilis, Escherichia coli, Salmonella)*, in combination for *Helicobacter pylori*, gram-positive bacilli *(Corynebacterium diphtheriae, Listeria monocytogenes)*; β-lactamase-negative organisms

USES: Infections of respiratory tract, skin, GI tract, GU tract, otitis media, meningitis, septicemia, sinusitis, and bacterial endocarditis prophylaxis in combination with other products used for treatment of *Helicobacter pylori*

Unlabeled uses: Lyme disease, anthrax treatment and prophylaxis

CONTRAINDICATIONS:
Hypersensitivity to penicillins

Precautions: Pregnancy **B**, breastfeeding, neonates, hypersensitivity to cephalosporins, severe renal disease, acute lymphocytic leukemia, mononucleosis, phenylketonuria

DOSAGE AND ROUTES
Renal disease
Adult: PO CCr 10-30 ml/min 250-500 mg q12hr; CCr <10 ml/min 250-500 mg q24hr; do not use 775, 875 mg strength if CCr <30 ml/min

Systemic infections, severe
Adult: PO 750 mg-1.75 g daily in divided doses q8hr or q12hr
Child: PO 20-50 mg/kg/day in divided doses q8hr or q12hr

Gonorrhea
Adult: PO 3 g given with 1 g probenecid as a single dose; followed by tetracycline or erythromycin

Chlamydia trachomatis
Adult: PO 500 mg/day × 1 wk

❦ Canada only   Adverse effects: *italics* = common; **bold** = life-threatening

Bacterial endocarditis prophylaxis
Adult: PO 2 g 1 hr prior to procedure
Child: PO 50 mg/kg/hr 1 hr prior to procedure, max 2 g

Helicobacter pylori
Adult: PO 1000 mg bid given with lansoprazole 30 mg bid, clarithromycin 500 mg bid × 2 wk; or 1000 mg bid given with omeprazole 20 mg bid, clarithromycin 500 mg bid × 2 wk; or 1000 mg tid given with lansoprazole 30 mg tid × 2 wk

Available forms: Caps 250, 500 mg; chewable tabs 125, 200, 250, 400 mg; tabs 250, 500, 875 mg; ext rel tab (Moxatag) 775 mg; susp 125, 200, 250, 400 mg/5 ml

Implementation
PO route
• Give in even doses around the clock; if GI upset occurs, give with food; product must be given for 10-14 days to ensure organism death and prevent superinfection; store in tight container
• The caps may be opened and contents taken with fluids
• **Suspension:** shake well before each dose, may be used alone or mixed in drinks, use immediately; susp may be stored in refrigerator for 14 days
• **Extended release:** do not crush, chew, or break

ADVERSE EFFECTS
CNS: Headache, **seizures,** agitation, confusion, dizziness, insomnia
GI: *Nausea, vomiting, diarrhea,* increased AST, ALT, abdominal pain, glossitis, colitis, **pseudomembranous colitis,** jaundice, cholestasis
HEMA: Anemia, increased bleeding time, **bone marrow depression, granulocytopenia, hemolytic anemia**
INTEG: *Urticaria, rash*
SYST: Anaphylaxis, respiratory distress, serum sickness, Stevens-Johnson syndrome, toxic epidermal necrolysis, exfoliative dermatitis

Pharmacokinetics
Absorption	Well absorbed (90%)
Distribution	Readily in body tissues, fluids, CSF; crosses placenta
Metabolism	Liver (30%)
Excretion	Breast milk, kidney, unchanged (70%)
Half-life	1-1.3 hr

Pharmacodynamics
Onset	$1/2$ hr
Peak	2 hr
Duration	Unknown

INTERACTIONS
Individual drugs
Methotrexate: increased methotrexate levels
Probenecid: increased amoxicillin levels, decreased renal excretion
Warfarin: increased anticoagulant effects

Drug classifications
Contraceptives (oral): decreased contraceptive effectiveness

Drug/lab test
Increase: AST/ALT, alk phos, LDH
False positive: direct Coombs' test

NURSING CONSIDERATIONS
Assessment
• Assess patient for previous sensitivity reaction to penicillins or other cephalosporins; cross-sensitivity between penicillins and cephalosporins is common
• Assess patient for signs and symptoms of **infection,** including characteristics of wounds, sputum, urine, stool, WBC >10,000/mm³, earache, fever; obtain baseline information and monitor symptoms during treatment
• Obtain C&S before beginning product therapy to identify if correct treatment has been initiated
• Assess for allergic reactions during treatment: rash, urticaria, pruritus, chills, fever, joint pain; angioedema may occur a few days after therapy begins; epinephrine and resuscitation equipment should be available for **anaphylactic reactions**
• Identify urine output; if decreasing, notify prescriber (may indicate nephrotoxicity); also, increased BUN, creatinine, urinalysis, protein, blood
• Monitor blood studies: AST, ALT, CBC, Hct, bilirubin, LDH, alkaline phosphatase, Coombs' test monthly if patient is on long-term therapy
• Monitor electrolytes: potassium, sodium, chloride monthly if patient is on long-term therapy
• Assess bowel pattern daily; diarrhea, cramping, blood in stools; if severe diarrhea occurs, notify prescriber; product should be discontinued; **pseudomembranous colitis** may occur
• Monitor for bleeding: ecchymosis, bleeding gums, hematuria, stool guaiac daily if on long-term therapy

- Assess for overgrowth of infection: perineal itching, fever, malaise, redness, pain, swelling, drainage, rash, diarrhea, change in cough, sputum

Nursing diagnoses
- Diarrhea (side effects)
- Infection, risk for (uses)
- Injury, risk for (side effects)
- Knowledge, physical deficient (teaching)
- Noncompliance (teaching)

Patient/family education
⚠ Teach patient to report sore throat, bruising, bleeding, joint pain; may indicate blood dyscrasias (rare)
- Advise patient to contact prescriber if vaginal itching, loose foul-smelling stools, diarrhea, sore throat, fever, fatigue, furry tongue occur; may indicate **superinfection** or **agranulocytopenia**
- Instruct patient to take all medication prescribed for the length of time ordered; not to double dose; chew form is available
- Advise patient to notify prescriber of diarrhea with blood or pus, abdominal pain, which may indicate **pseudomembranous colitis**

Evaluation
Positive therapeutic outcome
- Absence of signs/symptoms of infection (WBC <10,000/mm³, temp WNL, absence of red draining wounds or earache)
- Prevention of endocarditis
- Resolution of ulcer symptoms

TREATMENT OF ANAPHYLAXIS: Withdraw product, maintain airway, administer epinephrine, aminophylline, O₂, **IV** corticosteroids

---

amoxicillin/clavulanate (Rx)
(a-mox-i-sill'in)
Amoclan, Apo-Amoxi Clav ✚,
Augmentin, Augmentin XR,
Clavulin ✚
Func. class.: Broad-spectrum antiinfective (extended spectrum)
Chem. class.: Aminopenicillin-β-lactamase inhibitor
Pregnancy category B

Do not confuse:
Augmentin/amoxicillin

ACTION: Interferes with cell wall replication of susceptible organisms; the cell wall, rendered osmotically unstable, swells and bursts from osmotic pressure; lysis mediated by bacterial cell wall autolytic enzymes, combination increases spectrum of activity against β-lactamase resistance organisms

Therapeutic outcome: Bactericidal effects for the following organisms: *Escherichia coli, Proteus mirabilis, Haemophilus influenzae, Streptococcus faecalis, Streptococcus pneumoniae;* and β-lactamase–producing organisms: *Neisseria gonorrhoeae, Neisseria meningitidis, Shigella, Salmonella, Enterococcus, Streptococcus*

USES: Infections of lower respiratory tract, skin, GU tract; otitis media, sinusitis, pneumonia, and endocarditis prophylaxis

CONTRAINDICATIONS:
Hypersensitivity to penicillins, severe renal disease, dialysis, jaundice

Precautions: Pregnancy **B,** breastfeeding, neonates, children, hypersensitivity to cephalosporins, GI/renal disease, asthma, colitis, diabetes, eczema, leukemia, mononucleosis, viral infections, phenylketonuria

DOSAGE AND ROUTES
Adult: PO 250-500 mg q8hr or 500-875 mg q12hr depending on severity of infection
Child ≤40 kg: PO 20-90 mg/kg/day in divided doses q8-12hr

Renal dose
Adult: PO CCr 10-30 ml/min dose q12hr; CCr <10 ml/min dose q24hr; do not use 875 mg strength if CCr <30 ml/min; Augmentin XR is contraindicated in renal disease

Available forms: Tabs 250, 500, 875 mg/125 mg clavulanate; chewable tabs 200/28.5, 400/57 mg; powder for oral susp 125, 250/28.5, 200/28.5, 400/57, 600/42.9 mg/5 ml; (XR) ext rel tabs 1000 mg amoxicillin/62.5 mg clavulanate; (ES) powder for oral susp 600 mg amoxicillin; 42.9 mg clavulanate 5 ml

Implementation
PO route
- Give in even doses around the clock; if GI upset occurs, give with food; product must be taken for 10-14 days to ensure organism death and prevent superinfection; store in tight container; cap can be opened and mixed with food or liquid; chewable tabs should be chewed

• Administer only as directed; two 250-mg tabs not equivalent to one 500-mg tab due to strength of clavulanate
• Shake susp well before each dose; may be used alone or mixed in drinks, use immediately; susp may be stored in refrigerator for 10 days

ADVERSE EFFECTS

CNS: Headache, fever, **seizures,** agitation, insomnia
GI: *Nausea, diarrhea, vomiting,* increased AST, ALT, abdominal pain, glossitis, colitis, black tongue, **pseudomembranous colitis**
GU: Oliguria, proteinuria, hematuria, *vaginitis, moniliasis,* **glomerulonephritis**
HEMA: Anemia, **bone marrow depression, granulocytopenia, leukopenia, eosinophilia,** thrombocytopenic purpura
INTEG: Rash, urticaria, dermatitis, **toxic epidermal necrolysis**
META: Hyperkalemia, hypokalemia, alkalosis, hypernatremia
SYST: Anaphylaxis, respiratory distress, serum sickness, superinfection, Stevens-Johnson syndrome, candidiasis

Pharmacokinetics

Absorption	Well absorbed (90%)
Distribution	Readily in body tissues, fluids, CSF; crosses placenta
Metabolism	Liver (30%)
Excretion	Breast milk; kidney, unchanged (70%), removed by hemodialysis
Half-life	1-1.3 hr

Pharmacodynamics

Onset	$\frac{1}{2}$ hr
Peak	2 hr
Duration	Unknown

INTERACTIONS

Individual drugs
Allopurinol: increased skin rash
Probenecid: increased amoxicillin levels
Warfarin: increased anticoagulant effect

Drug classifications
Contraceptives (oral): decreased contraceptive effectiveness

Drug/food
High-fat meal: decreased absorption

Drug/lab test
Increased: AST/ALT, alk phos, LDH
False positive: direct Coombs' test

NURSING CONSIDERATIONS

Assessment
• Assess patient for previous sensitivity reaction to penicillins or other cephalosporins; cross-sensitivity between penicillins and cephalosporins is common
• Assess patient for signs and symptoms of **infection,** including characteristics of wounds, sputum, urine, stool, WBC >10,000/mm³, earache, fever; obtain baseline information and during treatment
• Complete C&S before beginning product therapy to identify if correct treatment has been initiated
• Assess for **anaphylaxis:** rash, urticaria, pruritus, chills, dyspnea, laryngeal edema, fever, joint pain; angioedema may occur a few days after therapy begins; epinephrine and resuscitation equipment should be available for anaphylactic reaction
• Identify urine output; if decreasing, notify prescriber (may indicate **nephrotoxicity**)
• Monitor renal studies: urinalysis, protein, blood, BUN, creatinine
• Monitor blood studies: AST, ALT, CBC, Hct, bilirubin, LDH, alkaline phosphatase, Coombs' test monthly if patient is on long-term therapy
• Monitor electrolytes: potassium, sodium, chloride monthly if patient is on long-term therapy
• Assess bowel pattern daily; diarrhea, cramping, blood in stools, report to prescriber; if severe diarrhea occurs, product should be discontinued; may indicate **pseudomembranous colitis**
• Monitor for bleeding: ecchymosis, bleeding gums, hematuria, stool guaiac daily if on long-term therapy
• Assess for **overgrowth of infection:** perineal itching, fever, malaise, redness, pain, swelling, drainage, rash, diarrhea, change in cough, sputum

Nursing diagnoses
• Diarrhea (side effects)
• Infection, risk for (uses)
• Injury, risk for (side effects)
• Knowledge, deficient (teaching)
• Noncompliance (teaching)

Patient/family education
⚠ **Teach patient to report sore throat, bruising, bleeding, joint pain; may indicate blood dyscrasias (rare)**
• Advise patient to contact prescriber if vaginal itching, loose foul-smelling stools occur; may indicate **superinfection**

⚠ Nurse Alert

- Instruct patient to take all medication prescribed for the length of time prescribed
- Advise patient to notify prescriber of diarrhea with blood or pus, which may indicate **pseudomembranous colitis**
- Advise patient to use alternative contraceptive measures if using oral contraceptives

Evaluation
Positive therapeutic outcome
- Absence of signs/symptoms of infection (WBC <10,000/mm^3, temp WNL)
- Reported improvement in symptoms of infection

TREATMENT OF ANAPHYLAXIS: Withdraw product, maintain airway, administer epinephrine, aminophylline, O$_2$, **IV** corticosteroids

AMPHOTERICIN B

amphotericin B lipid based (Rx)
Abelcet
amphotericin B liposome (Rx)
AmBisome
Func. class.: Antifungal
Chem. class.: Amphoteric polyene
Pregnancy category B

ACTION: Increased cell membrane permeability in susceptible organisms by binding sterols in fungal cell membrane, causing leakage of cell components and cell death

Therapeutic outcome: Fungistatic against histoplasmosis, blastomycosis, coccidioidomycosis, cryptococcosis, aspergillosis, zygomycosis, candidiasis, sporotrichosis, cryptococcal meningitis, mucormycosis caused by mucormycosis, *Rhizopus, Absidia, Entomorphthera, Basidobolus*

USES: Treatment of severe, possibly fatal fungal infections (**IV**); treatment of topical fungal infections

Unlabeled uses: Candiduria (bladder irrigation), funguria

CONTRAINDICATIONS:
Hypersensitivity, severe bone marrow depression

Precautions: Pregnancy **B,** breastfeeding, children, renal disease, anemia, hypokalemia, hypomagnesium, infections

BLACK BOX WARNING: Fungal infection

DOSAGE AND ROUTES
Abelcet
Adult and child: IV 5 mg/kg/day as a 1 mg/ml as a single INF given at 2.5 mg/kg/hr

AmBisome

Fungal infections
Adult and child: IV 3-5 mg/kg q24hr
Visceral leishmaniasis: 3-4 mg/kg q24hr days 1-5 and days 14, 21 (immunocompetent) and days 10, 17, 24, 31, 38 (immunocompromised)

Available forms: Amphotericin deoxycholate: inj 50-mg vial, oral susp 100 mg/ml; cream, ointment, lotion 3%; amphotericin B cholesteryl: powder for inj 50 mg/20 ml, 100 mg/50 ml; amphotericin B lipid complex: susp for inj 100 mg/20 ml vial; amphotericin B liposome: powder for inj 50 mg vial

Implementation
Topical route
- Provide enough medication to cover lesions completely; do not cover with occlusive dressing; apply liberally and rub thoroughly into affected area; administer after cleansing with soap, water before each application; dry well (as ordered); wear gloves during application
- Store at room temperature in dry place

Cholesteryl
Liposomal complex
IV route
- Reconstitute with 12 ml sterile water/50 ml vial (4 mg/ml), shake, use 5-mcm filter, dilute in D$_5$W (1-2 mg/ml), flush IV line with D$_5$W before use, or use separate IV line; use filter ≥1 micron, give over 2 hr

Y-site compatibilities: Acyclovir, amifostine, aminophylline, anidulafungin, atropine, azithromycin, bivalirudin, bumetanide, buprenorphine, busulfan, butorphanol, CARBOplatin, carmustine, ceFAZolin, cefoxitin, ceftizoxime, cefTRIAXone, cefuroxime, cimetidine, clindamycin, cyclophosphamide, cytarabine, DACTINomycin, DAPTOmycin, dexamethasone, dexmedetomidine, diphenhydrAMINE, doxacurium, enalaprilat, ePHEDrine, EPINEPHrine, eptifibatide, ertapenem, esmolol, etoposide, famotidine, fenoldopam, fentaNYL, fludarabine, fluorouracil, fosphenytoin, furosemide, granisetron, haloperidol, heparin, hydrocortisone, HYDROmorphone, ifosfamide, isoproterenol, ketorolac, levorphanol, lidocaine, linezolid, mesna, methotrexate, methylPREDNISolone,

Adverse effects: *italics* = common; **bold** = life-threatening

metoprolol, milrinone, mitomycin, nesiritide, nitroglycerin, nitroprusside, octreotide, oxaliplatin, oxytocin, palonosetron, pancuronium, pantoprazole, pemetrexed, PENTobarbital, PHENobarbital, phenylephrine, piperacillin/tazobactam, potassium chloride, procainamide, ranitidine, SUFentanil, tacrolimus, theophylline, thiopental, thiotepa, ticarcillin/clavulanate, tigecycline, trimethoprim/sulfamethoxazole, vasopressin, vinCRIStine, voriconazole, zidovudine

Lipid complex

IV route
• Shake vial until dissolved, withdraw dose using 18-G needle, replace needle from syringe with product using 5-mcm filter needle (use needle for 4 vials or less), empty contents in IV of D$_5$W (1 mg/ml), give at 2.5 mg/kg/hr, use infusion pump

Y-site compatibilities: Anidulafungin, ertapenem, octreotide

ADVERSE EFFECTS

CNS: *Headache, fever, chills,* peripheral nerve pain, paresthesias, peripheral neuropathy, **seizures,** dizziness
CV: Bradycardia, hypotension, **cardiac arrest**
EENT: Tinnitus, deafness, diplopia, blurred vision
GI: *Nausea, vomiting, anorexia,* diarrhea, cramps, **hemorrhagic gastroenteritis, acute liver failure**
GU: *Hypokalemia,* axotemia, hyposthenuria, **renal tubular acidosis,** nephrocalcinosis, **permanent renal impairment, anuria, oliguria**
HEMA: Normochromic and normocytic anemia, **thrombocytopenia, agranulocytosis, leukopenia, eosinophilia,** hypokalemia, hyponatremia, hypomagnesemia
INTEG: *Burning, irritation,* pain, necrosis at inj site with extravasation, flushing, dermatitis, skin rash (topical route)
MS: *Arthralgia, myalgia,* generalized pain, weakness, weight loss
SYST: **Stevens-Johnson syndrome, toxic epidermal necrolysis, exfoliative dermatitis,** anaphylaxis

Pharmacokinetics

Absorption	Complete bioavailability (**IV**), rapidly absorbed (TOP)
Distribution	Body tissues
Metabolism	Liver
Excretion	Kidneys, detectable for several weeks
Half-life	Terminal lipid complex mean 7 days, liposomal mean 4-6 days

Pharmacodynamics

	IV	Top
Onset	Immediate	Unknown
Peak	1-2 hr	Unknown
Duration	Unknown	Unknown

INTERACTIONS

Individual drugs
CISplatin, cycloSPORINE, polymyxin B, vancomycin: increased nephrotoxicity
Digoxin: increased hypokalemia

Drug classifications
Nephrotoxic antibiotics: increased nephrotoxicity
Glucocorticoids, thiazides, skeletal muscle relaxants: increased hypokalemia

NURSING CONSIDERATIONS

Assessment
• Monitor VS q15-30min during first inf; note changes in pulse, B/P
• Monitor blood studies: Hgb, Hct, potassium, sodium, calcium, magnesium q2wk; BUN, creatinine weekly; decreased Hgb, Hct, and magnesium are common with increased potassium
• Monitor weight weekly; if weight increases over 2 lb/wk, edema is present; renal damage should be considered
• Monitor for **renal toxicity:** increasing BUN, serum creatinine; if BUN is >40 mg/dl or if serum creatinine >3 mg/dl, product may be discontinued or dosage reduced; I&O ratio: watch for decreasing urinary output, change in specific gravity; discontinue product to prevent permanent damage to renal tubules; provide hydration of 2-3 L/day
• Monitor for **hepatotoxicity:** increasing AST, ALT, alkaline phosphatase, bilirubin
• Monitor for allergic reaction: dermatitis, rash; product should be discontinued, antihistamines (mild reaction) or EPINEPHrine (severe

reaction) administered; check inj site for throm-bophlebitis
• Monitor for **hypokalemia:** anorexia, drowsiness, weakness, decreased reflexes, dizziness, increased urinary output, increased thirst, paresthesias; if these occur, product should be decreased or discontinued and potassium administered
• Monitor for ototoxicity: tinnitus, ringing, roaring in the ears, vertigo; loss of hearing (rare)
Topical route
• Monitor for allergic reaction: burning, stinging, swelling, redness

Nursing diagnoses
• Infection, risk for (uses)
• Injury, risk for (adverse reaction)
• Knowledge, deficient (teaching)

Patient/family education
Topical route
• Teach patient that skin and clothing may become discolored; to use asepsis (hand washing) before, after each application to prevent further infection
• Instruct patient to apply with glove to prevent further infection; not to cover with occlusive dressing; to continue even if condition improves
• Teach patient to avoid use of OTC creams, ointments, lotions, unless directed by prescriber
• Instruct patient to report increased itching, burning, rash, redness; ointment may irritate most hairy areas; to report if condition worsens
IV route
• Advise patient that long-term therapy may be needed to clear infection (2 wk-3 mo depending on type of infection)
• Teach patient side effects and when to notify prescriber

Evaluation
Positive therapeutic outcome
• Decrease in size, number of lesions (TOP)
• Decreased fever, malaise, rash
• Negative C&S for infecting organism

ampicillin (Rx)
(am-pi-sill'in)
NovoAmpicillin ✦
Func. class.: Broad-spectrum antiinfective
Chem. class.: Aminopenicillin
Pregnancy category B

Do not confuse:
Omnipen/imipenem

ACTION: Interferes with cell wall replication of susceptible organisms; the cell wall, rendered osmotically unstable, swells and bursts from osmotic pressure, lysis mediated by cell wall autolysis

Therapeutic outcome: Bactericidal effects for the following organisms: effective for gram-positive cocci *(Streptococcus aureus, Streptococcus pyogenes, Streptococcus faecalis, Streptococcus pneumoniae)*, gram-negative cocci *(Neisseria meningitidis)*, gram-negative bacilli *(Haemophilus influenzae, Proteus mirabilis, Salmonella, Shigella, Listeria monocytogenes)*, gram-positive bacilli

USES: Infections of respiratory tract, skin, skin structures, GI/GU tract; otitis media, meningitis, septicemia, sinusitis, and endocarditis prophylaxis

CONTRAINDICATIONS:
Hypersensitivity to penicillins, antimicrobial resistance

Precautions: Pregnancy **B,** breastfeeding, neonates, hypersensitivity to cephalosporins, renal disease, mononucleosis

DOSAGE AND ROUTES
Renal dose
Adult and child: CCr 10-50 ml/min extend to q6-12hr; CCr <10 ml/min dose q12-16hr

Systemic infections
Adult and child ≥40 kg (88 lb): PO 250-500 mg q6hr; **IV/IM** 2-8 g daily in divided doses q4-6hr
Child <40 kg: PO 50-100 mg/kg/day in divided doses q6-8hr; **IV/IM** 100-200 mg/kg/day in divided doses q6-8hr

Bacterial meningitis
Adult/adolescent: IM/**IV** 150-200 mg/kg/day in divided doses, q3-4hr; IDSA IV 12 g divided q4hr
Infant/child: IM/**IV** 150-200 mg/kg/day in divided doses q3-4hr; IDSA dose IV 300 mg/kg/day divided q6hr
Neonates >7 days and >2000 g: IM/**IV** 200 mg/kg/day divided q6hr; IDSA dose IV 200 mg/kg/day divided q6-8hr

Gonorrhea (urethritis)
Adult and child ≥ 45 kg (99 lb): PO 3.5 g given with 1 g probenecid as a single dose (not recommended by CDC)

Prevention of bacterial endocarditis
Adult: IM/IV 2 g 30 min before procedure
Child: IM/IV 50 mg/kg 30 min before procedure, max 2 g

GI/GU infections other than caused by *N. gonorrhoeae*
Adult and child >20 kg: PO 250-500 mg q6hr, may use larger dose for more serious infections
Child ≤20 kg: PO 50-100 mg/kg/day in divided doses q6hr

Available forms: Powder for inj 125, 250, 500 mg, 1, 2, 10 g; IV inf 500 mg, 1, 2 g; caps 250, 500 mg; powder for oral susp, 125, 250, 500 mg/5 ml

Implementation
PO route
• Give in even doses around the clock; product must be taken for 10-14 days to ensure organism death and prevent superinfection; store caps in tight container
• Tabs may be crushed or caps opened and mixed with water
• Shake susp well before each dose; store for 2 wk in refrigerator or 1 wk at room temperature
IM route
• Reconstitute with 125 mg/0.9-1.2 ml; 250 mg/0.9-1.9 ml; 500 mg/1.2-1.8 ml; 1 g/2.4-7.4 ml; 2 g/6.8 ml
• Give deep in large muscle mass

IV route
• Reconstitute with 125 mg/0.9-1.2 ml; 250 mg/0.9-1.9 ml; 500 mg/1.2-1.8 ml; 1 g/2.4-7.4 ml; 2 g/6.8 ml
Direct IV route
• Give over 3-5 min in lower dosages (125-500 mg) or over 15 min in higher dosages (1-2 g)
Intermittent IV infusion route
• Give after diluting with 0.9% NaCl, LR, D₅W, D₅/0.45% NaCl; use 50 ml of sol and dilute to concentration of <30 mg/ml

Y-site compatibilities: Acyclovir, amifostine, allopurinol, aztreonam, cyclophosphamide, DOXOrubicin liposome, enalaprilat, esmolol, famotidine, filgrastim, fludarabine, foscarnet, granisetron, heparin, regular insulin, labetalol, magnesium sulfate, melphalan, meperidine, morphine, multivitamins, oflaxacin, perphenazine, phytonadione, potassium chloride, propofol, remifentanil, thiotepa, tolazoline, vit B with C

Y-site incompatibilities: Calcium gluconate, EPINEPHrine, fluconazole, hetastarch,

HYDROmorphone, hydrALAZINE, ondansetron, sargramostim, verapamil, vinorelbine

ADVERSE EFFECTS
CNS: Lethargy, hallucinations, anxiety, depression, twitching, **coma, seizures**
GI: *Nausea, vomiting, diarrhea,* **pseudomembranous colitis,** stomatitis
GU: Oliguria, proteinuria, hematuria, *vaginitis, moniliasis,* **glomerulonephritis**
HEMA: Anemia, increased bleeding time, **bone marrow depression, granulocytopenia, leukopenia, eosinophilia, hemolysis**
INTEG: *Rash,* urticaria, **toxic epidermal necrolysis,** erythema, multiforme
SYST: **Anaphylaxis, serum sickness, Stevens-Johnson syndrome**

Pharmacokinetics

Absorption	Moderate, in duodenum (35%-50%)
Distribution	Readily in body tissues, fluids, CSF; crosses placenta
Metabolism	Liver (30%)
Excretion	Breast milk; kidney unchanged (70%), removed by dialysis
Half-life	50-110 min

Pharmacodynamics

	PO	IM	IV
Onset	Rapid	Rapid	Rapid
Peak	2 hr	1 hr	Infusion's end
Duration	Unknown	Unknown	Unknown

INTERACTIONS
Individual drugs
Allopurinol: increased ampicillin-induced skin rash
Probenecid: increased ampicillin levels, decreased renal excretion

Drug classifications
Contraceptives (oral): decreased contraceptive effectiveness

Drug/lab test
Increased: AST, ALT
Decreased: conjugated estrone in pregnancy, conjugated estriol
False positive: urine glucose, direct Coombs' test

NURSING CONSIDERATIONS
Assessment
- Assess patient for previous sensitivity reaction to penicillins or other cephalosporins; cross-sensitivity between penicillins and cephalosporins is common
- Assess patient for signs and symptoms of **infection**, including characteristics of wounds, sputum, urine, stool, WBC >10,000/mm^3, earache, fever; obtain baseline information and during treatment
- Obtain C&S before beginning product therapy to identify if correct treatment has been initiated
- Assess for **allergic reactions:** rash, urticaria, pruritus, chills, fever, joint pain; angioedema may occur a few days after therapy begins; epinephrine and resuscitation equipment should be on unit for anaphylactic reaction; also, check for ampicillin rash: pruritic, red, raised
- ⚠ **Identify urine output, hematuria; if decreasing, notify prescriber (may indicate nephrotoxicity)**
- Monitor renal studies: urinalysis, protein, blood, BUN, creatinine
- Monitor blood studies: AST, ALT, CBC, Hct, bilirubin, LDH, alkaline phosphatase, Coombs' test monthly if patient is on long-term therapy
- Monitor electrolytes: potassium, sodium, chloride monthly if patient is on long-term therapy
- Assess bowel pattern daily; if severe diarrhea occurs, product should be discontinued; may indicate pseudomembranous colitis
- Assess for **overgrowth of infection:** perineal itching, fever, malaise, redness, pain, swelling, drainage, rash, diarrhea, change in cough, sputum

Nursing diagnoses
- Diarrhea (side effects)
- Infection, risk for (uses)
- Injury, risk for (side effects)
- Knowledge, deficient (teaching)
- Noncompliance (teaching)

Patient/family education
- ⚠ **Teach patient to report sore throat, bruising, bleeding, joint pain; may indicate blood dyscrasias (rare)**
- Advise patient to contact prescriber if vaginal itching, loose foul-smelling stools, furry tongue occur; may indicate **superinfection**
- Instruct patient to take all medication prescribed for the length of time ordered
- Advise patient to notify prescriber of diarrhea with blood or pus, which may indicate **pseudomembranous colitis**

- Tab may be crushed; cap may be opened and mixed with water

Evaluation
Positive therapeutic outcome
- Absence of signs/symptoms of infection (WBC <10,000, temp WNL)
- Reported improvement in symptoms of infection

TREATMENT OF ANAPHYLAXIS:
Withdraw product, maintain airway, administer epinephrine, aminophylline, O$_2$, **IV** corticosteroids

---

ampicillin/sulbactam (Rx)
(am-pi-sill′in/sul-bak′tam)
Unasyn
Func. class.: Broad-spectrum antiinfective
Chem. class.: Aminopenicillin
Pregnancy category B (ampicillin)

ACTION: Interferes with cell wall replication of susceptible organisms; the cell wall, rendered osmotically unstable, swells and bursts from osmotic pressure; lysis due to cell wall autolytic enzymes; this combination extends the spectrum of activity and inhibits β-lactamase that may inactivate ampicillin

Therapeutic outcome: Bactericidal against *Staphylococcus aureus, Klebsiella, Bacteroides fragilis, Enterobacter, Acinetobacter calcoaceticus, Pneumococcus, Enterococcus, Streptococcus, Escherichia coli, Proteus mirabilis, Neisseria meningitidis, Neisseria gonorrhoeae, Shigella, Salmonella,* and *Haemophilus influenzae* organisms; use only with β-lactamase–producing strain of infection

USES: Skin infections, intraabdominal infections, pneumonia, gynecologic infections, meningitis, septicemia

CONTRAINDICATIONS:
Hypersensitivity to penicillins, ampicillin, or sulbactam

Precautions: Pregnancy B, breastfeeding, neonates, hypersensitivity to cephalosporins, renal disease, mononucleosis, viral infections, syphilis

DOSAGE AND ROUTES
Adult and child >40 kg: IM/**IV** 1 g ampicillin and 0.5 g sulbactam to 2 g ampicillin, and 1 g sulbactam q6hr, not to exceed 4 g/day sulbactam

---

Child <40 kg: IV 100-200 mg/kg/day (ampicillin component) divided q6hr, max 4 g/day

Renal dose
Adult ≥40 kg: IM/IV CCr 15-29 ml/min dose q12hr; CCr 5-14 ml/min dose q24hr

Available forms: Powder for inj 1.5 g (1 g ampicillin, 0.5 g sulbactam), 3 g (2 g ampicillin, 1 g sulbactam), 10 g (10 g ampicillin, 5 g sulbactam)

Implementation
IM route
- Reconstitute by adding 3.2 ml/1.5 g or 6.4 ml/3 g; use sterile water, 0.5% or 2% lidocaine; give within 1 hr of preparation; give deep in large muscle mass, aspirate
- Give after C&S completed; on empty stomach

IV direct route
- Give IV after diluting 1.5 g/3.2 ml sterile water for inj; or 3 g/6.4 ml (250 mg ampicillin/125 mg sulbactam); allow to stand until foaming stops; give directly over 10-15 min

Intermittent IV infusion route
- Dilute further in 50 ml or more of D_5W, D_5/10.45% NaCl, 10% invert sugar in water, LR, 6% sodium lactate, isotonic NaCl; administer within 1 hr after reconstitution; give as an intermittent inf over 15-30 min

Y-site compatibilities: Amifostine, aminocaproic acid, anidulafungin, atenolol, bivalirudin, bleomycin, CARBOplatin, cefepime, CISplatin, codeine, cyclophosphamide, cytarabine, DAPTOmycin, dexmedetomidine, docetaxel, doxacurium, eptifibatide, etoposide, fenoldopam, filgrastim, fludarabine, fluorouracil, gallium, gatifloxacin, gemcitabine, granisetron, hetastarch, irinotecan, levofloxacin, linezolid, methotrexate, metroNIDAZOLE, octreotide, oxaliplatin, paclitaxel, palonosetron, pamidronate, pancuronium, pantoprazole, pemetrexed, remifentanil, riTUXimab, rocuronium, tacrolimus, teniposide, thiotepa, tigecycline, tirofiban, TNA, TPN, trastuzumab, vecuronium, vinCRIStine, voriconazole

Y-site incompatibilities: IDArubicin, ondansetron, sargramostim

ADVERSE EFFECTS
CNS: Lethargy, hallucinations, anxiety, depression, twitching, **coma, seizures**
GI: *Nausea, vomiting, diarrhea,* increased AST, ALT, abdominal pain, glossitis, colitis, **pseudomembranous colitis, hepatic necrosis/failure**

GU: Oliguria, proteinuria, hematuria, *vaginitis, moniliasis,* **glomerulonephritis,** dysuria
HEMA: Anemia, increased bleeding time, **bone marrow depression, granulocytopenia, leukopenia, eosinophilia, hemolysis**
INTEG: Injection site reactions, rash, edema, urticaria
SYST: Anaphylaxis, serum sickness, toxic epidermal necrolysis, Stevens-Johnson syndrome

Pharmacokinetics
Absorption	Well absorbed (IM)
Distribution	Readily in body tissues, fluids, CSF; crosses placenta
Metabolism	Liver (10%-50%)
Excretion	Breast milk; kidney unchanged (75%)
Half-life	50-110 min (ampicillin)

Pharmacodynamics
	IM	IV
Onset	Rapid	Immediate
Peak	1 hr	Infusion's end
Duration	Unknown	Unknown

INTERACTIONS
Individual drugs
Allopurinol: ampicillin-induced skin rash
Disulfiram: increased ampicillin level
Methotrexate: increased methotrexate level
Probenecid: increased ampicillin levels, decreased renal excretion

Drug classifications
Contraceptives (oral): decreased contraceptive effectiveness

Drug/lab test
False positive: urine glucose, urine protein

NURSING CONSIDERATIONS
Assessment
- Assess patient for previous sensitivity reaction to penicillins or cephalosporins; cross-sensitivity between penicillins and cephalosporins is common
- Assess patient for signs and symptoms of **infection,** including characteristics of wounds, sputum, urine, stool, WBC $>10,000/mm^3$, earache, fever; obtain baseline information and during treatment; complete C&S before beginning product therapy to identify if correct treatment has been initiated

• Assess for **allergic reactions:** rash, urticaria, pruritus, chills, fever, joint pain; angioedema may occur a few days after therapy begins; epinephrine and resuscitation equipment should be on unit for anaphylactic reaction

⚠ **Identify urine output; if decreasing, notify prescriber (may indicate nephrotoxicity)**

• Assess renal studies: urinalysis, protein, BUN, creatinine

• Monitor blood studies: AST, ALT, CBC, Hct, bilirubin, LDH, alkaline phosphatase, Coombs' test monthly if patient is on long-term therapy

• Monitor electrolytes: potassium, sodium, chloride monthly if patient is on long-term therapy

• Assess bowel pattern daily; if severe diarrhea occurs, product should be discontinued; may indicate **pseudomembranous colitis**

• Monitor for bleeding: ecchymosis, bleeding gums, hematuria, stool guaiac daily if on long-term therapy

• Assess for superinfection: perineal itching, fever, malaise, redness, pain, swelling, drainage, rash, diarrhea, change in cough, sputum

Nursing diagnoses
• Diarrhea (adverse reactions)
• Infection, risk for (uses)
• Injury, risk for (adverse reactions)
• Knowledge, deficient (teaching)
• Noncompliance (teaching)

Patient/family education
• Teach patient to report sore throat, bruising, bleeding, joint pain, persistent diarrhea; may indicate blood dyscrasias (rare) or superinfection

• Advise patient to contact prescriber if vaginal itching, loose foul-smelling stools, furry tongue occur; may indicate superinfection

• Instruct patient to use another form of contraception other than oral contraceptives

⚠ **To report immediately pseudomembranous colitis: fever, diarrhea with pus, blood, or mucus; may occur up to 4 wk after treatment**

• To wear or carry emergency ID if allergic to penicillin products

Evaluation
Positive therapeutic outcome
• Absence of signs/symptoms of infection (WBC <10,000/mm^3, temp WNL, absence of red draining wounds, earache)
• Reported improvement in symptoms of infection

TREATMENT OF OVERDOSE:
Withdraw product, maintain airway, administer epinephrine, aminophylline, O_2, **IV** corticosteroids for anaphylaxis

anagrelide (Rx)
(a-na′gre-lide)
Agrylin, Gen-Anagrelide ✹, PMS-Anagrelide ✹, Sandoz Anagrelide ✹
Func. class.: Antiplatelet
Chem. class.: Imidazoquinazolinone
Pregnancy category C

ACTION: Reduces platelet count (mechanism not clear) and prevents early platelet shape changes in response to aggregating agents, thus inhibiting platelet aggregation

Therapeutic outcome: Inhibition of platelet aggregation

USES: Chronic myelogenous leukemia (CML), thrombocytosis, polycythemia vera

CONTRAINDICATIONS:
Hypersensitivity

Precautions: Pregnancy **C**, breastfeeding, child <16 yr, cardiac/renal/hepatic disease, hypotension, abrupt discontinuation, females

DOSAGE AND ROUTES
Adult/child ≥7 yr: PO 0.5 mg qid or 1 mg bid, may be adjusted after 1 wk, max 10 mg/day or 2.5 mg single dose; maintenance: titrate to lowest dose to maintain platelets <600,000/mcl; dosage range 1.5-3 mg/day

Available forms: Caps 0.5, 1.0 mg

Implementation
• May give with food, monitor closely for dosage adjustment, there is better absorption on empty stomach
• Store at room temperature

ADVERSE EFFECTS
CNS: *Headache, dizziness,* **seizures,** paresthesia, **CVA,** fever
CV: *Postural hypotension,* tachycardia, palpitations, **CHF, MI, cardiomyopathy, cardiomegaly, complete heart block, atrial fibrillation, arrhythmia,** chest pain
EENT: Amblyopia, diplopia, tinnitus
GI: Diarrhea, abdominal pain, nausea, flatulence, vomiting, anorexia, constipation, pancreatitis

GU: Dysuria
HEMA: Anemia, **thrombocytopenia, ecchymosis, lymphadenoma**
INTEG: *Rash,* photosensitivity
MISC: Edema, pain
MS: Asthenia, back pain
RESP: Dyspnea

Pharmacokinetics

Absorption	Unknown
Distribution	Unknown
Metabolism	Liver, extensively
Excretion	Feces/urine
Half-life	Terminal half-life 3-4 days

Pharmacodynamics

Onset	Unknown
Peak	1 hr
Duration	>24 hr

INTERACTIONS

Individual drugs
Abciximab, antithymocyte globulin, aspirin, cimetidine, ciprofloxacin, eptifibatide, tirofiban, ticlopidine: increased bleeding risk
Sucralfate: decreased absorption, decreased plasma concentrations

Drug classifications
Anticoagulants, antineoplastics, NSAIDs, SSRIs, thrombolytics: increased bleeding risk

Drug/herb
DHEA, feverfew, fish oils, ginger, ginkgo, green tea, garlic, horse chestnut: increased bleeding risk

Drug/food
Grapefruit or grapefruit juice: avoid use
Decreased: absorption

NURSING CONSIDERATIONS

Assessment
• Monitor B/P, pulse baseline, during treatment until stable; take B/P with patient lying, standing; orthostatic hypotension is common
• Assess cardiac status: chest pain, what aggravates or ameliorates condition
• **Blood dyscrasias:** monitor platelet counts q2days × 1 wk, and qwk thereafter, response should begin after 1-2 wk; Hgb, WBC

Nursing diagnoses
• Cardiac output, decreased (uses)
• Knowledge, deficient (teaching)

Patient/family education
• Teach patient that this medication is not a cure
• Advise patient that product may have to be taken continuously in evenly spaced doses only as directed; if a dose is missed, take one when remembered up to 4 hr; do not double doses
• Inform patient that it is necessary to quit smoking to prevent excessive vasoconstriction
• Advise patient to rise slowly from sitting or lying down to prevent orthostatic hypotension
• Caution patient not to use alcohol or OTC medication unless approved by prescriber; avoid grapefruit or juice
• Caution patient to avoid hazardous activities until stabilized on medication; dizziness may occur
• Teach patient to report cardiac reactions, increased bruising/bleeding
• Advise patient to use contraception (female, child-bearing age)
• Teach patient to inform health care provider before surgery of product use
• Advise patient not to double dose; if dose is missed, take as soon as remembered; if close to next dose, omit dose

Evaluation
Positive therapeutic outcome
• Absence of thrombocythemia

anakinra (Rx)
(an-ah-kin′rah)
Kineret
Func. class.: Antirheumatic agent (disease modifying), immunomodulator
Chem. class.: Recombinant form of human interleukin-1 receptor antagonist (IL-1Ra)
Pregnancy category B

ACTION: A form of human interleukin-1 receptor antagonist (IL-1Ra) produced by DNA technology; blocks activity of IL-1, resulting in decreased inflammation, cartilage degradation, bone resorption

Therapeutic outcome: Decreased pain, inflammation

USES: Reduction in signs and symptoms of moderate to severe active rheumatoid arthritis in patients 18 years of age or older who have not responded to other disease-modifying agents

CONTRAINDICATIONS:
Hypersensitivity to *Escherichia coli*–derived proteins or this product, sepsis, latex

Precautions: Pregnancy **B**, breastfeeding, children, geriatric, renal impairment, active infections, immunosuppression, neoplastic disease, asthma

DOSAGE AND ROUTES
Adult: SUBCUT 100 mg daily

Renal dose
Adult: CCr <30 ml/min; SUBCUT 100 mg every other day

Available forms: Inj, 100 mg/0.67 ml prefilled glass syringe

Implementation
• Do not use if cloudy or discolored or if particulate is present; protect from light
• Do not admix with other sol or medications, do not use filter

ADVERSE EFFECTS
CNS: Headache
CV: Cardiac arrest
EENT: Sinusitis
GI: Abdominal pain, nausea, diarrhea
HEMA: Neutropenia
INTEG: Rash, *inj site reaction*, allergic reaction
MISC: Flulike symptoms, infection
MS: *Worsening of RA, arthralgia*
RESP: *URI*

Pharmacokinetics

Absorption	Well absorbed (SUBCUT)
Distribution	Unknown
Metabolism	Unknown
Excretion	Urine
Half-life	4-6 hr

Pharmacodynamics

Onset	Unknown
Peak	3-7 hr
Duration	Unknown

INTERACTIONS
Individual drugs
Rilonacept: do not give, use

Drug classifications
Antibody reactions: decreased
Etanercept, TNF-blocking agents: increased risk of severe infection
Vaccines: do not coadminister; immunizations should be brought up to date before treatment

NURSING CONSIDERATIONS
Assessment
• **Rheumatoid arthritis:** assess pain, stiffness, ROM, swelling of joints during treatment
• Assess for inj site pain, swelling; usually occur after 2 inj (4-5 days)
• Assess for **infections**, stop treatment if present

Nursing diagnoses
• Injury, risk for (side effects)
• Knowledge, deficient (teaching)
• Mobility, impaired physical (uses)
• Pain, chronic (uses)

Patient/family education
• Teach patient about self-administration if appropriate: inj should be made in thigh, abdomen, upper arm; rotate sites at least 1 in from old site
• Advise patient to notify prescriber if pregnancy is planned or suspected, avoid breastfeeding
• Advise patient not to receive vaccines while taking this product, update vaccines before treatment

Evaluation
Positive therapeutic outcome
• Decreased inflammation, pain in joints

---

anastrozole (Rx)
(an-ass-stroh'zole)
Arimidex
Func. class.: Antineoplastic
Chem. class.: Aromatase inhibitor
Pregnancy category X

ACTION: Highly selective nonsteroidal aromatase inhibitor that lowers serum estradiol concentrations; many breast cancers have strong estrogen receptors

Therapeutic outcome: Prevention of rapidly growing malignant cells

USES: Advanced breast carcinoma that has not responded to other therapy in estrogen-receptor-positive patients (usually postmenopausal); patients with advanced disease on tamoxifen, adjunct therapy in early breast cancer

CONTRAINDICATIONS:
Pregnancy **X**, hypersensitivity, breastfeeding

Precautions: Children, geriatric, cardiac/hepatic disease, premenopausal females, osteoporosis

---

Adverse effects: *italics* = common; **bold** = life-threatening

DOSAGE AND ROUTES
Adult: PO 1 mg daily; continue for 5 yr in ERT early breast cancer who have already received 2-3 yr of tamoxifen and are switched to anastrozole

Available forms: Tabs 1 mg

Implementation
• Do not break, crush, or chew enteric products
• Give with food or fluids for GI upset; repeat dose may be needed if vomiting occurs
• Store in light-resistant container at room temperature

ADVERSE EFFECTS
CNS: Hot flashes, headache, light-headedness, depression, dizziness, confusion, insomnia, anxiety, fatigue
CV: Chest pain, hypertension, **thrombophlebitis**, edema, **MI, CVA, cerebral infarction**, angina, vasodilation
GI: Nausea, vomiting, altered taste leading to anorexia, diarrhea, constipation, abdominal pain, dry mouth
GU: Vaginal bleeding, pruritus vulvae, vaginal dryness, pelvic pain, UTI
HEMA: Leukopenia
INTEG: *Rash,* Stevens-Johnson syndrome
MISC: Hypercholesterolemia
MS: Bone pain, myalgia, asthenia, bone loss, osteoporosis, arthralgia, fractures
RESP: Cough, sinusitis, dyspnea, **pulmonary embolism**

Pharmacokinetics

Absorption	Adequately absorbed
Distribution	Unknown
Metabolism	Liver
Excretion	Feces, urine
Half-life	50 hr

Pharmacodynamics

Onset	Unknown
Peak	4-7 hr
Duration	Unknown

INTERACTIONS
Drug/drug
• Do not use with oral contraceptives, estrogen, tamoxifen, androstenedione, DHEA

Drug/lab test
Increased: GGT, AST, ALT, alkaline phosphatase, cholesterol, LDL

NURSING CONSIDERATIONS
Assessment
• Monitor bone mineral density, cholesterol, lipid panel periodically
• Assess **serious skin reactions:** Stevens-Johnson syndrome

Nursing diagnoses
• Injury, risk for (adverse reactions)
• Knowledge, deficient (teaching)

Patient/family education
• Instruct patient to report any complaints, side effects to health care prescriber; if dose is missed, do not double next dose
• Advise patient that vaginal bleeding, pruritus, hot flashes, can occur and are reversible after discontinuing treatment
• Teach patient to take adequate calcium, vitamin D; risk of bone loss/fractures
• Inform patient that rash or lesions are temporary and may become large during beginning therapy

Evaluation
Positive therapeutic outcome
• Decreased spread of malignant cells in breast cancer

---

anidulafungin (Rx)
(a-nid-yoo-luh-fun′jin)
Eraxis
Func. class.: Antifungal, systemic
Chem. class.: Echinocandin
Pregnancy category C

ACTION: Inhibits fungal enzyme synthesis; causes direct damage to fungal cell wall

Therapeutic outcome: Decreased symptoms of candida infection, negative culture

USES: Esophageal candidiasis, *Candida albicans, Candida glabrata, Candida parapsilosis, Candida tropicalis*

CONTRAINDICATIONS: Hypersensitivity to this product or other echinocandins

Precautions: Pregnancy **C**, breastfeeding, children, severe hepatic disease

---

DOSAGE AND ROUTES

Candidemia and other candidal infections

Adult: IV loading dose 200 mg on day 1, then 100 mg/day until 14 days or more since last positive culture

Esophageal candidiasis

Adult: IV loading dose 100 mg on day 1, then 50 mg/day for at least 14 days and for at least 7 days after symptoms are resolved

Available forms: Powder for injection, lyophilized 50, 100 mg

Implementation

IV route

• **Reconstitution:** If dehydrated alcohol diluents are supplied, use supplied diluent (dehydrated alcohol in water for inj); reconstitute each 50 mg vial/15 ml of diluents or 100 mg/30 ml (3.33 mg/ml); if diluents are not supplied, reconstitute each 50 mg vial/15 ml sterile water for inj or 100 mg vial/30 ml of sterile water for inj (3.33 mg/ml)

• **Dilution: 200 mg loading dose inf with vials (dehydrated alcohol);** withdraw contents of 4 (50 mg reconstituted vials) or 2 (100 mg reconstituted vials)/500 ml of D₅W or 0.9% NaCl (0.36 mg/ml); **200 mg loading dose inf with vials (sterile water for inj),** withdraw contents of 4 (50 mg reconstituted vials) or 2 (100 mg reconstituted vials)/200 ml of D₅W or 0.9% NaCl, total volume 260 ml; **100 mg daily inf with vials (dehydrated alcohol),** withdraw contents of 1 (100 mg reconstituted vial) or 1 (50 mg reconstituted vial) and add to 250 ml D₅W or 0.9% NaCl (0.36 mg/ml); **100 mg daily inf with vials (sterile water),** withdraw contents of 1 (100 mg reconstituted vial) or 2 (50 mg reconstituted vials)/100 ml D₅W or 0.9% NaCl (total volume 130 ml); **50 mg daily inf (dehydrated alcohol),** withdraw 50 mg reconstituted vial/100 ml of D₅W or 0.9% NaCl (0.43 mg/ml); **50 mg daily inf (dehydrated alcohol),** withdraw contents of 1 (50 mg reconstituted vial)/100 ml D₅W or 0.9% NaCl final conc (0.43/ml)

• Inf rate max 1.1 mg/min (dehydrated alcohol); inf rate 1.4 mg/min (sterile water) or 84 ml/hr

• Give only as IV inf, not for IV bolus

• Do not use if cloudy or precipitated; do not admix

• Store at room temperature, away from light, do not freeze; diluted sol must be used within 24 hr

IV compatibilities: Acyclovir, alemtuzumab, alfentanil, allopurinol, amifostine, amikacin, aminocaproic acid, aminophylline, amiodarone hydrochloride, amphotericin B lipid complex, amphotericin B liposome, ampicillin, ampicillin sulbactam, argatroban, arsenic trioxide, atenolol, atracurium, azithromycin, aztreonam, bivalirudin, bleomycin, bumetanide, buprenorphine, busulfan, butorphanol, calcium chloride/gluconate, CARBOplatin, carmustine, caspofungin, ceFAZolin, cefepime, cefotaxime, cefotetan, cefoxitin, ceftazidime, ceftizoxime, cefTRIAXone, cefuroxime, chloramphenicol, chlorproMAZINE, cimetidine, ciprofloxacin, cisatracurium, CISplatin, clindamycin, cyclophosphamide, cycloSPORINE, cytarabine, dacarbazine, DACTINomycin, DAUNOrubicin, DAUNOrubicin liposome, dexamethasone, dexmedetomidine, dexrazoxane, diazepam, digoxin, diltiazem, diphenhydrAMINE, DOBUTamine, docetaxel, dolasetron, DOPamine, doripenem, doxacurium, DOXOrubicin, DOXOrubicin liposomal, doxycycline, droperidol, enalaprilat, ePHEDrine, EPINEPHrine, epirubicin, eptifibatide, erythromycin, esmolol, etoposide, etoposide phosphate, famotidine, fenoldopam, fentaNYL, fluconazole, fludarabine, fluorouracil, foscarnet, fosphenytoin, furosemide, gallium, ganciclovir, gatifloxacin, gemcitabine, gentamicin, glycopyrrolate, granisetron, haloperidol, heparin, hydrALAZINE, hydrocortisone, HYDROmorphone, hydrOXYzine, IDArubicin, ifosfamide, imipenem-cilastatin, inamrinone, insulin (regular), irinotecan, isoproterenol, ketorolac, labetalol, leucovorin, levofloxacin, lidocaine, linezolid injection, LORazepam, mannitol, mechlorethamine, melphalan, meperidine, meropenem, mesna, metaraminol, methotrexate, methyldopate, methylPREDNISolone, metoclopramide, metoprolol, metroNIDAZOLE, midazolam, milrinone, mitomycin, mitoxantrone, mivacurium, morphine, moxifloxacin, mycophenolate mofetil, nafcillin, naloxone, nesiritide, niCARdipine, nitroglycerin, nitroprusside, norepinephrine, octreotide, ondansetron, oxaliplatin, oxytocin, paclitaxel, palonosetron, pamidronate, pancuronium, pantoprazole, pentamidine, pentazocine, PENTobarbital, PHENobarbital, phentolamine, phenylephrine, piperacillin-tazobactam, polymyxin B, potassium acetate/chloride, procainamide, prochlorperazine, promethazine, propranolol, quiNIDine, quinupristin-dalfopristin, ranitidine, remifentanil, rocuronium, sodium acetate, streptozocin, succinylcholine, SUFentanil citrate, sulfamethoxazole-trimethoprim, tacrolimus, teniposide, theophylline, thiopental, thiotepa, ticarcillin,

ticarcillin-clavulanate, tirofiban, tobramycin, topotecan, trimethobenzamide, vancomycin, vasopressin, vecuronium, verapamil, vinBLAStine, vinCRIStine, vinorelbine, voriconazole, zidovudine, zoledronic acid

ADVERSE EFFECTS

Candidemia/other candida infections
CNS: Seizures, dizziness, *headache*
CV: Deep vein thrombosis, **atrial fibrillation, right bundle branch block,** hypotension, **QT prolongation, sinus arrhythmia, thrombophlebitis superficial, ventricular extrasystoles (rare)**
GI: *Nausea; anorexia; vomiting; diarrhea; increased AST, ALT*
META: Hypokalemia

Esophageal candidiasis
CNS: *Headache*
GI: *Nausea, anorexia, vomiting, diarrhea,* **hepatic necrosis**
HEMA: Neutropenia, thrombocytopenia, leukopenia, coagulopathy
INTEG: *Rash,* urticaria, itching, flushing
META: Hypocalcemia, hyperglycemia, hyperkalemia, hypernatremia, hypomagnesemia (rare)
MS: *Back pain, rigors*

Pharmacokinetics

Absorption	Unknown
Distribution	Steady state after loading dose, protein binding 84%
Metabolism	Unknown
Excretion	Unknown
Half-life	Distribution 0.5-1 hr, terminal 40-50 hr

Pharmacodynamics
Unknown

INTERACTIONS

Individual drugs
CycloSPORINE: increased plasma concentrations

Drug/lab test
Increased: amylase, bilirubin, CPK, creatinine, ECG, lipase
Decreased: platelets, magnesium, potassium, transferase, urea

NURSING CONSIDERATIONS

Assessment
• Assess for **infection**, clearing of cultures during treatment; obtain culture at baseline and throughout; product may be started as soon as culture is taken
• **Blood dyscrasias (rare):** monitor CBC (RBC, Hct, Hgb), differential, platelet count periodically; notify prescriber of results
• Monitor hepatic studies before and during treatment: bilirubin, AST, ALT, alk phosphatase; uric acid, as needed
• Assess for **bleeding:** hematuria, hemepositive stools, bruising or petechiae, mucosa or orifices; blood dyscrasias can occur
• Assess for GI symptoms: frequency of stools, cramping, if severe diarrhea occurs, electrolytes may need to be given

Nursing diagnoses
• Infection, risk for (uses)
• Injury, risk for (adverse reactions)
• Knowledge, deficient (teaching)

Patient/family education
• Advise patient to notify prescriber if pregnancy is suspected or planned; use nonhormonal form of contraception while taking this product
• Instruct patient to avoid breastfeeding while taking this product
• Advise patient to inform prescriber of kidney or liver disease
• Advise patient to report bleeding
• Teach patient to report signs of infection: increased temp, sore throat, flulike symptoms
• Teach patient to notify prescriber of nausea, vomiting, diarrhea, jaundice, anorexia, clay-colored stools, dark urine; heptatotoxicity may occur

Evaluation
Positive therapeutic outcome
• Decreased symptoms of candidal infection, negative culture

⚠ HIGH ALERT

antihemophilic factor VIII (AHF) (Rx)
(an-tee-hee-moe-fill′ik)
Advate, Alphanate, Helixate FS, Hemofil M, Humate-P, Koate-DVI, Kogenate, Kogenate FS, Monarc-M, Monoclate-P, Recombinate, Xyntha
Func. class.: Hemostatic, blood factor
Chem. class.: Factor VIII
Pregnancy category C

Do not confuse:
Kogenate/Kogenate-2

ACTION: Necessary for clotting. Activates factor X in conjunction with activated factor IX; transforms prothrombin to thrombin

Therapeutic outcome: Control of hemorrhage or excessive bleeding in factor VIII deficiency

USES: Hemophilia A, patients with acquired circulating factor VIII inhibitors, factor VIII deficiency; prevention of surgical bleeding, risk of thrombosis (von Willebrand's disease)

CONTRAINDICATIONS:
Hypersensitivity to mouse, hamster, bovine, porcine protein, breastfeeding, HIV

Precautions: Pregnancy C, neonates/infants, hepatic disease, blood types A, B, AB, factor VIII inhibitor, viral infection

DOSAGE AND ROUTES
Depends on severity of deficiency and level of antihemophilic factor

Massive hemorrhage (general dosing)
Adult and child: IV 30-50 units/kg to achieve peak factor VIII at 60%-100% normal

Moderate hemorrhage
Adult and child: IV 10-30 units/kg to achieve peak factor VIII at 20%-60% normal

Minor hemorrhage
Adult and child: IV 10-15 units/kg to achieve peak factor VIII at 20%-30% of normal

Available forms: Inj 250, 500, 1000, 1500 units/vial (number of units noted on label)

Implementation
• Give hepatitis A/B vaccination at birth when hemophilia is diagnosed

IV route
• Administer after dilution with warm 0.9% NaCl, D₅W, LR; give within 3 hr
• To prepare, administer factor VIII concentrates at first sign of danger; rotate gently to mix
• Warm to room temperature using plastic syringe to reconstitute

IV infusion route
• Administer by IV inf: give at ≤2 ml/min if concentration >34 units/ml, or over 3 min if concentration is <34 units/ml; filter before using
• Store in refrigerator; do not freeze; after reconstitution, do not refrigerate; give within 3 hr

• Do not mix with other products in sol or syringe

ADVERSE EFFECTS
CNS: Headache, *lethargy, chills, fever, flushing,* loss of consciousness
CV: *Hypotension,* tachycardia
GI: Nausea, vomiting, abdominal cramps, jaundice, constipation, diarrhea, anorexia, **viral hepatitis**
HEMA: Thrombosis, hemolysis, risk of hepatitis B, risk of HIV, antibody formation
INTEG: Rash, flushing, *urticaria,* stinging at inj site
MISC: Anaphylaxis, blurred vision, back pain
RESP: Bronchospasm, rhinitis, dyspnea, nosebleeds, wheezing, **pulmonary embolism**

Pharmacokinetics

Absorption	Complete availability
Distribution	Plasma
Metabolism	Not metabolized
Excretion	No excretion
Half-life	Biphasic 4 hr, 15 hr

Pharmacodynamics

Onset	Immediate
Peak	Unknown
Duration	12 hr

NURSING CONSIDERATIONS
Assessment
• Monitor blood studies (coagulation factors assay by % normal): 5% prevents spontaneous hemorrhage, 30%-50% for surgery, 80%-100% for severe hemorrhage; blood group of patient, donors (if applicable; most factor VIII not from specific blood group donors)
• Monitor I&O, urine color; notify prescriber if urine becomes orange, red; change in urine color signifying hemolytic reaction; patients other than blood type O are more at risk
• Monitor pulse: discontinue infusion if significant increase
• Obtain test for factor VIII inhibitors before starting treatment, may require concomitant antiinhibitor coagulant complex therapy; Hct, Coombs' test with blood types A, B, AB
• Assess for **allergy:** fever, rash, itching, jaundice, wheezing, tachycardia, nausea, vomiting; give diphenhydrAMINE (Benadryl); continue therapy if reaction is mild, discontinue if severe; notify prescriber

⚠ Monitor bleeding at ankles, knees, elbows, other joints; check for rebleeding after 15-30 min

Nursing diagnoses
• Injury, risk for (uses, adverse reactions)
• Knowledge, deficient (teaching)
• Tissue perfusion, ineffective (uses)

Patient/family education
• Advise patient to report any signs of bleeding: gums, under skin, urine, stools, emesis; review methods to prevent bleeding; to be checked q2-3mo for HIV screen
• Instruct patient to avoid salicylates/NSAIDs; increases bleeding tendencies, decreases clotting
• Instruct patient to prepare, administer factor VIII concentrates at first sign of danger
• Instruct patient to advise health professionals of treatment for hemophilia
• Advise patient that immunization for hepatitis B may be given first
• Instruct patient to report hives, urticaria, chest tightness, hypotension; may be monoclonal antibody–derived factor VII; signs of viral hepatitis, AIDS
• Advise patient to carry/wear emergency ID describing disease process, products used

Evaluation
Positive therapeutic outcome
• Absence of bleeding
• Prevention of rebleeding

apraclonidine ophthalmic
See Appendix B

aprepitant (Rx)
(ap-re′pi-tant)
Emend
fosaprepitant
Emend
Func. class.: Antiemetic
Chem. class:. Miscellaneous
Pregnancy category B

ACTION: Selective antagonist of human substance P/neurokinin 1 (NK_1) receptors, decreasing emetic reflex

Therapeutic outcome: Decreased nausea, vomiting during chemotherapy

USES: Prevention of nausea, vomiting associated with cancer chemotherapy (highly emetogenic/moderately emetogenic) including high-dose cisplatin; used in combination with other antiemetics; postop nausea, vomiting

CONTRAINDICATIONS:
Hypersensitivity

Precautions: Pregnancy **B**, breastfeeding, children, geriatric, hepatic disease

DOSAGE AND ROUTES
Highly emetogenic (aprepitant)
Adult: PO day 1 (1 hr prior to chemotherapy) aprepitant 125 mg with 12 mg 1st dose of aprepitant on day 1 of regimen (fosaprepitant)

Moderately emetogenic
Adult: PO day 1 dexamethasone 12 mg 125 mg aprepitant with PO, with PO ondansetron 8 mg × 2; days 2 and 3 PO 80 mg aprepitant only (aprepitant); **IV** inf 115 mg over 15 min, 30 min prior to chemotherapy as an alternative to the 1st dose of aprepitant on day 1 of regimen (fosaprepitant)

Prevention of postop nausea/ vomiting
Adult: PO 40 mg within 3 hr of induction of anesthesia

Available forms: Caps 40, 80, 125 mg; powder for inj 115 mg; combo pack cap 80-125 mg

Implementation
PO route
• Give PO on 3-day schedule
• Take first dose 1 hr prior to chemotherapy
• Store at room temperature

IV route
• Only approved as a substitute for the 1st dose of aprepitant in 3-day regimen
• Reconstitution: use aseptic technique; inject 5 ml 0.9% NaCl into the vial, directing stream to wall of vial to prevent foam; swirl; do not shake
• Prepare inf bag with 110 ml 0.9% NaCl; do not dilute or reconstitute with any divalent cations such as calcium, magnesium, including LR, Hartmann's sol
• Withdraw the entire volume from vial and transfer to inf bag; total volume 115 ml (1 mg/ 1 ml)
• Gently invert bag 2-3 times; reconstituted sol is stable for 24 hr at lower room temperature or <25° C
• Visually inspect for particulates and discoloration
• Infuse over 15 min

ADVERSE EFFECTS

CNS: *Headache, dizziness,* insomnia, anxiety, depression, confusion, peripheral neuropathy

CV: Bradycardia, tachycardia, DVT, hypertension, hypotension

GI: *Diarrhea; constipation;* abdominal pain; anorexia; gastritis; increased AST, ALT; *nausea;* vomiting; heartburn

GU: Increased BUN, serum creatine, proteinuria, dysuria

HEMA: Anemia, **thrombocytopenia, neutropenia**

INTEG: Pruritus, rash, urticaria

MISC: Asthenia, fatigue, dehydration, fever, hiccups, tinnitus, alopecia

SYST: Anaphylaxis

Pharmacokinetics

Absorption	Unknown
Distribution	95% protein bound
Metabolism	Liver (CYP3A4 enzymes to an active metabolite)
Excretion	Not in kidneys
Half-life	10-12 hr

Pharmacodynamics

Unknown

INTERACTIONS

Individual drugs

Paroxetine: decreased action of both products

Drug classifications

CYP2C9 substrates (phenytoin, TOLBUTamide, warfarin), oral contraceptives: decreased action

CYP3A4 inhibitors (clarithromycin, diltiazem, itraconazole, ketoconazole, nefazodone, nelfinavir, ritonavir, troleandomycin): increased aprepitant action

CYP3A4 inducers (carbamazepine, phenytoin, rifampin): decreased aprepitant action

CYP3A4 substrates (alprazolam, cisapride, dexamethasone, docetaxel, etoposide, ifosfamide, imatinib, irinotecan, methylPREDNISolone, midazolam, paclitaxel, pimozide, triazolam, vinBLAStine, vinCRIStine, vinorelbine): increased action

Drug/food

Grapefruit juice: decreased effect

NURSING CONSIDERATIONS

Assessment

• Assess for hypersensitivity reactions: pruritus, rash, urticaria, anaphylaxis

• Assess for absence of nausea, vomiting during chemotherapy

Nursing diagnoses

• Knowledge, deficient (teaching)

Patient/family education

• Teach to report diarrhea, constipation
• Advise to take only as prescribed
• Advise to report all medication to prescriber prior to taking this medication
• Instruct to use nonhormonal form of contraception while taking this agent
• Advise those on warfarin to have clotting monitored closely during 2-wk period following administration of aprepitant
• Teach to avoid breastfeeding

Evaluation

Positive therapeutic outcome
• Absence of nausea, vomiting during cancer chemotherapy

---

arformoterol (Rx)

(ar-for-moe'ter-ole)
Brovana
Func. class.: Long-acting adrenergic β_2-agonist, sympathomimetic, bronchodilator
Pregnancy category C

ACTION: Causes bronchodilation by action on β_2 (pulmonary) receptors by increasing levels of cyclic AMP, which relaxes smooth muscle; produces bronchodilation, CNS, and cardiac stimulation, and increased diuresis and gastric acid secretion; longer acting than isoproterenol

Therapeutic outcome: Absence of dyspnea, wheezing after 1 hr, improved airway exchange, improved ABGs

USES: COPD, including chronic bronchitis, emphysema

CONTRAINDICATIONS:

Hypersensitivity to sympathomimetics, this product, or racemic formoterol; tachydysrhythmias, severe cardiac disease, heart block, children, monotherapy in asthma

BLACK BOX WARNING: Actively deteriorating COPD

Precautions: Pregnancy C, breastfeeding, cardiac disorders, hyperthyroidism, diabetes mellitus, hypertension, prostatic hypertrophy, closed-angle glaucoma, seizures, hypoglycemia

---

Adverse effects: *italics* = common; **bold** = life-threatening

DOSAGE AND ROUTES
COPD
Adult: NEB 15 mcg, bid, AM, PM

Available forms: Inh sol 15 mcg/2 ml

Implementation
• Must be used by nebulization
• Store in refrigerator

ADVERSE EFFECTS
CNS: *Tremors, anxiety,* insomnia, headache, dizziness, stimulation, *restlessness,* hallucinations, flushing, irritability
CV: Palpitations, **tachycardia,** hypo/hypertension, angina, **dysrhythmias**
EENT: Dry nose, irritation of nose and throat
GI: Heartburn, nausea, vomiting
MISC: Flushing, sweating, anorexia, bad taste/smell changes, hypokalemia, **anaphylaxis**
MS: Muscle cramps
RESP: Cough, wheezing, dyspnea, **bronchospasm,** dry throat

Pharmacokinetics

Absorption	Unknown
Distribution	Crosses placenta, protein binding 52%-65%
Metabolism	Direct conjugation by CYP2D6, CYP2C19, extensively
Excretion	Urine 63%, feces 11%
Half-life	Terminal (COPD) 26 hr

Pharmacodynamics

Onset	5 min
Peak	1-1½ hr
Duration	4-6 hr

INTERACTIONS
Individual drugs
Oxytoxics: increased severe hypotension
Theophylline: increased toxicity

Drug classifications
Adrenergics, MAOIs, tricyclics: increased action of arformoterol; do not use together
Nebulized bronchodilators: increased action of nebulized bronchodilators
Other β-blockers: decreased arformoterol action, asthma-related death
Potassium-losing diuretics: increased ECG changes/hypokalemia

Drug/herb
Caffeine (kola nut, green/black tea, guarana, yerba maté, coffee, chocolate): increased stimulation

NURSING CONSIDERATIONS
Assessment

> **BLACK BOX WARNING:** Assess respiratory function: vital capacity, forced expiratory volume, ABGs; lung sounds, heart rate and rhythm, B/P, sputum (baseline and peak); actively deteriorating COPD may occur

• Determine that patient has not received theophylline therapy or other bronchodilators before giving dose
• Assess patient's ability to self-medicate
• Assess for allergic reactions; **anaphylaxis** may occur
• Assess **paradoxical bronchospasm;** hold medication, notify prescriber if bronchospasm occurs

Nursing diagnoses
• Airway clearance, ineffective (uses)
• Knowledge, deficient (teaching)

Patient/family education
• Teach patient to use exactly as prescribed, that death has resulted from asthma with products similar to this one
• Advise patient not to use OTC medications; excess stimulation may occur

Evaluation
Positive therapeutic outcome
• Absence of dyspnea, wheezing after 1 hr, improved airway exchange, improved ABGs

---

▲ HIGH ALERT
argatroban (Rx)
(are-ga-troe′ban)
Argatroban
Func. class.: Anticoagulant
Chem. class.: Thrombin inhibitor
Pregnancy category B

Do not confuse:
argatroban/Aggrastat

ACTION: Direct inhibitor of thrombin that is derived from L-arginine; it reversibly binds to the thrombin active site

Therapeutic outcome: Absence or decrease of thrombosis

USES: Thrombosis prophylaxis or treatment; anticoagulation prevention/treatment of thrombosis in heparin-induced thrombocytopenia (HIT); percutaneous coronary intervention (PCI) in those with a history of HIT

CONTRAINDICATIONS:
Hypersensitivity, overt major bleeding

Precautions: Pregnancy **B**, breastfeeding, children, intracranial bleeding, impaired renal function, hepatic disease, severe hypertension, after lumbar puncture, spinal anesthesia, major surgery, congenital or acquired bleeding, GI ulcers

DOSAGE AND ROUTES

DVT, pulmonary embolism
Adult: CONT **IV** inf 2 mcg/kg/min; adjust dose until steady-state aPPT is 1.5-3 × initial baseline, not to exceed 100 sec, max dose 10 mcg/kg/min

Percutaneous coronary intervention (PCI) in HIT
Adult: **IV** inf 25 mcg/kg/min and a bol of 350 mcg/kg given over 3-5 min, check ACT 5-10 min after bol is completed, proceed if ACT >300 sec; if ACT <300 sec, give another 150 mcg/kg bol and increase infusion rate to 30 mcg/kg/min; recheck ACT in 5-10 min; if ACT >450 sec, decrease infusion rate to 15 mcg/kg/min; recheck ACT in 5-10 min; once ACT is therapeutic, continue for duration of procedure

Hepatic dose
Adult: Cont inf 0.5 mcg/kg/min, adjust rate based on APTT

Available forms: Inj 100 mg/ml (2.5 ml) (must dilute 100-fold)

Implementation
• Avoid all IM inj that may cause bleeding

IV, direct route
• **For PCL:** 350 mg/kg bol, and continuous inf of 25 mcg/kg/min, check ACT 5-10 min after bolus

Intermittent IV INF route
• **Dilute** in 0.9% NaCl, D₅, LR to a final conc 1 mg/ml; **dilute** each 2.5-ml vial 100-fold by mixing with 250 ml of diluent, mix by repeated inversion of the diluent bag for 1 min; may be slightly hazy briefly
• Dosage adjustment may be made after review of aPTT, not to exceed 10 mcg/kg/min

ADVERSE EFFECTS
CNS: Fever, **intracranial bleeding,** headache
CV: **Atrial fibrillation, ventricular tachycardia, coronary thrombosis, MI, myocardial ischemia, coronary occlusion, bradycardia,** chest pain, hypotension
GI: Nausea, vomiting, abdominal pain, diarrhea, **GI bleeding**

GU: Hematuria, abnormal kidney function, UTI
HEMA: Hemorrhage
MISC: *Back pain, headache,* infection
RESP: Pneumonia, dyspnea, coughing, hemoptysis
SYST: Sepsis

Pharmacokinetics

Absorption	Unknown
Distribution	To extracellular fluid, 54% plasma protein binding
Metabolism	Liver
Excretion	Feces
Half-life	39-51 min

Pharmacodynamics
Unknown

INTERACTIONS

Individual drugs
Clopidogrel, dipyridamole, heparin, ticlodipine, warfarin: increased bleeding risk

Drug classifications
Antiplatelets, glycoprotein IIb/IIIa antagonists (abciximab, eptifibatide, tirofiban), NSAIDs, other anticoagulants, salicylates, thrombolytics (alteplase, reteplase, tenecteplase, urokinase): increased risk of bleeding

NURSING CONSIDERATIONS

Assessment
• Obtain baseline aPTT before treatment; do not start treatment if aPTT ratio ≥2.5, then aPTT 4 hr after initiation of treatment and at least daily thereafter; if aPTT above target, stop inf for 2 hr, then restart at 50%, take aPTT in 4 hr; if below target, increase inf rate by 20%, take aPTT in 4 hr, do not exceed inf rate of 0.21 mg/kg/hr without checking for coagulation abnormalities
• Monitor aPTT, which should be 1.5-3 × control
⚠ **Assess for bleeding gums, petechiae, ecchymosis, black tarry stools, hematuria/ epistaxis, B/P, vaginal bleeding, and possible hemorrhage**
• Fever, skin rash, urticaria
• **Anaphylaxis:** assess for dyspnea, rash during treatment

Nursing diagnoses
• Cardiac output, decreased (uses)
• Diarrhea (adverse reactions)
• Knowledge, deficient (teaching)

Patient/family education
• Advise patient to use soft-bristle toothbrush to avoid bleeding gums, avoid contact sports, use electric razor, avoid IM inj
• Instruct patient to report any signs of bleeding: gums, under skin, urine, stools

Evaluation
Positive therapeutic outcome
• Absence or decrease of thrombosis

aripiprazole (Rx)
(a-rip-ip-pra'zol)
Abilify, Abilify Discmelt
Func. class.: Antipsychotic/neuroleptic
Pregnancy category C

ACTION: Exact mechanism unknown; may be mediated through both dopamine type 2 (D_2) and serotonin type 2 ($5\text{-}HT_2$) antagonism

Therapeutic outcome: Decreased excitement, hallucinations, delusions, paranoia, reorganization of patterns of thought, speech

USES: Schizophrenia and bipolar disorder (adults and adolescents), agitation, mania, major depressive disorder, short-term mania or mixed episodes of bipolar disorder, irritability in autism

CONTRAINDICATIONS:
Hypersensitivity, breastfeeding, seizure disorders

Precautions: Pregnancy **C**, geriatric, renal/cardiac/hepatic disease

> **BLACK BOX WARNING:** Children, dementia, suicidal ideation

DOSAGE AND ROUTES
Schizophrenia
Adult: PO 10-15 mg/day; if needed, dosage may be increased to 30 mg daily after 2 wk; maintenance 15 mg/day, periodically reassess
Adolescent 13-17 yr: 2 mg/day, may increase to 5 mg after 2 days, then 10 mg after 2 more days, max 30 mg/day

Major depressive disorder
Adult: PO 2-5 mg/day as an adjunct to other antidepressant treatment; adjust by 5 mg at ≥1 wk (range, 2-15 mg/day)

Agitation in bipolar disorder/schizophrenia
Adult: IM 9.75 mg as a single dose; may start with a lower dose, max 30 mg/day

Bipolar disorder
Adult: 15 mg/day, may increase to 30 mg/day if needed (monotherapy): adjunctive to lithium or valproate PO 10-15 mg qd, may increase to 30 mg as needed
Child ≥10 yr/adolescents: PO 2 mg, titrate to 5 mg/day after 2 days to a target of 10 mg/day after another 2 days

Irritability associated with autism
Child ≥6 yr, adolescents: PO 2 mg/day, increase to 5 mg/day after 1 wk, may increase to 10-15 mg/day if needed, dose changes should not occur more frequently than q1wk

Potential CYP2D6 inhibitor, strong CYP3A4 inhibitors
Adult: PO reduce to 50% of usual dose, increase dose when CYP2D6, CYP3A4 inhibitor is withdrawn

Combination of strong CYP3A4/CYP2D6 inhibitors
Adult: PO reduce to 25% of usual dose
Available forms: Tabs 2, 5, 10, 15, 20, 30 mg; inj 9.75 mg/1.3 ml; orally disintegrating tab 10, 15 mg; oral sol 1 mg/ml

Implementation
• Administer reduced dose in geriatric
• Decreased stimulus by dimming lights, avoiding loud noises
• Supervise ambulation until patient is stabilized on medication; do not involve in strenuous exercise program because fainting is possible; patient should not stand still for a long time
• Store in tight, light-resistant container

ADVERSE EFFECTS
CNS: *Drowsiness, insomnia, agitation, anxiety, headache,* **seizures, neuroleptic malignant syndrome,** *lightheadedness, akathisia, asthenia, tremor,* **stroke, suicidal ideation,** dystonia
CV: Orthostatic hypotension, **tachycardia**
EENT: Blurred vision, rhinitis
GI: Constipation, *nausea,* vomiting, jaundice, weight gain
INTEG: *Rash*
META: Hypoglycemia
RESP: *Cough*
SYST: **Death in geriatric patients with dementia**

A

Pharmacokinetics

Absorption	Unknown
Distribution	Protein binding, 90%
Metabolism	Liver, extensively to major active metabolism
Excretion	Unknown
Half-life	Unknown

Pharmacodynamics

Unknown

INTERACTIONS

Individual drugs

Alcohol: increased sedation

Carbamazepine: decreased effects of aripiprazole

Erythromycin, fluoxetine, ketoconazole, quinidine, paroxetine: increased effects of aripiprazole, reduce dose

Famotidine, valproate: decreased aripiprazole level

Lithium: increased EPS

Drug classifications

Antipsychotics: increased EPS

CNS depressants: increased sedation

CYP3A4/CYP2D6 inhibitors: increased effects of aripiprazole, reduce dose

CYPA34 inducers: decreased effects of aripiprazole; increase dose

Drug/herb

St. John's wort: decreased aripiprazole effect

NURSING CONSIDERATIONS

Assessment

> **BLACK BOX WARNING:** Assess mental status before initial administration, children/young adults may exhibit suicidal thoughts/behaviors, the smallest amount of product should be given; do not use in elderly, dementia may occur

• Check for swallowing of PO medication; check for hoarding or giving of medication to other patients

• Monitor I&O ratio; palpate bladder if urinary output is low

• Monitor bilirubin, CBC, liver function tests qmo

• Assess affect, orientation, LOC, reflexes, gait, coordination, sleep pattern disturbances

• Monitor B/P standing and lying; also pulse, respirations; take q4hr during initial treatment; establish baseline before starting treatment; report drops of 30 mm Hg; watch for ECG changes

• Assess for dizziness, faintness, palpitations, tachycardia on rising

• Assess for EPS, including akathisia (inability to sit still, no pattern to movements), tardive dyskinesia (bizarre movements of the jaw, mouth, tongue, extremities), pseudoparkinsonism (rigidity, tremors, pill rolling, shuffling gait)

⚠ Assess for neuroleptic malignant syndrome: hyperthermia, increased CPK, altered mental status, muscle rigidity

• Assess skin turgor daily

• Assess for constipation, urinary retention daily; if these occur, increase bulk and water in diet

Nursing diagnoses

• Knowledge, deficient (teaching)
• Noncompliance (teaching)
• Sensory perception, disturbed (uses)
• Thought processes, disturbed (uses)

Patient/family education

• Advise patient that orthostatic hypotension may occur and to rise from sitting or lying position gradually

• Advise patient to avoid hot tubs, hot showers, tub baths; hypotension may occur

• Instruct patient to avoid abrupt withdrawal of this product; EPS may result; product should be withdrawn slowly

• Teach patient to avoid OTC preparations (cough, hayfever, cold) unless approved by prescriber, because serious product interactions may occur; avoid use with alcohol, CNS depressants; increased drowsiness may occur

• Advise patient to avoid hazardous activities if drowsy or dizzy

• Explain importance of compliance with product regimen

• Advise patient, family to report impaired vision, tremors, muscle twitching, urinary retention

• Instruct patient to take extra precautions to stay cool in hot weather, that heat stroke may occur

> **BLACK BOX WARNING:** Teach patient to report suicidal thoughts/behaviors immediately

Evaluation

Positive therapeutic outcome

• Decreased emotional excitement, hallucinations, delusions, paranoia; reorganization of patterns of thought, speech

TREATMENT OF OVERDOSE:

Lavage if orally ingested; provide airway; *do not induce vomiting*

ascorbic acid (vitamin C) (OTC, Rx)
(as-kor'bic)

Acerda C, Apo-C ✸, Ascor L-500, Cenolate, Equaline Vitamin C, Walgreens Gold Seal, and many more

Func. class.: Vitamin C, water-soluble vitamin

Pregnancy category C

ACTION: Needed for wound healing, collagen synthesis, antioxidant, carbohydrate metabolism

Therapeutic outcome: Replacement and supplementation of vit C

USES: Vit C deficiency, scurvy, delayed wound and bone healing, chronic disease, before gastrectomy, dietary supplement

Unlabeled uses: Common cold prevention

CONTRAINDICATIONS:
Tartrazine, sulfite sensitivity; G6PD deficiency

Precautions: Pregnancy C, gout, diabetes, renal calculi (large doses)

DOSAGE AND ROUTES
RDA
Neonates and up to 6 mo: PO 30 mg/day
Infants: PO 40-50 mg/day
Child 1-3 yr: PO 15 mg/day
Child 4-8 yr: PO 25 mg/day
Child 9-13 yr: PO 45 mg/day
Child 14-18 yr: PO 65 mg/day (females), 75 mg/day (males)
Adult: PO 50-500 mg/day

Scurvy
Adult: PO/SUBCUT/IM/**IV** 100 mg-250 mg daily × 2 wk, then 50 mg or more daily
Child: PO/SUBCUT/IM/**IV** 100-300 mg daily × 2 wk, then 35 mg or more daily

Wound healing/chronic disease/ fracture
May be given with zinc
Adult: SUBCUT/IM/**IV**/PO 200-500 mg daily for 1-2 mo
Child: SUBCUT/IM/**IV**/PO 100-200 mg added doses for 1-2 mo

Urine acidification
Adult: 4-12 g daily in divided doses
Child: 500 mg q6-8hr

Available forms: Tabs 25, 50, 100, 250, 500, 1000, 1500 mg; effervescent tabs 1000 mg; chewable tabs 100, 250, 500 mg; time-release tabs 500, 750, 1000, 1500 mg; time-release caps 500 mg; crystals 4 g/tsp; powder 4 g/tsp; liquid 35 mg/0.6 ml; sol 100 mg/ml; syr 20 mg/ml, 500 mg/5 ml; inj SUBCUT, IM, **IV** 100, 250, 500 mg/ml

Implementation
PO route
• Swallow time rel tabs or caps whole; do not break, crush, or chew
• Mix oral sol with foods or fluids
IM route
• Not to be diluted; give deep in large muscle mass

IV, direct route
• Give undiluted by *direct* **IV** 100 mg over at least 1 min, rapid inf may cause fainting

Intermittent IV infusion route
• Give by intermittent inf after diluting with D_5W, $D_{10}W$, 0.9% NaCl, 0.45% NaCl, LR, Ringer's sol, dextrose/saline, dextrose/Ringer's combinations; temp will increase pressure in ampules; wrap with gauze before breaking

Syringe compatibilities: Metoclopramide, aminophylline, theophylline

Syringe incompatibilities: CeFAZolin, doxapram

Y-site compatibilities: Warfarin

ADVERSE EFFECTS
CNS: Headache, insomnia, dizziness, fatigue, flushing
GI: Nausea, vomiting, diarrhea, anorexia, heartburn, cramps
GU: Polyuria, urine acidification, oxalate or urate renal stones, dysuria
HEMA: Hemolytic anemia in patients with G6PD
INTEG: Inflammation at inj site

Pharmacokinetics

Absorption	Readily absorbed (PO)
Distribution	Widely distributed; crosses placenta
Metabolism	Oxidation
Excretion	Kidneys, inactive; breast milk
Half-life	Unknown

Pharmacodynamics
Unknown

INTERACTIONS

Drug/lab test

False positive: negative in glucose tests (Clinitest, Tes-Tape)

False negative: occult blood (large dose), urine bilirubin, leukocyte determination

NURSING CONSIDERATIONS

Assessment

• Assess nutritional status for inclusion of foods high in vit C: citrus fruits, cantaloupe, tomatoes

• Assess for vit C deficiency before, during, and after treatment; scurvy (gingivitis, bleeding gums, loose teeth); poor bone development

• Monitor I&O ratio, polyuria; in patients receiving large doses, renal stones may occur; urine pH (acidification)

• Monitor ascorbic acid levels throughout treatment if continued deficiency is suspected

• Assess inj sites for inflammation, pain, redness, thrombophlebitis if in large doses

Nursing diagnoses

• Knowledge, deficient (teaching)

• Nutrition, impaired: less than body requirements, imbalanced (uses)

Patient/family education

• Teach patient necessary foods to be included in diet that are rich in vit C: citrus fruits, cantaloupe, tomatoes, chili peppers (red)

• Teach patient that smoking decreases vit C levels; not to exceed prescribed dose; increases will be excreted in urine, except time release

• Teach patient not to exceed RDA recommended dose, urinary stones may occur

• Teach patient using ascorbic acid for acidification of urine to test urine pH periodically

Evaluation

Positive therapeutic outcome

• Absence of anorexia, irritability, pallor, joint pain, hyperkeratosis, petechiae, poor wound healing

• Reversal of scurvy: bleeding gums, gingivitis, loose teeth

asenapine (Rx)

(a-sen'a-peen)

Saphris

Func. class.: Antipsychotic, atypical

Chem. class.: Benzisoxazole derivative

Pregnancy category C

ACTION: Unknown; may be mediated through both dopamine type 2 (D_2) and serotonin type 2 (5-HT_{2A}) antagonism

Therapeutic outcome: Decrease in delusions, hallucinations

USES: Bipolar 1 disorder, schizophrenia

CONTRAINDICATIONS:

Breastfeeding, hypersensitivity

Precautions: Pregnancy C, children, geriatric patients, cardiac/renal/hepatic disease, breast cancer, Parkinson's disease, dementia, seizure disorder, CNS depression, agranulocytosis, QT prolongation, torsades de pointes, suicidal ideation, substance abuse

> **BLACK BOX WARNING:** Dementia

DOSAGE AND ROUTES

Schizophrenia

Adult: SL 5 mg bid, max 20 mg/day

Bipolar 1 disorder

Adult: SL 10 mg bid, may decrease to 5 mg bid as needed, max 20 mg/day

Available forms: SL tab 5, 10 mg

Implementation

PO route

• Give anticholinergic agent for EPS

• Avoid use with CNS depressants

• **SL tab:** remove tab, place tab under tongue; after it dissolves, swallow; advise not to chew, crush or swallow tabs, not to eat or drink for 10 min

• Supervise ambulation until patient is stabilized on medication; do not involve in strenuous exercise program because fainting is possible; patient should not stand still for a long time

• Increase fluids to prevent constipation

• Store in tight, light-resistant container

ADVERSE EFFECTS

CNS: *EPS, pseudoparkinsonism, akathisia, dystonia, tardive dyskinesia, drowsiness, insomnia, agitation, anxiety, headache,* **seizures, neuroleptic malignant syndrome,** dizziness

CV: Orthostatic hypotension, **sinus tachycardia, heart failure, QT prolongation, stroke, bundle branch block**

GI: *Nausea,* vomiting, *constipation,* weight gain, increased appetite; oral hypoesthesia/parasthesia (SL)

GU: Hyperprolactinemia, hyperglycemia, hyponatremia

HEMA: Thrombocytopenia

INTEG: Serious allergic reaction

Pharmacokinetics

Absorption	Unknown
Distribution	Protein binding 95%
Metabolism	Liver
Excretion	Unknown
Half-life	Terminal 24 hr

Pharmacodynamics

Onset	Unknown
Peak	$^{1}/_{2}$-$1^{1}/_{2}$ hr
Duration	Unknown

INTERACTIONS

Individual drugs
Alcohol: increased sedation
Chloroquine, clarithromycin, droperidol, erythromycin, haloperidol, methadone, pentamidine: increased QT prolongation
CarBAMazepine: increased asenpine excretion

Drug classifications
Other CNS depressants: increased sedation
CYP2D6 inhibitors/substrates (SSRIs), other antipsychotics: increased EPS
Class IA/ III antidysrhythmics, some phenothiazines, β-agonists, local anesthetics, tricyclics: increased QT prolongation
CYP2D6 inducers (carbamazepine, barbiturates, phenytoin, rifampin): decreased asenapine action

Drug/herb
Kava: increased CNS depression, increased EPS
Betel palm: increased EPS

Drug/lab test
Increase: prolactin levels

NURSING CONSIDERATIONS

Assessment
⚠ **Assess mental status before initial administration; watch for suicidal thoughts and behaviors; dementia and death may occur in the elderly**
• Assess for affect, orientation, LOC, reflexes, gait, coordination, sleep pattern disturbances
• Monitor B/P standing and lying, pulse, respirations; take these q4hr during initial treatment; establish baseline before starting treatment; report drops of 30 mm Hg; watch for ECG changes; QT prolongation may occur
• Monitor for dizziness, faintness, palpitations, tachycardia on rising
• Assess for **EPS,** including akathisia, tardive dyskinesia (bizarre movements of the jaw,

mouth, tongue, extremities), pseudoparkinsonism (rigidity, tremors, pill rolling, shuffling gait)
• Assess for **neuroleptic malignant syndrome:** hyperthermia, increased CPK, altered mental status, muscle rigidity
• Assess for constipation daily; increase bulk and water in diet if needed
• Assess for weight gain, hyperglycemia, metabolic changes in diabetes

Nursing diagnoses
• Knowledge, deficit (teaching)
• Noncompliance (teaching)

Patient/family education
• Caution patient that orthostatic hypotension may occur and to rise from sitting or lying position gradually
• Teach patient to avoid hot tubs, hot showers, tub baths; hypotension may occur
• Advise patient to avoid abrupt withdrawal of this product; EPS may result; product should be withdrawn slowly
• Advise patient to avoid OTC preparations (cough, hay fever, cold) unless approved by prescriber, serious product interactions may occur; avoid use of alcohol, increased drowsiness may occur
• Advise patient to avoid hazardous activities if drowsy or dizzy
• Advise patient about compliance with product regimen
• Advise patient that heat stroke may occur in hot weather; take extra precautions to stay cool
• Advise patient to use contraception, inform prescriber if pregnancy is planned or suspected
• Advise patient to report suicidal thoughts/ behaviors immediately

Evaluation
Positive therapeutic outcome
• Therapeutic response: decrease in emotional excitement, hallucinations, delusions, paranoia; reorganization of patterns of thought, speech

TREATMENT OF OVERDOSE:
Lavage if orally ingested; provide airway; *do not induce vomiting*

aspirin (OTC)
(as'pir-in)
APC-ASA Coated Aspirin ✿, **A.S.A., Ascriptin Enteric, Aspergum, Aspirin** ✿, **Aspir-Low, Aspirtrin** ✿, **Bayer Aspirin, Bayer Children's Aspirin, Bufferin, Ecotrin, Equaline, Good Sense Aspirin, Halfprin, PMS-ASA** ✿, **St. Joseph Children's, St. Joseph's Adult, Walgreens Aspirin Adult**
Func. class.: Nonopioid analgesic
Chem. class.: Salicylate
Pregnancy category D (3rd trimester)

ACTION: Blocks pain impulses in CNS, reduces inflammation by inhibition of prostaglandin synthesis; antipyretic action results from vasodilatation of peripheral vessels; decreases platelet aggregation

Therapeutic outcome: Decreased pain, inflammation, fever; absence of MI, transient ischemic attacks, thrombosis

USES: Mild to moderate pain or fever including rheumatoid arthritis, osteoarthritis, thromboembolic disorders, transient ischemic attacks, rheumatic fever, post-MI, prophylaxis of MI, ischemic stroke, angina; acute MI

Unlabeled uses: Prevention of cataracts (long-term use), prevention of pregnancy loss in women with clotting disorders

CONTRAINDICATIONS:
Pregnancy **D** (3rd trimester), breastfeeding, children <12 yr, children with flulike symptoms, hypersensitivity to salicylates, tartrazine (FDC yellow dye #5), GI bleeding, bleeding disorders, vit K deficiency, peptic ulcer, acute bronchospasm, agranulocytosis, increased intracranial pressure, intracranial bleeding, nasal polyps, urticaria

Precautions: Abrupt discontinuation, acetaminophen/NSAIDs hypersensitivity, acid/base imbalance, alcoholism, ascites, asthma, bone marrow suppression, geriatric patients, dehydration, G6PD deficiency, gout, heart failure, anemia, renal/hepatic disease, pre/postoperatively, gastritis

DOSAGE AND ROUTES
Arthritis
Adult: PO 3 g/day in divided doses q4-6hr
Child >25 kg (55 lb): PO or RECT 90-130 mg/kg/day in divided doses

Kawasaki's disease (unlabeled)
Child: PO 80-100 mg/kg/day in 4 divided doses, maintenance 3-5 mg/kg/day

MI, stroke prophylaxis
Adult: PO 50-325 mg/day

Pain/fever
Adult: PO/RECT 325-650 mg q4hr prn, max 4 g/day
Child 2-11 yr: PO 10-15 mg/kg/dose q4hr, max 4 g/day

Thromboembolic disorders
Adult: PO 325-650 mg/day or bid

Transient ischemic attacks (risk)
Adult: PO 50-325 mg/day (grade 1A)

Prevention of recurrent MI
Adult: PO 75-162 mg/day

CABG
Adult: PO 325 mg/day starting 6 hr post-procedure, continue for 1 yr

PTCA
Adult: PO 325 mg 2 hr presurgery

Evolving MI with ST segment elevation (STEMI)
Adult: PO 160-325 mg nonenteric, chewed and swallowed immediately, maintenance 75-162 mg qd

Available forms: Tabs 81, 325, 500, 650, 800 mg; chewable tabs 81 mg; supp 300, 600, mg; gum 227 mg; enteric coated tabs 81, 325, 500, 975 mg; ext rel 800 mg; del rel tabs 325, 500 mg

Implementation
PO route
• Do not break, crush, or chew enteric product
• Administer to patient crushed or whole; chewable tab should be chewed
• Give with food or milk to decrease gastric symptoms; separate by 2 hr of enteric product; absorption may be slowed
• Give antacids 1-2 hr after enteric products
• Give with 8 oz of water and have patient sit upright for 30 min after dose; discard tabs if vinegar-like smell is present; avoid if allergic to tartrazine
• Give ½ hr before planned exercise

Adverse effects: *italics* = common; **bold** = life-threatening

ADVERSE EFFECTS

CNS: Stimulation, drowsiness, dizziness, confusion, **seizures,** headache, flushing, hallucinations, **coma**
CV: Rapid pulse, pulmonary edema
EENT: Tinnitus, hearing loss
ENDO: Hypoglycemia, hyponatremia, hypokalemia
GI: *Nausea, vomiting,* **GI bleeding,** diarrhea, heartburn, anorexia, **hepatitis**
HEMA: Thrombocytopenia, agranulocytosis, leukopenia, neutropenia, hemolytic anemia, increased PT, PTT, bleeding time
INTEG: *Rash,* urticaria, bruising
RESP: Wheezing, hyperpnea
SYST: Reye's syndrome (children), anaphylaxis, laryngeal edema

Pharmacokinetics

Absorption	Well absorbed, small intestine (PO); erratic (enteric); slow (RECT)
Distribution	Rapidly, widely distributed; crosses placenta, protein binding 90%
Metabolism	Liver, extensively
Excretion	Inactive metabolites, kidney; breast milk
Half-life	15-20 min (low doses); 9 hr (high doses)

Pharmacodynamics

	PO	RECT
Onset	15-30 min	Slow
Peak	1-2 hr	4-5 hr
Duration	4-6 hr	6-7 hr

INTERACTIONS

Individual drugs

Alcohol, cefamandole, clopidogrel, eptifibatide, heparin, plicamycin, ticlopidine, tirofiban: increased risk of bleeding
Ammonium chloride, nizatidine: increased salicylate level
Insulin, methotrexate, phenytoin, valproic acid, warfarin: increased effects of each specific product
Nitroglycerin: increased hypotension
Probenecid: decreased effects of probenecid
Spironolactone, sulfinpyrazone: decreased effects

Drug classifications

ACE inhibitors: decreased antihypertensive effect
Antacids (high doses), corticosteroids, urinary alkalizers: decreased effects of aspirin
Anticoagulants, thrombolytics: increased risk of bleeding
Diuretics (loop), sulfonylamides, NSAIDs, β-blockers: decreased effect of each specific product
NSAIDs, antiinflammatories, steroids: increased gastric ulcers
Penicillins, oral hypoglycemics, sulfonamides, thrombolytic agents: increased effects of each specific product
Salicylates: decreased blood glucose levels
Urinary acidifiers: increased salicylate levels

Drug/herb

Feverfew, garlic, ginger, ginkgo, ginseng *(Panax),* horse chestnut: increased risk of bleeding

Drug/food

Foods acidifying urine may increase aspirin levels
Fish oil (omega-3-fatty acids): increased risk of bleeding

Drug/lab test

Increased: coagulation studies, liver function studies, serum uric acid, amylase, CO_2, urinary protein
Decreased: serum potassium, cholesterol
Interference: VMA, 5-HIAA, xylose tolerance test, TSH, pregnancy test

NURSING CONSIDERATIONS

Assessment

• Assess for **pain:** character, location, intensity, ROM before and 1 hr after administration
• Monitor liver function studies: AST, ALT, bilirubin, creatinine if patient is on long-term therapy
• Monitor renal function studies: BUN, urine creatinine if patient is on long-term therapy
• Monitor blood studies: CBC, Hct, Hgb, PT if patient is on long-term therapy
• Check I&O ratio; decreasing output may indicate renal failure (long-term therapy)
⚠ **Assess hepatotoxicity: dark urine, clay-colored stools, yellowing of the skin and sclera, itching, abdominal pain, fever, diarrhea if patient is on long-term therapy**
• Assess for **allergic reactions:** rash, urticaria; if these occur, product may have to be discontinued; in patients with asthma, nasal polyps, allergies, severe allergic reactions may occur
• Assess for **ototoxicity:** tinnitus, ringing, roaring in ears; audiometric testing needed before, after long-term therapy

• Monitor **salicylate level:** therapeutic level 150-300 mcg/ml for chronic inflammation
• Check edema in feet, ankles, legs
• Identify prior product history; there are many product interactions

Nursing diagnoses
• Injury, risk for (side effects)
• Knowledge, deficient (teaching)
• Mobility, impaired physical (uses)
• Pain, acute (uses)
• Pain, chronic (uses)

Patient/family education
• Teach patient to report any symptoms of renal/hepatic toxicity, visual changes, ototoxicity, allergic reactions, bleeding (long-term therapy)
• Instruct patient to take with 8 oz of water and sit upright for 30 min after dose to facilitate product passing into the stomach; to discard tabs if vinegar-like smell is present; to avoid if allergic to tartrazine
• Instruct patient not to exceed recommended dosage; acute poisoning may result
• Advise patient to read label on other OTC products; many contain aspirin
• Inform patient that the therapeutic response takes 2 wk (arthritis)
• Teach patient to report tinnitus, confusion, diarrhea, sweating, hyperventilation
• Advise patient to avoid alcohol ingestion; GI bleeding may occur
• Advise patient with allergies, nasal polyps, asthma, that allergic reactions may develop
• Instruct patient to read labels on other OTC products: may contain salicylates
• Teach patient not to give to children or teens with flulike symptoms or chicken pox; Reye's syndrome may develop

Evaluation
Positive therapeutic outcome
• Decreased pain
• Decreased inflammation
• Decreased fever
• Absence of MI
• Absence of transient ischemic attacks, thrombosis

TREATMENT OF OVERDOSE:
Lavage, activated charcoal; monitor electrolytes, VS

---

atazanavir (Rx)
(at-a-za-na′veer)
Reyataz
Func. class.: Antiretroviral
Chem. class.: Protease inhibitor
Pregnancy category B

ACTION: Inhibits human immunodeficiency virus (HIV-1) protease, which prevents maturation of the infectious virus

Therapeutic outcome: Decreasing symptoms of HIV

USES: HIV-1 infection in combination with other antiretroviral agents

CONTRAINDICATIONS:
Hypersensitivity

Precautions: Pregnancy **B,** breastfeeding, children, geriatric, liver disease, alcoholism, antimicrobial resistance, AV block, diabetes, dialysis, elderly, women, hemophilia, hypercholesterolemia, immune reconstitution syndrome, lactic acidosis, pancreatitis

DOSAGE AND ROUTES
Antiretroviral-naive patients
Adult: PO 400 mg daily
Child ≥6 yr/adolescent ≤40 kg: PO 300 mg with ritonavir 100 mg qd
Child ≥6 yr/adolescent 20 to <40 kg: PO 200 mg with ritonavir 100 mg qd
Child ≥6 yr/adolescent 15 to <20 kg: PO 150 mg with ritonavir 80 mg qd

Antiretroviral-experienced patients
Adult: PO 300 mg daily and ritonavir 100 mg daily
Pregnant adult/adolescent (2nd/3rd trimester) with H₂ blocker or tenofovir: PO 400 mg with ritonavir 100 mg qd
Child ≥6 yr/adolescent ≥40 kg: PO 300 mg with ritonavir 100 mg qd
Child ≥6 yr/adolescent 20 to <40 kg: PO 200 mg with ritonavir 100 mg qd

Hepatic dose
Adult: PO (Child-Pugh B) 300 mg daily; (Child-Pugh C) do not use

Available forms: Caps 100, 150, 200, 300 mg

Implementation
• Administer with food; take 2 hr before or 1 hr after antacid or didanosine; swallow cap whole

---

ADVERSE EFFECTS

CNS: Headache, depression, dizziness, insomnia, peripheral neuropathy
GI: *Diarrhea, abdominal pain, nausea,* vomiting, **hepatotoxicity**
INTEG: *Rash,* **Stevens-Johnson syndrome,** *photosensitivity*
MISC: Fatigue, fever, arthralgia, back pain, cough, lipodystrophy, pain, gynecomastia, nephrolithiasis, **lactic acidosis, hyperbilirubinemia** (pregnancy, females, obesity)

Pharmacokinetics

Absorption	Rapid, increased with food
Distribution	86% protein bound
Metabolism	Liver extensively by CYP3A4
Excretion	27% excreted unchanged in urine/feces (minimal)
Half-life	7 hr

Pharmacodynamics

Onset	Unknown
Peak	2 hr
Duration	Unknown

INTERACTIONS

Individual drugs

Chlorazepate, clarithromycin, cycloSPORINE, diazepam, irinotecan, midazolam, pimozide, sildenafil, sirolimus, tacrolimus, triazolam, warfarin: increased levels resulting in toxicity
Didanosine, efavirenz, rifampin: decreased atazanavir levels
Indinavir: increased hyperbilirubinemia

Drug classifications

Antacids, H_2-receptor antagonists, proton pump inhibitors, CYP3A4 inducers: decreased atazanavir levels
Antidepressants (tricyclics), antidysrhythmics, ergots, calcium channel blockers, HMG-CoA reductase inhibitors, immunosuppressants, other protease inhibitors: increased levels resulting in increased toxicity
Contraceptives (oral), estrogens: increased effects
CYP3A4 substrates, CYP3A4 inhibitors: increased atazanavir levels

Drug/herb

Red yeast rice: myopathy, rhabdomyolysis
St. John's wort: decreased atazanavir levels

Drug/lab test

Increased: AST, ALT, total bilirubin, amylase, lipase, CK
Decreased: Hgb, neutrophils, platelets

NURSING CONSIDERATIONS

Assessment

⚠ **Assess for hepatic failure**
• Assess for signs of infection, anemia
• Monitor liver function studies: ALT, AST, bilirubin
• Monitor bowel pattern before, during treatment; if severe abdominal pain with bleeding occurs, product should be discontinued; monitor hydration
• Monitor viral load, CD4 count throughout treatment
• Assess skin eruptions, rash, urticaria, itching
• Identify allergies before treatment, reaction of each medication; place allergies on chart

Nursing diagnoses

• Injury, risk for (uses, adverse reactions)
• Knowledge, deficient (teaching)

Patient/family education

• Advise to take as prescribed with other antiretrovirals as prescribed; if dose is missed, take as soon as remembered up to 1 hr before next dose; do not double dose; do not share with others
• Teach that product must be taken daily to maintain blood levels for duration of therapy
• Teach that photosensitivity may occur; use protective clothing or stay out of the sun
• Instruct to notify prescriber if diarrhea, nausea, vomiting, rash occur; dizziness, lightheadedness; ECG may be altered
• Inform that product interacts with many products and St. John's wort; advise prescriber of all products, herbal products used
• Advise that redistribution of body fat may occur; the effect is not known
• Teach that product does not cure HIV-1 infection or prevent transmission to others, only controls symptoms
• Advise that if taking sildenafil with atazanavir, there may be an increased risk of phosphodiesterase type 5 inhibitor–associated adverse events, including hypotension and prolonged penile erection; notify physician promptly of these symptoms

Evaluation

Positive therapeutic outcome
• Increasing CD4 counts; decreased viral load, resolution of symptoms of HIV-1 infection

atenolol (Rx)
(a-ten'oh-lole)
**CO Atenolol ✤, Gen-Atenolol ✤,
PMS-Atenolol ✤, RAN Atenolol ✤,
ratio-Atenolol ✤, Sandoz
Atenolol ✤, Tenormin**
Func. class.: Antihypertensive
Chem. class.: β-Blocker; β₁-, β₂-blocker (high doses)
Pregnancy category D

Do not confuse:
atenolol/albuterol/Altenol,
Tenormin/thiamine/Imuran

ACTION: Competitively blocks stimulation of β-adrenergic receptor within vascular smooth muscle; produces negative chronotropic activity (decreases rate of SA node discharge, increases recovery time), slows conduction of AV node, decreases heart rate, negative inotropic activity, decreases O_2 consumption in myocardium; also decreases renin-aldosterone-angiotensin system at high doses, inhibits β₂-receptors in bronchial system at higher doses

Therapeutic outcome: Decreased B/P, heart rate, prevention of angina pectoris, MI

USES: Mild to moderate hypertension; prophylaxis of angina pectoris; suspected or known MI (**IV** use), MI prophylaxis

CONTRAINDICATIONS:
Pregnancy **D**, hypersensitivity to β-blockers, cardiogenic shock, 2nd- or 3rd-degree heart block, sinus bradycardia, cardiac failure, Raynaud's disease, pulmonary edema

Precautions: Major surgery, breastfeeding, diabetes mellitus, renal disease, thyroid disease, CHF, COPD, asthma, well-compensated heart failure, dialysis, myasthenia gravis

> **BLACK BOX WARNING:** Abrupt discontinuation

DOSAGE AND ROUTES
Adult: PO 25-50 mg daily, increasing q1-2wk to 100 mg daily; may increase to 200 mg daily for angina or up to 100 mg for hypertension
Child: PO 0.8-1 mg/kg/dose initially, range 0.8-1.5 mg/kg/day, max 2 mg/kg/day
Geriatric: PO 25 mg/day initially

Chronic stable angina
Adult: PO 50 mg q day, then 100 mg/day prn after 7 days, max 200 mg/day

Post MI, MI prophylaxis
Adult: PO 1000 mg/day, in 1-2 divided doses, may need for 1-3 yr post MI

Renal dose
Adult: PO CCr 15-35 ml/min, max 50 mg/day; CCr <15 ml/min max 25 mg/day; hemodialysis 25-50 mg after dialysis

Available forms: Tabs 25, 50, 100 mg

Implementation
PO route
• Given before meals, at bedtime; tablet may be crushed or swallowed whole; give with food to prevent GI upset; reduced dosage in renal dysfunction; take at same time each day
• Store protected from light, moisture; place in cool environment

ADVERSE EFFECTS
CNS: *Insomnia, fatigue, dizziness, mental changes,* memory loss, hallucinations, depression, lethargy, drowsiness, strange dreams, catatonia
CV: Profound hypotension, bradycardia, CHF, *cold extremities, postural hypotension, 2nd- or 3rd-degree heart block*
EENT: Sore throat, dry burning eyes, blurred vision, stuffy nose
ENDO: Increased hypoglycemic response to insulin
GI: *Nausea, diarrhea,* vomiting, **mesenteric arterial thrombosis, ischemic colitis**
GU: Impotence, decreased libido
HEMA: Agranulocytosis, thrombocytopenia, purpura
INTEG: Rash, fever, alopecia
RESP: Bronchospasm, dyspnea, wheezing, pulmonary edema

Pharmacokinetics

Absorption	50%-60% (PO)
Distribution	Crosses placenta; protein binding (5%-15%)
Metabolism	Not metabolized
Excretion	Breast milk, kidneys (50%), feces (50%—unabsorbed product)
Half-life	6-9 hr

Pharmacodynamics

	PO
Onset	1 hr
Peak	2-4 hr
Duration	24 hr

INTERACTIONS

Individual drugs
Digoxin, diltiazem, hydralazine, methyldopa, prazosin, reserpine, verapamil: increased hypotension, bradycardia

EPHEDrine, pseudoephedrine: increased hypertension

Dopamine, insulin, theophylline: decreased effect of each of these drugs

Drug classifications
Amphetamines: increased hypertension

Anticholinergics, antihypertensives: cardiac glycosides, increased hypotension, bradycardia

Antidiabetic agents (oral) MAOIs: decreased effect of each of these drugs

Sympathomimetics (cough, cold preparations): mutual inhibition

Drug/herb
Hawthorn: increased atenolol effect

Ephedra (ma huang): decreased atenolol effect

Drug/lab test
Increased: uric acid, potassium, triglyceride, blood glucose, BUN, ANA titer

NURSING CONSIDERATIONS

Assessment
• Monitor B/P during beginning treatment, periodically thereafter; pulse q4hr; note rate, rhythm, quality: apical/radial pulse before administration; notify prescriber of any significant changes (pulse <50 bpm); ECG
• Check for baselines in renal, liver function tests before therapy begins
• Assess for edema in feet, legs daily; monitor I&O, daily weight; check for jugular vein distention, crackles bilaterally, dyspnea (CHF)

Nursing diagnoses
• Cardiac output, decreased (uses)
• Injury, risk for (side effects)
• Knowledge, deficient (teaching)
• Noncompliance (teaching)

Patient/family education
⚠ Teach patient not to discontinue product abruptly; taper over 2 wk (angina) as directed; may cause precipitate angina if stopped abruptly; take at same time each day

• Teach patient not to use OTC products containing α-adrenergic stimulants (such as nasal decongestants, OTC cold preparations); to limit alcohol, smoking; to limit sodium intake as prescribed
• Teach patient how to take pulse and B/P at home; advise when to notify prescriber
• Instruct patient to comply with weight control, dietary adjustments, modified exercise program
• Advise patient to carry/wear emergency ID for products, allergies, conditions being treated; tell patient product controls symptoms but does not cure
• Caution patient to avoid hazardous activities if dizziness, drowsiness is present
• Teach patient to report symptoms of CHF: difficult breathing, especially on exertion or when lying down, night cough, swelling of extremities or bradycardia, dizziness, confusion, depression, fever
• Teach patient to take product as prescribed, not to double doses, skip doses; take any missed doses as remembered if at least 6 hr until next dose
• Advise to change position slowly
• Advise patient that product may mask symptoms of hypoglycemia in diabetic patients
• Advise patient to use contraception while taking this product

Evaluation
Positive therapeutic outcome
• Decreased B/P in hypertension (after 1-2 wk)
• Absence of dysrhythmias
• Absence of MI
• Decreased angina/pain
• Increased activity tolerance

TREATMENT OF OVERDOSE:
Lavage, IV atropine for bradycardia, IV theophylline for bronchospasm, digoxin, O$_2$, diuretic for cardiac failure, hemodialysis, IV glucose for hyperglycemia, IV diazepam (or phenytoin) for seizures

atomoxetine (Rx)
(at-o-mox′eh-teen)
Strattera
Func. class.: Psychotherapeutic—miscellaneous
Pregnancy category C

ACTION: A selective norepinephrine reuptake inhibitor; may inhibit the presynaptic norepinephrine transporter; exact mechanism of action is unknown

Therapeutic outcome: Decreased hyperactivity, impulsivity, increased attention, organization, ability to complete tasks

USES: Attention deficit hyperactivity disorder

CONTRAINDICATIONS:
Hypersensitivity, closed-angle glaucoma, arteriosclerosis, cardiac disease, cardiomyopathy, heart failure, jaundice, MAOI therapy, history of pheochromocytoma

Precautions: Pregnancy C, breastfeeding, hypertension, hepatic disease, angioedema, bipolar disorder, dysrhythmias, CAD, hypo/hypertension

> **BLACK BOX WARNING:** Children <6 yr, suicidal ideation

DOSAGE AND ROUTES
Child ≤70 kg, <6 yr: PO 0.5 mg/kg/day, increase after 3 days to a target daily dose of 1.2 mg/kg in AM or evenly divided doses AM, late afternoon; max 1.4 mg/kg/day or 100 mg daily, whichever is less
Adult and child >70 kg: PO 40 mg daily, increase after 3 days to a target daily dose of 80 mg in AM or evenly divided doses AM, late afternoon; max 100 mg daily

Maintenance
Adolescent ≤15 yr and child ≥6 yr: PO 1.2-1.8 mg/kg/day

Initial dosage titration with strong CYP2D6 inhibitors
Adult and child >6 yr weighing >70 kg: PO 40 mg/day each AM or 2 evenly divided doses, titrate to target of 80 mg/day if symptoms do not improve after 4 wk and dose is well tolerated

Hepatic dose
Child-Pugh B: reduce dose by 50%
Child-Pugh C: reduce dose by 75%

Available forms: Caps 10, 18, 25, 40, 60, 80, 100 mg

Implementation
• Swallow whole; do not break, crush, or chew
• Give without regard to food
• Provide gum, hard candy, frequent sips of water for dry mouth

ADVERSE EFFECTS
CNS: *Insomnia,* dizziness, headache, irritability, crying, mood swings, fatigue, hypoesthesia, lethargy, paresthesia

CV: *Palpitations,* hot flushes, tachycardia, increased B/P
ENDO: Growth retardation
GI: Dyspepsia, nausea, anorexia, dry mouth, weight loss, vomiting, diarrhea, constipation, **hepatic injury**
GU: Urinary hesitancy, retention, dysmenorrhea, erectile disturbance, ejaculation failure, impotence, prostatitis, abnormal orgasm, male pelvic pain
INTEG: Exfoliative dermatitis, sweating, rash
MISC: Cough, rhinorrhea, dermatitis, ear infection

Pharmacokinetics
Absorption	Unknown
Distribution	Protein binding, 98%
Metabolism	Liver
Excretion	Kidneys
Half-life	Unknown

Pharmacodynamics
Unknown

INTERACTIONS
Individual drug
Albuterol: increased cardiovascular effects

Drug classifications
CYP2D6 inhibitors (amiodarone, cimetidine [weak], citalopram, clomiPRAMINE, delavirdine, escitalopram, FLUoxetine, gefitinib, imatinib, paroxetine, propafenone, quiNIDine [potent], ritonavir, sertraline, thioridazine, venlafaxine): increased effects of atomoxetine
⚠ MAOIs or within 14 days of MAOIs, vasopressors: hypertensive crisis
Pressor agents: increased cardiovascular effects

NURSING CONSIDERATIONS
Assessment
• Monitor VS, B/P; check patients with cardiac disease more often for increased B/P
• Monitor height, growth rate q3mo in children; growth rate may be decreased

> **BLACK BOX WARNING:** Assess mental status: mood, sensorium, affect, stimulation, insomnia, aggressiveness, suicidal ideation in children/young adults

• Assess appetite, sleep, speech patterns
• Assess for attention span, decreased hyperactivity in ADHD persons

Adverse effects: *italics* = common; **bold** = life-threatening

Nursing diagnoses
- Coping, ineffective (uses)
- Coping, compromised family (uses)
- Knowledge, deficient (teaching)
- Thought processes, disturbed (uses)

Patient/family education
- Advise patient to avoid OTC preparations unless approved by prescriber
- Advise patient to avoid alcohol ingestion
- Advise patient to avoid hazardous activities until stabilized on medication
- Advise patient to get needed rest; patients will feel more tired at end of day; do not take dose late in day, insomnia may occur

> **BLACK BOX WARNING:** Advise to report suicidal ideation

Evaluation
Positive therapeutic outcome
- Decreased hyperactivity (ADHD)

---

atorvastatin (Rx)
(a-tore′va-stat-in)
Lipitor
Func. class.: Antilipidemic
Chem. class.: HMG-CoA reductase inhibitor
Pregnancy category X

ACTION: Inhibits HMG-CoA reductase enzyme, which reduces cholesterol synthesis, high doses lead to plaque regression

Therapeutic outcome: Decreased cholesterol levels and LDLs, increased HDLs

USES: As an adjunct in primary hypercholesterolemia (types Ia, Ib), dysbetalipoproteinemia, elevated triglyceride levels; prevention of cardiovascular disease by reduction of heart risk in those with mildly elevated cholesterol

CONTRAINDICATIONS:
Pregnancy **X**, breastfeeding, hypersensitivity, active liver disease

Precautions: Past liver disease, alcoholism, severe acute infections, trauma, severe metabolic disorders, electrolyte imbalance

DOSAGE AND ROUTES
Adult: PO 10-20 mg daily, usual range 10-80 mg, dosage adjustments may be made in 2-4 wk intervals, max 80 mg/day; patients requiring

>45% reduction in LDL may be started at 40 mg daily

Available forms: Tabs 10, 20, 40, 80 mg

Implementation
- Administer total daily dose at any time of day
- Store in cool environment in airtight, light-resistant container

ADVERSE EFFECTS
CNS: Headache, asthenia, **Lou Gehrig's disease (ALS)**
EENT: Lens opacities
GI: *Abdominal cramps, constipation, diarrhea, heartburn,* nausea, dyspepsia, *flatus,* **liver dysfunction, pancreatitis,** increased serum transaminase
GU: Impotence
INTEG: Rash, pruritus, alopecia, photosensitivity (rare)
MISC: Hypersensitivity
MS: Myalgia, **rhabdomyolysis,** arthralgia
RESP: Pharyngitis, sinusitis

Pharmacokinetics
Absorption	Unknown
Distribution	Unknown
Metabolism	Liver
Excretion	Bile, feces, kidneys
Half-life	14 hr

Pharmacodynamics
Unknown

INTERACTIONS

Individual drugs
Clofibrate, cycloSPORINE, erythromycin, gemfibrozil, niacin: increased risk of rhabdomyolysis
Colestipol: decreased action of atorvastatin
Digoxin: increased action of digoxin
Erythromycin: increased levels of atorvastatin
Warfarin: increased action of warfarin

Drug classifications
Antifungals (azole): possible rhabdomyolysis
Contraceptives (oral): increased levels

Drug/herb
St. John's wort: decreased effect

Drug/food
Grapefruit juice: possible toxicity
Oat bran may reduce effectiveness

Drug/lab test
Increased: bilirubin, alkaline phosphatase, ALT, AST, CK
Interference: thyroid function tests

NURSING CONSIDERATIONS

Assessment
• **Hypercholesterolemia:** assess nutrition: fat, protein, carbohydrates; nutritional analysis should be completed by dietitian before treatment; assess for muscle pain, tenderness; obtain CPK if these occur, product may need to be discontinued; monitor triglycerides, cholesterol at baseline and throughout treatment; LDL and VLDL should be watched closely; if increased, product should be discontinued
• Monitor bowel pattern daily; diarrhea may be a problem
• Monitor liver function studies q1-2mo during the first 1^1/$_2$ yr of treatment; AST, ALT, liver function tests may be increased
• Monitor renal studies in patients with compromised renal system: BUN, I&O ratio, creatinine
• Assess eyes via ophthalmic exam 1 mo after treatment begins, annually

Nursing diagnoses
• Diarrhea (adverse reactions)
• Knowledge, deficient (teaching)
• Noncompliance (teaching)

Patient/family education
• Inform patient that compliance is needed for positive results to occur, not to double doses
• Teach patient that risk factors should be decreased: high-fat diet, smoking, alcohol consumption, absence of exercise
• Advise patient to notify prescriber if the GI symptoms of diarrhea, abdominal or epigastric pain, nausea, vomiting; chills, fever, sore throat; muscle pain, weakness occur
• Advise patient that treatment will take several years
• Advise patient that blood work and eye exam will be necessary during treatment
• Advise not to take if pregnant (pregnancy **X**) or breastfeeding
• Advise patient to stay out of the sun, use protective clothing, or use sunscreen to prevent photosensitivity (rare)

Evaluation
Positive therapeutic outcome
• Decreased cholesterol levels, serum triglyceride
• Improved HDL:LDL ratio

atovaquone (Rx)
(a-toe′va-kwon)
Mepron
Func. class.: Antiprotozoal
Chem. class.: Aromatic diamide derivative; analog of ubiquinone
Pregnancy category C

ACTION: Interferes with DNA/RNA synthesis in protozoa

Therapeutic outcome: Antiprotozoal for *Pneumocystis jiroveci* only

USES: *P. jiroveci* infections in patients intolerant of trimethoprim/sulfamethoxazole (co-trimoxazole), prophylaxis, *Toxoplasma gondii,* toxoplasmosis

CONTRAINDICATIONS:
Hypersensitivity or history of developing life-threatening allergic reactions to any component of the formulation, benzyl alcohol sensitivity

Precautions: Pregnancy **C**, breastfeeding, GI/hepatic disease, neonates, respiratory insufficiency

DOSAGE AND ROUTES

Acute, mild, moderate Pneumocystis jiroveci *pneumonia (PCP)*
Adult and adolescent 13-16 yr: PO 750 mg tid with food for 21 days

Pneumocystis jiroveci *pneumonia prophylaxis*
Adult and adolescent: PO 1500 mg daily with meal

Available forms: Susp 750 mg/5 ml

Implementation
• Give with food (preferably fatty); to increase absorption of the product and higher plasma concentrations; give tid × 3 wk
• Give oral suspension after shaken
• Take all contents of foil pouch

ADVERSE EFFECTS
CNS: *Dizziness, headache, anxiety,* insomnia, asthenia, fever
CV: Hypotension
GI: *Nausea, vomiting, diarrhea,* anorexia, increased AST and ALT, **acute pancreatitis,** constipation, abdominal pain
HEMA: Anemia, **neutropenia**
INTEG: Pruritus, urticaria, *rash*

META: Hyperkalemia, hypoglycemia, hyponatremia
OTHER: Cough, dyspnea

Pharmacokinetics

Absorption	Poor; increased when taken with fatty foods
Distribution	Unknown
Metabolism	Hepatic recycling
Excretion	Feces, unchanged (94%)
Half-life	2-3 days

Pharmacodynamics

Onset	Unknown
Peak	1-8 hr
Duration	Unknown

INTERACTIONS

Individual drugs
Rifampin, rifabutin, tetracycline: decreased effectiveness of atovaquone
Zidovudine: increased level of zidovudine

Drug/lab test
Increase: AST, ALT, alk phos
Decrease: glucose, neutrophils, Hgb, sodium

NURSING CONSIDERATIONS

Assessment
• Assess for *Pneumocystis jiroveci:* monitor WBC, bilateral lung sounds, sputum for C&S; these should be checked before, periodically during, after treatment; after collection of 1st sputum, therapy may begin
• Monitor for signs of **infection;** anemia; monitor bowel pattern before, during treatment
• Monitor respiratory status: rate, character, wheezing, dyspnea; ABGs, chest films
• Assess for dizziness, confusion, hallucination
• Assess for allergies before treatment, reaction of each medication; place allergies on chart; notify all people giving products

Nursing diagnoses
• Diarrhea (adverse reactions)
• Infection, risk for (uses)
• Knowledge, deficient (teaching)

Patient/family education
• Instruct patient to take with food, preferably fatty foods, to increase plasma concentrations
• Advise patient to take product exactly as prescribed

Evaluation
Positive therapeutic outcome
• Decreased temperature
• Ability to breathe
• Three negative sputum cultures

⚠ HIGH ALERT

atropine (Rx)
(a′troe-peen)
Atreza, AtroPen, Sal-Tropine
Func. class.: Antidysrhythmic, anticholinergic parasympatholytic, antimuscarinic
Chem. class.: Belladonna alkaloid
Pregnancy category C

Do not confuse:
atropine/Akarpine

ACTION: Blocks acetylcholine at parasympathetic neuroeffector sites; increases cardiac output, heart rate by blocking vagal stimulation in heart; dries secretions by blocking vagus

Therapeutic outcome: Drying of secretions, increased heart rate, cycloplegia, mydriasis

USES: Bradycardia <40-50 bpm, bradydysrhythmia, reversal of anticholinesterase agents, insecticide poisoning, blocking cardiac vagal reflexes, decreasing secretions before surgery, antispasmodic with GU and biliary surgery, bronchodilator, AV heart block

CONTRAINDICATIONS:
Hypersensitivity to belladonna alkaloids, closed-angle glaucoma, GI obstructions, myasthenia gravis, thyrotoxicosis, ulcerative colitis, prostatic hypertrophy, tachycardia/tachydysrhythmias, asthma, acute hemorrhage, severe hepatic disease, myocardial ischemia, paralytic ileus

Precautions: Pregnancy C, breastfeeding, child <6 yr, geriatric, renal disease, CHF, hyperthyroidism, COPD, hypertension, intraabdominal infections, Down syndrome, spastic paralysis, gastric ulcer

DOSAGE AND ROUTES

Bradycardia/bradydysrhythmias
Adult: IV bol 0.5-1 mg given q3-5min, not to exceed 3 mg
Child: IV bol 0.01-0.03 mg/kg up to 0.4 mg or 0.3 mg/m^2; may repeat q4-6hr, min dose 0.1

mg to avoid paradoxical reaction, max single dose 0.5 mg

Organophosphate poisoning
Adult and child: IM (AtroPen)/**IV** 1-2 mg qhr until muscarinic symptoms disappear; may need 6 mg qhr
Adult and child ≥90 lb, usually >10 yr: 2 mg IM (AtroPen)
Child 40-90 lb, usually 4-10 yr: 1 mg IM (AtroPen)
Child 15-40 lb, 6 mo-4 yr: 0.5 mg IM (AtroPen)
Infant <15 lb: IM/IV 0.05 mg/kg q5-20min

Presurgery
Adult and child >20 kg: SUBCUT/IM/ **IV** 0.4-0.6 mg 30-60 min before anesthesia
Child <20 kg: IM/SUBCUT 0.01 mg/kg up to 0.4 mg 1/2-1 hr preop, max 0.6 mg/dose

Available forms: Inj 0.05, 0.1, 0.4, 0.5, 0.8, 1 mg/ml; tabs 0.4 mg; inj prefilled autoinjectors (AtroPen) 0.5, 1, 2 mg

Implementation
PO route
• PO 30 min before meals
• Give increased bulk, water in diet if constipation occurs (anticholinergic effect)
IM route
• Expect atropine flush 15-20 min after inj; it may occur in children and is not harmful
AtroPen
• Use no more than 3 AtroPen injections unless under the supervision of trained provider
• Use as soon as symptoms appear (tearing, wheezing, muscle fasciculations, excessive oral secretions)

IV route
• Give **IV** undiluted or diluted with 10 ml sterile water; give at a rate of 0.6 mg/min; give through Y-tube or 3-way stopcock; do not add to **IV** sol; may cause paradoxical bradycardia lasting 2 min

Y-site compatibilities: Amrinone, etomidate, famotidine, heparin, hydrocortisone sodium succinate, meropenem, nafcillin, potassium chloride, SUFentanil, vit B/C

ADVERSE EFFECTS
CNS: Headache, dizziness, involuntary movement, confusion, psychosis, anxiety, **coma,** flushing, drowsiness, insomnia, weakness, delirium (geriatric)
CV: Hypo/hypertension, paradoxical bradycardia, angina, PVCs, **tachycardia,** ectopic ventricular beats

EENT: Blurred vision, photophobia, glaucoma, eye pain, pupil dilatation, nasal congestion
GI: Dry mouth, nausea, vomiting, abdominal pain, anorexia, constipation, **paralytic ileus,** abdominal distention, altered taste
GU: Retention, hesitancy, impotence, dysuria
INTEG: Rash, urticaria, contact dermatitis, dry skin, flushing
MISC: Suppression of breastfeeding, decreased sweating

Pharmacokinetics

Absorption	Well absorbed (PO, SUBCUT, IM)
Distribution	Crosses blood-brain barrier, placenta
Metabolism	Liver
Excretion	Kidneys, unchanged (70%-90%); breast milk
Half-life	13-40 hr

Pharmacodynamics

	PO	IM/ SUB-CUT	IV	Ophth
Onset	1/2 hr	15 min	2-4 min	1/2 hr
Peak	1/2-1 hr	30 min	2-4 min	30-60 min
Duration	4-6 hr	4-6 hr	4-6 hr	1-2 wk

INTERACTIONS

Individual drugs
Amantadine: increased anticholinergic effects
Ketoconazole, levodopa: decreased absorption
Potassium chloride (oral): increased mucosal lesions

Drug classifications
Antacids: decreased absorption of atropine
Antidepressants (tricyclic), antiparkinson agents: increased anticholinergic effect

NURSING CONSIDERATIONS
Assessment
• Monitor I&O ratio; check for urinary retention and daily output in geriatric or postoperative patients
• Monitor ECG for ectopic ventricular beats, PVC, tachycardia in cardiac patients
• Monitor for bowel sounds; check for constipation; abdominal distention and constipation may occur
• Monitor respiratory status: rate, rhythm, cyanosis, wheezing, dyspnea, engorged neck veins

• Monitor cardiac rate: rhythm, character, B/P continuously
• Monitor allergic reaction: rash, urticaria

Nursing diagnoses
• Cardiac output, decreased (uses)
• Constipation (adverse reactions)
• Knowledge, deficient (teaching)

Patient/family education
• Advise patient not to perform strenuous activity in high temperatures; heat stroke may result
• Instruct patient to take as prescribed; not to skip doses
• Instruct patient to report change in vision; blurring or loss of sight; trouble breathing; sweating; flushing, chest pain, allergic reactions, constipation, urinary retention
• Caution patient not to operate machinery if drowsiness occurs
• Advise patient not to take OTC products without approval of physician

Evaluation
Positive therapeutic outcome
• Decreased dysrhythmias
• Increased heart rate
• Decreased secretions, GI, GU spasms
• Bronchodilatation

TREATMENT OF OVERDOSE:
O_2, artificial ventilation, ECG; administer DOPamine for circulatory depression; administer diazepam or thiopental for seizure; assess need for antidysrhythmics

atropine ophthalmic
See Appendix B

⚠ HIGH ALERT
azaCITIDine (Rx)
(a-za-sie-ti′deen)
Vidaza
Func. class.: Antineoplastic hormone
Chem. class.: DNA demethylation agent
Pregnancy category D

Do not confuse:
azaCITIDine/azaTHIOprine

ACTION: Cytotoxic by producing damage to double-strand DNA during DNA synthesis

Therapeutic outcome: Improved blood counts in refractor anemia

USES: Myelodysplastic syndrome (MDS)

CONTRAINDICATIONS:
Pregnancy **D**, hypersensitivity to this product or mannitol, advanced malignant hepatic tumors

Precautions: Breastfeeding, children, geriatric, renal/hepatic disease; baseline albumin <30 g/L; a man should not father a child while taking this product

DOSAGE AND ROUTES
Adult: SUBCUT 75 mg/m^2 daily × 7 days, q4wk, premedicate with antiemetic; dose may be increased to 100 mg/m^2 if no response is seen after 2 treatment cycles; minimum treatment 4 cycles

Available forms: Powder for inj, 100 mg

Implementation
• Increase patient's fluid intake to 2-3 L/day to prevent dehydration, unless contraindicated
• Assist patient with rinsing of mouth tid-qid with water, club soda; brushing of teeth bid-tid with soft brush or cotton-tipped applicator for stomatitis; use unwaxed dental floss
• Provide a nutritious diet with iron, vitamin supplement, low fiber, few dairy products
• Use cytotoxic handling procedures
SUBCUT route
• **Reconstitute** with 4 ml sterile water for inj (25 mg/ml), **inject** diluents slowly into vial, **invert** vial 2-3 times and gently rotate; sol will be cloudy, use immediately; divide doses >4 ml into two syringes; invert the contents 2-3 times and gently roll syringe between the palms for 30 sec immediately before administration; rotate inj site

IV intermittent INF route
• **Reconstitute** each vial with 4 ml sterile water for inj, **shake** well until all solids are dissolved, (10 mg/ml) withdraw sol and **inject** in 50-100 NS or LR, **infuse** over 10-40 min

ADVERSE EFFECTS
CNS: Anxiety, depression, dizziness, fatigue, headache, fever, insomnia
CV: Cardiac murmur, hypotension, tachycardia, peripheral edema, chest pain
GI: Diarrhea, nausea, vomiting, anorexia, constipation, abdominal pain, distention, tenderness, hemorrhoids, mouth hemorrhage, tongue ulceration, stomatitis, dyspepsia, **hepatotoxicity, hepatic coma**
GU: Real failure, renal tubular acidosis, dysuria, UTI

⚠ Nurse Alert

HEMA: Leukopenia, anemia, thrombo-cytopenia, neutropenia, ecchymosis, febrile neutropenia, petechiae
INTEG: Irritation at site, rash, sweating, pyrexia, pruritus
META: Hypokalemia
MS: Weakness, arthralgia, muscle cramps, myalgia, back pain
RESP: Cough, dyspnea, pharyngitis, **pleural effusion**

Pharmacokinetics

Absorption	Rapid
Distribution	Unknown
Metabolism	Liver
Excretion	Urine
Half-life	35-49 min

Pharmacodynamics

Onset	Unknown
Peak	$1/2$ hr
Duration	Unknown

INTERACTIONS
Drug classifications
Antineoplastics, other: increased bone marrow depression

NURSING CONSIDERATIONS
Assessment
• Assess for CNS symptoms: fever, headache, chills, dizziness
• Monitor **bone marrow suppression** with patients with baseline WBC 3×10^9/L, absolute neutrophil count (ANC) = 1.5×10^9/L, and platelets = 75×10^9/L, adjust dose; ANC < 0.5×10^9/L, platelets < 25×10^9/L, give 50% dose next course; ANC 0.5-1.5 $\times 10^9$/L, platelets 25-50 $\times 10^9$/L, give 67% next course
• Assess buccal cavity q8hr for dryness, sores, or ulceration, white patches, oral pain, bleeding, dysphagia
• Assess for bruising, bleeding, blood in stools, urine, sputum, emesis; myelodysplastic syndrome (MDS), splenomegaly

Nursing diagnoses
• Body image, disturbed (adverse reactions)
• Infection, risk for (adverse reactions)
• Injury, risk for (adverse reactions)
• Knowledge, deficient (teaching)

Patient/family education
• Instruct patient to avoid foods with citric acid or hot or rough texture if stomatitis is present; to drink adequate fluids

• Instruct patient to report stomatitis, any bleeding, white spots, ulcerations in mouth; tell patient to examine mouth daily, report symptoms
• Instruct patient to avoid crowds, persons with known infections; not to receive immunizations
• Advise patient to use contraception during and for several months after therapy, pregnancy **D** not to breastfeed, not to father a child while receiving this product

Evaluation
Positive therapeutic outcome
• Improvement in blood counts in refractory anemia, or refractory anemia with excess blasts

---

azaTHIOprine (Rx)
(ay-za-thye'oh-preen)
Apo-Azathioprine ✦, **Azasan,**
Gen-Azathioprine ✦, **Imuran**
Func. class.: Immunosuppressant
Chem. class.: Purine antagonist
Pregnancy category D

Do not confuse:
Imuran/Imferon/Elmiron/IMDUR/Enduron/Tenormin, **azaTHIOprine**/azaCITIDine

ACTION: Produces immunosuppression by inhibiting purine synthesis in cells

Therapeutic outcome: Absence of graft rejection, slowing of rheumatoid arthritis

USES: Renal transplants to prevent graft rejection, refractory rheumatoid arthritis

Unlabeled uses: Myasthenia gravis, chronic ulcerative colitis, Crohn's disease, Behçet's syndrome

CONTRAINDICATIONS:
Pregnancy **D**, breastfeeding, hypersensitivity

Precautions: Severe renal/hepatic disease, geriatric, thiopurine methyltransferase deficiency, infection

> **BLACK BOX WARNING:** Bone marrow suppression, neoplastic disease; must be used by experienced clinician

DOSAGE AND ROUTES
Renal dose
CCr 10-50 ml/min 75% of dose; CCr <10 ml/min 50% of dose

Adverse effects: *italics* = common; **bold** = life-threatening

Prevention of rejection
Adult and child: IV 3-5 mg/kg/day, then maintenance (PO) of at least 1-3 mg/kg/day

Refractory rheumatoid arthritis
Adult: PO 1 mg/kg/day; may increase dosage after 2 mo by 0.5 mg/kg/day and then q4wk; not to exceed 2.5 mg/kg/day

Available forms: Tabs 50, 75, 100 mg; inj **IV** 100 mg

Implementation
PO route
- Give with meals to reduce GI upset; nausea is common

IV route
- Prepare in biological cabinet using gown, gloves, mask

Direct, IV route
- **Dilute** to 10 mg/ml with 0.9% NaCl, 0.45% NaCl, D₅W, **give** over 5 min

Intermittent IV INF route
- **Reconstitute** 100 mg/10 ml of sterile water for inj; rotate to dissolve; **further dilute** with 50 ml or more saline or glucose in saline, **give** over ¹/₂-1 hr

Y-site compatibilities: Alfentanil, atracurium, atropine, benztropine, calcium gluconate, cycloSPORINE, enalaprilat, epoetin alfa, erythromycin, fentaNYL, fluconazole, folic acid, furosemide, glycopyrrolate, heparin, insulin, mannitol, mechlorethamine, metoprolol, naloxone, nitroglycerin, oxytocin, penicillin G, potassium chloride, propranolol, protamine, SUFentanil, trimetaphan, vasopressin

Solution compatibilities: D₅W, NaCl 0.9%, NaCl 0.45%

ADVERSE EFFECTS
GI: Nausea, vomiting, stomatitis, esophagitis, **pancreatitis, hepatotoxicity, jaundice**
HEMA: Leukopenia, thrombocytopenia, anemia, pancytopenia, bleeding
INTEG: Rash, alopeia
MISC: Raynaud's symptoms, **serum sickness,** secondary malignancy, infection
MS: Arthralgia, muscle wasting

Pharmacokinetics

Absorption	Readily (PO)
Distribution	Crosses placenta
Metabolism	Liver to mercaptopurine
Excretion	Kidney, minimal
Half-life	3 hr

Pharmacodynamics

	PO	IV
Onset	Unknown	Unknown
Peak	4 hr	Unknown
Duration	Unknown	Unknown

INTERACTIONS
Individual drugs
Do not admix with other products
Allopurinol: increased action of azaTHIOprine
CycloSPORINE: increased myelosuppression
Sulfamethoxazole-trimethoprim: increased leukopenia
Warfarin: decreased action of warfarin

Drug classifications
ACE inhibitors: increased leukopenia
Antineoplastics: increased myelosuppression
Toxoids, vaccines: decreased immune response

Drug/lab test
Increased: liver function tests
Decreased: uric acid
Interference: CBC, diff count

NURSING CONSIDERATIONS
Assessment
- Assess symptoms of **rheumatoid arthritis:** pain in joints, stiffness, poor range of motion, mobility, inflammation before and during treatment
- Monitor **blood studies:** Hgb, WBC, platelets during treatment monthly; if leukocytes are <3000/mm³ or platelets <100,000/mm³, product should be discontinued or reduced; decreased Hgb level may indicate bone marrow suppression
- **Bone marrow suppression:** severe leukopenia, pancytopenia, thrombocytopenia
- Monitor liver function studies: alkaline phosphatase, AST, ALT, amylase, bilirubin; and for **hepatotoxicity:** dark urine, jaundice, itching, light-colored stools; product should be discontinued
- Monitor I&O, weight daily, report decreasing urine output, toxicity may occur
- Assess for **infection:** increased temp, WBC; sputum, urine

Nursing diagnoses
- Infection, risk for (uses)
- Knowledge, deficient (teaching)
- Mobility, impaired physical (uses)

Patient/family education
- Teach patient to take as prescribed, do not miss doses; if dose is missed on daily regimen,

skip dose; if on multiple dosing/day, take as soon as remembered
• Teach patient that therapeutic response may take 3-4 mo in rheumatoid arthritis, to continue with prescribed exercise, rest, other medications; that product is needed for life in renal transplant
• Instruct patient to report fever, rash, severe diarrhea, chills, sore throat, fatigue, since serious **infections** may occur; or clay-colored stools and cramping (**hepatotoxicity**)
• Advise patient to use contraceptive measures during treatment for 16 wk after ending therapy; product is teratogenic, (pregnancy **D**)
• Advise patient to avoid vaccinations
• Tell patient to avoid crowds and persons with known infections to reduce risk of infection
• Instruct patient not to use OTC medications without approval of prescriber
• Advise patient to use soft-bristled toothbrush to prevent bleeding

Evaluation
Positive therapeutic outcome
• Absence of graft rejection
• Immunosuppression in autoimmune disorders
• Increased joint mobility without pain in rheumatoid arthritis

azelaic acid topical
See Appendix B

azelastine (Rx)
(ay′ze-lass-teen)
Optivar
Func. class.: Leukotriene synthesis inhibitor
Chem. class.: Phthalazinone derivative
Pregnancy category C

ACTION: Inhibits the synthesis and release of leukotrienes; antagonizes action of acetylcholine, histamine, serotonin

Therapeutic outcome: Decreased nasal stuffiness, itching, swollen eyes

USES: Seasonal allergic rhinitis

CONTRAINDICATIONS:
Hypersensitivity

Precautions: Pregnancy **C**

DOSAGE AND ROUTES
Adult and child ≥12 yr: NASAL 2 sprays/nostril bid

Available forms: Spray 137 mcg/actuation

Implementation
• Remove cap/safety clip from spray pump
• Prime pump if using for first time, push 4 times quickly, away from face, blow your nose, then place tip of pump into one nostril, while holding other nostril closed, tilt head forward, and spray into nostril
• Put cover/safety clip back on

ADVERSE EFFECTS
CNS: Sedation (more common with increased dosages), drowsiness
MISC: Weight increase, myalgia

Pharmacokinetics
Absorption	Unknown
Distribution	Unknown
Metabolism	Liver, extensively
Excretion	Feces
Half-life	25-42 hr

Pharmacodynamics
Onset	Unknown
Peak	4-5 hr
Duration	Unknown

INTERACTIONS
Individual drugs
Alcohol: increased CNS depression

Drug classifications
CNS depressants, opioids, sedative/hypnotics: increased CNS depression

NURSING CONSIDERATIONS
Assessment
• Assess respiratory status: rate, rhythm, increase in bronchial secretions, wheezing, chest tightness; provide fluids to 2 L/day to decrease secretion thickness

Nursing diagnoses
• Airway clearance, ineffective (uses)
• Knowledge, deficient (teaching)
• Noncompliance (teaching, overuse)

Patient/family education
• Teach patient all aspects of product uses; to notify prescriber if confusion, sedation occur; to avoid driving and other hazardous activity if drowsiness occurs; to avoid alcohol and other CNS depressants that may potentiate effect

• Caution patient not to exceed recommended dosage; dysrhythmias may occur

Evaluation
Positive therapeutic outcome
• Absence of runny or congested nose

azelastine nasal agent
See Appendix B

azelastine ophthalmic
See Appendix B

azilsartan
(ay-zil-sar′tan)
Edarbi
(Pronunciation)
Func. class.: Antihypertensive
Chem class.: Angiotensin II receptor antagonist
Pregnancy category D

ACTION:
Antagonizes angiotensin II at the AT_1 receptor in tissues like vascular smooth muscle and the adrenal gland. Two angiotensin II receptors, AT_1 and AT_2, have been identified; azilsartan exhibits more than a 10,000-fold greater affinity for the AT_1 receptor than the AT_2 receptor.

Therapeutic outcome: Decreased B/P

USES: Hypertension, alone or in combination with other antihypertensives

CONTRAINDICATIONS:

BLACK BOX WARNING: Pregnancy **D** (2nd/3rd trimesters)

Precautions: Angioedema, African descent, renal disease, renal artery stenosis, children, geriatrics, heart failure, hypovolemia, breastfeeding, pregnancy C 1st trimester

DOSAGE AND ROUTES:
Adult: PO 80 mg/day, may give an initial dose of 40 mg/day in patients receiving high-dose diuretic therapy

Available forms: Tabs 40, 80 mg

Implementation
• May administer without regard to food
• Use original package to protect from light, moisture, and heat

ADVERSE EFFECTS
CNS: Dizziness, fatigue, asthenia
CV: Hypotension, orthostatic hypotension
GI: Nausea, diarrhea
HEMA: Anemia
INTEG: Angioedema
MS: Muscle cramps
RESP: Cough
SYST: Secondary malignancy

Pharmacokinetics

Absorption	Absolute bioavailability (60%) not affected by food; steady state within 5 days and no accumulation in plasma occurs with once-daily dosing; hydrolyzed to the active metabolite, azilsartan, in GI tract during absorption, rapidly absorbed
Distribution	Protein binding, >99%, to serum albumin
Metabolism	Metabolized by CYP2C9
Excretion	55% eliminated (feces), 42% (urine)
Half-life	Elimination half-life 11 hr

Pharmacodynamics

Onset	Unknown
Peak	1.5-3 hr
Duration	Unknown

INTERACTIONS
Individual drugs
CycloSPORINE: in those with poor renal function, increased renal failure risk: monitor closely
Lithium: increased lithium toxicity
Sodium phosphate monobasic monohydrate: sodium phosphate dibasic anhydrous: increased phosphate nephropathy

Drug classifications
Antidiabetics: increased hypoglycemia
NSAIDs in those with poor renal function: monitor closely: Increased renal failure risk
Other antihypertensives, other angiotensin receptor antagonists, MAOIs: increased hypotensive effect

Drug/herb
Ephedra: decreased antihypertensive effect
Hawthorn: increased antihypertensive effect

NURSING CONSIDERATIONS

Assessment
• **Angioedema:** Assess for facial swelling, difficulty breathing

> **BLACK BOX WARNING:** Pregnancy **D** (2nd/3rd trimester), can cause fetal death

• Response and adverse reactions especially in renal disease
• B/P, pulse during beginning therapy and periodically thereafter; note rhythm, rate, quality; obtain electrolytes before beginning therapy

Patient/family education
• To comply with dosage schedule even if feeling better
• To notify prescriber of facial swelling; if pregnancy is planned or suspected (D 2nd/3rd trimester)
• That diarrhea, dehydration, excessive perspiration, vomiting, may lead to fall in B/P, to consult prescriber if these occur
• To rise slowly from lying or sitting to minimize orthostatic hypotension; that product may cause dizziness
• To avoid OTC medications unless approved by prescriber; to inform all health care providers of product use
• To use proper technique for obtaining B/P

Evaluation
• Therapeutic response: decreased B/P

---

azithromycin (Rx)
(ay-zi-thro-my′sin)
CO-Azithromycin ✦, ratio-Azithromycin ✦, Sandoz Azithromycin ✦, Zithromax, Zmax
Func. class.: Antiinfective
Chem. class.: Macrolide (azalide)
Pregnancy category B

Do not confuse:
azithromycin/erythromycin, Zithromax/Zinacef

ACTION: Binds to 50S ribosomal subunits of susceptible bacteria and suppresses protein synthesis; much greater spectrum of activity than erythromycin; more effective against gram-negative organisms

Therapeutic outcome: Bacteriostatic against the following susceptible organisms: *Moraxella catarrhalis, Streptococcus pneumoniae, Streptococcus pyogenes, Staphylococcus aureus, Streptococcus agalactiae,* *Haemophilus influenzae, Clostridium, Legionella pneumophila, Chlamydia trachomatis, Mycoplasma;* no effect on methicillin-resistant *S. aureus;* in children: acute otitis media *(H. influenzae, M. catarrhalis, S. pneumoniae)* PO, acute pharyngitis/tonsillitis (group A streptococcal) PO; acute skin/soft tissue infections (PO); community-acquired pneumonia *(C. pneumoniae, H. influenzae, M. pneumoniae, S. pneumoniae)* PO; pharyngitis/tonsillitis *(S. pyogenes)*

USES: Mild to moderate infections of the upper respiratory tract, in children: acute otitis media, lower respiratory tract; uncomplicated skin and skin structure infections, nongonococcal urethritis, or cervicitis; prophylaxis of disseminated *Mycobacterium avium* complex (MAC)

CONTRAINDICATIONS:
Hypersensitivity to azithromycin, erythromycin, or any macrolide

Precautions: Pregnancy **B,** breastfeeding, child <6 mo for otitis media, child <2 yr for pharyngitis, geriatric, renal/hepatic/cardiac disease, tonsillitis

DOSAGE AND ROUTES

Most infections
Adult: PO 500 mg on day 1, then 250 mg daily on days 2-5 for a total dose of 1.5 g
Child 2-15 yr: PO 10 mg/kg on day 1, then 5 mg/kg × 4 days

Pelvic inflammatory disease
Adult: PO/IV 500 mg **IV** q24hr × 2 doses, then 500 mg PO q24hr × 7-10 days

Cervicitis, chlamydia, chancroid, nongonococcal urethritis, syphilis
Adult: PO 1 g single dose

Gonorrhea
Adult: PO 2 g single dose

Endocarditis prophylaxis
Adult: PO 500 mg 1 hr prior to procedure
Child: PO 15 mg/kg 1 hr prior to procedure

Community-acquired pneumonia
Adult: PO 500 mg on day 1, then 250 mg PO once daily on days 2-5
Adolescent/child, infant ≥6 mo: Susp PO 10 mg/kg on day 1, then 5 mg/kg/day on days 2-5
Adult/adolescent, child ≥34 kg: Ext Rel Susp PO 2 g as a single dose (≥1 hr before or 2 hr after a meal)

Infant ≥6 mo and children weighing 5 to <34 kg and adolescents weighing <34 kg: Ext Rel Susp PO 60 mg/kg as a single dose (≥1 hr before or 2 hr after a meal)

Adult and adolescent ≥16 years: Initially, 500 mg **IV** infusion as a single daily dose × 2 days or more then 500 mg PO/day to complete a 7-10 day course

Adolescent <16 yr, child, infant ≥3 mo: IV 10 mg/kg, max 500 mg qd × 2 days, then conversion to oral therapy as soon as possible to complete a 5-day course. After **IV** loading doses have been given, oral dosage is 5 mg/kg/day, max 250 mg/dose

Disseminated MAC infections
Adult: PO 600 mg/day in combination with ethambutol 15 mg/kg/day

Lower respiratory tract infections
Adult: PO 500 mg day 1, then 250 mg × 4 days
Child: PO 5-12 mg/kg/day × 5 days

Acute otitis media
Child >6 months: PO 30 mg/kg as a single dose or 10 mg/kg daily × 3 days or 10 mg/kg as a single dose on day 1, max 500 mg/day, then 5 mg/kg on days 2-5, max 250 mg/day

Prevention of acute otitis media
Child: PO 10 mg/kg qwk × 6 mo

Available forms: Tabs 250, 500, 600 mg; powder for inj 500 mg; powder for oral susp 1 g/packet; susp 100, 200 mg/5 ml

Implementation
PO route
• Provide adequate intake of fluids (2 L) during diarrhea episodes
• Give with a full glass of water; give susp 1 hr before or 2 hr after meals; tabs may be taken without regard to food; do not give with fruit juices
• Store at room temperature
• Reconstitute 1 g packet for susp with 60 ml water, mix, rinse glass with more water and have patient drink to consume all medication; packets not for pediatric use
• Do not take aluminum/magnesium-containing antacids or food simultaneously with this product

Intermittent IV infusion route
• **Reconstitute** 500 mg product/4.8 ml sterile water for inj (100 mg/ml), shake, **dilute** with ≥ 250 ml 0.9% NaCl, 0.45% NaCl, or LR to 1-2 mg/ml; diluted solution is stable for 24 hr or 7 days if refrigerated
• **Give** 1 mg/ml sol over 3 hr or 2 mg/ml sol over 1 hr, never give IM or as a bolus

ADVERSE EFFECTS
CNS: Dizziness, headache, vertigo, somnolence, myasthenia gravis
CV: Palpitations, chest pain
EENT: Hearing loss, tinnitus, loss of smell (anosmia)
GI: *Nausea, vomiting, diarrhea,* **hepatotoxicity,** abdominal pain, stomatitis, heartburn, dyspepsia, flatulence, melena, **cholestatic jaundice, pseudomembranous colitis,** tongue discoloration
GU: Vaginitis, moniliasis, nephritis
HEMA: Anemia
INTEG: Rash, urticaria, pruritus, photosensitivity
SYST: Angioedema, Stevens-Johnson syndrome, toxic epidermal necrolysis

Pharmacokinetics

Absorption	Rapid, (PO) up to 50%
Distribution	Widely distributed
Metabolism	Unknown, minimal metabolism
Excretion	Unchanged (bile); kidneys, minimal
Half-life	11-70 hr

Pharmacodynamics

	PO	IV
Onset	Unknown	Unknown
Peak	2-4 hr	End of infusion
Duration	24 hr	24 hr

INTERACTIONS
Individual drugs
Bromocriptine, carBAMazepine, cycloSPORINE, digoxin, disopyramide, methylPREDNISolone, nelfinavir, phenytoin, tacrolimus, theophylline, triazolam: increased effects of specific products
Ergotamine: toxicity
⚠ **Pimozide: Increased dysrhythmias; fatal reaction**
Triazolam: decreased clearance of triazolam

Drug classifications
Aluminum, magnesium antacids: decreased levels of azithromycin
Anticoagulants (orals): increased effect of oral anticoagulants

Drug/lab test
Increased: bilirubin, alkaline phosphatase, CPK, BUN, creatinine, AST, ALT

NURSING CONSIDERATIONS

Assessment

- Assess for signs and symptoms of **infection**: drainage, fever, increased WBC >10,000/mm^3, urine culture positive, sore throat, sputum culture positive
- Monitor respiratory status: rate, character, wheezing, tightness in chest; discontinue product if these occur
- Monitor allergies before treatment, reaction of each medication; place allergies on chart, notify all people giving products; skin eruptions, itching
- Monitor I&O ratio, renal studies; report hematuria, oliguria in renal disease; check urinalysis, protein, blood
- Monitor liver studies: AST, ALT, bilirubin, LDH, alkaline phosphatase; CBC with diff
- Monitor C&S before product therapy; product may be taken as soon as culture is taken; C&S may be repeated after treatment
- Assess for **serious skin reactions**: Stevens-Johnson syndrome, toxic epidermal necrolysis, angioedema, discontinue if rash occurs
- Assess for **pseudomembranous colitis**: blood or pus in diarrhea stool, abdominal pain, fever, fatigue, anorexia; obtain CBC, serum albumin
- Assess for **superinfection**: sore throat, mouth, tongue; fever, fatigue, diarrhea, anogenital pruritus

Nursing diagnoses

- Diarrhea (adverse reactions)
- Infection, risk for (uses)
- Knowledge, deficient (teaching)

Patient/family education

- Instruct patient to report sore throat, black furry tongue, fever, loose foul-smelling stool, vaginal itching, discharge, fatigue; may indicate **superinfection**
- Caution patient not to take aluminum/magnesium-containing antacids or food simultaneously with this product; blood levels of azithromycin will be decreased
- Instruct patient to notify prescriber of diarrhea stools, dark urine, pale stools, yellow discoloration of eyes or skin, severe abdominal pain; **cholestatic jaundice** is a severe adverse reaction
- Teach patient to complete dosage regimen; to notify prescriber if symptoms continue
- Teach patient to notify prescriber if pregnancy is suspected
- Inform patient that sunburns may occur; wear protective clothing and sunscreen

Evaluation

Positive therapeutic outcome

- C&S negative for infection
- WBC within 5000-10,000/mm^3

azithromycin ophthalmic

See Appendix B

bacitracin topical

See Appendix B

baclofen (Rx)

(bak′loe-fen)
Apo-Baclofen ✦, **Gen-Baclofen** ✦, **Lioresal, PMS-Baclofen** ✦, **ratio-Baclofen** ✦
Func. class.: Skeletal muscle relaxant, central acting
Chem. class.: GABA, chlorophenyl derivative
Pregnancy category C

Do not confuse:

Lioresal/Lotensin

ACTION: Inhibits synaptic responses in CNS by stimulating GABA$_B$ receptor subtype, which decreases neurotransmitter function, decreasing frequency, severity of muscle spasms

Therapeutic outcome: Decreased spasticity of muscles

USES: Spasticity in spinal cord injury, multiple sclerosis

CONTRAINDICATIONS:

Hypersensitivity

Precautions: Pregnancy **C**, breastfeeding, geriatric, peptic ulcer, renal/hepatic disease, stroke, seizure disorder, diabetes mellitus

> **BLACK BOX WARNING:** Abrupt discontinuation

DOSAGE AND ROUTES

Adult: PO 5 mg tid × 3 days, then 10 mg tid × 3 days, then 15 mg tid × 3 days, then 20 mg tid × 3 days, then titrated to response, max 80 mg/day; IT use implantable IT inf pump; use screening trial of 3 separate bol doses if needed 24 hr apart (50 mcg/ml, 75 mcg/1.5 ml, 100 mcg/2 ml); patients who do not respond to 100 mcg should not be considered for chronic

Adverse effects: *italics* = common; **bold** = life-threatening

IT therapy; initial double screening dose that produced result and give over 24 hr, increase by 10%-30% q24hr only; maintenance 1200-1500 mcg/day

Child 2-7 yr: PO 10-15 mg/day divided q8hr; titrate every 3 days by 5-15 mg/day to max 40 mg/day

Child ≥8 yr: As above, max 60 mg/day

Child: IT initial test dose same as adult; for small children, initial dose of 25 mcg/dose may be used; 25-1200 mcg/day inf, titrated to response in screening phase

Geriatric: PO 5 mg bid-tid

Available forms: Tabs 10, 20 mg; IT inj 10 mg/20 ml (500 mcg/ml), 10 mg/5 ml (2000 mcg/ml); pharmacy can prepare extemporaneous liquid preparations

Implementation
PO route
• Give with meals for GI symptoms; gum, frequent sips of water for dry mouth
• Store in airtight container at room temperature

IT route
• **For screening,** dilute to a concentration of 50 mcg/ml with NaCl for inj (preservative free); give test over 1 min; watch for decreasing muscle tone, frequency of spasm; if inadequate, use two more test doses q24hr; **maintenance inf** via implantable pump of 500-2000 mcg/ml dosage because individual titration is required
• Do not give IT dose by inj, **IV,** IM, SUBCUT, epidural

ADVERSE EFFECTS
CNS: *Dizziness, weakness, fatigue, drowsiness,* headache, disorientation, insomnia, paresthesias, tremors, **seizures, coma; life-threatening CNS depression, CNS infection (IT)**

CV: Hypotension, chest pain, palpitations, edema; **cardiovascular collapse (IT)**

EENT: Nasal congestion, blurred vision, mydriasis, tinnitus

GI: *Nausea,* constipation, vomiting, increased AST, alkaline phosphatase, abdominal pain, dry mouth, anorexia

GU: Urinary frequency, hematuria

INTEG: Rash, pruritus

RESP: Dyspnea, respiratory failure (IT)

Absorption	Good (PO)
Distribution	Widely, crosses placenta
Metabolism	Liver, partially
Excretion	Kidney, unchanged 70%-80%
Half-life	$2^{1}/_{2}$-4 hr

Pharmacodynamics

	PO/IT
Onset	0.5-1 hr
Peak	4 hr
Duration	4-8 hr

INTERACTIONS
Individual drugs
Alcohol: CNS depression

Drug classifications
Antidepressants (tricyclics), barbiturates, MAOIs, opioids, sedative/hypnotics: increased CNS depression
Antihypertensives: increased hypotension

Drug/herb
Kava, valerian: increased CNS depression

Drug/lab test
Increased: AST, ALT, alkaline phosphatase, blood glucose

NURSING CONSIDERATIONS
Assessment
• **Multiple sclerosis:** spasms, spasticity, ataxia, mobility, improvement should occur
• Monitor B/P, weight, blood glucose, and hepatic function periodically
• Check for increased **seizure** activity in patients with epilepsy; this product decreases seizure threshold, monitor ECG
• Check I&O ratio; check for urinary retention, frequency, hesitancy
• Allergic reactions: rash, fever, respiratory distress; severe weakness, numbness in extremities
• Assess CNS depression: dizziness, drowsiness, psychiatric symptoms
• Check dosage, as individual titration is required
• Assess for **withdrawal symptoms:** CNS depression, dizziness, drowsiness, psychiatric symptoms
• **Intrathecal:** Have emergency equipment nearby; assess test dose and titration, if there is no response, check pump and catheter for proper functioning

Nursing diagnoses
* Injury, risk for (adverse reactions)
* Knowledge, deficient (teaching)
* Mobility, impaired physical (uses)

Patient/family education
* Advise patient not to discontinue medication quickly; hallucinations, spasticity, tachycardia will occur; product should be tapered off over 1-2 wk
* Advise patient not to take with alcohol, other CNS depressants
* Teach patient to avoid hazardous activities if drowsiness, dizziness occurs; to rise slowly to prevent orthostatic hypotension
* Teach patient to avoid using OTC medications: cough preparations, antihistamines, unless directed by prescriber
* Teach patient to notify prescriber if nausea, headache, tinnitus, insomnia, confusion, constipation, or inadequate, painful urination continues
* May require 1-2 mo for full response

Evaluation
Positive therapeutic outcome
* Decreased pain, spasticity

TREATMENT OF OVERDOSE:
Induce emesis of conscious patient, activated charcoal, dialysis, physostigmine to reduce life-threatening CNS side effects

balsalazide (Rx)
(ball-sal′a-zide)
Colazal
Func. class.: GI antiinflammatory
Chem. class.: Salicylate derivative
Pregnancy category B

Do not confuse:
Colazal/Clozaril

ACTION: Delivered intact to the colon, bioconverted to 5-ASA, may block production of arachidonic acid metabolites in the colon, topical rather than systemic acid

Therapeutic outcome: Decreased inflammation in colon

USES: Active, mild to moderate ulcerative colitis (adult and child)

CONTRAINDICATIONS:
Hypersensitivity to salicylates/5-aminosalicylates

Precautions: Pregnancy **B**, breastfeeding, child <5 yr, pyloric stenosis, renal disease, colitis, hepatitis

DOSAGE AND ROUTES
Adult: PO 2250 mg (three 750 mg cap) tid × 8-12 wk, max 6.75 g/day
Adolescent and child 5-12 yr: PO 2250 mg (three 750 mg cap) tid × 8 wk

Available forms: Caps 750 mg

Implementation
* Give with food in evenly divided doses; swallow tab whole or open cap, sprinkle on applesauce
* Use with resuscitative equipment available; severe allergic reactions may occur
* Give total daily dose evenly spaced to minimize GI intolerance
* Store in tight, light-resistant container at room temperature

ADVERSE EFFECTS
CNS: Headache, insomnia, fatigue, fever, dizziness
EENT: Dry eyes, rhinitis, sinusitis, blurred vision
GI: Nausea, vomiting, abdominal pain, diarrhea, anorexia, constipation, dyspepsia, flatulance, **GI bleeding, hepatic failure/necrosis, hepatitis**
MS: Arthralgia, back pain, myalgia
RESP: Cough, pharyngitis
SYST: Anaphylaxis

Pharmacokinetics
Absorption	Low, variable
Distribution	Protein binding 99%
Metabolism	Unknown
Excretion	Feces, as metabolites
Half-life	Unknown

Pharmacodynamics
Unknown

INTERACTIONS
Individual drugs
Azathioprine, warfarin: increased effect
Mercaptopurine: increased myelosuppression
Thioguanine: decreased effect
Varicella virus, live: avoid use

Drug/lab test
Increased: AST, ALT, GGT, LDH, bilirubin, alkaline phosphatase
False positive: urinary glucose test

NURSING CONSIDERATIONS
Assessment
• Monitor kidney function studies: BUN, creatinine, urinalysis (long-term therapy)
• Assess for allergic reaction: rash, dermatitis, urticaria, pruritus, dyspnea, bronchospasm
• Assess for myelosuppression: CBC

Nursing diagnoses
• Injury, risk for (uses)
• Knowledge, deficient (teaching)

Patient/family education
• Advise patient to notify prescriber if symptoms do not improve, if colitis symptoms worsen, if rash, hives, or respiratory problems occur

Evaluation
Positive therapeutic outcome
• Absence of fever, mucus in stools; resolution of symptoms of ulcerative colitis

---

⚠ HIGH ALERT

basiliximab (Rx)
(bas-ih-liks′ih-mab)
Simulect
Func. class.: Immunosuppressant
Chem. class.: Murine/human monoclonal antibody (interleukin-2) receptor antagonist
Pregnancy category B

ACTION: Binds to and blocks the IL-2 receptor, which is selectively expressed on the surface of activated T-lymphocytes; impairs the immune system to antigenic challenges

Therapeutic outcome: Prevention of graft rejection

USES: Acute allograft rejection in renal transplant patients when used with cycloSPORINE and corticosteroids

CONTRAINDICATIONS:
Hypersensitivity to mannitol/murine, exposure to viral infections, breastfeeding

Precautions: Pregnancy **B**, children, geriatric, human anti-murine antibody

> **BLACK BOX WARNING:** Infections

DOSAGE AND ROUTES
Adult/child ≥35 kg: IV 20 mg × 2 doses; first dose within 2 hr before transplant surgery;

second dose given 4 days after transplantation
Child <35 kg: IV 10 mg × 2 doses; first dose within 2 hr before transplant surgery; second dose given 4 days after transplantation

Available forms: Powder for inj 10, 20 mg

Implementation
Intermittent IV INF route
• **Reconstitute** 10 mg vial/2.5 ml or 20 mg vial in 5 ml sterile water for inj; shake gently to dissolve, **dilute** reconstituted sol in 25 ml (10 mg vial) or 50 ml (20 mg vial) with 0.9% NaCl or D$_5$, gently invert bag, do not shake, **give** over $^1/_2$ hr, do not admix

ADVERSE EFFECTS
CNS: *Pyrexia, chills, tremors, headache, insomnia, weakness,* dizziness
CV: *Chest pain,* angina, **cardiac failure,** hypo/hypertension, edema
GI: *Vomiting, nausea, diarrhea,* constipation, abdominal pain, GI bleeding, gingival hyperplasia, stomatitis
INTEG: *Acne,* pruritus, impaired wound healing
META: Acidosis, hypercholesterolemia, hyperuricemia, hypo/hyperkalemia, hypocalcemia, hypophosphatemia
MISC: Infection, moniliasis, **anaphylaxis,** anemia, allergic reaction, dysuria, CMV infection, candidiasis
MS: Arthralgia, myalgia
RESP: *Dyspnea, wheezing, cough,* **pulmonary edema**

Pharmacokinetics
Absorption	Unknown
Distribution	Unknown
Metabolism	Unknown
Excretion	Unknown
Half-life	7 days (adult)
	9$^1/_2$ days (child)

Pharmacodynamics
Onset	Unknown
Peak	$^1/_2$ hr (adults)
Duration	Unknown

INTERACTIONS
Drug classifications
Immunosuppressants: increased immunosuppression

Drug/lab test
Increased: BUN, cholesterol, uric acid, creatinine, potassium, calcium, blood glucose, Hgb, Hct

---

Decreased: Hgb, Hct, platelets, magnesium, phosphate

NURSING CONSIDERATIONS
Assessment

> **BLACK BOX WARNING:** Assess for infection, increased temp, WBC, sputum, urine, may be fatal (bacterial, protozoal, fungal)

• Monitor blood studies: Hgb, WBC, platelets during treatment qmo; if leukocytes are <3000/mm^3, product should be discontinued
• Monitor liver function studies: alkaline phosphatase, AST, ALT, bilirubin
• Assess hepatotoxicity: dark urine, jaundice, itching, light-colored stools; product should be discontinued
⚠ **Assess for anaphylaxis, hypersensitivity: dyspnea, wheezing, rash, pruritus, hypotension, tachycardia; if severe hypersensitivity reactions occur, product should not be used again**

Nursing diagnoses
• Infection, risk for (adverse reactions)
• Knowledge, deficient (teaching)

Patient/family education

> **BLACK BOX WARNING:** Instruct patient to report fever, chills, sore throat, fatigue, since serious infection may occur; avoid crowds, persons with known upper respiratory infections; use contraception during treatment

Evaluation
Positive therapeutic outcome
• Absence of graft rejection

beclomethasone (Rx)
(be-kloe-meth′a-sone)
Apo-Beclomethasone ✹, **QVAR**
Func. class.: Synthetic glucocorticoid (long acting)
Chem. class.: Beclomethasone diester
Pregnancy category C

Do not confuse:
beclomethasone/betamethasone

ACTION: Prevents inflammation by suppression of migration of polymorphonuclear leukocytes, fibroblasts, reversal of increased capillary permeability and lysosomal stabilization; does not suppress hypothalamus and pituitary function

Therapeutic outcome: Decreased inflammation and normal immunity

USES: Seasonal, perennial allergic/vasomotor rhinitis, nasal polyps, chronic steroid-dependent asthma

CONTRAINDICATIONS:
Hypersensitivity, status asthmaticus (primary treatment)

Precautions: Pregnancy **C**, breastfeeding, child <12, nasal disease/surgery, nonasthmatic bronchial disease, bacterial, fungal, viral infections of mouth, throat, lungs, HPA suppression, osteoporosis, Cushing's syndrome, diabetes mellitus, measles, cataracts, corticosteroid hypersensitivity, glaucoma, herpes infection

DOSAGE AND ROUTES
Adult and child >12 yr: Oral inh 48-80 mcg bid (alone) or 40-160 mcg bid (with inhaled corticosteroids), max 320 bid
Child 5-12 yr: Oral inh 40 mcg bid, max 80 mcg bid

Available forms: Oral inh 40, 80, 250 ✹ mcg /metered spray

Implementation
Oral route
• Give PO, using a spacer device for proper dose
• Shake oral aerosol well, use spacer
• Use after cleaning aerosol top daily with warm water; dry thoroughly
• Store in cool environment; do not puncture or incinerate container
Nasal route
• Shake inhaler, invert, tilt head backward, insert nozzle into nostril, away from septum; hold other nostril closed and depress activator, inhale through nose, exhale through mouth

ADVERSE EFFECTS
CNS: *Headache*
EENT: *Candidal infection of oral cavity, hoarseness,* sore throat, dysgeusia, loss of taste/smell
ENDO: Hypothalamic-pituitary (HPA) suppression
GI: Dry mouth, dyspepsia
MISC: Angioedema, **adrenal insufficiency,** facial edema, Churg-Strauss syndrome (rare)
RESP: **Bronchospasm,** wheezing, cough

Pharmacokinetics

Absorption	Locally only
Distribution	Not distributed
Metabolism	Lungs, liver (by CYP3A)
Excretion	Feces, urine
Half-life	2.8 hr

Pharmacodynamics

	Inh	Nasal
Onset	1-4 wk	10 min
Peak	Unknown	Unknown
Duration	Unknown	Unknown

NURSING CONSIDERATIONS

Assessment

• Assess adrenal suppression: 17-KS, plasma cortisol for decreased levels, adrenal function periodically for HPA axis suppression during prolonged therapy; monitor growth and development

• Assess blood studies, neutrophils, decreased platelets; WBC with diff at baseline and q3mo; if neutrophils are <1000/mm³, discontinue treatment

• Check nasal passages during long-term treatment for changes in mucus; check for burning, stinging; assess for glucocorticoid withdrawal: dizziness, hypotension, fatigue, muscle/joint pain; notify prescriber immediately

• Assess respiratory status: rest, rhythm, characteristics; auscultate lung bilaterally before and throughout treatment

• Assess for fungal infections in mucous membranes

Nursing diagnoses

• Airway clearance, ineffective (uses)
• Knowledge, deficient (teaching)
• Noncompliance (teaching)
• Oral mucous membrane, impaired (adverse reactions)

Patient/family education

• Teach patient to gargle/rinse mouth after each use to prevent oral fungal infections

• Teach patient that in times of stress, systemic corticosteroids may be needed to prevent adrenal insufficiency; do not discontinue oral product abruptly, taper slowly

• Teach patient to continue using product even if mild nasal bleeding occurs; is usually transient

• Teach patient method of administration after providing written instructions from manufacturer

• Clean inhaler by wiping with dry cloth

• Teach patient the symptoms of **adrenal insufficiency:** nausea, anorexia, fatigue, dizziness, dyspnea, weakness, joint pain, depression

Evaluate

Positive therapeutic outcome

• Decrease in runny nose, improved symptoms of bronchial asthma

beclomethasone nasal agent
See Appendix B

belatacept (Rx)
(bel-a-ta′sept)
Nulojix
Func. class.: Biologic response modifier
Chem. class.: Fusion protein
Pregnancy category C

ACTION: Activated T lymphocytes are the mediators of immunologic rejection, and this product is a selective T-cell costimulation blocker; blocks the CD28 mediated costimulation of T lymphocytes by binding to CD80 and CD86 on antigen-presenting cells; inhibits T lymphocyte proliferation and the production of the cytokines interleukin-2, interferon-gamma, interleukin-4, and TNF-alpha.

Therapeutic outcome: Absence of kidney transplant rejection

USES: Kidney transplant rejection prophylaxis given with basiliximab induction, mycophenolate mofetil, corticosteroids

CONTRAINDICATIONS: Hypersensitivity

> **BLACK BOX WARNING:** Infection, organ transplant, requires an experienced clinician, secondary malignancy, post-transplant lymphoproliferation disorder (PTLD)

Precautions: Breastfeeding, child/infant/neonate, pregnancy C, diabetes mellitus, progressive multifocal leukoencephalopathy, immunosuppression, sunlight exposure, TB

DOSAGE AND ROUTES

Adult: IV 10 mg/kg rounded to nearest 12.5 mg increment give over 30 min the day of transplantation (day 1) but before transplantation, on day 5 approximately 96 hours after the day 1 dose 1, at the end of wk 2, at the end of wk 4, at the end of wk 8, and at the end of wk

12; maintenance dosage is 5 mg/kg rounded to nearest 12.5 mg increment given over 30 min at the end of wk 16 and q4wk ± 3 days thereafter; doses should be calculated on actual body weight on the transplantation day unless the patient's weight varies by >10%

Available forms:
Powder for inj 250 mg

Implementation

> **BLACK BOX WARNING:** Only providers skilled in the use of immunosuppressant and management of transplant should use these products

IV route
• Visually inspect products for particulate matter, discoloration whenever solution/ container permit, discard if present
• Calculate the number of drug vials required to provide total infusion dose
• Reconstitute each vial/10.5 ml of sterile water for injection, 0.9% sodium chloride, D₅W using the silicone-free disposable syringe provided with each vial and an 18G to 21G needle. If silicone-free disposable syringe is dropped or becomes contaminated, use a new silicone-free disposable syringe from inventory. If you need additional silicone-free disposable syringes, call 1-888-685-6549. If the powder is accidentally reconstituted using a different syringe than the one provided, the solution may develop a few translucent particles. Discard any solutions prepared using siliconized syringes.
• Using aseptic technique, inject the diluent into the vial and direct the stream of diluent to the glass wall of the vial. To minimize foaming, rotate the vial and invert with gentle swirling until the contents are dissolved. Do not shake when reconstituted (25 mg/ml), should be clear to slightly opalescent and colorless to pale yellow. Do not use if opaque particles, discoloration, or other foreign particles are present.
• Calculate the total volume of the reconstituted 25 mg/ml sol required to provide the total inf dose. Further dilute this volume with a volume of inf fluid equal to the volume of the reconstituted drug sol required to provide the prescribed dose. Use either NS or D₅W if drug was reconstituted with SWFI; use NS if drug was reconstituted with NS; use D₅W if drug was reconstituted with D₅W. With the same silicone-free disposable syringe used for reconstitution, withdraw the required amount of belatacept sol from the vial, inject it into the inf container, gently rotate the inf container to ensure mixing; final concentration in inf container should range

(2-10 mg/ml). Volume of 100 ml will be appropriate for most patients and doses, but total inf volumes ranging from 50-250 ml may be used. Discard any unused drug solution remaining in the vials; after reconstitution, immediately transfer the reconstituted sol from the vial to the inf bag or bottle; complete within 24 hr.

IV INF route
• Give over 30 min, use an infusion set and a sterile, nonpyrogenic low-protein-binding filter (0.2-1.2 mm), use a separate line

ADVERSE EFFECTS
CNS: Guillain-Barré syndrome, anxiety, dizziness, fever, insomnia, tremor
EENT: Pharyngitis, stomatitis
GI: Abdominal pain, constipation, diarrhea, nausea, vomiting
GU: Renal tubular necrosis, renal failure, proteinuria, urinary incontinence
HEMA: Anemia, neutropenia, leukopenia, leukoencephalopathy
INTEG: Acne, alopecia
META: Hypercholesterolemia, hyperglycemia, hyper/hypokalemia, hypocalcemia, hypophosphatemia, hypomagnesemia
MS: Arthralgia
SYST: Secondary malignancy, post-transplant lymphoproliferative disorder (PTLD), wound dehiscence, BK-virus associated neuropathy

Pharmacokinetics

Absorption	Unknown
Distribution	Steady-state by week 8 after transplantation and by month 6 during the maintenance phase
Metabolism	Unknown
Excretion	Unknown
Half-life	Half life range 6.1-15.1 days during receipt of 10 mg/kg IV doses; 3.1-11.9 days during receipt of 5 mg/kg IV doses

Pharmacodynamics

Onset	Unknown
Peak	Unknown
Duration	Unknown

INTERACTIONS

Individual drugs
Basiliximab induction, mycophenolate mofetil: increased effect

Drug classifications

Corticosteroids: increased belatacept effect
Vaccines: avoid concurrent use
Immunosuppressives: avoid increased dose

NURSING CONSIDERATIONS
Assessment

> **BLACK BOX WARNING:** Transplant rejection: flu-like symptoms, decreasing urinary output, malaise; some may experience pain in area (rare; monitor BUN/Creatinine)

> **BLACK BOX WARNING:** Infection: Monitor for fever, chills, increased WBC, wound dehiscences

> **BLACK BOX WARNING:** Post-transplant lymphoproliferation disorder (PTLD): May lead to secondary malignancy (lymphoma) or infectious mononucleosis-like lesions; may be treated with antivirals or immunosuppressant may need to be discontinued

• Hyperlipidemia: Monitor cholesterol, triglycerides; an antilipidemic may be needed
• Store refrigerated, protected from light ≤24 hr; max 4 hr of the total 24 hr can be at room temperature and room light

Evaluate

• Therapeutic response: Absence of renal transplant rejection

Patient/family education

• Teach reason for product and expected result
• Teach to avoid exposure to sunlight, tanning beds, risk of secondary malignancy
• Teach to avoid crowds, persons with known infections
• Advise that repeated lab test will be needed
• Advise to avoid with vaccines
• Advise that immunosuppressants will be needed for life to prevent rejection; teach symptoms of rejection and to call provider immediately

belimumab (Rx)

(be-lim′ue-mab)
Benlysta
Func. class.: Monoclonal antibody
Chem. class.: Disease-modifying antirheumatic drugs (DMARDs)
Pregnancy category C

ACTION: Inhibits B lymphocyte stimulator (BLyS), which is needed for B-cell survival; normally, soluble BLyS binds to its receptors on B cells and allows B-cell survival; binds BLyS and prevents binding to its receptors on B cells

Therapeutic outcome: Decreasing symptoms of SLE: decreased fever, malaise, joint pains, myalgias, fatigue

USES: Active, autoantibody-positive, systemic lupus erythematosus (SLE) in combination with standard therapy

CONTRAINDICATIONS:
Hypersensitivity

Precautions: African descent patients, depression, children/infants, immunosuppression, infection, pregnancy C, breastfeeding, suicidal ideation, vaccination, geriatrics, secondary malignancy, cardiac disease, requires experienced clinician

DOSAGE AND ROUTES
Adult: 10 mg/kg IV over 1 hr q2wk for the first 3 doses, then q4wk

Available forms: Powder for injection 120, 400 mg

Implementation

• Use only by health care providers prepared to manage anaphylaxis should administer this product, may give premedication for prophylaxis against infusion and hypersensitivity reactions

Intermittent IV infusion route

• Visually inspect particulate matter and discoloration whenever solution and container permits
• Give as IV infusion only, do not give IV bolus or push, give over 1 hr and slow or stop if infusion reactions occur
• Do not give with any other agents in the same IV line
• Allow to stand at room temperature for 10-15 min before using
• Reconstitute with the appropriate amount of sterile water for injection to a final concentration 80 mg/ml; add 1.5 ml of sterile water/120 mg vial or 4.8 ml of sterile water/400 mg vial
• When reconstituting, direct the stream of sterile water toward the side of the vial to minimize foaming; gently swirl the vial for 60 sec and allow to sit at room temperature during reconstitution, gently swirling the vial for 60 secs q5min until the powder is dissolved; do not shake; reconstitution is complete in 10 to 30 min
• If a mechanical reconstitution device (swirler) is used to reconstitute, max 500 rpm swirled for ≤30 min

- The solution should be opalescent and colorless to pale yellow, and without particles; Small air bubbles are expected; protect from sunlight
- Dilution: Only dilute in 0.9% sodium chloride inj; dilute reconstituted solution with enough 0.9% sodium chloride injection (normal saline) to a total volume of 250 ml. From a 250-ml infusion bag or bottle of normal saline, withdraw and discard a volume equal to the volume of the reconstituted solution required for the patient's dose; add the required volume of the reconstituted solution the infusion bag/bottle; gently invert to mix the solution
- Discard any unused solution that remains in the vials
- *Storage:* In refrigerator or room temperature; total time from reconstitution to completion of infusion max 8 hr

ADVERSE EFFECTS
CNS: Anxiety, depression, dizziness, fever, headache, insomnia, migraine, suicidal ideation
CV: Bradycardia, hypotension
GI: Diarrhea, nausea
MISC: Bronchitis, cystitis, dyspnea, leukopenia, myalgia, nasopharyngitis, pharyngitis, rash
SYST: Anaphylaxis, angioedema, antibody formation, infection, influenza, secondary malignancy

Pharmacokinetics

Absorption	Unknown
Distribution	Unknown
Metabolism	Unknown
Excretion	Unknown
Half-life	Terminal half-life 19.4 days; distribution half-life 1.75 days

Pharmacodynamics

Onset	Unknown
Peak	Unknown
Duration	Unknown

INTERACTIONS
Individual drugs
IV cyclophosphamide, biologic therapies (rituximab, ofatumumab): avoid concurrent use

Drug classifications
Vaccines: avoid concurrent use

NURSING CONSIDERATIONS
Assessment
- **SLE:** Monitor for decreasing fever, malaise, fatigue, joint pain, myalgias

- **Suicidal ideation:** More common in those with preexisting depression
- **Infection:** Determine if a chronic or acute infection is present, may be fatal when used with this product; do not begin therapy if any products are being used for a chronic infection; leucopenia may occur with this product and susceptibility to infections increased
- **Anaphylaxis, infusion site reactions:** If these occur, stop infusion
- **African descent patients:** Use cautiously in these patients, may not respond to this product
- Cardiac disease: Monitor closely for cardiovascular side effects, bradycardia, hypotension
- Pregnancy: Determine if pregnant or if pregnancy is planned or suspected

Nursing diagnoses
- Injury, risk for (uses, adverse reactions)

Patient/family education
- Teach patient to notify prescriber if pregnancy is planned or suspected, use reliable contraception during and for 4 mo after final treatment, to avoid breastfeeding
- Advise patient to seek treatment immediately for serious hypersensitive reactions
- Advise patient not to receive vaccinations during treatment

Evaluation
- Decreasing symptoms of SLE: decreasing fatigue, fever, malaise

benazepril (Rx)
(ben-a'za-pril)
Lotensin
Func. class.: Antihypertensive
Chem. class.: ACE inhibitor
Pregnancy category D

ACTION: Selectively suppresses renin-angiotensin-aldosterone system; inhibits ACE, preventing conversion of angiotensin I to angiotensin II

Therapeutic outcome: Decreased B/P in hypertension

USES: Hypertension, alone or in combination with thiazide diuretics

Unlabeled uses: CHF

CONTRAINDICATIONS:
Breastfeeding, children, hypersensitivity to ACE inhibitors, angioedema

BLACK BOX WARNING: Pregnancy D

Adverse effects: *italics* = common; **bold** = life-threatening

Precautions: Impaired renal/liver function, dialysis patients, hypovolemia, blood dyscrasias, CHF, COPD, asthma, geriatric, bilateral renal artery stenosis

DOSAGE AND ROUTES

Adult: PO 10 mg daily initially, then 20-40 mg/day divided bid or daily (without a diuretic); 5 mg PO daily (with a diuretic); max 80 mg daily
Geriatric: PO based on clinical response

Renal dose
Adult: PO 5 mg daily with CCr <30 ml/min; increase as needed to max of 40 mg/day

Available forms: Tabs 5, 10, 20, 40 mg

Implementation
• Store in air-tight container at 86° F (30° C) or less
• Severe hypotension may occur after 1st dose of this medication; decreased hypotension may be prevented by reducing or discontinuing diuretic therapy 3 days before beginning benazepril therapy

ADVERSE EFFECTS

CNS: Anxiety, hypertonia, insomnia, paresthesia, headache, dizziness, fatigue
CV: Hypotension, postural hypotension, syncope, palpitations, angina
GI: Nausea, constipation, vomiting, gastritis, diarrhea, melena
GU: Increased BUN, creatinine, decreased libido, impotence, urinary tract infection
HEMA: Agranulocytosis, neutropenia
INTEG: Rash, flushing, sweating
META: Hyperkalemia, hyponatremia
MISC: Angioedema
MS: Arthralgia, arthritis, myalgia
RESP: Cough, asthma, bronchitis, dyspnea, sinusitis

Pharmacokinetics

Absorption	<40%
Distribution	Unknown; crosses placenta
Metabolism	Liver metabolites; protein binding 97%
Excretion	Kidney, breast milk (minimal)
Half-life	10-11 hr (metabolite); increased in renal disease

Pharmacodynamics

Onset	Unknown
Peak	$1/2$-1 hr
Duration	Unknown

INTERACTIONS

Individual drugs
Alcohol: increased hypotension (large amounts)
Azathioprine: increased myelosuppression
Digoxin, lithium: increased serum levels

Drug classifications
Antihypertensives, diuretics, nitrates, phenothiazines: increased hypotension
Diuretics (potassium-sparing), potassium supplements: increased hyperkalemia
NSAIDs: decreased hypotensive effects

Drug/herb
Hawthorn: increased antihypertensive effect

Drug/lab test
Increased: AST, ALT, alkaline phosphatase, bilirubin, uric acid, blood glucose
False positive: ANA titer
Positive: ANA titer

NURSING CONSIDERATIONS

Assessment
• **Hypertension:** B/P, pulse baseline and periodically; monitor B/P at peak/trough level of product, check for orthostatic hypotension, syncope; if changes occur, dosage change may be required; notify prescriber of changes; monitor compliance
• Monitor **blood dyscrasias:** neutrophils, decreased platelets; WBC with differential at baseline, q3mo; if neutrophils <1000/mm³, discontinue treatment
• Monitor renal studies: protein, BUN, creatinine; watch for increased levels that may indicate nephrotic syndrome and renal failure; monitor urine for protein; monitor renal symptoms: polyuria, oliguria, frequency, dysuria
• Establish baselines in renal, liver function tests before therapy begins
• Check potassium levels throughout treatment, although hyperkalemia rarely occurs
• Assess for allergic reactions: rash, fever, pruritus, urticaria; product should be discontinued if antihistamines fail to help

Nursing diagnoses
• Cardiac output, decreased (uses)
• Injury, risk for (side effects)
• Knowledge, deficient (teaching)
• Noncompliance (teaching)

Patient/family education
• Instruct patient not to discontinue product abruptly; advise patient to tell all persons associated with care

---

⚠ Nurse Alert

B

• Teach patient not to use OTC products (cough, cold, allergy) unless directed by prescriber; serious side effects can occur; xanthines such as coffee, tea, chocolate, cola can prevent action of product

• Emphasize the importance of complying with dosage schedule, even if feeling better; to continue with medical regimen to decrease B/P: exercise, cessation of smoking, decreasing stress, diet modifications

• Emphasize the need to rise slowly to sitting or standing position to minimize orthostatic hypotension, not to exercise in hot weather because increased hypotension can occur

• Teach patient to notify prescriber of mouth sores, sore throat, fever, swelling of hands or feet, irregular heartbeat, chest pain, coughing, shortness of breath

• Caution patient to report excessive perspiration, dehydration, vomiting, diarrhea; may lead to fall in B/P

• Caution patient that product may cause dizziness, fainting, light-headedness; may occur during first few days of therapy; to avoid activities that may be hazardous

• Teach patient how to take B/P; teach normal readings for age group; ensure patient takes own B/P

> **BLACK BOX WARNING:** Advise patient to notify prescriber of pregnancy (**D**), product will need to be discontinued

Evaluation
Positive therapeutic outcome
• Decreased B/P in hypertension

TREATMENT OF OVERDOSE:
0.9% NaCl **IV** inf, hemodialysis

> **⚠ HIGH ALERT**

bendamustine (Rx)
(ben-da-muss'teen)
Treanda
Func. class.: Antineoplastic alkylating agent
Chem. class.: Nitrogen mustard
Pregnancy category D

ACTION: Cross-linking DNA, which causes single strand and double strand breaks, inhibits several mitotic checkpoints, combines alkylating and antimetabolite properties

Therapeutic outcome: Improvement in blood counts and morphology

USES: Chronic lymphocytic leukemia, non-Hodgkin's lymphoma

CONTRAINDICATIONS:
Pregnancy **D**, fetal harm may occur; hypersensitivity to this product or mannitol, children, hepatic disease, renal impairment, breastfeeding

Precautions: Hyperuricemia, infusion-related reactions, myelosuppression, infection, skin reactions

DOSAGE AND ROUTES
Chronic lymphocytic leukemia
Adult: **IV** inf 100 mg/m^2 over 30 min on days 1, 2, q28days up to 6 cycles

Non-Hodgkin's lymphoma
Adult: **IV** inf 120 mg/m^2 over 60 min on days 1, 2, q21days up to 8 cycles

Renal/hepatic dose
Adult: **IV** inf CCr <40 ml/min, do not use; AST or ALT 2.5-10 × upper limit normal (ULN) or bilirubin 1.5-3 × ULN, do not use

Available forms: Powder for inj 25, 100 mg

Implementation
• Give blood transfusions or RBC colony-stimulating factors to counter anemia

• Give antiemetic 30-60 min before giving product to prevent vomiting

• Give all medications PO, if possible avoid IM inj if platelets are <100,000/mm^3

• Store reconstituted sol in refrigerator for 24 hr, or room temperature for 3 hr; protect from light; store vials at room temperature

Intermittent IV inf route
• Prepare in biological cabinet wearing gown, gloves, mask; avoid contact with skin; can cause burning and stain the skin brown; use cytotoxic handling procedures

• After reconstituting 100 mg product/20 ml or 25 mg/5 ml sterile water for inj (5 mg/ml), sol should be clear, colorless to pale yellow, completely dissolve in 5 min; if particulate is present, do not use

• Use within 30 min of reconstitution, withdraw the volume needed and **further dilute** in 500 ml NS or D$_{2.5\%/0.45\%}$ NS to a final conc 0.2-0.6 mg/ml; doses ≤100 mg/m^2, **give** over 30 min; doses >100 mg/m^2, **give** over 60 min

• Monitor for infusion reaction, may use antihistamines or corticosteroids in grade 1, 2 reaction; if grade 3 or 4, discontinue if needed

---

ADVERSE EFFECTS
CNS: Asthenia, fatigue, fever, headache, chills
CV: Hypertension, **hypertensive crisis**
GI: *Nausea, vomiting,* diarrhea, hyperbilirubinemia, constipation, stomatitis, anorexia
GU: Renal failure
HEMA: Thrombocytopenia, leukopenia, anemia, lymphocytopenia, neutropenia, secondary malignancy, toxic epidermal necrolysis, tumor lysis syndrome
INTEG: Bulbous rash, pruritus, extravasation
META: Hyperuricemia
SYST: Anaphylaxis, infection, dehydration, **severe skin toxicities, tumor lysis syndrome, Stevens-Johnson syndrome**

Pharmacokinetics

Absorption	Unknown
Distribution	Protein binding 95%
Metabolism	Hydrolysis via cytochrome P450 1A2; two metabolites are produced
Excretion	90% unchanged (feces)
Half-life	40 min

Pharmacodynamics
Unknown

INTERACTIONS
Individual drugs
Aspirin: Increased risk of bleeding
Clozapine: do not use owing to risk of agranulocytosis

Drug classifications
Anticoagulants, NSAIDs, platelet inhibitors, thrombolytics: increased risk of bleeding
Antineoplastics (other), radiation: increased toxicity
CYP1A2 inducers (barbiturates, carbamazepine, rifampin): decreased bendamustine
CYP1A2 inhibitors (atazanavir, cimetidine, ciprofloxacin, enoxacin, ethyl estradiol, fluvoxamine, mexiletine, norfloxacin, tacrine, thiabendazole, zileuton): increased bendamustine
Myelosuppressive agents: increased myelosuppression
Vaccines (live): increased adverse reactions, decreased antibody reaction

Drug/lab test
Increased: LFTs

NURSING CONSIDERATIONS
Assessment
• **Blood dyscrasias:** assess CBC, differential, platelet count weekly; withhold product if WBC is <1000 or platelet count is <75,000; notify prescriber of results
• Monitor hepatic studies: AST, ALT, bilirubin
• Monitor renal studies: BUN, serum uric acid, urine CCr before, during therapy; I&O ratio; report fall in urine output of 30 ml/hr; electrolytes
• Assess for cold, cough, fever (may indicate beginning infection)
• Assess bleeding: hematuria, guaiac, bruising, petechiae, mucosa, orifices q8hr
• **Serious skin toxicities:** assess for toxic epidermal necrolysis, Stevens-Johnson syndrome, product should be discontinued
• **Tumor lysis syndrome:** monitor uric acid, potassium, may occur during first treatment cycle, use allopurinol in those at high risk for TLS, usually during the first 2 wk, provide adequate hydration

Nursing diagnoses
• Infection, risk for (adverse reactions)
• Injury, risk for (adverse reactions)
• Knowledge, deficient (teaching)
• Nutrition, impaired, less than body requirements, imbalanced (adverse reactions)

Patient/family education
• Advise patient to avoid use of aspirin, ibuprofen, razors, commercial mouthwash
• Instruct patient to report signs of anemia (fatigue, irritability, shortness of breath, faintness)
• Instruct patient to report signs of infection
• Teach patient to use contraception during therapy and for 3 mo after (pregnancy **D**)
• Advise patient to report signs of infection, myelosuppression, skin toxicities

Evaluation
Positive therapeutic outcome
• Improvement in blood counts and morphology

benzocaine topical
See Appendix B

benztropine (Rx)
(benz′troe-peen)
Apo-Benztropin ✦, Cogentin
Func. class.: Cholinergic blocker, antiparkinson agent
Chem. class.: Tertiary amine
Pregnancy category C

ACTION: Blockade of central acetylcholine receptors in the CNS; neurotransmitters are balanced

Therapeutic outcome: Decreased involuntary movements

USES: Parkinsonian symptoms, EPS associated with neuroleptic products, acute dystonia, hypersalivation

CONTRAINDICATIONS:
Hypersensitivity, closed-angle glaucoma, myasthenia gravis, GI/GU obstruction, child <3 yr, peptic ulcer, megacolon, prostate hypertrophy, dementia, tardive dyskinesia

Precautions: Pregnancy C, breastfeeding, children, geriatric, tachycardia, renal/hepatic disease, product abuse history, dysrhythmias, hypo/hypertension, psychiatric patients

DOSAGE AND ROUTES
Drug-induced extrapyramidal symptoms
Adult: IM/IV 1-4 mg daily/bid; give PO dose as soon as possible; PO 1-2 mg bid/tid; increase by 0.5 mg q5-6days
Child >3 yr: IM/IV 0.02-0.05 mg/kg/dose 1-2 ×/day
Geriatric: PO 0.5 mg daily-bid, increase by 0.5 mg q5-6days; max 4 mg/day

Parkinsonian symptoms
Adult: PO 1-2 mg daily, in 1-2 divided doses; increased 0.5 mg q5-6days titrated to patient response; max 6 mg daily

Acute dystonic reactions
Adult: IM/IV 1-2 mg, may increase to 1-2 mg bid (PO)

Available forms: Tabs 0.5, 1, 2 mg; inj 1 mg/ml

Implementation
PO route
• Give with or after meals to prevent GI upset; may give with fluids other than water; hard candy, frequent drinks, gum to relieve dry mouth
• Give at bedtime to avoid daytime drowsiness in patient with parkinsonism
• May be crushed and mixed with food
• Store at room temperature
IM route
• Give in large muscle mass for dystonic symptoms
IV direct route
• Give parenteral dose with patient recumbent to prevent postural hypotension; give undiluted 1 mg/1 min

Syringe compatibilities: ChlorproMAZINE, fluphenazine, metoclopramide, perphenazine, thiothixene

Y-site compatibilities: Fluconazole, tacrolimus

ADVERSE EFFECTS
CNS: Confusion, anxiety, restlessness, irritability, delusions, hallucinations, headache, sedation, depression, incoherence, dizziness, memory loss; delirium (geriatric)
CV: Palpitations, tachycardia, hypotension, bradycardia
EENT: Blurred vision, photophobia, dilated pupils, difficulty swallowing, dry eyes, mydriasis, increased intraocular tension, closed-angle glaucoma
GI: *Dryness of mouth, constipation,* nausea, vomiting, abdominal distress, **paralytic ileus,** epigastric distress, xerostomia
GU: Hesitancy, retention, dysuria
INTEG: Rash, urticaria, dermatoses
MISC: Increased temperature, flushing, decreased sweating, **hyperthermia, heat stroke,** numbness of fingers
MS: Muscular weakness, cramping

Pharmacokinetics
Absorption	Good (PO, IM), complete (**IV**)
Distribution	Unknown
Metabolism	Unknown
Excretion	Unknown
Half-life	Unknown

Pharmacodynamics
	IM/IV	PO
Onset	15 min	1 hr
Peak	Unknown	Unknown
Duration	6-10 hr	6-10 hr

INTERACTIONS
Individual drugs
Bethanechol: decreased cholinergic effects
Disopyramide, quinidine: increased anticholinergic effects

Drug classifications
Antidepressants (tricyclic), antihistamines, phenothiazines: increased anticholinergic effects
Antidiarrheals, antacids: decreased absorption

NURSING CONSIDERATIONS
Assessment
• Assess for **parkinsonism**, EPS: shuffling gait, muscle rigidity, involuntary movements, loss of balance, pill rolling, muscle spasms, drooling before and during treatment
• Monitor I&O ratio; retention commonly causes decreased urinary output, distention, frequency, incontinence
• Monitor for urinary hesitancy, retention; palpate bladder if retention occurs
• Monitor for constipation, cramping, pain in abdomen, abdominal distention; increase fluids, bulk, exercise if this occurs
• Assess for tolerance over long-term therapy; dosage may have to be increased or changed
• Assess for mental status: affect, mood, CNS depression, worsening of mental symptoms during early therapy
• Assess for benztropine "buzz" or "high," patients may imitate EPS

Nursing diagnoses
• Knowledge, deficient (teaching)
• Mobility, impaired physical (uses)
• Noncompliance (teaching)

Patient/family education
• Teach patient to use caution in hot weather; product may increase susceptibility to stroke since perspiration is decreased; patient should remain indoors
• Advise patient not to discontinue this product abruptly; to taper off over 1 wk to prevent withdrawal symptoms (insomnia, involuntary movements, anxiety, tachycardias), to take as directed, not to double doses
• Caution patient to avoid driving or other hazardous activities; drowsiness, dizziness may occur
• Teach patient to avoid OTC medication: cough, cold preparations with alcohol, antihistamines, antacids, or antidiarrheals within 2 hr unless directed by prescriber; increased CNS depression may occur
• Advise patient to rise from sitting or recumbent position slowly to minimize orthostatic hypotension
• Teach patient to use good oral hygiene; to use sugarless gum, hard candy, frequent sips of water to decrease dry mouth; if dry mouth continues, saliva substitutes may be prescribed
• Instruct patient that doses should not be doubled, but missed dose may be taken up to 2 hr before next dose

Evaluation
Positive therapeutic outcome
• Absence of involuntary movements (pill rolling, tremors, muscle spasms) after 2 days of treatment

betamethasone (Rx)
(bay-tah-meth'ah-sone)
Celestone
Func. class.: Corticosteroid, synthetic; glucocorticoid, long acting
Pregnancy category C

Do not confuse:
betamethasone/beclomethasone

ACTION: Decreases inflammation by suppression of migration of polymorphonuclear leukocytes, fibroblasts, reversal of increased capillary permeability and lysosomal stabilization

Therapeutic outcome: Decreased inflammation and normal immunity

USES: Immunosuppression, severe inflammation, graft-versus-host disease (GVHD)

CONTRAINDICATIONS: Psychosis, hypersensitivity, idiopathic thrombocytopenia, acute glomerulonephritis, amebiasis, fungal infections, nonasthmatic bronchial disease, child <2 yr, AIDS, TB, threadworm, high doses in traumatic brain injury

Precautions: Pregnancy **C**, breastfeeding, diabetes mellitus, glaucoma, osteoporosis, seizure disorders, ulcerative colitis, CHF, myasthenia gravis, renal disease, esophagitis, peptic ulcer

DOSAGE AND ROUTES
Adult: PO 0.6-7.2 mg daily; IM/IV 0.6-7.2 mg daily in joint or soft tissue (sodium phosphate)
Child: PO 17.5-250 mcg/kg/day in 3 divided doses; IM 17.5-250 mcg/kg/day in 3 divided doses every 3rd day or 5.8-8.75 mcg/kg/day as a single dose (adrenal insufficiency)

Acute GVHD
Adult/adolescent/child: IM (sodium phosphate and acetate combinate) 0.5-9 mg/day, range is $^1/_3$-$^1/_2$ normal corticosteroid dose q12hr

Nonsuppurative thyroiditis
Adult/adolescents: PO 0.6-7.2 mg/day, as a single or divided doses; IM 0.5-9 mg/day in divided doses

Child: PO 62.5-250 mcg/kg/day or 1.875-7.5 mg/m²/day in 3-4 divided doses; IM 0.5-9 mg/day individual doses

Other uses
Child: PO 62.5-250 mcg/kg/day in 3 divided doses; IM 20.8-125 mcg/kg/day of the base q12-24hr

Available forms: Tabs 500, 600 mcg; effervescent tabs 500 mcg ✤; syr 600 mcg/5 ml; ext rel tab 1 mg; susp for inj (phosphate/acetate) 6 mg/ml

Implementation
PO route
• Give with food or milk to decrease GI symptoms
IM route
• Give IM inj deep in large mass, rotate sites, avoid deltoid, use 21-G needle; in one dose in AM to prevent adrenal suppression; avoid SUBCUT administration; may damage tissue
Inhalation route
• Give inh with water to decrease possibility of fungal infections; titrated dose; use lowest effective dose
• Use after cleaning aerosol *top* daily with warm water; dry thoroughly
• Store in cool environment; do not puncture or incinerate container
Topical route
• Apply only to affected areas; do not get in eyes; apply medication, then cover with occlusive dressing (only if prescribed), seal to normal skin, change q12hr; systemic absorption may occur
• Apply only to dermatoses; do not use on weeping, denuded, or infected area
• Cleanse before applying product; use treatment for a few days after area has cleared
• Store at room temperature

ADVERSE EFFECTS
CNS: *Depression, flushing, sweating,* headache, bruising, mood changes
CV: *Hypertension,* **circulatory collapse, thromboembolism,** tachycardia, **necrotizing angiitis, CHF**
EENT: Fungal infections, increased intraocular pressure, blurred vision
GI: *Diarrhea, nausea, abdominal distention,* **GI hemorrhage,** increased appetite, **pancreatitis**
HEMA: **Thrombocytopenia**
INTEG: *Acne, poor wound healing,* ecchymosis, *bruising,* petechiae
MS: Fractures, osteoporosis, weakness, myopathy

Pharmacokinetics
Absorption	Well absorbed (PO); systemic (TOP)
Distribution	Crosses placenta
Metabolism	Liver, extensively
Excretion	Kidney, breast milk
Half-life	3-5 hr, adrenal suppression 3-4 days

Pharmacodynamics
	PO	IM	IV	Top
Onset	1-2 hr	Unknown	Rapid	Unknown
Peak	2 hr	4-8 hr	4-8 hr	Unknown
Duration	3 days	1-1½ days	1-1½ days	Unknown

INTERACTIONS
Individual drugs
Alcohol, indomethacin: increased GI bleeding
Amphotericin B, piperacillin, ticarcillin: increased hypokalemia
CYP3A4 inhibitors (erythromycin, ketoconazole, indinavir, itraconazole, ritonavir, saquinavir): increased effects of betamethasone
Insulin: increased need for insulin
Isoniazid: decreased effect
Phenytoin, rifampin: decreased action; increased metabolism
Somatrem, somatropin: decreased effects

Drug classifications
Anticoagulants, antidiabetics: decreased effect
Barbiturates: decreased action; increased metabolism
Fluoroquinolones: increased tendon rupture
Hypoglycemic agents: increased need for hypoglycemic agents
NSAIDs, salicylates: increased GI bleeding
Salicylates, oral contraceptives: decreased effects
Thiazides, loop diuretics: increased hypokalemia
Toxoids/vaccines: decreased immune response

Drug/food
Grapefruit juice should be avoided

Drug/lab test
Increased: cholesterol, sodium, blood glucose, uric acid, calcium, urine glucose
Decreased: calcium, potassium, T_4, T_3, thyroid ^{131}I uptake test, urine 17-OHCS, 17-KS, PBI
False negative: skin allergy tests

Adverse effects: *italics* = common; **bold** = life-threatening

NURSING CONSIDERATIONS
Assessment
Systemic route
• **Adrenal insufficiency crisis:** decreased B/P, nausea/vomiting, anorexia, weakness, weight loss, confusion, lethergy
• Monitor potassium, blood glucose, urine glucose while on long-term therapy; hypokalemia and hyperglycemia; check weight daily; notify prescriber of weekly gain >5 lb
• Monitor B/P, pulse; notify prescriber if chest pain occurs
• Monitor I&O ratio; be alert for decreasing urinary output and increasing edema
• Check plasma cortisol levels during long-term therapy (normal level: 138-635 nmol/L [SI units] when drawn at 8 AM); adrenal function periodically for HPA axis suppression
• Assess for symptoms of **infection:** increased temp, WBC even after withdrawal of medication; product masks infection symptoms
• Assess for symptoms of **potassium depletion:** paresthesias, fatigue, nausea, vomiting, depression, polyuria, dysrhythmias, weakness
• Monitor for edema, hypo/hypertension, cardiac symptoms
• Assess for mental status: affect, mood, behavioral changes, aggression
Topical route
• Check temp; if fever develops, product should be discontinued
• Assess for systemic absorption: increased temp, inflammation, irritation

Nursing diagnoses
• Infection, risk for (adverse reactions)
• Knowledge, deficient (teaching)
• Noncompliance (teaching)

Patient/family education
Systemic route
• Advise patient that long-term therapy may be needed to clear infection (1-2 mo depending on type of infection); that emergency ID as corticosteroid user should be carried or worn; dosage adjustment may be needed
⚠ **Instruct patient to notify prescriber if therapeutic response decreases; caution patient not to discontinue abruptly; adrenal crisis can result**
• Instruct patient to avoid OTC products unless directed by prescriber, avoid vaccines without prescriber approval
• Teach patient all aspects of product use, including cushingoid symptoms, to report to prescriber immediately black, tarry stools or abdominal pain

• Teach patient symptoms of **adrenal insufficiency:** nausea, anorexia, fatigue, dizziness, dyspnea, weakness, joint pain
Topical route
• Caution patient to avoid sunlight on affected area; burns may occur

Evaluation
Positive therapeutic outcome
• Ease of respirations, decreased inflammation (systemic)
• Absence of severe itching, patches on skin, flaking (topical)

betamethasone topical
See Appendix B

betamethasone (augmented) topical
See Appendix B

betaxolol ophthalmic
See Appendix B

bethanechol (Rx)
(be-than′e-kol)
Urecholine
Func. class.: Urinary tract stimulant, cholinergic
Chem. class.: Synthetic choline ester
Pregnancy category C

ACTION: Stimulates muscarinic acetylcholine receptors directly; mimics effects of parasympathetic nervous system stimulation; stimulates gastric motility, micturition; increases lower esophageal sphincter pressure

Therapeutic outcome: Absence of continued urinary retention

USES: Urinary retention (postoperative, postpartum), neurogenic atony of bladder with retention

Unlabeled uses: Ileus

CONTRAINDICATIONS: Hypersensitivity, severe bradycardia, asthma, severe hypotension, hyperthyroidism, peptic ulcer, parkinsonism, seizure disorders, CAD, COPD, coronary occlusion, mechanical obstruction, peritonitis, recent urinary or GI surgery, GI/GU obstruction

Precautions: Pregnancy **C**, breastfeeding, child <8 yr, hypertension

DOSAGE AND ROUTES
Adult: PO 10-50 mg bid-qid
Child: PO 0.3-0.6 mg/kg/day divided in 3-4 doses/day

Ileus (unlabeled)
Adult: PO/SUBCUT 10-20 mg tid-qid; before meals (PO)

Available forms: Tabs 5, 10, 25, 50 mg

Implementation
PO route
• Give increased doses as prescribed if tolerance occurs
• To avoid nausea and vomiting, take on an empty stomach; 1 hr before or 2 hr after meals
• Store at room temperature

ADVERSE EFFECTS
CNS: Dizziness, headache, malaise
CV: Hypotension, bradycardia, reflex tachycardia, **cardiac arrest, circulatory collapse**
EENT: Miosis, increased salivation, lacrimation, blurred vision
GI: *Nausea, bloody diarrhea, belching, vomiting, cramps, fecal incontinence*
GU: Urgency
INTEG: Rash, urticaria, flushing, increased sweating
RESP: Acute asthma, dyspnea, bronchoconstriction

Pharmacokinetics
Absorption	Poor (PO)
Distribution	Does not cross blood-brain barrier
Metabolism	Unknown
Excretion	Kidneys
Half-life	Unknown

Pharmacodynamics
	PO	SUBCUT
Onset	30-90 min	5-15 min
Peak	1 hr	15-30 min
Duration	1-6 hr	2 hr

INTERACTIONS
Individual drugs
Procainamide, quinidine: decreased action of procainamide and quinidine

Drug classifications
Anticholinergics: decreased action
Anticholinesterase agents, cholinergic agonists: increased action, increased toxicity
Ganglionic blockers: increased severe hypotension

Drug/lab test
Increased: AST, lipase/amylase, bilirubin

NURSING CONSIDERATIONS
Assessment
• Assess **urinary patterns:** retention, urgency
• Monitor B/P, pulse, respirations; observe after parenteral dose for 1 hr
• Check I&O ratio; check for urinary retention or incontinence; if bladder emptying does not occur, notify prescriber; catheterization may be needed
• Assess for **toxicity:** bradycardia, hypotension, bronchospasm, headache, dizziness, seizures, sweating, cramping, respiratory depression; product should be discontinued if toxicity occurs; administer atropine

Nursing diagnoses
• Injury, risk for (adverse reactions)
• Knowledge, deficient (teaching)
• Urinary elimination, impaired (uses)

Patient/family education
• Instruct patient to take product exactly as prescribed; 1 hr before meals or 2 hr after meals; do not double doses; if dose is missed, take within 1 hr of scheduled dose
• Caution patient to make position changes slowly; orthostatic hypotension may occur
• Instruct patient to report cramping, diarrhea with blood, flushing to prescriber

Evaluation
Positive therapeutic outcome
• Absence of urinary retention
• Absence of abdominal distention

TREATMENT OF OVERDOSE:
Administer atropine 0.6-1.2 mg IV or IM (adult)

⚠ HIGH ALERT

bevacizumab (Rx)
(beh-va-kiz′you-mab)
Avastin
Func. class.: Antineoplastic—miscellaneous
Chem. class.: Monoclonal antibody
Pregnancy category C

Do not confuse:
Avastin/Astelin

ACTION: DNA-derived monoclonal antibody selectively binds to and inhibits activity of human vascular endothelial growth factor to

Adverse effects: *italics* = common; **bold** = life-threatening

reduce microvascular growth and inhibition of metastatic disease progression

Therapeutic outcome: Decreased tumor size

USES: Metastatic carcinoma of the colon or rectum in combination with 5-FU **IV**, renal cell carcinoma, glioblastoma, non–small cell lung cancer

Unlabeled uses: Adjunctive in breast, renal/pancreatic/neovascular/ovarian cancer, (wet) macular degeneration

CONTRAINDICATIONS:
Hypersensitivity

Precautions: Pregnancy **C**, breastfeeding, children, geriatric, CHF, blood dyscrasias, CV disease, hypertension, surgery, thromboembolic disease, hamster protein/murine hypersensitivity

> **BLACK BOX WARNING:** GI perforation, wound dehiscence

DOSAGE AND ROUTES
Colorectal cancer
Adult: **IV** INF 5 mg/kg q14days given over 90 min; if well tolerated, the next infusion may be given over 60 min; if 60 min infusions are well tolerated, subsequent infusions may be given over 30 min

Non–small cell lung cancer
Adult: **IV** 15 mg/kg over 60-90 min with CARBOplatin and paclitaxel

Metastatic renal cell carcinoma
Adult: **IV** 15 mg/kg q2wk with interferon alfa 9 million units SUBCUT 3 × per wk, up to 52 wk

Available forms: Inj 25 mg/ml

Implementation
IV intermittent infusion route
- Do not give by **IV** bolus or **IV** push
- Give as **IV** inf over 90 min for first dose and 60 min thereafter, if well tolerated

> **BLACK BOX WARNING: Wound dehiscence:** do not give for ≥28 days after surgery, make sure wounds are healed prior to use

ADVERSE EFFECTS
CNS: *Asthenia, dizziness,* **intracranial hemorrhage (malignant glioma),** headache, fatigue, confusion

CV: Deep vein thrombosis, hypo/hypertension, **hypertensive crisis**

GI: Nausea, vomiting, anorexia, diarrhea, constipation, abdominal pain, colitis, stomatitis, **GI hemorrhage/perforation**

GU: Proteinuria, urinary frequency/urgency, **nephrotic syndrome,** ovarian failure

HEMA: Leukopenia, neutropenia, thrombocytopenia, microangiopathic hemolytic anemia, thromboembolism, bleeding

META: Bilirubinemia, hypokalemia

MISC: Exfoliative dermatitis, hemorrhage, non-GI fistula formation, alopecia, *impaired wound healing,* **osteonecrosis of the jaw**

RESP: Dyspnea, upper respiratory infection

Pharmacokinetics
Absorption	Unknown
Distribution	Steady state 100 days
Metabolism	Unknown
Excretion	Unknown
Half-life	20 days

Pharmacodynamics
Onset	Unknown
Peak	Unknown
Duration	Steady state 100 days

INTERACTIONS
Individual drugs
Sunitab: avoid concurrent use; microangiopathic hemolytic anemia may occur, avoid concurrent use

NURSING CONSIDERATIONS
Assessment
- Monitor B/P q3-4wk
- Assess for symptoms of infection; may be masked by product
- Monitor **CNS reaction:** dizziness, confusion
- Assess for **CHF:** crackles, jugular vein distention, dyspnea during treatment
- Assess **GU status** (proteinuria); nephrotic syndrome may occur; monitor urinalysis for increasing protein level; products should be held if protein ≥2 g/24 hr

⚠ Assess for GI perforation, serious bleeding, nephrotic syndrome, hypertensive crisis; product should be discontinued permanently; for surgery, product should be discontinued temporarily

Nursing diagnoses
- Body image, disturbed (adverse reactions)
- Infection, risk for (adverse reactions)

- Injury, risk for (adverse reactions)
- Knowledge, deficient (teaching)

Patient/family education
- Instruct patient to avoid hazardous tasks, since confusion, dizziness may occur
- Instruct patient to report signs of infection: sore throat, fever, diarrhea, vomiting
- Advise patient not to become pregnant while taking this product, or for several months after discontinuing treatment
- Advise patient to notify prescriber if pregnant or planning a pregnancy

Evaluation
Positive therapeutic outcome
- Decrease in size of tumors

bicalutamide (Rx)
(bi-kal-yut'ah-mide)
**Casodex, Co-Bicalutamide ✤,
PMS-Bicalutamide ✤, ratio-
Bicalutamide ✤, Sandoz
Bicalutamide**
Func. class.: Antineoplastic hormone
Chem. class.: Nonsteroidal antiandrogen
Pregnancy category X

Do not confuse:
Casadex/Kapidex

ACTION: Competitively inhibits the action of androgens by binding to cytosol androgen receptors in target tissue

Therapeutic outcome: Prevention of growth of malignant cells

USES: Stage D-2 metastatic prostate cancer in combination with luteinizing hormone–releasing hormone (LHRH) analog

CONTRAINDICATIONS:
Pregnancy **X**, women, hypersensitivity

Precautions: Breastfeeding, geriatric, renal/hepatic disease, diabetes mellitus

DOSAGE AND ROUTES
Adult: PO 50 mg daily with LHRH

Available forms: Tabs 50 mg

Implementation
- Give at same time each day (for both products) either AM or PM with or without food
- Give only with LHRH treatment

ADVERSE EFFECTS
CNS: Dizziness, paresthesia, insomnia, anxiety, neuropathy, headache
CV: Hot flashes, hypertension, chest pain, **CHF,** edema
GI: *Diarrhea, constipation, nausea,* vomiting, increased liver enzyme test, anorexia, dry mouth, melena, abdominal pain, **hepatitis**
GU: Nocturia, hematuria, UTI, impotence, gynecomastia, urinary incontinence, frequency, dysuria, retention, urgency, breast tenderness, decreased libido
INTEG: Rash, sweating, dry skin, pruritus, alopecia
MISC: Infection, anemia, dyspnea, bone pain, headache, asthenia, *back pain,* flulike symptoms

Pharmacokinetics
Absorption	Well absorbed
Distribution	Unknown
Metabolism	Liver
Excretion	Urine, feces
Half-life	5.2 days

Pharmacodynamics
Onset	Unknown
Peak	$31\frac{1}{2}$ hr
Duration	Unknown

INTERACTIONS
Drug classifications
Anticoagulants: increased anticoagulation
CYP3A4 inhibitors (amiodarone, antiretrovirals, protease inhibitors, clarithromycin, dalfopristin, quinupristin, delavirdine, efavirenz, erythromycin, fluoxetine, fluvoxamine, imatinib, mifepristone, RU-486, nefazodone, some azole antifungals): increased bicalutamide effects
CYP3A4 inducers (barbiturates, bosentan, carBAMazepine, dexamethasone, nevirapine, oxcarbazepine, phenytoins, rifabutin, rifampin, rifapentine): decreased bicalutamide effects

Drug/herb
St. John's wort: may require dosage change

Drug/food
Grapefruit juice: do not use together

Drug/lab test
Increased: AST, ALT, bilirubin, BUN, creatinine
Decreased: Hgb, WBC

Adverse effects: *italics* = common; **bold** = life-threatening

NURSING CONSIDERATIONS

Assessment
• Assess for diarrhea, constipation, nausea, vomiting
• Assess for hot flashes, gynecomastia; assure patient that these are common side effects
• Monitor prostate-specific antigen (PSA) liver function tests

Nursing diagnoses
• Injury, risk for (uses, adverse reactions)
• Knowledge, deficient (teaching)

Patient/family education
• Teach patient to recognize and report signs of anemia, renal/hepatic toxicity
• Advise patient that hair may be lost, but loss is reversible after therapy is discontinued
• Advise patient not to use other products unless approved by prescriber
• Advise patient to use contraception

Evaluation
Positive therapeutic outcome
• Decreased tumor size, spread of malignancy

---

bimatoprost ophthalmic
See Appendix B

bisacodyl (Rx, OTC)
(bis-a-koe′dill)
Alophen, APC-Bisacodyl ✤, Apo-Bisacodyl ✤, Bisac-Evac, Corrective, Correctol, Dacodyl, Dulcolax, Ex-Lax Ultra Tab, Femilax, Feminine, Femitrol, Good Sense Women's, Leader Laxative, ratio-Bisacodyl ✤, Top Care Laxative, Veracolate, Walgreens Gentle, Walgreens Women's
Func. class.: Laxative, stimulant
Chem. class.: Diphenylmethane
Pregnancy category C

ACTION: Acts directly on intestine by increasing motor activity; thought to irritate colonic intramural plexus; increases water in the colon

Therapeutic outcome: Decreased constipation

USES: Short-term treatment of constipation, bowel or rectal preparation for surgery, examination

CONTRAINDICATIONS:
Hypersensitivity, rectal fissures, abdominal pain, nausea, vomiting, appendicitis, acute surgical abdomen, ulcerated hemorrhoids, acute hepatitis, fecal impaction, intestinal/biliary tract obstruction

Precautions: Pregnancy C, breastfeeding

DOSAGE AND ROUTES
Adult ≥12 yr: PO 5-15 mg in PM or AM; may use up to 30 mg for bowel or rectal preparation; RECT 10 mg (single dose), 30 ml enema
Child 6-11 yr: PO 5 mg as a single dose; RECT 5 mg as a single dose

Available forms: Tabs 5 mg; enteric coated tabs 5 mg; supp 5, 10 mg; enema 10 mg/30 ml

Implementation
Oral route
• Swallow tabs whole; do not break, crush, or chew
• Give alone with water only for better absorption; do not take within 1 hr of antacids, milk
• Administer in AM or PM (oral dose)
Rectal route
• Lubricate before insertion, patient should retain for $^1/_2$ hr

ADVERSE EFFECTS
CNS: Muscle weakness
GI: *Nausea, vomiting, anorexia, cramps,* diarrhea, rectal burning (supp)
META: Protein-losing enteropathy, alkalosis, hypokalemia, **tetany,** electrolyte and fluid imbalances

Pharmacokinetics
Absorption	Poor
Distribution	Unknown
Metabolism	Liver, minimally
Excretion	Kidneys
Half-life	Unknown

Pharmacodynamics
	PO	Rect
Onset	6-10 hr	15-60 min
Peak	Unknown	Unknown
Duration	Unknown	Unknown

INTERACTIONS
Drug classifications
Antacids, gastric acid pump inhibitors, H$_2$-blockers: increased gastric irritation

---

⚠ Nurse Alert

Drug/herb
Flax, lily of the valley, pheasant's eye, senna, squill: increased laxative action

Drug/food
Milk: increased gastric irritation

NURSING CONSIDERATIONS

Assessment
• Monitor blood, urine electrolytes if used often by patient; check I&O ratio to identify fluid loss
• Assess **GI symptoms:** cramping, rectal bleeding, nausea, vomiting; if these symptoms occur, product should be discontinued; identify cause of constipation; identify whether fluids, bulk, or exercise are missing from lifestyle

Nursing diagnoses
• Constipation (uses)
• Diarrhea (side effects)
• Knowledge, deficient (teaching)
• Noncompliance (teaching)

Patient/family education
• Discuss with the patient that adequate fluid and bulk consumption is necessary
• Advise patient that normal bowel movements do not always occur daily
• Teach patient not to use in presence of abdominal pain, nausea, vomiting; tell patient to notify prescriber if constipation is unrelieved or if symptoms of electrolyte imbalance occur: muscle cramps, pain, weakness, dizziness, excessive thirst

Evaluation
Positive therapeutic outcome
• Decreased constipation within 3 days

---

bismuth subsalicylate (OTC)
(bis'meth sub-sa-li'si-late)
Bismatrol, Equaline Stomach Relief, Good Sense Stomach Relief, Kao-Tin, Leader Pink Bismuth, Maalox Total Stomach Relief, Peptic Relief, Pepto-Bismol, Pink Bismuth, Top Care Stomach Relief, Walgreens Soothe
Func. class.: Antidiarrheal/weak antacid
Chem. class.: Salicylate
Pregnancy category C

Do not confuse:
Kaopectate/Kayoxalate

ACTION: Inhibits prostaglandin synthesis responsible for GI hypermotility, intestinal inflammation; stimulates absorption of fluid and electrolytes; binds toxins produced by *Escherichia coli*

Therapeutic outcome: Absence of loose, watery stools

USES: Diarrhea (cause undetermined); prevention of diarrhea when traveling; may be included to treat *Helicobacter pylori,* heartburn, indigestion, nausea

CONTRAINDICATIONS:
Child <3 yr; flulike symptoms; history of GI bleeding; renal disease, varicella, hypersensitivity to this product or salicylates

Precautions: Pregnancy **C,** breastfeeding, geriatric, anticoagulant therapy, gout, diabetes mellitus, immobility, bleeding disorders, previous hypersensitivity to NSAIDs, *Clostridium difficile*–associated diarrhea when used with antiinfectives for *H. pylori*

DOSAGE AND ROUTES
Antidiarrheal
Adult: PO 2 tab or 30 ml/15 ml extra/max strength q30min or 2 tabs q6min, max 4.2 g/24 hr

Antiulcer (unlabeled)
Adult: PO 524 mg q30-60min or 1048 mg q1hr, max 4.2 g/24 hr; given with metronidazole or tetracycline

Available forms: Tabs 262 mg; chewable tabs 262, mg; susp 87 mg/5 ml, 130 mg/15 ml, 262 mg/15 ml, 525 mg/15 ml

Implementation
• **Suspension:** Shake susp before use; chewable tabs should not be swallowed whole

ADVERSE EFFECTS
CNS: Confusion, twitching, **neurotoxicity (high dose)**
EENT: Hearing loss, tinnitus, metallic taste, blue gums, black tongue (chew tabs)
GI: Increased fecal impaction (high doses), dark stools, constipation, diarrhea, nausea
HEMA: Increased bleeding time

Pharmacokinetics
Absorption	Salicylate >90%
Distribution	None
Metabolism	None
Excretion	Feces (unchanged)
Half-life	Unknown

Adverse effects: *italics* = common; **bold** = life-threatening

Pharmacodynamics

Onset	1 hr
Peak	2 hr
Duration	4 hr

INTERACTIONS

Individual drugs
Methotrexate: increased toxicity
Tetracycline: decreased absorption

Drug classifications
Anticoagulants (oral): increased effect of anticoagulants
Antidiabetics (oral): increased effect of antidiabetics
Quinolones: decreased absorption of quinolones
Salicylates: increased risk of salicylate toxicity

Drug/lab test
Interference: radiographic studies of GI system

NURSING CONSIDERATIONS

Assessment
• **Diarrhea:** Assess bowel pattern (frequency, consistency, shape, volume, color) before product therapy, after treatment; check weight, bowel sounds; identify factors contributing to diarrhea (bacteria, diet, medications, tube feedings)
• Monitor skin turgor; dehydration may occur in severe diarrhea; monitor electrolytes (potassium, sodium, chloride) if diarrhea is severe or continues long term

Nursing diagnoses
• Constipation (adverse reactions)
• Diarrhea (uses)
• Knowledge, deficient (teaching)

Patient/family education
• Teach patient to stop use if symptoms do not improve within 2 days or become worse, or if diarrhea is accompanied by high fever
• Teach patient to increase fluids for rehydration
• Tell patient to chew or dissolve chewable tabs in mouth; do not swallow whole; shake susp before using
• Tell patient to avoid other salicylates unless directed by prescriber; not to give to children because of possibility of Reye's syndrome
• Tell patient that stools may turn gray; tongue may darken; impaction may occur in debilitated patients

Evaluation

Positive therapeutic outcome
• Decreased diarrhea or absence of diarrhea when traveling; resolution of ulcers

---

bisoprolol (Rx)
(bis-oh'pro-lole)
Apo-Bisoprolol ✦, PMS-Bisoprolol ✦, Sandoz Bisoprolol ✦, Zebeta
Func. class.: Antihypertensive
Chem. class.: β_1-Blocker (selective)
Pregnancy category C

Do not confuse:
Zebeta/Diabeta/Zetia

ACTION: Preferentially and competitively blocks stimulation of β_1-adrenergic receptor within cardiac muscle (decreases rate of SA node discharge, increases recovery time), slows conduction of AV node, decreases heart rate, which decreases O_2 consumption in myocardium; decreases renin-aldosterone-angiotensin system; inhibits β_2-receptors in bronchial and vascular smooth muscle at high doses

Therapeutic outcome: Decreased B/P, heart rate

USES: Mild to moderate hypertension

Unlabeled uses: Stable angina, stable CHF

CONTRAINDICATIONS:
Hypersensitivity to β-blockers, cardiogenic shock, heart block (2nd or 3rd degree), sinus bradycardia, CHF, cardiac failure

Precautions: Pregnancy C, breastfeeding, children, major surgery, diabetes mellitus, renal/hepatic/thyroid/peripheral vascular/aortic/mitral valve disease, COPD, asthma, well-compensated heart failure, myasthenia gravis

> **BLACK BOX WARNING:** Abrupt discontinuation

DOSAGE AND ROUTES

Renal/hepatic dose
Adult: PO CCr <40 ml/min 2.5 mg, titrate upward

Hypertension
Adult: PO 2.5-5 mg/day, may increase if necessary to 20 mg once daily, max 20 mg/day; may need to reduce dose in presence of renal or hepatic impairment

Angina (unlabeled)
Adult: PO 5-20 mg/day

Heart failure (unlabeled)
Adult: PO 1.25 mg/day × 48 hr, then 2.5 mg/day for 1st mo, then 5 mg/day, max 10 mg/day

Available forms: Tabs 5, 10 mg

Implementation
• Give daily; give with food to prevent GI upset; may be crushed
• Store protected from light, moisture; place in cool environment

ADVERSE EFFECTS
CNS: Vertigo, headache, insomnia, fatigue, dizziness, mental changes, memory loss, hallucinations, depression, lethargy, drowsiness, strange dreams, catatonia, peripheral neuropathy
CV: Ventricular dysrhythmias, profound hypotension, bradycardia, CHF, cold extremities, postural hypotension, **2nd- or 3rd-degree heart block**
EENT: Sore throat, dry burning eyes
ENDO: Increased hypoglycemic response to insulin
GI: Nausea, diarrhea, vomiting, **mesenteric arterial thrombosis,** ischemic colitis, flatulence, gastritis, gastric pain
GU: Impotence, decreased libido
HEMA: Agranulocytosis, thrombocytopenia, purpura, **eosinophilia**
INTEG: Rash, flushing, alopecia, pruritus, sweating
MISC: Facial swelling, weight gain, decreased exercise tolerance
MS: Joint pain, arthralgia
RESP: Bronchospasm, dyspnea, wheezing, cough, nasal stuffiness

Pharmacokinetics

Absorption	Well absorbed
Distribution	Unknown; protein binding (30%)
Metabolism	Liver, inactive metabolites
Excretion	Urine, unchanged (50%)
Half-life	9-12 hr

Pharmacodynamics

Onset	Unknown
Peak	2-4 hr
Duration	24 hr

INTERACTIONS
Individual drugs
Amiodarone, digoxin: increased bradycardia
Guanethidine, reserpine: increased hypotension

Drug classifications
ACE inhibitors, α-blockers, calcium channel blockers, diuretics: increased antihypertensive effect
Antidiabetics: increased antidiabetic effect
Calcium channel blockers: increased myocardial depression
Ergots: increased peripheral ischemia
NSAIDs, salicylates: decreased antihypertensive effects

Drug/herb
Hawthorn: increased β-blocking effect
Ephedra: decreased β-blocking effect

Drug/lab test
Increased: AST, ALT, blood glucose, BUN, uric acid, potassium, lipoprotein, ANA titer
Interference: glucose/insulin tolerance tests

NURSING CONSIDERATIONS
Assessment
• **Hypertension:** Monitor B/P during beginning treatment, periodically thereafter; pulse: note rate, rhythm, quality; apical/radial pulse before administration; notify prescriber of any significant changes (pulse <50 bpm)
• Check for baselines in renal, liver function tests before therapy begins
• **CHF:** assess for edema in feet, legs daily, monitor I&O, daily weight; check for jugular vein distention, crackles, bilaterally, dyspnea (CHF)
• Monitor skin turgor, dryness of mucous membranes for hydration status, especially geriatric

Nursing diagnoses
• Cardiac output, decreased (uses)
• Injury, risk for (side effects)
• Knowledge, deficient (teaching)
• Noncompliance (teaching)

Patient/family education

> **BLACK BOX WARNING:** Teach patient not to discontinue product abruptly; may cause precipitate angina if stopped abruptly; evaluate noncompliance

• Teach patient not to use OTC products containing α-adrenergic stimulants (such as nasal decongestants, cold preparations); to avoid alcohol, smoking; to limit sodium intake as prescribed
• Teach patient how to take pulse and B/P at home; advise when to notify prescriber
• Instruct patient to comply with weight control, dietary adjustments, modified exercise program

• Tell patient to carry/wear emergency ID to identify product being taken, allergies; tell patient product controls symptoms but does not cure

• Caution patient to avoid hazardous activities if dizziness, drowsiness present

• Teach patient to take product as prescribed, not to double doses, skip doses; take any missed doses as soon as remembered if at least 8 hr until next dose

• Advise patient to report bradycardia, dizziness, confusion, depression, fever, cold extremities

• Teach diabetic patient drug may mask signs of hypoglycemia or alter blood glucose levels

Evaluation

Positive therapeutic outcome
• Decreased B/P in hypertension (after 1-2 wk)

TREATMENT OF OVERDOSE:

Lavage, **IV** atropine for bradycardia, **IV** theophylline for bronchospasm, digoxin, O_2, diuretic for cardiac failure, hemodialysis, **IV** glucose for hypoglycemia, **IV** diazepam (or phenytoin) for seizures

---

⚠ HIGH ALERT

bivalirudin (Rx)
(bye-val-i-rue′din)
Angiomax
Func. class.: Anticoagulant
Chem. class.: Thrombin inhibitor
Pregnancy category B

ACTION: Direct inhibitor of thrombin that is highly specific; able to inhibit free and clot-bound thrombin

Therapeutic outcome: Anticoagulation in percutaneous transluminal coronary angioplasty (PTCA), used with aspirin; heparin-induced thrombocytopenia with thrombosis syndrome

USES: Unstable angina in patients undergoing PTCA, used with aspirin; heparin-induced thrombocytopenia; heparin-induced thrombocytopenia with thrombosis syndrome

CONTRAINDICATIONS:

Hypersensitivity, active bleeding, cerebral aneurysm, intracranial hemorrhage, recent surgery, CVA

Precautions: Pregnancy **B**, breastfeeding, children, geriatric, renal function impairment, hepatic disease, asthma, blood dyscrasias, thrombocytopenia, GI ulcers, hypertension

DOSAGE AND ROUTES

PCI/PTCA
Adult: **IV** bol 0.75 mg/kg, then **IV** inf 1.75 mg/kg/hr for 4 hr; another **IV** inf may be used at 0.2 mg/kg/hr for ≤20 hr; this product is intended to be used with aspirin (325 mg daily) adjusted to body weight

HIT/HITTS
Adult: **IV** bol 0.75 mg/kg, then cont INF 1.75 mg/kg/hr for duration of procedure

Renal dose
Adult: **IV** GFR 30-59 ml/min, give 1.75 mg/kg/hr; GFR 10-29 ml/min, give 1 mg/kg/hr; dialysis-dependent patients, give 0.25 mg/kg/hr

Available forms: Inj, lyophilized 250 mg vial

Implementation
• Prior to PTCA, give with aspirin, 325 mg **IV** direct 1 mg/kg as a bolus; then intermittent infusion

Intermittent IV infusion route
• To each 250-mg vial add 5 ml of sterile water for inj, swirl until dissolved, further dilute reconstituted vial with 50 ml of D_5W or 0.9% NaCl (5 mg/ml); the dose is adjusted to body weight, run at 2.5 mg/kg/hr, do not admix before or during administration
• Give reduced dose in renal impairment

Y-site compatibilities: Abciximab, acyclovir, alfentanil, allopurinol, amifostine, amikacin, aminocaproic acid, aminophylline, amphotericin B liposome, ampicillin, ampicillin-sulbactam, anidulafungin, argatroban, arsenic trioxide, atenolol, atracurium, atropine, azithromycin, aztreonam, bleomycin, bumetanide, buprenorphine, busulfan, butorphanol, calcium chloride/gluconate, capreomycin, CARBOplatin, carmustine, ceFAZolin, cefepime, cefoperazone, cefotaxime, cefotetan, cefoxitin, ceftazidime, ceftizoxime, cefTRIAXone, cefuroxime, chloramphenicol, cimetidine hydrochloride, ciprofloxacin, cisatracurium, CISplatin, clindamycin, cyclophosphamide, cycloSPORINE, cytarabine, dacarbazine, DACTINomycin, DAPTOmycin, DAUNOrubicin, DAUNOrubicin liposome, dexamethasone, dexmedetomidine, dexrazoxane, digoxin, diltiazem, diphenhydrAMINE, docetaxel, dolasetron, DOPamine, DOXOrubicin, DOXOrubicin liposomal, doxycycline, droperidol, enalaprilat, ePHEDrine, EPINEPHrine, epirubicin, epoprostenol, eptifibatide, ertapenem,

erythromycin, esmolol, etoposide, etoposide
phosphate, famotidine, fenoldopam, fentaNYL,
fluconazole, fludarabine, fluorouracil, foscarnet,
fosphenytoin, furosemide, gallium, ganciclovir,
gatifloxacin, gemcitabine, gentamicin, glycopyrrolate, granisetron, haloperidol, heparin, hydrALAZINE, hydrocortisone, HYDROmorphone,
hydrOXYzine, IDArubicin, ifosfamide, imipenem-
cilastatin, inamrinone, insulin, irinotecan,
isoproterenol, ketorolac, labetalol, leucovorin,
levofloxacin, lidocaine, linezolid, LORazepam,
magnesium, mannitol, mechlorethamine,
melphalan, meperidine, meropenem, mesna,
methohexital, methotrexate, methyldopate,
methylPREDNISolone, metoclopramide, metoprolol, metroNIDAZOLE, midazolam, milrinone,
mitomycin, mitoxantrone, mivacurium, morphine, moxifloxacin, mycophenolate, nafcillin,
nalbuphine, naloxone, nesiritide, niCARdipine,
nitroglycerin, nitroprusside, norepinephrine,
octreotide, ofloxacin, ondansetron, oxaliplatin,
oxytocin, paclitaxel, palonosetron, pamidronate,
pancuronium, pemetrexed, PENTobarbital,
PHENobarbital, phenylephrine, piperacillin,
piperacillin-tazobactam, polymyxin B, potassium
acetate/chloride/phosphates, procainamide,
promethazine, propranolol, ranitidine, remifentanil, rocuronium, sodium acetate/bicarbonate/
phosphates, streptozocin, succinylcholine,
SUFentanil, sulfamethoxazole-trimethoprim,
tacrolimus, teniposide, theophylline, thiopental,
thiotepa, ticarcillin, ticarcillin-clavulanate,
tigecycline, tirofiban, tobramycin, topotecan, vasopressin, vecuronium, verapamil, vinBLAStine,
vinCRIStine, vinorelbine, voriconazole, warfarin,
zidovudine, zoledronic acid

ADVERSE EFFECTS
CNS: *Headache, insomnia, anxiety, nervousness*
CV: *Hypo/hypertension, bradycardia*
GI: *Nausea, vomiting, abdominal pain, dyspepsia*
HEMA: **Hemorrhage, thrombocytopenia**
MISC: Pain at inj site, pelvic pain, urinary retention, fever
MS: *Back pain*

Pharmacokinetics
Absorption	Unknown
Distribution	No protein binding
Metabolism	Unknown
Excretion	Kidneys
Half-life	25 min

Pharmacodynamics
Onset	Unknown
Peak	Unknown
Duration	1 hr

INTERACTIONS
Individual drugs
Aspirin, treprostinil: increased risk of bleeding

Drug classifications
Anticoagulants, thrombolytics: increased risk of bleeding

Drug/herb
Agrimony, alfalfa, angelica, anise, bilberry, black haw, bogbean, buchu, cat's claw, chamomile, chondroitin, devil's claw, dong quai, evening primrose, fenugreek, feverfew, fish oils, garlic, ginger, ginkgo, ginseng, horse chestnut, Irish moss, kava, kelp, kelpware, khella, licorice, lovage, lungwort, meadowsweet, motherwort, mugwort, nettle, papaya, parsley (large amounts), pau d'arco, pineapple, poplar, prickly ash, red clover, safflower, saw palmetto, senega, skullcap, tonka bean, turmeric, wintergreen, yarrow: increased risk of bleeding
Coenzyme Q10, flax, glucomannan, goldenseal, guar gum: decreased anticoagulant effect

NURSING CONSIDERATIONS
Assessment
⚠ Assess for fall in B/P or Hct that may indicate hemorrhage
• Assess for fever, skin rash, urticaria
• Assess **bleeding:** check arterial and venous sites, IM inj sites, catheters; all punctures should be minimized

Nursing diagnoses
• Cardiac output, decreased (uses)
• Knowledge, deficient (teaching)

Patient/family education
• Explain reason for product and expected results

Evaluation
Positive therapeutic outcome
• Anticoagulation in PTCA

⚠ HIGH ALERT

bleomycin (Rx)

(blee-oh-mye'sin)

Blenoxane ✦

Func. class.: Antineoplastic, antibiotic
Chem. class.: Glycopeptide
Pregnancy category D

ACTION: Inhibits synthesis of DNA, RNA, protein; derived from *Streptomyces verticillus;* phase specific in the G_2 and M phases; a nonvesicant, sclerosing agent

Therapeutic outcome: Prevention of rapidly growing malignant cells

USES: Cancer of head, neck, penis, cervix, vulva of squamous cell origin, Hodgkin's/non-Hodgkin's disease, testicular carcinoma, as a sclerosing agent for malignant pleural effusion

CONTRAINDICATIONS:

Pregnancy **D,** breastfeeding, hypersensitivity, prior idiosyncratic reaction

Precautions: Renal/hepatic/respiratory disease, patients >70 yr old

> **BLACK BOX WARNING:** Idiosyncratic reaction, pulmonary fibrosis

DOSAGE AND ROUTES

Adult and child: IM/SUBCUT/**IV** 0.25-0.5 units/kg q1-2wk or 10-20 units/m²; then 1 unit/ day or 5 units/wk; may also be given by cont INF; max total dose, 400 units in lifetime

Hodgkin's disease (test dose)

Adult and child (unlabeled): IM/**IV**/SUBCUT <2 units for first 2 doses followed by 24 hr observation

Malignant pleural effusion

Adult: 60 units diluted in 100 ml of 0.9% NaCl intrapleural inj given through a thoracotomy tube following drainage of excess pleural fluid and complete lung expansion, remove after 4 hr

Renal Dose

Adult/child: CCr 40-50 ml/min reduce dose by 30%; CCr 30-39 ml/min reduce dose by 40%; CCr 20-29 ml/min reduce dose by 45%; CCr 10-19 ml/min reduce dose by 55%; CCr 5-10 ml/ min reduce dose by 60%

Available forms: Powder for inj 15, 30 units/vial

Implementation

• Avoid contact with skin; very irritating; wash completely to remove
• Give fluids **IV** or PO before chemotherapy to hydrate patient
• Give antacid before oral agent; give antiemetic 30-60 min before giving product and prn to prevent vomiting; give antibiotics for prophylaxis of infection
• Provide liquid diet: carbonated beverages, gelatin may be added if patient is not nauseated or vomiting
• Rinse mouth tid-qid with water, club soda; brush teeth bid-qid with soft brush or cotton-tipped applicators for stomatitis; use unwaxed dental floss

IM/SUBCUT route

• IM test dose in lymphoma
• Reconstitute with 1-5 ml sterile water for inj; D_5W, 0.9% NaCl, rotate inj sites

INTRAPLEURAL route

• Give 60 units/50-100 ml of 0.9% NaCl, administered by physician through thoracotomy tube

IV route

• Product should be prepared by experienced personnel using proper precautions
• Two test doses 2-5 units before initial dose in lymphoma; monitor for anaphylaxis
• Give by direct **IV** after reconstituting 15 units or less/5 ml or more of D_5W or 0.9% NaCl; give 15 units or less/10 min through Y-tube or 3-way stopcock initial dose; monitor for anaphylaxis

Intermittent IV infusion route

• Administer after diluting 50-100 ml 0.9% NaCl, D_5W and giving at prescribed rate

Y-site compatibilities: Acyclovir, alfentanil, allopurinol, amifostine, amikacin, aminocaproic acid, aminophylline, amiodarone, ampicillin, ampicillin-sulbactam, anidulafungin, atenolol, atracurium, azithromycin, aztreonam, bivalirudin, bumetanide, buprenorphine, busulfan, butorphanol, calcium chloride/gluconate, CARBOplatin, carmustine, caspofungin, ceFAZolin, cefepime, cefotaxime, cefotetan, cefoxitin, ceftazidime, ceftizoxime, cefTRIAXone, cefuroxime, chloramphenicol, chlorproMAZINE, cimetidine, ciprofloxacin, cisatracurium, CISplatin, clindamycin, codeine, cyclophosphamide, cycloSPORINE, cytarabine, dacarbazine, DACTINomycin, DAPTOmycin, DAUNOrubicin, dexamethasone, dexmedetomidine, dexrazoxane, digoxin, diltiazem, diphenhydrAMINE, DOBUTamine, docetaxel, DOPamine, doxacurium, DOXOrubicin, DOXOrubicin liposomal, doxycycline, droperidol, enalaprilat, ePHEDrine, EPINEPHrine, epirubicin, ertapenem, erythromycin, esmolol, etoposide, famotidine, fenoldopam, fentaNYL, filgrastim, fluconazole, fludarabine, fluorouracil, foscarnet, fosphenytoin, furosemide, ganciclovir, gatifloxacin, gemcitabine, gentamicin, glycopyrrolate, granisetron, haloperidol, heparin, hydrALAZINE, hydrocortisone sodium succinate, HYDROmorphone, hydrOXYzine, IDArubicin, ifosfamide, imipenem-cilastatin, inamrinone, insulin (regular), irinotecan, isoproterenol, ketorolac, labetalol, leucovorin, levofloxacin, levorphanol, lidocaine, linezolid, LORazepam, magnesium sulfate, mannitol, mechlorethamine, melphalan, meperidine, meropenem, mesna, metaraminol, methohexital, methotrexate, methyldopate, methylPREDNISolone, metoclopramide, metoprolol, metroNIDAZOLE, midazolam, milrinone, minocycline, mitomycin, mitoxantrone, mivacurium, morphine, nafcillin, nalbuphine, naloxone, nesiritide, niCARdipine, nitroglycerin, nitroprusside, norepinephrine, octreotide, ondansetron, oxaliplatin, palonosetron, pamidronate, pancuronium, pantoprazole, pemetrexed, pentamidine, pentazocine, PENTobarbital, PHENobarbital, phenylephrine, piperacillin, piperacillin-tazobactam, polymyxin B, potassium chloride, potassium phosphates, procainamide, prochlorperazine, promethazine, propranolol, quiNIDine, ranitidine, remifentanil, riTUXimab, rocuronium, sargramostim, sodium acetate, sodium bicarbonate, sodium phosphates, succinylcholine, SUFentanil, sulfamethoxazole-trimethoprim, tacrolimus, teniposide, theophylline, thiopental, thiotepa, ticarcillin, ticarcillin-clavulanate, tirofiban, tobramycin, tolazoline, trastuzumab, trimethobenzamide, vancomycin, vasopressin, vecuronium, verapamil, vinBLAStine, vinCRIStine, vinorelbine, voriconazole, zidovudine

ADVERSE EFFECTS
CNS: Pain at tumor site, headache, confusion
CV: *MI*, stroke
GI: *Nausea, vomiting, anorexia, stomatitis, weight loss,* ulceration of mouth, lips
GU: Hemolytic-uremic syndrome
IDIOSYNCRATIC REACTION: Hypotension, confusion, fever, chills, wheezing
INTEG: *Rash, hyperkeratosis, nail changes, alopecia,* pruritus, acne, striae, peeling, hyperpigmentation
RESP: Fibrosis, pneumonitis, wheezing, pulmonary toxicity
SYST: Anaphylaxis, radiation recall, Raynaud's phenomenon

Pharmacokinetics

Absorption	Well absorbed (IM, SUBCUT, intrapleural, intraperitoneal)
Distribution	Widely distributed
Metabolism	Liver, 30%
Excretion	Kidneys, unchanged (50%)
Half-life	2 hr; increased in renal disease

Pharmacodynamics
Unknown

INTERACTIONS
Individual drugs
Filgrastim, sargramostim: increased toxicity
Fosphenytoin, phenytoin: decreased phenytoin levels
Radiation: increased toxicity, bone marrow suppression

Drug classifications
Anesthetics (general), antineoplastics: increased toxicity
Live virus vaccines: avoid concurrent use

Drug/lab test
Increased: uric acid

NURSING CONSIDERATIONS
Assessment
• Assess buccal cavity q8hr for dryness, sores or ulceration, white patches, oral pain, bleeding, dysphagia; obtain prescription for viscous lidocaine (Xylocaine)
⚠ Assess symptoms indicating anaphylaxis: rash, pruritus, urticaria, purpuric skin lesions, itching, flushing, wheezing, hypotension; have emergency equipment available

> **BLACK BOX WARNING: Pulmonary toxicity/ fibrosis:** Assess pulmonary function tests; chest x-ray before, during therapy; monitor q2wk during treatment; pulmonary diffusion capacity for carbon monoxide (DL_{CO}) monthly; if <40% of pretreatment value, stop treatment; assess for dyspnea, crackles, unproductive cough, chest pain, tachypnea, fatigue, increased pulse, pallor, lethargy

• Monitor CBC, differential, platelet count weekly; withhold product for WBC <4000/ mm^3 or platelet count <100,000/mm^3; notify prescriber of results for WBC <20,000/mm^3, platelets <150,000/mm^3

B

Adverse effects: *italics* = common; **bold** = life-threatening

• Monitor temp q4hr (may indicate beginning of infection)
• Monitor liver function tests before, during therapy (bilirubin, AST, ALT, LDH) as needed or monthly
• Assess for bleeding: hematuria, stool guaiac, bruising or petechiae, mucosa or orifices q8hr; inflammation of mucosa, breaks in skin
• Treat pulmonary infection prior to treatment; identify dyspnea, crackles, unproductive cough, chest pain, tachypnea
• Identify effects of alopecia on body image; discuss feelings about body changes; if edema in feet, joint pain, stomach pain, shaking present, prescriber should be notified; identify inflammation of mucosa, breaks in skin

Nursing diagnoses
• Body image, disturbed (adverse reactions)
• Infection, risk for (adverse reactions)
• Injury, risk for (adverse reactions)
• Knowledge, deficient (teaching)

Patient/family education
• Teach patient to avoid use of products containing aspirin or ibuprofen, razors, commercial mouthwash; bleeding may occur; to report symptoms of bleeding (hematuria, tarry stools)
• Instruct patient to report signs of anemia (fatigue, headache, irritability, faintness, shortness of breath)
• Instruct patient to report any changes in breathing or coughing even several months after treatment; to avoid crowds and persons with respiratory tract or other infections
• Inform patient that hair may be lost during treatment; a wig or hairpiece may make patient feel better; new hair may be different in color, texture
• Caution patient not to have any vaccinations without the advice of the prescriber; serious reactions can occur
• Advise patient contraception is needed during treatment and for several months after completion of therapy, pregnancy **D**

Evaluation
Positive therapeutic outcome
• Prevention of rapid division of malignant cells

boceprevir
(boe-se′pro-vir)
Victrelis
Func. class.: Antiviral, anti-hepatitis agents
Pregnancy category X

ACTION: Prevents hepatitis C viral (HCV) replication by blocking the activity of HCV NS3/4A serine protease. Hepatitis C virus NS3/4A serine protease is an enzyme responsible for the conversion of HCV encoded polyproteins to mature/functioning viral proteins. These mature proteins, NS4A, NS4B, NS5A, and NS5B, are needed for viral replication.

Theurapeutic outcome: Resolution of hepatitis C infection

USES: Hepatitis C infection

CONTRAINDICATIONS
Pregnancy (X), male partners of women who are pregnant

Precautions: Breastfeeding, anemia, neutropenia, thrombocytopenia, HIV, hepatitis B, decompensated hepatic disease, in liver or other organ transplants, neonates, infants, children, adolescents <18 years of age

DOSAGE AND ROUTES

Chronic hepatitis C infection (genotype 1) compensated liver disease (in those without cirrhosis, previously untreated with interferon and ribavirin therapy)
Adult: PO Before starting therapy with boceprevir, give peginterferon alfa and ribavirin for 4 wk, then add boceprevir 800 mg (four 200-mg capsules) PO tid (every 7-9 hr). Treatment length is determined by HCV RNA concentrations at treatment wk 4, 8, 12, and 24. If the patient has undetectable HCV RNA concentrations at wk 8 and 24, discontinue all three medications at week 28. If HCV RNA is detectable at wk 8 but undetectable at wk 24, continue the three-drug regimen through wk 36, then give only peginterferon alfa and ribavirin through treatment wk 48. If the patient has a poor response to peginterferon alfa and ribavirin during the initial 4 wk, continue treatment with all three medications for a total of 48 wks. Discontinue the three-drug regimen if the HCV RNA concentration >100 IU/ml at treatment wk 12 or a detectable HCA RNA concentration at treatment wk 24.

Chronic hepatitis C Infection (genotype 1) compensated liver disease (in those without cirrhosis, previous partial responders/relapsers to interferon and ribavirin therapy)

Adult: PO Before starting therapy with boceprevir, peginterferon alfa and ribavirin must be given for 4 wk; then add boceprevir 800 mg (four 200-mg capsules) PO tid (every 7-9 hr). Treatment length is determined by the HCV RNA concentrations at treatment wk 8, 12, and 24. If the patient has undetectable HCV RNA concentrations at wk 8 and 24, discontinue all three medications at wk 36. If HCV RNA is detectable at wk 8 but undetectable at wk 24, continue the three-drug regimen through wk 36 and then administer only peginterferon alfa and ribavirin through treatment wk 48. Discontinue the three-drug regimen if the patient has an HCV RNA concentration >100 IU/ml at treatment wk 12 or a detectable HCA RNA concentration at treatment wk 24. It is recommended to continue all three medications through wk 48 if the response to prior treatment with peginterferon alfa and ribavirin was <2-log reduction in HCV RNA at wk 12.

Chronic hepatitis C infection (genotype 1) compensated liver disease with cirrhosis

Adult: PO Before starting therapy with boceprevir, peginterferon alfa and ribavirin must be given for 4 wk; then add boceprevir 800 mg (four 200-mg capsules) PO tid (q7-9 hr) to peginterferon alfa and ribavirin for an additional 44 wk (48 wk total)

Available forms: Cap 200 mg

Implementation

• Only use in combination with peginterferon alfa and ribavirin; never give as monotherapy
• Discontinue in hepatitis C virus (HCV) RNA concentrations ≥100 IU/ml at wk 12 or a confirmed detectable HCV RNA concentrations at wk 24
• Any contraindication to peginterferon alfa or ribavirin also applies to boceprevir. See ribavirin or peginterferon alfa monographs for additional information regarding contraindications and warning associated with these products
• Give with food

ADVERSE EFFECTS

When used in combination with peginterferon/ribavarin

CNS: *Asthenia, chills,* dizziness, *fatigue,* insomnia, irritability

GI: Diarrhea, decreased appetite, dysgeusia, nausea, vomiting, xerostomia
HEMA: Anemia (Hgb <10 g/dl), neutropenia, thrombocytopenia
INTEG: *Alopecia, rash,* xerosis
MISC: *Arthralgia, exertional dyspnea*

Pharmacokinetics

Absorption	Unknown
Distribution	75% protein binding
Metabolism	By the enzyme aldoketoreductase (AKR) to a ketone-reduced metabolite; undergoes oxidative metabolism by the hepatic isoenzyme CYP3A4/5 and is a substrate for the drug efflux transporter, P-glycoprotein (PGP)
Excretion	Feces (79%), urine (9%)
Half-life	3.4 hrs

Pharmacodynamics

Onset	Unknown
Peak	2 hrs
Duration	Unknown

INTERACTIONS

Individual drugs

Alfuzosin, cisapride, ezetimibe, lovastatin, niacin with simvastatin and boceprevir, oral midazolam, pimozide, sildenafil, simvastatin, tadalafil (pulmonary arterial hypertension), triazolam: Increased, life-threatening reactions of each product: do not use concurrently

Acetaminophen, alfentanil, aliskiren, almotriptan, alosetron, ALPRAZolam, aminophylline, amiodarone, amitriptyline, amLODIPine, aripiprazole, astemizole, atorvastatin, bepridil, boceprevir, bosentan, budesonide, bupivacaine, buprenorphine, busPIRone, carvedilol, cevimeline, chloroquine, cilostazol, cinacalcet, citalopram, clarithromycin, clomipramine, clonazePAM, clopidogrel, clozapine, colchicine, cyclobenzaprine, cycloSPORINE, dapsone, DAUNOrubicin, desipramine, desloratadine, dexamethasone, dexlansoprazole, dextromethorphan, diazepam, diclofenac, digoxin, diltiazem, disopyramide, disulfiram, docetaxel, dolasetron, donepezil, DOXOrubicin, droperidol, dutasteride, ebastine, eletriptan, eplerenone, erlotinib, erythromycin, estazolam, eszopiclone, ethosuximide, etoposide, exemestane,

felodipine, fentaNYL, fexofenadine, finasteride, flecainide, flunitrazepam, flurazepam, galantamine, gefitinib, glyburide, granisetron, halofantrine, haloperidol, HYDROcodone, ifosfamide, imipramine, indiplon, irinotecan, isradipine, itraconazole, ivermectin, ixabepilone, ketoconazole, lansoprazole, lidocaine, loperamide, loratadine, losartan, maraviroc, mefloquine, meloxicam, mirtazapine, mitomycin, montelukast, morphine, nateglinide, niCARdipine, NIFEdipine, nisoldipine, nortriptyline, omeprazole, ondansetron, oxybutynin, oxyCODONE, paclitaxel, palonosetron, paricalcitol, plicamycin, posaconazole, prasugrel, praziquantel, propafenone, quazepam, QUEtiapine, quinacrine, quiNIDine, ramelteon, repaglinide, rifabutin, risperidone, ropivacaine, salmeterol, selegiline, sertraline, sibutramine, silodosin, sirolimus, sitaxsentan, solifenacin, SUFentanil, sunitinib, systemic corticosteroids, tacrolimus, telithromycin, teniposide, terfenadine, testosterone, theophylline, tiaGABine, tinidazole, tolterodine, tolvaptan, traMADol, traZODone, vardenafil, venlafaxine, verapamil, vinBLAStine, vinCRIStine, voriconazole, warfarin, and others: increased effect, adverse reactions of each product; use cautiously; may need to reduce dose
Drosperinone: increased hyperkalemia
Ethinyl estradiol: decreased estrogen levels
Methadone: decreased effect of this product
Efavirenz, ritonavir, atazanavir, lopinavir with ritonavir: possible treatment failure

Drug classifications
Ergots (dihydroergotamine, ergotamine, ergonovine, methylergonovine): do not use concurrently
Phosphodiesterase type 5 (PDE5) inhibitors (for erectile dysfunction): increased effect, adverse reactions of each product
CYP3A4 inhibitors (phenytoin, carBAMazepine, PHENobarbital, rifampin): decreased boceprevir effect

Drug/herb
Do not use with St. John's wort

NURSING CONSIDERATIONS
Assessment
• **Pregnancy: Obtain a pregnancy test prior to, monthly during, and for 6 months after treatment is completed; those who are not willing to practice strict contraception should not receive treatment with these products; report any cases of prenatal ribavirin exposure to the Ribavirin**

Pregnancy registry at (800) 593-2214
• **Anemia:** Monitor hemoglobin prior to, at treatment wks 4, 8, and 12, and as needed. If Hgb is less than 10 g/dl, decrease ribavirin dosage; if Hgb is less than 8.5 g/dl, discontinuation of therapy is recommended; boceprevir dosage should not be altered based on adverse reactions; Anemia may be managed through ribavirin dose modifications; never alter the dose of boceprevir. If anemia persists despite a reduction in ribavirin dose, consider discontinuing boceprevir. If management of anemia requires permanent discontinuation of ribavirin, treatment with boceprevir MUST also be permanently discontinued. Once boceprevir has been discontinued, it must not be restarted; monitor CBC with differential at treatment wks 4, 8, 12, and at other treatment points as needed

Nursing diagnoses
• Risk for injury (uses, adverse reactions)
• Knowledge deficit (teaching)

Patient/family education
• **To use 2 forms of effective contraception (intrauterine devices and barrier methods)**

Evaluation
Positive therapeutic outcome
• Resolution of hepatitis C infection

boric acid otic
See Appendix B

bortezomib (Rx)
(bor-tez′oh-mib)
Velcade
Func. class.: Antineoplastic—miscellaneous
Chem. class.: Proteasome inhibitor
Pregnancy category D

ACTION: Reversible inhibitor of chymotrypsin-like activity in mammalian cells;causes a delay in tumor growth by disrupting normal homeostatic mechanisms

Therapeutic outcome: Decreased growth and spread of malignant cells

USES: Multiple myeloma previously untreated or when at least two other treatments have failed; mantle cell lymphoma

CONTRAINDICATIONS:
Pregnancy **D**, breastfeeding, hypersensitivity to this product, boron, or mannitol

Precautions: Peripheral neuropathy, children, geriatric, renal/hepatic disease, hypotension, tumor lysis syndrome, thrombocytopenia, infection, diabetes mellitus, bone marrow suppression

DOSAGE AND ROUTES

Multiple myeloma (previously untreated)

Adult: IV bol Give for 9 6-wk cycles; cycle 1-4, 1.3 mg/m^2/dose given on days 1, 4, 8, 11, then a 10-day rest period (days 12-21) and again on days 22, 25, 29, 32, then a 10-day rest period (days 33-42) given with melphalan (9 mg/m^2/day on days 1-4) and predniSONE (60 mg/m^2/day on days 1-4); this 6-wk cycle is considered one course; in cycles 5-9, give bortezomib 1.3 mg/m^2/dose on days 1, 8, 22, 29 with melphalan (9 mg/m^2/day on days 1-4) and predniSONE (60 mg/m^2/day on days 1-4); this 6-wk cycle is considered one course; at least 72 hr should elapse between consecutive doses

Mantle cell lymphoma

Adult: IV bol 1.3 mg/m^2/dose (days 1, 4, 8, 11) followed by 10-day rest period (days 12 to 21); max 8 cycles

Neuropathic pain

Grade 1 with pain or grade 2, reduce to 1 mg/m^2; grade 2 with pain or grade 3, hold product until toxicity resolves, then start at 0.7 mg/m^2 qwk; grade 4 hematologic toxicities, withhold use

Hepatic dose

Adult: IV bilirubin >1.5 × ULN reduce to 0.7 mg/m^2 in cycle 1, consider dose escalation to 1 mg/m^2 or further reduction to 0.5 mg/m^2 in next cycles based on tolerability

Available forms: Lyophilized powder for inj 3.5 mg

Implementation

IV direct
• **Reconstitute** each vial with 3.5 ml 0.9% NaCl (1 mg/ml), sol should be clear/colorless; **inject** bol over 3-5 sec
• Use protective clothing during handling, preparation; avoid contact with skin

ADVERSE EFFECTS

CNS: Anxiety, insomnia, dizziness, headache, peripheral neuropathy, rigors, paresthesia
CV: Hypotension, edema, **CHF**
GI: Abdominal pain, constipation, diarrhea, dyspepsia, nausea, vomiting, anorexia

HEMA: Anemia, neutropenia, thrombocytopenia
MISC: Dehydration, weight loss, herpes zoster, rash, pruritus, blurred vision
MS: Fatigue, malaise, weakness, arthralgia, bone pain, muscle cramps, myalgia, back pain, tumor lysis syndrome
RESP: Cough, pneumonia, dyspnea, URI

Pharmacokinetics

Absorption	Unknown
Distribution	Protein binding 83%
Metabolism	P450 enzymes (3A4, 2D6, 2C19, 2C9, 1A2)
Excretion	Unknown
Half-life	9-15 hr

Pharmacodynamics

Unknown

INTERACTIONS

Individual drugs

Amiodarone, amprenavir, chloramphenicol, cisplatin, colchicine, cycloSPORINE, dapsone, didanosine, disulfiram, docetaxel, gold salts, INH, iodoquinal, isoniazid, lamivudine, metronidazole, nitrofurantoin, oxaliplatin, paclitaxel, penicillamine, phenytoin, ritonavir, stavudine, sulfasalazine, thalidomide, vinBLAStine, vinCRIStine, zacatabine, zidovudine, and others: increased peripheral neuropathy

Drug classifications

Anticoagulants, NSAIDs, platelet inhibitors, salicylates, thrombolytics: increased bleeding risk

Antihypertensives: increased hypotension

Antivirals, statins, HMG-CoA reductase inhibitors: increased peripheral neuropathy

Hematopoietic pregenitor cells (sargramostim, filgrastim): do not use within 24 hr of chemotherapy

Oral hypoglycemics: increased hypo/hyperglycemia

Products that induce or inhibit CYP3A4: increased toxicity or decreased efficacy

Drug/herb

St. John's wort: toxicity or decreased efficacy

NURSING CONSIDERATIONS

Assessment

• Assess hematologic status: platelets, CBC throughout treatment
• Monitor for extravasation at inj site

Adverse effects: *italics* = common; **bold** = life-threatening

Nursing diagnoses
• Injury, risk for (uses, adverse reactions)
• Knowledge, deficient (teaching)

Patient/family education
• Teach to use contraception while on this product, avoid breastfeeding
• Advise diabetic to monitor blood glucose levels
• Instruct to contact prescriber if new or worsening peripheral neuropathy, severe vomiting, diarrhea
• Advise to avoid driving, operating machinery until effect is known
• Advise to avoid using other medications unless approved by prescriber

Evaluation
Positive therapeutic outcome
• Improvement of multiple myeloma symptoms

---

bosentan (Rx)
(boh-sen-tan)
Tracleer
Func. class.: Vasodilator
Chem. class.: Endothelin receptor antagonist
Pregnancy category X

ACTION: Peripheral vasodilation occurs via antagonism of the effect of endothelin on endothelium and vascular smooth muscle

Therapeutic outcome: Decreased pulmonary arterial hypertension

USES: Pulmonary arterial hypertension with WHO class III, IV symptoms

Unlabeled uses: Septic shock to improve microcirculatory blood flow

CONTRAINDICATIONS:
Pregnancy **X**, hypersensitivity, CVA, CAD

Precautions: Breastfeeding, children, geriatric, mitral stenosis, impaired hepatic function

> **BLACK BOX WARNING:** Hepatic disease

DOSAGE AND ROUTES
Adult >40 kg and child >12 yr: PO 62.5 mg bid × 4 wk, then 125 mg bid
Adult <40 kg and child >12 yr: PO 62.5 mg bid

Adults taking a protease inhibitor for ≥10 days
Adult: PO 62.5 mg qday or every other day based on tolerance

Available forms: Tabs 62.5, 125 mg

Implementation
• Store at room temperature

ADVERSE EFFECTS
CNS: Headache, flushing, fatigue, fever
CV: *Hypo/hypertension,* palpitations, edema of lower limbs
GI: Abnormal liver function, dyspepsia, **hepatotoxicity,** diarrhea
HEMA: Anemia, leukopenia, neutropenia, lymphopenia, thrombocytopenia
INTEG: Pruritus, **Stevens-Johnson syndrome, toxic epidermal necrolysis,** rash
MISC: Anaphylaxis, oligospermia, tumor lysis syndrome
SYST: Secondary malignancy

Pharmacokinetics
Absorption	50% absorbed
Distribution	Protein binding >98%
Metabolism	Liver (metabolites); metabolized CYP2C9, CYP3A4, and possibly CYP2C19; steady state 3-5 days
Excretion	Biliary
Half-life	5 hr

Pharmacodynamics
Unknown

INTERACTIONS

Individual drugs
CycloSPORINE A, glyBURIDE: do not coadminister
CycloSPORINE A, ketoconazole: increased bosentan level
CycloSPORINE: decreased cycloSPORINE level
GlyBURIDE: glyBURIDE level decreased significantly, bosentan also decreased, increased liver function tests
Ketoconazole: increased bosentan level
Simvastatin: decreased effects
Warfarin: decreased anticoagulation

Drug classifications
Contraceptives (hormonal), statins: decreased effects
CYP2C9, CYP3A4 inhibitors: increased bosentan effects

Drug/lab test
Increased: ALT, AST
Decreased: Hgb, Hct

NURSING CONSIDERATIONS
Assessment
• **Serious skin toxicities:** Stevens-Johnson syndrome, toxic epidermal necrolysis
• Assess B/P, pulse during treatment until stable
• Assess hepatic toxicity: AST, ALT, bilirubin; liver enzymes may increase; if ALT/AST >3 and ≤5 × ULN, decrease dose or interrupt treatment and monitor AST/ALT q2wk; if >2 × ULN, and bilirubin >2 × ULN or signs of hepatitis, hepatic disease, stop treatment; vomiting, jaundice; product should be discontinued
• Assess blood studies: Hct, Hgb may be decreased

Nursing diagnoses
• Knowledge, deficient (teaching)
• Tissue perfusion, ineffective (uses)

Patient/family education
• Instruct patient to report jaundice, dark urine, joint pain, fatigue, malaise, bruising, easy bleeding; may indicate blood dyscrasias
• Caution patient to avoid pregnancy; to use nonhormonal form of contraception

Evaluation
Positive therapeutic outcome
• Decrease in pulmonary hypertension

brentuximab (Rx)
(bren-tak′see-mab)
Adcetris
Func. class.: Monoclonal antibody; antineoplastic
Pregnancy category D

ACTION: The anticancer activity is due to the binding of the ADC to CD30-expressing cells, followed by the internalization and transportation of the ADC-CD30 complex to lysosomes, and the release of MMAE via selective proteolytic cleavage. MMAE binds to tubulin and disrupts the microtubule network within the cell, inducing cell cycle arrest and apoptotic death of the cells

Therapeutic outcome: Decreasing symptoms of Hodgkin's disease (increased lymph nodes, night sweats, weight loss, splenomegaly, hepatomegaly)

USES: For the treatment of Hodgkin's disease after failure of autologous stem cell transplant (ASCT) or after failure of at least 2 prior multi-agent chemotherapy regimens in patients who are not ASCT candidates; For the treatment of non-Hodgkin's lymphoma (NHL): For the treatment of systemic anaplastic large cell lymphoma (sALCL) after failure of at least one prior multi-agent chemotherapy regimen

CONTRAINDICATIONS:
Hypersensitivity, pregnancy D

> **BLACK BOX WARNING:** Progressive multifocal leukoencephalopathy (PML)

Precautions: Breastfeeding, children, infants, neonates, neutropenia, peripheral neuropathy, tumor lysis syndrome (TLS)

DOSAGE AND ROUTES
Adult: IV 1.8 mg/kg IV over 30 minutes every 3 weeks until a maximum of 16 cycles, disease progression, or unacceptable toxicity. For patients >100 kg, max weight used for dosage calculation should be 100 kg, which translates to no more than 180 mg/dose

Dose adjustments for toxicity due to peripheral neuropathy:
For Grade <3: No dosage adjustments are recommended; For new or worsening grade 2/3: Interrupt treatment until toxicity resolves to grade ≤1; when resuming treatment, reduce dosage to 1.2 mg/kg IV q 3 wks; For Grade 4: Discontinue treatment

Dose adjustments for toxicity due to neutropenia:
For neutropenia Grade <3: No dosage adjustments; For Grade 3/4 neutropenia: Interrupt treatment until toxicity resolves to baseline or grade ≤2; consider the use of growth factors (CSFs) for subsequent cycles of therapy; For Grade 4 neutropenia despite the use of growth factors: Discontinue treatment or reduce the dose to 1.2 mg/kg IV q 3 weeks

Available forms: Powder for injection 50 mg

Implementation:
Intermittent IV infusion route
• Visually inspect for particulate matter and discoloration whenever solution and container permit
• Give only as an IV infusion, do not give as an IV push or bolus
• Use cytoxic handling procedures
• Do not mix with, or administer as an infusion with, other IV products

• Calculate the dose (mg) and the number of vials required. For patients weighing >100 kg, use 100 kg to calculate the dose; reconstitute each 50 mg vial/10.5 ml of sterile water for injection (5 mg/ml)
• Direct the stream of sterile water toward the wall of the vial and not directly at the cake or powder; gently swirl the vial to aid in dissolution, do not shake
• Discard any unused portion left in the vial
• After reconstitution, dilute immediately with ≥100 ml of 0.9% sodium chloride, 5% dextrose, or lactated ringers solution to a final concentration (0.4 mg/ml-1.8 mg/ml)
• Use the diluted solution immediately or store in refrigerator for ≤24 hrs after reconstitution; do not freeze
• Infuse over 30 min

ADVERSE EFFECTS

CNS: Headache, dizziness, fever, peripheral neuropathy, anxiety, chills, confusion, fatigue, paresthesias, insomnia, night sweats
CV: Peripheral edema, supraventricular arrhythmia
GI: Abdominal pain, nausea, vomiting, constipation, diarrhea, weight loss
INTEG: Rash, pruritus, alopecia, xerosis
RESP: Pneumothorax, pneumonitis, pulmonary embolism, dyspnea, cough
SYST: Anaphylaxis, tumor lysis syndrome, antibody formation, Stevens-Johnson syndrome

Pharmacokinetics

Absorption	Unknown
Distribution	Protein binding, 68%-82%
Metabolism	Small amount, potent inhibitors or inducers of CYP3A4, may alter action
Excretion	Unknown
Half-life	Terminal 4-6 days; three components are released: MMAE (monomethyl auristatin E), ADC, and the total antibody; the half-life of MMAE a component is 3.43-3.6 days

Pharmacodynamics

Onset	Unknown
Peak	ADC: End of infusion MME: 1-3 days
Duration	Unknown

INTERACTIONS

Individual drugs

Boceprevir, dalfopristin; delavirdine, isoniazid, indinavir, itraconazole, ketoconazole, quinupristin, rifampin, ritonavir, telithromycin, tipranavir: increased brentuximab component action:
Bleomycin: increased non-infectious pulmonary toxicity; do not use together

Drug/herb

St. John's wort: increased brentuximab component action

NURSING CONSIDERATIONS

Assessment

• **Tumor lysis syndrome (TLS): Assess for hyperkalemia, hyperphosphatemia, hypocalcemia; may develop renal failure may use allopurinol or rasburicase to prevent TLS; monitor serum BUN/Creatinine**
• Pregnancy: determine if pregnancy is planned or suspected, pregnancy D
• Peripheral neuropathy:
• **Progressive multifocal leukoencephalopathy (PML): Assess for weakness, or paralysis, vision loss, impaired speech, and cognitive deterioration; often fatal**
• Monitor CBC

Nursing diagnoses

• Risk for injury (uses, adverse reactions)
• Knowledge deficit (teaching)

Patient/family education

• **Teach patient to report immediately weakness, change in vision, impaired speech**
• **Advise patient to use reliable contraception, pregnancy D; avoid breastfeeding**

Evaluation

Positive therapeutic outcome
• Decreasing symptoms of Hodgkin's disease (increased lymph nodes, night sweats, weight loss, splenomegaly, hepatomegaly)

brimonidine ophthalmic
See Appendix B

brinzolamide ophthalmic
See Appendix B

bromfenac ophthalmic
See Appendix B

bromocriptine (Rx)
(broe-moe-krip′teen)
**Apo-Bromocriptine ✝, Cycloset,
Parlodel, PMS-Bromocriptine**
Func. class.: Antiparkinsonian agent;
DOPamine receptor agonist
Chem. class.: Ergot alkaloid derivative
Pregnancy category B

Do not confuse:
Parlodel/pindolol/Provera

ACTION: Inhibits prolactin release by activating postsynaptic dopamine receptors; activation of striatal dopamine receptors may be reason for improvement in Parkinson's disease

Therapeutic outcome: Decreased involuntary movements in Parkinson's disease; decreased breastfeeding; decreased hormone levels in acromegaly; absence of amenorrhea in hyperprolactinemia

USES: Parkinson's disease, amenorrhea/galactorrhea caused by hyperprolactinemia, infertility, acromegaly, pituitary adenomas, adjunct in type 2 diabetes

Unlabeled uses: Neuroleptic malignant syndrome, alcoholism, premenstrual syndrome, mastalgia, cocaine withdrawal, premenstrual breast syndromes

CONTRAINDICATIONS:
Hypersensitivity to ergot, bromocriptine; severe ischemic disease, severe peripheral vascular disease, uncontrolled hypertension, preeclampsia, migraine

Precautions: Pregnancy **B**, breastfeeding, children, hepatic/renal disease, pituitary tumors, peptic ulcer disease, sulfite hypersensitivity, pulmonary fibrosis, dementia, GI bleeding, bipolar disorder

DOSAGE AND ROUTES
Hyperprolactinemia
Adult: PO 1.25-2.5 mg with meals; may increase by 2.5 mg q3-7days; usual dosage 2.5-15 mg/day

Acromegaly
Adult: PO 1.25-2.5 mg/day × 3 days at bedtime; may increase by 1.25-2.5 mg q3-7days; usual range 20-30 mg/day; max 100 mg/day

Type 2 diabetes (Cycloset only)
Adult: PO (initially) 0.8 mg qd in AM within 2hr of waking, titrate by 0.8 mg/day no more than qwk to max 1.6-4.8 mg/day

Parkinson's disease
Adult: PO 1.25 mg bid with meals; may increase q2-4wk by 2.5 mg/day; not to exceed 100 mg/day, levodopa should be continued while bromocriptine is being instituted

Pituitary adenoma
Adult: PO 1.25 mg bid-tid, may increase over several weeks to 10-20 mg/day

Neuroleptic malignant syndrome (unlabeled)
Adult: PO 2.5-10 mg tid

Cocaine withdrawal (unlabeled)
Adult: PO 0.625 mg qid × 42 days

Alcoholism (unlabeled)
Adult: PO 7.5 mg/day

Mastalgia (unlabeled)
Adult: PO 2.5-7.5 bid, starting 10-14 days prior to menses, discontinue when menses begins

Available forms: Caps 5 mg; tabs 2.5 mg; Cycloset tabs 0.8 mg

Implementation
• Give with meals or milk to prevent GI symptoms; crush tab if patient has swallowing difficulty
• Give at bedtime so dizziness, orthostatic hypotension do not occur
• Store at room temperature in air-tight container

ADVERSE EFFECTS
CNS: *Headache,* depression, restlessness, anxiety, nervousness, confusion, **seizures,** hallucinations, *dizziness,* fatigue, drowsiness, abnormal involuntary movements, psychosis
CV: *Orthostatic hypotension,* decreased B/P, palpitations, extrasystole, **shock,** dysrhythmias, bradycardia, **MI**
EENT: Blurred vision, diplopia, burning eyes, nasal congestion
GI: *Nausea, vomiting, anorexia,* cramps, constipation, diarrhea, dry mouth, GI hemorrhage
GU: Frequency, retention, incontinence, diuresis
INTEG: *Rash on face, arms,* alopecia, coolness, pallor of fingers, toes, peripheral edema

Adverse effects: *italics* = common; **bold** = life-threatening

Pharmacokinetics

Absorption	Poorly absorbed
Distribution	Unknown
Metabolism	Liver, completely
Excretion	85%-98% feces
Half-life	4 hr (initial); 50 hr (terminal)

Pharmacodynamics

Onset	$1/2$-$1^1/2$ hr
Peak	1-3 hr
Duration	8-12 hr

INTERACTIONS

Individual drugs
Alcohol: increased disulfiram-like reaction
Haloperidol, loxapine, methyldopa, meto-
clopramide, reserpine: decreased levels of
bromocriptine
Levodopa: increased neurologic effects

Drug classifications
Antihypertensives: increased hypotension
Contraceptives (oral), estrogens, MAOIs,
phenothiazines, progestins: decreased levels
of bromocriptine

Drug/herb
Horehound: increased serotonin effect

Drug/lab test
Increased: growth hormone, AST, ALT, BUN, CK,
uric acid, alkaline phosphatase

NURSING CONSIDERATIONS

Assessment
• Assess symptoms of **Parkinson's disease**
(EPS): shuffling gait, muscle rigidity, involuntary
movements, pill rolling, muscle spasms, drooling before, during treatment
• Assess for resolution of symptoms of **neuroleptic malignant syndrome:** decreased temp,
seizures, sweating, pulse
• Monitor for change in size of soft tissue
volume in acromegaly
• Monitor B/P; establish baseline, compare
with other readings; this product decreases B/P;
patient should remain recumbent for 2-4 hr
after first dose; supervise ambulation

Nursing diagnoses
• Knowledge, deficient (teaching)
• Mobility, impaired physical (uses)

Patient/family education
• Advise patient to change position slowly to
prevent orthostatic hypotension

• Tabs may be crushed and mixed with food
• Caution patient to use contraceptives during
treatment with this product; pregnancy may occur; to use methods other than oral contraceptives
• Teach patient that therapeutic effect for Parkinson's disease may take 2 mo: galactorrhea,
amenorrhea
• Caution patient to avoid hazardous activity if
dizziness, drowsiness occurs during treatment
start-up
• Advise patient to avoid alcohol and OTC
medication unless approved by prescriber
• Teach patients with acromegaly to notify prescriber immediately if severe headache, nausea,
vomiting, blurred vision occur; indicates change
in or enlargement of tumor
• Advise patient to report symptoms of MI immediately

Evaluation
Positive therapeutic outcome
• Parkinson's disease: decreased slow move-
ments, decreased drooling
• Decreased breast engorgement with accompa-
nied pain, tenderness
• Acromegaly: decreased growth hormone levels

budesonide (Rx)
(byoo-des'oh-nide)
**Entocort EC, Gen-
Budesonide AQ ❖, Pulmicort,
Pulmicort Flexhaler, Rhinocort Aqua**
Func. class.: Glucocorticoid
Pregnancy category C

ACTION: Prevents inflammation by
depression of migration of polymorphonuclear
leukocytes, fibroblasts, reversal of increased
capillary permeability and lysosomal stabilization; does not suppress hypothalamus and
pituitary function

USES: Rhinitis; prophylaxis for asthma;
Crohn's disease

CONTRAINDICATIONS:
Hypersensitivity, status asthmaticus

Precautions: Pregnancy **C**; inhaled form
pregnancy **B**; breastfeeding, children, TB, fungal, bacterial, systemic viral infections, ocular
herpes simplex, nasal septal ulcers; hepatic
disease (caps)

DOSAGE AND ROUTES

Rhinitis (Rhinocort Aqua)
Adult and child >6 yr: Spray/inh 256 mcg/day (2 sprays in each nostril AM, PM, or 4 sprays in each nostril AM)

Asthma
Adult and child ≥6 yr: INH 400-1200 mcg/day

Crohn's disease
Adult: PO 9 mg daily AM × 8 wk

Available forms: Dry powder for INH 90, 180, 200 mg/actuation (Pulmicort Flexhaler); 32 mcg/actuation (Rhinocort Aqua)

Implementation
PO route (Crohn's disease)
• Swallow caps whole; do not break, crush, or chew
• May repeat 8-wk course if needed; may taper to 6 mg/day for 2 wk before cessation
INH route (asthma)
• Use scissors to open pouch
• Store at 59°-86° F (15°-30° C); keep away from heat, open flame

ADVERSE EFFECTS
CNS: *Headache,* insomnia, hypertonia, syncope, dizziness, drowsiness
CV: Chest pain, hypertension, sinus tachycardia, palpitation
EENT: *Sinusitis, pharyngitis,* rhinitis, oral candidiasis
ENDO: Adrenal insufficiency, growth suppression in children
GI: Dry mouth, dyspepsia, nausea, vomiting, abdominal pain
MISC: Ecchymosis, fever, *hypersensitivity,* flulike symptoms, epistaxis, dysuria
MS: Back pain, myalgias, fractures
RESP: Nasal irritation, cough, nasal bleeding, *respiratory infections,* **bronchospasm**

Pharmacokinetics

Absorption	39%
Distribution	In airways, protein binding 85%-90%
Metabolism	Liver
Excretion	In urine (60%), small amounts in feces, enters breast milk
Half-life	2-3.6 hr

Pharmacodynamics

Onset	Respules 2-8 days, Rhinocort Aqua 10 hr
Peak	Respules 4-6 wk, Rhinocort Aqua 2 wk
Duration	Unknown

INTERACTIONS
Avoid using with products metabolized by CYP3A4 inhibition

Individual drugs
Cimetidine, ketoconazole: decreased budesonide metabolism
Varicella live vaccine: avoid concurrent use in pediatric patients

NURSING CONSIDERATIONS

Assessment
• Assess respiratory status: rate, rhythm, increase in bronchial secretions, wheezing, chest tightness; provide fluids to 2 L/day to decrease thickness of secretions; check for oral candidiasis
• For **bronchospasm**, stop treatment and give bronchodilator
• With viral infections, corticosteroid use can mask infections
• For increased intraocular pressure, discontinue use if increase occurs

Nursing diagnoses
• Airway clearance, ineffective (uses)
• Injury, risk for (uses)
• Knowledge, deficient (teaching)

Patient/family education
• Teach patient to notify prescriber of pharyngitis, nasal bleeding, oral candidiasis
• Instruct patient not to exceed recommended dosage; adrenal suppression may occur
• Teach patient to carry/wear emergency ID identifying steroid use
• Instruct patient to read and follow package directions
• Instruct patient to prevent exposure to infections, especially viral
• Advise to use good oral hygiene if using by nebulizer or inhaler
• Teach patient to avoid breastfeeding

Evaluation
Positive therapeutic outcome
• Absence of asthma, rhinitis

budesonide nasal agent
See Appendix B

Adverse effects: *italics* = common; **bold** = life-threatening

bumetanide (Rx)

(byoo-met'a-nide)

Func. class.: Loop diuretic, antihypertensive

Chem. class.: Sulfonamide derivative

Pregnancy category C

ACTION: Acts on the ascending loop of Henle in the kidney to inhibit the reabsorption of the electrolytes sodium and chloride

Therapeutic outcome: Decreased edema in lung tissue and peripherally; decreased B/P

USES: Edema in congestive heart failure, renal/hepatic disease, ascites, heart failure

CONTRAINDICATIONS:

Hypersensitivity to sulfonamides, anuria, hepatic coma

> **BLACK BOX WARNING:** Electrolyte imbalance

Precautions: Pregnancy **C**, breastfeeding, neonates, severe renal disease, ascites, hepatic cirrhosis, blood dyscrasias, ototoxicity, hyperuricemia, hypokalemia, hyperglycemia, oliguria, hypomagnesemia, hypovolemia

> **BLACK BOX WARNING:** Dehydration

DOSAGE AND ROUTES

Adult/adolescent: PO 0.5-2 mg daily may give 2nd or 3rd dose at 4-5 hr intervals; max 10 mg/day; may be given on alternate days or intermittently; IM/IV 0.5-1 mg; may give 2nd or 3rd dose at 2-3 hr intervals; max 10 mg/day

Child (unlabeled): PO/IM/IV 0.015-0.1 mg/kg q day or every other day, max 10 mg/day

Available forms: Tabs 0.5, 1, 2 mg; inj 0.25 mg/ml

Implementation

• Give in AM to avoid interference with sleep

• Potassium replacement if potassium level is <3.0 mg/dl whole, or use oral solutions; product may be crushed if patient is unable to swallow

PO route

• With food, if nausea occurs; absorption may be reduced; the safest dosage schedule is on alternate days

IV route

• Do not use solution that is yellow or has a precipitate or crystals

IV, direct route

• Give undiluted through Y-tube or 3-way stopcock; give 20 mg or less/min

Intermittent IV infusion route

• May be added to 0.9% NaCl, D_5W, $D_{10}W$, $D_{20}W$, invert sugar 10% in electrolyte #1, LR, sodium lactate $^1/_6$ mol/L; use within 24 hr to ensure compatibility; give through Y-tube or 3-way stopcock; give at 4 mg/min or less; use infusion pump

Syringe compatibility: Doxapram

Y-site compatibilities: Acyclovir, alfentanil, allopurinol, amifostine, amikacin, aminocaproic acid, aminophylline, amiodarone, amoxicillin, amphotericin B lipid complex (Abelcet), amphotericin B liposome (AmBisome), anidulafungin, ascorbic acid injection, atenolol, atracurium, atropine, aztreonam, benztropine, bivalirudin, bleomycin, buprenorphine, butorphanol, calcium chloride/gluconate, CARBOplatin, caspofungin, cefamandole, ceFAZolin, cefepime, cefmetazole, cefonicid, cefoperazone, cefotaxime, cefotetan, cefoxitin, ceftazidime, ceftizoxime, ceftobiprole, cefTRIAXone, cefuroxime, cephalothin, cephapirin, chloramphenicol, cimetidine, cisatracurium, CISplatin, cladribine, clarithromycin, clindamycin, codeine, cyanocobalamin, cyclophosphamide, cycloSPORINE, cytarabine, DACTINomycin, DAPTOmycin, dexamethasone, dexmedetomidine, digoxin, diltiazem, diphenhydrAMINE, DOBUTamine, docetaxel, DOPamine, doripenem, doxacurium, DOXOrubicin, doxycycline, enalaprilat, ePHEDrine, EPINEPHrine, epirubicin, epoetin alfa, eptifibatide, ertapenem, erythromycin, esmolol, etoposide, famotidine, fentaNYL, filgrastim, fluconazole, fludarabine, fluorouracil, folic acid, furosemide, gatifloxacin, gemcitabine, gentamicin, glycopyrrolate, granisetron, heparin, hydrocortisone sodium succinate, HYDROmorphone, hydrOXYzine, IDArubicin, ifosfamide, imipenem-cilastatin, indomethacin, insulin (regular), irinotecan, isoproterenol, ketorolac, labetalol, levofloxacin, lidocaine, linezolid, LORazepam, magnesium sulfate, mannitol, mechlorethamine, melphalan, meperidine, metaraminol, methotrexate, methoxamine, methyldopa, methylPREDNISolone, metoclopramide, metoprolol, metroNIDAZOLE, mezlocillin, micafungin, miconazole, milrinone, mitoxantrone, morphine, moxalactam, multiple vitamins injection, mycophenolate, nafcillin, nalbuphine, naloxone, netilmicin, nitroglycerin, nitroprusside, norepinephrine, octreotide, ondansetron, oxacillin, oxaliplatin, oxytocin, palonosetron, pamidronate, pancuronium, pantoprazole, pemetrexed, penicillin G potassium/sodium, pentazocine, PENTobarbital, PHENobarbital, phenylephrine, phytonadione, piperacillin, piperacillin-tazobactam, polymyxin B, potassium chloride, procainamide, promethazine, propofol, propranolol, protamine, pyridoxine, quiNIDine, ranitidine, remifentanil, rifampin, ritodrine, riTUXimab, rocuronium, sodium acetate, sodium bicarbonate, succinylcholine, SUFentanil, tacrolimus, teniposide, theophylline, thiamine, thiotepa, ticarcillin, ticarcillin-clavulanate, tigecycline, tirofiban, TNA, tobramycin, tolazoline, TPN, tramadol, trastuzumab, trimetaphan, urokinase, vancomycin, vasopressin, vecuronium, verapamil, vinCRIStine, vinorelbine, voriconazole

ADVERSE EFFECTS

CNS: Headache, fatigue, weakness, vertigo, encephalopathy
CV: *Hypotension*, chest pain, ECG changes, **circulatory collapse**, dehydration
EENT: Loss of hearing
ELECT: *Hypokalemia, hypochloremic alkalosis, hypomagnesemia, hyperuricemia, hypocalcemia, hyponatremia*
ENDO: *Hyperglycemia*
GI: *Nausea*, diarrhea, dry mouth, vomiting, anorexia, cramps, **acute pancreatitis**, upset stomach, abdominal pain, **jaundice**
GU: *Polyuria*, **renal failure**, *glycosuria*, premature ejaculation, hypercholesterolemia
HEMA: **Thrombocytopenia, leukopenia, granulocytopenia, hemoconcentration**
INTEG: *Rash, pruritus, purpura*, **Stevens-Johnson syndrome**, sweating, photosensitivity
MS: Muscular cramps, stiffness, arthritis

Pharmacokinetics

	PO/IM
Absorption	Rapidly, completely absorbed
	PO/IM/IV
Distribution	Crosses placenta, protein binding >91%
Metabolism	Liver (30%-40%)
Excretion	Breast milk, urine (50% unchanged), feces (20%)
Half-life	1-1½ hr; 6-15 hr neonates

Pharmacodynamics

	PO	IM	IV
Onset	½-1 hr	40 min	5 min
Peak	1-2 hr	1-2 hr	½ hr
Duration	3-6 hr	4-6 hr	3-6 hr

INTERACTIONS

Individual drugs

Digoxin: increased toxicity
Indomethacin: decreased diuretic and antihypertensive effects of bumetanide
Lithium: decreased renal clearance causing increased toxicity
Metolazone: increased diuresis, electrolyte loss
Probenecid: decreased diuretic effect

Drug classifications

Aminoglycosides: increased ototoxicity
Antidiabetics: decreased antidiabetic effects
NSAIDs: decreased diuretic effect
Potassium-wasting products: increased hypokalemia

Drug/herb

Hawthorn, horse chestnut: increased diuretic effect

NURSING CONSIDERATIONS

Assessment

• Assess patient for tinnitus, hearing loss, ear pain; periodic testing of hearing is needed when high doses of this product are given by **IV** route
• Assess fluid volume status: I&O ratio and record, distended red veins, crackles in lung, color, quality and specific gravity of urine, skin turgor, adequacy of pulses, moist mucous membranes, bilateral lung sounds, peripheral pitting edema; dehydration symptoms of decreasing output, thirst, hypotension, dry mouth and mucous membranes should be reported; if urinary output decreases or azotemia occurs, product should be discontinued
• Monitor for electrolyte imbalances: potassium, sodium, calcium, magnesium; also include BUN, blood pH, ABGs, uric acid, CBC, blood glucose; severe electrolyte imbalances should be corrected before starting treatment
• Assess B/P before and during therapy with patient lying, standing, and sitting as appropriate; orthostatic hypotension can occur rapidly
• Monitor for **digoxin toxicity** (anorexia, nausea, vomiting, confusion, paresthesia, muscle cramps) in patients taking digoxin; lithium toxicity in those taking lithium

Nursing diagnoses

• Fluid volume, deficient (side effects)
• Fluid volume, excess (uses)
• Knowledge, deficient (teaching)
• Urinary elimination, impaired (side effects)

Patient/family education

• Teach patient to take the medication early in the day to prevent nocturia

- Instruct the patient to take with food or milk if GI symptoms of nausea and anorexia occur
- Teach patient to maintain weekly record of weight and notify prescriber of weight loss of >5 lb
- Caution the patient that this product causes a loss of potassium, so food rich in potassium should be added to the diet; refer to a dietitian for assistance in planning
- Caution the patient not to exercise in hot weather or stand for prolonged periods since orthostatic hypotension will be enhanced
- Teach patient not to use alcohol or any OTC medications without prescriber's approval; serious product reactions may occur
- Emphasize the need to contact prescriber immediately if muscle cramps, weakness, nausea, dizziness, or numbness occur
- Teach patient to take own B/P and pulse and record
- Caution the patient that orthostatic hypotension may occur; patient should rise slowly from sitting or reclining positions and lie down if dizziness occurs
- Teach patient to continue taking medication even if feeling better; this product controls symptoms but does not cure the condition
- Advise the patient with hypertension to continue other medical treatment (exercise, weight loss, relaxation techniques, cessation of smoking)

Evaluation
Positive therapeutic outcome
- Decreased edema
- Decreased B/P
- Increased diuresis

---

buprenorphine (Rx)
(byoo-pre-nor′feen)
Buprenex, Butrans, Subutex
Func. class.: Opioid analgesic, partial agonist
Chem. class.: Thebaine derivative
Pregnancy category C
Controlled substance schedule V
(parenteral); schedule III (tablet)

Do not confuse:
Buprenex/Bumex

ACTION: Depresses pain impulse transmission at the spinal cord level by interacting with opioid receptors

Therapeutic outcome: Relief of pain

USES: Moderate to severe pain, opiate agonist withdrawal

Unlabeled uses: Cocaine

CONTRAINDICATIONS:
Hypersensitivity, ileus

Precautions: Pregnancy **C,** breastfeeding, substance abuse/alcoholism, increased intracranial pressure, MI (acute), severe heart disease, respiratory depression, renal/hepatic/pulmonary disease, hypothyroidism, Addison's disease

> **BLACK BOX WARNING:** QT prolongation, use of heating pad

DOSAGE AND ROUTES
Adult: IM/IV 0.3 mg q6hr prn; may repeat; reduce dosage in geriatric, may repeat after 30-60 min; EPIDURAL (unlabeled) 4 mcg/kg or 2 mcg/kg (epidural injection), remove over 48 hr; TD: each patch is worn for 7 days (moderate-severe pain); **opioid-naive patients** (those taking <30 mg oral morphine or equivalent prior to beginning treatment with TD buprenorphine), 5 mcg/hr q7days, overestimating dose can be fatal; **conversion from other opiate agonist therapy,** titrate from other opioids for up to 7 days to no more than 30 mg oral morphine or equivalent prior to beginning TD therapy, begin with 5 mcg/hr q7days; for those with daily dose of 30-80 mg oral morphine or equivalent, start with 10 mcg/hr q7days; for those >80 mg oral morphine or equivalent start with 20 mcg/hr q7days
Child 2-12 yr: IM/IV 2-6 mcg/kg q4-6hr

Opiate dependence
Adult/adolescent ≥16 yr: SL 8 mg day 1, 16 mg day 2, then maintenance 16 mg daily

Available forms: Inj 0.3 mg/ml (1-ml vials); SL tab 2, 8 mg as base, TD system 5, 10, 20 mcg/hr (weekly)

Implementation
- Give by inj (IM, **IV**), only with resuscitative equipment available; give slowly to prevent rigidity
- Long-term use is not recommended
Transdermal route
- Apply to clean, dry, intact skin, each patch should be worn for 7 days

> **BLACK BOX WARNING:** Do not apply direct heat source to patch

- Apply to upper outer arm, upper chest/back, or side of chest

---

IM route
- **Give** deep in large muscle mass; rotate sites of inj

IV route
- **Give IV** direct undiluted over 3-5 min (0.3 mg/2 min); give slowly
- With antiemetic if nausea, vomiting occur
- When pain is beginning to return; determine dosage interval by patient response

Syringe compatibilities: Glycopyrrolate, haloperidol, heparin, midazolam

Y-site compatibilities: Acyclovir, alfentanil, allopurinol, amifostine, amikacin, aminocaproic acid, amphotericin B liposome (AmBisone), anidulafungin, ascorbic acid injection, atenolol, atracurium, atropine, aztreonam, benztropine, bivalirudin, bleomycin, bumetanide, butorphanol, calcium chloride/gluconate, CARBOplatin, cefamandole, ceFAZolin, cefepime, cefmetazole, cefonicid, cefoperazone, cefotaxime, cefotetan, cefoxitin, ceftazidime, ceftizoxime, cefTRIAXone, cefuroxime, cephalothin, cephapirin, chloramphenicol, chlorproMAZINE, cimetidine, cisatracurium, CISplatin, cladribine, clindamycin, cyanocobalamin, cyclophosphamide, cycloSPORINE, cytarabine, D₅W-dextrose 5%, DACTINomycin, DAPTOmycin, dexamethasone, dexmedetomidine, digoxin, diltiazem, diphenhydrAMINE, DOBUTamine, docetaxel, DOPamine, doxacurium, DOXOrubicin HCl, doxycycline, enalaprilat, ePHEDrine, EPINEPHrine, epirubicin, epoetin alfa, eptifibatide, ertapenem, erythromycin, esmolol, etoposide, famotidine, fenoldopam, fentaNYL, filgrastim, fluconazole, fludarabine, gatifloxacin, gemcitabine, gentamicin, glycopyrrolate, granisetron, heparin, hydrocortisone, hydrOXYzine, IDArubicin, ifosfamide, imipenem-cilastatin, inamrinone, insulin (regular), irinotecan, isoproterenol, ketorolac, labetalol, lactated Ringer's injection, levofloxacin, lidocaine, linezolid, LORazepam, magnesium sulfate, mannitol, mechlorethamine, melphalan, meperidine, metaraminol, methicillin, methotrexate, methoxamine, methyldopa, methylPREDNISolone, metoclopramide, metoprolol, metroNIDAZOLE, mezlocillin, miconazole, midazolam, milrinone, minocycline, mitoxantrone, morphine, moxalactam, multiple vitamins injection, mycophenolate mofetil, nafcillin, nalbuphine, naloxone, nesiritide, netilmicin, nitroglycerin, nitroprusside, norepinephrine, octreotide, ondansetron, oxacillin, oxaliplatin, oxytocin, palonosetron, pamidronate, pancuronium, papaverine, pemetrexed, penicillin G potassium/sodium, pentamidine, pentazocine, phenylephrine, phy-

tonadione, piperacillin, piperacillin-tazobactam, polymyxin B, potassium chloride, procainamide, prochlorperazine promethazine, propofol, propranolol, protamine, pyridoxine, quiNIDine, ranitidine, remifentanil, Ringer's injection, ritodrine, riTUXimab, rocuronium, sodium acetate, succinylcholine, SUFentanil, tacrolimus, teniposide, theophylline, thiamine, thiotepa, ticarcillin, ticarcillin-clavulanate, tigecycline, tirofiban, TNA (3-in-1), tobramycin, tolazoline, TPN, trastuzumab, trimetaphan, urokinase, vancomycin, vasopressin, vecuronium, verapamil, vinCRIStine, vinorelbine, voriconazole

Additive compatibilities: Atropine, bupivacaine, diphenhydrAMINE, droperidol, glycopyrrolate, haloperidol, hydrOXYzine, promethazine, scopolamine

Additive incompatibilities: Diazepam, floxacillin, furosemide, LORazepam

ADVERSE EFFECTS
CNS: *Drowsiness, dizziness, confusion, headache, sedation, euphoria,* **increased intracranial pressure,** amnesia
CV: Palpitations, bradycardia, change in B/P, tachycardia
EENT: Tinnitus, blurred vision, *miosis,* diplopia
GI: *Nausea,* vomiting, anorexia, constipation, cramps, dry mouth
GU: Dysuria, urinary retention
INTEG: *Rash,* urticaria, bruising, flushing, diaphoresis, pruritus
RESP: **Respiratory depression,** dyspnea, hypo/hyperventilation

Pharmacokinetics

Absorption	Well absorbed (IM)
Distribution	Crosses placenta
Metabolism	Liver, extensively by CYP3A4
Excretion	Kidneys, feces, breast milk
Half-life	2.2 hr (**IV**); 37 hr (SL)

Pharmacodynamics

	IM	IV
Onset	15 min	Immediate
Peak	1 hr	5 min
Duration	6 hr	6 hr

INTERACTIONS

Individual drugs
Alcohol: increased respiratory depression, hypotension, sedation

Drug classifications

> **BLACK BOX WARNING:** Antidysrhythmics (class IA, III): increased QT prolongation

Antihistamines, antipsychotics, CNS depressants, MAOIs, sedatives/hypnotics, skeletal muscle relaxants: increased respiratory depression, hypotension
CYP3A4 inducers (carBAMazepine, PHENobarbital, phenytoin, rifampin): decreased buprenorphine effect
CYP3A4 inhibitors (erythromycin, indinavir, ketoconazole, ritonavir, saquinavir): increased buprenorphine effect
Opioids: increased CNS depression

Drug/herb
St. John's wort: increased CNS depression

NURSING CONSIDERATIONS
Assessment
• Assess **pain characteristics:** location, intensity, type, severity before medication administration and after treatment

> **BLACK BOX WARNING: QT prolongation:** Assess often in those taking class Ia, III antidysrhythmics; patients with hypokalemia or cardiac instability (TD)

• Monitor VS after parenteral route; note muscle rigidity, product history, liver, kidney function tests, respiratory dysfunction: respiratory depression, character, rate, rhythm; notify prescriber if respirations are <10/min
• Monitor CNS changes: dizziness, drowsiness, hallucinations, euphoria, LOC, pupil reaction; withdrawal in opioid-dependent persons; if dependence occurs within 2 wk of discontinuing product, **withdrawal symptoms** will occur
• Monitor allergic reactions: rash, urticaria
• Monitor bowel pattern; severe constipation can occur

Nursing diagnoses
• Breathing pattern, ineffective (adverse reactions)
• Knowledge, deficient (teaching)
• Pain, acute (uses)
• Pain, chronic
• Sensory perception, disturbed (adverse reactions)

Patient/family education
• Instruct patient to report any symptoms of CNS changes, allergic reactions
• Caution patients to avoid CNS depressants: alcohol, sedative/hypnotics for at least 24 hr after taking this product
• Advise that tolerance may result when used for extended periods, but long-term use is not recommended
• Advise to avoid driving, other hazardous activities until reaction is known
• Discuss with patient that dizziness, drowsiness, and confusion are common; to avoid getting up without assistance; to avoid hazardous activities
• Discuss in detail all aspects of the product

Evaluation
Positive therapeutic outcome
• Relief of pain

TREATMENT OF OVERDOSE:
Naloxone 0.4 mg ampule diluted in 10 ml 0.9% NaCl, give by direct **IV** push 0.02 mg q2min (adult)

buPROPion (Rx)
(byoo-proe'pee-on)
Aplenzin, Budeprion SR, Buproban, Sandoz Bupropion ✦, Wellbutrin, Wellbutrin SR, Wellbutrin XL, Zyban
Func. class.: Antidepressant—miscellaneous, smoking deterrent
Chem. class.: Aminoketone
Pregnancy category C

Do not confuse:
buPROPion/busPIRone, Zyban/Diovan/Zagam

ACTION: Inhibits reuptake of dopamine

Therapeutic outcome: Decreased symptoms of depression after 2-3 wk

USES: Depression (Wellbutrin), smoking cessation (Zyban); seasonal affective disorder

Unlabeled uses: Neuropathic pain, enhancement of weight loss, attention-deficit/hyperactivity disorder (ADHD)

CONTRAINDICATIONS:
Hypersensitivity, eating disorders, seizure disorder

Precautions: Pregnancy **C**, breastfeeding, geriatric, renal/hepatic disease, recent MI, cranial trauma, seizure disorders

> **BLACK BOX WARNING:** Children <18 yr, suicidal thinking/behavior (young adults)

DOSAGE AND ROUTES

Depression

Adult: PO 100 mg bid initially, then increase after 3 days to 100 mg tid if needed; may increase after 1 mo to 150 mg tid; ER/SR, initially 150 mg AM, increase to 300 mg/day if initial dose is tolerated; Aplenzin 174 mg qAM; may increase to 348 mg qAM on day 4; may increase to 522 mg after several weeks if needed

Geriatric: PO 50-100 mg/day, may increase by 50-100 mg q3-4days

Smoking cessation (Zyban)

Adult: SR 150 mg q day × 3 days, then 150 mg bid for remainder of treatment, initiate 1-2 wk before targeted "quit day," continue for 7-12 wk; in combination with nicotine TD, 150 mg q day × 3 days, then 150 mg bid for remainder of treatment, give ≥8 hr apart, max 300 mg/day, initiate 1-2 wk before targeted "quit day," continue for 7-12 wk, may be continued for 8-20 wk

Available forms: Tabs 75, 100 mg; sus rel tabs (SR) 150 mg; ext rel tab (XL) 100, 150, 300 mg (SR-12 hr, XL-24 hr); ext rel tab (Aplenzin) 174, 348, 522 mg

Implementation

• Give with food or milk for GI symptoms
• Give sugarless gum, hard candy, or frequent sips of water for dry mouth
• **When switching to Aplenzin from Wellbutrin, Wellbutrin SR, or XL use these equivalents: 174 buPROPion HBr = 150 mg buPROPion HCl; 348 mg buPROPion HBr = 300 mg buPROPion HCl; 522 mg buPROPion HBr = 450 mg buPROPion HCl**
• **Wellbutrin immediate rel,** separate by ≥6 hr, give in 3 divided doses; **Wellbutrin SR,** if multiple doses are used, separate by ≥8 hr; **Wellbutrin XL,** give q day in AM; Zyban SR, give in 2 divided doses ≥8 hr apart; **Aplenzin ER,** give q day in AM, a larger dose of Aplenzin is needed because these products are not equivalent
• Store at room temperature; do not freeze

ADVERSE EFFECTS

CNS: *Headache, agitation, confusion,* **seizures,** delusions, *insomnia, sedation, tremors,* dizziness, akinesia, bradykinesia, **suicidal ideation**
CV: **Dysrhythmias,** *hypertension,* palpitations, *tachycardia,* hypotension, **complete AV block, QRS prolongation (overdose)**
EENT: *Blurred vision, auditory disturbance*

GI: *Nausea, vomiting, dry mouth,* anorexia, diarrhea, increased appetite, *constipation,* altered taste
GU: Impotence, frequency, retention, *menstrual irregularities*
INTEG: *Rash,* pruritus, *sweating,* **Stevens-Johnson syndrome**
MISC: *Weight loss or gain*

Pharmacokinetics

Absorption	Well absorbed; bioavailability poor
Distribution	Unknown
Metabolism	Liver extensively
Excretion	Kidneys
Half-life	14 hr, steady state 1½-5 wk

Pharmacodynamics

Onset	Up to 4 wk
Peak	Unknown
Duration	Unknown

INTERACTIONS

Individual drugs

Alcohol, levodopa, theophylline: increased risk of seizures
CarBAMazepine, cimetidine, phenobarbitol, phenytoin: decreased buPROPion effect
Cimetidine: increased buPROPion levels
Ritonavir: increased buPROPion toxicity
Tamoxifen: decreased effect of tamoxifen

Drug classifications

Antidepressants, benzodiazepines, MAOIs, phenothiazines, steroids (systemic): increased risk of seizures
CYP2D6/CYP2B6 inhibitors: increased buPROPion effect
CYP450, CYP2D6 products: decreased buPROPion effects
CYP2D6, CYP2B6 inducers: decreased buPROPion effect
MAOIs: acute toxicity

Drug/herb

Kava, valerian: increased CNS depression

NURSING CONSIDERATIONS

Assessment

• Monitor B/P (with patient lying, standing), pulse q4hr; if systolic B/P drops 20 mm Hg hold product, notify prescriber; take vital signs q4hr in patients with CV disease
• Assess smoking cessation progress after 7-12 wk, if progress has not been made, product should be discontinued

- Assess for increased risk of seizures; if patient has used CNS depressant or CNS stimulants, dosage of buPROPion should not be exceeded
- Monitor blood studies: CBC, leukocytes, differential, cardiac enzymes if patient is receiving long-term therapy
- Monitor hepatic studies: AST, ALT, bilirubin if on long-term treatment
- Check weight weekly; appetite may increase with product
- Assess ECG for flattening of T wave, bundle branch block, AV block, dysrhythmias in cardiac patients
- Assess for EPS primarily in geriatric: rigidity, dystonia, akathisia

> **BLACK BOX WARNING:** Assess mental status: mood, sensorium, affect, suicidal tendencies; increase in psychiatric symptoms: depression, panic

- Monitor urinary retention, constipation; constipation is more likely to occur in children or geriatric
- Identify alcohol consumption; if alcohol was consumed, hold dose

Nursing diagnoses
- Coping, ineffective (uses)
- Injury, risk for (side effects)
- Knowledge, deficient (teaching)
- Noncompliance (teaching)

Patient/family education
- Teach patient that therapeutic effects may take 2-3 wk; not to increase dose without prescriber's approval; that treatment for smoking cessation lasts 7-12 wk
- Teach patient to use caution in driving or other activities requiring alertness because of drowsiness, dizziness, blurred vision; to avoid rising quickly from sitting to standing, especially geriatric
- Teach patient to avoid alcohol ingestion; alcohol may increase risk of seizures, obtain approval for other products
- Teach patient to increase fluids, bulk in diet if constipation, urinary retention occur, especially geriatric; notify prescriber immediately if urinary retention occurs
- Teach patient to take gum, hard sugarless candy, or frequent sips of water for dry mouth
- Advise patient not to use with nicotine patches unless directed by prescriber, may increase B/P

> **BLACK BOX WARNING:** Teach patient that risk of seizures increases when dose is exceeded or if patient has seizure disorder; suicidal ideas, behavior, hostility, depression may occur in children or young adults

- Teach patient to notify prescriber if pregnancy is suspected or planned

Evaluation
Positive therapeutic outcome
- Decrease in depression
- Absence of suicidal thoughts
- Smoking cessation

TREATMENT OF OVERDOSE:
ECG monitoring, induce emesis, lavage, activated charcoal, administer anticonvulsant

---

busPIRone (Rx)
(byoo-spye'rone)
Apo-Buspirone ❀**, BuSpar, BuSpar Dividose, CO Buspirone** ❀**, Gen-Buspirone** ❀**, PMS-Buspirone** ❀
Func. class.: Antianxiety, sedative
Chem. class.: Azaspirodecanedione
Pregnancy category B

Do not confuse:
busPIRone/buPROPion

ACTION: Acts by inhibiting the action of serotonin (5-HT) by binding to serotonin and dopamine receptors; also increases norepinephrine metabolism; has shown little potential for abuse, a good choice in substance abuse

Therapeutic outcome: Decreased anxiety

USES: Management and short-term relief of generalized anxiety disorders

CONTRAINDICATIONS:
Hypersensitivity, child <18 yr

Precautions: Pregnancy **B,** breastfeeding, geriatric, impaired renal/hepatic function

DOSAGE AND ROUTES
Adult: PO 7.5 mg tid; may increase by 5 mg/day q2-3days; max 60 mg/day

Renal/hepatic dose
Adult: PO reduce by 25%-50% in mild to moderate hepatic disease, do not use in severe hepatic disease, CCr 11-70 ml/min reduce dose by 25%-50%, CCr <10 ml/min do not use

Available forms: Tabs 5, 7.5, 10, 15, 30 mg

Implementation
• Give with food or milk for GI symptoms (avoid grapefruit juice); sugarless gum, hard candy, frequent sips of water for dry mouth
• May be crushed

ADVERSE EFFECTS
CNS: *Dizziness, headache, depression, stimulation, insomnia, nervousness, light-headedness, numbness, paresthesia, incoordination, tremors,* excitement, involuntary movements, confusion, akathisia, nightmares, hostility
CV: *Tachycardia, palpitations,* hypo/hypertension, **CVA, CHF, MI**
EENT: *Sore throat, tinnitus, blurred vision, nasal congestion,* red, itching eyes, change in taste, smell
GI: *Nausea, dry mouth, diarrhea, constipation,* flatulence, increased appetite, rectal bleeding
GU: Frequency, hesitancy, menstrual irregularity, change in libido
INTEG: *Rash,* edema, pruritus, alopecia, dry skin
MISC: *Sweating,* fatigue, weight gain, fever
MS: *Pain, weakness,* muscle cramps, spasms
RESP: Hyperventilation, chest congestion, shortness of breath

Pharmacokinetics	
Absorption	Rapid
Distribution	Protein binding 86%
Metabolism	Liver, extensively
Excretion	Feces
Half-life	2-3 hr

Pharmacodynamics	
Onset	Unknown
Peak	40-90 min
Duration	Unknown

INTERACTIONS
Individual drugs
Alcohol: increased CNS depression; avoid use

Drug classifications
Products metabolized by CYP3A4 (erythromycin, itraconazole, nefazodone, ketoconazole, ritonavir, several other protease inhibitors): increased busPIRone levels
MAOIs, procarbazine: increased B/P, do not use together

Products induced by CYP3A4 (rifampin, phenytoin, PHENobarbital, carBAMazepine, dexamethasone): decreased busPIRone action
Psychotropics: increased CNS depression, avoid use
Selective serotonin reuptake inhibitors (SNRIs, serotonin receptor agonists): increase serotonin syndrome

Drug/food
Grapefruit juice: increased peak concentration of busPIRone

NURSING CONSIDERATIONS
Assessment
• Assess anxiety reaction: inability to sleep, apprehension, dread, foreboding, or uneasiness related to unidentified source of danger
• Assess for previous product dependence or tolerance; if patient is product dependent or tolerant, amount of medication should be restricted
• Monitor B/P (lying, standing), pulse; if systolic B/P drops 20 mm Hg, hold product, notify prescriber; check I&O; may indicate renal dysfunction
• Monitor mental status: mood, sensorium, affect, sleeping patterns, drowsiness, dizziness, suicidal tendencies; withdrawal symptoms when dose is reduced or product discontinued
• Assess for CNS reaction, some reactions may be unpredictable

Nursing diagnoses
• Anxiety (uses)
• Knowledge, deficient (teaching)
• Noncompliance (teaching)

Patient/family education
• Teach patient that product may be taken consistently with or without food; if dose is missed take as soon as remembered; do not double doses
• Caution patient to avoid OTC preparations unless approved by the prescriber; to avoid alcohol ingestion and other psychotropic medications unless prescribed; that 1-2 wk of therapy may be required before therapeutic effects occur; to avoid large amounts of grapefruit juice
• Caution patient to avoid driving and activities requiring alertness since drowsiness may occur; until medication response is known, tell patient that drowsiness may worsen at beginning of treatment
• Instruct patient not to discontinue medication abruptly after long-term use; if dose is missed, do not double

- Advise patient to rise slowly or fainting may occur, especially in geriatric

Evaluation
Positive therapeutic outcome
- Increased well-being
- Decreased anxiety, restlessness, sleeplessness, dread

> **⚠ HIGH ALERT**

busulfan (Rx)
(byoo-sul'fan)
Busulfex, Myleran
Func. class.: Antineoplastic alkylating agent
Chem. class.: Bifunctional alkylating agent
Pregnancy category D

Do not confuse:
Myleran/Leukeran

ACTION: Changes essential cellular ions to covalent bonding with resultant alkylation; this interferes with normal biological function of DNA; activity is not phase specific; action is due to myelosuppression

Therapeutic outcome: Prevention of rapid growth of malignant cells in chronic myelocytic leukemia

USES: Chronic myelocytic leukemia, bone marrow ablation, stem cell transplant preparation in CML

CONTRAINDICATIONS:
Pregnancy **D** (3rd trimester), breastfeeding, radiation, chemotherapy, blastic phase of chronic myelocytic leukemia, hypersensitivity

Precautions: Child-bearing-age men and women, leukopenia, thrombocytopenia, anemia, hepatotoxicity, renal toxicity, seizures, tumor lysis syndrome, hyperkalemia, hyperphosphatemia, hypocalcemia, hyperuricemia

> **BLACK BOX WARNING:** Neutropenia, secondary malignancy, thrombocytopenia

DOSAGE AND ROUTES
Chronic myelocytic leukemia
Adult: PO 4-8 mg/day or 1.8-4 mg/m²/day initially; reduce dosage if WBC levels reach 30,000-40,000/mm³; stop if WBC ≤20,000/mm³; maintenance 1-3 mg/day

Child: PO 0.06-0.12 mg/kg/day or 1.8-4.6 mg/m²/day, reduce if WBC is 30,000-40,000/mm³; discontinue if WBC ≤20,000/mm³

Allogenic hemopoietic stem cell transplantation in chronic myelogenous leukemia
Adult: IV 0.8 mg/kg over 2 hr, q6hr × 4 days (total 16 doses); give cyclophosphamide **IV** 60 mg/kg over 1 hr/day for 2 days, starting after 16th dose of busulfan

Available forms: Tabs 2 mg; sol for inj 6 mg/ml

Implementation
- Give 1 hr before or 2 hr after meals to lessen nausea and vomiting; give at same time daily
- Increased fluid intake to 2-3 L/day to prevent urate deposits, calculus formation
- Administer antibiotics for prophylaxis of infection; may be prescribed since infection potential is high
- Store in tight container

Intermittent IV infusion route
- Prepared in biologic cabinet using gloves, gown, mask; **dilute** with 10 times volume of product with D₅W or 0.9% NaCl, (0.5 mg/ml); when withdrawing product, use needle with 5-micron filter provided, remove amount needed, remove filter and **inject** product into diluent; always add product to diluent, not vice versa; stable for 8 hr at room temperature (using D₅W) or 12 hr refrigerated; **give** by central venous catheter over 2 hr q6hr × 4 days, use infusion pump, do not admix
- Give antiemetics before **IV** route, on schedule
- In those with history of seizures give phenytoin before **IV** route, to prevent seizures (using 0.9% NaCl)

Y-site compatibilities: Acyclovir, amphotericin B lipid complex, amphotericin B liposome, anidulafungin, atenolol, bivalirudin, bleomycin, caspofungin, codeine, DAPTOmycin, dexmedetomidine, diltiazem, docetaxel, ertapenem, fenoldopam, gatifloxacin, granisetron, HYDROmorphone, levofloxacin, linezolid, LORazepam, meperidine, metroNIDAZOLE, milrinone, nesiritide, octreotide acetate, ondansetron, palonosetron, pancuronium, piperacillin-tazobactam, riTUXimab, sodium acetate, tacrolimus, tigecycline, tirofiban, trastuzumab, vasopressin

ADVERSE EFFECTS
PO route
CV: *Hypotension, thrombosis, chest pain,* **tachycardia, atrial fibrillation, heart block,**

---

pericardial effusion, cardiac tamponade (high dose with cyclophosphamide)
GI: Anorexia, constipation, dry mouth, nausea, vomiting, *diarrhea*
RESP: Alveolar hemorrhage, atelectasis, cough, hemoptysis, hypoxia, pleural effusion, pneumonia, sinusitis, **pulmonary fibrosis**
IV route
CNS: Cerebral hemorrhage, coma, seizures, *anxiety, depression, dizziness, headache,* encephalopathy, weakness, mental changes
EENT: *Pharyngitis, epistaxis, cataracts*
GI: *Diarrhea, nausea, vomiting, weight loss*
GU: Impotence, sterility, amenorrhea, gynecomastia, **renal toxicity,** hyperuremia, adrenal insufficiency–like syndrome
HEMA: Thrombocytopenia, leukopenia, pancytopenia, severe bone marrow depression
INTEG: Dermatitis, hyperpigmentation, alopecia
MISC: Chromosomal aberrations
RESP: Irreversible pulmonary fibrosis, pneumonitis

Pharmacokinetics

Absorption	Rapidly absorbed
Distribution	Unknown; crosses placenta
Metabolism	Liver, extensively
Excretion	Kidneys, breast milk
Half-life	2.5 hr

Pharmacodynamics

Unknown

INTERACTIONS
Individual drugs
Acetaminophen, itraconazole: decreased busulfan clearance
Cyclophosphamide: cardiac tamponade
Phenytoin: decreased busulfan level
Radiation: increased toxicity, bone marrow suppression
Thioguanine: hepatotoxicity

Drug classifications
Anticoagulants, salicylates: increased risk of bleeding
Antineoplastics: increased toxicity, bone marrow suppression
Live virus vaccines: decreased antibody reaction

Drug/lab test
False positive: breast, bladder, cervix, lung cytology tests

NURSING CONSIDERATIONS
Assessment
• Monitor CBC, differential, platelet count weekly; withhold product for WBC <15,000/mm³ or platelets <150,000/mm³; notify prescriber of results; institute thrombocytopenia precautions, levels to withhold product are different in children

> **BLACK BOX WARNING:** Assess bone marrow status prior to chemotherapy, bone marrow suppression may be prolonged (up to 2 mo); seizure history

• **Pulmonary fibrosis:** Monitor pulmonary function tests, chest x-ray films before, during therapy; chest film should be obtained q2wk during treatment; check for dyspnea, crackles, nonproductive cough, chest pain, tachypnea; pulmonary fibrosis may occur up to 10 yr after treatment with busulfan
• Assess for increased uric acid levels, swelling, joint pain primarily in extremities; patient should be well hydrated to prevent urate deposits
• Monitor renal function studies: BUN, serum uric acid, urine CCr before, during therapy; I&O ratio; report fall in urine output of 30 ml/hr; check for hyperuricemia
• Monitor for cold, fever, sore throat (may indicate beginning infection); identify edema in feet, joint or stomach pain, shaking; prescriber should be notified
• Assess for bleeding: hematuria, guaiac, bruising or petechiae, mucosa or orifices q8hr; no rectal temps

> **BLACK BOX WARNING:** Assess for secondary malignancy within 5-8 yr of chronic oral therapy, long-term follow-up may be required

Nursing diagnoses
• Body image, disturbed (adverse reactions)
• Infection, risk for (adverse reactions)
• Injury, risk for (adverse reactions)
• Knowledge, deficient (teaching)

Patient/family education
• Teach patient to avoid use of products containing aspirin or ibuprofen, razors, commercial mouthwash since bleeding may occur; to report symptoms of bleeding (hematuria, tarry stools)
• Instruct patient to report signs of anemia (fatigue, headache, irritability, faintness, shortness of breath); symptoms of **infection** (fever, sore throat, cough); jaundice; congestion; skin pigmentation; darkening of skin; sudden

weakness, weight loss **(may resemble adrenal insufficiency)**
• Instruct patient to report any changes in breathing or coughing even several months after treatment; to avoid crowds and persons with respiratory tract or other infections
• Teach patient that hair loss may occur; discuss the use of wigs or hair pieces
• Caution patient not to have any vaccinations without the advice of the prescriber; serious reactions can occur
• Advise patient that contraception is needed during treatment and for ≥3 months after the completion of therapy (pregnancy **D**); avoid breastfeeding

Evaluation
Positive therapeutic outcome
• Decreased leukocytes to normal limits
• Absence of sweating at night
• Increased appetite, increased weight

butoconazole vaginal antifungal
See Appendix B

butorphanol (Rx)
(byoo-tor'fa-nole)
Apo-Butorphanol ✦, PMS-Butorphanol ✦
Func. class.: Mixed opiate analgesic
Chem. class.: Opioid antagonist, partial agonist
Pregnancy category C
Controlled substance schedule IV

Do not confuse:
Stadol/Haldol/Sotalol

ACTION: Depresses pain impulse transmission at the spinal cord level by interacting with opioid receptors

Therapeutic outcome: Relief of pain

USES: Moderate to severe pain, general anesthesia induction/maintenance, headache, migraine, preanesthesia

CONTRAINDICATIONS:
Hypersensitivity to this product or preservative, addiction (opioid)

Precautions: Pregnancy **C**, breastfeeding, child <18 yr, addictive personality, increased ICP, respiratory depression, renal/hepatic disease, bowel impaction, CHF, MI

DOSAGE AND ROUTES
Moderate to severe pain
Adult: IM 1-4 mg q3-4hr prn; **IV** 0.5-2 mg q3-4hr prn; **nasal** spray in 1 nostril; may give another dose 1-1½ hr later; may repeat if needed in q3-4hr after last dose
Geriatric: **IV** ½ adult dose at 2× the interval; **intranasal** if no relief in 90-120 min, may repeat with 1 spray

Severe pain
Adult: INTRANASAL 1 spray in each nostril q3-4hr

Renal dose
Adult: INTRANASAL max 1 mg, followed by 1 mg in 90-120 min; IM/IV give 50% of dose (0.5 mg **IV**, 1 mg IM); do not repeat within 6 hr

Available forms: Inj 1, 2 mg/ml; INTRANASAL 10 mg/ml

Implementation
• Store in light-resistant container at room temperature
IM route
• Give deeply in large muscle mass; rotate inj sites
Intranasal route
• Give 1 spray in nostril
• Remove clip and cover, prime before using until spray appears; pump must be reprimed q48hr; close nostril with finger and spray once quickly; have patient sniff
IV direct route
• Give **IV** undiluted at a rate of ≤2 mg/>3-5 min; titrate to patient response

Syringe compatibilities: Atropine, chlorproMAZINE, cimetidine, diphenhydrAMINE, droperidol, fentanyl, hydrOXYzine, meperidine, methotrimeprazine, metoclopramide, midazolam, morphine, pentazocine, perphenazine, prochlorperazine, promethazine, scopolamine, thiethylperazine

Syringe incompatibilities: DimenhyDRINATE, PENTobarbital

Y-site compatibilities: Acyclovir, alfentanil, allopurinol, amifostine, amikacin, aminocaproic acid, aminophylline, amphotericin B liposome (AmBisome), anidulafungin, ascorbic acid injection, atenolol, atracurium, atropine, aztreonam, benztropine, bivalirudin, bleomycin, bumetanide, buprenorphine, calcium chloride/gluconate, CARBOplatin, caspofungin, cefamandole, ceFAZolin, cefepime, cefmetazole, cefonicid, cefoperazone, cefotaxime, cefotetan, cefoxitin, ceftazidime, ceftizoxime, cefTRIAXone, cefuroxime, cephalothin, chlorproMAZINE, cimetidine, cisatracurium, CISplatin, cladribine, clindamycin, cyanocobalamin, cyclophosphamide, cycloSPORINE, cytarabine, DACTINomycin, DAPTOmycin, dexamethasone phosphate, dexmedetomidine, digoxin, diltiazem, diphenhydrAMINE, DOBUTamine, docetaxel, DOPamine, doxacurium, DOXOrubicin, DOXOrubicin liposomal, doxycycline, enalaprilat, ePHEDrine, EPINEPHrine, epirubicin, epoetin alfa, eptifibatide, ertapenem, erythromycin, esmolol, etoposide, famotidine, fenoldopam, fentaNYL, filgrastim, fluconazole, fludarabine, fluorouracil, gatifloxacin, gemcitabine, gentamicin, glycopyrrolate, granisetron, heparin, hydrocortisone, hydrOXYzine, IDArubicin, ifosfamide, imipenem-cilastatin, irinotecan, isoproterenol, ketorolac, labetalol, lactated Ringer's injection, levofloxacin, lidocaine, linezolid injection, LORazepam, magnesium, mannitol, mechlorethamine, melphalan, meperidine, metaraminol, methicillin, methotrexate, methoxamine, methyldopate, methylPREDNISolone, metoclopramide, metoprolol, metroNIDAZOLE, mezlocillin, miconazole, milrinone, minocycline, mitoxantrone, morphine, moxalactam, multiple vitamins injection, mycophenolate mofetil, nafcillin, nalbuphine, naloxone, nesiritide, netilmicin, niCARdipine, nitroglycerin, nitroprusside, norepinephrine, octreotide, ondansetron, oxacillin, oxaliplatin, oxytocin, palonosetron, pamidronate, pancuronium, papaverine, pemetrexed, penicillin G potassium/sodium, pentazocine, PHENobarbital, phenylephrine, phytonadione, piperacillin, piperacillin-tazobactam, polymyxin B, potassium chloride, procainamide, prochlorperazine, promethazine, propofol, propranolol, protamine, pyridoxine, quiNIDine, ranitidine, remifentanil, Ringer's injection, ritodrine, riTUXimab, rocuronium, sargramostim, sodium acetate, succinylcholine, SUFentanil, tacrolimus, teniposide, theophylline, thiamine, thiotepa, ticarcillin, ticarcillin-clavulanate, tigecycline, tirofiban, TNA, tobramycin, tolazoline, TPN, trastuzumab, trimetaphan, urokinase, vancomycin, vasopressin, vecuronium, verapamil, vinCRIStine, vinorelbine, voriconazole

ADVERSE EFFECTS

CNS: *Drowsiness, dizziness, confusion, headache, sedation, euphoria, weakness, hallucinations,* insomnia (nasal)
CV: Palpitations, bradycardia, hypotension
EENT: Tinnitus, blurred vision, miosis, diplopia, nasal congestion, unpleasant taste
GI: *Nausea, vomiting, anorexia, constipation, cramps*

GU: Dysuria, urinary retention
INTEG: Rash, urticaria, bruising, flushing, diaphoresis, pruritus
RESP: Respiratory depression, upper respiratory infection, sinusitis

Pharmacokinetics

Absorption	Well absorbed (IM, nasal); complete (**IV**)
Distribution	Crosses placenta, protein binding 80%
Metabolism	Liver, extensively
Excretion	Feces (10%-15%); kidneys, unchanged (small amounts)
Half-life	2-9 hr

Pharmacodynamics

	IM	IV	Nasal
Onset	5-15 min	1 min	15 min
Peak	30-60 min	4-5 min	1-2 hr
Duration	3-4 hr	2-4 hr	4-5 hr

INTERACTIONS

Individual drugs
Alcohol: increased respiratory depression, hypotension, sedation

Drug classifications
Antipsychotics, CNS depressants, opioids, sedative/hypnotics, skeletal muscle relaxants: increased respiratory depression, hypotension
MAOIs: do not use 2 wk before butorphanol, fatal reaction

NURSING CONSIDERATIONS

Assessment
• Monitor VS after parenteral administration; note muscle rigidity, product history, liver, kidney function tests, respiratory dysfunction: respiratory depression, character, rate, rhythm; notify prescriber if respirations are <10/min
• Monitor CNS changes: dizziness, drowsiness, hallucinations, euphoria, LOC, pupil reaction
• Monitor allergic reactions: rash, urticaria
• Assess for withdrawal symptoms in opioid-dependent patient; pulmonary embolism, vascular occlusion, abscesses, ulcerations

Nursing diagnoses
• Injury, risk for (adverse reactions)
• Knowledge, deficient (teaching)
• Pain, acute (uses)
• Pain, chronic (uses)
• Sensory perception, disturbed (adverse reactions)

Patient/family education
• Instruct patient to report any symptoms of CNS changes, allergic reactions; to avoid CNS depressants: alcohol, sedative/hypnotics for at least 24 hr after taking this product
• Discuss with patient that dizziness, drowsiness, and confusion are common; to avoid getting up without assistance, hazardous activities
• Discuss in detail all aspects of the product
Nasal route
• Teach patient to blow nose to clear both nostrils before using
• Patient should replace clip and cover after use; caution patient not to shake medication

Evaluation
Positive therapeutic outcome
• Pain relief

TREATMENT OF OVERDOSE:
Narcan 0.2-0.8 **IV**, O$_2$, **IV** fluids, vasopressors

---

cabazitaxel (Rx)
(ka-baz′i-tax′el)
Jevtana
Func. class.: Antineoplastic
Chem. class.: Taxane
Pregnancy category D

ACTION: A taxane that binds to tubulin, inhibits microtubule depolymerization, cell division, cell cycle arrest (G2/M) phase, cell proliferation; unlike other taxanes, this product may be useful for treating multidrug resistant tumors.

Therapeutic outcome: Decreased tumor size, spread of malignancy

USES: Hormone-refractory prostate cancer in combination with prednisone in patients that have been previously treated with a docetaxel-containing regimen

CONTRAINDICATIONS:
Hypersensitivity to this product, pregnancy **D**

> **BLACK BOX WARNING:** Hypersensitivity to polysorbate 80, neutropenia (ANC ≤1500/ mm^3)

Precautions: Breastfeeding, children, diarrhea, elderly, hepatic disease, renal disease, sepsis, vomiting

DOSAGE AND ROUTES
Adult: IV INF 25 mg/m^2 over 1 hr on day 1 with predniSONE 10 mg/day continuously; give q3wk cycles for up to 10 cycles

Hepatic dose
Adult: **IV INF:** do not use if total bilirubin ULN ≥ or AST and/or ALT >1.5 times ULN

Available forms: Solution for injection 60 mg/1.5 ml

Implementation
• Use cytotoxic handling procedures
• Obtain neutrophil counts prior to administration, count should be >1500/ mm^3
• Do not use PVC infusion containers or polyurethane infusion sets for preparation or administration
• Premedicate with diphenhydramine 25 mg **IV** or equivalent, dexamethasone 8 mg or equivalent and raniditine 50 mg or equivalent and antiemetics
• Do not use solution if it is discolored or if particulate is present; solution should be clear, yellow to brownish, discard if first or second dilution is not clear, remove immediately if solution comes in contact with skin

Intermittent IV infusion
• Two dilutions are required, both product and dilution are overfilled; first dilution: mix each vial of product (60 mg/1.5 ml) with the entire contents of supplied diluent (10 mg/ml); when transferring diluent, direct needle on side of vial and inject slowly to limit foaming; remove syringe and needle and gently mix by several inversions, do not shake; let stand for a few mins; *Second dilution:* withdraw the required dose, further dilute the withdrawn product with 0.9% NaCL or D5 in a PVC free container, remove syringe and needle, mix by gently inverting the bag/bottle (final concentration 0.1-0.2 6 mg/ ml), if a dose of ≥65 mg use a larger volume of infusion solution, so the concentration is max 0.26 mg/ml; do not mix with other drugs, solution may crystallize over time, discard if this occurs, us solution within 8 hrs (room temperature), 24 hrs (refrigerated); give over 1 hr, use 0.22 micrometer in-line filter

ADVERSE EFFECTS
CNS: *Peripheral neuropathy, dysgeusia, dizziness, headache, fatigue, fever*
CV: *Dysrhythmia,* peripheral edema, hypotension
GI: *Diarrhea, nausea, vomiting, constipation, abdominal pain, dyspepsia, anorexia, mucosal inflammation*

⚠ Nurse Alert

GU: Renal failure, dehydration, hematuria, urinary tract infection, dysuria, **obstructive uropathy,** infertility
HEMA: Neutropenia, febrile neutropenia, anemia, leucopenia, thrombocytopenia
MS: Back pain, arthralgia, muscle spasms
RESP: Cough, dyspnea
SYST: Fatal infections, sepsis, anaphylaxis

Pharmacokinetics

Absorption	89-92% protein binding, primarily bound to albumin and lipoproteins
Distribution	Equally distributed between blood and plasma
Metabolism	Extensively metabolized by CYP3A4/5 in the liver and CYP2C8 to a lesser extent
Excretion	80% eliminated within 2 wks mainly in feces
Half-life	Half-life alpha, beta, gamma of 4 mins, 2 hrs, 95 hrs respectively

Pharmacodynamics

Unknown

INTERACTIONS
Individual drugs
Radiation: increased bone marrow depression

Drug classifications
Other antineoplastics: increased bone marrow depression
Strong CYP3A4 inhibitors (conivaptan, chloramphenicol, danazol, dalfopristin, delavirdine, ethinyl estradiol, fluvoxamine, imatinib, isoniazid, tipranavir, troleadomycin, zafirlukast, ketoconazole, itraconazole, clarithromycin, atazanavir, indinavir, nefazodone, nelfinavir, ritonavir, saquinavir, telithromycin, voriconazole); mild or moderate CYP3A4 inhibitors (basiliximab, fluoxetine, niCARdipine, ranolazine, amiodarone, darunavir, diltiazem, miconazole, mifepristone [RU-486], posaconazole, propoxyphene, tamoxifen, erythromycin, verapamil, fluconazole): increased cabazitaxel concentrations
CYP3A4 inducers (rifampin, phenytoin, carBAMazepine, rifabutin, rifapentine): decreased cabazitaxel concentrations
Vaccines: decreased immune response

NURSING CONSIDERATIONS
Assessment
• **Assess for symptoms of anaphylaxis:** hypotension, dyspnea, generalized urticaria, bronchospasm, discontinue immediately; keep emergency equipment near; usually occurs during the first or second infusion, do not use this product again, after severe hypersensitivity reactions
• Check infusion site for reactions: if given by regular **IV,** not port (redness, inflammation, warmth)
• **Assess for bone marrow depression:** monitor CBC with differential, prior to and after one week, withhold if WBC <1500/mm³ or platelets <100,000/mm³. May not be a concern if an erythropoietin agent is given
• Assess for neurological side effects: peripheral neuropathy, dizziness, headache. During infusion of product, ice on extremities periodically, may prevent peripheral neuropathy
• Assess for musculoskeletal reactions: back pain, arthralgia, muscle spasms
• **Monitor for renal failure:** monitor BUN, creatinine and serum electrolytes; usually associated with sepsis, dehydration or obstructive uropathy; renal failure has been fatal
• **Assess for bleeding:** bruising, petechiae, hematuria, blood in emesis or stools; check mucosa orifices for stomatitis, obtain order for vicious xylocaine if needed
• Monitor temp periodically, increased temperature may indicate beginning infection
• Monitor hepatic studies: AST, ALT, bilirubin, LDH, prior to and periodically; jaundice of skin, eyes, clay-colored stools, dark urine, itching skin, abdominal pain, fever, diarrhea
• Identify effects of alopecia on body image, discuss feelings about body changes

Nursing diagnoses
• Risk for infection (adverse reactions)
• Risk for injury (adverse reactions)
• Knowledge deficit (teaching)

Patient/family education
• **Instruct patient to use a non hormonal form of contraception,** to notify prescriber if pregnancy is planned or suspected, pregnancy category (D); not to breastfeed
• Advise patient that hair may be lost during treatment, a wig or hairpiece may make the patient feel better, new hair will be different in color, texture
• Instruct patient to avoid receiving vaccinations while using this product

• **Teach patient to report signs of infection:** fever, sore throat, flu-like symptoms, avoid persons with known respiratory infections

Evaluation
Positive therapeutic outcome
• Decreased size, spread of malignancy

---

calcitonin (rDNA) (Rx)
(kal-sih-toh′nin)
Apo-Calcitonin ✦, **Fortical, Sandoz Calcitonin** ✦
calcitonin (salmon) (Rx)
Miacalcin
Func. class.: Parathyroid agents (calcium regulator)
Chem. class.: Polypeptide hormone
Pregnancy category C

ACTION: Decreases bone resorption, blood calcium levels; increases deposits of calcium in bones; opposes parathyroid hormone

Therapeutic outcome: Lowered calcium level, decreasing symptoms of Paget's disease

USES: Paget's disease, postmenopausal osteoporosis, hypercalcemia

CONTRAINDICATIONS: Hypersensitivity to this product or fish

Precautions: Pregnancy **C**, breastfeeding, children, renal disease, osteogenic sarcoma, pernicious anemia

DOSAGE AND ROUTES
rDNA
Paget's disease
Adult: SUBCUT 0.5 mg/day initially; may require 0.5 mg bid × 6 mo, then decrease until symptoms reappear

Salmon
Postmenopausal osteoporosis
Adult: SUBCUT/IM 100 international units/day; nasal 200 international units (1 spray) alternating nostrils daily, activate pump before 1st dose

Paget's disease
Adult: SUBCUT/IM 100 international units daily, maintenance 50-100 international units daily or every other day, or 3 × per wk

Hypercalcemia
Adult: SUBCUT/IM 4 international units/kg q12hr, increase to 8 international units/kg q12hr if response is unsatisfactory

Available forms: Inj 200 international units/ml; nasal spray 200 international units/actuation

Implementation
• Store at <77° F (25° C); protect from light
SUBCUT route (human)
• **Give** by SUBCUT route only; rotate inj sites; use within 6 hr of reconstitution; **give** at bedtime to minimize nausea, vomiting
IM route (salmon)
• **Give** after test dose of 10 international units/ml, 0.1 ml intradermally; watch 15 min; **give** only with EPINEPHrine and emergency meds available
• IM inj in deep muscle mass slowly; rotate sites; preferred route if volume is >2 ml
Nasal route
• Use alternating nostrils for nasal spray; allow to warm to room temperature, prime to get full spray

ADVERSE EFFECTS
CNS: Headache, **tetany,** chills, weakness, dizziness, fever
CV: Chest pressure
EENT: Nasal congestion, eye pain
GI: Nausea, diarrhea, vomiting, anorexia, abdominal pain, salty taste, epigastric pain
GU: Diuresis, nocturia, urine sediment, frequency
INTEG: Rash, flushing, pruritus of earlobes, edema of feet, inj site reaction
MS: Swelling, tingling of hands, backache
RESP: Dyspnea
SYST: Anaphylaxis

Pharmacokinetics
Absorption	Completely absorbed
Distribution	Unknown
Metabolism	Rapid; kidneys, tissue, blood
Excretion	Kidneys, inactive metabolite
Half-life	1 hr

Pharmacodynamics
	SUBCUT
Onset	15 min
Peak	4 hr
Duration	8-24 hr

INTERACTIONS
Individual drugs
Lithium: decreased lithium effect

⚠ Nurse Alert

NURSING CONSIDERATIONS

Assessment

• **Anaphylaxis, hypersensitivity:** inabilities to breathe, rash, fever; have emergency equipment nearby

• Assess for GI symptoms, polyuria, flushing, head swelling, tingling, headache; may indicate hypercalcemia; nervousness, irritability, twitching, seizures, spasm, paresthesia indicate hypocalcemia during beginning of treatment

• Identify nutritional status; check diet for sources of vit D (milk, some seafood), calcium (dairy products, dark green vegetables), phosphates

• Monitor BUN, creatinine, uric acid, chloride, electrolytes, urine pH, urinary calcium, magnesium, phosphate, urinalysis (calcium should be kept at 9-10 mg/dl; vit D 50-135 international units/dl), alkaline phosphatase baseline and q3-6mo; check urine sediment for casts throughout treatment; monitor urine hydroxyproline in Paget's disease, biochemical markers of bone formation/absorption, radiologic evidence of fracture; bone density (osteoporosis)

• **Toxicity (can occur rapidly):** Assess for increased product level, since toxic reactions occur rapidly; have parenteral calcium or gluconate on hand if calcium level drops too low; check for tetany (irritability, paresthesia, nervousness, muscle twitching, seizure, tetanic spasm)

Nursing diagnoses

• Injury, risk for (adverse reactions)
• Knowledge, deficient (teaching)
• Pain, chronic (uses)

Patient/family education

• Teach method of inj if patient will be responsible for self-medication

• Instruct patient to notify prescriber for hypercalcemic relapse: renal calculi, nausea, vomiting, thirst, lethargy, deep bone or flank pain

• Teach patient that warmth and flushing occur and last 1 hr

• Provide a low-calcium diet as prescribed (Paget's disease, hypercalcemia)

• Advise patients with osteoporosis to increase calcium and vit D in diet and to continue with moderate exercise to prevent continued bone loss

• Advise patients to report difficulty swallowing or change in side effects to prescriber immediately

Evaluation

Positive therapeutic outcome

• Calcium levels 9-10 mg/dl
• Decreasing symptoms of Paget's disease, including pain
• Decreased bone loss in osteoporosis

calcitriol (Rx)

(kal-si-tree′ole)
Calcijex, Rocaltrol
Func. class.: Parathyroid agent (calcium regulator)
Chem. class.: Vitamin D hormone
Pregnancy category C

Do not confuse:
calcitriol/Calciferol

ACTION: Increases intestinal absorption of calcium, provides calcium for bones, increases renal tubular resorption of phosphate

Therapeutic outcome: Calcium at normal level

USES: Hypocalcemia in chronic renal disease, hyperparathyroidism, pseudohypoparathyroidism

CONTRAINDICATIONS: Hypersensitivity, hyperphosphatemia, hypercalcemia, vit D toxicity

Precautions: Pregnancy **C**, breastfeeding, renal calculi, CV disease

DOSAGE AND ROUTES

Hypocalcemia (stage 5 chronic kidney disease, on dialysis)
Adult and child ≥6 yr: PO 0.25 mcg/day **IV** 0.5 mcg tid, initially; may increase by 0.25 every other day q4-8wk
Child 1-5 yr: PO 0.25-2 mcg/day

Renal osteodystrophy
Adult and child ≥3 yr: PO 0.25 mcg/day, may increase to 0.5 mcg/day
Child <3 yr: PO 0.01-0.015 mcg/kg/day

Hypoparathyroidism
Adult and child ≥6 yr: PO 0.25 mcg/day, may increase q2-4wk, maintenance 0.5-2 mcg/day
Child 1-5 yr: PO 0.25-0.75 mcg daily
Child <1 yr: PO 0.04-0.08 mcg/kg/day

Available forms: Caps 0.25, 0.5 mcg; inj 1 mcg/ml; oral sol 1 mcg/ml

Implementation
PO route
- Do not break, crush, or chew caps
- Give with meals for GI symptoms

IV route
- Give by direct **IV** over 1 min

ADVERSE EFFECTS
CNS: Drowsiness, headache, vertigo, fever, lethargy, hallucinations
CV: Palpitations, hypertension
EENT: Blurred vision, photophobia
GI: Nausea, diarrhea, vomiting, jaundice, anorexia, dry mouth, constipation, cramps, metallic taste
GU: Polyuria, hypercalciuria, hyperphosphatemia, hematuria, thirst
MS: Myalgia, arthralgia, decreased bone development, weakness
SYST: Anaphylaxis

Pharmacokinetics

Absorption	Well absorbed
Distribution	To liver, crosses placenta
Metabolism	Liver
Excretion	Bile
Half-life	3-6 hr, undergoes hepatic recycling, excreted in bile

Pharmacodynamics

Onset	2-6 hr
Peak	10-12 hr
Duration	Up to 5 days

INTERACTIONS
Individual drugs
Cholestyramine, mineral oil: decreased absorption of calcitriol
Phenytoin: increased vit D metabolism
Verapamil: increased dysrhythmias

Drug classifications
Antacids (magnesium): increased hypermagnesemia
Calcium supplements, diuretics (thiazide): increased hypercalcemia
Cardiac glycosides: increased dysrhythmias
Vitamin D products: increased toxicity
Vitamins (fat-soluble): decreased calcitriol absorption

Drug/food
Large amounts of high-calcium foods may cause hypercalcemia

Drug/lab test
False: increased cholesterol
Interference: alkaline phosphatase, electrolytes

NURSING CONSIDERATIONS
Assessment
- Assess GI symptoms, polyuria, flushing, head swelling, tingling, headache; may indicate hypercalcemia
- **Hypercalcemia:** dry mouth, metallic taste, polyuria, bone pain, muscle weakness, headache, fatigue, change in LOC, dysrhythmias, increased respirations, anorexia, nausea, vomiting, cramps, diarrhea, constipation; paresthesia, twitching, Chvostek's/Trousseau's sign, **hypocalcemia**
- Identify nutritional status; check diet for sources of vit D (milk, some seafood), calcium (dairy products, dark green vegetables), phosphates
- Monitor BUN, creatinine, uric acid, chloride, electrolytes, urine pH, urinary calcium, magnesium, phosphate, urinalysis (calcium should be kept at 9-10 mg/dl; vit D 50-135 international units/dl), alkaline phosphatase baseline and q3-6mo

Nursing diagnoses
- Injury, risk for (adverse reactions)
- Knowledge, deficient (teaching)
- Pain, chronic (uses)

Patient/family education
- Teach patient the symptoms of hypercalcemia (renal stones, nausea, vomiting, anorexia, lethargy, thirst, bone or flank pain) and about foods rich in calcium
- Advise patient to avoid products with sodium: cured meats, dairy products, cold cuts, olives, beets, pickles, soups, meat tenderizers in chronic renal failure
- Advise patient to avoid products with potassium: oranges, bananas, dried fruit, peas, dark green leafy vegetables, milk, melons, beans in chronic renal failure
- Advise patient to avoid OTC products containing calcium, potassium, or sodium in chronic renal failure
- Instruct patient to avoid all preparations containing vit D
- Instruct patient to monitor weight weekly; maintain fluid intake

Evaluation
Positive therapeutic outcome
- Calcium levels 9-10 mg/dl

calcium carbonate (Rx) (PO-OTC, Rx)

Acid Free, Alka-Mints, Amitone, Apo-Cal ✽, Calcarb, Calci-Chew, Calci-Mix, Calcite ✽, Cal-Gest, Caltrate, Equaline Calcium, Leader Calcium, Maalox Antacid, Os-Cal 500, PMS-Calcium ✽, Rolaids Extra Strength Soft-chew, Tums, Tums E-X, Walgreens Calcium

Func. class.: Antacid, calcium supplement
Chem. class.: Calcium product

calcium acetate (OTC)

(kal'see-um ass'e-tate)
Calphron, Eliphos, PhosLo
Pregnancy category C

Do not confuse:
Os-Cal/Asacol

ACTION: Neutralizes gastric acidity

Therapeutic outcome: Neutralized gastric acidity; calcium at normal levels

USES: Antacid, calcium supplement; not suitable for chronic therapy, hyperphosphatemia, hypertension in pregnancy, osteoporosis, prevention/treatment of hypocalcemia, hypoparathyroidism

CONTRAINDICATIONS:

Hypersensitivity, hypercalcemia, hyperparathyroidism, bone tumors

Precautions: Pregnancy C, breastfeeding, geriatric, fluid restriction, decreased GI motility, GI obstruction, dehydration, renal disease

DOSAGE AND ROUTES

Nutritional supplement including osteoporosis prophylaxis
Adult ≥51 yr: PO 1000-1500 mg/day elemental calcium (2500-3750 calcium carbonate)
Adult 19-50 yr: PO 1000 mg/day elemental calcium (2500 mg calcium carbonate)

Chronic hypocalcemia
Adult: PO 2-4 g/day elemental calcium (5-10 g calcium carbonate) in 3-4 divided doses
Child: PO 45-65 mg/kg/day elemental calcium (112.5-162.5 mg/kg calcium carbonate) in 4 divided doses
Neonate: PO 50-150 mg/kg/day elemental calcium (125-375 mg/kg/day in 4-6 divided doses, max 1 g/day)

Supplementation
Adolescent and child 9-18 yr: PO 1300 mg elemental calcium (3250 mg calcium carbonate)
Child 4-8 yr: PO 800 mg/day elemental calcium (2000 mg calcium carbonate)
Child 1-3 yr: PO 500 mg/day elemental calcium (1250 mg calcium carbonate)
Infant 6-12 mo: PO 270 mg/day elemental calcium based on total intake
Nenates and infants <6 mo: PO 210 mg/day elemental calcium based on total intake

Hyperphosphatemia
Adult: PO Individualized on response

Heartburn, dyspepsia, hyperacidity (OTC)
Adult: PO 1-2 tabs q2hr, max 9 tabs/24 hr (Alka-mints); chew 2-4 tab q1hr prn, max 16 tabs (Tums regular strength); chew 2-4 tab q1hr prn, max 10 tabs (Tums E-X); chew 2-3 tabs q1hr prn, max 10 tabs/24 hr (Tums Ultra); chew 2 tabs q2-3hr, max 19 tabs/24 hr (Titralac Extra Strength)

Available forms: Calcium carbonate: chewable tabs 350, 420, 450, 500, 750, 1000, 1250 mg; tabs 500, 600, 650, 667, 1000, 1250, 1500 mg; gum 300, 450 500 mg; susp 1250 mg/5 ml; caps 1250 mg; powder 6.5 g/packet; **calcium acetate:** tabs 250 mg (65 mg Ca), 667 mg (169 mg Ca), 668 mg (169 mg Ca), 1 g (250 mg Ca); caps 500 mg (125 mg Ca)

Implementation
PO route
• Administer as antacid 1 hr after meals and at bedtime
• Administer as supplement 1$\frac{1}{2}$ hr after meals and at bedtime
• Administer only with regular tablets or capsules; do not give with enteric-coated tablets
• Administer laxatives or stool softeners if constipation occurs

ADVERSE EFFECTS

GI: *Constipation,* anorexia, nausea, vomiting, flatulence, diarrhea, rebound hyperacidity, eructation
GU: Calculi, hypercalciuria

Pharmacokinetics

Absorption	$1/3$ absorbed by small intestines, must have adequate vit D for absorption
Distribution	Unknown
Metabolism	Unknown
Excretion	Feces, urine, crosses placenta
Half-life	Unknown

Pharmacodynamics

Onset	20 min
Peak	Unknown
Duration	20-180 min

INTERACTIONS
Individual drugs
Atenolol, etidronate, phenytoin, risedronate, ketoconazole: decreased levels of each drug
Digoxin: increased toxicity from hypercalcemia
QuiNIDine: increased quiNIDine levels

Drug classifications
Amphetamines: increased levels of amphetamines
Calcium channel blockers, fluoroquinolones, iron products, salicylates, tetracyclines: decreased levels of each specific product
Thiazide diuretics: increased hypercalcemia

Drug/lab test
False increase: chloride
False decrease: magnesium, oxylate, lipase
False positive: benzodiazepines

NURSING CONSIDERATIONS
Assessment
• Monitor Ca^+ (serum, urine); Ca^+ should be 8.5-10.5 mg/dl, urine Ca^+ should be 150 mg/day, monitor weekly
⚠ **Assess for milk-alkali syndrome: nausea, vomiting, disorientation, headache**
• Assess for constipation; increase bulk in the diet if needed
• Assess for **hypercalcemia:** headache, nausea, vomiting, confusion; hypocalcemia: paresthesia, twitching, colic, dysrhythmias, Chvostek's/Trousseau's sign
• Assess those taking digoxin for toxicity
• Assess those taking for abdominal pain, heartburn, indigestion before, after administration

Nursing diagnoses
• Knowledge, deficient (teaching)
• Nutrition, impaired less than body requirements, imbalanced (uses)

Patient/family education
• Advise patient to increase fluids to 2 L unless contraindicated, to add bulk to diet for constipation; notify prescriber of constipation
• Advise patient not to switch antacids unless directed by prescriber, not to use as antacid for >2 wk without approval by prescriber
• Teach patient that therapeutic dose recommendations are figured as elemental calcium
• Advise to avoid excessive use of alcohol, caffeine, tobacco
• Teach to avoid spinach, cereals, dairy products in large amounts

Evaluation
Positive therapeutic outcome
• Absence of pain, decreased acidity
• Decreased hyperphosphatemia in renal failure (Acetate)

CALCIUM SALTS
calcium chloride (Rx)
calcium gluceptate (Rx)
calcium gluconate (Rx)
calcium lactate (PO-OTC, IV-Rx)
Func. class.: Electrolyte replacement—calcium product
Pregnancy category C

ACTION: Cation needed for maintenance of nervous, muscular, skeletal systems, enzyme reactions, normal cardiac contractility, coagulation of blood; affects secretory activity of endocrine, exocrine glands

Therapeutic outcome: Calcium at normal level, absence of increased magnesium, potassium

USES: Prevention and treatment of hypocalcemia, hypermagnesemia, hypoparathyroidism, neonatal tetany, cardiac toxicity caused by hyperkalemia, lead colic, hyperphosphatemia, vit D deficiency, osteoporosis prophylaxis, calcium antagonist toxicity (calcium channel blocker toxicity)

CONTRAINDICATIONS: Hypercalcemia, digoxin toxicity, ventricular fibrillation, renal calculi

Precautions: Pregnancy **C,** breastfeeding, children, renal disease, respiratory disease, cor pulmonale, digitalized patient, respiratory failure, diarrhea, dehydration

DOSAGE AND ROUTES

Calcium chloride
Adult: IV 500 mg-1 g q1-3days as indicated by serum calcium levels; give at <1 ml/min; IV 200-800 mg injected in ventricle of heart

Calcium gluceptate
Adult: IV 5-20 ml; IM 2-5 ml

Calcium gluconate
Adult: PO 0.5-2 g bid-qid; IV 0.5-2 g at 0.5 ml/min (10% sol); max IV dose 3 g
Child: PO/IV 500 mg/kg/day in divided doses

Calcium lactate
Adult: PO 325 mg-1.3 g tid with meals
Child: PO 500 mg/kg/day in divided doses

Available forms: Many; check product listings

Implementation
PO route
• Give PO with or following meals to enhance absorption
• Store at room temperature

IV route
• Administer IV undiluted or diluted with equal amounts of 0.9% NaCl for inj to a 5% sol; give 0.5-1 ml/min
• Give through small-bore needle into large vein; if extravasation occurs, necrosis will result (IV); IM inj may cause severe burning, necrosis, and tissue sloughing; warm sol to body temp before administering (only gluconate/gluceptate)
• Provide seizure precautions: padded side rails, decreased stimuli (noise, light); place airway suction equipment, padded mouth gag if calcium levels are low
• Patient should remain recumbent 30 min after IV dose

Calcium chloride
Syringe compatibilities: Milrinone

Y-site compatibilities: DOBUTamine, EPINEPHrine, esmolol, inamrinone, morphine, paclitaxel

Additive compatibilities: Amikacin, amphotericin B, ampicillin, ascorbic acid, bretylium, cefTRIAXone, cephapirin, chloramphenicol, DOPamine, hydrocortisone, isoproterenol, lidocaine, methicillin, norepinephrine, penicillin G potassium, penicillin G sodium, PENTobarbital, PHENobarbital, verapamil, vit B/C

Calcium gluceptate
Additive compatibilities: Ascorbic acid inj, isoproterenol, lidocaine, norepinephrine, phytonadione, sodium bicarbonate

Calcium gluconate
Syringe compatibilities: Aldesleukin, allopurinol, amifostine, aztreonam, ceFAZolin, cefepime, ciprofloxacin, cladribine, DOBUTamine, enalaprilat, EPINEPHrine, famotidine, filgrastim, granisetron, heparin/hydrocortisone, labetalol, melphalan, midazolam, netilmicin, piperacillin/tazobactam, potassium chloride, prochlorperazine, propofol, sargramostim, tacrolimus, teniposide, thiotepa, tolazoline, vinorelbine, vit B/C

Additive compatibilities: Amikacin, aminophylline, ascorbic acid inj, bretylium, cephapirin, chloramphenicol, corticotropin, dimenhyDRINATE, erythromycin, furosemide, heparin, hydrocortisone, lidocaine, magnesium sulfate, methicillin, norepinephrine, penicillin G potassium, penicillin G sodium, PHENobarbital, potassium chloride, tobramycin, vancomycin, verapamil, vit B/C

ADVERSE EFFECTS
CV: **Shortened QT interval, heart block,** hypotension, bradycardia, dysrhythmias; **cardiac arrest (IV)**
GI: Vomiting, nausea, constipation
HYPERCALCEMIA: Drowsiness, lethargy, muscle weakness, headache, constipation, **coma,** anorexia, nausea, vomiting, polyuria, thirst
INTEG: Pain, burning at IV site, severe venous thrombosis, necrosis, extravasation

Pharmacokinetics
Absorption	Complete bioavailability (IV)
Distribution	Readily extracellular; crosses placenta, protein binding 40%-50%
Metabolism	Liver
Excretion	Feces (80%), kidney (20%), breast milk
Half-life	Unknown

Pharmacodynamics
	PO	IV
Onset	Unknown	Immediate
Peak	Unknown	Rapid
Duration	Unknown	$1/2$-$1^1/_2$ hr

Adverse effects: *italics* = common; **bold** = life-threatening

INTERACTIONS

Individual drugs
Atenolol: decreased effect
Phenytoin, tetracyclines, thyroid: decreased absorption when calcium is taken PO
Verapamil: decreased effects, increased toxicity

Drug classifications
Antacids: milk-alkali syndrome (renal disease)
Digoxin glycosides: increased dysrhythmias
Diuretics (thiazide): increased hypercalcemia
Fluoroquinolones: decreased absorption of fluoroquinolones when calcium is taken PO
Iron salts: decreased absorption of iron when calcium is taken PO

Drug/herb
Lily of the valley, pheasant's eye, shark cartilage, squill: increased side effects, action

Drug/lab test
False: decreased magnesium
Decreased: 17-OHCS
Increased: 11-OHCS

NURSING CONSIDERATIONS

Assessment
• Monitor ECG for decreased QT interval and T-wave inversion: in hypercalcemia, product should be reduced or discontinued
• Monitor calcium levels during treatment (9-10 mg/dl is normal level), urine calcium if hypercaluria occurs
• Assess cardiac status: rate, rhythm, CVP (PWP, PAWP if being monitored directly)
• Assess digitalized patients closely, an increase in calcium increases digoxin toxicity risk
• **Hypocalcemia:** muscle twitching, paresthesia, dysrhythmias, laryngospasm

Nursing diagnoses
• Injury, risk for (uses, adverse reactions)
• Knowledge, deficient (teaching)

Patient/family education
• Caution patient to add food high in vit D content; to add calcium-rich foods to diet: dairy products, shellfish, dark green leafy vegetables; decrease oxalate-rich and zinc-rich foods: nuts, legumes, chocolate, spinach, soy
• Advise patient to prevent injuries, avoid immobilization

Evaluation
Positive therapeutic outcome
• Decreased twitching, paresthesias, muscle spasms
• Absence of tremors, seizures, dysrhythmias, dyspnea, laryngospasm, negative Chvostek's sign, negative Trousseau's sign

candesartan (Rx)
(can-deh-sar'tan)
Atacand
Func. class.: Antihypertensive
Chem. class.: Angiotensin II receptor (type AT_1)
**Pregnancy category
C (1st trimester),
D (2nd/3rd trimesters)**

ACTION: Blocks the vasoconstrictor and aldosterone-secreting effects of angiotensin II; selectively blocks the binding of angiotensin II to the AT_1 receptor found in tissues

Therapeutic outcome: Decreased B/P

USES: Hypertension, alone or in combination; CHF NYHA Class II-IV and ejection fraction ≤40%

CONTRAINDICATIONS:
Hypersensitivity

> **BLACK BOX WARNING:** Pregnancy **D** (2nd/3rd trimesters)

Precautions: Pregnancy **C** (1st trimester), breastfeeding, children, geriatric, hypersensitivity to ACE inhibitors, volume depletion, renal/hepatic impairment

DOSAGE AND ROUTES
Adult: PO (single agent) 16 mg daily initially in patients who are not volume depleted, range 8-32 mg/day; with diuretic or volume depletion, 2-32 mg/day as a single dose or divided dose
Adult and child ≥6 yr and weight >50 kg: PO 8-16 mg q day or divided bid, adjust to B/P, usual range 4-32 mg/day max 30 mg/day
Child ≥6 yr and weight <50 kg: PO 4-8 mg/day or divided bid, adjust to B/P
Child ≥1 yr and <6 yr: PO 0.2 mg/kg/day in 1 dose or divided in 2 doses/day, adjust B/P, max 0.4 mg/kg/day

Heart failure
Adult: PO 4 mg q day, may be doubled ≥2 wk, target dose 32 mg q day

Renal/hepatic dose
Adult: PO ≤8 mg/day in severe renal disease/moderate hepatic disease, adjust dose as needed

Available forms: Tabs 4, 8, 16, 32 mg

Implementation
• Administer without regard to meals

ADVERSE EFFECTS
CNS: *Dizziness,* fatigue, headache
CV: Chest pain, peripheral edema, hypotension
EENT: Sinusitis, rhinitis, pharyngitis
GI: *Diarrhea,* nausea, abdominal pain, vomiting
GU: Renal failure
MS: Arthralgia, pain
RESP: *Cough, upper respiratory infection*
SYST: Angioedema

Pharmacokinetics

Absorption	Well absorbed
Distribution	Bound to plasma proteins
Metabolism	Extensive
Excretion	Feces, urine, breast milk
Half-life	9 hr

Pharmacodynamics

Onset	Unknown
Peak	2 hr
Duration	24 hr

INTERACTIONS
Individual drugs
Lithium: increased lithium level
Potassium: increased hypokalemia

Drug classifications
α-Blockers, ACE inhibitors, β-blockers, calcium channel blockers: increased hypotension
Diuretics (potassium sparing): increased hypokalemia
NSAIDs, salicylates: decreased effect

Drug/herb
Astragalus, cola tree: increased or decreased antihypertensive effect
Ephedra: decreased antihypertensive effect
Hawthorn: increased antihypertensive effect

NURSING CONSIDERATIONS
Assessment
• **Serious hypersensitivity reactions:** Assess for angioedema, anaphylaxis; facial swelling, difficulty breathing (rare)
• **Heart failure:** Assess for jugular vein distention, weight, edema, dyspnea, crackles
• Assess B/P, pulse q4hr; note rate, rhythm, quality
• Monitor electrolytes: potassium, sodium, chloride; total CO_2
• Obtain baselines in renal, liver function tests before therapy begins
• Assess blood studies: BUN, creatinine, liver function tests before treatment

• Monitor for edema in feet, legs daily
• Assess for skin turgor, dryness of mucous membranes for hydration status; for angio-edema: facial swelling, dyspnea

> **BLACK BOX WARNING:** Assess for pregnancy; this product can cause fetal death when given in pregnancy (**D**), 2nd/3rd trimester

• Assess for adverse reactions, especially in renal disease

Nursing diagnoses
• Fluid volume, deficient (side effects)
• Knowledge, deficient (teaching)
• Noncompliance (teaching)

Patient/family education
• Teach patient not to take the product if breastfeeding or pregnant, or having had an allergic reaction to this product
• If a dose is missed, instruct patient to take as soon as possible, unless it is within 1 hour before next dose
• Advise patient to comply with dosage schedule, even if feeling better
• Teach patient to notify prescriber of fever, swelling of hands or feet, irregular heartbeat, chest pain
• Advise patient excessive perspiration, dehydration, diarrhea may lead to fall in blood pressure—consult prescriber if these occur
• Inform patient that product may cause dizziness, fainting; light-headedness may occur
• Caution patient to rise slowly to sitting or standing position to minimize orthostatic hypotension
• Advise patient to avoid all OTC medications unless approved by prescriber; to inform all health care providers of medication use
• Teach proper technique for obtaining B/P and acceptable parameters

> **BLACK BOX WARNING:** Teach patient to notify prescriber immediately if pregnant, not to use if breastfeeding

Evaluation
Positive therapeutic outcome
• Decreased B/P

capecitabine (Rx)

(cap-eh-sit'ah-bean)

Xeloda

Func. class.: Antineoplastic, antimetabolite

Chem. class.: Fluoropyrimidine carbamate

Pregnancy category D

Do not confuse:
Xeloda/Xenical

ACTION: Competes with physiologic substrate of DNA synthesis, thus interfering with cell replication in the S phase of cell cycle (before mitosis); also interferes with RNA and protein synthesis; product is converted to 5-fluorouracil (5-FU)

Therapeutic outcome: Decreasing symptoms of breast cancer

USES: Monotherapy for paclitaxel-anthracycline-resistant metastatic breast, colorectal cancer when 5-FU monotherapy is preferred; treatment of patients with colorectal cancer who have undergone complete resection of their primary tumor

CONTRAINDICATIONS:

Pregnancy **D**, infants, hypersensitivity to 5-FU, severe renal impairment (CCr <30 ml/min), DPD deficiency

Precautions: Renal/hepatic disease, breastfeeding, children, geriatric

DOSAGE AND ROUTES:

Metastatic breast cancer resistant to both paclitaxel and anthracycline or resistant to paclitaxel and when further anthracycline therapy is not indicated

Adult: PO 2500 mg/m^2/day divided q12hr after meal ×2 wk, repeat q3wk

Breast cancer (locally advanced/metastatic) with docetaxel, previously treated with anthracycline

Adult: PO 2500 mg/m^2/day divided q12hr after a meal on days 1-14, with docetaxel 75 mg/m^2 IV on day 1

Advanced/metastatic breast cancer (HER2 positive), who have received anthracycline, taxane, and trastuzumab

Adult: PO 2000 mg/m^2/day divided q12hr after a meal on days 1-14 with lapatinib 1250 mg q day on days 1-21, repeat q21days

Metastatic/locally advanced breast cancer, resistant to anthracycline, and a taxane or taxane resistant and when further anthracycline is contraindicated

Adult: PO 2000 mg/m^2/day divided q12hr on days 1-14 with ixabepilone 40 mg/m^2 IV over 3 hr, repeat q3wk

As an adjuvant in Dukes C colorectal cancer with a complete resection when fluoropyrimidine alone is preferred

Adult: PO 2500 mg/m^2/day divided q12hr within 30 min of a meal ×2 wk, repeat q3wk for 8 cycles

First-line in metastatic colorectal cancer when fluoropyrimidine alone is preferred

Adult: PO 2500 mg/m^2/day divided q12hr after a meal ×2 wk repeat q3wk

Renal dose

Adult: PO CCr 30-50 ml/min; decrease initial dose to 75% of usual dose; CCr < 30 ml/min contraindicated

Available forms: Tabs 150, 500 mg

Implementation

• **Dosage adjustments of capecitabine monotherapy based on the most severe toxicity OR when used in combination with ixabepilone based on nonhematologic toxicity:** *Grade 1 toxicity:* Maintain current dosage; *Grade 2 toxicity (1st appearance):* interrupt therapy until toxicity is resolved to grade 0–1; do not replace missed doses, begin the next cycle with 100% of the starting dose; *Grade 2 toxicity (2nd appearance):* interrupt therapy until toxicity is resolved to grade 0–1; do not replace missed doses, begin the next cycle with 75% of the starting dose; *Grade 2 toxicity (3rd appearance):* interrupt therapy until toxicity is resolved to grade 0–1; do not replace missed doses, begin the next cycle with 50% of the starting dose; *Grade 2 toxicity (4th appearance):* discontinue treatment permanently; *Grade 3 toxicity (1st appearance):* interrupt therapy until toxicity is resolved to grade 0-1

• Help patient to rinse mouth tid-qid with water or club soda, brush teeth bid-qid with soft brush

ACTION: Exact mechanism unknown; appears to decrease polysynaptic responses and block posttetanic potentiation

Therapeutic outcome: Absence of seizures; decreased trigeminal neuralgia pain

USES: Tonic-clonic, complex-partial, mixed seizures; trigeminal neuralgia; bipolar disorder

Unlabeled uses: Neurogenic pain, psychotic behavior with dementia, diabetic neuropathy, agitation, hiccups

CONTRAINDICATIONS:
Pregnancy **D**, hypersensitivity to carBAMazepine or tricyclics, AV or bundle branch block

> **BLACK BOX WARNING:** Bone marrow depression

Precautions: Glaucoma, renal/hepatic/cardiac disease, psychosis, breastfeeding, child <6 yr, alcoholism, hepatic porphyria

> **BLACK BOX WARNING:** Hematologic disease, agranulocytosis, leukopenia, neutropenia, thrombocytopenia, Asian patients

DOSAGE AND ROUTES

Seizures
Adult and child >12 yr: PO 200 mg bid; may be increased by 200 mg/day in weekly intervals, give in divided doses q6-8hr; maintenance 800-1200 mg/day; max 1600 mg/day (adult); max child 12-15 yr 1000 mg/day; max child >15 yr 1200 mg/day; adjustment is needed to minimum dose to control seizures; EXT REL give bid; RECT administration of oral SUSP 200 mg/10 ml or 6 mg/kg as a single dose
Child 6-12 yr: PO tabs 100 mg bid or SUSP 50 mg qid; may increase by <100 mg qwk, max 1000 mg/day; EXT REL tabs daily-bid
Child <6 yr: PO 10-20 mg/kg/day in 2-3 divided doses, may increase qwk

Trigeminal neuralgia
Adult: PO 100 mg/bid; may increase 100 mg q12hr until pain subsides; max 1200 mg/day; maintenance is 200-400 mg bid

Bipolar disorder
Adult: PO (Equetro only) 200 mg bid, may adjust dose by 200 mg daily to desired response; max 1600 mg/day

Agitation due to dementia (unlabeled)
Adult: PO 100 mg bid, may increase to 250-300 mg/day

Hiccups (unlabeled)
Adult: PO 200 mg tid

Available forms: Chewable tabs 100, 200 mg; tabs 200 mg; oral susp 100 mg/5 ml; ext rel tabs 100, 200, 400 mg; ext rel caps (Carbatrol) 200, 300 mg

Implementation
• Do not break, crush, or chew ext rel tabs and caps: ext rel caps may be opened and beads mixed with food; chewable tabs should be chewed, not swallowed whole
• Give with food for GI symptoms
• Shake oral susp before use
• Mix an equal amount of water, D5W, 0.9% NaCl when giving by NG tube, flush tube with 100 ml of above sol

ADVERSE EFFECTS
CNS: *Drowsiness*, dizziness, confusion, fatigue, **paralysis**, headache, hallucinations, **worsening of seizures**, unsteadiness, speech disturbances, **suicidal ideation**
CV: Hypertension, CHF, hypotension, aggravation of CAD, dysrhythmias, **AV block**
EENT: Tinnitus, dry mouth, blurred vision, diplopia, nystagmus, conjunctivitis
ENDO: Syndrome of inappropriate antidiuretic hormone (SIADH) (geriatric)
GI: *Nausea, constipation, diarrhea,* anorexia, vomiting, abdominal pain, stomatitis, glossitis, increased liver enzymes, **hepatitis, hepatic porphyria**
GU: Frequency, retention, albuminuria, glycosuria, impotence, increased BUN, **renal failure**
HEMA: Thrombocytopenia, leukopenia, **agranulocytosis, leukocytosis, aplastic anemia, eosinophilia,** increased pro-time
INTEG: *Rash,* **Stevens-Johnson syndrome,** urticaria, photosensitivity, **toxic epidermal necrolysis**
RESP: Pulmonary hypersensitivity (fever, dyspnea, pneumonitis)

Pharmacokinetics

Absorption	Slow; completely absorbed
Distribution	Widely distributed; protein binding 76%
Metabolism	Extensively, liver, metabolized by CYP3A4
Excretion	Urine, feces, breast milk
Half-life	18-65 hr, then 8-29 hr after first month

or cotton-tipped applicators for stomatitis, use unwaxed dental floss

ADVERSE EFFECTS
CNS: Dizziness, headache, *paresthesia, fatigue,* insomnia
CV: Venous thrombosis
GI: *Nausea, vomiting, anorexia, diarrhea, stomatitis, abdominal pain, constipation, dyspepsia,* **intestinal obstruction, necrotizing enterocolitis,** hyperbilirubinemia, **hepatic failure**
HEMA: Neutropenia, lymphopenia, thrombocytopenia, anemia
INTEG: *Hand and foot syndrome,* dermatitis, nail disorder
MISC: Eye irritation, edema, myalgia, limb pain, *pyrexia,* dehydration
RESP: *Cough,* **dyspnea, pulmonary embolism**

Pharmacokinetics

Absorption	Readily absorbed, decreased with food
Distribution	Unknown
Metabolism	Liver, extensively
Excretion	Kidneys
Half-life	45 min

Pharmacodynamics

Onset	Unknown
Peak	$1\frac{1}{2}$ hr
Duration	Unknown

INTERACTIONS

Individual drugs
Leucovorin: increased toxicity
Phenytoin: increased phenytoin level

Drug classifications
Antacids (aluminum, magnesium): increased capecitabine

> **BLACK BOX WARNING:** Anticoagulants: increased risk of bleeding

Food/drug
Increased absorption; give within 30 min of a meal

NURSING CONSIDERATIONS

Assessment
• **Bone marrow suppression:** Monitor CBC, differential, platelet count weekly; withhold product if WBC <4000/mm^3 or platelet count is <75,000/mm^3 or RBC, HCT, Hgb is low; notify

prescriber of results; frequently monitor INR in those receiving warfarin
• Assess buccal cavity q8hr for dryness, sores or ulceration, white patches, pain, bleeding, dysphagia; obtain prescription for viscous lidocaine (Xylocaine)
• Assess symptoms indicating severe allergic reaction: rash, pruritus, urticaria, purpuric skin lesions, itching, flushing; product should be discontinued
• Monitor temp q4hr (may indicate beginning of infection)
• Assess for **hand/foot syndrome:** paresthesia, tingling, painful/painless swelling, blistering, erythema with severe pain of hands/feet
• Assess for **toxicity:** severe diarrhea, nausea, vomiting, stomatitis
• Assess **GI symptoms:** frequency of stools, cramping; if severe diarrhea occurs, fluids/electrolytes may need to be given
• Monitor liver function tests before and during therapy (bilirubin, AST, ALT, LDH) as needed or monthly; note jaundice of skin or sclera, dark urine, clay-colored stools, itchy skin, abdominal pain, fever, diarrhea
• Assess for bleeding: hematuria, stool guaiac, bruising or petechiae, mucosa or orifices q8hr; inflammation of mucosa, breaks in skin

Nursing diagnoses
• Body image, disturbed (adverse reactions)
• Infection, risk for (adverse reactions)
• Injury, risk for (adverse reactions)
• Knowledge, deficient (teaching)

Patient/family education
• Advise patient to avoid use of products containing aspirin or ibuprofen, razors, commercial mouthwash, since bleeding may occur; to report symptoms of bleeding (hematuria, tarry stools)
• Instruct patient to report signs of **anemia** (fatigue, headache, irritability, faintness, shortness of breath); **infection:** increased temp, sore throat, flulike symptoms
• Advise patient not to become pregnant while taking this product; to avoid using while breastfeeding
• Advise patient not to double dose, if dose is missed
• Advise patient to report immediately severe diarrhea, vomiting, stomatitis, fever ≥100° F, hand/foot syndrome, anorexia

Evaluation
Positive therapeutic outcome
• Prevention of rapid division of malignant cells

captopril (Rx)

(kap'toe-pril)

Apo-Capto ✦, **Capoten, Gen-Captopril** ✦, **PMS-Captopril** ✦

Func. class.: Antihypertensive

Chem. class.: Angiotensin-converting enzyme (ACE) inhibitor

Pregnancy category D

Do not confuse:

captopril/Capitrol/carvedilol

ACTION: Selectively suppresses renin-angiotensin-aldosterone system; inhibits ACE; prevents conversion of angiotensin I to angiotensin II

Therapeutic outcome: Decreased B/P in hypertension; decreased preload, afterload in CHF

USES: Hypertension, CHF, left ventricular dysfunction (LVD) after MI, diabetic nephropathy

CONTRAINDICATIONS:

Breastfeeding, children, hypersensitivity, heart block, potassium-sparing diuretics, bilateral renal artery stenosis, angioedema

BLACK BOX WARNING: Pregnancy D

Precautions: Dialysis patients, hypovolemia, leukemia, scleroderma, LE, blood dyscrasias, CHF, diabetes mellitus, renal/hepatic disease, thyroid disease, COPD, asthma

DOSAGE AND ROUTES

Hypertension

Adult: Initial dose: PO 12.5-25 mg bid-tid; may increase to 50 mg bid-tid at 1-2 wk intervals; usual range 25-150 mg bid-tid; max 450 mg/day

Child: PO 0.3-0.5 mg/kg/dose, titrate up to 6 mg/kg/day in 2-4 divided doses

Neonate: PO 0.05-0.1 mg/kg bid-tid, may increase as needed

CHF

Adult: PO 25 mg tid; may increase to 50 mg bid-tid; after 14 days may increase to 150 mg tid if needed

Diabetic nephropathy

Adult: PO 25 mg tid

Renal dose

Adult: PO CCr >50 ml/min, no change; CCr 10-50 ml/min, decrease dose by 25%; CCr <10 ml/min, decrease dose by 50%

Available forms: Tabs 12.5, 25, 50, 100 mg

Implementation

• Store in air-tight container at 86° F (30° C) or less

• Severe hypotension may occur after first dose of this medication; decreasing hypotension may be prevented by reducing or discontinuing diuretic therapy 3 days before beginning captopril therapy

• Administer 1 hr before or 2 hr after meals

• **Oral sol:** May crush tab and dissolve in water, give within ½ hr, make sure tab is completely dissolved

ADVERSE EFFECTS

CNS: Fever, chills

CV: *Hypotension,* postural hypotension, *tachycardia,* angina

GI: Loss of taste, increased liver function tests

GU: Impotence, dysuria, nocturia, proteinuria, **nephrotic syndrome, acute reversible renal failure,** polyuria, oliguria, frequency

HEMA: **Neutropenia, agranulocytosis, pancytopenia, thrombocytopenia,** anemia

INTEG: Rash, pruritus

MISC: **Angioedema,** hyperkalemia

RESP: **Bronchospasm,** *dyspnea, cough*

Pharmacokinetics

Absorption	Well absorbed
Distribution	Widely distributed; crosses placenta, excreted in breast milk (small amounts)
Metabolism	Liver (50%)
Excretion	Kidneys, unchanged (50%)
Half-life	2 hr increase in renal disease

Pharmacodynamics

Onset	¼-1 hr
Peak	1 hr
Duration	6-12 hr

INTERACTIONS

Individual drugs

Alcohol (acute ingestion): increased hypotension (large amounts)

Digoxin, lithium: increased serum levels, toxicity

Insulin: increased hypoglycemia

Drug classifications

Antacids, NSAIDs, salicylates: decreased captopril effect

Antidiabetics (oral): increased hypoglycemia

Antihypertensives, diuretics, nitrates, phenothiazines: increased hypotension

Diuretics (potassium-sparing), potassium supplements: increased toxicity, do not use

Sympathomimetics: do not use

Drug/herb

Ephedra: decreased antihypertensive effect

Hawthorn: increased antihypertensive effect

Drug/food

• Food: decreased absorption of captopril

Drug/lab test

Increased: AST, ALT, alkaline phosphatase, bilirubin, uric acid, glucose

False positive: urine acetone, ANA titer

NURSING CONSIDERATIONS

Assessment

• **Blood dyscrasias:** Monitor blood studies: decreased platelets; WBC with diff baseline, periodically q3mo, if neutrophils are <1000/mm³, discontinue treatment

• **Hypertension:** Monitor B/P, check for orthostatic hypotension, syncope; if changes occur, dosage change may be required

• Monitor renal studies: protein, BUN, creatinine; watch for increased levels that may indicate nephrotic syndrome and renal failure; monitor renal symptoms: polyuria, oliguria, frequency, dysuria

• Establish baselines in renal, liver function tests before therapy begins and check periodically; monitor for increased liver function studies; watch for increased uric acid, glucose

• Check potassium levels throughout treatment, although hyperkalemia rarely occurs

• **CHF:** Assess for edema, dyspnea, wet crackles, increased B/P, weight gain

• Assess for allergic reactions: rash, fever, pruritus, urticaria; product should be discontinued if antihistamines fail to help

Nursing diagnoses

• Cardiac output, decreased (uses)

• Injury, risk for (side effects)

• Knowledge, deficient (teaching)

• Noncompliance (teaching)

Patient/family education

• Caution patient not to discontinue product abruptly; advise patient to tell all persons associated with care

• Teach patient not to use OTC products (cough, cold, allergy) unless directed by prescriber; serious side effects can occur; xanthines such as coffee, tea, chocolate, cola can prevent action of product

• Teach patient importance of complying with dosage schedule, even if feeling better; to continue with medical regimen to decrease B/P: exercise, smoking cessation, decreasing stress, diet modifications

• Emphasize the need to rise slowly to sitting or standing position to minimize orthostatic hypotension; not to exercise in hot weather or increased hypotension can occur

• Teach patient to notify prescriber of mouth sores, sore throat, fever, swelling of hands or feet, irregular heartbeat, chest pain, coughing, shortness of breath

• Caution patient to report excessive perspiration, dehydration, vomiting, diarrhea; may lead to fall in B/P

• Caution patient that product may cause dizziness, fainting, light-headedness; may occur during first few days of therapy; to avoid activities that may be hazardous

• Teach patient how to take B/P, and teach normal readings for age-group; ensure patient takes regularly

BLACK BOX WARNING: Advise patient to tell prescriber if pregnancy is suspected or planned

Evaluation

Positive therapeutic outcome

• Decreased B/P in hypertension

TREATMENT OF OVERDOSE:

0.9% NaCl **IV** infusion, hemodialysis

carbachol ophthalmic

See Appendix B

carBAMazepine (Rx)

(kar-ba-maz'e-peen)

Apo-Carbamazepine ✦, **Carbatrol, Epitol, Equetro, Gen-Carbamazepine CR** ✦, **PMS-Carbamazepine** ✦, **Sandoz-Carbamazepine** ✦, **Taro-Carbamazepine** ✦, **Tegretol, Tegretol-XR**

Func. class.: Anticonvulsant

Chem. class.: Iminostilbene derivative

Pregnancy category D

Do not confuse:

Tegretol/Toradol

Pharmacodynamics

Onset	Slow
Peak	4-5 hr
Duration	Unknown

INTERACTIONS

Individual drugs

Benzodiazepines, darunavir, delavirdine, doxy-cycline, felbamate, haloperidol, nefazodone, oxcarbazepine, PHENobarbitol, phenytoin, primidone: decreased effect of these products

Cimetidine, clarithromycin, danzol, diltiazem, erythromycin, fluoxetine, fluvoxamine, isonia-zid, propoxyphene, valproic acid, verapamil, voriconazole: increased carBAMazepine levels

CISplatin, darunavir, delavirdine, DOXOrubicin, felbamate, nefazodone, oxcarbazepine, PHE-Nobarbitol, phenytoin, primidone, rifampin, theophylline: decreased carBAMazepine levels

Contraceptives (oral): decreased effect of oral contraceptives

Desmopressin, lithium, hypressin, vasopressin: increased effects of each specific product

Doxycycline: decreased effect of doxycycline

Lithium: increased CNS toxicity

Phenytoin: increased and decreased plasma levels; decreased carbamazepine plasma levels

Thyroid hormones: decreased effect of thyroid hormones

Warfarin: decreased effect of warfarin

Drug classifications

CYP3A4 inducers: decreased carbamazepine levels

CYP3A4 inhibitors: increased carbamazepine levels

⚠ **MAOIs: fatal reaction; do not use together**

Drug/herb

Echinacea: decreased carBAMazepine metabolism, increased levels

St. John's wort: decreased anticonvulsant action

Drug/food

Grapefruit juice: increased peak concentration of carBAMazepine

NURSING CONSIDERATIONS

Assessment

> **BLACK BOX WARNING:** Serious skin reactions: Asian patient, obtain genetic test prior to administration

• Assess for **seizures:** character, location, duration, intensity, frequency, presence of aura
• Assess for **trigeminal neuralgia:** facial pain

including location, duration, intensity, character, activity that stimulates pain
• Monitor liver function tests (AST, ALT) and urine function tests, BUN, urine protein periodically during treatments
• **Bone marrow depression:** Assess blood studies: RBC, Hct, Hgb, reticulocyte counts qwk for 4 wk then q3-6mo if on long-term therapy; if myelosuppression occurs, product should be discontinued
• Check blood levels during treatment or when changing dose; therapeutic level 4-12 mcg/ml
• Assess for **blood dyscrasias:** fever, sore throat, bruising, rash, jaundice, epistaxis (long-term treatment only)
⚠ **Assess mental status: mood, sensorium, affect, behavioral changes, suicidal thoughts/behaviors**
• **Toxicity:** Assess for bone marrow depression, nausea, vomiting, ataxia, diplopia, CV collapse, Stevens-Johnson syndrome

Nursing diagnoses

• Injury, risk for (side effects)
• Knowledge, deficient (teaching)

Patient/family education

• Teach patient to carry/wear emergency ID stating patient's name, products taken, condition, prescriber's name, phone number
• Caution patient to avoid driving, other activities that require alertness until stabilized on medication
• Teach patient not to discontinue medication quickly after long-term use
• Teach patient to use a nonhormonal type of contraception to prevent harm to the fetus
• Advise patient to use sunscreen to prevent burns
• Teach patient to take exactly as prescribed; do not double or omit doses
• Teach patient to report immediately chills, rash, light-colored stools, dark urine, yellowing of skin/eyes, abdominal pain, sore throat, mouth ulcers, bruising, blurred vision, dizziness

Evaluation

Positive therapeutic outcome
• Decreased seizure activity

TREATMENT OF OVERDOSE:

Lavage, VS

Adverse effects: *italics* = common; **bold** = life-threatening

carbidopa-levodopa (Rx)
(kar-bi-doe′pa lee-voe-doe′pa)
Apo-Levocarb ✦, Atamet, Parcopa, Sinemet, Sinemet CR
Func. class.: Antiparkinsonism agent
Chem. class.: Catecholamine
Pregnancy category C

ACTION: Decarboxylation of levodopa in periphery is inhibited by carbidopa; more levodopa is made available for transport to brain and conversion to dopamine in the brain

Therapeutic outcome: Absence of involuntary movements

USES: Parkinson's disease, parkinsonism resulting from carbon monoxide, chronic manganese intoxication, cerebral arteriosclerosis

Unlabeled uses: Restless legs syndrome

CONTRAINDICATIONS:
Hypersensitivity, malignant melanoma, history of malignant melanoma, or undiagnosed skin lesions resembling melanoma

Precautions: Pregnancy C, breastfeeding, diabetes, renal/cardiac/hepatic/respiratory disease, MI with dysrhythmias, open-angle glaucoma, seizures, peptic ulcer, depression

DOSAGE AND ROUTES
Beginning therapy for those not taking levodopa
Adult: PO 25 mg carbidopa/100 mg levodopa tid, may increase daily or every other day by 1 tab to desired response (8 tabs/day); EXT REL tabs carbidopa 50 mg/levodopa 200 mg bid

For those not taking levodopa ER
Adult: PO 50 mg carbidopa/200 mg levodopa bid

For those taking levodopa ER
Adult: Begin treatment with 10% more levodopa/day given PO q4-8hr, may increase or decrease dose q3days

For those taking levodopa <1.5 g/day
Adult: PO 25 mg carbidopa/100 mg levodopa tid-qid, may increase daily to desired response

For those taking levodopa >1.5 g/day
Adult: PO 25 mg carbidopa/250 mg levodopa tid-qid, may increase daily to desired response

Restless legs syndrome (RLS) (unlabeled)
Adult: PO carbidopa 25 mg/levodopa 100 mg, 1 tab at bedtime, may repeat if awakening within 2 hr or 50 mg carbidopa/200 mg levodopa SUS REL tab 1-2 tabs 1 hr before bedtime

Available forms: Tabs 10 mg carbidopa/100 mg levodopa, 25 mg carbidopa/100 mg levodopa, 25 mg carbidopa/250 mg levodopa; ext rel tab 25 mg/100 mg, 50 mg/200 mg carbidopa/levodopa (Sinemet CR); oral disintegrating tab (Parcopa) 10 mg carbidopa/100 mg levodopa, 25 mg carbidopa/100 mg levodopa, 25 mg carbidopa/250 mg levodopa

Implementation
PO route
• Swallow **ext rel tabs** whole; do not break, crush, or chew
• **Oral disintegrating tab:** gently remove from bottle, place on tongue, swallow with saliva; after it dissolves, liquid is not necessary
• Give product until NPO before surgery; check with prescriber for continuing product
• Adjust dosage depending on patient response
• Give with meals or after meals to prevent GI symptoms; limit protein taken with product
• Give only after MAOIs have been discontinued for 2 wk; if previously on levodopa, discontinue for at least 8 hr before change to levodopa-carbidopa

ADVERSE EFFECTS
CNS: *Involuntary choreiform movements, hand tremors, fatigue, headache, anxiety, twitching, numbness, weakness, confusion, agitation, insomnia, nightmares,* psychosis, hallucination, hypomania, severe depression, dizziness, impulsive behaviors, **neuroleptic malignant syndrome**
CV: *Orthostatic hypotension,* tachycardia, hypertension, palpitation
EENT: Blurred vision, diplopia, dilated pupils
GI: *Nausea, vomiting, anorexia, abdominal distress, dry mouth, flatulence, dysphagia, bitter taste, diarrhea, constipation*
HEMA: Hemolytic anemia, leukopenia, agranulocytosis
INTEG: Rash, sweating, alopecia
MISC: Urinary retention, incontinence, weight change, dark urine

Pharmacokinetics

Absorption	Well absorbed (PO); ER dose slowly absorbed
Distribution	Widely distributed
Metabolism	Liver, extensively
Excretion	Kidneys, metabolites
Half-life	Levodopa (1 hr); carbidopa (1-2 hr)

Pharmacodynamics

	PO	PO-ER
Onset	Unknown	Unknown
Peak	1 hr	2¹/₂ hr
Duration	6-24 hr	Unknown

INTERACTIONS

Individual drugs
Metoclopramide: increased effects of levodopa
Papaverine, pyridoxine: decreased effects of levodopa

Drug classifications
Antacids: increased effects of levodopa
Anticholinergics, antipsychotics, benzodiazepines, hydantoins: decreased effects of levodopa
MAOIs: hypertensive crisis

Drug/food
Protein: decreased absorption of levodopa

Drug/lab test
Increased: AST, ALT, bilirubin, LDH, alkaline phosphatase, BUN, serum glucose
Decreased: BUN, creatinine, uric acid
False increase: urine protein
False positive: urine ketones (dipstick), Coombs' test
False negative: urine glucose

NURSING CONSIDERATIONS

Assessment
• Assess for **parkinsonism:** shuffling gait, muscle rigidity, involuntary movements, pill rolling, muscle spasms, drooling before and during treatment
• Assess B/P, respiration, orthostatic B/P
• Monitor I&O ratio; retention commonly causes decreased urinary output, distention, frequency, incontinence; palpate bladder if retention occurs
• Assess for muscle twitching, blepharospasm that may indicate **toxicity**
• Monitor renal, liver, hematopoietic studies; also for diabetes, acromegaly during long-term therapy
• Monitor for constipation, cramping, pain in abdomen, abdominal distention; increase fluids, bulk, exercise if this occurs
• Assess for tolerance over long-term therapy; dose may have to be increased or changed
• Assess for mental status: affect, mood, CNS depression, worsening of mental symptoms during early therapy

Nursing diagnoses
• Knowledge, deficient (teaching)
• Mobility, impaired physical (uses)

Patient/family education
• Teach patient to change positions slowly to prevent orthostatic hypotension
• Teach patient to report side effects: twitching, eye spasms, grimacing, protrusion of tongue, personality changes that indicate overdose
• Instruct patient to use product exactly as prescribed; if product is discontinued abruptly, parkinsonian crisis may occur; do not double doses; take missed dose as soon as remembered up to 2 hr before next dose
• Teach patient that urine, sweat may darken and is harmless
• Advise patient to use physical activities to maintain mobility and lessen spasms
• Instruct patient that OTC medications should not be used unless approved by prescriber
• Advise patient that drowsiness, dizziness are common; to avoid hazardous activities until response is known
• Explain that sips of water, hard candy, or gum may lessen dry mouth
• Teach patient to take with meals to prevent GI symptoms; to limit protein intake, which impairs product's absorption

Evaluation
Positive therapeutic outcome
• Decrease in akathisia
• Improved mood
• Decreased involuntary movements

⚠ HIGH ALERT

CARBOplatin (Rx)
(kar′boe′pla-tin)
Func. class.: Antineoplastic alkylating agent
Chem. class.: Platinum coordination compound
Pregnancy category D

Do not confuse:
CARBOplatin/CISplatin, **Paraplatin**/platinol

ACTION: Produces interstrand DNA cross-links and to a lesser extent DNA-protein cross-links; activity is not cell cycle phase specific

Therapeutic outcome: Prevention of rapidly growing malignant cells

USES: Initial treatment of advanced ovarian cancer in combination with other agents; palliative treatment of recurrent ovarian carcinoma after treatment with other antineoplastic agents

CONTRAINDICATIONS:
Pregnancy **D,** hypersensitivity to this product, breastfeeding, significant bleeding, aluminum products used to prepare or administer carboplatin

> **BLACK BOX WARNING:** Severe bone marrow depression, platinum compound hypersensitivity

Precautions: Geriatric patients, radiation therapy within 1 mo, other cancer, chemotherapy within 1 mo, renal disease, liver disease

> **BLACK BOX WARNING:** Anemia, infection

DOSAGE AND ROUTES
(single agent)
Adult: IV INF initially 300 mg/m^2 on day 1 with cyclophosphamide, 600 mg/m^2 **IV** on day 1, repeat q4wk × 6 cycles; refractory tumors 360 mg/m^2 single dose, may repeat q4wk as needed; do not repeat until neutrophils are >2000 mm^3 and platelets are >100,000/mm^3

Renal dose
Adult: IV INF CCr 41-59 ml/min 250 mg/m^2, CCr 16-40 ml/min 200 mg/m^2; do not use in CCr <15 ml/min

Available forms: Lyophilized powder for inj 50, 150, 450 mg vials; aqueous sol for inj 50 mg/5 ml vial, 150 mg/15 ml vial, 450 mg/45 mg vial, 600 mg/60 ml vial

Implementation
• Antiemetic 30-60 min before giving product to prevent vomiting, and prn

IV route
• Use cytotoxic handling procedures
• **Reconstitute** CARBOplatin 50, 150, or 450 mg with 5, 15, or 45 ml respectively of sterile water for inj, D$_5$W, or NaCl (10 mg/ml); then further **dilute** with the same sol to 0.5-4 mg/ml; **give** over 15 min or more (**intermittent INF**)

• **Continuous IV INF** over 24 hr; do not use needles or IV administration sets containing aluminum; may cause precipitate or loss of potency
• Store protected from light at room temperature; reconstituted sol is stable for 8 hr at room temperature

Y-site compatibilities: Acyclovir, alfentanil, allopurinol, amifostine, amikacin, aminocaproic acid, aminophylline, amiodarone, amphotericin B lipid complex, amphotericin B liposome, ampicillin, ampicillin sulbactam, anidulafungin, atenolol, atracurium, azithromycin, aztreonam, bivalirudin, bleomycin, bumetanide, buprenorphine, butorphanol, calcium chloride/gluconate, caspofungin, ceFAZolin, cefepime, cefoperazone, cefotaxime, cefotetan, cefoxitin, ceftazidime, ceftizoxime, cefTRIAXone, cefuroxime, cimetidine, ciprofloxacin, cisatracurium, CISplatin, cladribine, clindamycin, codeine, cyclophosphamide, cycloSPORINE, cytarabine, DAPTOmycin, DAUNOrubicin, dexamethasone, dexmedetomidine, dexrazoxane, digoxin, diltiazem, diphenhydrAMINE, DOBUTamine, docetaxel, DOPamine, doripenem, doxacurium, DOXOrubicin, DOXOrubicin liposomal, doxycycline, droperidol, enalaprilat, ePHEDrine, EPINEPHrine, epirubicin, ertapenem, erythromycin, esmolol, etoposide, famotidine, fenoldopam, fentaNYL, filgrastim, fluconazole, fludarabine, fluorouracil, foscarnet, fosphenytoin, furosemide, ganciclovir, gatifloxacin, gemcitabine, gentamicin, granisetron, haloperidol, heparin, hydrocortisone, HYDROmorphone, hydrOXYzine, IDArubicin, ifosfamide, imipenem-cilastatin, inamrinone, insulin (regular), irinotecan, isoproterenol, ketorolac, labetalol, levofloxacin, levorphanol, lidocaine, linezolid injection, LORazepam, magnesium sulfate, mannitol, melphalan, meperidine, meropenem, mesna, methohexital, methotrexate, methylPREDNISolone, metoclopramide, metoprolol, metroNIDAZOLE, micafungin, midazolam, milrinone, minocycline, mitoxantrone, mivacurium, morphine, nafcillin, nalbuphine, naloxone, nesiritide, niCARdipine, nitroglycerin, nitroprusside, norepinephrine, octreotide, ofloxacin, ondansetron, oxaliplatin, paclitaxel, palonosetron, pamidronate, pancuronium, pantoprazole, pemetrexed, pentamidine, PENTobarbital, PHENobarbital, phentolamine, piperacillin, piperacillin-tazobactam, potassium chloride, potassium phosphates, prochlorperazine, promethazine, propofol, propranolol, ranitidine, remifentanil, riTUXimab, rocuronium, sargramostim, sodium acetate, sodium bicarbonate, sodium phosphates, succinylcholine, SUFentanil, sulfamethoxazole-trimethoprim, tacrolimus, teniposide, theophylline, thiotepa, ticarcillin, ticarcillin-clavulanate, tigecycline, tirofiban, TNA, tobramycin, topotecan, TPN, trastuzumab, trimethobenzamide, vancomycin, vasopressin, vecuronium, verapamil, vinBLAStine, vinCRIStine, vinorelbine, voriconazole, zidovudine

Solution compatibilities: D₅/0.2% NaCl, D₅/0.45% NaCl, D₅/0.9% NaCl, 0.9% NaCl, D₅W, sterile water for inj

Solution incompatibilities: Sodium bicarbonate

ADVERSE EFFECTS
CNS: Seizures, central neurotoxicity, peripheral neuropathy, dizziness, confusion
CV: Cardiac abnormalities (fatal CV events), stroke
EENT: Tinnitus, hearing loss, *vestibular toxicity*, visual changes
GI: Severe nausea, vomiting, diarrhea, weight loss, mucositis, anorexia, constipation, taste change
HEMA: Thrombocytopenia, leukopenia, pancytopenia, neutropenia, anemia, bleeding
INTEG: Alopecia, dermatitis, rash, erythema, pruritus, urticaria
META: Hypomagnesemia, hypocalcemia, hypokalemia, hyponatremia, hyperuremia
SYST: Anaphylaxis

Pharmacokinetics

Absorption	Complete
Distribution	Unknown
Metabolism	Liver
Excretion	Kidneys
Half-life	Initial 1-2 hr; postdistribution 2¹/₂-6 hr; increased in renal disease

Pharmacodynamics

Onset	¹/₂ hr
Peak	Unknown
Duration	4-6 hr

INTERACTIONS
Individual drugs
Amphotericin B: increased nephrotoxicity or ototoxicity
Aspirin: increased risk of bleeding
Phenytoin: decreased levels
Radiation: increased toxicity, bone marrow suppression

Drug classifications
Aminoglycosides: ototoxicity, increased nephrotoxicity
Antineoplastics, bone marrow–suppressing products: increased bone marrow suppression
Myelosuppressives: increased myelosuppression
NSAIDs: increased risk of bleeding
Thrombolytic agents: increased risk of bleeding

Drug/lab test
Increased: AST, BUN, alkaline phosphatase, bilirubin, creatinine

NURSING CONSIDERATIONS
Assessment

> **BLACK BOX WARNING: Bone marrow depression:** Monitor CBC, differential, platelet count weekly; withhold product if neutrophil count is <2000/mm³ or platelet count is <100,000/mm³; notify prescriber of results, calcium, magnesium, phosphate, potassium, sodium, uric adic

• Assess for **anaphylaxis:** pruritus, wheezing, tachycardia; notify physician after discontinuing products; resuscitation equipment should be available
• Monitor renal function studies: BUN, creatinine, serum uric acid, urine CCr before, during therapy; I&O ratio; report fall in urine output to <30 ml/hr
• Monitor temp q4hr (may indicate beginning of infection)
• Monitor liver function tests before, during therapy (bilirubin, AST, ALT, LDH) as needed or monthly; note jaundice of skin or sclera, dark urine, clay-colored stools, itchy skin, abdominal pain, fever, diarrhea
• Assess for **bleeding:** hematuria, stool guaiac, bruising or petechiae, mucosa or orifices q8hr; inflammation of mucosa, breaks in skin
• Identify dyspnea, crackles, unproductive cough, chest pain, tachypnea
• Identify effects of alopecia on body image; discuss feelings about body changes

Nursing diagnoses
• Body image, disturbed (adverse reactions)
• Infection, risk for (adverse reactions)
• Injury, risk for (adverse reactions)
• Knowledge, deficient (teaching)

Patient/family education
• Advise patient to report ringing/roaring in the ears, numbness, tingling in face, extremities, weight gain

• Teach patient to avoid use of products containing aspirin or ibuprofen, NSAIDs, alcohol, razors, commercial mouthwash, since bleeding may occur; to report symptoms of bleeding (hematuria, tarry stools)
• Instruct patient to report signs of **anemia** (fatigue, headache, irritability, faintness, shortness of breath); sore throat, bleeding, bruising, chills, back pain, blood in stools, dyspnea
• Instruct patient to report any changes in breathing or coughing even several months after treatment; to avoid crowds and persons with respiratory tract or other infections
• Advise patient that hair may be lost during treatment; a wig or hairpiece may make patient feel better; new hair may be different in color, texture
• Caution patient not to have any vaccinations without the advice of the prescriber; serious reactions can occur
• Teach patient that contraception is needed during treatment and for several months after the completion of therapy; not to breastfeed during treatment; to notify prescriber if pregnancy is planned or suspected
• Teach patient to notify prescriber immediately of fever, fatigue, sore throat, bleeding, bruising, chills, back pain, blood in stools, dyspnea

Evaluation
Positive therapeutic outcome
• Prevention of rapid division of malignant cells

carboprost (Rx)
(kar'boe-prost)
Hemabate
Func. class.: Oxytocic, abortifacient
Chem. class.: Prostaglandin
Pregnancy category C

ACTION: Stimulates uterine contractions, causing complete abortion in approximately 16 hr

Therapeutic outcome: Loss of fetus; decreased postpartum bleeding

USES: Abortion between 13 and 20 wk gestation; postpartum hemorrhage caused by uterine atony not controlled by other methods

CONTRAINDICATIONS:
Hypersensitivity to this product or benzyl alcohol, severe renal/hepatic/cardiac/respiratory disease, PID

Precautions: Pregnancy **C**, asthma, anemia, jaundice, diabetes mellitus, seizure disorders, past uterine surgery

DOSAGE AND ROUTES
To induce abortion
Adult: IM 100 mcg (0.4 ml) test dose, then IM 250 mcg, then 250 mcg q1^1/$_2$-3^1/$_2$ hr, may increase to 500 mcg if no response, max 12 mg total dose

Postpartum hemorrhage
Adult: IM 250 mcg, repeat at 15-90 min intervals, max total dosage 2 mg

Available forms: Inj 250 mcg/ml

Implementation
• Give IM inj in deep muscle mass; rotate inj sites if additional doses are given
• Have crash cart available on unit

ADVERSE EFFECTS
CNS: *Fever, chills,* headache
GI: *Nausea, vomiting, diarrhea*

Pharmacokinetics
Absorption	Well absorbed (nasal)
Distribution	Widely distributed (extracellular fluid)
Metabolism	Liver, rapidly
Excretion	Kidneys
Half-life	3-9 min

Pharmacodynamics
Onset	Unknown
Peak	16 hr
Duration	Unknown

INTERACTIONS
Drug classifications
Oxytocics: increased effects

NURSING CONSIDERATIONS
Assessment
• Monitor B/P, pulse; watch for change that may indicate hemorrhage
• Monitor respiratory rate, rhythm, depth; notify physician of abnormalities
• For length, duration of contraction; notify physician of contractions lasting >1 min or absence of contractions
• Assess for incomplete abortion; pregnancy must be terminated by another method; product is teratogenic

Nursing diagnoses
• Knowledge, deficient (teaching)

Patient/family education
• Advise patient to report increased blood loss, abdominal cramps, increased temp, or foul-smelling lochia

Evaluation
Positive therapeutic outcome
• Loss of fetus
• Control of bleeding

---

carisoprodol (Rx)
(kar-i-soe-proe′dole)
Soma
Func. class.: Skeletal muscle relaxant, central acting
Chem. class.: Meprobamate congener
Pregnancy category C

Do not confuse:
Soma/Soma compound

ACTION: Depresses CNS by blocking interneuronal activity in descending reticular formation of spinal cord, producing sedation

Therapeutic outcome: Relaxation of skeletal muscles

USES: Relieving pain, stiffness in musculoskeletal disorders

CONTRAINDICATIONS:
Hypersensitivity, intermittent porphyria

Precautions: Pregnancy **C**, breastfeeding, geriatric, renal/hepatic disease, addictive personality, Asian patients

DOSAGE AND ROUTES
Adult and child ≥16 yr: PO 250-350 mg tid and at bedtime, max 3 wk of use

Available forms: Tabs 350 mg

Implementation
• Give with meals for GI symptoms
• Have patient use gum, frequent sips of water for dry mouth
• Store in tight container at room temperature
• Use for short term (2-3 wk), potential for habituation

ADVERSE EFFECTS
CNS: *Dizziness, weakness, drowsiness,* headache, tremor, depression, insomnia, ataxia, irritability, **seizures**

CV: Postural hypotension, tachycardia
EENT: Diplopia, temporary loss of vision
GI: Nausea, vomiting, hiccups, epigastric discomfort
HEMA: Eosinophilia
INTEG: Rash, pruritus, fever, facial flushing, **erythema multiforme**
RESP: Asthmatic attack
SYST: Angioedema, anaphylaxis

Pharmacokinetics
Absorption	Well absorbed
Distribution	Crosses placenta
Metabolism	Liver, extensively, substrate of CYP2C19
Excretion	Kidney, unchanged; breast milk
Half-life	8 hr

Pharmacodynamics
Onset	$1/2$ hr
Peak	4 hr
Duration	4-6 hr

INTERACTIONS
Individual drugs
Alcohol: increased CNS depression
Meprobamate: do not use together

Drug classifications
Antidepressants (tricyclic), barbiturates, opioids, sedative/hypnotics: increased CNS depression

Drug/herb
Kava, valerian: increased CNS depression
St. John's wort: increased metabolism of carisoprodol

Drug/lab test
Increased: AST, alkaline phosphatase, blood glucose

NURSING CONSIDERATIONS
Assessment
• **Pain:** Monitor ROM, atrophy, stiffness, and pain in muscles; assess throughout treatment
• Monitor **ECG in seizure patients;** poor seizure control has occurred with patients taking this product
• Assess for **idiosyncratic reaction** within a few min or 1 hr of administration (disorientation, restlessness, weakness, euphoria, blurred vision); patient should be reassured that reaction is temporary
• Check for **allergic reactions:** rash, fever

• **CNS depression:** Assess for dizziness, drowsiness, psychiatric symptoms, abuse potential

Nursing diagnoses
• Injury, risk for (adverse reactions)
• Knowledge, deficient (teaching)
• Mobility, impaired physical (uses)

Patient/family education
• Caution patient not to take with alcohol, other CNS depressants
• Advise patient to avoid altering activities while taking this product
• Caution patient to avoid hazardous activities if drowsiness or dizziness occurs
• Caution patient to avoid using OTC medication such as cough preparations, antihistamines, unless directed by prescriber
• Teach patient to report **allergic reactions** immediately: rash, swelling of tongue/lips, hives, dyspnea

Evaluation
Positive therapeutic outcome
• Decreased pain, spasticity

TREATMENT OF OVERDOSE:
Activated charcoal, lavage, dialysis

⚠ **HIGH ALERT**

carmustine (Rx)
(kar-mus'teen)
BiCNU, Gliadel
Func. class.: Antineoplastic alkylating agent
Chem. class.: Nitrosourea
Pregnancy category D

ACTION: Alkylates DNA, RNA; inhibits enzymes that allow synthesis of amino acids in proteins; also responsible for cross-linking DNA strands; activity is not cell cycle phase specific

Therapeutic outcome: Prevention of rapidly growing malignant cells

USES: Brain tumors such as glioblastoma, medulloblastoma, astrocytoma, ependymoma, brain stem glioma, metastic brain tumors; multiple myeloma (with prednisone), non-Hodgkin's, Hodgkin's disease, other lymphomas; GI, breast, bronchogenic, and renal carcinomas; wafer, as adjunct to surgery/radiation in newly diagnosed high-grade malignant glioma patients

Unlabeled uses: Malignant melanoma

CONTRAINDICATIONS:
Pregnancy **D**, breastfeeding, hypersensitivity, leukopenia, thrombocytopenia

Precautions: Dental disease, extravasation, females, infection, leukopenia, neutropenia, secondary malignancy, thrombocytopenia

> **BLACK BOX WARNING:** Bone marrow suppression, pulmonary fibrosis

DOSAGE AND ROUTES
Carmustine should not be given until platelets $>100,000/mm^3$ and WBC $>4000/mm^2$
Adult: IV 75-100 mg/m^2 over 1-2 hr × 2 days or 150-200 mg/m^2 × 1 dose q6-8wk or 40 mg/m^2/day × 5 days q6wk
Adult: Intracavitary up to 8 wafers inserted into resection cavity

Available forms: Powder for inj 100 mg; wafer 7.7 mg intracavitary

Implementation
• RBC colony-stimulating factors to counter anemia may be required
• Give fluids IV or PO before chemotherapy to hydrate patient
• Provide antiemetic 30-60 min before giving product to prevent vomiting, and prn; antibiotics for prophylaxis of infection
• Give all medications PO, if possible; avoid IM inj if platelets are $<100,000/mm^3$
Wafer route
• Foil pouches may be kept at room temperature for 6 hr, if unopened
• If wafers are broken into several pieces, do not use

Intermittent IV infusion route
• Prepare in biologic cabinet wearing gown, gloves, mask; avoid contact with skin
• Administer after **diluting** 100 mg/3 ml ethyl alcohol (provided); then **further dilute** 27 ml sterile water for inj; **then dilute** with 100-500 ml 0.9% NaCl or D$_5$W; **give** over 1 hr or more; use only glass containers; reduce rate if discomfort is felt
• Flush IV line after carmustine with 10 ml 0.9% NaCl to prevent irritation at site
• Store reconstituted sol in refrigerator for 24 hr or room temperature for 8 hr

Y-site compatibilities: Amifostine, amphotericin B lipid complex, amphotericin B liposome, anidulafungin, aztreonam, bivalirudin, bleomycin, caspofungin, cefepime, codeine, DAPTOmycin, dexmedetomidine, docetaxel, ertapenem, etoposide, fenoldopam, filgrastim, fludarabine, gemcitabine, granisetron, levo-floxacin, melphalan, meperidine, mitoxantrone, nesiritide, octreotide, ondansetron, paclitaxel, palonsetron, pamidronate, pantoprazole, peme-trexed, piperacillin-tazobactam, riTUXimab, sargramostim, sodium acetate, tacrolimus, teni-poside, thiotepa, tigecycline, tirofiban, trastu-zumab, vinCRIStine, vinorelbine, voriconazole

ADVERSE EFFECTS

GI: *Nausea, vomiting, anorexia, stomatitis,* **hepatotoxicity**
GU: *Azotemia,* **renal failure**
HEMA: **Thrombocytopenia, leukopenia, myelosuppression, anemia**
INTEG: Pain, burning, hyperpigmentation at inj site
RESP: **Fibrosis, pulmonary infiltrate**
SYST: **Secondary malignant neoplastic disease**

Pharmacokinetics

Absorption	Completely absorbed
Distribution	Readily penetrates CSF
Metabolism	Liver, rapid
Excretion	Kidneys, breast milk
Half-life	Unknown

Pharmacodynamics

Unknown

INTERACTIONS

Individual drugs
Aspirin: increased risk of bleeding
Cimetidine, radiation: increased toxicity
Digoxin: decreased effects of digoxin
Phenytoin: decreased effects of phenytoin

Drug classifications
Anticoagulants: increased risk of bleeding
Antineoplastics: increased toxicity
Live vaccines: increased adverse reactions; decreased antibody reaction
Myelosuppressive agents: increased myelosup-pression

NURSING CONSIDERATIONS

Assessment
• Assess buccal cavity q8hr for dryness, sores or ulceration, white patches, pain, bleeding, dys-phagia; obtain prescription for viscous lidocaine (Xylocaine)
• Assess symptoms indicating severe allergic reaction: rash, pruritus, urticaria, purpuric skin lesions, itching, flushing; product should be discontinued

• **Bone marrow depression:** Monitor CBC, differential, platelet count weekly; withhold product if WBC <4000/mm³ or platelet count is <100,000/mm³; notify prescriber of results
• Monitor renal function studies: BUN, creatinine, urine CCr before and during therapy; I&O ratio; report fall in urine output to <30 ml/hr
• Monitor temp q4hr (may indicate beginning of infection)
• Monitor liver function tests before, during therapy (bilirubin, AST, ALT, LDH) as needed or monthly; note yellowing of skin or sclera, dark urine, clay-colored stools, itchy skin, abdominal pain, fever, diarrhea; hepatotoxicity can be serious and fatal
• Assess for **bleeding:** hematuria, stool guaiac, bruising or petechiae, mucosa or orifices q8hr; inflammation of mucosa, breaks in skin
• **Pulmonary fibrosis/infiltrate:** Monitor pulmonary function tests, chest x-ray films before, during therapy; chest film should be obtained q2wk during treatment; monitor for dyspnea, cough, pulmonary fibrosis; infiltrate occurs after high doses or several low-dose courses
• Identify effects of alopecia on body image; discuss feelings about body changes

Nursing diagnoses
• Body image, disturbed (adverse reactions)
• Infection, risk for (adverse reactions)
• Injury, risk for (adverse reactions)
• Knowledge, deficient (teaching)

Patient/family education
• Teach patient to avoid use of products containing aspirin or ibuprofen, razors, commercial mouthwash, since bleeding may occur; to report symptoms of bleeding (hematuria, tarry stools)
• Advise patient to avoid foods with citric acid, hot flavor, or rough texture if stomatitis is present
• Instruct patient to report signs of anemia (fatigue, headache, irritability, faintness, shortness of breath); avoid smoking
• Advise patient that hair may be lost during treatment; a wig or hairpiece may make patient feel better; new hair may be different in color, texture
• Caution patient not to have any vaccinations without the advice of the prescriber; serious reactions can occur
• Advise patient that contraception is needed during treatment and for several months after completion of therapy; product has teratogenic properties

Evaluation
Positive therapeutic outcome
• Prevention of rapid division of malignant cells

carteolol ophthalmic
See Appendix B

carvedilol (Rx)
(kar-veh'dee-lol)
Apo-Carvedilol ✦, Coreg, Coreg CR, PMS-Carvedilol ✦, RAN-Carvedilol ✦, ratio-Carvedilol ✦
Func. class.: Antihypertensive α/β-blocker
Pregnancy category C

Do not confuse:
carvedilol/Captopril/Carteolol

ACTION: A mixture of nonselective β-blocking and α-blocking activity; decreases cardiac output, exercise-induced tachycardia, reflex orthostatic tachycardia; causes reduction in peripheral vascular resistance and vasodilatation

Therapeutic outcome: Decreased B/P in hypertension

USES: Essential hypertension alone or in combination with other antihypertensives, CHF, LV dysfunction following MI, cardiomyopathy

CONTRAINDICATIONS:
Hypersensitivity, asthma, class IV decompensated cardiac failure, 2nd- or 3rd-degree heart block, cardiogenic shock, severe bradycardia, pulmonary edema

Precautions: Pregnancy C, breastfeeding, children, geriatric, cardiac failure, hepatic injury, peripheral vascular disease, anesthesia, major surgery, diabetes mellitus, thyrotoxicosis, emphysema, chronic bronchitis, renal disease

> **BLACK BOX WARNING:** Abrupt discontinuation

DOSAGE AND ROUTES
Essential hypertension
Adult: PO 6.25 mg bid × 7-14 days if tolerated well, then increase to 12.5 mg bid × 7-14 days if tolerated well, may be increased if needed to 25 mg bid, max 50 mg daily; EXT REL cap 20 mg/day, may increase after 7-14 days to 40 mg/day

Congestive heart failure
Adult: PO 3.125 mg bid × 2 wk; if well tolerated, give 6.25 mg bid × 2 wk, then double q2wk to max dose 25 mg bid <85 kg or 80 mg bid >85 kg; EXT REL cap (Coreg CR) 10 mg/day × 2 wk, increase to 20, 40, 80 mg/day over successive intervals of 2 wk

Postmyocardial infarction
Adult: PO 6.25 mg bid with food ×3-10 days, a lower starting dose may be used if indicated, titrate upward as tolerated, may increase to 12.5 mg bid, then titrate to 25 mg bid; PO EXT REL 20 mg q day with food, a lower starting dose of 10 mg q day and titrate upwards after 3-10 days, increase to 40 mg q day as required

Available forms: Tabs 3.125, 6.25, 12.5, 25 mg; ext rel cap 10, 20, 40, 80 mg

Implementation
• Give PO before meals, at bedtime; tablets may be crushed or swallowed whole, give with food to decrease orthostatic hypotension; do not break, crush, or chew ext rel cap
• Administer reduced dosage in renal dysfunction

> **BLACK BOX WARNING:** Do not discontinue prior to surgery

ADVERSE EFFECTS
CNS: *Dizziness,* somnolence, insomnia, ataxia, hyperesthesia, paresthesia, vertigo, depression, fatigue, weakness, headache
CV: *Bradycardia, postural hypotension,* dependent edema, peripheral edema, **AV block, extrasystoles,** hypo/hypertension, palpitations, peripheral ischemia, **CHF, pulmonary edema**
GI: *Diarrhea,* abdominal pain, increased alkaline phosphatase, increased ALT/AST
GU: Decreased libido, *impotence,* UTI
INTEG: Rash
MISC: Injury, back pain, viral infection, hypertriglyceridemia, **thrombocytopenia,** *hyperglycemia*
RESP: Rhinitis, pharyngitis, dyspnea, **bronchospasm,** cough

Pharmacokinetics

Absorption	Readily and extensively absorbed
Distribution	>98% protein binding
Metabolism	Extensively liver
Excretion	Via bile into feces
Half-life	Terminal half-life 7-10 hr, increased in the geriatric, hepatic disease

Pharmacodynamics
Unknown

INTERACTIONS
Individual drugs
Alcohol (acute ingestion), cimetidine: increased toxicity

Clonidine: decreased heart rate, B/P

Digoxin: increased concentrations of digoxin

Reserpine, levodopa: increased hypotension, bradycardia

Rifampin: decreased levels of carvedilol

Drug classifications
Antihypertensives, nitrates: increased toxicity

Antidiabetic agents: increased hypoglycemia

Calcium channel blockers: increased conduction disturbance

MAOIs: increased bradycardia, hypotension

NSAIDs, thyroid hormones: decreased levels of carvedilol

Drug/herb
Ephedra: decreased antihypertensive effect

Hawthorn: increased antihypertensive effect

Drug/lab test
Increased: blood glucose, potassium, triglycerides, uric acid

NURSING CONSIDERATIONS
Assessment
• Monitor I&O, weight daily

• **Hypertension:** Monitor B/P during beginning treatment and periodically thereafter; pulse q4hr, note rate, rhythm, quality

• Monitor apical/radial pulse before administration; notify prescriber of significant changes, pulse <50 bpm hold product, notify prescriber

• **CHF:** Assess for edema in feet and legs daily, fluid overload: dyspnea, weight gain, jugular vein distention, fatigue, crackles

Nursing diagnoses
• Cardiac output, decreased (uses)

• Injury, risk for (adverse reactions)

• Knowledge, deficient (teaching)

• Noncompliance (teaching)

Patient/family education
• Teach patient not to break, crush, or chew ext rel cap

• Instruct patient to comply with dosage schedule even if feeling better, that improvement may take several weeks

• Teach patient to rise slowly to sitting or standing position to minimize orthostatic hypotension

• Encourage patient to report bradycardia, dizziness, confusion, depression, fever, weight gain, shortness of breath, cold extremities, rash, sore throat, bleeding, bruising

• Teach patient to take pulse at home; advise when to notify prescriber

⚠ **Encourage patient not to discontinue product abruptly, taper over 1-2 wk, life-threatening dysrhythmias may occur**

• Advise patient to avoid hazardous activities until stabilized on medication; dizziness may occur

• Advise patient to avoid all OTC medications unless approved by prescriber

• Advise patient to carry/wear emergency ID with product name, prescriber at all times

• Advise patient to inform all health care providers of products, supplements taken

Evaluation
Positive therapeutic outcome
• Decreased B/P

• Decreased symptoms of CHF or angina

cefaclor
See cephalosporins—2nd generation

cefadroxil
cefazolin
See cephalosporins—1st generation

cefdinir
cefditoren pivoxil
cefepime
cefotaxime
See cephalosporins—3rd generation

cefotetan
cefoxitin
See cephalosporins—2nd generation

cefpodoxime
See cephalosporins—3rd generation

cefprozil
See cephalosporins—2nd generation

ceftaroline (Rx)

(sef-tar'oh-leen)
Teflaro
Func. class.: Cephalosporin
Pregnancy category B

ACTION: Inhibits cell wall synthesis through binding to essential penicillin-binding protein (PBP)

Therapeutic outcome: Negative C&S, resolution of symptoms of infection

USES: Acute bacterial skin/skin structure infections (ABSSI), bacterial community acquired pneumonia

CONTRAINDICATIONS:

Cephalosporin hypersensitivity

Precautions: Antimicrobial resistance, breastfeeding, carbapenem/penicillin hypersensitivity, child/infant/neonate, coagulopathy, colitis, dialysis, diarrhea, geriatrics, GI disease, hypoprothrombinemia, IBS, pregnancy **B**, pseudomembraneous colitis, renal disease, ulcerative colitis, viral infection, vitamin K deficiency

DOSAGE AND ROUTES

Adult: **IV** 600 mg q 12 hrs × 5-14 days (skin/skin structure infections), × 5-7 days (bacterial community acquired pneumonia)

Renal dose
Adult: **IV** CCr >30-≤50 ml/min 400 mg q 12 hrs; CCr ≥15-≤30 ml/min 300 mg q 12 hrs, CCr ≤15 ml/min 200 mg q 12 hrs

Available forms: Powder for injection 400 mg, 600 mg

Implementation
• Visually inspect for particulate matter or discoloration if solution or container permit
• **Reconstitute:** add 20 ml of sterile water to 400 or 600 mg vial (20 ml/ml for 400 mg), (30 mg/ml for 600 mg), mix gently until dissolved: **Dilute:** in 250 ml of 0.9% NaCl, 0.45% NaCl, LR, D5, D2.5, give over 1 hr, do not admix, use within 6 hrs at room temperature or 24 hrs refrigerated
• Store reconstituted solution in the refrigerator

ADVERSE EFFECTS
CV: Phlebitis
ENDO: Hypokalemia

GI: Diarrhea, nausea, vomiting, constipation, abdominal pain, **pseudomembranous colitis (rare)**, elevated hepatic enzymes
INTEG: Rash, **anaphylaxis**

Pharmacokinetics

Absorption	Unknown
Distribution	Unknown
Metabolism	Not hepatically metabolized
Excretion	In urine 88%, feces 6%
Half-life	2.66 hrs

Pharmacodynamics
Unknown

INTERACTIONS

Drug classifications
Anticoagulants: increased prothrombin time risk

NURSING CONSIDERATIONS

Assessment
• **Assess for infection:** vital signs, sputum, WBC prior to and during therapy
• **Assess for hypersensitivity:** prior to use, obtain a history of hypersensitivity reactions to cephalosporins, carbapenems, penicillins; cross sensitivity may occur
• Obtain specimens for culture and sensitivity before beginning therapy. Begin dose and specimens are obtained
• **Assess for anaphylaxis (rare):** rash, pruritus, laryngeal edema, dyspnea, wheezing; discontinue and notify health care provider immediately, keep emergency equipment nearby
• **Monitor for pseudomembraneous colitis:** diarrhea, abdominal pain, fever, bloody stools; report immediately if these occur, may occur several weeks after terminating therapy

Nursing diagnoses
• Risk for infection (uses)

Patient/family education
• Explain reason for treatment and expected result
• Instruct patient to report immediately rash, itching, difficulty breathing, bloody diarrhea, fever, abdominal pain

Evaluation
Positive therapeutic outcome
• Negative C&S, resolution of symptoms of infection

ceftazidime
ceftibuten
ceftizoxime
ceftriaxone
See cephalosporins—3rd generation

cefuroxime
See cephalosporins—2nd generation

⚠ HIGH ALERT

celecoxib (Rx)
(cel-eh-cox′ib)
Celebrex
Func. class.: Nonsteroidal antiinflammatory, antirheumatic
Chem. class.: COX-2 inhibitor
Pregnancy category C (1st/2nd trimesters), D (3rd trimester)

Do not confuse:
CeleBREX/Celexa/Cerebra/Cerebyx

ACTION: Inhibits prostaglandin synthesis by selectively inhibiting cyclooxygenase 2 (COX-2), an enzyme needed for biosynthesis

Therapeutic outcome: Decreased pain, inflammation

USES: Acute, chronic rheumatoid arthritis, osteoarthritis, acute pain, primary dysmenorrhea, ankylosing spondylitis, juvenile rheumatoid arthritis (JRA)

Unlabeled uses: Colorectal adenoma prophylaxis

CONTRAINDICATIONS:
Pregnancy **D** (3rd trimester), hypersensitivity to salicylates, iodides, other NSAIDs, sulfonamides

BLACK BOX WARNING: CABG

Precautions: Pregnancy **C** (1st/2nd trimester), breastfeeding, children <18 yr, geriatric, renal/hepatic disease, hypertension, severe dehydration, bleeding, GI, cardiac disorders, PVD, asthma

BLACK BOX WARNING: GI bleeding/perforation, peptic ulcer disease, MI, stroke

DOSAGE AND ROUTES
Do not exceed recommended dose, deaths have occurred

Acute pain/primary dysmenorrhea
Adult: PO 400 mg initially, then 200 mg if needed on first day, then 200 mg bid prn on subsequent days, if needed; start with ½ dose in poor CYP2C9 metabolizers
Geriatric: PO use lowest possible dose

Osteoarthritis
Adult: PO 200 mg/day as a single dose or 100 mg bid; start with ½ dose in poor CYP2C9 metabolizers

Rheumatoid arthritis
Adult: PO 100-200 mg bid; start with ½ dose in poor CYP2C9 metabolizers

Ankylosing spondylitis
Adult: PO 200 mg daily or in divided dose (bid); start with ½ dose in poor CYP2C9 metabolizers

Juvenile rheumatoid arthritis (JRA)
Adolescent and child ≥2 yr (>25 kg): PO 100 mg bid; start with ½ dose in poor CYP2C9 metabolizers
Child ≥2 yr (10-25 kg): PO 50 mg bid; start with ½ dose in poor CYP2C9 metabolizers

Colorectal adenoma prophylaxis (unlabeled)
Adult: PO 400 mg bid × 6 mo

Hepatic dose

(Child-Pugh class II)
Adult: PO reduce dose by 50%

Available forms: Caps 50, 100, 200, 400 mg

Implementation
• Do not break, crush, chew, or dissolve caps; caps may be opened and mixed with applesauce, ingest immediately with water
• Administer with food or milk to decrease gastric symptoms
• Do not increase dose

ADVERSE EFFECTS
CNS: *Fatigue, anxiety, depression, nervousness, paresthesia,* dizziness, insomnia
CV: **Stroke, MI, tachycardia, CHF,** angina, palpitations, dysrhythmias, hypertension, fluid retention
EENT: Tinnitus, hearing loss, blurred vision, glaucoma, cataract, conjunctivitis, eye pain
GI: *Nausea, anorexia, vomiting, constipation, dry mouth,* diverticulitis, gastritis, gastro-

enteritis, hemorrhoids, hiatal hernia, stomatitis, **GI bleeding/ulceration**
GU: Nephrotoxicity: dysuria, hematuria, oliguria, azotemia, cystitis, UTI, renal papillary necrosis
HEMA: Blood dyscrasias, epistaxis, bruising, anemia, **platelet aggregation**
INTEG: Purpura, rash, pruritus, sweating, erythema, petechiae, photosensitivity, alopecia, **serious sometimes fatal Stevens-Johnson syndrome, toxic epidermal necrolysis**
RESP: Pharyngitis, shortness of breath, pneumonia, coughing

Pharmacokinetics

Absorption	Well absorbed (PO)
Distribution	Crosses placenta, protein binding ~97%
Metabolism	Liver by CYP2C9
Excretion	Feces/kidneys, small amount
Half-life	11 hr

Pharmacodynamics

Onset	Unknown
Peak	3 hr
Duration	Unknown

INTERACTIONS

Individual drugs
Aspirin: decreased effectiveness; increased adverse reactions
Fluconazole: increased celecoxib level
Furosemide: decreased effect of furosemide
Lithium: increased toxicity
Warfarin: increased anticoagulant effects

Drug classifications
ACE inhibitors: may decrease effects of ACE inhibitors
Anticoagulants, antiplatelets, SSRIs, salicylates, thrombolytics: increased risk of bleeding
Antineoplastics: increased risk of hematologic toxicity
Bisphosphonates: increased toxicity
Glucocorticoids, NSAIDs: increased adverse reactions
Thiazide diuretics: decreased effectiveness of diuretics

Drug/herb
Feverfew: decreased effect of feverfew
Garlic, ginger, gingko: increased bleeding risk

Drug/lab test
Increased: ALT, AST, BUN

NURSING CONSIDERATIONS

Assessment
• Assess for **pain** of rheumatoid arthritis, osteoarthritis; check ROM, inflammation of joints, characteristics of pain

> **BLACK BOX WARNING:** Assess for cardiac disease that may be worse after taking this product; MI, stroke, do not use in coronary artery bypass graft (CABG)

• Monitor CBC during therapy; watch for decreasing platelets; if low, therapy may need to be discontinued, restarted after hematologic recovery; LFTs, serum creatinine BUN, stool guaiac

> **BLACK BOX WARNING:** Assess for blood dyscrasias (thrombocytopenia): bruising, fatigue, bleeding, poor healing

• Assess for **GI toxicity:** black, tarry stools; abdominal pain
⚠ **Assess for serious skin disorders: Stevens-Johnson syndrome, toxic epidermal necrolysis; may be fatal**

Nursing diagnoses
• Injury, risk for (side effects)
• Knowledge, deficient (teaching)
• Mobility, impaired physical (uses)
• Pain, acute (uses)
• Pain, chronic (uses)

Patient/family education
⚠ **Do not exceed recommended dose; notify prescriber, immediately of chest pain, skin eruptions, stop product**
• Teach patient that product must be continued for prescribed time to be effective; to avoid other NSAIDs, sulfonamides
• Caution patient to report bleeding, bruising, fatigue, malaise, since blood abnormalities do occur; to report GI symptoms: black tarry stools, cramping
• Teach patient to take with a full glass of water to enhance absorption
• Teach patient to check with prescriber to determine when product should be discontinued before surgery; advise patient to notify prescriber if pregnancy is planned or suspected
• Advise patient to report possible respiratory infection: fever, shortness of breath, coughing, painful swallowing

Evaluation
Positive therapeutic outcome
• Decreased pain in arthritic conditions

⚠ Nurse Alert

- Decreased inflammation in arthritic conditions
- Decreased number of polyps (FAP)

cephalexin
See cephalosporins—1st generation

CEPHALOSPORINS— 1ST GENERATION

cefadroxil (Rx)
(sef-a-drox'ill)
Apo-Cefadroxil ❦
cefazolin (Rx)
(sef-a'zoe-lin)
cephalexin (Rx)
(sef-a-lex'in)
Keflex, Panixine
Pregnancy category B

Do not confuse:
cephalexin/cefaclor

ACTION: Inhibits bacterial cell wall synthesis, rendering cell wall osmotically unstable, leading to cell death by binding to cell wall membrane, lysis mediated by cell wall autolytic enzymes

cefadroxil

Therapeutic outcome: Bactericidal effects for the following: gram-negative bacilli *Escherichia coli, Proteus mirabilis, Klebsiella* (UTI only); gram-positive organisms *Streptococcus pneumoniae, Streptococcus pyogenes, Staphylococcus aureus*

USES: Upper, lower respiratory tract, urinary tract, skin infections; otitis media; tonsillitis, UTI

cefazolin

Therapeutic outcome: Bactericidal effects for the following: gram-negative organisms *Haemophilus influenzae, Escherichia coli, Proteus mirabilis, Klebsiella;* gram-positive organisms *Staphylococcus aureus*

USES: Upper, lower respiratory tract, urinary tract, skin infections; bone, joint, biliary, genital infections; endocarditis, surgical prophylaxis, septicemia

cephalexin

Therapeutic outcome: Bactericidal effects for the following: gram-negative organisms *Haemophilus influenzae, Escherichia coli, Proteus mirabilis, Klebsiella;* gram-positive organisms *Streptococcus pneumoniae, Streptococcus pyogenes, Staphylococcus aureus*

USES: Upper, lower respiratory tract, urinary tract, skin, bone infections; otitis media

CONTRAINDICATIONS:
Hypersensitivity to cephalosporins, infants <1 mo

Precautions: Pregnancy **B,** breastfeeding, hypersensitivity to penicillins, renal disease

DOSAGE AND ROUTES
cefadroxil
Adult: PO 1-2 g daily or q12hr in divided doses, give a loading dose of 1 g initially
Child: PO 30 mg/kg/day in divided doses bid, max 2 g/day

Renal dose
Adult: PO CCr 25-50 ml/min, 500 mg q12hr; CCr 10-24 ml/min 500 mg q24hr, CCr <10 ml/min 500 mg q36hr

Available forms: Caps 500 mg; tabs 1 g; oral susp 125, 250, 500 mg/5 ml

cefazolin

Life-threatening infections
Adult: IM/IV 1-2 g q6-8hr, max 12 g/day
Child >1 mo: IM/IV 75-100 mg/kg in 3-4 divided doses, max 6 g/day

Mild/moderate infections
Adult: IM/IV 250 mg-1 g q8hr, max 12 g/day
Child >1 mo: IM/IV 25-50 mg/kg in 3-4 equal doses, max 6 g/day or 2 g as a single dose

Renal dose
Adult: IM/IV following loading dose CCr 35-54 ml/min dose q8hr; CCr 10-34 ml/min 50% of dose q12hr; CCr <10 ml/min 50% of dose q18-24hr
Child: IM/IV CCr >70 ml/min, no dosage adjustment; CCr 40-70 ml/min following loading dose, reduce dose to 7.5-30 mg/kg q12hr; CCr 20-39 ml/min, give 3.125-12.5 mg/kg after loading dose q12hr; CCr 5-19 ml/min, 2.5-10 mg/kg after loading dose q24hr

Available forms: Inj 250, 500 mg, 1, 5, 10, 20 g; infusion 500 mg, 1 g/50 ml vial

cephalexin

Moderate infections
Adult: PO 250-500 mg q6hr, max 4 g/day
Child: PO 25-50 mg/kg/day in 4 equal doses, max 4 g/day

Adverse effects: *italics* = common; **bold** = life-threatening

Moderate skin infections
Adult: PO 500 mg q12hr

Endocarditis prophylaxis
2 g 1 hr before procedure

Severe infections
Adult: PO 500 mg-1 g q6hr
Child: PO 50-100 mg/kg/day in 4 equal doses, max 4 g/day

Renal dose
Adult: PO CCr 10-40 ml/min 250-500 mg, then 250-500 mg q8-12hr; CCr <10 mg/min 250-500 mg, then 250-500 mg q12-24hr

Available forms: Caps 250, 500 mg; tabs 250, 500 mg, 1 g; oral susp 125, 250 mg/5 ml

cefadroxil

Implementation
• Give in even doses around the clock; if GI upset occurs, give with food; product must be given for 10-14 days to ensure organism death and prevent superinfection
• Shake susp, refrigerate, discard after 2 wk

cefazolin

Implementation
IM route
• Reconstitute 250-500 mg of product with 2 ml sterile or bacteriostatic water for inj, or 0.9% NaCl; reconstitute 1 g of product with 2.5 ml; give deep in large muscle mass, massage

IV route
• Check for irritation, extravasation, phlebitis daily, change site q72hr
• For direct IV dilute in 10 ml of sterile water for inj; give over 5 min
• For intermittent inf dilute reconstituted sol (500 mg or 1 mg) in 50-100 ml D$_5$W, D$_{10}$W, D$_5$/0.25% NaCl, D$_5$/0.45% NaCl, D$_5$/0.9% NaCl, D$_5$/LR, or LR, 0.9% NaCl; give over 30-60 min; may be refrigerated up to 96 hr or stored 24 hr at room temperature

Syringe compatibilities: Heparin, vit B complex

Syringe incompatibilities: Ascorbic acid inj, cimetidine, lidocaine, vit B/C

Y-site compatibilities: Acyclovir, alfentanil, allopurinol, alprostadil, amifostine, amikacin, aminocaproic acid, aminophylline, amphotericin B liposome, anidulafungin, ascorbic acid injection, atenolol, atracurium, atropine, aztreonam, benztropine, bivalirudin, bleomycin, bumetanide, buprenorphine, butorphanol, calcium gluconate, CARBOplatin, cefamandole, cefmetazole, cefonicid, cefoperazone, cefotetan, cefoxitin, cefpirome, ceftazidime, ceftizoxime, cefTRIAXone, cefuroxime, cephalothin, cephapirin, chloramphenicol, cimetidine, CISplatin, clindamycin, codeine, cyanocobalamin, cyclophosphamide, cycloSPORINE, cytarabine, DACTINomycin, DAPTOmycin, dexamethasone, dexmedetomidine, digoxin, diltiazem, docetaxel, doxacurium, doxapram, DOXOrubicin liposomal, enalaprilat, ePHEDrine, EPINEPHrine, epirubicin, epoetin alfa, eptifibatide, esmolol, etoposide, fenoldopam, fentaNYL, filgrastim, fluconazole, fludarabine, fluorouracil, folic acid (as sodium salt), foscarnet, furosemide, gallium, gatifloxacin, gemcitabine, gentamicin, glycopyrrolate, granisetron, heparin, hydrocortisone, hydrOXYzine, IDArubicin, ifosfamide, imipenem-cilastatin, indomethacin, insulin (regular), irinotecan, isoproterenol, ketorolac, lidocaine, linezolid, LORazepam, LR's injection, mannitol, mechlorethamine, melphalan, meperidine, metaraminol, methicillin, methotrexate, methoxamine, methyldopate, methylPREDNISolone, metoclopramide, metoprolol, metroNIDAZOLE, mezlocillin, miconazole, midazolam, milrinone, morphine, moxalactam, multiple vitamins injection, nafcillin, nalbuphine, naloxone, nesiritide, niCARdipine, nitroglycerin, nitroprusside, norepinephrine, octreotide, ondansetron, oxacillin, oxaliplatin, oxytocin, paclitaxel, palonosetron, pamidronate, pancuronium, pantoprazole, penicillin G potassium/sodium, peritoneal dialysis solution, perphenazine, PHENobarbital, phenylephrine, phytonadione, piperacillin, Plasma-Lyte M in dextrose 5%, polymyxin B, potassium chloride, procainamide, propofol, propranolol, ranitidine, remifentanil, Ringer's injection, ritodrine, riTUXimab, sargramostim, sodium acetate, sodium bicarbonate, succinylcholine, SUFentanil, tacrolimus, teniposide, tenoxicam, theophylline, thiamine, thiotepa, ticarcillin, ticarcillin-clavulanate, tigecycline, tirofiban, TNA, tolazoline, trastuzumab, trimetaphan, urokinase, vasopressin, vecuronium, verapamil, vinCRIStine, vitamin B complex with C, voriconazole, warfarin

Y-site incompatibilities: Amiodarone, hetastarch, HYDROmorphone, IDArubicin, vinorelbine tartrate

cephalexin

Implementation
• Do not break, crush, or chew caps
• Give in even doses around the clock; if GI upset occurs, give with food; product must be

taken for 10-14 days to ensure organism death and prevent superinfection
• Shake susp, refrigerate, discard after 2 wk

ADVERSE EFFECTS
CNS: Headache, dizziness, weakness, paresthesia, fever, chills, **seizures** (high doses)
GI: Nausea, vomiting, *diarrhea, anorexia,* pain, glossitis, bleeding; increased AST, ALT, bilirubin, LDH, alkaline phosphatase; abdominal pain, **pseudomembranous colitis**
GU: Proteinuria, vaginitis, pruritus, candidiasis, increased BUN, **nephrotoxicity, renal failure**
HEMA: **Leukopenia, thrombocytopenia, agranulocytosis,** anemia, **neutropenia, lymphocytosis, eosinophilia, pancytopenia, hemolytic anemia**
INTEG: Rash, urticaria, dermatitis
RESP: Dyspnea
SYST: **Anaphylaxis, serum sickness,** superinfection, **Stevens-Johnson syndrome**

cefadroxil
Pharmacokinetics

Absorption	Well absorbed
Distribution	Widely distributed; crosses placenta
Metabolism	Not metabolized
Excretion	Unchanged by kidneys; enters breast milk
Half-life	$1^1/_2$-2 hr

Pharmacodynamics

	PO
Onset	Rapid
Peak	$1^1/_2$-2 hr
Duration	12-24 hr

cefazolin
Pharmacokinetics

Absorption	Well absorbed
Distribution	Widely distributed; crosses placenta
Metabolism	Not metabolized
Excretion	Unchanged by kidneys; enters breast milk
Half-life	$1^1/_2$-$2^1/_2$ hr

Pharmacodynamics

	IM	IV
Onset	Rapid	10 min
Peak	1-2 hr	Infusion's end
Duration	6-12 hr	Unknown

cephalexin
Pharmacokinetics

Absorption	Well absorbed
Distribution	Widely distributed; crosses placenta
Metabolism	Not metabolized
Excretion	Kidneys, unchanged; enters breast milk
Half-life	$1/_2$-1 hr; increased in renal disease

Pharmacodynamics

Onset	15-30 min
Peak	1 hr
Duration	6-12 hr

INTERACTIONS
Individual drugs
Probenecid: increased toxicity

Drug classifications
Aminoglycosides, diuretics (loop): increased toxicity
Anticoagulants: increased protime; use cautiously

Drug/lab test
Increased: AST, ALT, alkaline phosphatase, LDH, BUN, creatinine, bilirubin
False positive: urinary protein, direct Coombs' test, urine glucose
Interference: cross-matching

NURSING CONSIDERATIONS
Assessment
• Assess patient for previous sensitivity reaction to penicillins or other cephalosporins; cross-sensitivity between penicillins and cephalosporins is common
• Assess patient for signs and symptoms of **infection** including characteristics of wounds, sputum, urine, stool, WBC >10,000/mm³, earache, fever; obtain baseline information and during treatment
• Obtain C&S before beginning product therapy to identify if correct treatment has been initiated
• Assess for **anaphylaxis:** rash, urticaria, pruritus, chills, fever, joint pain; angioedema may occur a few days after therapy begins; epinephrine and resuscitation equipment should be available for anaphylactic reaction
• Identify urine output; if decreasing, notify prescriber (may indicate **nephrotoxicity**); also check for increased BUN, creatinine

Adverse effects: *italics* = common; **bold** = life-threatening

• Monitor blood studies: AST, ALT, CBC, Hct, bilirubin, LDH, alkaline phosphatase, Coombs' test monthly if patient is on long-term therapy
• Monitor electrolytes: potassium, sodium, chloride monthly if patient is on long-term therapy
• Assess bowel pattern daily; if severe diarrhea occurs, product should be discontinued; may indicate **pseudomembranous colitis**
• Monitor for bleeding: ecchymosis, bleeding gums, hematuria, stool guaiac daily if on long-term therapy
• Assess for **superinfection:** perineal itching, fever, malaise, redness, pain, swelling, drainage, rash, diarrhea, change in cough, sputum

Nursing diagnoses
• Diarrhea (side effects)
• Fluid volume, risk for deficient (side effects)
• Infection, risk for (uses)
• Injury, risk for (side effects)
• Knowledge, deficient (teaching)
• Noncompliance (teaching)

Patient/family education
• Teach patient to report sore throat, bruising, bleeding, joint pain; may indicate **blood dyscrasias** (rare)
• Advise patient to contact prescriber if vaginal itching, loose foul-smelling stools, furry tongue occur; may indicate superinfection
• Instruct patient to take all medication prescribed for the length of time ordered
• Advise patient to notify prescriber of diarrhea with blood, pus, mucus, which may indicate **pseudomembranous colitis**

Evaluation
Positive therapeutic outcome
• Absence of signs/symptoms of infection (WBC <10,000/mm^3, temp WNL, absence of red draining wounds, earache)
• Reported improvement in symptoms of infection
• Negative C&S

TREATMENT OF ANAPHYLAXIS: EPINEPHrine, antihistamines, resuscitate if needed

CEPHALOSPORINS— 2ND GENERATION
cefaclor (Rx)
(sef'a-klor)
Ceclor, Raniclor
cefotetan (Rx)
(sef'oh-tee-tan)
Cefotan
cefoxitin (Rx)
(se-fox'i-tin)
Mefoxin
cefprozil (Rx)
(sef-proe'zill)
Cefzil
cefuroxime (Rx)
(sef-yoor-ox'eem)
Ceftin, Cefuroxime, Zinacef
Func. class.: Antiinfective
Chem. class.: Cephalosporin (2nd generation)
Pregnancy category B

Do not confuse:
cefaclor/cephalexin, **Cefotan**/Ceftin, cefprozil/cefazolin/cefuroxime, **Cefzil**/Ceftin

ACTION: Inhibits bacterial cell wall synthesis, rendering cell wall osmotically unstable, leading to cell death by binding to cell wall membrane

cefaclor
Therapeutic outcome: Bactericidal effects for the following: gram-negative bacilli *Haemophilus influenzae, Escherichia coli, Proteus mirabilis, Klebsiella*; gram-positive organisms *Streptococcus pneumoniae, Streptococcus pyogenes, Staphylococcus aureus*

USES: Upper and lower respiratory tract, urinary tract, skin infections; otitis media; bone, joint infections

cefotetan
Therapeutic outcome: Bactericidal effects for the following: gram-negative organisms *Citrobacter, Haemophilus influenzae, Escherichia coli, Enterobacter aerogenes, Proteus mirabilis, Klebsiella, Salmonella, Shigella, Acinetobacter, Bacteroides fragilis, Neisseria, Serratia*; gram-positive organisms *Streptococcus pneumoniae, Streptococcus pyogenes, Staphylococcus aureus*

USES: Serious upper or lower respiratory tract, urinary tract, gynecologic, skin, bone, joint, gonococcal, intraabdominal infections

cefoxitin

Therapeutic outcome: Bactericidal effects for the following: gram-negative bacilli *Bacteroides fragilis, Haemophilus influenzae, Escherichia coli, Proteus, Klebsiella, Neisseria gonorrhoeae*; gram-positive organisms *Streptococcus pneumoniae, Streptococcus pyogenes, Staphylococcus aureus*; anaerobes including *Clostridium*

USES: Lower respiratory tract, urinary tract, skin, bone, gynecologic, gonococcal infections; septicemia, peritonitis

cefprozil

Therapeutic outcome: Bactericidal effects for the following: gram-negative bacilli *Haemophilus influenzae, Escherichia coli*; gram-positive organisms *Streptococcus pneumoniae, Streptococcus pyogenes, Staphylococcus aureus*

USES: Pharyngitis/tonsillitis, otitis media, secondary bacterial infection of acute bronchitis, and acute bacterial exacerbation of chronic bronchitis and uncomplicated skin and skin structure infections; acute sinusitis

cefuroxime

Therapeutic outcome: Bactericidal effects for the following: gram-negative bacilli *Haemophilus influenzae, Escherichia coli, Neisseria, Proteus mirabilis, Klebsiella*; gram-positive organisms: *Streptococcus pneumoniae, Streptococcus pyogenes, Staphylococcus aureus*

USES: Serious lower respiratory tract, urinary tract, skin, bone, joint, gonococcal infections; septicemia, meningitis

CONTRAINDICATIONS:

Hypersensitivity to cephalosporins or related antibiotics, seizures

Precautions: Pregnancy **B**, breastfeeding, children, renal/GI disease

DOSAGE AND ROUTES

cefaclor
Adult: PO 250-500 mg q8hr, max 4 g/day
Child >1 mo: PO 20-40 mg/kg daily in divided doses q8hr, or total daily dose may be divided and given q12hr, max 1 g/day

Available forms: Caps 250, 500 mg; oral susp 125, 187, 250, 375 mg/5 ml; chew tabs (Raniclor) 250, 375 mg

cefotetan
Adult: IV/IM 1-2 g q12hr × 5-10 days

Renal dose
Adult: IM/IV CCr 10-30 ml/min q24hr or ½ dose q12hr; CCr <10 ml/min q48hr or ½ dose q24hr

Perioperative prophylaxis
Adult: IV 1-2 g ½-1 hr before surgery

Available forms: Inj 1, 2, 10 g

cefoxitin
Adult: IM/IV 1-2 g q6-8hr

Uncomplicated gonorrhea (outpatient)
Adult/adolescent/child ≥45 kg: IM 2 g as single dose with 1 g PO probenecid at same time

Renal dose
Adult: IM/IV after loading dose CCr 30-50 ml/min 1-2 g q8-12hr; CCr 10-29 ml/min 1-2 g q12-24hr; CCr <10 ml/min 0.5-1 g q12-24hr

Severe infections
Adult: IM/IV 2 g q4hr
Child ≥3 mo: IM/IV 80-160 mg/kg/day divided q4-6hr; max 12 g/day

Available forms: Powder for inj 1, 2, 10 g

cefprozil

Renal dose
CCr <30 ml/min 50% of dose

Upper respiratory infections
Adult: PO 500 mg q24hr × 10 days

Otitis media
Child 6 mo-12 yr: PO 15 mg/kg q12hr × 10 days

Lower respiratory infections
Adult: PO 500 mg q12hr × 10 days

Skin/skin structure infections
Adult: PO 250-500 mg q12hr × 10 days

Available forms: Tabs 250, 500 mg; susp 125, 250 mg/5 ml

cefuroxime
Adult and child: PO 250 mg q12hr; may increase to 500 mg of q12hr in serious infections
Adult: IM/IV 750 mg-1.5 g q8hr for 5-10 days

Urinary tract infections
Adult: PO 125 mg q12hr; may increase to 250 mg q12hr if needed

Otitis media
Child <2 yr: PO 125 mg bid
Child >2 yr: PO 250 mg bid

Surgical prophylaxis
Adult: IV 1.5 g ¹/₂-1 hr preop

Severe infections
Adult: IM/IV 1.5 g q6hr; may give up to 3 g q8hr for bacterial meningitis
Child >3 mo: IM/IV 50-100 mg/kg/day; or IM in divided doses q6-8hr

Uncomplicated gonorrhea
Adult: 1.5 g IM as single dose with oral pro-benecid in 2 separate sites

Renal dose
• Dosage reduction indicated in severe renal impairment (CCr <20 ml/min)

Available forms: Tabs 125, 250, 500 mg; inj 150, 750 mg, 1.5, 7.5 g; inj 750 mg; 1.5 g powder, susp 125, 250 mg/5 ml

Implementation

cefaclor
• Do not break, crush, chew, or cut ext rel tabs
• Give in even doses around the clock; if GI upset occurs, give with food; product must be given for 10-14 days to ensure organism death and prevent superinfection
• Shake susp, refrigerate, discard after 2 wk

cefotetan
IM route
• Reconstitute 1 g/2 ml or 2 g/3 ml of sterile or bacteriostatic water for inj; may be diluted with 0.5% of 1% lidocaine to prevent pain; give deep in large muscle mass, massage

IV route
• May be stored 96 hr refrigerated or 24 hr at room temperature
• Check for irritation, extravasation, phlebitis daily; change site q72hr
• For direct IV dilute in 1 g/10 ml or more and give over 5 min
• For intermittent inf further dilute in 50-100 ml of 0.9% NaCl or D₅W; give over 3-5 min; discontinue primary line while running intermittent inf

Y-site compatibilities: Allopurinol, amifostine, aztreonam, diltiazem, famotidine, filgrastim, fluconazole, fludarabine, heparin, regular insulin, melphalan, meperidine, morphine, paclitaxel, sargramostim, tacrolimus, teniposide, theophylline, thiotepa

cefoxitin
IM route
• Reconstitute 1 g/2 ml of sterile water for inj; may be diluted with 0.5% or 1% lidocaine to prevent pain; give deep in large muscle mass, massage

IV route
• Check for irritation, extravasation, phlebitis daily; change site q72hr
• For direct IV, dilute 1 g/10 ml or 2 g/20 ml of sterile water for inj; shake, let stand until clear; give over 3-5 min
• For intermittent inf further dilute with 50-100 ml of D₅W, D₁₀W, D₅/0.25% NaCl, D₅/0.45% NaCl, D₅/0.9% NaCl, 0.9% NaCl D₅/LR, D₅/0.02%, sodium bicarbonate, Ringer's, or LR; give over 15-30 min; may store 96 hr refrigerated or 24 hr room temperature
• For cont inf dilute in 500-1000 ml; give over prescribed rate

Syringe compatibilities: Heparin, insulin

Y-site compatibilities: Acyclovir, amifostine, aztreonam, cyclophosphamide, diltiazem, famotidine, fluconazole, foscarnet, HYDROmorphone, magnesium sulfate, meperidine, morphine, ondansetron, perphenazine, temiposide, thiotepa

Y-site incompatibilities: Hetastarch

cefprozil
IM route
• Reconstitute with 1 g/2 ml or 2 g/3 ml of sterile or bacteriostatic water for inj; may be diluted with 0.5% or 1% lidocaine to prevent pain; give deep in large muscle mass, massage

IV route
• Check for irritation, extravasation, phlebitis daily; change site q72hr
• For direct IV, dilute 1 g/10 ml or more and give over 5 min
• For intermittent inf further dilute with 50-100 ml of 0.9% NaCl or D₅W; give over 3-5 min; discontinue primary line while running intermittent inf

Syringe incompatibilities: Doxapram

Y-site compatibilities: Famotidine, fluconazole, fludarabine, regular insulin, meperidine, morphine, sargramostim

Additive incompatibilities: Aminoglycosides, tetracyclines, heparin

cefuroxime
• Give for 10-14 days to ensure organism death, prevent superinfection

- Give with food if needed for GI symptoms
- Five after C&S obtained

ADVERSE EFFECTS

CNS: Dizziness, headache, fatigue, paresthesia, fever, chills, confusion

GI: *Diarrhea,* nausea, vomiting, anorexia, dysgeusia, glossitis, bleeding; increased AST, ALT, bilirubin, LDH, alkaline phosphatase; abdominal pain, loose stools, flatulence, heartburn, stomach cramps, colitis, jaundice, **pseudomembranous colitis**

GU: Vaginitis, pruritus, candidiasis, increased BUN, **nephrotoxicity, renal failure,** pyuria, dysuria, reversible interstitial nephritis

HEMA: **Leukopenia, thrombocytopenia, agranulocytosis,** anemia, **neutropenia,** lymphocytosis, **eosinophilia, pancytopenia, hemolytic anemia, leukocytosis, granulocytopenia**

INTEG: Rash, urticaria, dermatitis, **Stevens-Johnson syndrome**

RESP: Dyspnea

SYST: **Anaphylaxis, serum sickness,** superinfection

cefaclor

Pharmacokinetics

Absorption	Well absorbed
Distribution	Widely distributed; crosses placenta
Metabolism	Not metabolized
Excretion	Unchanged by kidneys (60%-80%); enters breast milk
Half-life	36-54 min; increased in renal disease

Pharmacodynamics

Onset	15 min
Peak	$^1/_2$-1 hr
Duration	Unknown

cefotetan

Pharmacokinetics

Absorption	Well absorbed (IM)
Distribution	Widely distributed; crosses placenta
Metabolism	Not metabolized
Excretion	Kidneys, unchanged; enters breast milk
Half-life	5 hr; increased in renal disease

Pharmacodynamics

	IM	IV
Onset	Rapid	Immediate
Peak	1-3 hr	Infusion's end
Duration	Unknown	Unknown

cefoxitin

Pharmacokinetics

Absorption	Well absorbed (IM)
Distribution	Widely distributed; crosses placenta
Metabolism	Not metabolized
Excretion	Kidneys, unchanged; enters breast milk
Half-life	$^1/_2$-1 hr; increased in renal disease

Pharmacodynamics

	IM	IV
Onset	Rapid	Immediate
Peak	$^1/_2$ hr	Infusion's end
Duration	Unknown	Unknown

cefprozil

Pharmacokinetics

Absorption	Well absorbed
Distribution	Widely distributed; crosses placenta
Metabolism	Not metabolized
Excretion	Kidneys (60%), unchanged; enters breast milk
Half-life	1.3 hr (normal renal function); 2 hr (hepatic disease); $5^1/_4$-6 hr (end-stage renal disease)

Pharmacodynamics

Unknown

INTERACTIONS

Individual drugs

Antacids: decreased absorption of cephalosporins

Furosemide: increased effect/toxicity

Plicamycin, valproic acid: increased bleeding

Probenecid: decreased excretion of product and increased blood levels/toxicity

Drug classifications

Aminoglycosides: increased effect/toxicity

Anticoagulants, antiplatelets, NSAIDs, thrombolytics: increased bleeding (cefotetan)

H_2-blockers: decreased effects of cephalosporins

Drug/lab test
False: increased creatinine (serum urine), urinary 17-KS
False positive: urinary protein, direct Coombs' test, urine glucose (Clinitest)
Interference: cross-matching

NURSING CONSIDERATIONS

Assessment
• Assess patient for previous sensitivity reaction to penicillins or other cephalosporins; cross-sensitivity between penicillins and cephalosporins is common
• Assess patient for signs and symptoms of **infection** including characteristics of wounds, sputum, urine, stool, WBC $>10,000/mm^3$, earache, fever; obtain baseline information and during treatment
• Obtain C&S before beginning product therapy to identify if correct treatment has been initiated
• Assess for **anaphylaxis:** rash, urticaria, pruritus, dyspnea, chills, fever, joint pain; angioedema may occur a few days after therapy begins; epinephrine and resuscitation equipment should be available for anaphylactic reaction
• Identify urine output; if decreasing, notify prescriber (may indicate **nephrotoxicity**); also check for increased BUN, creatinine
• Monitor blood studies: AST, ALT, CBC, Hct, bilirubin, LDH, alkaline phosphatase, Coombs' test monthly if patient is on long-term therapy
• Monitor electrolytes: potassium, sodium, chloride monthly if patient is on long-term therapy
• Assess bowel pattern daily; if severe diarrhea occurs, product should be discontinued; may indicate **pseudomembranous colitis**
• Monitor for bleeding: ecchymosis, bleeding gums, hematuria, stool guaiac daily if on long-term therapy
• Assess for **overgrowth of infection:** perineal itching, fever, malaise, redness, pain, swelling, drainage, rash, diarrhea, change in cough, sputum

Nursing diagnoses
• Diarrhea (side effects)
• Fluid volume, risk for, deficient (side effects)
• Infection, risk for (uses)
• Injury, risk for (side effects)
• Knowledge, deficient (teaching)
• Noncompliance (teaching)

Patient/family education
• Teach patient to report sore throat, bruising, bleeding, joint pain; may indicate **blood dyscrasias** (rare)

• Advise patient to contact prescriber if vaginal itching, loose foul-smelling stools, furry tongue occur; may indicate **superinfection**
• Instruct patient to take all medication prescribed for the length of time ordered; to use yogurt or buttermilk to maintain intestinal flora, decrease diarrhea
• Advise patient to notify prescriber of diarrhea with blood or pus, which may indicate **pseudomembranous colitis**

Evaluation
Positive therapeutic outcome
• Absence of signs/symptoms of infection (WBC $<10,000/mm^3$, temp WNL, absence of red draining wounds, earache)
• Reported improvement in symptoms of infection
• Negative C&S

TREATMENT OF ANAPHYLAXIS: EPINEPHrine, antihistamines, resuscitate if needed

CEPHALOSPORINS— 3RD/4TH GENERATION

cefdinir (Rx)
(sef′dih-ner)
Omnicef

cefditoren pivoxil (Rx)
(sef-dit′oh-ren pih-vox′il)
Spectracef

(4th generation) cefepime (Rx)
(sef′e-peem)
Maxipime

cefixime (Rx)
(sef-iks′ime)
Cefixime, Suprax

cefotaxime (Rx)
(sef-oh-taks′eem)
Claforan

cefpodoxime (Rx)
(sef-poe-docks′eem)
Vantin

ceftazidime (Rx)
(sef′tay-zi-deem)
Ceptaz, Fortaz, Tazicef, Tazidime

ceftibuten (Rx)
(sef-ti-byoo′tin)
Cedax

ceftizoxime (Rx)
(sef-ti-zox′eem)
Cefizox

cefTRIAXone (Rx)
(sef-try-ax′one)
Rocephin
Func. class.: Broad-spectrum antibiotic
Chem. class.: Cephalosporin (3rd generation)
Pregnancy category B

Do not confuse:
ceftazidime/ceftizoxime, **Vantin/**Ventolin

ACTION: Inhibits bacterial cell wall synthesis, rendering cell wall osmotically unstable, leading to cell death

cefdinir

Therapeutic outcome: Bactericidal effects for the following: gram-negative organisms *Haemophilus influenzae, Haemophilus parainfluenzae, Moraxella catarrhalis;* gram-positive organisms *Streptococcus pneumoniae, Streptococcus pyogenes, Staphylococcus aureus*

USES: Uncomplicated skin and skin structure infections, community-acquired pneumonia, acute exacerbations of chronic bronchitis, acute maxillary sinusitis, pharyngitis, otitis media

cefditoren pivoxil

Therapeutic outcome: Bactericidal effects for the following organisms: *Haemophilus influenzae, Haemophilus parainfluenzae, Streptococcus pneumoniae, Moraxella catarrhalis, Streptococcus pyogenes, Staphylococcus aureus*

USES: Acute bacterial exacerbation of chronic bronchitis, pharyngitis/tonsillitis; uncomplicated skin, skin structure infections, community-acquired pneumonia

cefepime

Therapeutic outcome: Bactericidal effects for the following: gram-negative bacilli *Escherichia coli, Proteus, Klebsiella;* gram-positive organisms *Streptococcus pneumoniae, Streptococcus pyogenes, Staphylococcus aureus*

USES: Lower respiratory tract, urinary tract, skin, bone, febrile neutropenia, intraabdominal infection

cefixime

Therapeutic outcome: Bactericidal effects for the following organisms: *Escherichia coli, Proteus mirabilis, Streptococcus pyogenes, Haemophilus influenzae, Moraxella catarrhalis, Streptococcus pneumoniae*

USES: Uncomplicated UTI, pharyngitis/tonsillitis, otitis media, acute bronchitis, exacerbations of chronic bronchitis, uncomplicated gonorrhea

cefotaxime

Therapeutic outcome: Bactericidal effects for the following: gram-negative organisms *Haemophilus influenzae, Haemophilus parainfluenzae, Escherichia coli, Enterococcus faecalis, Neisseria gonorrhoeae, Neisseria meningitidis, Proteus mirabilis, Klebsiella, Citrobacter, Serratia, Salmonella, Shigella Pseudomonas;* gram-positive organisms

Streptococcus pneumoniae, Streptococcus pyogenes, Staphylococcus aureus

USES: Lower serious respiratory tract, urinary tract, skin, bone, gonococcal infections; bacteremia, septicemia, meningitis, skin, skin structure infections, CNS infections, perioperative prophylaxis

cefpodoxime

Therapeutic outcome: Bactericidal effects for the following: gram-negative organisms *Neisseria gonorrhoeae, Haemophilus influenzae, Escherichia coli, Proteus mirabilis, Klebsiella*; gram-positive organisms *Streptococcus pneumoniae, Streptococcus pyogenes, Staphylococcus aureus*

USES: Upper and lower respiratory tract, urinary tract, skin infections; otitis media, STDs

ceftazidime

Therapeutic outcome: Bactericidal effects for the following: gram-negative organisms *Haemophilus influenzae, Escherichia coli, Enterobacter aerogenes, Proteus mirabilis, Klebsiella, Citrobacter, Enterobacter, Salmonella, Serratia, Pseudomonas aeruginosa, Shigella, Acinetobacter, Bacteroides fragilis, Neisseria*; gram-positive organisms *Streptococcus pneumoniae, Streptococcus pyogenes, Staphylococcus aureus*

USES: Serious upper or lower respiratory tract, urinary tract, skin, gynecologic, bone, joint, intraabdominal infections; septicemia, meningitis, febrile neutropenia

ceftibuten

Therapeutic outcome: Bactericidal effects for the following: gram-negative bacilli *Haemophilus influenzae, Escherichia coli*; gram-positive organisms *Streptococcus pneumoniae, Streptococcus pyogenes, Staphylococcus aureus*

USES: Pharyngitis, tonsilitis, otitis media, secondary bacterial infection of acute bronchitis

ceftizoxime

Therapeutic outcome: Bactericidal effects for the following: gram-negative organisms *Haemophilus influenzae, Escherichia coli, Enterobacter aerogenes, Proteus mirabilis, Klebsiella, Enterobacter*; gram-positive organisms *Streptococcus pneumoniae, Strepto-*

coccus pyogenes, Staphylococcus aureus, Neisseria gonorrhoeae

USES: Serious lower respiratory tract, urinary tract, skin, intraabdominal infections; septicemia, meningitis; bone, joint infections, PID

cefTRIAXone

Therapeutic outcome: Bactericidal effects on the following: gram-negative organisms *Haemophilus influenzae, Escherichia coli, Enterobacter aerogenes, Proteus mirabilis, Klebsiella, Citrobacter, Enterobacter, Salmonella, Shigella, Acinetobacter, Bacteroides fragilis, Neisseria, Serratia*; gram-positive organisms *Streptococcus pneumoniae, Streptococcus pyogenes, Staphylococcus aureus*

USES: Serious lower respiratory tract, urinary tract, skin, gonococcal, intraabdominal infections; septicemia, meningitis; bone, joint infections, otitis media, PID

CONTRAINDICATIONS:
Hypersensitivity to cephalosporins, infants <1 mo

Precautions: Pregnancy **B,** breastfeeding, children, hypersensitivity to penicillins, renal/GI disease

DOSAGE AND ROUTES

cefdinir

Uncomplicated skin and skin structure infections/community-acquired pneumonia
Adult and child ≥13 yr: PO 300 mg q12hr × 10 days
Child 6 mo-12 yr: PO 7 mg/kg q12hr or 14 mg/kg q24hr × 10 days

Acute exacerbations of chronic bronchitis/acute maxillary sinusitis
Adult and child ≥13 yr: PO 300 mg q12hr or 600 mg q24hr × 10 days or 300 mg bid × 5 days in some infections

Pharyngitis/tonsillitis
Adult and child ≥13 yr: PO 300 mg q12hr or 600 mg q24hr × 10 days
Child 6 mo-12 yr: PO 7 mg/kg q12hr × 5-10 days or 14 mg/kg q24hr × 10 days

Renal dose
CCr <30 ml/min 300 mg daily (adult); 7 mg/kg daily (child)

Available forms: Caps 300 mg, oral susp 125 mg/5 ml, 250 mg/5 ml

cefditoren pivoxil
Adult: PO 200-400 mg bid × 10 days

Renal dose
Adult: PO CCr 30-50 ml/min, max 200 mg bid; CCr <30 ml/min, max 200 mg daily

Available forms: Tabs 200 mg

cefepime

Febrile neutropenia
Adult/adolescent >16 yr/child ≥40 kg: IV 2 g q3hr × 7 days or until neutropenia resolves
Infants ≥2 mo/children/adolescents ≤16 yr and weighing up to 40 kg: IV 50 mg/kg/dose q8hr × 7-10 days or until resolution

Urinary tract infections (mild to moderate)
Adult: IV/IM 0.5-1 g q12hr × 7-10 days

Urinary tract infections (severe)
Adult/adolescent >16 yr/child ≥40 kg: IV 2 g q12hr × 10 days

Pneumonia (moderate to severe)
Adult: IV 1-2 g q12hr × 10 days
Dosage reduction indicated in renal impairment (CCr <50 ml/min)

Uncomplicated gonorrhea
Adult: IM 2 g as a single dose with 1 g PO probenecid at the same time

Available forms: Powder for inj 500 mg, 1, 2 g; 1 g/50 ml, 2 g/100 ml

cefixime
Adult: PO 400 mg/day as a single dose or 200 mg q12hr
Child >50 kg or >12 yr: PO use adult dosage
Child <50 kg or <12 yr: PO 8 mg/kg/day as a single dose or 4 mg/kg q12hr

Renal dose
CCr 21-60 ml/min give 75% of dose; CCr <20 ml/min give 50% of dose

Available forms: Tabs 400 mg; powder for oral susp 100 mg/5 ml

cefotaxime
Adult: IM/IV 1-2 g q12hr
Child 1 mo-12 yr: IM/IV 50-180 mg/kg/day divided q6hr

Severe infections
Adult: IM/IV 2 g q4hr, max 12 g/day
Child 1 mo-12 yr: IM/IV 50-180 mg/kg in 4-6 divided doses

Uncomplicated gonorrhea
Adult: IM 1 g; dosage reduction indicated for severe renal impairment (CCr <30 ml/min)

Available forms: Powder for inj 500 mg, 1, 2, 10 g; 1, 2 g premixed frozen

cefpodoxime

Pneumonia
Adult >13 yr: PO 200 mg q12hr for 14 days

Uncomplicated gonorrhea
Adult >13 yr: PO 200 mg single dose

Skin and skin structure
Adult >13 yr: PO 400 mg q12hr for 7-14 days

Pharyngitis and tonsillitis
Adult >13 yr: PO 100 mg q12hr for 10 days
Child 5 mo-12 yr: PO 5 mg/kg q12hr (max 100 mg/dose or 200 mg/day) × 5-10 days

Uncomplicated UTI
Adult >13 yr: PO 100 mg q12hr for 7 days; dosing interval increased in presence of severe renal impairment

Acute otitis media
Child 5 mo-12 yr: PO 5 mg/kg q12hr for 10 days

Available forms: Tabs 100, 200 mg; granules for susp 50, 100 mg/5 ml

ceftazidime
Adult: IV/IM 1-2 g q8-12hr × 5-10 days
Child: IV 30-50 mg/kg q8hr, max 6 g/day
Neonate: IV 30-50 mg/kg q12hr

Renal dose
Adult: IV CCr <50 ml/min q12hr; CCr 10-30 ml/min q24hr; CCr <10 ml/min q48hr, CCr <10 ml/min give q48-72hr

Available forms: Inj 250, 500 mg, 1, 2, 6 g

ceftibuten
Adult: PO 400 mg daily × 10 days
Child 6 mo-12 yr: PO 9 mg/kg daily × 10 days

Renal dose
Adult: PO CCr 30-49 ml/min 200 mg q24hr; CCr 5-29 ml/min 100 mg q24hr

Available forms: Caps 400 mg; susp 90, 180 mg/5 ml

ceftizoxime
Adult: IM/IV 1-2 g q8-12hr, may give up to 4 g q8hr in life-threatening infections
Child >6 mo: IM/IV 50 mg/kg q6-8hr

Renal dose
Adult: IM/IV CCr 50-80 ml/min 500-1500 mg q8hr; CCr 5-49 ml/min 250-1000 mg q12hr

PID
Adult: IV 2 g q8hr, may increase to 4 g q8hr in severe infections

Adverse effects: *italics* = common; **bold** = life-threatening

Available forms: Powder for inj 500 mg, 1, 2, 10 g; premixed 1 g, 2 g/50 ml

cefTRIAXone
Adult: IM/IV 1-2 g daily, max 2 g q12-24hr
Child: IM/IV 50-75 mg/kg/day in equal doses q12hr

Uncomplicated gonorrhea
Adult: 250 mg IM as single dose
Reduce dosage in severe renal impairment (CCr <10 ml/min)

Meningitis
Adult and child: IM/IV 100 mg/kg/day in equal doses q12hr, max 4 g/day

Surgical prophylaxis
Adult: IV 1 g ½-2 hr preop

Available forms: Inj 250, 500 mg, 1, 2, 10 g

Implementation
cefdinir
PO route
• Give oral susp after adding 39 ml water to the 60 ml bottle; 65 ml water to the 12.0 ml bottle; discard unused portion after 10 days, give without regard to food, do not give within 2 hr of antacids, iron supplements

cefditoren pivoxil
• Give for 10 days to ensure organism death, prevent superinfection
• Give with food if needed for GI symptoms, do not give with antacids
• Give after C&S is completed

cefepime
IV route
• Check for irritation, extravasation, phlebitis daily; change site q72hr
• For **intermittent inf** dilute with 50-100 ml of D_5W, give over 30 min

Solution compatibilities: 0.9% NaCl, D_5, 0.5, 1.0% lidocaine, bacteriostatic water for inj with parabens/benzyl alcohol

cefixime
• Do not break, crush, or chew tab
• Give for 10-14 days to ensure organism death, prevent superinfection

cefotaxime
IV route
• **Dilute** 1 g/10 ml D_5W, NS, sterile water for inj and **give** over 3-5 min by Y-tube or 3-way stopcock; may be **diluted further** with 50-100 ml of 0.9% NaCl or D_5W; **run** over ½-1 hr; discontinue primary inf during administration; or may be diluted in larger volume of sol and given as a cont inf over 6-24 hr
• Give for 10-14 days to ensure organism death, prevent superinfection
• Thaw frozen container at room temperature or refrigeration, do not force thaw by immersion or microwave; visually inspect container for leaks

Syringe compatibilities: Heparin, oflaxacin

Y-site compatibilities: Acyclovir, alfentanil, alprostadil, amifostine, amikacin, aminocaproic acid, aminophylline, anidulafungin, ascorbic acid injection, atenolol, atracurium, atropine, aztreonam, benztropine, bivalirudin, bleomycin, bumetanide, buprenorphine, butorphanol, caffeine, calcium chloride/gluconate, CARBOplatin, cefamandole, cefmetazole, cefonicid, cefoperazone, cefotetan, cefoxitin, ceftazidime (L-arginine), cefTRIAXone sodium, cefuroxime, cimetidine, CISplatin, clindamycin, codeine, cyanocobalamin, cyclophosphamide, cycloSPORINE, cytarabine, DACTINomycin, DAPTOmycin, dexamethasone, dexmedetomidine, digoxin, diltiazem, docetaxel, DOPamine, doxacurium, doxycycline, enalaprilat, ePHEDrine, EPINEPHrine, epirubicin, epoetin alfa, eptifibatide, erythromycin, esmolol, etoposide, famotidine, fenoldopam, fentaNYL, fludarabine, fluorouracil, folic acid, furosemide, gatifloxacin, gentamicin, glycopyrrolate, granisetron, heparin, hydrocortisone, HYDROmorphone, ifosfamide, imipenem-cilastatin, insulin (regular), isoproterenol, ketorolac, lidocaine, linezolid, LORazepam, LR, magnesium sulfate, mannitol, mechlorethamine, melphalan, meperidine, metaraminol, methicillin, methotrexate, methoxamine, methyldopate, metoclopramide, metoprolol, metroNIDAZOLE, mezlocillin, miconazole, midazolam, milrinone, minocycline, mitoxantrone, morphine, moxalactam, multiple vitamins, mycophenolate, nafcillin, nalbuphine, naloxone, nesiritide, netilmicin, nitroglycerin, nitroprusside, norepinephrine, normal saline, octreotide, ofloxacin, ondansetron, ornidazole, oxacillin, oxaliplatin, oxytocin, paclitaxel, palonosetron, pamidronate, pancuronium, pantoprazole, papaverine, pefloxacin, pemetrexed, penicillin G potassium/sodium, pentamidine, pentazocine, PENTobarbital, peritoneal dialysis solution, perphenazine, PHENobarbital, phenylephrine, phenytoin, phytonadione, piperacillin, polymyxin B, potassium chloride, procainamide, prochlorperazine, promethazine, propofol, propranolol, protamine, quiNIDine, quinupristin, ranitidine, remifentanil, Ringer's injection, ritodrine, riTUXimab, rocuronium, sargramostim, sodium acetate/bicarbonate, sodium fusidate, sodium lactate, succinylcholine, SUFentanil, sulfamethoxazole-trimethoprim, tacrolimus, teniposide, theophylline, thiamine, thiotepa, ticarcillin, ticarcillin-clavulanate, tigecycline, tirofiban, TNA, tobramycin, tolazoline, TPN, trastuzumab, trimetaphan, urokinase, vancomycin, vasopressin, vecuronium, verapamil, vinorelbine, voriconazole

cefpodoxime
PO route
• Do not break, crush, or chew tabs due to taste
• Give for 10-14 days to ensure organism death, prevent superinfection
• With food for better absorption, do not give within 2 hr of antacids, H_2 receptor antagonists

ceftazidime
IM route
• **Fortaz, Tazidime vials:** Reconstitute 500 mg or 1 g with 1.5 or 3 ml, respectively, of sterile or bacteriostatic water for injection, or 0.5%-1% lidocaine (approx. 280 mg/ml)
• **Tazicef vials:** Reconstitute 1 g/3 ml sterile water for injection (approx. 280 mg/ml)
• **Ceptaz vials:** Reconstitute 1 g/3 ml sterile or bacteriostatic water for injection or 0.5%-1% lidocaine (approx. 250 mg/ml)
• Withdraw the dose, making sure the needle remains in the vial; ensure that no CO_2 bubbles are present; inject deeply in large muscle mass; aspirate prior to injection

IV route
• If possible, visually inspect for particulate matter and discoloration
• **Fortaz, Tazicef, Tazidime packs:** Reconstitute 1 or 2 g/100 ml sterile water for injection or other compatible IV sol (10 or 20 mg/ml, respectively). Reconstitution is done in two stages. First, inject 10 ml of the diluents into the pack and shake well to dissolve and become clear; CO_2 pressure inside the container will occur; insert a vent needle to release the pressure; add remaining diluents and remove vent needle
• **Fortaz, Tazicef, Tazidime vials:** Reconstitute 500 mg, 1 g, 2 g with 5, 10, 10 ml, respectively, of sterile water for injection or other compatible IV sol (100, 95-100, or 170-180 mg/ml, respectively); shake well to dissolve
• **Fortaz, Tazidime-ADD-Vantage vials** (for IV only): Reconstitute 1 or 2 g with NS, $^1/_2$ NS, D_5W in either 50 or 100 ml flexible diluents container; to release CO_2 pressure, insert a vent needle after dissolving; remove vent before using

• **Ceptaz packs:** Reconstitute 1 or 2 g/100 ml sterile water for injection or compatible IV sol (10 or 20 mg/ml, respectively). Reconstitution is done in two stages. First, inject 10 ml of the diluent into the pack and shake well to dissolve; add the remaining diluents; insert as vent needle before giving
• **Ceptaz vials:** Reconstitute 1 or 2 g/10 ml of sterile water for injection or compatible IV sol (90-95, or 170-180 mg/ml, respectively)
• **Ceptaz ADD-Vantage vials** (for IV infusion only): Reconstitute 1 or 2 g with NS, $^1/_2$ NS, or D_5W in either 50 or 100 ml diluent container as appropriate
Direct intermittent IV infusion route
• **Vials:** Withdraw the correct dose, making sure the needle opening remains in the solution; make sure there are no CO_2 bubbles in the syringe before injection; inject directly over 3-5 min or slowly into the tubing of a free-flowing compatible IV solution
Intermittent IV infusion route
• **Vials:** Withdraw the correct dose, making sure the needle opening remains in the solution; make sure there are no CO_2 bubbles in the syringe before injection; infusion packs and ADD-Vantage systems are ready for infusion after reconstitution; infuse over 15-30 min

ceftibuten
• Administer for 10 days to ensure organism death, prevent superinfection
• Administer after C&S

ceftizoxime
IM route
• Reconstitute 250 mg/0.9 ml, 500 mg/1.8 ml, 1 g/3.6 ml, 2 g/7.2 ml; may be diluted with 0.5% or 1% lidocaine to prevent pain; give deep in large muscle mass, massage

IV route
• Check for irritation, extravasation, phlebitis daily; change site q72hr
• For intermittent inf reconstitute 250 mg/2.4 ml, 500 mg/4.8 ml, 1 g/9.6 mg/2 g/19.2 ml sterile water for inj, D_5W, or 0.9% NaCl; do not use sol with benzyl alcohol for neonates; may be further diluted in 50-100 ml of D_5W, D_{10}W, 0.9% NaCl, or LR; give over 30-60 min
• May store 96 hr refrigerated, 24 hr room temperature

Y-site compatibilities: Acyclovir, allopurinol, amifostine, aztreonam, enalaprilat, esmolol, famotidine, fludarabine, foscarnet, HYDROmorphone, labetalol, melphalan, meperidine, morphine, ondansetron, sargramostim, teniposide, thiotepa, vinorelbine

Additive compatibilities: Clindamycin, metroNIDAZOLE

Additive incompatibilities: Aminoglycosides

cefTRIAXone
- Give IM inj deep in large muscle mass
- Give for 10-14 days to ensure organism death, prevent superinfection

IV route
- Give **IV** after diluting 250 mg/2.4 ml of D$_5$W, water for inj, 0.9% NaCl; may be further diluted with 50-100 ml of 0.9% NaCl, D$_5$W, D$_{10}$W, shake; run over ^{1}/$_2$-1 hr
- Do not mix with calcium salts

Y-site compatibilities: Acyclovir, allopurinol, aztreonam, cisatracurium, diltiazem, DOXOrubicin liposome, fludarabine, foscarnet, heparin, melphalan, meperidine, methotrexate, morphine, paclitaxel, remifentanil, sargramostim, tacrolimus, teniposide, theophylline, vinorelbine, warfarin, zidovudine

Additive compatibilities: Amino acids or sodium bicarbonate, metroNIDAZOLE

ADVERSE EFFECTS
CNS: Headache, dizziness, weakness, paresthesia, fever, chills, **seizures,** dyskinesia (cefdinir)
CV: Heart failure, syncope (cefdinir)
EENT: *Oral candidiasis*
GI: *Nausea, vomiting, diarrhea, anorexia,* pain, glossitis, **bleeding;** increased AST, ALT, bilirubin, LDH, alkaline phosphatase; abdominal pain, **pseudomembranous colitis,** cholestasis (cefotaxime)
GU: Proteinuria, vaginitis, pruritus, *candidiasis,* increased BUN, **nephrotoxicity, renal failure**
HEMA: Leukopenia, thrombocytopenia, agranulocytosis, anemia, **neutropenia, lymphocytosis, eosinophilia, pancytopenia, hemolytic anemia**
INTEG: Rash, urticaria, dermatitis
RESP: Dyspnea
SYST: Anaphylaxis, serum sickness, Stevens-Johnson syndrome, toxic epidermal necrolysis

cefdinir
Pharmacokinetics
Absorption	Well absorbed
Distribution	Widely distributed; crosses placenta
Metabolism	Not metabolized
Excretion	Kidneys, unchanged; enters breast milk
Half-life	1.7 hr

Pharmacodynamics
Unknown

cefditoren pivoxil
Pharmacokinetics
Absorption	Well absorbed after it is broken down (prodrug)
Distribution	Widely
Metabolism	Unknown
Excretion	Unknown
Half-life	100 mins

Pharmacodynamics
Onset	Rapid
Peak	0.5-3 hr
Duration	12 hrs

cefepime
Pharmacokinetics
Absorption	Well absorbed (IM)
Distribution	Widely distributed; crosses placenta
Metabolism	Not metabolized
Excretion	Kidneys, unchanged; enters breast milk
Half-life	2 hr; increased in renal disease

Pharmacodynamics
	IM	IV
Onset	Rapid	Immediate
Peak	79 min	Infusion's end
Duration	Unknown	Unknown

cefixime
Pharmacokinetics
Absorption	Unknown
Distribution	Protein binding 65%-70%
Metabolism	Unknown
Excretion	Urine, bile
Half-life	3-4 hr

Pharmacodynamics

Onset	Unknown
Peak	2-6 hr
Duration	Unknown

cefotaxime

Pharmacokinetics

Absorption	Widely distributed
Distribution	Breast milk, small amounts
Metabolism	Liver, active metabolites
Excretion	40%-65% unchanged, kidney
Half-life	1 hr

Pharmacodynamics

	IV	IM
Onset	5 min	30 min
Peak	Unknown	Unknown
Duration	Unknown	Unknown

cefpodoxime

Pharmacokinetics

Absorption	Well absorbed
Distribution	Widely distributed; crosses placenta, protein binding 21%-29%
Metabolism	Not metabolized
Excretion	Kidneys, unchanged; enters breast milk
Half-life	3 hr, increased in renal disease

Pharmacodynamics

Unknown

ceftazidime

Pharmacokinetics

Absorption	Well absorbed (IM)
Distribution	Widely distributed; crosses placenta
Metabolism	Not metabolized
Excretion	Kidneys, unchanged; enters breast milk
Half-life	1-2 hr; increased in renal disease

Pharmacodynamics

	IM	IV
Onset	Rapid	Immediate
Peak	1 hr	Infusion's end

ceftibuten

Pharmacokinetics

Absorption	Well absorbed
Distribution	Widely distributed; crosses placenta
Metabolism	Not metabolized
Excretion	Kidneys, unchanged; enters breast milk
Half-life	1-1½ hr; increased in renal disease

Pharmacodynamics

Unknown

ceftizoxime

Pharmacokinetics

Absorption	Well absorbed (IM)
Distribution	Widely distributed; crosses placenta, protein binding 30%
Metabolism	Not metabolized
Excretion	Kidneys, unchanged; enters breast milk
Half-life	1½-2 hr; increased in renal disease

Pharmacodynamics

	IM	IV
Onset	Rapid	Immediate
Peak	1 hr	Infusion's end

cefTRIAXone

Pharmacokinetics

Absorption	Well absorbed
Distribution	Widely distributed; crosses placenta; enters CSF, protein binding 58%-96%
Metabolism	Liver
Excretion	Kidneys, partly
Half-life	6-9 hr

Pharmacodynamics

	IM	IV
Onset	Rapid	Immediate
Peak	1 hr	Infusion's end

INTERACTIONS

Individual drugs

Furosemide, probenecid: increased toxicity
Iron: decreased absorption of cefdinir
Plicamycin, valproic acid: increased bleeding

Drug classifications
Aminoglycosides: increased toxicity
Anticoagulants, NSAIDs, thrombolytics: increased bleeding

Drug/food
Iron-rich cereal, infants' formula: decreased absorption

Drug/lab test
Increased: ALT, AST, alkaline phosphatase, LDH, bilirubin, BUN, creatinine
False increase: creatinine (serum urine), urinary 17-KS
False positive: urinary protein, direct Coombs' test, urine glucose
Interference: cross-matching

NURSING CONSIDERATIONS

Assessment
• Assess patient for previous sensitivity reaction to penicillins or other cephalosporins; cross-sensitivity between penicillins and cephalosporins is common
• Assess patient for signs and symptoms of **infection** including characteristics of wounds, sputum, urine, stool, WBC >10,000/mm³, fever; obtain baseline information and during treatment
• Obtain C&S before beginning product therapy to identify if correct treatment has been initiated
• Assess for **anaphylaxis:** rash, urticaria, pruritus, chills, fever, joint pain; angioedema may occur a few days after therapy begins; epinephrine and resuscitation equipment should be available for anaphylactic reaction
• Identify urine output; if decreasing, notify prescriber (may indicate **nephrotoxicity**); also check for increased BUN, creatinine
• Monitor blood studies: AST, ALT, CBC, Hct, bilirubin, LDH, alkaline phosphatase, Coombs' test monthly if patient is on long-term therapy
• Monitor electrolytes: potassium, sodium, chloride monthly if patient is on long-term therapy
• Assess bowel pattern daily; if severe diarrhea occurs, product should be discontinued; may indicate **pseudomembranous colitis**
• Monitor for **bleeding:** ecchymosis, bleeding gums, hematuria, stool guaiac daily if on long-term therapy
• Assess for **overgrowth of infection:** perineal itching, fever, malaise, redness, pain, swelling, drainage, rash, diarrhea, change in cough, sputum

Nursing diagnoses
• Diarrhea (side effects)
• Infection, risk for (uses)
• Injury, risk for (side effects)
• Knowledge, deficient (teaching)

Patient/family education
• Teach patient to report sore throat, bruising, bleeding, joint pain; may indicate blood dyscrasias (rare)
• Advise patient to contact prescriber if vaginal itching, loose foul-smelling stools, furry tongue occur; may indicate superinfection
• Advise patient to notify prescriber of diarrhea with blood or pus, may indicate pseudomembranous colitis
• Cefditoren can be taken with oral contraceptives

Evaluation
Positive therapeutic outcome
• Absence of signs/symptoms of infection (WBC <10,000/mm³, temp WNL, absence of red draining wounds, earache)
• Reported improvement in symptoms of infection
• Negative C&S

TREATMENT OF ANAPHYLAXIS: EPINEPHrine, antihistamines, resuscitate if needed

cephradine
See cephalosporins—1st generation

certolizumab pegol (Rx)
(ser'tue-liz'oo-mab) (pegh'ol)
Cimzia
Func. class.: Biologic response modifier
Chem. class.: Anti-TNF (tissue necrosis factor) agent
Pregnancy category B

ACTION: Monoclonal antibody that neutralizes the activity of tumor necrosis factor-α (TNF-α) found in Crohn's disease; decreased infiltration of inflammatory cells

Therapeutic outcome: Absence of fever, mucus in stools

USES: Crohn's disease (moderate-severe) that has not responded to conventional therapy, rheumatoid arthritis (moderate-severe)

CONTRAINDICATIONS:
Influenza, **IV** administration, sepsis, hypersensitivity

> **BLACK BOX WARNING:** Infection

Precautions: Pregnancy **B,** breastfeeding, children, geriatric patients, AIDS, coagulopathy, diabetes, fungal infection, heart failure, hepatitis, human anti-chimertic antibody, immunosuppression, leukopenia, MS, cancer, neurologic disease, surgery, thrombocytopenia, TB, vaccinations, renal disease

DOSAGE AND ROUTES
Crohn's disease (moderate-severe)
Adult: SUBCUT 400 mg given as 2 inj at wk 0, 2, 4; if clinical response occurs, give 400 mg q4wk

Rheumatoid arthritis (moderate-severe)
Adult: SUBCUT 400 mg q2wk × 3 doses, then 200 mg q2wk; given with methotrexate

Available forms: Powder for inj 400 mg kit

Implementation
• Store in refrigerator; do not freeze
SUBCUT route
• Give by SUBCUT only
• Allow reconstitution to warm to room temp; add 1 ml sterile water for inj to each vial; two vials will be needed for Crohn's disease
• Gently swirl; do not shake; full reconstitution may take up to 30 min; reconstituted product may remain at room temp for up to 2 hr or refrigerated up to 24 hr
• Warm to room temperature if reconstituted product has been refrigerated
• Use 2 syringes and 2 20-G needles
• Withdraw reconstituted sol from each vial into separate syringes; each will contain 200 mg; switch 20-G to 23-G needle; inject into 2 separate sites in abdomen or thigh

ADVERSE EFFECTS
CNS: *Dizziness,* syncope, peripheral neuropathy, fever, **seizures, demyelinating disease of CNS**
CV: Hypotension, **heart failure, MI, cardiac dysrhythmia**
EENT: Optic neuritis, retinal hemorrhage, uveitis
GI: Increased LFTs, **hepatitis, bowel obstruction**
GU: UTI, renal disease

HEMA: Anemia, aplastic anemia, pancytopenia, thrombocytopenia
INTEG: *Rash, urticaria,* angioedema
RESP: Dyspnea, URI
SYST: Anaphylaxis, malignancies, serum sickness, bleeding, antibody formation, infection, lupus-like symptoms, lymphadenopathy, arthralgia, **suicidal ideation**

Pharmacokinetics
Absorption	Unknown
Distribution	Unknown
Metabolism	Unknown
Excretion	Unknown
Half-life	Terminal 14 days

Pharmacodynamics
Onset	Unknown
Peak	54-171 hr
Duration	Unknown

INTERACTIONS
Individual drugs
Abatacept, adalimumab, anakinra, etanercept, infliximab, do not use concurrently, rilonacept: increased possible infections
Adalimumab, etanercept, infliximab: increased possible malignancies

Drug classifications
Immunosuppressive agents: increased possible infections, do not use concurrently
Live vaccines, toxoids: do not administer concurrently

NURSING CONSIDERATIONS
Assessment
• Monitor antibody test (ANA), hepatitis B serology, CBC
• Assess for rheumatoid arthritis, ROM, pain
• Assess GI symptoms: nausea, vomiting, abdominal pain, hepatitis, increased LFTs
• Monitor periodic blood counts (CBC)
• Assess CV status: B/P, pulse, chest pain
⚠ Assess for allergic reaction, anaphylaxis: rash, dermatitis, urticaria, dyspnea, hypotension, fever, chills; discontinue if severe, administer epinephrine, corticosteroids, antihistamines; assess for allergies to murine proteins before starting therapy

> **BLACK BOX WARNING:** Assess **infections:** discontinue if infection occurs; do not administer to patients with active infections

- Identify TB, risk for HBV before beginning treatment; a TB test should be obtained; if present, TB should be treated prior to receiving infliximab

Nursing diagnoses
- Diarrhea (uses)
- Knowledge, deficient (teaching)
- Mobility, impaired physical (uses)

Patient/family education
- Instruct patient not to breastfeed while taking this product
- Advise patient to notify prescriber of GI symptoms, hypersensitivity reactions, infections, fluid retention, redness, pain, swelling at injection site
- Caution patient not to operate machinery, drive if dizziness, vertigo occur

Evaluation
Positive therapeutic outcome
- Absence of fever, mucus in stools

---

cetirizine (Rx)
(se-tear'i-zeen)
All Day Allergy, All Day Allergy Children's, Apo-Cetirizine ✤, GNP All Day Allergy, GNP Children's All Day Allergy, Good Sense All Day Allergy, Good Sense Children's All Day Allergy, Publix Allergy Children's, Reactine ✤, Top Care Children's All Day Allergy, Zyrtec, Zyrtec Children's
Func. class.: Antihistamine, peripherally selective (2nd generation)
Chem. class.: Piperazine, H_1 histamine antagonist
Pregnancy category B

Do not confuse:
Zyrtec/Xanax/Zantac

ACTION: Acts on blood vessels, GI, respiratory system by competing with histamine for H_1-receptor site; decreases allergic response by blocking pharmacologic effects of histamine; minimal anticholinergic/sedative action

Therapeutic outcome: Absence of allergy symptoms, rhinitis, and chronic idiopathic urticaria

USES: Rhinitis, allergy symptoms, and chronic idiopathic urticaria

CONTRAINDICATIONS:
Hypersensitivity to this product or hydrOXYzine, breastfeeding, newborn or premature infants, severe hepatic disease

Precautions: Pregnancy **B**, children, geriatric, respiratory disease, closed-angle glaucoma, prostatic hypertrophy, bladder neck obstruction, asthma

DOSAGE AND ROUTES
Perennial/seasonal allergic rhinitis or idiopathic urticaria
Adult and child ≥6 yr: PO 5-10 mg daily
Child 2-5 yr: PO 2.5 mg daily, may increase to 5 mg daily or 2.5 mg bid
Child 1-2 yr: PO 2.5 mg daily, may increase to 2.5 mg q12hr
Child 6-11 mo: PO 2.5 mg daily
Geriatric: PO 5 mg daily, may increase to 10 mg/day

Self-treatment of hay fever/other respiratory allergies
Adult/adolescent/child ≥6 yr: PO 10 mg/day, oral SOL 5-10 mg/day

Renal dose
Adult: PO CCr 11-31 ml/min 5 mg daily

Hemodialysis
Adult: PO 5 mg/day

Hepatic dose
Adult: PO 5 mg daily

Available forms: Tabs 5, 10 mg; syr 5 mg/5 ml; prefilled spoons 1 mg/ml; oral sol 5 mg/5 ml; liquid filled cap 10 mg; chew tab 5, 10 mg

Implementation
- Give without regard to meals
- **Caps:** swallow whole, do not break, cut, chew, crush
- **Chew tabs:** chew before swallowing, may use without or with water
- **Oral liquid:** use calibrated measuring device
- Store in tight, light-resistant container

ADVERSE EFFECTS
CNS: *Headache*, stimulation, *drowsiness*, sedation, *fatigue*, confusion, blurred vision, tinnitus, restlessness, tremors, parodoxical excitation in children or geriatric
GI: *Dry mouth*, increased liver function tests, constipation
INTEG: Rash, eczema, photosensitivity, urticaria

RESP: *Thickening of bronchial secretions;* dry nose, throat

Pharmacokinetics

Absorption	Well absorbed, rapid
Distribution	Protein binding 93%
Metabolism	Liver
Excretion	Kidneys
Half-life	8.3 hr, decreased in children, increased in renal/hepatic disease

Pharmacodynamics

Onset	$^1/_2$ hr
Peak	1-2 hr
Duration	24 hr

INTERACTIONS

Individual drugs
Alcohol: increased CNS depression
Ritonavir: increased cetirizine effect

Drug classifications
CNS depressants, opioids, sedative/hypnotics: increased CNS depression
MAOIs: increased anticholinergic effect

Drug/food
Prolongs absorption by 1.7 hr

Drug/lab test
False negative: skin allergy tests (discontinue antihistamine 3 days before testing)

NURSING CONSIDERATIONS

Assessment
• Assess respiratory status: rate, rhythm; increase in bronchial secretions, wheezing, chest tightness; provide fluids to 2 L/day to decrease secretion thickness
• Assess for **allergy symptoms:** pruritus, urticaria, watering eyes, baseline, during treatment

Nursing diagnoses
• Airway clearance, ineffective (uses)
• Injury, risk for (side effects)
• Knowledge, deficient (teaching)
• Noncompliance (teaching overuse)

Patient/family education
• Teach all aspects of product uses; to notify prescriber if confusion, sedation, hypotension occur; to avoid driving or other hazardous activity if drowsiness occurs; to avoid alcohol or other CNS depressants that may potentiate effect
• Instruct patient to take without regard to meals

• Instruct patient not to exceed recommended dose; dysrhythmias may occur
• Advise patient to avoid using if breastfeeding
• Advise patient to avoid exposure to sunlight; burns may occur
• Advise patient to use sugarless gum, candy, frequent sips of water to minimize dry mouth
• Advise patient to avoid alcohol, OTC antihistamines, other CNS depressants

Evaluation
Positive therapeutic outcome
• Absence of runny or congested nose, rashes

TREATMENT OF OVERDOSE:
Lavage, diazepam, vasopressors, phenytoin IV

cetrorelix (Rx)
(set-roe-ree′lix)
Cetrotide
Func. class.: Gonadotropin-releasing
Chem. class.: Synthetic decapeptide
Pregnancy category X

ACTION: Inhibitor of pituitary gonadotropin secretion; initially increases LH and FSH, induces a rapid suppression of gonadotropin secretion

Therapeutic outcome: Pregnancy

USES: For inhibition of premature LH surges in women undergoing controlled ovarian hyperstimulation

CONTRAINDICATIONS:
Pregnancy **X,** breastfeeding, hypersensitivity, latex allergy, renal disease

Precautions: Geriatric

DOSAGE AND ROUTES

Single-dose regimen
Adult: SUBCUT 3 mg when serum estradiol level is at appropriate stimulation response, usually on stimulation day 7; if hCG has not been given within 4 days after inj of 3 mg cetrorelix, give 0.25 mg daily until day of hCG administration

Multiple-dose regimen
Adult: SUBCUT 0.25 mg is given on stimulation day 5 (either morning or evening) or 6 (morning) and continued daily until day hCG is given

Available forms: Inj 0.25, 3 mg

Implementation
SUBCUT route
• Give SUBCUT using abdomen, 1 inch away from navel, or upper thigh; swab inj area with disinfectant, clean a 2-in circle and allow to dry, pinch up area between thumb and finger, insert needle at 45-90 degrees to surface; if blood is drawn into the syringe, reposition needle without removing it; rotate inj sites
• Do not administer if patient is pregnant
• Protect from light

ADVERSE EFFECTS
CNS: Headache
CV: Edema
ENDO: Ovarian hyperstimulation syndrome, abdominal pain (gyn)
GI: Nausea, vomiting, diarrhea
INTEG: Pain on inj; local site reactions, bruising, pruritus
OTHER: Rapid weight gain
RESP: Shortness of breath
SYST: Fetal death, anaphylaxis

Pharmacokinetics

Absorption	Unknown
Distribution	Protein binding 86%
Metabolism	Liver to metabolites
Excretion	Feces/urine
Half-life	Depends on dosage

Pharmacodynamics
Unknown

NURSING CONSIDERATIONS
Assessment
• Assess for suspected pregnancy; product should not be used, pregnancy X
• Assess for **latex allergy;** product should not be used
• Monitor ALT, AST, GGT, alkaline phosphatase, serum progesterone, LH; ovarian ultrasound days 7-14
• Assess for **anaphylaxis** during first infusion

Nursing diagnoses
• Knowledge, deficient (teaching)

Patient/family education
• Instruct to report abdominal pain, vaginal bleeding, nausea, vomiting, diarrhea, shortness of breath, peripheral edema
• Teach self-administration technique if needed

Evaluation
Positive therapeutic outcome
• Pregnancy

cetuximab (Rx)
(se-tux′i-mab)
Erbitux
Func. class.: Antineoplastic— miscellaneous, monoclonal antibody
Chem. class.: Epidermal growth factor receptor inhibitor
Pregnancy category C

ACTION: Not fully understood; binds to epidermal growth factor receptors (EGFRs); inhibits phosphorylation and activation of receptor-associated kinase resulting in inhibition of cell growth

Therapeutic outcome: Decrease in tumor size

USES: Alone or in combination with irinotecan for EGFR expressing metastatic colorectal carcinoma, head/neck cancer

CONTRAINDICATIONS:
Hypersensitivity to this product or murine proteins

Precautions: Pregnancy **C**, breastfeeding, child, geriatric, CV/renal/hepatic disease, ocular, pulmonary disorders

> **BLACK BOX WARNING:** Arrhythmias, CAD, infusion-related reactions, radiation

DOSAGE AND ROUTES
Adult: **IV** INF 400 mg/m^2 loading dose given over 120 min, max INF rate 5 ml/min, weekly maintenance dose (all other infusions) is 250 mg/m^2 given over 60 min, max INF rate 5 ml/min (10 mg/min); premedicate with an H_1 antagonist (diphenhydrAMINE 50 mg **IV**); dosage adjustments are made for INF reactions or dermatologic toxicity; other protocols are used

Available forms: Sol for inj 100 mg/50 ml, 200 mg/100 ml

Implementation
Intermittent infusion route
• Administer by **IV** infusion only, do not give by **IV** push or bolus
• Do not shake or dilute
• **Infusion pump:** draw up volume of a vial using appropriate syringe/needle (a vented spike or other appropriate transfer device); fill Erbitux into sterile evacuated container/bag, repeat until calculated volume has been put into the container. Use a new needle for each vial;

⚠ Nurse Alert

give through in-line filter (low protein binding 0.22-micrometer); affix inf line and prime before starting inf, max rate 5 ml/min; flush line at end of inf with 0.9% NaCl
• **Syringe pump:** Draw up volume of a vial using appropriate syringe/needle (a vented spike); place syringe into syringe driver of a syringe pump and set rate; use an in-line filter 0.22 micrometer (low protein binding); connect inf line and start inf after priming; repeat until calculated volume has been given
• Use a new needle and filter for each vial, max 5 ml/min rate; use 0.9% NaCl to flush line after inf
• Do not piggyback to patient inf line
• Observe patient for adverse reactions for 1hr after inf
• Inf reactions: if mild (grade 1 or 2) reduce all doses by 50%; if severe (grade 3 or 4) permanently discontinue
• Store refrigerated 36°-46° F, discard unused portions

ADVERSE EFFECTS

CNS: *Headache, insomnia, depression,* **aseptic meningitis**
GI: *Nausea, diarrhea, vomiting, anorexia, mouth ulceration, dehydration, constipation, abdominal pain*
HEMA: **Leukepenia, anemia**
INTEG: Rash, pruritus, acne, dry skin, **toxic epidermal necrolysis, angioedema,** *blepharitis, cheilitis, cellulitis, cysts, alopecia, skin/nail disorder,* **acute infusion reactions, other skin toxicities**
MISC: *Conjunctivitis, asthma, malaise, fever,* **renal failure,** hypomagnesemia
MS: *Back pain*
RESP: **Interstitial lung disease,** *cough, dyspnea,* **pulmonary embolus,** *peripheral edema*
SYST: **Anaphylaxis, sepsis, infection**

Pharmacokinetics

Absorption	Unknown
Distribution	Unknown
Metabolism	Unknown
Excretion	Unknown
Half-life	114 hrs

Pharmacodynamics

Onset	Unknown
Peak	168-235 g/ml, trough 41-85 g/ml
Duration	Steady state by 3rd weekly infusion

Drug/lab test
Increase: LFTs

NURSING CONSIDERATIONS

Assessment
⚠ **Monitor pulmonary changes: lung sounds, cough, dyspnea; interstitial lung disease may occur, may be fatal; discontinue therapy if confirmed**
⚠ **Assess for toxic epidermal necrosis, angioedema, anaphylaxis**
• Assess GI symptoms: frequency of stools, dehydration, abdominal pain, stomatitis
• Obtain **K-RAS mutation** in metastatic colorectal carcinoma; if K-RAS mutation in codon 12 or 13 is detected, then patient should not receive anti-EGFR antibody therapy

Nursing diagnoses
• Body image, disturbed (adverse reactions)
• Infection, risk for (adverse reactions)
• Injury, risk for (adverse reactions)
• Knowledge, deficient (teaching)

Patient/family education
• Instruct patient to report adverse reactions immediately: SOB, severe abdominal pain, skin eruptions
• Explain reason for treatment, expected results
• Instruct patient to use contraception during treatment
• Advise patient to wear sunscreen and hat to limit sun exposure; sun exposure can exacerbate any skin reactions

Evaluation
Positive therapeutic outcome
• Decrease growth, spread of EGFR expressing metastatic colorectal carcinoma

---

charcoal, activated (OTC)
Actidose-Aqua, Actidose with Sorbitol, Charcoal Plus, Charcoal Plus DS, Charcocaps, EZ Char
Func. class.: Antiflatulent/antidote
Pregnancy category D

ACTION: Binds poisons, toxins, irritants; increases adsorption in GI tract; inactivates toxins and binds until excreted

Therapeutic outcome: Prevention of toxicity and death resulting from absorption of products

USES: Poisoning, overdose

Unlabeled uses: Diarrhea, flatulence

CONTRAINDICATIONS:
Pregnancy **D,** hypersensitivity to this product, unconsciousness, semiconsciousness, poisoning of cyanide, mineral acids, alkalis, gag reflex, depression, ethanol intoxication, intestinal obstruction, absent bowel sounds

Precautions: Pregnancy **(C),** hypersensitivity to quinidine, quinine

DOSAGE AND ROUTES
Poisoning
Children should not get more than 1 dose of products with sorbitol
• Tabs/caps should not be used in poisonings
Adult/adolescents: PO (activated charcoal aqueous susp) 5-10 × estimated weight of drug/chemical ingested or 50-100 g dose, may repeat q4-6hr as needed; (activated charcoal with sorbitol susp) 50 g as a single dose, do not use multiple dosing
Child: PO (activated charcoal aqueous susp) 1-2 g/kg/dose or 25-50 g dose, may repeat as needed q4-6hr
Infant: PO (activated charcoal aqueous susp) 1 g/kg/dose, may repeat as needed q4-6hr

Available forms: Powder 15, 25🍁, 30, 40, 120, 125, 240 g/container; oral susp 12.5 g/60 ml, 15 g/72 ml, 15 g/120 ml, 25 g/120 ml, 30 g/120 ml, 50 g/240 ml; 🍁15 g/120 ml, 25 g/125 ml, 50 g/225 ml, 50 g/250 ml

Implementation
• Give after inducing vomiting unless vomiting is contraindicated (i.e., cyanide or alkalis); mix with 8 oz of water or fruit juice to form thick syrup; do not use dairy products to mix charcoal; repeat dose if vomiting occurs soon after dose
• Space at least 2 hr before or after other products, or absorption will be decreased; use a laxative to promote elimination; constipation occurs often
• If patient unable to swallow, dilute to a less thick sol; keep container tightly closed to prevent absorption of gases
• Give through a nasogastric tube if patient is unable to swallow

ADVERSE EFFECTS
GI: *Nausea, black stools,* vomiting, constipation, diarrhea, abdominal pain
OTHER: Pulmonary aspiration

Absorption	None
Distribution	None
Metabolism	None
Excretion	Feces (unchanged)
Half-life	Unknown

Onset	1 min
Peak	Unknown
Duration	4-12 hr

INTERACTIONS
Individual drugs
Acetylcysteine: inactivation
Acarbose, carBAMazepine, digoxin, ipecac, phenytoin: decreased effects

NURSING CONSIDERATIONS
Assessment
• Assess neurologic status including LOC, pupil reactivity, cough reflex, gag reflex, and swallowing ability before administration; do not give if neurologic status is impaired; aspiration may occur unless a protected airway is present
• Assess toxin, poison ingested, time of ingestion, and amount
• Monitor respiration, pulse, B/P to determine charcoal effectiveness if taken for barbiturate/opioid poisoning, serum electrolytes

Nursing diagnoses
• Injury, risk for (uses)
• Knowledge, deficient (teaching)
• Poisoning, risk for (uses)

Patient/family education
• Tell patient stools will be black
• Teach patient about overdose/poison prevention and about keeping poison control chart available

Evaluation
Positive therapeutic outcome
• Alert, PERL (poisoning)
• Absence of distention
• Absence of odor in wounds

chloral hydrate (Rx)
(klor'al hye'drate)
Chloral hydrate ODAN ✤, Somnote
Func. class.: Sedative/hypnotic, non-barbiturate
Chem. class.: Chloral derivative
Pregnancy category C
Controlled substance schedule IV (USA), schedule F (Canada)

ACTION: Reduced to product trichloroethanol, which produces mild cerebral depression, causing sleep; generalized CNS depression

Therapeutic outcome: Ability to sleep, sedation

USES: Sedation, short-term treatment of insomnia, alcohol withdrawal, anxiety

CONTRAINDICATIONS:
Hypersensitivity to this product or triclofos, severe renal/hepatic disease, GI disorders (oral forms), gastritis

Precautions: Pregnancy **C,** breastfeeding, geriatric, severe cardiac disease, depression, suicidal individuals, asthma, intermittent porphyria, esophagitis, gastric/duodenal ulcers, gastritis

DOSAGE AND ROUTES
Sedation
Adult: PO/RECT 250 mg tid after meals; max 2 g/day
Child: PO 25-50 mg/kg tid, max 500 mg tid

Alcohol withdrawal
Adult: PO/RECT 500 mg-1 g q6hr, max 2 g/day

Postop pain adjunct
Adult: PO 250 mg tid, after meals, max 2 g/day

Insomnia
Adult: PO/RECT 500 mg-1 g 30 min before bedtime; max 2 g/day
Child: PO/RECT 50-75 mg/kg (one dose)

Renal disease
Adult: PO/RECT CCr <50 ml/min avoid use

Available forms: Caps 500 mg; SYR 250, 500 mg/5 ml; SUPP 325, 650 mg

Implementation
• Regulate environmental stimuli (light, noise, temperature), remove foods and fluids that interfere with sleep

• Place side rails up after giving medication for hypnotic; remove cigarettes/matches from patient's environment to prevent fires
PO route
• Do not break, crush, or chew caps
• Give $^1/_2$-1 hr before bedtime for sleeplessness; give on empty stomach with full glass of water or juice for best absorption and to decrease corrosion (do not chew); after meals to decrease GI symptoms if used for sedation; dilute syr in 4 oz water or juice, chilling syrup may mask unpleasant taste
⚠ Check dose of syrup carefully, fatal overdoses have occurred
Rectal route
• Store supp in dark container, in refrigerator; remove outer wrapper before insertion

ADVERSE EFFECTS
CNS: *Drowsiness,* dizziness, stimulation, nightmares, ataxia, hangover (rare), light-headedness, headache, paranoia, hallucinations
CV: Hypotension, **dysrhythmias**
GI: *Nausea, vomiting, flatulence, diarrhea,* unpleasant taste, **gastric necrosis,** abdominal pain
HEMA: Eosinophilia, leukopenia
INTEG: Rash, urticaria, **angioedema,** fever, purpura, eczema
RESP: Depression

Pharmacokinetics
Absorption	Well absorbed (PO, RECT)
Distribution	Widely distributed; crosses placenta
Metabolism	Liver to trichloroethanol
Excretion	Kidneys (inactive metabolite), feces, breast milk
Half-life	8-10 hr; active metabolite

Pharmacodynamics
	PO	RECT
Onset	$^1/_2$-1 hr	Slow
Peak	Unknown	Unknown
Duration	4-8 hr	4-8 hr

INTERACTIONS
Individual drugs
Alcohol: increased action of both products
Furosemide: increased action of furosemide
Phenytoin: decreased effect of phenytoin

Drug classifications
Anticoagulants (oral): increased action of anticoagulants

Adverse effects: *italics* = common; **bold** = life-threatening

CNS depressants: increased action of both products

Drug/lab test
Interferences: urine catecholamines, urinary 17-OHCS

NURSING CONSIDERATIONS
Assessment
• Assess patient's sleep pattern and note physical (sleep apnea, obstructed airway, pain/discomfort, urinary frequency) and psychological (fear, anxiety) circumstances that interrupt sleep
• Assess patient's bedtime routine, presleep cues/props
• Assess potential for abuse; this product may lead to physical and psychological dependency; amount of product should be limited
• Monitor mental status: mood, sensorium, affect, memory (long, short)
• Monitor **physical dependency:** more frequent requests for medication, shakes, anxiety, pinpoint pupils
• Monitor **respiratory dysfunction:** respiratory depression, character, rate, rhythm; hold product if respirations are <10/min or if pupils are dilated (rare)
• Assess previous history of substance abuse, cardiac disease, or gastritis

Nursing diagnoses
• Anxiety (uses)
• Knowledge, deficient (teaching)
• Noncompliance (teaching)
• Insomnia (uses)

Patient/family education
• Caution patient to avoid driving and other activities requiring alertness; to avoid alcohol ingestion or CNS depressants; serious CNS depression may result plus tachycardia, flushing, headache, hypotension
• Instruct patient not to discontinue medication quickly after long-term use; product should be tapered over 1-2 wk, delirium may occur; that benefits may take 2 nights to be noticed; withdrawal symptoms include tremors, anxiety, hallucinations, delirium
• Teach patient alternative measures to improve sleep (reading, exercise several hours before bedtime, warm bath, warm milk, TV, self-hypnosis, deep breathing)
• Instruct the patient about factors that contribute to sleep pattern disturbances (lifestyle, shift work, long work hours, environmental factors, frequent napping)

• Teach patient to take product as prescribed, not to double doses
• Avoid breastfeeding

Evaluation
Positive therapeutic outcome
• Ability to sleep at night
• Decreased amount of early morning awakening if taking product for insomnia
• Sedation

TREATMENT OF OVERDOSE:
Lavage, activated charcoal; monitor electrolytes, VS

---

chlorambucil (Rx)
(klor-am′byoo-sil)
Leukeran
Func. class.: Antineoplastic alkylating agent
Chem. class.: Nitrogen mustard
Pregnancy category D

Do not confuse:
Leukeran/leucovorin/Leukine

ACTION: Alkylates DNA, RNA; inhibits enzymes that allow synthesis of amino acids in proteins; activity is not cell cycle phase specific

Therapeutic outcome: Prevention of rapidly growing malignant cells

USES: Chronic lymphocytic leukemia, non-Hodgkin's/Hodgkin's disease, other lymphomas

Unlabeled uses: Macroglobulinemia, ovarian, testicular carcinoma, Behçet's syndrome, nephrotic syndrome

CONTRAINDICATIONS:
Breastfeeding, radiation therapy within 1 mo, chemotherapy within 1 mo, thrombocytopenia, recent smallpox vaccination

BLACK BOX WARNING: Pregnancy **D**

Precautions: *Pneumococcus* vaccination, children, tumor lysis syndrome

BLACK BOX WARNING: Bone marrow suppression, infertility, secondary malignancy

DOSAGE AND ROUTES
Adult: PO 0.1-0.2 mg/kg/day × 3-6 wk initially, then 4-10 mg/day maintenance
Geriatric: PO initially ≤2-4 mg/day

---

d crowds and persons with
r other infections
air loss is common; discuss
hairpieces
to drink 2-3 L of fluid daily
cated
not to have any vaccinations
of the prescriber; serious
ur

RNING: Advise patient
needed during treatment and
s after the completion of
se irreversible gonadal sup-
ncy **D**

utic outcome
of tumor
ad of malignancy
l values
ating at night
tite, increased weight

henicol (Rx)
ole)

ntiinfective—miscellaneous
ichloroacetic acid deriva-

egory C

nds to 50S ribosomal subunit,
ith or inhibits protein

outcome: Bactericidal
*influenzae, Salmonella
Neisseria, Staphylococcus,
cherichia coli,* mycoplasma,

gitis, bacteremia, abdominal,
fections; not to be used if less
n be used

DICATIONS:
evere renal/hepatic disease,
labor, influenza, tympanic
ation

Pregnancy **C**, breastfeeding,
renal/hepatic disease, ulcer-
lomembraneous colitis

RNING: Bone marrow depres-
uced)

DOSAGE AND ROUTES

Adult and child: PO/**IV** 50 mg/kg/day in
divided doses q6hr; 100 mg/kg/day (for meningitis only); max 100 g/day
Premature infant and neonate: IV 20 mg
loading dose, then 25 mg/kg/day divided q6hr,
12 hr after loading dose

Available forms: Inj **IV** 1 g; caps 250 mg

Implementation
PO route
⚠ Do not break, crush, or chew caps
• Give oral form on empty stomach with full
glass of water
• Store cap in airtight container at room tem-
perature

Intermittent IV infusion route
• Give after **diluting** 1 g/10 ml of sterile water
for inj or D₅W (10% sol); give >1 min
• May be **further diluted** in 50-100 ml of
D₅W; give through Y-tube, 3-way stopcock, or
additive inf set; **run** over ¹/₂-1 hr; store reconstituted sol at room temperature for up to 30 days

Syringe compatibilities: Ampicillin,
cloxacillin, heparin, methicillin, penicillin G
sodium

Y-site compatibilities: Acyclovir,
alfentanil, amikacin, aminophylline, anidulafungin, atenolol, atracurium, atropine,
aztreonam, bivalirudin, bleomycin, bumetanide,
buprenorphine, calcium chloride/gluconate,
cefamandole, ceFAZolin, cefmetazole, cefonicid,
cefoperazone, cefotetan, cefoxitin, cefuroxime,
cephalothin, cephapirin, clindamycin, corticotropin, cyanocobalamin, cyclophosphamide,
cycloSPORINE, DACTINomycin, DAPTOmycin,
dexamethasone, digoxin, docetaxel, enalaprilat, ePHEDrine, EPINEPHrine, epoetin alfa,
ertapenem, etoposide, fenoldopam, fentaNYL,
fludarabine, folic acid, foscarnet, furosemide,
glycopyrrolate, granisetron, heparin, hydrocortisone, HYDROmorphone, imipenem-cilastatin,
indomethacin, insulin (regular), isoproterenol,
ketorolac, lidocaine, linezolid, LORazepam, LR,
magnesium sulfate, mannitol, methicillin, methylPREDNISolone, metoclopramide, metoprolol,
metroNIDAZOLE, mezlocillin, miconazole, milrinone, mitoxantrone, morphine, moxalactam,
multiple vitamins injection, naloxone, nesiritide,
niCARdipine, nitroglycerin, nitroprusside, norepinephrine, octreotide, oxacillin, oxaliplatin,
oxytocin, paclitaxel, palonosetron, pamidronate,
pancuronium, penicillin G potassium/sodium,
PENTobarbital, perphenazine, PHENobarbital,
phenylephrine, phytonadione, piperacillin,

Child: PO 0.1-0.2 mg/kg/day (4.5 mg/m²/day) in divided doses or 4.5 mg/m²/day as 1 dose or in divided doses × 3-6 wk

Nephrotic syndrome (unlabeled)
Child: PO 0.1-0.2 mg/kg daily with predniSONE × 8-12 wk

Available forms: Tabs 2 mg

Implementation
• Give 1 hr before or 2 hr after meals to lessen nausea and vomiting or antacid before oral agent, give product after evening meal, before bedtime or 1 hr before breakfast; antiemetic 30-60 min before giving product to prevent vomiting

• Give allopurinol to maintain uric acid levels, alkalinization of urine; increase fluid intake to 2-3 L/day to prevent urate deposits, calculus formation

• Antibiotics for prophylaxis of infection may be prescribed, since infection potential is high

• Give all products PO if possible, avoid IM inj when platelets are <100,000/mm³

• Store in tight container

ADVERSE EFFECTS
CNS: Seizures, tremors, confusion, agitation, ataxia, hallucinations
GI: *Nausea, vomiting, diarrhea, weight loss, hepatotoxicity, jaundice*
GU: Hyperuremia
HEMA: **Thrombocytopenia, leukopenia, pancytopenia (prolonged use), permanent bone marrow suppression**
INTEG: Alopecia (rare), dermatitis, rash, **Stevens-Johnson syndrome**
RESP: Fibrosis, pneumonitis

Pharmacokinetics

Absorption	Rapidly, completely absorbed
Distribution	Crosses placenta
Metabolism	Liver, extensively
Excretion	Kidneys
Half-life	2 hr

Pharmacodynamics

Unknown

INTERACTIONS

Individual drugs
Filgrastim, sargramostim: contraindicated 24 hr prior to or after chemotherapy
Nalidixic acid: do not use in combination
Radiation: increased toxicity, bone marrow suppression

Drug...
Antic...
ble...
Antin...
pre...
Live v...

NU...

Ass...

BLA...
pres...
coun...
<20...
mm³...
<20...

• **Pne...**
functi...
therap...
durin...
unpro...

• Ass...
ing, j...
shoul...
its

• Mo...
uric a...
ratio;...
monit...

• Ass...
clay-c...
fever,...

• Mo...
indica...
feet, j...
shoul...

• Ass...
ing or...
rectal...

Nurs...
• Boo...
• Infe...
• Inju...
• Kno...

Patie...
• Tea...
taining...
mouth...
sympt...

• Inst...
(fatig...
ness o...

• Inst...
breath...

treatment; to avo...
respiratory tract...
• Advise patient...
the use of wigs o...
• Instruct patien...
unless contraind...
• Caution patien...
without the advic...
reactions can oc...

BLACK BOX WA...
contraception is...
for several mon...
therapy; may ca...
pression, pregn...

Evaluation
Positive therap...
• Decreased siz...
• Decreased sp...
• Improved bloo...
• Absence of sw...
• Increased app...

chloramp...
(klor-am-fen'i...
Pentamyceti...
Func. class.: A...
Chem. class.: ...
tive
Pregnancy ca...

ACTION: B...
which interferes...
synthesis

Therapeutic...
for *Haemophilu...*
typhi, Rickettsi...
Streptococcus, ...
Bacteroides

USES: Meni...
skin, soft tissue...
toxic products c...

CONTRAI...
Hypersensitivity,...
minor infections...
membrane perfo...

Precautions...
infants, children...
ative colitis, pse...

BLACK BOX W...
sion (product-in...

---

treatment; to avoid crowds and persons with respiratory tract or other infections
• Advise patient hair loss is common; discuss the use of wigs or hairpieces
• Instruct patient to drink 2-3 L of fluid daily unless contraindicated
• Caution patient not to have any vaccinations without the advice of the prescriber; serious reactions can occur

> **BLACK BOX WARNING:** Advise patient contraception is needed during treatment and for several months after the completion of therapy; may cause irreversible gonadal suppression, pregnancy **D**

Evaluation
Positive therapeutic outcome
• Decreased size of tumor
• Decreased spread of malignancy
• Improved blood values
• Absence of sweating at night
• Increased appetite, increased weight

---

chloramphenicol (Rx)
(klor-am-fen′i-kole)
Pentamycetin ✦
Func. class.: Antiinfective—miscellaneous
Chem. class.: Dichloroacetic acid derivative
Pregnancy category C

ACTION: Binds to 50S ribosomal subunit, which interferes with or inhibits protein synthesis

Therapeutic outcome: Bactericidal for *Haemophilus influenzae, Salmonella typhi, Rickettsia, Neisseria, Staphylococcus, Streptococcus, Escherichia coli,* mycoplasma, *Bacteroides*

USES: Meningitis, bacteremia, abdominal, skin, soft tissue infections; not to be used if less toxic products can be used

CONTRAINDICATIONS:
Hypersensitivity, severe renal/hepatic disease, minor infections, labor, influenza, tympanic membrane perforation

Precautions: Pregnancy **C**, breastfeeding, infants, children, renal/hepatic disease, ulcerative colitis, pseudomembraneous colitis

> **BLACK BOX WARNING:** Bone marrow depression (product-induced)

DOSAGE AND ROUTES
Adult and child: PO/IV 50 mg/kg/day in divided doses q6hr; 100 mg/kg/day (for meningitis only); max 100 g/day
Premature infant and neonate: IV 20 mg loading dose, then 25 mg/kg/day divided q6hr, 12 hr after loading dose

Available forms: Inj IV 1 g; caps 250 mg

Implementation
PO route
⚠ **Do not break, crush, or chew caps**
• Give oral form on empty stomach with full glass of water
• Store cap in airtight container at room temperature

Intermittent IV infusion route
• Give after **diluting** 1 g/10 ml of sterile water for inj or D₅W (10% sol); give >1 min
• May be **further diluted** in 50-100 ml of D₅W; give through Y-tube, 3-way stopcock, or additive inf set; **run** over ¹/₂-1 hr; store reconstituted sol at room temperature for up to 30 days

Syringe compatibilities: Ampicillin, cloxacillin, heparin, methicillin, penicillin G sodium

Y-site compatibilities: Acyclovir, alfentanil, amikacin, aminophylline, anidulafungin, atenolol, atracurium, atropine, aztreonam, bivalirudin, bleomycin, bumetanide, buprenorphine, calcium chloride/gluconate, cefamandole, ceFAZolin, cefmetazole, cefonicid, cefoperazone, cefotetan, cefoxitin, cefuroxime, cephalothin, cephapirin, clindamycin, corticotropin, cyanocobalamin, cyclophosphamide, cycloSPORINE, DACTINomycin, DAPTOmycin, dexamethasone, digoxin, docetaxel, enalaprilat, ePHEDrine, EPINEPHrine, epoetin alfa, ertapenem, etoposide, fenoldopam, fentaNYL, fludarabine, folic acid, foscarnet, furosemide, glycopyrrolate, granisetron, heparin, hydrocortisone, HYDROmorphone, imipenem-cilastatin, indomethacin, insulin (regular), isoproterenol, ketorolac, lidocaine, linezolid, LORazepam, LR, magnesium sulfate, mannitol, methicillin, methylPREDNISolone, metoclopramide, metoprolol, metroNIDAZOLE, mezlocillin, miconazole, milrinone, mitoxantrone, morphine, moxalactam, multiple vitamins injection, naloxone, nesiritide, niCARdipine, nitroglycerin, nitroprusside, norepinephrine, octreotide, oxacillin, oxaliplatin, oxytocin, paclitaxel, palonosetron, pamidronate, pancuronium, penicillin G potassium/sodium, PENTobarbital, perphenazine, PHENobarbital, phenylephrine, phytonadione, piperacillin,

Child: PO 0.1-0.2 mg/kg/day (4.5 mg/m²/day) in divided doses or 4.5 mg/m²/day as 1 dose or in divided doses × 3-6 wk

Nephrotic syndrome (unlabeled)
Child: PO 0.1-0.2 mg/kg daily with predniSONE × 8-12 wk

Available forms: Tabs 2 mg

Implementation
• Give 1 hr before or 2 hr after meals to lessen nausea and vomiting or antacid before oral agent, give product after evening meal, before bedtime or 1 hr before breakfast; antiemetic 30-60 min before giving product to prevent vomiting
• Give allopurinol to maintain uric acid levels, alkalinization of urine; increase fluid intake to 2-3 L/day to prevent urate deposits, calculus formation
• Antibiotics for prophylaxis of infection may be prescribed, since infection potential is high
• Give all products PO if possible, avoid IM inj when platelets are <100,000/mm³
• Store in tight container

ADVERSE EFFECTS
CNS: *Seizures,* tremors, confusion, agitation, ataxia, hallucinations
GI: *Nausea, vomiting, diarrhea, weight loss,* **hepatoxicity,** *jaundice*
GU: Hyperuremia
HEMA: **Thrombocytopenia, leukopenia, pancytopenia** (prolonged use), **permanent bone marrow suppression**
INTEG: Alopecia (rare), dermatitis, rash, **Stevens-Johnson syndrome**
RESP: **Fibrosis, pneumonitis**

Pharmacokinetics

Absorption	Rapidly, completely absorbed
Distribution	Crosses placenta
Metabolism	Liver, extensively
Excretion	Kidneys
Half-life	2 hr

Pharmacodynamics

Unknown

INTERACTIONS
Individual drugs
Filgrastim, sargramostim: contraindicated 24 hr prior to or after chemotherapy
Nalidixic acid: do not use in combination
Radiation: increased toxicity, bone marrow suppression

Drug classifications
Anticoagulants, salicylates: increased risk of bleeding
Antineoplastics: increased bone marrow suppression; increased toxicity
Live virus vaccines: do not use together

NURSING CONSIDERATIONS
Assessment

> **BLACK BOX WARNING: Bone marrow depression:** Monitor CBC, differential, platelet count weekly; withhold product if WBC is <2000/mm³ or granulocyte count <1000/mm³; notify prescriber of results if WBC <20,000/mm³, platelets <50,000/mm³

• **Pneumoniti/fibrosis:** Monitor pulmonary function tests, chest x-ray films before, during therapy; chest film should be obtained q2wk during treatment; check for dyspnea, crackles, unproductive cough, chest pain, tachypnea
• Assess for increased uric acid levels, swelling, joint pain primarily in extremities; patient should be well hydrated to prevent urate deposits
• Monitor renal function studies: BUN, serum uric acid, urine CCr before, during therapy; I&O ratio; report fall in urine output of 30 ml/hr; monitor for decreased hyperuricemia
• Assess for jaundice of skin, sclera, dark urine, clay-colored stools, itchy skin, abdominal pain, fever, diarrhea
• Monitor for cold, fever, sore throat (may indicate beginning infection); identify edema in feet, joint, stomach pain, shaking; prescriber should be notified
• Assess for bleeding: hematuria, guaiac, bruising or petechiae, mucosa or orifices q8hr, no rectal temp

Nursing diagnoses
• Body image, disturbed (adverse reactions)
• Infection, risk for (adverse reactions)
• Injury, risk for (adverse reactions)
• Knowledge, deficient (teaching)

Patient/family education
• Teach patient to avoid use of products containing aspirin or ibuprofen, razors, commercial mouthwash, since bleeding may occur; to report symptoms of bleeding (hematuria, tarry stools)
• Instruct patient to report signs of **anemia** (fatigue, headache, irritability, faintness, shortness of breath)
• Instruct patient to report any changes in breathing or coughing even several mo after

piperacillin-tazobactam, potassium chloride, propranolol hydrochloride, ranitidine, Ringer's injection, ritodrine, sodium bicarbonate, succinylcholine, SUFentanil, tacrolimus, teniposide, theophylline, thiotepa, ticarcillin, ticarcillin-clavulanate, tirofiban, tobramycin, TPN, urokinase, vasopressin, voriconazole

Y-site incompatibilities: Fluconazole

ADVERSE EFFECTS

CNS: Headache, *depression,* confusion, peripheral neuritis
CV: Gray baby syndrome in newborns: failure to feed, pallor, cyanosis, abdominal distention, irregular respiration, vasomotor collapse
EENT: Optic neuritis, blindness
GI: *Nausea, vomiting, diarrhea,* abdominal pain, xerostomia, glossitis, colitis, pruritus ani
HEMA: Anemia, thrombocytopenia, aplastic anemia, granulocytopenia, leukopenia, acute generalized exanthematous pustulosis (AGEP) (rare)
INTEG: Itching, urticaria, contact dermatitis, rash

Pharmacokinetics

Absorption	Well absorbed (PO), completely absorbed (**IV**)
Distribution	Wide
Metabolism	Liver
Excretion	Kidneys, unchanged
Half-life	$1^{1}/_{2}$-4 hr

Pharmacodynamics

	PO	IV
Onset	15 min	Rapid
Peak	1-2 hr	Inf end
Duration	Unknown	Unknown

INTERACTIONS

Individual drugs
Folic acid: decreased action of folic acid
Hydantoins: increased action of hydantoins
Iron: increased action of iron
Rifampin: decreased action of rifampin
Vitamin B_{12}: decreased action of vit B_{12}

Drug classifications
Anticoagulants: increased PTT
Antidiabetics: increased action of antidiabetics
Barbiturates: increased levels of barbiturates
Penicillins: decreased action of penicillins
Sulfonylureas: increased action of sulfonylureas

NURSING CONSIDERATIONS
Assessment
• Assess patient for previous sensitivity reaction to other antiinfectives; cross-sensitivity between penicillins and cephalosporins is common
• Assess patient for signs and symptoms of **infection** including characteristics of wounds, sputum, urine, stool, WBC >10,000/mm³, fever; obtain baseline information and during treatment
• Perform C&S testing before starting product therapy to identify if correct treatment has been initiated
• Monitor product level in impaired renal/hepatic systems; peak 10-25 microgram/ml, draw 90 min after IV dose, trough 5-15 microgram/ml before next dose

> **BLACK BOX WARNING:** Monitor blood studies: platelets, CBC, WBC, RBC, Hct, Hgb, serum, iron, reticulocytes; product should be discontinued if **bone marrow depression** occurs

• Assess bowel pattern daily; if severe diarrhea occurs, product should be discontinued
• Monitor for bleeding: ecchymosis, bleeding gums, hematuria, stool guaiac daily if on long-term therapy
• Assess for **overgrowth of infection:** perineal itching, fever, malaise, redness, pain, swelling, drainage, rash, diarrhea, change in cough, sputum
• Assess neonates for beginning **gray baby syndrome:** cyanosis, abdominal distention, irregular respiration, failure to feed; product should be discontinued immediately

Nursing diagnoses
• Diarrhea (adverse reaction)
• Infection, risk for (uses)
• Injury, risk for (side effects)
• Knowledge, deficient (teaching)
• Noncompliance (teaching)

Patient/family education
• Teach patient all aspects of product therapy; need to complete entire course of medication to ensure organism death (10-14 days); culture may be taken after complete course of medication
• Advise patient to report sore throat, fever, fatigue, unusual bleeding, or bruising; could indicate bone marrow depression (may occur weeks or months after termination of product)
• Tell patient that product must be taken at regular intervals around the clock to maintain blood levels

Evaluation
Positive therapeutic outcome
• Decreased symptoms of infection

chloramphenicol ophthalmic
See Appendix B

chloramphenicol otic
See Appendix B

chlordiazePOXIDE (Rx)
(klor-dye-az-e-pox′ide)
Apo-Chlordiazepoxide ✦, Librium
Func. class.: Antianxiety
Chem. class.: Benzodiazepine, long-acting
Pregnancy category D
Controlled substance schedule IV

Do not confuse:
Librium/Librax

ACTION: Potentiates the actions of GABA, an inhibitory neurotransmitter, especially in the limbic system, reticular formation, which depresses the CNS

Therapeutic outcome: Decreased anxiety, successful alcohol withdrawal, relaxation

USES: Short-term management of anxiety, acute alcohol withdrawal, preoperative relaxation

CONTRAINDICATIONS:
Pregnancy **D**, breastfeeding, child <6 yr, hypersensitivity to benzodiazepines, closed-angle glaucoma, psychosis

Precautions: Geriatric, debilitated, renal/hepatic disease, suicidal ideation, abrupt discontinuation

DOSAGE AND ROUTES
Mild anxiety
Adult: PO 5-10 mg tid-qid
Geriatric: PO 5 mg bid initially, increase as needed
Child >6 yr: PO 5 mg bid-qid, max 10 mg bid-tid

Severe anxiety
Adult: PO 20-25 mg tid-qid

Preoperatively
Adult: PO 5-10 mg tid-qid on day before surgery

Alcohol withdrawal
Adult: PO 50-100 mg q4-6hr prn, max 300 mg/day

Renal disease
Adult: PO CCr <10 ml/min give 50% dose

Available forms: Caps 5, 25 mg

Implementation
PO route
• Give with food or milk for GI symptoms, crushed if patient is unable to swallow medication whole; do not open capsules; provide sugarless gum, hard candy, frequent sips of water for dry mouth

ADVERSE EFFECTS
CNS: *Dizziness, drowsiness,* confusion, headache, anxiety, tremors, stimulation, fatigue, depression, insomnia, hallucinations
CV: *Orthostatic hypotension,* **ECG changes, tachycardia,** hypotension, edema
EENT: *Blurred vision,* tinnitus, mydriasis
GI: Constipation, dry mouth, nausea, vomiting, anorexia, diarrhea
GU: Irregular periods, decreased libido
HEMA: Agranulocytosis
INTEG: Rash, dermatitis, itching

Pharmacokinetics

Absorption	Well absorbed (PO); slow, erratic (IM)
Distribution	Widely distributed; crosses placenta, blood-brain barrier
Metabolism	Liver extensively
Excretion	Kidneys, breast milk
Half-life	5-30 hr (increased in geriatric)

Pharmacodynamics

	PO	IM	IV
Onset	30 min	15-30 min	1-5 min
Peak	Within 2 hr	Unknown	Unknown
Duration	4-6 hr	Unknown	Up to 1 hr

INTERACTIONS
Individual drugs
Alcohol: increased CNS depression
Cimetidine, disulfiram, fluoxetine, isoniazid, ketoconazole, metoprolol, propranolol, valproic acid: increased action of chlordiazePOXIDE
Levodopa: decreased action of levodopa

⚠ Nurse Alert

Drug classifications
CNS depressants: increased CNS depression
Contraceptives (oral): increased effect of chlordiazePOXIDE
CYP3A4 inhibitors (barbiturates, protease inhibitors, rifamycins): decreased effect of chlordiazePOXIDE

Drug/lab test
False increase: 17-OHCS
False positive: pregnancy test (some methods)

NURSING CONSIDERATIONS

Assessment
• Assess **anxiety reaction:** inability to sleep, apprehension, dread, foreboding, or uneasiness related to unidentified source of danger
• Assess for previous **product dependence** or tolerance; if product dependent or tolerant, amount of medication should be restricted
• Monitor B/P (with patient lying, standing), pulse; if systolic B/P drops 20 mm Hg, hold product, notify prescriber
• Monitor blood studies: CBC during long-term therapy; **blood dyscrasias** have occurred rarely
• Monitor hepatic studies: AST, ALT, bilirubin, creatinine, LDH, alkaline phosphatase during long-term therapy
• Monitor mental status: mood, sensorium, affect, sleeping patterns, drowsiness, dizziness, suicidal tendencies, paradoxical reactions such as excitement, stimulation, acute rage
• Assess for pregnancy, product should not be used during pregnancy **D**

Nursing diagnoses
• Anxiety (uses)
• Knowledge, deficient (teaching)
• Noncompliance (teaching)

Patient/family education
• Instruct patient that product may be taken with food; if dose is missed take as soon as remembered; do not double doses
• Tell patient to avoid OTC preparations unless approved by prescriber; to avoid alcohol ingestion or other psychotropic medications unless directed by a prescriber
• Caution patient to avoid driving and activities requiring alertness, since drowsiness may occur; until medication response is known, tell patient that drowsiness may worsen at beginning of treatment
• Instruct patient not to discontinue medication abruptly after long-term use; product should be tapered over 1 wk

• Caution patient to rise slowly or fainting may occur, especially in geriatric
• Advise patient that product should be avoided during pregnancy
• Advise patient to report immediately suicidal thoughts/behaviors

Evaluation
Positive therapeutic outcome
• Increased well being
• Decreased anxiety, restlessness, sleeplessness, dread
• Successful alcohol withdrawal

TREATMENT OF OVERDOSE:
Lavage, VS, supportive care

chloroquine (Rx)
(klor'oh-kwin)
Aralen, Novo-chloroquine ✚
Func. class.: Antimalarial
Chem. class.: Synthetic 4-aminoquinoline derivative
Pregnancy category C

ACTION: Inhibits parasite replications, transcription of DNA to RNA by forming complexes with DNA of parasite

Therapeutic outcome: Decreased symptoms of malaria, amebiasis

USES: Malaria caused by *Plasmodium vivax, Plasmodium malariae, Plasmodium ovale, Plasmodium falciparum* (some strains), amebiasis

CONTRAINDICATIONS:
Hypersensitivity, retinal field changes

Precautions: Pregnancy **C,** breastfeeding, children, blood dyscrasias, severe GI disease, neurologic disease, alcoholism, hepatic disease, G6PD deficiency, psoriasis, eczema, seizures, preexisting auditory damage, infection, torsades de pointes

> **BLACK BOX WARNING:** Infection

DOSAGE AND ROUTES
Acute malaria attacks
Adult: PO 1000 mg (600 mg base), then 500 mg (300 mg base) in 6-8 hr, then 500 mg (300 mg base) q day × 2 days for a total of 2.5 g (1.5 g base) in 3 days

---

Adult/adolescent of low body weight, child/ infant: **PO** 16.5 mg (10 mg base)/kg, max 600 mg base, then 8.3 mg (5 mg base)/kg max 300 mg base, 6 hr after 1st dose, then 8.3 mg (5 mg base)/kg, max 300 mg base 24 hr after 1st dose, then 8.3 mg (5 mg base)/kg max 300 mg base 36 hr after 1st dose

Malaria prophylaxis (in areas with chloroquine–sensitive *P. falci- parum)*

Adult: **PO** 500 mg (300 mg base) q wk on same day of each wk, starting 2 wk before travel and 8 wk after leaving

Extraintestinal amebiais

Adult: **PO** 1 g (600 mg base) q day × 2 days, then 500 mg (300 mg base) for ≥2-3 wk
Child (unlabeled): **PO** 16.6 mg (10 mg base)/ kg (max 300 mg base) q day × 2-3wk

Available forms: Tabs 250 mg (150 mg base), 500 mg (300 mg base) phosphate

Implementation
PO route
• Give with meals to decrease GI symptoms; better to take on empty stomach 1 hr before or 2 hr after meals
• Give antiemetic if vomiting occurs
• Give after C&S is completed; monthly to detect resistance
IM route
• Give IM after aspirating to prevent inj into bloodstream

Additive compatibility: Promethazine

ADVERSE EFFECTS
CNS: Headache, stimulation, fatigue, **seizure,** psychosis, hallucinations, insomnia
CV: Hypotension, **heart block, asystole with syncope,** ECG changes, cardiomyopathy
EENT: *Blurred vision, corneal changes, retinal changes, difficulty focusing,* tinnitus, vertigo, deafness, photophobia, corneal edema
GI: *Nausea, vomiting, anorexia,* diarrhea, cramps
HEMA: **Thrombocytopenia, agranulocyto- sis, hemolytic anemia, leukopenia**
INTEG: Pruritus, pigmentary changes, skin eruptions, lichen planus–like eruptions, eczema, **exfoliative dermatitis**

Pharmacokinetics

Absorption	Well absorbed
Distribution	Widely
Metabolism	Liver
Excretion	Kidneys, feces
Half-life	3-5 days

Pharmacodynamics

	PO	IM
Onset	Rapid	Rapid
Peak	1-3 hr	30 min
Duration	6-8 hr	Unknown

INTERACTIONS
Individual drugs
Ampicillin, rabies vaccine (ID): decreased effects
Cimetidine: decreased oral clearance, metabo- lism
Kaolin: decreased absorption
Magnesium: decreased action of chloroquine

Drug classifications
CYP2D6 inhibitors (amiodarone, chlorpheni- ramine, fluoxetine, haloperidol, ritonavir, paroxetine, terbinafine, ticlopidine), CYP3A4 inhibitors (clarithromycin, diltiazem, doxycy- cline, erythromycin, itraconazole, ketocon- azole, verapamil): increased effects
Antacids (aluminum): decreased absorption
Class IA, III antidysrhythmics: increased QT prolongation, torsades de pointes

NURSING CONSIDERATIONS
Assessment

> **BLACK BOX WARNING:** Assess for **infection:** resistance is common, not to be used for *P. falciparum* acquired in areas of resistance or where prophylaxis has failed

• Monitor **ECG** during therapy; watch for de- pression of T waves, widening of QRS complex
• Assess for **allergic reactions:** pruritus, rash, urticaria
• Assess for **ototoxicity:** tinnitus, vertigo, change in hearing; audiometric testing should be done before, after treatment
• Assess for **blood dyscrasias:** malaise, fever, bruising, bleeding (rare)
• Assess mental status often: affect, mood, behavioral changes; psychosis may occur

- Assess for **toxicity:** blurring vision, difficulty focusing, headache, dizziness, decreased knee and ankle reflexes, product should be discontinued immediately

Nursing diagnoses
- Diarrhea (side effects)
- Infection, risk for (uses)
- Injury, risk for (side effects)
- Knowledge, deficient (teaching)
- Noncompliance (teaching)

Patient/family education
- Advise patient that compliance with dosage schedule, duration is necessary
- Instruct patient that scheduled appointments must be kept or relapse may occur
- Caution patient to avoid alcohol while taking product
- Instruct diabetic to use blood glucose monitor to obtain correct result
- Teach patient to report weakness, fatigue, loss of appetite, nausea, vomiting, yellowing of skin or eyes, tingling/numbness of hands/feet
- Advise patient that urine may turn rust brown color
- Instruct patient to use sunglasses in bright sunlight to prevent photophobia

Evaluation
Positive therapeutic outcome
- Decreased symptoms of malaria

TREATMENT OF OVERDOSE:
Induce vomiting, gastric lavage, administer barbiturate (ultrashort-acting), vasopressor; tracheostomy may be necessary

chlorothiazide (Rx)
(klor-oh-thye′a-zide)
Diuril
Func. class.: Diuretic, antihypertensive
Chem. class.: Thiazide; sulfonamide derivative
Pregnancy category C

Do not confuse:
chlorothiazide/chlorproMAZINE/chlorproPAMIDE/chlorthalidone

ACTION: Acts on the distal tubule and thick ascending limb of the loop of Henle in the kidney, increasing excretion of sodium, water, chloride, magnesium, and potassium

Therapeutic outcome: Decreased B/P, decreased edema in tissues peripherally, diuresis

USES: Hypertension, diuresis, CHF, edema, nephrotic syndrome

CONTRAINDICATIONS:
Hypersensitivity to thiazides or sulfonamides, anuria, renal decompensation, breastfeeding, hepatic coma

Precautions: Pregnancy C, geriatric, hypokalemia, renal/hepatic disease, gout, COPD, LE, diabetes mellitus, hyperlipidemia

DOSAGE AND ROUTES
Hypertension
Adult: PO/IV 500 mg-1 g daily; may divide bid, max 2 g/day in divided doses

Edema
Adult: IV 250 mg q6-12hr
Child >6 mo: PO 10-20 mg/kg/day may divide bid
Child <6 mo: PO 10-20 mg/kg/day in 2 doses

Renal dose
Adult: PO/IV CCr <30 ml/min; do not use

Available forms: Tabs 250, 500 mg; oral susp 250 mg/5 ml; powder for inj 500 mg

Implementation
- Give in AM to avoid interference with sleep
- Potassium replacement if potassium level is 3.0 mg/dl
- Give whole, or use oral sol; product may be crushed if patient is unable to swallow
PO route
- Give with food; if nausea occurs, absorption may be increased
IV route
- Do not use sol that is yellow or has a precipitate or crystals
IV direct/IV infusion route
- May be given undiluted over 5 min or as an infusion
- Reconstitute: add 18 ml of sterile water for injection to the vial (28 mg/ml)

Additive compatibilities: Cimetidine, lidocaine, nafcillin, sodium bicarbonate

Additive incompatibilities: Amikacin, blood, blood products, chlorproMAZINE, codeine, hydrALAZINE, insulin, levorphanol, methadone, morphine, multivitamins, norepinephrine, polymyxin B, procaine, prochlorperazine, promazine, promethazine, streptomycin, tetracycline, triflupromazine, vancomycin

ADVERSE EFFECTS

CNS: Paresthesia, headache, *dizziness, fatigue*
CV: Irregular pulse, orthostatic hypotension, volume depletion
EENT: Blurred vision
ELECT: *Hypokalemia,* hypercalcemia, hyponatremia, hypochloremia, hypomagnesemia, hyperuricemia
GI: Nausea, vomiting, anorexia, constipation, diarrhea, pancreatitis, GI irritation, **hepatitis**
GU: *Frequency,* polyuria, incontinence, ED
HEMA: Aplastic anemia, hemolytic anemia, leukopenia, agranulocytosis, thrombocytopenia, neutropenia
INTEG: Rash, urticaria, purpura, photosensitivity, alopecia, fever, **exfoliative dermatitis**
META: Hyperglycemia, *hyperuricemia,* increased creatinine, BUN
SYST: Anaphylaxis

Pharmacokinetics

	PO
Absorption	GI tract (10%-20%)
Distribution	Extracellular spaces; crosses placenta
Metabolism	Liver
Excretion	Urine, unchanged; breast milk
Half-life	1-2 hr

Pharmacodynamics

	PO	IV
Onset	2 hr	15 min
Peak	4 hr	½ hr
Duration	6-12 hr	2 hr

INTERACTIONS

Individual drugs

Alcohol: increased hypotension
Allopurinol, digoxin, lithium: increased toxicity
Amphotericin, mezlocillin, piperacillin, ticarcillin: increased hypokalemia
Cholestyramine, colestipol: decreased absorption of thiazides

Drug classifications

Antihypertensives: increased antihypertensive effect
Glucocorticoids: increased hypokalemia
Nitrates: increased hypotension
NSAIDs: decreased diuretic action
Nondepolarizing skeletal muscle relaxants: increased toxicity

Drug/herb

Ephedra: decreased antihypertensive
Hawthorn, horse chestnut: increased antihypertensive effect

Drug/lab test

Increased: calcium, amylase, parathyroid test, CPK
Decreased: PBI
False negative: tyramine tests
Interference: urine steroid tests

NURSING CONSIDERATIONS

Assessment

• Monitor improvement in CVP q8hr
• Check for rashes, temp elevation daily
• Assess for confusion, especially in geriatric; take safety precautions if needed
• Monitor electrolytes: potassium, sodium, calcium, magnesium; also include BUN, blood pH, ABGs, uric acid, CBC, blood glucose
• Assess B/P before, during therapy with patient lying, standing, and sitting as appropriate; orthostatic hypotension can occur rapidly

Nursing diagnoses

• Fluid volume, deficient
• Fluid volume, excess (uses)
• Knowledge, deficient (teaching)
• Urinary elimination, impaired (adverse reactions)

Patient/family education

• Teach patient to take medication early in the day to prevent nocturia
• Instruct patient to take with food or milk if GI symptoms of nausea and anorexia occur
• Teach patient to maintain a weekly record of weight and notify prescriber of weight loss >5 lb
• Caution patient that this product causes a loss of potassium, so food rich in potassium should be added to the diet; refer to a dietitian for assistance in planning
• Caution patient not to exercise in hot weather or stand for prolonged periods, since orthostatic hypotension will be enhanced; to use sunscreen to prevent burning
• Teach patient not to use alcohol or any OTC medications without prescriber's approval; serious product reactions may occur
• Emphasize the need to contact prescriber immediately if muscle cramps, weakness, nausea, dizziness, or numbness occur
• Teach patient to take own B/P and pulse and record

• Caution patient that orthostatic hypotension may occur; patient should rise slowly from sitting or reclining positions and lie down if dizziness occurs

• Teach patient to continue taking medication even if feeling better; this product controls symptoms but does not cure the condition

• Advise the patient with hypertension to continue other medical treatment (exercise, weight loss, relaxation techniques, cessation of smoking)

Evaluation
Positive therapeutic outcome
• Decreased edema
• Decreased B/P
• Increased diuresis

TREATMENT OF OVERDOSE:
Lavage if taken orally, monitor electrolytes; administer dextrose in saline; monitor hydration, CV, renal status

---

chlorpheniramine (OTC, Rx)
(klor-fen-ir'a-meen)
AHIST, Aller-Chlor, Allergy, Chlor-Pheniton, Chlor-Trimeton, Diabetic Tussin Allergy Relief, ED-Chlor-Tann, Equaline Allergy, Equate Chlortabs Allergy, Good Sense Allergy, Leader Allergy, P-Tann, Select Brand Chlorpheniramine, Tana Hist-PD, Teldrin, Top Care Allergy, Wal-finate Allergy
Func. class.: Antihistamine (1st generation, nonselective)
Chem. class.: Alkylamine, H_1-receptor antagonist
Pregnancy category B

Do not confuse:
Teldrin/Tedral

ACTION: Acts on blood vessels, GI, respiratory system by competing with histamine for H_1-receptor site; decreases allergic response by blocking histamine

Therapeutic outcome: Absence of allergy symptoms and rhinitis

USES: Allergy symptoms, rhinitis, conjunctivitis (allergic)

CONTRAINDICATIONS:
Newborns/neonates

Precautions: Pregnancy **B**, breastfeeding, geriatric, increased intraocular pressure, renal/cardiac disease, hypertension, bronchial asthma, seizure disorder, hyperthyroidism, prostatic hypertrophy, GI obstruction, peptic ulcer disease, emphysema, hypersensitivity to H_1-receptor antagonists, lower respiratory tract disease, stenosed peptic ulcers, bladder neck obstruction, closed-angle glaucoma, children

DOSAGE AND ROUTES
Adult/child ≥12 yr: PO 4 mg tid-qid, max 24 mg/day; EXT REL 8-12 mg bid-tid, max 24 mg/day
Child 6-12 yr: PO 2 mg q4-6hr, max 12 mg/day; EXT REL 8 mg at bedtime or daily; EXT REL not recommended for child <6 yr
Child 2-5 yr: PO (syr) 1 mg q4-6hr, max 4 mg/day

For self-treatment of hay fever or other upper respiratory allergies
Adult/adolescent/child ≥12 yr: PO 4 mg q4-6hr, max 24 mg/24 hr
Child 6-11 yr: PO 2 mg q4-6hr, max 12 mg/24 hr

Available forms: Chewable tabs 2 mg; tabs 4, 8, 12 mg; ext rel tabs 8, 12 mg; ext rel caps 8, 12 mg; syr 1, 2, 2.5 mg/5 ml

Implementation
PO route
• Swallow time rel tabs and caps whole
• Do not break, crush, chew, or open time rel tabs
• Chewable tabs should be chewed and not swallowed whole
• Avoid use in children ≤2 yr
• May give with food to decrease GI upset
• Store in tight, light-resistant container
IM/SUBCUT route
• Use only 20 and 100 mg/ml strengths; does not need to be reconstituted or diluted

IV route
Give undiluted by direct **IV** (10 mg/ml strength only); administer 10 mg over 1 min or more

Additive incompatibilities: Calcium chloride, kanamycin, norepinephrine, pentobarbital

ADVERSE EFFECTS
CNS: *Dizziness, drowsiness,* poor coordination, fatigue, anxiety, euphoria, confusion, paresthesia, neuritis

---

Adverse effects: *italics* = common; **bold** = life-threatening

EENT: Blurred vision, dilated pupils, tinnitus, nasal stuffiness, dry nose, throat, mouth
GI: Nausea, anorexia, diarrhea
GU: *Retention,* dysuria, frequency
HEMA: Thrombocytopenia, agranulocytosis, hemolytic anemia
INTEG: Photosensitivity
RESP: Increased thick secretions, wheezing, chest tightness

Pharmacokinetics

Absorption	Well absorbed (PO, SUBCUT, IM, **IV**)
Distribution	Widely distributed; crosses blood-brain barrier
Metabolism	Liver, mostly
Excretion	Kidneys, metabolite; breast milk (minimal)
Half-life	12-15 hr

Pharmacodynamics

	PO	PO-ER	SUB-CUT	IM	IV
Onset	15-30 min	Un-known	Un-known	Un-known	Un-known
Peak	1-2 hr	Un-known	Un-known	Un-known	Un-known
Duration	4-12 hr	8-24 hr	4-12 hr	4-12 hr	4-12 hr

INTERACTIONS

Individual drugs
Alcohol: increased CNS depression
Atropine, haloperidol, quinidine: increased anticholinergic reactions

Drug classifications
Barbiturates, CNS depressants, opiates, sedative/hypnotics, tricyclics: increased CNS depression
MAOIs: increased effect of chlorpheniramine
Phenothiazines: increased anticholinergic reactions

Drug/lab test
False negative: skin allergy tests (discontinue antihistamines 3 days before testing)

NURSING CONSIDERATIONS

Assessment
• Assess respiratory status: rate, rhythm, increase in bronchial secretions, wheezing, chest tightness; provide fluids to 2 L/day to decrease secretion thickness

• Monitor I&O ratio: be alert for urinary retention, frequency, dysuria, especially geriatric; product should be discontinued if these occur
• **IV** administration may result in rapid drop in B/P, sweating, dizziness, especially in geriatric

Nursing diagnoses
• Airway clearance, ineffective (uses)
• Injury, risk for (side effects)
• Knowledge, deficient (teaching)
• Noncompliance (teaching, overuse)

Patient/family education
• Teach all aspects of product use; to notify prescriber if confusion, sedation, hypotension, or difficulty voiding occurs; to avoid driving and other hazardous activity if drowsiness occurs; to avoid alcohol and other CNS depressants that may potentiate effect
• Teach patient not to exceed recommended dosage; dysrhythmias may occur
• Advise patient hard candy, gum, frequent rinsing of mouth may be used for dryness

Evaluation
Positive therapeutic outcome
• Absence of running or congested nose, rashes, conjunctivitis

TREATMENT OF OVERDOSE:
Administer lavage, diazepam, vasopressors, phenytoin IV

chlorproMAZINE (Rx)
(klor-proe'ma-zeen)
Novo-Chlorpromazine ✦
Func. class.: Antipsychotic/neuroleptic/antiemetic
Chem. class.: Phenothiazine, aliphatic
Pregnancy category C

Do not confuse:
chlorproMAZINE/chlorothiazide/
chlorproPAMIDE/chlorthalidone/
prochlorperazine

ACTION: Depresses cerebral cortex, hypothalamus, limbic system, which control activity, aggression; blocks neurotransmission produced by dopamine at synapse; exhibits a strong α-adrenergic, anticholinergic blocking action; mechanism for antipsychotic effects is unclear

Therapeutic outcome: Decreased signs and symptoms of psychosis; control of nausea, vomiting, intractable hiccups, decreased anxiety preoperatively

USES: Psychotic disorders, Tourette's syndrome, mania, schizophrenia, anxiety, intractable hiccups (adults), nausea, vomiting, preoperative relaxation, acute intermittent porphyria, behavioral problems in children, nonpsychotic patients with dementia

Unlabeled uses: Vascular headache

CONTRAINDICATIONS:
Hypersensitivity, circulatory collapse, liver damage, cerebral arteriosclerosis, coronary disease, severe hypo/hypertension, blood dyscrasias, coma, child <6 mo, brain damage, bone marrow depression, alcohol and barbiturate withdrawal, closed-angle glaucoma

Precautions: Pregnancy **C**, breastfeeding, geriatric, seizure disorders, hypertension, hepatic/cardiac disease, prostateenlargement, pulmonary/Parkinson's disease

> **BLACK BOX WARNING:** Dementia

DOSAGE AND ROUTES
Psychosis
Adult: PO 10-50 mg q1-4hr initially, then increase up to 2 g/day if necessary; IM 10-50 mg q1-4hr, usual dose 300-800 mg/day
Geriatric: PO 10-25 mg daily-bid, increased by 10-25 mg/day q4-7day, max 800 mg/day
Child >6 mo: PO 0.55 mg/kg q4-6hr; IM 0.5 mg/kg q6-8hr

Nausea and vomiting
Adult: PO 10-25 mg q4-6hr prn; IM 25-50 mg q3hr prn; max 400 mg/day; **IV** 25-50 mg daily-qid
Child ≥6 mo: PO 0.55 mg/kg q4-6hr; IM q6-8hr; IM ≤5 yr or ≤22.7 kg 40 mg; max IM 5-10 yr or 22.7-45.5 kg 75 mg

Intractable hiccups
Adult: PO 25-50 mg tid-qid; IM 25-50 mg (used only if PO dose does not work); **IV** 25-50 mg in 500-1000 ml saline (only for severe hiccups)

Available forms: Tabs 10, 25, 50, 100; inj 25 mg/ml

Implementation
PO route
⚠ Do not break, crush, or chew time rel caps
• Give product in liquid form mixed in glass of juice or cola if hoarding is suspected
• Periodically attempt dosage reduction in patients with behavioral problems

• Give with full glass of water, milk; or give with food to decrease GI upset
• Store in tight, light-resistant container, oral sol in amber bottle
IM route
• Inject in deep muscle mass; do not give SUBCUT; may be diluted with 0.9% NaCl, 2% procaine as prescribed; do not administer sol with a precipitate
• Remain lying down after IM inj for at least 30 min
Rectal route
• Give after placing in refrigerator for 30 min if too soft to insert; this route is used for nausea, vomiting, hiccups
Direct IV
• Give by direct **IV** by diluting with 0.9% NaCl to a concentration of 1 mg/1 ml; administer at a rate of 1 mg/2 min, never give undiluted
• Give by continuous IV infusion diluting 50 mg/500-1000 ml of D_5W, $D_{10}W$, 0.9% NaCl, 0.45% NaCl, LR, Ringer's or combinations (used for intractable hiccups)

Syringe compatibilities: Atropine, benztropine, butorphanol, diphenhydrAMINE, doxapram, droperidol, fentaNYL, glycopyrrolate, HYDROmorphone, hydrOXYzine, meperidine, metoclopramide, midazolam, morphine, pentazocine, perphenazine, prochlorperazine, promazine, promethazine, scopolamine

Syringe incompatibilities: Cimetidine, dimenhyDRINATE, heparin, PENTobarbital, thiopental

Y-site compatibilities: Alfentanil, amikacin, amphotericin B lipid complex, amsacrine, anidulafungin, ascorbic acid injection, atenolol, atracurium, atropine, benztropine, bleomycin sulfate, buprenorphine, butorphanol, calcium chloride/gluconate, caspofungin, cimetidine, cisatracurium, CISplatin, cladribine, codeine, cyanocobalamin, cyclophosphamide, cycloSPORINE, cytarabine, DACTINomycin, DAPTOmycin, dexmedetomidine, digoxin, diltiazem, diphenhydrAMINE, DOBUTamine, docetaxel, DOPamine, doxacurium, DOXOrubicin, DOXOrubicin liposomal, doxycycline, enalaprilat, ePHEDrine, EPINEPHrine, epirubicin, erythromycin, esmolol, etoposide, famotidine, fenoldopam, fentaNYL, filgrastim, fluconazole, gatifloxacin, gemcitabine, gentamicin, glycopyrrolate, granisetron, hydrocortisone, HYDROmorphone, hydrOXYzine, IDArubicin, isofosfamide, isoproterenol, labetalol, levofloxacin, lidocaine, LORazepam, LR, magnesium sulfate, mannitol, mechlorethamine, meperidine, methicillin,

methoxamine, methyldopa, methylPREDNISolone, metoclopramide, metoprolol, metroNI-
DAZOLE, miconazole, midazolam, milrinone,
minocycline, mitoxantrone, morphine, multiple
vitamins injection, mycophenolate mofetil,
nafcillin, nalbuphine, naloxone, netilmicin,
nitroglycerin, norepinephrine, octreotide, ondansetron, oxacillin, oxaliplatin, palonosetron,
pamidronate, pancuronium, papaverine, penicillin G potassium, pentamidine, pentazocine,
phytonadione, polymyxin B, potassium chloride,
procainamide, prochlorperazine, promethazine, propofol, propranolol, protamine sulfate,
pyridoxine, quiNIDine, quinupristin-dalfopristin,
ranitidine, Ringer's injection, ritodrine,
riTUXimab, rocuronium, sodium acetate, succinylcholine, SUFentanil, tacrolimus, teniposide,
theophylline, thiamine, thiotepa, tirofiban, TNA,
tolazoline, TPN, trimetaphan, vancomycin, vasopressin, vecuronium, verapamil, vinCRIStine,
vinorelbine, vitamin B complex with C, voriconazole, zoledronic acid

ADVERSE EFFECTS

CNS: **Neuroleptic malignant syndrome,**
dizziness, *extrapyramidal symptoms: pseudoparkinsonism, akathisia, dystonia, tardive
dyskinesia,* **seizures,** *headache*
CV: *Orthostatic hypotension,* hypertension,
cardiac arrest, ECG changes, **tachycardia**
EENT: Blurred vision, glaucoma, dry eyes
ENDO: SIADH
GI: *Dry mouth, nausea, vomiting, anorexia,
constipation,* diarrhea, cholestatic jaundice,
weight gain
GU: Urinary retention, enuresis, impotence,
amenorrhea, gynecomastia, breast engorgement
HEMA: Anemia, **leukopenia, leukocytosis,
agranulocytosis**
INTEG: *Rash,* photosensitivity, dermatitis
RESP: **Laryngospasm,** dyspnea, **respiratory
depression**
SYST: **Death in geriatric patients with
dementia**

Pharmacokinetics

Absorption	Variable (PO); well ab-sorbed (IM)
Distribution	Widely distributed; crosses placenta
Metabolism	Liver, GI mucosa extensively
Excretion	Kidneys
Half-life	30 hr

Pharmacodynamics

	PO	RECT	IM	IV
Onset	$1/2$-1 hr	12 hr	Unknown	Rapid
Peak	Unknown	Unknown	Unknown	Unknown
Duration	4-6 hr*	3-4 hr	4-8 hr	Unknown

*Duration PO ext rel is 10-12 hr.

INTERACTIONS

Individual drugs

Alcohol: increased effects of both products, oversedation
Aluminum hydroxide, magnesium hydroxide: decreased absorption
Bromocriptine, levodopa: decreased antiparkinsonian activity
EPINEPHrine: increased toxicity
Lithium: decreased chlorproMAZINE levels
Valproic acid: increased valproic acid level
Warfarin: decreased anticoagulant effect

Drug classifications

Antacids: decreased absorption
Anticholinergics, antidepressants, antiparkinsonian agents: increased anticholinergic effects
Anticonvulsants: decreased seizure threshold
Antidepressants, antihistamines, barbiturate anesthetics, opioids, sedative/hypnotics: increased CNS depression
Antithyroid agents: increased agranulocytosis
Barbiturates: decreased serum chlorproMAZINE
β-Adrenergic blockers: increased effect of both products

Drug/lab test

Increased: liver function tests, cardiac enzymes, cholesterol, blood glucose, prolactin, bilirubin, PBI, cholinesterase, alkaline phosphatase, leukocytes, granulocytes, platelets, [131]I
Decreased: hormones (blood and urine)
False positive: pregnancy tests, PKU
False negative: urinary steroids, 17-OHCS

NURSING CONSIDERATIONS

Assessment

• Assess mental status: orientation, mood, behavior, presence of hallucinations, and type before initial administration and monthly; this product should significantly reduce psychotic behavior
• Assess any potentially reversible cause of behavior problems in geriatric before, during therapy

⚠ Nurse Alert

- Check for swallowing of PO medication; check for hoarding or giving of medication to other patients
- Monitor I&O ratio; palpate bladder if low urinary output occurs, especially in geriatric; urinalysis recommended before, during prolonged therapy
- Monitor bilirubin, CBC, liver function studies, ocular exam; agranulocytosis, glaucoma, cholestatic jaundice may occur
- Assess affect, orientation, LOC, reflexes, gait, coordination, sleep pattern disturbances
- Monitor B/P with patient sitting, standing, lying; take pulse and respirations q4hr during initial treatment; establish baseline before starting treatment; report drops of 30 mm Hg; obtain baseline ECG, Q wave, and T wave changes
- Check for dizziness, faintness, palpitations, tachycardia on rising; severe orthostatic hypotension is common
⚠ Identify for neuroleptic malignant syndrome: hyperpyrexia, muscle rigidity, increased CPK, altered mental status; product should be discontinued
- Assess for **EPS** including akathisia (inability to sit still, no pattern to movements), tardive dyskinesia (bizarre movements of the jaw, mouth, tongue, extremities), pseudoparkinsonism (rigidity, tremors, pill rolling, shuffling gate); an antiparkinsonian product should be prescribed
- Assess for constipation, urinary retention daily; if these occur, increase bulk, water in diet

Nursing diagnoses
- Coping, ineffective (uses)
- Knowledge, deficient (teaching)
- Noncompliance (teaching)
- Thought processes, disturbed (uses)

Patient/family education
- Teach patient to use good oral hygiene; frequent rinsing of mouth, sugarless gum, candy, or ice chips for dry mouth
- Caution patient to avoid hazardous activities until product response is determined; dizziness, blurred vision may occur
- Inform patient that orthostatic hypotension occurs often and to rise from sitting or lying position gradually, to remain lying down after IM inj for at least 30 min; tell patient to avoid hot tubs, hot showers, tub baths, since hypotension may occur; tell patient that in hot weather heat stroke may occur; take extra precautions to stay cool
- Advise patient to avoid abrupt withdrawal of this product, or extrapyramidal symptoms may result; product should be withdrawn slowly

- Teach patient to avoid OTC preparations (cough, hay fever, cold) unless approved by prescriber, since serious product interactions may occur; avoid use with alcohol, CNS depressants, since increased drowsiness may occur
- Caution patient to use sunscreen and sunglasses to prevent burns
- Teach patient about extrapyramidal symptoms and necessity of meticulous oral hygiene, since oral candidiasis may occur
- Instruct patient to take antacids 2 hr before or after taking this product
- Instruct patient to report sore throat, malaise, fever, bleeding, mouth sores; if these occur, CBC should be drawn and product discontinued
- Teach that urine may turn pink or reddish-brown
- Teach patient to use contraceptive measures

Evaluation
Positive therapeutic outcome
- Decrease in emotional excitement, hallucinations, delusions, paranoia
- Reorganization of patterns of thought, speech
- Increase in target behaviors

TREATMENT OF OVERDOSE:
Lavage if orally ingested; provide airway, *do not induce vomiting or use epinephrine*

chlorthalidone (Rx)
(klor-tha′li-doan)
Apo-Chlorthalidone ✦, Hygroton, Thalitone, Uridon ✦
Func. class.: Diuretic, antihypertensive
Chem. class.: Thiazide-like phthalimidine derivative
Pregnancy category B

Do not confuse:
chlorthalidone/chlorothiazide/
chlorproMAZINE/chlorproPAMIDE,
Hygroton/Regroton, **Uridon ✦**/Vicodin

ACTION: Acts on the distal tubule and thick ascending limb of the loop of Henle in the kidney, increasing excretion of sodium, water, chloride, magnesium, potassium, and bicarbonate; possible arteriolar dilatation

Therapeutic outcome: Decreased B/P, decreased edema in lung tissues and peripherally, diuresis

USES: Edema, hypertension, edema in congestive heart failure

CONTRAINDICATIONS:
Hypersensitivity to thiazides or sulfonamides, anuria, renal decompensation, breastfeeding

Precautions: Pregnancy **B**, geriatric, hypokalemia, renal/hepatic disease, gout, diabetes mellitus, hyperlipidemia, SLE, hypotension, CCr <25 ml/min

DOSAGE AND ROUTES
Adult: PO 12.5-100 mg q day

Available forms: Tabs 25, 50, 100 mg

Implementation
• Brand names Thalitone/Hygroton should not be used interchangeably
• Give in AM to avoid interference with sleep
• Provide potassium replacement if potassium level is 3.0 mg/dl; give whole, or use oral solutions lightly; product may be crushed if patient is unable to swallow
• Give with food if nausea occurs; may crush tab and mix with fluids or applesauce for swallowing

ADVERSE EFFECTS
CNS: Paresthesia, headache, *dizziness, fatigue, weakness,* fever
CV: Hypertension, orthostatic hypotension, palpitations, volume depletion
EENT: Blurred vision
ELECT: *Hypokalemia,* hypercalcemia, hyponatremia, hypochloremia, hypomagnesemia
GI: *Nausea, vomiting, anorexia,* constipation, diarrhea, pancreatitis, GI irritation, jaundice
GU: *Frequency,* polyuria, **uremia,** glucosuria, impotence
HEMA: Aplastic anemia, hemolytic anemia, leukopenia, agranulocytosis, thrombocytopenia, neutropenia
INTEG: Rash, urticaria, purpura, photosensitivity
META: *Hyperglycemia, hyperuricemia,* increased creatinine, BUN, gout

Pharmacokinetics

Absorption	Well absorbed
Distribution	Extracellular spaces; crosses placenta
Metabolism	Liver
Excretion	Urine, unchanged (30%-60%)
Half-life	40 hr

Pharmacodynamics

Onset	2 hr
Peak	6 hr
Duration	24-72 hr

INTERACTIONS
Individual drugs
Alcohol: increased hypotensive effect
Allopurinol, lithium: increased toxicity
Amphotericin B: increased hypokalemia
Cholestyramine, colestipol: decreased absorption of thiazides
Diazoxide: increased hyperglycemia, hypotension

Drug classifications
Glucocorticoids: increased hypokalemia
Nondepolarizing skeletal muscle relaxants: increased toxicity

Drug/herb
Ephedra: decreased antihypertensive effect
Hawthorn, horse chestnut: increased hypotension

Drug/lab test
Increased: triglycerides, calcium, amylase, cholesterol, bilirubin, creatinine, low-density lipoproteins, serum/urine glucose (diabetics), uric acid
Decreased: PBI, parathyroid test, magnesium, potassium, sodium, urinary calcium

NURSING CONSIDERATIONS
Assessment
• Monitor for **hypokalemia;** *CV:* hypotension, broad T wave, U wave, ectopy, tachycardia, weak pulse; *GI:* anorexia, nausea, cramps, constipation, distention, paralytic ileus; *NEURO:* muscle weakness, altered LOC, drowsiness, apathy, lethargy, confusion, depression; *RENAL:* acidic urine, reduced urine, osmolality, nocturia; *RESP:* hypoventilation, respiratory muscle weakness
• Assess fluid volume status: I&O ratios and record, weight, distended red veins, crackles in lung, color, quality, and specific gravity of urine, skin turgor, adequacy of pulses, moist mucous membranes, bilateral lung sounds, peripheral pitting edema; dehydration symptoms of decreasing output, thirst, hypotension, dry mouth, and mucous membranes should be reported
• Monitor electrolytes: potassium, sodium, calcium, magnesium; also include BUN, blood pH, ABGs, uric acid, CBC, blood glucose
• **Hypertension:** Assess B/P before and during therapy with patient lying, standing, and sitting

as appropriate; orthostatic hypotension can occur rapidly
• Assess for signs of **metabolic alkalosis:** drowsiness, restlessness

Nursing diagnoses
• Fluid volume, deficient (adverse reactions)
• Fluid volume, excess (uses)
• Knowledge, deficient (teaching)
• Urinary elimination, impaired (side effect)

Patient/family education
• Teach patient to take the medication early in the day to prevent nocturia
• Instruct patient to take with food or milk if GI symptoms of nausea and anorexia occur
• Teach patient to maintain weekly record of weight and notify prescriber of weight loss >5 lb
• Caution patient that this product causes a loss of potassium, so foods rich in potassium should be added to the diet; refer to a dietitian for assistance in planning
• Caution the patient not to exercise in hot weather or stand for prolonged periods, since orthostatic hypotension will be enhanced; to use sunscreen to prevent burns
• Teach patient not to use alcohol, or any OTC medications without prescriber's approval; serious product reactions may occur
• Emphasize the need to contact prescriber immediately if muscle cramps, weakness, nausea, dizziness, or numbness occur
• Teach patient to take own B/P and pulse and record
• Caution patient that orthostatic hypotension may occur; patient should rise slowly from sitting or reclining positions and lie down if dizziness occurs
• Teach patient to continue taking medication even if feeling better; this product controls symptoms but does not cure the condition
• Advise patient with hypertension to continue other medical treatment (exercise, weight loss, relaxation techniques, cessation of smoking)

Evaluation
Positive therapeutic outcome
• Decreased edema
• Decreased B/P
• Increased diuresis

TREATMENT OF OVERDOSE:
Lavage if taken orally, monitor electrolytes; administer dextrose in saline; monitor hydration, CV, renal status

cholecalciferol
See vitamin D

cholestyramine (Rx)
(koe-less-tear'a-meen)
PMS-Cholestyramine, Prevalite, Questran, Questran Light
Func. class.: Antilipemic
Chem. class.: Bile acid sequestrant
Pregnancy category C

Do not confuse:
Questran/Quarzan

ACTION: Absorbs, combines with bile acids to form an insoluble complex that is excreted through feces; loss of bile acids lowers LDL, cholesterol levels

Therapeutic outcome: Decreasing cholesterol levels and low-density lipoproteins, decreased pruritus

USES: Primary hypercholesterolemia (especially type IIa/IIb hyperlipoproteinemia), pruritus associated with biliary obstruction

Unlabeled uses: Diarrhea caused by excess bile acid

CONTRAINDICATIONS:
Hypersensitivity; biliary obstruction; hyperlipidemia III, IV, V

Precautions: Pregnancy **C**, breastfeeding, children

DOSAGE AND ROUTES
Adult: PO 4 g daily-bid, max 24 g/day
Child: PO 240 mg/kg/day in 3 divided doses; administer with food or drink, max 8 g/day, titrated up over several weeks to decrease GI effects

Available forms: Powder for susp 4 g/ cholestyramine/packet or scoop; tab 1 g

Implementation
• Give product daily-bid, at bedtime; give all other medications 1 hr before cholestyramine or 4-6 hr after cholestyramine to avoid poor absorption; do not take dry; mix product with applesauce or stir into beverage (2-6 oz); let stand for 2 min; do not mix with carbonated beverages; avoid inhaling powder, avoid GI tube administration
• Provide supplemental doses of vit A, D, E, K if levels are low

ADVERSE EFFECTS

CNS: Headache, dizziness, drowsiness, vertigo, tinnitus, anxiety

GI: *Constipation, abdominal pain, nausea,* fecal impaction, hemorrhoids, flatulence, vomiting, steatorrhea, peptic ulcer

HEMA: Bleeding, increased pro-time

INTEG: Rash, irritation of perianal area, tongue, skin

META: Decreased vit A, D, K, red cell folate content, **hyperchloremic acidosis**

MS: Muscle, joint pain

Pharmacokinetics

Absorption	Not absorbed
Distribution	Not distributed
Metabolism	Not metabolized; LDL lowered in 4-7 days, serum cholesterol lowered in 1 mo
Excretion	Binds with bile acids, feces
Half-life	Unknown

Pharmacodynamics

Onset	24-48 hr
Peak	1-3 wk
Duration	2-4 wk

INTERACTIONS

Individual drugs

Acetaminophen, amiodarone, clofibrate, gemfibrozil, glipizide, iron, penicillin G, propranolol, thyroid hormones, warfarin: decreased absorption of each specific product

Drug classifications

Cardiac glycosides, corticosteroids, tetracyclines, thiazides, vit A, D, E, K: decreased absorption

Drug/lab test

Increased: AST, ALT, alkaline phosphatase
Decreased: Na, K

NURSING CONSIDERATIONS

Assessment

• Assess nutrition: fat, protein, carbohydrates, nutritional analysis should be completed by dietitian

• Assess skin integrity after patient has been receiving product; itching, pruritus often occur from bile deposits on skin

• Monitor cardiac glycoside level if both products are being administered; cardiac glycoside levels will be decreased

• **Hypercholesterolemia:** Monitor for signs of vit A, D, E, K deficiency; fasting LDL, HDL, total cholesterol, triglyceride levels, electrolytes if on extended therapy, diet history

• Monitor bowel pattern daily; increase bulk, water in diet if constipation develops

• **Pruritus:** Assess for itching

Nursing diagnoses

• Constipation (adverse reactions)
• Knowledge, deficient (teaching)
• Noncompliance (teaching)

Patient/family education

⚠ Teach patient symptoms of hypoprothrombinemia: bleeding mucous membranes, dark tarry stools, hematuria, petechiae; report immediately

• Teach patient importance of compliance

• Teach patient that risk factors should be decreased: high-fat diet, smoking, alcohol consumption, absence of exercise

• Have patient mix product with 6 oz of milk, water, fruit juice; do not mix with carbonated beverages; rinse glass to make sure all medication is taken or may mix product in applesauce; allow to stand for 2 min before mixing

Evaluation

Positive therapeutic outcome

• Decreased cholesterol level (hyperlipidemia)
• Decreased diarrhea, pruritus (excess bile acids)

choline/magnesium salicylates (Rx)

Func. class.: Nonopioid analgesic
Chem. class.: Salicylate
Pregnancy category C

ACTION: Blocks pain impulses in CNS that occur in response to inhibition of prostaglandin synthesis; antipyretic action results from inhibition of hypothalamic heat-regulating center to produce vasodilatation to allow heat dissipation

Therapeutic outcome: Decreased pain, inflammation, fever

USES: Mild to moderate pain or fever including arthritis, juvenile rheumatoid arthritis

CONTRAINDICATIONS:

Hypersensitivity to salicylates, GI bleeding, bleeding disorders, children <3 yr, vit K deficiency, children with flulike symptoms, Reye's syndrome

Precautions: Pregnancy **C,** breastfeeding, anemia, renal/hepatic disease, Hodgkin's disease

DOSAGE AND ROUTES
Adult: PO 1500 mg bid
Child >37 kg: PO 2.2 g of salicylate/day divided bid
Child <37 kg: PO 50 mg of salicylate/kg/day divided bid

Available forms: Tabs 500, 750, 1000 mg; liquid 500 mg/5 ml

Implementation
• Administer to patient crushed or whole
• Give with food or milk to decrease gastric symptoms; give 30 min before or 2 hr after meals; absorption may be slowed; sit upright for 30 min after dose
• Give antacids 1-2 hr after enteric products

ADVERSE EFFECTS
CNS: Stimulation, drowsiness, dizziness, confusion, **seizure**, headache, flushing, hallucinations, **coma**
CV: Rapid pulse, pulmonary edema
EENT: Tinnitus, hearing loss
ENDO: Hypoglycemia, hyponatremia, hypokalemia
GI: *Nausea, vomiting, GI bleeding, diarrhea, heartburn,* anorexia, **hepatitis, hepatotoxicity**
HEMA: **Thrombocytopenia, agranulocytosis, leukopenia, neutropenia, hemolytic anemia,** increased pro-time
INTEG: *Rash,* urticaria, bruising, sweating
RESP: Wheezing, hyperpnea, hyperventilation

Pharmacokinetics

Absorption	Well absorbed
Distribution	Widely distributed; crosses placenta
Metabolism	Liver, extensively
Excretion	Kidney, active metabolites; breast milk
Half-life	2-3 hr (low doses); 9-17 hr (high doses)

Pharmacodynamics

Onset	15-30 min
Peak	1-3 hr
Duration	3-6 hr

INTERACTIONS
Individual drugs
Alcohol, aspirin, heparin, plicamycin: increased bleeding
Ammonium chloride, nizatidine: increased salicylate levels

Insulin, methotrexate, penicillins, phenytoin, valproic acid: increased effects
Probenecid, spironolactone, sulfinpyrazone: decreased effects

Drug classifications
Antacids (high doses), corticosteroids, steroids, urinary alkalizers: decreased effects of choline salicylate
Anticoagulants, hypoglycemics (oral), sulfonamides, thrombolytics: increased effects
Antiinflammatories, NSAIDs, steroids: increased gastric ulcers
β-Blockers, NSAIDs, sulfonamides: decreased effects
Urinary acidifiers: increased salicylate levels

Drug/lab test
Increased: coagulation studies, liver function studies, serum uric acid, amylase, CO_2, urinary protein
Decreased: serum potassium, cholesterol
Interference: VMA, TSH, 5-HIAA

NURSING CONSIDERATIONS
Assessment
• Monitor **pain:** location, duration, type, intensity, before dose and 1-2 hr after
• Monitor musculoskeletal status: ROM before dose
• Identify fever, length of time and related symptoms
• Monitor liver function studies: AST, ALT, bilirubin, creatinine if patient is on long-term therapy
• Monitor renal function studies: BUN, urine creatinine if patient is on long-term therapy; check I&O ratio; decreasing output may indicate renal failure
• Monitor blood studies: CBC, Hct, Hgb, pro-time if patient is on long-term therapy
⚠ Assess hepatotoxicity: dark urine, clay-colored stools, yellowing of the skin and sclera, itching, abdominal pain, fever, diarrhea if patient is on long-term therapy
• Assess for allergic reactions: rash, urticaria; if these occur, product may have to be discontinued
• Assess for ototoxicity: tinnitus, ringing, roaring in ears; audiometric testing needed before, after long-term therapy
• Check edema in feet, ankles, legs
• Identify prior product history; there are many product interactions

Nursing diagnoses
• Injury, risk for (side effects)
• Knowledge, deficient (teaching)

- Mobility, impaired physical (uses)
- Pain, acute (uses)
- Pain, chronic (uses)

Patient/family education
- Teach patient to report any symptoms of **hepatotoxicity, renal toxicity,** vision changes, **ototoxicity,** allergic reactions, bleeding (long-term therapy)
- Advise patient to take with 8 oz of water
- Caution patient not to exceed recommended dosage; acute poisoning may result
- Caution patient to read label on other OTC products; many contain aspirin products
- Inform patient that the therapeutic response takes 2 wk (arthritis)
- Teach patient to report tinnitus, confusion, diarrhea, sweating, hyperventilation
- Caution patient to avoid alcohol ingestion; GI bleeding may occur
- Teach patient that patients who have allergies may develop allergic reactions
- Caution patient to avoid buffered or effervescent products
- Teach patient not to give to children; Reye's syndrome may develop

Evaluation
Positive therapeutic outcome
- Decreased pain
- Decreased inflammation
- Decreased fever
- Increased mobility

TREATMENT OF OVERDOSE:
Lavage, activated charcoal, monitor electrolytes, VS

cidofovir (Rx)
(si-doh-foh'veer)
Vistide
Func. class.: Antiviral
Chem. class.: Nucleotide analog
Pregnancy category C

ACTION: Suppresses cytomegalovirus (CMV) replication by selective inhibition of viral DNA synthesis

Therapeutic outcome: Decreased symptoms of CMV

USES: CMV retinitis in patients with HIV, used with probenecid

CONTRAINDICATIONS:
Hypersensitivity to this product or probenecid; sulfa products, direct intraocular injection

> **BLACK BOX WARNING:** Proteinuria, renal disease/failure

Precautions: Pregnancy C, breastfeeding, children <6 mo, geriatric, preexisting cytopenias, renal function impairment, platelet count <25,000/mm^3

> **BLACK BOX WARNING:** Neutropenia, infertility, secondary malignancy

DOSAGE AND ROUTES
Adult: **IV** 5 mg/kg qwk × 2 wk; then 3 mg/kg q2wk, give with probenecid

Renal dose
Adult: **IV** CCr ≤55 ml/min, do not use; SCr increase of 0.3-0.4 mg/dl above baseline, decrease dose to 3 mg/kg; SCr increase of ≥0.5 mg/dl above baseline or ≥2+ proteinuria, discontinue

Available forms: Inj 75 mg/ml

Implementation
Intermittent IV infusion route
- **Dilute** in 100 ml 0.9% NaCl sol before administration; probenecid must be given PO 2 g 3 hr before the cidofovir INF and 1 g at 2 and 8 hr after ending the cidofovir INF; **give** 1 L of 0.9% NaCl sol **IV** with each INF of cidofovir, **give** saline INF over 1-2 hr period immediately before cidofovir; patient should be given a second L if the patient can tolerate the fluid load (second L given at time of cidofovir or immediately afterward and should be given over a 1-3 hr period)
- **Mix** under strict aseptic conditions using gloves, gown, and mask and using precautions for antineoplastics
- **Administer** after diluting in 100 ml of 0.9% NaCl
- **Give** slowly; do not give by BOL **IV, IV,** SUB-CUT inj
- **Use** diluted sol within 24 hr, do not refrigerate or freeze; do not use sol with particulate matter or discoloration, allow to warm to room temperature before using

ADVERSE EFFECTS
CNS: *Fever, chills,* **coma,** confusion, abnormal thought, *dizziness,* bizarre dreams, *headache,* psychosis, tremors, somnolence, paresthesia, *amnesia, anxiety, insomnia,* **seizures**

CV: **Dysrhythmias,** hypo/hypertension
EENT: Retinal detachment in CMV retinitis
GI: Abnormal liver function tests, *nausea, vomiting, anorexia, diarrhea,* abdominal pain, hemorrhage
GU: **Hematuria,** increased creatinine, BUN, **nephrotoxicity**
HEMA: **Granulocytopenia, thrombocytopenia, irreversible neutropenia, anemia,** eosinophilia
INTEG: *Rash, alopecia, pruritus, acne,* urticaria, pain at inj site, phlebitis
RESP: Dyspnea

Pharmacokinetics

Absorption	Unknown
Distribution	Unknown
Metabolism	Unknown
Excretion	Unknown
Half-life	Terminal 2.6 hr

Pharmacodynamics

Unknown

INTERACTIONS
Individual drugs
Amphotericin B, foscarnet, pentamidine **IV:** increased nephrotoxicity; wait 7 days after use to begin cidofovir

Drug classifications
Aminoglycosides, NSAIDs, salicylates: increased nephrotoxicity; wait 7 days after use to begin cidofovir

NURSING CONSIDERATIONS
Assessment
• Obtain culture before treatment is initiated; cultures of blood, urine, and throat may all be taken; CMV is not confirmed by this method; the diagnosis is made by an ophthalmic exam

BLACK BOX WARNING: Monitor renal, liver function, increased hematopoietic studies and BUN; serum creatinine, AST, ALT, creatinine, CCr, A-G ratio, baseline and drip treatment, blood counts should be done q2wk; watch for decreasing granulocytes, Hgb; if low, therapy may have to be discontinued and restarted after hematologic recovery; blood transfusions may be required

• Assess for GI symptoms: severe nausea, vomiting, diarrhea; severe symptoms may necessitate discontinuing product

• Assess electrolytes and minerals: calcium, phosphorous, magnesium, sodium, potassium; watch closely for tetany during first administration
• Assess for symptoms of **blood dyscrasias** (anemia, granulocytopenia); bruising, fatigue, bleeding, poor healing; assess for leukopenia, neutropenia, thrombocytopenia: WBCs, platelets q2day during 2 ×/day dosing and qwk thereafter; check for leukopenias, with daily WBC count in patients with prior leukopenia, with other nucleoside analogs, or for whom leukopenia counts are <1000 cells/mm^3 at start of treatment
• Assess allergic reactions: flushing, rash, urticaria, pruritus
• Monitor serum creatinine or CCr at least q2wk; give only to those with creatinine levels ≤1.5 mg/dl, CCr >55 ml/min, urine protein <100 mg/dl

Nursing diagnoses
• Infection, risk for (uses)

Patient/family education

BLACK BOX WARNING: Advise to notify prescriber if sore throat, swollen lymph nodes, malaise, fever occur; may indicate other infections

• Advise to report perioral tingling, numbness in extremities, and paresthesias; report rash immediately
• Teach that serious product interactions may occur if OTC products are ingested; check first with prescriber
• Teach that product is not a cure, but will control symptoms
• Advise that regular ophthalmic exams must be continued
• Advise that major toxicities may necessitate discontinuing product
• Advise to use contraception during treatment and that infertility may occur; men should use barrier contraception for 90 days after treatment

Evaluation
Positive therapeutic outcome
• Decreased symptoms of CMV

TREATMENT OF OVERDOSE:
Discontinue product; use hemodialysis, and increase hydration

cilastatin
See imipenem/cilastatin

cilostazol (Rx)

(sih-los′tah-zol)
Pletal
Func. class.: Platelet aggregation inhibitor
Chem. class.: Quinolinone derivative
Pregnancy category C

Do not confuse:
Pletal/Plendil

ACTION: Reversibly inhibits cellular phosphodiesterase; inhibits platelet aggregation induced by thrombin, ADP, collagen, arachidonic acid, epinephrine, stress

Therapeutic outcome: Increased walking distance

USES: Intermittent claudication

CONTRAINDICATIONS:

Hypersensitivity, acute MI, active bleeding conditions, hemostatic conditions

> **BLACK BOX WARNING:** CHF

Precautions: Pregnancy C, breastfeeding, children, geriatric, past liver disease, renal/cardiac disease, increased bleeding risk, low platelet count, platelet dysfunction

DOSAGE AND ROUTES

Adult: PO 100 mg bid taken ≥30 min before or 2 hr after breakfast and dinner or 50 mg bid, if using products that inhibit CYP3A4 and CYP2C19; 12 wk of treatment may be needed for beneficial effect

Available forms: Tabs 50, 100 mg

Implementation
• Give bid ≥1 hr before or 2 hr after meals; do not give with grapefruit juice

ADVERSE EFFECTS

CNS: *Dizziness,* headache
CV: *Palpitations, tachycardia,* **nodal dysrhythmia,** postural hypotension
EENT: Blindness, diplopia, ear pain, tinnitus, retinal hemorrhage
GI: *Nausea, vomiting, diarrhea, GI discomfort,* colitis, cholelithiasis, ulcer, esophagitis, gastritis, anorexia, *flatulence, dyspepsia*
GU: Cystitis, frequency, vaginitis, **vaginal hemorrhage,** hematuria
HEMA: **Bleeding (epistaxis, hematuria, retinal hemorrhage, GI bleeding),** thrombocytopenia, anemia, polycythemia; **aplastic anemia**
INTEG: *Rash,* urticaria, dry skin, **Stevens-Johnson syndrome**
MISC: *Back pain,* headache, *infection, myalgia, peripheral edema,* chills, fever, malaise, diabetes mellitus
RESP: *Cough, pharyngitis, rhinitis,* asthma, pneumonia

Pharmacokinetics

Absorption	Unknown
Distribution	95%-98% protein binding
Metabolism	Hepatic extensively by CYP450 enzymes
Excretion	Urine (74%), feces (20%)
Half-life	11-13 hr

Pharmacodynamics

Unknown

INTERACTIONS

Individual drugs
Abciximab, eptifibatide, ticlopidine, tirofiban: increased bleeding tendencies
Clarithromycin, diltiazem, erythromycin, omeprazole, verapamil: increased cilostazol levels
Fluconazole, fluoxetine, fluvoxamine, gemfibrozil, isoniazid, itraconazole, ketoconazole, omeprazole, voriconazole: may increase cilostazol levels; exercise caution when coadministering and reduce dose to 50 mg bid

Drug classifications
Anticoagulants, NSAIDs, thrombolytics: may increase bleeding tendencies
CYP3A4 inducers: decreased cilostazol
Protease inhibitors, CYP3A4 inhibitors, CYP2C19 inhibitors: increased cilostazol levels

Drug/food
Grapefruit juice: do not use; toxicity may occur

NURSING CONSIDERATIONS

Assessment
• Assess for underlying CV disease since CV risk is great; for severe headache, signs of toxicity
• Assess for CV lesions with repeated oral administration
• Assess for CHF
• Monitor blood studies: CBC, Hct, Hgb, pro-time if patient is on long-term therapy; thrombocytopenia, neutropenia may occur

Nursing diagnoses
- Injury, risk for (uses)
- Knowledge, deficient (teaching)

Patient/family education
- Advise patient to report any unusual bleeding to prescriber
- Caution patient to report side effects such as diarrhea, skin rashes, subcutaneous bleeding
- Teach patient that effects may take 2-4 wk, treatment of up to 12 wk may be required for necessary effect
- Teach patients with CHF about potential risks
- Advise patient to take ≥1 hr before or 2 hr after meals
- Advise patient that reading patient package insert is necessary
- Advise patient to discontinue tobacco use
- Advise that there are many drug and herb interactions; obtain approval by prescriber before use

Evaluation
Positive therapeutic outcome
- Increased walking distance and duration
- Decreased pain

---

cimetidine (OTC, Rx)
(sye-met′i-deen)
Acid Reducer, Apo-Cimetidine ✸, Equaline Acid Reducer, Gen-Cimetidine ✸, Good Sense Heartburn Relief, Leader Cimetidine, Nu-Cimet ✸, Select Brand Cimetidine, Tagamet, Tagamet HB, Top care Heartburn Relief, Walgreens Cimetidine
Func. class.: H$_2$-receptor antagonist
Chem. class.: Imidazole derivative
Pregnancy category B

ACTION: Inhibits histamine at H$_2$-receptor site in the gastric parietal cells, which inhibits gastric acid secretion

Therapeutic outcome: Healing of duodenal or gastric ulcers; prevention of duodenal ulcers; decreases symptoms of gastroesophageal reflux disease (GERD) and Zollinger-Ellison syndrome

USES: Short-term treatment of duodenal and gastric ulcers and maintenance; management of GERD, Zollinger-Ellison syndrome; prevention of upper GI bleeding; prevent, relieve heartburn, acid indigestion, upper GI bleeding

Unlabeled uses: Prevention of aspiration pneumonitis, stress ulcers

CONTRAINDICATIONS:
Hypersensitivity

Precautions: Pregnancy **B,** breastfeeding, child <16 yr, geriatric, organic brain syndrome, renal/hepatic disease

DOSAGE AND ROUTES
Treatment of active ulcers
Adult: PO 300 mg qid with meals, at bedtime × 8 wk or 400 mg bid, 800 mg at bedtime; after 8 wk give at bedtime dose only; **IV BOL** 300 mg/20 ml 0.9% NaCl over 1-2 min q6hr; **IV INF** 300 mg/50 ml D$_5$W over 15-20 min; **IM** 300 mg q6hr, max 2400 mg
Child: PO 20-40 mg/kg/day; IM/IV 5-10 mg/kg q6-8hr

Prophylaxis of duodenal ulcer
Adult and child >16 yr: 400 mg at bedtime or 300 mg bid

GERD
Adult: PO 800-1600 mg/day in divided doses

Hypersecretory conditions (Zollinger-Ellison syndrome)
Adult: PO/IM/IV 300-600 mg q6hr; may increase to 12 g/day if needed; OTC use up to 200 mg daily or bid, max 2 ×/wk

Upper GI bleeding prophylaxis
Adult: IV 50 mg/hr; lowered in renal disease

Aspiration pneumonitis prophylaxis (unlabeled)
Adult: IM/IV 300 mg IM 1 hr before anesthesia, then 300 mg IV q4hr until patient is alert, max 2400 mg/day

Renal dose
Adult: PO/IV CCr <30 ml/min 300 mg q12hr

Available forms: Tabs 100, 200, 300, 400, 800 mg; liquid 200, 300 mg/5 ml; inj 300 mg/2 ml, 300 mg/50 ml 0.9% NaCl

Implementation
PO route
- Give with meals for lengthened product effect; antacids 1 hr before or 1 hr after cimetidine

IV route
- Give by **direct IV** after diluting 300 mg/20 ml of 0.9% NaCl for inj; give over 5 min or more
- Give **intermittent IV** by diluting 300 mg/50 ml of D$_5$W; run over 15-20 min

---

• Give by **cont inf** after using total daily dose (900 mg) diluted in 100-1000 ml D₅W given over 24 hr
• Store diluted sol at room temperature up to 48 hr

Y-site incompatibilities: Amsacrine

Y-site compatibilities: Acyclovir, alfentanil, amifostine, amikacin, aminocaproic acid, aminophylline, amphotericin B lipid complex/liposome, anakinra, anidulafungin, ascorbic acid injection, atenolol, atracurium, atropine, aztreonam, benztropine, bivalirudin, bleomycin, bumetanide, buprenorphine, butorphanol, calcium chloride/gluconate, CARBOplatin, caspofungin, cefamandole, ceFAZolin, cefmetazole, cefonicid, cefotaxime, cefotetan, cefoxitin, ceftazidime, ceftizoxime, cefTRIAXone, cefuroxime, cephalothin, cephapirin, chlorproMAZINE, cisatracurium, CISplatin, cladribine, clarithromycin, clindamycin, codeine, cyanocobalamin, cyclophosphamide, cycloSPORINE, cytarabine, DACTINomycin, DAPTOmycin, dexamethasone, dexmedetomidine, digoxin, diltiazem, diphenhydrAMINE, DOBUTamine, docetaxel, DOPamine, doripenem, doxacurium, doxapram, DOXOrubicin, DOXOrubicin liposome, enalaprilat, ePHEDrine, EPINEPHrine, epirubicin, epoetin alfa, eptifibatide, ertapenem, erythromycin, esmolol, etoposide, famotidine, fenoldopam, fentaNYL, filgrastim, fluconazole, fludarabine, fluorouracil, folic acid, foscarnet, gallium, gatifloxacin, gemcitabine, gentamicin, glycopyrrolate, granisetron, heparin, hydrocortisone, HYDROmorphone, hydrOXYzine, IDArubicin, ifosfamide, imipenem-cilastatin, irinotecan, isoproterenol, ketorolac, labetalol, levofloxacin, lidocaine, linezolid, LORazepam, LR, magnesium sulfate, mannitol, mechlorethamine, melphalan, meperidine, metaraminol, meropenem, methicillin, methotrexate, methoxamine, methyldopate, methylPREDNISolone, metoclopramide, metoprolol, metroNIDAZOLE, mezlocillin, miconazole, midazolam, milrinone, minocycline, mitoxantrone, morphine, moxalactam, multiple vitamins injection, mycophenolate, nafcillin, nalbuphine, naloxone, nesiritide, netilmicin, niCARdipine, nitroglycerin, nitroprusside, norepinephrine, octreotide, ondansetron, oxacillin, oxaliplatin, oxytocin, paclitaxel, palonosetron, pamidronate, pancuronium, pantoprazole, papaverine, pemetrexed, penicillin G sodium/potassium, pentamidine, pentazocine, phenylephrine, phytonadione, piperacillin, piperacillin/tazobactam, polymyxin B, potassium chloride, procainamide, prochlorperazine, promethazine, propofol, propranolol, protamine, pyridoxine, quiNIDine, quinupristin-dalfopristin, ranitidine, remifentanil, Ringer's ritodrine, riTUXimab, rocuronium, sargramostim, sodium acetate/bicarbonate, succinylcholine, SUFentanil, tacrolimus, teniposide, theophylline, thiamine, thiotepa, ticarcillin, ticarcillin-clavulanate, tigecycline, tirofiban, TNA, tobramycin, tolazoline, topotecan, TPN, trastuzumab, trimetaphan, urokinase, vancomycin, vasopressin, vecuronium, verapamil, vinCRIStine, vinorelbine, voriconazole, zidovudine, zoledronic acid

ADVERSE EFFECTS
CNS: *Confusion, headache,* depression, dizziness, anxiety, weakness, psychosis, tremors, **seizures**
CV: Bradycardia, tachycardia, **dysrhythmias**
GI: *Diarrhea,* abdominal cramps, **paralytic ileus,** *jaundice*
GU: Gynecomastia, galactorrhea, impotence, increase in BUN, creatinine
HEMA: Agranulocytosis, thrombocytopenia, neutropenia, aplastic anemia, increase in pro-time
INTEG: Urticaria, rash, alopecia, sweating, flushing, **exfoliative dermatitis**
RESP: Pneumonia

Pharmacokinetics

Absorption	Well absorbed (PO, IM); completely absorbed (**IV**)
Distribution	Widely distributed; crosses placenta
Metabolism	Liver (30%)
Excretion	Kidneys, unchanged (70%); breast milk
Half-life	1½-2 hr; increased in renal disease

Pharmacodynamics

	PO	IM/IV
Onset	½ hr	10 min
Peak	45-90 min	½ hr
Duration	4-5 hr	4-5 hr

INTERACTIONS
Individual drugs
CarBAMazepine, chloroquine, lidocaine, metronidazole, moricizine, phenytoin, quiNIDine, quinine, valproic acid, warfarin: increased toxicity (CYP450 pathway)
Itraconazole: decreased absorption of itraconazole

Ketoconazole: decreased absorption of ketoconazole

Sucralfate: decreased cimetidine absorption

Drug classifications
Antacids: decreased absorption of cimetidine

Antidepressants (tricyclic), benzodiazepines, β-
adrenergic blockers, calcium channel blockers, phenytoins, sulfonylureas, theophyllines:
increased toxicity (CYP450 pathway)

Drug/lab test
Increased: alkaline phosphatase, AST, creatinine, prolactin

False positive: Hemoccult, Gastroccult tests

False negative: TB skin tests

NURSING CONSIDERATIONS

Assessment
• Assess patient with ulcers or suspected ulcers:
epigastric or abdominal pain, hematemesis,
occult blood in stools, blood in gastric aspirate
before and/or throughout treatment; monitor
gastric pH (≥5 should be maintained)

• Monitor I&O ratio, BUN, creatinine, CBC with
differential periodically

Nursing diagnoses
• Knowledge, deficient (teaching)

• Pain, acute (uses)

Patient/family education
• Advise patient that any gynecomastia or impotence that develops is reversible after treatment
is discontinued

• Caution patient to avoid driving, other hazardous activities until stabilized on this medication;
drowsiness or dizziness may occur

• Advise patient to avoid black pepper, caffeine,
alcohol, harsh spices, extremes in temperature
of food; tell patient to avoid OTC preparations:
aspirin, cough, cold preparations; condition
may worsen

• Advise patient that smoking decreases the
effectiveness of the product; smoking cessation
should be considered

• Teach patient that product must be continued
for prescribed time to be effective and taken exactly as prescribed; doses are not to be doubled;
to take missed dose when remembered up to 1
hr before next dose

• Instruct patient to report bruising, fatigue,
malaise; blood dyscrasias may occur

• Have patient report to prescriber immediately
any diarrhea, black tarry stools, sore throat,
dizziness, confusion, or delirium

Evaluation
Positive therapeutic outcome
• Decreased pain in abdomen
• Healing of ulcers
• Absence of gastroesophageal reflux
• Gastric pH of ≥5

cinacalcet (Rx)
(sin-a-kal′set)

Sensipar

Func. class.: Calcium receptor agonist

Chem. class.: Polypeptide hormone

Pregnancy category C

ACTION: Directly lowers PTH levels by increasing sensitivity of calcium sensing receptors
to extracellular calcium

Therapeutic outcome: Decreased
symptoms of hypercalcemia

USES: Hypercalcemia in parathyroid
carcinoma, secondary hyperparathyroidism
in chronic kidney disease on dialysis, primary
hyperparathyroidism

CONTRAINDICATIONS:
Hypersensitivity, hypocalcemia

Precautions: Pregnancy C, breastfeeding,
children, seizure disorders, hepatic disease

DOSAGE AND ROUTES

Parathyroid carcinoma
Adult: PO 30 mg bid, titrate q2-4wk, with sequential doses of 30 mg bid, 60 mg bid, 90 mg
bid, 90 mg tid-qid to normalize calcium levels

Secondary hyperparathyroidism
Adult: PO 30 mg daily, titrate no more frequently than 2-4 wks with sequential doses of
30, 60, 90, 120, 180 mg daily

Available forms: Tabs 30, 60, 90 mg

Implementation
• Swallow tabs whole; do not break, crush,
chew, or divide tabs
• Can be used alone or in combination with vit
D sterols and/or phosphate binders
• Take with food or shortly after meal

ADVERSE EFFECTS
CNS: Dizziness, asthenia, **seizures,** tetany,
hallucinations, depression

CV: Hypertension, dysrhythmia exacerbation

GI: Nausea, diarrhea, vomiting, anorexia

MISC: Access infection, noncardiac chest pain, hypocalcemia
MS: Myalgia

Pharmacokinetics

Absorption	93%-97% bound to plasma
Distribution	Unknown
Metabolism	Proteins metabolized by CYP3A4, 2D6, 1A2
Excretion	Renal (80% renal, 15% feces)
Half-life	30-40 hr

Pharmacodynamics

Unknown

INTERACTIONS

Individual drugs
Ketoconazole, erythromycin, itraconazole (products metabolized by CYP3A4); flecainide, vinBLAStine, thioridazine: adjustments may be necessary

Drug classifications
Tricyclics (metabolized by CYP2D6): adjustments may be necessary

Drug/food
High-fat meal: increased action

NURSING CONSIDERATIONS

Assessment
• Assess for **hypocalcemia:** cramping, seizures, tetany, myalgia, paresthesia
• Monitor calcium, phosphorous within 1 wk and iPTH 1-4 wk after initiation or dosage adjustment when maintenance is established; measure calcium, phosphorus monthly; iPTH q1-3mo, target range 150-300 pg/ml for iPTH level; biochemical markers of bone formation/resorption, radiologic evidence of fracture
• If calcium <8.4 mg/dl, do not start therapy

Nursing diagnoses
• Injury, risk for (uses)
• Knowledge, deficient (teaching)

Secondary hyperthyroidism
• Titrate q2-4wk to target iPTH consistent with National Kidney Foundation—Kidney Disease Outcomes Quality Initiative (NKF-K/DOQI) for chronic kidney disease patient on dialysis of 150-300 pg/ml; if iPTH drops below 150-300 pg/ml, reduce dose of cinacalcet and/or vit D sterols or discontinue treatment
• Store at <77° F (25° C)

Patient/family education
• Instruct patient to take with food or shortly after a meal
• Instruct patient to immediately report cramping, seizures, muscle pain, tingling, tetany

Evaluation
Positive therapeutic outcome
• Calcium levels 9-10 mg/dl, decreasing symptoms of hypercalcemia

ciprofloxacin (Rx)
(sip-ro-floks'a-sin)
**Cipro, Cipro XR, CO Ciprofloxacin ✦,
PMS-Ciprofloxacin✦, ProQuin
XR, RAN Ciprofloxacin ✦,
ratio-Ciprofloxacin ✦,
Sandoz Ciprofloxacin ✦, Taro
Ciprofloxacin ✦**
Func. class.: Antiinfectives, broad-spectrum
Chem. class.: Fluoroquinolone
Pregnancy category C

Do not confuse:
ciprofloxacin/cephalexin

ACTION: Interferes with conversion of intermediate DNA fragments into high-molecular-weight DNA in bacteria; DNA gyrase inhibitor

Therapeutic outcome: Bactericidal action against the following: gram-positive organisms *Staphylococcus epidermidis,* methicillin-resistant strains of *Staphylococcus aureus;* gram-negative organisms *Escherichia coli, Klebsiella* species, *Enterobacter, Salmonella, Proteus vulgaris, Pseudomonas aeruginosa, Serratia, Campylobacter jejuni*

USES: Adult urinary tract infections (including complicated); chronic bacterial prostatitis; acute sinusitis; infectious diarrhea; typhoid fever; complicated intraabdominal infections; nosocomial pneumonia; exposure to inhalation anthrax

CONTRAINDICATIONS:
Hypersensitivity to quinolones

Precautions: Pregnancy **C**, breastfeeding, children, geriatric, renal disease, epilepsy, QT prolongation, hypokalemia

> **BLACK BOX WARNING:** Tendon pain/rupture, tendonitis

DOSAGE AND ROUTES

Uncomplicated urinary tract infections
Adult: PO 250 mg q12hr × 3 days or 500 mg q24hr × 3 days

Complicated/severe urinary tract infections
Adult: PO 500 mg q12hr or 1000 mg q24hr × 7-14 days; **IV** 400 mg q12hr

Respiratory, bone, skin, joint infections
Adult: PO 500-750 mg q12hr × 7-14 days; **IV** 400 mg q12hr

Nosocomial pneumonia
Adult: **IV** 400 mg q8hr × 10-14 days

Intraabdominal infections, complicated
Adult: PO 500 mg q12hr × 7-14 days, **IV** 400 mg q12hr × 7-14 days, usually given with metroNIDAZOLE

Acute sinusitis, mild/moderate
Adult: PO 500 mg q12hr × 10 days; **IV** 400 mg q12hr × 10 days

Inhalational anthrax (postexposure)
Adult: PO 500 mg q12hr × 60 days; **IV** 400 mg q12hr × 60 days
Child: PO 15 mg/kg/dose q12hr × 60 days, max 500 mg/dose; **IV**, 10 mg/kg q12hr, max 400 mg/dose

Infectious diarrhea
Adult: PO 500 mg q12hr × 5-7 days

Chronic bacterial prostatitis
Adult: PO 500 mg q12hr × 28 days; **IV** 400 mg q12hr × 28 days

Pyelonephritis, acute uncomplicated
Adult: PO 1000 mg q24hr × 7-14 days, q4-6wk

Renal dose
Adult: PO CCr 30-50 ml/min PO 250-500 mg q12hr; CCr 5-29 ml/min PO 250-500 mg q18hr; IV 200-400 mg q18-24hr

Available forms: Tabs 100, 250, 500, 750 mg; ext rel tabs (XR) 500, 1000 mg; inj 200 mg/20 ml, 400 mg/40 ml, 200 mg/100 ml D₅, 400 mg/200 ml D₅; oral susp 250, 500 mg/5 ml

Implementation
PO route
• Give around the clock to maintain proper blood levels

• Administer 2 hr before or 2 hr after antacids, zinc, iron, calcium
• Do not give oral sup by GI tube

IV route
• Check for irritation, extravasation, phlebitis daily
• For **intermittent inf**, dilute to 1-2 mg/ml of D₅W, 0.9% NaCl; give over 60 min; it will remain stable under refrigeration for 2 wk

Y-site incompatibilities: Heparin, mezlocillin
• Limit intake of alkaline soda, products with milk, dairy products, alkaline antacids, sodium bicarbonate

ADVERSE EFFECTS
CNS: *Headache,* dizziness, fatigue, insomnia, depression, *restlessness,* **seizures,** confusion
GI: *Nausea,* increased ALT, AST, flatulence, heartburn, *vomiting, diarrhea,* oral candidiasis, dysphagia, **pseudomembranous colitis,** dry mouth
HEMA: **Bone marrow depression**
INTEG: *Rash,* pruritus, urticaria, photosensitivity, flushing, fever, chills, **toxic epidermal necrolysis**
MISC: **Anaphylaxis, Stevens-Johnson syndrome,** visual impairment, QT prolongation
MS: Tremor, arthralgia, tendon rupture

Pharmacokinetics
Absorption	Well absorbed (75%) (PO)
Distribution	Widely distributed
Metabolism	Liver (15%)
Excretion	Kidneys (40%-50%)
Half-life	3-4 hr; increased in renal disease

Pharmacodynamics
	PO	IV
Onset	Rapid	Immediate
Peak	1 hr	Infusion's end

INTERACTIONS
Individual drugs
Alfuzosin, arsenic trioxide, astemizole, chloroquine, clopazine, cyclobenzapine, dasatinib, dolasetron, droperidol, flecainide, haloperidol, lapatinib, levomethadyl, methadone, octreotide, ondansetron, paliperidone, palonosetron, pentamidine, probucol, propafenone, ranolazine, risperidone, sertindole, sunitinib, tacrolimus, terfenadine, vardenafil, vorinostat, ziprasidone: increased QT prolongation

Adverse effects: *italics* = common; **bold** = life-threatening

Calcium, enteral feeding, iron, sucralfate, zinc sulfate: decreased ciprofloxacin absorption
CycloSPORINE: increased nephrotoxicity
Probenecid: increased blood levels of cipro-floxacin, increased toxicity
Theophylline: increased theophylline levels, monitor blood levels
Warfarin: increased warfarin effect, monitor blood levels

Drug classifications
Antacids (containing magnesium, aluminum), iron salts: decreased absorption of cipro-floxacin
β-agonists, class IA/III antidysrhythmics, halogenated anesthetics, local anesthetics, macrolides, phenothiazines, tetracyclines, tricyclics: increased QT prolongation

Drug/food
Dairy products, food: decreased absorption

Drug/lab test
Increased: AST, ALT, bilirubin, BUN, creatinine, alkaline phosphatase, LDH, glucose, protein-uria, albuminuria
Decreased: WBC, glucose

NURSING CONSIDERATIONS
Assessment
• Assess patient for previous sensitivity reaction
• Assess patient for signs and symptoms of **infection** including characteristics of wounds, sputum, urine, stool, WBC >10,000/mm³, fever; obtain baseline information before, during treatment
• Obtain C&S before beginning product therapy to identify if correct treatment has been initiated
• Assess for **anaphylaxis:** rash, urticaria, dyspnea, pruritus, chills, fever, joint pain; may occur a few days after therapy begins; epinephrine and resuscitation equipment should be available for anaphylactic reaction
• Identify urine output; if decreasing, notify prescriber (may indicate nephrotoxicity); also check for increased BUN, creatinine
• Monitor blood studies: AST, ALT, CBC, Hct, bilirubin, LDH, alkaline phosphatase, Coombs' test monthly if patient is on long-term therapy
• Monitor electrolytes: potassium, sodium, chloride monthly if patient is on long-term therapy
• Assess for **CNS symptoms:** headache, dizziness, fatigue, insomnia, depression
• Monitor for bleeding: ecchymosis, bleeding gums, hematuria, stool guaiac daily if on long-term therapy

• Assess for **overgrowth of infection:** perineal itching, fever, malaise, redness, pain, swelling, drainage, rash, diarrhea, change in cough, sputum

> **BLACK BOX WARNING:** Assess for tendon pain, especially in children

Nursing diagnoses
• Diarrhea (side effects)
• Infection, risk for (uses)
• Injury, risk for (side effects)
• Knowledge, deficient (teaching)
• Noncompliance (teaching)

Patient/family education
• Teach patient to report sore throat, bruising, bleeding, joint pain; may indicate blood dyscrasias (rare)
• Teach patient to contact prescriber if adverse reaction occurs or if inflammation or pain in tendon occurs
• Instruct patient to take all medication prescribed for the length of time ordered; product must be taken around the clock to maintain blood levels; do not give medication to others
• Teach patient to report tendon pain, chest pain, palpitations
• Advise patient to rinse mouth frequently, use sugarless candy or gum for dry mouth

Evaluation
Positive therapeutic outcome
• Absence of signs/symptoms of infection (WBC <10,000/mm³, temp WNL, absence of red draining wounds)
• Reported improvement in symptoms of infection

ciprofloxacin ophthalmic
See Appendix B

cisatracurium (Rx)
(sis-a-tra-cyoor'ee-um)
Nimbex
Func. class.: Neuromuscular blocker (nondepolarizing)
Pregnancy category B

ACTION: Inhibits transmission of nerve impulses by binding with cholinergic receptor sites, antagonizing action of acetylcholine

Therapeutic outcome: Paralysis of body for administration of anesthesia

USES: Facilitation of endotracheal intubation, skeletal muscle relaxation during mechanical ventilation surgery, or general anesthesia

CONTRAINDICATIONS:
Hypersensitivity

Precautions: Pregnancy **B**, breastfeeding, children <2 yr, electrolyte imbalances, dehydration, cardiac/neuromuscular/respiratory disease

DOSAGE AND ROUTES
Adult: **IV** 0.15 and 0.2 mg/kg depending on desired time to intubate and length of surgery: use peripheral nerve stimulation to evaluate dosage
Child 2-12 yr: **IV** 0.1 mg/kg over 5-10 sec with halothane or opioid anesthesia

Available forms: Inj 2, 10 mg/ml

Implementation
IV route
• Use nerve stimulator by anesthesiologist to determine neuromuscular blockade
• Give anticholinesterase to reverse neuromuscular blockade
• Give by slow **IV** only by qualified person; do not administer IM
• Store in light-resistant area
• Reassure if communication is difficult during recovery from neuromuscular blockage

ADVERSE EFFECTS
CV: Bradycardia, tachycardia; increased, decreased B/P
EENT: Increased secretions
INTEG: Rash, flushing, pruritus, urticaria
RESP: Prolonged apnea, bronchospasm, cyanosis, respiratory depression

Pharmacokinetics	
Unknown	

Pharmacodynamics	
Onset	1-3 min
Peak	2-5 min
Duration	30-40 min

INTERACTIONS
Individual drugs
CarBAMazepine, phenytoin: decreased duration of neuromuscular blockade
Isoflurane, lithium: increased neuromuscular blockade
Succinylcholine: decreased neuromuscular blockade

Drug classifications
Aminoglycosides, antibiotics (polymix), β-adrenergic blockers, opioids: increased neuromuscular blockade

NURSING CONSIDERATIONS
Assessment
• Assess for electrolyte imbalances (K, Mg), may lead to increased action of this product
• Assess vital signs (B/P, pulse, respirations, airway) until fully recovered; rate, depth, pattern of respirations; strength of handgrip
• Assess I&O ratio: check for urinary retention, frequency, hesitancy
• Assess recovery: decreased paralysis of face, diaphragm, legs, arms, rest of body
• Assess allergic reactions: rash, fever, respiratory distress, pruritus; product should be discontinued

Nursing diagnoses
• Breathing pattern, ineffective (uses)
• Communication, impaired verbal (adverse reactions)
• Knowledge, deficient (teaching)

Evaluation
Positive therapeutic outcome
• Paralysis of jaw, eyelid, head, neck, rest of body

TREATMENT OF OVERDOSE:
Edrophonium or neostigmine, atropine, monitor VS; mechanical ventilation

> ⚠ **HIGH ALERT**
>
> ## CISplatin (Rx)
> (sis′pla-tin)
> *Func. class.:* Antineoplastic alkylating agent
> *Chem. class.:* Inorganic heavy metal
> **Pregnancy category D**

Do not confuse:
CISplatin/carboplatin, **Platinol**/Paraplatin

ACTION: Alkylates DNA, RNA; inhibits enzymes that allow synthesis of amino acids in proteins; activity is not cell cycle phase specific

Therapeutic outcome: Prevention of rapidly growing malignant cells

USES: Advanced bladder cancer; adjunctive in metastatic testicular cancer and metastatic ovarian cancer; osteosarcoma; soft tissue sarcomas; head, neck, esophageal, prostatic, lung, and cervical cancer; lymphoma

CONTRAINDICATIONS:

Pregnancy **D**, breastfeeding, radiation therapy within 1 mo, chemotherapy within 1 mo, thrombocytopenia, recent smallpox vaccination, aluminum products used to prepare or administer cisplatin

> **BLACK BOX WARNING:** Bone marrow suppression, platinum compound hypersensitivity, renal disease/failure, preexisting hearing impairment

Precautions: Geriatric patients, pneumococcal vaccination

DOSAGE AND ROUTES
Dosage protocols may vary

Metastatic testicular cancer
Adult: **IV** 20 mg/m^2 daily $\times$ 5 days, repeat q3wk for 2 cycles or more, depending on response

Advanced bladder cancer
Adult: **IV** 50-70 mg/m^2 q3-4wk

Metastatic ovarian cancer
Adult: **IV** 100 mg/m^2 q4wk or 75-100 mg/m^2 q3wk with cyclophosphamide therapy; mix with 2 L of NaCl and 37.5 g mannitol over 6 hr

Available forms: Inj 0.5 mg/ml ✿, 1 mg/ml

Implementation
• Hydrate patient with 0.9% NaCl over 8-12 hr before treatment
• Give all medications PO, if possible; avoid IM inj when platelets <100,000/mm^3
• Give EPINEPHrine, antihistamines, corticosteroids for hypersensitivity reaction; antiemetic 30-60 min before giving product to prevent vomiting, and prn; allopurinol or sodium bicarbonate to maintain uric acid level, alkalinization of urine; antibiotics for prophylaxis of infection; diuretic (furosemide 40 mg **IV**) or mannitol after infusion
• Prepare in biological cabinet using gown, gloves, mask; do not allow product to come in contact with skin; use soap and water if contact occurs

Intermittent IV infusion route
• Give after **diluting** 10 mg/10 ml or 50 mg/50 ml sterile water for inj; **withdraw** prescribed dose, **dilute** $^1\!/_2$ dose with 1000 ml D$_5$ 0.2 NaCl or D$_5$ 0.45 NaCl with 37.5 g mannitol; **IV** inf is

given over 3-4 hr; use a 0.45 μm filter; total dose 2000 ml over 6-8 hr; check site for irritation, phlebitis; do not use equipment containing aluminum

Continuous IV infusion route
• Give over 24 hr $\times$ 5 days

Syringe compatibilities: Bleomycin, cyclophosphamide, doxapram, droperidol, fluorouracil, furosemide, heparin, leucovorin, methotrexate, metoclopramide, vinBLAStine, vinCRIStine

Y-site compatibilities: Acyclovir, alfentanil, allopurinol, amikacin, aminophylline, amiodarone, ampicillin, ampicillin-sulbactam, anidulafungin, atenolol, atracurium, azithromycin, aztreonam, bivalirudin, bleomycin, bumetanide, buprenorphine, butorphanol, calcium chloride/gluconate, caspofungin, ceFAZolin, cefoperazone, cefotaxime, cefotetan, cefoxitin, ceftazidime, ceftizoxime, cefTRIAXone, cefuroxime, chlorproMAZINE, cimetidine, ciprofloxacin, cisatracurium, cladribine, clindamycin, codeine, cyclophosphamide, cycloSPORINE, cytarabine, DACTINomycin, DAPTOmycin, DAUNOrubicin, dexamethasone, dexmedetomidine, dexrazoxane, digoxin, diltiazem, diphenhydrAMINE, DOBUTamine, docetaxel, DOPamine, doripenem, doxacurium, DOXOrubicin, DOXOrubicin liposomal, doxycycline, droperidol, enalaprilat, ePHEDrine, EPINEPHrine, epirubicin, ertapenem, erythromycin, esmolol, etoposide, famotidine, fenoldopam, fentaNYL, filgrastim, fluconazole, fludarabine, fluorouracil, foscarnet, fosphenytoin, furosemide, ganciclovir, gatifloxacin, gemcitabine, gentamicin, glycopyrrolate, granisetron, haloperidol, heparin, hydrocortisone, HYDROmorphone, IDArubicin, ifosfamide, imipenem-cilastatin, inamrinone, indomethacin, irinotecan, isoproterenol, ketorolac, labetalol, leucovorin, levofloxacin, levorphanol, lidocaine, linezolid, LORazepam, magnesium sulfate, mannitol, melphalan, meperidine, meropenem, methohexital, methotrexate, methylPREDNISolone, metoclopramide, metoprolol, metroNIDAZOLE, midazolam, milrinone, minocycline, mitomycin, mitoxantrone, mivacurium, nafcillin, naloxone, nesiritide, niCARdipine, nitroglycerin, nitroprusside, norepinephrine, octreotide, ofloxacin, ondansetron, oxaliplatin, paclitaxel, palonosetron, pamidronate, pancuronium, pemetrexed, pentamidine, pentazocine, PENTobarbital, PHENobarbital, phenylephrine, phenytoin, piperacillin, polymyxin B, potassium chloride/phosphates, procainamide, prochlorperazine, promethazine, propofol, propranolol, quiNIDine, quinupristin-dalfopristin, ranitidine, remifentanil, riTUXimab, sargramostim, sodium acetate/bicarbonate/phosphates, succinylcholine, SUFentanil, sulfamethoxazole-trimethoprim, tacrolimus, teniposide, theophylline, thiopental, ticarcillin, ticarcillin-clavulanate, tigecycline, tirofiban, TNA, tobramycin, topotecan, trastuzumab, vancomycin, vasopressin, vecuronium, verapamil, vinBLAStine, vinCRIStine, vinorelbine, voriconazole, zidovudine, zoledronic acid

Additive compatibilities: CARBOplatin, cyclophosphamide, floxuridine, hydrOXYzine, ifosfamide, leucovorin, magnesium sulfate, mannitol, ondansetron

Additive incompatibilities: Fluorouracil, mesna, thiotepa

Solution compatibilities: $D_5/0.225\%$ NaCl, $D_5/0.45\%$ NaCl, $D_5/0.9\%$ NaCl, $D_5/0.45\%$ NaCl with mannitol 1.875%, $D_5/0.33\%$ NaCl with mannitol 1.875%, $D_5/0.33\%$ NaCl with KCl 20 mEq and mannitol 1.875%, 0.9% NaCl, 0.45% NaCl, 0.3% NaCl, 0.225% NaCl, water

Solution incompatibilities: Sodium bicarbonate 5%, 0.1% NaCl, water

ADVERSE EFFECTS
CNS: **Seizures**, peripheral neuropathy
CV: Cardiac abnormalities
EENT: *Tinnitus, hearing loss, vestibular toxicity*, blurred vision, altered color perception
GI: *Severe nausea, vomiting, diarrhea, weight loss*
GU: **Renal tubular damage**, renal insufficiency, impotence, sterility, amenorrhea, gynecomastia, hyperuremia
HEMA: **Thrombocytopenia, leukopenia, pancytopenia**
INTEG: *Alopecia*, dermatitis
META: Hypomagnesemia, hypocalcemia, hypokalemia, hypophosphatemia
RESP: **Fibrosis**
SYST: **Anaphylaxis**

Pharmacokinetics

Absorption	Complete
Distribution	Widely distributed, accumulates in body tissues for several months
Metabolism	Liver
Excretion	Kidneys
Half-life	30-100 hr

Pharmacodynamics
Unknown

INTERACTIONS
Individual drugs
Alcohol, aspirin: increased risk of bleeding
Bumetanide, ethacrynic acid, furosemide: ototoxicity
Phenytoin: decreased phenytoin effect

Drug classifications
Aminoglycosides, diuretics (loop), salicylates: increased nephrotoxicity
Myelosuppressive agents, radiation: increased myelosuppression
NSAIDs: increased risk of bleeding
Vaccines, live virus: decreased antibody response

Drug/lab test
Increased: uric acid, BUN, creatinine
Decreased: CCr, calcium, phosphate, potassium, magnesium
Positive: Coombs' test

NURSING CONSIDERATIONS
Assessment

> **BLACK BOX WARNING:** Monitor for **bone marrow depression:** CBC, differential, platelet count weekly; withhold product if WBC count is $<4000/mm^3$ or platelet count is $<100,000/mm^3$; notify prescriber of results if WBC $<20,000/mm^3$, platelets $<150,000/mm^3$

> **BLACK BOX WARNING:** Monitor renal function studies: BUN, creatinine, serum uric acid, urine CCr before, during therapy; I&O ratio; report fall in urine output to <30 ml/hr; dose should not be given if BUN <25 mg/dl; creatinine <1.5 mg/dl

• Assess for **anaphylaxis:** wheezing, tachycardia, facial swelling, fainting; discontinue product and report to prescriber; resuscitation equipment should be nearby
• Monitor temp q4hr (may indicate beginning of infection)
• Monitor liver function tests before, during therapy (bilirubin, AST, ALT, LDH) as needed or monthly; note yellowing of skin or sclera, dark urine, clay-colored stools, itchy skin, abdominal pain, fever, diarrhea
• Assess for increased uric acid levels, swelling, joint pain primarily in extremities; patient should be well hydrated to prevent urate deposits
• Assess for **bleeding:** hematuria, stool guaiac, bruising or petechiae, mucosa or orifices q8hr; note inflammation of mucosa, breaks in skin

- Identify dyspnea, crackles, nonproductive cough, chest pain, tachypnea
- Identify effects of alopecia on body image; discuss feelings about body changes
- Identify edema in feet, joint pain, stomach pain, shaking; prescriber should be notified

Nursing diagnoses
- Body image, disturbed (adverse reactions)
- Infection, risk for (adverse reactions)
- Injury, risk for (adverse reactions)
- Knowledge, deficient (teaching)

Patient/family education
- Teach patient to avoid use of products containing aspirin or ibuprofen, NSAIDs, alcohol (may cause GI bleeding), razors, commercial mouthwash; to report symptoms of bleeding (hematuria, tarry stools, bruising, petechiae)
- Advise patient to report numbness, tingling in face or extremities, poor hearing or joint pain, swelling
- Instruct patient to report signs of anemia (fatigue, headache, irritability, faintness, shortness of breath)
- Instruct patient to report any changes in breathing or coughing even several months after treatment; to avoid crowds and persons with respiratory tract or other infections
- Advise patient that hair may be lost during treatment; a wig or hairpiece may make patient feel better; new hair may be different in color, texture
- Tell patient not to have any vaccinations without the advice of the prescriber; serious reactions can occur
- Caution patient contraception is needed during treatment and for 4 months after the completion of therapy, pregnancy **D**

Evaluation
Positive therapeutic outcome
- Prevention of rapid division of malignant cells

---

citalopram (Rx)
(sigh-tal′oh-pram)
Apo-Citalopram ✦, **Celexa, CO Citalopram** ✦, **Gen-Citalopram** ✦, **PMS-Citalopram** ✦, **RAN-Citalopram** ✦, **ratio-Citalopram** ✦, **Sandoz Citalopram** ✦
Func. class.: Antidepressant
Chem. class.: Selective serotonin reuptake inhibitor (SSRI)
Pregnancy category C

Do not confuse:
Celexa/Celebrex/Cerebyx/Cerebra

ACTION: Inhibits CNS neuron uptake of serotonin but not of norepinephrine; weak inhibitor of CYP450 enzyme system, making it more appealing than other products

Therapeutic outcome: Decreased symptoms of depression after 2-3 wk

USES: Major depressive disorder

Unlabeled uses: Premenstrual disorders, panic disorder, social phobia, impulsive aggression in children, obsessive-compulsive disorder in adolescents, treatment of psychotic symptoms in nondepressed demented patients, anxiety, hot flashes, menopause, adjunct in schizophrenia, PTSD

CONTRAINDICATIONS:
Hypersensitivity

Precautions: Pregnancy **C**, breastfeeding, geriatric, renal/hepatic disease, seizure disorder, hypersensitivity to escitalopram

> **BLACK BOX WARNING:** Children, suicidal ideation

DOSAGE AND ROUTES
Depression
Adult: PO 20 mg daily AM or PM, may increase if needed to 40 mg/day after 1 wk; maintenance: after 6-8 wk of initial treatment, continue for 24 wk (32 wk total), reevaluate long-term usefulness (max 60 mg/day)

Hepatic dose/geriatric
Adult: PO 20 mg/day, may increase to 40 mg/day if no response

Panic disorder (unlabeled)
Adult: PO 20-60 mg/day

Premenstrual dysphoria, social phobia

Adult: PO 10-30 mg/day used intermittently in premenstrual dysphoria

Available forms: Tabs 10, 20, 40 mg; oral SOL 10 mg/5 ml

Implementation

- Give with food or milk for GI symptoms
- Give dosage at bedtime if oversedation occurs during day
- Leave orally disintegrating tabs on tongue and allow to dissolve before swallowing
- Store at room temperature; do not freeze

ADVERSE EFFECTS

CNS: *Headache, nervousness, insomnia, drowsiness, anxiety, tremor, dizziness, fatigue, sedation, poor concentration, abnormal dreams, agitation,* **seizures,** apathy, euphoria, hallucinations, delusions, psychosis, **suicidal attempts, malignant neuroleptic-like syndrome reactions**

CV: *Hot flashes, palpitations,* angina pectoris, **hemorrhage,** hypertension, tachycardia, 1st-degree AV block, bradycardia, **MI,** thrombophlebitis

EENT: Vision changes, ear/eye pain, photophobia, tinnitus

GI: *Nausea, diarrhea, dry mouth, anorexia, dyspepsia, constipation, cramps, vomiting, taste changes, flatulence, decreased appetite*

GU: *Dysmenorrhea, decreased libido, urinary frequency, urinary tract infection,* amenorrhea, cystitis, impotence, urine retention

INTEG: *Sweating, rash, pruritus,* acne, alopecia, urticaria

MS: *Pain,* arthritis, twitching

RESP: *Infection, pharyngitis, nasal congestion, sinus headache, sinusitis, cough, dyspnea, bronchitis,* asthma, hyperventilation, pneumonia

SYST: *Asthenia, viral infection, fever, allergy, chills,* hyponatremia (geriatric patients), **serotonin syndrome**

Pharmacokinetics

Absorption	Well absorbed
Distribution	Unknown
Metabolism	Liver, by CYP1A2, CYP2D6
Excretion	Kidneys, steady state 28-35 days
Half-life	Unknown

Pharmacodynamics

Unknown

INTERACTIONS

Individual drugs

Alcohol: increased CNS depression

CarBAMazepine, clonidine: decreased citalopram levels

Lithium, tramadol, trazodone: increased serotonin syndrome

Pimoside, ziprasidone: increased QTc interval; do not use together

Drug classifications

Anticoagulants, antiplatelets, NSAIDs, salicylates, thrombolytics: increased risk of bleeding

Antidepressants (tricyclics): increased effect, use cautiously

Antifungals (azole), macrolides: increased citalopram levels

β-Adrenergic blockers: increased plasma levels of β-blockers

Barbiturates, benzodiazepines, CNS depressants, sedatives/hypnotics: increased CNS depression

MAOIs: hypertensive crisis, seizures, fatal reactions; do not use together

Quinolones: increased QTc interval; do not use together

Serotonin receptor agonists, SNRIs, SSRIs: increased serotonin syndrome

Drug/herb

SAM-e, St. John's wort: serotonin syndrome; do not use with citalopram; fatal reaction may occur

Yohimbe: increased CNS stimulation

Drug/lab test

Increased: serum bilirubin, blood glucose, alkaline phosphatase

Decreased: VMA, 5-HIAA

False increase: increased urinary catecholamines

NURSING CONSIDERATIONS

Assessment

- Monitor B/P (lying, standing), pulse q4hr; if systolic B/P drops 20 mm Hg, hold product and notify prescriber; take vital signs q4hr in patients with cardiovascular disease
- Monitor blood studies: CBC, leukocytes, differential, cardiac enzymes if patient is receiving long-term therapy; check platelets; bleeding can occur
- Monitor hepatic studies: AST, ALT, bilirubin
- Check weight qwk; appetite may increase with product
- Assess ECG for flattening of T wave, bundle branch block, AV block, dysrhythmias in cardiac patients

Adverse effects: *italics* = common; **bold** = life-threatening

- Assess EPS primarily in geriatric: rigidity, dystonia, akathisia
- Assess mental status: mood, sensorium, affect, suicidal tendencies; increase in psychiatric symptoms: depression, panic
- Monitor urinary retention, constipation; constipation is more likely to occur in children or geriatric
- Assess for **serotonin syndrome:** increased heart rate, sweating, dilated pupils, tremors, twitching, hyperthermia, agitation
- Identify patient's alcohol consumption; if alcohol is consumed, hold dose until AM

Nursing diagnoses
- Coping, ineffective (uses)
- Injury, risk for (side effects)
- Knowledge, deficient (teaching)
- Noncompliance (teaching)

Patient/family education
- Teach patient that therapeutic effects may take 4-6 wk
- Instruct patient to use caution in driving or other activities requiring alertness because of drowsiness, dizziness, blurred vision; to avoid rising quickly from sitting to standing, especially geriatric patients
- Advise that suicidal ideas, behavior may occur in children or young adults
- Caution patient to avoid alcohol ingestion, other CNS depressants
- Instruct patient to increase fluids, bulk in diet if constipation, urinary retention occur, especially geriatric
- Advise patient to take gum, hard sugarless candy, or frequent sips of water for dry mouth
- Teach patient how to use orally disintegrating tabs
- Teach patient to report **serotonin syndrome:** sweating, dilated pupils, tremors, twitching, extreme heat, agitation

Evaluation
Positive therapeutic outcome
- Decrease in depression
- Absence of suicidal thoughts

clarithromycin (Rx)
(clare-i-thro-mye′sin)
Biaxin, Biaxin Filmtab, Biaxin XL
Func. class.: Antiinfective
Chem. class.: Macrolide
Pregnancy category C

ACTION: Binds to 50S ribosomal subunits of susceptible bacteria and suppresses protein synthesis

Therapeutic outcome: Bactericidal action against the following: *Streptococcus pneumoniae, Streptococcus pyogenes, Mycoplasma pneumoniae, Corynebacterium diphtheriae, Bordetella pertussis, Listeria monocytogenes, Haemophilus influenzae, Staphylococcus aureus, Mycobacterium avium (MAC), Legionella pneumophila, Moxarella catarrhalis, Neisseria gonorrhoeae,* complex infections in AIDS patients, *Helicobacter pylori* in combination with omeprazole, *Helicobacter parainfluenzae*

USES: Mild to moderate infections of the upper respiratory tract, lower respiratory tract; uncomplicated skin and skin structure infections

CONTRAINDICATIONS:
Hypersensitivity to this product or other macrolides

Precautions: Pregnancy **C**, breastfeeding, geriatric, renal/hepatic disease, QT prolongation

DOSAGE AND ROUTES
Acute exacerbation of chronic bronchitis
Adult: PO 250-500 mg q12hr × 7-14 days or 1000 mg/day × 7 days (XL)

Pharyngitis/tonsillitis
Adult: PO 250 mg q12hr × 10 days

Community-acquired pneumonia
Adult: PO 250 mg q12hr × 7-14 days or 1000 mg/day × 7 days (XL)

Endocarditis prophylaxis
Adult: PO 500 mg 1 hr before procedure

MAC prophylaxis/treatment
Adult: PO 500 mg bid, will require an additional antiinfective for active infection

H. pylori infection
Adult: PO 500 mg/bid plus omeprazole 2 × 20 mg qAM (days 1-14), then omeprazole 20 mg qAM (days 15-28)

⚠ Nurse Alert

Acute maxillary sinusitis
Adult: PO 500 mg q12hr × 14 days

Most infections
Child: PO 7.5 mg/kg q12hr × 10 days, max 500 mg/dose for MAC

Renal dose
Adult: PO CCr <30 ml/min reduce dose by 50%

Available forms: Tabs 250, 500 mg; oral susp 125, 250 mg/5 ml; ext rel tab (XL) 500 mg

Implementation
- Do not break, crush, or chew ext rel tab
- Ensure adequate fluid intake (2 L) during diarrhea episodes
- Give q12hr to maintain serum level

ADVERSE EFFECTS
CV: Ventricular dysrhythmias, QT prolongation
GI: Nausea, vomiting, diarrhea, **hepatotoxicity**, abdominal pain, stomatitis, heartburn, anorexia, abnormal taste, **pseudomembranous colitis**
GU: Vaginitis, moniliasis
HEMA: Leukopenia, thrombocytopenia, increased INR
INTEG: Rash, urticaria, pruritus, **Stevens-Johnson syndrome, toxic epidermal necrolysis**
MISC: Headache, hearing loss

Pharmacokinetics

Absorption	50%
Distribution	Widely distributed
Metabolism	Liver
Excretion	Kidneys, unchanged (20%-30%)
Half-life	4-6 hr

Pharmacodynamics

Onset	Unknown
Peak	2 hr
Duration	Unknown

INTERACTIONS

Individual drugs
Alprazolam, busPIRone, carBAMazepine, cycloSPORINE, digoxin, disopyramide, felodipine, fluconazole, omeprazole, tacrolimus, theophylline: increased levels, increased toxicity
CarBAMazepine: increased toxicity, from increased levels of carBAMazepine, increased oral anticoagulants effect

Cisapride, pimozide: increased effect, increased dysrhythmias
Digoxin: increased blood levels of digoxin, increased digoxin effects, increased oral anticoagulants effect
Midazolam, tacrolimus: increased effects
Rifabutin, rifampin: decreased levels
Theophylline: increased toxicity from increased levels of theophylline, increased oral anticoagulants effect
Zidovudine: increased or decreased action

Drug classifications
All products metabolized by CYP3A enzyme system: increased action, risk of toxicity
Calcium channel blockers, benzodiazepines: increased effects
Class IA, III antidysrhythmics: increased QT prolongation
Ergots: increased levels, increased toxicity
HMG-CoA reductase inhibitors: increased levels
Oral anticoagulants: increased effects of oral anticoagulants

Drug/lab test
Increased: 17-OHCS/17-KS, AST, ALT, BUN, creatinine, LDH, total bilirubin
Decreased: folate assay, WBC

NURSING CONSIDERATIONS

Assessment
- Assess patient for signs and symptoms of **infection** including characteristics of wounds, sputum, urine, stool, WBC >10,000/mm^3, earache, fever; obtain baseline information before, during treatment; obtain C&S before beginning product therapy to identify if correct treatment has been initiated, product may be given as soon as culture is taken, repeat after treatment
- Monitor blood studies: AST, ALT, CBC, Hct, bilirubin, LDH, alkaline phosphatase, Coombs' test monthly if patient is on long-term therapy
- Assess bowel pattern daily; if severe diarrhea occurs, product should be discontinued
- Assess for overgrowth of infection: perineal itching, fever, malaise, redness, pain, swelling, drainage, rash, diarrhea, change in cough, sputum
- Assess for **QT prolongation, ventricular dysrhythmias:** monitor ECG, cardiac status in those with cardiac abnormalities
- Assess for **serious skin reaction:** Stevens-Johnson syndrome, toxic epidermal necrolysis, product should be discontinued immediately

Nursing diagnoses
- Diarrhea (side effects)
- Infection, risk for (uses)

- Knowledge, deficient (teaching)
- Noncompliance (teaching)

Patient/family education
- Advise patient to contact physician if vaginal itching, loose foul-smelling stools, furry tongue occur; may indicate superinfection
- Instruct patient to take all medication prescribed for the length of time ordered
- Advise prescriber if pregnancy is planned or suspected
- Teach patient to notify prescriber of diarrhea, dark urine, pale stools, yellowing of eyes/skin, severe abdominal pain

Evaluation
Positive therapeutic outcome
- Absence of signs/symptoms of infection: WBC <10,000/mm^3, temp WNL, absence of red draining wounds
- Reported improvement in symptoms of infection

clavulanate
See amoxicillin/clavulanate, ticarcillin/clavulanate

clevidipine (Rx)
(klev-id'i-peen)
Cleviprex
Func. class.: Calcium channel blocker (L-type)
Chem. class.: Dihydropyridine
Pregnancy category C

ACTION: L-type calcium channels mediate the influx of calcium during depolarization in arterial smooth muscle; reduces mean arterial B/P by decreasing systemic vascular resistance

Therapeutic outcome: Decreased B/P

USES: Treatment of hypertension when oral therapy is not feasible

CONTRAINDICATIONS:
Hypersensitivity to this product, eggs, or soya lecithin; defective lipid metabolism; severe aortic stenosis; pancreatitis

Precautions: Pregnancy **C**, breastfeeding, children <18 yr, heart failure, hyperlipidemia, hypertension, labor, phenochromocytoma

DOSAGE AND ROUTES
Adult: CONT **IV** 1-2 mg/hr; dose may be doubled q90sec initially; as B/P reaches goal, adjust dose less frequently (5-10 min) with

smaller increases in dose; most patients require 4-6 mg/hr, max 32 mg/hr; no more than 1000 ml should be infused per 24 hr period due to lipid load restrictions

Available forms: Single dose vial 50, 100 ml (0.5 mg/ml), intravenous emulsion

Implementation
Intermittent IV infusion route
- Do not give through same line as other medications, do not dilute
- Gently invert several times before use; do not use if discolored or if particulate matter is present
- Give through central or peripheral line at 1-2 mg/hr, use infusion device
- Store vials in refrigerator, do not freeze; leave vials in carton until use; product is photosensitive, however protection from light during administration is not required

ADVERSE EFFECTS
CNS: Headache
CV: Hypotension, **MI, sinus tachycardia,** syncope, **reflex tachycardia, atrial fibrillation**
GI: Nausea, vomiting
GU: Renal failure

Pharmacokinetics

Absorption	Unknown
Distribution	Protein binding >99%
Metabolism	By esterases in blood, extravascular tissues
Excretion	Urine 63%-74%, feces 7%-22%
Half-life	Initially 1 min; terminal 15 min; increased in hepatic disease

Pharmacodynamics

Onset	2-4 min
Peak	6-12 hr
Duration	Unknown

NURSING CONSIDERATIONS
Assessment
- Assess cardiac status: B/P, pulse, respiration, ECG; some patients have developed severe angina, acute MI after calcium channel blockers if obstructive CAD is severe; if not transitioned to other antihypertensive therapies following clevidipine infusion, patients should be monitored ≥8 hr for rebound hypertension; monitor for rebound hypertension following drug stoppage
- **Renal failure:** Monitor I&O ratio, weight daily; peripheral edema, dyspnea, jugular vein

distention, crackles (perioperative hypertensive patients)

Nursing diagnoses
- Knowledge, deficient (teaching)
- Noncompliance (teaching)

Patient/family education
- Instruct patient to notify prescriber immediately if neurological symptoms, visual changes, or symptoms of CHF occur
- Instruct patient to continue follow up for hypertension
- Teach patient to notify prescriber if pregnancy is planned or suspected or if breastfeeding

Evaluation
Positive therapeutic outcome
- Decreased B/P

---

clindamycin HCl (Rx)
(klin-dah-my′sin)
Cleocin HCl
clindamycin palmitate (Rx)
Cleocin Pediatric
clindamycin phosphate (Rx)
Cleocin Phosphate
Func. class.: Antiinfective—miscellaneous
Chem. class.: Lincomycin derivative
Pregnancy category B

ACTION: Binds to 50S subunit of bacterial ribosomes; suppresses protein synthesis

Therapeutic outcome: Absence of infection

USES: Infections caused by staphylococci, streptococci, *Rickettsia, Fusobacterium, Actinomyces, Peptococcus, Bacteroides, Pneumocystis jiroveci*

CONTRAINDICATIONS:
Hypersensitivity to this product or lincomycin, tartrazine dye, ulcerative colitis/enteritis

> **BLACK BOX WARNING:** Pseudomembranous colitis

Precautions: Pregnancy **B**, breastfeeding, geriatric, renal/liver/GI disease, asthma, allergy

> **BLACK BOX WARNING:** Diarrhea

DOSAGE AND ROUTES
Adults: PO 150-450 mg q6hr, max 1.8 g/day; IM/IV 1.2-2.7 g/day in 2-4 divided doses q6-12hr, max 4800 mg/day
Child >1 mo: PO 8-25 mg/kg/day in divided doses q6-8hr; IM/IV 20-40 mg/kg/day in divided doses q6-8hr in 3-4 equal doses
Neonates: 15-20 mg/kg/day divided q6-8hr

PID
Adult: IV 900 mg q8hr plus gentamicin

Bacterial endocarditis prophylaxis
Adult: 600 mg 1 hr before procedure

P. jiroveci pneumonia (unlabeled)
Adult: PO 1200-1800 mg/day in divided doses with 15-30 mg primaquine/day × 21 days

Available forms: Phosphate: inj 150, 300, 600 mg base/4 ml; 900 mg base/ml; inj inf in D$_5$ 300, 600, 900 mg; HCl: caps 75, 150, 300 mg; palmitate: oral sol 75 mg/5 ml

Implementation
PO route
- Do not break, crush, or chew caps
- Give with 8 oz of water; give with meals for GI symptoms
- Shake liquids well
- Do not refrigerate oral preparations; stable at room temperature for 2 wk

IM route
- If more than 600 mg must be given, divide into 2 inj
- Give deeply in large muscle mass; rotate sites

Intermittent IV infusion route
- Give by inf only; do not administer BOL dose; dilute 300 mg or 600 mg dose/50 ml or more of D$_5$W, 0.9% NaCl, give over 10 or 20 min, respectively

Rapid IV injection route
- Dilute as above, administer as a rapid first dose only, then give as **continuous IV infusion** rate based on clindamycin levels; 900 and 1200 mg doses/100 ml of compatible diluent and give over 30 or 40 min, respectively, final conc ≤12 mg/ml; if using ADD-Vantage vials dilute container with NS, D$_5$W and give over 10-60 min at max 30 mg/min or 1.2 g/hr

Syringe compatibilities: Amikacin, aztreonam, gentamicin, heparin

Syringe incompatibilities: Tobramycin

Y-site compatibilities: Acyclovir, alfentanil, amifostine, amikacin, aminocaproic acid, aminophylline, amiodarone, amphotericin B cholesteryl, amphotericin B lipid complex,

---

amsacrine, anakinra, anidulafungin, ascorbic acid injection, atenolol, atracurium, atropine, aztreonam, benztropine, bivalirudin, bleomycin, bumetanide, buprenorphine, butorphanol, calcium chloride/gluconate, CARBOplatin, cefamandole, ceFAZolin, cefmetazole, cefonicid, cefoperazone, cefotaxime, cefotetan, cefoxitin, cefpirome, ceftazidime, ceftizoxime, ceftobiprole, cefuroxime, cephalothin, cephapirin, chloramphenicol, cimetidine, cisatracurium, CISplatin, codeine, cyanocobalamin, cyclophosphamide, cycloSPORINE, cytarabine, DACTINomycin, DAPTOmycin, dexamethasone, dexmedetomidine, digoxin, diltiazem, diphenhydrAMINE, docetaxel, DOPamine, doxacurium, DOXOrubicin, DOXOrubicin liposomal, doxycycline, enalaprilat, ePHEDrine, EPINEPHrine, epirubicin, epoetin alfa, eptifibatide, esmolol, etoposide, famotidine, fenoldopam, fentaNYL, fludarabine, fluorouracil, folic acid, foscarnet, furosemide, gatifloxacin, gemcitabine, gemtuzumab, gentamicin, glycopyrrolate, granisetron, heparin, hydrocortisone, HYDROmorphone, ifosfamide, imipenem-cilastatin, indomethacin, insulin (regular), irinotecan, isoproterenol, ketorolac, levofloxacin, lidocaine, linezolid, LORazepam, LR, magnesium sulfate, mannitol, mechlorethamine, melphalan, meperidine, metaraminol, methicillin, methotrexate, methoxamine, methyldopate, methylPREDNISolone, metoclopramide, metoprolol, metroNIDAZOLE, mezlocillin, miconazole, milrinone, morphine, moxalactam, multiple vitamins injection, nafcillin, nalbuphine, naloxone, nesiritide, netilmicin, niCARdipine, nitroglycerin, nitroprusside, norepinephrine, octreotide, ondansetron, oxacillin, oxaliplatin, oxytocin, paclitaxel, palonosetron, pamidronate, pancuronium, pantoprazole, pemetrexed, penicillin G potassium/sodium, pentazocine, perphenazine, PHENobarbital, phenylephrine, phytonadione, piperacillin, piperacillin-tazobactam, potassium chloride, procainamide, propofol, propranolol, protamine, pyridoxine, ranitidine, remifentanil, Ringer's, ritodrine, riTUXimab, rocuronium, sargramostim, sodium acetate/bicarbonate, succinylcholine, SUFentanil, tacrolimus, teniposide, theophylline, thiamine, thiotepa, ticarcillin, ticarcillin-clavulanate, tigecycline, tirofiban, TNA, tobramycin, tolazoline, TPN, trimetaphan, urokinase, vancomycin, vasopressin, vecuronium, verapamil, vinCRIStine, vinorelbine, vitamin B complex/C, voriconazole, zidovudine, zoledronic acid

Y-site incompatibilities: IDArubicin

ADVERSE EFFECTS

GI: *Nausea, vomiting, abdominal pain, diarrhea,* **pseudomembranous colitis,** *anorexia, weight loss,* increased AST, ALT, bilirubin, alkaline phosphatase, jaundice
GU: *Vaginitis,* urinary frequency
INTEG: Rash, urticaria, pruritus, erythema, pain, abscess at inj site
SYST: Stevens-Johnson syndrome, exfoliative dermatitis

Pharmacokinetics

Absorption	Well absorbed (PO, IM), minimal (TOP)
Distribution	Widely distributed; crosses placenta
Metabolism	Liver, extensively
Excretion	Kidneys, breast milk
Half-life	$2^{1}/_{2}$ hr

Pharmacodynamics

	PO	IM	IV
Onset	Rapid	Rapid	Rapid
Peak	$^{1}/_{2}$-1 hr	$1^{1}/_{2}$ hr	Infusion's end

INTERACTIONS

Individual drugs
Erythromycin, chloramphenicol: decreased action of clindamycin
Kaolin: decreased absorption

Drug classifications
Neuromuscular blockers: increased neuromuscular blockade

Drug/lab test
Increased: alkaline phosphatase, bilirubin, CPK, AST, ALT

NURSING CONSIDERATIONS

Assessment
• Assess any patient with compromised renal system; product is excreted slowly in poor renal system function; toxicity may occur rapidly
• Assess patient for signs and symptoms of infection including characteristics of wounds, sputum, urine, stool, WBC >10,000/mm³, fever; obtain baseline information before, during treatment; complete C&S testing before beginning product therapy; this will identify if correct treatment has been initiated, give product as soon as culture is taken
• Assess for allergic reactions: rash, urticaria, pruritus, chills, fever, joint pain; may occur a few days after therapy begins; epinephrine and

resuscitation equipment should be available in case of an anaphylactic reaction
• Identify urine output; if decreasing, notify prescriber (may indicate nephrotoxicity); also look for increased BUN and creatinine levels
• Monitor blood studies: AST, ALT, CBC, Hct, bilirubin, LDH, alkaline phosphatase, Coombs' test monthly if patient is on long-term therapy
• Monitor electrolytes: potassium, sodium, chloride monthly if patient is on long-term therapy

> **BLACK BOX WARNING:** Assess bowel pattern daily; if severe diarrhea occurs, product should be discontinued; may indicate **pseudomembranous colitis**

• Monitor for bleeding: ecchymosis, bleeding gums, hematuria, stool guaiac daily if on long-term therapy
• Assess for overgrowth of infection: perineal itching, fever, malaise, redness, pain, swelling, drainage, rash, diarrhea, change in cough, sputum
• Assess for **serious skin infections:** Stevens-Johnson syndrome, exfoliative dermatitis

Nursing diagnoses
• Diarrhea (adverse reactions)
• Infection, risk for (uses)
• Injury, risk for (adverse reaction)
• Knowledge, deficient (teaching)
• Noncompliance (teaching)

Patient/family education
• Tell patient to take oral product with full glass of water; may take with food if GI symptoms occur; antiperistaltic products may worsen diarrhea
• Teach patient aspects of product therapy: need to complete entire course of medication to ensure organism death (10-14 days); culture may be taken after medication course has been completed
• Advise patient to report sore throat, fever, fatigue; may indicate **superinfection**
• Advise patient that product must be taken at equal intervals around clock to maintain blood levels

> **BLACK BOX WARNING:** Teach patient to report diarrhea with pus, mucus

Evaluation
Positive therapeutic outcome
• Decreased temp, negative C&S

TREATMENT OF HYPERSENSITIVITY: Withdraw product; maintain airway; administer epinephrine, aminophylline, O_2, **IV** corticosteroids

clindamycin topical
See Appendix B

clobetasol topical
See Appendix B

clomiPHENE (Rx)
(kloe′mi-feen)
Clomid, Scrophene
Func. class.: Ovulation stimulant
Chem. class.: Nonsteroidal antiestrogenic
Pregnancy category X

Do not confuse:
clomiPHENE/clomiPRAMINE

ACTION: Increases LH, FSH release from the pituitary, which increases maturation of ovarian follicle, ovulation, development of corpus luteum

Therapeutic outcome: Pregnancy

USES: Female infertility (ovulatory failure)

CONTRAINDICATIONS:
Pregnancy **X,** hypersensitivity, hepatic disease, undiagnosed uterine bleeding, uncontrolled thyroid or adrenal dysfunction, intracranial lesion, ovarian cysts, endometrial carcinoma

Precautions: Hypertension, depression, seizures, diabetes mellitus, abnormal ovarian enlargement, ovarian hyperstimulation

DOSAGE AND ROUTES
Adult: PO 50-100 mg daily × 5 days or 50-100 mg daily beginning on day 5 of the menstrual cycle; may be repeated until conception occurs or 3 cycles of therapy have been completed

Available forms: Tabs 50 mg

Implementation
• Give after discontinuing estrogen therapy
• Give at same time daily to maintain product level; begin on 5th day of menstrual cycle

ADVERSE EFFECTS
CNS: *Headache, depression,* restlessness, anxiety, nervousness, fatigue, insomnia, dizziness, flushing

---

CV: Vasomotor flushing, phlebitis, **deep vein thrombosis**
EENT: Blurred vision, diplopia, photophobia
GI: *Nausea, vomiting, constipation,* abdominal pain, bloating
GU: Polyuria, frequency of urination, **birth defects, spontaneous abortions,** multiple ovulation, breast pain, oliguria, abnormal uterine bleeding, ovarian cyst, hypertrophy of ovary
INTEG: *Rash, dermatitis,* urticaria, alopecia

Pharmacokinetics

Absorption	Well distributed
Distribution	Unknown
Metabolism	Liver, extensively
Excretion	Feces
Half-life	5 days

Pharmacodynamics
Unknown

INTERACTIONS
Drug/lab test
Increased: FSH/LH, BSP, thyroxine, TBG

NURSING CONSIDERATIONS
Assessment
• Determine liver function tests before therapy: AST, ALT, alkaline phosphatase
• Monitor serum progesterone, urinary excretion of pregnanediol to identify occurrence of ovulation
• Pelvic exam should be done to determine ovary size, condition of cervix
• Endometrial biopsy may be done in women over 35 to rule out endometrial carcinoma

Nursing diagnoses
• Knowledge, deficient (teaching)
• Sexual dysfunction (uses)

Patient/family education
• Advise patient that multiple births are common after product is taken
• Instruct patient to notify prescriber immediately if low abdominal pain occurs; may indicate ovarian cyst, cyst rupture
• Advise patient to notify prescriber of photophobia, blurred vision, diplopia, abnormal bleeding, hot flashes, nausea, vomiting, headache
• Teach patient if dose is missed, double at next time; if more than one dose is missed, call prescriber
• Instruct patient that response usually occurs 4-10 days after last day of treatment

• Teach patient method for taking, recording basal body temp to determine whether ovulation has occurred; if ovulation can be determined (there is a slight decrease in temp, then a sharp increase for ovulation), to attempt coitus 3 days before and every other day until after ovulation
• Teach patient if pregnancy is suspected, to notify prescriber immediately

Evaluation
Positive therapeutic outcome
• Fertility

clomiPRAMINE (Rx)
(klom-ip´ra-meen)
Anafranil
Func. class.: Tricyclic antidepressant
Chem. class.: Tertiary amine
Pregnancy category C

Do not confuse:
clomiPRAMINE/clomiPHENE/desipramine/Norpramin

ACTION: Potentiates serotonin and norepinephrine uptake; moderate anticholinergic effect

Therapeutic outcome: Decreased signs and symptoms of obsessive-compulsive disorder, decreased depression

USES: Obsessive-compulsive disorder

Unlabeled uses: Dysphoria, anxiety, agoraphobia and other phobias

CONTRAINDICATIONS:
Hypersensitivity, immediately after MI

Precautions: Pregnancy C, breastfeeding, geriatric, seizures, cardiac disease, glaucoma, prostatic hypertrophy, urinary retention

> **BLACK BOX WARNING:** Suicidal ideation, children

DOSAGE AND ROUTES
Obsessive-compulsive disorder
Adult: PO 25 mg at bedtime; increase gradually over 4 wk to a dosage of 75-250 mg/day in divided doses
Child 10-18 yr: PO 25 mg/day gradually increased max 3 mg/kg/day or 200 mg/day, whichever is smaller

Available forms: Caps 25, 50, 75 mg

Implementation
- Do not break, crush, or chew caps
- Give with food or milk for GI symptoms
- Store at room temperature; do not freeze

ADVERSE EFFECTS
CNS: *Dizziness, tremors, mania,* **seizures,** aggressiveness, drowsiness, headache, EPS, **neuroleptic malignant syndrome,** insomnia, agitation
CV: Hypotension, tachycardia, **cardiac arrest**
EENT: Blurred vision
ENDO: Galactorrhea, hyperprolactinemia
GI: *Constipation, dry mouth, nausea, dyspepsia,* weight gain, **hepatic toxicity**
GU: *Delayed ejaculation, anorgasmia,* retention, decreased libido
HEMA: **Agranulocytosis, neutropenia, pancytopenia**
INTEG: Diaphoresis, photosensitivity
META: Hyponatremia
SYST: **Suicide in children/adolescents**

Pharmacokinetics

Absorption	Well absorbed
Distribution	Widely distributed
Metabolism	Liver, extensively
Excretion	Kidneys, breast milk
Half-life	19-37 hr; steady state 1-2 wk

Pharmacodynamics

Onset	≥ 2 wk
Peak	2-6 hr
Duration	Unknown

INTERACTIONS
Individual drugs
Alcohol: increased CNS depression
CarBAMazepine: decreased clomiPRAMINE action
Cimetidine, fluoxetine, fluvoxamine, sertraline: increased clomiPRAMINE level; do not use together
Clonidine, EPINEPHrine, norepinephrine: severe hypertension; avoid use
Clonidine, haloperidol, levodopa: decreased effect of these products
Phenytoin: decreased clomiPRAMINE action

Drug classifications
Barbiturates: decreased clomiPRAMINE levels
CNS depressants, general anesthetics: increased effects; do not use together
CYP1A2, CYP2D6: increased clomiPRAMINE level

MAOIs: hypertensive crisis, seizures; do not use together
Other tricyclics, phenothiazines, quinolones: QT prolongation
Skeletal muscle relaxants, opiates: decreased action of these products

Drug/herb
SAM-e, St. John's wort: serotonin syndrome, do not use together

Drug/lab test
Increased: prolactin, TBG, AST, ALT, blood glucose
Decreased: serum thyroid hormone (T_3, T_4)

NURSING CONSIDERATIONS
Assessment
- Monitor B/P (with patient lying, standing), pulse q4hr; if systolic B/P drops 20 mm Hg hold product, notify prescriber; take VS q4hr in patients with cardiovascular disease
- Monitor blood studies: CBC, leukocytes, differential, cardiac enzymes if patient is receiving long-term therapy
- Assess for **neuroleptic malignant syndrome:** hyperpyrexia, rigidity, irregular pulse, diaphoresis
- Monitor hepatic studies: AST, ALT, bilirubin
- Check weight weekly; appetite may increase with product
- Assess **ECG** for flattening of T wave, QTc prolongation bundle branch block, AV block, dysrhythmias in cardiac patients
- Assess for EPS primarily in geriatric: rigidity, dystonia, akathisia
- Assess mental status: mood, sensorium, affect, suicidal tendencies; increase in psychiatric symptoms: depression, panic, frequency of obsessive-compulsive behaviors
- Monitor urinary retention, constipation; constipation is more likely to occur in children or geriatric
- Assess for **withdrawal symptoms:** headache, nausea, vomiting, muscle pain, weakness; do not usually occur unless product was discontinued abruptly
- Identify alcohol consumption; if alcohol is consumed, hold dose until morning

Nursing diagnoses
- Coping, ineffective (uses)
- Injury, risk for (side effects)
- Knowledge, deficient (teaching)
- Noncompliance (teaching)

Patient/family education
• Teach patient that therapeutic effects may take 4-6 wk
• Teach patient to use caution in driving or other activities requiring alertness because of drowsiness, dizziness, blurred vision; to avoid rising quickly from sitting to standing, especially geriatric
• Teach patient to avoid alcohol ingestion, other CNS depressants
• Teach patient not to discontinue medication quickly after long-term use: may cause nausea, headache, malaise
• Teach patient to wear sunscreen or large hat, since photosensitivity occurs
• Teach patient to increase fluids, bulk in diet if constipation, urinary retention occur, especially geriatric
• Teach patient to take gum, hard sugarless candy, or frequent sips of water for dry mouth
• Advise patient to notify prescriber if pregnancy is planned or suspected
• Teach patient that suicidal ideas, behavior may occur in children/young adults

Evaluation
Positive therapeutic outcome
• Decrease in depression
• Absence of suicidal thoughts

TREATMENT OF OVERDOSE:
ECG monitoring, induce emesis, lavage, activated charcoal, administer anticonvulsant

---

clonazePAM (Rx)
(kloe-na'zi-pam)
Apo-Clonazepam ✤, **CO Clonazepam** ✤, **Gen-Clonazepam** ✤, **Klonopin, PMS-Clonazepam, ratio-Clonazepam** ✤, **Sandoz Clonazepam** ✤
Func. class.: Anticonvulsant
Chem. class.: Benzodiazepine derivative
Pregnancy category D
Controlled substance schedule IV

Do not confuse:
clonazePAM/LORazepam/clorazepate, Klonopin/cloNIDine

ACTION: Inhibits spike, wave formation in absence seizures (petit mal), decreases amplitude, frequency, duration, spread of discharge in minor motor seizures

Therapeutic outcome: Decreased frequency, severity of seizures

USES: Absence, atypical absence, akinetic, myoclonic seizures, Lennox-Gastaut syndrome, panic disorder

CONTRAINDICATIONS:
Pregnancy **D**, hypersensitivity to benzodiazepines, acute closed-angle glaucoma, psychosis, severe liver disease

Precautions: Open-angle glaucoma, chronic respiratory disease, renal/hepatic disease, breastfeeding, geriatric

DOSAGE AND ROUTES
Adult: PO max 1.5 mg/day in 3 divided doses; may be increased 0.5-1 mg q3day until desired response; max 20 mg/day
Child <10 yr or <30 kg: PO 0.01-0.03 mg/kg/day in divided doses q8hr, max 0.05 mg/kg/day; may be increased 0.25-0.5 mg q3day until desired response; max 0.1-0.2 mg/kg/day
Geriatric: PO 0.25 daily-bid initially, increase by 0.25 daily q7-14day as needed

Available forms: Tabs 0.5, 1, 2 mg; orally disintegrating tabs 0.125, 0.25, 0.5, 1, 2 mg

Implementation
PO route
• Give on empty stomach for best absorption
Rectal route
• IV sol may be used rectally, 1 ml syringe inserted 3 cm into rectum
• Oral susp may be used rectally (1 mg/ml of product with 1 ml of water), use plastic tube (volume 2.2-3.3 ml)

ADVERSE EFFECTS
CNS: *Drowsiness,* dizziness, confusion, behavioral changes, tremors, insomnia, headache, **suicidal tendencies,** slurred speech, anterograde amnesia
CV: Palpitations, bradycardia, tachycardia
EENT: *Increased salivation, nystagmus, diplopia,* abnormal eye movements
GI: *Nausea, constipation,* polyphagia, anorexia, xerostomia, diarrhea, gastritis, sore gums
GU: Dysuria, enuresis, nocturia, retention, libido changes
HEMA: **Thrombocytopenia, leukocytosis, eosinophilia**
INTEG: Rash, alopecia, hirsutism
RESP: **Respiratory depression,** dyspnea, congestion

⚠ Nurse Alert

Pharmacokinetics

Absorption	Well absorbed
Distribution	Crosses blood-brain barrier, placenta
Metabolism	Liver, protein binding 85%
Excretion	Kidneys
Half-life	18-50 hr

Pharmacodynamics

Onset	$^1/_2$-1 hr
Peak	1-2 hr
Duration	6-12 hr

INTERACTIONS

Individual drugs
Alcohol: increased CNS depression
CarBAMazepine: decreased clonazePAM effect
Cimetidine, clarithromycin, diltiazem, erythromycin, fluoxetine: increased clonazePAM effect
PHENobarbitol: decreased clonazePAM effect
Phenytoin: decreased clonazePAM levels

Drug classifications
Anticonvulsants, antidepressants, barbiturates, general anesthetics, opiates, sedative/hypnotics: increased CNS depression
Azoles, oral contraceptives: increased clonazePAM effect
CYP3A4 inducers: decreased clonazePAM effect

Drug/herb
Ginkgo, melatonin: increased clonazePAM effect
Ginseng, St. John's wort: decreased clonazePAM effect
Kava, chamomile, valerian: increased sedative effect

Drug/lab test
Increased: AST, alkaline phosphatase

NURSING CONSIDERATIONS

Assessment
• Assess for **blood dyscrasias:** fever, sore throat, bruising, rash, jaundice, epistaxis (long-term treatment only)
• Assess **seizures:** duration, type, intensity, with or without aura
⚠ Assess mental status: mood, sensorium, affect, memory (long, short), especially geriatric; behavioral changes, suicidal thoughts/behaviors
• Assess seizure activity including type, location, duration, and character; provide seizure precaution

• Assess renal studies: urinalysis, BUN, urine creatinine
• Monitor blood studies: RBCs, Hct, Hgb, reticulocyte counts weekly for 4 wk, then monthly
• Monitor hepatic studies: ALT, AST, bilirubin, creatinine
• Assess for signs of physical withdrawal if medication suddenly discontinued
• Assess eye problems: need for ophthalmic examinations before, during, after treatment (slit lamp, fundoscopy, tonometry)
• Assess allergic reaction: red raised rash; if this occurs, product should be discontinued
• Monitor for **toxicity:** bone marrow depression, nausea, vomiting, ataxia, diplopia, cardiovascular collapse; monitor drug levels during initial treatment (therapeutic 20-80 ng/ml)

Nursing diagnoses
• Injury, risk for (side effects)
• Knowledge, deficient (teaching)

Patient/family education
• Teach patient to carry/wear emergency ID card stating patient's name, products taken, condition, physician's name, phone number
• Caution patient to avoid driving, other activities that require alertness
• Caution patient to avoid alcohol ingestion or CNS depressants; increased sedation may occur
• Teach patient not to discontinue medication quickly after long-term use; taper off over several weeks
• Teach patient to notify prescriber of yellowing skin/eyes, pale stools, bleeding, fever, extreme fatigue, sore throat, suicidal thoughts/behaviors

Evaluation
Positive therapeutic outcome
• Decreased seizure activity

TREATMENT OF OVERDOSE:
Lavage, activated charcoal, VS, flumazenil, monitor electrolytes

Adverse effects: *italics* = common; **bold** = life-threatening

cloNIDine (Rx)
(klon'i-deen)
Apo-Clonidine ❀**, Catapres, Catapres-TTS, Duraclon, Kapvay**
Func. class.: Antihypertensive, centrally acting analgesic
Chem. class.: Centrally acting α-adrenergic agonist
Pregnancy category C

Do not confuse:
cloNIDine/Klonopin/clonazePAM,
Catapres/Cataflam/catarase

ACTION: Inhibits sympathetic vasomotor center in CNS, which reduces impulses in sympathetic nervous system; B/P, pulse rate, cardiac output decreased; prevents pain signal transmission in CNS by α-adrenergic receptor stimulation of the spinal cord

Therapeutic outcome: Decreased B/P in hypertension

USES: Mild to moderate hypertension, used alone or in combination; severe pain in cancer patients (epidural)

Unlabeled uses: Opioid withdrawal, prevention of vascular headaches, treatment of menopausal symptoms, dysmenorrhea, attention-deficit/hyperactivity disorder (ADHD), autism, cycloSPORINE nephrotoxicity prophylaxis, diabetic neuropathy, ethanol withdrawal, Tourette's syndrome, hypertensive emergency

CONTRAINDICATIONS:
Hypersensitivity; (epidural) bleeding disorders, anticoagulants

Precautions: Pregnancy C, breastfeeding, child <12 yr (transdermal), geriatric, MI (recent), diabetes mellitus, chronic renal failure, Raynaud's disease, thyroid disease, depression, COPD, asthma, noncompliant patients

BLACK BOX WARNING: Labor

DOSAGE AND ROUTES
Hypertension
Adult: PO/TD 0.1 mg bid, then increase by 0.1-0.2 mg/day at weekly intervals, until desired response; range 0.2-0.6 mg/day in divided doses
Geriatric: PO 0.1 mg at bedtime, may increase gradually

Child: PO 5-10 mcg/kg/day in divided doses q8-12hr, max 0.9 mg/day

Opioid withdrawal (unlabeled)
Adult: PO 0.3-1.2 mg/day; may decrease by 50% × 3 days, then decrease by 0.1-0.2 mg/day or discontinue

Severe pain
Adult: CONT EPIDURAL INF 30 mcg/hr
Child: CONT EPIDURAL INF 0.5 mcg/kg/hr, then titrate to response

Menopausal symptoms (unlabeled)
Adult: TD 0.1 mg patch q1wk; PO 0.05-0.4 mg daily

ADHD/tic disorders in children/autism (unlabeled)
Child: PO 0.05 mg/kg/day in 3-4 divided doses × 8 wk, max 0.4 mg/day (unlabeled) Kapvay 0.1 mg at bedtime, increase dose by 0.1 mg/day up to 0.4 mg/day

Tourette's syndrome (unlabeled)
Adult: PO 0.15-0.2 mg/day

Available forms: Tabs 0.025 ❀, 0.1, 0.2, 0.3 mg; transdermal sys 2.5, 5, 7.5 mg delivering 0.1, 0.2, 0.3 mg/24 hr, respectively; inj 100, 500 mcg/ml, ext rel tab 0.1 mg (Kapvay)

Implementation
PO route
• Give last dose at bedtime
• Do not crush, cut, chew, or break ER tabs
Transdermal route
• Apply patch weekly; remove old patch and wash off residue; apply to site without hair; best absorption over chest or upper arm; rotate sites with each application; clean site before application; apply firmly, especially around edges
• Store patches in cool environment, tabs in tight container

ADVERSE EFFECTS
CNS: *Drowsiness, sedation, headache, fatigue,* nightmares, insomnia, mental changes, anxiety, depression, hallucinations, delirium
CV: *Orthostatic hypotension, palpitations,* CHF, ECG abnormalities, sinus tachycardia
EENT: Taste change, parotid pain
ENDO: Hyperglycemia
GI: *Nausea, vomiting, malaise,* constipation, *dry mouth*
GU: Impotence, dysuria, *nocturia,* gynecomastia
INTEG: *Rash,* alopecia, facial pallor, pruritus, hives, edema, burning papules, excoriation (TD patches)

MISC: *Withdrawal symptoms*
MS: Muscle, joint pain, leg cramps

Pharmacokinetics

Absorption	Well absorbed (PO, TD)
Distribution	Widely distributed; crosses blood-brain barrier
Metabolism	Liver, extensively
Excretion	Kidneys, unchanged (30%)
Half-life	12-21 hr

Pharmacodynamics

	PO	TD
Onset	$1/2$-1 hr	3 days
Peak	2-4 hr	Unknown
Duration	8-12 hr	8 hr (after removal)

INTERACTIONS

Individual drugs
Alcohol: increased CNS depression
Levodopa: decreased levodopa effect
Prazosin: decreased hypotensive effects
Verapamil: AV block

Drug classifications
Amphetamines, appetite suppressants, MAOIs, tricyclics: decreased hypotensive effects
Anesthetics, opiates, sedatives/hypnotics: increased CNS depression
Antidepressants (tricyclic), β-adrenergic blockers: life-threatening increase in B/P
Diuretics, nitrates: increased hypotensive effects

Drug/herb
Aconite: increased toxicity, death
Ephedra, ginseng: decreased antihypertensive effect
Hawthorn: increased antihypertensive effect

Drug/lab test
Increased: blood glucose
Decreased: VMA, urinary catecholamines, aldosterone

NURSING CONSIDERATIONS

Assessment
• Assess **cancer pain:** location, intensity, character, alleviating, aggravation factors, baseline and frequency
• Perform blood studies: neutrophils, decreased platelets
• Perform renal studies: protein, BUN, creatinine; watch for increased levels that may indicate nephrotic syndrome: polyuria, oliguria, frequency

• Monitor baselines for renal/liver function tests before therapy begins; check potassium levels, although hyperkalemia rarely occurs
• Monitor B/P, pulse if the product is being used for **hypertension;** notify prescriber of changes
• Assess for **opiate withdrawal** (unlabeled) in patients receiving the product for opioid withdrawal, including fever, diarrhea, nausea, vomiting, cramps, insomnia, shivering, dilated pupils, weakness
• Check for edema in feet, legs daily; monitor I&O; check for decreasing output
• Assess **allergic reaction:** rash, fever, pruritus, urticaria; product should be discontinued if antihistamines fail to help
• Assess for symptoms of **CHF:** edema; dyspnea, wet crackles, B/P, weight gain, report significant changes

Nursing diagnoses
• Injury, risk for (side effects)
• Knowledge, deficient (teaching)
• Noncompliance (teaching)

Patient/family education
• Instruct patient not to discontinue product abruptly, or **withdrawal symptoms** may occur: anxiety, increased B/P, headache, insomnia, increased pulse, tremors, nausea, sweating
• Caution patient not to use OTC (cough, cold, or allergy) products unless directed by prescriber
• Teach patient to comply with dosage schedule even if feeling better; product controls symptoms, does not cure
• Caution patient to change position slowly, to rise slowly to sitting or standing position to minimize orthostatic hypotension, especially geriatric
• Instruct patient to notify physician of mouth sores, sore throat, fever, swelling of hands or feet, irregular heartbeat, chest pain, signs of **angioedema,** increased weight
• Teach patient about excessive perspiration, dehydration, vomiting; diarrhea may lead to fall in B/P; consult prescriber if these occur
• Tell patient that product may cause dizziness, fainting; light-headedness may occur during first few days of therapy; use hard candy, saliva product, or frequent rinsing of mouth for dry mouth
• Advise patient that compliance is necessary; not to skip or stop product unless directed by prescriber
• Teach patient that product may cause skin rash or impaired perspiration

- Teach patient that response may take 2-3 days if product is given TD; instruct on administration of patch; return demonstration
- Teach patient to avoid hazardous activities, since product may cause drowsiness, dizziness
- Teach patient to administer 1 hr before meals

Evaluation
Positive therapeutic outcome
- Decrease in B/P in hypertension
- Decrease in withdrawal symptoms
- Decrease in pain
- Decrease in vascular headaches
- Decrease in dysmenorrhea
- Decrease in menopausal symptoms

TREATMENT OF OVERDOSE:
Supportive treatment; administer tolazoline, atropine, DOPamine prn

---

clopidogrel (Rx)
(klo-pid′oh-grel)
Plavix
Func. class.: Platelet aggregation inhibitor
Chem. class.: Thienopyridine derivative
Pregnancy category B

Do not confuse:
Plavix/Paxil/Elavil

ACTION: Inhibits first and second phases of ADP-induced effects in platelet aggregation

Therapeutic outcome: Decreased possibility of stroke, MI by decreasing platelet aggregation

USES: Reducing the risk of stroke, MI, vascular death, peripheral arterial disease in high-risk patients, acute coronary syndrome, transient ischemic attack (TIA), unstable angina

CONTRAINDICATIONS:
Hypersensitivity, active bleeding

Precautions: Pregnancy **B**, breastfeeding, children, past liver disease, increased bleeding risk, neutropenia, agranulocytosis, renal disease, Asian/Black/Caucasian patients

BLACK BOX WARNING: CYP2C19 allele (poor metabolizers)

DOSAGE AND ROUTES
Recent MI, stroke, peripheral arterial disease
Adult: PO 75 mg daily with or without aspirin

Acute coronary syndrome
Adult: PO loading dose 300 mg then 75 mg daily with aspirin

Available forms: Tabs 75, 300 mg

Implementation
- Give with food to decrease gastric symptoms

ADVERSE EFFECTS
CNS: Headache, dizziness, depression, syncope, hyperesthesia, neuralgia
CV: Edema, hypertension, chest pain
GI: Nausea, vomiting, diarrhea, GI discomfort, **GI bleeding, pancreatitis,** hepatic failure
GU: Glomerulonephritis
HEMA: *Epistaxis,* purpura, **bleeding, neutropenia, aplastic anemia, agranulocytosis, thrombotic thrombocytopenic purpura**
INTEG: Rash, pruritus
MISC: UTI, hypercholesterolemia, chest pain, fatigue, **intracranial hemorrhage, toxic epidermal necrolysis, Stevens-Johnson syndrome,** flu-like syndrome, **anaphylaxis**
MS: Arthralgia, back pain
RESP: Upper respiratory tract infection, dyspnea, rhinitis, bronchitis, cough, **bronchospasm**

Pharmacokinetics

Absorption	Rapidly absorbed
Distribution	Unknown
Metabolism	Liver, extensively, protein binding 95%
Excretion	Kidneys, unchanged product
Half-life	8 hr

Pharmacodynamics

Onset	Unknown
Peak	1-3 hr
Duration	Unknown

INTERACTIONS
Individual drugs
Abciximab, aspirin, eptifibatide, rifampin, ticlopidine, tirofiban, treprostinil: increased bleeding tendencies
Fluvastatin, phenytoin, tamoxifen, TOLBUTamide, torsemide, warfarin: increased action of each specific product

Drug classifications
Anticoagulants, NSAIDs, SSRIs, thrombolytics: increased bleeding tendencies

---

⚠ Nurse Alert

CYP3A4 inhibitors/substrates (atorvastatin, cerivistatin, esomeprazole, omeprazole, simvistatin): decreased effects
CYP2C19 inhibitors: avoid use
NSAIDs: increased action of some NSAIDs
Proton pump inhibitors (PPIs): decreased clopidogrel effect

Drug/herb
Bilberry, saw palmetto: decreased clopidogrel effect
Feverfew, fish oil, garlic, ginger, ginkgo biloba, green tea, horse chestnut, omega-3 fatty acids: increased clopidogrel effect

Drug/lab test
Increased: AST, ALT, bilirubin, uric acid, total cholesterol, nonprotein nitrogen (NPN)

NURSING CONSIDERATIONS
Assessment
• Assess for symptoms of stroke, MI during treatment
• Assess for thrombotic/thrombocytic purpura; fever, thrombocytopenia, neurolytic anemia
• Monitor liver function tests: AST, ALT, bilirubin, creatinine if patient is on long-term therapy (4 mo or more)
• Monitor blood studies: CBC, Hct, Hgb, protime, cholesterol if patient is on long-term therapy; thrombocytopenia, neutropenia may occur

Nursing diagnoses
• Injury, risk for (uses)
• Knowledge, deficient (teaching)

Patient/family education
• Advise patient that blood work will be necessary during treatment
• Advise patient to report any unusual bleeding to prescriber, that it may take longer to stop bleeding
• Instruct patient to take with food or just after eating to minimize GI discomfort
• Caution patient to report diarrhea, skin rashes, subcutaneous bleeding, chills, fever, sore throat
• Teach patient to tell all health care providers that clopidogrel is used

Evaluation
Positive therapeutic outcome
• Absence of stroke

clorazepate (Rx)
(klor-az'e-pate)
APO-Clorazepate ✦, Novo-Clopate ✦, Tranxene
Func. class.: Antianxiety, anticonvulsant, sedative/hypnotic
Chem. class.: Benzodiazepine, long-acting
Pregnancy category D
Controlled substance schedule IV

Do not confuse:
clorazepate/clonazePAM

ACTION: Potentiates the actions of GABA; especially in limbic system, reticular formation has anticonvulsant effects

Therapeutic outcome: Decreased anxiety, restlessness, insomnia

USES: Anxiety, acute alcohol withdrawal, adjunct in seizure disorders

Unlabeled uses: Insomnia

CONTRAINDICATIONS:
Pregnancy **D**, breastfeeding, children <9 yr, hypersensitivity to benzodiazepines, closed-angle glaucoma, psychosis

Precautions: Geriatric, debilitated, renal/hepatic disease, suicidal ideation, dependency problems

DOSAGE AND ROUTES
Anxiety
Adult: PO 15-60 mg/day in divided doses or 7.5 mg tid
Geriatric: PO 7.5 mg daily bid

Alcohol withdrawal
Adult: Day 1, PO 30 mg then 30-60 mg in divided doses; day 2, 45-90 mg in divided doses; day 3, 22.5-45 mg in divided doses; day 4, 15-30 mg in divided doses; then gradually reduce daily dose to 7.5-15 mg

Seizure disorders
Adult and child >12 yr: PO 7.5 mg tid; may increase by 7.5 mg/wk or less, max 90 mg/day
Child 9-12 yr: PO 3.75-7.5 mg bid; may increase by 3.75 mg/wk or less, max 60 mg/day

Insomnia (unlabeled)
Adult: PO 7.5-15 mg at bedtime
Geriatric: PO 3.75-7.5 mg at bedtime, max 15 mg at bedtime

Available forms: Tabs 3.75, 7.5, 15 mg

Implementation
- Give with food or milk for GI symptoms
- Give crushed if patient cannot swallow whole (tab only)
- Use sugarless gum, hard candy, frequent sips of water for dry mouth
- Check to see PO medication has been swallowed

ADVERSE EFFECTS
CNS: *Dizziness, drowsiness,* confusion, headache, anxiety, tremors, stimulation, fatigue, depression, insomnia, hallucinations, lethargy
CV: *Orthostatic hypotension,* **ECG changes, tachycardia,** hypotension, chest pain
EENT: *Blurred vision,* tinnitus, mydriasis
GI: Constipation, dry mouth, nausea, vomiting, anorexia, diarrhea
INTEG: Rash, dermatitis, itching

Pharmacokinetics
Absorption	Well absorbed
Distribution	Widely distributed, crosses placenta, 97% protein binding
Metabolism	Liver
Excretion	Kidneys, breast milk
Half-life	30-200 hr

Pharmacodynamics
Onset	1 hr
Peak	1-2 hr
Duration	Up to 24 hr

INTERACTIONS
Individual drugs
Alcohol: increased CNS depression
Cimetidine, disulfiram, fluoxetine, isoniazid, ketoconazole, propoxyphene, valproic acid: increased effects of clorazepate
Rifampin: decreased action of clorazepate

Drug classifications
Antidepressants, β-blockers (some), CYP3A4 inhibitors, MAOIs, oral contraceptives: increased clorazepate action
Barbiturates: decreased clorazepate effect
CNS depressants: increased CNS depression

Drug/lab test
Increased: AST/ALT
Decreased: Hct

NURSING CONSIDERATIONS
Assessment
- Assess **seizures:** duration, location, intensity, aura
- Monitor B/P (with patient lying, standing), pulse; if systolic B/P drops 20 mm Hg, hold product, notify prescriber
- Monitor blood studies: CBC during long-term therapy; blood dyscrasias have occurred rarely
- Monitor hepatic studies: AST, ALT, bilirubin, creatinine, LDH, alkaline phosphatase
- Monitor I&O; may indicate renal dysfunction
- Monitor **mental status:** mood, sensorium, affect, sleeping pattern, drowsiness, dizziness, **physical dependency; withdrawal symptoms:** headache, nausea, vomiting, muscle pain, weakness after long-term use; **suicidal tendencies**
- Assess for **physical dependency withdrawal symptoms:** headache, nausea, vomiting, muscle pain/weakness after long-term use

Nursing diagnoses
- Coping, ineffective (uses)
- Knowledge, deficient (teaching)
- Noncompliance (teaching)

Patient/family education
- Teach patient that product may be taken with food
- Teach patient not to use for everyday stress or longer than 4 mo, unless directed by a prescriber; not to take more than prescribed amount; may be habit forming
- Caution patient to avoid OTC preparations unless approved by a prescriber
- Caution patient to avoid driving, activities that require alertness; drowsiness may occur, especially in geriatric
- Advise patient to avoid alcohol ingestion or other psychotropic medications, unless prescribed
- Advise patient not to discontinue medication abruptly after long-term use; restlessness, insomnia, irritability may occur
- Advise patient to rise slowly; fainting may occur
- Teach patient that drowsiness may worsen at beginning of treatment
- Teach patient that those using for seizures should carry ID with condition, medications used
- Advise patient to notify prescriber if pregnancy is planned or suspected (pregnancy D)
- Advise patients to notify all providers of medication use

Evaluation
Positive therapeutic outcome
• Decreased anxiety, restlessness
• Decreased seizure activity

TREATMENT OF OVERDOSE:
Lavage, VS, supportive care, flumazenil

clotrimazole topical
See Appendix B

clotrimazole vaginal anti-fungal
See Appendix B

clozapine (Rx)
(kloz´a-peen)
clozapine, Clozaril, Fazaclo
Func. class.: Antipsychotic
Chem. class.: Tricyclic dibenzodiazepine derivative
Pregnancy category B

Do not confuse:
Clozaril/Clinoril/Colazal

ACTION: Interferes with dopamine receptor binding with lack of EPS and tardive dyskinesia; also acts as an adrenergic, cholinergic, histaminergic, serotoninergic antagonist

Therapeutic outcome: Decreased psychotic behavior

USES: Management of psychotic symptoms in schizophrenic patients for whom other antipsychotics have failed, recurrent suicidal behavior; orally disintegrating tabs are not used for recurrent suicidal behavior

Unlabeled uses: Agitation, bipolar disorder, dementia, tremor in Parkinson's disease

CONTRAINDICATIONS:
Hypersensitivity, severe granulocytopenia (WBC <3500/mm³ before therapy), coma

BLACK BOX WARNING: Myeloproliferative disorders, severe CNS depression, agranulocytosis, leukopenia, neutropenia, seizure disorders

Precautions: Pregnancy **B,** breastfeeding, children <16 yr, geriatric, renal/hepatic/cardiac/CV/pulmonary disease, seizures, prostatic enlargement, closed-angle glaucoma, stroke

BLACK BOX WARNING: Bone marrow suppression, dementia, hypotension, myocarditis, orthostatic hypotension, seizures

DOSAGE AND ROUTES
Adult: PO 12.5 mg daily or bid; may increase by 25-50 mg/day; normal range 300-450 mg/day after 2 wk; do not increase dosage more than 2 times/wk; max 900 mg/day; use lowest dosage to control symptoms

Tremor in Parkinson's disease (unlabeled)
Adult: PO 40 mg at bedtime

Dementia with multiple behavioral disturbances (unlabeled)
Geriatric: PO 12.5 mg qd at bedtime, may increase by 12.5 mg every other day; max 50 mg/day

Available forms: Tabs 25, 50, 100, 200 mg; orally disintegrating tabs 25, 100 mg; Fazaclo: 125, 150, 200 mg

Implementation
• Decrease dosage in geriatric since metabolism is slowed
• Give with full glass of water, milk; or give with food to decrease GI upset
• Store in tight, light-resistant container; oral sol in amber bottle
• Patient-specific registration is required before administration; if WBC <3500 cells/mm³ or ANC <2000 cells/mm², therapy should not be started
• **Orally disintegrating tab:** do not push through foil, leave in foil blister until ready to take, peel back foil, place tab in mouth, allow to dissolve, swallow, water is not needed

ADVERSE EFFECTS
CNS: *Sedation, salivation, dizziness, headache, tremors, sleep problems, akinesia, fever,* **seizures,** *sweating, akathisia, confusion, fatigue, insomnia, depression, slurred speech, anxiety,* **neuroleptic malignant syndrome,** agitation, dystonia, obsessive-compulsive symptoms
CV: *Tachycardia, hypo/hypertension,* chest pain, ECG changes, orthostatic hypotension
EENT: Blurred vision
GI: *Drooling or excessive salivation, constipation, nausea, abdominal discomfort, vomiting, diarrhea,* anorexia, weight gain, dry mouth, heartburn, dyspepsia, gastroesophageal reflux

GU: *Urinary abnormalities,* incontinence, ejaculation dysfunction, frequency, urgency, retention, dysuria
HEMA: Leukopenia, neutropenia, agranulocytosis, eosinophilia
MS: Weakness; pain in back, neck, legs; spasm; rigidity
RESP: Dyspnea, nasal congestion, lower respiratory tract infection
OTHER: Diaphoresis
SYST: Death in geriatric patients with dementia, aggravation of diabetes mellitus

Pharmacokinetics

Absorption	Well absorbed
Distribution	Widely distributed; crosses blood-brain barrier, placenta; 95% protein binding
Metabolism	Liver, CYP1A2, 2D6, 3A4
Excretion	Kidneys (50%), feces (30%) (metabolites)
Half-life	8-12 hr

Pharmacodynamics

Onset	Unknown
Peak	Unknown
Duration	8-12 hr

INTERACTIONS

Individual drugs

Alcohol: increased CNS depression
Caffeine, citalopram, erythromycin, fluoxetine, fluvoxamine, ketoconazole, risperidone, ritonavir, sertraline: increased clozapine levels
CarBAMazepine, omeprazole, PHENobarbital, rifampin: decreased clozapine level
Digoxin: increased plasma concentration of digoxin
Warfarin: increased plasma concentrations

Drug classifications

Benzodiazepines: increased hypotension, respiratory, cardiac arrest, collapse
CNS depressants, psychoactives: increased CNS depression
CYP1A2 inducers: decreased clozapine levels
CYP1A2 inhibitors, CYP3A4 inhibitors: increased clozapine level
Highly protein-bound products: increased plasma concentrations

Drug/food

Caffeine: increased clozapine levels

Drug/lab test

Increased: liver function tests, cardiac enzymes, cholesterol, blood glucose, bilirubin, PBI, cholinesterase, ^{131}I
False positive: pregnancy tests, PKU
False negative: urinary steroids, 17-OHCS

NURSING CONSIDERATIONS

Assessment

• Assess for **myocarditis** if suspected, discontinue; myocarditis usually occurs during first month of treatment
• Assess for **seizures;** usually occurs with higher doses
• Assess mental status: orientation, mood, behavior, presence of hallucinations, and type before initial administration and monthly; this product should significantly reduce psychotic behavior
• Check for swallowing of PO medication; check for hoarding or giving of medication to other patients
• Monitor I&O ratio; palpate bladder if low urinary output occurs, especially in geriatric; urinalysis recommended before, during prolonged therapy

> **BLACK BOX WARNING: Bone marrow depression:** Monitor bilirubin, CBC, liver function test monthly; discontinue treatment if WBC <3000/mm^3 or if ANC <1500/mm^3; test qwk; may resume when normal; if WBC <2000/mm^3 or ANC <1000/mm^3, discontinue

• Assess affect, orientation, LOC, reflexes, gait, coordination, sleep pattern disturbances

> **BLACK BOX WARNING: Hypotension:** Monitor B/P with patient sitting, standing, and lying; take pulse and respirations q4hr during initial treatment; establish baseline before starting treatment; report drops of 30 mm Hg

• Check for dizziness, faintness, palpitations, tachycardia on rising
• Assess for **neuroleptic malignant syndrome:** hyperpyrexia, muscle rigidity, increased CPK, altered mental status; product should be discontinued
• Assess for **EPS** including akathisia (inability to sit still, no pattern to movements), tardive dyskinesia (bizarre movements of the jaw, mouth, tongue, extremities), pseudoparkinsonism (rigidity, tremors, pill rolling, shuffling gate)
• Assess for constipation, urinary retention daily; if these occur, increase bulk, water in diet

Nursing diagnoses
- Coping, ineffective (uses)
- Knowledge, deficient (teaching)
- Noncompliance (teaching)
- Thought processes, disturbed (uses)

Patient/family education
- Teach patient to use good oral hygiene; frequent rinsing of mouth, sugarless gum for dry mouth
- Caution patient to avoid hazardous activities until product response is determined
- Inform patient that orthostatic hypotension occurs often and to rise from sitting or lying position gradually
- Caution patient to avoid hot tubs, hot showers, tub baths, since hypotension may occur
- Teach patient to avoid OTC preparations (cough, hay fever, cold) unless approved by prescriber, since serious product interactions may occur; avoid use with alcohol, CNS depressants; increased drowsiness may occur
- Teach patient about EPS and necessity of meticulous oral hygiene, since oral candidiasis may occur
- Teach patient to report sore throat, malaise, fever, bleeding, mouth sores; if these occur, CBC should be performed and product discontinued
- Advise patient that in hot weather, heat stroke may occur; take extra precautions to stay cool

> **BLACK BOX WARNING:** Teach patient symptoms of agranulocytosis and need for blood test qwk for 6 mo, then q2wk; report flulike symptoms

Evaluation
Positive therapeutic outcome
- Decrease in emotional excitement, hallucinations, delusions, paranoia
- Reorganization of patterns of thought, speech

TREATMENT OF ANAPHYLAXIS:
Withdraw product, maintain airway; if diabetic, check blood glucose levels

codeine (Rx)
(koe′deen)
Paveral ✤
Func. class.: Opiate, phenanthrene derivative
Pregnancy category C
Controlled substance schedule II, III, IV, V (depends on content)

Do not confuse:
codeine/Lodine/Iodine/Cardene

ACTION: Depresses pain impulse transmission at the spinal cord level by interacting with opioid receptors; decreases cough reflex, GI motility

Therapeutic outcome: Pain relief, decreased cough, decreased diarrhea depending on route

USES: Moderate to severe pain

Unlabeled uses: Diarrhea, nonproductive cough

CONTRAINDICATIONS:
Hypersensitivity to opiates, respiratory depression, increased intracranial pressure, seizure disorders, severe respiratory disorders, breastfeeding

Precautions: Pregnancy C, geriatric, cardiac dysrhythmias,prostatic hypertrophy, bowel impacton

DOSAGE AND ROUTES
Pain
Adult: PO IM/SUBCUT 15-60 mg q4hr prn
Child: PO 6-17 yr 3 mg/kg/day in divided doses q4hr prn

Cough
Adult: PO 10-20 mg q4-6hr, max 120 mg/day

Renal dose
Adult: PO CCr 10-50 ml/min 75% of dose; CCr <10 ml/min 50% of dose

Diarrhea (unlabeled)
Adult: PO 30 mg; may repeat qid prn

Available forms: Inj tab 30, 60 mg; tabs 15, 30, 60 mg; inj 15, 30 mg/ml

Implementation
- Give with antiemetic if nausea, vomiting occur
- Administer when pain is beginning to return, determine dosage interval by patient response;

Adverse effects: *italics* = common; **bold** = life-threatening

continuous dosing of medication is more effective given prn; explain analgesic effect
• Medication should be slowly withdrawn after long-term use to prevent withdrawal symptoms
• Store in light-resistant container at room temp

PO route
• May be given with food or milk to lessen GI upset

IM/SUBCUT route
• Do not give if cloudy, or a precipitate has formed

Direct IV route
• Give slowly by direct inj

Syringe compatibilities: DimenhyDRINATE, glycopyrrolate, hydrOXYzine

IV compatibilities: Amifostine, amikacin, aminophylline, ammonium, ampicillin, aztreonam, bleomycin, bumetanide, busulfan, calcium, CARBOplatin, carmustine, ceFAZolin, cefotaxime, cefotetan, cefoxitin, ceftazidime, ceftizoxime, cefTRIAXone, cefuroxime, chlorproMAZINE, cimetidine, ciprofloxacin, CISplatin, clindamycin, cyclophosphamide, cycloSPORINE, cytarabine, DACTINomycin, DAUNOrubicin, dexamethasone, dexrazoxane, digoxin, diphenhydrAMINE, DOBUTamine, docetaxel, DOPamine, DOXOrubicin, doxycycline, droperidol, enalaprilat, etoposide, etoposide phosphate, famotidine, floxuridine, fluconazole, fludarabine, fluorouracil, gemcitabine, gentamicin, haloperidol, heparin, hydrocortisone phosphate, hydrocortisone succinate, hydrOXYzine, IDArubicin, ifosfamide, imipenem-cilastatin, leucovorin, levofloxacin, magnesium, mesna, metoclopramide, metroNIDAZOLE, mezlocillin, minocycline, mitomycin, mitoxantrone, netilmicin, ofloxacin, ondansetron, paclitaxel, plicamycin, potassium, prochlorperazine, promethazine, ranitidine, sodium bicarbonate, streptozocin, teniposide, theophylline, thiotepa, ticarcillin, tobramycin, topotecan, trimethobenzamide, vancomycin, vinBLAStine, vinCRIStine, vinorelbine tartrate, zidovudine

Additive incompatibilities: Aminophylline, amobarbital, chlorothiazide, heparin, methicillin, pentobarbital, phenobarbital, phenytoin, secobarbital, thiopental

ADVERSE EFFECTS

CNS: *Drowsiness, sedation,* dizziness, agitation, dependency, lethargy, restlessness, euphoria, **seizures,** hallucinations, headache, confusion
CV: Bradycardia, palpitations, orthostatic hypotension, tachycardia, **circulatory collapse**

GI: *Nausea, vomiting, anorexia, constipation,* dry mouth
GU: Urinary retention
INTEG: Flushing, rash, urticaria, pruritus
RESP: Respiratory depression, respiratory paralysis, dyspnea
SYST: Anaphylaxis

Pharmacokinetics

Absorption	Bioavailability 60%-90%
Distribution	Widely distributed; crosses placenta, protein binding 7%
Metabolism	Liver, extensively by CYP3A4; altered in ethnic groups
Excretion	Kidneys (up to 15%), breast milk
Half-life	3-4 hr

Pharmacodynamics

	PO	IM	SUBCUT
Onset	30-60 min	30-60 min	15-30 min
Peak	1-2 hr	30-60 min	Unknown
Duration	4 hr	4 hr	4 hr

INTERACTIONS

Individual drugs
Alcohol: increased CNS depression

Drug classifications
Antipsychotics, CYP2D6, sedative, hypnotics, opiates, skeletal muscle relaxants: increased CNS depression
MAOIs: increased toxicity; use cautiously

Drug/lab test
Increased: amylase, lipase

NURSING CONSIDERATIONS

Assessment
• Assess **pain:** intensity, type, alleviating factors, type, location, need for pain medication, tolerance, use pain scoring
• Assess GI function: nausea, vomiting, constipation
• Assess **cough:** type, duration, ability to raise secretion for productive cough; do not use to suppress a productive cough
• Monitor VS after parenteral route; note muscle rigidity, product history, renal/hepatic function tests, respiratory dysfunction: respiratory depression, character, rate, rhythm; notify prescriber if respirations are <10/min
• Monitor CNS changes: dizziness, drowsiness, hallucinations, euphoria, LOC, pupil reaction
• Monitor allergic reactions: rash, urticaria

• Respiratory dysfunction: respiratory depression, character, rate, rhythm; notify prescriber if respirations are <10/min, shallow

Nursing diagnoses
• Breathing pattern, ineffective (adverse reactions)
• Knowledge, deficient (teaching)
• Pain, acute (uses)
• Sensory perception, disturbed (adverse reactions)

Patient/family education
• Teach patient to report any symptoms of CNS changes, allergic reactions; to avoid CNS depressants: alcohol, sedative/hypnotics for at least 24 hr after taking this product
• Discuss with patient that dizziness, drowsiness, and confusion are common
• Advise patient to avoid getting up without assistance
• Discuss in detail with patient all aspects of the product
• Advise patient not to breastfeed
• Teach patient that physical dependency may result after extended periods
• Advise patient to use sugarless gum, rinse mouth after, for dry mouth

Evaluation
Positive therapeutic outcome
• Decreased pain
• Decreased cough
• Decreased diarrhea

TREATMENT OF OVERDOSE:
Naloxone 0.4 ampule diluted in 10 ml 0.9% NaCl and given by direct **IV** push 0.02 mg q2min (adult)

---

colchicine (Rx)
(kol′chih-seen)
Colcrys
Func. class.: Antigout agent
Chem. class.: *Colchicum autumnale* alkaloid
Pregnancy category C

ACTION: Inhibits microtubule formation of lactic acid in leukocytes, which decreases phagocytosis and inflammation in joints

Therapeutic outcome: Decreased pain, inflammation of joints

USES: Gout, gouty arthritis (prevention, treatment); to arrest progression of neurologic disability in multiple sclerosis

Unlabeled uses: Hepatic cirrhosis, familial Mediterranean fever, pericarditis, amyloidosis, Behçet's syndrome, biliary cirrhosis, dermatitis herpetiformis, idiopathic thrombocytopenic purpura, Paget's disease, pseudogout, pulmonary fibrosis

CONTRAINDICATIONS:
Pregnancy **D** (injectable), hypersensitivity; serious GI disorders, severe renal/hepatic/cardiac disorders

Precautions: Pregnancy **C** (**PO**), breastfeeding, children, geriatric, blood dyscrasias, hepatic disease

DOSAGE AND ROUTES
Gout prevention
Adult: PO 0.6-1.8 mg daily depending on severity

Gout treatment
Adult: 1.2 mg initially, then 0.6 mg 1 hr later (1.8 mg); those on strong CYP3A4 inhibitor (past 14 days) 0.6 mg initially, then 0.3 mg 1 hr later

Renal dose
Adult: PO CCr <30 ml/min for acute gout, do not repeat course for 2 wk, familial Mediterranean fever 0.3 mg daily, increase cautiously

Available forms: Tabs 0.5, 0.6, 1 mg ♣

Implementation
PO route
• Give with food for GI symptoms
• Cumulative doses ≤4 mg, renal patients ≤2 mg, when reached, administer only for 3 wks

ADVERSE EFFECTS
GI: *Nausea, vomiting, anorexia, malaise,* metallic taste, cramps, peptic ulcer, diarrhea
GU: Hematuria, **oliguria, renal damage**
HEMA: Agranulocytosis, thrombocytopenia, aplastic anemia, pancytopenia
INTEG: Chills, dermatitis, pruritus, purpura, erythema
MISC: Myopathy, alopecia, reversible azoospermia, peripheral neuritis

Pharmacokinetics
Absorption	Well absorbed
Distribution	WBCs
Metabolism	Deacetylates in liver
Excretion	Feces (metabolites/active product)
Half-life	4.4 hr

Adverse effects: *italics* = common; **bold** = life-threatening

Pharmacodynamics

	PO
Onset	Unknown
Peak	$^{1}/_{2}$-2 hr
Duration	Unknown

INTERACTIONS

Individual drugs
CycloSPORINE, radiation: increased bone marrow depression
Clarithromycin, cycloSPORINE, erythromycin: toxicity
Ethanol: increased GI effects
Vitamin B_{12}: decreased action of vit B_{12}; may cause reversible malabsorption

Drug classifications
Bone marrow depressants: increased bone marrow depression
NSAIDs: increased GI effects

Drug/lab test
Increased: alkaline phosphatase, AST
False positive: urine Hgb
Interference: urinary 17-hydroxycorticosteroids

NURSING CONSIDERATIONS

Assessment
• Assess pain and mobility of joints, uric acid levels returning to normal
• Monitor I&O ratio; observe for decrease in urinary output; CBC, platelets, reticulocytes before, during therapy (q3mo); may cause aplastic anemia, agranulocytosis, decreased platelets
• Assess for **toxicity:** weakness, abdominal pain, nausea, vomiting, diarrhea, product should be discontinued, report symptoms immediately

Nursing diagnoses
• Knowledge, deficient (teaching)
• Mobility, impaired (uses)
• Pain, chronic (uses)

Patient/family education
• Caution patient to avoid alcohol, OTC preparations that contain alcohol
• Instruct patient to report any pain, redness, or hard area, usually in legs; rash, sore throat, fever, bleeding, bruising, weakness, numbness, tingling, nausea, vomiting, abdominal pain
• Teach patient importance of complying with medical regimen (diet, weight loss, product therapy); bone marrow depression may occur
• Advise patient to tell all providers of product use, surgery may increase possibility of acute gout symptoms

Evaluation
Positive therapeutic outcome
• Decreased stone formation on x-ray
• Decreased pain in kidney region
• Absence of hematuria
• Decreased pain in joints

TREATMENT OF OVERDOSE:
Discontinue medication, may need opioids to treat diarrhea

colesevelam (Rx)
(coal-see-vel′am)
Welchol
Func. class.: Antilipemic
Chem. class.: Bile acid sequestrant
Pregnancy category B

ACTION: Absorbs, combines with bile acids to form insoluble complex that is excreted through feces; loss of bile acids lowers cholesterol levels

Therapeutic outcome: Decreasing LDL cholesterol

USES: Elevated LDL cholesterol, alone or in combination with HMG-coA reductase inhibitor; type 2 diabetes (adjunct)

CONTRAINDICATIONS:
Hypersensitivity, biliary obstruction; dysphagia, bowel disease, primary biliary cirrhosis, triglycerides >300 mg/dl, fat-soluble vitamin deficiency

Precautions: Pregnancy **B,** breastfeeding, children

DOSAGE AND ROUTES

Monotherapy
Adult: PO 3 625 mg tabs bid with meals or 6 tabs daily with a meal; may increase to 7 tabs if needed

Combination therapy
Adult: PO 3 tabs bid with meals or 6 tabs daily with a meal given with an HMG-coA reductase inhibitor

Type 2 diabetes, adjunct (to improve glycemic control)
Adult and geriatric: PO approx 3.8 g (6 tabs)/day or approx 1.9 g (3 tabs) bid

Heterozygous familial hypercholesterolemia
Females (postmenarchal and >10 yr) and males ≥10 yr: PO 1.875 g packet bid or 3.75 g packet q day dissolved in 4-8 oz of water with a meal

Available forms: Tabs 625 mg, powder for oral susp 3.75 g

Implementation
• Give product daily, bid with meals; give all other medications 1 hr before colesevelam or 4 hr after colesevelam to avoid poor absorption; take with liquid
• Give supplemental doses of vit A, D, K if levels are low

ADVERSE EFFECTS
CNS: Headache, dizziness, drowsiness, vertigo, tinnitus
GI: *Constipation, abdominal pain, nausea,* fecal impaction, hemorrhoids, flatulence, vomiting, **GI obstruction**
INTEG: Rash, irritation of perianal area, tongue, skin
MISC: Hypertriglycerides, hypoglycemia
MS: Muscle, joint pain

Pharmacokinetics

Absorption	Unknown
Distribution	Unknown
Metabolism	Unknown
Excretion	Feces
Half-life	Unknown

Pharmacodynamics
LDL decreased in 4-7 days

INTERACTIONS
Individual drugs
Digoxin, diltiazem, gemfibrozil, glyBURide, iron, mycophenolate, penicillin G, phenytoin, propanolol, warfarin: decreased absorption of each specific product
Thyroid hormones: decreased absorption of thyroid

Drug classifications
Corticosteroids: decreased corticosteroid action
Oral contraceptives: decreased action of oral contraceptives
Tetracyclines: decreased absorption of tetracyclines
Thiazides: decreased absorption of thiazides
Vitamins (fat-soluble): decreased absorption of fat-soluble vitamins

Drug/lab test
Increased: liver function tests

NURSING CONSIDERATIONS
Assessment
• Assess cardiac glycoside level if both products are being administered
• Assess for signs of vit A, D, K deficiency
• Monitor fasting LDL, HDL, total cholesterol, triglyceride levels, electrolytes if on extended therapy
• Monitor bowel pattern daily; increase bulk, H_2O in diet for constipation

Nursing diagnoses
• Constipation (adverse reactions)
• Knowledge, deficient (teaching)
• Noncompliance (teaching)

Patient/family education
• Teach the importance of compliance; toxicity may result if doses missed
• Teach that risk factors should be decreased: high-fat diet, smoking, alcohol consumption, absence of exercise

Evaluation
Positive therapeutic outcome
• Decreased cholesterol level (hyperlipidemia); diarrhea, pruritus (excess bile acids)

colestipol (Rx)
(koe-les'ti-pole)
Colestid
Func. class.: Antilipemic
Chem. class.: Bile acid sequestrant
Pregnancy category B

ACTION: Absorbs, combines with bile acids to form an insoluble complex that is excreted through feces; loss of bile acids lowers cholesterol levels

Therapeutic outcome: Decreasing cholesterol levels and low-density lipoproteins, decreased pruritus

USES: Primary hypercholesterolemia, xanthomas

Unlabeled uses: Digoxin toxicity/overdose, pruritus, diarrhea due to increased bile acids after surgery

CONTRAINDICATIONS:
Hypersensitivity, biliary obstruction

Precautions: Pregnancy **B**, breastfeeding, children, bleeding disorders

DOSAGE AND ROUTES
Adult: PO tabs 2 g daily-bid, may increase by 1 g/mo, max 16 g/day; powder 5-30 g mixed with liquid daily or in divided doses

Available forms: Powder/packet/scoop (granules) 5 g; tabs 1 g

Implementation
• Swallow tabs whole; do not break, crush, or chew
• Give product daily or bid; give all other medications 1 hr before or 4 hr after colestipol to avoid poor absorption; give product mixed with applesauce or stirred into beverage (2-6 oz), let stand for 2 min; rinse glass to make sure all medication is taken; do not take dry, use of powdered products may not be bioequivalent with other products
• Provide supplemental doses of vit A, D, E, K if levels are low

ADVERSE EFFECTS
GI: *Constipation, abdominal pain, nausea,* fecal impaction, hemorrhoids, flatulence, vomiting, steatorrhea, peptic ulcer
HEMA: Bleeding, increased pro-time
INTEG: *Rash,* irritation of perianal area, tongue, skin
META: *Decreased vit A, D, K,* red folate content; **hyperchloremic acidosis**

Pharmacokinetics
Absorption	Not absorbed
Distribution	Not distributed
Metabolism	Not metabolized
Excretion	Binds with bile acids, feces
Half-life	Unknown

Pharmacodynamics
Onset	24-48 hr
Peak	30 days
Duration	30 days

INTERACTIONS
Individual drugs
Atorvastatin, bexarotene, calcifediol, calcitriol, digoxin, ezetimibe, fenofibric acid, gemfibrozil, glipiZIDE, iron, mycophenolate, penicillin G, propranolol, tetracycline, thyroid agents, vancomycin, warfarin: decreased action of each specific product
Phenytoin, TOLBUTamide: decreased effect of each specific product

Drug classifications
Corticosteroids, NSAIDs, phosphorous salts: decreased effect of each specific product
Diuretics (thiazide): decreased absorption
Vitamins A, D, E, K: decreased absorption

Drug/lab test
Increased: Cl, PO_4, AST, ALT, alkaline phosphatase
Decreased: Na, K, Ca

NURSING CONSIDERATIONS
Assessment
• **Hypercholesterolemia:** Assess nutrition: fat, protein, carbohydrates; nutritional analysis should be completed by dietitian
• Assess skin integrity after patient has been receiving product; itching, pruritus often occur from bile deposits on skin
• Monitor cardiac glycoside level, if both products are being administered; cardiac glycoside levels will be decreased
• Monitor for signs of vit A, D, E, K deficiency; check serum cholesterol, triglyceride levels, electrolytes if on extended therapy
• **Diarrhea:** Monitor bowel pattern daily; increase bulk, water in diet if constipation develops

Nursing diagnoses
• Constipation (adverse reactions)
• Knowledge, deficient (teaching)
• Noncompliance (teaching)

Patient/family education
⚠ Teach patient symptoms of hypoprothrombinemia: bleeding mucous membranes, dark, tarry stools, hematuria, petechiae; report immediately
• Teach patient importance of compliance, not to miss or double doses
• Teach patient that risk factors should be decreased: high-fat diet, smoking, alcohol consumption, absence of exercise
• Tell patient to mix product with 6 oz of milk, water, fruit juice; may be mixed with carbonated beverages; rinse glass to make sure all medication is taken or may mix product in applesauce; allow to stand for 2 min before mixing

Evaluation
Positive therapeutic outcome
• Decreased cholesterol level (hyperlipidemia)

conivaptan (Rx)
(kon-ih-vap'-tan)
Vaprisol
Func. class.: Vasopressin receptor antagonist
Pregnancy category C

ACTION: Dual arginine vasopressin (AVP) antagonist with affinity for V_{1A}, V_2 receptors; level of AVP in circulating blood is critical for regulation of water, electrolyte balance and is usually elevated in euvolemic/hypervolemic hyponatremia

Therapeutic outcome: Correct serum sodium levels

USES: Euvolemia hyponatremia in those hospitalized, not indicated for CHF, hypervolemia, hyponatremia

CONTRAINDICATIONS: Hypersensitivity, hypovolemia

Precautions: Pregnancy **C**, breastfeeding, orthostatic/renal disease, heart failure, rapid correction of serum sodium

DOSAGE AND ROUTES
Adult: IV INF loading dose 20 mg given over 30 min, then CONT **IV** over 24 hr; after 1 day, give for an additional 1-3 days as a CONT INF of 20 mg/day total, can be titrated up to 40 mg/day if serum sodium is not rising at the desired rate; max time 4 days

Hepatic/renal dose
Adult: IV Child-Pugh A-C or CCr 30-60 ml/min: Give **IV** loading dose over 10 min, then cont **IV** INF 10 mg over 24 hr × 2-4 days

Available forms: 5 mg/ml (20 mg/4 ml) in single-use ampule; 20 mg/100 ml in D_5W for injection

Implementation
IV route
• Withdraw 4 ml (20 mg) of conivaptan, add to 100 ml D_5W, gently invert several times to mix, give over 30 min

Continuous IV infusion route
• Withdraw 4 ml (20 mg) of conivaptan, add to 250 ml D_5W, gently invert several times to mix, give over 24 hr; or 40 mg in 250 ml D_5W, gently invert several times to mix, give over 24 hr

ADVERSE EFFECTS
CNS: Headache, confusion, insomnia
CV: *Atrial fibrillation,* hypo/hypertension, orthostatic hypotension, phlebitis
GI: Nausea, vomiting, constipation, dry mouth
GU: Hematuria, polyuria, UTI, pollakiuria
HEMA: Anemia
INTEG: Erythemia, inj site reaction
META: Dehydration, hypo/hyperglycemia, hypokalemia, hypomagnesia, hyponatremia
MISC: Oral candidiasis, pain, peripheral edema, pneumonia

Pharmacokinetics
Absorption	Unknown
Distribution	Protein binding 99%
Metabolism	By CYP3A4
Excretion	Unknown
Half-life	Terminal 5 hr

Pharmacodynamics
Unknown

INTERACTIONS
Drug classifications
CYP3A4 substrates (alfuzosin, aripiprazole, bexarolene, bortezomib, bosentan, bupivacaine, buprenorphine, carBAMazepine, cevimeline, cilostazol, cinacalcet, clopidogrel, colchicine, cyclobenzaprine, dapsone, darifenacin, disopyramide, docetaxel, donepezil, DOXOrubicin, dutasteride, eletriptan, eplerenone, ergots, erlotinib, eszopiclone, ethinyl estradiol, ethosuximide, etoposide, fentaNYL, galantamine, gefitinib, halofantrine, ifosfamide, irinotecan, levobupivacaine, levomethadyl, lidocaine, loperamide, loratadine, mefloquine, methadone, modafinil, paclitaxel, pimozide, praziquantel, quiNIDine, quiNINE, ramelteon, reboxetine, repaglinide, rifabutin, sibutramine, sildenafil, sirolimus, SUFentanil, sunitinib, tacrolimus, tamoxifen, teniposide, testosterone, tiagabine, tinidazole, trimetrexate, vardenafil, vinca alkaloids, ziprasidone, zolpidem, zonisamide): increased effects, do not use concurrently

NURSING CONSIDERATIONS
Assessment
• Monitor renal/hepatic function
• Assess frequent sodium volume status; overly rapid correction of sodium concentration (>12 mEq/L per 24 hr) may result in osmotic demyelination syndrome
• Assess neurologic status: confusion, headache

• Assess CV status: atrial fibrillation, hyper/hypotension, orthostatic hypotension; monitor B/P, pulse
• Monitor other electrolytes (magnesium and potassium)

Nursing diagnoses
• Injury, risk for (uses)
• Knowledge, deficient (teaching)

Patient/family education
• Advise patient to avoid pregnancy, breastfeeding while taking this product
• Advise patient to report neurologic changes: headache, insomnia, confusion
• Teach patient administration procedure and expected result
• Advise patient to report inj site pain, redness, swelling

Evaluation
Positive therapeutic outcome
• Correction of serum sodium levels

CONTRACEPTIVES, HORMONAL

MONOPHASIC, ORAL

ethinyl estradiol/desogestrel (Rx)
Apri, Cesia, Desogen, Kariva, Mircette, Ortho-Cept, Reclipsen, Solia, Velivet

ethinyl estradiol/drospirenone (Rx)
Yasmin, Yaz 28

ethinyl estradiol/ethynodiol (Rx)
Kelnor 1/35, Zovia

ethinyl estradiol/levonorgestrel (Rx)
Alesse, Aviane-28, Enpresse, Jolessa, Lessina, Levlen, Levlite, Levora, Lutera, Nordette, Portia, Quasense, Seasonique, Sronyx

ethinyl estradiol/norethindrone (Rx)
Brevicon, Genora 0.5/35, Genora 1/35, Junel 21 1/20, Junel 21 1.5/20, Loestrin 21 1.5/30, Loestrin 21 1/20, Microgestin, Modicon, N.E.E 1/35, Nelova 0.5/35E, Nelova 1/35E, Norcept-E 1/35, Norethin 1/35E, Norinyl 1+35, Norlestrin 1/50, Norlestrin 2.5/50, Nortrel

ethinyl estradiol/norgestimate (Rx)
MonoNessa, Ortho-Cyclen, Previfem, Sprintec

ethinyl estradiol/norgestrel (Rx)
Cryselle, Lo/Ovral, Low-Ogestrel, Ogestrel, Ovral

mestranol/norethindrone (Rx)
Genora 1/50, Nelova 1/50m, Norethin 1/50m, Norinyl 1+50, Ortho-Novum 1/50

BIPHASIC, ORAL

ethinyl estradiol/norethindrone (Rx)
Nelova 10/11, Ortho-Novum 10/11

TRIPHASIC, ORAL

ethinyl estradiol/desogestrel (Rx)
Cyclessa

ethinyl estradiol/ norethindrone (Rx)
Necor 7/7/7, Nortrel 7/7/7, Ortho-Novum 7/7/7, Tri-Norinyl

ethinyl estradiol/ norgestimate (Rx)
Ortho Tri-Cyclen, Ortho Tri-Cyclen Lo

ethinyl estradiol/ levonorgestrel (Rx)
Enpresse, Tri-Levlen, Triphasil

EXTENDED CYCLE, ORAL
ethinyl estradiol/ levonorgestrel (Rx)
Seasonale

PROGESTIN, ORAL
norethindrone (Rx)
Errin, Ortho Micronor, Camila, Jolivette, Nor-Q D

PROGRESSIVE ESTROGEN, ORAL
ethinyl estradiol/ norethindrone acetate (Rx)
Estrostep, Estrostep Fe

EMERGENCY
levonorgestrel/ethinyl estradiol (Rx)
Preven
levonorgestrel (Rx)
Plan B
medroxyprogesterone (Rx)
Depo-Provera

INTRAUTERINE
levonorgestrel (Rx)
Mirena

IMPLANT
etonogestrel (Rx)
Implanon

VAGINAL RING
ethinyl estradiol/etonoges-trel (Rx)
Nuva Ring

TRANSDERMAL
ethinyl estradiol/norel-gestromin (Rx)
Ortho Evra

ACTION: Prevents ovulation by contraceptives suppressing FSH, LH; *monophasic:* estrogen/progestin (fixed dose) used during a 21-day cycle; ovulation is inhibited by suppression of FSH and LH; thickness of cervical mucus and endometrial lining prevents pregnancy; *biphasic:* ovulation is inhibited by suppression of FSH and LH; alteration of cervical mucus, endometrial lining prevents pregnancy; *triphasic:* ovulation is inhibited by suppression of FSH and LH; change of cervical mucus, endometrial lining prevents pregnancy; variable doses of estrogen/progestin combinations may be similar to natural hormonal fluctuations; *extended cycle:* estrogen/progestin continuous for 84 days, off for 7 days, result 4 menstrual periods/yr; *progressive estrogen:* constant progestin with 3 progressive doses of estrogen; *progestin-only pill, implant, intrauterine:* change of cervical mucus and endometrial lining prevents pregnancy; ovulation may be suppressed

Therapeutic outcome: Prevention of pregnancy, decreased severity of endometriosis, hypermenorrhea

USES: To prevent pregnancy, regulation of menstrual cycle, treatment of acne in women >14 yr that other treatment has failed, emergency contraception; *injection:* inhibits gonadotropin secretion, ovulation, follicular maturation; *emergency:* inhibits ovulation and fertilization, decreases transport of sperm and egg from fallopian tube to uterus; *vaginal ring, transdermal:* inhibits ovulation, prevents sperm entry into uterus; *antiacne:* may decrease sex hormone binding globulin, results in decreased testosterone

CONTRAINDICATIONS: Pregnancy **X**, breastfeeding, women 40 yr and over, reproductive cancer, thrombophlebitis, MI, hepatic tumors, hepatic disease, CAD, CVA

Precautions: Depression, hypertension, renal disease, seizure disorders, lupus erythematosus, rheumatic disease, migraine headache, amenorrhea, irregular menses, breast cancer (fibrocystic), gallbladder disease, diabetes mellitus, heavy smoking, acute mononucleosis, sickle cell disease

DOSAGE AND ROUTES
Monophasic
Adult: PO take first tab on Sunday after start of menses × 21 days; skip 7 days; then repeat cycle; start on 1st day of menses × 21 days;

skip 7 days, then repeat cycle; may contain 7 placebo tabs, where 1 tab is taken daily

Biphasic
Adult: PO Take 10 days of small progestin, then large progestin; estrogen is the same during cycle; skip 7 days, then repeat cycle; may contain 7 placebo tabs, where 1 tab is taken daily

Triphasic
Adult: PO estrogen dose remains constant, progestin changes throughout 21 day cycle, some products contain 28 tabs per month

Extended cycle
Adult: PO start taking on first day of menses; continue for 84 days of active tab, then 7 days of placebo; repeat cycle

Progestin
Adult: PO start on 1st day of menses, then daily and continuously

Progressive estrogen
Adult: PO progestin dose remains constant, estrogen increases q7days throughout 21-day cycle, may include 7 placebo tabs for 28-day cycle

Emergency
Adult and adolescent: Give within 72 hr of intercourse, repeat 12 hr later; Plan B 1 tab, then 1 tab 12 hr later; Preven 2 tab, then 2 tab 12 hr later; Ovral (unlabeled) 2 white tabs; Lo/Ovral (unlabeled) 4 white tabs; Levlen (unlabeled), Nordette (unlabeled) 4 orange tabs; Triphasil (unlabeled), Tri-Levlen (unlabeled) 4 yellow tabs

Injectable
Adult: IM (Depo-Provera) 150 mg within 5 days of start of menses, or within 5 days postpartum (must not be breastfeeding); if breastfeeding, give 6 wk postpartum, repeat q3mo

Intrauterine
Adult: To be inserted using the levonorgestrel-releasing intrauterine system (LRIS) by those trained in procedure; inserted into uterine cavity within 7 days of the onset of menstruation; use should not exceed 5 years per implant

Vaginal ring
Adult: VAG insert 1 ring on or prior to day 5 of cycle, leave in place 3 wk; remove for 1 wk, then repeat

Transdermal
Adult: Transdermal apply patch within 7 days of menses, change weekly × 3 wk; no patch wk 4, repeat cycle

Implant
Adult: Subdermal in inner side of upper arm on days 1-5 of menses, replace q3yr

Acne
Adult: PO (Ortho Tri-Cyclen) take daily × 21 days, off 7 days

Implementation
PO route
• If GI symptoms occur, medication may be taken with food; take at same time each day
Implant route
• Inject 6 cap subdermally
• Implant is effective for 5 yr, should be removed after that
IM route
• Administer inj deep in large muscle mass after shaking susp well; ensure pregnancy has not occurred if inj are 2 wk or more apart

ADVERSE EFFECTS
CNS: Depression, fatigue, dizziness, nervousness, anxiety, headache
CV: Increased B/P, **cerebral hemorrhage, thrombosis, pulmonary embolism,** fluid retention, edema
EENT: Optic neuritis, retinal thrombosis, cataracts
ENDO: Decreased glucose tolerance, increased TBG, PBI, T_4, T_3
GI: *Nausea*, vomiting, cramps, diarrhea, bloating, constipation, change in appetite, **cholestatic jaundice**
GU: Breakthrough bleeding, amenorrhea, spotting, dysmenorrhea, galactorrhea, endocervical hyperplasia, vaginitis, cystitis-like syndrome, breast change
HEMA: Increased fibrinogen, clotting factor
INTEG: *Chloasma, melasma,* acne, rash, urticaria, erythema, pruritus, hirsutism, alopecia, photosensitivity

Pharmacokinetics

Absorption	Unknown
Distribution	Unknown
Metabolism	Unknown
Excretion	Breast milk
Half-life	Unknown

Pharmacodynamics
Unknown

INTERACTIONS
Individual drugs
Griseofulvin, rifampin: decreased effectiveness of oral contraceptive

Drug classifications

Analgesics, antibiotics, anticonvulsants, antihistamines: decreased action of oral contraceptives

Anticoagulants (oral): decreased action of oral anticoagulants

Drug/herb

Black cohosh: altered action

Saw palmetto, St. John's wort: decreased oral contraceptive effect

Drug/food

Grapefruit juice: increased peak level

Drug/lab test

Increased: pro-time; clotting factors VII, VIII, IX, X; TBG, PBI, T_4, platelet aggregation, BSP, triglycerides, bilirubin, AST, ALT

Decreased: T_3, antithrombin III, folate, metyrapone test, GTT, 17-OHCS

NURSING CONSIDERATIONS

Assessment

• Assess for reproductive changes: change in breasts, tumors, positive Pap smear; product should be discontinued if changes occur

• Monitor glucose, thyroid function, liver function tests, B/P

Nursing diagnoses

• Body image, disturbed (adverse reactions)

• Injury, risk for (adverse reactions)

• Knowledge, deficient (teaching)

• Noncompliance (teaching)

Patient/family education

• Teach patient about detection of clots using Homans' sign; teach monitoring technique for heat, redness, pain, swelling

• Teach patient to use sunscreen or to avoid sunlight; photosensitivity can occur

• Teach patient to take at same time each day to ensure equal product level; to take another tab as soon as possible if one is missed

• Teach patient that after product is discontinued, pregnancy may not occur for several mo

• Instruct patient to report GI symptoms that occur after 4 mo

• Advise patient to use another birth control method during first 3 wk of oral contraceptive use

• Teach patient to report abdominal pain, change in vision, shortness of breath, change in menstrual flow, spotting, breakthrough bleeding, breast lumps, swelling, headache, severe leg pain, mental changes; that continuing medical care is needed: Pap smear and gynecologic exam q6mo

• Teach patient to notify physicians and dentist of oral contraceptive use

Evaluation

Positive therapeutic outcome

• Absence of pregnancy

• Decreased severity of endometriosis

• Decreased severity of hypermenorrhea

---

cortisone (Rx)

(kor′ti-sone)

Cortone ✤

Func. class.: Corticosteroid, synthetic

Chem. class.: Short-acting glucocorticoid

Pregnancy category D

ACTION: Decreases inflammation by suppression of migration of polymorphonuclear leukocytes and fibroblasts, reversal of increased capillary permeability, and lysosomal stabilization; suppresses adrenal function with long-term use

Therapeutic outcome: Replacement of cortisol in adrenal insufficiency

USES: Inflammation, severe allergy, adrenal insufficiency; collagen, respiratory, dermatologic, rheumatic disorders, CLL, ALL, Hodgkin's/non-Hodgkin's lymphoma, endocrine system disorders, eye disorders, Crohn's/ulcerative colitis, hypercalcemia of malignancy, mycosis fungoides, nephrotic syndrome, TB of meninges

CONTRAINDICATIONS: Pregnancy **D**, child <2 yr, psychosis, hypersensitivity, idiopathic thrombocytopenia, acute glomerulonephritis, amebiasis, fungal infections, nonasthmatic bronchial disease, AIDS, TB, measles, varicella

Precautions: Breastfeeding, diabetes mellitus, glaucoma, osteoporosis, seizure disorders, ulcerative colitis, CHF, myasthenia gravis, renal/hepatic disease, esophagitis, peptic ulcer

DOSAGE AND ROUTES

Adult: PO 25-300 mg daily or q2day, titrated to patient response

Available forms: Tabs 25 mg

Implementation

PO route

• Administer in AM with food or milk to decrease GI symptoms

ADVERSE EFFECTS

CNS: *Depression, flushing, sweating,* headache, mood changes, insomnia
CV: *Hypertension,* **circulatory collapse, thrombophlebitis, embolism,** tachycardia, **necrotizing angiitis, CHF,** edema
EENT: Fungal infections, increased intraocular pressure, blurred vision, cataracts, glaucoma
GI: *Diarrhea, nausea, abdominal distention,* **GI hemorrhage,** increased appetite, **pancreatitis,** ulcerative esophagitis
HEMA: Thrombocytopenia
INTEG: Acne, poor wound healing, ecchymosis, bruising, petechiae, hirsutism
META: Sodium fluid retention; potassium loss, diabetes
MS: Fractures, osteoporosis, weakness, loss of muscle mass

Pharmacokinetics

Absorption	Slowly (IM)
Distribution	Widely, crosses placenta
Metabolism	Liver
Excretion	Unknown
Half-life	8-12 hr

Pharmacodynamics

	PO
Onset	Unknown
Peak	2 hr
Duration	$1^1/_2$ days

INTERACTIONS

Individual drugs

Alcohol: increased side effects
Amphotericin B: increased hypokalemia
CycloSPORINE, tacrolimus: increased effect of each product
Ketoconazole: increased cortisone action
PHENobarbital, phenytoin: decreased effectiveness of cortisone
Rifampin, theophylline: decreased cortisone action

Drug classifications

Acetylcholinesterases, barbiturates: decreased cortisone action
Anticoagulants: increased or decreased anticoagulant effect
Antidiabetics: decreased antidiabetic effect
Antiinfectives (macrolide), estrogens: increased cortisone action
Barbiturates: decreased cortisone action
Contraceptives (hormonal): increased action of cortisone

Diuretics (potassium-wasting): increased side effects
Fluoroquinolones: increased tendon rupture
NSAIDs, salicylates: increased GI symptoms, increased cortisone effects, increased side effects; decreased salicylate effect
Thiazide/loop diuretics: increased hypokalemia
Toxoids: decreased toxoid effect
Vaccines: decreased vaccine effect

Drug/lab test

Increased: cholesterol, sodium, blood glucose, uric acid, calcium, urine glucose
Decreased: calcium, potassium, T_4, T_3, thyroid ^{131}I uptake test, urine 17-OHCS, 17-KS
False negative: skin allergy tests

NURSING CONSIDERATIONS

Assessment

• Assess for **adrenal insufficiency** symptoms: weakness, nausea, vomiting, confusion, anxiety, restlessness, decreased B/P, weight loss; check before, during treatment
• Monitor potassium, blood glucose for patient on long-term therapy; hypokalemia and hyperglycemia can occur
• Check B/P, pulse; notify prescriber if chest pain occurs
• Monitor I&O ratio and weight daily; be alert for decreasing urinary output and increasing edema with bilateral crackles, dyspnea, weight gain
• Monitor plasma cortisol levels during long-term therapy (normal level: 138-635 nmol/L if checked at 8 AM)
• Assess for symptoms of **infection:** increased temp, WBC even after withdrawal of medication; product masks symptoms of infection
• Monitor for potassium depletion: paresthesias, fatigue, nausea, vomiting, depression, polyuria, dysrhythmias, weakness, edema, hypertension, cardiac symptoms, weight daily; notify prescriber of weekly gain >5 lb
• Assess for mental changes: affect, mood, behavioral changes, aggression; depression, psychosis may occur
• **Growth inhibition:** monitor children receiving long-term therapy

Nursing diagnoses

• Infection, risk for (adverse reactions)
• Injury, risk for (adverse reactions)
• Knowledge, deficient (teaching)

Patient/family education

• Advise patient to carry/wear emergency ID as corticosteroid user at all times

• Instruct patient to notify prescriber if therapeutic response decreases; dosage adjustment may be needed; teach not to discontinue this medication abruptly or **adrenal crisis** can result; teach all aspects of product usage, including cushingoid symptoms

• Caution patient to avoid all OTC products: salicylates, potassium, alcohol in cough products, cold preparations unless directed by prescriber; avoid high-sodium foods

• Teach patient symptoms of **adrenal insufficiency:** nausea, anorexia, fatigue, dizziness, dyspnea, weakness, joint pain, tarry stools, bruising, blurred vision

• Advise patient to avoid persons with known infections; report probable infection rapidly; product masks infection

• Caution patient that diet modification is necessary if on long-term treatment: increased calcium, potassium, and protein; also low sodium and carbohydrates

• Advise the patient to avoid exposure to chickenpox, measles

• Advise the patient to take PO dose in AM with food or fluid (milk)

• Advise patient to report immediately black, tarry stools, or abdominal pain; also report swelling, bruising, back pain, visual changes, or mood changes

Evaluation
Positive therapeutic outcome
• Decreased inflammation

---

cotrimoxazole
See trimethoprim/sulfamethoxazole

---

crizotinib
(kriz-oh'ti-nib)
XALKORI
Func. class.: Antineoplastic; biologic response modifiers
Pregnancy category D

ACTION: An inhibitor of receptor tyrosine kinases (anaplastic lymphoma kinase (ALK), hepatocyte growth factor receptor (HGFR, c-Met), recepteur d'origine nantais (RON).

Therapeutic outcome: Decreased spread of malignancy

USES: Locally advanced or metastatic non–small-cell lung cancer (NSCLC) that is anaplastic lymphoma kinase (ALK)-positive as detected by an FDA-approved test

CONTRAINDICATIONS:
Pregnancy D, breastfeeding

Precautions: Pneumonitis, severe hepatic disease, congenital long QT syndrome, neonates, infants, children, adolescents, severe renal impairment, end-stage renal disease, vision disorders

DOSAGE AND ROUTES
Adult: PO 250 mg bid; continue as long as is beneficial

Dose adjustments for hematologic toxicities
For Grade 1-2: No dosage adjustment needed

For Grade 3: Interrupt treatment until toxicity resolves to grade ≤2, then, continue with the same dosage schedule. In case of recurrence after a grade 4 event with dose reduction, interrupt treatment until toxicity resolves to grade ≤2; when resuming treatment, reduce dosage to 250 mg PO daily

For Grade 4: Interrupt treatment until toxicity resolves to grade ≤2; when resuming treatment, reduce dosage to 200 mg PO bid. In case of grade 4 recurrence, permanently discontinue treatment

Dose adjustment for hepatic laboratory abnormalities
For Grade 1: No dosage adjustment necessary:

For Grade 2 ALT/AST elevations with grade ≤1 total bilirubin elevations: No dosage adjustment necessary

For Grade 3-4 ALT/AST elevations with grade ≤1 total bilirubin elevations: Interrupt treatment until toxicity resolves to grade ≤1 or baseline; when resuming treatment, reduce dosage to 200 mg PO bid; in case of recurrence, interrupt treatment until toxicity resolves to grade ≤1, and when resuming treatment, reduce dosage to 250 mg PO daily; permanently discontinue treatment in case of further recurrence

For Grade 2-4 ALT/AST elevations with concurrent Grade 2-4 total bilirubin elevations (in the absence of cholestasis or hemolysis): Permanently discontinue treatment

Dose adjustment for pneumonitis not attributable to NSCLC progression, other pulmonary disease, infection, or radiation effect
For any grade pneumonitis: Permanently discontinue

Dose adjustment for QTc prolongation:

For Grade 1–2 QTc prolongation: No dosage adjustment necessary

For Grade 3 QTc prolongation: Interrupt treatment until toxicity resolves to grade ≤1; when resuming treatment, reduce dosage to 200 mg PO bid; in case of recurrence, interrupt treatment until toxicity resolves to grade ≤1 and when resuming treatment, reduce dosage to 250 mg PO daily; permanently discontinue in case of further recurrence

For Grade 4 QTc prolongation: Permanently discontinue

Available forms: Caps 200, 250 mg

Implementation

• May be taken orally with or without food
• Have the patient swallow capsule whole; do not crush or chew
• If a dose is missed, it can be taken up to 6 hr before the next dose is due to maintain the twice daily regimen. Do not take both doses at the same time
• Store capsules at room temperature

ADVERSE EFFECTS

CNS: Dizziness, balance disorder, presyncope, neuropathy (motor and sensory), burning sensation, dysesthesia, hyperesthesia, hypoesthesia, neuralgia, paresthesias, peripheral neuropathy (motor and sensory), headache, insomnia

CV: QT prolongation, disseminated intravascular coagulation (DIC), septic shock, bradycardia

EENT: Diplopia, photopsia, photophobia, blurred vision, visual field defect, vitreous floaters, visual brightness, reduced visual acuity, esophageal disorders, dyspepsia, dysphagia, epigastric discomfort/pain, burning, esophagitis, **esophageal obstruction/pain/spasm, esophageal ulceration,** gastroesophageal reflux, odynophagia, and reflux esophagitis

GI: Nausea, diarrhea, vomiting, constipation, decreased appetite, dysgeusia, abdominal pain, abdominal discomfort/pain, stomatitis, oral ulceration, elevated hepatic enzymes, hyperbilirubinemia, glossodynia, glossitis, cheilitis, mucosal inflammation, oropharyngeal pain/discomfort, oral pain, esophageal disorder

HEMA: Grade 3/4 neutropenia, thrombocytopenia, lymphopenia

MISC: Fatigue, fever, edema, localized/peripheral edema, chest pain (unspecified), chest discomfort, musculoskeletal chest pain, arthralgia, back pain, rash

RESP: Severe, life-threatening pneumonitis, pneumonia, hypoxia, acute respiratory distress syndrome (ARDS), dyspnea, empyema, **pulmonary hemorrhage, pulmonary embolism,** upper respiratory tract infection (nasopharyngitis, pharyngitis, rhinitis), cough

Pharmacokinetics

Absorption	43%
Distribution	Steady state 15 days, protein binding 91%, distribution tissue, plasma
Metabolism	By 3YPA4/5, oxidation to metabolites
Excretion	63% feces, unchanged 53%; 22% urine, unchanged 2, 3%
Half-life	Terminal 42 hr

Pharmacodynamics

Onset	Unknown
Peak	4-6 hr
Duration	Unknown

INTERACTIONS

Drug classifications

β-agonists, Class IA antiarrhythmics (disopyramide, procainamide, quiNIDine), Class III antiarrhythmics (amiodarone, dofetilide, ibutilide, sotalol), halogenated anesthetics, local anesthetics, tricyclic antidepressants: increased QT prolongation, torsades de pointes

CYP3A4 inhibitors (ketoconazole, atazanavir, indinavir, itraconazole, nefazodone, nelfinavir, ritonavir, voriconazole, boceprevir, delavirdine, isoniazid, dalfopristin, quinupristin, tipranavir: increased crizotinib

CYP3A4 inducers (rifampin, carBAMazepine, PHENobarbital, phenytoin, rifabutin); antacids, H2-blockers, proton pump inhibitors (PPIs): decreased crizotinib

CYP3A4 substrates (alfentanil, cycloSPORINE, ergotamine, dihydroergotamine fentaNYL, sirolimus, colchicine): avoid concurrent use

Individual drugs

Abarelix, alfuzosin, amoxapine, apomorphine, arsenic trioxide, asenapine, chloroquine, ciprofloxacin, citalopram, clarithromycin, clozapine, cyclobenzaprine, dasatinib, dolasetron, dronedarone, droperidol, eribulin, erythromycin, ezogabine, flecainide, fluconazole, gatifloxacin, gemifloxacin, grepafloxacin, halofantrine, haloperidol, iloperidone, indacaterol, lapatinib, levofloxacin, levomethadyl, lopinavir/ritonavir, magnesium

sulfate, maprotiline, mefloquine, methadone, moxifloxacin, nilotinib, norfloxacin, octreotide, ofloxacin, olanzapine, ondansetron, paliperidone, palonosetron, pentamidine, certain phenothiazines (chlorpromazine, mesoridazine, thioridazine, fluphenazine, perphenazine, prochlorperazine, trifluoperazine), pimozide, posaconazole, potassium sulfate, probucol, propafenone, QUEtiapine, quiNIDine, ranolazine, rilpivirine, risperidone, saquinavir, sodium, sparfloxacin, sunitinib, tacrolimus, telavancin, telithromycin, tetrabenazine, troleandomycin, vardenafil, vemurafenib, venlafaxine, vorinostat, ziprasidone: increased QT prolongation, torsades de pointes
Midazolam: increased midazolam action

Drug/herb
Do not use with St. John's Wort

Drug/food
Do not use with grapefruit juice

NURSING CONSIDERATIONS

Assessment
• **Severe, life-threatening, or fatal treatment-related pneumonitis:** All cases occurred within 2 months of treatment initiation; monitor for pulmonary symptoms that may indicate pneumonitis and other causes of pneumonitis should be excluded; permanently discontinue in patients with treatment-related pneumonitis
• **Hepatic disease:** Liver function test (LFT) abnormalities, altered bilirubin levels, may occur during treatment; monitor LFTs and bilirubin levels prior to treatment, then monthly; more frequent testing is needed in those presenting with grade 2 or greater toxicities; Laboratory alterations should be managed with dose reduction, treatment interruption, or discontinuation
• **QT prolongation**: has been reported with the use of crizotinib; crizotinib should be avoided in these patients. Monitor ECG and electrolytes in those with CHF, bradycardia, electrolyte imbalance (hypokalemia, hypomagnesemia), or in those who are taking concomitant medications known to prolong the QT interval; treatment interruption, dosage adjustment, or treatment discontinuation may be needed in those who develop QT prolongation
• **Vision disorders:** Generally started within 2 weeks of the start of therapy; ophthalmologic evaluation should be considered, particularly if patients experience photopsia or new/ increased vitreous floaters; caution should be used when driving or operating machinery by patients who experience vision disorders
• **Pregnancy/breastfeeding:** Identify if pregnancy is planned or suspected; pregnancy category D, avoid breastfeeding

Nursing diagnoses
• Risk for injury (uses, adverse reactions)

Patient/family education
• Missed doses can be taken up to 6 hr before the next dose is due to maintain the twice daily regimen
• Teach patient to use reliable contraception; both women and men of childbearing age should use adequate contraceptive methods during therapy and for at least 90 days after completing treatment; pregnancy D
• Teach patient to report immediately shortness of breath, cough, fatigue

Evaluation
Positive therapeutic outcome
• Decreased spread of malignancy

---

cyclobenzaprine (Rx)
(sye-kloe-ben'za-preen)
Amrix, Apo-Cyclobenzaprine ✤, Fexmid, Flexeril, Gen Cyclobenzaprine ✤, PMS-Cyclobenzaprine ✤, ratio-Cyclobenzaprine ✤
Func. class.: Skeletal muscle relaxant, central acting
Chem. class.: Tricyclic amine salt
Pregnancy category B

Do not confuse:
cyclobenzaprine/cyproheptadine

ACTION: Reduction of tonic muscle activity at the brain stem; may be related to antidepressant effects

Therapeutic outcome: Relaxation of skeletal muscle

USES: Adjunct for relief of muscle spasm and pain in musculoskeletal conditions

Unlabeled uses: Fibromyalgia

CONTRAINDICATIONS:
Acute recovery phase of MI, dysrhythmias, heart block, CHF, hypersensitivity, child <12 yr, intermittent porphyria, thyroid disease

---

Adverse effects: *italics* = common; **bold** = life-threatening

Precautions: Pregnancy **B**, breastfeeding, geriatric, renal/hepatic disease, addictive personality

DOSAGE AND ROUTES
Musculoskeletal disorders
Adult/adolescent ≥15 yr: PO 5 mg tid × 1 wk, max 30 mg/day × 3 wk
Adult: EXT REL 15 mg q day, max 30 mg q day × 3 wk
Geriatric: PO 5 mg tid

Hepatic dose
Adult (mild hepatic disease): PO 5 mg, titrate slowly

Fibromyalgia (unlabeled)
Adult: PO 10 mg at bedtime, titrated up

Available forms: Tabs 5, 10 mg; ext rel tab 15, 30 mg

Implementation
• Give without regard to meals
• Store in airtight container at room temperature

ADVERSE EFFECTS
CNS: *Dizziness, weakness, drowsiness,* headache, tremor, depression, insomnia, confusion, paresthesia, nervousness
CV: Postural hypotension, tachycardia, **dysrhythmias**
EENT: Diplopia, temporary loss of vision
GI: *Nausea,* vomiting, hiccups, dry mouth, constipation, hepatitis
GU: Urinary retention, frequency, change in libido
INTEG: Rash, pruritus, fever, facial flushing, sweating

Pharmacokinetics
Distribution	Well
Metabolism	Liver, partially
Excretion	Kidney (unchanged)
Half-life	1-3 days

Pharmacodynamics
Onset	1 hr
Peak	3-8 hr
Duration	12-24 hr

INTERACTIONS
Individual drugs
Alcohol: increased CNS depression
Erythromycin, levaquin: increased QT interval
TraMADol: do not use within 14 days

Drug classifications
Antidepressants (tricyclic), barbiturates, opiates, sedative/hypnotics: increased CNS depression
MAOIs: do not use within 14 days

Drug/herb
Kava: increased CNS depression

NURSING CONSIDERATIONS
Assessment
• Assess pain periodically: location, duration, mobility, stiffness, baseline
• Monitor ECG in epileptic patients; poor seizure control has occurred in patients taking this product
• Check for allergic reactions: rash, fever, respiratory distress
• Check for severe weakness, numbness, in extremities
• Assess for CNS depression: dizziness, drowsiness, psychiatric symptoms

Nursing diagnoses
• Injury, risk for (adverse reactions)
• Knowledge, deficient (teaching)
• Mobility, impaired physical (uses)

Patient/family education
• Teach patient not to discontinue medication quickly; insomnia, nausea, headache, spasticity, tachycardia will occur; product should be tapered off over 1-2 wk
• Caution patient not to take with alcohol, other CNS depressants
• Advise to avoid altering activities while taking this product
• Caution patient to avoid hazardous activities if drowsiness/dizziness occurs
• Caution patient to avoid using OTC medication: cough preparations, antihistamines, unless directed by prescriber
• Teach patient to use gum, frequent sips of water for dry mouth

Evaluation
Positive therapeutic outcome
• Decreased pain, spasticity; muscle spasms of acute, painful musculoskeletal conditions are generally short term; long-term therapy is seldom warranted

TREATMENT OF OVERDOSE:
Empty stomach with emesis, gastric lavage, then administer activated charcoal; use anticonvulsants if indicated; monitor cardiac function

---

⚠ Nurse Alert

cyclopentolate ophthalmic
See Appendix B

⚠ HIGH ALERT

cyclophosphamide (Rx)
(sye-kloe-foss'fa-mide)
Cytoxan, Procytox ✤
Func. class.: Antineoplastic alkylating agent
Chem. class.: Nitrogen mustard
Pregnancy category D

Do not confuse:
cyclophosphamide/cycloSPORINE,
Cytoxan/Cytosar/Cytotec/Cytarabine

ACTION: Alkylates DNA; responsible for cross-linking DNA strands; activity is not cell cycle phase specific

Therapeutic outcome: Prevention of rapidly growing malignant cells

USES: Hodgkin's disease, lymphomas, leukemia, multiple myeloma, neuroblastoma, retinoblastoma, Ewing's sarcoma, cancer of female reproductive tract, breast, lung, prostate; disseminated neuroblastoma, nephrotic syndrome

CONTRAINDICATIONS:
Pregnancy **D,** breastfeeding, severely depressed bone marrow function, hypersensitivity, prostatic hypertrophy, bladder neck obstruction

Precautions: Radiation therapy, cardiac disease

DOSAGE AND ROUTES
Adult: PO initially 1-5 mg/kg over 2-5 days; maintenance 1-5 mg/kg; IV initially 40-50 mg/kg in divided doses over 2-5 days; maintenance 10-15 mg/kg q7-10days, or 3-5 mg/kg q3day
Child: PO/IV 2-8 mg/kg or 60-250 mg/m² in divided doses × 6 or more days; maintenance IV 10-15 mg/kg q7-10 days or 30 mg/kg q3-4wk; dose should be reduced by half when bone marrow suppression occurs

Neuroblastoma
Child and infant: PO 150 mg/m²/day, days 1-7 with DOXOrubicin (IV 35 mg/m² on day 5) q21days × 5 cycles
Child: IV 70 mg/kg/day with hydration on days 1 and 2 with DOXOrubicin and vinCRIStine q21days for courses 1, 2, 4, 6, alternating with

CISplatin and etoposide q21days for courses 3, 5, 7

Breast cancer
Adult: PO 100-200 mg/m²/day or 2 mg/kg/day × 4-14 days; IV 500-1000 mg/m² on day 1 in combination with fluorouracil and methotrexate or DOXOrubicin, or DOXOrubicin alone; also cyclophosphamide 600 mg/m², may be given dose-dense on day 1 of q14day with DOXOrubicin (60 mg/m²) with growth factor support

Operable node-positive breast cancer
IV (TAC regimen) Adult: 500 mg/m² with DOXOrubicin (50 mg/m² IV) then docetaxel (75 mg/m²) IV given 1 hr later × 6 cycles q3wk

Nephrotic syndrome
Adult: PO 2-3 mg/kg/day for up to 12 wk when corticosteroids are unsuccessful

Available forms: Inj IV 100, 200, 500 mg, 1, 2 g; tabs 25, 50 mg

Implementation
• Give fluids IV or PO before chemotherapy to hydrate patient
• Give antacid before oral agent, after PM meals, before bedtime; antiemetic 30-60 min before giving product to prevent vomiting and prn; antibiotics for prophylaxis of infection
• Give top or syst analgesics for pain; give in AM so product can be eliminated before bedtime

PO route
• To be taken on empty stomach; do not crush, break, chew tab
• May be taken as a single dose or divided doses
• Take in AM or afternoon, avoid evening

Intermittent IV infusion route
• Use cytotoxic handling procedures
• Give IV after diluting 100 mg/5 ml of sterile or bacteriostatic water; shake; let stand until clear; may be further diluted in up to 250 ml D₅ 0.9% NaCl, 0.45% NaCl, LR, Ringer's; give 100 mg or less/min through 3-way stopcock of glucose or saline inf
• Use 21-, 23-, or 25-G needle; check site for irritation, phlebitis

Syringe compatibilities: Bleomycin, CISplatin, doxapram, DOXOrubicin, droperidol, fluorouracil, furosemide, heparin, leucovorin, methotrexate, metoclopramide, mitomycin, mitoxantrone, vinBLAStine, vinCRIStine

Y-site compatibilities: Amifostine, amikacin, ampicillin, azlocillin, aztreonam, bleomycin, cefamandole, ceFAZolin, cefepime,

C

Adverse effects: *italics* = common; **bold** = life-threatening

cefoperazone, cefotaxime, cefoxitin, cefuroxime, cephalothin, cephapirin, chloramphenicol, chlorproMAZINE, cimetidine, CISplatin, cladribine, clindamycin, dexamethasone, diphenhydrAMINE, DOXOrubicin, doxycycline, droperidol, erythromycin, famotidine, filgrastim, fludarabine, fluorouracil, furosemide, gallium, ganciclovir, gentamicin, granisetron, heparin, HYDROmorphone, IDArubicin, kanamycin, leucovorin, LORazepam, melphalan, methotrexate, methylPREDNISolone, metoclopramide, metroNIDAZOLE, mezlocillin, minocycline, mitomycin, moxalactam, nafcillin, ondansetron, oxacillin, paclitaxel, penicillin G potassium, piperacillin, piperacillin/tazobactam, prochlorperazine, promethazine, propofol, ranitidine, sargramostim, sodium bicarbonate, teniposide, tetracycline, thiotepa, ticarcillin, ticarcillin-clavulanate, tobramycin, trimethoprim-sulfamethoxazole, vancomycin, vinBLAStine, vinCRIStine, vinorelbine

Solution compatibilities: Amino acids 4.25%/D_{25}, D_5/0.9% NaCl, D_5W, 0.9% NaCl

ADVERSE EFFECTS
CNS: Headache, dizziness
CV: Cardiotoxicity (high doses), myocardial fibrosis
ENDO: Syndrome of inappropriate antidiuretic hormone (SIADH), gonadal suppression
GI: *Nausea, vomiting, diarrhea, weight loss,* colitis, **hepatotoxicity**
GU: Hemorrhagic cystitis, hematuria, neoplasms, amenorrhea, azoospermia, sterility, ovarian fibrosis
HEMA: Thrombocytopenia, leukopenia, pancytopenia, myelosuppression
INTEG: *Alopecia,* dermatitis
META: Hyperuricemia
MISC: Secondary neoplasms, **anaphylaxis**
RESP: Pulmonary fibrosis, interstitial pneumonia

Pharmacokinetics
Absorption	Well absorbed (PO)
Distribution	Widely distributed; crosses placenta, blood-brain barrier (50%)
Metabolism	Liver to active product
Excretion	Kidneys, unchanged (30%)
Half-life	4-6$^1/_2$ hr

Pharmacodynamics
Unknown

INTERACTIONS
Individual drugs
Allopurinol: increased bone marrow suppression
Chloramphenicol: decreased cyclophosphamide effect
Digoxin: decreased digoxin levels
Insulin: increased hypoglycemia
Succinylcholine: increased neuromuscular blockade
Warfarin: increased warfarin action

Drug classifications
Diuretics (thiazides): increased bone marrow suppression
Barbiturates: increased toxicity of cyclophosphamide
Corticosteroids: decreased cyclophosphamide effect
Live virus vaccines: decreased antibody reaction

Drug/herb
St. John's wort: increased toxicity

Drug/lab test
Increased: uric acid
Decreased: pseudocholinesterase
False positive: Pap smear
False negative: PPD, mumps trichophytin, *Candida*, *Trichophyton*, Pap smear

NURSING CONSIDERATIONS
Assessment
⚠ **Assess symptoms indicating severe allergic reaction: rash, pruritus, urticaria, purpuric skin lesions, itching, flushing**
• Assess for tachypnea, ECG changes, dyspnea, edema, fatigue
• **Bone marrow suppression:** Monitor CBC, differential, platelet count weekly; withhold product if WBC count is <2500/mm³ or platelet count is <75,000/mm³; notify prescriber of results
• Assess for **hemorrhagic cystitis:** renal function studies including BUN, creatinine, serum uric acid, urine CCr before, during therapy; I&O ratio; report fall in urine output to <30 ml/hr
• Monitor temp q4hr (elevated temp may indicate beginning of infection)
• **Hepatotoxicity:** Monitor liver function tests before, during therapy (bilirubin, AST, ALT, LDH) as needed or monthly; note jaundice of skin or sclera, dark urine, clay-colored stools, itchy skin, abdominal pain, fever, diarrhea
• Assess for **bleeding:** hematuria, stool guaiac, bruising or petechiae, mucosa or orifices q8hr

• Identify dyspnea, crackles, unproductive cough, chest pain, tachypnea
• Identify effects of alopecia on body image; discuss feelings about body changes

Nursing diagnoses
• Body image, disturbed (adverse reactions)
• Infection, risk for (adverse reactions)
• Injury, risk for (adverse reactions)
• Knowledge, deficient (teaching)

Patient/family education
• Teach patient to avoid use of products containing aspirin or ibuprofen, razors, commercial mouthwash, since bleeding may occur; to report symptoms of bleeding (hematuria, tarry stools, bruising)
• Instruct patient to report signs of anemia (fatigue, headache, irritability, faintness, shortness of breath)
• Teach patient to report any changes in breathing or coughing even several months after treatment
• Advise patient that hair may be lost during treatment; a wig or hairpiece may make patient feel better; new hair may be different in color, texture
• Teach patient not to have any vaccinations without the advice of the prescriber; serious reactions can occur
• Advise patient contraception is needed during treatment and for several months after the completion of therapy

Evaluation
Positive therapeutic outcome
• Prevention of rapid division of malignant cells
• Increased appetite, increased weight

---

cycloSPORINE (Rx)
(sye-kloe-spor'een)
Gengraf, Neoral, Pulminiq, Sandimmune
Func. class.: Immunosuppressant
Chem. class.: Fungus-derived peptide
Pregnancy category C

Do not confuse:
cycloSPORINE/CycloSERINE/cyclophosphamide

ACTION: Produces immunosuppression by inhibiting T lymphocytes

Therapeutic outcome: Absence of transplant rejection

USES: Organ transplants (liver, kidney, heart) to prevent rejection, rheumatoid arthritis, psoriasis

Unlabeled uses: Recalcitrant ulcerative colitis, aplastic anemia, Crohn's disease, GVHD, thrombocytopenia purpura, lupus, nephritis, myasthenia gravis, psoriatic arthritis

CONTRAINDICATIONS:
Hypersensitivity to polyxyethylated castor oil (inj only), psoriasis or rheumatoid arthrits in renal disease (Neoral/Gengraf), Gengraf/Neoral used with PUVA/UVB; methotrexate, coal tar, breastfeeding, ocular infections

> **BLACK BOX WARNING:** Neoplastic disease, sunlight (UV) exposure, renal disease/failure, uncontrolled, malignant hypertension; radiation in psoriasis

Precautions: Pregnancy **C**, geriatric, severe renal/hepatic disease

DOSAGE AND ROUTES
Prevention of transplant rejection (unmodified)
Adult and child: PO 15 mg/kg several hr before surgery, daily for 2 wk, reduce dosage by 2.5 mg/kg/wk to 5-10 mg/kg/day; **IV** 5-6 mg/kg several hr before surgery, daily, switch to PO form as soon as possible

Prevention of transplant rejection (modified)
Adult and child: PO 4-12 mg/kg/day divided q12hr, depends on organ transplanted

Rheumatoid arthritis (Neoral/Gengraf)
Adult: PO 2.5 mg/kg/day divided bid, may increase 0.5-0.75 mg/kg/day after 8-12 wk, max 4 mg/kg/day

Psoriasis (Neoral/Gengraf)
Adult: PO 2.5 mg/kg/day divided bid × 4 wk, then increase by 0.5 mg/kg/day q2wk, max 4 mg/kg/day

Idiopathic thrombocytopenia purpura (unlabeled)
Adult: PO 1.25-2.5 mg/kg bid

Severe aplastic anemia (unlabeled)
Adult and child: PO 12 mg/kg/day or 15 mg/kg/day (child) with antithymocyte globulin (ATG)

Available forms: Oral sol (Neoral) 100 mg/ml; soft gel cap 25, 50, 100 mg; inj 50 mg/ml; inh sol 300 mg/4.8 ml

Implementation
PO route
- Do not break, crush, or chew caps
- Use pipette provided to draw up oral sol; may mix with milk or juice, wipe pipette, do not wash
- Give for several days before transplant surgery with corticosteroids
- Microemulsion products (Neoral) and other products are not interchangeable
- Give with meals for GI upset or place product in chocolate milk
- Give with oral antifungal for *Candida* infections

Intermittent IV infusion route
- Give **IV** after diluting each 50 mg/20-100 ml of 0.9% NaCl or D₅W; run over 2-6 hr; use an inf pump, glass inf bottles only

Continuous IV infusion route
- May run over 24 hr
- **For Sandimmune parenteral:** give 1/3 of PO dose, initial dose 4-12 hr prior to transplantation as a single **IV** dose 5-6 mg/kg/day, continue the single daily dose until PO can be used

Additive compatibilities: Ciprofloxacin

Y-site compatibilities: Abciximab, alatrofloxacin, alfentanil, amikacin, aminocaproic acid, aminophylline, amphotericin B lipid complex, anidulafungin, argatroban, ascorbic acid injection, atenolol, atracurium, atropine, azaTHIOprine, aztreonam, benztropine, bivalirudin, bleomycin, bretylium, bumetanide, buprenorphine, butorphanol, calcium chloride/gluconate, CARBOplatin, carmustine, caspofungin, cefamandole, ceFAZolin, cefmetazole, cefonicid, cefoperazone, cefotaxime, cefotetan, cefoxitin, ceftaroline, ceftazidime, ceftizoxime, ceftobiprole, cefTRIAXone, cefuroxime, cephalothin, cephapirin, chloramphenicol, chlorproMAZINE, cimetidine, ciprofloxacin, CISplatin, clindamycin, codeine, cyanocobalamin, cyclophosphamide, cytarabine, DACTINomycin, DAPTOmycin, DAUNOrubicin, dexamethasone, dexmedetomidine, digoxin, diltiazem, diphenhydrAMINE, DOBUTamine, docetaxel, DOPamine, doripenem, doxacurium, DOXOrubicin, doxycycline, enalaprilat, ePHEDrine, EPINEPHrine, epirubicin, epoetin alfa, eptifibatide, ertapenem, erythromycin, esmolol, etoposide, famotidine, fenoldopam, fentaNYL, fluconazole, fludarabine, fluorouracil, folic acid, furosemide, gallium, ganciclovir, gatifloxacin, gemcitabine, gentamicin, glycopyrrolate, granisetron, heparin, hydrocortisone, HYDROmorphone, hydrOXYzine, ifosfamide, imipenem-cilastatin, indomethacin, irinotecan, isoproterenol, ketorolac, labetalol, lansoprazole, levofloxacin, lidocaine, linezolid, LORazepam, mannitol, mechlorethamine, meperidine, meropenem, methicillin, methotrexate, methoxamine, methyldopate, methylPREDNISolone, metoclopramide, metoprolol, metroNIDAZOLE, mezlocillin, micafungin, miconazole, midazolam, milrinone, minocycline, mitoxantrone, morphine, moxalactam, multiple vitamins injection, nafcillin, naloxone, nesiritide, netilmicin, nitroglycerin, nitroprusside, norepinephrine, octreotide, ondansetron, oxacillin, oxaliplatin, oxytocin, paclitaxel, palonosetron, pamidronate, pancuronium, pantoprazole, papaverine, pemetrexed, penicillin G potassium/sodium, pentamidine, pentazocine, phentolamine, phenylephrine, phytonadione, piperacillin, piperacillin-tazobactam, polymyxin B, potassium acetate/chloride, procainamide, prochlorperazine, promethazine, propofol, propranolol, protamine, pyridoxine, quiNIDine, quinupristin-dalfopristin, ranitidine, ritodrine, sargramostim, sodium acetate/bicarbonate, succinylcholine, SUFentanil, tacrolimus, teniposide, theophylline, thiamine, thiotepa, ticarcillin, ticarcillin-clavulanate, tigecycline, tirofiban, tobramycin, trimetaphan, urokinase, vancomycin, vasopressin, vecuronium, verapamil, vinCRIStine, vinorelbine, zoledronic acid

Solution compatibilities: D₅W, NaCl 0.9%

ADVERSE EFFECTS
CNS: *Tremors, headache,* **seizures,** confusion
GI: Nausea, vomiting, diarrhea, *oral candida, gum hyperplasia,* **hepatotoxicity,** pancreatitis
GU: **Albuminuria, hematuria, proteinuria, renal failure**
INTEG: Rash, acne, *hirsutism,* pruritus
META: Hyperkalemia, hypomagnesemia, hyperlipidemia, hyperuricemia
MISC: *Infection, hypertension*

Pharmacokinetics

Absorption	Poorly absorbed (PO)
Distribution	Crosses placenta
Metabolism	Liver to mercaptopurine
Excretion	Kidney, minimal
Half-life	Biphasic 1.2 hr, 25 hr

Pharmacodynamics

	PO
Onset	Unknown
Peak	4 hr
Duration	Unknown

INTERACTIONS

Individual drugs

Allopurinol, amiodarone, amphotericin B, bromocriptine, carvedilol, cimetidine, colchicine, foscarnet, imipenem-cilastatin, melphalan, metoclopramide: increased action, cycloSPORINE toxicity

Digoxin: increased digoxin level

Etoposide: increased etoposide level

Methotrexate: increased methotrexate level

Nafcillin, orlistat, phenobarbital, phenytoin, terbinafine, ticlopidine, trimethoprim/sulfamethoxazole: decreased cycloSPORINE action

Sirolimus: increased sirolimus level

Tacrolimus: increased tacrolimus level

Drug classifications:

Androgens, antifungals (azole), β-blockers, calcium channel blockers, contraceptives (oral), corticosteroids, fluoroquinolones, macrolides, NSAIDs, selective serotonin reuptake inhibitors: increased cycloSPORINE levels, toxicity

Anticonvulsants, rifamycins: decreased cycloSPORINE levels

HMG-CoA reductase inhibitors, diuretics (potassium-sparing): increased effects of each product

Live virus vaccines: decreased antibody reaction

Drug/food

Grapefruit juice, food: increased slowed metabolism of product

NURSING CONSIDERATIONS

Assessment

• **Encephalopathy:** Assess for impaired cognition, seizures, vision changes including blindness, loss of motor function, movement disorders, psychiatric changes; dosage reduction or discontinuation may be needed in severe cases

• Monitor renal studies: BUN, creatinine at least monthly during treatment, 3 mo after treatment

• Monitor liver function studies: alkaline phosphatase, AST, ALT, bilirubin

• Monitor product blood levels during treatment

• Assess for **hepatotoxicity:** dark urine, jaundice, itching, light-colored stools; product should be discontinued

• Assess for **nephrotoxicity:** 6 wk postop, CyA trough level >200 ng/ml, intracapsular pressure <40 mm Hg, rise in creatinine 0.15 mg/dl/day

Nursing diagnoses

• Infection, risk for (uses)
• Knowledge, deficient (teaching)
• Mobility, impaired physical (uses)

Patient/family education

• Advise patient to report fever, rash, severe diarrhea, chills, sore throat, fatigue, since serious infections may occur; also to report clay-colored stools, cramping (may indicate hepatotoxicity); tremors, bleeding gums, increased B/P

> **BLACK BOX WARNING:** Advise patient to limit UV exposure

• Caution patient to use contraceptive measures during treatment and for 12 wk after ending therapy; product is teratogenic, to notify prescriber if pregnancy is planned or suspected

• Caution patient to avoid crowds and persons with known infections to reduce risk of infection

• Teach patient to take at the same time of day, every day; do not skip or double a missed dose; not to use with grapefruit juice or receive vaccines; there are many drug interactions, do not add or discontinue products without prescriber approval

• Teach patient that treatment is lifelong to prevent rejection; to identify signs of rejection

• Advise patient to report severe diarrhea as drug loss may result

• **Nephrotoxicity:** Teach patient to notify prescriber of increased B/P, tremors of the hands, change in gums, increased hair on body/face

• Advise patient to continue with lab work and follow-up appointment

• Teach patient types of products are not interchangeable

Evaluation

Positive therapeutic outcome

• Absence of graft rejection

cyproheptadine (Rx)

(si-proe-hep'ta-deen)

PMS-Cyproheptadine

Func. class.: Antihistamine, H_1-receptor antagonist

Chem. class.: Piperidine

Pregnancy category B

Do not confuse:
cyproheptadine/cyclobenzaprine

ACTION: Acts on blood vessels, GI, respiratory system by competing with histamine for H_1-receptor site; decreases allergic response by blocking histamine

Therapeutic outcome: Absence of allergy symptoms and rhinitis

USES: Allergy symptoms, rhinitis, pruritus, common cold, urticaria

Unlabeled uses: Appetite stimulant, management of vascular headache, nightmares, posttraumatic stress disorder

CONTRAINDICATIONS:
Breastfeeding, hypersensitivity to H_1-receptor antagonist, closed-angle glaucoma, peptic ulcers, bladder neck obstruction, prostatic hypertrophy, neonates/infants

Precautions: Pregnancy **B**, cardiac disease, geriatric patients, asthma, ileus, urinary retention, COPD

DOSAGE AND ROUTES
Adult: PO 4 mg tid-qid, max 0.5 mg/kg/day
Geriatric: PO 4 mg bid, may increase if needed
Child 6-14 yr: PO 4 mg bid-tid, max 16 mg/day
Child 2-6 yr: PO 2 mg bid-tid, max 12 mg/day

Available forms: Tabs 4 mg; syr 2 mg/5 ml

Implementation
• May give with food to decrease GI upset
• Syrup may be used for patients with difficulty swallowing or children
• Store in tight, light-resistant container

ADVERSE EFFECTS
CNS: *Dizziness, drowsiness,* poor coordination, fatigue, anxiety, euphoria, confusion, paresthesia, neuritis
CV: Hypotension, palpitations, tachycardia
EENT: *Blurred vision,* dilated pupils; tinnitus; nasal stuffiness; dry nose, throat, mouth

GI: *Constipation, dry mouth,* nausea, vomiting, anorexia, diarrhea, weight gain, increased appetite
GU: *Urinary retention,* dysuria, urinary frequency
HEMA: Hemolytic anemia, leukopenia, thrombocytosis, agranulocytosis
INTEG: Rash, urticaria, photosensitivity
MISC: Anaphylaxis
RESP: Increased thick secretions, wheezing, chest tightness

Pharmacokinetics

Absorption	Well absorbed
Distribution	Unknown
Metabolism	Liver, complete
Excretion	Urine (65%-75%); feces (25%-35%)
Half-life	Unknown

Pharmacodynamics

Onset	15-60 min
Peak	1-2 hr
Duration	8 hr

INTERACTIONS

Individual drugs
Alcohol: increased CNS depression

Drug classifications
Antidepressants (tricyclics), barbiturates, CNS depressants, opiates, sedative/hypnotics: increased CNS depression
MAOIs: increased anticholinergic effect

Drug/herb
Corkwood, henbane leaf: increased anticholinergic effect
Hops, Jamaican dogwood, kava, khat, senega: increased CNS depression

Drug/lab test
False negative: skin allergy tests (discontinue antihistamine 3 days before testing)

NURSING CONSIDERATIONS
Assessment
• Assess respiratory status: rate, rhythm, increase in bronchial secretions, wheezing, chest tightness; provide fluids to 2 L/day to decrease secretion thickness
• Monitor I&O ratio: be alert for urinary retention, frequency, dysuria, especially geriatric; product should be discontinued if these occur; monitor food intake, weight if using as an appetite stimulant

Nursing diagnoses
• Airway clearance, ineffective (uses)
• Injury, risk for (side effects)
• Knowledge, deficient (teaching)
• Noncompliance (teaching, overuse)

Patient/family education
• Teach all aspects of product uses; tell patient to notify prescriber if confusion, sedation, hypotension occur; to avoid driving and other hazardous activity if drowsiness occurs; to avoid alcohol and other CNS depressants that may potentiate effect
• Caution patient not to exceed recommended dosage; dysrhythmias may occur
• Teach patient hard candy, gum, frequent rinsing of mouth may be used for dryness
• Advise patient to avoid breastfeeding

Evaluation
Positive therapeutic outcome
• Absence of runny or congested nose, rashes

TREATMENT OF OVERDOSE:
Administer lavage, diazepam, vasopressors, phenytoin IV

⚠ HIGH ALERT

cytarabine (Rx)
(sye-tare'a-been)
Ara-C, Cytosar ✤, Cytosar-U

cytarabine liposomal (Rx)
Depo Cyt
Func. class.: Antineoplastic, antimetabolite
Chem. class.: Pyrimidine nucleoside
Pregnancy category D

Do not confuse:
Cytosar ✤/Cytovene/Cytoxan

ACTION: Competes with physiologic substrate of DNA synthesis, thus interfering with cell replication in the S phase of the cell cycle (before mitosis)

Therapeutic outcome: Prevention of rapidly growing malignant cells

USES: Acute myelocytic leukemia, acute lymphocytic leukemia, chronic myelocytic leukemia, lymphomatous meningitis (IT/intraventricular)

Unlabeled uses: Hodgkin's/non-Hodgkin's lymphoma

CONTRAINDICATIONS:
Pregnancy **D**, hypersensitivity

Precautions: Renal/hepatic disease, breastfeeding, children, tumor lysis syndrome, infection, hyperkalemia, hyperphosphatemia, hyperuricemia, hypocalcemia

BLACK BOX WARNING: Bone marrow suppression

DOSAGE AND ROUTES
Acute myelogenous leukemia (AML)
Adult: cont **IV** infusion 100 mg/m²/day × 7 days q2 wk as a single agent or 2-3 divided doses × 5-10 days until remission used in combination; maintenance 70-200 mg/m²/day × 2-5 days qmo; **SUBCUT** maintenance 100 mg/m²/day × 5 days q28days

Meningeal leukemia
Adult and child: Intrathecal 5-70 mg/m² variable daily × 4 days to q2-7day

Carcinomatous meningitis (liposoma)
Adult: Intrathecal 50 mg over 1-5 min q14days, during induction and consolidation wk 1, 3, 5, 7, 9, give another 50 mg wk 13; maintenance 50 mg q28days on wk 17, 21, 25, 29 use with dexamethasone 4 mg PO/IV × 5 days on each day of cytarabine

Renal dose
Adult CCr ≤60 ml/min, serum creatinine 1.5-1.9 mg/dl or increase of 0.5-1.2 mg/dl from baseline: during treatment reduce to 1 g/m²/dose; **serum creatinine ≥2 mg/dl or change from baseline serum creatinine was 1.2 mg/dl** reduce to 100 mg/m²/day

Available forms: Powder for inj 100, 500 mg, 1, 2 g; sus rel (Depo Cyt) liposomal for intrathecal use 10 mg/ml

Implementation
• Avoid contact with skin; very irritating; wash completely to remove
• Give fluids **IV** or PO before chemotherapy to hydrate patient
• Give antiemetic 30-60 min before giving product to prevent vomiting, and prn; antibiotics for prophylaxis of infection
• Increase fluids to 3 L/day
• Give top or syst analgesics for pain
• Give in AM so product can be eliminated before bedtime
• Use cytotoxic handling precautions

IM/SUBCUT route
- **Reconstitute** 100 mg/5 ml or 500 mg/10 ml with bacteriostatic water for inj with benzyl alcohol 0.9%; do not use sol with precipitate; stable for 48 hr

Intrathecal route
- **Liposomal: withdraw** product immediately before use; **use** within 4 hr, do not save unused portions or use in-line filter; **give** directly into CSF by intraventricular reservoir or by direct inj into lumbar site
- **Give** slowly over 1-5 min; follow with lumbar puncture; instruct patient to lie flat; **give** dexamethasone 4 mg bid PO or **IV** × 5 days beginning on day of liposomal inj

Direct IV route
- **Dilute** 100 mg/5 ml of sterile water for inj, **give** over 1-3 min through a free-flowing IV

Intermittent IV infusion route
- May be further diluted in 50-100 ml NS or D$_5$W and **give** over 30 min-24 hr, depending on dose

Continuous IV infusion route
- May be given as continuous IV infusion

Syringe compatibilities: Metoclopramide

Y-site compatibilities: Acyclovir, alfentanil, amifostine, amikacin, aminocaproic acid, aminophylline, amphotericin B lipid complex, amphotericin B liposome, ampicillin, ampicillin-sulbactam, amsacrine, anidulafungin, atenolol, atracurium, azithromycin, aztreonam, bivalirudin, bleomycin, bumetanide, buprenorphine, butorphanol, calcium chloride/gluconate, CARBOplatin, ceFAZolin, cefepime, cefoperazone, cefotaxime, cefotetan, cefoxitin, ceftazidime, ceftizoxime, cefTRIAXone, cefuroxime, chlorproMAZINE, cimetidine, ciprofloxacin, cisatracurium, CISplatin, cladribine, clindamycin, codeine, cyclophosphamide, cycloSPORINE, DAUNOrubicin, dexamethasone, dexmedetomidine, dexrazoxane, digoxin, diltiazem, diphenhydrAMINE, DOBUTamine, docetaxel, dolasetron, DOPamine, doxacurium, DOXOrubicin, DOXOrubicin liposomal, doxycycline, droperidol, enalaprilat, ePHEDrine, EPINEPHrine, ertapenem, erythromycin, esmolol, etoposide, famotidine, fenoldopam, fentaNYL, filgrastim, fluconazole, fludarabine, foscarnet, fosphenytoin, furosemide, gatifloxacin, gemcitabine, gemtuzumab, gentamicin, granisetron, haloperidol, heparin, hydrocortisone, HYDROmorphone, hydrOXYzine, IDArubicin, ifosfamide, imipenem-cilastatin, inamrinone, insulin (regular), irinotecan, isoproterenol, ketorolac, labetalol, leucovorin, levofloxacin, levorphanol, lidocaine, linezolid, LORazepam, magnesium sulfate, mannitol, melphalan, meperidine, meropenem, mesna, methohexital, methotrexate, methyl-PREDNISolone, metoclopramide, metoprolol, metroNIDAZOLE, midazolam, milrinone, minocycline, mitoxantrone, mivacurium, morphine, nalbuphine, naloxone, nesiritide, niCARdipine, nitroglycerin, nitroprusside, norepinephrine, octreotide, ofloxacin, ondansetron, oxaliplatin, paclitaxel, palonosetron, pamidronate, pancuronium, pantoprazole, pemetrexed, pentamidine, PENTobarbital, PHENobarbital, phenylephrine, piperacillin, piperacillin-tazobactam, potassium chloride/phosphates, procainamide, prochlorperazine, promethazine, propofol, propranolol, quinupristin-dalfopristin, ranitidine, rapacuronium, remifentanil, riTUXimab, rocuronium, sargramostim, sodium acetate/bicarbonate/phosphates, succinylcholine, SUFentanil, sulfamethoxazole-trimethoprim, tacrolimus, teniposide, theophylline, thiopental, thiotepa, ticarcillin, ticarcillin-clavulanate, tigecycline, tirofiban, TNA, tobramycin, trastuzumab, trimethobenzamide, vancomycin, vasopressin, vecuronium, verapamil, vinCRIStine, vinorelbine, voriconazole, zidovudine, zoledronic acid

Additive compatibilities: Corticotropin, DAUNOrubicin with etoposide, etoposide, hydrOXYzine, lincomycin, mitoxantrone, potassium chloride, prednisoLONE, ondansetron, sodium bicarbonate, vinCRIStine

Additive incompatibilities: Carbenicillin, fluorouracil, heparin, regular insulin, nafcillin, oxacillin, penicillin G sodium

Solution compatibilities: Amino acids, 4.25%/D$_{25}$, D$_5$/LR, D$_5$/0.2% NaCl, D$_5$/0.9% NaCl, D$_{10}$/0.9% NaCl, D$_5$W, invert glucose 10% in electrolyte #1, Ringer's LR, 0.9% NaCl, sodium lactate 1/6 mol/L, TPN #57

ADVERSE EFFECTS

CNS: Neuritis, dizziness, headache, cerebellar syndrome, personality changes, ataxia, mechanical dysphasia, **coma; chemical arachnoiditis** (IT)

CV: Chest pain, **cardiopathy**

CYTARABINE SYNDROME: Fever, myalgia, bone pain, chest pain, rash, conjunctivitis, malaise (6-12 hr after administration)

EENT: Sore throat, conjunctivitis

GI: *Nausea, vomiting, anorexia, diarrhea, stomatitis,* **hepatotoxicity,** abdominal pain, hematemesis, **GI hemorrhage**

⚠ Nurse Alert

C

gism, CSF pleocytosis;
y dexamethasone
yspnea, edema, fatigue;
kles, unproductive cough,
pulmonary edema may be

bine syndrome 6-12 hr
, myalgia, bone pain,
njunctivitis, malaise;
be ordered
ppression: Monitor CBC,
ount weekly; withhold
is <1000/mm³ or platelet
n³
d uric acid levels, swell-
ily in extremities; patient
ed to prevent urate depos-

tion studies: BUN, creati-
, urine CCr before and dur-
; report fall in urine output

(may indicate beginning

Monitor liver function tests
erapy (bilirubin, AST, ALT,
LDH) as needed or monthly; note yellowing of skin or sclera, dark urine, clay-colored stools, pruritus, abdominal pain, fever, diarrhea; an antispasmodic may be used for GI symptoms

• Assess for bleeding: hematuria, stool guaiac, bruising or petechiae, mucosa or orifices q8hr; identify inflammation of mucosa, breaks in skin

Individual drugs

Digoxin oral: decreased digoxin effects
Filgrastim, G-CSF, GM-CSF, sargramostim: do not use within 24 hr
Flucytosine, methotrexate: increased toxicity, immunosuppression
Gentamicin: decreased effects
Radiation: increased toxicity, bone marrow suppression

Drug classifications

Anticoagulants, NSAIDs, platelet inhibitors, salicylates, thrombolytics: increased bleeding risk
Immunosuppressants, antineoplastics: increased toxicity, bone marrow suppression
Live virus vaccines: do not use together

NURSING CONSIDERATIONS

Assessment

• Assess buccal cavity q8hr for dryness, sores or ulceration, white patches, pain, bleeding, dysphagia; obtain prescription for viscous lidocaine (Xylocaine)
• Assess symptoms indicating **anaphylaxis:** rash, pruritus, urticaria, purpuric skin lesions, itching, flushing; resuscitation equipment should be nearby
A Assess for chemical arachnoiditis (IT): headache, nausea, vomiting, fever; neck

Nursing diagnoses

• Body image, disturbed (adverse reactions)
• Infection, risk for (adverse reactions)
• Injury, risk for (adverse reactions)
• Knowledge, deficient (teaching)

Patient/family education

• Advise patient that contraceptive measures are recommended during and 4 mo after therapy
• Teach patient to avoid use of products containing aspirin or ibuprofen, NSAIDs, razors, commercial mouthwash, since bleeding may occur; to report symptoms of bleeding (hematuria, tarry stools)
• Advise that fever, headache, nausea, vomiting are likely to occur but to continue using dexamethasone with IT administration
• Provide liquid diet: carbonated beverages; gelatin may be added if patient is not nauseated or vomiting
• Provide rinsing of mouth tid-qid with water, club soda; brushing of teeth bid-qid with soft brush or cotton-tipped applicators for stomatitis; use unwaxed dental floss

• Advise patient to report signs of anemia (fatigue, headache, irritability, faintness, shortness of breath)

• Advise patient to avoid foods with citric acid, hot flavor, or rough texture if stomatitis is present, to use sponge brush and rinse with water after each meal; to report stomatitis: any bleeding, white spots, ulcerations in mouth; tell patient to examine mouth daily, report any symptoms

• Instruct patient to report any changes in breathing or coughing even several months after treatment; to avoid crowds and persons with respiratory tract or other infections; neurotoxicity

• Caution patient not to have any vaccinations without the advice of the prescriber; serious reactions can occur

• Advise patient to take 3 L/day fluids to prevent renal damage

Evaluation
Positive therapeutic outcome
• Prevention of rapid division of malignant cells

dabigatran (Rx)
(da-bye-gat'ran)
Pradaxa
Func. class.: Anticoagulant-thrombin inhibitor
Pregnancy category C

ACTION: Direct thrombin inhibitor that inhibits both free and clot-bound thrombin, prevents thrombin-induced platelet aggregation and thrombus formation by preventing conversion of fibrinogen to fibrin

Therapeutic outcome: Decreased thrombus formation/extension, absence of emboli, post-thrombotic effects

USES: Stroke/systemic embolism prophylaxis with non-valvular atrial fibrillation

CONTRAINDICATIONS:
Hypersensitivity, bleeding

Precautions: Abrupt discontinuation, anticoagulant therapy, breastfeeding, pregnancy C, children, geriatrics, labor, obstetric delivery, renal disease, surgery

DOSAGE AND ROUTES
Stroke prophylaxis
Adult: PO 150 mg bid

For conversion from an alternative anticoagulant to dabigatran
• When converting from warfarin to dabigatran, discontinue warfarin and initiate dabigatran therapy when the INR is <2.0. When converting from a parenteral anticoagulant to dabigatran, initiate dabigatran 0-2 hr before the time of the next scheduled anticoagulant dose or at the time of discontinuation of a continuously administered anticoagulant (e.g., intravenous unfractionated heparin)

For conversion from dabigatran to warfarin
Adult: CCr >50 ml/min start warfarin 3 days before discontinuing dabigatran; CCr 31-50 ml/min start warfarin 2 days before discontinuing dabigatran; CCr 15-30 ml/min start warfarin 1 day before discontinuing dabigatran

For conversion from dabigatran to parenteral anticoagulants
Adult: PO discontinue dabigatran, start parenteral anticoagulant 12 hr (CCR ≥30 ml/min), 24 hr (CCR <30 ml/min) after the last dabigatran dose

Renal dose
Adult: PO CCr 15-30 ml/min 75 mg bid

Deep vein thrombus (DVT)/pulmonary embolism prophylaxis (unlabeled)
Adult: PO 220 mg or 150 mg q day × 28-35 days, starting with ½ dose 1-4 hr after surgery

Available forms: Cap 75, 150 mg

Implementation
• Do not crush break, chew, or empty contents of capsule

• If dose is missed take as soon as remembered if on the same day, do not administer if <6 hr before next dose

• Take without regard to food

• Store in original package until time of use at room temperature, discard after 30 days, protect from moisture

ADVERSE EFFECTS
CV: Myocardial infarction
CNS: Intracranial bleeding
GI: Abdominal pain, dyspepsia, peptic ulcer, esophagitis, GERD, gastritis, **GI bleeding**
HEMA: Bleeding
INTEG: Rash, pruritus
SYST: Anaphylaxis (rare)

GU: Urinary retention, renal failure, hyperuricemia
HEMA: Thrombophlebitis, bleeding, thrombocytopenia, leukopenia, myelosuppression, anemia
INTEG: *Rash, fever,* freckling, cellulitis
META: Hyperuricemia
RESP: Pneumonia, dyspnea, pulmonary edema (high doses)
SYST: Anaphylaxis

Pharmacokinetics

Absorption	Complete
Distribution	Widely distributed; crosses blood-brain barrier, placenta
Metabolism	Liver, extensively
Excretion	Kidneys
Half-life	Distribution 10 min; elimination 1-3 hr; IT 100-236 hr

Pharmacodynamics

Unknown

INTERACTIONS

Individual drugs

Digoxin oral: decreased digoxin effects
Filgrastim, G-CSF, GM-CSF, sargramostim: do not use within 24 hr
Flucytosine, methotrexate: increased toxicity, immunosuppression
Gentamicin: decreased effects
Radiation: increased toxicity, bone marrow suppression

Drug classifications

Anticoagulants, NSAIDs, platelet inhibitors, salicylates, thrombolytics: increased bleeding risk
Immunosuppressants, antineoplastics: increased toxicity, bone marrow suppression
Live virus vaccines: do not use together

NURSING CONSIDERATIONS

Assessment

• Assess buccal cavity q8hr for dryness, sores or ulceration, white patches, pain, bleeding, dysphagia; obtain prescription for viscous lidocaine (Xylocaine)
• Assess symptoms indicating **anaphylaxis:** rash, pruritus, urticaria, purpuric skin lesions, itching, flushing; resuscitation equipment should be nearby
⚠ **Assess for chemical arachnoiditis (IT):** headache, nausea, vomiting, fever; neck rigidity/pain, meningism, CSF pleocytosis; may be decreased by dexamethasone
• Assess tachypnea, dyspnea, edema, fatigue; identify dyspnea, crackles, unproductive cough, chest pain, tachypnea; pulmonary edema may be fatal (rare)
⚠ **Assess for cytarabine syndrome 6-12 hr after infusion: fever, myalgia, bone pain, chest pain, rash, conjunctivitis, malaise; corticosteroid may be ordered**
• **Bone marrow suppression:** Monitor CBC, differential, platelet count weekly; withhold product if WBC count is <1000/mm³ or platelet count is <50,000/mm³
• Assess for increased uric acid levels, swelling, joint pain primarily in extremities; patient should be well hydrated to prevent urate deposits
• Monitor renal function studies: BUN, creatinine, serum uric acid, urine CCr before and during therapy; I&O ratio; report fall in urine output to <30 ml/hr
• Monitor temp q4hr (may indicate beginning of infection)
• **Hepatotoxicity:** Monitor liver function tests before and during therapy (bilirubin, AST, ALT, LDH) as needed or monthly; note yellowing of skin or sclera, dark urine, clay-colored stools, pruritus, abdominal pain, fever, diarrhea; an antispasmodic may be used for GI symptoms
• Assess for bleeding: hematuria, stool guaiac, bruising or petechiae, mucosa or orifices q8hr; identify inflammation of mucosa, breaks in skin

Nursing diagnoses

• Body image, disturbed (adverse reactions)
• Infection, risk for (adverse reactions)
• Injury, risk for (adverse reactions)
• Knowledge, deficient (teaching)

Patient/family education

• Advise patient that contraceptive measures are recommended during and 4 mo after therapy
• Teach patient to avoid use of products containing aspirin or ibuprofen, NSAIDs, razors, commercial mouthwash, since bleeding may occur; to report symptoms of bleeding (hematuria, tarry stools)
• Advise that fever, headache, nausea, vomiting are likely to occur but to continue using dexamethasone with IT administration
• Provide liquid diet: carbonated beverages; gelatin may be added if patient is not nauseated or vomiting
• Provide rinsing of mouth tid-qid with water, club soda; brushing of teeth bid-qid with soft brush or cotton-tipped applicators for stomatitis; use unwaxed dental floss

• Advise patient to report signs of anemia (fatigue, headache, irritability, faintness, shortness of breath)

• Advise patient to avoid foods with citric acid, hot flavor, or rough texture if stomatitis is present, to use sponge brush and rinse with water after each meal; to report stomatitis: any bleeding, white spots, ulcerations in mouth; tell patient to examine mouth daily, report any symptoms

• Instruct patient to report any changes in breathing or coughing even several months after treatment; to avoid crowds and persons with respiratory tract or other infections; neurotoxicity

• Caution patient not to have any vaccinations without the advice of the prescriber; serious reactions can occur

• Advise patient to take 3 L/day fluids to prevent renal damage

Evaluation
Positive therapeutic outcome
• Prevention of rapid division of malignant cells

dabigatran (Rx)
(da-bye-gat′ran)
Pradaxa
Func. class.: Anticoagulant-thrombin inhibitor
Pregnancy category C

ACTION: Direct thrombin inhibitor that inhibits both free and clot-bound thrombin, prevents thrombin-induced platelet aggregation and thrombus formation by preventing conversion of fibrinogen to fibrin

Therapeutic outcome: Decreased thrombus formation/extension, absence of emboli, post-thrombotic effects

USES: Stroke/systemic embolism prophylaxis with non-valvular atrial fibrillation

CONTRAINDICATIONS:
Hypersensitivity, bleeding

Precautions: Abrupt discontinuation, anticoagulant therapy, breastfeeding, pregnancy C, children, geriatrics, labor, obstetric delivery, renal disease, surgery

DOSAGE AND ROUTES

Stroke prophylaxis
Adult: PO 150 mg bid

For conversion from an alternative anticoagulant to dabigatran
• When converting from warfarin to dabigatran, discontinue warfarin and initiate dabigatran therapy when the INR is <2.0. When converting from a parenteral anticoagulant to dabigatran, initiate dabigatran 0-2 hr before the time of the next scheduled anticoagulant dose or at the time of discontinuation of a continuously administered anticoagulant (e.g., intravenous unfractionated heparin)

For conversion from dabigatran to warfarin
Adult: CCr >50 ml/min start warfarin 3 days before discontinuing dabigatran; CCr 31-50 ml/min start warfarin 2 days before discontinuing dabigatran; CCr 15-30 ml/min start warfarin 1 day before discontinuing dabigatran

For conversion from dabigatran to parenteral anticoagulants
Adult: PO discontinue dabigatran, start parenteral anticoagulant 12 hr (CCR ≥30 ml/min), 24 hr (CCR <30 ml/min) after the last dabigatran dose

Renal dose
Adult: PO CCr 15-30 ml/min 75 mg bid

Deep vein thrombus (DVT)/pulmonary embolism prophylaxis (unlabeled)
Adult: PO 220 mg or 150 mg q day × 28-35 days, starting with ½ dose 1-4 hr after surgery

Available forms: Cap 75, 150 mg

Implementation
• Do not crush break, chew, or empty contents of capsule
• If dose is missed take as soon as remembered if on the same day, do not administer if <6 hr before next dose
• Take without regard to food
• Store in original package until time of use at room temperature, discard after 30 days, protect from moisture

ADVERSE EFFECTS
CV: Myocardial infarction
CNS: Intracranial bleeding
GI: Abdominal pain, dyspepsia, peptic ulcer, esophagitis, GERD, gastritis, **GI bleeding**
HEMA: Bleeding
INTEG: Rash, pruritus
SYST: Anaphylaxis (rare)

Pharmacokinetics

Absorption	Protein binding 35%
Distribution	Unknown
Metabolism	Unknown
Excretion	Unknown
Half-life	12-17 hr (extended in renal disease)

Pharmacodynamics

Onset	Unknown
Peak	1 hr; high-fat meal delays peak
Duration	Unknown

INTERACTIONS

Individual drugs
Amiodarone, clopidogrel, ketoconazole, quiNIDine, verapamil: increased bleeding risk
Rifampin: decreased dabigatran effect

Drug classifications
Anticoagulants, thrombolytics: increased bleeding risk

NURSING CONSIDERATIONS

Assessment
• **Assess for bleeding:** blood in urine or emesis, dark tarry stools, lower back pain. Caution with arterial/venous punctures, catheters, NG tubes. Monitor vital signs frequently. The elderly are more prone to serious bleeding
• **Assess for thrombosis/MI/emboli:** swelling, pain, redness, difficulty breathing, chest pain, tachypnea, cough, coughing up blood, cyanosis
• **Assess for post-thrombotic syndrome:** pain, heaviness, itching/tingling, swelling, varicose veins, brownish/reddish skin discoloration, ulcers; ambulation, compression stockings and adequate anticoagulation can prevent this syndrome
• Monitor serum creatinine

Nursing diagnoses
• Risk of injury (uses, adverse reactions)

Patient/family education
• Explain the purpose and expected results of this product
• Instruct patient to report if bleeding is present

Evaluation
Positive therapeutic outcome
• Decreased thrombus formation/extension, absence of emboli, post-thrombotic effects

---

⚠ HIGH ALERT

dacarbazine (Rx)
(da-kar′ba-zeen)
dacarbazine, DTIC ✦, DTIC-Dome
Func. class.: Antineoplastic— miscellaneous agent
Chem. class.: Imidazole
Pregnancy category C

ACTION: Alkylates DNA, RNA; inhibits RNA, DNA synthesis; also responsible for breakage, cross-linking DNA strands; activity is not cell cycle phase specific

Therapeutic outcome: Prevention of rapidly growing malignant cells

USES: Hodgkin's disease, malignant melanoma

Unlabeled uses: Malignant pheochromocytoma in combination with cyclophosphamide and vinCRIStine, metastatic soft tissue sarcoma in combination with other agents, carcinoma meningitis, neuroblastoma

CONTRAINDICATIONS:
Hypersensitivity, breastfeeding

Precautions: Renal disease

> **BLACK BOX WARNING:** Pregnancy **C** (1st trimester), radiation therapy, hepatic disease, bone marrow suppression, secondary malignancy

DOSAGE AND ROUTES

Metastatic malignant melanoma
Adult: IV 2-4.5 mg/kg daily × 10 days or 100-250 mg/m² daily × 5 days; repeat q3wk depending on response

Hodgkin's disease
Adult: IV 150 mg/m² daily × 5 days with other agents, repeat q4wk or 375 mg/m² on days 1 and 15 when given in combination, repeat q28day

Osteogenic sarcoma (unlabeled)
Adult and child: IV 250 mg/m²/day as a cont INF × 4 days q28day

Soft tissue sarcoma (unlabeled)
Adult and child: IV 250-300 mg/m²/day as a cont INF × 3 days q21-28day

---

Adverse effects: *italics* = common; **bold** = life-threatening

Carcinoma meningitis (unlabeled)
Adult: Intrathecal 5-30 mg in a fixed dose 2-3 × wk until disease controlled

Available forms: Powder for inj 10, 100, 200 mg

Implementation
• Give fluids **IV** or PO before chemotherapy to hydrate patient
• Give antiemetic 30-60 min before giving product to prevent vomiting, and prn; antibiotics for prophylaxis of infection
• Provide liquid diet: carbonated beverages; gelatin may be added if patient is not nauseated or vomiting

Direct IV route
• After diluting 100 mg/9.9 ml of sterile water for inj (10 mg/ml), give by direct **IV** over 1 min through Y-tube or 3-way stopcock

Intermittent IV infusion route
• May be further diluted in 50-250 ml of D_5W or normal saline for inj and given over 30 min
• Watch for extravasation; give 3-5 ml of mixture of 4 ml sodium thiosulfate 10% plus 5 ml of sterile water SUBCUT as prescribed

Y-site compatibilities: Amifostine, aztreonam, filgrastim, fludarabine, granisetron, melphalan, ondansetron, paclitaxel, sargramostim, teniposide, thiotepa, vinorelbine

ADVERSE EFFECTS
CNS: Facial paresthesia, flushing, fever, malaise, confusion, headache, **seizures, cerebral hemorrhage,** blurred vision (high doses)
GI: *Nausea, anorexia, vomiting,* **hepatotoxicity** (rare)
HEMA: **Thrombocytopenia, leukopenia,** anemia
INTEG: *Alopecia,* dermatitis, pain at inj site, photosensitivity, severe sun reactions (high doses)
MISC: Flulike symptoms, malaise, fever, myalgia, hypotension
SYST: Anaphylaxis

Pharmacokinetics

Absorption	Complete bioavailability (**IV**)
Distribution	Widely distributed; concentrates in liver
Metabolism	Liver (50%, 5% protein bound)
Excretion	Kidneys, unchanged (50%)
Half-life	Initial 35 min, terminal 5 hr

Pharmacodynamics
Unknown

INTERACTIONS
Individual drugs
PHENobarbital, phenytoin: increased metabolism; decreased dacarbazine effect
Radiation: bone marrow suppression, toxicity

Drug classifications
Aminoglycosides: increased nephrotoxicity
Anticoagulants, salicylates: increased risk of bleeding
Antineoplastics, bone marrow–suppressing products: increased toxicity, bone marrow suppression
Diuretics, loop: increased ototoxicity
Live virus vaccines: increased adverse reactions; decreased antibody reaction

NURSING CONSIDERATIONS
Assessment
• **Assess symptoms indicating severe allergic reaction:** rash, pruritus, urticaria, purpuric skin lesions, itching, flushing; product should be discontinued

> **BLACK BOX WARNING: Assess for bone marrow suppression:** Monitor CBC, differential, platelet count weekly; withhold product if WBC is <4000/mm³ or platelet count is <75,000/mm³

• Monitor renal function tests: BUN, creatinine, urine CCr before, during therapy; I&O ratio; report fall in urine output to <30 ml/hr
• Monitor temp q4hr (may indicate beginning of infection)

> **BLACK BOX WARNING: Assess for hepatic disease:** Monitor liver function tests before, during therapy (bilirubin, AST, ALT, LDH) as needed or monthly; note jaundice of skin or sclera, dark urine, clay-colored stools, itchy skin, abdominal pain, fever, diarrhea; hepatotoxicity can be serious and fatal

• Assess for bleeding: hematuria, stool guaiac, bruising or petechiae, mucosa or orifices q8hr; check for inflammation of mucosa, breaks in skin
• Identify effects of alopecia on body image; discuss feelings about body changes

Nursing diagnoses
• Body image, disturbed (adverse reactions)
• Infection, risk for (adverse reactions)
• Injury, risk for (adverse reactions)
• Knowledge, deficient (teaching)

⚠ Nurse Alert

Patient/family education
• Teach patient to avoid use of products containing aspirin or ibuprofen, razors, commercial mouthwash, since bleeding may occur; to report symptoms of bleeding (hematuria, tarry stools)
• Instruct patient to report signs of **anemia** (fatigue, headache, irritability, faintness, shortness of breath)
• Advise patient that hair may be lost during treatment; a wig or hairpiece may make patient feel better; new hair may be different in color, texture
• Caution patient not to have any vaccinations without the advice of prescriber; serious reactions can occur

BLACK BOX WARNING: Advise patient contraception is needed during treatment and for several months after the completion of therapy; product has teratogenic properties

• Teach patient to report signs of **infection:** fever, sore throat, flulike symptoms

Evaluation
Positive therapeutic outcome
• Prevention of rapid division of malignant cells

▲ HIGH ALERT

DACTINomycin (Rx)
(dak-ti-noe-mye′sin)
Cosmegen
Func. class.: Antineoplastic, antibiotic
Pregnancy category D

Do not confuse:
DACTINomycin/DAPTOmycin

ACTION: Inhibits DNA, RNA, protein synthesis; derived from *Streptomyces parvulus;* replication is decreased by binding to DNA, which causes strand splitting; cell cycle nonspecific; a vesicant

Therapeutic outcome: Prevention of rapidly growing malignant cells, immunosuppression

USES: Sarcomas, trophoblastic tumors in women, testicular cancer, Wilms' tumor, rhabdomyosarcoma

Unlabeled uses: Kaposi's sarcoma, malignant melanoma, osteogenic sarcoma, ovarian cancer, soft tissue sarcoma

CONTRAINDICATIONS:
Hypersensitivity, herpes infections, child <6 mo

BLACK BOX WARNING: Pregnancy **D**

Precautions: Breastfeeding, renal/hepatic disease, bone marrow suppression, tumor lysis syndrome, infection

BLACK BOX WARNING: Accidental exposure, extravasation, secondary malignancy

DOSAGE AND ROUTES
Adult: IV 500 mcg/m^2/day × 5 days; stop product for 2-4 wk, then repeat cycle
Child: IV 15 mcg/kg/day × 5 days, max 500 mcg/day; stop product until bone marrow recovery, then repeat cycle

Choriocarcinoma/hydatidiform mole
Adult: IV 1250 mcg/m^2 q14days × 4 cycles

Wilms' tumor/childhood rhabdomyosarcoma/Ewing's sarcoma
Adult and child: IV 15 mcg/kg/day × 5 days

Germ cell testicular cancer
Adult and child: IV 1000 mcg/m^2 as a single dose on day 1

Available forms: Inj 0.5 mg/vial

Implementation
• Provide antacid before oral agent; give product after meals PM, before bedtime; antiemetic 30-60 min before giving product to prevent vomiting, and prn; antibiotics for prophylaxis of infection
• Provide liquid diet: carbonated beverages; gelatin may be added if patient is not nauseated or vomiting
• Help patient rinse mouth tid-qid with water, club soda, brush teeth bid-qid with soft brush or cotton-tipped applicators for stomatitis, use unwaxed dental floss
• Drug should be prepared by experienced personnel using proper precautions

Direct IV route
• Give after diluting 0.5 mg/1.1 ml of sterile water for inj without preservative; use 2.2 ml (0.25 mg/ml), give by direct **IV** at 0.5 mg or less/min through Y-tube or 3-way stopcock of inf in progress
• Increase fluids to 3 L/day

Intermittent IV infusion route
• May be further diluted in 50 ml of D$_5$W or 0.9% NaCl for inf; run over 10-15 min

• Give hydrocortisone, sodium thiosulfate to infiltration area, and ice compress after stopping inf
• Store in darkness in cool environment

Y-site compatibilities: Acyclovir, alfentanil, allopurinol, amifostine, amikacin, aminophylline, amiodarone, amphotericin B colloidal, amphotericin B lipid complex, amphotericin B liposome, ampicillin, ampicillin-sulbactam, anidulafungin, atenolol, atracurium, aztreonam, bivalirudin, bleomycin, bumetanide, buprenorphine, butorphanol, calcium chloride/gluconate, caspofungin, ceFAZolin, cefepime, cefoperazone, cefotaxime, cefotetan, cefoxitin, ceftazidime, ceftizoxime, cefTRIAXone, cefuroxime, chloramphenicol, chlorproMAZINE, cimetidine, ciprofloxacin, cisatracurium, CISplatin, clindamycin, codeine, cyclophosphamide, cycloSPORINE, DAPTOmycin, DAUNOrubicin, dexamethasone, dexmedetomidine, dexrazoxane, digoxin, diltiazem, diphenhydrAMINE, DOBUTamine, docetaxel, DOPamine, DOXOrubicin, doxycycline, droperidol, enalaprilat, ePHEDrine, EPINEPHrine, ertapenem, erythromycin, esmolol, etoposide, famotidine, fenoldopam, fentaNYL, fluconazole, fludarabine, foscarnet, fosphenytoin, furosemide, ganciclovir, gatifloxacin, gemcitabine, gentamicin, glycopyrrolate, granisetron, haloperidol, heparin, hydrALAZINE, hydrocortisone, HYDROmorphone, hydrOXYzine, IDArubicin, ifosfamide, imipenem-cilastatin, inamrinone, insulin (regular), isoproterenol, ketorolac, labetalol, leucovorin, levofloxacin, levorphanol, lidocaine, linezolid, LORazepam, magnesium sulfate, mannitol, melphalan, meperidine, meropenem, mesna, metaraminol, methohexital, methotrexate, methyldopa, methylPREDNISolone, metoclopramide, metoprolol, metroNIDAZOLE, midazolam, milrinone, minocycline, mitomycin, mitoxantrone, morphine, nafcillin, nalbuphine, naloxone, nesiritide, nitroglycerin, nitroprusside, norepinephrine, octreotide, ofloxacin, ondansetron, oxaliplatin, paclitaxel, palonosetron, pancuronium, pemetrexed, pentamidine, pentazocine, PENTobarbital, PHENobarbital, phenylephrine, piperacillin, piperacillin-tazobactam, polymyxin B, potassium chloride/phosphates, procainamide, prochlorperazine, promethazine, propranolol, quiNIDine, quinupristin-dalfopristin, ranitidine, remifentanil, riTUXimab, sargramostim, sodium acetate/bicarbonate/phosphates, succinylcholine, SUFentanil, sulfamethoxazole-trimethoprim, tacrolimus, teniposide, theophylline, thiopental, thiotepa, ticarcillin, ticarcillin-clavulanate, tigecycline, tirofiban, tobramycin, tolazoline, topotecan, trastuzumab, trimethobenzamide, vancomycin, vasopressin, vecuronium, verapamil, vinBLAStine, vinCRIStine, vinorelbine, voriconazole, zidovudine, zoledronic acid

ADVERSE EFFECTS
CNS: Malaise, fatigue, lethargy, fever
EENT: Cheilitis, dysphagia, esophagitis
GI: *Nausea, vomiting, anorexia, stomatitis,* **hepatotoxicity,** abdominal pain, diarrhea
HEMA: Thrombocytopenia, leukopenia, aplastic anemia
INTEG: *Rash,* alopecia, pain at inj site, folliculitis, acne, desquamation, **extravasation**
MS: Myalgia

Pharmacokinetics

Absorption	Complete bioavailability
Distribution	Widely distributed; crosses placenta
Metabolism	Unknown
Excretion	Bile; feces, unchanged (50%); kidneys (10%)
Half-life	36 hr

Pharmacodynamics
Unknown

INTERACTIONS
Individual drugs
Radiation: increased toxicity

Drug classifications
Antineoplastics: increased toxicity

Drug/lab test
Increased: uric acid

NURSING CONSIDERATIONS
Assessment
• Assess buccal cavity q8hr for dryness, sores or ulceration, white patches, pain, bleeding, dysphagia; obtain prescription for viscous lidocaine (Xylocaine)
⚠ **Assess symptoms indicating severe allergic reaction: rash, pruritus, urticaria, purpuric skin lesions, itching, flushing; product should be discontinued**
• **Assess for bone marrow suppression:** Monitor CBC, differential, platelet count weekly; withhold product if WBC is <4000/mm³ or platelet count is <75,000/mm³; notify prescriber of results if WBC <20,000/mm³, platelets <150,000/mm³
• Monitor renal function studies: BUN, creatinine, serum uric acid, urine CCr before, during

therapy; I&O ratio; report fall in urine output to
<30 ml/hr
• Monitor temp q4hr (may indicate beginning
of infection)
• Monitor liver function tests before and during
therapy (bilirubin, AST, ALT, LDH) as needed or
monthly; note jaundice of skin or sclera, dark
urine, clay-colored stools, itchy skin, abdominal
pain, fever, diarrhea
• Assess for bleeding: hematuria, stool guaiac,
bruising or petechiae, mucosa or orifices q8hr;
check for inflammation of mucosa, breaks in
skin
• Identify effects of alopecia on body image;
discuss feelings about body changes

Nursing diagnoses
• Body image, disturbed (adverse reactions)
• Infection, risk for (adverse reactions)
• Injury, risk for (adverse reactions)
• Knowledge, deficient (teaching)
• Oral mucous membranes, impaired (adverse
reactions)

Patient/family education
• Teach patient to avoid use of products containing aspirin or ibuprofen, razors, commercial
mouthwash, since bleeding may occur; to report
symptoms of bleeding (hematuria, tarry stools)
• Instruct patient to report signs of anemia (fatigue, headache, irritability, faintness, shortness
of breath)
• Advise patient that hair may be lost during
treatment; a wig or hairpiece may make patient
feel better; new hair may be different in color,
texture
• Caution patient not to have any vaccinations
without the advice of the prescriber, serious
reactions can occur
• Advise patient that contraception is needed
during treatment and for 4-6 mo after the
completion of therapy (pregnancy **D**); do not
breastfeed
• Advise patient to increase fluids to 3 L/day

Evaluation
Positive therapeutic outcome
• Prevention of rapid division of malignant cells

dalfampridine (Rx)
(dal-fam′pri-deen)
Ampyra
Func. class.: Neurological agent—MS
Chem. class.: Broad-spectrum potassium
channel blocker
Pregnancy category C

ACTION: Mechanism of action is not
fully understood, a broad-spectrum potassium
channel blocker inhibits potassium channels
and increased action potential conduction in
demyelinated axons

Therapeutic outcome: Ability to walk at
improved speed in MS

USES: For improved walking in patients
with multiple sclerosis

CONTRAINDICATIONS:
Renal failure (CCr <50 ml/min), seizures

Precautions: Pregnancy **C**, breastfeeding,
renal disease, elderly

DOSAGE AND ROUTES
Adult: PO 10 mg q12hr

Renal dose
Adult: PO CCr 51-80 ml/min no dosage adjustment needed; seizure risk is unknown; CCr
≤50 ml/min, do not use

Available forms: Ext rel tab 10 mg

Implementation
• Do not break, crush, or chew; give without
regard to meals
• Do not give closer together than q12hr,
seizures may occur
• Do not double doses, if a dose is missed, skip
it

ADVERSE EFFECTS
CNS: **Seizures,** paresthesias, headache, dizzi-
ness, asthenia, insomnia
GI: Nausea, constipation, dyspepsia
GU: Urinary tract infection
MS: Back pain

Pharmacokinetics

Absorption	Bioavailability 96%
Distribution	Largely unbound to plasma proteins
Metabolism	Unknown
Excretion	96% is recovered in the urine
Half-life	Unknown

Pharmacodynamics

Onset	Unknown
Peak	3-4 hr (fasting), longer if taken with food
Duration	Unknown

INTERACTIONS

Individual drugs
Fampridine: do not use together

Drug classifications
4-aminopyridine (4-AP)-containing products: do not use together

NURSING CONSIDERATIONS

Assessment
• **Multiple sclerosis:** assess walking, including speed
• **Assess for seizures:** more common in those with previous seizure disorder

Nursing diagnoses
• Activity intolerance (uses)
• Injury, risk for (adverse reactions)

Patient/family education
• Advise patient to notify prescriber if pregnancy is planned or suspected, do not breastfeed
• Teach patient about expected results, side effects including seizures

Evaluation
Positive therapeutic outcome
• Ability to walk at improved speed in MS

⚠ HIGH ALERT

dalteparin (Rx)
(dahl'ta-pear-in)
Fragmin
Func. class.: Anticoagulant
Chem. class.: Low-molecular-weight heparin
Pregnancy category B

ACTION: Inhibits factor Xa/IIa (thrombin), resulting in anticoagulation

Therapeutic outcome: Absence of deep vein thrombosis

USES: Unstable angina/non-Q-wave MI; prevention of deep vein thrombosis in abdominal surgery, hip replacement patients or those with restricted mobility during acute illness; pulmonary embolism

Unlabeled uses: Antiphospholipid antibody, arterial thromboembolism (after heart valve surgery), cerebral thromboembolism

CONTRAINDICATIONS:
Hypersensitivity to this product, heparin, pork products, benzyl alcohol; active major bleeding, hemophilia, leukemia with bleeding, thrombocytopenic purpura, cerebrovascular hemorrhage, cerebral aneurysm, those undergoing regional anesthesia for unstable angina, non–Q-wave MI, dalteparin-induced thrombocytopenia

Precautions: Pregnancy **B**, recent childbirth, breastfeeding, child, geriatric, hepatic disease, severe renal/cardiac disease, blood dyscrasias, bacterial endocarditis, acute nephritis, peptic ulcer disease, pericarditis, pericardial effusion, recent lumbar puncture, vasculitis, other diseases where bleeding is possible, uncontrolled hypertension; recent brain, spine, eye surgery; congenital or acquired disorders; hemorrhagic stroke, history of HIT

> **BLACK BOX WARNING:** Epidural anesthesia

DOSAGE AND ROUTES

Hip replacement surgery/DVT prophylaxis
Adult: SUBCUT 2500 international units 2 hr before surgery and 2nd dose in the evening the day of surgery (4-8 hr postop), then 5000 international units SUBCUT 1st postop day and daily 5-10 days

Unstable angina/non-Q-wave MI
Adult: SUBCUT 120 international units/kg q12hr × 5-8 days; max 10,000 international units q12hr × 5-8 days with concurrent aspirin, continue until stable

Deep vein thrombosis, prophylaxis for abdominal surgery
Adult: SUBCUT 2500 international units 1-2 hr prior to abdominal surgery and repeat daily × 5-10 days; in high-risk patients 5000 international units should be used

---

Deep vein thrombosis/pulmonary embolism in cancer patients

Adult: SUBCUT 200 international units/kg q day during 1st month (max single dose 18,000 international units), then 150 IU/kg q day in month 2-6 (max single dose 18,000 international units), use prefilled syringe that is closest to calculated dose; if platelets are 50,000-100,000/mm³ reduce dose by 2500 international units until platelets ≥100,000/mm³; if platelets <50,000/mm³ discontinue until >50,000/mm³

Renal dose

Adult: SUBCUT cancer patient with CCr <30 ml/min, monitor antifactor Xa in extended

Available forms: Prefilled syringes, 2500, 5000 international units/0.2 ml; 7500 international units/0.3 ml, 10,000 international units/ml

Implementation

SUBCUT route

• Cannot be used interchangeably unit for unit with unfractionated heparin or LMWHs
• Do not give IM or **IV** product route; approved in SUBCUT only; do not mix with other inj or sol
• Give by SUBCUT only; have patient sit or lie down; SUBCUT inj may be 2 in from umbilicus in a U-shape, upper outer side of thigh, around navel, or upper outer quadrangle of the buttocks; rotate inj sites
• Changing needles is not recommended; change inj site daily, use at same time of day

ADVERSE EFFECTS

CNS: Intracranial bleeding
HEMA: Thrombocytopenia
INTEG: Pruritus, superficial wound infection
SYST: Hypersensitivity, **hemorrhage, anaphylaxis** possible

Pharmacokinetics

Absorption	87%
Distribution	Unknown
Metabolism	Liver
Excretion	Kidney
Half-life	3-5 hr elimination

Pharmacodynamics

Onset	Unknown
Peak	4 hr
Duration	Unknown

INTERACTIONS

Individual drugs
Aspirin: increased bleeding risk

Drug classifications
Anticoagulants, NSAIDs, platelet inhibitors, salicylates, thrombolytics: increased risk of bleeding

NURSING CONSIDERATIONS

Assessment
• Assess for bleeding (Hct, occult blood in stools) during treatment since bleeding can occur
A Assess for bleeding gums, petechiae, ecchymosis, black tarry stools, hematuria, epistaxis, decrease in Hct, B/P; may indicate bleeding, possible hemorrhage; notify prescriber immediately; product should be discontinued
• **Assess for hypersensitivity:** fever, skin rash, urticaria; notify prescriber immediately
• Assess for needed dosage change q1-2wk; dosage may need to be decreased if bleeding occurs

Nursing diagnoses
• Injury, risk for (uses, adverse reactions)
• Knowledge, deficient (teaching)

Patient/family education
• Advise patient to avoid OTC preparations that contain aspirin, other anticoagulants; serious product interaction may occur
• Advise patient to use soft-bristle toothbrush to avoid bleeding gums, avoid contact sports, use electric razor, avoid IM inj
• Instruct patient to report any signs of bleeding: gums, under skin, urine, stools; unusual bruising

Evaluation
Positive therapeutic outcome
• Absence of deep vein thrombosis

TREATMENT OF OVERDOSE:

Protamine sulfate 1% given **IV**; 1 mg protamine/100 anti-Xa international units of dalteparin given

dantrolene (Rx)
(dan'troe-leen)
Dantrium, Revonto
Func. class.: Skeletal muscle relaxant, direct acting
Chem. class.: Hydantoin
Pregnancy category C

Do not confuse:
Dantrium/danazol

ACTION: Interferes with intracellular release from the sarcoplasmic reticulum of calcium necessary to initiate contraction; slows catabolism in malignant hyperthermia

Therapeutic outcome: Decreased muscle spasticity; absence of malignant hyperthermia

USES: Spasticity in multiple sclerosis, stroke, spinal cord injury, cerebral palsy, prevention and treatment of malignant hyperthermia

Unlabeled uses: Neuroleptic malignant syndrome

CONTRAINDICATIONS:
Hypersensitivity, compromised pulmonary function, active hepatic disease, impaired myocardial function

> **BLACK BOX WARNING:** Active hepatic disease

Precautions: Pregnancy C, breastfeeding, geriatric, peptic ulcer disease, renal/cardiac/hepatic, stroke, seizure disorder, diabetes mellitus, ALS, COPD, MS, mannitol/gelatin hypersensitivity, labor, lactase deficiency, extravasation

> **BLACK BOX WARNING:** Females

DOSAGE AND ROUTES
Spasticity
Adult: PO 25 mg/day; may increase to 25-100 mg bid-qid, max 400 mg/day
Child: PO 0.5 mg/kg/day given in divided doses bid; may increase gradually; max 400 mg daily

Malignant hyperthermia
Adult and child: IV 1 mg/kg; may repeat to total dose of 10 mg/kg; PO 4-8 mg/kg/day in 4 divided doses × 3 days to prevent further hyperthermia; postcrisis follow-up 4-8 mg/kg/day for 1-3 days

Prevention of malignant hyperthermia
Adult and child: PO 4-8 mg/kg/day in 3-4 divided doses × 1-2 days before procedures; give last dose 4 hr preoperatively; IV 2.5 mg/kg prior to anesthesia

Neuroleptic malignant syndrome (unlabeled)
Adult: PO 100-300 mg/day in divided doses, IV 1.25-1.5 mg/kg

Available forms: Caps 25, 50, 100 mg; powder for inj 20 mg/vial

Implementation
PO route
• Do not crush or chew caps; caps may be opened and mixed with juice and swallowed; drink immediately after mixing
• Give with meals for GI symptoms
• Store in airtight container at room temperature

IV route
• Administer **IV** after diluting 20 mg/60 ml sterile water for inj without bacteriostatic agent (333 mcg/ml); shake until clear; give by rapid **IV** push through Y-tube or 3-way stopcock; follow by prescribed doses immediately; may also give by intermittent inf over 1 hr before anesthesia; assess site for extravasation, phlebitis
• Protect diluted sol from light; use reconstituted sol within 6 hr
• Considered incompatible in sol or syringe, compatibility unknown

ADVERSE EFFECTS
CNS: *Dizziness, weakness, fatigue, drowsiness,* headache, disorientation, insomnia, paresthesias, tremors, **seizures**
CV: Hypotension, chest pain, palpitations
EENT: Nasal congestion, blurred vision, mydriasis
GI: Hepatic injury, *nausea,* constipation, vomiting, increased AST and alkaline phosphatase, abdominal pain, dry mouth, anorexia, hepatitis, dyspepsia
GU: Urinary frequency, nocturia, impotence, crystalluria
HEMA: Eosinophilia, aplastic anemia, leukopenia
INTEG: Rash, pruritus, photosensitivity, extravasation (tissue necrosis)
RESP: Pleural effusion

Pharmacokinetics

Absorption	PO (30%-35%), poor
Distribution	Unknown
Metabolism	Liver, extensively
Excretion	Kidney
Half-life	9 hr

Pharmacodynamics

	PO	IV
Onset	Unknown	Immediate
Peak	5 hr	5 hr
Duration	Dose related	Dose related

INTERACTIONS

• Considered incompatible in sol or syringe; compatibility unknown

Individual drugs
Alcohol: increased CNS depression
Verapamil: increased dysrhythmias

Drug classifications
Antidepressants (tricyclic), antihistamines, barbiturates, opiates, sedative/hypnotics: increased CNS depression
Estrogens, hepatotoxic agents: increased hepatotoxicity

NURSING CONSIDERATIONS

Assessment
• Monitor I&O ratio; check for urinary retention, frequency, hesitancy, especially geriatric
• **Seizures:** Monitor ECG in epileptic patients; poor seizure control has occurred with patients taking this product; assess for increased seizure activity in epilepsy patient

> **BLACK BOX WARNING: Active hepatic disease:** Monitor hepatic function by frequent determination of AST, ALT, bilirubin, alkaline phosphatase, GGTP; renal function studies; CBC

• Assess for allergic reactions: rash, fever, respiratory distress
• Monitor for severe weakness, numbness in extremities
• Assess for CNS depression: dizziness, drowsiness, psychiatric symptoms

> **BLACK BOX WARNING: Assess for signs of hepatotoxicity:** Jaundice, yellow sclera, pain in abdomen, nausea, fever; product should be discontinued if these signs and symptoms occur

Nursing diagnoses
• Injury, risk for (adverse reactions)
• Knowledge, deficient (teaching)
• Mobility, impaired physical (uses)
• Pain, chronic (uses)

Patient/family education
• Caution patient not to discontinue product quickly, hallucinations, spasticity, tachycardia will occur; product should be tapered over 1-2 wk; notify prescriber of abdominal pain, jaundiced sclera, clay-colored stools, change in color of urine, rash, itching
• Caution patient not to take with alcohol, other CNS depressants; severe CNS depression can occur; avoid using OTC medication (cough preparations, antihistamines, alcohol, other CNS depressants), unless directed by prescriber
• Tell patient that if improvement does not occur within 6 wk, prescriber may discontinue
• Caution patient to avoid hazardous activities if drowsiness, dizziness, blurred vision occurs; wait several days to identify patient response to medication
• Teach patient to use sunscreen, protective clothing for photosensitivity
• Instruct patient to take medication as prescribed; do not double doses; take missed dose within 1 hr of scheduled time

Evaluation
Positive therapeutic outcome
• Decreased pain, spasticity
• Absence or decreased symptoms of malignant hyperthermia

TREATMENT OF OVERDOSE:
Activated charcoal, supportive care

dapiprazole ophthalmic
See Appendix B

daptomycin (Rx)
(dap′toe-mye-sin)
Cubicin
Func. class.: Antiinfective—miscellaneous
Chem. class.: Lipopeptides
Pregnancy category B

ACTION: New class of antiinfective; binds to the bacterial membrane and results in a rapid depolarization of the membrane potential, leading to inhibition of DNA, RNA, and protein synthesis

Therapeutic outcome: Absence of infections

USES: Complicated skin, skin structure infections caused by *Staphylococcus aureus,* including methicillin-resistant strains, *Streptococcus pyogenes, S. agalactiae, S. dysgalactiae, Enterococcus faecalis* (vancomycin-susceptible strains only)

CONTRAINDICATIONS:
Hypersensitivity

Precautions: Pregnancy **B**, breastfeeding, children, geriatrics, GI/renal disease, myopathy, ulcerative/pseudomembranous colitis, rhabdomyolysis, eosinophilic pneumonia

DOSAGE AND ROUTES
Adult: IV INF 4-6 mg/kg over ½ hr diluted in 0.9% NaCl, give q24hr × 7-14 days
Adolescent/child/infant ≥5 mo (unlabeled): IV 4-6 mg/kg/day

Renal dose
Adult: IV CCr <30 ml/min; hemodialysis, CAPD 4 mg/kg q48hr

Available forms: Lyophilized powder for inj 500 mg

Implementation
Intermittent IV infusion route
• Give after reconstitution with 5 ml 0.9% NaCl (250 mg/5 ml) or 10 ml 0.9% NaCl (500 mg/10 ml), further dilution is needed with 0.9% NaCl; infuse over ½ hr

Direct IV route
• Give reconstituted sol (50 mg/ml) by direct IV inj over 2 min

Y-site compatibilities: Alfentanil, amifostine, amikacin, aminocaproic acid, aminophylline, amiodarone, amphotericin B liposome, ampicillin, ampicillin-sulbactam, argatroban, arsenic trioxide, atenolol, atracurium, azithromycin, aztreonam, bivalirudin, bleomycin, bumetanide, buprenorphine, busulfan, butorphanol, calcium chloride/gluconate, CARBOplatin, carmustine, caspofungin, ceFAZolin, cefepime, cefotaxime, cefotetan, cefoxitin, ceftazidime, ceftizoxime, cefTRIAXone, cefuroxime, chloramphenicol, chlorproMAZINE, cimetidine, ciprofloxacin, cisatracurium, CISplatin, clindamycin, cyclophosphamide, cycloSPORINE, dacarbazine, DACTINomycin, DAUNOrubicin, dexamethasone, dexmedetomidine, dexrazoxane, diazepam, digoxin, diltiazem, diphenhydrAMINE, DOBUTamine, docetaxel, dolasetron, DOPamine, doripenem, doxacurium, DOXOrubicin, DOXOrubicin liposomal, doxycycline, droperidol, enalaprilat, ePHEDrine, EPINEPH-rine, epirubicin, eptifibatide, ertapenem, erythromycin, esmolol, etoposide, famotidine, fenoldopam, fentaNYL, fluconazole, fludarabine, fluorouracil, foscarnet, fosphenytoin, furosemide, ganciclovir, gentamicin, glycopyrrolate, granisetron, haloperidol, heparin, hydrALAZINE, hydrocortisone, HYDROmorphone, hydrOXYzine, IDArubicin, ifosfamide, inamrinone, insulin (regular), irinotecan, isoproterenol, ketorolac, labetalol, leucovorin, levofloxacin, lidocaine, linezolid, LORazepam, magnesium sulfate, mannitol, mechlorethamine, melphalan, meperidine, meropenem, mesna, metaraminol, methyldopate, methylPREDNISolone, metoclopramide, metoprolol, midazolam, milrinone, mitoxantrone, mivacurium, morphine, moxifloxacin, mycophenolate mofetil, nafcillin, nalbuphine, naloxone, niCARdipine, nitroprusside, norepinephrine, octreotide, ondansetron, oxaliplatin, oxytocin, paclitaxel, palonosetron, pamidronate, pancuronium, pemetrexed, pentamidine, PHENobarbital, phenylephrine, piperacillin-tazobactam, polymyxin B, potassium acetate/chloride/phosphates, procainamide, prochlorperazine, promethazine, propranolol, quinupristin-dalfopristin, ranitidine, rocuronium, sodium acetate/bicarbonate/citrate/phosphates, succinylcholine, sulfamethoxazole-trimethoprim, tacrolimus, teniposide, theophylline, thiotepa, ticarcillin, ticarcillin-clavulanate, tigecycline, tirofiban, tobramycin, topotecan, trimethobenzamide, vasopressin, vecuronium, verapamil, vinBLAStine, vinCRIStine, vinorelbine, voriconazole, zidovudine, zoledronic acid

Solution compatibilities: 0.9% NaCl, LR

ADVERSE EFFECTS
CNS: Headache, insomnia, dizziness, confusion, anxiety, fatigue, fever
CV: Hypo/hypertension, **heart failure,** chest pain
GI: Nausea, constipation, diarrhea, vomiting, dyspepsia, **pseudomembranous colitis,** abdominal pain
GU: Nephrotoxicity: increased BUN
HEMA: Leukocytosis, anemia, thrombocytopenia
INTEG: Rash, pruritus
MISC: Fungal infections, UTI, anemia
MS: Muscle pain or weakness, arthralgia, pain, **rhabdomyolysis**
RESP: Cough, **eosinophilic pneumonia**
SYST: Anaphylaxis

Nurse Alert

Pharmacokinetics

Absorption	Unknown
Distribution	Protein binding 92%
Metabolism	Unknown
Excretion	Unknown
Half-life	Unknown

Pharmacodynamics

Unknown

INTERACTIONS

Drug classifications
HMG-CoA reductase inhibitors: myopathy

Drug/lab test
Increase: CPK, AST, ALT, BUN, creatinine, albumin

NURSING CONSIDERATIONS

Assessment
• Assess signs of infection, C&S, product may be given as soon as culture is taken
• Monitor I&O ratio: report hematuria, oliguria; nephrotoxicity may occur
⚠ **Nephrotoxicity: Monitor any patient with compromised renal system: BUN, creatinine; toxicity may occur**
• **Eosinophilic pneumonia:** Assess for dyspnea, fever, cough, shortness of breath, if left untreated can lead to respiratory failure and death
• Monitor blood tests: CBC
• Monitor C&S, product may be given as soon as culture is taken
• Monitor B/P during administration; hypo/hypertension may occur
• Assess respiratory status: rate, character, wheezing
• Identify allergies before treatment, reaction of each medication

Nursing diagnoses
• Infection, risk for (uses)
• Knowledge, deficient (teaching)

Patient/family education
• Teach all aspects of product therapy
• Advise to report sore throat, fever, fatigue; could indicate **superinfection**

Evaluation
Positive therapeutic outcome
• Negative culture

darbepoetin (Rx)
(dar'bee-poh'-eh-tin)
Aranesp
Func. class.: Hematopoietic agent
Chem. class.: Recombinant human erythropoietin
Pregnancy category C

ACTION: Stimulates erythropoiesis by the same mechanism as endogenous erythropoietin; in response to hypoxia, erythropoietin is produced in the kidney and released into the bloodstream, where it interacts with progenitor stem cells to increase red cell production

Therapeutic outcome: Decreased anemia with increased RBCs

USES: Anemia associated with chronic renal failure in patients on and not on dialysis and anemic in nonmyeloid malignancies receiving coadministered chemotherapy

CONTRAINDICATIONS:
Hypersensitivity to mammalian cell–derived products or human albumin, uncontrolled hypertension, red cell aplasia

Precautions: Pregnancy C, breastfeeding, children, seizure disorder, porphyria, hypertension, sickle cell disease, vit B_{12}, folate deficiency, chronic renal failure, dialysis, latex hypersensitivity, CABG, angina, anemia

> **BLACK BOX WARNING:** Hgb >12 g/dl, surgery

DOSAGE AND ROUTES

Correction of anemia in chronic renal failure
Adult: SUBCUT/IV 0.45 mcg/kg as a single inj, titrate max target Hgb of 12 g/dl

Chemotherapy treatment
Adult: SUBCUT 2.5 mcg/kg/wk or 500 mcg q3wk

Epoetin alfa to darbepoetin conversion
Adult: SUBCUT/IV (epoetin alfa <2500 units/wk) 6.25 mcg/wk; (epoetin alfa 2500-4999 units/wk) 12.5 mcg/wk; (epoetin alfa 5000-10,999 units/wk) 25 mcg/wk; (epoetin alfa 11,000-17,999 units/wk) 40 mcg/wk; (epoetin alfa 18,000-33,999 units/wk) 60 mcg/wk; (epoetin alfa 34,000-89,999 units/wk) 100 mcg/wk; (epoetin alfa >90,000 units/wk) 200 mcg/wk

Adverse effects: *italics* = common; **bold** = life-threatening

Available forms: Sol for inj 25, 40, 60, 100, 150, 200, 300, 500 mcg/ml

Implementation
IV/SUBCUT
• Do not shake, do not dilute, do not mix with other products or solutions
• Check for discoloration, particulate matter; do not use if present; discard unused portion; do not pool unused portion

ADVERSE EFFECTS
CNS: **Seizures**, sweating, headache, dizziness, **stroke**
CV: *Hypo/hypertension,* **cardiac arrest,** *angina pectoris,* **thrombosis, CHF, acute MI, dysrhythmias,** chest pain, transient ischemic attacks, edema
GI: *Diarrhea, vomiting, nausea, abdominal pain, constipation*
HEMA: **Red cell aplasia**
MISC: *Infection, fatigue, fever,* **death,** *fluid overload,* **vascular access hemorrhage,** dehydration, sepsis
MS: *Bone pain, myalgia, limb pain, back pain*
RESP: *Upper respiratory infection, dyspnea, cough, bronchitis,* **pulmonary embolism**
SYST: Allergic reactions, **anaphylaxis**

Pharmacokinetics
Absorption	Slow, rate-limiting (SUBCUT)
Distribution	Vascular space
Metabolism	Metabolized in body (**IV**), extent unknown
Excretion	Unknown
Half-life	49 hr

Pharmacodynamics
Onset	Onset of increased reticulocyte count 1-6 wk
Peak	34 hr
Duration	Unknown

INTERACTIONS
Individual drugs
⚠ Do not use epoetin alfa with this product

Drug classifications
Androgens: increased darbepoetin alfa effect

Drug/lab test
Increased: WBC, platelets
Decreased: bleeding time

NURSING CONSIDERATIONS
Assessment
• **Assess for serious allergic reactions:** rash, urticaria; if anaphylaxis occurs, stop product, administer emergency treatment (rare)

> **BLACK BOX WARNING:** Assess blood studies: ferritin, transferrin monthly; transferrin sat ≥20%, ferritin ≥100 ng/ml; Hgb 2 ×/wk until stabilized in target range (30%-33%), then at regular intervals; those with endogenous erythropoietin levels of <500 units/L respond to this agent

• Assess renal studies: urinalysis, protein, blood, BUN, creatinine
• Assess B/P, Hct; check for rising B/P as Hct rises; antihypertensives may be needed
⚠ **Assess CV status: hypertension may occur rapidly, leading to hypertensive encephalopathy; Hgb >12 g/dl may lead to death**
• Assess I&O ratio; report drop in output to <50 ml/hr
• Assess for **seizures** if Hgb is increased within 2 wk by 4 points
• Assess CNS symptoms: cold sensation, sweating, pain in long bones
• Assess **dialysis patients** for thrill, bruit of shunts; monitor for circulation impairment

Nursing diagnoses
• Activity intolerance (uses)
• Fatigue (uses)
• Knowledge, deficient (teaching)

Patient/family education
• Caution patient to avoid driving or hazardous activity during beginning of treatment
• Advise patient to monitor B/P, Hgb
• Advise patient to take iron supplements, vit B$_{12}$, folic acid as directed
• Advise patient to report side effects to prescriber, to comply with treatment regimen
• Teach patient that menses may return, use contraception
• Teach home administration and review information for patients and caregivers if home administration is deemed appropriate

Evaluation
Positive therapeutic outcome
• Increased reticulocyte count, Hgb/Hct
• Increased appetite
• Enhanced sense of well-being

TREATMENT OF OVERDOSE:
If polycythemia occurs, discontinue product

temporarily; perform phlebotomy if clinically indicated

darunavir (Rx)

(dar-ue′na vir)
Prezista
Func. class.: Antiretroviral
Chem. class.: Protease inhibitor
Pregnancy category B

ACTION: Inhibits human immunodeficiency virus (HIV-1) protease; this prevents maturation of virus

Therapeutic outcome: Decreased viral load, increase in CD4 counts

USES: HIV-1 in combination with ritonavir and other antiretrovirals

CONTRAINDICATIONS:

Hypersensitivity

Precautions: Pregnancy **B**, breastfeeding, children, renal/hepatic disease, history of renal stones, diabetes, hypercholesterolemia, sulfonamide hypersensitivity, antimicrobial resistance, bleeding, elderly, immune reconstitution syndrome, pancreatitis

DOSAGE AND ROUTES

Treatment-naive patients
Adult: PO 800 mg with ritonavir 100 mg qd

Treatment-experienced patients
Adult/adolescent >40 kg/child ≥6 yr: PO 600 mg with ritonavir 100 mg qd; 800 qd with ritonavir 100 mg with food (without darunavir resistance)
Child ≥6 yr/adolescents ≥30 kg, <40 kg: PO 450 mg bid with ritonavir 60 mg bid
Child ≥6 yr/adolescent ≥20 kg, <30 kg: PO 375 mg with ritonavir 50 mg bid
Child 3 to <6 yr (14 to <15 kg): PO 280 mg (with ritonavir 48 mg) bid with food
Child 3 to <6 yr (13 to <14 kg): PO 260 mg (with ritonavir 40 mg) bid with food
Child 3 to <6 yr (12 to <13 kg): PO 240 mg (with ritonavir 40 mg) bid with food
Child 3 to <6 yr (11 to <12 kg): PO 220 mg (with ritonavir 32 mg) bid with food
Child 3 to <6 yr (10 to <11 kg): PO 200 mg (with ritonavir 32 mg) bid with food

Available forms: Tabs 75, 150, 400, 600 mg

Implementation

- Give with food and ritonavir
- Give water to 1.5 L/day minimum to prevent nephrolithiasis
- Tab should be swallowed whole

ADVERSE EFFECTS

CNS: *Headache, insomnia,* dizziness, somnolence
GI: *Diarrhea, abdominal pain, nausea, vomiting,* anorexia, dry mouth, **hepatitis, hepatotoxicity**
GU: Nephrolithiasis
INTEG: Rash, angioedema, **Stevens-Johnson syndrome,** toxic epidermal necrolysis
MS: Pain
OTHER: Asthenia, **insulin-resistant hyperglycemia,** hyperlipidemia, **ketoacidosis,** lipodystrophy

Pharmacokinetics

Absorption	Unknown
Distribution	Protein binding 95%
Metabolism	By CYP3A4
Excretion	Feces 79.5%, urine 13.9%
Half-life	Terminal 15 hr

Pharmacodynamics

Onset	Unknown
Peak	2.5-4 hr
Duration	Unknown

INTERACTIONS

Individual drugs

Atorvastatin, lovastatin, simvastatin: increased myopathy
CarBAMazepine, efavirenz, fluconazole, fosphenytoin, nevirapine, PHENobarbital, phenytoin: decreased darunavir levels
Clarithromycin, zidovudine: increased levels of both products
Delavirdine, itraconazole, ketoconazole: increased darunavir levels
Isoniazid: increased levels of isoniazid
⚠ **Midazolam, pimozide, rifampin, triazolam: life-threatening dysrhythmias**

Drug classifications

⚠ **Ergots: life-threatening dysrhythmias; do not use concurrently**
Oral contraceptives: increased levels of oral contraceptives
Rifamycins: decreased darunavir levels

Drug/herb

Red yeast rice: increased myopathy, rhabdomyolysis

St. John's wort: decreased darunavir levels; avoid concurrent use

Drug/food
Darunavir: increased absorption

NURSING CONSIDERATIONS

Assessment
• Assess for complaints of lower back, flank pain; indicates kidney stones
• Assess for signs of infection, anemia, the presence of other STDs
• **Serious skin reaction:** angioedema, Stevens-Johnson syndrome, toxic epidermal necrolysis; discontinue immediately, notify prescriber
• **Hepatotoxicity:** Monitor liver function tests: ALT, AST, bilirubin, amylase; all may be elevated in those with underlying liver disease
• Monitor viral load, CD4 during treatment; viral load should be decreasing, CD4 increasing
• Assess bowel pattern before, during treatment; if severe abdominal pain with bleeding occurs, product should be discontinued; monitor hydration
• Assess skin eruptions: rash, urticaria, itching
• Assess allergies before treatment, reaction of each medication; place allergies on chart
• **Hyperlipidemia:** Cholesterol, triglycerides, LDL may be elevated, monitor serum cholesterol, lipid panel throughout treatment

Nursing diagnoses
• Infection, risk for (uses)
• Knowledge, deficient (teaching)
• Noncompliance (teaching)

Patient/family education
• Teach patient to use nonhormonal birth control, do not breastfeed
• Instruct patient to take as prescribed; if dose is missed, take as soon as remembered up to 1 hr before next dose; do not double dose
• Advise patient that product must be taken at same time of day to maintain blood levels for duration of therapy
⚠ Advise patient that hyperglycemia may occur; watch for increased thirst, weight loss, hunger; dry, itchy skin; notify prescriber
• Teach patient to increase fluids to prevent kidney stones; if stone formation occurs, treatment may need to be interrupted
• Teach patient that product does not cure AIDS, only controls symptoms; do not donate blood, do not share, notify all health care providers of use, do not use with any other products without prescriber's approval

Evaluation
Positive therapeutic outcome
• Decreased viral load, increased CD4 counts

dasatinib (Rx)
(da-si′ti-nib)
Sprycel
Func. class.: Miscellaneous antineoplastic
Chem. class.: Protein-tyrosine kinase inhibitor
Pregnancy category D

ACTION: Inhibits BCR-ABL, SRC, LCK, YES, FYN, C-KIT, EPHA$_2$, and PDGFR-β tyrosine kinase created in chronic myeloid leukemia (CML)

Therapeutic outcome: Decrease in number of leukemic cells or size of tumor

USES: Treatment of accelerated, chronic blast phase CML or acute lymphoblastic leukemia (ALL); chronic phase CML with resistance or intolerance to prior therapy; Philadelphia chromosome–positive CML in chronic phase

CONTRAINDICATIONS:
Pregnancy **D**, hypersensitivity

Precautions: Breastfeeding, children, geriatric, QT prolongation, infection, thrombocytopenia, accidental exposure, edema, infertility, lactase deficiency, neutropenia

DOSAGE AND ROUTES

Accelerated or myeloid/lymphoid blast phase CML with resistance/intolerance to prior therapy
Adult: PO 140 mg daily, titrated up to 180 mg bid in those resistant to therapy

Chronic phase CML with resistance/intolerance to prior therapy
Adult: PO 100 mg daily either AM or PM

Dosage reduction for those taking a strong CYP3A4 inhibitor
Adult: 20 mg daily

Available forms: Tabs 20, 50, 70, 100 mg

Implementation
• Do not break, crush, or chew tab
• Give after meal and with large glass of water
• Give nutritious diet with iron, vitamin supplement
• Store at 25° C (77° F)

ADVERSE EFFECTS

CNS: **CNS hemorrhage,** headache, dizziness, insomnia, neuropathy, asthenia
CV: **Dysrhythmias,** chest pain, **CHF, pericardial effusion,** congestive cardiomyopathy; decreased injection fraction, QT prolongation
GI: *Nausea, vomiting, anorexia, abdominal pain,* constipation, diarrhea, GI bleeding, muscositis, stomatitis
HEMA: **Neutropenia, thrombocytopenia, bleeding**
INTEG: *Rash, pruritus*
META: Fluid retention, edema, hypocalcemia, hypophosphatemia
MISC: Increased/decreased weight
MS: Pain, arthralgia, myalgia
RESP: Cough, dyspnea, pulmonary edema/hypertension, pneumonia, URI, **pleural effusion**

Pharmacokinetics

Absorption	Unknown
Distribution	Protein binding 96%
Metabolism	By CYP3A4
Excretion	Feces 85%, urine 4%
Half-life	Terminal 1.3-5 hr

Pharmacodynamics

Onset	0.5-6 hr
Peak	Unknown
Duration	Unknown

INTERACTIONS

Individual drugs

Clarithromycin, erythromycin, itraconazole, ketoconazole, nefazodone, telithromycin: increased dasatinib concentrations
Simvastatin: increased concentrations of this product

Drug classifications

Class IA/III antidysrhythmics and other products that increase QT prolongation: increased QT prolongation
CYP3A4 inducers (dexamethasone, phenytoin, carBAMazepine, rifampin, PHENobarbital), H₂ blockers (famotidine), proton pump inhibitors (omeprazole): decreased dasatinib concentrations
CYP3A4 substrates (alfentanil, cycloSPORINE, ergots, fentaNYL, pimozide, quiNIDine, sirolimus, tacrolimus): altered action
Protease inhibitors: increased dasatinib concentrations

Drug/herb

St. John's wort: decreased dasatinib concentration

NURSING CONSIDERATIONS

Assessment

• **Myelosuppression:** Monitor ANC and platelets; in chronic phase if ANC is $<1 \times 10^9/L$ and/or platelets $<50 \times 10^9/L$, stop until ANC $>1.5 \times 10^9/L$ and platelets $>75 \times 10^9/L$; in accelerated phase/blast crisis if ANC $<0.5 \times 10^9/L$ and/or platelets $<10 \times 10^9/L$, determine whether cytopenia is related to biopsy/aspirate, if not, reduce dose by 200 mg, if cytopenia continues, reduce dose by another 100 mg; if cytopenia continues for 4 wk, stop product until ANC $\geq 1 \times 10^9/L$
• Assess for hepatotoxicity: monitor liver function tests before treatment and qmo; if liver transaminases $>5 \times$ IULN, withhold until transaminase levels return to $<2.5 \times$ IULN
• **Monitor for signs of fluid retention, edema:** weigh, monitor lung sounds, assess for edema, some fluid retention is dose dependent, may result in CHF, congestive cardiomyopathy, decreased injection fraction

Nursing diagnoses

• Infection, risk for (adverse reactions)
• Knowledge, deficient (teaching)
• Nutrition: less than body requirements, imbalanced (adverse reactions)

Patient/family education

• Instruct patient to report adverse reactions immediately: SOB, swelling of extremities, bleeding
• Teach patient reason for treatment, expected result
• Teach patient to use contraception, pregnancy **D,** avoid breastfeeding

Evaluation

Positive therapeutic outcome
• Decrease in number of leukemic cells

⚠ HIGH ALERT

DAUNOrubicin (Rx)
(daw-noe-roo′bi-sin)
Cerubidine

DAUNOrubicin citrate liposome (Rx)
DaunoXome
Func. class.: Antineoplastic, antibiotic
Chem. class.: Anthracycline glycoside
Pregnancy category D

Do not confuse:
DAUNOrubicin/DOXOrubicin

ACTION: Inhibits DNA synthesis, primarily; derived from *Streptomyces coeruleorubidus;* replication is decreased by binding to DNA, which causes strand splitting; cell cycle specific (S phase); a vesicant

Therapeutic outcome: Prevention of rapidly growing malignant cells; immunosuppression

USES: Acute lymphocytic leukemia (ALL), acute myelogenous leukemia (AML); liposomal Kaposi's sarcoma

CONTRAINDICATIONS: Pregnancy **D,** breastfeeding, hypersensitivity, systemic infections, cardiac disease, bone marrow depression

Precautions: Renal/hepatic disease, gout, tumor lysis syndrome, MI, infection, thrombocytopenia

> **BLACK BOX WARNING:** Bone marrow suppression, cardiac disease, extravasation, renal failure

DOSAGE AND ROUTES
Use decreased dose for those >60 yr

DAUNOrubicin

In combination
Adult: IV 45-60 mg/m^2/day × 3 days, then 2 days of subsequent courses in combination, max 400-600 mg/m^2 total cumulative dose
Child: IV 25-60 mg/m^2 depending on cycle (AML); ≤2 yr or <0.5 m^2: 1 mg/kg on day 1 weekly in combination with vinCRIStine and predniSONE, base dose on body weight, not surface area (ALL); >2 yr or 0.5 m^2: 25 mg/m^2 day 1 q wk in combination with vinCRIStine and predniSONE (ALL)

DAUNOrubicin citrate liposome
Adult: IV 40 mg/m^2 q2wk (Kaposi's sarcoma); 100 mg/m^2 q3wk (multiple myeloma, unlabeled); IV 100-140 mg/m^2 q3wk (non-Hodgkin's lymphoma, unlabeled; metastatic breast cancer, unlabeled; IV escalating doses of 75, 100, 125, 135, 150 mg/m^2/day × 3 days (AML, unlabeled)

Renal dose
Adult: IV serum Cr >3 mg/dl reduce dose by 50%

Hepatic dose
Adult: IV serum bilirubin 1.2-3 mg/dl reduce dose by 50%; bilirubin >3 mg/dl reduce dose by 75%; bilirubin > 5 mg/dl omit dose

Available forms: Inj 20 mg powder/vial, sol for inj 5 mg/ml (DaunoXome); liposome: dispersion for inj 2 mg/ml

Implementation
- Avoid contact with skin; very irritating; wash completely to remove
- Give fluids **IV** or PO before chemotherapy to hydrate patient; give antiemetic 30-60 min before giving product to prevent vomiting, and prn; antibiotics for prophylaxis of infection
- Provide liquid diet: carbonated beverages; gelatin may be added if patient is not nauseated or vomiting
- Help patient rinse mouth tid-qid with water, club soda, brush teeth bid-qid with soft brush or cotton-tipped applicators for stomatitis, use unwaxed dental floss
- Product should be prepared by experienced personnel using proper precautions
- Do not give by IM/SUBCUT inj

Cerubidine

IV route
- Give after diluting 20 mg/4 ml sterile water for inj (5 mg/ml); rotate; further dilute in 10-15 ml 0.9% NaCl; give over 3-5 min by direct **IV** through Y-tube or 3-way stopcock of inf of D$_5$W or 0.9% NaCl

Intermittent IV infusion route
- Dilute further in 50-100 ml 0.9% NaCl, LR, D$_5$W; give over 15 min (50 ml), 30 min (100 ml)

Y-site compatibilities: Amifostine, anidulafungin, atenolol, bivalirudin, bleomycin, CARBOplatin, caspofungin, CISplatin, codeine, cyclophosphamide, cytarabine, DACTINomycin, DAPTOmycin, dexmedetomidine, etoposide, fenoldopam, filgrastim, gemcitabine, gemtuzumab, granisetron, melphalan, meperidine, methotrexate, nesiritide, octreotide, ondansetron, oxaliplatin, paclitaxel, palonosetron, quinupristin-dalfopristin, riTUXimab, sodium acetate/bicarbonate, teniposide, thiotepa, tigecycline, trastuzumab, vinCRIStine, vinorelbine, voriconazole, zoledronic acid

Y-site incompatibilities: Fludarabine

Solution compatibilities: D$_{3.3}$/0.3% NaCl, D$_5$W, Normosol-R, Ringer's, 0.9% NaCl

DaunoXome

IV route
- Dilute with D$_5$W (1 mg/ml), give over 60 min, do not use in-line filter, reconstituted sol may be stored ≤6 hr refrigerated; do not admix

ADVERSE EFFECTS

DAUNOrubicin

CNS: Fever, chills

CV: **CHF, pericarditis, myocarditis,** peripheral edema, fatal myocarditis, left ventricular failure, QT prolongation, ST-T wave changes, QRS voltage changes, tachycardia, SVT, PVCs

GI: *Nausea, vomiting, anorexia, mucositis,* **hepatotoxicity**

GU: Impotence, sterility, amenorrhea, gynecomastia

HEMA: **Thrombocytopenia, leukopenia, anemia**

INTEG: *Rash, extravasation,* dermatitis, reversible alopecia, cellulitis, thrombophlebitis at inj site

MISC: **Anaphylaxis, tumor lysis syndrome**

DAUNOrubicin citrate liposome

CNS: Fatigue, headache, depression, insomnia, dizziness, malaise, neuropathy

CV: Chest pain, edema

GI: Abdominal pain, nausea, vomiting, *diarrhea,* constipation, stomatitis

INTEG: *Alopecia,* sweating, *pruritus*

MISC: *Allergic reactions, chest pain, fever,* edema, flulike symptoms

MS: *Rigors,* arthralgia, back pain

RESP: *Cough, dyspnea, rhinitis, sinusitis*

Pharmacokinetics

Absorption	Complete
Distribution	Widely distributed; crosses placenta
Metabolism	Liver, extensively
Excretion	Biliary (40%-50%)
Half-life	$18^1/_2$ hr, liposome $55^1/_2$ hr

Pharmacodynamics

Unknown

INTERACTIONS

Arsenic trioxide, chloroquine, clarithromycin, dasatinib, dolasetron, droperidol, erythromycin, flecainide, halofantrine, haloperidol, levomethadyl, methadone, ondansetron, palonosetron, pentamide, propafenone, risperidone, sparfloxacin, vorinstat, ziprasidone: Increase QT prolongation, torsades de pointes

Individual drugs

Cyclophosphamide, radiation: increased toxicity

Drug classifications

Antineoplastics: increased toxicity
Class IA/III antidysrhythmics, some phenothiazines, tricyclic antidepressants (high doses): increased QT prolongation, torsades de pointes

Live virus vaccines: decreased antibody reaction

NSAIDs, salicylates: increased risk of bleeding, anticoagulants, platelet inhibitors, thrombolytics

Hematopoietic progenitor cells: given within 24 hr: decreased DAUNOrubicin given within 24 hr

Drug/lab test

Increased: uric acid

NURSING CONSIDERATIONS

Assessment

• Assess buccal cavity q8hr for dryness, sores or ulceration, white patches, pain, bleeding, dysphagia; obtain prescription for viscous lidocaine (Xylocaine)

• Assess symptoms indicating severe allergic reaction: rash, pruritus, urticaria, purpuric skin lesions, itching, flushing; product should be discontinued

> **BLACK BOX WARNING:** Assess chest x-ray, echocardiography, radionuclide angiography, MUGA, ECG; watch for ST-T wave changes, low QRS and T, QT prolongation possible, dysrhythmias (sinus tachycardia, heart block, PVCs); watch for CHF (jugular vein distention, weight gain, edema, crackles), may occur after 2-6 mo of treatment

> **BLACK BOX WARNING:** Monitor CBC, differential, platelet count weekly, leukocyte nadir within 2 wk after administration, recovery within 3 wk; do not administer if absolute granulocyte count is <750/mm^3 (liposome)

• Assess for increased uric acid levels, swelling, joint pain primarily in extremities; patient should be well hydrated to prevent urate deposits

• **Acute renal failure, uric acid nephropathy:** Monitor renal function tests: BUN, creatinine, serum uric acid, urine CCr baseline and before each dose; I&O ratio; report fall in urine output to <30 ml/hr, provide aggressive alkalinization of the urine as use of allopurinol can prevent urate nephropathy

• Monitor temp q4hr (may indicate beginning of infection)

• **Hepatotoxicity:** Monitor liver function tests baseline and before each dose (bilirubin, AST, ALT, LDH) as needed or monthly; note jaundice of skin or sclera, dark urine, clay-colored

stools, itchy skin, abdominal pain, fever, diarrhea; hepatotoxicity can be severe
• Assess for bleeding: hematuria, stool guaiac, bruising or petechiae, mucosa or orifices q8hr; check for inflammation of mucosa, breaks in skin
• Identify effects of alopecia on body image; discuss feelings about body changes
• **Tumor lysis syndrome:** hyperkalemia, hyperphosphatemia, hyperuricemia, hypocalcemia

---

BLACK BOX WARNING: Extravasation:
swelling, pain, decreased blood return, if extravasation occurs stop infusion, remove tubing, attempt to aspirate the drug prior to removing the needle, elevate area, treat with ice

---

Nursing diagnoses
• Body image, disturbed (adverse reactions)
• Cardiac output, decreased (adverse reactions)
• Infection, risk for (adverse reactions)
• Injury, risk for (adverse reactions)
• Knowledge, deficient (teaching)

Patient/family education
• Teach patient to avoid use of products containing aspirin or ibuprofen, razors, commercial mouthwash, since bleeding may occur; to report symptoms of bleeding (hematuria, tarry stools)
• Instruct patient to report signs of **anemia** (fatigue, headache, irritability, faintness, shortness of breath); signs of **infection;** bleeding, bruising, shortness of breath, swelling, change in heart rate; to avoid crowds, those with known infections
• Advise patient that hair may be lost during treatment; a wig or hairpiece may make patient feel better; new hair may be different in color, texture
• Caution patient not to have any vaccinations without the advice of the prescriber; serious reactions can occur
• Advise patient that contraception is needed during treatment and for 4 mo after the completion of therapy, pregnancy **D**
• Advise patient to avoid alcohol, aspirin, NSAIDs
• Inform patient that urine and other body fluids may be red-orange for 48 hr
• Teach patient to avoid crowds, those with known infections

Evaluation
Positive therapeutic outcome
• Prevention of rapid division of malignant cells

decitabine (Rx)
(de-sit′-a-been)
Dacogen
Func. class.: Antineoplastic, antimetabolite
Chem. class.: Pyrimidine analog
Pregnancy category D

ACTION: Incorporated into DNA and inhibits DNA methylation, halting growth of rapid proliferation of blasts

Therapeutic outcome: Decreasing blast count

USES: Treatment of naïve and experienced myelodysplasic syndrome

CONTRAINDICATIONS:
Pregnancy **D**, breastfeeding, children, hypersensitivity to this product, severe neurotoxicity, severe blood dyscrasias

Precautions: Severe renal/hepatic disease, men (men should not father a child while receiving treatments or for 2 months after treatment ends), dental work, infections, thrombocytopenia

DOSAGE AND ROUTES
Adult: CONT **IV** first treatment cycle: 15 mg/m^2 over 3 hr, q8hr $\times$ 3 days; subsequent treatment cycles: repeat above cycle q6wk for at least 4 cycles; a partial or complete response may take more than 4 cycles

Available forms: Powder for injection, lyophilized 50 mg, in single-dose vial

Implementation
• Use cytotoxic handling procedures
• Rinse mouth tid-qid with water or club soda; brush teeth tid with soft toothbrush or cotton-tipped applicator for stomatitis; use unwaxed dental floss
• Store at room temperature, away from light

ADVERSE EFFECTS
CNS: Headache, anxiety, dizziness, hypoesthesia, insomnia, confusion
CV: Edema, murmur, hypotension
GI: Nausea, anorexia, vomiting, diarrhea, constipation, stomatitis, abdominal pain, dyspepsia
HEMA: Neutropenia, thrombocytopenia, leukopenia, anemia

INTEG: *Alopecia, ecchymosis, erythema, pallor, petechiae, pruritus, rash, swelling face, urticaria,* hematoma, cellulitis
META: *Decreased potassium, sodium, magnesium, albumin; increased bilirubin, increased/decreased glucose*
MS: *Myalgia, arthralgia, back pain, chest wall pain, pain in limbs*
RESP: *Cough, crackles,* **hypoxia,** *pharyngitis,* **pneumonia, pulmonary edema**

Pharmacokinetics

Absorption	Unknown
Distribution	Protein binding <1%
Metabolism	Liver, granulocytes, intestinal epithelium, whole blood
Excretion	Unknown
Half-life	Terminal 0.2-0.8 hr

Pharmacodynamics
Unknown

INTERACTIONS
Drug classifications
Do not use with live virus vaccines

NURSING CONSIDERATIONS
Assessment
• **Bone marrow suppression:** Monitor CBC (RBC, Hct, Hgb), differential, platelet count weekly; withhold product if WBC <4000/mm³, platelets <75,000/mm³, or RBC, Hct, Hgb is low; notify prescriber of results
• Monitor renal studies: BUN, serum uric acid, urine CCr, electrolytes before, during therapy
• Monitor temp q4hr; fever may indicate beginning infection; no rectal temps
• Monitor hepatic studies before, during treatment: bilirubin, AST, ALT, alkaline phosphatase, as needed or monthly
• Assess for **bleeding:** hematuria, heme-positive stools, bruising or petechiae, mucosa or orifices daily; blood dyscrasias can occur
• Assess for dyspnea, crackles, unproductive cough, chest pain, tachypnea, fatigue, increased pulse, pallor, lethargy, personality changes
• Assess buccal cavity daily for dryness, ulceration, white patches, oral pain, bleeding, dysphagia
• Assess GI symptoms: frequency of stools, cramping; if severe diarrhea occurs, electrolytes may need to be given

Nursing diagnoses
• Injury, risk for (uses)
• Knowledge, deficient (teaching)

Patient/family education
• Advise patient to report **bleeding;** not to use commercial mouthwashes, razors
• Teach patient to report signs of **infection:** increased temp, sore throat, flulike symptoms
• Teach patient to report signs of **anemia:** fatigue, headache, faintness, shortness of breath, irritability
• Advise patient to avoid citric acid, rough textured foods, if stomatitis is present
• Instruct patient not to operate machinery or perform other hazardous activities while taking this product
• Teach patient to notify prescriber if pregnancy is planned or suspected; use contraception while taking this product; men should not father a child while taking this product, pregnancy category **D;** to avoid breastfeeding while taking this product
• Teach patient to inform prescriber of kidney or liver disease
• Teach patient not to receive vaccinations while taking this product
• Advise to drink 2-3 L of fluids/day unless contraindicated

Evaluation
Positive therapeutic outcome
• Decreased blast count

delavirdine (Rx)
(de-la-veer′deen)
Rescriptor
Func. class.: Antiretroviral
Chem. class.: Nonnucleoside reverse transcriptase inhibitor (NNRTI)
Pregnancy category C

ACTION: Binds directly to reverse transcriptase and blocks RNA, DNA-dependent polymerase activities causing a disruption of the enzyme's site

Therapeutic outcome: Improvement of HIV-1 infection

USES: HIV-1 in combination with at least 2 other antiretrovirals

CONTRAINDICATIONS:
Hypersensitivity

Precautions: Pregnancy **C,** breastfeeding, children, hepatic disease, exfoliative dermatitis, hepatitis, immune reconstitution syndrome, achlorhydria, antimicrobial resistance

DOSAGE AND ROUTES
Adult and child ≥16 yr: PO 400 mg tid; max 1200 mg/day

Available forms: Tabs 100, 200 mg

Implementation
- Add 4 tabs/3-4 oz of water, let stand, stir, swallow, rinse glass, swallow; use only 100 mg tabs for dispersion
- Do not give within 1 hr of antacids or didanosine
- Take in equal intervals around the clock

ADVERSE EFFECTS
CNS: Headache, fatigue, anxiety, insomnia, fever
GI: Diarrhea, anorexia, abdominal pain, nausea, vomiting, dyspepsia, **hepatotoxicity**
GU: Nephrotoxicity
HEMA: Neutropenia, leukopenia, thrombocytopenia, anemia, granulocytopenia
INTEG: Rash, pruritus
MISC: Cough
MS: Pain, myalgia
SYST: Stevens-Johnson syndrome, immune reconstitution syndrome (combination therapy)

Pharmacokinetics
Absorption	Well
Distribution	98% protein bound
Metabolism	Liver, extensively by CYP3A4
Excretion	Kidneys, feces
Half-life	2-11 hr

Pharmacodynamics
Onset	Unknown
Peak	1 hr
Duration	8 hr

INTERACTIONS
Individual drugs
Alprazolam, amprenavir, atorvastatin, clarithromycin, dapsone, felodipine, indinavir, lovastatin, midazolam, NIFEdipine, saquinavir, simvastatin: increased level of each specific product
Alprazolam, astemizole, cisapride, midazolam, pimozide, sildenafil, terfenadine, triazolam: life-threatening reactions; do not combine
Clarithromycin, quiNIDine, warfarin: increased level of both products
Didanosine: decreased delavirdine levels, decreased action of didanosine

Fluoxetine, ketoconazole: increased level of delavirdine

Drug classifications
Amphetamines, antidysrhythmics, benzodiazepines, calcium channel blockers, ergots, sedative/hypnotics, opiates: increased serious life-threatening adverse reaction
Antacids, anticonvulsants, protease inhibitors, rifamycins: decreased delavirdine levels
Contraceptives (oral): decreased action of oral contraceptives
CYP3A4, 2D6 inhibitors: increased levels
Ergots: increased levels of ergots

Drug/herb
St. John's wort: decreased delavirdine level

NURSING CONSIDERATIONS
Assessment
- Assess CBC, blood chemistry, plasma HIV RNA, absolute $CD4^+/CD8^+$/cell counts/%, serum β_2 microglobulin, serum ICD+24 antigen levels
- Assess signs of infection, anemia
- Assess liver function tests: ALT, AST; renal studies
- Assess C&S before product therapy; product may be taken as soon as culture is taken; repeat C&S after treatment; determine the presence of other STDs
- Assess bowel pattern before, during treatment; if severe abdominal pain with bleeding occurs, product should be discontinued; monitor hydration
- Assess allergies before treatment, reaction to each medication; place allergies on chart
- Assess plasma delavirdine concentrations (trough 10 mcm)
- HIV: Obtain hepatitis B virus (HBV) screening to ensure proper treatment, if co-infected, a fully suppressive antiretroviral regimen with productions against both
- **Serious skin reactions: Stevens-Johnson syndrome;** any rash may occur within 1-3 wk of beginning treatment; if rash is not severe, manage with diphenhydrAMINE, hydrOXYzine, topical corticosteroids
- Immune reconstitution syndrome: When treated with combination therapy; development of opportunistic infections (*Mycobacterium avium* complex [MAC]), cytomegalovirus (CMV), *Pneumocystis jiroveci* pneumonia (PCP), or TB
- **Delavirdine toxicity:** severe nausea, vomiting, maculopapular rash

⚠ Nurse Alert

Nursing diagnoses
- Diarrhea (side effects)
- Infection, risk for (uses)
- Knowledge, deficient (teaching)

Patient/family education
- Advise patient to take as prescribed; if dose is missed, take as soon as remembered up to 1 hr before next dose; do not double dose
- Advise patient that product must be taken in equal intervals around the clock to maintain blood levels for duration of therapy
- Advise patient that tabs may be dissolved; drink right away, rinse cup with water, and drink that to get all medication
- Instruct patient to make sure health care provider knows of all the medications being taken
- Advise patient that if severe rash, mouth sores, swelling, aching muscles/joints, or eye redness occur, stop taking and notify health care provider
- Advise patient not to breastfeed if taking this product
- Teach patient that this product is not a cure, only controls symptoms

Evaluation
Positive therapeutic outcome
- Increased CD4⁺ cell count
- Decreased viral load
- Improvement in symptoms of HIV

demecarium ophthalmic
See Appendix B

denileukin diftitox (Rx)
(den-ih-loo′kin dif′tih-tox)
Ontak
Func. class.: Antineoplastic—miscellaneous agent
Pregnancy category C

ACTION: A recombinant DNA–derived cytotoxic protein that interacts with high-affinity IL-2 receptors on the cell surface and inhibits cellular protein synthesis

Therapeutic outcome: Prevention of rapidly growing malignant cells

USES: Cutaneous T-cell lymphoma that expresses CD25 component of the IL-2 receptor

Unlabeled uses: Non-Hodgkin's lymphoma, psoriasis

CONTRAINDICATIONS:
Hypersensitivity to denileukin, diphtheria toxin, interleukin-2

Precautions: Pregnancy C, breastfeeding, children, geriatric, CAD, *E. coli,* protein hypersensitivity, immunosuppression, peripheral vascular disease

> **BLACK BOX WARNING:** Capillary leak syndrome, infection-related reactions, visual disturbances

DOSAGE AND ROUTES
Adult: IV 9-18 mcg/kg/day given for 5 days q21day, give over ≥15 min

Available forms: sol for inj, frozen 150 mcg/ml

Implementation
- Give fluids **IV** or PO before chemotherapy to hydrate patient
- Give antiemetic 30-60 min before giving product to prevent vomiting, and prn; antibiotics for prophylaxis of infection
- Premedicate with acetaminophen or NSAID and diphenhydrAMINE 15-30 min before infusion; use dexamethasone (20 mg PO or 8 mg **IV**)
- Provide liquid diet: carbonated beverages; gelatin may be added if patient is not nauseated or vomiting

Intermittent IV infusion route
- Use cytotoxic handling procedures
- Bring to room temperature, after thawing, a haze may be visible, should be clear at room temperature
- Draw calculated dose from vial, inject into empty **IV** infusion bag; for each 1 ml of product removed from vial, no more than 9 ml of sterile saline without preservative should be added to **IV** bag; infuse over ≥15 min; do not give by BOL; do not admix with other products; do not use a filter, do not shake vigorously, mix gently by swirling
- Prepare and hold sol in plastic syringes or soft plastic **IV** bags only
- Use within 6 hr, discard unused portions

> **BLACK BOX WARNING:** Watch for extravasation; give 3-5 ml of mixture of 4 ml sodium thiosulfate 10% plus 5 ml sterile water SUBCUT as prescribed

ADVERSE EFFECTS

CNS: *Dizziness, paresthesia, nervousness, confusion, insomnia*

CV: *Hypo/hypertension, vasodilatation, tachycardia, thrombosis, dysrhythmia, hypertension,* **capillary leak syndrome**

EENT: Persistent visual impairment

GI: *Nausea, anorexia, vomiting, diarrhea, constipation, dyspepsia, dysphagia*

GU: *Hematuria,* albuminuria, pyuria, creatinine increase

HEMA: **Thrombocytopenia, leukopenia,** anemia

INTEG: *Rash, pruritus, sweating*

META: Hypoalbuminemia, edema, hypocalcemia, weight decrease, dehydration, hypokalemia

MISC: *Fever, chills, asthenia, infection, pain, headache, chest pain,* flulike symptoms, **serious infection, capillary leak syndrome**

MS: Myalgia, arthralgia

RESP: *Dyspnea, cough, pharyngitis, rhinitis*

Pharmacokinetics

Absorption	Complete bioavailability (**IV**)
Distribution	Widely distributed; concentrates in liver/kidneys
Metabolism	Proteolytic degradation
Excretion	Unknown
Half-life	Unknown

Pharmacodynamics

Unknown

INTERACTIONS

Drug classifications

Antineoplastics, bone marrow–suppressing products, radiation: increased bone marrow suppression

Live virus vaccines: increased adverse reactions; decreased antibody reaction

NURSING CONSIDERATIONS

Assessment

• Assess symptoms indicating severe allergic reaction: rash, pruritus, urticaria, purpuric skin lesions, itching, flushing; product should be discontinued

> **BLACK BOX WARNING:** Assess for **vascular leak syndrome** after 2 wk of treatment: hypotension, edema, hypoalbuminemia; monitor weight, B/P, serum albumin, edema

• Obtain CD25 expression on skin biopsy samples

> **BLACK BOX WARNING:** Assess for **infusion-related reactions,** may be fatal; vision disturbances may be permanent, monitor visual acuity, color vision

• Monitor CBC, differential, platelet count weekly; withhold product if WBC count is $<4000/mm^3$ or platelet count is $<100,000/mm^3$

• Monitor renal function studies: BUN, creatinine, urine CCr before, during therapy; I&O ratio; report fall in urine output to <30 ml/hr

• Monitor temp q4hr (may indicate beginning of infection)

• Monitor liver function tests before, during therapy (bilirubin, AST, ALT, LDH) as needed or monthly; note jaundiced skin or sclera, dark urine, clay-colored stools, itchy skin, abdominal pain, fever, diarrhea; hepatotoxicity can be serious and fatal

• Assess for bleeding: hematuria, stool guaiac, bruising or petechiae, mucosa or orifices q8hr; check for inflammation of mucosa, breaks in skin

Nursing diagnoses

• Body image, disturbed (adverse reactions)
• Infection, risk for (adverse reactions)
• Injury, risk for (adverse reactions)
• Knowledge, deficient (teaching)

Patient/family education

• Teach patient to avoid use of products containing aspirin or NSAIDs, razors, commercial mouthwash, since **bleeding** may occur; to report symptoms of bleeding (hematuria, tarry stools)

• Instruct patient to report signs of **anemia** (fatigue, headache, irritability, faintness, shortness of breath)

• Advise patient to report signs of **infection:** fever; sore throat, flu-like symptoms

• Caution patient not to have any vaccinations without the advice of prescriber; serious reactions can occur

• Advise patient contraception is needed during treatment and for several months after the completion of therapy; product has teratogenic properties

Evaluation

Positive therapeutic outcome

• Prevention of rapid division of malignant cells

⚠ Nurse Alert

denosumab (Rx)

(den-oh'sue-mab)
Prolia, Xgeva
Func. class.: Bone resorption inhibitor
Chem. class.: Monoclonal antibody, bone resorption
Pregnancy category C

ACTION: Neutralizes activity of receptor activator nuclear factor kappa-B ligand (RANKL) by binding to it and blocking its interaction with cell surface receptors, use of a RANKL inhibitor may reduce bone turnover and decrease tumor burden

Therapeutic outcome: Increased/maintained bone density

USES: Osteoporosis in postmenopausal women at high risk for fractures, prevention of skeletal-related events in bone metastases from solid tumors

CONTRAINDICATIONS:

Hypersensitivity, hypocalcemia

Precautions: Anemia, breastfeeding, child/infant/neonate, coagulopathy, diabetes mellitus, dialysis, eczema, hypoparathyroidism, immunosuppression, latex hypersensitivity, malabsorption syndrome, neonates, neoplastic disease, pancreatitis, parathyroid disease, pregnancy C, dental/renal/thyroid disease, TB, Vitamin D deficiency

DOSAGE AND ROUTES

Postmenopausal osteoporosis
Adult female: Subcut 60 mg q6mo with 1000 mg calcium and 400 international units vitamin D, max 60 mg q6mo

Bone metastases from solid tumors
Adult: SUBCUT 120 mg q4wk, max 120 mg q4wk; administer with calcium and vitamin D as necessary to prevent hypocalcemia

Prevention of skeletal-related events in bone metastases from solid tumors
Adult: SUBCUT (Xgeva): 120 mg q4wk

Available forms: Solution for injection 60 mg/ml (Prolia); 120 mg/1.7 ml (Xgeva)

Implementation
SUBCUT route
• Give acetaminophen before and for 72 hr after to decrease pain

• Do not use if particulate matter or discoloration is present; solution is clear and colorless to slightly yellow with small white/opalescent particles, remove from refrigerator and allow to warm to room temperature (15-30 min)
• **Use of prefilled syringe with needle safety guard:** Leave green guard in original position until after administration, remove and discard needle cap immediately before injection, give by SUBCUT injection in upper arm, thigh, or abdomen; after injection, point needle away from people and slide green guard over needle
• **Use of single-use vials:** Use 27G needle, give in upper arm/thigh, or abdomen, do not re-insert needle in vial, discard supplies as appropriate
• Avoid direct sunlight/heat, do not freeze, use within 14 days after removal from refrigerator, store unopened containers in refrigerator

ADVERSE EFFECTS
CNS: Chills, fever, flushing, headache, vertigo, neuropathic pain
CV: Angina, **atrial fibrillation**
GI: Abdominal pain, constipation, *diarrhea*, flatulence, GERD, *vomiting, nausea*
GU: Cystitis, lactation suppression
HEMA: Anemia, neutropenia
INTEG: Atopic dermatitis, pruritus
META: Hypercholesterolemia, hypocalcemia, hypophosphatemia
MS: Back/bone pain, MS pain, myalgia, **osteonecrosis of the jaw**
RESP: Cough, *dyspnea*
SYST: Infection, secondary malignancy

Pharmacokinetics

Absorption	Bioavailability 62%
Distribution	Unknown
Metabolism	Unknown
Excretion	Unknown
Half-life	25.4 days

Pharmacodynamics

Onset	Unknown
Peak	Maximum serum concentration 3-21 days
Duration	Steady state 6 months

INTERACTIONS

Drug classifications
Immunosuppressives, corticosteroids: possible increased infection
Antineoplastics, corticosteroids: possible increased osteonecrosis of the jaw

NURSING CONSIDERATIONS

Assessment
• **Assess for acute acute-phase reaction:** fever, myalgia, headache, flulike symptoms, for 72 hr after injection, usually resolves after 72 hr
• Monitor blood tests: serum calcium/creatinine/BUN/magnesium/phosphate
• **Assess for hypocalcemia:** paresthesia, twitching, laryngospasm, Chvostek's/Trousseau's signs; preexisting hypocalcemia prior to treatment; patient with vitamin D deficiency may require higher doses of vitamin D
• **Assess for hypercalcemia:** nausea, vomiting, anorexia, weakness, thirst, constipation, dysrhythmias
• **Monitor dental status:** correct dental complications prior to product use, good oral hygiene should be maintained; if dental work is to be performed, antiinfectives should be given to prevent osteonecrosis of the jaw
• **Assess for infection:** Do not start treatment in those with active infections, infections should be resolved first

Nursing diagnoses
• Electrolyte imbalance, risk for (uses)

Patient/family education
• Advise patient to report hypercalcemic relapse: nausea, vomiting, bone pain, thirst
• Teach patient to continue with dietary recommendations including additional calcium and vitamin D
• Advise patient to avoid use in pregnancy and breastfeeding, notify prescriber if pregnancy is planned or suspected
• Instruct patient to use acetaminophen prior to and for 72 hrs after injection to lessen bone pain
• Explain the purpose of this product and expected results
• Advise patient to avoid OTC, Rx, or herbs and supplements unless approved by prescriber
• Teach patient to use regular exercise, stop smoking, and avoid alcohol to maintain bone health
• Advise patient to inform all health care providers of product use, avoid dental procedures/surgery if possible, practice good oral hygiene
• Teach patient that lab tests and follow-up exams will be required

Evaluation
Positive therapeutic outcome
• Increased/maintained bone density

---

desipramine (Rx)
(dess-ip′ra-meen)
Apo-Desipramine ✶, Norpramin, PMS-Desipramine ✶
Func. class.: Antidepressant, tricyclic
Chem. class.: Dibenzazepine, secondary amine
Pregnancy category C

ACTION: Blocks reuptake of norepinephrine, serotonin into nerve endings, increasing action of norepinephrine, serotonin in nerve cells

Therapeutic outcome: Decreased depression

USES: Depression

Unlabeled uses: Chronic pain, ADHD, bulimia, diabetic neuropathy, panic disorder, social phobia

CONTRAINDICATIONS:
Hypersensitivity to tricyclics, closed-angle glaucoma, acute MI

Precautions: Pregnancy **C,** breastfeeding, geriatric, severe depression, increased intraocular pressure, seizure disorder, CV disease, urinary retention, cardiac dysrhythmias, cardiac conduction disturbances, family history of sudden death, prostatic hypertrophy, thyroid disease

> **BLACK BOX WARNING:** Suicidal patients, children <18 yr

DOSAGE AND ROUTES
Major depression
Adult: PO 50-75 mg/day in 1-4 divided doses; titrate by 25-50 mg qwk up to 300 mg/day in single or divided doses
Geriatric: PO 25 mg/day at bedtime, titrate qwk; may increase to 150 mg/day
Child >12 yr: PO 25-50 mg/day in divided doses, max 150 mg/day
Child 6-12 yr: PO 1-3 mg/kg/day in divided doses, give >3 mg/kg/day with close medical monitoring; max 5 mg/kg/day

Available forms: Tabs 10, 25, 50, 75, 100, 150 mg

Implementation
• Increase fluids, bulk in diet for constipation, especially in geriatric
• Take with food or milk for GI symptoms

• Crush if patient is unable to swallow medication whole
• Give dosage at bedtime if oversedation occurs during day; may take entire dose at bedtime; geriatric may not tolerate once a day dosing
• Give gum, hard candy, frequent sips of water for dry mouth
• Store at room temperature
• Provide assistance with ambulation during beginning of therapy for drowsiness/dizziness
• Provide safety measures, primarily in the geriatric
• Check to see that PO medication is swallowed

ADVERSE EFFECTS

CNS: *Dizziness, drowsiness,* confusion, headache, anxiety, tremors, stimulation, weakness, insomnia, nightmares, EPS (geriatric), increased psychiatric symptoms, paresthesia, suicidal ideation
CV: *Orthostatic hypo/hypertension, ECG changes, tachycardia, palpitations*
EENT: *Blurred vision,* tinnitus, mydriasis, ophthalmoplegia
GI: *Diarrhea, dry mouth,* nausea, vomiting, **paralytic ileus**, increased appetite, cramps, epigastric distress, jaundice, **hepatitis**, stomatitis, constipation, weight gain
GU: *Retention,* **acute renal failure**
HEMA: Agranulocytosis, thrombocytopenia, eosinophilia, leukopenia
INTEG: Rash, urticaria, sweating, pruritus, photosensitivity

Pharmacokinetics

Absorption	Well
Distribution	Widely, protein binding 92%
Metabolism	Extensively, liver
Excretion	Unknown
Half-life	12-24 hr

Pharmacodynamics

Unknown

INTERACTIONS

Individual drugs

Alcohol: increased CNS depression
Cimetidine, diltiazem, fluvoxamine, fluoxetine, paroxetine, sertraline, verapamil: increased desipramine level
CloNIDine: increased life-threatening B/P elevations, do not use concurrently
EPINEPHrine, norepinephrine: increased hypertension

Gatifloxacin, levofloxacin, moxifloxacin, sparfloxacin, sunitinib, vorinostat, ziprasidone: increased serotonin syndrome, neuroleptic malignant syndrome

Drug classifications

Barbiturates, opioids, CNS depressants: increased CNS depression
MAOIs: increased hyperpyrexia, seizures, excitation; do not use within 14 days of MAOIs
SSRIs, SNRIs, serotonin-receptor agonists, other tricyclic antidepressants: increased serotonin syndrome, neuroleptic malignant syndrome
Class IA/III dysrhythmics, tricyclic antidepressants: increased QT interval

Drug/herb

Kava, valerian: increased CNS depression
St. John's wort: may increase serotonin syndrome; avoid concurrent use

Drug/lab test

Increase: serum bilirubin, blood glucose, alkaline phosphatase

NURSING CONSIDERATIONS

Assessment

• Monitor B/P (lying, standing), pulse q4hr; if systolic B/P drops 20 mm Hg, hold product, notify prescriber; take vital signs q4hr in patients with CV disease
• Monitor blood studies: CBC, leukocytes, differential, cardiac enzymes if patient is receiving long-term therapy
• Monitor hepatic studies: AST, ALT, bilirubin
• Check weight qwk; appetite may increase with this product
• Monitor ECG for flattening T wave, bundle branch block, AV block, dysrhythmias in cardiac patients
• Assess for EPS primarily in geriatric: rigidity, dystonia, akathisia
• Assess for **seizure activity** in those with a history of seizures
• Assess mental status: mood, sensorium, affect, **suicidal tendencies,** increase in psychiatric symptoms: depression, panic
• Assess for urinary retention, constipation; constipation most likely in children
• Assess for **withdrawal symptoms:** headache, nausea, vomiting, muscle pain, weakness; not usual unless product is discontinued abruptly
• Assess for alcohol consumption; if consumed, hold dose until morning

Nursing diagnoses
• Coping, ineffective (uses)
• Knowledge, deficient (teaching)
• Noncompliance (teaching)

Patient/family education
• Advise patient that therapeutic effects may take 2-3 wk
• Teach patient that suicidal thoughts and behavior may occur, notify prescriber immediately
• Advise patient to use caution in driving, other activities requiring alertness because of drowsiness, dizziness, blurred vision
• Teach patient to avoid alcohol ingestion, other CNS depressants
• Teach patient not to discontinue medication quickly after long-term use; may cause nausea, headache, malaise
• Teach patient to wear sunscreen or large hat, since photosensitivity occurs

Evaluation
Positive therapeutic outcome
• Decreased depression

TREATMENT OF OVERDOSE:
ECG monitoring; induce emesis; lavage, activated charcoal; administer anticonvulsant

---

desloratadine (Rx)
(des-lor-at'ah-deen)
Clarinex, Clarinex RediTabs
Func. class.: Antihistamine, 2nd generation
Chem. class.: Selective histamine (H_1) receptor antagonist
Pregnancy category C

ACTION: Binds to peripheral histamine receptors, providing antihistamine action without sedation

Therapeutic outcome: Decreased nasal stuffiness, itching, swollen eyes

USES: Seasonal/perennial allergic rhinitis, chronic idiopathic urticaria

CONTRAINDICATIONS:
Hypersensitivity, infants/neonates

Precautions: Pregnancy C, bronchial asthma, renal/hepatic impairment, child, breastfeeding

DOSAGE AND ROUTES
Adult and child ≥12 yr: PO 5 mg daily
Child 6-11 yr: PO 2.5 mg daily

Child 1-5 yr: PO 1.25 mg daily
Child 6-11 mo: PO 1 mg daily (urticaria only)

Renal/hepatic dose
Adult: PO 5 mg every other day

Available forms: Tabs 5 mg; orally disintegrating (Reditabs) 2.5, 5 mg; syr 0.5 mg/ml

Implementation
• May administer without regard to meals
• Store in airtight container at room temperature

ADVERSE EFFECTS
CNS: Sedation (more common with increased dosages), headache, psychomotor hyperactivity, **seizures,** fatigue
GI: Hepatitis, nausea, dry mouth
MISC: Flulike symptoms

Pharmacokinetics
Absorption	Unknown
Distribution	Bound to plasma proteins (82%-87%)
Metabolism	Liver (active metabolites)
Excretion	Urine, feces (metabolites)
Half-life	$8^1/_2$-28 hr

Pharmacodynamics
Onset	1 hr, relief in 1 day
Peak	$1^1/_2$ hr
Duration	24 hr

INTERACTIONS

Drug/drug
Alcohol: increased CNS depression (rare)
Etravirine, nilotinib: increased desloratadine effect

Drug classification
Anxiolytics, antipsychotics, H_1 blockers, opiates, sedative/hypnotics, tricyclics, antidepressants: increased CNS depression (rare)

NURSING CONSIDERATIONS

Assessment
• Assess for **allergy:** hives, rash, rhinitis; monitor respiratory status; test interaction, antigen skin test

Nursing diagnoses
• Airway clearance, ineffective (uses)
• Knowledge, deficient (teaching)
• Noncompliance (teaching, overuse)

Patient/family education
• Advise patient to avoid driving, other hazardous activities if drowsiness occurs; to observe caution until product's effects are known
• Advise patient that product may cause photosensitivity; use sunscreen or stay out of the sun to prevent burns
• Caution patient to avoid use of other CNS depressants
• Teach not to remove Reditabs from blister until ready to use; to place Reditab directly on tongue; may take with or without water

Evaluation
Positive therapeutic outcome
• Absence of running or congested nose, other allergy symptoms

---

desmopressin (Rx)
(des-moe-press'in)
Apo-Desmopressin, DDAVP, Minirin, Octostim ✦, Stimate
Func. class.: Pituitary hormone
Chem. class.: Synthetic antidiuretic hormone
Pregnancy category B

ACTION: Promotes reabsorption of water by action on renal tubular epithelium in the kidney; causes smooth muscle constriction and increase in plasma factor VIII levels, which increases platelet aggregation resulting in vasopressor effect; similar to vasopressin

Therapeutic outcome: Prevention of nocturnal enuresis, decreased bleeding in hemophilia A, von Willebrand's disease type 1, control and stabilization of water in diabetes insipidus

USES: Hemophilia A, von Willebrand's disease type 1, nonnephrogenic diabetes insipidus, symptoms of polyuria/polydipsia caused by pituitary dysfunction, nocturnal enuresis

CONTRAINDICATIONS:
Hypersensitivity, nephrogenic diabetes insipidus, severe renal disease

Precautions: Pregnancy **B**, breastfeeding, CAD, hypertension, cystic fibrosis, thrombus

DOSAGE AND ROUTES
Primary nocturnal enuresis
Adult and child ≥6 yr: INTRANASAL 0.2 mg (half in each nostril) at bedtime, may increase to 40 mcg; PO 0.2 mg at bedtime, may be increased to max 0.6 mg at bedtime

Diabetes insipidus
Adult: Intranasal 0.1-0.4 ml daily in divided doses (1-4 sprays with pump); SUBCUT/IV 0.5-1 ml daily in divided doses
Child 3 mo-12 yr: INTRANASAL 0.05-0.3 ml daily in divided doses

Hemophilia/von Willebrand's disease
Adult and child >3 mo: IV 0.3 mcg/kg in NaCl over 15-30 min; may repeat if needed

Antihemorrhagic
Adult and child >3 mo: IV 0.3 mcg/kg
Adult and child <50 kg: Intranasal 1 spray in one nostril
Adult and child >50 kg: 1 spray each nostril

Available forms: Inj 4, 15 mcg/ml, Rhinal Tube delivery 2.5 mg/vial (0.1 mg/ml); tabs 0.1, 0.2 mg; nasal spray pump 10 mcg/spray (0.1 mg/ml); nasal sol 1.5 mg/ml (150 mcg/dose)

Implementation
• Draw medication into tube, insert tube into nostril to instill product and blow on other end to deliver sol into nasal cavity; rinse after use
• Store in refrigerator or cool environment

IV, direct route
• Give undiluted over 1 min in diabetes insipidus

Intermittent IV infusion route
• Give single dose diluted in 50 ml of 0.9% NaCl (adult and child >10 kg); a single dose/10 ml as an IV inf over 15-30 min in von Willebrand's disease or hemophilia A

ADVERSE EFFECTS
CNS: Drowsiness, headache, lethargy, flushing, **seizures**
CV: Increased B/P, palpitations, tachycardia
EENT: Nasal irritation, congestion, rhinitis
GI: Nausea, heartburn, cramps
GU: *Vulval pain*
META: Hyponatremia, hyponatremia-induced seizures
SYST: Anaphylaxis (IV)

Pharmacokinetics

Absorption	Nasal (up to 20%)
Distribution	Unknown
Metabolism	Unknown
Excretion	Unknown; breast milk
Half-life	8 min (initial), 76 min (terminal)

Pharmacodynamics

	PO	Intra-nasal	SUBCUT/IV
Onset	1 hr	1 hr	Rapid
Peak	4-7 hr	1-4 hr	15-30 min
Duration	Unknown	8-20 hr	3 hr

INTERACTIONS

Individual drugs

Alcohol, demeclocycline, EPHINEPHrine (large doses), heparin, lithium: decreased antidiuretic action

CarBAMazepine, chlorpropamide, clofibrate: increased antidiuretic action

NURSING CONSIDERATIONS

Assessment

• Monitor I&O ratio, urine osmolality, specific gravity, weight daily; check for edema in extremities; if water retention is severe, diuretic may be prescribed; check pulse, B/P when giving product **IV** or SUBCUT

• Assess for **water intoxication:** lethargy, behavioral changes, disorientation, neuromuscular excitability, dehydration, poor skin turgor, severe thirst, dry skin, tachycardia

• Assess intranasal use: nausea, congestion, cramps, headache; usually decreased with decreased dosage

• Monitor for enuresis during treatment (**nocturnal enuresis**)

• Assess for allergic reaction, including anaphylaxis (**IV route**)

• Assess for nasal mucosa changes: congestion, edema, discharge, scarring (nasal route)

• Monitor urine volume osmolality and plasma osmolality (diabetes insipidus)

• Monitor factor VIII coagulant activity before using for hemostasis

Nursing diagnoses

• Fluid volume, deficient (uses)
• Fluid volume, excess (side effects)
• Knowledge, deficient (teaching)

Patient/family education

• Use demonstration, return demonstration to teach technique for nasal instillation

• Teach patient to notify prescriber of dyspnea, vomiting, cramping, drowsiness, headache, nasal congestion

• Caution patient to avoid OTC products (cough, hay fever), since these preparations may contain epinephrine and decrease product response; do not use with alcohol

• Advise patient to carry/wear emergency ID or other identification specifying disease and medication used

• Advise patient if dose is missed, take when remembered, up to 1 hr before next dose; do not double doses; avoid fluids from 1 hr to up to 8 hr after PO dose

• Teach patient to report upper respiratory infection, nasal congestion

Evaluation
Positive therapeutic outcome

• Absence of severe thirst
• Decreased urine output, osmolality
• Absence of bleeding (hemophilia)

desonide topical
See Appendix B

desoximetasone topical
See Appendix B

desoxyephedrine nasal agent
See Appendix B

desoxyribonuclease
See fibrinolysin/desoxyribonuclease

desvenlafaxine (Rx)
Pristiq
Func. class.: Antidepressant, serotonin-receptor norepinephrine reuptake inhibitor (SNRI)
Pregnancy category C

ACTION: May work by blocking the central presynaptic reuptake of 5-HT and NE, resulting in an increased sustained level of these neurotransmitters.

Therapeutic outcome: Decreased depression, increased sense of well-being and renewed interest in activities

USES: Major depressive disorder

Unlabeled uses: Vasomotor symptoms (hot flashes) associated with menopause

CONTRAINDICATIONS:
Hypersensitivity to this product or venlafaxine, MAOI therapy

Precautions: CNS depression, abrupt discontinuation, hypertension, hepatic/renal disease, hyponatremia, geriatric patients, pregnancy C, labor and delivery, breastfeeding, angina, bleeding, cardiac dysrhythmias, MI, stroke, mania, hypovolemia, dehydration

> **BLACK BOX WARNING:** Children, suicidal ideation

DOSAGE AND ROUTES
Adult: PO Initially, 50 mg daily; max 400 mg/day with adjustments as needed

Vasospastic effects of menopause (unlabeled)
Adults: PO 100-150 mg/day

Available forms: Ext rel tabs 50, 100 mg

ADVERSE EFFECTS
CNS: *Dizziness,* drowsiness, *headache,* tremor, paresthesias, asthenia, worsening of depression, **suicidal thoughts and behaviors, seizures,** fatigue, chills, yawning, hot flashes, flushing, *irritability, insomnia, anxiety, abnormal dreams, fatigue*
CV: Palpitations, sinus tachycardia, increased blood pressure, orthostatic hypotension
EENT: Blurred vision, mydriasis, tinnitus
GI: *Nausea,* xerostomia, *diarrhea,* constipation, vomiting, anorexia, weight loss, dysgeusia, hypercholesterolemia, hypertriglyceridemia
GU: Urinary retention/hesitancy, orgasm dysfunction, decreased libido, impotence, proteinuria
HEMA: Impaired platelet aggregation
INTEG: Photosensitivity, hyperhidrosis, diaphoresis
SYST: Serotonin syndrome, neuroleptic malignant syndrome-like symptoms, toxic epidermal necrolysis, rash, Stevens-Johnson syndrome, erythema multiforme, angioedema; neonatal abstinence syndrome (fetal exposure)

Pharmacokinetics
Absorption	Unknown
Distribution	Protein binding 30%; enters breast milk
Metabolism	Liver, 55%
Excretion	Urine, unchanged, 45%
Half-life	Elimination 11 hr, increased in hepatic/renal disease

Pharmacodynamics
Onset	Unknown
Peak	7.5 hr
Duration	24 hr

INTERACTIONS
Individual drugs
Dexfenfluramine, dexmethylphenidate, dextromethorphan, fenfluramine, linezolid, lithium, nefazodone, meperidine, methylphenidate, mirtazapine, pentazocine, phentermine, promethazine, sibutramine, sumatriptan, trazodone, tryptophan: do not administer concurrently; increased serotonin syndrome, neuroleptic malignant syndrome-like reactions
Zolpidem: increased hallucinations, delusions, disorientation

Drug classifications
Anticoagulants, NSAIDs, platelet inhibitors, salicylates, thrombolytics: increased bleeding risk
Alcohol, antihistamines, opioids, sedatives/hypnotics: increased CNS depression
Ergots, MAOIs, serotonin receptor agonists (almotriptan, eletriptan, frovatriptan, naratriptan, rizatriptan, sumatriptan, zolmitriptan), SSRIs, other SNRIs, TCAs: do not administer concurrently; increased serotonin syndrome, neuroleptic malignant syndrome-like reactions

Drug/herb
Kava kava, valerian: increased desvenlafaxine action

NURSING CONSIDERATIONS
Assessment
• **Suicidal thoughts/behaviors: Assess mental status and mood, identify suicidal ideation**
• **Serotonin syndrome, neuroleptic malignant syndrome-like symptoms:** Assess for nausea/vomiting, sedation, dizziness,

diaphoresis (sweating), facial flush, hallucinations, mental status changes, myoclonia, restlessness, shivering, elevated blood pressure, hyperthermia, muscle rigidity, autonomic instability, and mental status changes; if serotonin syndrome occurs discontinue desvenlafaxine, and any other serotonergic agents
• Monitor B/P baseline and periodically during treatment
• Assess appetite and nutritional intake, weight loss is common, change diet as need to support weight

Nursing diagnoses
• Ineffective coping (uses)
• Risk for injury (adverse reactions)

Patient/family education
• Teach patient to take as directed, not to double or skip doses; if a dose is missed, take as soon as remembered unless close to next dose, do not discontinue abruptly, decreased gradually
• Advise patient report immediately suicidal thoughts or behaviors, have family members look for symptoms of suicidal ideation
• Inform patient not to operate machinery or engage in hazardous activities until reaction ins known, may cause dizziness, drowsiness
• Teach patient to avoid all others products unless approval by prescriber
• Teach patient to report if pregnancy is planned or suspected, pregnancy C, or if breastfeeding
• Teach patient to report immediately allergic reactions including, rash, hives, difficulty breathing, or swelling of face, lips
• Advise patient that continuing follow-up exams will be needed

Evaluation
Positive therapeutic outcome
• Decreased depression, increased sense of well-being and renewed interest in activities

dexamethasone (Rx)
(dex-ah-meth′ah-sone)
Apo-Dexamethasone ✦, **Baycadvor, Decadron, Dexasone** ✦, **Dex Pak, Maxidex** ✦, **PMS-Dexamethasone** ✦, **ratio-Dexamethasone** ✦, **Zena-Pak**
dexamethasone sodium phosphate (Rx)
Func. class.: Corticosteroid, synthetic
Chem. class.: Glucocorticoid, long-acting
Pregnancy category C

Do not confuse:
Decadron/Percodan

ACTION: Decreases inflammation by suppressing migration of polymorphonuclear leukocytes, fibroblasts, reversing increased capillary permeability and lysosomal stabilization

USES: Inflammation, allergies, neoplasms, cerebral edema, septic shock, collagen disorders

CONTRAINDICATIONS:
Psychosis, hypersensitivity to corticosteroids or benzyl alcohol, idiopathic thrombocytopenia, acute glomerulonephritis, amebiasis, fungal infections, nonasthmatic bronchial disease, child <2 yr, AIDS, TB, glaucoma, ocular infection

Precautions: Pregnancy C, breastfeeding, diabetes mellitus, osteoporosis, seizure disorders, ulcerative colitis, CHF, myasthenia gravis, renal disease, peptic ulcer, esophagitis

DOSAGE AND ROUTES
Inflammation
Adult: PO 0.75-9 mg/day, in divided doses q6-12hr; or phosphate IM 0.5-9 mg/day divided q6-12hr
Child: PO 0.024-0.34 mg/kg/day in divided doses q6-12hr

Shock
Adult: IV (phosphate) single dose 1-6 mg/kg or IV 40 mg q2-6hr as needed up to 72 hr

Cerebral edema
Adult: IV (phosphate) 10 mg, then 4-6 mg IM q6hr × 2-4 days, then taper over 1 wk
Child: PO/IM/IV loading dose 1-2 mg/kg, then 1-1.5 mg/kg/day, max 16 mg/day divided q4-6hr for 2-4 days, then taper down qwk

Adrenocortical insufficiency
Adult: PO 0.75-9 mg/day in divided doses
Child: PO 0.03-0.3 mg/kg/day divided in 2-4 doses

Suppression test
Adult: PO 1 mg at 11 PM or 0.5 mg q6hr × 48 hr

Croup (unlabeled)
Child: PO 0.024-0.34 mg/kg/day or 0.66-10 mg/m^2/day in 2-4 divided doses; a single dose of 0.6 mg/kg has been used for mild to moderate croup; IM/IV 0.06-0.3 mg/kg/day or 1.2-10 mg/m^2/day in divided doses q6-12hr; a single dose of 0.6 mg/kg IM has been used for severe croup

Available forms: Dexamethasone: tabs 0.25, 0.5, 0.75, 1, 1.5, 2, 4, 6 mg; elix 0.5 mg/5 ml; oral sol 0.5 mg/5 ml, 1 mg/ml; **phosphate** 4, 10, 20, 24 mg/ml

Implementation
PO route
• Give with food or milk to decrease GI symptoms
• Provide assistance with ambulation in patient with bone tissue disease to prevent fractures
IM route
• IM inj deep in large muscle mass; rotate sites; avoid deltoid; use 21-G needle
• In one dose in AM to prevent adrenal suppression; avoid SUBCUT administration, may damage tissue

Direct IV route
• IV undiluted direct over 1 min or less
• After shaking susp (parenteral); do not give susp IV
• Titrated dose; use lowest effective dose
Intermittent IV infusion route
• Diluted with 0.9% NaCl or D$_5$W and give as an IV inf at prescribed rate

Dexamethasone sodium phosphate

Syringe compatibilities: Caffeine, dimenhydrAMINE, furosemide, granisetron, ketamine, metoclopramide, octreotide, oxy-CODONE, palonosetron, ranitidine, SUFentanil, tramadol

Y-site compatibilities: Acyclovir, alfentanil, allopurinol, amifostine, amikacin, aminocaproic acid, aminophylline, amphotericin B cholesteryl, amphotericin B lipid complex, amphotericin B liposome, amsacrine, anidulafungin, ascorbic acid injection, atenolol, atracurium, atropine, aztreonam, benztropine, bivalirudin, bleomycin, bumetanide, buprenor-phine, butorphanol, caffeine, CARBOplatin, cefamandole, ceFAZolin, cefepime, cefmetazole, cefonicid, cefoperazone, cefotaxime, cefotetan, cefoxitin, cefpirome, ceftazidime, ceftizoxime, ceftobiprole, cefTRIAXone, cephalothin, cephapirin, chloramphenicol, cimetidine, cisatracurium, CISplatin, cladribine, clindamycin, codeine, cyanocobalamin, cyclophosphamide, cycloSPORINE, cytarabine, DACTINomycin, DAPTOmycin, dexmedetomidine, digoxin, diltiazem, docetaxel, DOPamine, doripenem, doxacurium, DOXOrubicin, DOXOrubicin liposomal, enalaprilat, ePHEDrine, EPINEPHrine, epoetin alfa, eptifibatide, ertapenem, etoposide, famotidine, fentaNYL, filgrastim, fluconazole, fludarabine, fluorouracil, folic acid, foscarnet, furosemide, ganciclovir, gatifloxacin, gemcitabine, glycopyrrolate, granisetron, heparin, hydrocortisone, HYDROmorphone, ifosfamide, imipenem-cilastatin, indomethacin, insulin (regular), irinotecan, isoproterenol, ketorolac, lansoprazole, levofloxacin, lidocaine, linezolid, LORazepam, LR, mannitol, mechlorethamine, melphalan, meropenem, metaraminol, methadone, methicillin, methoxamine, methyldopa, methylPREDNISolone, metoclopramide, metoprolol, metroNIDAZOLE, mezlocillin, miconazole, milrinone, morphine, moxalactam, multiple vitamins injection, nafcillin, nalbuphine, naloxone, nitroglycerin, nitroprusside, norepinephrine, octreotide, ondansetron, oxacillin, oxaliplatin, oxyCODONE, oxytocin, paclitaxel, palonosetron, pamidronate, pancuronium, pemetrexed, penicillin G potassium/sodium, PENTobarbital, PHENobarbital, phenylephrine, phytonadione, piperacillin, piperacillin-tazobactam, potassium chloride, procainamide, propofol, propranolol, pyridoxine, ranitidine, remifentanil, Ringer's, ritodrine, riTUXimab, sargramostim, sodium acetate/bicarbonate, succinylcholine, SUFentanil, tacrolimus, teniposide, theophylline, thiamine, thiotepa, ticarcillin, ticarcillin-clavulanate, tigecycline, tirofiban, TNA, tolazoline, topotecan, trastuzumab, trimetaphan, urokinase, vancomycin, vasopressin, vecuronium, verapamil, vinCRIStine, vinorelbine, vitamin B complex/C, voriconazole, zidovudine, zoledronic acid

ADVERSE EFFECTS
CNS: *Depression, flushing, sweating,* headache, mood changes, euphoria, psychosis, **seizures,** insomnia
CV: *Hypertension,* circulatory collapse, **thrombophlebitis, embolism,** tachycardia, edema, cardiomyopathy
EENT: Fungal infections, increased intraocular pressure, blurred vision, cataracts, glaucoma

ENDO: Hypothalmic-pituitary-adrenal axis suppression, hyperglycemia, sodium, fluid retention
GI: *Diarrhea, nausea, abdominal distention,* **GI hemorrhage,** *increased appetite,* **pancreatitis**
HEMA: **Thrombocytopenia,** transient leukocytosis, **thromboembolism**
INTEG: Acne, poor wound healing, ecchymosis, petechiae, hirsutism
META: Hypokalemia
MS: Fractures, osteoporosis, weakness, arthralgia, myopathy

Pharmacokinetics

Absorption	Unknown
Distribution	Unknown
Metabolism	Liver
Excretion	Kidneys
Half-life	36-54 hr

Pharmacodynamics

	PO	IM
Onset	1 hr	Unknown
Peak	1-2 hr	8 hr
Duration	2½ days	6 days-3 wk

INTERACTIONS

Individual drugs
Alcohol, amphotericin B, cycloSPORINE, digoxin, indomethacin: increased side effects
Ambemonium, isoniazid, neostigmine, sometrem: decreased effects of each specific product
Cholestyramine, colestipol, ephedrine, phenytoin, rifampin, theophylline: decreased action of dexamethasone
CycloSPORINE, tacrolimus: increased effect of each drug
Ketoconazole: increased action of dexamethasone

Drug classifications
Antacids, barbiturates: decreased action of dexamethasone
Antibiotics (macrolide), contraceptives (hormonal), estrogens, salicylates: increased action of dexamethasone
Anticholinesterases, anticoagulants, anticonvulsants, antidiabetics, salicylates, toxoids/vaccines: decreased effects of each specific product
Antidiabetics: increased effect of these products
Diuretics, NSAIDs, salicylates: increased side effects

Quinolones: increased risk of tendinitis, tendon rupture

Drug/lab test
Increased: cholesterol, Na, blood glucose, uric acid, Ca, urine glucose
Decreased: Ca, K, T_4, T_3, thyroid ^{131}I uptake test, urine 17-OHCS, 17-KS, PBI
False negative: skin allergy tests

NURSING CONSIDERATIONS

Assessment
• Monitor K, blood, urine glucose while on long-term therapy; hypokalemia and hyperglycemia
• Monitor weight daily; notify prescriber of weekly gain >5 lb
• Monitor B/P q4hr, pulse; notify prescriber of chest pain
• Monitor I&O ratio; be alert for decreasing urinary output, increasing edema
• Monitor plasma cortisol levels during long-term therapy (normal: 138-635 nmol/L when assessed at 8 AM), prolonged use can cause **cushingoid symptoms**
• **Assess infection:** fever, WBC even after withdrawal of medication; product masks infection
• **Assess potassium depletion:** paresthesias, fatigue, nausea, vomiting, depression, polyuria, dysrhythmias, weakness
• Assess edema, hypertension, cardiac symptoms
• Assess mental status: affect, mood, behavioral changes, aggression

Nursing diagnoses
• Infection, risk for (adverse reaction)
• Knowledge, deficient (teaching)
• Mobility, impaired physical (uses)

Patient/family education
• Advise that emergency ID as corticosteroid user should be carried or worn
• Teach to notify prescriber if therapeutic response decreases; dosage adjustment may be needed
• Teach not to discontinue abruptly or **adrenal crisis** can result
• Teach to avoid OTC products: salicylates, alcohol in cough products, cold preparations unless directed by prescriber
• Instruct patient to contact prescriber if surgery, trauma, stress occurs, dosage may need to be adjusted
• Teach patient all aspects of product use, including cushingoid symptoms
• Instruct patient to notify prescriber of infection

• Teach symptoms of adrenal insufficiency: nausea, anorexia, fatigue, dizziness, dyspnea, weakness, joint pain
• Advise patient to avoid exposure to chickenpox or measles, persons with infections

Evaluation
Positive therapeutic outcome
Decreased inflammation

dexamethasone ophthalmic
See Appendix B

dexamethasone topical
See Appendix B

dexlansoprazole (Rx)
(dex-lan-so-prey′zole)
Dexilant
Func. class.: Anti-ulcer–proton pump inhibitor
Chem. class.: Benzimidazole
Pregnancy category B

ACTION: Suppresses gastric secretion by inhibiting hydrogen/potassium ATPase enzyme system in gastric parietal cell; characterized as gastric acid pump inhibitor, since it blocks final step of acid production

Therapeutic outcome: Reduction in gastric pain, swelling, fullness

USES: Gastroesophageal reflux disease (GERD), severe erosive esophagitis, heartburn

CONTRAINDICATIONS:
Hypersensitivity

Precautions: Pregnancy **B**, breastfeeding, children, proton-pump hypersensitivity, gastric cancer, hepatic disease, vit B_{12} deficiency

DOSAGE AND ROUTES
Erosive esophagitis
Adult: PO 60 mg qd for up to 8 wk; maintenance: PO 30 mg qd for up to 6 mo

GERD
Adult: **PO:** 30 mg qd × 4 wk

Available forms: Del rel caps 30, 60 mg

Implementation
• Swallow del rel cap whole; do not break, crush, chew; caps may be opened and contents sprinkled on food, use immediately; do not chew contents of caps, give without regard to food

ADVERSE EFFECTS
CNS: Headache, dizziness, confusion, agitation, amnesia, depression, **anxiety, seizures,** insomnia
CV: Chest pain, angina, bradycardia, palpitations, **CVA,** hypertension, **MI**
EENT: Tinnitus
GI: Diarrhea, abdominal pain, vomiting, nausea, constipation, flatulence, colitis, dysgeusia
HEMA: Anemia, **neutropenia, thrombocytopenia, pernicious anemia, thrombosis**
INTEG: Rash, urticaria, pruritus
META: Gout
MS: Arthralgia, myalgia
RESP: Upper respiratory infections, cough, epistaxis, dyspnea
SYST: **Anaphylaxis, Stevens-Johnson syndrome, toxic epidermal necrolysis, exfoliative dermatitis, pneumonia**

Pharmacokinetics

Absorption	57%-64%
Distribution	Protein binding 97%
Metabolism	Liver extensively
Excretion	Urine, feces; clearance decreased in geriatric, renal/hepatic disease
Half-life	Plasma 1-2 hr, 4-5 hr

Pharmacodynamics
Unknown

INTERACTIONS
Individual drugs
Ampicillin, calcium carbonate, delavirdine, iron, itraconazole, ketoconazole: decreased absorption of each specific product

Drug classifications
CYP2C19, CYP3A4 (fluvoxamine, voriconazole): increased dexlansoprazole effect
Sucralfate: delayed absorption of dexlansoprazole

NURSING CONSIDERATIONS
Assessment
• Assess GI system: bowel sounds q8hr, abdomen for pain, swelling, anorexia; monitor serum magnesium
• **Anaphylaxis, serious skin disorders** requiring emergency intervention
• **Hepatotoxicity:** Hepatitis, jaundice, monitor liver enzymes (AST, ALT, alkaline phosphatase)

during treatment if hepatic adverse reactions occur

Nursing diagnoses
• Knowledge, deficient (teaching)
• Pain, chronic (uses)

Patient/family education
• Instruct patient to report severe diarrhea; product may have to be discontinued
• Inform diabetic patient that hypoglycemia may occur
• Encourage patient to avoid hazardous activities; dizziness may occur
• Tell patient to avoid alcohol, salicylates, ibuprofen; may cause GI irritation

Evaluation
Positive therapeutic outcome
• Absence of gastric pain, swelling, fullness

dexmedetomidine (Rx)
(deks-med-ee-tome′a-dine)
Precedex
Func. class.: Sedative, α_2-adrenoceptor agonist
Pregnancy category C

ACTION: Produces α_2-agonist activity as seen at low and moderate doses; also, α_1 at high doses

USES: Sedation in mechanically ventilated, intubated patients in ICU

CONTRAINDICATIONS:
Hypersensitivity, chronic hypertension

Precautions: Pregnancy **C**, breastfeeding, children, geriatric, respiratory depression, severe respiratory disorders, cardiac dysrhythmias, hypovolemia, diabetes, CV/renal/hepatic disease

DOSAGE AND ROUTES
Adult: **IV** loading dose of 1 mcg/kg over 10 min, then 0.2-0.7 mcg/kg/hr, do not use for more than 24 hr

Available forms: Inj 100 mcg/ml

Implementation
Continuous IV infusion route
• Give after diluting with 0.9% NaCl; withdraw 2 ml of product and add to 48 ml of 0.9% NaCl to a total of 50 ml (4 mcg/ml); shake gently to mix well; use controlled infusion device
• Give only with resuscitative equipment available

• Give loading dose over 10 min by continuous **IV** infusion, do not give by bol or rapid **IV** inj, use for ≤24 hr
• Give only by qualified persons trained in management of ICU sedation

Solution compatibilities: LR, D_5W, 0.9% NaCl, 20% mannitol

Y-site compatibilities: Acyclovir, alfentanil, allopurinol, amifostine, amikacin, aminocaproic acid, aminophylline, amiodarone, amphotericin B liposome, ampicillin, ampicillin-sulbactam, anidulafungin, atenolol, atracurium, atropine, azithromycin, aztreonam, bivalirudin, bleomycin, bumetanide, buprenorphine, busulfan, butorphanol, calcium chloride/gluconate, CARBOplatin, carmustine, caspofungin, ceFAZolin, cefepime, cefoperazone, cefotaxime, cefotetan, cefoxitin, ceftazidime, ceftizoxime, cefTRIAXone, cefuroxime, chlorproMAZINE, cimetidine, ciprofloxacin, cisatracurium, CISplatin, clindamycin, cyclophosphamide, cycloSPORINE, cytarabine, dacarbazine, DACTINomycin, DAPTOmycin, DAUNOrubicin, dexamethasone, dexrazoxane, digoxin, diltiazem, diphenhydrAMINE, DOBUTamine, docetaxel, dolasetron, DOPamine, doxacurium, DOXOrubicin, doxycycline, droperidol, enalaprilat, ePHEDrine, EPINEPHrine, ertapenem, erythromycin, esmolol, etomidate, etoposide, famotidine, fenoldopam, fentaNYL, fluconazole, fludarabine, fluorouracil, foscarnet, fosphenytoin, furosemide, ganciclovir, gatifloxacin, gemcitabine, gentamicin, glycopyrrolate, granisetron, haloperidol, heparin, hydrocortisone, HYDROmorphone, hydrOXYzine, IDArubicin, ifosfamide, imipenem-cilastatin, inamrinone, insulin (regular), isoproterenol, ketorolac, labetalol, leucovorin, levofloxacin, levorphanol, lidocaine, linezolid, LORazepam, magnesium sulfate, mannitol, mechlorethamine, meperidine, meropenem, mesna, methohexital, methotrexate, methylPREDNISolone, metoclopramide, metoprolol, metroNIDAZOLE, midazolam, milrinone, minocycline, mitomycin, mitoxantrone, mivacurium, morphine, mycophenolate mofetil, nalbuphine, naloxone, nesiritide, niCARdipine, nitroglycerin, nitroprusside, norepinephrine, octreotide, oflaxacin, ondansetron, oxaliplatin, oxytocin, paclitaxel, palonosetron, pamidronate, pancuronium, pemetrexed, pentamidine, PENTobarbital, PHENobarbital, phenylephrine, piperacillin, piperacillin-tazobactam, potassium chloride/phosphates, procainamide, prochlorperazine, promethazine, propofol, propranolol, quinupristin-dalfopristin, ranitidine, rapacuronium, remifentanil, rocuronium, sodium acetate/bicarbonate/phosphates, succinylcholine, SUFentanil, sulfamethoxazole-trimethoprim, tacrolimus, teniposide, theophylline, thiopental, thiotepa, ticarcillin, ticarcillin-clavulanate, tigecycline, tirofiban, tobramycin, topotecan, vancomycin, vasopressin, vecuronium, verapamil, vinBLAStine, vinCRIStine, vinorelbine, voriconazole, zidovudine, zoledronic acid

ADVERSE EFFECTS

CV: *Bradycardia, hypo/hypertension,* **atrial fibrillation, infarction, cardiac arrest**
GI: *Nausea,* thirst
GU: Oliguria
HEMA: Leukocytosis, anemia
MISC: Hyperkalemia
RESP: Pulmonary edema, pleural effusion, hypoxia, respiratory acidosis

Pharmacokinetics

Absorption	Rapid
Distribution	Protein binding 94%
Metabolism	Liver
Excretion	Urine
Half-life	2 hr

Pharmacodynamics

Unknown

INTERACTIONS

Individual drugs
Alcohol: increased CNS depression

Drug classifications
Anesthetics (inhalational), antipsychotics, opiates, sedative/hypnotics, skeletal muscle relaxants: increased CNS depression
Antihypertensives: increased hypotension

NURSING CONSIDERATIONS

Assessment
• Assess inj site: phlebitis, burning, stinging
• Monitor ECG for changes: atrial fibrillation; monitor geriatric more closely
• Assess CNS changes: movement, jerking, tremors, dizziness, LOC, pupil reaction
• Assess respiratory dysfunction: respiratory depression, character, rate, rhythm; notify prescriber if respirations are <10/min
• Assess cardiac status: B/P, heart rate

Nursing diagnoses
• Injury, risk for (uses)

Patient/family education
• Explain reason for treatment, expected results

Evaluation
Positive therapeutic outcome
• Induction of sedation

dexmethylphenidate (Rx)
(dex′meth-ul-fen′ih-dayt)
Focalin, Focalin XR
Func. class.: Central nervous system (CNS) stimulant, psychostimulant
Pregnancy category C
Controlled substance schedule II

ACTION: Increases release of norepinephrine and dopamine into the extraneuronal space, also blocks reuptake of norepinephrine and dopamine into the presynaptic neuron; mode of action in treating attention-deficit-hyperactivity disorder (ADHD) is unknown

Therapeutic outcome: Increased alertness, decreased fatigue, ability to stay awake (narcolepsy), increased attention span, decreased hyperactivity (ADHD)

USE: ADHD

CONTRAINDICATIONS:
Hypersensitivity to methylphenidate, anxiety, history of Tourette's syndrome; children <6 yr, glaucoma, concurrent treatment with MAOIs or within 14 days of discontinuing treatment with MAOIs, breastfeeding, tics, psychosis

Precautions: Pregnancy **C**, hypertension, depression, seizures, CV disorders, alcoholism

BLACK BOX WARNING: Substance abuse

DOSAGE AND ROUTES
Adult: PO EXT REL 10 mg/day, may adjust to 20 mg/day in 10 mg increments
Child >6 yr: PO 2.5 mg bid with doses at least 4 hr apart, gradually increase to a max of 20 mg/day (10 mg bid); for those taking methylphenidate, use $^1/_2$ of methylphenidate dose initially, then increase as needed to max 20 mg/day; EXT REL 5 mg/day, may adjust to 20 mg/day in 5 mg increments

Available forms: Tabs 2.5, 5, 10 mg; ext rel caps (Focalin XR) 5, 10, 20 mg

Implementation
• Do not break, crush, or chew ext rel caps
• Twice daily at least 4 hr apart; ext rel once a day
• Without regard to meals

ADVERSE EFFECTS

CNS: Dizziness, headache, drowsiness, nervousness, insomnia, **toxic psychosis, neuroleptic malignant syndrome (rare),** Tourette's syndrome
CV: Palpitations, B/P changes, angina, **dysrhythmias, tachycardia, MI, stroke**
GI: *Nausea, anorexia*, abnormal liver function, **hepatic coma,** *abdominal pain*
HEMA: **Leukopenia, anemia, thrombocytopenic purpura**
INTEG: **Exfoliative dermatitis,** urticaria, rash, erythema multiforme
MISC: *Fever,* arthralgia, scalp hair loss

Pharmacokinetics

Absorption	Readily absorbed
Distribution	Unknown
Metabolism	Liver
Excretion	Kidneys
Half-life	2.2 hr

Pharmacodynamics

	PO	EXT REL
Onset	$^{1}/_{2}$-1 hr	Unknown
Peak	1-1 $^{1}/_{2}$ hr	4 hr
Duration	4 hr	8 hr

INTERACTIONS

Drug classifications

Anticoagulants (coumarin), anticonvulsants, selective serotonin reuptake inhibitors, tricyclics: increased effects
Antihypertensives: decreased effects
Decongestants, vasoconstrictors: increased sympathomimetic effect
MAOIs: hypertensive crisis if coadministered or given within 14 days
Vasopressors: hypertensive crisis

Drug/herb

Melatonin: increased synergistic effect

NURSING CONSIDERATIONS

Assessment

BLACK BOX WARNING: Assess for previous or current substance abuse

• Assess VS, B/P; may reverse antihypertensives; check patients with cardiac disease more often for increased B/P
• Assess CBC, differential, platelet counts during long-term therapy, urinalysis; in diabetes: blood/urine glucose; insulin changes may have to be made, since eating will decrease

• Assess height, growth rate q3mo in children; growth rate may be decreased
• Assess mental status: mood, sensorium, affect, stimulation, insomnia, aggressiveness
⚠ Assess withdrawal symptoms: headache, nausea, vomiting, muscle pain, weakness
• Assess appetite, sleep, speech patterns
• Assess for attention span, decreased hyperactivity in persons with ADHD

Nursing diagnoses

• Coping, disabled family (uses)
• Coping, ineffective (uses)
• Knowledge, deficient (teaching)

Patient/family education

• Advise patient to decrease caffeine consumption (coffee, tea, cola, chocolate); may increase irritability, stimulation
• Advise patient to avoid OTC preparations unless approved by prescriber
• Caution patient to taper off product over several wk to avoid depression, increased sleeping, lethargy
• Caution patient to avoid alcohol ingestion
• Caution patient to avoid hazardous activities until stabilized on medication
• Advise patient to get needed rest; patients will feel more tired at end of day
• Notify all health providers including school nurse of medication and schedule
• Discuss information instructions provided in patient information section

Evaluation

Positive therapeutic outcome
• Decreased hyperactivity or ability to stay awake

TREATMENT OF OVERDOSE:

Administer fluids; hemodialysis or peritoneal dialysis; antihypertensive for increased B/P; administer short-acting barbiturate before lavage

dextroamphetamine (Rx)

(dex-troe-am-fet'a-meen)
Dexedrine, ProCentra
Func. class.: Cerebral stimulant
Chem. class.: Amphetamine
Pregnancy category C
Controlled substance schedule II

ACTION: Increases release of norepinephrine, dopamine in cerebral cortex to reticular activating system

Therapeutic outcome: Increased alertness, decreased fatigue, ability to stay awake (narcolepsy); increased attention span, decreased hyperactivity (ADHD)

USES: Narcolepsy, attention-deficit disorder with hyperactivity

Unlabeled use: Obesity

CONTRAINDICATIONS:
Hypersensitivity to sympathomimetic amines, hyperthyroidism, hypertension, glaucoma, severe arteriosclerosis, drug abuse, anxiety, anorexia nervosa, tartrazine dye hypersensitivity

> **BLACK BOX WARNING:** Symptomatic CV disease, substance abuse

Precautions: Pregnancy **C**, breastfeeding, child <3 yr, Gilles de la Tourette's disorder, depression, cardiomyopathy, bipolar disorder

DOSAGE AND ROUTES
Narcolepsy
Adult: PO 5 mg bid, titrate daily dose by no more than 10 mg/wk, max 60 mg/day
Child 6-12 yr: PO 5 mg daily increasing by no more than 5 mg/day at weekly intervals

ADHD
Adult: PO 5-60 mg/day in divided doses
Child 6-12 yr: PO 5 mg daily-bid increasing by 5 mg/day at weekly intervals
Child 3-5 yr: PO 2.5 mg daily increasing by 2.5 mg/day at weekly intervals (max 40 mg/day)

Available forms: Tabs 5, 10 mg, oral sol 5 mg/5 ml

Implementation
• Give at least 6 hr before bedtime to avoid sleeplessness; titrate to patient's response; lowest dosage should be used to control symptoms
• Give gum, hard candy, frequent sips of water for dry mouth at beginning of treatment; these symptoms tend to lessen with time

ADVERSE EFFECTS
CNS: *Hyperactivity, insomnia, restlessness, talkativeness,* dizziness, headache, chills, stimulation, dysphoria, irritability, aggressiveness, tremor, dependence, addiction
CV: *Palpitations, tachycardia,* hypertension, decrease in heart rate, **dysrhythmias**
GI: *Anorexia,* dry mouth, diarrhea, constipation, weight loss, metallic taste
GU: Impotence, change in libido
INTEG: Urticaria

Pharmacokinetics
Absorption	Well absorbed
Distribution	Widely distributed; crosses placenta
Metabolism	Liver
Excretion	Kidneys, pH dependent: increased pH, increased reabsorption
Half-life	10-30 hr; increased when urine is alkaline

Pharmacodynamics
Onset	$1/2$ hr
Peak	1-3 hr
Duration	4-10 hr

INTERACTIONS
Individual drugs
AcetaZOLAMIDE, sodium bicarbonate: increased effect of dextroamphetamine
Ammonium chloride, ascorbic acid, guanethidine: decreased effect of dextroamphetamine
Haloperidol: increased CNS effect
Phenytoin: decreased absorption of phenytoin

Drug classifications
Adrenergic blockers: decreased adrenergic blocking effect
Antacids: increased effect of dextroamphetamine
Antidepressants (tricyclic), phenothiazines: increased CNS effect
Antidiabetics: decreased antidiabetic effect
Antihistamines: decreased antihistamine effect
Antihypertensives: decreased antihypertensive effect
Barbiturates: decreased absorption of barbiturate
MAOIs: hypertensive crisis if used within 14 days
SSRIs, SNRIs: increased serotonin syndrome, increased neuroleptic malignant syndrome, do not use concurrently

Drug/herb
Eucalyptus: decreased stimulant effect
St. John's wort: increased serotonin syndrome

Drug/food
Caffeine (cola, coffee, tea [green/black]): increased amine effect

Drug/lab test
Increase: plasma corticosteroids, urinary steroids

NURSING CONSIDERATIONS
Assessment

> **BLACK BOX WARNING:** Monitor VS, B/P, since this product may reverse antihypertensives; check patients with cardiac disease more often for increased B/P

• Monitor CBC, urinalysis; for diabetic patients monitor blood, urine glucose; insulin changes may be required, since eating will decrease
• Monitor height and weight q3mo since growth rate in children may be decreased; appetite is suppressed so weight loss is common during the first few months of treatment
• Monitor mental status: mood, sensorium, affect, stimulation, insomnia; aggressiveness may occur; depression with crying spells may occur after product has worn off
• Assess for **physical dependency;** should not be used for extended time except in ADHD; dosage should be decreased gradually to prevent withdrawal symptoms
• Assess for **narcoleptic symptoms** before medication and after; ability to stay awake should increase significantly
• In children or adults with ADHD, monitor for improved organizational skills, attention span, attending to tasks, impulse control, socialization, and ability to get along better with others
• Assess for **withdrawal symptoms:** headache, nausea, vomiting, muscle pain, weakness; product tolerance develops after long-term use; dosage should not be increased if tolerance develops; this medication has a high abuse potential

Nursing diagnoses
• Coping, ineffective family (uses)
• Coping, ineffective (uses)
• Knowledge, deficient (teaching)

Patient/family education
• Advise patient to decrease caffeine consumption (coffee, tea, cola, chocolate), which may increase irritability and stimulation; to avoid OTC preparations unless approved by prescriber; to avoid alcohol ingestion; these may cause serious drug interactions
• Advise patient to take before meals (obesity)
• Caution patient to taper off product over several weeks, or depression, increased sleeping, lethargy may occur
• Caution patient to avoid hazardous activities until patient is stabilized on medication
• Instruct patient not to double doses if medication is missed; prescriber may suggest product holidays (ADHD) during the school year to assess progress and determine continued need for product
• Instruct patient/family to notify prescriber if significant side effects occur: tremors, insomnia, palpitations, restlessness, product changes may be needed
• Inform patient that if dry mouth occurs, to use frequent sips of water, sugarless gum, hard candy during beginning therapy; dry mouth lessens with continued treatment
• Advise patient to get needed rest; patients will feel more tired at end of day; to give last dose at least 6 hr before bedtime to avoid insomnia

Evaluation
Positive therapeutic outcome
• Decreased activity in ADHD
• Absence of sleeping during day in narcolepsy

TREATMENT OF OVERDOSE:
Administer fluids, hemodialysis, peritoneal dialysis, antihypertensives for increased B/P; ammonium chloride for increased excretion

dextromethorphan (OTC)
(dex-troe-meth-or′fan)
Balminil ✲, Benlyn ✲, Buckley's DM, Buckley's Mixture, Cough Suppressant Long-Acting, Delsym 12-Hour, ElixSure Cough, Koffex, PediaCare Children's Long-Acting Cough, PediaCare Long-Acting Cough, Robafan, Robitussin, Robitussin Cough with Honey, Robitussin Maximum Strength, Scot-Tussin Diabetes CF, Silphen-DM, Top Care Day Time Cough, Top Care Tussin Cough Suppressant Long Acting, Triaminic Long-Acting Cough, Tylenol Children's Simply Cough, Vicks Formula 44 Cough Relief, Wal-Tussin
Func. class.: Antitussive, nonopioid
Chem. class.: Levorphanol derivative
Pregnancy category C

ACTION: Depresses cough center in medulla by direct effect related to levorphanol

Therapeutic outcome: Absence of cough

USES: Nonproductive cough carried by minor respiratory tract infections or irritants that might be inhaled

CONTRAINDICATIONS:
Hypersensitivity

Precautions: Pregnancy **C,** fever, hepatic disease, asthma/emphysema, chronic cough

DOSAGE AND ROUTES
Adult and child ≥12 yr: PO 10-20 mg q4hr, or 30 mg q6-8hr, max 120 mg/day; SUS REL LIQUID 60 mg q12hr, max 120 mg/day
Child 6-12 yr: PO 5-10 mg q4hr; SUS REL LIQUID 30 mg bid, max 60 mg/day; LOZENGE 5-10 mg q1-4hr, max 60 mg/day
Child 4-6 yr: PO 2.5-7.5 mg q4-8hr, max 30 mg/day, SUS REL LIQ 15 ml bid
Child <4 yr: PO: not recommended

Available forms: Liquid 7.5, 15 mg/5 ml; syr 15 mg/15 ml, 10 mg/5 ml; 15 mg/5 ml, 30 mg/15 ml; caps 15 mg; gel caps 15 mg; EXT REL SUSP 30 mg/5 ml

Implementation
• Give **chew tabs:** chew well; **syrup:** use calibrated measuring device; **ext rel susp:** shake well, use calibrated measuring device
• Administer decreased dosage to geriatric patients; their metabolism may be slowed; do not provide water within 30 min of administration because it dilutes product
• Shake susp before administration

ADVERSE EFFECTS
CNS: *Dizziness,* sedation, confusion, ataxia, fatigue
GI: *Nausea*

Pharmacokinetics
Absorption	Rapid (PO); slow (SUS REL)
Distribution	Unknown
Metabolism	Liver
Excretion	Kidneys
Half-life	Terminal 11 hr

Pharmacodynamics
	PO	PO-sus
Onset	15-30 min	Unknown
Peak	Unknown	Unknown
Duration	3-6 hr	12 hr

INTERACTIONS
Individual drugs
Alcohol: increased CNS depression
Amiodarone, quiNIDine, sibutramine: increased adverse reactions

Furazolidone, linezolid, procarbazine: increased hypotension, hyperpyrexia; do not give within 2 wk (MAOI activity)

Drug classifications
Antihistamines, antidepressants, opiates, sedative-hypnotics: increased CNS depression
MAOIs: increased hypotension, hyperpyrexia, do not give within 2 wk of MAOIs
Serotonin receptor agonists, SSRIs: increased serotonin syndrome

NURSING CONSIDERATIONS
Assessment
• Assess **cough:** type, frequency, character including sputum; provide adequate hydration to 2 L/day to decrease viscosity of secretions

Nursing diagnoses
• Airway clearance, ineffective (uses)
• Knowledge, deficient (teaching)

Patient/family education
• Caution patient to avoid driving or other hazardous activities until stabilized on this medication; may cause drowsiness, dizziness in some individuals
• Advise patient to avoid smoking, smoke-filled rooms, perfumes, dust, environmental pollutants, cleaners, which increase cough; may use gum, hard candy to prevent dry mouth
• Advise patient to avoid alcohol or other CNS depressants while taking this medication; drowsiness will be increased
• Caution patient that any cough lasting over a few days should be assessed by prescriber

Evaluation
Positive therapeutic outcome
• Absence of dry, irritating cough

dextrose (D-glucose) (Rx)
Func. class.: Caloric agent

ACTION: Needed for adequate utilization of amino acids; decreases protein, nitrogen loss; prevents ketosis

Therapeutic outcome: Provides calories, prevents severe hypoglycemia

USES: Increases intake of calories; increases fluids in patients unable to take adequate fluids, calories orally; acute hypoglycemia

Adverse effects: *italics* = common; **bold** = life-threatening

CONTRAINDICATIONS:

Hyperglycemia, delirium tremens, hemorrhage (cranial/spinal), CHF, anuria, allergy to corn products

Precautions: Renal/ liver/cardiac disease, diabetes mellitus, carbohydrate intolerance

DOSAGE AND ROUTES

Adult and child: IV, depends on individual requirements

Hypoglycemia
Adult: PO/IV 10-25 mg

Available forms: Inj IV 2.5%, 5%, 10%, 20%, 25% 30%, 38.5%, 40%, 50%, 60%, 70%; oral gel 40%; chewable tabs 5 g

Implementation
PO route
• Oral glucose preparations (gel, chewable tabs) are to be used for conscious patients only; serum blood glucose should be monitored after first oral dose; if glucose has not increased by 20 mg/100 ml in 20-30 min, dose should be repeated and serum glucose checked again

IV route
• Give only protein (4%) and dextrose (up to 12.5%) via peripheral vein; stronger sol requires central IV administration
• May be given undiluted via prepared sol; give 10% sol (5 ml/15 sec), 20% sol (1000 ml/3 hr or more), 50% sol (500 ml/30-60 min); too rapid IV administration may cause fluid overload and hyperglycemia
• After changing IV catheter, change dressing q24hr with aseptic technique

ADVERSE EFFECTS

CNS: Confusion, loss of consciousness, dizziness
CV: Hypertension, CHF, pulmonary edema, intracranial hemorrhage
ENDO: Hyperglycemia, rebound hypoglycemia, hyperosmolar syndrome, hyperglycemic nonketolytic syndrome, aluminum toxicity, hypokalemia, hypomagnesium
GI: Nausea
GU: *Glycosuria, osmotic diuresis*
INTEG: Chills, flushing, warm feeling, rash, urticaria, extravasation necrosis
RESP: Pulmonary edema

Pharmacokinetics

Absorption	Well absorbed (PO); completely absorbed (**IV**)
Distribution	Widely distributed
Metabolism	Unknown
Excretion	Unknown
Half-life	Unknown

Pharmacodynamics

	PO	IV
Onset	Rapid	Immediate
Peak	Rapid	Immediate
Duration	Rapid	Immediate

INTERACTIONS

Drug classifications
Corticosteroids: increased fluid retention/electrolyte excretion

NURSING CONSIDERATIONS

Assessment
• Assess I&O, skin turgor, edema, electrolytes (potassium, sodium, calcium, chloride, magnesium), blood glucose, ammonia, phosphate
• Monitor inj site for extravasation: redness along vein, edema at site, necrosis, pain, hard tender area; site should be changed immediately
• Monitor temp q4hr for increased fever, indicating infection; if infection suspected, inf is discontinued and tubing, bottle, catheter tip cultured
• Monitor serum glucose in patients receiving hypertonic glucose 5% and over
• Assess nutritional status: calorie count by dietitian; GI system function

Nursing diagnoses
• Fluid volume, excess (adverse reactions)
• Knowledge, deficient (teaching)
• Nutrition, less than body requirements, imbalanced (uses)

Patient/family education
• Teach patient reason for dextrose infusion
• Provide literature and information on when and how to use oral products for hypoglycemia
• Review hypo/hyperglycemia symptoms
• Review blood glucose monitoring procedure

Evaluation
Positive therapeutic outcome
• Increased weight
• Blood glucose level at normal limits for patient
• Adequate hydration

⚠ Nurse Alert

diazepam (Rx)

(dye-az′e-pam)

Apo-Diazepam ✦, Diastat, Valium

Func. class.: Antianxiety, anticonvulsant, skeletal muscle relaxant, central acting

Chem. class.: Benzodiazepine, long-acting

Pregnancy category D

Controlled substance schedule IV

Do not confuse:
diazepam/Ditropan/LORazepam

ACTION: Potentiates the actions of GABA, especially in limbic system, reticular formation; enhances presympathetic inhibition, inhibits spinal polysynaptic afferent paths

Therapeutic outcome: Decreased anxiety, restlessness, insomnia

USES: Anxiety, acute alcohol withdrawal, adjunct in seizure disorders; preoperative skeletal muscle relaxation; rectally for acute repetitive seizures

CONTRAINDICATIONS:

Pregnancy **D**, hypersensitivity to benzodiazepines, closed-angle glaucoma, coma, myasthenia gravis, ethanol intoxication, hepatic disease, sleep apnea

Precautions: Breastfeeding, geriatric, debilitated, addiction, child <6 mo, asthma, renal disease, bipolar disorder, COPD, CNS depression, labor, Parkinson's disease, neutropenia, psychosis, seizures, substance abuse, smoking

DOSAGE AND ROUTES

Anxiety/convulsive disorders

Adult: PO 2-10 mg bid-qid; IM/IV 2-10 mg q3-4hr

Geriatric: PO 1-2 mg daily-bid, increase slowly as needed

Child >6 mo: IM/IV 0.04-0.3 mg/kg/dose q2-4hr, max 0.6 mg/kg in an 8-hr period

Precardioversion

Adult: IV 5-15 mg 5-10 min precardioversion

Preendoscopy

Adult: IV 2.5-20 mg, IM 5-10 mg ½ hr preendoscopy

Muscle relaxation

Adult: PO 2-10 mg tid-qid or EXT REL 15-30 mg daily; IM/IV 5-10 mg repeat in 2-4 hr

Geriatric: PO 2-5 mg bid-qid; IM/IV 2-5 mg, may repeat in 2-4 hr

Tetanic muscle spasms

Child >5 yr: IM/IV 5-10 mg q3-4hr prn

Infants >30 days: IM/IV 1-2 mg q3-4hr prn

Status epilepticus

Adult: IM/IV 5-10 mg, 2 mg/min, may repeat q10-15min; max 30 mg; may repeat in 2-4 hr if seizures reappear

Child >5 yr: IV 1 mg slowly; IM 1 mg q2-5min

Child 1 mo-5 yr: IV 0.2-0.5 mg slowly; IM 0.2-0.5 mg slowly q2-5min up to 5 mg; may repeat in 2-4 hr prn

Seizures other than status epilepticus

Adult: RECT 0.2 mg/kg, may repeat 4-12 hr later

Child 6-11 yr: RECT 0.3 mg/kg, may repeat 4-12 hr later

Child 2-5 yr: RECT 0.5 mg/kg, may repeat 4-12 hr later

Alcohol withdrawal

Adult: IV 10 mg initially, then 5-10 mg q3-4hr prn

Available forms: Tabs 2, 5, 10 mg; inj 5 mg/ml; oral sol 5 mg/5 ml, 5 mg/ml; gel, rectal delivery system 10 mg, twin packs; ext rel cap 15 mg

Implementation
PO route

• Give with food or milk for GI symptoms

• Crush tab if patient is unable to swallow medication whole

• Use sugarless gum, hard candy, frequent sips of water for dry mouth

• Reduce opioid dosage by one third if given concomitantly with diazepam

• Check to see if PO medication has been swallowed

• Concentrate: use calibrated dropper only; mix with water, juice, pudding, applesauce; consume immediately

Rectal route

• Do not use more than 5 ×/mo or for an episode q5day

Direct IV route

• Administer **IV** into large vein; do not dilute or mix with any other product; give **IV** 5 mg or less/min or total dose over 3 min or more (children, infants); cont inf is not recommended; inject closest vein insertion as possible; do not dilute or mix with other products

• Check IV site for thrombosis or phlebitis, which may occur rapidly

Adverse effects: *italics* = common; **bold** = life-threatening

Sterile emulsion for injection route
• Use **IV** only, within 6 hr, flush line after use and after 6 hr

Y-site compatibilities: Daptomycin, DAUNOrubicin, docetaxel, fentaNYL, methadone, piperacillin/tazobactam, teniposide

Y-site incompatibilities: Acetaminophen, acyclovir, alemtuzumab, alfentanil, amikacin, aminophylline, amphotericin B cholesteryl, amphotericin B colloidal, amphotericin B liposome, ampicillin, ampicillin/sulbactam, anidulafungin, ascorbic acid, atracurium, atropine, azaTHIOprine, aztreonam, bivalirudin, bumetanide, buprenorphine, butorphanol, calcium chloride/gluconate, CARBOplatin, caspofungin, ceFAZolin, cefepime, cefonicid, cefoperazone, cefotaxime, cefotetan, cefoxitin, ceftazidime, ceftizoxime, cefTRIAXone, cefuroxime, chloramphenicol, chlorproMAZINE, cimetidine, CISplatin, clindamycin, cyanocobalamin, cyclophosphamide, cycloSPORINE, cytarabine, DACTINomycin, dantrolene, dexamethasone, dexmedetomidine, diazoxide, digoxin, diltiazem, diphenhydrAMINE, DOPamine, doripenem, doxacurium, DOXOrubicin, doxycycline, enalaprilat, ePHEDrine, EPINEPHrine, epirubicin, epoetin alfa, eptifibatide, erythromycin, esmolol, etoposide, etoposide phosphate, famotidine, fenoldopam, fluconazole, fludarabine, fluorouracil, folic acid, foscarnet, furosemide, ganciclovir, gemcitabine, gentamicin, glycopyrrolate, granisetron, haloperidol, heparin, hydrALAZINE, hydrocortisone, hydrOXYzine, IDArubicin, ifosfamide, imipenem/cilastatin, inamrinone, indomethacin, insulin, isoproterenol, ketorolac, labetalol, levofloxacin, lidocaine, linezolid, magnesium chloride, mannitol, mechlorethamine, meperidine, meropenem, metaraminol, methotrexate, methoxamine, methyldopate, methylPREDNISolone, metoclopramide, metoprolol, metroNIDAZOLE, midazolam, milrinone, mitoxantrone, multivitamin, nalbuphine, naloxone, nesiritide, nitroglycerin, nitroprusside, norepinephrine, octreotide, oxacillin, oxaliplatin, oxytocin, paclitaxel, palonosetron, pancuronium, pantoprazole, papaverine, pemetrexed, penicillin G, pentamidine, pentazocine, PENTobarbital, PHENobarbital, phentolamine, phenylephrine, phenytoin, phytonadione, potassium chloride, procainamide, prochlorperazine, promethazine, propofol, propranolol, protamine, pyridoxime, quinupristin/dalfopristin, ranitidine, rocuronium, sodium acetate, sodium bicarbonate, succinylcholine, tacrolimus, theophylline, thiamine, thiotepa, ticarcillin/clavulanate, tigecycline, tirofiban, tobramycin, tolazoline, trimetaphan, trimethoprim/sulfamethoxazole, urokinase, vancomycin, vasopressin, vecuronium, verapamil, vinCRIStine, vinorelbine, vitamin B complex with C, voriconazole, zoledronic acid

ADVERSE EFFECTS
CNS: *Dizziness, drowsiness,* confusion, headache, anxiety, tremors, stimulation, fatigue, depression, insomnia, hallucinations, ataxia, fatigue
CV: *Orthostatic hypotension,* **ECG changes, tachycardia,** hypotension
EENT: *Blurred vision,* tinnitus, mydriasis, nystagmus
GI: Constipation, dry mouth, nausea, vomiting, anorexia, diarrhea
HEMA: Neutropenia
INTEG: Rash, dermatitis, itching
RESP: Respiratory depression

Pharmacokinetics

Absorption	Rapid (PO); erratic (IM)
Distribution	Widely distributed; crosses blood-brain barrier, placenta; protein binding 99%
Metabolism	Liver, extensively, CYP2C19, CYP3A4
Excretion	Kidneys, breast milk
Half-life	20-80 hr

Pharmacodynamics

	PO	IM	IV
Onset	1/2 hr	15 min	Immediate
Peak	1-2 hr	1/2-1 1/2 hr	15 min
Duration	2-3 hr	1-1 1/2 hr	15 min-1 hr

INTERACTIONS
Individual drugs
Alcohol: increased CNS depression
Cimetidine, valproic acid: increased toxicity
CYP3A4 inducers (carBAMazepine, ethetoin, fosphenytoin, phenytoins, rifampin): decreased diazepam effect
Disulfiram, isoniazid, propranolol, valproic acid: decreased metabolism of diazepam

Drug classifications
Barbiturates, CNS depressants, CYP3A4 inhibitors, SSRIs: increased toxicity
CNS depressants: increased CNS depression
CYP3A4 inducers (barbiturates): decreased diazepam effect
Oral contraceptives: decreased metabolism of diazepam

Drug/lab test
Increased: AST/ALT, serum bilirubin
Decreased: radioactive iodine uptake
False increase: 17-OHCS

NURSING CONSIDERATIONS
Assessment
• **Assess degree of anxiety;** what precipitates anxiety and whether product controls symptoms; other signs of anxiety: dilated pupils, inability to sleep, restlessness, inability to focus
• **Assess for alcohol withdrawal symptoms,** including hallucinations (visual, auditory), delirium, irritability, agitation, fine to coarse tremors
• Monitor B/P (with patient lying, standing), pulse, respiratory rate; if systolic B/P drops 20 mm Hg, hold product, notify prescriber; monitor respirations q5-15min if given **IV**
• Monitor blood studies: CBC during long-term therapy; blood dyscrasias have occurred (rarely); hepatic studies: ALT, AST
• **Monitor for seizure control:** type, duration, and intensity of seizures; what precipitates seizures
• Monitor hepatic studies: AST, ALT, bilirubin, creatinine, LDH, alkaline phosphatase
• Assess mental status: mood, sensorium, affect, sleeping pattern, drowsiness, dizziness, **suicidal tendencies,** and ability of product to control these symptoms; check for tolerance, **withdrawal symptoms:** headache, nausea, vomiting, muscle pain, weakness after long-term use
• Assess for muscle spasms, pain relief

Nursing diagnoses
• Anxiety (uses)
• Coping, ineffective (uses)
• Injury, risk for (uses, adverse reactions)
• Knowledge, deficient (teaching)
• Noncompliance (teaching)

Patient/family education
• Advise patient that product may be taken with food; that product is not to be used for everyday stress or used longer than 4 mo unless directed by prescriber; take no more than prescribed amount; may be habit forming
• Caution patient to avoid OTC preparations unless approved by a prescriber; to avoid alcohol, other psychotropic medications unless prescribed; that smoking may decrease diazepam effect by increasing diazepam metabolism; not to discontinue medication abruptly after long-term use, gradually taper

• Inform patient to avoid driving, activities that require alertness; drowsiness may occur; to rise slowly or fainting may occur, especially in geriatric
• Advise patient not to become pregnant while using this product
• Inform patient that drowsiness may worsen at beginning of treatment

Evaluation
Positive therapeutic outcome
• Decreased anxiety, restlessness, insomnia

TREATMENT OF OVERDOSE:
Lavage, VS, supportive care, flumazenil

dibucaine topical
See Appendix B

diclofenac ophthalmic
See Appendix B

diclofenac epolamine (Rx)
(dye-kloe′fen-ak)
Flector
diclofenac potassium (Rx)
Cambia, Cataflam, Voltaren Rapide ✦, Zipsor
diclofenac sodium (Rx)
Apo-Dilo ✦, Novo-Difenac ✦, Nu-Diclo ✦, Pennsaid, Sandoz Diclofenac ✦, Solaraze Topical Gel, Voltram Topical Gel, Voltaren, Voltaren XR
Func. class.: Nonsteroidal antiinflammatory drug (NSAID), nonopioid analgesic
Chem. class.: Phenylacetic acid
Pregnancy category C

Do not confuse:
Cataflam/Catapres

ACTION: Inhibits COX-1, COX-2 by blocking arachidonate, resulting in analgesic, antiinflammatory, antipyretic properties

Therapeutic outcome: Decreased pain, inflammation

USES: Acute, chronic rheumatoid arthritis, osteoarthritis, ankylosing spondylitis, analgesia, primary dysmenorrhea; patch: mild to moderate pain

CONTRAINDICATIONS:

Hypersensitivity to aspirin, iodides, other NSAIDs; asthma, serious CV disease, pregnancy **D** 3rd trimester

> **BLACK BOX WARNING:** Treatment of perioperative pain in CABG surgery

Precautions: Pregnancy **C** (1st trimester), not recommended in 2nd half of pregnancy, breastfeeding, children, bleeding disorders, GI/cardiac disorders, hypersensitivity to other antiinflammatory agents, CCr <30 ml/min

> **BLACK BOX WARNING:** GI bleeding, MI, stroke

DOSAGE AND ROUTES

Osteoarthritis

Adult: PO (Cataflam) 50 mg bid-tid, max 150 mg/day; DEL REL (Voltaren) 50 mg bid-tid or 75 mg bid, max 150 mg/day; EXT REL (Voltaren-XR) 100 mg daily, max 150 mg/day; TOP gel 1% (Voltaren gel) 4 g for each lower extremity qid, max 16 g/day; 2 g for each upper extremity qid, max 8 g/day; TOP SOL (Pennsaid) apply 40 drops to each affected knee qid, apply 10 drops at a time, spread over entire knee

Rheumatoid arthritis

Adult: PO (Cataflam) 50 mg tid-qid, max 200 mg/day; DEL REL (Voltaren) 50 mg tid-qid or 75 mg bid, max 200 mg/day; EXT REL (Voltaren-XR) 100 mg qd, may increase to 200 mg/day, max 200 mg/day

Ankylosing spondylitis

Adult: PO DEL REL (Voltaren) 25 mg qid and 25 mg at bedtime, max 125 mg/day

Acute migraine with/without aura

Adult: PO (powder for oral SOL) (Cambia) 50 mg as a single dose; mix contents of packet in 1-2 oz water

Mild to moderate pain

Adult: PO (Zipsor) 25 mg qid

Dysmenorrhea or nonrheumatic inflammatory conditions

Adult: PO (Cataflam) 50 mg tid or 100 mg initially, then 50 mg tid, max 200 mg 1st day, then 150 mg/day

Pain of strains/sprains

Adult: TOP patch (Flector) apply patch to area bid

Actinic keratosis

Adult: TOP gel (Solaraze) apply to area bid

Renal dose

Avoid use of top gel, patch, sol, potassium oral tab in advanced renal disease

Available forms: Epolamine: topical patch 1.3%; potassium: tabs 50 mg tabs liquid filled 25 mg; sodium: del rel tabs (enteric-coated) 25, 50, 75, 100 mg; Pennsaid: top sol 1.5%; oral powder for sol 50 mg; ext rel 100 mg; topical gel 1%, 3%

Implementation
PO route

- Do not break, crush, chew, or dissolve enteric-coated or ext rel tabs
- Administer with food or milk to decrease gastric symptoms
- Remain upright for $1/2$ hr

Topical route (patch) (Flector)

- Wash hands before handling patch
- Remove and release liner before administering
- Use only on normal, intact skin
- Remove before bath, shower, swimming
- Discard removed patch in trash away from children, pets

Topical route (gel)

- Apply to intact skin
- Use only for osteoarthritis: mild-moderate pain

Ophthalmic route

- Administer with patient recumbent or tilting head back; pull down on lower lid; when conjunctival sac is exposed, instill 1 drop; wait a few minutes before instilling other drops

ADVERSE EFFECTS

CNS: *Dizziness, headache,* drowsiness, fatigue, tremors, confusion, insomnia, anxiety, depression, nervousness, paresthesia, muscle weakness

CV: **CHF,** tachycardia, peripheral edema, palpitations, dysrhythmias, hypo/hypertension, fluid retention, **MI, stroke**

EENT: Tinnitus, hearing loss, blurred vision, **laryngeal edema**

GI: Nausea, anorexia, vomiting, diarrhea, **jaundice, cholestatic hepatitis,** constipation, flatulence, cramps, dry mouth, peptic ulcer, GI bleeding, **hepatotoxicity**

GU: **Nephrotoxicity: dysuria, hematuria, oliguria, azotemia, cystitis, UTI**

HEMA: **Blood dyscrasias,** epistaxis, bruising

INTEG: Purpura, rash, pruritus, sweating, erythema, petechiae, photosensitivity, alopecia

RESP: Dyspnea, hemoptysis, pharyngitis, bronchospasm, rhinitis, shortness of breath
SYST: Anaphylaxis

Pharmacokinetics

Absorption	Well absorbed (PO, ophth)
Distribution	Crosses placenta; 99% bound to plasma proteins
Metabolism	Liver (50%)
Excretion	Breast milk
Half-life	2.5 hr

Pharmacodynamics

	PO	Ophth	TOP (Patch)
Onset	Unknown	Unknown	Unknown
Peak	2-3 hr	Unknown	12 hr
Duration	Unknown	Unknown	Unknown

INTERACTIONS

Individual drugs
Aspirin: increased GI side effects
CycloSPORINE, lithium, methotrexate, phenytoin: increased toxicity

Drug classifications
ACE inhibitors, β-blockers, diuretics: decreased antihypertensive effect
Anticoagulants, NSAIDs, platelet inhibitors, salicylates, SSRIs, thrombolytics: increased risk of bleeding
Antidiabetic agents: increased need for dosage adjustment
Diuretics (potassium-sparing): hyperkalemia
NSAIDs, bisphosphonates, corticosteroids: increased GI side effects

NURSING CONSIDERATIONS

Assessment
• **Assess for pain of rheumatoid arthritis, osteoarthritis, ankylosing spondylitis;** check ROM, inflammation of joints, characteristics of pain
• Assess ophthalmic patients for pain, inflammation, redness, swelling
• Assess for asthma, aspirin hypersensitivity, nasal polyps; may develop hypersensitivity
• Monitor liver function tests (may be elevated) and uric acid (may be decreased in serum, increased in urine) periodically; also BUN, creatinine, electrolytes (may be elevated)
⚠ **Monitor for blood dyscrasias (thrombocytopenia): bruising, fatigue, bleeding, poor healing; monitor blood counts during**
therapy; watch for decreasing platelets; if low, therapy may need to be discontinued, restarted after hematologic recovery; stool guaiac

Nursing diagnoses
• Injury, risk for (side effects)
• Knowledge, deficient (teaching)
• Mobility, impaired physical (uses)
• Pain, chronic (uses)

Patient/family education
• Teach patient that product must be continued for prescribed time to be effective; to avoid aspirin, NSAIDs, acetaminophen, or other OTC medications unless approved by prescriber, alcoholic beverages; to contact prescriber before surgery regarding when to discontinue this product
• Caution patient to report bleeding, bruising, fatigue, malaise, since **blood dyscrasias** do occur
• Advise patient to report **hepatotoxicity:** flulike symptoms, nausea, vomiting, jaundice, pruritus, lethargy
• Instruct patient to use sunscreen to prevent photosensitivity
• Teach patient to avoid use in 3rd trimester of pregnancy
• Instruct patient to use caution when driving; drowsiness, dizziness may occur
• Teach patient to take with a full glass of water to enhance absorption; remain upright for ½ hr; if dose is missed, take as soon as remembered within 2 hr if taking 1-2 ×/day; do not double doses
• Teach to report respiratory difficulty, trouble swallowing
• Advise to notify all providers that product is being used

Evaluation
Positive therapeutic outcome
• Decreased pain in arthritic conditions
• Decreased inflammation in arthritic conditions
• Decreased ocular irritation

didanosine (Rx)

(dye-dan'oh-seen)
ddl, Pediatric Videx, Videx EC
Func. class.: Antiretroviral
Chem. class.: Synthetic purine nucleoside
reverse transcriptase inhibitor (NRTI)
Pregnancy category B

ACTION: Nucleoside analog incorporating into cellular DNA by viral reverse transcriptase, thereby terminating the cellular DNA chain and preventing viral replication

Therapeutic outcome: Antiviral against the retroviruses, primarily HIV-1

USES: HIV-1 infection in combination with at least 2 other antiretrovirals

CONTRAINDICATIONS:

Hypersensitivity, lactic acidosis, pancreatitis, phenylketonuria

Precautions: Pregnancy **B**, breastfeeding, children, renal disease, sodium-restricted diets, elevated amylase, preexistent peripheral neuropathy, hyperuricemia, gout, CHF, noncirrhotic portal hypertension

> **BLACK BOX WARNING:** Hepatic disease, lactic acidosis, pancreatitis

DOSAGE AND ROUTES

Adult: PO >60 kg, DEL REL caps 400 mg daily; 200 mg bid preferred; <60 kg, DEL REL caps 250 mg daily; 125 mg bid preferred
Child: PO (child BSA 1.1-1.4 m²); reconstituted pediatric powder 125 mg q8-12hr; PO (child BSA 0.8-1 m²); reconstituted pediatric powder 94 mg q8-12hr; PO (child BSA 0.5-0.7 m²); reconstituted pediatric powder 62 mg q8-12hr; PO (child BSA <0.4 m²); reconstituted pediatric powder 31 mg q8-12hr

Videx EC cap
Renal dose
Adult >60 kg: PO CCr 30-59 ml/min 200 mg/day; CCr 10-29 ml/min 125 mg/day; CCr <10 ml/min 125 mg/day
Adult <60 kg: PO CCr 30-59 ml/min 125 mg/day; CCr 10-29 ml/min 125 mg/day; CCr <10 ml/min, avoid use

Available forms: Powder for oral sol 10 mg/ml; del rel caps 125, 200, 250, 400 mg

Implementation
• Give on empty stomach 1 hr before or 2 hr after meals q12hr; food decreases effectiveness of product; adjust dose in renal impairment
• Pediatric powder for oral sol should be prepared in the pharmacy; shake before using
• Packets for oral sol must be mixed with ½ glass of water, not fruit juice; stir until dissolved; drink immediately
• Store caps in tightly closed bottle at room temperature; store oral sol after dissolving at room temperature ≤4 hr
• Do not take dapsone at same time as ddl

ADVERSE EFFECTS
CNS: Peripheral neuropathy, seizures, confusion, *anxiety,* hypertonia, abnormal thinking, asthenia, *insomnia, CNS depression,* pain, dizziness, chills, fever
CV: Hypertension, vasodilatation, **dysrhythmia,** syncope, **CHF,** palpitations
EENT: Ear pain, otitis, photophobia, visual impairment, retinal depigmentation
GI: Pancreatitis, *diarrhea, nausea,* vomiting, *abdominal pain,* constipation, stomatitis, dyspepsia, liver abnormalities, flatulence, taste perversion, dry mouth, oral thrush, melena, increased ALT, AST, alkaline phosphatase, amylase, **hepatic failure,** noncirrhotic portal hypertension
GU: Increased bilirubin, uric acid
HEMA: Leukopenia, granulocytopenia, thrombocytopenia, anemia
INTEG: *Rash, pruritus,* alopecia, ecchymosis, hemorrhage, petechiae, sweating
MS: Myalgia, arthritis, myopathy, muscular atrophy
RESP: Cough, pneumonia, dyspnea, asthma, epistaxis, hypoventilation, sinusitis
SYST: Lactic acidosis, anaphylaxis

Pharmacokinetics

Absorption	Rapidly absorbed (up to 40%)
Distribution	Unknown
Metabolism	Not metabolized
Excretion	Kidneys (55%), feces
Half-life	0.8-1.6 hr, shorter in children

Pharmacodynamics

Onset	Unknown
Peak	Up to 1 hr, del rel 2 hr
Duration	Unknown

INTERACTIONS
Individual drugs
Allopurinol, tenofovir: increased didanosine level; do not use together

Dapsone, ketoconazole: decreased absorption of each specific product

Gatifloxacin, gemifloxacin, grepafloxacin, levofloxacin, lomefloxacin, moxifloxacin, norfloxacin, sparfloxacin, trovafloxacin: Do not use didanosine with these products (PO)

Itraconazole: decreased concentrations

Methadone: decreased didanosine level

Drug classifications
Aluminum, antacids, magnesium: increased side effects

Antiretrovirals, other: decreased concentration

Fluoroquinolones, tetracyclines: decreased concentrations of each specific product

Drug/food
Do not use with acidic juices

Decreased: absorption 50%

NURSING CONSIDERATIONS
Assessment
• **Assess for peripheral neuropathy:** tingling or pain in hands and feet, distal numbness; onset usually occurs 2-6 mo after beginning treatment; if these occur during therapy, product may be decreased or discontinued

• **Assess for pancreatitis:** abdominal pain, nausea, vomiting, elevated liver enzymes; product should be discontinued since condition can be fatal

• Assess children by dilated retinal examination q6mo to rule out retinal depigmentation

• Monitor CBC, differential, platelet count monthly; withhold product if WBC is <4000/mm^3 or platelet count is <75,000 mm^3, viral load, CD4$^+$ count; notify prescriber of results

• Monitor renal function studies: BUN, serum uric acid, urine CCr before, during therapy; these may be elevated throughout treatment

• **Assess for anaphylaxis, lactic acidosis**

• Monitor temp q4hr; may indicate beginning of infection

• Monitor liver function tests before, during therapy (bilirubin, AST, ALT, amylase, alkaline phosphatase) as needed or monthly

Nursing diagnoses
• Infection, risk for (uses)
• Injury, risk for (adverse reactions)
• Knowledge, deficient (teaching)

Patient/family education
• Advise patient to take on empty stomach; not to mix powder with fruit juice; to drink powder immediately after mixing; to use exactly as prescribed

• Instruct patient to report signs of **infection:** increased temp, sore throat, flulike symptoms; to avoid crowds and those with known infections

• Instruct patient to report signs of **anemia:** fatigue, headache, faintness, shortness of breath, irritability

• Advise patient to report numbness/tingling in extremities

• Instruct patient to report **bleeding;** avoid use of razors and commercial mouthwash

• Advise patient that hair may be lost during therapy; a wig or hairpiece may make patient feel better

• Caution patient to avoid OTC products and other medications without approval of prescriber; to avoid alcohol

• Teach patient not to have any sexual contact without use of a condom; needles should not be shared; blood from infected individual should not come in contact with another's mucous membranes

Evaluation
Positive therapeutic outcome
• Absence of opportunistic infection, symptoms of HIV

---

difenoxin with atropine
See diphenoxylate with atropine

⚠ HIGH ALERT

digoxin (Rx)
(di-jox'in)
Apo-Digoxin ✦, PMS-Digoxin ✦, Lanoxin
Func. class.: Inotropic antidysrhythmic, cardiac glycoside
Chem. class.: Digitalis preparation
Pregnancy category C

Do not confuse:
Lanoxin/Lasix/Lonox/Lomotil/Xanax/Levoxine

ACTION: Inhibits sodium-potassium ATPase, which makes more calcium available for contractile proteins, resulting in increased cardiac output; increases force of contraction (positive inotropic effect); decreases heart rate (negative chronotropic effect); decreases AV conduction speed

Therapeutic outcome: Decreased edema, pulse, respiration, crackles

USES: Rapid digitalization in acute and chronic CHF, atrial fibrillation, atrial flutter, atrial tachycardia; cardiogenic shock, paroxysmal atrial tachycardia

CONTRAINDICATIONS:

Hypersensitivity to digoxin, ventricular fibrillation, ventricular tachycardia, carotid sinus syndrome, 2nd- or 3rd-degree heart block

Precautions: Pregnancy C, breastfeeding, geriatric, renal disease, acute MI, AV block, severe respiratory disease, hypothyroidism, sinus nodal disease, hypokalemia

DOSAGE AND ROUTES

Loading dose (IV or oral dosage—capsules)
• **Adult: PO/IV** 10-15 mcg/kg in 3 divided doses q6-8hr, with 1st dose equaling about $^{1}/_{2}$ the total
• **Child >10 yr: PO/IV** 8-12 mcg/kg divided in 3 or more doses with the 1st dose equaling about $^{1}/_{2}$ the total, give other doses q6-8hr
• **Child 6-10 yr: PO/IV** 15-30 mcg/kg divided in 3 or more doses with the 1st dose equaling about $^{1}/_{2}$ the total, give other doses q6-8hr
• **Child 2-5 yr: PO/IV** 25-35 mcg/kg divided in 3 or more doses with the 1st dose equaling about $^{1}/_{2}$ the total, give other doses q6-8hr
• **Child <2 yr and infant: PO/IV** 30-50 mcg/kg divided in 3 or more doses with the 1st dose equaling about $^{1}/_{2}$ the total, give other doses q6-8hr
• **Full-term neonate: PO/IV** 20-30 mcg/kg divided in 3 or more doses with the 1st dose equaling about $^{1}/_{2}$ the total, give other doses q6-8hr
• **Premature neonate: PO/IV** 15-25 mcg/kg divided in 3 or more doses with the 1st dose equaling about $^{1}/_{2}$ the total, give other doses q6-8hr

Maintenance dose (IV or oral dosage—capsules)
• **Adult: PO/IV** 125-350 mcg depending on CCr and lean body weight in 1 or 2 divided doses
• **Child >10 yr: PO/IV** 2-3 mcg/kg/day in single daily dose
• **Child 5-10 yr: PO/IV** 4-8 mcg/kg/day in 2 daily doses
• **Child 2-5 yr: PO/IV** 6-9 mcg/kg/day in 2 daily doses
• **Child <2 yr and infant: PO/IV** 7.5-12 mcg/kg/day in 2 daily doses
• **Full-term neonate: PO/IV** 5-8 mcg/kg/day in 2 daily doses
• **Preterm neonate: PO/IV** 4-6 mcg/kg/day in 2 daily doses

Loading dose (oral dosage—elixir or tablets)
• **Adult, adolescent, child >10 yr: PO** 10-15 mcg/kg divided in 3 or more doses with the 1st dose equaling about $^{1}/_{2}$ the total, give other doses q6-8hr
• **Child 5-10 yr: PO** 20-35 mcg/kg divided in 3 doses q6-8hr
• **Child 2-5 yr: PO** 30-40 mcg/kg divided in 3 doses q6-8hr
• **Child <2 yr and infant: PO** 35-60 mcg/kg divided in 3 doses q6-8hr
• **Full-term neonate: PO** 25-35 mcg/kg divided in 3 doses q6-8hr
• **Premature neonate: PO** 20-30 mcg/kg divided in 3 doses q6-8hr

Maintenance dose (oral dosage—elixir or tablets)
• **Adult: PO** 125-500 mcg q day depending on CCr and lean body weight
• **Child >10 yr: PO** 2.5-5 mcg/kg q day
• **Child 5-10 yr: PO** 5-10 mcg/kg/day in 2 divided doses
• **Child 2-5 yr: PO** 7.5-10 mcg/kg/day in 2 divided doses
• **Child <2 yr and infant: PO** 10-15 mcg/kg/day in 2 divided doses
• **Full-term neonate: PO** 6-10 mcg/kg/day in 2 divided doses
• **Preterm neonate: PO** 5-7.5 mcg/kg/day in 2 divided doses

Renal dose

Oral dosage (capsules) or IV
• **PO/IV** CCr 50-59 ml/min LBW 50-69 kg: 150 mcg q day
• **PO/IV** CCr 50-59 ml/min LBW 70-89 kg: 200 mcg q day
• **PO/IV** CCr 20-49 ml/min LBW 50-59 kg: 100 mcg q day

Oral dosage (elixir or tablets)
• **PO** CCr 50-59 ml/min LBW 50-69 kg: 188 mcg q day
• **PO** CCr 50-59 ml/min LBW 70-89 kg: 250 mcg q day
• **PO** CCr 20-49 ml/min LBW 50-59 kg: 125 mcg q day

Available forms: Caps 0.05, 0.1, 0.2 mg; elix 0.05 mg/ml; tabs 0.125, 0.25, 0.5 mg; inj 0.5 ✿, 0.25 mg/ml; pediatric inj 0.1 mg/ml

Implementation
- Do not give at same time as antacids or other products that decrease absorption

PO route
- Give PO with or without food; may crush tabs
- Give medication at same time each day
- Give potassium supplements if ordered for potassium levels <3, or give foods high in potassium: bananas, orange juice

IV route
- Give **IV** undiluted or 1 ml of product/4 ml sterile water, D_5, or 0.9% NaCl; give over >5 min through Y-tube or 3-way stopcock; during digitalization, close monitoring is necessary
- Store protected from light

Syringe compatibilities: Heparin, milrinone

Syringe incompatibility: Doxapram

Y-site compatibilities: Amrinone, cefmetazole, ciprofloxacin, cisatracurium, diltiazem, famotidine, meperidine, meropenem, midazolam, milrinone, morphine, potassium chloride, propofol, remifentanil, tacrolimus, vit B/C

Y-site incompatibilities: Fluconazole, foscarnet

Additive compatibilities: Bretylium, cimetidine, floxacillin, furosemide, lidocaine, ranitidine, verapamil

Additive incompatibility: DOBUTamine

ADVERSE EFFECTS
CNS: *Headache,* drowsiness, apathy, confusion, disorientation, fatigue, depression, hallucinations
CV: **Dysrhythmias,** hypotension, bradycardia, **AV block**
EENT: Blurred vision, yellow-green halos, photophobia, diplopia
GI: Nausea, vomiting, anorexia, abdominal pain, diarrhea

Pharmacokinetics

Absorption	Unknown
Distribution	Widely distributed; 20%-25% protein bound
Metabolism	Liver, small amount; also intestinal bacteria
Excretion	Urine
Half-life	$1^{1}/_{2}$ days

Pharmacodynamics

	PO	IV
Onset	$^{1}/_{2}$-$1^{1}/_{2}$ hr	5-30 min
Peak	2-6 hr	1-5 hr
Duration	After steady state	6-8 days

INTERACTIONS
Individual drugs
Amiodarone, diltiazem, NIFEdipine, propantheline, quiNIDine, verapamil: increased digoxin levels
Amphotericin B, carbenicillin, ticarcillin: increased hypokalemia, increased toxicity
Calcium IV: increased hypercalcemia, hypomagnesemia, digoxin toxicity
Cholestyramine, colestipol, metoclopramide, thyroid hormones: decreased digoxin levels
Kaolin/pectin: decreased absorption

Drug classifications
Antacids: decreased digoxin absorption
Anticholinergics: increased digoxin blood levels
Antidysrhythmics, β-adrenergic blockers: increased bradycardia
Diuretics (thiazide) corticosteroids: increased hypokalemia, hypercalcemia, hypomagnesemia, digoxin toxicity
Sympathomimetics: increased cardiac dysrhythmia risk

Drug/lab test
Increased: CPK

NURSING CONSIDERATIONS
Assessment
- Assess and document apical pulse for 1 min before giving product; if pulse <60 in adult or <90 in an infant or is significantly different, take again in 1 hr; if <60 in adult, call prescriber; note rate, rhythm, character
- Monitor electrolytes: potassium, sodium, chloride, magnesium, calcium; renal function studies: BUN, creatinine; other blood studies: ALT, AST, bilirubin, Hct, Hgb, product levels (therapeutic level 0.5-2 ng/ml) before initiating treatment and periodically thereafter
- Monitor I&O ratio, daily weights; monitor turgor, lung sounds, edema
- Monitor cardiac status: apical pulse, character, rate, rhythm; resolution of atrial dysrhythmias by ECG; if tachydsrhythmia develops, hold product; delay cardioversion while product levels are determined
- **Monitor ECG continuously** during parenteral loading doses and for patients with suspected toxicity; provide hemodynamic

monitoring for patients with heart failure or administer multiple cardiac products

Nursing diagnoses
• Cardiac output, decreased (uses)
• Gas exchange, impaired (adverse reactions)
• Knowledge, deficient (teaching)

Patient/family education
• Advise patient not to stop abruptly; teach all aspects of product
• Caution patient to avoid OTC medications including cough, cold, allergy preparations, antacids, since many adverse product interactions may occur; do not take antacid at same time
• Instruct patient to notify prescriber of any loss of appetite, lower stomach pain, diarrhea, weakness, drowsiness, headache, blurred or yellow-green vision, rash, depression; teach toxic symptoms of this product and when to notify prescriber
• Advise patient to maintain a sodium-restricted diet as ordered; to take potassium supplements as ordered to prevent toxicity
• Instruct patient to report shortness of breath, difficulty breathing, weight gain, edema, persistent cough
• Teach patient purpose of product is to regulate the heart's functioning
• Teach patient as outpatient to check and record pulse for 1 min before taking dose; if there is a change of >15 bpm from usual pulse, prescriber should be notified
• Teach patient to take medication at the same time each day, take missed doses within 12 hr; do not double doses; notify prescriber if doses are missed for 2 days or more; how to monitor heart rate
• Teach patient toxic symptoms and when to notify prescriber
• Advise patient to carry/wear emergency ID describing dosage and reason for digoxin

Evaluation
Positive therapeutic outcome
• Decreased weight, edema, pulse, respiration, crackles
• Increased urine output
• Serum digoxin level 0.5-2 ng/ml

TREATMENT OF OVERDOSE:
Discontinue product, administer potassium, monitor ECG, administer an adrenergic blocking agent, digoxin immune FAB

digoxin immune FAB (ovine) (Rx)
(di-jox'in)
DigiFab
Func. class.: Antidote, digoxin specific
Pregnancy category C

ACTION: Antibody fragments bind to free digoxin or to reverse toxicity by not allowing digoxin or digitoxin to bind to sites of action

Therapeutic outcome: Correction of digoxin toxicity

USES: Reversal of life-threatening digoxin or digitoxin toxicity, including severe bradycardia, ventricular tachycardia/fibrillation, severe hypertension

CONTRAINDICATIONS:
Mild digoxin toxicity, hypersensitivity to this product, papain, or ovine protein

Precautions: Pregnancy **C**, breastfeeding, children, geriatric, cardiac/renal disease, hypocalcemia, heart failure, allergy to ovine proteins

DOSAGE AND ROUTES
1 (38 mg) vial binds 0.5 mg digoxin, 1 (40 mg) DigiFab binds 0.5 mg digoxin

Digoxin toxicity (known amount) (tabs, oral sol, IM)
Adult and child: IV dose (mg) = dose ingested (mg) $\times$ 0.8/1000 $\times$ 38 or 40 mg vial

Toxicity (known amount) (cap, IV)
Adult and child: IV dose = dose ingested (mg)/0.5 $\times$ 38 or 40 mg vial

Toxicity (known amount) by serum digoxin concentrations (SDCs)
Adult and child: IV SDC (nanograms/ml) $\times$ kg of weight/100 $\times$ 38 or 40 mg vial

Digoxin toxicity (unknown amount)
Adult and child >20 kg: IV 228 mg (6 vials)
Infant and child <20 kg: IV 38 mg (1 vial)

Acute ingestion
Adult: IV 10 vials (380 mg)

Life-threatening ingestion
Adult: IV 20 vials (760 mg)

Skin test
Adult: ID 9.5 mcg

Available forms: Inj 38 mg/vial (binds 0.5 mg of digoxin), 40 mg/vial (binds 0.5 mg digoxin)

Implementation

• Test doses have proved to be ineffective in the general population; only use test dose in those with known allergies or those previously treated with digoxin immune FAB

• **For test dose** dilute 0.1 ml or reconstituted product (9.5 mg/ml) in 9.9 ml sterile isotonic saline, inj 0.1 ml (1:100 dilution) ID and observe for wheal with erythema; read in 20 min

• **For scratch test,** place 1 drop of sol on skin and make a scratch through the drop with a sterile needle; read in 20 min

• Give after diluting 40 mg/4 ml of sterile water (10 mg/ml), mix gently; may be further diluted with 0.9% NaCl; sol should be clear, colorless

• Give by BOL if cardiac arrest is imminent or **IV** over 30 min using a 0.22-μm filter

• Store reconstituted sol for up to 4 hr in refrigerator; do not freeze DigiFab

ADVERSE EFFECTS

CV: CHF, *ventricular rate increase,* atrial fibrillation, *low cardiac output,* hypotension
INTEG: *Hypersensitivity,* allergic reactions, facial swelling, redness, phlebitis
META: *Hypokalemia*
MISC: Anaphylaxis (rare)
RESP: Impaired respiratory function, rapid respiratory rate

Pharmacokinetics

Absorption	Complete
Distribution	Widely distributed into plasma, interstitial fluids
Metabolism	Unknown
Excretion	Kidneys
Half-life	Biphasic (14-20 hr); increased in renal disease

Pharmacodynamics

Onset	30 min (variable)
Peak	Unknown
Duration	Unknown

INTERACTIONS

Individual drugs
Considered incompatible with all products in syringe or sol

Drug/lab test
Interference: immunoassay (digoxin)

NURSING CONSIDERATIONS

Assessment

• **Assess for CHF:** dyspnea, crackles, peripheral edema, B/P, volume overload

• **Assess for hypokalemia:** ST depression, flat T waves, presence of U wave, ventricular dysrhythmias

• Obtain information on previous allergies: previous exposure to sheep (ovine) proteins; scratch test may be performed before use of this product; hypersensitive reactions are more common in persons with previous exposure

• Monitor VS before, during, after infusion

• Monitor heart rate, B/P q10min during inf and after completion until stabilized; hemodynamic monitoring is used for unstable or hypotensive patients; check potassium levels until toxicity is resolved

• Assess for oxygen or perfusion deficit: hypotension, chest pain, dizziness, loss of consciousness

• Assess respiratory status: auscultate lung fields for bibasilar crackles in patients with advanced CHF, B/P, volume overload

Nursing diagnoses

• Injury, risk for (uses)
• Knowledge, deficient (teaching)

Patient/family education

• Teach that purpose of medication is to bind excess digoxin and reduce high blood levels

• Instruct patients to report fever, chills, itching, sweating, dyspnea, delayed hypersensitivity

• Advise other prescribers that this medication has been used previously

Evaluation
Positive therapeutic outcome
• Correction of digoxin toxicity
• Digoxin blood level 0.5-2 ng/ml
• Digitoxin blood level 9-25 ng/ml

dihydroergotamine
See ergotamine

dihydrotachysterol (Rx)
(dye-hye-droh-tak-iss′ter-ole)
DHT Intensol ✦, Hytakerol
Func. class.: Parathyroid agent (calcium regulator)
Chem. class.: Vitamin D analog
Pregnancy category C

ACTION: Increases intestinal absorption of calcium, increases renal tubular absorption of phosphorus; is able to regulate calcium levels by regulation of calcitonin, parathyroid hormone

Therapeutic outcome: Prevention of continued calcium loss in bones

USES: Hypoparathyroidism, pseudohypoparathyroidism, postoperative tetany

CONTRAINDICATIONS:
Hypersensitivity, renal disease, hyperphosphatemia, hypercalcemia, hypervitaminosis D

Precautions: Pregnancy **C**, breastfeeding, renal calculi, CV disease

DOSAGE AND ROUTES
Hypoparathyroidism/pseudohypoparathyroidism
Adult: PO 0.75-2.5 mg daily × 4 days, maintenance 0.2-1 mg daily regulated by serum calcium levels

Neonate: PO 0.05-0.1 mg/day
Child/infant: PO 1-5 mg qd × 4 days then 0.5-1.5 mg qd

Rickets (vit D resistant)
Child: PO 0.25-1 mg/day

Available forms: Tabs 0.125, 0.2, 0.4 mg; caps 0.125 mg; oral sol 0.2, 0.25 mg/5 ml, 0.2 mg/ml ✦ (Intensol)

Implementation
• Do not break, crush, or chew caps
• May be increased q4wk depending on blood level; give with meals for GI symptoms
• Store in tight, light-resistant containers at room temperature
• Restrict sodium, potassium if required
• Restriction of fluids may be required for chronic renal failure

ADVERSE EFFECTS
CNS: Drowsiness, headache, vertigo, fever, lethargy, depression
CV: Dysrhythmias, hypertension
EENT: Tinnitus
GI: Nausea, diarrhea, vomiting, jaundice, anorexia, dry mouth, constipation, cramps, metallic taste, thirst
GU: Polyuria, hypercalciuria, hyperphosphatemia, **hematuria,** nocturia, renal calculi
MS: Myalgia, arthralgia, decreased bone development, weakness, ataxia

Pharmacokinetics
Absorption	Well absorbed from small intestine
Distribution	Liver, fat
Metabolism	Liver
Excretion	Feces (inactive, active metabolites)
Half-life	Unknown

Pharmacodynamics
Onset	2 wk
Peak	2 wk
Duration	2-9 wk

INTERACTIONS
Individual drugs
Cholestyramine, colestipol, mineral oil: decreased absorption of dihydrotachysterol
Phenytoin: decreased effect of dihydrotachysterol
Verapamil: increased dysrhythmias

Drug classifications
Barbiturates, corticosteroids: decreased effect of dihydrotachysterol
Calcium supplements, diuretics (thiazide): increased hypercalcemia
Cardiac glycosides: increased dysrhythmias

Drug/lab test
False increase: cholesterol

NURSING CONSIDERATIONS
Assessment
• Monitor BUN, urinary calcium, AST, ALT, cholesterol, alkaline phosphatase, creatinine, uric acid, chloride, magnesium, electrolytes, urine pH, phosphate; may increase calcium; should be kept at 9-10 mg/dl; keep vit D at 50-135 international units/dl, phosphate at 70 mg/dl; these tests should be checked before and throughout treatment
• Monitor for increased blood level, since toxic reaction may occur rapidly
• Monitor for dry mouth, metallic taste, polyuria, bone pain, muscle weakness, headache, fatigue, tinnitus, change in LOC, irregular pulse, dysrhythmias, increased respirations, anorexia, nausea, vomiting, cramps, diarrhea, constipation; may indicate hypercalcemia; if these occur, discontinue product, give laxatives, low-calcium diet
• Monitor renal status: decreased urinary output (oliguria, anuria), edema in extremities, weight gain >5 lb, periorbital edema

• Assess nutritional status; check diet for sources of vit D (milk, some seafood), calcium (dairy products, dark green vegetables); phosphates (dairy products) must be avoided

Nursing diagnoses
• Knowledge, deficient (teaching)
• Nutrition: less than body requirements, imbalanced (uses)

Patient/family education
• Teach symptoms of hypercalcemia and when to report symptoms to prescriber
• Teach patient about foods rich in calcium, vit D; provide list of calcium-rich foods; renal failure patients are given a renal diet
• Caution patient not to double doses, take exactly as prescribed

Evaluation
Positive therapeutic outcome
• Prevention of bone deficiencies
• Calcium, phosphorus at normal levels

▲ HIGH ALERT

diltiazem (Rx)
(dil-tye′a-zem)
Cardizem, Cardizem CD, Cardizem LA, Cartia XT, Dilacor-XR, Dilt-CD, Diltia XR, Diltia XT, Diltzac, Gen-Diltiazem ✦, ratio-Diltiazem ✦, Sandoz Diltiazem ✦, Taztia XT, Tiamate, Tiazac
Func. class.: Calcium channel blocker, antianginal, antiarrhythmic class IV, antihypertensive
Chem. class.: Benzothiazepine
Pregnancy category C

Do not confuse:
Cardizem/Cardene

ACTION: Inhibits calcium ion influx across cell membrane during cardiac depolarization, produces relaxation of coronary vascular smooth muscle, dilates coronary arteries, slows SA/AV node conduction times, dilates peripheral arteries

Therapeutic outcome: Decreased angina pectoris, dysrhythmias, B/P

USES
Oral: Angina pectoris due to hypertension, coronary artery spasm

Parenteral: Atrial fibrillation, flutter; paroxysmal supraventricular tachycardia

CONTRAINDICATIONS:
Sick sinus syndrome, 2nd- or 3rd-degree heart block, hypotension less than 90 mm Hg systolic, acute MI, pulmonary congestion, cardiogenic shock

Precautions: Pregnancy **C**, breastfeeding, children, CHF, aortic stenosis, bradycardia, GERD, hepatic disease, hiatal hernia, ventricular dysfunction, elderly

DOSAGE AND ROUTES
Hypertension
Adult: PO 60-120 mg bid (SUS REL) (Cardizem SR), max 540 mg/day, or 120-240 mg (EXT REL) daily

Prinzmetal's or variant angina, chronic stable angina
Adult: PO 30 mg qid, increasing dose gradually to 180-360 mg/day in divided doses or (SR) 60-120 mg bid; may increase to 240-360 mg/day or 120 or 180 mg EXT REL (LA, CD, XT, XR products) PO daily

Atrial fibrillation, flutter, paroxysmal supraventricular tachycardia
Adult: IV 0.25 mg/kg as BOL over 2 min initially, then 0.35 mg/kg may be given after 15 min; if no response, may give CONT INF 5-15 mg/hr for up to 24 hr

Available forms: Tabs 30, 60, 90, 120 mg; ext rel tab 120, 180, 240, 300, 360, 420 mg; ext rel caps 60, 90, 120, 180, 240, 300, 360, 420 mg; inj 5 mg/ml (5, 10 ml)

Implementation
PO route
• **Cardiazem LA ext rel tab 24 hr:** give daily, either AM or PM, without regard to meals
• **Dilacor XR/Diltia XT ext rel cap 24 hr** give daily, take on empty stomach, swallow whole, do not cut, crush, chew, open
• **Tiazac, Tiztia XT:** give daily without regard to meals
• **Conventional regular-rel tab:** give before meals and at bedtime
• **Cardizem CD or equivalent (Cartia XT) generic ext rel cap 24 hr:** give daily, without regard to meals
• Give with meals for GI symptoms; may crush and sprinkle (reg tab) on applesauce
• Store in airtight container at room temperature

Oral suspension (unlabeled)
• Grind 16, 90 mg diltiazem reg rel tab into fine powder
• In separate container, mix 60 ml Ora-Sweet and 60 ml Ora-Plus
• Add small amount of sol to powder to form paste, add geometric amounts of base to achieve desired vol, place in amber container

Direct IV route
• Give direct **IV** undiluted over 2 min

Continuous IV infusion route
• **Dilute** 125 mg/100 ml (1.25 mg/ml) or 250 mg/250 ml (1 mg/ml) or 250 mg/500 ml (0.5 mg/ml) of D$_5$W, 0.9% NaCl, D$_5$/0.45% NaCl; give 10 mg/hr; may increase by 5 mg/hr to 15 mg/hr; may continue inf up to 24 hr

Y-site compatibilities: Albumin, amikacin, amphotericin B, aztreonam, bretylium, bumetanide, ceFAZolin, cefotaxime, cefotetan, cefoxitin, ceftazidime, cefTRIAXone, cefuroxime, cimetidine, ciprofloxacin, clindamycin, digoxin, DOBUTamine, DOPamine, doxycycline, EPINEPHrine, erythromycin, esmolol, fentaNYL, fluconazole, gentamicin, hetastarch, HYDROmorphone, imipenem-cilastatin, labetalol, lidocaine, LORazepam, meperidine, metoclopramide, metroNIDAZOLE, midazolam, milrinone, morphine, multivitamins, niCARdipine, nitroglycerin, norepinephrine, oxacillin, penicillin G potassium, pentamidine, piperacillin, potassium chloride, potassium phosphates, ranitidine, sodium nitroprusside, theophylline, ticarcillin, ticarcillin/clavulanate, tobramycin, trimethoprim-sulfamethoxazole, vancomycin, vecuronium

ADVERSE EFFECTS
CNS: *Headache, fatigue, drowsiness,* dizziness, depression, weakness, insomnia, tremor, paresthesia
CV: Dysrhythmia, *edema,* CHF, bradycardia, hypotension, palpitations, **heart block**
GI: *Nausea,* vomiting, diarrhea, gastric upset, *constipation,* increased LFTs
GU: Nocturia, polyuria, **acute renal failure**
INTEG: *Rash,* pruritus at inj site, flushing, photosensitivity, burning
RESP: Rhinitis, dyspnea, pharyngitis

Pharmacokinetics

Absorption	Well absorbed
Distribution	Not known
Metabolism	Liver, extensively
Excretion	Metabolites (96%)
Half-life	3$\frac{1}{2}$-9 hr

Pharmacodynamics

	PO	PO–sus rel	IV
Onset	$\frac{1}{2}$ hr	Unknown	Unknown
Peak	2-3 hr	Unknown	Unknown
Duration	6-8 hr	12 hr	Unknown

INTERACTIONS
Individual drugs
CarBAMazepine, lithium, lovastatin, methylPREDNISolone: increased effects of each specific product
Cimetidine: increased effects of diltiazem
CycloSPORINE: increased cycloSPORINE effect
Digoxin: increased digoxin effect
Theophylline: increased effect, toxicity

Drug classifications
Anesthetics: increased effects of anesthetics
β-Adrenergic blockers: increased bradycardia, CHF, increased β-blocker effect
Benzodiazepines: increased effect of benzodiazepines
HMG-CoA reductase inhibitors: increased effects

Drug/food
Grapefruit juice: increased hypotension

NURSING CONSIDERATIONS
Assessment
• **CHF:** monitor for dyspnea, weight gain, edema, jugular vein distention, rales; monitor I&O ratios daily, weight
• **Angina:** location, duration, alleviating factors, activity when pain starts
• **Dysrhythmias:** monitor B/P and pulse, respiration, ECG and intervals (PR, QRS, QT); PCWP, CVP often during infusion; if B/P drops 30 mm Hg, stop infusion and call prescriber

Nursing diagnoses
• Cardiac output, decreased (uses)
• Knowledge, deficient (teaching)

Patient/family education
• Caution patient to avoid hazardous activities until stabilized on product and dizziness is no longer a problem
• Instruct patient to limit caffeine consumption; to avoid grapefruit juice; to avoid alcohol and OTC products unless directed by prescriber
⚠ Tell patient to comply in all areas of medical regimen; diet, exercise, stress reduction, product therapy; to notify prescriber of irregular heartbeat, shortness of breath, swelling of feet and hands, pronounced dizziness, constipation, nausea, hypotension

- Teach patient to use as directed even if feeling better; may be taken with other cardiovascular products (nitrates, β-blockers); how to take pulse, B/P before taking product; to change position slowly
- Teach patient not to discontinue abruptly

Evaluation
Positive therapeutic outcome
- Decreased anginal pain
- Decreased B/P
- Absence of dysrhythmias

TREATMENT OF OVERDOSE:
Atropine for AV block, vasopressor for hypotension

---

dinoprostone (Rx)
(dye-noe-prost′one)
Cervidil, Prepidil, Prostin E-Z
Func. class.: Oxytocic, abortifacient
Chem. class.: Prostaglandin E_2
Pregnancy category C

Do not confuse:
Prepidil/bepridil

ACTION: Stimulates uterine contractions similar to labor by myometrium stimulation, causing abortion; acts within 30 hr for complete abortion

Therapeutic outcome: Beginning of labor, fetal expulsion

USES: Abortion during 2nd trimester, benign hydatidiform mole, expulsion of uterine contents in fetal deaths to 28 wk, missed abortion, cervical effacement and dilatation in term pregnancy when they have not occurred spontaneously

CONTRAINDICATIONS:
Hypersensitivity, C-section, surgery

Precautions: Pregnancy **C,** renal/hepatic/cardiac disease, asthma, anemia, jaundice, diabetes mellitus, seizure disorders, hypertension, glaucoma, uterine fibrosis, cervical stenosis, pelvic surgery, PID, respiratory disease

---

BLACK BOX WARNING: Hypotension, diarrhea, fever, vomiting

DOSAGE AND ROUTES

Abortifacient/2nd trimester/missed abortion/benign hydatidiform mole/intrauterine fetal death
Adult: VAG SUPP 20 mg; repeat q3-5hr until abortion occurs; max dose 240 mg

Cervical ripening
Adult: GEL warm to room temperature; choose correct length shielded catheter (10 or 20 mm); fill catheter by pushing plunger; have patient recumbent for 15-30 min; insert one 10 mg insert

Available forms: Vag supp 20 mg; gel 0.5 mg/3 g (prefilled syringe); vag insert 10 mg

Implementation
Suppository route
- Warm supp by running warm water over package; insert high in vagina, wear gloves to prevent absorption; have patient recumbent for at least 10 min

Gel route
- Do not allow to come in contact with skin; use soap and water to wash after use
- Gel should be at room temperature
- Place patient in dorsal or lithotomy position to insert gel into cervical canal; remove catheter; discard all items after use; keep supine 15-30 min

ADVERSE EFFECTS
CNS: *Headache,* dizziness, chills, fever, flushing
CV: Hypotension, **dysrhythmias,** DIC
EENT: Blurred vision
GI: *Nausea, vomiting, diarrhea*
GU: Vaginitis, vaginal pain, vulvitis, vaginismus
INTEG: Rash, skin color changes
MS: *Leg cramps, joint swelling,* weakness
SYST: Anaphylactoid syndrome of pregnancy
Insert: Uterine hyperstimulation, fever, nausea, vomiting, diarrhea, abdominal pain
Gel: Uterine contractile abnormality, GI side effects, back pain, fever
Fetal: Bradycardia (i.e., deceleration)
Suppository: Uterine rupture, anaphylaxis

Pharmacokinetics	
Absorption	Rapidly absorbed
Distribution	Unknown
Metabolism	Enzymes
Excretion	Kidneys
Half-life	Unknown

Adverse effects: *italics* = common; **bold** = life-threatening

Pharmacodynamics

	Gel	Supp
Onset	Rapid	10 min
Peak	30-45 min	Unknown
Duration	Unknown	2-3 hr

INTERACTIONS

Individual drugs
Alcohol: decreased oxytoxic effect

Drug classifications
Other oxytocics: increased effect

NURSING CONSIDERATIONS

Assessment
• **Cervical ripening:** assess dilatation and effacement of the cervix, uterine contractions, fetal heart tones; watch for contractions lasting over 1 min, hypertonus, fetal distress; product should be slowed or discontinued
• Assess for fever that occurs approximately 30 min after supp insertion (abortion)
• Monitor for nausea, vomiting, diarrhea; these may require medication
• **Assess for hypersensitivity reaction:** dyspnea, rash, chest discomfort
• Assess respiratory rate, rhythm, depth; notify prescriber of abnormalities in pulse, B/P
• **Check vaginal discharge;** itching, irritation indicates vaginal infection

Nursing diagnoses
• Injury, risk for (side effects)
• Knowledge, deficient (teaching)

Patient/family education
• Teach patient all aspects of treatment including purpose of medication and expected results
• Tell patient that gel may produce warmth in her vagina
• Caution patient that if contractions are longer than 1 min to notify nurse or prescriber
• Advise patient to notify prescriber of cramping, pain, increased bleeding, chills, increased temp, or foul-smelling discharge; these symptoms may indicate uterine infection
• Advise patient to remain supine 10-15 min after insertion of suppository, 2 hr after insert, 15-30 min after gel

Evaluation
Positive therapeutic outcome
• Progression of labor
• Abortion

---

diphenhydrAMINE
(OTC, Rx)
(dye-fen-hye′dra-meen)
Allerdryl ✳, AllerMax ✳, Altaryl, Banophen, Benadryl, Benadryl Allergy, Benadryl Allergy Dye Free, Benadryl Children's Allergy, Buckley's Bedtime, Diphedryl, Diphenhist, Dytan, ElixSure Allergy, Equaline Allergy, Equaline Children's Allergy, Equate Allergy, Equate Children's Allergy, Genahist, Good Sense Children's Allergy Relief, Good Sense Diphedryl, Leader Complete Allergy, Nytol, PediaCare Children's Allergy, PediaCare Nighttime Cough, Q-Dryl Allergy, Select Brand Allergy, Siladryl, Silphen, Simply Sleep, Sleepinal, Sleep Tabs, Sominex, Top Care Allergy, Top Care Children's Allergy, Unisom ✳, Valu-Dryl, Wal-dryl Allergy, Wal-dryl Allergy Dye Free, Wal-dryl Children's Allergy, Walgreen's Sleep Aid, Walgreen's Sleep II, Wal-Som

Func. class.: Antihistamine (1st generation, nonselective), antitussive
Chem. class.: Ethanolamine derivative, H_1-receptor antagonist
Pregnancy category B

Do not confuse:
diphenhydrAMINE/dicyclomine/dimenhyDRINATE

ACTION: Acts on blood vessels, GI, respiratory system by competing with histamine for H_1-receptor site; decreases allergic response by blocking histamine

Therapeutic outcome: Absence of allergy symptoms and rhinitis, decreased dystonic symptoms, absence of motion sickness, absence of cough, ability to sleep

USES: Allergy symptoms, rhinitis, motion sickness, antiparkinsonism, nighttime sedation, infant colic, nonproductive cough, insomnia in children

CONTRAINDICATIONS:
Hypersensitivity to H_1-receptor antagonist, acute asthma attack, lower respiratory tract disease, neonates

---

⚠ Nurse Alert

Precautions: Pregnancy **B,** breastfeeding, children <2 yr, increased intraocular pressure, renal/cardiac disease, hypertension, bronchial asthma, seizure disorder, stenosed peptic ulcers, hyperthyroidism, prostatic hypertrophy, bladder neck obstruction

DOSAGE AND ROUTES
Adult and child >12 yr: PO 25-50 mg q4-6hr, max 300 mg/day; IM/IV 10-50 mg, max 300 mg/day
Child 6-12 yr: PO/IM/IV 5 mg/kg/day in 4 divided doses, max 300 mg/day

Nighttime sleep aid
Adult and child ≥12 yr: PO 25-50 mg at bedtime

Antitussive (syrup only)
Adult and child ≥12 yr: 25 mg q4hr, max 150 mg/24 hr
Child 6-12 yr: 12.5 mg q4hr, max 75 mg/24 hr

Renal dosage
Adult: PO CCr >50 ml/min give dose q6hr; CCr 10-50 ml/min dose q6-12hr; CCr <10 ml/min dose q12-18hr

Available forms: Caps 25, 50 mg; tabs 25, 50 mg; chew tabs 12.5 mg; elix 12.5 mg/5 ml; syr 12.5 mg/5 ml; inj 10, 50 mg/ml; orally disintegrating tabs 12.5, 25 mg

Implementation
• Avoid use in children <2 yr, death has occurred; overdose has occurred in topical gel taken orally (adult/child)
• Give 20 min before bedtime if using for sleep aid
PO route
• Give with meals if GI symptoms occur; absorption rate may be slightly decreased; cap may be opened and product mixed with food/fluids for patients with swallowing difficulties
IM route
• Give IM inj in large muscle mass; aspirate to avoid IV administration; rotate sites

Direct IV route
• Give IV undiluted 25 mg/min
Intermittent IV infusion route
May be diluted with 0.9% NaCl, D₅W, D₁₀W, 0.45% NaCl, D₅/0.9% NaCl, D₅/0.45% NaCl, D₅/0.25% NaCl, LR, Ringer's; give 25 mg/min or less

Syringe compatibilities: Atropine, butorphanol, chlorproMAZINE, cimetidine, cisatracurium, dimenhyDRINATE, DOXOrubicin liposome, droperidol, fentaNYL, fluphenazine, glycopyrrolate, HYDROmorphone, hydrOXYzine, meperidine, metoclopramide, midazolam, morphine, nalbuphine, pentazocine, perphenazine, prochlorperazine, promazine, promethazine, ranitidine, remifentanil, scopolamine, SUFentanil

Syringe incompatibilities: PENTobarbital, phenytoin, thiopental

Y-site compatibilities: Abciximab, aldesleukin, alfentanil hydrochloride, amifostine, amikacin sulfate, aminocaproic acid, amphotericin B lipid complex (Abelcet), amphotericin B liposome (AmBisome), amsacrine, anidulafungin, argatroban, ascorbic acid injection, atenolol, atracurium besylate, atropine sulfate, azithromycin, benztropine mesylate, bivalirudin, bleomycin, bumetanide, buprenorphine, butorphanol, calcium chloride/gluconate, CARBOplatin, caspofungin, ceftazidime, ceftizoxime, chlorproMAZINE, cimetidine, ciprofloxacin, cisatracurium, CISplatin, cladribine, clindamycin, codeine, cyanocobalamin, cyclophosphamide, cycloSPORINE, cytarabine, DACTINomycin, DAPTOmycin, digoxin, diltiazem, DOBUTamine, docetaxel, DOPamine, doripenem, doxacurium, DOXOrubicin, DOXOrubicin liposomal, doxycycline, enalaprilat, ePHEDrine, EPINEPHrine, epirubicin, epoetin alfa, eptifibatide, ertapenem, erythromycin, esmolol, etoposide, famotidine, fenoldopam, fentaNYL, filgrastim, fluconazole, fludarabine, folic acid, gallium, gatifloxacin, gemcitabine, gemtuzumab, gentamicin, glycopyrrolate, granisetron, HYDROmorphone, hydrOXYzine, IDArubicin, ifosfamide, imipenem-cilastatin, irinotecan, isoproterenol, labetalol, levofloxacin, lidocaine, linezolid, LORazepam, LR, magnesium sulfate, mannitol, mechlorethamine, melphalan, meperidine, meropenem, metaraminol, methadone, methicillin, methotrexate, methoxamine, methyldopate, metoclopramide, metoprolol, metroNIDAZOLE, miconazole, midazolam, minocycline, mitoxantrone, morphine, multiple vitamins injection, mycophenolate, nalbuphine, naloxone, nesiritide, netilmicin, nitroglycerin, norepinephrine, octreotide, ondansetron, oxaliplatin, oxytocin, paclitaxel, palonosetron, pamidronate, pancuronium, papaverine, pemetrexed, penicillin G potassium/sodium, pentamidine, pentazocine, phenylephrine, phytonadione, piperacillin, piperacillin-tazobactam, polymyxin B, potassium chloride, procainamide, prochlorperazine, promethazine, propofol, propranolol, protamine, pyridoxine, quiNIDine, quinupristin-dalfopristin, ranitidine, remifentanil, Ringer's, ritodrine, riTUXimab, rocuronium, sargramostim, sodium acetate, succinylcholine, SUFentanil, tacrolimus, teniposide, theophylline, thiamine, thiotepa, ticarcillin, ticarcillin-clavulanate, tigecycline, tirofiban, TNA, tobramycin, tolazoline, TPN, trastuzumab, trimetaphan, urokinase, vancomycin, vasopressin, vecuronium, verapamil, vinCRIStine, vinorelbine, vitamin B complex/C, voriconazole, zoledronic acid

Y-site incompatibilities: Foscarnet

ADVERSE EFFECTS

CNS: *Dizziness, drowsiness,* poor coordination, fatigue, anxiety, euphoria, confusion, paresthesia, neuritis, **seizures**
CV: Hypotension, palpitations
EENT: Blurred vision, dilated pupils, tinnitus, nasal stuffiness, dry nose, throat, mouth
GI: Nausea, anorexia, diarrhea
GU: *Retention,* dysuria, frequency
HEMA: Thrombocytopenia, agranulocytosis, hemolytic anemia
INTEG: Photosensitivity
MISC: Anaphylaxis
RESP: Increased thick secretions, wheezing, chest tightness

Pharmacokinetics

Absorption	Well absorbed (PO, IM); completely absorbed (**IV**)
Distribution	Widely distributed; crosses placenta
Metabolism	Liver (95%)
Excretion	Kidneys, breast milk
Half-life	$2^{1}/_{2}$-7 hr

Pharmacodynamics

	PO	IM	IV
Onset	15-60 min	30 min	Immediate
Peak	1-4 hr	1-4 hr	Unknown
Duration	4-8 hr	4-8 hr	4-8 hr

INTERACTIONS

Individual drugs
Alcohol: increased CNS depression

Drug classifications
Antidepressants (tricyclic), barbiturates, CNS depressants, opiates, sedative/hypnotics: increased CNS depression
MAOIs: increased effect of diphenhydrAMINE

Drug/lab test
False negative: skin allergy tests (discontinue antihistamines 3 days before testing)

NURSING CONSIDERATIONS

Assessment
• Assess respiratory status: rate, rhythm, increase in bronchial secretions, wheezing, chest tightness; provide fluids to 2 L/day to decrease secretion thickness
• Monitor I&O ratio: be alert for urinary retention, frequency, dysuria, especially geriatric; product should be discontinued if these occur
• Monitor CBC during long-term therapy; blood dyscrasias may occur but are rare
• If giving for dystonic reactions, assess type of involuntary movements and evaluate response to this medication
• Assess cough characteristics including type, frequency, thickness of secretions; evaluate response to this medication if using for cough

Nursing diagnoses
• Injury, risk for (side effects)
• Knowledge, deficient (teaching)
• Sleep deprivation (uses)

Patient/family education
• Tell patient that a false-negative result may occur with skin testing; these procedures should not be scheduled until 3 days after discontinuing use
• Caution patient to avoid hazardous activities and activities requiring alertness, since dizziness may occur; instruct patient to request assistance with ambulation
• Teach patient to use sunscreen to prevent photosensitivity
• Advise patient to avoid alcohol, other depressants; may potentiate effect; CNS depression may occur
• Teach all aspects of product uses; to notify prescriber if confusion, sedation, hypotension occur; to avoid driving and other hazardous activity if drowsiness occurs; to avoid alcohol or other CNS depressants that may potentiate effect
• Advise patient to avoid breastfeeding

Evaluation
Positive therapeutic outcome
• Absence of motion sickness
• Absence of nausea, vomiting
• Ability to sleep
• Absence of cough
• Decrease in involuntary movements

TREATMENT OF OVERDOSE:
• Administer lavage, diazepam, vasopressors, phenytoin **IV**

diphenoxylate with atropine (Rx)
(dye-fen-ox′i-late)
Lomotil, Lonox
difenoxin/atropine (Rx)
(dye-fen-ox′in/a′troe-peen)
Motofen
Func. class.: Antidiarrheal
Chem. class.: Phenylpiperidine derivative, opiate agonist
Pregnancy category C
Controlled substance schedule V diphenoxylate/atropine; IV difenoxin/atropine (US)

Do not confuse:
Lomotil/Lamictal/Lamasil/Lanoxin/Lasix/Ludomil

ACTION: Inhibits gastric motility by acting on mucosal receptors responsible for peristalsis

Therapeutic outcome: Decreased loose stools

USES: Acute nonspecific and acute exacerbations of chronic functional diarrhea

CONTRAINDICATIONS:
Hypersensitivity, pseudomembranous colitis, child <2 yr, severe electrolyte imbalances, diarrhea associated with organisms that penetrate intestinal mucosa

Precautions: Pregnancy **C**, breastfeeding, hepatic disease, ulcerative colitis, severe hepatic disease, substance abuse, dehydration

DOSAGE AND ROUTES
diphenoxylate/atropine
Adult: PO 5 mg qid, titrated to patient response, max 8 tabs/24 hr
Child 2-12 yr: PO (liquid only) 0.3-0.4 mg/kg/day in 4 divided doses

difenoxin/atropine
Adult: PO initially 2 tabs, then 1 tab after each loose stool or q3-4hr prn, max 8 tabs/day

Available forms: diphenoxylate/atropine: tab 2.5 mg diphenoxylate/0.025 mg atropine; liq 2.5 mg diphenoxylate/0.025 mg atropine/5 ml; difenoxin/atropine: tabs 1 mg difenoxin/0.025 atropine

Implementation
• Give for 48 hr only; tabs may be given with food, crushed and mixed with fluids; liquid should be measured accurately

ADVERSE EFFECTS
CNS: *Dizziness, drowsiness, light-headedness, headache,* fatigue, nervousness, insomnia, confusion
EENT: Blurred vision, burning eyes
GI: *Nausea, vomiting, dry mouth, epigastric distress,* constipation, **paralytic ileus, toxic megacolon**
MISC: **Anaphylaxis, angioedema**
RESP: **Respiratory depression**

Pharmacokinetics
Absorption	Well absorbed
Distribution	Unknown
Metabolism	Liver, active metabolite
Excretion	Kidneys
Half-life	$2\frac{1}{2}$ hr

Pharmacodynamics
Onset	45-60 min
Peak	2 hr
Duration	3-4 hr

INTERACTIONS
Individual drugs
Alcohol: increased action of alcohol
Amantadine, amoxapine, diphenhydrAMINE, clemastine, clozapine, cyclobenzaprine, disopyramide, loperamide, maprotiline, olanzapine: decreased GI motility, possible toxic megacolon

Drug classifications
Anticholinergics: increased anticholinergic effect
Antimuscarinics, phenothiazines, tricyclics: decreased GI motility, possible toxic megacolon
Barbiturates: increased action of barbiturates
CNS depressants: increased action of CNS depressants
MAOIs: hypertensive crisis; do not use together
Opiates: increased action of opioids

NURSING CONSIDERATIONS
Assessment
• Monitor electrolytes (potassium, sodium, chloride) if on long-term therapy; fluid status, skin turgor
• Assess bowel pattern before, during treatment; check for rebound constipation after termination of medication; check bowel sounds

Adverse effects: *italics* = common; **bold** = life-threatening

• Check response after 48 hr; if no response, product should be discontinued and other treatment initiated
• **Assess for abdominal distention and toxic megacolon,** which may occur in ulcerative colitis
• Assess hepatic function if on long-term therapy

Nursing diagnoses
• Constipation (adverse reactions)
• Diarrhea (uses)
• Knowledge, deficient (teaching)
• Noncompliance (teaching)

Patient/family education
• Advise patient to avoid alcohol and OTC products unless directed by prescriber; may cause increased CNS depression
• Caution patient not to exceed recommended dosage; that product may be habit forming
• Advise patient that product may cause drowsiness; to avoid hazardous activities until response to product is determined
• Teach patient that dry mouth can be decreased by frequent sips of water, hard candy, sugarless gum

Evaluation
Positive therapeutic outcome
• Decreased diarrhea

dipivefrin ophthalmic
See Appendix B

dipyridamole (Rx)
(dye-peer-id′a-mole)
Apo-Dipyridamole ✦, Persantine
Func. class.: Coronary vasodilator, antiplatelet agent
Chem. class.: Nonnitrate
Pregnancy category B

ACTION: Inhibits adenosine uptake, which produces coronary vasodilatation; increases oxygen saturation in coronary tissues, coronary blood flow; acts on small vessels with little effect on vascular resistance; may increase development of collateral circulation; decreased platelet aggregation by the inhibition of phosphodiesterases (enzymes)

Therapeutic outcome: Inhibition of platelet aggregation; absence of ischemic attacks, reinfarction

USES: Prevention of transient ischemic attacks, inhibition of platelet adhesion to prevent myocardial reinfarction, thromboembolism, with warfarin in prosthetic heart valves, prevention of coronary bypass graft occlusion with aspirin; **IV** form used to evaluate coronary artery disease; used as alternative to exercise in thallium myocardial perfusion imaging to evaluate coronary artery disease

CONTRAINDICATIONS:
Hypersensitivity

Precautions: Pregnancy **B,** breastfeeding, hypotension

DOSAGE AND ROUTES
Inhibition of platelet adhesion
Adult: PO 75-100 mg qid in combination with aspirin or warfarin

Thallium myocardial perfusion imaging
Adult: IV 570 mcg/kg

Transient ischemic attacks with aspirin (unlabeled)
Adult: PO 225-400 mg/day, max 400 mg daily

Available forms: Tabs 25, 50, 75 mg; inj 10 mg/2 ml

Implementation
PO route
• Give with 8 oz of water; to improve absorption give on an empty stomach; if GI symptoms occur may give with meals
• Tabs may be crushed, mixed with food or fluids for swallowing difficulty, or swallowed whole
• Store at room temperature

Intermittent IV infusion route
• Give by **IV** after diluting to at least 1:2 ratio using D$_5$W, 0.45% NaCl, or 0.9% NaCl; 20-50 ml should be given; give over 4 min; do not give undiluted

ADVERSE EFFECTS
CNS: *Headache, dizziness, weakness, fainting, syncope;* **IV**: transient cerebral ischemia, weakness
CV: *Postural hypotension;* **IV**: MI
GI: *Nausea, vomiting,* anorexia, diarrhea
INTEG: *Rash,* flushing
RESP: **IV: Bronchospasm**

Pharmacokinetics

Absorption	30%-50% (PO)
Distribution	Widely distributed; crosses placenta
Metabolism	Liver
Excretion	Bile, undergoes enterohepatic recirculation; enters breast milk
Half-life	10 hr

Pharmacodynamics

	PO	IV
Onset	Unknown	Unknown
Peak	1.25 hr	6 min
Duration	6 hr	$\frac{1}{2}$ hr
Therapeutic effect	Several mo	

INTERACTIONS

Individual drugs
Aspirin, cefamandole, cefotetan, cefoperazone, plicamycin, sulfinpyrazone, valproic acid: increased risk of bleeding

Digoxin: increased digoxin effect

Theophylline: prevention of coronary vasodilation

Drug classifications
Anticoagulants, NSAIDs, salicylates, thrombolytics: increased risk of bleeding

NURSING CONSIDERATIONS

Assessment
• Monitor B/P, pulse baseline and during treatment until stable; take B/P with patient lying, standing; orthostatic hypotension is common
• Assess cardiac status: chest pain, what aggravates or ameliorates condition
• If using by **IV** route, monitor VS before, during, and after infusion; monitor for chest pain, bronchospasm; use ECG for identifying dysrhythmias; use aminophylline up to 250 mg **IV** for bronchospasm and chest pain; if chest pain is unrelieved with the 250 mg dose of aminophylline, give SL dose of nitroglycerin

Nursing diagnoses
• Cardiac output, decreased (uses)
• Knowledge, deficient (teaching)
• Pain, acute (uses)

Patient/family education
• Teach patient that this medication is not a cure; that product may have to be taken continuously in evenly spaced doses only as directed; if a dose is missed, take one when remembered up to 4 hr; do not double doses
• Advise patient to rise slowly from sitting or lying down to prevent orthostatic hypotension
• Caution patient not to use alcohol or OTC medication unless approved by prescriber
• Caution patient to avoid hazardous activities until stabilized on medication; dizziness may occur

Evaluation
Positive therapeutic outcome
• Absence of reinfarction, ischemic attacks

TREATMENT OF OVERDOSE:
Administer **IV** phenylephrine

disopyramide (Rx)
(dye-soe-peer′a-mide)
Norpace, Norpace CR, Rhythmodan ✽
Func. class.: Antidysrhythmic (class IA)
Chem. class.: Nonnitrate
Pregnancy category C

Do not confuse:
Disopyramide/desipramine

ACTION: Decreases myocardial conduction, velocity, excitability, and contraction by inhibiting the influx of sodium by fast channels in myocardial cell membrane with increased recovery after repolarization

Therapeutic outcome: Suppression of supraventricular dysrhythmias

USES: PVCs, ventricular tachycardia, supraventricular tachycardia

Unlabeled uses: Atrial flutter, fibrillation

CONTRAINDICATIONS:
Hypersensitivity, 2nd- or 3rd-degree heart block, cardiogenic shock, CHF (uncompensated), sick sinus syndrome

> **BLACK BOX WARNING:** QT prolongation

Precautions: Pregnancy **C**, breastfeeding, children, geriatric patients, diabetes mellitus, renal/hepatic disease, myasthenia gravis, closed-angle glaucoma, cardiomyopathy, conduction abnormalities, potassium imbalance

> **BLACK BOX WARNING:** Arrhythmias, MI, torsades de pointes

DOSAGE AND ROUTES

Adult >18 yr and >50 kg: PO 150-200 mg q6hr; EXT REL cap 300-400 mg q12hr

Adult >18 yr and <50 kg: PO 100 mg q6hr; EXT REL cap 200 mg q12hr

Adolescent 12-18 yr: PO 6-15 mg/kg/day, in divided doses q6hr

Child 5-12 yr: PO 10-15 mg/kg/day in divided doses q6hr

Child 1-4 yr: PO 10-20 mg/kg/day in divided doses q6hr

Child <1 yr: PO 10-30 mg/kg/day, in divided doses q6hr

Renal dose

Adult: PO CCr >40 ml/min 100 mg q6hr or 200 mg q12hr (EXT REL); CCr 30-40 ml/min dose q8hr; CCr 15-30 ml/min dose q12hr; CCr <15 ml/min dose q24hr

Hepatic dose

Adult: PO 400 mg/day in divided doses (q6hr for regular release, q12hr for EXT REL)

Available forms: Caps 100, 150 mg; cont rel caps 100, 150 mg; sus rel tabs 150 mg ✤

Implementation

- Do not break, crush, or chew sus rel tabs
- Give 1 hr before or 2 hr after meals
- If changing from regular release to sus rel cap, give sus rel 6 hr after last dose of regular release

ADVERSE EFFECTS

CNS: *Headache, dizziness,* psychosis, fatigue, depression, paresthesias, insomnia

CV: *Hypotension, bradycardia,* angina, PVCs, tachycardia, increases in QRS and QT segments, **cardiac arrest,** edema, weight gain, AV block, CHF, syncope, chest pain, **torsades de pointes**

EENT: *Blurred vision, dry nose, throat, eyes,* closed-angle glaucoma

GI: *Dry mouth, constipation,* nausea, anorexia, flatulence, diarrhea, vomiting

GU: *Retention, hesitancy,* impotence

HEMA: **Thrombocytopenia, agranulocytosis,** anemia (rare), decreased Hgb, Hct

INTEG: Rash, pruritus, urticaria

META: Hypoglycemia, hypokalemia

MS: Weakness, pain in extremities

Pharmacokinetics

Absorption	Well absorbed
Distribution	Widely distributed
Metabolism	Liver
Excretion	Kidneys
Half-life	4-10 hr

Pharmacodynamics

	PO	PO–Sus Rel
Onset	$^{1}/_{2}$-$3^{1}/_{2}$ hr	Unknown
Peak	2 hr	Unknown
Duration	$1^{1}/_{2}$-8 hr	12 hr

INTERACTIONS

Individual drugs

Atenolol, erythromycin, lidocaine, procainamide, propranolol, quinidine: increased effects of disopyramide

PHENobarbital, phenytoin, rifampin: decreased effects of disopyramide

Drug classifications

Anticholinergics: increased side effects, urinary retention

Antidysrhythmics: increased disopyramide effect

Drug/lab test

Increased: liver enzymes, lipids, BUN, creatinine

Increased: QT prolongation: Class IA/IC/III antidysrhythmics, arsenic trioxide, chloroquine, droperidol, grepafloxacin, halofantrine, levomethadyl, methadone, pentamidine, some phenothiazines, pimozide, probucol, sparfloxacin, ziprasidone

Decreased: Hgb/Hct, blood glucose

NURSING CONSIDERATIONS

Assessment

- **CHF:** Assess respiratory status: auscultate lung fields for bibasilar crackles
- Monitor I&O ratio and electrolytes: potassium, sodium, chloride; watch for decreasing urinary output, possible retention
- Monitor liver function tests: AST, ALT, bilirubin, alkaline phosphatase

> **BLACK BOX WARNING: QT prolongation:** monitor ECG to determine product effectiveness, measure PR, QRS, QT intervals; check for PVCs, other dysrhythmias; monitor B/P for hypotension; check for prolonged widening QT intervals, QRS complex; if QT or QRS increase by 50% or more, withhold next dose, notify prescriber

- Monitor for dehydration or hypovolemia
- Monitor for CNS symptoms: psychosis, numbness, depression; if these occur, product should be discontinued

Nursing diagnoses

- Cardiac output, decreased (uses)
- Knowledge, deficient (teaching)

Patient/family education

• Teach patient to report side effects immediately to prescriber; to take exactly as prescribed; if dose is missed take when remembered if within 3-4 hr of next dose; do not double doses, may take with food or milk to prevent gastric upset

• Teach patient to avoid alcohol or severe hypotension may occur; to avoid OTC products or serious drug interactions may occur

• Advise patient to avoid hazardous activities if dizziness or blurred vision occurs, use a medical alert bracelet

• Teach patient to complete follow-up appointment with prescriber including pulmonary function tests, chest x-ray

• Instruct patient that dry mouth may be relieved by frequent sips of water, hard candy, sugarless gum

• Caution patient to make position changes from lying to standing slowly to prevent orthostatic hypotension

Evaluation
Positive therapeutic outcome
• Decreased PVCs, ventricular tachycardia

TREATMENT OF OVERDOSE:
Administer O_2, artificial ventilation, ECG; administer DOPamine for circulatory depression; administer diazepam or thiopental for seizures, isoproterenol

---

divalproex sodium
See valproate

DOBUTamine (Rx)
(doe-byoo′ta-meen)
DOBUTamine
Func. class.: Adrenergic direct-acting β_1-agonist, inotropic agent, cardiac stimulant
Chem. class.: Catecholamine
Pregnancy category B

Do not confuse:
DOBUTamine/DOPamine

ACTION: Causes increased contractility, increased cardiac output without marked increase in heart rate by acting on β_1-receptors in heart; minor α/β_2 effects

Therapeutic outcome: Cardiac output increased with decreased fatigue and dyspnea

USES: Cardiac decompensation due to organic heart disease or cardiac surgery

Unlabeled uses: Cardiogenic shock in children, congenital heart disease in children undergoing cardiac catherization

CONTRAINDICATIONS:
Hypersensitivity, idiopathic hypertrophic subaortic stenosis

Precautions: Pregnancy **B**, breastfeeding, children, hypertension, CAD, MI, hypovolemia, dysrhythmias

DOSAGE AND ROUTES
Adult and child: IV INF 2-20 mcg/kg/min; may increase to 40 mcg/kg/min if needed

Available forms: Inj 12.5 mg/ml, 250 mg/20 ml

Implementation
IV route
• Reconstitute 250 mg/10 ml of D_5W or sterile water for inj; may add another 10 ml to dissolve completely if needed, then dilute in 50 ml or more of D_5W, 0.9% NaCl, 0.45% NaCl, D_5/0.45% NaCl, D_5/0.9% NaCl, D_5/LR, LR; titrate to patient response; use infusion pump for correct dose
• Use a CVP catheter or large peripheral vein, use infusion pump, titrate to patient response
• Change **IV** site q48hr

Syringe compatibilities: Heparin, ranitidine

Syringe incompatibility: Doxapram

Y-site compatibilities: Alfentanil, alprostadil, amifostine, amikacin, aminocaproic acid, amiodarone, anidulafungin, argatroban, ascorbic acid injection, atenolol, atracurium, atropine, aztreonam, benztropine, bleomycin, bumetanide, buprenorphine, butorphanol, calcium chloride/gluconate, CARBOplatin, caspofungin, chlorproMAZINE, cimetidine, ciprofloxacin, cisatracurium, CISplatin, cladribine, clarithromycin, cloNIDine, codeine, cyanocobalamin, cyclophosphamide, cycloSPORINE, cytarabine, DACTINomycin, DAPTOmycin, dexmedetomidine, digoxin, diltiazem, diphenhydrAMINE, docetaxel, DOPamine, doripenem, doxacurium, DOXOrubicin, DOXOrubicin liposomal, doxycycline, enalaprilat, ePHEDrine, EPINEPHrine, epirubicin, epoetin alfa, eptifibatide, erythromycin, esmolol, etoposide, famotidine, fenoldopam, fentaNYL, fluconazole, fludarabine, gatifloxacin, gemcitabine, gentamicin, glycopyrrolate, granisetron, HYDROmorphone, hydrOXYzine, IDArubicin, ifosfamide, irinotecan, isoproterenol, labetalol, levofloxacin, lidocaine, linezolid, LORazepam, LR, magnesium sulfate, mannitol, mechloretamine, meperidine, meropenem, metaraminol, methoxamine, methyldopate, methylPREDNISolone, metoclopramide, metoprolol, metroNIDAZOLE, miconazole, milrinone, minocycline, mitoxantrone, morphine, multiple vitamins injection, mycophenolate mofetil, nafcillin, nalbuphine, naloxone, netilmicin, niCARdipine, nitroglycerin, norepinephrine, octreotide, ondansetron, oxaliplatin, oxytocin, paclitaxel, palonosetron, pamidronate, pancuronium, papaverine, pentamidine, pentazocine, phenylephrine, polymyxin B, potassium chloride, procainamide, prochlorperazine, promethazine, propofol, propranolol, protamine, pyridoxine, quiNIDine, ranitidine, remifentanil, Ringer's, ritodrine, riTUXimab, rocuronium, sodium acetate, succinylcholine, SUFentanil, tacrolimus, temocillin, teniposide, theophylline, thiamine, thiotepa, tigecycline, tirofiban, TNA, tobramycin, tolazoline, TPN, trastuzumab, trimetaphan, urokinase, vancomycin, vasopressin, vecuronium, verapamil, vinCRIStine, vinorelbine, voriconazole, zidovudine, zoledronic acid

Y-site incompatibilities: Acyclovir, alteplase, aminophylline, foscarnet, phytonadione

ADVERSE EFFECTS
CNS: *Anxiety,* headache, dizziness, fatigue
CV: Palpitations, tachycardia, hypo/hypertension, PVCs, angina
ENDO: Hypokalemia
GI: Heartburn, nausea, vomiting
MS: Muscle cramps (leg)
RESP: Dyspnea

Pharmacokinetics

Absorption	Complete
Distribution	Unknown
Metabolism	Liver
Excretion	Kidneys
Half-life	2 min

Pharmacodynamics

Onset	1-5 min
Peak	10 min
Duration	<10 min

INTERACTIONS
Individual drugs
Atomoxetine: increased pressor effect, dysrhythmias
Bretylium, oxytocin: increased dysrhythmias

Guanethidine: increased severe hypertension
Oxytocin: increased pressor effects

Drug classifications
Anesthetics (general): increased dysrhythmias
Antidepressants (tricyclic), COMT inhibitors, MAOIs, oxytocics: increased pressor response, dysrhythmias
β-Blockers: decreased action of DOBUTamine

NURSING CONSIDERATIONS
Assessment
• **Assess for hypovolemia;** if present, correct before beginning treatment with DOBUTamine; avoid use in patients with atrial fibrillation before digitalization
• **Monitor ECG for dysrhythmias, ischemia** during treatment; some patients may not need continuous ECG monitoring; also monitor PCWP, CVP, CO_2, urinary output; notify prescriber if <30 ml/hr
• **Assess for heart failure:** bibasilar crackles, S_3 gallop, dyspnea, neck vein distention in patients with cardiomyopathy or CHF
• Assess for oxygenation or perfusion deficit: decreased B/P, chest pain, dizziness, loss of consciousness
• Monitor B/P and pulse q5min during infusion; if B/P drops 30 mm Hg, stop infusion and call prescriber
• Monitor ALT, AST, bilirubin daily
• **Monitor for sulfite sensitivity,** which may be life threatening

Nursing diagnoses
• Cardiac output, decreased (uses)
• Knowledge, deficient (teaching)

Patient/family education
• Teach patient reason for medication and expected results, reason for all monitoring and procedures
• Advise patient to report dyspnea, headache, **IV** site discomfort, chest pain, numbness of extremities

Evaluation
Positive therapeutic outcome
• Increased cardiac output
• Decreased PCWP, adequate CVP
• Decreased dyspnea, fatigue, edema, ECG
• Increased urine output

TREATMENT OF OVERDOSE:
Discontinue product, support circulation

docetaxel (Rx)

(doe-se-tax'el)
Taxotere
Func. class.: Antineoplastic, miscellaneous
Pregnancy category D

Do not confuse:
Taxotere/Taxol

ACTION: Inhibits the reorganization of the microtubule network needed for interphase and mitotic cellular functions; also causes abnormal bundles of microtubules during cell cycle and multiple esters of microtubules during mitosis

Therapeutic outcome: Prevention of rapidly growing malignant cells

USES: Locally advanced or metastatic breast cancer, non–small cell lung cancer, androgen-independent metastatic prostate cancer, postsurgery operable node-positive breast cancer, induction treatment of locally advanced squamous cell cancer of the head/neck, adjuvant treatment of breast cancer with carboplatin and trastuzumab, gastric adenocarcinoma

CONTRAINDICATIONS:

Pregnancy **D**, breastfeeding, hypersensitivity to this product, severe hepatic disease, bilirubin exceeding upper normal limit, or severely elevated ALT, AST, alkaline phosphatase

> **BLACK BOX WARNING:** Hypersensitivity to other products with polysorbate 80, neutropenia (neutrophils <1500/mm³)

Precautions: Children, CV disease, pulmonary disorders, bone marrow depression, herpes zoster, pleural effusion

> **BLACK BOX WARNING:** Edema, hepatic disease, lung cancer, taxane hypersensitivity

DOSAGE AND ROUTES
• Other regimens are used

Locally advanced or metastatic breast cancer after failure of other chemotherapy
Adult: IV 60-100 mg/m² given over 1 hr q3wk; if neutrophil count is <500/mm³ for >1 wk, reduce dose by 25%

Operable node-positive breast cancer
Adult: IV (TAC regimen) 75 mg/m² 1 hr after DOXOrubicin 50 mg/m² and cyclophosphamide 500 mg/m² q3wk for 6 cycles

Adjuvant treatment of operable stage I-III invasive breast cancer in combination with cyclophosphamide
Adult: IV (TAC) regimen docetaxel 75 mg/m² with cyclophosphamide 600 mg/m² q21day × 4 cycles

Locally advanced or metastatic non–small cell lung cancer after failure of CISplatin chemotherapy
Adult: IV 75 mg/m² over 1 hr q3wk; if neutrophil count is <500/mm³ for >1 wk, reduce dose to 55 mg/m²; if patient develops grade 3 peripheral neuropathy, stop product

Unresectable, locally advanced or metastatic non–small cell lung cancer previously treated with chemotherapy
Adult: IV 75 mg/m² over 1 hr, then CISplatin 75 mg/m² IV given over 30-60 min q3wk; reduce dose to 65 mg/m² in those with hematologic or nonhematologic toxicities

Androgen-independent metastatic prostate cancer
Adult: IV 75 mg/m² given over 1 hr q3wk, with 5 mg predniSONE PO bid continuously; give dexamethasone 8 mg PO at 12 hr, 3 hr, and 1 hr prior to docetaxel; if neutrophil count is <500 cells/mm³ for more than 1 wk or other toxicities occur, reduce dose to 60 mg/m²

Adjuvant postsurgery treatment of operable node-positive breast cancer
Adult: IV 75 mg/m² over 1 hr, given 1 hr after DOXOrubicin 50 mg/m², cyclophosphamide 500 mg/m² q3wk × 6 cycles

Squamous cell cancer of head/neck
Adult: IV 75 mg/m² over 1 hr, then CISplatin 75 mg/m² over 1 hr on day 1, then 5-FU 750 mg/m²/day CONT INF × 5 days, repeat cycle q3wk

Gastric adenocarcinoma
Adult: IV 75 mg/m² q3wk, given with CISplatin, fluorouracil

Available forms: Inj 20 mg/0.5 ml, 20 mg/ml, 80 mg/2 ml, 80 mg/4 ml

Implementation
- Give top or systemic analgesics for pain to lessen effects of stomatitis
- Give liquid diet: carbonated beverages; gelatin may be added if patient is not nauseated or vomiting

Intermittent IV infusion route
- Use gloves and cytotoxic handling precautions
- Allow vials to warm to room temperature, withdraw all diluent and inject in vial of docetaxel, rotate gently to mix, allow to stand to decrease foaming, then withdraw the required amount (10 mg/ml) and inject in 250 ml of 0.9% NaCl or D₅W, mix gently, give over 1 hr

Y-site compatibilities: Acyclovir, alfentanil, allopurinol, amifostine, amikacin, aminocaproic acid, aminophylline, amiodarone, amphotericin B lipid complex, ampicillin, ampicillin-sulbactam, anidulafungin, atenolol, atracurium, azithromycin, aztreonam, bivalirudin, bleomycin, bumetanide, buprenorphine, busulfan, butorphanol, calcium chloride/gluconate, CARBOplatin, carmustine, caspofungin, ceFAZolin, cefepime, cefonicid, cefoperazone, cefotaxime, cefotetan, cefoxitin, ceftazidime, ceftizoxime, cefTRIAXone, cefuroxime, cephapirin, chloramphenicol, chlorproMAZINE, cimetidine, ciprofloxacin, cisatracurium, CISplatin, clindamycin, codeine, cyclophosphamide, cycloSPORINE, cytarabine, dacarbazine, DACTINomycin, DAPTOmycin, dexamethasone, dexmedetomidine, dexrazoxane, diazepam, digoxin, diltiazem, diphenhydrAMINE, DOBUTamine, DOPamine, doripenem, doxacurium, DOXOrubicin, doxycycline, droperidol, enalaprilat, ePHEDrine, EPINEPHrine, epirubicin, ertapenem, erythromycin, esmolol, etoposide, famotidine, fenoldopam, fentaNYL, fluconazole, fludarabine, fluorouracil, foscarnet, fosphenytoin, furosemide, ganciclovir, gatifloxacin, gemcitabine, gentamicin, glycopyrrolate, granisetron, haloperidol, heparin, hydrALAZINE, hydrocortisone, HYDROmorphone, hydrOXYzine, ifosfamide, imipenem-cilastatin, inamrinone, insulin (regular), irinotecan, isoproterenol, ketorolac, labetalol, leucovorin, levofloxacin, levorphanol, lidocaine, linezolid, LORazepam, LR, magnesium sulfate, mannitol, meperidine, meropenem, mesna, methotrexate, methyldopate, metoclopramide, metoprolol, metroNIDAZOLE, midazolam, milrinone, minocycline, mitoxantrone, mivacurium, morphine, nafcillin, naloxone, nesiritide, netilmicin, niCARdipine, nitroglycerin, nitroprusside, norepinephrine, octreotide, ofloxacin, ondansetron, oxaliplatin, palonosetron, pamidronate, pancuronium, pantoprazole, pemetrexed, pentamidine, pentazocine, PENTobarbital, PHENobarbital, phenylephrine, piperacillin, piperacillin-tazobactam, polymyxin B, potassium chloride/phosphates, procainamide, prochlorperazine, promethazine, propranolol, quiNIDine, quinupristin-dalfopristin, ranitidine, remifentanil, riTUXimab, rocuronium, sodium acetate/bicarbonate/phosphates, succinylcholine, SUFentanil, sulfamethoxazole-trimethoprim, tacrolimus, teniposide, theophylline, thiopental, thiotepa, ticarcillin, ticarcillin-clavulanate, tigecycline, tirofiban, tobramycin, tolazoline, trastuzumab, trimethobenzamide, vancomycin, vasopressin, vecuronium, verapamil, vinCRIStine, vinorelbine, voriconazole, zidovudine, zoledronic acid

ADVERSE EFFECTS
CNS: Seizures
CV: *Hypotension,* fluid retention, peripheral edema, flushing, MI, sinus tachycardia
GI: *Nausea, vomiting, diarrhea,* hepatotoxicity, stomatitis, colitis
HEMA: Neutropenia, leukopenia, thrombocytopenia, anemia, bleeding, infections, myelosuppression
INTEG: *Alopecia,* nail pain, rash, skin eruptions
MISC: Amenorrhea, fever of unknown origin, secondary malignancy, Stevens-Johnson syndrome
MS: *Arthralgia, myalgia,* back pain
NEURO: *Peripheral neuropathy*
RESP: Dyspnea, pulmonary edema, fibrosis, embolism
SYST: Hypersensitivity reactions, AML, death

Pharmacokinetics
Absorption	Completely absorbed
Distribution	Unknown
Metabolism	Liver, extensively
Excretion	Fecal
Half-life	11.1 hr

Pharmacodynamics
Onset	Rapid
Peak	Unknown
Duration	Unknown

INTERACTIONS
Individual drugs
CycloSPORINE, erythromycin, ketoconazole, troleadomycin: altered metabolism of docetaxel

Drug classifications

Antineoplastics, radiation: increased myelosuppression

Live virus vaccines: decreased immune response

NURSING CONSIDERATIONS

Assessment

• **Assess CNS changes:** confusion, paresthesias, dysethenia, pain, weakness: if severe, product should be discontinued

• Check buccal cavity q8hr for dryness, sores or ulceration, white patches, oral pain, bleeding, dysphagia; obtain prescription for viscous lidocaine (Xylocaine) to use in mouth

• **Assess symptoms indicating severe allergic reaction, anaphylaxis:** rash, pruritus, urticaria, purpuric skin lesions, itching, flushing

> **BLACK BOX WARNING:** Monitor CBC, differential, platelet count weekly; withhold product if WBC is <1500/mm³ or platelet count is <100,000/mm³, notify prescriber of results

• Monitor renal function tests: BUN, creatinine, serum uric acid, urine CCr before, during therapy; check I&O ratio; report fall in urine output to <30 ml/hr

• Monitor temp q4hr (may indicate beginning of infection)

> **BLACK BOX WARNING: Hepatic disease:** Monitor liver function tests before, during therapy (bilirubin, AST, ALT, LDH) as needed or monthly; check for jaundice of skin and sclera, dark urine, clay-colored stools, itchy skin, abdominal pain, fever, diarrhea

> **BLACK BOX WARNING: Assess for bone marrow depression/bleeding:** hematuria, stool guaiac, bruising or petechiae, mucosa or orifices q8hr; check for inflammation of mucosa, breaks in skin

• Assess effects of alopecia on body image; discuss feelings about body changes

Nursing diagnoses

• Body image, disturbed (adverse reactions)
• Infection, risk for (adverse reactions)
• Injury, risk for (adverse reactions)
• Knowledge, deficient (teaching)

Patient/family education

• Inform patient that nonhormonal contraceptive measures are recommended during therapy and >4 mo after; teratogenic effects are possible, pregnancy **D**

• Teach patient to avoid use of products containing aspirin or ibuprofen, razors, commercial mouthwash, since bleeding may occur; to report symptoms of bleeding (hematuria, tarry stools)

• Instruct patient to report signs of **anemia** (fatigue, headache, irritability, faintness, shortness of breath) and CNS reactions (confusion, psychosis, nightmares, seizures, severe headaches)

• Instruct patient to report signs of **infection:** fever, sore throat, flulike symptoms

• Inform patient that hair may be lost during treatment; a wig or hairpiece may make patient feel better; new hair may be different in color and texture

• Inform patient that receiving vaccinations during therapy may cause serious reactions

• Instruct patient to rinse mouth tid-qid with water, club soda; brush teeth bid-qid with soft brush or cotton-tipped applicators for stomatitis; use unwaxed dental floss

Evaluation
Positive therapeutic outcome

• Prevention of rapid division of malignant cells

---

docosanol topical
See Appendix B

---

docusate calcium (OTC)
(dok′yoo-sate cal′see-um)
**Kao-Tin, ratio-Docusate Calcium ✤,
Stool Softener DC, Sur-Q-Lax,
Walgreen's Stool Softener**
docusate sodium (OTC)
**Apo-Docusate ✤, Colace, Correctol,
Diocto, Doc-Q-Lace, Docu DOK,
Doculace, Enemeez, Equaline Stool
Softener, Good Sense Stool Softener,
Leader Stool Softener, Phillip's Stool
Softener, ratio-Docusate Sodium ✤,
Regulex ✤, Select Brand Docusate
Sodium, Selex ✤, Silace, Soflax ✤,
Top Care Stool Softener, Walgreen's
Stool Softener**
Func. class.: Laxative, emollient
Chem. class.: Anionic surfactant
Pregnancy category C

ACTION: Increases water, fat penetration in intestine; allows for easier passage of stool

Therapeutic outcome: Passage of softened stool, absence of constipation

---

Adverse effects: *italics* = common; **bold** = life-threatening

USES: Prevent hard, dry stools, prevent constipation, soften fecal impaction (rectal route)

CONTRAINDICATIONS:
Hypersensitivity, obstruction, fecal impaction, nausea/vomiting

Precautions: Pregnancy **C**, breastfeeding

DOSAGE AND ROUTES
Adult: PO 50-300 mg/day (docusate sodium) or 240 mg (docusate calcium) prn enema 4 ml (docusate sodium)
Child >12 yr: Enema 2 ml (docusate sodium)
Child 6-12 yr: PO 40-150 mg/day (docusate sodium) in divided doses
Child 3-6 yr: PO 20-60 mg/day (docusate sodium) in divided doses
Child <3 yr: PO 10-40 mg/day (docusate sodium) in divided doses

Available forms: Docusate calcium: caps 240 mg; **docusate sodium:** caps 50, 100, 250 mg; tabs 100 mg; syr 20 mg/5 ml, 50 mg/15 ml, 100 mg/30 ml, 150 mg/15 ml; oral sol 10, 50 mg/ml; enema 283 mg/3.9 g cap

Implementation
PO route
• Dilute oral sol in juice or other fluid to disguise taste
• Give tabs or caps with 8 oz of liquid; give on empty stomach for increased absorption, results

ADVERSE EFFECTS
EENT: Bitter taste, throat irritation
GI: Nausea, anorexia, cramps, diarrhea
INTEG: Rash

Pharmacokinetics

Absorption	Minimal (PO)
Distribution	Unknown
Metabolism	Not metabolized
Excretion	Bile
Half-life	Unknown

Pharmacodynamics

	PO	RECT
Onset	24-72 hr	4-6 hr
Peak	Unknown	Unknown
Duration	Unknown	Unknown

INTERACTIONS
Individual drugs
Mineral oil: toxicity

Drug/herb
Flax, senna: increased laxative action

NURSING CONSIDERATIONS
Assessment
• Assess cramping, rectal bleeding, nausea, vomiting; if these symptoms occur, product should be discontinued; identify cause of constipation; identify fluids, bulk, or exercise is missing from lifestyle

Nursing diagnoses
• Constipation (uses)
• Diarrhea (side effects)
• Knowledge, deficient (teaching)
• Noncompliance (teaching)

Patient/family education
• Discuss with patient that adequate fluid consumption is as necessary as bulk, exercise for adequate bowel function
• Teach patient that normal bowel movements do not always occur daily
• Advise patient not to use in presence of abdominal pain, nausea, vomiting; tell patient to notify prescriber if unrelieved constipation or if symptoms of electrolyte imbalance occur: muscle cramps, pain, weakness, dizziness, excessive thirst
• Advise patient that product may take up to 3 days to soften stools
• Instruct patient to take oral preparation with a full glass of water and increase fluid intake unless on fluid restrictions
• Caution patients with heart disease to avoid using the Valsalva maneuver to expedite evacuation

Evaluation
Positive therapeutic outcome
• Decreased constipation within 3 days

dofetilide
(doff-ee-till'-lide)
Tikosyn
Func. class.: Antidysrhythmic (Class III)
Pregnancy category C

ACTION: Blocks cardiac ion channel carrying the rapid component of delayed potassium current, no effect on sodium channels

Therapeutic outcome: Absence of atrial fibrillation

USES: Atrial fibrillation, flutter, maintenance of normal sinus rhythm

CONTRAINDICATIONS:
Hypersensitivity, digoxin toxicity, aortic stenosis, pulmonary hypertension, children, severe renal disease

> **BLACK BOX WARNING:** QT prolongation, torsades de pointes, renal failure

Precautions: Pregnancy **C**, breastfeeding, AV block, bradycardia, electrolyte imbalance

> **BLACK BOX WARNING:** Renal disease, arrhythmias

DOSAGE AND ROUTES
Adult: PO 125-500 mcg bid depending on CCr; initial dose is based on renal function and QTc; may be adjusted q2-3hr to get appropriate increase in QTc
Renal dose: PO initial dose for CCr >60 mg/ml 500 mcg bid; CCr 40-60 mg/min 250 mcg bid; CCr 20-39 mg/min 125 mcg bid; CCr <20 mg/min do not use

Available forms: Caps 125, 250, 500 mcg

Implementation
• Give for 3 days with patient hospitalized
• Give dofetilide after withholding class I or III antidysrhythmic for 3 half-lives of dofetilide before starting dofetilide

ADVERSE EFFECTS
CNS: *Syncope, dizziness,* headache
CV: *Hypotension, postural hypotension, bradycardia,* angina, PVCs, substernal pressure, precipitation of angina, transient hypertension, **QT prolongation, torsades de pointes, ventricular dysrhythmias**
GI: *Nausea, vomiting,* severe diarrhea, anorexia
RESP: Dyspnea, respiratory infections

Pharmacokinetics
Absorption	>90%
Distribution	Steady state 2-3 days
Metabolism	Not metabolized
Excretion	Kidneys 80%
Half-life	10 hr

Pharmacodynamics
Unknown

INTERACTIONS
Arsenic trioxide, chloroquine, clarithromycin, droperidol, erythromycin, halofantrine, haloperidol, levomethadyl, methadone, pentamidine, ziprasidone: increased QT prolongation, torsades de pointes

Individual drugs
Amiloride, entecavir, lamivudine, memantine, metFORMIN, procainamide, triamterene, trospium: increased toxicity
Cimetidine, hydrochlorothiazide, ketoconazole, megestrol, metformin, prochlorperazine, triamterene, trimethoprim/sulfamethoxazole, verapamil: do not use together

Drug classifications
Antiretroviral protease inhibitors: increased dofetilide levels
Class IA/III antidysrhythmics, some phenothiazines: increased QT prolongation, torsades de pointes
Diuretics, potassium depletion: increased hypokalemia

Drug/food
• Do not use with grapefruit juice

NURSING CONSIDERATIONS
Assessment

> **BLACK BOX WARNING:** Monitor ECG continuously for a minimum of 3 days or 12 hr after conversion to determine product effectiveness; measure PR, QRS, QT intervals; check for PVCs, other dysrhythmias; renal function, QTc baseline, reassess QTc interval 2-3 hr after each dose; if QTc is >440 msec or 500 msec if ventricular conduction disturbance, discontinue until QTc is at starting level; this product is available only to facilities that have been educated in its administration; patient must be hospitalized

Nursing diagnoses
• Cardiac output, decreased (uses)
• Gas exchange, impaired (adverse reactions)
• Knowledge, deficient (teaching)

Patient/family education
• Instruct patient to notify prescriber if fast heartbeats with fainting or dizziness occur
• Instruct patient to notify all prescribers of all medications and supplements taken
• Teach patient that if a dose is missed, do not double, take next dose at usual time

Evaluation
Positive therapeutic outcome
• Increased control in atrial fibrillation

dolasetron (Rx)

(do-la´se-tron)

Anzemet

Func. class.: Antiemetic

Chem. class.: 5-HT receptor antagonist

Pregnancy category B

ACTION: Prevents nausea, vomiting by blocking serotonin peripherally, centrally, and in the small intestine

Therapeutic outcome: Control of nausea, vomiting

USES: Prevention of nausea, vomiting associated with cancer chemotherapy and prevention of postoperative nausea, vomiting

Unlabeled uses: Radiotherapy-induced nausea/vomiting

CONTRAINDICATIONS:

Hypersensitivity

Precautions: Pregnancy **B,** breastfeeding, children, geriatric, hypokalemia, electrolyte imbalances, granisetron, ondansetron, palonosetron hypersensitivity, QT prolongation

DOSAGE AND ROUTES

Prevention of nausea/vomiting associated with cancer chemotherapy

Adult and child 2-16 yr: IV 1.8 mg/kg as a single dose $1/2$ hr before chemotherapy, max 40 mcg/kg

Adult: PO 100 mg 1 hr before chemotherapy

Child 2-16 yr: PO 1.8 mg/kg 1 hr before chemotherapy, max 100 mg

Prevention of postoperative nausea/vomiting

Adult: IV 12.5 mg as a single dose 15 min before cessation of anesthesia; PO 100 mg 2 hr before surgery (prevention only)

Child 2-16 yr: IV 0.35 mg/kg as a single dose 15 min before cessation of anesthesia; PO 1.2 mg/kg within 2 hr before surgery (prevention only)

Available forms: Tabs 50, 100 mg; inj 20 mg/ml (12.5 mg/0.625 ml)

Implementation

PO route

• Do not mix product for oral administration in juice until immediately before administration; apple or apple-grape diluted can be kept for 2 hr at room temperature

Intermittent IV infusion route

• Administer by inj 100 mg/30 sec or less or diluted in 50 ml of compatible sol; give over 15 sec

• Store at room temperature for 24 hr after dilution

Y-site compatibilities: Anidulafungin, atenolol, azithromycin, bivalirudin, caspofungin, cyclophosphamide, cytarabine, DAPTOmycin, dexmedetomidine, doxacurium, DOXOrubicin, epirubicin, eptifibatide, ertapenem, fenoldopam, ifosfamide, irinotecan, levofloxacin, linezolid, mechlorethamine, meperidine, mycophenolate, nesiritide, octreotide, oxaliplatin, oxytocin, pamidronate, pancuronium, pemetrexed, quinupristin-dalfopristin, rocuronium, sodium acetate, tacrolimus, tigecycline, tirofiban, vecuronium, vinCRIStine, voriconazole, zoledronic acid

ADVERSE EFFECTS

CNS: *Headache,* dizziness, fatigue, drowsiness

CV: **Dysrhythmias,** ECG changes, hypo/hypertension, tachycardia, bradycardia, **QT prolongation, torsades de pointes, ventricular tachycardia/fibrillation, cardiac arrest (IV)**

GI: *Diarrhea,* constipation, increased AST, ALT, abdominal pain, anorexia

GU: Urinary retention, oliguria

MISC: Rash, **bronchospasm**

Pharmacokinetics

Absorption	Completely absorbed
Distribution	Unknown
Metabolism	Liver, extensively
Excretion	Kidneys
Half-life	Unknown

Pharmacodynamics

Unknown

INTERACTIONS

Individual drugs

Arsenic trioxide, chloroquine, clarithromycin, droperidol, erythromycin, halofantrine, haloperidol, levomethadyl, methadone, pentamidine, ziprasidone: increased QT prolongation

Cimetidine: increased dolasetron levels

Rifampin: decreased dolasetron levels

Drug classifications

Antidysrhythmics: increased dysrhythmias

Class IA/III antidysrhythmics, some phenothiazines, loop diuretics, thiazide: increased QT prolongation

---

⚠ Nurse Alert

NURSING CONSIDERATIONS

Assessment
- Assess for absence of nausea, vomiting during chemotherapy
- **Assess for hypersensitivity reaction:** rash, bronchospasm
- Assess for cardiac conduction conditions; electrolyte imbalances or dysrhythmias

Nursing diagnoses
- Knowledge, deficient (teaching)
- Noncompliance (teaching)

Patient/family education
- Instruct patient to report diarrhea, constipation, rash, or changes in respirations; may cause headache; use analgesic
- Teach patient reason for medication and expected results

Evaluation
Positive therapeutic outcome
- Absence of nausea, vomiting during cancer chemotherapy

donepezil (Rx)
(don-ep-ee′zill)
Aricept, Aricept ODT
Func. class.: Anti-Alzheimer's agent
Chem. class.: Reversible cholinesterase inhibitor
Pregnancy category C

ACTION: Elevates acetylcholine concentrations (cerebral cortex) by slowing degradation of acetylcholine released in cholinergic neurons; does not alter underlying dementia

Therapeutic outcome: Decreased symptoms of Alzheimer's disease

USES: Treatment of mild to severe dementia in Alzheimer's disease

Unlabeled uses: Subcortical vascular dementia, dementia with Lewy bodies

CONTRAINDICATIONS:
Hypersensitivity to this product or piperidine derivatives

Precautions: Pregnancy **C**, breastfeeding, children, sick sinus syndrome, history of ulcers, GI bleeding, hepatic disease, bladder obstruction, asthma, seizures, COPD, abrupt discontinuation, AV block, GI obstruction, Parkinson's disease, surgery

DOSAGE AND ROUTES
Adult: PO 5 mg/day at bedtime; may increase to 10 mg/day after 4-6 wk, may increase to 23 mg/day after 3 mo of 10 mg/day

Available forms: Tabs 5, 10, 23 mg; oral sol 1 mg/ml; orally disintegrating tabs 5, 10 mg (Aricept ODT)

Implementation
PO route
- Give between meals; may be given with meals for GI symptoms
- Administer dosage adjusted to response no more than q4-6wk, oral dosage forms are interchangeable
- Provide assistance with ambulation during beginning therapy; dizziness, ataxia may occur
- Oral sol: measure with calibrated oral syringe or other calibrated device
- Orally disintegrating tabs: allow to dissolve on tongue before swallowing

ADVERSE EFFECTS
CNS: Dizziness, insomnia, somnolence, headache, fatigue, abnormal dreams, syncope, **seizures,** drowsiness, agitation, depression, confusion, fever, hallucinations
CV: **Atrial fibrillation,** hypo/hypertension, **sinus bradycardia, AV block**
GI: *Nausea, vomiting,* anorexia, *diarrhea,* abdominal pain, weight loss, **GI bleeding**
GU: Frequency, UTI, incontinence
INTEG: Rash, flushing, diaphoresis, bruising
META: Hyperlipidemia
MS: Cramps, arthritis, arthralgia
RESP: Rhinitis, URI, cough, pharyngitis

Pharmacokinetics
Absorption	Well
Distribution	Unknown
Metabolism	Liver to metabolites
Excretion	Unknown
Half-life	10 hr (single dose)

Pharmacodynamics
Unknown

INTERACTIONS
Individual drugs
CarBAMazepine, dexamethasone, PHENobarbital, phenytoin, rifampin: decreased donepezil effect
Succinylcholine: synergistic effects

Drug classification

Anticholinergics: decreased activity

Cholinergic agonists, cholinesterase inhibitors:
synergistic effects

NSAIDs: increased gastric acid secretions

CYP2D6, CYP3A4 inducers: decreased donepezil
effects

CYP2D6, CYP3A4 inhibitors: increased donepezil
effects

Drug/herb

St. John's wort: decreased donepezil effect

NURSING CONSIDERATIONS

Assessment

- Monitor B/P, heart rate: hypo/hypertension
- Assess mental status: affect, mood, behavioral
changes, depression, complete suicide assessment
- Assess GI status: nausea, vomiting, anorexia,
diarrhea
- Assess GU status: urinary frequency, incontinence

Nursing diagnoses

- Memory, impaired (uses)

Patient/family education

- Advise patient to report side effects: twitching,
nausea, vomiting, sweating, dizziness; indicates
overdose
- Advise patient to use product exactly as
prescribed
- Advise patient to notify prescriber of nausea,
vomiting, diarrhea (dose increase or beginning
treatment), or rash
- Advise patient not to increase or abruptly
decrease dosage, serious consequences may
result
- Instruct patient that product is not a cure

Evaluation

Positive therapeutic outcome

- Decrease in confusion; improved mood

⚠ HIGH ALERT

DOPamine (Rx)

(doe′pa-meen)

Func. class.: Agonist, vasopressor, inotropic agent

Chem. class.: Catecholamine

Pregnancy category C

Do not confuse:

DOPamine/DOBUTamine

ACTION: Causes increased cardiac output;
acts on β_1- and α-receptors, causing vasoconstriction in blood vessels; when low doses are
administered, causes renal and mesenteric vasodilatation; β_1 stimulation produces inotropic
effects with increased cardiac output

Therapeutic outcome: Increased B/P,
cardiac output

USES: Shock; to increase perfusion; hypotension, cardiogenic/septic shock

CONTRAINDICATIONS:

Hypersensitivity, ventricular fibrillation, tachydysrhythmias, pheochromocytoma, hypovolemia

Precautions: Pregnancy **C**, breastfeeding,
geriatric, arterial embolism, peripheral vascular
disease, sulfite hypersensitivity, acute MI

BLACK BOX WARNING: Extravasation

DOSAGE AND ROUTES

Shock

Adult: **IV** INF 2-5 mcg/kg/min, titrate upward
5-10 mcg/kg/min, max 50 mcg/kg/min; titrate to
patient's response

Child: **IV** 1-5 mcg/kg/min initially; usual dosage range 2-20 mcg/kg/min

COPD

Adult: **IV** 4 mcg/kg/min

CHF

Adult: **IV** 3-10 mcg/kg/min

Available forms: Inj 40, 80, 160 mg/ml;
conc for **IV** inf 0.8, 1.6, 3.2 mg/ml in 250, 500
ml D_5W

Implementation

Continuous infusion route

- Dilute 200-400 mg/250-500 ml of D_5W, 0.9%
NaCl, D_5/LR, $D_5/0.45\%$ NaCl, $D_5/0.9\%$ NaCl, LR;
do not use discolored sol; sol is stable for 24

---

hr; give 0.5-5 mcg/kg/min; may increase by 1-4 mcg/kg/min q15-30min until desired patient response; use infusion pump

Y-site compatibilities: Alfentanil, alprostadil, amifostine, amikacin, aminocaproic acid, aminophylline, amiodarone, anidulafungin, argatroban, ascorbic acid injection, atenolol, atracurium, atropine, aztreonam, benztropine, bivalirudin, bleomycin, bumetanide, buprenorphine, butorphanol, calcium chloride/gluconate, CARBOplatin, caspofungin, cefamandole, cefmetazole, cefonicid, cefotaxime, cefotetan, cefoxitin, cefpirome, ceftazidime, ceftizoxime, cefTRIAXone, cefuroxime, chlorproMAZINE, cimetidine, ciprofloxacin, cisatracurium, CISplatin, cladribine, clarithromycin, clindamycin, cloNIDine, codeine, cyanocobalamin, cyclophosphamide, cycloSPORINE, cytarabine, DACTINomycin, DAPTOmycin, dexamethasone, dexmedetomidine, digoxin, diltiazem, diphenhydrAMINE, DOBUTamine, docetaxel, doripenem, doxacurium, DOXOrubicin, DOXOrubicin liposomal, doxycycline, droperidol, enalaprilat, ePHEDrine, EPINEPHrine, epirubicin, epoetin alfa, eptifibatide, ertapenem, erythromycin, esmolol, etoposide, famotidine, fenoldopam, fentaNYL, fluconazole, fludarabine, fluorouracil, folic acid, foscarnet, gatifloxacin, gemcitabine, gemtuzumab, gentamicin, glycopyrrolate, granisetron, heparin, hydrocortisone, HYDROmorphone, hydrOXYzine, IDArubicin, ifosfamide, imipenem-cilastatin, irinotecan, isoproterenol, ketorolac, labetalol, levofloxacin, lidocaine, linezolid, LORazepam, LR, magnesium sulfate, mannitol, mechlorethamine, meperidine, metaraminol, methicillin, methoxamine, methyldopate, methylPREDNISolone, metoclopramide, metoprolol, metroNIDAZOLE, mezlocillin, micafungin, miconazole, midazolam, milrinone, minocycline, mitoxantrone, morphine, moxalactam, multiple vitamins injection, mycophenolate, nafcillin, nalbuphine, naloxone, netilmicin, niCARdipine, nitroglycerin, nitroprusside, norepinephrine, octreotide, ondansetron, oxacillin, oxaliplatin, oxytocin, paclitaxel, palonosetron, pamidronate, pancuronium, pantoprazole, papaverine, pemetrexed, penicillin G potassium/sodium, pentamidine, pentazocine, PENTobarbital, PHENobarbital, phenylephrine, phytonadione, piperacillin, piperacillin-tazobactam, polymyxin B, potassium chloride, procainamide, prochlorperazine, promethazine, propofol, propranolol, protamine, pyridoxine, quiNIDine, ranitidine, remifentanil, Ringer's, ritodrine, riTUXimab, rocuronium, sargramostim, sodium acetate, succinylcholine, SUFentanil, tacrolimus,

temocillin, teniposide, theophylline, thiamine, thiotepa, ticarcillin, ticarcillin-clavulanate, tigecycline, tirofiban, TNA, tobramycin, tolazoline, TPN, trastuzumab, trimetaphan, urokinase, vancomycin, vasopressin, vecuronium, verapamil, vinCRIStine, vinorelbine, vitamin B complex/C, voriconazole, warfarin, zidovudine, zoledronic acid

ADVERSE EFFECTS

CNS: *Headache,* anxiety
CV: *Palpitations,* **tachycardia,** *hypertension,* **ectopic beats,** *angina,* **wide QRS complex,** peripheral vasoconstriction, hypotension
GI: *Nausea, vomiting, diarrhea*
INTEG: Necrosis, tissue sloughing with extravasation, **gangrene**
RESP: Dyspnea

Pharmacokinetics

Absorption	Complete
Distribution	Widely
Metabolism	Liver
Excretion	Kidney, plasma
Half-life	2 min

Pharmacodynamics

Onset	2-5 min
Peak	Unknown
Duration	<10 min

INTERACTIONS

Individual drugs
Phenytoin: bradycardia, hypotension

Drug classifications
α-Adrenergic blockers, β-adrenergic blockers: decreased action of DOPamine
Anesthetics (general): increased dysrhythmias
Antidepressants (tricyclic): increased pressor response
Ergots: severe hypertension
MAOIs: increased hypertension (severe), do not use within 2 wk; increased pressor effect; hypertensive crisis may result
Oxytocics: increased B/P

Drug/lab test
Increased: urinary catecholamine, serum glucose

NURSING CONSIDERATIONS

Assessment
• Monitor ECG for dysrhythmias, ischemia during treatment; some patients may not need continuous ECG monitoring; also monitor PCWP,

CVP, CO_2, urinary output; notify prescriber if
<30 ml/hr
• **Assess for heart failure:** bibasilar crackles,
S_3 gallop, dyspnea, neck vein distention in
patients with cardiomyopathy or CHF
• **Assess for oxygenation or perfusion
deficit:** decreased B/P, chest pain, dizziness,
loss of consciousness
• Monitor B/P and pulse q5min during inf; if
B/P drops 30 mm Hg, stop inf and call prescriber
• Check for extravasation: if this occurs, administer phentolamine mixed with 0.9% NaCl

Nursing diagnoses
• Cardiac output, decreased (uses)
• Fluid volume, excess (uses)
• Knowledge, deficient (teaching)

Patient/family education
• Teach patient reason for medication, expected
results, reason for all monitoring and procedures
• Advise patient to report all side effects

Evaluation
Positive therapeutic outcome
• Increased cardiac output

TREATMENT OF OVERDOSE:
Discontinue product, support circulation; give a
short-acting α-blocker

---

doripenem (Rx)
(dore-i-pen′em)
Doribax
Func. class.: Antiinfective, miscellaneous
Chem. class.: Carbapenem
Pregnancy category B

ACTION: Bactericidal, interferes with
cell wall replication of susceptible organisms;
osmotically unstable cell wall swells, bursts from
osmotic pressure

Therapeutic outcome: Negative C&S;
decreasing symptoms and signs of infection

USES: Serious infections caused by *Acinetobacter baumannii, Bacteroides caccae,
Bacteroides fragilis, Bacteroides thetaiotaomicron, Bacteroides uniformis, Bacteroides vulgatus, Escherichia coli, Klebsiella
pneumoniae, Peptostreptococcus micros,
Proteus mirabilis, Pseudomonas aeruginosa,
Streptococcus contellatus, Streptococcus
intermedius;* complicated UTIs, pyelonephritis,
complicated intraabdominal infections

CONTRAINDICATIONS:
Hypersensitivity to carbapenems (meropenem,
doripenem, imipenem), penicillin, β-lactam;
viral infection

Precautions: Pregnancy **B**, breastfeeding,
geriatric, renal disease, seizure disorder, pseudomembranous colitis, nebulizer or inhalation
use

DOSAGE AND ROUTES
Adult: IV 500 mg every 8 hr × 5-14 days; if
improvement occurs after 3 days, switch to an
appropriate oral product

Renal dose
Adult: IV CCr 30-50 ml/min 250 mg over 1 hr
q8hr; CCr >10 to <30 ml/min 250 mg over 1
hr q12hr; CCr ≤10 ml/min no data

Available forms: Powder for inj 500 mg

Implementation
Intermittent IV infusion route
• Give after C&S is taken
• **When giving 500-mg dose using 500 mg
vial:** constitute vial with 10 ml of sterile water
for inj or NaCl 0.9%; gently shake; (50 mg/ml);
sol must be further diluted using a 21-G needle;
withdraw susp and add to 100-ml infusion bag
of D_5W; gently shake until clear
• **When giving 250-mg dose using 500-mg
vial:** constitute vial with 10 ml of sterile water
for inj or NaCl 0.9%; gently shake; (50 mg/ml);
sol must be further diluted using a 21-G needle;
withdraw susp and add to 100-ml infusion bag
of D_5W; gently shake; remove 55 ml of solution;
discard; the remaining sol contains 250 mg
doripenem (4.5 mg/ml)
• **When giving 250-mg dose using 250-mg
vial:** constitute vial with 10 ml of sterile water
for inj or 0.9% NaCl; gently shake (25 mg/ml);
the solution must be further diluted using a 21-G
needle; withdraw suspension and add to 50 or
100 ml of D_5W or 0.9% NaCl, gently shake (4.2
mg/ml for 50 ml infusion bag, 2.3 mg/ml for
100 ml infusion bag)
• Infuse over 1 hr
• Storage: constituted solution may be held in
vial for ≤1 hr prior to transfer/dilution in infusion bag; diluted infusion solutions are stable
for ≤12 hr in 0.9% NaCl, 4 hr D_5W at room
temperature, 72 hr in 0.9% NaCl, 24 hr in D_5W
refrigerated, do not freeze constituted sol; if
Baxter min bag infusion bags are used, consult
instructions from Baxter
• Do not mix with or physically add to solution
containing other drugs

⚠ Nurse Alert

Solution compatibilities: D_5W, 0.9% NaCl, sterile water for inj

Y-site compatibilities: Acyclovir, amikacin, aminophylline, amiodarone, anidulafungin, atropine, azithromycin, bumetanide, calcium gluconate, CARBOplatin, caspofungin, ceftobiprole, cimetidine, ciprofloxacin, CISplatin, cyclophosphamide, cycloSPORINE, DAPTOmycin, dexamethasone, digoxin, diltiazem, diphenhydrAMINE, DOBUTamine, docetaxel, DOPamine, DOXOrubicin, enalaprilat, esmolol, esomeprazole, etoposide, famotidine, fentaNYL, fluconazole, fluorouracil, foscarnet, furosemide, gemcitabine, gentamicin, granisetron, heparin, hydrocortisone, HYDROmorphone, ifosfamide, insulin (regular), labetalol, levofloxacin, linezolid, LORazepam, magnesium sulfate, mannitol, meperidine, methotrexate, methylPREDNISolone, metoclopramide, metroNIDAZOLE, micafungin, midazolam, milrinone, morphine, moxifloxacin, norepinephrine, ondansetron, paclitaxel, pantoprazole, PHENobarbital, phenylephrine, potassium chloride, ranitidine, sodium bicarbonate/phosphates, tacrolimus, tigecycline, tobramycin, vancomycin, voriconazole, zidovudine

ADVERSE EFFECTS

CNS: Seizures, headache
GI: Diarrhea, nausea, vomiting, **pseudomembranous colitis, hepatitis**
HEMA: Neutropenia, leukopenia, anemia
INTEG: *Rash*, urticaria, phlebitis, erythema at inj site, **Stevens-Johnson syndrome, toxic epidermal necrolysis**, pruritus
SYST: Anaphylaxis

Pharmacokinetics

Absorption	Unknown
Distribution	To most body fluids/tissue
Metabolism	Unknown
Excretion	Mainly unchanged in urine, 70% recovered in 48 hr
Half-life	1 hr, extended in renal disease

Pharmacodynamics

Unknown

INTERACTIONS

Individual drugs
Probenecid: increased doripenem plasma levels
Divalproex sodium, valproic acid: decreased effects

Drug/lab test
Increased: AST, ALT, LDH, BUN, alkaline phosphatase, bilirubin, creatinine
False positive: direct Coombs' test

NURSING CONSIDERATIONS

Assessment
• Assess sensitivity to carbapenem antibiotics, penicillins
• Monitor renal disease: lower dose may be required
• Monitor bowel pattern daily; if severe diarrhea occurs, product should be discontinued; may indicate pseudomembranous colitis
• **Monitor for infection:** temp, sputum, characteristics of wound, before, during, and after treatment
⚠ **Monitor for allergic reactions, anaphylaxis: rash, urticaria, pruritus; may occur few days after therapy begins**
• **Monitor overgrowth of infection:** perineal itching, fever, malaise, redness, pain, swelling, drainage, rash, diarrhea, change in cough, sputum

Nursing diagnoses
• Infection, risk for (uses)
• Knowledge, deficient (teaching)

Patient/family education
• Instruct patient to report severe diarrhea; may indicate pseudomembranous colitis
• Instruct patient to report sore throat, bruising, bleeding, joint pain; may indicate blood dyscrasias (rare)
• Instruct patient to report overgrowth of infection: black, furry tongue; vaginal itching; foul-smelling stools
• Advise patient to avoid breastfeeding; product is excreted in breast milk

Evaluation
Positive therapeutic outcome
• Negative C&S
• Absence of symptoms and signs of infection

TREATMENT OF HYPERSENSITIVITY: EPINEPHrine, antihistamines; resuscitate if needed (anaphylaxis)

dorzolamide ophthalmic

See Appendix B

doxazosin (Rx)

(dox-ay′zoe-sin)
Cardura, Cardura XL
Func. class.: Peripheral α-adrenergic
blocker, antihypertensive
Chem. class.: Quinazoline
Pregnancy category C

Do not confuse:
Cardura/Coumadin/Cardene/Ridaura

ACTION: Peripheral blood vessels are
dilated, peripheral resistance lowered; reduction in B/P results from peripheral α-adrenergic
receptors being blocked

Therapeutic outcome: Decreased
B/P, decreased symptoms of benign prostatic
hypertrophy (BPH)

USES: Hypertension, urinary outflow
obstruction, symptoms of benign prostatic
hyperplasia

CONTRAINDICATIONS:

Hypersensitivity to quinazolines

Precautions: Pregnancy C, breastfeeding,
children, hepatic disease

DOSAGE AND ROUTES

BPH
Adult: PO 1 mg/day, increase in stepwise
manner to 2, 4, 8 mg/day as needed at 1-2 wk
intervals, max 8 mg

Hypertension
Adult: PO 1 mg/day, increasing up to 16 mg
daily if required; usual range 4-16 mg/day
Geriatric: PO 0.5 mg nightly, gradually
increase

Available forms: Tabs 1, 2, 4, 8 mg; ext rel
tabs 4, 8 mg

Implementation
PO route
• **Tabs** broken, crushed, or chewed; chewed
tabs taste bitter; do not break, crush, chew **XL
tabs**
• **Immediate release tab:** give without regard
to meals; **EXT REL tabs:** give with breakfast;
when switching from immediate release to EXT

REL, the final evening dose of immediate release
should be taken
• Store in tight container at 86° F (30° C) or
less
• May be used in combination with other
antihypertensives
• May be given with food to prevent GI symptoms

ADVERSE EFFECTS

CNS: *Dizziness,* headache, drowsiness,
anxiety, depression, vertigo, weakness, fatigue,
asthenia
CV: Palpitations, *orthostatic hypotension,*
tachycardia, edema, **dysrhythmias,** chest pain
EENT: Epistaxis, tinnitus, dry mouth, red
sclera, pharyngitis, rhinitis
GI: Nausea, vomiting, diarrhea, constipation,
abdominal pain
GU: Incontinence, polyuria, priapism

Pharmacokinetics

Absorption	Well absorbed
Distribution	Not known; 98% plasma protein bound
Metabolism	Liver, extensively ($<$63%)
Excretion	Kidneys
Half-life	22 hr

Pharmacodynamics

Onset	2 hr
Peak	2-6 hr
Duration	6-12 hr

INTERACTIONS

Individual drugs
Alcohol, sildenafil, vardenafil: increased hypo-
tensive effects
CloNIDine: decreased antihypertensive effect

Drug classifications
Other antihypertensives, nitrates: increased
hypotensive effects

NURSING CONSIDERATIONS

Assessment
• **Hypertension:** monitor B/P (lying, standing)
and pulse, syncope; check for edema in feet,
legs daily; I&O; monitor for weight daily; notify
prescriber of changes
• **BPH:** urinary pattern changes (hesitancy,
dribbling, incomplete bladder emptying, dysuria, urgency, nocturia, urgency incontinence,
intermittency before and during treatment
• Assess for orthostatic hypotension; tell patient
to rise slowly from sitting or lying position;

assess pulse, jugular venous distention q4hr, crackles, dyspnea, orthopnea with B/P

Nursing diagnoses
• Cardiac output, decreased (uses)
• Injury, risk for (side effects)
• Knowledge, deficient (teaching)
• Noncompliance (teaching)

Patient/family education
• Teach patient not to discontinue product abruptly; emphasize the importance of complying with dosage schedule, even if feeling better; if dose is missed take as soon as remembered; take at same time each day
• Teach patient not to use OTC products (cough, cold, allergy) unless directed by prescriber; also to avoid large amounts of caffeine
• Emphasize the need to rise slowly to sitting or standing position to minimize orthostatic hypotension
• Teach patient to notify prescriber of mouth sores, sore throat, fever, swelling of hands or feet, irregular heartbeat, chest pain
• Caution patient to report excessive perspiration, dehydration, vomiting, diarrhea; may lead to fall in B/P
• Caution patient that product may cause dizziness, fainting, light-headedness; may occur during 1st few days of therapy; to avoid hazardous activities
• Teach patient how to take B/P, and normal readings for age-group; to take B/P q7days
• Inform patient that fainting occasionally occurs after 1st dose; do not drive or operate machinery for 4 hr after 1st dose or after dosage increase or take 1st dose at bedtime; may take 1-2 wk in BPH

Evaluation
Positive therapeutic outcome
• Decreased B/P in hypertension
• Decreased symptoms of BPH

TREATMENT OF OVERDOSE:
Administer volume expanders or vasopressors; discontinue product; place in supine position

doxepin (Rx)
(dox′e-pin)
Apo-Doxepin, Prudoxin Cream, Silenor ✤, Zonolon Topical Cream
Func. class.: Antidepressant, tricyclic; antianxiety
Chem. class.: Dibenzoxepin, tertiary amine
Pregnancy category
B (Topical)
C (PO)

ACTION: Blocks reuptake of norepinephrine, serotonin into nerve endings, increasing action of norepinephrine, serotonin in nerve cells; has anticholinergic effects

Therapeutic outcome: Decreased symptoms of depression after 2-3 wk

USES: Major depression, anxiety, topical: lichen simplex, atopic dermatitis, eczema

Unlabeled uses: Insomnia, migraine prophylaxis; topical: pruritus

CONTRAINDICATIONS:
Hypersensitivity to tricyclics, urinary retention, closed-angle glaucoma, prostatic hypertrophy, acute recovery from MI

Precautions: Pregnancy **C** (PO), **B** (topical), breastfeeding, geriatric, seizures

> **BLACK BOX WARNING:** Suicidal patients, children

DOSAGE AND ROUTES
Depression/anxiety
Adult: PO 50-75 mg/day, may increase to 300 mg/day for severely ill, give in divided doses if >150 mg/day
Geriatric: PO 25-50 mg at bedtime, increase qwk by 25-50 mg to desired dose, max 150 mg/day

Pruritus
Adult: PO 10 mg at bedtime, may increase to 25 mg at bedtime; TOP apply a thin film qid ≥3 hr apart

Available forms: Caps 10, 25, 50, 75, 100, 150 mg; oral conc 10 mg/ml; cream 5%; tabs (Silenor) 3, 6 mg

Implementation
• **Oral conc** should be diluted with 120 ml of water, milk, or orange, grapefruit, tomato,

prune, pineapple juice; do not mix with grape juice
• Give with food or milk for GI symptoms; do not give with carbonated beverages
• Give dose at bedtime if oversedation occurs during day; may take entire dose at bedtime; geriatric may not tolerate once/day dosing
• Store at room temperature; do not freeze
• Provide safety measures, primarily for geriatric
• **Topical:** apply to affected area; rub slightly, do not use occlusive dressing

ADVERSE EFFECTS

CNS: *Dizziness, drowsiness,* confusion, headache, anxiety, tremors, stimulation, weakness, insomnia, nightmares, EPS (geriatric), increased psychiatric symptoms, paresthesia, **suicidal ideation**
CV: *Orthostatic hypotension, ECG changes,* **tachycardia,** *hypertension,* palpitations, **dysrhythmias**
EENT: *Blurred vision,* tinnitus, mydriasis, ophthalmoplegia, glossitis
GI: *Diarrhea, dry mouth,* nausea, vomiting, **paralytic ileus,** increased appetite, cramps, epigastric distress, jaundice, **hepatitis,** stomatitis, constipation
GU: *Retention,* **acute renal failure**
HEMA: **Agranulocytosis, thrombocytopenia, eosinophilia, leukopenia,** pancytopenia, purpuric disorder
INTEG: Rash, urticaria, sweating, pruritus, photosensitivity

Pharmacokinetics

Absorption	Well absorbed
Distribution	Widely distributed; crosses placenta
Metabolism	Liver, extensively
Excretion	Kidneys, breast milk
Half-life	8-24 hr

Pharmacodynamics

Unknown

INTERACTIONS

Individual drugs

Alcohol: increased CNS depression
Cimetidine, fluoxetine, fluvoxamine, paroxetine, sertraline: increased doxepin effect
CloNIDine: increased hypertensive crisis; do not use together
EPINEPHrine, norepinephrine: increased hypertensive action

Drug classifications

Antiarrhythmics, 1C (propafenone, flecainide), class III, quinolones: increased QT interval
Anticholinergics: increased anticholinergic effect
Barbiturates, benzodiazepines, CNS depressants, sedative/hypnotics: increased CNS depression
MAOIs: hypertensive crisis, seizures, hyperpyretic crisis
SSRIs, SNRIs, serotonin receptor agonists: increased toxicity

Drug/herb

St. John's wort: increased serotonin syndrome

Drug/lab test

Increased: serum bilirubin, blood glucose, alkaline phosphatase, LFTs

NURSING CONSIDERATIONS

Assessment

• **Assess chronic pain:** location, severity, type, alleviating/aggravating factors before and during treatment
• Monitor B/P (with patient lying, standing), pulse q4hr; if systolic B/P drops 20 mm Hg, hold product, notify prescriber; take VS q4hr in patients with CV disease
• Monitor blood studies: CBC, leukocytes, differential, cardiac enzymes if patient is receiving long-term therapy
• Monitor liver function tests: AST, ALT, bilirubin
• Check weight weekly; appetite may increase with product
• **Assess ECG** for flattening of T wave, bundle branch block, AV block, dysrhythmias in cardiac patients; product should be discontinued gradually several days before surgery
• Assess for EPS primarily in geriatric: rigidity, dystonia, akathisia
• **Assess depression:** mood, sensorium, affect, **suicidal tendencies;** increase in psychiatric symptoms
• Monitor urinary retention, constipation; constipation is more likely to occur in children or geriatric
• **Assess for withdrawal symptoms:** headache, nausea, vomiting, muscle pain, weakness; do not usually occur unless product was discontinued abruptly
• Identify alcohol consumption; if alcohol is consumed, hold dose until AM

Nursing diagnoses

• Coping, ineffective (uses)
• Injury, risk for (side effects)
• Knowledge, deficient (teaching)

Patient/family education
• Tell patient that therapeutic effects of decreased depression may take 2-3 wk, antianxiety effects sooner; to use caution in driving and other activities requiring alertness because of drowsiness, dizziness, blurred vision
• Advise patient to avoid rising quickly from sitting to standing, especially geriatric
• Teach patient to avoid alcohol ingestion, other CNS depressants: may potentiate effects; not to discontinue medication quickly after long-term use: may cause nausea, headache, malaise
• Teach patient to wear sunscreen or large hat, since photosensitivity occurs
• Teach patient that clinical worsening and suicidal ideation may occur
• Teach patient to increase fluids, bulk in diet if constipation occurs, especially geriatric; to take gum, hard sugarless candy, or frequent sips of water for dry mouth
• Teach patient to report urinary retention immediately

Evaluation
Positive therapeutic outcome
• Decrease in depression
• Absence of suicidal thoughts

TREATMENT OF OVERDOSE:
ECG monitoring, induce emesis, lavage, activated charcoal, administer anticonvulsant

doxercalciferol (Rx)
(dox-er-kal'-cif-er-ol)
Hectorol
Func. class.: Parathyroid agent (calcium regulator)
Chem. class.: Vitamin D hormone
Pregnancy category C

ACTION: Synthetic vit D analog, reduces parathyroid hormone

Therapeutic outcome: Calcium at normal level

USES: To lower high parathyroid hormone levels in patients undergoing chronic kidney dialysis and those in stages 3 or 4 of chronic renal disease prior to dialysis

CONTRAINDICATIONS:
Hypersensitivity, hyperphosphatemia, hypercalcemia, vit D toxicity

Precautions: Pregnancy **C**, breastfeeding, renal calculi, CV disease, hepatic disease

DOSAGE AND ROUTES
Stage 5 chronic kidney disease on dialysis
Adult: **PO** 10 mcg 3×/wk at dialysis (iPTH >400 pg/ml) max 20 mcg 3×/wk; **IV BOL** 4 mcg 3×/wk end of dialysis (iPTH >400 pg/ml), max 6 mcg 3×/wk (initially); if iPTH decreases by <50% and are >300 pg/ml, increase dose by 2.5 mcg **PO** or 1-2 mcg **IV** q8wk as needed; if iPTH decreases by >50% and are <300 pg/ml, maintain **IV** dose; if iPTH are 150-300 pg/ml, maintain dose; if iPTH 100-149 pg/ml 2.5 mcg **PO** or 1 mcg **IV**, lower than previous dose

Available forms: Caps 0.5, 1, 2.5 mcg; inj 2 mcg/ml

Implementation
• Do not break, crush, or chew caps
• Give with meals for GI symptoms

ADVERSE EFFECTS
CNS: Drowsiness, headache, lethargy
GI: Nausea, diarrhea, vomiting, anorexia, dry mouth, constipation, cramps, metallic taste
GU: Polyuria, hypercalciuria, hyperphosphatemia, hematuria
MS: Myalgia, arthralgia, decreased bone development
RESP: Shortness of breath

Pharmacokinetics	
Absorption	Unknown
Distribution	Unknown
Metabolism	Liver
Excretion	Unknown
Half-life	32-37 hr, terminal

Pharmacodynamics	
Peak	11-12 hr

INTERACTIONS
Individual drugs
Cholestyramine, magnesium antacids, mineral oil: decreased doxercalciferol levels, do not use together

NURSING CONSIDERATIONS
Assessment
• Assess GI symptoms, polyuria, flushing, head swelling, tingling, headache; may indicate hypercalcemia
• Identify nutritional status; check diet for sources of vit D (milk, some seafood), calcium

(dairy products, dark green vegetables), phosphates
• Monitor BUN, creatinine, uric acid, chloride electrolytes, urine pH, urinary calcium, magnesium, phosphate, urinalysis (calcium should be kept at 9-10 mg/dl; vit D 50-135 international units/dl), alkaline phosphatase baseline and q3-6mo

⚠ Assess for increased drug level, since toxic reactions occur rapidly; have calcium chloride on hand if calcium level drops too low; check for tetany

Nursing diagnoses
• Injury, risk for (adverse reactions)
• Knowledge, deficient (teaching)
• Pain, chronic (uses)

Patient/family education
• Teach patient the symptoms of hypercalcemia and about foods rich in calcium
• Advise patient to avoid products with sodium: cured meats, dairy products, cold cuts, olives, beets, pickles, soups, meat tenderizers in chronic renal failure
• Advise patient to avoid products with potassium: oranges, bananas, dried fruit, peas, dark green leafy vegetables, milk, melons, beans in chronic renal failure
• Advise patient to avoid OTC products containing calcium, potassium, sodium, or antacids in chronic renal failure
• Instruct patient to avoid all preparations containing vit D
• Instruct patient to monitor weight weekly

Evaluation
Positive therapeutic outcome
• Calcium levels 9-10 mg/dl

⚠ HIGH ALERT

DOXOrubicin (Rx)
(dox-oh-roo'bi-sin)
Adriamycin, Adriamycin PFS ✽, Caelyx ✽
DOXOrubicin liposome (Rx)
Doxil
Func. class.: Antineoplastic, antibiotic
Chem. class.: Anthracycline glycoside
Pregnancy category D

Do not confuse:
DOXOrubicin/DAUNOrubicin/IDArubicin/idamycin, Adriamycin/Aredia/Idamycin

ACTION: Inhibits DNA synthesis primarily; derived from *Streptomyces peucetius;* replication is decreased by binding to DNA, which causes strand splitting; active throughout entire cell cycle; a vesicant

Therapeutic outcome: Prevention of rapidly growing malignant cells

USES: Wilms' tumor; bladder, breast, liver, lung, ovarian, stomach, testicular, thyroid cancer; Hodgkin's disease; acute lymphoblastic leukemia; myeloblastic leukemia; neuroblastomas; lymphomas; sarcomas; *Doxil:* AIDS-related Kaposi's sarcoma, metastatic ovarian carcinoma

CONTRAINDICATIONS:
Pregnancy **D** (1st trimester), breastfeeding, hypersensitivity, systemic infections, cardiac disorders

Precautions: Renal/cardiac disease, gout

> **BLACK BOX WARNING:** Hepatic disease, bone marrow suppression (severe), extravasation, heart failure, secondary malignancy

DOSAGE AND ROUTES
DOXOrubicin
ALL
Adult and child: IV 30 mg/m^2 q wk × 4 wk or 30 mg/m^2 on day 1, 2, 14 of induction or 20 mg/m^2 on 15, 16, 17 as part multiregimen

AML
Adult and child: IV 30 mg/m^2/day × 3 days, may repeat q4wk

Ovarian cancer
Adult: IV 40-50 mg/m^2 q mo

Hepatic dose
Adult: IV Bilirubin 1.2-3 mg/dl give 50% of dose; bilirubin 3.1-5 mg/dl give 25% of dose

DOXOrubicin liposome
Kaposi's sarcoma
Adult: IV 20 mg/m^2 q3wk

Available forms: Inj 10, 20, 50, 100, 150 mg; liposomal dispersion for inj: (Doxil) 2 mg/ml

Implementation
• Use cytotoxic handling procedures; avoid contact with skin; very irritating; wash completely to remove; give fluids IV or PO before chemotherapy to hydrate patient

- Give antiemetic 30-60 min before giving product to prevent vomiting and prn; give antibiotics for prophylaxis of infection
- Provide liquid diet: carbonated beverages; gelatin may be added if patient is not nauseated or vomiting
- Do not interchange DOXOrubicin with DOXOrubicin liposome

Direct IV route (DOXOrubicin)
- Give **IV** after diluting 10 mg/5 ml of NaCl for inj; another 5 ml of diluent/10 mg is recommended; shake; give over 3-5 min; give through Y-tube or 3-way stopcock through free-flowing D₅ inf or 0.9% NaCl

Y-site compatibilities: Alemtuzumab, alfentanil, amifostine, amikacin, anidulafungin, argatroban, aztreonam, bivalirudin, bleomycin, bumetanide, buprenorphine, butorphanol, calcium chloride, calcium gluconate, CARBOplatin, carmustine, caspofungin, ceftizoxime, chlorproMAZINE, cimetidine, ciprofloxacin, CISplatin, cladribine, clindamycin, cyclophosphamide, cycloSPORINE, cytarabine, DACTINomycin, DAPTOmycin, dexamethasone, dexmedetomidine, dexrazoxane, diltiazem, diphenhydrAMINE, DOBUTamine, docetaxel, dolasetron, DOPamine, doripenem, doxycycline, droperidol, enalaprilat, ePHEDrine, EPINEPHrine, erythromycin, esmolol, etoposide, etoposide phosphate, famotidine, fenoldopam, fentaNYL, filgrastim, fluconazole, fludarabine, gemcitabine, gentamicin, granisetron, haloperidol, hydrocortisone, HYDROmorphone, ifosfamide, imipenem-cilastatin, inamrinone, isoproterenol, ketorolac, labetalol, leucovorin calcium, levorphanol, lidocaine, linezolid, LORazepam, mannitol, mechlorethamine, melphalan, meperidine, mesna, methotrexate, metoclopramide, metoprolol, metroNIDAZOLE, midazolam, milrinone, mitomycin, morphine, nalbuphine, naloxone, nesiritide, niCARDipine, nitroglycerin, nitroprusside, octreotide, ofloxacin, ondansetron, oxaliplatin, paclitaxel, palonosetron, pancuronium, phenylephrine, potassium chloride, procainamide, prochlorperazine, promethazine, propranolol, quinupristin/dalfopristin, ranitidine, sargramostim, sodium acetate, tacrolimus, teniposide, theophylline, thiotepa, ticarcillin/clavulanate, tigecycline, tirofiban, tobramycin, topotecan, trastuzumab, trimethobenzamide, vancomycin, vasopressin, vecuronium, verapamil, vinBLAStine, vinCRIStine, vinorelbine, zidovudine, zoledronic acid

Y-site incompatibilities: Acyclovir, allopurinol, aminophylline, amiodarone, amphotericin B cholesteryl, amphotericin B colloidal, amphotericin B lipsosome, ampicillin, ampicillin/sulbactam, ceFAZolin, cefepime, cefoperazone, cefotaxime, cefotetan, cefoxitin, ceftazidime, cefTRIAXone, cefuroxime, diazepam, digoxin, ertapenem, foscarnet, fosphenytoin, ganciclovir, magnesium sulfate, meropenem, methohexital, minocycline, pantoprazole, pemetrexed, pentamidine, PENTobarbital, PHENobarbital, phenytoin, piperacillin/tazobactam, potassium phosphates, propofol, riTUXimab, sodium phosphates, thiopental, TPN (2 in 1), TPN (3 in 1), trimethoprim/sulfamethoxazole, voriconazole

Intermittent IV infusion route (DOXOrubicin liposomal)
- Dilute dose up to 90 mg/250 ml of D₅W, give over ¹/₂ hr; do not admix with other solution medications
- **Dose modifications for HFS: Toxicity grade 1,** redose unless patient has experienced previous grade 3 or 4; **grade 2,** delay dosing up to 2 wk, or until resolved to grades 0 or 1; **grade 3,** delay dosing up to 2 wk or until resolved to grades 0 or 1; resume dose at 25% decrease, return to original dosing after interval; **grade 4,** delay dosing up to 2 wk or until grades 0 or 1; resume dose at 25% decrease, then return to original dose; if after 2 wk there is no resolution, discontinue

Y-site compatibilities: Acyclovir, allopurinol, aminophylline, ampicillin, aztreonam, bleomycin, butorphanol, calcium gluconate, CARBOplatin, ceFAZolin, cefepime, cefoxitin, ceftizoxime, cefTRIAXone, chlorproMAZINE, cimetidine, ciprofloxacin, CISplatin, clindamycin, cyclophosphamide, cytarabine, dacarbazine, dexamethasone, diphenhydrAMINE, DOBUTamine, DOPamine, droperidol, etoposide, famotidine, fluconazole, fluorouracil, furosemide, ganciclovir, gentamicin, granisetron, haloperidol, heparin, hydrocortisone, HYDROmorphone, ifosfamide, leucovorin, LORazepam, magnesium sulfate, mesna, methotrexate, methylPREDNISolone, metroNIDAZOLE, ondansetron, piperacillin, potassium chloride, prochlorperazine, ranitidine, ticarcillin/clavulanate, tobramycin, trimethoprim/sulfamethoxazole, vancomycin, vinBLAStine, vinCRIStine, vinorelbine, zidovudine

Y-site incompatibilities: Amphotericin B, amphotericin B cholesteryl sulfate, buprenorphine, cefoperazone, ceftazidime, docetaxel, mannitol, meperidine, metoclopramide, mitoxantrone, morphine, oflaxacin, paclitaxel, piperacillin/tazobactam, promethazine, sodium bicarbonate

ADVERSE EFFECTS
CV: Increased B/P, **sinus tachycardia, PVCs,** chest pain, **bradycardia, extrasystole**
GI: Nausea, vomiting, anorexia, mucositis, **hepatotoxicity**
GU: Impotence, sterility, amenorrhea, gynecomastia, hyperuricemia
HEMA: Thrombocytopenia, leukopenia, anemia
INTEG: *Rash, necrosis at inj site,* dermatitis, reversible alopecia, cellulitis, thrombophlebitis at inj site

Pharmacokinetics
Absorption	Complete bioavailability
Distribution	Widely distributed; crosses placenta
Metabolism	Liver, extensively
Excretion	Bile (40%-50%)
Half-life	12 min; $3\frac{1}{2}$ hr; $29\frac{2}{3}$ hr

Pharmacodynamics
Unknown

INTERACTIONS
Individual drugs
Cyclophosphamide: increased cardiotoxicity, increased hemorrhagic cystitis risk
Mercaptopurine, radiation: increased hepatotoxicity
Radiation: increased toxicity

Drug classifications
Antineoplastics: increased toxicity, bone marrow suppression
Hematopoietic progenitor cell: decreased antineoplastic effect, do not use 24 hr before or after treatment
Live virus vaccines: decreased antibody response

Drug/lab test
Increased: uric acid

NURSING CONSIDERATIONS
Assessment

> **BLACK BOX WARNING:** Dysrhythmias: monitor ECG; watch for ST-T wave changes, low QRS and T; possible dysrhythmias (sinus tachycardia, heart block, PVCs); signs of irreversible cardiomyopathy, can occur up to 6 mo after treatment begins

• Assess buccal cavity q8hr for dryness, sores or ulceration, white patches, pain, bleeding, dysphagia; obtain prescription for viscous lidocaine (Xylocaine)

> **BLACK BOX WARNING: Bone marrow depression:** monitor CBC, differential, platelet count weekly; withhold product if WBC is <4000/mm³ or platelet count is <75,000/mm³; notify prescriber of results

• Assess for increased uric acid levels, swelling, joint pain, primarily extremities; patient should be well hydrated to prevent urate deposits
• Monitor renal function studies: BUN, creatinine, serum uric acid, urine CCr before, during therapy; I&O ratio; report fall in urine output to <30 ml/hr
• Monitor temp q4hr (may indicate beginning of infection)

> **BLACK BOX WARNING: Hepatotoxicity:** monitor liver function tests before, during therapy (bilirubin, AST, ALT, LDH) as needed or monthly; note jaundice of skin or sclera, dark urine, clay-colored stools, itchy skin, abdominal pain, fever, diarrhea

• Assess for bleeding: hematuria, stool guaiac, bruising or petechiae, mucosa or orifices q8hr; inflammation of mucosa, breaks in skin
• Identify effects of alopecia on body image; discuss feelings about body changes

> **BLACK BOX WARNING: Extravasation:** local irritation, redness, swelling, a vesicant; if extravasation occurs, stop drug, restart at another site, apply ice, elevate extremity to reduce swelling; if resolution does not occur, surgical débridement may be required

Nursing diagnoses
• Body image, disturbed (adverse reactions)
• Infection, risk for (adverse reactions)
• Injury, risk for (adverse reactions)
• Knowledge, deficient (teaching)

Patient/family education
• Help patient to rinse mouth tid-qid with water or club soda, brush teeth bid-qid with soft brush or cotton-tipped applicators for stomatitis, use unwaxed dental floss
• Advise patient to add 2-3 L of fluids unless contraindicated prior to and for 24-48 hr after, to decrease possible hemorrhagic cystitis
• Tell patient that urine and other body fluids may be red-orange for 48 hr; contraceptive measures are recommended during and 4 mo after therapy; product is teratogenic to fetus
• Advise patient to avoid use of products containing aspirin or ibuprofen, razors, commercial mouthwash, since bleeding may occur; to report symptoms of bleeding (hematuria, tarry stools)

• Instruct patient to report signs of anemia (fatigue, headache, irritability, faintness, shortness of breath)

• Inform patient that hair may be lost during treatment; a wig or hairpiece may make patient feel better; new hair may be different in color, texture

• Caution patient not to have any vaccinations without the advice of the prescriber; serious reactions can occur

Evaluation
Positive therapeutic outcome
• Prevention of rapid division of malignant cells

---

doxycycline (Rx)
(dox-i-sye′kleen)
Adoxa, Apo-Doxy ✦, Doryx, Doxy, Doxycaps, Doxycin ✦, doxycycline calcium, doxycycline hyclate, doxycycline monohydrate, Monodox, Oracea, Periostat, Vibramycin, Vibra-Tabs
Func. class.: Antiinfective
Chem. class.: Tetracycline
Pregnancy category D

Do not confuse:
doxycycline/doxepin/dicyclomine

ACTION: Inhibits protein synthesis, phosphorylation in microorganisms by binding to 30S ribosomal subunits, reversibly binding to 50S ribosomal subunits; bacteriostatic

Therapeutic outcome: Bactericidal action against the following: gram-positive pathogens: *Bacillus anthracis, Clostridium perfringens, Clostridium tetani, Listeria monocytogenes, Nocardia, Propionibacterium acnes, Actinomyces israelii;* gram-negative pathogens *Haemophilus influenzae, Legionella pneumophila, Yersinia enterocolitica, Yersinia pestis, Neisseria gonorrhoeae, Neisseria meningitidis, Mycoplasma, Chlamydia*

USES: Syphilis, gonorrhea, *Chlamydia, Rickettsia,* lymphogranuloma venereum, uncommon gram-negative or gram-positive organisms, malaria prophylaxis, acne, anthrax, chronic periodontitis, Lyme disease

Unlabeled uses: Traveler's diarrhea, prevention of chronic bronchitis

CONTRAINDICATIONS:
Pregnancy **D**, children <8 yr, esophageal ulceration, hypersensitivity to tetracyclines

Precautions: Hepatic disease, breastfeeding, pseudomembranous colitis, ulcerative colitis

DOSAGE AND ROUTES
Most infections
Adult: PO/**IV** 100 mg q12hr on day 1, then 100 mg/day; **IV** 200 mg in 1-2 INF on day 1, then 100-200 mg/day
Child >8 yr (≥45 kg): PO/**IV** 100 mg q12hr on day 1, then 100 mg q day; severe infections 100 mg q12hr; **IV** 200 mg on day 1, then 100-200 mg q day, give 200 mg dose as 1 or 2 infusions
Child ≥8 yr, <45 kg: PO 2.2 mg/kg q12hr on day 1, then 2.2 mg/kg/day, severe infections 2.2 mg/kg q12hr; **IV** 4.4 mg/kg on day 1, then 2.2-4.4 mg/kg/day in 1-2 divided doses

Gonorrhea (uncomplicated) (patients allergic to penicillin)
Adult: PO 100 mg q12hr × 7 days, or 300 mg followed 1 hr later by another 300 mg

Malaria prophylaxis
Adult: 100 mg/day 1-2 days before travel, daily during travel, and 4 wk after return
Adolescent/child ≥8 yr <45 kg: PO 2 mg/kg (up to 100 mg q day) begin 1-2 days before travel, continue for 4 wk after return

Chlamydia trachomatis
Adult: PO 100 mg bid × 7 days

Syphilis
Adult: PO 100 mg bid × 14 days

Anthrax
Adult and child >8 yr and ≥45 kg: **IV** 100 mg q12hr, change to PO when able × 60 days
Adolescent/child ≥8 yr and <45 kg: PO 2.2 mg/kg q12hr × 60 days; **IV** 100 mg q12hr, change to PO when able × 60 days

Lyme disease
Adult: PO 100 mg bid × 14-21 days

Periodontitis
Adult: 20 mg bid after sealing and root planing for ≤9 mo; give close to meal AM or PM

Available forms: Doxycycline: cap 40 mg; doxycycline calcium: syrup 50 mg/5 ml; doxycycline hyclate: cap 50, 100 mg; pellet caps 75, 100 mg; inj 42.5, 100, 200 mg; tabs 20, 100, mg; doxycycline monohydrate: caps 50, 100 mg; tabs 50, 75, 100 mg; oral susp 25 mg/5 ml

---

Adverse effects: *italics* = common; **bold** = life-threatening

Implementation
PO route
- Do not break, crush, or chew caps
- Give around the clock to maintain proper blood levels; give with food to increase absorption of product; do not give within 3 hr of other agents; product reactions may occur
- Give with 8 oz of water 1 hr before bedtime to prevent ulceration
- Shake liquid preparation well before giving; use calibrated device for proper dosing
- Do not give with iron, calcium, magnesium products or antacids, which decrease absorption and form insoluble chelate

Intermittent IV infusion route
- Check for irritation, extravasation, phlebitis daily
- Dilute each 100 mg/10 ml of 0.9% NaCl, sterile water for inj; further dilute in at least 100 ml of 0.9% NaCl, D$_5$W, Ringer's, LR, D$_5$/LR; protect from direct light; keep at room temperature; give over 1-4 hr; **IV** sol stable for 12 hr at room temperature, 72 hr refrigerated, discard if precipitate forms

Y-site compatibilities: Acyclovir, alemtuzumab, alfentanil, amifostine, amikacin, aminophylline, amiodarone, anidulafungin, ascorbic acid, atracurium, atropine, aztreonam, bivalirudin, bumetanide, buprenorphine, butorphanol, calcium chloride, calcium gluconate, CARBOplatin, caspofungin, cefonicid, cefotaxime, cefTRIAXone, chlorproMAZINE, cimetidine, cisatracurium, CISplatin, clindamycin, codeine, cyanocobalamin, cyclophosphamide, cycloSPORINE, cytarabine, DACTINomycin, DAPTOmycin, dexmedetomidine, digoxin, diltiazem, diphenhydrAMINE, DOBUTamine, docetaxel, DOPamine, doxacurium, DOXOrubicin, enalapril, ePHEDrine, EPINEPHrine, epirubicin, epoetin alfa, eftifibitide, ertapenem, esmolol, etoposide, etoposide phosphate, famotidine, fenoldopam, fentaNYL, filgrastim, fluconazole, fludarabine, gemcitabine, gentamicin, glycopyrrolate, granisetron, HYDROmorphone, IDArubicin, ifosfamide, imipenem/cilastatin, insulin, isoproterenol, labetalol, levofloxacin, lidocaine, linezolid, LORazepam, magnesium sulfate, mannitol, mechlorethamine, melphalan, meperidine, metaraminol, methoxamine, methyldopa, metoclopramide, metoprolol, metroNIDAZOLE, miconazole, midazolam, milrinone, mitoxantrone, morphine, multivitamins, nalbuphine, naloxone, nesiritide, netilmicin, nitroglycerin, nitroprusside, norepinephrine, octreotide, ondansetron, oxaliplatin, oxytocin, paclitaxel, pancuronium, pantoprazole, papaverine, pentamidine, pentazocine, perphenazine, phentolamine, phenylephrine, phytonadione, potassium chloride, procainamide, prochlorperazine, promethazine, propofol, propranolol, protamine, pyridoxine, quinupristin/dalfopristin, ranitidine, remifentanil, ritodrine, riTUXimab, rocuronium, sargramostim, sodium acetate, streptokinase, succinylcholine, SUFentanil, tacrolimus, telavancin, teniposide, theophylline, thiamine, thiotepa, tirofiban, tobramycin, tolazoline, TPN (2 in 1), trastuzumab, trimetaphan, urokinase, vancomycin, vasopressin, vecuronium, verapamil, vinCRIStine, vinorelbine, voriconazole, zoledronic acid

Y-site incompatibilities: Allopurinol, amphotericin B colloidal, amphotericin B liposome, ampicillin, ampicillin/sulbactam, azaTHIOprine, ceFAZolin, cefoperazone, cefotetan, cefoxitin, ceftizoxime, cefuroxime, chloramphenicol, dantrolene, dexamethasone, diazepam, diazoxide, erythromycin, fluorouracil, folic acid, furosemide, ganciclovir, heparin, hydrocortisone, inamrinone, indomethacin, ketorolac, methotrexate, methylPREDNISolone, mezlocillin, moxalactam, nafcillin, oxacillin, palonosetron, pemetrexed, penicillin G, PENTobarbital, PHENobarbital, phenytoin, piperacillin/tazobactam, potassium acetate, sodium bicarbonate, trimethoprim/sulfamethoxazole

ADVERSE EFFECTS
CNS: Fever
CV: Pericarditis
EENT: Dysphagia, glossitis, decreased calcification of deciduous teeth, oral candidiasis, tooth discoloration
GI: *Nausea, abdominal pain, vomiting, diarrhea,* anorexia, enterocolitis, **hepatotoxicity,** flatulence, abdominal cramps, gastric burning, stomatitis
GU: *Increased BUN*
HEMA: **Eosinophilia, neutropenia, thrombocytopenia, hemolytic anemia**
INTEG: Rash, urticaria, photosensitivity, increased pigmentation, **exfoliative dermatitis,** pruritus
MS: Bone growth retardation (child <8 yr)
SYST: **Stevens-Johnson syndrome, angioedema**

Pharmacokinetics

Absorption	Well absorbed
Distribution	Widely distributed, crosses placenta
Metabolism	Some hepatic recycling
Excretion	Bile, feces; kidneys unchanged (20%-40%), enters breast milk
Half-life	14-17 hr; increased in severe renal disease

Pharmacodynamics

	PO	IV
Onset	$1^{1}/_{2}$-4 hr	Immediate
Peak	$1^{1}/_{2}$-4 hr	Infusion's end

INTERACTIONS

Individual drugs

Bismuth, calcium, carBAMazepine, cimetidine, cholestyramine, colestipol, kaolin/pectin, magnesium, NaHCO$_3$, phenytoin, rifampin, sucralfate, zinc: decreased effect of doxycycline

Digoxin: increased or decreased effect of digoxin

Iron: forms chelates, decreased absorption

Penicillins: decreased effects of penicillins

Warfarin: increased effect of warfarin

Drug classifications

Alkali products, antacids, barbiturates: decreased effect of doxycycline

Anticoagulants (oral): increased effect of anticoagulants

Contraceptives (oral): decreased effect of oral contraceptive

Drug/food

Decreased: absorption with dairy products

Drug/lab test

Increased: BUN, alkaline phosphatase, bilirubin, amylase, ALT, AST, eosinophils, WBC

False increase: urinary catecholamines

NURSING CONSIDERATIONS

Assessment

• Assess patient for previous sensitivity reaction

• **Assess patient for signs and symptoms of infection** including characteristics of wounds, sputum, urine, stool, WBC >10,000/mm^3, fever; obtain baseline information before, during treatment

• Obtain C&S before beginning product therapy to identify if correct treatment has been initiated

• **Assess for allergic reactions:** rash, urticaria, pruritus, chills, fever, joint pain; angioedema may occur a few days after therapy begins

• Assess bowel pattern daily; if severe diarrhea occurs, product should be discontinued

• Monitor for bleeding: ecchymosis, bleeding gums, hematuria, stool guaiac daily if on long-term therapy; blood dyscrasias may occur

• **Assess for overgrowth of infection:** perineal itching, fever, malaise, redness, pain, swelling, drainage, rash, diarrhea, change in cough, sputum

Nursing diagnoses

• Diarrhea (side effects)
• Infection, risk for (uses)
• Injury, risk for (side effects)
• Knowledge, deficient (teaching)
• Noncompliance (teaching)

Patient/family education

• Teach patient to report sore throat, bruising, bleeding, joint pain; may indicate blood dyscrasias (rare)

• Advise patient to contact prescriber if vaginal itching, loose foul-smelling stools, furry tongue occur; may indicate superinfection; report itching, rash, pruritus, urticaria

• Instruct patient to take all medication prescribed for the length of time ordered; product must be taken around the clock to maintain blood levels; do not give medication to others

• Advise patient to notify prescriber of diarrhea with blood or pus

Evaluation

Positive therapeutic outcome

• Absence of signs/symptoms of infection (WBC <10,000/mm^3, temp WNL, absence of red draining wounds)

• Reported improvement in symptoms of infection

⚠ HIGH ALERT

dronedarone (Rx)

(drone-da-rone)

Multaq

Func. class.: Antidysrhythmic (Class III)
Chem. class.: Iodinated benzofuran derivative

Pregnancy category X

ACTION: Prolongs action potential duration and effective refractory period, noncompetitive α- and β-adrenergic inhibition; increases PR and QT intervals, decreases sinus rate, decreases peripheral vascular resistance

Therapeutic outcome: Decreased amount and severity of ventricular dysrhythmias

USES: Atrial fibrillation, atrial flutter

CONTRAINDICATIONS:
Pregnancy **X**, breastfeeding, severe sinus node dysfunction, 2nd- or 3rd-degree AV block; bradycardia, hypersensitivity, heart failure, hepatic disease, QT prolongation

> **BLACK BOX WARNING:** NYHA class IV heart failure or class II-III with recent decompensation requiring hospitalization, permanent atrial fibrillation (cannot restore sinus rhythm)

Precautions: Children, electrolyte imbalances, elderly, Asian patients, females, atrial fibrillation/flutter

DOSAGE AND ROUTES
Adult: **PO** 400 mg bid; discontinue class I, III antidysrhythmias or strong CYP3A4 inhibitors prior to beginning treatment; max 800 mg/day

Available forms: Tabs 400 mg

Implementation
• Start with patient hospitalized and monitored
PO route
• Give reduced dosage slowly with ECG monitoring only
• Give loading dose with food to decrease nausea

ADVERSE EFFECTS
CV: *Bradycardia,* **heart failure, QT prolongation, torsades de pointes**
ENDO: Hypo/hyperthyroidism
GI: Nausea, vomiting, diarrhea, abdominal pain, **severe hepatic injury, hepatic failure**
INTEG: Rash, photosensitivity

Pharmacokinetics

Absorption	Slow, variable (PO) up to 65%
Distribution	Body tissues; crosses placenta
Metabolism	Liver
Excretion	Bile, kidney (minimal)
Half-life	15-100 day

Pharmacodynamics

	PO
Onset	1-3 wk
Peak	Unknown
Duration	Up to months

INTERACTIONS
Individual drugs
CycloSPORINE, dextromethorphan, digoxin, disopyramide, flecainide, methotrexate, phenytoin, procainamide, quiNIDine, theophylline: increased blood levels, increased toxicity
Dabigatran, warfarin: increased anticoagulant effect

Drug classifications
β-Adrenergic blockers, calcium channel blockers: increased bradycardia
CYP3A4 inhibitors, CYP2D6 inhibitors: increased dronedarone levels
CYP3A, CYP2D6 inducers: decreased dronedarone levels
CYP3A, CYP2D6 substrates: increased levels

Drug/herb
St. John's wort: decreased effect
Yohimbine: increased anticoagulant effect

Drug/food
Grapefruit juice: increased dronedarone effect, avoid use

Drug/lab test
Increased: T4

NURSING CONSIDERATIONS
Assessment
• Monitor I&O ratio; monitor electrolytes: potassium, creatinine, magnesium
• Monitor liver function studies: AST, ALT, bilirubin, alkaline phosphatase
• Monitor **ECG** to determine product effectiveness; measure PR, QRS, QT intervals; check for PVCs, other dysrhythmias; monitor B/P continuously for hypo/hypertension; check for rebound hypertension after 1-2 hr
• Monitor serum creatine, potassium, magnesium
• Monitor for dehydration or hypovolemia
• **Assess for hypothyroidism:** lethargy, dizziness, constipation, enlarged thyroid gland, edema of extremities, cool, pale skin
• **Monitor hyperthyroidism:** restlessness, tachycardia, eyelid puffiness, weight loss, frequent urination, menstrual irregularities, dyspnea, warm, moist skin
• Monitor cardiac rate, respiration: rate, rhythm, character, chest pain, ventricular tachycardia, supraventricular tachycardia or fibrillation
• Assess sight and vision before treatment and throughout therapy; microdeposits on the cornea may cause blurred vision, halos, and photophobia

Nursing diagnoses
- Cardiac output, decreased (uses)
- Gas exchange, impaired (adverse reactions)
- Knowledge, deficient (teaching)

Patient/family education
- Instruct patient to report weight gain, edema, difficulty breathing immediately to prescriber
- Instruct patient to use sunscreen and protective clothing to prevent burning associated with photosensitivity
- Instruct patient to take medication as prescribed, not to double doses, avoid use with all other products without approval of prescriber, do not use grapefruit juice
- Instruct patient to complete follow-up appointment with health care provider, including pulmonary function studies, chest x-ray
- Teach patient to use effective contraception during treatment, pregnancy **X**, do not breastfeed

Evaluation
Positive therapeutic outcome
- Decreased dysrhythmias

TREATMENT OF OVERDOSE:
Administer O_2, artificial ventilation, ECG, DOPamine for circulatory depression, diazepam or thiopental for seizures, isoproterenol

---

⚠ HIGH ALERT

droperidol (Rx)
(droe-per′i-dole)
Func. class.: Sedative-hypnotic
Chem. class.: Butyrophenone derivative
Pregnancy category C

ACTION: Acts on CNS at subcortical levels, producing tranquilization, sleep; antiemetic; mild α-blockade

Therapeutic outcome: Maintenance of anesthesia

USES: Premedication for surgery; induction, maintenance in general anesthesia; postoperatively for nausea and vomiting

CONTRAINDICATIONS:
Hypersensitivity, breastfeeding, child <2 yr

BLACK BOX WARNING: QT prolongation, torsades de pointes

Precautions: Pregnancy **C**, geriatric, CV disease (hypotension, bradydysrhythmias), renal/hepatic disease, Parkinson's disease, pheochromocytoma, CHF, hypokalemia, hypomagnesemia, cardiac hypertrophy

DOSAGE AND ROUTES

D

Induction, adjunct
Adult: IV/IM 1.25-2.5 mg, may give additional 1.25 mg with caution
Child 2-12 yr: IV 0.05-0.1 mg/kg titrate to response

Premedication
Adult: IM 2.5 mg $^1/_2$-1 hr before surgery, may give 1.25-2.5 mg additionally
Child 2-12 yr: IM 0.05-0.1 mg/kg

Available forms: Inj 2.5 mg/ml

Implementation
- Protect from light
IM route
- Give deeply in large muscle mass

Direct IV route
- Give undiluted; give through Y-tube or 3-way stopcock at 10 mg or less/min; titrate to patient response

Intermittent IV infusion route
- May be given by adding dose to 250 ml of LR, D_5W, 0.9% NaCl; give slowly, titrate to patient response
- Give anticholinergics (benztropine, diphenhydrAMINE) for extrapyramidal reaction
- Give only with resuscitative equipment nearby

Syringe compatibilities: Atropine, bleomycin, butorphanol, chlorproMAZINE, cimetidine, CISplatin, cyclophosphamide, dimenhyDRINATE, diphenhydrAMINE, DOXOrubicin, fentaNYL, glycopyrrolate, hydrOXYzine, meperidine, metoclopramide, midazolam, mitomycin, morphine, nalbuphine, pentazocine, perphenazine, prochlorperazine, promazine, promethazine, scopolamine, vinBLAStine, vinCRIStine

Syringe incompatibilities: Fluorouracil, furosemide, heparin, leucovorin, methotrexate, pentobarbital

Y-site compatibilities: Amifostine, aztrenonam, bleomycin, cisatracurium, CISplatin, cladribine, cyclophosphamide, cytarabine, DOXOrubicin, DOXOrubicin liposome, famotidine, filgrastim, fluconazole, fludarabine, granisetron, hydrocortisone sodium succinate, IDArubicin, melphalan, meperidine, metoclopramide, mitomycin, ondansetron, paclitaxel,

---

potassium chloride, propofol, remifentanil, sargramostim, teniposide, thiotepa, vinBLAStine, vinCRIStine, vinorelbine, vit B/C

Y-site incompatibilities: Fluorouracil, foscarnet, furosemide, leucovorin, methotrexate, nafcillin

Additive incompatibilities: Barbiturates

ADVERSE EFFECTS

CNS: EPS: Dystonia, akathisia, flexion of arms, fine tremors; dizziness, anxiety, drowsiness, restlessness, hallucinations, depression, **seizures, neuroleptic malignant syndrome**
CV: Tachycardia, *hypotension,* **QT prolongation, torsades de pointes**
EENT: Upward rotation of eyes, oculogyric crisis
INTEG: *Chills, facial sweating, shivering*
RESP: Laryngospasm, bronchospasm

Pharmacokinetics

Absorption	Well absorbed (IM)
Distribution	Crosses blood-brain barrier, placenta
Metabolism	Liver
Excretion	Kidneys, unchanged (10%)
Half-life	2-3 hr

Pharmacodynamics

	IM/IV
Onset	3-10 min
Peak	30 min
Duration	3-6 hr

INTERACTIONS

Individual drugs
Alcohol: increased CNS depression
Lithium: increased side effects of lithium

Drug classifications
Antihistamines, antipsychotics, barbiturates, CNS depressants, opiates: increased CNS depression
Antihypertensives, nitrates: increased hypotension
Class IA/III antiarrhythmics, some phenothiazines, some quinolones, tricyclics, others: QT prolongation

Drug/herb
Chamomile, hops, kava, valerian: increased action

NURSING CONSIDERATIONS
Assessment
⚠ **Check VS q10min during IV administration, q30min after IM dose; for increasing heart rate or decreasing B/P, notify prescriber at once; do not place patient in Trendelenburg's position, sympathetic blockade may occur, causing respiratory arrest**
• Assess extrapyramidal reactions: dystonia, akathisia, extended neck, restlessness, tremors; if these occur, an anticholinergic should be given
• If given for nausea or vomiting, monitor for significant loss of fluids, bowel sounds before, during administration

> **BLACK BOX WARNING:** ECG prior to and 2-3 hr after administration for serious arrhythmias

Nursing diagnoses
• Injury, risk for (adverse reactions)
• Knowledge, deficient (teaching)

Patient/family education
• Advise patient that orthostatic hypotension is common; to rise from lying or sitting position slowly; to avoid ambulation without assistance
• Caution patient that drowsiness, dizziness may occur; to call for assistance for ambulation

Evaluation
Positive therapeutic outcome
• Decreased anxiety
• Absence of vomiting during and after surgery

drotrecogin alfa (Rx)
(droh'treh-koh-jin al'fah)
Xigris
Func. class.: Biological response modifier
Chem. class.: Recombinant human activated protein C
Pregnancy category C

ACTION: Activated protein C exerts an antithrombotic effect by inhibiting factor Va/VIIIa

Therapeutic outcome: Reduction of mortality in adult patients with severe sepsis who have a high risk of death

USES: Severe sepsis (sepsis associated with acute organ dysfunction)

CONTRAINDICATIONS:
Hypersensitivity, internal active bleeding, intraspinal surgery, CNS neoplasms, ulcerative colitis,

hypocoagulation, within 3 mo of hemorrhagic stroke, epidural catheter in place, cerebral embolism/thrombosis/hemorrhage, within 2 mo of major surgery, trauma

Precautions: Pregnancy **C,** breastfeeding, children, within 6 wk of GI bleeding, prothrombin time INR >3, use >96 hr, hepatic disease, within 3 mo of ischemic stroke

DOSAGE AND ROUTES
Adult: **IV** INF 24 mcg/kg/hr × 96 hr; based on actual body weight

Available forms: Powder for inj, lyophilized, 5 mg, 20 mg

Implementation
• Store in refrigerator at 2°-8° C (36°-46° F); do not freeze
• Protect unreconstituted vials from light; keep in carton until time of use

Intermittent IV infusion route
• Reconstitute 5 mg vial/2.5 ml; 20 mg vial/10 ml sterile water for inj to a concentration of 2 mg/ml; slowly add sterile water for inj; do not shake or invert; gently swirl until dissolved
• Further dilute with 0.9% NaCl, slowly withdraw prescribed amount and add to bag of 0.9% NaCl, direct stream to side of bag, gently invert bag; do not transport infusion bag between locations using mechanical delivery systems
• Use immediately after reconstituting; may be held for only 3 hr at controlled room temperature 59°-86° F, must complete inf within 12 hr after preparation
• Do not use if discolored or if particulate is present
• If using an infusion pump, usual concentration is 100-200 mcg/ml; if using a syringe pump, usual concentration is 100-1000 mcg/ml
• Y-site incompatibilities: Use a dedicated **IV** line, or dedicated lumen of central venous catheter, may use only 0.9% NaCl, LR, dextrose, or dextrose/saline mixtures through same line
• Do not expose to heat or direct sunlight
• Discontinue 2 hr prior to invasive surgery or procedures introducing risk of bleeding

ADVERSE EFFECTS
HEMA: Decreased Hct, **bleeding**
SYST: **GI, GU, intracranial, intraabdominal, intrathoracic, retroperitoneal bleeding;** surface bleeding

Pharmacokinetics
Absorption	Rapid
Distribution	Plasma
Metabolism	Unknown
Excretion	Unknown
Half-life	Unknown

Pharmacodynamics
Onset	Within 2 hr of beginning infusion
Peak	96 hr
Duration	2 hr postinfusion

INTERACTIONS
Individual drugs
Asprin, cilostazol, clopidogrel, dipyridamole, indomethacin, phenylbutazone, ticlopidine: increased bleeding risk

Drug classifications
Anticoagulants, glycoprotein IIb/IIIa inhibitors, thrombolytics, other NSAIDs: increased bleeding risk

NURSING CONSIDERATIONS
Assessment
⚠ **Assess for bleeding during treatment; hematuria, hematemesis, bleeding from mucous membranes, epistaxis, ecchymosis; may require transfusion (rare), continue to assess for bleeding**
• Assess blood studies (Hct, platelets, PTT, protime, TT, aPTT) before starting therapy; pro-time or aPTT must be less than 2 × control before starting therapy; PTT or pro-time q3-4hr during treatment
• Assess VS, B/P, pulse, respirations, neurologic signs, temp q4hr; temp >104° F (40° C) indicates internal bleeding; systolic pressure increase >25 mm Hg should be reported to prescriber
⚠ **Assess for neurologic changes that may indicate intracranial bleeding**
⚠ **Assess for retroperitoneal bleeding: back pain, leg weakness, diminished pulses**

Nursing diagnoses
• Knowledge, deficient (teaching)

Evaluation
Positive therapeutic outcome
• Decreasing symptoms of sepsis, lack of mortality

DULoxetine (Rx)
(du-lox'uh-teen)
Cymbalta
Func. class.: Antidepressant, miscellaneous
Chem. class: Serotonin, norepinephrine reuptake inhibitor (SNRI)
Pregnancy category C

ACTION: Unknown, may potentiate serotoninergic, noradrenergic activity in the CNS. In studies duloxetine is a potent inhibitor of neuronal serotonin and norepinephrine reuptake

Therapeutic outcome: Decreased depression, decreased neuropathic pain

USES: Major depressive disorder (MDD), neuropathic pain associated with diabetic neuropathy, generalized anxiety disorder, fibromyalgia, chronic low back pain, osteoarthritis pain

CONTRAINDICATIONS:
Hypersensitivity, closed-angle glaucoma, alcohol intoxication, alcoholism, hepatic disease, hepatitis, jaundice

Precautions: Pregnancy C, breastfeeding, geriatric, mania, hypertension, cardiac/renal/hepatic disease, seizures, increased intraocular pressure, anorexia nervosa, bleeding, dehydration, diabetes, hyponatremia, hypotension, hypovolemia, orthostatic hypotension, abrupt drug withdrawal

> **BLACK BOX WARNING:** Children, suicidal ideation

DOSAGE AND ROUTES

Depression
Adult: PO 40-60 mg/day as a single dose or 2 divided doses

Diabetic neuropathy
Adult: PO 60 mg qday

Generalized anxiety disorder
Adult: PO 60 mg/day, may start with 30 mg/day × 1 wk, then increase to 60 mg/day, maintenance 60-120 mg q day

Fibromyalgia
Adult: PO 30 mg/day × 1 wk, then 60 mg/day

Musculoskeletal pain
Adult: PO 60 mg/day

Renal dose
Adult: PO Start with 20 mg, gradually increase; avoid use in severe renal disease

Available forms: Caps 20, 30, 60 mg

Implementation
• Swallow caps whole; do not break, crush, or chew; do not sprinkle on food or mix with liquid
• Give without regard to food
• Store in tight container at room temperature; do not freeze
• Provide assistance with ambulation during beginning therapy, since drowsiness, dizziness occur
• Check to see if PO medication was swallowed

ADVERSE EFFECTS
CNS: Insomnia, anxiety, dizziness, tremor, somnolence, fatigue, decreased appetite, decreased weight, agitation, diaphoresis, hallucinations, **neuroleptic malignant syndrome–like reaction,** aggression, **seizures,** headache
CV: Thrombophlebitis, peripheral edema, palpitations, hypertension, **supraventricular dysrhythmia**
EENT: *Abnormal vision*
ENDO: Hypoglycemia
GI: Constipation, diarrhea, dysphagia, *nausea,* vomiting, anorexia, dry mouth, colitis, gastritis, abdominal pain, **hepatic failure**
GU: Abnormal ejaculation, urinary hesitation, ejaculation delayed, erectile dysfunction, urinary frequency/retention, gyn bleeding
INTEG: Photosensitivity, bruising, sweating, **Stevens-Johnson syndrome**
MS: Gait disturbances, muscle spasm, restless legs syndrome
SYST: Anaphylaxis, angioedema, serotonin syndrome

Pharmacokinetics

Absorption	Well absorbed
Distribution	90% protein binding
Metabolism	Extensively metabolized (CYP2D6, CYP1A2) in the liver to an active metabolite
Excretion	70% of product recovered in urine, 20% in feces
Half-life	12 hr

Pharmacodynamics
Unknown

INTERACTIONS
Individual drugs
Alcohol: increased ALT, bilirubin

⚠ Nurse Alert

Drug classifications
⚠ MAOIs: coadministration (or within 14 days of MAOIs use) is contraindicated: hyperthermia, rigidity, rapid fluctuations of VS, mental status changes, neuroleptic malignant syndrome

Anticoagulants, antiplatelets, salicylates, NSAIDs: increased bleeding risk

Opioids, antihistamines, sedative/hypnotics: increased CNS depression

CYP1A2 inhibitors (fluvoxamine, quinolone antiinfectives); CYP2D6 inhibitors (fluoxetine, quinidine, paroxetine): increased action of DULoxetine

CYP2D6 extensively metabolized products (flecainide, phenothiazines, propafenone, tricyclics, thioridazine): narrow therapeutic index

SSRIs serotonin receptor agonists: increased serotonin syndrome, neuroleptic malignant syndrome

Drug/herb
Kava: increased CNS depression
St. John's wort: serotonin syndrome

Drug/lab test
Increased: blood glucose

NURSING CONSIDERATIONS
Assessment

> **BLACK BOX WARNING: Depression:** Assess mental status: mood, sensorium, affect, **suicidal tendencies,** increase in psychiatric symptoms; depression, panic

- Assess B/P lying, standing; pulse q4hr; if systolic B/P drops 20 mm Hg, hold product, notify prescriber; take VS q4hr in patients with CV disease
- Monitor hepatic studies: AST, ALT, bilirubin
- Monitor weight qwk; weight loss or gain; appetite may increase; peripheral edema may occur
- Offer sugarless gum, hard candy, frequent sips of water for dry mouth
- Assess for withdrawal symptoms: headache, nausea, vomiting, muscle pain, weakness; not usual unless product is discontinued abruptly
- ⚠ Assess for neuroleptic malignant syndrome–like reaction
- **Serotonin syndrome:** assess for nausea, vomiting, dizziness, facial flushing, shivering, sweating
- **Sexual dysfunction:** ejaculation dysfunction, erectile dysfunction, decreased libido, orgasm dysfunction

Nursing diagnoses
- Injury, risk for (uses)
- Knowledge, deficient (teaching)
- Noncompliance (teaching)

Patient/family education
- Advise that product is dispensed in small amounts because of suicide potential, especially in the beginning of therapy
- Teach patient/family to use caution when driving or other activities requiring alertness because of drowsiness, dizziness, blurred vision
- Advise patient to avoid alcohol ingestion, other CNS depressants, MAOIs
- **Abrupt discontinuation:** Advise patient not to discontinue medication quickly after long-term use; may cause nausea, headache, malaise
- Advise patient to wear sunscreen or large hat, since photosensitivity may occur
- Advise patient to notify prescriber if pregnancy is planned or suspected or if breastfeeding
- Tell patient that improvement may occur in 4-8 wk; up to 12 wk (geriatric patients)

> **BLACK BOX WARNING:** Advise that clinical worsening and suicide risk may occur

Evaluation
Positive therapeutic outcome
- Decreased depression

---

dutasteride (Rx)
(doo-tass′ter-ide)
Avodart
Func. class.: Sex hormone, 5α-reductase inhibitor
Chem. class.: Synthetic 4-azasteroid compound
Pregnancy category X

ACTION: Inhibits both types 1 and 2 forms of a steroid enzyme that converts testosterone to 5 μ-dihydrotestosterone (DHT), which is responsible for the initial growth of prostatic tissue

Therapeutic outcome: Decreased symptoms of benign prostatic hyperplasia (BPH)

USES: Treatment of symptomatic BPH in men with an enlarged prostate gland, or may be used in combination with tamsulosin

Unlabeled uses: Alopecia

CONTRAINDICATIONS:
Pregnancy **X,** breastfeeding, children, women, hypersensitivity

Precautions: Hepatic disease

DOSAGE AND ROUTES

Benign prostatic hyperplasia (BPH)
Adult: PO 0.5 mg/day

Alopecia (unlabeled)
Adult: PO 0.5-2.5 mg/day

Available forms: Caps 0.5 mg

Implementation
• Swallow caps whole: do not break, crush, chew, or open
• May be given without regard to meals

ADVERSE EFFECTS
GU: Decreased libido, impotence, gynecomastia, ejaculation disorders (rare), mastalgia, teratogenesis
INTEG: Serious skin infections

Pharmacokinetics

Absorption	Absolute bioavailability ~60%
Distribution	Protein binding 99%
Metabolism	Liver (CYP3A4)
Excretion	Feces
Half-life	5 wk at steady state

Pharmacodynamics

Onset	Rapid
Peak	2-3 hr
Duration	Levels detectable 4-6 mo posttreatment

INTERACTIONS

Individual drugs
Cimetidine, ciprofloxacin, diltiazem, ketoconazole, ritonavir, verapamil: increased dutasteride concentrations

Drug classifications
Antiretroviral protease inhibitors or other CYP3A4-metabolized products: increased dutasteride concentrations

Drug/lab test
Decreased: PSA

NURSING CONSIDERATIONS

Assessment
• **Assess for decreasing symptoms in BPH:** decreasing urinary retention, frequency, urgency, nocturia

• Assess PSA levels, digital rectal exam, urinary obstruction; determine the absence of urinary cancer before starting treatment
• Assess liver function tests: ALT, AST, bilirubin; blood studies: CBC with differential, serum creatitine, serum electrolytes

Nursing diagnoses
• Body image, disturbed (adverse reactions)
• Knowledge, deficient (teaching)

Patient/family education
• Advise patient to notify prescriber if therapeutic response decreases, if edema occurs
• Caution patient not to discontinue product abruptly
• Inform patient about changes in sex characteristics
• Caution patient not to donate blood for at least 6 mo after last dose to prevent possible blood administration to pregnant woman
• Advise patient and family that caps should not be handled by pregnant women or those who may become pregnant since this product can be absorbed through the skin
• Inform patient that ejaculate volume may decrease during treatment, that product rarely interferes with sexual function
• Advise patient to read patient information leaflet before starting therapy and reread it upon prescription renewal

Evaluation
Positive therapeutic outcome
• Decreased levels of DHT (5 α-dihydrotestosterone)
• Decreased urinary frequency
• Decreased urinary retention
• Decreased urinary urgency
• Decreased nocturia

⚠ Nurse Alert

econazole topical
See Appendix B

ecothiophate ophthalmic
See Appendix B

efavirenz (Rx)
(ef-ah-veer′enz)
Sustiva
Func. class.: Antiretroviral
Chem. class.: Nonnucleoside reverse
transcriptase inhibitor (NNRTI)
Pregnancy category D

ACTION: Binds directly to reverse
transcriptase and blocks RNA polymerase and
DNA polymerase, causing a disruption of the
enzyme's site

Therapeutic outcome: Improvement of
HIV-1 infection

USES: HIV-1 in combination with other
antiretrovirals

CONTRAINDICATIONS:
Pregnancy **D**, hypersensitivity

Precautions: Liver disease, breastfeeding,
children <3 yr, renal disease, myelosuppression, depression, seizures

DOSAGE AND ROUTES
Given in combination with protease inhibitor or
nucleoside analog reverse transcriptase inhibitors (NRTIs)
Adult and child >40 kg: PO 600 mg/day at
bedtime
Child:
10-14.9 kg: PO 200 mg/day at bedtime
15-19.9 kg: PO 250 mg/day at bedtime
20-24.9 kg: PO 300 mg/day at bedtime
25-32.4 kg: PO 350 mg/day at bedtime
32.5-39.9 kg: PO 400 mg/day at bedtime

Available forms: Caps 50, 100, 200 mg;
tabs 600 mg

Implementation
• Give at bedtime to decrease CNS side effects,
give on empty stomach

ADVERSE EFFECTS
CNS: Headache, dizziness, fatigue, impaired
cognition, insomnia, abnormal dreams, depression, anxiety, drowsiness
GI: *Diarrhea,* abdominal pain, *nausea,*
hyperlipidemia, constipation, increased liver
function tests
GU: Hematuria, kidney stones
INTEG: *Rash,* **erythema multiforme,
Stevens-Johnson syndrome, toxic epidermal necrosis**

Pharmacokinetics

Absorption	Well absorbed, concentra-tions higher in females, Africans, Asians, Hispanics
Distribution	Highly protein bound (99%)
Metabolism	Liver
Excretion	Kidneys, feces
Half-life	Terminal 52-76 hr

Pharmacodynamics

Onset	Unknown
Peak	3-5 hr
Duration	Unknown

INTERACTIONS
Individual drugs
Alcohol: increased CNS depression
CarBAMazepine: decreased efavirenz levels
Cisapride, midazolam, triazolam: do not give
together
Clarithromycin, indinavir, methadone, saquina-
vir: decreased level of each specific product
Midazolam, triazolam: Do not use together
Ritonavir: increased levels of both products

Drug classifications
Anticonvulsants, ergots, statins (except pravas-
tatin, fluvastatin): increased levels of each
specific product
Antidepressants, antihistamines, opioids:
increased CNS depression
Benzodiazepines, ergots: do not give together
CYP3A4 inhibitors (conivaptan, ambrisentan,
sorafenib): decreased efavirenz metabolism
CYP3A4 inducers (carBAMazepine, rifamycins):
decreased efavirenz effect
Estrogens: increased level of both products
Rifamycins: decreased efavirenz action

Drug/herb
St. John's wort: decreased efavirenz level; do not
use together

Drug/food
Increased: absorption of high-fat foods

Drug/lab test
Increased: ALT
False positive: cannabinoids

Adverse effects: *italics* = common; **bold** = life-threatening

NURSING CONSIDERATIONS

Assessment
- Assess signs of infection, anemia
- **HIV:** Assess CBC, blood chemistry, plasma HIV RNA, absolute $CD4^+/CD8^+$/cell counts/%, serum β_2 microglobulin, serum ICD+24 antigen levels, cholesterol, hepatic enzymes
- **Serious skin reactions:** Stevens-Johnson syndrome, toxic epidermal necrolysis
- Assess bowel pattern before, during treatment; if severe abdominal pain with bleeding occurs, product should be discontinued; monitor hydration
- **Assess for signs of toxicity:** severe nausea/vomiting, maculopapular rash

Nursing diagnoses
- Diarrhea (side effects)
- Infection, risk for (uses)
- Knowledge, deficient (teaching)

Patient/family education
- Advise patient to take as prescribed; if dose is missed, take as soon as remembered; do not double dose; take on empty stomach with water/juice
- Instruct patient to make sure health care provider knows of all the medications being taken, supplements, herbs, OTC products
- Advise patient that if severe rash occurs, stop taking and notify health care provider
- Advise patient not to breastfeed or become pregnant (pregnancy **D**) if taking this product
- Advise patient that adverse reactions (rash, dizziness, abnormal dreams, insomnia) lessen after a month
- Teach patient to avoid hazardous activities if dizziness, drowsiness occurs
- Teach patient that product does not cure disease but controls symptoms; HIV can be transmitted to others even while taking this product
- Advise patient to continue safer-sex practices

Evaluation
Positive therapeutic outcome
- Increased CD4, cell counts
- Decreased viral load
- Improvement in symptoms and progression of HIV-1 infection

eletriptan (Rx)
(el-ee-trip'tan)
Relpax
Func. class.: Antimigraine agent
Pregnancy category C

ACTION: Binds selectively to the vascular 5-HT_1-receptor subtype, exerts antimigraine effect; causes vasoconstriction in cranial arteries

Therapeutic outcome: Decreased severity of migraine

USES: Acute treatment of migraine with or without aura

CONTRAINDICATIONS:
Uncontrolled hypertension, hypersensitivity, basilar or hemiplegic migraine, ischemic bowel disease, severe renal/hepatic disease, coronary artery vasospasm, peripheral vascular disease, heart disease, acute MI, stroke, angina, CV disease

Precautions: Pregnancy **C,** breastfeeding, children, geriatric, postmenopausal women, men >40 yr, risk factors of CAD, MI, or other cardiac disease, hypercholesterolemia, obesity, diabetes, impaired renal/hepatic function

DOSAGE AND ROUTES
Adult: PO 20 or 40 mg, may increase if needed, max 40 mg (single dose); may repeat in 2 hr if headache improves but returns, max 80 mg/24 hr

Available forms: Tabs 20, 40 mg

Implementation
- Swallow tabs whole; do not break, crush, or chew
- Provide quiet, calm environment with decreased stimulation from noise, bright light, excessive talking

ADVERSE EFFECTS
CNS: *Dizziness,* headache, anxiety, paresthesia, asthenia, somnolence, flushing, fatigue, hot/cold sensation, chills, vertigo, hypertonia, seizures, serotonin syndrome
CV: Chest pain, palpitations, hypertension, MI, sinus tachycardia, stroke, ventricular fibrillation/tachycardia, atrial fibrillation, AV block, bradycardia, chest pressure syndrome, coronary vasospasm
GI: Nausea, dry mouth
MS: *Weakness,* back pain
RESP: Chest tightness, pressure

Pharmacokinetics

Absorption	Unknown
Distribution	Unknown
Metabolism	Liver
Excretion	Urine, feces
Half-life	Unknown

Pharmacodynamics

Onset	Of pain relief 2 hr
Peak	Unknown
Duration	Unknown

INTERACTIONS

Individual drugs

Clarithromycin, erythromycin, itraconazole, ketoconazole, nelfinavir, propanolol, ritonavir: increased plasma concentration of eletriptan

Drug classifications

CYP3A4 inhibitors: increased concentration of ergots, eletriptan

SSRIs, SNRIs, serotonin-receptor agonists: increased serotonin syndrome

NURSING CONSIDERATIONS

Assessment

• **Migraine:** pain location, character, intensity, nausea, vomiting, aura

• Monitor B/P; signs/symptoms of coronary vasospasms

• Assess for tingling, hot sensation, burning, feeling of pressure, numbness, flushing

• Assess stress level, activity, recreation, coping mechanisms

• Assess neurologic status: LOC, blurring vision, nausea, vomiting, tingling in extremities preceding headache

• Identify ingestion of tyramine foods (pickled products, beer, wine, aged cheese), food additives, preservatives, colorings, artificial sweeteners, chocolate, caffeine, which may precipitate these types of headaches

Nursing diagnoses

• Knowledge, deficient (teaching)
• Pain, acute (uses)

Patient/family education

• Have patient report any side effects to prescriber

• Teach patient to use contraception while taking product

• Teach patient to have dark, quiet environment

• Teach patient that product does not prevent or reduce number of migraine attacks

Evaluation

Positive therapeutic outcome
• Decreased severity of migraine

eltrombopag
Promacta
See Appendix A, Selected New Drugs

emedastine ophthalmic
See Appendix B

emtricitabine (Rx)
(em-tri-sit′uh-bean)
Emtriva
Func. class.: Antiretroviral
Chem. class.: Nucleoside reverse transcriptase inhibitor (NRTI)
Pregnancy category B

ACTION: Synthetic nucleoside analog of cytosine; inhibits replication of HIV virus by competing with the natural substrate and then becoming incorporated into cellular DNA by viral reverse transcriptase, thereby terminating cellular DNA chain

Therapeutic outcome: Decreasing symptoms of HIV

USES: HIV-1 infection with other antiretrovirals

Unlabeled uses: HBV (hepatitis B virus) infection

CONTRAINDICATIONS:
Hypersensitivity

BLACK BOX WARNING: Lactic acidosis

Precautions: Pregnancy **B**, breastfeeding, children, geriatric, renal disease

BLACK BOX WARNING: Hepatic insufficiency, chronic hepatitis B virus (HBV) infection

DOSAGE AND ROUTES

Oral cap and sol are not interchangeable

Adult: PO (caps) 200 mg/day; oral SOL 240 mg (24 ml) daily

Adolescent/child >33 kg: PO (caps) 200 mg/day

Child 3 mo-17 yr: oral SOL 6 mg/kg/day, max 240 mg (24 ml)

Infants <3 mo: PO oral SOL 3 mg/kg daily, do not use caps

Renal dose
Adult: PO CCr 30-49 ml/min 200 mg q48hr, SOL 120 mg q24hr; caps CCr 15-29 ml/min 200 mg q72hr, SOL 80 mg q24hr; caps CCr <15 ml/min 200 mg q96hr, SOL 60 mg q24hr

Available forms: Caps 200 mg; oral sol 10 mg/ml; oral cap and sol are not interchangeable

Implementation
• Give without regard to meals
• Store at 25° C (77° F)
• Take at same time every day
• Oral cap and sol are not interchangeable

ADVERSE EFFECTS
CNS: Headache, abnormal dreams, depression, dizziness, insomnia, neuropathy, paresthesia, *asthenia*
GI: *Nausea, vomiting, diarrhea, anorexia, abdominal pain, dyspepsia,* **hepatomegaly with stenosis (may be fatal)**
INTEG: Rash, skin discoloration
MS: Arthralgia, myalgia
RESP: Cough
SYST: Change in body fat distribution, **lactic acidosis**

Pharmacokinetics

Absorption	Rapidly, extensively absorbed
Distribution	Protein binding <4%
Metabolism	Unknown
Excretion	Excreted unchanged in urine (86%), feces (14%)
Half-life	10 hr

Pharmacodynamics

Onset	Unknown
Peak	1-2 hr
Duration	Unknown

INTERACTIONS
Efavirenz, lamivudine, tenofovir: Do not use together, treatment duplication
Ribavirin: Complex interactions

Drug classifications
Interferons: Decreased emtricitabine level

NURSING CONSIDERATIONS

Assessment
• Monitor liver, renal function tests: AST, ALT, bilirubin, amylase, lipase, triglycerides periodically during treatment

---

> **BLACK BOX WARNING:** Assess for lactic acidosis, severe hepatomegaly with steatosis; if lab reports confirm these conditions, discontinue treatment; more common in females, obese; monitor serum lactate levels, liver function tests

> **BLACK BOX WARNING:** Confirm that patient is free of HBV (hepatitis B virus) before starting treatment

Nursing diagnoses
• Infection, risk for (uses)
• Injury, risk for (adverse reactions)
• Knowledge, deficient (teaching)

Patient/family education
• Teach that GI complaints resolve after 3-4 wk of treatment
• Advise patient to report planned or suspected pregnancy, not to breastfeed while taking this product
• Instruct that product must be taken at same time of day to maintain blood level
• Advise that product will control symptoms, but is not a cure for HIV; patient is still infectious, may pass HIV virus on to others
• Instruct that other products may be necessary to prevent other infections
• Advise that changes in body fat distribution may occur

> **BLACK BOX WARNING:** Lactic acidosis: notify prescriber immediately of fatigue, muscle aches/pains, abdominal pain, difficulty breathing, nausea, vomiting, change in heart rate

> **BLACK BOX WARNING:** Hepatotoxicity: notify prescriber of dark urine, yellowing of skin/eyes, clay-colored stools, anorexia, nausea, vomiting

Evaluation
Positive therapeutic outcome
• Decrease in signs/symptoms of HIV
• Decrease viral load, increase CD4 counts

---

enalapril/enalaprilat (Rx)
(e-nal′a-pril/e-nal′a-pril-at)
Vasotec
Func. class.: Antihypertensive
Chem. class.: Angiotensin-converting enzyme (ACE) inhibitor
Pregnancy category D

Do not confuse:
enalapril/Eldepryl/ramipril/Anafranil

ACTION: Selectively suppresses renin-angiotensin-aldosterone system; inhibits ACE; prevents conversion of angiotensin I to angiotensin II, resulting in dilatation of arterial and venous vessels

Therapeutic outcome: Decreased B/P in hypertension; decreased preload, afterload in CHF

USES: Hypertension, CHF, left ventricular dysfunction

CONTRAINDICATIONS:
Hypersensitivity, history of angioedema

> **BLACK BOX WARNING:** Pregnancy D

Precautions: Breastfeeding, renal disease, hyperkalemia, hepatic failure, dehydration, bilateral renal artery stenosis

DOSAGE AND ROUTES
Hypertension
Adult: PO 2.5-5 mg/day, may increase or decrease to desired response, range 10-40 mg/day; **IV** 0.625-1.25 mg q6hr over 5 min
Child: PO 0.08 mg/kg/day in 1-2 divided doses, max 0.58 mg/kg/day; **IV** 5-10 mcg/kg/dose q8-24hr

CHF
Adult: PO 2.5-20 mg/day in 2 divided doses, max 40 mg/day in divided doses

Renal dose
Adult: PO CCr <30 ml/min 2.5 mg/day, increase gradually; **IV** CCr >30 ml/min 1.25 mg q6hr; CCr <30 ml/min 0.625 mg as one-time dose, increase as per B/P

Available forms: Enalapril: tabs 2.5, 5, 10, 20 mg; enalaprilat: inj 1.25 mg/ml

Implementation
PO route
• Store in air-tight container at 86° F (30° C) or less

• Severe hypotension may occur after 1st dose of this medication; hypotension may be prevented by reducing or discontinuing diuretic therapy 3 days before beginning benazepril therapy
• Give by **IV** inf of 0.9% NaCl (as ordered) to expand fluid volume if severe hypotension occurs

Direct IV route/ intermittent IV infusion
• Give undiluted over ≥5 min; use diluent provided or 50 ml D₅W, 0.9% NaCl, 0.9% NaCl in D₅W, or LR, give over ≥5 min, sol is stable for 24 hr

Y-site compatibilities: Acyclovir, alemtuzumab, alfentanil, allopurinol, amifostine, amikacin, aminophylline, amphotericin B liposome, anidulafungin, ascorbic acid, atracurium, atropine, azaTHIOprine, aztreonam, benztropine, bivalirudin, bretylium, bumetanide, buprenorphine, butorphanol, calcium chloride/gluconate, CARBOplatin, ceFAZolin, cefonicid, cefoperazone, cefotaxime, cefotetan, cefoxitin, ceftazidime, ceftizoxime, cefTRIAXone, cefuroxime, cephalothin, cephapirin, chloramphenicol, cimetidine, cisatracurium, cladribine, clindamycin, cyanocobalamin, cyclophosphamide, cycloSPORINE, cytarabine, DACTINomycin, DAPTOmycin, dexamethasone, dexmedetomidine, dextran 40, digoxin, diltiazem, diphenhydrAMINE, DOBUTamine, docetaxel, DOPamine, doripenem, doxacurium, DOXOrubicin, DOXOrubicin liposome, doxycycline, ePHEDrine, EPINEPHrine, epirubicin, epoetin, ertapenem, erythromycin, esmolol, etoposide, etoposide phosphate, famotidine, fenoldopam, fentaNYL, filgrastim, fluconazole, fludarabine, fluorouracil, folic acid, furosemide, ganciclovir, gemcitabine, gentamicin, granisetron, heparin, hydrocortisone, HYDROmorphone, ifosfamide, imipenem/cilastatin, indomethacin, insulin, isoproterenol, ketorolac, labetalol, levofloxacin, lidocaine, linezolid, LORazepam, magnesium sulfate, mannitol, mechlorethamine, melphalan, meperidine, meropenem, metaraminol, methicillin, methotrexate, methoxamine, methyldopate, methylPREDNISolone, metoclopramide, metoprolol, metroNIDAZOLE, mezlacillin, miconazole, midazolam, milrinone, minocycline, mitoxantrone, morphine, moxalactam, multiple vitamin infusion, nafcillin, nalbuphine, naloxone, netilmicin, niCARDipine, nitroglycerin, nitroprusside, norepinephrine, octreotide, ondansetron, oxacillin, oxaliplatin, oxytocin, paclitaxel, palonosetron, papaverine, pemetrexed, penicillin G potassium, pentamidine, pentazocine, PENTobarbital, PHENobarbital, phentol-

E

amine, phenylephrine, phytonadione, piperacillin/tazobactam, potassium chloride/phosphate, procainamide, prochlorperazine, promethazine, propofol, propranolol, protamine, pyridoxine, quinupristin/dalfopristin, ranitidine, remifentanil, ritodrine, riTUXimab, rocuronium, sodium acetate, sodium bicarbonate, succinylcholine, SUFentanil, tacrolimus, teniposide, tetracycline, theophylline, thiamine, thiotepa, ticarcillin/clavulanate, tigecycline, tirofiban, tobramycin, tolazoline, trastuzumab, trimetaphan, urokinase, vancomycin, vasopressin, vecuronium, verapamil, vinCRIStine, vinorelbine, voriconazole

Y-site incompatibilities: Amphotericin B cholesteryl sulfate, caspofungin, cefepime, dantrolene, diazepam, diazoxide, gemtuzumab, lansoprazole, phenytoin

Additive compatibilities: DOBUTamine, DOPamine, heparin, meropenem, nitroglycerin, nitroprusside, potassium chloride

ADVERSE EFFECTS

CNS: *Insomnia, dizziness,* paresthesias, headache, fatigue, anxiety
CV: *Hypotension,* chest pain, tachycardia, **dysrhythmias,** syncope, angina, **MI,** orthostatic hypotension
EENT: *Tinnitus,* visual changes, sore throat, double vision, dry burning eyes
GI: Nausea, vomiting, colitis, cramps, diarrhea, constipation, flatulence, dry mouth, loss of taste
GU: **Proteinuria, renal failure,** increased frequency of polyuria or oliguria
HEMA: **Agranulocytosis, neutropenia**
INTEG: Rash, purpura, alopecia, hyperhidrosis, photosensitivity
META: Hyperkalemia
RESP: Dyspnea, dry cough, crackles
SYST: Toxic epidermal necrolysis, **Stevens-Johnson syndrome, angioedema**

Pharmacokinetics

Absorption	Well absorbed (PO), complete (**IV**)
Distribution	Unknown
Metabolism	Liver (active metabolite—enalaprilat)
Excretion	Kidneys (60%—enalaprilat, 20%—enalapril)
Half-life	Enalaprilat 11 hr, increased in renal disease

Pharmacodynamics

	PO	IV
Onset	1 hr	5-15 min
Peak	4-6 hr	1-4 hr
Duration	24 hr	4-6 hr

INTERACTIONS

Individual drugs
Alcohol: increased hypotension (large amounts)
Allopurinol: increased hypersensitivity
CycloSPORINE, indomethacin: increased potassium levels
Digoxin, lithium: increased serum levels
Rifampin: decreased effects of enalapril

Drug classifications
Antacids: decreased effects of enalapril
Diuretics, general anesthesia, nitrates, other antihypertensives, phenothiazines: increased hypotension
Diuretics (potassium-sparing), potassium supplements, salt substitutes: increased potassium levels

Drug/lab test
Increased: ALT, AST, bilirubin, alkaline phosphatase, glucose, uric acid
False positive: ANA titer

NURSING CONSIDERATIONS

Assessment
• **Bone marrow depression (rare):** monitor blood studies: neutrophils, decreased platelets with differential baseline and q3mo; if neutrophils <1000/mm^3, discontinue treatment
• **Hypertension:** monitor B/P, orthostatic hypotension, syncope; if changes occur, dosage change may be required; obtain peak/trough levels
• **CHF:** monitor for increased weight, rales, jugular vein distention, edema, difficulty breathing
• Monitor electrolytes: K, Na, Cl during 1st 2 wk of therapy
• Monitor renal studies: protein, BUN, creatinine; increased levels may indicate nephrotic syndrome and renal failure
• Monitor renal symptoms: polyuria, oliguria, frequency, dysuria
• Establish baselines in renal, liver function tests before therapy begins and 1 wk into therapy
• Check potassium levels throughout treatment, although hyperkalemia rarely occurs
• Check for edema in feet, legs daily

• Assess for allergic reactions: rash, fever, pruritus, urticaria; product should be discontinued if antihistamines fail to help

Nursing diagnoses
• Cardiac output, decreased (uses)
• Injury, risk for (adverse reactions)
• Knowledge, deficient (teaching)
• Noncompliance (teaching)

Patient/family education
• Advise patient not to discontinue product abruptly; advise patient to tell all persons associated with health care that product is being taken
• Teach patient not to use OTC products (cough, cold, allergy medications) unless directed by physician, to avoid potassium, salt substitutes; serious side effects can occur; xanthines, such as coffee, tea, chocolate, cola, can prevent action of product
• Instruct patient on the importance of complying with dosage schedule, even if feeling better; to continue with medical regimen to decrease B/P: exercise, cessation of smoking, decreasing stress, diet modifications
• Emphasize the need to rise slowly to sitting or standing position to minimize orthostatic hypotension; not to exercise in hot weather, which can cause increased hypotension
• Advise patient to notify prescriber of mouth sores, sore throat, fever, swelling of hands or feet, irregular heartbeat, chest pain, coughing, shortness of breath
• Caution patient to report excessive perspiration, dehydration, vomiting, diarrhea; may lead to fall in B/P
• Caution patient that product may cause skin rash or impaired perspiration; that angioedema may occur and to discontinue if it occurs
• Caution patient that product may cause dizziness, fainting, light-headedness; may occur during 1st few days of therapy; to avoid activities that may be hazardous
• Teach patient how to take B/P, normal readings for age-group

> **BLACK BOX WARNING:** Teach patient to use contraception during treatment, pregnancy **D**

Evaluation
Positive therapeutic outcome
• Decreased B/P in hypertension

TREATMENT OF OVERDOSE:
Lavage, **IV** atropine for bradycardia; **IV** theophylline for bronchospasm, digoxin, O_2; diuretic for cardiac failure, hemodialysis

enfuvirtide (Rx)
(en-fyoo′vir-tide)
Fuzeon
Func. class.: Antiretroviral
Chem. class.: Fusion inhibitor
Pregnancy category B

ACTION: Inhibitor of the fusion of HIV-1 with CD4+ cells

Therapeutic outcome: Decreasing symptoms of HIV

USES: Treatment of HIV-1 infection in combination with other antiretrovirals

CONTRAINDICATIONS:
Breastfeeding, hypersensitivity

Precautions: Pregnancy **B**, children <6 yr, liver disease, myelosuppression, infections

DOSAGE AND ROUTES
Adult: SUBCUT 90 mg (1 ml) bid
Child 6-16 yr and <42.6 kg: SUBCUT 2 mg/kg bid, max 90 mg bid; 11-15.5 kg 27 mg/0.3 ml bid; 15.6-20 kg 36 ml/0.4 ml bid; 20.1-24.5 kg 45 mg/0.5 ml bid; 24.6-29 kg 54 mg/0.6 ml bid; 29.1-33.5 kg 63 mg/0.7 ml bid; 33.6-38 kg 72 mg/0.8 ml bid; 38.1-42.5 kg 81 mg/0.9 ml bid

Available forms: Powder for inj, lyophilized 108 mg (90 mg/ml when reconstituted)

Implementation
• Give SUBCUT, bid; rotate sites; preferred sites are upper arm, anterior thigh, abdomen

ADVERSE EFFECTS
CNS: Anxiety, peripheral neuropathy, taste disturbance, **Guillain-Barré syndrome,** insomnia, depression
GI: Abdominal pain, anorexia, constipation, pancreatitis
GU: Glomerulonephritis, renal failure
HEMA: Thrombocytopenia, neutropenia
INTEG: Inj site reactions
MISC: Influenza, cough, conjunctivitis, lymphadenopathy, myalgias, hyperglycemia, pneumonia, rhinitis, fatigue

Pharmacokinetics

Absorption	Well absorbed
Distribution	92% protein binding
Metabolism	Undergoes catabolism
Excretion	Unknown
Half-life	Terminal 3.8 hr

Pharmacodynamics

Onset	Unknown
Peak	8 hrs
Duration	Unknown

NURSING CONSIDERATIONS

Assessment
• Assess for signs of infection, inj site reactions
• Monitor renal studies: BUN, creatinine, renal failure may occur
• Monitor bowel pattern before, during treatment; if severe abdominal pain or constipation occurs, notify prescriber; monitor hydration
• Assess skin eruptions, rash, urticaria, itching
• Identify allergies before treatment, reaction to each medication
• CBC, blood chemistry, plasma HIV RNA, absolute CD4/CD8 cell counts/%, serum β_2 microglobulin, serum ICD+24 antigen levels, cholesterol

Nursing diagnoses
• Infection, risk for (uses)
• Injury, risk for (adverse reactions)
• Knowledge, deficient (teaching)

Patient/family education
• Instruct to notify prescriber if pregnancy is suspected or if breastfeeding
• Advise that pneumonia may occur, to contact prescriber if cough, fever occur
• Teach that hypersensitive reactions may occur: rash, pruritus; stop product, contact prescriber
• Teach that this product is not a cure for HIV-1 infection but controls symptoms; HIV-1 can still be transmitted to others
• Teach that this product is to be used in combination only with other antiretrovirals

Evaluation
Positive therapeutic outcome
• Increased CD4 cell counts; decreased viral load; slowing progression of HIV-1 infection

---

⚠ HIGH ALERT

enoxaparin (Rx)
(ee-nox'a-par-in)
Lovenox
Func. class.: Anticoagulant, antithrombotic
Chem. class.: Unfractionated porcine heparin (low-molecular-weight heparin)
Pregnancy category B

Do not confuse:
enoxaparin/enoxacin, **Lovenox**/Lotronex

ACTION: Binds to antithrombin III inactivating factors Xa/IIa resulting in higher ratio of anti-factor Xa to anti-factor IIa

Therapeutic outcome: Prevention of deep vein thrombosis

USES: Prevention of DVT (inpatient or outpatient), pulmonary emboli (inpatient) in hip and knee replacement, abdominal surgery at risk for thrombosis; unstable angina/non–Q-wave MI

CONTRAINDICATIONS:
Hypersensitivity to this product, benzyl alcohol, heparin, or pork; hemophilia; leukemia with bleeding; peptic ulcer disease; thrombocytopenic purpura, heparin-induced thrombocytopenia, active major bleeding

Precautions: Pregnancy **B**, breastfeeding, children, geriatric, severe renal/hepatic disease, blood dyscrasias, severe hypertension, subacute bacterial endocarditis, acute nephritis, recent burn, spinal surgery, indwelling catheters, low weight (men <57 kg, women <45 kg)

BLACK BOX WARNING: Lumbar puncture, epidural/spinal anesthesia

---

DOSAGE AND ROUTES

DVT prevention before hip/knee surgery
Adult: SUBCUT 30 mg bid given 12-24 hr postoperatively for 7-10 days until DVT risk is diminished

DVT prevention before hip replacement
Adult: SUBCUT 40 mg/day started 9-15 hr preop or 30 mg q12hr started 12-24 hr postop, continued until DVT risk is diminished or patient is adequately on anticoagulant

DVT prophylaxis before abdominal surgery
Adult: SUBCUT 40 mg/day × 7-10 days to prevent thromboembolic complications, start 24 hr before surgery

Treatment of DVT/PE
Adult: SUBCUT (outpatient without PE) 1 mg/kg q12hr or 1.5 mg/kg/day (outpatient/inpatient); warfarin should be started within 72 hr and continued ≥5 days until INR is 2-3 (usually 7 days)

Prevention of ischemic complications in unstable angina/non–Q-wave MI with aspirin
Adult: SUBCUT/IV 1 mg/kg q12hr until stable with aspirin 100-325 mg/day × ≥2 days

Renal dose
Adult: SUBCUT <30 ml/min 30 mg q day (thrombosis prophylaxis)

Available forms: Prefilled syringes/inj 30 mg/0.3 ml, 40 mg/0.4 ml, 60 mg/0.6 ml, 80 mg/0.8 ml, 100 mg/1 ml, 120 mg/0.8 ml, 150 mg/ml; multidose vials 100 mg/ml (3 ml)

Implementation
• Give at same time each day to maintain steady blood levels
SUBCUT route
• Administer SUBCUT deeply; do not give IM, begin 1 hr before surgery, do not aspirate, do not expel bubble from syringe before administration; sol is clear to yellow; do not use sol with precipitate; apply gentle pressure for 1 min
• Give to recumbent patient, rotate sites (left/right anterolateral, left/right posterolateral abdominal wall)
• Leave vascular access sheath in place for 6 hr after dose, then give next dose 6 hr after sheath removed

Direct IV route
• Use multidose vial for **IV** administration; use TB syringe or other graduated syringe to measure dose; give **IV** BOL through **IV** line; flush after
• If withdrawing from multidose vial, use TB syringe for proper measurement
• Prefilled syringes (30, 40 mg) are not graduated; do not use for partial doses
• Do not mix with other products or infusion fluids
⚠ Give only this product when ordered; not interchangeable with heparin or LMWHs

ADVERSE EFFECTS
CNS: Fever, confusion
GI: Nausea
HEMA: Hemorrhage, hypochromic anemia, thrombocytopenia, bleeding
INTEG: Ecchymosis, inj site hematoma
META: Hyperkalemia in renal failure
SYST: Edema, peripheral edema

Absorption	Well absorbed (90%)
Distribution	Unknown
Metabolism	Unknown
Excretion	Kidneys
Half-life	$4^{1}/_{2}$ hr

Pharmacodynamics

Onset	Unknown
Peak	3-5 hr
Duration	Unknown

INTERACTIONS
Drug classifications
Anticoagulants, antiplatelets, NSAIDs, salicylates, thrombolytics: increased bleeding

Drug/lab test
Increased: AST/ALT
Decreased: platelets

NURSING CONSIDERATIONS
Assessment
• Monitor blood studies (Hct, CBC, coagulation studies, occult blood in stools), anti-Xa levels q3mo; platelet count q2-3day; thrombocytopenia may occur
• Assess patient for bleeding gums, petechiae, ecchymosis, black tarry stools, hematuria, epistaxis, decrease in B/P; indicate bleeding and possible hemorrhage; notify prescriber immediately

BLACK BOX WARNING: Assess for neuro-symptoms in patients who have received spinal anesthesia

Nursing diagnoses
• Injury, risk for (uses, adverse reactions)
• Knowledge, deficient (teaching)
• Tissue perfusion, ineffective (uses)

Patient/family education
• Warn patient to avoid OTC preparations unless directed by prescriber because they could cause serious product interactions
• Instruct patient to use soft-bristled toothbrush to avoid bleeding gums; to avoid contact sports; to use electric razor; to avoid IM inj
• Advise patient to report any signs of bleeding, bruising: gums, under skin, urine, stools

Evaluation
Positive therapeutic outcome
• Absence of DVT

entacapone (Rx)

(en-ta'-ka-pone)

Comtan

Func. class.: Antiparkinsonian agent
Chem. class.: COMT

Pregnancy category C

ACTION: Inhibits COMT (catechol *O*-methyltransferase) and alters the plasma pharmacokinetics of levodopa; given with levodopa/carbidopa

Therapeutic outcome: Decreased symptoms of Parkinson's disease (involuntary movements)

USES: Parkinsonism in those experiencing end of dose, decreased effect as an adjunct to levodopa/carbidopa

CONTRAINDICATIONS:

Hypersensitivity

Precautions: Pregnancy **C**, breastfeeding, children, renal/hepatic disease, affective disorders, psychosis

DOSAGE AND ROUTES

Adult: PO 200 mg given with carbidopa/levodopa, max 1600 mg/day; may allow 25% dosage reduction in levodopa therapy

Available forms: Tabs 200 mg film coated

Implementation

• Adjust dosage to patient response
• Give with meals to decrease GI upset; limit protein taken with product
• Give only after MAOIs have been discontinued for 2 wk

ADVERSE EFFECTS

CNS: *Involuntary choreiform movements, dyskinesia, hypokinesia, hyperkinesia, hand tremors, fatigue, headache, anxiety, twitching, numbness, weakness, confusion, agitation, nightmares,* psychosis, hallucinations, hypomania, severe depression, dizziness, **neuroleptic malignant syndrome**

CV: *Orthostatic hypotension*

GI: *Nausea, vomiting, anorexia, abdominal distress, dry mouth, flatulence,* gastritis, GI disorder, *diarrhea, constipation,* bitter taste

INTEG: Rash, sweating, alopecia

MISC: Dark urine and other body fluids, back pain, dyspnea, purpura, fatigue, asthenia, infection-bacterial, **rhabdomyolysis**

Pharmacokinetics

Absorption	Well absorbed
Distribution	Protein binding 98%
Metabolism	Liver extensively
Excretion	Kidneys, feces; breast milk
Half-life	0.5 hr initial, 2.5 hr second

Pharmacodynamics

Onset	Unknown
Peak	Unknown
Duration	≤8 hr

INTERACTIONS

Individual drugs

Ampicillin, chloramphenicol, erythromycin, probenecid, rifampin: decreased excretion of entacapone

Bitolterol, DOBUTamine, DOPamine, EPHINEPHrine, isoetharine, methyldopa, norepinephrine: increased CV reactions; avoid use

Drug classifications

MAOIs: prevent catecholamine metabolism; do not use together

Drug/herb

Kava: decreased effect
Ma huang: increased B/P

NURSING CONSIDERATIONS

Assessment

• **Assess for neuroleptic malignant syndrome:** high temp, increased CPK, rigidity, change in consciousness, usually during rapid withdrawal
• Monitor B/P, respiration during initial treatment; hypotension should be reported
• Assess mental status: affect, mood, behavioral changes, depression; complete suicide assessment
• Monitor liver function enzymes: AST, ALT, alkaline phosphatase; also check LDH, bilirubin, CBC
• **Assess for involuntary movements in parkinsonism:** akinesia, tremors, staggering gait, muscle rigidity, drooling; these symptoms should improve with therapy when given with levodopa/carbidopa
• **Rhabdomyolysis:** Assess for muscle pain, tenderness, weakness, swelling of affected muscles, may lead to decreased B/P, shock

Nursing diagnoses

• Injury, risk for (uses)
• Knowledge, deficient (teaching)

- Mobility, impaired physical (uses)
- Noncompliance (teaching)

Patient/family education
- Advise patient that hallucinations, mental changes, nausea, dyskinesia can occur
- Caution patient to change positions slowly to prevent orthostatic hypotension; not to drive or operate machinery until stabilized on medication and mental performance is not affected
- Instruct patient to use product exactly as prescribed; if dose is missed, take as soon as remembered, up to 2 hr before next dose, not to discontinue abruptly, withdraw gradually
- Inform patient that urine, sweat may darken
- Instruct patient to notify prescriber if pregnancy is suspected; if breastfeeding, product is excreted in breast milk

Evaluation
Positive therapeutic outcome
- Decreased akathisia, other involuntary movements when used with levodopa/carbidopa
- Increased mood when used with levodopa/carbidopa

---

entecavir (Rx)
(en-te′ka-veer)
Baraclude
Func. class.: Antiretroviral nucleoside reverse transcriptase inhibitors (NRTIs)
Chem. class.: Guanosine nucleoside analog
Pregnancy category C

ACTION: Inhibits hepatitis B virus DNA polymerase by competing with natural substrates and by causing DNA termination after its incorporation into viral DNA; causes viral DNA death

Therapeutic outcome: Improved liver function tests in chronic hepatitis B (HBV)

USES: Chronic hepatitis B (HBV)

CONTRAINDICATIONS:
Hypersensitivity

Precautions: Pregnancy **C**, breastfeeding, child, geriatric, severe renal disease

> **BLACK BOX WARNING:** Hepatic disease, hepatitis, lactic acidosis, HIV

DOSAGE AND ROUTES
Chronic hepatitis B (nucleoside treatment–naive)
Adult and adolescent ≥16 yr: PO 0.5 mg/day

Chronic hepatitis B with compensated liver disease and history of hepatitis B viremia, while receiving lamivudine/telbivudine or known lamivudine resistance mutations
Adult and adolescent ≥16 yr: PO 1 mg/day

Renal dose
Adult: PO CCr ≥50 ml/min 0.5 mg/day; CCr 30-49 ml/min 0.25 mg daily, 0.5 mg/day or 1 mg q48hr for lamivudine refractory patient; CCr 10-29 ml/min 0.15/day, 0.3 for lamivudine refractory patient; CCr <10 ml/min 0.05 mg PO/day, 0.1 mg/day or 1 mg q7days for lamivudine refractory patient

Available forms: Tabs, film coated 0.5, 1 mg; oral sol 0.05 mg/ml

Implementation
- After hemodialysis give by mouth on empty stomach 2 hr before or after food
- **Oral liquid:** Use calibrated oral dosing spoon provided, may be used interchangeably with tabs
- Store in cool environment; protect from light

ADVERSE EFFECTS
CNS: *Headache*, fatigue, dizziness, insomnia
ENDO: Hyperglycemia
GI: *Dyspepsia*, nausea, vomiting, diarrhea, elevated liver function enzymes, **hepatotoxicity with steatosis**
INTEG: Alopecia, rash
SYST: Lactic acidosis

Pharmacokinetics
Absorption	100%
Distribution	Extensively to tissues, protein binding 13%
Metabolism	Unknown
Excretion	Unchanged 62%-73% via kidneys
Half-life	Terminal 128-149 hr

Pharmacodynamics
Onset	Unknown
Peak	0.5-1.5 hr
Duration	Unknown

INTERACTIONS

Drug/food
High-fat meal: decreased absorption

Drug/lab test
Increased: ALT, AST, total bilirubin, amylase, lipase, creatinine, blood glucose, urine glucose
Decreased: platelets, albumin

NURSING CONSIDERATIONS

Assessment

> **BLACK BOX WARNING:** Assess for HIV before beginning treatment because HIV resistance may occur in patients with chronic hepatitis B infection; monitor HIV RNA

⚠ **Assess for lactic acidosis, severe hepatomegaly with stenosis: increased serum lactate, increased hepatic enzymes, palpate liver; discontinue product if these occur**
• Monitor geriatric patients more carefully; may develop renal, cardiac symptoms more rapidly
• Assess for exacerbations of hepatitis (jaundice, pruritus, fatigue) after discontinuing treatment; monitor liver function tests

Nursing diagnoses
• Infection, risk for (uses)
• Injury, risk for (uses, adverse reactions)

Patient/family education
• Teach patient not to take with food
• Teach patient to take exactly as prescribed
• Advise patient not to stop medication without approval of prescriber
• Advise that optimal duration of treatment is unknown
• Teach patient to avoid use with other medications unless approved by prescriber
• Teach patient to notify prescriber of decreased urinary output, blood in urine

> **BLACK BOX WARNING: Teach patient symptoms of lactic acidosis:** muscle pain, severe tiredness, weakness, trouble breathing, stomach pain with nausea/vomiting, coldness in arms/legs, fast/irregular heartbeat, dizziness

> **BLACK BOX WARNING: Teach patient symptoms of hepatotoxicity:** eyes/skin turns yellow, dark urine, light bowel movements, no appetite for days, nausea, stomach pain

• Advise patient that product does not cure, but lowers the amount of HBV in body

• Teach patient that product does not stop the spreading of HBV to others by sex, sharing needles, or being exposed to blood

Evaluation
Positive therapeutic outcome
• Decreased symptoms of chronic hepatitis B, improving liver function tests

ePHEDrine nasal agent
See Appendix B

epinastine ophthalmic
See Appendix B

⚠ HIGH ALERT

EPINEPHrine (Rx, OTC)
(ep-i-nef′rin)
Adrenaclick, Adrenalin, EpiPen, EpiPen Jr., Primatene Mist, Twinject, Walgreens Bronchial Mist
Func. class.: Bronchodilator, nonselective adrenergic agonist, cardiac stimulant, vasopressor
Chem. class.: Catecholamine
Pregnancy category C

Do not confuse:
EPINEPHrine/ePHEDrine

ACTION: β_1- and β_2-agonist causing increased levels of cyclic AMP producing bronchodilatation, cardiac and CNS stimulation; large doses cause vasoconstriction via α-receptors; small doses can cause vasodilation via β_2-vascular receptors

Therapeutic outcome: Vasoconstrictor, cardiac stimulator, bronchodilator, decreased aqueous humor

USES: Acute asthmatic attacks, hemostasis, bronchospasm, anaphylaxis, allergic reactions, cardiac arrest, adjunct in anesthesia, shock

CONTRAINDICATIONS:
Hypersensitivity to sympathomimetics, closed-angle glaucoma, nonanaphylactic shock during general anesthesia

Precautions: Pregnancy **C**, breastfeeding, cardiac disorders, hyperthyroidism, diabetes mellitus, prostatic hypertrophy, hypertension, organic brain syndrome, local anesthesia of certain areas, labor, cardiac dilatation, coronary insufficiency, cerebral arteriosclerosis, organic heart disease

DOSAGE AND ROUTES

Anaphylaxis/severe asthma exacerbation
Adult: IM/SUBCUT 0.3-0.5 mg, may repeat q10-15min (anaphylaxis) or q20min-4 hr (asthma)

Severe allergic reactions type 1
Adult/child ≥30 kg: IM 0.3 mg (EpiPen/EpiPen 2-Pak, 1:1000)
Child <30 kg: IM 0.15 mg (EpiPen Jr/EpiPen Jr 2-Pak 1:2000)
Adult/child ≥66 lb: IM/SUBCUT 0.3 mg (0.3 ml) initially (Twinject 1.1 ml 1:1000, 1 mg/ml, containing 2 doses of 0.3 mg)
Adult/child 33-66 lb: IM/SUBCUT 0.15 mg (0.15 ml) initially, may give another 0.15 mg after 10 min (Twinject 1.1 ml 1:1000 [1 mg/ml] containing 2 doses of 0.15 mg)

Status asthmaticus
Adult: IV 0.3-0.5 mg SUBCUT (0.3-0.5 ml 1:1000 inj) q20min ×3 doses
Infant/child: IV 0.01 mg/kg up to 0.5 mg SUBCUT q20min ×3 doses

Available forms: Nasal spray (sol) 1 mg/ml; sol for inj 1 mg/ml; 1:10,000, 1:1000; inh vapor (sol) 0.22 mg/acuation; pressurized inh (sol) 0.22 mg/actuation; sol for inj 0.15 mg/0.15 ml autoinjector, 0.3 mg/0.3 ml autoinjector, 0.15 mg/0.3 ml

Implementation
• Check for correct concentration, route, dosage before administration
• Use this medication before other medications and allow at least 5 min between each to prevent overstimulation
IM/SUBCUT route
• Rotate inj sites, massage well, do not use gluteal (IM) site
• Shake susp before using
Inhalation route
• Use 2.25% sol diluted in nebulizer/respirator
• Rinse mouth after inh
• 10 gtt of a 1% sol should be placed in nebulizer
• Dilute racepinephrine 2.25% sol
Endotracheal route
• Only used in intubated patient; use **IV** dose that should be injected by endotracheal tube into bronchi

IV route
• Give after diluting 1 mg of 1:1000 sol/10 ml or more; 0.9% NaCl yields 1:10,000 sol, give l mg/min
• Give by continuous inf after further diluting in 0.9% NaCl, D₅W, D₁₀W, D₅LR, LR via 3-way stopcock; for Y-site, use infusion pump, protect from light; increase dose of insulin in diabetic patients

Y-site compatibilities: Alfentanil, amikacin, amiodarone, amphotericin B liposome, anidulafungin, ascorbic acid, atracurium, aztreonam, benztropine, bivalirudin, bleomycin, bumetanide, buprenorphine, butorphanol, calcium chloride/gluconate, CARBOplatin, caspofungin, ceFAZolin, cefoperazone, cefotaxime, cefotetan, cefoxitin, ceftazidime, ceftizoxime, cefTRIAXone, cefuroxime, chloramphenicol, chlorproMAZINE, cimetidine, cisatracurium, CISplatin, clindamycin, cyanocobalamin, cyclophosphamide, cycloSPORINE, cytarabine, DACTINomycin, DAPTOmycin, dexamethasone, dexmedetomidine, digoxin, diltiazem, diphenhydrAMINE, DOBUTamine, docetaxel, DOPamine, DOXOrubicin, doxycycline, enalaprilat, epirubicin, epoetin alfa, ertapenem, erythromycin, esmolol, etoposide, etoposide phosphate, famotidine, fenoldopam, fentaNYL, fluconazole, fludarabine, folic acid, furosemide, gemcitabine, gentamicin, glycopyrrolate, granisetron, heparin, hydrocortisone, HYDROmorphone, ifosfamide, imipenem/cilastatin, isoproterenol, ketorolac, labetalol, levofloxacin, lidocaine, linezolid, LORazepam, magnesium sulfate, mannitol, mechlorethamine, meperidine, metaraminol, methicillin, methotrexate, methoxamine, methyldopa, methylPREDNISolone, metoclopramide, metoprolol, metroNIDAZOLE, midazolam, milrinone, minocycline, mitoxantrone, morphine, multiple vitamins, nafcillin, nalbuphine, naloxone, niCARdipine, nitroglycerin, nitroprusside, norepinephrine, octreotide, ondansetron, oxacillin, oxaliplatin, oxytocin, paclitaxel, palonosetron, pancuronium, pantoprazole, pemetrexed, penicillin G potassium, pentamidine, pentazocine, phentolamine, phenylephrine, phytonadione, piperacillin-tazobactam, potassium chloride, procainamide, prochlorperazine, promethazine, propofol, propranolol, protamine, pyridoxime, quinupristin/dalfopristin, ranitidine, remifentanil, ritodrine, rocuronium, sodium acetate, streptomycin, succinylcholine, SUFentanil, tacrolimus, teniposide, theophylline, thiamine, thiotepa, ticarcillin/clavulanate, tigecycline, tirofiban, tobramycin, tolazoline, trimethaphan, urokinase, vancomycin, vasopressin, vecuronium, verapamil, vinCRIStine, vinorelbine, vitamin B complex with C, voriconazole, warfarin, zoledronic acid

Y-site incompatibilities: Acyclovir, aminophylline, azaTHIOprine, carmustine, cephapirin, dantrolene, diazepam, diazoxide, fluorouracil, ganciclovir, gemtuzumab, indomethacin, micafungin, PENTobarbital, PHENobarbital, phenytoin, sodium bicarbonate, thiopental, sulfamethoxazole/trimethoprim

ADVERSE EFFECTS

CNS: *Tremors, anxiety,* insomnia, headache, dizziness, weakness, drowsiness, confusion, hallucinations, **cerebral hemorrhage**
CV: *Palpitations, tachycardia,* hypertension, *dysrhythmias,* increased T-wave
GI: *Anorexia, nausea, vomiting*
MISC: Sweating, dry eyes
RESP: *Dyspnea*

Pharmacokinetics

Absorption	Well absorbed (PO), complete (**IV**)
Distribution	Unknown, crosses placenta
Metabolism	Liver
Excretion	Breast milk
Half-life	Unknown

Pharmacodynamics

	SUB-CUT	IM	IV	INH
Onset	3-5 min	5-10 min	Immediate	1 min
Peak	Unknown	Unknown	Unknown	Unknown
Duration	1-4 hr	1-4 hr	Unknown	1-4 hr

INTERACTIONS

Drug classifications

β-Adrenergic blockers: decreased hypertensive effects
Antidepressants (tricyclics): increased chance of hypertensive crisis; do not use together
MAOIs: increased chance of hypertensive crisis, do not use together
Other sympathomimetics: toxicity

NURSING CONSIDERATIONS

Assessment

• **Asthma:** Monitor respiratory function: vital capacity, forced expiratory volume, ABGs, lung sounds, heart rate, rhythm (baseline); amount, color of sputum

• Monitor **ECG** during administration continuously; if B/P increases, product should be decreased; check B/P, pulse q5min after parenteral route; CVP, PCWP, SVR; inadvertent high arterial B/P can result in angina, aortic rupture, cerebral hemorrhage
• Check inj site for tissue sloughing; if this occurs, administer phentolamine mixed with 0.9% NaCl
• **Monitor for evidence of allergic reactions, paradoxical bronchospasm:** withhold dose, notify prescriber; **sulfite sensitivity,** which may be life threatening

Nursing diagnoses

• Airway clearance, ineffective (uses)
• Cardiac output, decreased (uses)
• Gas exchange, impaired (uses)
• Knowledge, deficient (teaching)

Patient/family education

• Tell patient not to use OTC medications; extra stimulation may occur; to use this medication before other medications and allow at least 5 min between each, to prevent overstimulation
• Teach patient that paradoxical bronchospasm may occur and to stop product immediately and notify prescriber; to limit caffeine products such as chocolate, coffee, tea, and colas
• Patient should rinse mouth after inh
• Patient should report blurred vision, irritation with ophth preparations

Evaluation
Positive therapeutic outcome

• Absence of dyspnea, wheezing
• Improved airway exchange, improved ABGs
• Decreased aqueous humor
• Stabilization of heart rate and cardiac output

TREATMENT OF OVERDOSE:

Administer a β$_2$-adrenergic blocker, vasodilators, α-blocker

EPINEPHrine/epinephryl borate ophthalmic
See Appendix B

EPINEPHrine nasal agent
See Appendix B

A HIGH ALERT

epirubicin (Rx)

(ep-i-roo'-bi-sin)

Ellence, Pharmorubicin ✸

Func. class.: Antineoplastic, antibiotic

Chem. class.: Anthracycline

Pregnancy category D

ACTION: Inhibits DNA synthesis primarily; replication is decreased by binding to DNA, which causes strand splitting; maximum cytotoxic effects at S and G_2 phases; a vesicant

Therapeutic outcome: Prevention of rapidly growing malignant cells

USES: Breast cancer as an adjuvant therapy, with axillary node involvement, after resection

Unlabeled uses: Used in combination for treatment of advanced forms of cancer

CONTRAINDICATIONS:

Pregnancy **D,** breastfeeding, hypersensitivity to this product, anthracyclines, anthracenediones, systemic infections, baseline neutrophil count <1500 cell/mm^3, severe myocardial insufficiency, recent MI

BLACK BOX WARNING: Severe hepatic disease

Precautions: Children, geriatric, renal/hepatic/cardiac disease, gout, previous anthracycline use

BLACK BOX WARNING: Bone marrow suppression (severe), heart failure, extravasation, secondary malignancy

DOSAGE AND ROUTES

Adult: IV INF 100-120 mg/m^2 initially given with other antineoplastics (cyclophosphamide, 5-fluorouracil); given in repeated 3-4 wk cycles

Epirubicin dosage adjustments

Adult: IV 100 mg/m^2 on day 1 of each cycle; toxicity nadir platelet counts $<50,000$ mm^3, ANC 250 mm^3, neutropenic fever or grade 3 or 4 nonhematologic toxicity; next cycle give 75% of day 1 dose; delay next cycle until platelets are $\geq100,000$ mm^3, ANC >1500 mm^3, and nonhematologic toxicities have recovered to $<$ grade 1

Hepatic dose

Adult: IV Bilirubin 1.2-3 mg/dl or AST 2-4 $\times$ normal upper limit, 50% of starting dose;

bilirubin >3 mg/dl or AST $>4 \times$ normal upper limit, 25% of starting dose

Available forms: Inj (2 mg/ml) 10 mg/5 ml, 50 mg/25 ml, 150 mg/75 ml, 200 mg/100 ml

Implementation

• Avoid contact with skin; very irritating; wash completely to remove; give fluids **IV** or PO before chemotherapy to hydrate patient

• Give antiemetic 30-60 min before giving product to prevent vomiting and prn

• Administer prophylactic antibiotic with a fluoroquinolone or trimethoprim/sulfamethoxazole if dose of epirubicin is 120 mg/m^2

• Provide liquid diet: carbonated beverages; gelatin may be added if patient is not nauseated or vomiting

IV route

• Product should be prepared by experienced personnel using proper precautions

• Reconstitute 50 mg and 200 mg powder for inj with 25 ml, 100 ml, respectively, of sterile water for inj (2 mg/ml), shake well

IV injection route

• Give into tubing of free-flowing **IV** inf 0.9% NaCl or D$_5$W over 3-5 min; do not admix with other products in syringe

Intermittent IV infusion route

• Dilute in appropriate dose of 0.9% NaCl or D$_5$W, infuse over 30-60 min

Y-site compatibilities: Alfentanil, amifostine, amikacin, aminocaproic acid, anidulafungin, atracurium, aztreonam, bivalirudin, bleomycin, bumetanide, buprenorphine, butorphanol, calcium chloride/gluconate, CARBOplatin, caspofungin, ceFAZolin, cefotaxime, ceftizoxime, chlorproMAZINE, cimetidine, ciprofloxacin, cisatracurium, CISplatin, clindamycin, cyclophosphamide, cycloSPORINE, DAPTOmycin, dexrazoxane, digoxin, diltiazem, diphenhydrAMINE, DOBUTamine, docetaxel, dolasetron, DOPamine, doxacurium, doxycycline, droperidol, enalaprilat, ePHEDrine, EPINEPHrine, erythromycin, etoposide, famotidine, fenoldopam, fentaNYL, fluconazole, gatifloxacin, gemcitabine, gentamicin, granisetron, haloperidol, hydrocortisone, HYDROmorphone, hydrOXYzine, ifosfamide, imipenem-cilastatin, inamrinone, insulin (regular), isoproterenol, labetalol, levofloxacin, levorphanol, lidocaine, linezolid, LORazepam, mannitol, meperidine, mesna, methotrexate, metoclopramide, metoprolol, metroNIDAZOLE, midazolam, milrinone, minocycline, mitomycin, mivacurium, morphine, nalbuphine, naloxone, nesiritide, niCARdipine, nitroglycerin, nitroprus-

E

side, norepinephrine, octreotide, ofloxacin, ondansetron, oxaliplatin, paclitaxel, palonosetron, pamidronate, pancuronium, pentamidine, pentazocine, phenylephrine, potassium chloride, procainamide, prochlorperazine, promethazine, propranolol, quinupristin-dalfopristin, ranitidine, remifentanil, rocuronium, sodium acetate, succinylcholine, SUFentanil, tacrolimus, teniposide, theophylline, thiotepa, tirofiban, tobramycin, trimethobenzamide, vancomycin, vasopressin, vecuronium, verapamil, vinBLAStine, vinCRIStine, vinorelbine, voriconazole, zidovudine, zoledronic acid

Y-site incompatibilities: Acyclovir, allopurinol, aminophylline, amphotericin B colloidal, amphotericin B lipid complex, amphotericin B liposome, ampicillin, ampicillin/sulbactam, azithromycin, cefepime, cefoperazone, cefotetan, cefoxitin, ceftazidime, cefTRIAXone, cefuroxime, dexamethasone, diazepam, ertapenem, fluorouracil, foscarnet, fosphenytoin, furosemide, ganciclovir, gemtuzumab, heparin, hydrocortisone, ketorolac, leucovorin, magnesium sulfate, meropenem, methohexital, methylPREDNISolone, nafcillin, pantoprazole, pemetrexed, PENTobarbital, PHENobarbital, phenytoin, piperacillin/tazobactam, potassium phosphates, sodium bicarbonate, sodium phosphates, thiopental, ticarcillin/clavulanate, tigecycline, sulfamethoxazole/trimethoprim

ADVERSE EFFECTS

CV: Increased B/P, **sinus tachycardia, PVCs,** chest pain, **bradycardia, extrasystole**
GI: Nausea, vomiting, diarrhea, anorexia, mucositis
GU: *Hot flashes, amenorrhea, hyperuricemia*
HEMA: **Thrombocytopenia, leukopenia, anemia, neutropenia, secondary AML**
INTEG: *Rash, necrosis, pain at inj site, reversible alopecia*
MISC: Infection, febrile neutropenia, lethargy, fever, conjunctivitis, tumor lysis syndrome

Pharmacokinetics

Absorption	Complete bioavailability
Distribution	Widely distributed, crosses placenta
Metabolism	Liver, extensively
Excretion	Bile (60%)
Half-life	3 min; 2.5 hr; 33 hr

Pharmacodynamics

Unknown

INTERACTIONS

Individual drugs
Cimetidine, radiation: increased toxicity

Drug classifications
Antineoplastics: increased toxicity
Live virus vaccines: decreased antibody response

NURSING CONSIDERATIONS

Assessment
• **Heart failure:** monitor left ventricular ejection fraction, multigated acquisition scan or echocardiogram, ECG; watch for ST-T wave changes, low QRS and T; possible dysrhythmias (sinus tachycardia, heart block, PVCs) may occur; assess tachypnea, ECG changes, dyspnea, edema, fatigue; cardiac status: B/P, pulse, character, rhythm, rate, ABGs
• Assess symptoms indicating severe allergic reaction: rash, pruritus, urticaria, purpuric skin lesions, itching, flushing; product should be discontinued

> **BLACK BOX WARNING: Bone marrow depression (severe):** monitor CBC, differential, platelet count weekly; withhold product if baseline neutrophil count is <1500/mm³; notify prescriber of results if WBC <20,000/mm³, platelets <150,000/mm³; leukocyte nadir occurs 10-14 days after administration; recovery by 21st day

• Assess for increased uric acid levels, swelling, joint pain, primarily extremities; patient should be well hydrated to prevent urate deposits
• Monitor renal function studies: BUN, creatinine, serum uric acid, urine CCr before, during therapy; I&O ratio; report fall in urine output to <30 ml/hr; dosage adjustment is needed for serum creatinine >5 mg/dl

> **BLACK BOX WARNING: Severe hepatic disease:** monitor liver function tests before, during therapy (bilirubin, AST, ALT, LDH) as needed or monthly; note jaundice of skin or sclera, dark urine, clay-colored stools, itchy skin, abdominal pain, fever, diarrhea

• Assess for bleeding: hematuria, stool guaiac, bruising or petechiae, mucosa or orifices q8hr; inflammation of mucosa, breaks in skin
• Identify effects of alopecia on body image; discuss feelings about body changes

> **BLACK BOX WARNING: Extravasation (vesicant):** Assess for local irritation, pain, burning, necrosis at injection site; discontinue and start at another site

Nursing diagnoses
* Body image, disturbed (adverse reactions)
* Infection, risk for (adverse reactions)
* Injury, risk for (adverse reactions)
* Knowledge, deficient (teaching)

Patient/family education
* Advise patient to avoid use of products containing aspirin or NSAIDs, razors, commercial mouthwash, since bleeding may occur; to report symptoms of bleeding (hematuria, tarry stools)
* Instruct patient to report signs of anemia (fatigue, headache, irritability, faintness, shortness of breath)
* Inform patient that hair may be lost during treatment; a wig or hairpiece may make patient feel better; new hair may be different in color, texture
* Caution patient not to have any vaccinations without the advice of the prescriber; serious reactions can occur
* Advise patient to use contraception during treatment and 4 mo afterward; pregnancy **D**
* Advise patient that urine may appear red for 2 days
* Instruct patient to avoid crowds, persons with known infection
* Caution patient to avoid OTC medications, supplements unless approved by prescriber

Evaluation
Positive therapeutic outcome
* Prevention of rapid division of malignant cells

---

eplerenone (Rx)
(ep-ler-ee'known)
Inspra
Func. class.: Antihypertensive
Pregnancy category B

ACTION: Binds to mineralocorticoid receptor and blocks the binding of aldosterone, a component of the renin-angiotensin aldosterone system (RAAS)

Therapeutic outcome: Absence of hypertension

USES: Hypertension, alone or in combination with thiazide diuretics, CHF, post-MI

CONTRAINDICATIONS:
Hypersensitivity, increased serum creatinine >2 mg/dl (male) or >1.8 mg/dl (female), potassium >5.5 mEq/L, type 2 diabetes with microalbuminuria, hepatic disease, CCr <30 ml/min, CCr <50 ml/min in hypertension

Precautions: Pregnancy **B**, breastfeeding, children, geriatric, impaired renal/hepatic function, hyperkalemia

DOSAGE AND ROUTES
Adult: PO 50 mg/day initially, may increase to 50 mg bid after 4 wk; start dose at 25 mg/day if patient is taking CYP3A4 inhibitors

CHF/post-MI
Adult: PO 25 mg/day initially, may increase to 50 mg/day max

Available forms: Tabs 25, 50 mg

Implementation
* Store in tight container at 86° F (30° C) or less

ADVERSE EFFECTS
CNS: Headache, dizziness, fatigue
CV: Angina, **MI**
GI: Increased GGT diarrhea, abdominal pain, increased ALT
GU: Increased BUN, creatinine, gynecomastia, mastodynia (males), abnormal vaginal bleeding
META: Hyperkalemia, hyponatremia, hypercholesteremia, hypertriglyceridemia, increased uric acid
RESP: Cough

Pharmacokinetics
Absorption	Unknown
Distribution	Protein binding 50%
Metabolism	Liver (CYP3A4 inhibitor)
Excretion	Urine, feces
Half-life	4-6 hr

Pharmacodynamics
Onset	Unknown
Peak	$1\frac{1}{2}$ hr
Duration	Unknown

INTERACTIONS

Individual drugs
Erythromycin, fluconazole, itraconazole, ketoconazole, saquinavir, verapamil: increased levels of eplerenone; reduce dose of eplerenone
Lithium: increased serum lithium levels

Drug classifications
ACE inhibitors, angiotensin II antagonists, diuretics (potassium-sparing), NSAIDs, potassium supplements: increased hyperkalemia
CYP3A4 inhibitors: increased levels of eplerenone; reduce dose of eplerenone
NSAIDs: decreased antihypertensive effect

E

Drug/herb
Decreased antihypertensive effect: ephedra

Drug/food
Grapefruit, grapefruit juice: increased product level by 25%
• Do not use salt substitutes with potassium

NURSING CONSIDERATIONS

Assessment
• **Hypertension:** monitor B/P at peak/trough level of product, orthostatic hypotension, syncope when used with diuretic
• Monitor renal studies: protein, BUN, creatinine; increased liver function tests; uric acid may be increased
• Monitor potassium levels, hyperkalemia may occur

Nursing diagnoses
• Cardiac output, decreased (uses)
• Diarrhea (side effects)
• Knowledge, deficient (teaching)
• Noncompliance (teaching)

Patient/family education
• Advise patient not to discontinue product abruptly
• Advise patient not to use OTC products (cough, cold, allergy) unless directed by prescriber; do not use salt substitutes containing potassium without consulting prescriber
• Teach patient the importance of complying with dosage schedule, even if feeling better
• Teach patient that product may cause dizziness, fainting, light-headedness; may occur during first few days of therapy
• Teach patient how to take B/P, normal readings for age-group

Evaluation
Positive therapeutic outcome
• Decrease in B/P

---

epoetin alfa (Rx)
(ee-poe′e-tin)
Epogen, EPO, Eprex ✤, Procrit
Func. class.: Antianemic, biologic modifier, hormone
Chem. class.: Amino acid polypeptide
Pregnancy category C

ACTION: Erythropoietin is one factor controlling rate of red cell production; product is developed by recombinant DNA technology

Therapeutic outcome: Decreased anemia with increased RBCs

USES: Anemia caused by reduced endogenous erythropoietin production, primarily end-stage renal disease; to correct hemostatic defect in uremia; anemia caused by AZT (zidovudine) treatment in HIV-positive patients; anemia caused by chemotherapy; reduction of allogeneic blood transfusion in surgery patients

Unlabeled uses: Anemia in premature preterm infants

CONTRAINDICATIONS:
Hypersensitivity to mammalian cell–derived products or human albumin; uncontrolled hypertension

Precautions: Pregnancy C, breastfeeding, children <1 mo, seizure disorder, porphyria, CV disease, hemodialysis, latex allergy, hypertension, history of CABG; multidose preserved formulation contains benzyl alcohol and should not be used in premature infants

> **BLACK BOX WARNING:** Hgb >12 g/dl, surgery, neoplastic disease

DOSAGE AND ROUTES

Anemia secondary to chemotherapy (nonmyeloid malignancies)
Adult: SUBCUT 150 units/kg 3 ×/wk, may increase after 2 mo up to 300 units/kg 3 ×/wk

Anemia in chronic renal failure
Adult: SUBCUT/IV 50-100 units/kg 3 ×/wk, then adjust to maintain the target Hct of 30%-36%
Child: IV/SUBCUT 50 units/kg 3 ×/wk

Anemia secondary to zidovudine treatment
Adult: SUBCUT/IV 100 units/kg 3 ×/wk × 2 mo; may increase by 50-100 units/kg q1-2mo, up to 300 units/kg 3 ×/wk

Surgery
Adult: SUBCUT 300 units/kg/day × 10 days before surgery, the day of surgery, and for 4 days postsurgery or 600 units/kg 3, 2, 1 wk before and on day of surgery

Available forms: Inj 2000, 3000, 4000, 10,000, 20,000, 40,000 units/ml

Implementation
SUBCUT route
• Before injecting, preservative-free, single-dose formulation may be admixed by using 0.9% NaCl, USP, with benzyl alcohol 0.9% at a 1:1 ratio to reduce injection site discomfort

---

Direct IV route
• Administer by direct route at end of dialysis by venous line, do not shake vial
• If Hct increases by 4% in 2 wk, decrease dose by 25 units/kg; increase dose if Hct does not increase by 5-6 points after 8 wk of therapy; suggested target Hct range 30%-36%
• Give additional heparin to lower chance of clots

Solution compatibilities: Do not dilute or administer with other solutions

ADVERSE EFFECTS
CNS: Seizures, coldness, sweating, headache
CV: *Hypertension,* **hypertensive encephalopathy, CHF,** edema, **DVT**
INTEG: Pruritus, rash, inj site reaction
MISC: Iron deficiency
MS: Bone pain
RESP: Cough

Pharmacokinetics

Absorption	Well absorbed (SUBCUT), completely absorbed (**IV**)
Distribution	Increased RBC count 2-6 wk
Metabolism	Unknown
Excretion	Unknown
Half-life	5-14 hr

Pharmacodynamics

	SUBCUT/IV
Onset	Unknown
Peak	Immediate
Duration	Unknown

INTERACTIONS
Drug classifications
Anticoagulants: need for increased heparin during hemodialysis

NURSING CONSIDERATIONS
Assessment
• Monitor renal studies: urinalysis, protein, blood, BUN, creatinine; I&O; report drop in output to <50 ml/hr

BLACK BOX WARNING: Monitor blood studies: ferritin, transferrin monthly, transferrin sat ≥20%; ferritin ≥100 ng/ml; Hct 2 ×/wk until stabilized in target range (30%-36%), then at regular intervals; those with endogenous erythropoietin levels of <500 units/L respond to this agent; check for symptoms of anemia: fatigue, pallor, dyspnea; monitor Hct 2 ×/wk in chronic renal failure; cancer patients and those being treated with zidovudine should be monitored weekly, then periodically after stabilization; death may occur in Hgb >12 g/dl

• Assess for CNS symptoms: coldness, sweating, pain in long bones
• Assess CV status: B/P before, during treatment; hypertension may occur rapidly, leading to hypertension encephalopathy; antihypertensives may be needed
• Assess patient during hemodialysis for bruits, thrills, or shunts; product prevents severe anemia in chronic renal failure; clotting may need to be treated with increased anticoagulant
• **Seizures:** place on seizure precautions; assess for seizures if Hct is increased within 2 wk by 4 points, increased B/P, more common in chronic renal failure in the first 90 days of treatment
• Monitor serum iron, ferritin, transferrin levels; iron therapy may be needed to prevent recurring anemia
• Monitor B/P, check for rising B/P as Hct rises
• Monitor blood studies: BUN, creatinine, uric acid, platelets, WBC, phosphorus, potassium, bleeding time; Hct, Hgb, RBCs, reticulocytes should be checked in chronic renal failure
• For hypersensitivity reactions: Skin rashes, urticaria (rare), antibody development does not occur
⚠ For pure cell aplasia (PRCA) in absence of other causes, evaluate by testing serum for recombinant erythropoietin antibodies; any loss of response to epoetin should be evaluated

Nursing diagnoses
• Activity intolerance (uses)
• Fatigue (uses)
• Knowledge, deficient (teaching)

Patient/family education
• Teach patient how to take B/P
• Advise patients to take iron supplements, vit B$_{12}$, folic acid as directed
• Teach patient to avoid driving or hazardous activity during treatment
• Teach patients with renal disease to include high-iron and low-potassium foods in their

diets (meat, dark green leafy vegetables, eggs, enriched breads)
• Teach patient the reason for treatment, expected results
• Advise patient to use contraception

Evaluation
Positive therapeutic outcome
• Increased appetite
• Enhanced sense of well-being
• Increase in reticulocyte count in 2-6 wk, Hgb, Hct

---

eprosartan (Rx)
(ep-roh-sar′tan)
Teveten
Func. class.: Antihypertensive
Chem. class.: Angiotensin II receptor antagonist (Subtype AT_1)
Pregnancy category C (1st trimester), D (2nd/3rd trimesters)

ACTION: Blocks the vasoconstrictor and aldosterone-secreting effects of angiotensin II; selectively blocks the binding of angiotensin II to the AT_1 receptor found in tissues

Therapeutic outcome: Decreased B/P

USES: Hypertension, alone or in combination with other antihypertensives

CONTRAINDICATIONS:
Hypersensitivity

> **BLACK BOX WARNING:** Pregnancy **D** (2nd/3rd trimesters)

Precautions: Pregnancy **C** (1st trimester), breastfeeding, children, geriatric, hypersensitivity to ACE inhibitors, renal/hepatic disease, angioedema

DOSAGE AND ROUTES
Adult: PO 600 mg/day; dose may be divided and given bid, with total daily doses ranging from 400-800 mg, max 900 mg/day

Available forms: Tabs 400, 600 mg

Implementation
• May be given without regard to meals

ADVERSE EFFECTS
CNS: *Dizziness,* depression, fatigue, headache
CV: Chest pain
EENT: Sinusitis
GI: *Diarrhea, dyspepsia,* abdominal pain

GU: UTI
INTEG: Pruritus, **angioedema**
META: Hypertriglyceridemia
MS: Myalgia, arthralgia, **rhabdomyolysis**
RESP: *Cough, upper respiratory infection,* rhinitis, pharyngitis, viral infection
SYST: Anaphylaxis

Pharmacokinetics

Absorption	Absolute bioavailability ~13%; food delays absorption
Distribution	Protein binding 98%
Metabolism	Moderate renal impairment increases product levels by 30%, hepatic impairment increases levels by 40%
Excretion	Urine, feces
Half-life	5-9 hr

Pharmacodynamics

Onset	Unknown
Peak	1-2 hr
Duration	Unknown

INTERACTIONS

Drug classifications
NSAIDs, salicylates: decreased antihypertensive effect

Drug/lab test
Increased: ALT, AST, alkaline phosphatase
Decreased: Hgb

NURSING CONSIDERATIONS

Assessment
• Assess B/P with position changes, pulse q4hr; note rate, rhythm, quality
• Assess electrolytes: K, Na, Cl
• Assess baselines in renal, liver function tests before therapy begins
• Assess for edema in feet, legs daily
• Assess skin turgor, dryness of mucous membranes for hydration status

Nursing diagnoses
• Fluid volume, deficient (adverse reactions)
• Injury, risk for (adverse reactions)
• Knowledge, deficient (teaching)
• Noncompliance (teaching)

Patient/family education
• Advise patient to comply with dosage schedule, even if feeling better
• Advise patient to notify prescriber of fever, swelling of hands or feet, chest pain

---

⚠ Nurse Alert

• Inform patient that excessive perspiration, dehydration, diarrhea may lead to fall in blood pressure; consult prescriber if these occur

• Inform patient that product may cause dizziness; advise to avoid hazardous activities until effect is known

> **BLACK BOX WARNING:** Advise patient not to take this medication if pregnant or breastfeeding, or if allergic reaction to this product has occurred

• Advise patient to take missed dose as soon as possible, unless within 1 hr of next dose

Evaluation
Positive therapeutic outcome
• Decreased B/P

⚠ HIGH ALERT

eptifibatide (Rx)
(ep-tih-fib′ah-tide)
Integrilin
Func. class.: Antiplatelet agent
Chem. class.: Glycoprotein IIb/IIIa inhibitor
Pregnancy category B

ACTION: Platelet glycoprotein antagonist; reversibly prevents fibrinogen, von Willebrand factor from binding to the glycoprotein IIb/IIIa receptor, inhibiting platelet aggregation

Therapeutic outcome: Decreased platelets

USES: Acute coronary syndrome, including those undergoing percutaneous coronary intervention (PCI)

CONTRAINDICATIONS:
Hypersensitivity, active internal bleeding, history of bleeding, stroke within 2 yr, major surgery with severe trauma, severe hypertension, history of intracranial bleeding, current or planned use of another parenteral GPIIb/IIIa inhibitor, dependence on renal dialysis, coagulopathy, AV malformation, aneurysm

Precautions: Pregnancy **B**, breastfeeding, children, geriatric, bleeding, renal function impairment

DOSAGE AND ROUTES
Acute coronary syndrome
Adult: **IV** BOL 180 mcg/kg as soon as diagnosed, max 22.6 mg; then **IV** CONT INF 2 mcg/kg/min until discharge or coronary artery bypass graft (CABG) up to 72 hr, max 15 mg/hr

PCI in patients without acute coronary syndrome
Adult: **IV** BOL 180 mcg/kg given immediately before PCI; then 2 mcg/kg/min × 18 hr and a 2nd 180 mcg/kg BOL, 10 min after 1st BOL; continue INF for up to 18-24 hr at a rate of 1 mcg/kg/min

Renal dose
Adult: **IV** BOL CCr <50 ml/min 2-4 mg/dl same loading dose, then ¹/₂ usual INF dose; CCr <10 ml/min contraindicated

Available forms: Sol for inj 2 mg/ml (10 ml), 0.75 mg/ml (100 ml)

Implementation
• Aspirin and heparin may be given with this product; check for bleeding

• Discontinue heparin before removing femoral artery sheath after PCI

Direct IV route
• After withdrawing the BOL dose from 10-ml vial, give **IV** push over 1-2 min

• Do not use discolored sol or sol with particulate

Continuous IV infusion route
• Follow BOL dose with cont inf using infusion pump, give product undiluted directly from the 100-ml vial, spike the 100-ml vial with a vented infusion set; use caution when centering the spike on the circle of the stopper top

Y-site compatibilities: Alfentanil, alteplase, amikacin, aminophylline, amphotericin B lipid complex, amphotericin B liposome, ampicillin, ampicillin-sulbactam, anidulafungin, argatroban, atenolol, atracurium, atropine, azithromycin, aztreonam, bivalirudin, bumetanide, buprenorphine, butorphanol, calcium chloride/gluconate, ceFAZolin, cefepime, cefoperazone, cefotaxime, cefotetan, cefoxitin, ceftazidime, ceftizoxime, cefTRIAXone, cefuroxime, cimetidine, ciprofloxacin, cisatracurium, clindamycin, cycloSPORINE, DAPTOmycin, dexamethasone, D₅/NaCl 0.9%, diazepam, diltiazem, diphenhydrAMINE, DOBUTamine, dolasetron, DOPamine, doxycycline, droperidol, enalaprilat, ePHEDrine, EPINEPHrine, ertapenem, erythromycin, esmolol, famotidine, fentaNYL, fluconazole, fosphenytoin, ganciclovir, gatifloxacin, gentamicin, granisetron, haloperidol, heparin, hydrocortisone, HYDROmorphone, hydrOXYzine, imipenem-cilastatin, inamrinone, isoproterenol, ketorolac, labetalol, leucovorin, levofloxacin, levorphanol, lidocaine, linezolid, LORazepam, magnesium sulfate, mannitol, meperidine, meropenem, methylPREDNISolone, metoclopramide, metoprolol, metroNIDAZOLE, micafungin, midazolam, milrinone, minocycline, mivacurium, morphine, nalbuphine, naloxone, niCARdipine, nitroglycerin, nitroprusside, NS, octreotide, ofloxacin, ondansetron, oxytocin, palonosetron, pancuronium, pemetrexed, PENTobarbital, PHENobarbital, phenylephrine, piperacillin, piperacillin-tazobactam, potassium chloride/phosphates, procainamide, prochlorperazine, promethazine, propranolol, ranitidine, remifentanil, rocuronium, sodium bicarbonate/phosphates, succinylcholine, SUFentanil, sulfamethoxazole-trimethoprim, teniposide, theophylline, ticarcillin, ticarcillin-clavulanate, tigecycline, tirofiban, tobramycin, trimethobenzamide, vancomycin, vecuronium, verapamil, zidovudine, zoledronic acid

Solution compatibilities: 0.9% NaCl, D_5/0.9% NaCl

• Discontinue product before CABG
• Give all medications PO if possible, avoid IM inj and catheters

ADVERSE EFFECTS
CV: Stroke, hypotension
GU: Hematuria
HEMA: Thrombocytopenia
SYST: Bleeding, anaphylaxis

Pharmacokinetics

Absorption	Unknown
Distribution	Protein binding 25%
Metabolism	Limited
Excretion	Kidneys
Half-life	1.5-2 hr

Pharmacodynamics

Onset	Within 1 hr

INTERACTIONS
Individual drugs
Abciximab, aspirin, clopidogrel, dipyridamole, heparin, ticlopidine, valproate: increased bleeding

Drug classifications
Anticoagulants, NSAIDs, thrombolytics: increased bleeding
Platelet receptor inhibitors IIb, IIIa: do not give together

Drug/herb
Arnica, chamomile, clove, dong quai, feverfew, garlic, ginger, ginkgo, Panax ginseng

NURSING CONSIDERATIONS
Assessment
• **Thrombocytopenia:** Monitor platelets, Hgb, Hct, creatinine, pro-time/APTT baseline, INR, within 6 hr of loading dose and daily thereafter; patients undergoing PCI should have ACT monitored; maintain APTT 50-70 sec unless PCI is to be performed; during PCI, ACT should be 200-300 sec; if platelets drop <100,000/mm³, obtain additional platelet counts; if thrombocytopenia is confirmed, discontinue product; also draw Hct, Hgb, serum creatinine
• **Assess for bleeding:** gums, bruising, ecchymosis, petechiae; from GI, GU tract, cardiac catheter sites, IM inj sites

Nursing diagnoses
• Knowledge, deficient (teaching)

Patient/family education
• Teach patient to report bruising, bleeding, chest pain immediately
• Inform patient of reason for medication and expected results

Evaluation
Positive therapeutic outcome
• Decreased platelets

ergocalciferol
See vitamin D

ergotamine (Rx)
(er-got'a-meen)
Ergomar
dihydroergotamine
(dy-hy'droh-er-got'ah-meen)
DHE 45, Migranal
Func. class.: α-Adrenergic blocker, vascular headache suppressant
Chem. class.: Ergot alkaloid–amino acid
Pregnancy category X

ACTION: Constricts smooth muscle in peripheral, cranial blood vessels; relaxes uterine muscle; blocks serotonin release

Therapeutic outcome: Absence of headache

USES: Vascular headache (migraine, histamine, cluster)

CONTRAINDICATIONS:
Pregnancy **X**, hypersensitivity to ergot preparations, occlusion (peripheral, vascular), renal/

hepatic disease, peptic ulcer, intermittent claudication, glaucoma, CVA

> **BLACK BOX WARNING:** CAD, hypertension, Raynaud's disease, peripheral vascular disease, angina

Precautions: Breastfeeding, children, geriatric, anemia, basilar/hemiplegic migraine

> **BLACK BOX WARNING:** MI, stroke, Buerger's disease, cardiac disease

DOSAGE AND ROUTES

ergotamine
Adult: SL 1 tab (2 mg), may use q30min, max 3 tabs (6 mg)/24 hr or 10 mg/wk

dihydroergotamine
Adult: SUBCUT/IM/**IV** 1 mg, may repeat in 1 hr to 3 mg, max 3 mg/day (IM, SUBCUT), 2 mg (**IV**) or 6 mg/ wk; Intranasal 1 spray in each nostril, repeat in 15 min, max 3 mg/24 hr, 4 mg/wk
Child ≥6 yr: SUBCUT/IM 0.5 mg, may repeat in 1 hr; **IV** 0.25 mg, may repeat in 1 hr

Available forms: Ergotamine: SL tab 2 mg; tabs 1 mg; dihydroergotamine: inj 1 mg/ml; nasal spray 4 mg/ml

Implementation
SL route
• Do not break, crush, chew, or swallow SL tab
• Place tab under tongue, do not drink, eat, or smoke until tab has dissolved
Inhalation route
• Teach patient how to use inhaler, protect ampules from heat, light
Direct IV route
• Give dihydroergotamine undiluted over 1 min

ADVERSE EFFECTS
CNS: *Numbness in fingers, toes,* headache, weakness
CV: Transient tachycardia, chest pain, bradycardia, edema, claudication, increase or decrease in B/P, **MI,** peripheral vascular ischemia
GI: Nausea, vomiting, diarrhea, abdominal cramps
MS: Muscle pain

Pharmacokinetics

Absorption	Erratic (PO), poor (SL), rapidly (SUBCUT, IM)
Distribution	Crosses blood-brain barrier
Metabolism	Liver, extensively
Excretion	Kidneys (metabolites)
Half-life	Biphasic 2.7 hr, 21 hr

Pharmacodynamics

	PO	SL	IM/SUBCUT	IV
Onset	1-2 hr	Unknown	Unknown	Unknown
Peak	$1/2$-3 hr	Unknown	Unknown	$1/4$-2 hr
Duration	Unknown	Unknown	8 hr	8 hr

INTERACTIONS
Individual drugs
Nicotine: increased vasoconstriction

Drug classifications
β-Blockers, contraceptives (oral), vasoconstrictors, other migraine agents: increased vasoconstriction
CYP450384 inhibitors (protease inhibitors, some macrolides, azole antifungals): increased ergot toxicity; do not use together

NURSING CONSIDERATIONS
Assessment
• **Assess characteristics of migraine:** duration, intensity, location, frequency, alleviating factors; also identify if halos, nausea, vomiting, blurred vision occur with headache; assess before, during treatment
• **Assess for ergotism or overdose:** nausea, vomiting, weakness, muscular pain, insensitivity to cold, paresthesia of extremities; product should be decreased or infusion discontinued
• **Check for hypertension:** B/P, pulse, monitor all peripheral pulses; if hypertension occurs, notify prescriber; also check for tachycardia or bradycardia

> **BLACK BOX WARNING: CAD, hypertension, Raynaud's disease, angina, MI, stroke:** Do not use in these patients

Nursing diagnoses
• Injury, risk for (adverse reactions)
• Knowledge, deficient (teaching)
• Pain, acute (uses)

Patient/family education
• Caution patient not to smoke during treatment to prevent excessive vasoconstriction
• Advise patient to avoid alcohol or OTC medications unless approved by prescriber
• Tell patient to inform prescriber if pregnancy occurs
• Advise patient to keep product out of children's reach; death may occur

Evaluation
Positive therapeutic outcome
• Decreasing headache

TREATMENT OF OVERDOSE:
Stop product, give vasodilators, heparin, dextran

---

eribulin (Rx)
(er'i-bue'lin)
Halaven
Func. class.: Antineoplastics, nontaxane
Pregnancy category D

ACTION: Potent antimitotic agent, different from taxes, vinca alkaloids, epothilones; blocks cell progression in G_2-M phase, inhibits the growth phase of microtubules and sequesters tubules, leading to disruption of mitotic spindles and apoptotic cell death

Therapeutic outcome: Decreased spread and size of tumor

USES: Metastatic breast cancer patients who have received at least 2 chemotherapy regimens

CONTRAINDICATIONS:
Hypersensitivity, pregnancy **D**

Precautions: Bradycardia, breastfeeding, children, electrolyte imbalances, heart failure, hepatic disease, hypokalemia, hypomagnesemia, infertility, neonates, neutropenia, peripheral neuropathy, QT prolongation, renal disease

DOSAGE AND ROUTES
Adult: **IV** 1.4 mg/m² over 2-5 min on days 1 and 8, repeat q21days

Recommendations for dose delay
• *For ANC < 1000/mm³, platelets ,75,000/ mm³, or grade 3 or 4 non-hematologic toxicities:* Do not administer; the day 8 dose may be delayed a maximum of 1 wk
• *For the day 8 dose, if toxicities do not resolve to ≤grade 2 by day 15:* Omit the dose

• *For the day 8 dose, if toxicities resolve or improve to ≤ grade 2 by day 15:* Administer eribulin at a reduced dose (see below) and initiate the next cycle no sooner than 2 wk later

Dosage adjustments for hematologic toxicity
• *ANC < 500/mm3 for >7 days or ANC <1000/mm³ with fever or infection:* Permanently reduce dosage to 1.1 mg/m²
• *Platelets <25,000/mm³ or <50,000/mm³ requiring transfusion:* Permanently reduce dosage to 1.1 mg/m²
• *If day 8 of previous cycle omitted or delayed:* Permanently reduce dosage to 1.1 mg/m²
• *While receiving 1.1 mg/m², if recurrence of hematologic event occurs, or if day 8 of previous cycle omitted or delayed:* Permanently reduce dosage to 0.7 mg/m²
• *While receiving 0.7 mg/m², if recurrence of hematologic event occurs, or if day 8 of previous cycle omitted or delayed:* Discontinue

Dose adjustments of eribulin for non-hematologic toxicity during treatment
• *Any grade 3 or 4 non-hematologic toxicity:* Permanently reduce dosage to 1.1 mg/m²
• *If day 8 of previous cycle omitted or delayed:* Permanently reduce dosage to 1.1 mg/m²
• *While receiving 1.1 mg/m², if recurrence of grade 3 or 4 non-hematologic toxicity occurs, or if day 8 of previous cycle omitted or delayed:* Permanently reduce dosage to 0.7 mg/ m²
• *While receiving 0.7 mg/m², if recurrence of grade 3 or 4 non-hematologic toxicity occurs, or if day 8 of previous cycle omitted or delayed:* Discontinue

Available forms: Solution for injection 1 mg/2 ml

Implementation
IV direct, intermittent route
• Visually inspect for particulate matter or discoloration as solution and container permit; withdraw required amount (0.5 mg/ml) from single-use vial, give undiluted over 2-5 min or diluted in 100 ml 0.9% NaCl and give as intermittent infusion, do not give through line with dextrose or any other product
• Store at room temperature for 4 hr or 24 hr refrigerated

ADVERSE EFFECTS
CNS: Depression, dizziness, fatigue, fever, headache, insomnia, peripheral neuropathy
CV: QT prolongation, peripheral edema

GI: Abdominal pain, anorexia, constipation, diarrhea, dyspepsia, nausea, vomiting, weight loss
HEMA: Anemia, neutropenia, thrombocytopenia
INTEG: Alopecia, rash, stomatitis
META: Hypokalemia
MS: Arthralgia, myalgia, bone/back pain
RESP: Cough, dyspnea
SYST: Infection

Pharmacokinetics

Absorption	Protein binding, 49-65%
Distribution	Unknown
Metabolism	Inhibits CYP3A4
Excretion	Feces 82%, urine 9%
Half-life	40 hr, increased levels in renal/hepatic disease

Pharmacodynamics

Unknown

INTERACTIONS

Individual drugs

Arsenic trioxide, astemizole, bepridil, chloroquine, cisapride, clarithromycin, dextromethorphan, dronedarone, droperidol, erythromycin, halofantrine, haloperidol, levomethadyl, methadone, pentamidine, pimozide, posaconazole, probucol, propafenone, quiNIDine, saquinavir, sparfloxacin, terfenadine, troleandomycin, and ziprasidone; also to a lesser degree abarelix, alfuzosin, amoxapine, apomorphine, artemether; lumefantrine, asenapine, ofloxacin, clozapine, cyclobenzaprine, dasatinib, dolasetron, flecainide, gatifloxacin, gemifloxacin, iloperidone, lapatinib, levofloxacin, lopinavir; ritonavir, magnesium sulfate; potassium sulfate; sodium sulfate, maprotiline, mefloquine, moxifloxacin, nilotinib, norfloxacin, octreotide, ciprofloxacin, OLANZapine, ondansetron, paliperidone, palonosetron, QUEtiapine, ranolazine, risperidone, sertindole, sunitinib, tacrolimus, telavancin, telithromycin, tetrabenazine, venlafaxine, vardenafil, vorinostat: increased QT prolongation

Drug classifications

Certain phenothiazines (chlorpromazine, mesoridazine, thioridazine), class IA antiarrhythmics (disopyramide, procainamide, quiNIDine), class III antiarrhythmics (amiodarone, bretylium, dofetilide, ibutilide, sotalol), also to a lesser degree, beta-agonists, halogenated anesthetics, local anesthetics, some phenothiazines (fluphenazine, perphenazine,

prochlorperazine, trifluoperazine), tricyclic antidepressants: increased QT prolongation

NURSING CONSIDERATIONS

Assessment

• **QT prolongation:** assess for drug interactions that may occur; monitor ECG, heart rate
• **Bone marrow depression:** CBC and differential, serum creatinine/bun/electrolytes, liver function tests, baseline and periodically, increased AST/ALT $>3 \times$ ULN or total bilirubin $>1.5 \times$ ULN are at a greater chance of grade 4 or febrile neutropenia

Nursing diagnoses

• Injury, risk for (adverse reactions)
• Infection, risk for (adverse reactions)

Patient/family education

• Teach patient reason for product and expected results
• Advise patient to report side effects to health care provider
• Advise patient to avoid other medications, supplements unless approved by provider, serious drug interactions may occur
• Discuss hair loss and use of wig or hairpiece
• Advise patient to notify prescriber if pregnancy is planned or suspected (pregnancy **D**), avoid breastfeeding

Evaluation
Positive therapeutic outcome
• Decreasing tumor spread and size

erlotinib (Rx)
(er-loe′tye-nib)
Tarceva
Func. class.: Misc. antineoplastic
Chem. class.: Epidermal growth factor receptor inhibitor
Pregnancy category D

ACTION: Not fully understood. Inhibits intracellular phosphorylation of cell surface receptors associated with epidermal growth factor receptors.

Therapeutic outcome: Decrease in tumor size

USES: Non–small cell lung cancer (NSCLC), pancreatic cancer

Unlabeled uses: Squamous cell, head and neck cancer

CONTRAINDICATIONS:
Pregnancy **D**, breastfeeding, hypersensitivity

Precautions: Renal, hepatic; ocular, pulmonary disorders; children; geriatric, tobacco smoking, radiation therapy, fever, dehydration, chemotherapy

DOSAGE AND ROUTES

CYP3A4 inducers concurrently (such as rifampin or phenytoin)
Dosage increase is advised

CYP3A4 inhibitors (atazanavir, clarithromycin, indinavir, itraconazole, ketoconazole, telithromycin, ritonavir, saquinavir, troleandomycin, nelfinavir)
Dosage reduction may be needed.

Non–small cell lung cancer (NSCLC)
Adult: PO 150 mg/day

Pancreatic cancer
Adult: PO 100 mg/day in combination with gemcitabine 1000 mg/m² cycle 1, days 1, 8, 15, 22, 29, 36, 43 of an 8-wk cycle; cycle 2 and subsequent cycles, days 1, 8, 15 of a 4-wk cycle

Available forms: Tabs 25, 100, 150 mg

Implementation
• Administer 1 hr before or 2 hr after food

ADVERSE EFFECTS
CNS: CVA, anxiety, depression, headache, rigors
CV: MI/ischemia
EENT: Ocular changes, *conjunctivitis, eye pain*
GI: *Nausea, diarrhea, vomiting, anorexia, mouth ulceration,* hepatic failure, GI perforation
GU: Renal impairment/failure
HEMA: DVT
INTEG: *Rash,* Stevens-Johnson–like skin reactions, toxic epidermal necrolysis
MISC: *Fatigue, infection*
RESP: Interstitial lung disease, *cough, dyspnea,* ARDS, pulmonary fibrosis
SYST: Hepatorenal syndrome

Pharmacokinetics

Absorption	Slowly absorbed
Distribution	Unknown
Metabolism	Metabolized by CYP3A4
Excretion	Feces (86%), urine (<4%)
Half-life	36 hr

Pharmacodynamics

Onset	Unknown
Peak	3-7 hr
Duration	Unknown

INTERACTIONS

Individual drugs
Metoprolol, warfarin: increased plasma concentrations
Smoking: decreased erlotinib level, dose may need to be increased

Drug classifications
CYP3A4 inducers (phenytoin, rifampin, carbamazepine, phenobarbital): decreased erlotinib levels
CYP3A4 inhibitors (clarithromycin, erythromycin, itraconazole, ketoconazole, telithromycin): increased erlotinib concentrations

Drug/herb
St. John's wort: decreased erlotinib levels

Drug/food
Grapefruit juice: increased effect of erlotinib

NURSING CONSIDERATIONS

Assessment
⚠ Assess for MI/ischemia, CVA in pancreatic cancer
⚠ Assess for pulmonary changes: lung sounds, cough, dyspnea; interstitial lung disease may occur, may be fatal; discontinue therapy if confirmed
• Assess for ocular changes: eye irritation, corneal erosion/ulcer, aberrant eyelash growth
• Assess for GI symptoms: frequency of stools; if diarrhea is poorly tolerated, therapy may be discontinued for up to 14 days
• Monitor blood studies: INR, LFTs, PT
• **Hepatic failure:** interrupt dosing if severe changes to liver function occur (total bilirubin >3× ULN and/or transaminases >5× ULN for normal pretreatment LFTs)

Nursing diagnoses
• Body image, disturbed (adverse reactions)
• Infection, risk for (adverse reactions)
• Injury, risk for (adverse reactions)
• Knowledge, deficient (teaching)

Patient/family education
⚠ Teach patient to report adverse reactions immediately: SOB, severe abdominal pain, persistent diarrhea or vomiting, ocular changes, skin eruptions
• Explain reason for treatment, expected results

- Advise patient to use contraception during treatment; pregnancy **D,** avoid breastfeeding

Evaluation
Positive therapeutic outcome
- Decrease non–small cell lung cancer cells

---

ertapenem (Rx)
(er-tah-pen′em)
Invanz
Func. class.: Antiinfective, miscellaneous
Chem. class.: Carbapenem
Pregnancy category B

Do not confuse:
Invanz/Aninza

ACTION: Interferes with cell wall replication of susceptible organisms; osmotically unstable cell wall swells, bursts from osmotic pressure

Therapeutic outcome: Bactericidal action against the following organisms: *Bacteroides fragilis, Bacteroides distasonis, Bacteroides ovatus, Bacteroides thetaiotaomicron, Bacteroides uniformis; Clostridium clostridioforme, Escherichia coli, Eubacterium lentum, Haemophilus influenzae* (β lactamase–negative), *Klebsiella pneumoniae, Moraxella catarrhalis, Peptostreptococcus* sp., *Porphyromonas asaccharolytica, Prevotella bivia, Staphylococcus aureus* (methicillin-susceptible); *Streptococcus agalactiae, Streptococcus pneumoniae* (penicillin-susceptible), *Streptococcus pyogenes*

USES: Adult patients with moderate to severe intraabdominal infections, complicated skin/skin structure infections, community-acquired pneumonia, complicated UTI, acute pelvic infections; infection prophylaxis prior to elective colorectal surgery

CONTRAINDICATIONS:
Hypersensitivity to this product or its components, to amide-type local anesthetics (IM only); anaphylactic reactions to β-lactams

Precautions: Pregnancy **B,** breastfeeding, children, geriatric, renal/hepatic/GI disease

DOSAGE AND ROUTES
Complicated intraabdominal infections
Adult: IM/IV 1 g/day × 5-14 days

Child 3 mo-12 yr: IM/IV 15 mg/kg bid (max 1 g/day) × 5-14 days

Complicated skin/skin structure infections
Adult: IM/IV 1 g/day × 7-14 days
Child 3 mo-12 yr: IM/IV 15 mg/kg bid × 7-14 days

Community-acquired pneumonia
Adult: IM/IV 1 g/day × 10-14 days
Child 3 mo-12 yr: IM/IV 15 mg/kg bid × 10-14 days

Complicated UTI
Adult: IM/IV 1 g/day × 10-14 days
Child 3 mo-12 yr: IM/IV 15 mg/kg bid × 10-14 days

Acute pelvic infections
Adult: IM/IV 1 g/day × 3-10 days
Child 3 mo-12 yr: IM/IV 15 mg/kg bid × 3-10 days

Surgical infection prophylaxis
Adult: IV 1 g as a single dose 1 hr prior to surgical incision

Available forms: Powder, lyophilized, 1 g

Implementation
- Administer by **IV** or IM
- Give after C&S is taken
IM route
- Reconstitute 1 g vial of ertapenem with 3.2 ml of 1% lidocaine HCl without EPINEPHrine, shake well
- Withdraw contents, administer IM deep in large muscle mass, use within 1 hr

Intermittent IV infusion route
- Do not co-infuse or mix with other medications; do not use diluents containing dextrose
- Reconstitute 1 g vial of ertapenem with either 10 ml of water for inj, 0.9% NaCl, or bacteriostatic water for inj (100 mg/ml)
- Shake well to dissolve, transfer contents of reconstituted vial to 50 ml 0.9% NaCl inj
- Complete inf within 6 hr

Y-site compatibilities: Acyclovir, alfentanil, amifostine, amikacin, aminocaproic acid, aminophylline, amphotericin B lipid complex, amphotericin B liposome, argatroban, arsenic trioxide, atenolol, atracurium, azithromycin, aztreonam, bivalirudin, bleomycin, bumetanide, buprenorphine, busulfan, butorphanol, calcium chloride/gluconate, CARBOplatin, carmustine, chloramphenicol, cimetidine, ciprofloxacin, cisatracurium, CISplatin, cyclophosphamide, cycloSPORINE, cytarabine, dacarbazine, DACTINomycin, DAPTOmycin, dexamethasone,

dexmedetomidine, dexrazoxane, digoxin, diltiazem, diphenhydrAMINE, docetaxel, dolasetron,
DOPamine, doxacurium, doxycycline, enalaprilat, ePHEDrine, EPINEPHrine, eptifibatide,
erythromycin, esmolol, etoposide, famotidine,
fenoldopam, fluconazole, fludarabine, fluorouracil, foscarnet, fosphenytoin, furosemide,
ganciclovir, gatifloxacin, gemcitabine, gemtuzumab, gentamicin, glycopyrrolate, granisetron,
haloperidol, heparin, hydrocortisone, HYDRO-
morphone, ifosfamide, inamrinone, insulin
(regular), irinotecan, isoproterenol, ketorolac,
labetalol, leucovorin, levofloxacin, lidocaine,
linezolid, LORazepam, magnesium sulfate, mannitol, mechlorethamine, melphalan, meperidine,
mesna, metaraminol, methotrexate, methyldopate, methylPREDNISolone, metoclopramide,
metroNIDAZOLE, milrinone, mitomycin, mivacurium, morphine, moxifloxacin, nalbuphine,
naloxone, nesiritide, nitroglycerin, nitroprusside, norepinephrine, octreotide, oxaliplatin,
oxytocin, paclitaxel, pamidronate, pancuronium,
pantoprazole, pemetrexed, PENTobarbital,
PHENobarbital, phentolamine, phenylephrine,
polymixin B, potassium acetate/chloride/
phosphates, procainamide, propranolol,
ranitidine, remifentanil, rocuronium, sodium
acetate/bicarbonate/phosphates, streptozocin,
succinylcholine, SUFentanil, sulfamethoxazole-
trimethoprim, tacrolimus, teniposide, theophylline, thiotepa, tigecycline, tirofiban, tobramycin,
trimethobenzamide, vancomycin, vasopressin,
vecuronium, vinBLAStine, vinCRIStine, vinorelbine, voriconazole, zidovudine

ADVERSE EFFECTS

CNS: Insomnia, **seizures,** dizziness, *head-
ache*
CV: Tachycardia
GI: *Diarrhea, nausea, vomiting,* **pseudo-
membranous colitis**
GU: *Vaginitis*
INTEG: *Rash,* urticaria, *pruritus,* pain at inj
site, *infused vein complication, phlebitis/
thrombophlebitis,* erythema at inj site
RESP: Dyspnea, cough, pharyngitis, crackles,
respiratory distress
SYST: Anaphylaxis

Pharmacokinetics

Absorption	Almost completely absorbed (IM); completely absorbed (**IV**)
Distribution	85%-95% plasma protein bound
Metabolism	Liver (IM, **IV**)
Excretion	Urine (80%), feces (10%), breast milk (IM, **IV**)
Half-life	4 hr (**IV**)

Pharmacodynamics

	IM	IV
Onset	Unknown	Immediate
Peak	2.3 hr	Dose-dependent
Duration	Unknown	Unknown

INTERACTIONS

Individual drugs
Probenecid: increased ertapenem plasma levels;
do not coadminister

Drug/lab test
Increased: hepatic enzymes

NURSING CONSIDERATIONS

Assessment
• Assess for renal disease: lower dose may be
required
• **Pseudomembranous colitis:** Assess bowel
pattern daily: if severe diarrhea occurs, product
should be discontinued
• **Assess for infection:** temp, sputum, characteristics of wound before, during, after treatment
⚠ Assess for allergic reactions, anaphylaxis: rash, urticaria, pruritus may occur a
few days after therapy begins; assess for
sensitivity to carbapenem antibiotics, other
β-lactam antibiotics, penicillins
• Assess for overgrowth of infection: perineal
itching, fever, malaise, redness, pain, swelling,
drainage, rash, diarrhea, change in cough or
sputum

Nursing diagnoses
• Diarrhea (adverse reaction)
• Infection, risk for (uses)
• Injury, risk for (adverse reactions)
• Knowledge, deficient (teaching)
• Noncompliance (teaching)

Patient/family education
• Advise patient to report severe diarrhea; may
indicate pseudomembranous colitis
• Advise patient to report overgrowth of
infection: black, furry tongue, vaginal itching,
foul-smelling stools

E

• Caution patient to avoid breastfeeding; product is excreted in breast milk

Evaluation
Positive therapeutic outcome
• Negative C&S, absence of signs and symptoms of infection

TREATMENT OF OVERDOSE:
Administer EPINEPHrine, antihistamines; resuscitate if needed (anaphylaxis)

---

erythromycin base (Rx)
(eh-rith-roh-my'sin)
Apo Erythro ✹, Ery-Tab, Novo-Rythro Encap ✹, PCE
erythromycin ethylsuccinate (Rx)
Apo-Erythro-ES ✹, EES, Ery Ped, Novo-Rythro ✹
erythromycin lactobionate (Rx)
Erythrocin
erythromycin stearate (Rx)
Apo-Erythro-S ✹, My-E, Novo-Rythro ✹
Func. class.: Antiinfective
Chem. class.: Macrolide
Pregnancy category B

Do not confuse:
erythromycin/azithromycin

ACTION: Binds to 50S ribosomal subunits of susceptible bacteria and suppresses protein synthesis

Therapeutic outcome: Bactericidal action against the following organisms: *Neisseria gonorrhoeae, Streptococcus pneumoniae, Mycoplasma pneumoniae, Corynebacterium diphtheriae, Bordetella pertussis, Borrelia burgdorferi, Listeria monocytogenes, Treponema pallidum;* streptococci, staphylocci; gram-negative pathogens: *Neisseria, Haemophilus influenzae* (when used with sulfonamides), *Legionella pneumophila, Chlamydia trachomatis*

USES: Mild to moderate respiratory tract, skin, soft tissue infections, Legionnaire's disease, syphilis

CONTRAINDICATIONS:
Hypersensitivity, preexisting liver disease (estolate)

Precautions: Pregnancy **B**, breastfeeding, geriatric, hepatic/GI disease, QT prolongation, seizure disorder, myasthenia gravis

DOSAGE AND ROUTES
Lower/upper respiratory infections
Adult: PO (base, stearate) 250-500 mg q6hr; **PO** (ethylsuccinate) 400-800 mg q6hr; **IV INF** (lactobionate) 15-20 mg/kg/day divided q6hr
Adolescent/child/infant: PO 20-50 mg/kg/day divided q6hr, max adult dose
Neonates >7 days, weighing ≥1200 g: PO 30 mg/day in divided doses q8hr
Neonates >7 days, weighing <1200 g: PO 20 mg/kg/day divided q12hr
Neonates ≤7 days: PO 20 mg/kg/day divided q12hr

N. gonorrhoeae/PID
Adult: **IV** 500 mg q6hr × 3 days (gluceptate, lactobionate), then PO 250 mg (base, estolate, stearate) or 400 mg (ethylsuccinate) q6hr × 1 wk

Pertussis (whooping cough) treatment/prophylaxis
Adult: PO 500 mg qid (2 g total) × 14 days
Infants, children, adolescents: PO 40-50 mg/kg/day, max 2 g/day in divided doses × 14 days

Syphilis
Adult: PO 500 mg qid × 14 days

Chlamydia
Adult: PO 500 mg q6hr × 1 wk or 250 mg qid × 2 wk
Infant: PO 50 mg/kg/day in 4 divided doses × 3 wk or more

Intestinal amebiasis
Adult: PO 250 mg q6hr × 10-14 days (base, estolate, stearate)
Child: PO 30-50 mg/kg/day in divided doses q6hr × 10-14 days (base, estolate, stearate)

Available forms: Base: enteric-coated tab 250, 333, 500 mg; film-coated tab 250, 500 mg; enteric-coated caps, 250, 333 mg; stearate: film-coated tabs, 250 mg, granules for oral susp: 200, 400 mg/5 ml powder for inj 500 mg, 1 g (lactobionate); 1 g (as gluceptate)

Implementation
PO route
• Give around the clock on an empty stomach, at least 1 hr before or 2 hr after meals; may be taken with food if GI upset occurs; do not take with juices; take dose with a full glass of water; use calibrated measuring device for drops or susp; shake well

---

Adverse effects: *italics* = common; **bold** = life-threatening

- Store susp in refrigerator
- Chewable tab may be crushed or chewed, not swallowed whole
- Do not crush or chew enteric-coated tab

IV route
- Add 10 ml of sterile water for inj without preservatives to 250- or 500-mg vials and 20 ml to 1-g vial; sol is stable for 1 wk after reconstitution if refrigerated

Intermittent IV infusion route
- Dilute further in 100-250 ml of 0.9% NaCl or D$_5$W
- Give over 20-60 min to avoid phlebitis; assess for pain along vein; slow inf if pain occurs; apply ice to site and notify prescriber if unable to relieve pain

Continuous infusion route
- May also be administered as an inf in a dilution of 1 g/L of 0.9% NaCl, D$_5$W, over 4 hr

Erythromycin lactobionate

Y-site compatibilities: Acyclovir, alfentanil, amikacin, aminocaproic acid, aminophylline, amiodarone, anidulafungin, atenolol, atosiban, atracurium, atropine, azaTHIOprine, benztropine, bivalirudin, bleomycin, bumetanide, buprenorphine, butorphanol, calcium chloride/gluconate, CARBOplatin, caspofungin, cefotaxime, ceftazidime, cefTRIAXone, cefuroxime, chlorproMAZINE, cimetidine, CISplatin, cyanocobalamin, cyclophosphamide, cycloSPORINE, cytarabine, DACTINomycin, DAPTOmycin, dexmedetomidine, digoxin, diltiazem, diphenhydrAMINE, DOBUTamine, docetaxel, DOPamine, doxacurium, doxapram, DOXOrubicin, enalaprilat, ePHEDrine, EPINEPHrine, epirubicin, epoetin alfa, eptifibatide, ertapenem, esmolol, etoposide, famotidine, fenoldopam, fentaNYL, fluconazole, fludarabine, fluorouracil, folic acid, foscarnet, gatifloxacin, gemcitabine, gentamicin, glycopyrrolate, granisetron, hydrocortisone, HYDROmorphone, hydrOXYzine, IDArubicin, ifosfamide, imipenem-cilastatin, insulin (regular), irinotecan, isoproterenol, labetalol, levofloxacin, lidocaine, LORazepam, LR, mannitol, mechlorethamine, meperidine, methicillin, methotrexate, methoxamine, methyldopate, methylPREDNISolone, metoclopramide, metroNIDAZOLE, miconazole, midazolam, milrinone, mitoxantrone, morphine, multiple vitamins injection, mycophenolate nafcillin, nalbuphine, naloxone, nesiritide, netilmicin, niCARdipine, nitroglycerin, norepinephrine, octreotide, ondansetron, oxacillin, oxaliplatin, oxytocin, paclitaxel, palonosetron, pamidronate, pancuronium, papaverine, pentamidine, pentazocine, perphenazine, phenylephrine, phytonadione, piperacillin, piperacillin-tazobactam, polymyxin B, procainamide, prochlorperazine, promethazine, propranolol, protamine, pyridoxine, quiNIDine, ranitidine, Ringer's, ritodrine, sodium acetate/bicarbonate, succinylcholine, SUFentanil, tacrolimus, temocillin, teniposide, theophylline, thiamine, thiotepa, tigecycline, tirofiban, TNA, tobramycin, tolazoline, TPN, trimetaphan, urokinase, vancomycin, vasopressin, vecuronium, verapamil, vinCRIStine, vinorelbine, vitamin B complex/C, voriconazole, zidovudine, zoledronic acid

ADVERSE EFFECTS
CNS: Seizures
CV: Dysrhythmias, QT prolongation
EENT: Hearing loss, tinnitus
GI: *Nausea, vomiting, diarrhea,* hepatotoxicity, abdominal pain, stomatitis, heartburn, anorexia, pruritus ani, pseudomembranous colitis
GU: *Vaginitis, moniliasis*
INTEG: Rash, urticaria, pruritus, thrombophlebitis (**IV** site)
SYST: Anaphylaxis

Pharmacokinetics

Absorption	Well absorbed (PO)
Distribution	Widely distributed; minimally distributed (CSF); crosses placenta
Metabolism	Liver, partially
Excretion	Bile, unchanged; kidneys (minimal), unchanged
Half-life	1-3 hr

Pharmacodynamics

	PO	IV
Onset	1 hr	Rapid
Peak	4 hr	Infusion's end
Duration	Unknown	Unknown

INTERACTIONS

Individual drugs
Alfentanil, alprazolam, bromocriptine, busPIRone, carBAMazepine, cilostazol, clindamycin, clopazine, cycloSPORINE, diazepam, digoxin, disopyramide, felodipine, methylPREDNISolone, midazolam, quiNIDine, rifabutin, sildenafil, tacrolimus, tadalafil, theophylline, triazolam, vardenafil, vinBLAStine, warfarin: increased toxicity, increased action
Diltiazem, itraconazole, ketoconazole, nefazodone, pimozide, verapamil: increased serious dysrhythmias, do not use together

Drug classifications
Ergots: increased action, toxicity
HMG-CoA reductase inhibitors: increased action, toxicity
Protease inhibitors: serious dysrhythmias

Drug/lab test
Increased: AST/ALT
Decreased: folate assay
False increase: 17-OHCS/17-KS

NURSING CONSIDERATIONS
Assessment
• Assess patient for previous sensitivity reaction
• **Assess patient for signs and symptoms of infection** including characteristics of wounds, sputum, urine, stool, WBC >10,000/mm³, earache, fever; obtain baseline information before, during treatment
• Obtain C&S test results before beginning product therapy to identify if correct treatment has been initiated
• Assess for allergic reactions: rash, urticaria may occur a few days after therapy begins
• Identify urine output; if decreasing, notify prescriber (may indicate nephrotoxicity); also monitor increases in BUN, creatinine
• Monitor blood studies: AST, ALT, CBC, Hct, bilirubin, LDH, alkaline phosphatase, Coombs' test monthly if patient is on long-term therapy
• Monitor electrolytes: potassium, sodium, chloride monthly if patient is on long-term therapy
• **Assess for overgrowth of infection:** perineal itching, fever, malaise, redness, pain, swelling, drainage, rash, diarrhea, change in cough, sputum
• **Pseudomembranous colitis:** assess for diarrhea with blood, mucus, abdominal pain, fever, product should be discontinued immediately
• **Anaphylaxis:** assess for generalized hives, itching, flushing, swelling of lips/tongue/throat, wheezing; have emergency equipment nearby
• **QT prolongation:** may occur (**IV** >15 mg/min), those with electrolyte imbalances, congenital QT prolongation, and the elderly are at greater risk; correct electrolyte imbalances prior to treatment; monitor ECG

Nursing diagnoses
• Diarrhea (adverse reactions)
• Infection, risk for (uses)
• Injury, risk for (adverse reactions)
• Knowledge, deficient (teaching)
• Noncompliance (teaching)

Patient/family education
• Teach patient to report sore throat, bruising, bleeding, joint pain; may indicate blood dyscrasias (rare)
• Advise patient to contact prescriber if vaginal itching, loose foul-smelling stools, furry tongue occur; may indicate superinfection
• Instruct patient to take all medication prescribed for the length of time ordered

Evaluation
Positive therapeutic outcome
• Absence of signs/symptoms of infection (WBC <10,000/mm³, temp WNL, absence of red, draining wounds, earache)
• Reported improvement in symptoms of infection

TREATMENT OF OVERDOSE:
Withdraw product, maintain airway, administer epinephrine, aminophylline, O₂, **IV** corticosteroids

erythromycin ophthalmic
See Appendix B

erythromycin topical
See Appendix B

escitalopram (Rx)
(es-sit-tal'oh-pram)
Lexapro
Func. class.: Antidepressant, selective serotonin reuptake inhibitor
Pregnancy category C

ACTION: Inhibits CNS neuron uptake of serotonin but not of norepinephrine

Therapeutic outcome: Decreased symptoms of depression

USES: General anxiety disorder; major depressive disorder in adults/adolescents

Unlabeled uses: Panic disorder, social phobia

CONTRAINDICATIONS:
Hypersensitivity to this product or citalopram

Precautions: Pregnancy **C,** breastfeeding, geriatric, renal/hepatic disease, history of seizures

BLACK BOX WARNING: Children ≤12 yr/adolescents, suicidal ideation

DOSAGE AND ROUTES
Adult: PO 10 mg/day in AM or PM; after 1 wk if no clinical improvement is noted, dosage may be increased to 20 mg/day PM; maintenance 10-20 mg/day; reassess to determine need for treatment

Geriatric/hepatic dose: PO 10 mg/day

Available forms: Tabs 5, 10, 20 mg; oral sol 5 mg (as base)/5 ml (contains sorbitol)

Implementation
• Give with food or milk for GI symptoms; give with full glass of water
• Give crushed if patient is unable to swallow medication whole
• Give dose at bedtime if oversedation occurs during the day
• Give gum, hard candy, frequent sips of water for dry mouth
• Oral sol: measure with calibrated device
• Store at room temperature; do not freeze
• Provide assistance with ambulation during therapy, because drowsiness, dizziness occur
• Provide safety measures primarily in geriatric
• Check to see if PO medication swallowed

ADVERSE EFFECTS
CNS: *Headache, nervousness, insomnia,* **suicidal ideation,** *drowsiness, anxiety, tremor, dizziness, fatigue, sedation, poor concentration, abnormal dreams, agitation,* **seizures,** apathy, euphoria, hallucinations, delusions, psychosis, **neuroleptic malignant syndrome–like reactions**

CV: *Hot flashes, palpitations,* angina pectoris, **hemorrhage,** hypertension, **tachycardia,** 1st-degree AV block, **bradycardia, MI, thrombophlebitis,** postural hypotension

EENT: Visual changes, ear/eye pain, photophobia, tinnitus

GI: *Nausea, diarrhea, dry mouth, anorexia, dyspepsia, constipation, cramps, vomiting, taste changes, flatulence, decreased appetite*

GU: *Dysmenorrhea, decreased libido, urinary frequency, UTI,* amenorrhea, cystitis, impotence, urine retention, ejaculation disorder

INTEG: *Sweating, rash, pruritus,* acne, alopecia, urticaria, photosensitivity

MS: *Pain,* arthritis, twitching

RESP: *Infection, pharyngitis, nasal congestion, sinus headache, sinusitis, cough, dyspnea, bronchitis,* asthma, hyperventilation, pneumonia

SYST: *Asthenia, viral infection, fever, allergy, chills,* **serotonin syndrome**

INTERACTIONS

Individual drugs
Alcohol: increased CNS depression
Amantadine, bromocriptine, busPIRone, lithium, tramadol, tryptophan: increased serotonin syndrome
BusPIRone: increased symptoms of OCD
CarBAMazepine, lithium, phenytoin, warfarin: increased levels or toxicity of each specific product
Cyproheptadine: decreased escitalopram effect
Diazepam: increased half-life of diazepam
Haloperidol: increased effect of haloperidol

Drug classifications
Antidepressants, opioids, sedatives: increased CNS depression
Antidysrhythmics, antipsychotics: increased levels, toxicity
Highly protein-bound products: increased side effects of escitalopram
MAOIs: do not use with or 14 days before escitalopram
NSAIDs, salicylates, anticoagulants, SSRIs, platelet inhibitors: increased bleeding risk
Phenothiazines: increased levels of phenothiazines
SSRIs, SNRIs, serotonin-receptor agonists, amphetamines: increased serotonin syndrome
Tricyclics: increased levels of tricyclics

Drug/herb
Kava: increased CNS effect
St. John's wort: do not use together

Drug/food
Grapefruit juice: increased escitalopram effect

Drug/lab test
Increased: serum bilirubin, blood glucose, alkaline phosphatase
Decreased: VMA, 5-HIAA
False increase: urinary catecholamines

NURSING CONSIDERATIONS
Assessment

> **BLACK BOX WARNING:** Assess mental status: mood, sensorium, affect, **suicidal tendencies,** increase in psychiatric symptoms, depression, panic

• Assess appetite in bulimia nervosa, weight daily, increase nutritious foods in diet, watch for bingeing and vomiting
• **Assess allergic reactions:** itching, rash, urticaria; product should be discontinued; may need to give antihistamine
• Monitor B/P (lying/standing), pulse q4hr; if systolic B/P drops 20 mm Hg, hold product, notify prescriber; take VS q4hr in patients with cardiovascular disease
• Monitor blood studies: CBC, leukocytes, differential, cardiac enzymes if patient is receiving long-term therapy; check platelets; bleeding can occur
• **Serotonin syndrome:** Assess for nausea, vomiting, sedation, dizziness, sweating, facial flushing, mental changes, shivering, increased B/P: discontinue, notify prescriber
• Monitor liver function tests: AST, ALT, bilirubin, creatinine; thyroid function studies
• Monitor weight qwk; appetite may decrease with product
• Monitor ECG for flattening of T wave, bundle branch, AV block, dysrhythmias in cardiac patients
• Monitor alcohol consumption; if alcohol is consumed, hold dose until AM

Nursing diagnoses
• Coping, ineffective (uses)
• Injury, risk for (uses/adverse reactions)
• Knowledge, deficient (teaching)

Patient/family education
• Teach patient that therapeutic effect may take 1-4 wk
• Advise patient to use caution in driving, other activities requiring alertness because of drowsiness, dizziness, blurred vision
• Advise patient to use sunscreen to prevent photosensitivity
• Advise patient to avoid alcohol ingestion, other CNS depressants
• Advise patient to notify prescriber if pregnant or plan to become pregnant or breastfeed
• Advise patient to change positions slowly; orthostatic hypotension may occur
• Teach patient to avoid all OTC products unless approved by prescriber
• Teach patient to report immediately signs of urinary retention

> **BLACK BOX WARNING:** Teach patient that clinical worsening and suicide risk may occur

• Teach patient using MedGuide provided
• Teach patient about drug interactions

Evaluation
Positive therapeutic outcome
• Decreased depression

TREATMENT OF OVERDOSE:
Activated charcoal, supportive care

esmolol (Rx)
(ez′moe-lole)
Brevibloc
Func. class.: β-Adrenergic blocker (antidysrhythmic II)
Pregnancy category C

Do not confuse:
esmolol/Osmitrol, Brevibloc/Brevital

ACTION: Competitively blocks stimulation of β_1-adrenergic receptors in the myocardium; produces negative chronotropic, inotropic activity (decreases rate of SA node discharge, increases recovery time), slows conduction of AV node, decreases heart rate, decreases O_2 consumption in myocardium; also decreases renin-aldosterone-angiotensin system at high doses; inhibits β_2-receptors in bronchial system at higher doses

Therapeutic outcome: Decreased supraventricular tachycardia

USES: Supraventricular tachycardias, noncompensatory sinus tachycardia, hypertensive crisis, intraoperative and postoperative tachycardia and hypertension

CONTRAINDICATIONS:
Heart block (2nd- or 3rd-degree), cardiogenic shock, CHF, cardiac failure, hypersensitivity, severe bradycardia

Precautions: Pregnancy C, breastfeeding, geriatric patients, hypotension, peripheral vascular disease, diabetes, hypoglycemia, thyrotoxicosis, renal disease, atrial fibrillation, bronchospasms, hyperthyroidism, myasthenia gravis

> **BLACK BOX WARNING:** Abrupt discontinuation

DOSAGE AND ROUTES

Adult: **IV** Loading dose 500 mcg/kg/min over 1 min; maintenance 50 mcg/kg/min for 4 min; if no response in 5 min, give 2nd loading dose; then increase INF to 100 mcg/kg/min for 4 min; if no response, repeat loading dose, then increase maintenance INF by 50 mcg/kg/min (max of 200 mcg/kg/min); titrate to patient response
Child: **IV** A total loading dose of 600 mcg/kg over 2 min, maintenance **IV** INF 200 mcg/kg/min, titrate upward by 50-100 mcg/kg/min q5-10min until B/P, heart rate reduced by >10%

Available forms: Inj 10 mg, 250 mg/ml

Implementation

IV route
• Check that correct concentration is being given
• The 10 mg/ml inj solution needs no dilution and may be used as an **IV** loading dose using handheld syringe

Continuous IV infusion route
• Ready-to-use bags premixed isotonic sol of 10 mg/ml and 20 mg/ml are available in 100, 250 ml bags; use controlled device, a central line is preferred, rate is based on patient's weight
• Store at room temperature for 24 hr; sol should be clear

Y-site compatibilities: Amikacin, aminophylline, ampicillin, amiodarone, atracurium, butorphanol, calcium chloride, ceFAZolin, cefmetazole, cefoperazone, ceftazidime, ceftizoxime, chloramphenicol, cimetidine, cisatracurium, clindamycin, diltiazem, DOPamine, enalaprilat, erythromycin, famotidine, fentaNYL, gentamicin, heparin, hydrocortisone, regular insulin, labetalol, magnesium sulfate, methyldopate, metronidazole, midazolam, morphine, nafcillin, nitroglycerin, norepinephrine, nitroprusside, pancuronium, penicillin G potassium, phenytoin, piperacillin, polymyxin B, potassium chloride, potassium phosphate, propofol, ranitidine, remifentanil, streptomycin, tacrolimus, tobramycin, trimethoprim/sulfamethoxazole, vancomycin, vecuronium, voriconazole, zoledronic acid

Y-site incompatibilities: Furosemide

ADVERSE EFFECTS

CNS: Confusion, light-headedness, paresthesia, somnolence, fever, dizziness, fatigue, headache, depression, anxiety, **seizures**
CV: Hypotension, bradycardia, chest pain, peripheral ischemia, shortness of breath, CHF, conduction disturbances 1st-, 2nd-, 3rd-degree heart block

GI: *Nausea,* vomiting, anorexia, gastric pain, flatulence, constipation, heartburn, bloating
GU: Urinary retention, impotence, dysuria
INTEG: *Induration, inflammation at inj site,* discoloration, edema, erythema, burning, pallor, flushing, rash, pruritus, dry skin, alopecia
RESP: Bronchospasm, dyspnea, cough, wheezing, nasal stuffiness, **pulmonary edema**

Pharmacokinetics

Absorption	Complete
Distribution	Unknown
Metabolism	Liver
Excretion	Kidneys
Half-life	9 min

Pharmacodynamics

Onset	Rapid
Peak	Unknown
Duration	1-2 min

INTERACTIONS

Individual drugs
Amphetamine, ephedrine, epinephrine, norepinephrine, phenylephrine, pseudoephedrine: increased α-adrenergic stimulation
Digoxin: increased digoxin levels
Thyroid hormones: decreased effect of esmolol, decreased action of thyroid hormone

Drug classifications
MAOIs: avoid use
General anesthetics: increased antihypertensive effect

Drug/herb
Ephedra, hawthorn: decreased antihypertensive effect

Drug/lab test
Interference: glucose/insulin tolerance test

NURSING CONSIDERATIONS

Assessment
• **Dysrhythmias:** Monitor B/P during beginning treatment, periodically thereafter; pulse q4hr; note rate, rhythm, quality; apical/radial pulse before administration; notify prescriber of any significant changes (pulse <50 bpm)
• Check for baselines in renal, liver function tests before therapy begins
• **CHF:** Assess for edema in feet, legs daily; monitor I&O, daily weight; check for jugular vein distention, crackles bilaterally, dyspnea
• **Bronchospasm:** Assess breath sounds and respiratory patterns

Nursing diagnoses
- Cardiac output, decreased (uses)
- Injury, risk for (adverse reactions)
- Knowledge, deficient (teaching)
- Noncompliance (teaching)

Patient/family education
- Teach patient need for medication and expected results
- Caution patient to rise slowly to prevent orthostatic hypotension
- Advise patient to notify if pain, swelling occurs at **IV** site

Evaluation
Positive therapeutic outcome
- Absence of dysrhythmias

TREATMENT OF OVERDOSE:
Defibrillation, vasopressor for hypotension

esomeprazole (Rx)
(es′oh-mep′rah-zohl)
Nexium
Func. class.: Anti-ulcer, proton pump inhibitor
Chem. class.: Benzimidazole
Pregnancy category B

ACTION: Suppresses gastric secretion by inhibiting hydrogen/potassium ATPase enzyme system in the gastric parietal cell; characterized as gastric acid pump inhibitor, since it blocks final step of acid production

Therapeutic outcome: Absence of duodenal ulcers; decreased gastroesophageal reflux

USES: Gastroesophageal reflux disease (GERD), adult/child/infant; severe erosive esophagitis; treatment of active duodenal ulcers in combination with antiinfectives for *Helicobacter pylori* infection; long-term use in hypersecretory conditions

CONTRAINDICATIONS:
Hypersensitivity to proton-pump inhibitors (PPIs)

Precautions: Pregnancy **B,** breastfeeding, children, geriatric

DOSAGE AND ROUTES
Active duodenal ulcers associated with *H. pylori*
Adult: PO 40 mg/day × 10 days in combination with clarithromycin 500 mg bid × 10 days and amoxicillin 1000 mg bid × 10 days

Hepatic dose
Adult: PO/IV max 20 mg/day (severe hepatic disease)

GERD/erosive gastritis
Adult: PO 20 or 40 mg/day × 4-8 wk; no adjustment needed in renal, liver failure, geriatric; **IV** 20 or 40 mg/day up to 10 days
Child and adolescent 12-17 yr: PO 20 or 40 mg/day 1 hr before meals up to 8 wk
Child 1-11 yr and ≥20 kg: PO 10 mg/day 1 hr before meals for up to 8 wk
Infant ≥ 1 mo: IV 0.5 mg/kg over 10-30 min
Infant 1-11 mo (>7.5-12 kg): PO 10 mg daily up to 6 wk
Infant 1-11 mo (5-7.5 kg): PO 5 mg daily up to 6 wk
Infant 1-11 mo (3-5 kg): PO 2.5 mg daily up to 6 wk

Available forms: Del rel caps 20, 40 mg; powder for **IV** inj 20, 40 mg/vial; del rel powder for oral susp 20, 40 mg

Implementation
- Swallow caps whole; do not crush or chew; cap may be opened and sprinkled over Tbsp of applesauce
- Same time daily, 1 hr before meal
- **Oral susp (del rel):** empty contents of packet into container with 1 Tbsp of water, let stand 2-3 min to thicken, restir, give within 30 min of mixing; any residual product should be flushed with more water, taken immediately
- **NG tube (del rel oral susp):** add 15 ml water to contents of packet in syringe, shake, leave 2-3 min to thicken, shake, inject through NG tube within 30 min

IV, direct route
- Reconstitute each vial with 5 ml 0.9% NaCl, D$_5$W, LR; give over 3 min

Intermittent IV INF route
- Dilute reconstituted sol to 50 ml, give over 30 min, do not admix, flush line with D$_5$W, 0.9% NaCl, LR after inf

Solution compatibilities: D$_5$W, LR, 0.9% NaCl

Y-site compatibilities: D$_5$W, doripenem, LR

ADVERSE EFFECTS
CNS: *Headache, dizziness*
GI: *Diarrhea, flatulence,* abdominal pain, constipation, dry mouth, **hepatic failure, hepatitis**
INTEG: *Rash,* dry skin
MISC: **Heart failure**

RESP: *Cough,* pneumonia
SYST: Stevens-Johnson syndrome, toxic epidermal necrolysis, exfoliative dermatitis

Pharmacokinetics

Absorption	Unknown
Distribution	97% plasma protein bound
Metabolism	Liver (metabolites)
Excretion	Urine (metabolites), feces (metabolites); in geriatric, elimination rate decreased, bioavailability increased
Half-life	1-1½ hr

Pharmacodynamics

Onset	Unknown
Peak	1½ hr
Duration	Unknown

INTERACTIONS

Individual drugs
Calcium carbonate, clopidogrel, dapsone, indinavir, iron, itraconazole, ketoconazole, vitamin B_{12}: decreased effect
Diazepam, digoxin, penicillins, saquinavir: increased effect, toxicity

Drug/lab test
Increase: creatinine, bilirubin, uric acid, alk phos, AST, ALT
Interference: sodium, potassium, Hgb, WBC, platelets, thyroxine

NURSING CONSIDERATIONS

Assessment
• Assess GI system: bowel sounds q8hr, abdomen for pain, swelling, anorexia
• **Hepatic failure, hepatitis:** monitor AST, ALT, alkaline phosphatase during treatment
• **Serious skin disorders: Stevens-Johnson syndrome,** toxic epidermal necrolysis, exfoliative dermatitis

Nursing diagnoses
• Knowledge, deficient (teaching)
• Pain, acute (uses)
• Pain, chronic (uses)

Patient/family education
• Instruct patient to report severe diarrhea; product may have to be discontinued
• Advise diabetic patients that hypoglycemia may occur
• Advise patient to avoid hazardous activities; dizziness may occur
• Advise patient to avoid alcohol, salicylates, ibuprofen; may cause GI irritation

Evaluation
Positive therapeutic outcome
• Absence of epigastric pain, swelling, fullness

---

estradiol (Rx)
(ess-tra-dye´ole)
Estrace, Femtrace, Gynodiol
estradiol cypionate (Rx)
Depo-Estradiol
estradiol topical emulsion (Rx)
Estrasorb
estradiol valerate (Rx)
Delestrogen
estradiol transdermal system (Rx)
Alora, Climara, Estraderm, Menostar, Vivelle
estradiol vaginal tablet (Rx)
Vagifem
estradiol vaginal ring (Rx)
Estring, Femring
estradiol gel (Rx)
Divigel, Elestrin, Estrogel
estradiol spray (Rx)
Evamist
Func. class.: Estrogen, progestin
Chem. class.: Nonsteroidal synthetic estrogen
Pregnancy category X

ACTION: Needed for adequate functioning of female reproductive system; affects release of pituitary gonadatropins, inhibits ovulation, promotes adequate calcium use in bone structure

Therapeutic outcome: Decreased tumor size in prostatic cancer; increased estrogen levels in menopause, female hypogonadism

USES: Vasomotor symptoms associated with menopause, inoperable breast cancer (selected cases), prostatic cancer, atrophic vaginitis, kraurosis vulvae, hypogonadism, primary ovarian failure, prevention of osteoporosis, castration

CONTRAINDICATIONS:
Pregnancy **X,** breastfeeding, reproductive cancer, genital bleeding (abnormal, undiagnosed)

BLACK BOX WARNING: Breast/endometrial cancer, thromboembolic disorders, MI, stroke

---

Precautions: Hypertension, asthma, blood dyscrasias, gallbladder disease, CHF, diabetes mellitus, bone disease, depression, migraine headache, seizure disorders, renal/hepatic disease, family history of cancer of breast or reproductive tract, history of smoking, uterine fibroids, vaginal irritation/infection, accidental exposure of topical products to children/pets

> **BLACK BOX WARNING:** Cardiac disease, dementia

DOSAGE AND ROUTES

Hormone replacement/menopause symptoms

Adult: TD 1 patch delivering 0.025, 0.0375, 0.05, 0.075, or 0.1 mg/day 2×/wk (Alora, Estraderm, Vivelle-Dot); 1 patch delivering 0.025, 0.0375, 0.05, 0.06, 0.075, or 0.1 mg/day replace q7days (Climara); 1 patch delivering 0.025 mg/day replace q7days, may increase to 2 patches after 4-6 wk; **GEL** apply entire unit dose packet to 5- × 7-inch area of upper thigh/day, alternate thighs; **SPRAY** (Evamist) 1 spray to inner surface of forearm/day in AM

Menopause/hypogonadism/ castration/ovarian failure

Adult: PO 1-2 mg/day 3 wk on, 1 wk off or 5 days on, 2 days off; IM 1-5 mg q3-4wk (cypionate), 1-5 mg q3-4wk; 10-20 mg q4wk (valerate); TOP Estraderm 0.05 mg/24 hr applied 2 ×/wk, Climara 0.05 mg/hr applied 1 ×/wk in a cyclic regimen; women with hysterectomy may use continuously

Prostatic cancer

Adult: IM 30 mg q1-2wk (valerate); PO 1-2 mg tid (oral estradiol)

Breast cancer (palliative treatment)

Adult: PO 10 mg tid × 3 mo or longer

Atropic vaginitis/kraurosis vulvae

Adult: VAG cream 2-4 g/day × 1-2 wk, then 1 g 1-3 ×/wk cycled; VAG tab 1/day × 2 wk, maintenance 1 tab 2 ×/wk; VAG ring inserted and left in place continuously for 3 mo

Vasomotor symptoms

Adult: TOP after cleaning and drying skin on left thigh, calf, rub in contents of pouch using both hands until completely absorbed; wash hands

Available forms: Estradiol: tabs 0.5, 1, 2 mg; **valerate:** inj 10, 20, 40 mg/ml; **transdermal** 0.025, 0.0375, 0.05, 0.075, 0.1 mg/24-hr release rate; **vag cream** 100 mcg/g; **vag**

ring 2 mg/90 days; **vag tab** 25 mcg; **topical emulsion:** 2.5 mg; **gel** 0.1% (Divigel); **spray** (Evamist) 1.53 mg/acuation

Implementation

PO route
- Give titrated dose, use lowest effective dose
- Give with food or milk to decrease GI symptoms

IM route
- Administer deeply in large muscle mass; product is painful
- Rotate syringe to mix oil and medication

Transdermal route
- Apply to area free of hair to ensure adhesion on trunk of body 2 ×/wk; press firmly and hold in place for 10 sec to ensure good contact
- Start transdermal dose 7 days before last PO dose if routes are to be changed

Topical route spray (Evamist)
- Use daily; spray to inner upper arm; may increase to 2-3 ×/day based on response; let dry for 2 min

Vaginal route
- Place cream in applicator by attaching tube to applicator; squeeze cream into tube to mark; insert with patient reclining
- Applicator should be washed after each use

ADVERSE EFFECTS

CNS: Dizziness, headache, migraine, depression, **seizures**

CV: Hypertension, thrombophlebitis, edema, **thromboembolism, stroke, pulmonary embolism, MI,** chest pain

EENT: Contact lens intolerance, increased myopia, astigmatism, throat swelling, eyelid edema

GI: *Nausea,* vomiting, diarrhea, anorexia, pancreatitis, cramps, constipation, increased appetite, increased weight, **cholestatic jaundice, hepatic adenoma**

GU: Amenorrhea, cervical erosion, breakthrough bleeding, dysmenorrhea, vaginal candidiasis, breast changes, *gynecomastia, testicular atrophy, impotence;* **increased risk of breast, endometrial cancer,** changes in libido; **toxic shock, vaginal wall ulceration/ erosion (vag ring)**

INTEG: Rash, urticaria, acne, hirsutism, alopecia, oily skin, seborrhea, purpura, melasma

META: Folic acid deficiency, hypercalcemia, hyperglycemia

Absorption	Well absorbed
Distribution	Widely distributed, crosses placenta
Metabolism	Unknown
Excretion	Unknown
Half-life	Unknown

	PO	IM	IV
Onset	Rapid	Slow	Rapid
Peak	Unknown	Unknown	Unknown
Duration	Unknown	Unknown	Unknown

INTERACTIONS

Individual drugs
Calcium, phenylbutazone, rifampin: decreased estradiol action
CycloSPORINE, dantrolene: increased toxicity
Tamoxifen: decreased tamoxifen action

Drug classifications
Anticoagulants: decreased action of anticoagulants
Anticonvulsants, barbiturates: decreased estradiol action
Corticosteroids: increased action of corticosteroids
Hypoglycemics (oral): decreased action of hypoglycemics

Drug/herb
Black cohosh, DHEA: altered estrogen effect
Saw palmetto, St. John's wort: decreased estrogen effect

Drug/food
Grapefruit juice: increased estrogen level

Drug/lab test
Increased: BSP retention test; PBI; T_4; serum sodium; platelet aggregation; thyroxine-binding globulin (TBS); prothrombin; factors VII, VIII, IX, X; triglycerides
Decreased: serum folate, serum triglyceride, T_3 resin uptake test, glucose tolerance test, antithrombin III, pregnanediol, metyrapone test
False positive: LE prep, ANA titer

NURSING CONSIDERATIONS

Assessment

> **BLACK BOX WARNING:** Assess for previous breast/endometrial cancer, thromboembolic disorders, MI, stroke, dementia

• Monitor blood glucose in patient with diabetes; hyperglycemia may occur
• Monitor B/P q4hr; watch for increase caused by water and sodium retention
• Monitor I&O ratio; be alert for decreasing urinary output and increasing edema; monitor weight daily; notify prescriber if weekly weight gain is >5 lb; if increased, diuretic may be ordered
• Obtain liver function tests baseline, periodically, including AST, ALT, bilirubin, alkaline phosphatase, periodic folic acid level
• Assess edema, hypertension, cardiac symptoms, jaundice
• Assess mental status: affect, mood, behavioral changes, aggression; depression may occur, product may need to be discontinued
• Assess female patient for intact uterus; if so, progesterone should be added to estrogen therapy to decrease risk of endometrial cancer

Nursing diagnoses
• Injury, risk for (adverse reactions)
• Sexual dysfunction (uses)

Patient/family education
• Tell patient to take exactly as prescribed; do not double doses
⚠ Advise patient that increased weight gain and symptoms of fluid retention should be reported to prescriber: edema of feet, ankles, sacral area; abnormal vaginal bleeding; breast lumps; hepatic disease (dark urine, clay-colored stools, jaundice of skin, sclera, pruritus); to report dermal rash with transdermal patch
⚠ Caution patient that thromboembolic symptoms should be reported: tenderness in legs, chest pain, dyspnea, headaches, blurred vision
• Inform patient to use sunscreen and protective clothing because sunburns may occur
• Advise patient to stop smoking; smokers have a greater chance of thromboembolic disorder
• Tell patient to use nonhormonal birth control and to notify prescriber if pregnancy is suspected

Evaluation
Positive therapeutic outcome
• Reversal of menopausal symptoms
• Decrease in tumor size in prostatic or breast cancer
• Decrease in itching, inflammation of vagina
• Absence of symptoms of osteoporosis

⚠ Nurse Alert

estrogens, conjugated (Rx)
Cenestin, Premarin
estrogens, conjugated synthetic B (Rx)
Enjuvia
Pregnancy category X

Do not confuse:
Premarin/Provera

ACTION: Needed for adequate functioning of female reproductive system; affects release of pituitary gonadotropins; inhibits ovulation; promotes adequate calcium use in bone structures

Therapeutic outcome: Decreased tumor size in prostatic cancer; increased estrogen levels in menopause, female hypogonadism

USES: Symptoms associated with menopause, inoperable breast cancer, prostatic cancer, abnormal uterine bleeding, hypogonadism, primary ovarian failure, prevention of osteoporosis, castration

CONTRAINDICATIONS:
Pregnancy **X,** breastfeeding, thromboembolic disorders, reproductive cancer, genital bleeding (abnormal, undiagnosed), hypersensitivity, MI, stroke, phlebitis

BLACK BOX WARNING: Endometrial cancer

Precautions: Hypertension, asthma, blood dyscrasias, gallbladder disease, CHF, diabetes mellitus, bone disease, depression, migraine headache, seizure disorders, renal/hepatic disease, family history of cancer of breast or reproductive tract, history of smoking, dementia, hypothyroidism, obesity, SLE

BLACK BOX WARNING: Cardiac disease, dementia

DOSAGE AND ROUTES
Estrogens, conjugated
Menopause
Adult: PO 0.3-1.25 mg/day 3 wk on, 1 wk off

Prevention of osteoporosis
Adult: PO 0.625 mg/day or in a cycle

Atrophic vaginitis
Adult: VAG cream 2-4 g/day × 21 days, off 7 days, repeat

Prostatic cancer
Adult: PO 1.25-2.5 mg tid

Advanced inoperable breast cancer
Adult: PO 10 mg tid × 3 mo or longer

Abnormal uterine bleeding
Adult: IV/IM 25 mg, repeat in 6-12 hr

Castration/primary ovarian failure
Adult: PO 1.25 mg/day 3 wk on, 1 wk off

Hypogonadism
Adult: PO 2.5-7.5 mg/day × 20 days/mo

Estrogens, conjugated synthetic B
Menopause
Adult: PO 0.625 mg/day initially, may increase based on response

Available forms: Tabs 0.3, 0.45, 0.625, 0.9, 1.25, 2.5 mg; inj 25 mg/vial; vag cream 0.625 mg/g; synthetic B: tabs 0.625, 1.25 mg

Implementation
PO route
• Give titrated dose, use lowest effective dose
• Give in 1 dose in AM for prostatic cancer, vaginitis, hypogonadism
• Give with food or milk to decrease GI symptoms
IM route
• Reconstitute after withdrawing at least 5 ml of air from container and inject sterile diluent on vial side, rotate to dissolve
• Give IM inj deeply in large muscle
Vaginal route
• Place cream in applicator by attaching tube to applicator, squeeze cream into tube to mark, insert with patient recumbent
• Applicator should be washed after each use
IV, direct route
• Reconstitute as for IM, inject into distal port of running IV line of D₅W, 0.9% NaCl, LR, at a rate of 5 mg/min or less

Y-site compatibilities: Heparin/hydrocortisone, potassium chloride, vit B/C

ADVERSE EFFECTS
CNS: Dizziness, headache, migraine, depression, **seizures,** mood disturbances
CV: Hypertension, thrombophlebitis, edema, **thromboembolism, stroke, pulmonary embolism, MI,** chest pain
EENT: Contact lens intolerance, increased myopia, astigmatism
GI: *Nausea,* vomiting, diarrhea, anorexia, pancreatitis, cramps, constipation, increased appetite, **cholestatic jaundice, hepatic adenoma,** weight gain/loss

GU: Amenorrhea, cervical erosion, breakthrough bleeding, dysmenorrhea, vaginal candidiasis, breast changes, *gynecomastia, testicular atrophy, impotence,* **increased risk of breast, endometrial cancer,** libido changes
INTEG: Rash, urticaria, acne, hirsutism, alopecia, oily skin, seborrhea, purpura, melasma
META: Folic acid deficiency, hypercalcemia, hyperglycemia

Pharmacokinetics

Absorption	Well absorbed (PO), completely absorbed (**IV**)
Distribution	Widely distributed, crosses placenta
Metabolism	Liver, exclusively; hepatic recirculation
Excretion	Kidney
Half-life	Unknown

Pharmacodynamics

	PO	IM	IV
Onset	Rapid	Slow	Immediate
Peak	Unknown	Unknown	Unknown
Duration	Unknown	Unknown	Unknown

INTERACTIONS

Individual drugs
CycloSPORINE, dantrolene: increased toxicity
Phenylbutazone, rifampin: decreased action of estrogens
Tamoxifen, thyroid: decreased tamoxifen action

Drug classifications
Anticoagulants: decreased action of anticoagulants
Anticonvulsants, barbiturates: decreased action of estrogens
Corticosteroids: increased action of corticosteroids
Oral hypoglycemics: decreased action of hypoglycemics

Drug/food
Grapefruit juice: increased estrogen level

Drug/lab test
Increased: BSP retention test; PBI, T_4; serum sodium; platelet aggregation; thyroxine-binding globulin (TBG); prothrombin; factors VII, VIII, IX, X; triglycerides
Decreased: serum folate, serum triglyceride, T_3 resin uptake test, glucose tolerance test, antithrombin III, pregnanediol, metyrapone test
False positive: LE prep, ANA titer

NURSING CONSIDERATIONS

Assessment
• Monitor blood glucose in patient with diabetes; hyperglycemia may occur
• Monitor B/P q4hr; watch for increase caused by water and sodium retention
• Monitor I&O ratio; be alert for decreasing urinary output and increasing edema; monitor weight daily; notify prescriber if weekly weight gain is >5 lb; if increased, diuretic may be ordered
• Obtain liver function tests, including AST, ALT, bilirubin, alkaline phosphatase
• Assess edema, hypertension, cardiac symptoms, jaundice
• Assess mental status: affect, mood, behavioral changes, aggression; depression may occur; product may need to be discontinued
• Assess female patient for intact uterus; if so, progesterone should be added to estrogen therapy to decrease risk of endometrial cancer; abnormal uterine bleeding, breast exam

Nursing diagnoses
• Injury, risk for (adverse reactions)
• Sexual dysfunction (uses)

Patient/family education
• Caution patient to take exactly as prescribed and not to double doses
⚠ Advise patient that increased weight gain and symptoms of fluid retention should be reported to prescriber: edema of feet, ankles, sacral area; abnormal vaginal bleeding; breast lumps; hepatic disease (dark urine, clay-colored stools, jaundice of skin, sclera, pruritus)
⚠ Caution patient that thromboembolic symptoms should be reported: pain, redness, tenderness in legs; chest pain, dyspnea, headaches, blurred vision
• Inform patient that sunburns may occur and to use sunscreen and protective clothing
• Advise patient to stop smoking; smokers have a greater chance of thromboembolic disorder
• Tell patient to use nonhormonal birth control and to notify prescriber if pregnancy is suspected
• Tell patient that vasomotor symptoms improve in 2 wk, max relief 8 wk

Evaluation
Positive therapeutic outcome
• Reversal of menopause symptoms
• Decrease in tumor size in prostatic, breast cancer
• Decrease in itching, inflammation of vagina
• Absence of symptoms of osteoporosis

⚠ Nurse Alert

eszopiclone (Rx)
(es-zop'i-klone)
Lunesta
Func. class.: Sedative-hypnotic, non-benzodiazepine
Chem. class.: Cyclopyrrolone
Pregnancy category C
Controlled substance schedule IV

ACTION: Interacts with GABA receptors

Therapeutic outcome: Ability to sleep and stay asleep throughout the night

USES: Insomnia

CONTRAINDICATIONS:
Hypersensitivity, ethanol intoxication

Precautions: Pregnancy C, breastfeeding, children, geriatric, severe hepatic disease, abrupt discontinuation, COPD, depression, labor, sleep apnea, substance abuse, suicidal ideation

DOSAGE AND ROUTES
Adult: PO 2 mg immediately before bed, may increase to 3 mg if needed

Hepatic dose/CYP3A4 inhibitors
Adult: PO 1 mg immediately before bed in severe hepatic disease

Available forms: Tabs 1, 2, 3 mg

Implementation
• Do not break, crush, or chew tab
• For short-term use only
• Give immediately before bedtime
• Avoid use with a high-fat meal
• Provide assistance with ambulation, nightlight, call bell within reach
• Check to see product is swallowed

ADVERSE EFFECTS
CNS: Worsening depression, hallucinations, headache, daytime drowsiness, **suicidal thoughts/actions,** migraine, restlessness, anxiety, sleep driving, sleep walking
CV: Peripheral edema, chest pain
GI: Dry mouth, bitter taste (dysgeusia)
GU: Gynecomastia, dysmenorrhea
INTEG: Rash, **angioedema**

Pharmacokinetics
Absorption	Unknown
Distribution	Unknown
Metabolism	Extensively in the liver by CYP3A4, CYP2E1; protein binding 52%-59%
Excretion	Via kidneys
Half-life	6 hr, geriatric 9 hr

Pharmacodynamics
Onset	Rapid
Peak	1 hr
Duration	6 hr

INTERACTIONS
Drug classifications
CNS depressants: increased CNS depression
CYP3A4 inhibitors (clarithromycin, itraconazole, ketoconazole, nefazodone, nelfinavir, ritonavir, troleandomycin): increased toxicity due to decreased eszopiclone elimination

Drug/food
High-fat meal: decreased product action

NURSING CONSIDERATIONS
Assessment
• **Assess sleep pattern:** ability to go to sleep, stay asleep; early morning awakenings; conservative methods used
• Monitor for abuse of this or other products

Nursing diagnoses
• Injury, risk for (adverse reactions)
• Knowledge, deficient (teaching)
• Sleep deprivation (uses)

Patient/family education
• Caution patient that daytime drowsiness may occur; not to engage in hazardous activities until effect is known, memory problems may occur
• Advise patient that all other medications and supplements should be avoided unless approved by prescriber
• Advise patient to notify prescriber if pregnancy is suspected or planned
• Discuss alternative methods to improve sleep: reading, quiet environment, warm bath, milk

Evaluation
Positive therapeutic outcome
• Ability to sleep and stay asleep throughout the night

etanercept (Rx)

(eh-tan′er-sept)

Enbrel

Func. class.: Antirheumatic agent (disease-modifying) (DMARDs)

Chem. class.: Anti-TNF agent

Pregnancy category B

ACTION: Binds to tumor necrosis factor (TNF), which decreases inflammation and immune response

Therapeutic outcome: Decreased pain, inflammation

USES: Acute, chronic rheumatoid arthritis that has not responded to other disease-modifying agents; polyarticular course juvenile rheumatoid arthritis (JRA), ankylosing spondylitis, plaque psoriasis, psoriatic arthritis

Unlabeled uses: Crohn's disease

CONTRAINDICATIONS:

Sepsis, active infections

> **BLACK BOX WARNING:** Hypersensitivity to this product, latex, needle cap, benzyl alcohol

Precautions: Pregnancy **B**, breastfeeding, children <4 yr, geriatric, malignancies, CHF, seizures, multiple sclerosis

> **BLACK BOX WARNING:** Infection, lymphoma, neoplastic disease

DOSAGE AND ROUTES

Rheumatoid/psoriatic arthritis, ankylosing spondylitis

Adult: SUBCUT 50 mg qwk or 25 mg 2×/wk, 3-4 days apart

Child 2-17 yr: SUBCUT 0.8 mg/kg/wk, max 50 mg/wk

Plaque psoriasis

Adult: SUBCUT 50 mg 2 ×/wk × 3 mo

Adolescent and child 4-17 yr (unlabeled): SUBCUT 0.8 mg/kg/wk, max 50 mg/wk

Juvenile rheumatoid arthritis (JRA)

Adolescent and child 2-17 yr: SUBCUT 0.8 mg/kg/wk, max 50 mg/wk

Available forms: Powder for inj 25 mg; inj 50 mg/ml; auto injector, single use

Implementation

• Administer after reconstituting 1 ml of supplied diluent, slowly inject diluent into vial; swirl contents, do not shake; sol should be clear/colorless, do not use if cloudy or discolored

• Do not admix with other sol or medications; do not use filter

• May be injected SUBCUT into upper arm, abdomen, thigh; rotate inj sites

ADVERSE EFFECTS

CNS: Headache, asthenia, dizziness

GI: Abdominal pain, dyspepsia, vomiting

HEMA: Pancytopenia, **anemia, thrombocytopenia, leukopenia, neutropenia**

INTEG: Rash, *inj site reaction*, keratoderma blenorrhagicum

RESP: Pharyngitis, rhinitis, *cough, URI,* non-URI sinusitis

SYST: Serious infections, sepsis, death, malignancies

Pharmacokinetics

Absorption	Rapidly absorbed (60%)
Distribution	Unknown
Metabolism	Unknown
Excretion	Unknown
Half-life	115 hr

Pharmacodynamics

Unknown

INTERACTIONS

Individual drugs

Anakinra, cyclophosphamide, rilonacept: avoid use

Sulfasalazine: increased neutropenia

Drug classifications

Immunizations: should be brought up to date before treatment

Immunizations, vaccines: do not give concurrently

NURSING CONSIDERATIONS

Assessment

• **Rheumatoid arthritis:** assess for pain; check ROM, inflammation of joints, characteristics of pain

• Assess inj site for pain, swelling; usually occurs after 2 inj (4-5 days)

> **BLACK BOX WARNING: Infection:** patients using immunosuppressives, corticosteroids, methotrexate are at greater risk, assess for fever

Nursing diagnoses
• Injury, risk for (side effects)
• Knowledge, deficient (teaching)
• Mobility, impaired physical (uses)
• Pain, chronic (uses)

Patient/family education
• Teach patient that product must be continued for prescribed time to be effective; to avoid aspirin, alcoholic beverages
• Instruct patient to use caution when driving; dizziness may occur
• Teach patient about self-administration, if appropriate: inj should be made in thigh, abdomen, upper arm; rotate sites at least 1 in from old site

Evaluation
Positive therapeutic outcome
• Decreased pain in arthritic conditions
• Decreased inflammation in arthritic conditions

ethambutol (Rx)
(e-tham′byoo-tole)
Etibi ✦, Myambutol
Func. class.: Antitubercular
Chem. class.: Diisopropylethylene diamide derivative
Pregnancy category B

Do not confuse:
ethambutol/Ethmozine

ACTION: Inhibits RNA synthesis, decreases tubercle bacilli replication

Therapeutic outcome: Resolution of TB infection

USES: Pulmonary TB, as an adjunct, other mycobacterial infections

CONTRAINDICATIONS:
Hypersensitivity, optic neuritis, child <13 yr

Precautions: Pregnancy **B**, breastfeeding, renal disease, diabetic retinopathy, cataracts, ocular defects, hepatic and hematopoietic disorders

DOSAGE AND ROUTES
Adult and child >13 yr: PO 15-25 mg/kg/day as a single dose or 50 mg/kg 2 ✕/wk or 25-30 mg/kg 3 ✕/wk

Renal dose
Adult: PO CCr 10-50 ml/min dose q24-36hr; CCr <10 ml/min dose q48hr

Retreatment
Adult: PO 25 mg/kg/day as single dose ✕ 2 mo with at least 1 other product, then decrease to 15 mg/kg/day as single dose, max 2.5 g/day
Child: PO 15 mg/kg/day

Available forms: Tabs 100, 400 mg

Implementation
• Give with meals to decrease GI symptoms, at same time each day to maintain blood level
• Give 2 hr before antacids
• Give antiemetic if vomiting occurs

ADVERSE EFFECTS
CNS: *Headache, confusion,* fever, malaise, dizziness, *disorientation,* hallucinations, peripheral neuropathy
EENT: Blurred vision, optic neuritis, photophobia, decreased visual acuity
GI: *Abdominal distress, anorexia, nausea, vomiting*
INTEG: Dermatitis, pruritus, **toxic epidermal necrolysis,** erythema multiforme
META: *Elevated uric acid, acute gout,* liver function impairment
MISC: **Thrombocytopenia,** joint pain, **anaphylaxis**

Pharmacokinetics

Absorption	Rapidly absorbed
Distribution	Widely distributed, crosses blood-brain barrier, placenta
Metabolism	Liver
Excretion	Kidneys, unchanged
Half-life	3 hr, increased in liver, kidney disease

Pharmacodynamics

Onset	Rapid
Peak	2-4 hr
Duration	Unknown

INTERACTIONS
Drug classifications
Aluminum, antacids: decreased absorption, separate by 4 hr
Neurotoxic agents, other: increased neurotoxicity

Adverse effects: *italics* = common; **bold** = life-threatening

NURSING CONSIDERATIONS
Assessment
• Obtain C&S tests including sputum tests before initiating treatment; monitor qmo to detect resistance
• Monitor liver function tests qwk × 2 wk, then q2mo: ALT, AST, bilirubin; renal studies: before, qmo: BUN, creatinine output, specific gravity, urinalysis, uric acid; decreased appetite, jaundice, dark urine, fatigue
• Assess patient's mental status often: affect, mood, behavioral changes; psychosis may occur with hallucinations, confusion
• Assess patient for vision disturbance that may indicate optic neuritis: blurred vision, change in color perception; may lead to blindness
• **Serious skin reaction:** toxic epidermal necrolysis

Nursing diagnoses
• Diarrhea (adverse reactions)
• Infection, risk for (uses)
• Knowledge, deficient (teaching)
• Noncompliance (teaching)

Patient/family education
• Advise patient that compliance with dosage schedule and duration is necessary to eradicate disease; to keep scheduled appointments, including ophthalmic appointments, or relapse may occur
• Caution patient to report weakness, fatigue, loss of appetite, nausea, vomiting, yellowing of skin or eyes, tingling/numbness of hands/feet, weight gain, or decreased urine output
• Instruct patient to report any vision changes; rash; hot, swollen, painful joints; numbness or tingling of extremities to physician
• Caution patient to inform prescriber if pregnancy is suspected

Evaluation
Positive therapeutic outcome
• Decreased symptoms of TB
• Decrease in acid-fast bacteria

etidronate (Rx)
(eh-tih-droe′nate)
Didronel
Func. class.: Bone resorption inhibitor
Chem. class.: Bisphosphonate
Pregnancy category C

Do not confuse:
etidronate/etomidate/etretinate

ACTION: Decreases bone resorption and new bone development (accretion)

Therapeutic outcome: Decreased bone reabsorption, calcium levels WNL

USES: Paget's disease, heterotopic ossification, hypercalcemia of malignancy

CONTRAINDICATIONS:
Achalasia, esophageal stricture, osteomalacia

Precautions: Pregnancy C, breastfeeding, children, renal disease, restricted vit D, calcium, colitis, vitamin D deficiency, anemia, esophagitis, pathologic fractures, asthma, coagulopathy, dental disease or work, hiatal hernia, hyperparathyroidism, infection, phosphate hypersensitivity, severe renal disease with creatinine >5 mg/dl, poor dentition

DOSAGE AND ROUTES
Paget's disease
Adult: PO 5-10 mg/kg/day, 2 hr before meals with water, max 20 mg/kg/day, max 6 mo or 11-20 mg/kg/day for max of 3 mo

Heterotopic ossification
Adult: PO 20 mg/kg/day × 2 wk, then 10 mg/kg/day for 10 wk, total 12 wk

Hypercalcemia
Adult: PO 20 mg/kg/day × 30 days

Heterotopic ossification/hip replacement
Adult: PO 20 mg/kg/day × 4 wk before and 3 mo after surgery (4 months total)

Available forms: Tabs 200, 400 mg

Implementation
PO route
• Administer on empty stomach to improve absorption (2 hr before meals); avoid simultaneous vitamins/minerals, antacids with calcium, iron, magnesium, or aluminum

ADVERSE EFFECTS
CNS: Headache
CV: Atrial fibrillation
GI: *Nausea,* constipation, gastritis, esophagitis
GU: Nephrotoxicity
MISC: Dyspnea; low magnesium, phosphorus, alopecia, **Stevens-Johnson syndrome, angioedema**
MS: *Bone pain,* hypocalcemia, decreased mineralization of nonaffected bones, **osteonecrosis of the jaw,** arthralgia, leg cramps

Pharmacokinetics

Absorption	Poorly absorbed (PO)
Distribution	50% bound to crystals in osteogenesis
Metabolism	None
Excretion	Feces (unabsorbed), kidney (unchanged)
Half-life	5-7 hr; in bone >3 mo

Pharmacodynamics

	PO
Onset	4 wk
Peak	Unknown
Duration	Up to 1 yr

INTERACTIONS

Individual drugs
Warfarin: increased pro-time

Drug classifications
Aluminum, antacids, calcium, iron products, or mineral supplements with magnesium: decreased absorption of etidronate

Drug/food
Dairy products: decreased absorption of etidronate

NURSING CONSIDERATIONS

Assessment
• Assess for GI symptoms, polyuria, flushing, head swelling, tingling, headache; may indicate hypercalcemia; nervousness, irritability, twitching, seizures, spasm, paresthesia: indicates hypocalcemia at start of treatment
• **Hypocalcemia:** assess for muscle spasm, laryngospasm, paresthesias, facial twitching, colic
• Identify nutritional status; evaluate diet for sources of vit D (milk, some seafood), calcium (dairy products, dark green vegetables), phosphates
• **Nephrotoxicity:** monitor BUN, creatinine, alk phos, calcium, phosphate, urinalysis (calcium: should be kept at 9-10 mg/dl), albumin, alkaline phosphatase baseline and q3-6mo; check urine sediment for casts throughout treatment; patients with renal failure should not use this product
• Assess for bone pain, weakness during treatment
• Assess for increased product level; toxic reactions occur rapidly; have calcium chloride or gluconate on hand if calcium level drops too low; check for tetany

• **Osteonecrosis of the jaw:** patients receiving dental procedures (extraction) should use antiinfectives if appropriate

Nursing diagnoses
• Injury, risk for (adverse reactions)
• Knowledge, deficient (teaching)
• Pain, chronic (uses)

Patient/family education
• Teach patient that therapeutic response may take 1-3 mo; persists for months after product is discontinued
• Advise to report onset of unexplained pain, restricted mobility, heat over bone's hypercalcemic relapse
• Caution patient to notify prescriber if hypercalcemia recurs: renal calculi, nausea, vomiting, thirst, lethargy, deep bone or flank pain, heat over bone, restricted mobility
• Teach patient that warmth and flushing occur and last 1 hr
• Teach patient to follow a low-calcium diet as prescribed (Paget's disease, hypercalcemia)
• Advise patient to notify prescriber of diarrhea, nausea; dose may be divided to lessen these symptoms
• Advise patient to continue with good dental hygiene

Evaluation
Positive therapeutic outcome
• Calcium levels 9-10 mg/dl
• Decreasing symptoms of Paget's disease including pain
• Decreased bone loss in osteoporosis

etodolac (Rx)
(ee-toe-doe'lak)
Lodine, Lodine XL
Func. class.: Nonsteroidal antiinflammatory, nonopioid analgesic
Pregnancy category C

Do not confuse:
Lodine/codeine/iodine

ACTION: Inhibits prostaglandin synthesis by decreasing enzyme needed for biosynthesis; analgesic, antiinflammatory properties

Therapeutic outcome: Decreased pain, inflammation

USES: Mild to moderate pain, osteoarthritis

CONTRAINDICATIONS:

Hypersensitivity; patients in whom aspirin, iodides, or other NSAIDs have produced asthma, rhinitis, urticaria, nasal polyps, angioedema, bronchospasm; avoid in 2nd half of pregnancy

Precautions: Pregnancy **C,** breastfeeding, children, geriatric, bleeding, GI/cardiac/renal/ hepatic disorders

DOSAGE AND ROUTES

Osteoarthritis

Adult: PO 800-1200 mg/day in divided doses q6-8hr initially, then adjust to 600-1200 mg/ day in divided doses; max 1200 mg/day; patients <60 kg max 20 mg/kg

Analgesia

Adult: PO 200-400 mg q6-8hr prn for acute pain; max 1200 mg/day; patients <60 kg max 20 mg/kg

Available forms: Caps 200, 300 mg; tabs 400, 500 mg; ext rel tabs 400, 600 mg

Implementation

- Do not break, crush, or chew ext rel tabs
- Administer with full glass of water to enhance absorption
- Administer with food or milk to decrease gastric symptoms; food will slow absorption slightly, will not decrease absorption

ADVERSE EFFECTS

CNS: Dizziness, headache, drowsiness, fatigue, tremors, confusion, insomnia, anxiety, depression, light-headedness, vertigo

CV: Tachycardia, peripheral edema, fluid retention, palpitations, dysrhythmias, CHF

EENT: Tinnitus, hearing loss, blurred vision, photophobia

GI: *Nausea, anorexia,* vomiting, diarrhea, jaundice, **cholestatic hepatitis,** constipation, flatulence, cramps, dry mouth, peptic ulcer, dyspepsia, **GI bleeding**

GU: **Nephrotoxicity, dysuria, hematuria, oliguria, azotemia, cystitis, UTI**

HEMA: **Blood dyscrasias**

INTEG: Erythema, urticaria, purpura, rash, pruritus, sweating, **Stevens-Johnson syndrome**

SYST: **Angioedema, anaphylaxis**

Pharmacokinetics

Absorption	Well absorbed
Distribution	Highly bound to plasma protein
Metabolism	Unknown
Excretion	Unknown
Half-life	7 hr

Pharmacodynamics

Onset	$1/2$ hr
Peak	1-2 hr
Duration	4-12 hr

INTERACTIONS

Individual drugs

Aspirin: may increase GI toxicity

CycloSPORINE, digoxin, lithium, methotrexate, phenytoin: increased toxicity

Drug classifications

Antacids: delayed etodolac effect

β-Adrenergic blockers: decreased effect

Diuretics: decreased effectiveness of diuretics

Drug/herb

Arginine, gossypol: increased gastric irritation

Bearberry, bilberry: increased NSAIDs action

Bogbean, chondroitin, saw palmetto, turmeric: increased bleeding risk

St. John's wort: severe photosensitivity

NURSING CONSIDERATIONS

Assessment

- Assess pain: location, frequency, characteristics; relief after medication
- Assess for GI bleeding: black stools, hematemesis
- Assess for asthma, aspirin hypersensitivity, nasal polyps that may be hypersensitive to etodolac
- Monitor blood counts during therapy; watch for decreasing platelets; if low, therapy may need to be discontinued, then restarted after hematologic recovery; watch for blood dyscrasia (thrombocytopenia): bruising, fatigue, bleeding, poor healing

Nursing diagnoses

- Injury, risk for (adverse reactions)
- Knowledge, deficient (teaching)
- Mobility, impaired physical (uses)
- Pain, acute (uses)
- Pain, chronic (uses)

Patient/family education

- Inform patient that product must be continued for prescribed time to be effective; to avoid aspirin, alcoholic beverages, NSAIDs

---

⚠ Nurse Alert

- Caution patient to report bleeding, bruising, fatigue, malaise because blood dyscrasias can occur
- Instruct patient to use caution when driving; drowsiness, dizziness may occur
- Teach patient to take with a full glass of water to enhance absorption

Evaluation
Positive therapeutic outcome
- Decreased pain
- Decreased inflammation
- Increased mobility

⚠ HIGH ALERT

etoposide (Rx)
(e-toe'poe-side)
Toposar
etoposide phosphate (Rx)
Etopophos
Func. class.: Antineoplastic—miscellaneous
Chem. class.: Semisynthetic podophyllotoxin

Pregnancy category D

ACTION: Inhibits mitotic activity through metaphase to mitosis; also inhibits cells from entering mitosis, depresses DNA, RNA synthesis, cell cycle specific S and G_2, binds to a complex of DNA and topoisomerase II

Therapeutic outcome: Prevention of rapid growth of malignant cells

USES: Leukemias, small cell carcinoma of the lung, testicular cancer

Unlabeled uses: Lymphomas

CONTRAINDICATIONS:
Pregnancy **D,** breastfeeding, hypersensitivity, severe renal/hepatic disease

Precautions: Children, renal/hepatic disease, gout

BLACK BOX WARNING: Bone marrow depression, infection, bleeding

DOSAGE AND ROUTES
Testicular cancer
Adult: IV 100 mg/m²/day on days 1, 2 in combination with methotrexate, leucovorin, actinomycin D, cyclophosphamide, and vinCRIStine (EMA-CO regimen) q2-3wk

Small cell carcinoma of the lung
Adult: IV 35 mg/m²/day × 4 days to 50 mg/m²/day × 5 days in combination; resected stage IB-IIII (unlabeled) with CISplatin IV 100 mg/m² on days 1-3 with CISplatin 100 mg/m² on day 1 q21 days × 4 cycles; PO 2 × the IV dose rounded to the nearest 50 mg, given once a day if total dose ≤400 mg/day or individual dose if >400 mg/day

Renal dose
Adult: IV CCr 45-60 ml/min reduce dose by 15%; CCr 30-44 ml/min reduce dose by 20%; CCr <30 ml/min reduce dose by 25%

Available forms: Inj 20 mg/ml, caps 50 mg

Implementation
PO route
- Caps need to be refrigerated
- Give without regard to food

Intermittent IV infusion route
- Use cytotoxic handling procedures

Etoposide
- Dilute 5 ml vial with D_5W or 0.9% NaCl (200-400 mcg/ml); give slowly over 30-60 min; do not give over <30 min, hypotension may occur
- 200 mcg/ml is stable for 96 hr; 400 mcg/ml 48 hr
- Use Luer-Lok tubing to prevent leakage; do not let sol come in contact with skin; if contact occurs, wash well with soap and water

Y-site compatibilities: Acyclovir, alfentanil, allopurinol, amifostine, amikacin, aminocaproic acid, aminophylline, amiodarone, amphotericin B colloidal, amphotericin B lipid complex, amphotericin B liposome, ampicillin, ampicillin-sulbactam, anidulafungin, atenolol, atracurium, aztreonam, bivalirudin, bleomycin, bumetanide, buprenorphine, butorphanol, calcium chloride/gluconate, CARBOplatin, caspofungin, ceFAZolin, cefoperazone, cefotaxime, cefotetan, cefoxitin, ceftazidime, ceftizoxime, cefTRIAXone, cefuroxime, chloramphenicol, chlorproMAZINE, cimetidine, ciprofloxacin, cisatracurium, CISplatin, cladribine, clindamycin, codeine, cyclophosphamide, cycloSPORINE, cytarabine, DACTINomycin, DAPTOmycin, DAUNOrubicin, dexamethasone, dexmedetomidine, dexrazoxane, digoxin, diltiazem, diphenhydrAMINE, DOBUTamine, docetaxel, DOPamine, doxacurium, DOXOrubicin, DOXOrubicin liposomal, doxycycline, droperidol, enalaprilat, ePHEDrine, EPINEPHrine, epirubicin, ertapenem, erythromycin, esmolol, famotidine, fenoldopam, fentaNYL, floxuridine, fluconazole,

Adverse effects: *italics* = common; **bold** = life-threatening

E

fludarabine, fluorouracil, foscarnet, fosphenytoin, furosemide, ganciclovir, gatifloxacin, gemcitabine, gentamicin, glycopyrrolate, granisetron, haloperidol, heparin, hydrALAZINE, hydrocortisone, HYDROmorphone, hydrOXYzine, ifosfamide, imipenem-cilastatin, inamrinone, insulin (regular), irinotecan, isoproterenol, ketorolac, labetalol, lansoprazole, leucovorin, levofloxacin, levorphanol, lidocaine, linezolid, LORazepam, magnesium sulfate, mannitol, mechlorethamine, melphalan, meperidine, meropenem, mesna, methohexital, methotrexate, methyldopate, methylPREDNISolone, metoclopramide, metoprolol, metroNIDAZOLE, micafungin, midazolam, milrinone, minocycline, mitoxantrone, mivacurium, morphine, nafcillin, nalbuphine, naloxone, nesiritide, nitroglycerin, nitroprusside, norepinephrine, NS, octreotide, ofloxacin, ondansetron, oxaliplatin, paclitaxel, palonosetron, pamidronate, pancuronium, pemetrexed, pentamidine, pentazocine, PENTobarbital, PHENobarbital, phenylephrine, piperacillin, piperacillin-tazobactam, polymyxin B, potassium chloride/phosphates, procainamide, prochlorperazine, promethazine, propranolol, quinupristin-dalfopristin, ranitidine, remifentanil, rocuronium, sargramostim, sodium acetate/bicarbonate/phosphates, succinylcholine, SUFentanil, sulfamethoxazole-trimethoprim, tacrolimus, teniposide, theophylline, thiotepa, ticarcillin, ticarcillin-clavulanate, tigecycline, tirofiban, tobramycin, topotecan, trimethobenzamide, vancomycin, vasopressin, vecuronium, verapamil, vinBLAStine, vinCRIStine, vinorelbine, voriconazole, zidovudine, zoledronic acid

Y-site incompatibility: IDArubicin

Additive compatibilities: CARBOplatin, CISplatin, cytarabine, floxuridine, fluorouracil, hydrOXYzine, ifosfamide, ondansetron

Intermittent IV INF route (etoposide phosphate)
• Reconstitute each vial with 5 or 10 ml of D_5W, 0.9% NaCl for a concentration of 20 mg/ml or 10 mg/ml, respectively; may give diluted or undiluted to concentration of as little as 0.1 mg/ml, give over 5-210 min

Y-site compatibilities: Acyclovir, alfentanil, amifostine, amikacin, aminocaproic acid, aminophylline, amiodarone, ampicillin, ampicillin-sulbactam, anidulafungin, atenolol, atracurium, aztreonam, bivalirudin, bleomycin, bumetanide, buprenorphine, butorphanol, calcium acetate/chloride/gluconate, CARBOplatin, carmustine, caspofungin, cefAZolin, cefonicid, cefoperazone, cefotaxime, cefotetan, cefoxitin, ceftazidime, ceftizoxime, cefTRIAXone, cefuroxime, chloramphenicol, cimetidine, ciprofloxacin, cisatracurium, CISplatin, clindamycin, codeine, cyclophosphamide, cycloSPORINE, cytarabine, dacarbazine, DACTINomycin, DAPTOmycin, DAUNOrubicin, dexamethasone, digoxin, diltiazem, diphenhydrAMINE, DOBUTamine, docetaxel, DOPamine, doripenem, doxacurium, DOXOrubicin, doxycycline, enalaprilat, ePHEDrine, EPINEPHrine, epirubicin, ertapenem, erythromycin, esmolol, famotidine, fenoldopam, fentaNYL, floxuridine, fluconazole, fludarabine, fluorouracil, foscarnet, fosphenytoin, furosemide, ganciclovir, gatifloxacin, gemcitabine, gentamicin, glycopyrrolate, granisetron, haloperidol, heparin, hydrALAZINE, hydrocortisone, HYDROmorphone, hydrOXYzine, IDArubicin, ifosfamide, inamrinone, insulin (regular), irinotecan, isoproterenol, ketorolac, labetalol, leucovorin, levofloxacin, levorphanol, lidocaine, linezolid, LORazepam, magnesium sulfate, mannitol, mechlorethamine, meperidine, meropenem, mesna, metaraminol, methotrexate, methyldopate, metoclopramide, metoprolol, metroNIDAZOLE, midazolam, milrinone, minocycline, mitoxantrone, mivacurium, morphine, nafcillin, nalbuphine, naloxone, nesiritide, netilmicin, nitroglycerin, nitroprusside, norepinephrine, octreotide, ofloxacin, ondansetron, oxaliplatin, paclitaxel, palonosetron, pamidronate, pancuronium, pemetrexed, pentamidine, pentazocine, PENTobarbital, PHENobarbital, phenylephrine, piperacillin, piperacillin-tazobactam, plicamycin, polymyxin B, potassium chloride/phosphates, procainamide, promethazine, propranolol, quiNIDine, quinupristin-dalfopristin, ranitidine, remifentanil, riTUXimab, rocuronium, sodium acetate/bicarbonate/phosphates, streptozocin, succinylcholine, SUFentanil, sulfamethoxazole-trimethoprim, tacrolimus, teniposide, theophylline, thiopental, thiotepa, ticarcillin, ticarcillin-clavulanate, tigecycline, tirofiban, tobramycin, tolazoline, trastuzumab, trimethobenzamide, vancomycin, vasopressin, vecuronium, verapamil, vinBLAStine, vinCRIStine, vinorelbine, voriconazole, zidovudine, zoledronic acid

ADVERSE EFFECTS
CNS: Headache, *fever,* peripheral neuropathy, paresthesia, confusion, chills, fever
CV: *Hypotension,* **MI,** dysrhythmia
GI: *Nausea, vomiting, anorexia,* **hepatotoxicity,** dyspepsia, diarrhea, constipation
GU: Nephrotoxicity
HEMA: Thrombocytopenia, leukopenia, myelosuppression, anemia

INTEG: *Rash, alopecia,* phlebitis at **IV** site, radiation recall, **Stevens-Johnson syndrome**
RESP: **Bronchospasm,** pleural effusion
SYST: **Anaphylaxis**

Pharmacokinetics

Absorption	Variably absorbed
Distribution	Rapidly absorbed, 97% protein binding, crosses placenta
Metabolism	Liver, some
Excretion	Kidneys, unchanged 50%; breast milk
Half-life	3 hr initially, 15 hr terminally

Pharmacodynamics

Unknown

INTERACTIONS

Individual drugs

Conivaptan, cycloSPORINE, imatinib, nilotinib, etravirine, telithromycin: increased etoposide effect, toxicity
Filgrastim, sargramostim: decreased etoposide effect, separate ≥24 hr
Radiation: increased bone marrow depression

Drug classifications

Other antineoplastics, immunosuppressives: increased bone marrow depression
Anticoagulants, NSAIDs, platelet inhibitors, thrombolytics, salicylates: increased bleeding risk
Live virus vaccines: increased adverse reactions

Drug/food

Grapefruit juice: decreased etoposide (PO)

NURSING CONSIDERATIONS

Assessment

• Monitor B/P (baseline and q15min) during administration

> **BLACK BOX WARNING: Bone marrow suppression:** monitor CBC, differential, platelet count weekly; withhold product if WBC is <4000/mm³ or platelet count is <75,000/mm³; notify prescriber of results; recovery will take 3 wk

• **Nephrotoxicity:** monitor renal function tests: BUN, urine CCr before, during therapy; I&O ratio; report fall in urine output of 30 ml/hr; for decreased hyperuricemia

• Monitor for cold, fever, sore throat (may indicate beginning of infection); notify prescriber if these occur

> **BLACK BOX WARNING:** Assess for bleeding: hematuria, guaiac, bruising or petechiae, mucosa or orifices q8hr; no rectal temp; avoid IM inj; use pressure to venipuncture sites

⚠ Assess for symptoms indicating severe allergic reactions: rash, pruritus, urticaria, itching, flushing, bronchospasm, hypotension; epinephrine and crash cart should be nearby

• **Geriatric patients:** assess for increased alopecia, GI effects, infection, nephrotoxicity, myelosuppression

Nursing diagnoses

• Body image, disturbed (adverse reactions)
• Infection, risk for (adverse reactions)
• Injury, risk for (adverse reactions)
• Knowledge, deficient (teaching)

Patient/family education

• Teach patient to avoid use of products containing aspirin or ibuprofen, razors, commercial mouthwash because bleeding may occur; to report symptoms of bleeding (hematuria, tarry stools)
• Instruct patient to report signs of anemia (fatigue, headache, irritability, faintness, shortness of breath)
• Teach patient to report any changes in breathing or coughing even several months after treatment
• Advise patient that contraception will be necessary during treatment because teratogenesis may occur
• Caution patient that hair loss may occur during treatment; a wig or hairpiece may make patient feel better; new hair will be different in color, texture
• Advise patient to avoid vaccinations during treatment because serious reactions may occur
• Teach patient to report signs/symptoms of infection: fever, chills, sore throat; patient should avoid crowds and persons with known infections

Evaluation

Positive therapeutic outcome

• Decreased spread of malignant, leukemic cells

E

Adverse effects: *italics* = common; **bold** = life-threatening

etravirine (Rx)

(e-tra'veer-een)

INTELENCE

Func. class.: Antiretroviral

Chem. class.: Non-nucleoside reverse transcriptase inhibitor (NNRTI)

Pregnancy category B

ACTION: Binds directly to reverse transcriptase, blocking the RNA- and DNA-dependent DNA polymerase action, causing a disruption of the enzyme's catalytic site

Therapeutic outcome: Increased CD4 count, decrease viral load

USES: In combination with other antiretroviral agents for HIV infection in treatment-experienced patients with evidence of HIV replication despite ongoing antiretroviral therapy

CONTRAINDICATIONS:

Hypersensitivity, breastfeeding

Precautions: Pregnancy **B**, impaired hepatic function, children, antimicrobial resistance, geriatric patients, hepatitis, hypercholesterolemia, hypertriglycerides, immune reconstitution syndrome

DOSAGES AND ROUTES

Adult: PO 200 mg bid after a meal, max 400 mg/day; not established in treatment-naïve patients

Available forms: Tabs 100, 200 mg

Implementation

• Give in combination with other antiretrovirals with food

• Store in cool environment; protect from light

ADVERSE EFFECTS

CNS: *Headache, insomnia,* amnesia, anxiety, confusion, fatigue, nightmares, peripheral neuropathy, **seizures, stroke,** tremor

CV: Atrial fibrillation, hypertension, MI

EENT: Blurred vision

GI: *Nausea, vomiting, diarrhea, anorexia,* abdominal pain, increased AST/ALT, constipation, flatulence, gastritis, GERD, **hematemesis, hepatitis,** hepatomegaly, **pancreatitis**

GU: Renal failure

HEMA: Hemolytic anemia, neutropenia, thrombocytopenia, anemia

INTEG: *Rash,* erythema multiforme, **angioedema, Stevens-Johnson syndrome**

MS: Rhabdomyolysis

OTHER: Diabetes mellitus, gynecomastia, hyperamylasemia, hypercholesterolemia, hyperglycemia, hyperlipidemia

RESP: Dyspnea, **bronchospasm**

Pharmacokinetics

Absorption	Unknown
Distribution	Plasma protein binding 99.9%
Metabolism	By CYP3A4, 2C9, 2C19
Excretion	Feces
Half-life	21-61 hr

Pharmacodynamics

Unknown

INTERACTIONS

Individual drugs

Amiodarone, atazanavir, clarithromycin, flecainide, fosamprenavir, lidocaine, mexiletine, propafenone, quiNIDine, sildenafil, tadalafil, vardenafil: decreased levels

Atazanavir, carBAMazepine, delavirdine, fosamprenavir, fosphenytoin, phenytoin, PHENobarbital, rifapentine, rifampin, tipranavir: do not use concurrently

Darunavir, dexamethasone, disopyramide, efavirenz, nevirapine, ritonavir, tipranavir: decreased etravirine levels

CycloSPORINE, sirolimus, tacrolimus: altered effect

Diazepam, rifampin, voriconazole, warfarin: increased levels

Fluconazole, itraconazole, ketoconazole, lopinavir, posaconazole, ritonavir, voriconazole: increased etravirine levels

Methadone: increased withdrawal symptoms

Drug classifications

HMG-CoA reductase inhibitors: increased myopathy, rhabdomyolysis

Drug/herb

St. John's wort: decreased etravirine

NURSING CONSIDERATIONS

Assessment

• **Assess symptoms of HIV and for possible infections;** increased temp

⚠ **Monitor for fatal hypersensitivity reactions: fever, rash, nausea, vomiting, fatigue, cough, dyspnea, diarrhea, abdominal discomfort; treatment should be discontinued and not restarted**

• **Assess blood dyscrasias** (anemia, granulocytopenia): bruising, fatigue, bleeding, poor healing

• **Renal failure:** monitor renal studies: BUN, serum uric acid, CCr before, during therapy; these may be elevated throughout treatment
• Monitor hepatic studies before, during therapy: bilirubin, AST, ALT, amylase, alk phos, creatine phosphokinase, creatinine, qmo
• **HIV:** monitor blood counts q2wk; monitor viral load and CD4 counts during treatment; watch for decreasing granulocytes, Hgb; if low, therapy may have to be discontinued and restarted after hematologic recovery; blood transfusions may be required; cholesterol/lipid profile

Nursing diagnoses
• Infection, risk for (uses)
• Knowledge, deficient (teaching)

Patient/family education
• Inform patient that product is not a cure but will control symptoms; patient is still infective, may pass AIDS virus on to others
• Instruct patient to notify prescriber of sore throat, swollen lymph nodes, malaise, fever; other infections may occur; to stop product and notify prescriber immediately if skin rash, fever, cough, shortness of breath, GI symptoms occur; advise all health care providers that allergic reaction has occurred with etravirine
• Advise patient that follow-up visits must be continued since serious toxicity may occur; blood counts must be done
• Instruct patient to use contraception during treatment; still able to transmit disease
• Give patient Medication Guide and Warning Card, discuss points on guide
• Inform patient that other products may be necessary to prevent other infections
• Advise patient to take medication following a meal

Evaluation
Positive therapeutic outcome
• Increased CD4 count, decreased viral load

---

everolimus (Rx)
(e-ve-ro′-li-mus)
Afinitor, Zortress
Func. class.: Antineoplastic (miscellaneous)
Chem. class.: Immunosuppressant, macrolide
Pregnancy category D

ACTION: Proliferation signal inhibitor that inhibits mammalian target of rapamycin (mTOR); this pathway is dysregulated in cancer

USES: Renal cell cancer in those with failed treatment with suritinib or sorafenib, kidney transplant rejection prophylaxis with cycloSPORINE, subependymal giant cell astrocytoma, progressive pancreatic neuroendocrine tumor (PNET) with unresectable locally advanced metastatic disease

Therapeutic outcome: Decreasing tumor size, decreasing spread of malignancy

CONTRAINDICATIONS:
Breastfeeding; hypersensitivity to this product, rapamine, and torisel; pregnancy **D**

Precautions: Children <13 yr, renal/hepatic disease, diabetes mellitus, infection, hyperlipidemia, plural effusion

> **BLACK BOX WARNING:** Immunosuppression, infection, renal artery thrombosis, renal impairment, renal vein thrombosis

DOSAGE AND ROUTES
Kidney transplant rejection prophylaxis (Zortress)
Adult: PO 0.75 mg q12hr with cycloSPORINE in combination with basiliximab corticosteroids, reduced doses of cycloSPORINE

Advanced renal cancer (Afinitor)
Adult: PO 10 mg qd as long as clinically beneficial; with strong CYP3A4 inducers 10 mg qd, may increase by 5-mg increments to 20 mg qd

Progressive neuroendocrine tumor (PNET) (Afinitor only)
Adult: PO 10 mg q day, reduce dose to 5 mg q day if intolerable adverse reactions occur

Subependymal giant cell astrocytoma (SEGA) (Afinitor only)
Adult/adolescent/child ≥3 yr: PO BSA ≥2.2 m³ give 7.5 mg q day; BSA 1.3-2.1 m³ give 5 mg q day; BSA 0.5-1.2 m² give 2.5 mg q day, adjust q2wk, based on trough, clinical response

Hepatic dose
Adult: PO (Child-Pugh B) Afinitor 5 mg qd; not to be used in Child-Pugh C

Available forms: Tabs 0.25, 0.5, 0.75, 2.5 (Zortress); 2.5, 5, 10 mg (Afinitor)

Implementation
• Swallow tabs whole with a full glass of water; do not chew, crush, or break
• Afinitor: take at same time of day without regard to food; if unable to swallow, disperse in 30 ml of water

---

Adverse effects: *italics* = common; **bold** = life-threatening

• Zortress: must take consistently with or without food, give at same time of day q12h with cycloSPORINE

• Follow procedure for proper handling of antineoplastics

• Give all medications PO if possible, avoiding IM inj; bleeding may occur

• Store protected from light, at room temperature

ADVERSE EFFECTS

CNS: *Headache, insomnia, paresthesia, chills,* fever

CV: Hypertension, *CHF,* peripheral edema

EENT: Blurred vision, photophobia

GI: Nausea, vomiting, diarrhea

GU: Renal failure

HEMA: Anemia, leukopenia, thrombocytopenia

INTEG: *Rash, acne*

META: Hyperglycemia, increased creatinine, *hyperlipemia,* hyperphosphatemia, weight loss

RESP: Pleural effusion, *dyspnea*

Pharmacokinetics

Absorption	Rapid
Distribution	Protein binding 74%
Metabolism	Extensively by CYP3A4
Excretion	Feces 80%, urine 5%
Half-life	30 hr, reduced by high-fat meal

Pharmacodynamics

Onset	Unknown
Peak	1-2 hr
Duration	Unknown

INTERACTIONS

Individual drugs

Cimetidine, cycloSPORINE, danazol, erythromycin: increased blood levels of these products

CarBAMazepine, PHENobarbital, phenytoin, rifamycin, rifapentine: decreased blood levels of everolimus

Drug classifications

Antifungals, calcium channel blockers, HIV-protease inhibitors: increased blood levels of these products

Vaccines: decreased effect

Drug/herb

St. John's wort: may decrease the effect of everolimus

Drug/food

Alters bioavailability; use consistently with or without food; do not use with grapefruit juice

NURSING CONSIDERATIONS

Assessment

• Monitor lipid profile: cholesterol, triglycerides, a lipid-lowering agent may be needed; blood glucose

> **BLACK BOX WARNING:** Monitor blood studies: Hgb, WBC, platelets during treatment qmo; if leukocytes <3000/mm^3 or platelets <100,000/mm^3, product should be discontinued or reduced; decreased hemoglobulin level may indicate bone marrow suppression

• Monitor hepatic studies: alk phos, AST, ALT, amylase, bilirubin, and for hepatotoxicity: dark urine, jaundice, itching, light-colored stools; product should be discontinued

Nursing Diagnoses

• Injury, risk for (adverse reactions)

• Infection, risk for (adverse reactions)

• Knowledge, deficient (teaching)

Patient/family education

• Advise to report fever, rash, severe diarrhea, chills, sore throat, fatigue; serious infections may occur; clay-colored stools, cramping (hepatotoxicity)

• Advise to avoid crowds, persons with known infections to reduce risk of infection

• Teach to use contraception before, during, and 12 wk after product has been discontinued, avoid breastfeeding

• Advise not to use with grapefruit juice

• Inform to avoid live virus vaccines

• Advise to take up to 6 hr after normally scheduled time if dose is missed

• Advise that product may decrease male/female fertility

• Teach that drinking alcohol is not recommended

Evaluation

Positive therapeutic outcome

• Decreasing size of tumor, decreasing spread of malignancy

exemestane (Rx)

(x-ee-mes′-tane)

Aromasin

Func. class.: Antineoplastic

Chem. class.: Aromatase inhibitor

Pregnancy category D

ACTION: Lowers serum estradiol concentrations; many breast cancers have strong estrogen receptors

Therapeutic outcome: Prevention of rapidly growing malignant cells

USES: Advanced breast carcinoma that has not responded to other therapy in estrogen receptor–positive patients (postmenopausal)

CONTRAINDICATIONS:
Pregnancy **X**, breastfeeding, hypersensitivity, premenopausal women

Precautions: Children, geriatric, renal/hepatic disease

DOSAGE AND ROUTES
Adult: PO 25 mg/day after meals; may need 50 mg/day if taken with a potent CYP3A4 inhibitor

Available forms: Tabs 25 mg

Implementation
• Give after food or fluids for GI upset
• Store in light-resistant container at room temperature

ADVERSE EFFECTS
CNS: Headache, fatigue, depression, insomnia, anxiety, hot flashes, diaphoresis
CV: Hypertension
GI: Nausea, vomiting, increased appetite, diarrhea, constipation, abdominal pain
HEMA: *Lymphopenia*
MS: Fracture, bone loss
RESP: Cough, dyspnea

Pharmacokinetics

Absorption	Rapidly absorbed
Distribution	Unknown
Metabolism	Liver
Excretion	Feces, urine
Half-life	24 hr

Pharmacodynamics
Unknown

INTERACTIONS
Drug classifications
CYP3A4 inducers, estrogens: decreased exemestane action

NURSING CONSIDERATIONS
Assessment
• Assess B/P; hypertension may occur
• Bone mineral density, x-ray of thoracic or lumbar spine if bone changes are suspected

Nursing diagnoses
• Injury, risk for (adverse reactions)
• Knowledge, deficient (teaching)

Patient/family education
• Instruct patient to report any complaints, side effects to prescriber; if dose is missed, do not double next dose
• Advise patient that hot flashes can occur and are reversible after discontinuing treatment
• Inform patient about who should be told about therapy
• Advise patient to use reliable contraception, pregnancy **X**, do not breastfeed

Evaluation
Positive therapeutic outcome
• Decreased spread of malignant cells in breast cancer

---

exenatide (Rx)
(ex-en′a-tide)
Byetta
Func. class.: Antidiabetic
Chem. class.: Incretin mimetic
Pregnancy category C

ACTION: Binds and activates known human GLP-1 receptor, mimics natural physiology for self-regulating glycemic control

Therapeutic outcome: Decreased polyuria, polydipsia, polyphagia; improved Hgb A1c

USES: Type 2 diabetes mellitus given in combination with metformin, sulfonylurea, or a thiazolidinedione

CONTRAINDICATIONS:
Hypersensitivity

Precautions: Pregnancy **C**, geriatric, severe renal/hepatic/GI disease

DOSAGE AND ROUTES
Adult: SUBCUT 5 mcg bid 1 hr before morning and evening meal; may increase to 10 mcg bid after 1 mo of therapy

Available forms: Inj 5, 10 mcg

Implementation
• Give SUBCUT only, do not give **IV/IM**
• Pen needles must be purchased separately and be compatible
• Prime prior to use
• Inject into thigh, abdomen, upper arm

• Give 1 hr before meals, approximately 6 hr apart; if patient is NPO, may need to hold dose to prevent hypoglycemia
• Store in refrigerator; unopened pen may be stored at room temperature after opening for up to 30 days

ADVERSE EFFECTS

CNS: *Headache, dizziness,* jittery feeling, restlessness, weakness
ENDO: Hypoglycemia
GI: Nausea, vomiting, diarrhea, dyspepsia, anorexia, gastroesophageal reflux, weight loss

Pharmacokinetics

Absorption	Unknown
Distribution	Unknown
Metabolism	Unknown
Excretion	Glomerular filtration
Half-life	Unknown

Pharmacodynamics

Onset	Unknown
Peak	2.1 hr
Duration	Unknown

INTERACTIONS

Individual drugs

Acetaminophen: may decrease the effect of acetaminophen
Acetaminophen (elixir), digoxin, lovastatin: decreased action of these products
Alcohol, disopyramide: increased hypoglycemia
Dextrothyroxine, niacin, triamterene: decreased hypoglycemia
Erythromycin, metoclopramide: do not use with exenatide

Drug classifications

ACE inhibitors, anabolic steroids, androgens, fibric acid derivatives, sulfonylureas: increased hypoglycemia
Corticosteroids, phenothiazines: increased hyperglycemia
Estrogens, MAOIs, oral contraceptives, progestins, thiazide diuretics: decreased hypoglycemia

NURSING CONSIDERATIONS

Assessment

• Monitor fasting blood, glucose, A1c levels, postprandial glucose during treatment to determine diabetes control
• Assess for hypo/hyperglycemic reaction that can occur soon after meals; for severe hypoglycemia give IV D₅W, then IV dextrose solution

• Assess for nausea, vomiting, ability to tolerate product

Nursing diagnoses

• Injury, risk for (uses)
• Knowledge, deficient (teaching)
• Noncompliance (teaching)

Patient/family education

• Teach patient symptoms of hypo/hyperglycemia, what to do about each; to have glucagon emergency kit available; to carry a glucose source (candy, sugar cube) to treat hypoglycemia
• Advise patient that product must be continued on daily basis; explain consequences of discontinuing product abruptly
• Teach patient that diabetes is a lifelong illness; product will not cure disease
• Advise that all food in diet plan must be eaten to prevent hypoglycemia
• Advise patient to carry emergency ID with prescriber and medications
• Advise patient to continue weight control, dietary restrictions, exercise, hygiene
• Inform patient that regular blood glucose monitoring and A1c testing is needed
• Advise patient to notify prescriber if pregnant or intend to become pregnant
• Advise patient to read "Information for the Patient" and "Pen User Manual"; provide education on self-injection

Evaluation

Positive therapeutic outcome
• Decrease in polyuria, polydipsia, polyphagia, clear sensorium; improved A1c, weight; absence of dizziness, stable gait

---

ezetimibe (Rx)
(ehz-eh-tim′bee)
Ezetrol ✦, Zetia
Func. class.: Antilipemic
Pregnancy category C

ACTION: Inhibits absorption of cholesterol by the small intestine

Therapeutic outcome: Decreased cholesterol levels

USES: Hypercholesterolemia, homozygous familial hypercholesterolemia (HoFH), homozygous sitosterolemia

CONTRAINDICATIONS: Hypersensitivity, severe hepatic disease

⚠ Nurse Alert

Precautions: Pregnancy **C**, breastfeeding, children, hepatic disease

DOSAGE AND ROUTES

Adult: **PO** 10 mg/day; may be given with HMG-CoA reductase inhibitor at same time; may be given with bile acid sequestrant; give ezetimibe 2 hr before or 4 hr after the bile acid sequestrant

Available forms: Tabs 10 mg

Implementation

• Give without regard to meals

ADVERSE EFFECTS

CNS: Fatigue, dizziness, headache
GI: Diarrhea, abdominal pain
MISC: Chest pain
MS: *Myalgias, arthralgias,* back pain, myopathy, **rhabdomyolysis**
RESP: Pharyngitis, sinusitis, cough, URI

Pharmacokinetics

Absorption	Unknown
Distribution	Unknown
Metabolism	Small intestine, liver
Excretion	Urine (11%), feces (78%)
Half-life	Unknown

Pharmacodynamics

Unknown

INTERACTIONS

Individual drugs

Cholestyramine: decreased ezetimibe action
CycloSPORINE: increased action of ezetimibe

Drug classifications

Antacids: decreased action of ezetimibe
Fibric acid derivatives: increased ezetimibe action

Drug/lab test

Increase: LFTs

NURSING CONSIDERATIONS

Assessment

• **Hypercholesterolemia:** obtain diet history; monitor fat content, lipid levels (triglycerides, LDL, HDL, total cholesterol), LFTs baseline and periodically during treatment
• **Myopathy/rhabdomyolysis:** monitor for increased CPK; myalgia, muscle cramps, musculoskeletal pain, lethargy, fatigue, fever; more common when combined with statins

Nursing diagnoses

• Knowledge, deficient (teaching)
• Noncompliance (teaching)

Patient/family education

• Teach patient that compliance is needed
• Advise that risk factors should be decreased: high-fat diet, smoking, alcohol consumption, absence of exercise
• Advise patient to notify prescriber if pregnancy is suspected or planned or if breastfeeding
• Advise patient to notify prescriber if unexplained weakness, or muscle pain is present
• Teach patient to notify prescriber of dietary/herbal supplements

Evaluation

Positive therapeutic outcome
• Decreased cholesterol

ezogabine (Rx)

(e-zog'a-been)
Potiga
Func. class.: Anticonvulsant

ACTION: The exact mechanism of anticonvulsant effects is not fully known. However, studies indicate that the drug enhances transmembrane potassium currents, which may stabilize the resting membrane potential and reduce brain excitability. May also augment GABA-mediated currents.

USES: Partial seizures

CONTRAINDICATIONS:

Hypersensitivity

Precautions: **Suicidal ideation/behavior,** prostatic hypertrophy, dementia, psychotic disorders, QT prolongation, congestive heart failure, ventricular hypertrophy, hypokalemia, hypomagnesemia, abrupt discontinuation, renal impairment, hepatic disease, geriatrics, pregnancy category C, breastfeeding, neonates, infants, children, adolescents

DOSAGE AND ROUTES

Adults and geriatric patients ≤65 years of age: **PO** Initially, 100 mg tid; increase by ≤50 mg tid per day at weekly intervals depending on response, up to a maintenance dose of 200-400 mg tid depending on response; max is 400 mg tid (1200 mg/day).
Geriatric patients >65 years of age: **PO** Initially, 50 mg tid; increase by ≤50 mg tid per day at weekly intervals depending on response; max 250 mg tid (750 mg/day).

Available forms: Film-coated tabs 50, 200, 300, 400 mg

Implementation
- Tabs should be swallowed whole without regard to meals
- Give in 3 equally divided doses

ADVERSE EFFECTS
CNS: Dizziness, drowsiness, memory impairment, tremor, vertigo, abnormal coordination, disturbance in attention, gait disturbance, aphasia, dysarthria, balance disorder, paresthesias, amnesia, dysphagia, myoclonia, hypokinesia, confusion, anxiety, hallucinations, **suicidal thoughts/behaviors,** fatigue, asthenia, malaise
EENT: *Diplopia, blurred vision*
GI: *Nausea, constipation, dyspepsia , xerostomia, constipation, weight gain, appetite stimulation*
GU: *Urinary retention, hydronephrosis, dysuria, urinary hesitation, hematuria, chromaturia*
MISC: *Influenza, dyspnea,* **QT prolongation**
MS: Muscle spasms, weakness

Pharmacokinetics

Absorption	Rapid, 60%
Distribution	Extensively in the body, 80% protein binding
Metabolism	Extensive (glucuronidation, acetylation), metabolite (N-glucuronides)
Excretion	Renal 36% (exogabine), 18% (NAMR), 24% (N-glucuronides); fecal 14%
Half-life	Elimination 7 hr, metabolite 11 hr

Pharmacodynamics

Onset	Unknown
Peak	0.5-2 hr, increased by high-fat food
Duration	Unknown

INTERACTIONS

Individual drugs
Amantadine: increased urinary retention
Arsenic trioxide, chloroquine, chlorproMAZINE, clarithromycin, dextromethorphan; dronedarone, droperidol, erythromycin, grepafloxacin, halofantrine, levomethadyl, mesoridazine, methadone, pentamidine, pimozide, posaconazole, probucol, propafenone, quiNIDine, saquinavir, sparfloxacin, terfenadine, thioridazine, troleandomycin, ziprasidone: **increased QT prolongation**

Buprenorphine, butorphanol, dronabinol, ethanol, mirtazapine, nabilone, nalbuphine, opiate agonists, pentazocine, pregabalin, tramadol, trazodone, ethanol: increased CNS depression
CarBAMazepine: decreased effect of ezogabine
Digoxin: increased effect of each product
Phenytoin: decreased effect of each product

Drug classifications
Antimuscarinics, H1-blockers: increased urinary retention
Class IA antiarrhythmics (disopyramide, procainamide, quiNIDine), Class III antiarrhythmics (amiodarone, dofetilide, ibutilide, sotalol): **increased QT prolongation**
Anxiolytics, hypnotics, opiate agonists, sedatives, skeletal muscle relaxants: increased CNS depression

NURSING CONSIDERATIONS

Assessment
- **Seizures:** Assess for type, duration, location, activity, presence of aura
- **QT prolongation:** Monitor in those with known QT prolongation, congestive heart failure, ventricular hypertrophy, hypokalemia, hypomagnesemia, and in patients receiving medications known to cause QT prolongation. QT prolongation can occur within 3 hrs of dose
- **Abrupt withdrawal:** Withdraw gradually to minimize increased seizure frequency
- **Suicidal thoughts/behaviors:** Assess for any unusual changes in moods or behaviors, including emotional lability or emerging or worsening depression and suicidal ideation

Patient/family education
- Instruct patient to avoid driving or operating machinery, or performing other tasks that require mental alertness until reaction is known
- Instruct patient to avoid concurrent use of alcohol
- Instruct patient to avoid abruptly discontinuing this medication
- **Suicidal thought/behaviors:** Advise patient to notify prescriber immediately for suicidal thought/behaviors

> ⚠ **HIGH ALERT**

factor VIIa, recombinant (Rx)

NovoSeven, NovoSeven RT
Func. class.: Antihemophilic
Pregnancy category C

ACTION: Promotes hemostasis by activating the intrinsic pathway of coagulation

Therapeutic outcome: Prevention of hemorrhage

USES: Bleeding in hemophilia A or B, with inhibitors to factor VIII or IX, acquired hemophilia, factor VII deficiency

Unlabeled uses: Coumarin toxicity

CONTRAINDICATIONS:
Hypersensitivity to this product or mouse, hamster, or bovine products

Precautions: Pregnancy C, breastfeeding, children, DIC, septicemia, intracranial hemorrhage

DOSAGE AND ROUTES

Bleeding prophylaxis or hemophilic with inhibitors to factor VIII/IX
Adult: IV BOL 90 mcg/kg q2hr until hemostasis occurs, or until therapy is deemed to be inadequate; posthemostatic doses q3-6hr may be required

Bleeding prophylaxis factor VII deficiency
Adult: IV BOL 15-30 mcg/kg over 2-5 min q4-6hr

Acquired hemophilia
Adult/adolescent/child: IV BOL 70-90 mcg/kg q2-3hr

Available forms: Lyophilized powder 1.2 mg/vial (1200 mcg/vial), 2.4 mg/vial (2400 mcg/vial), 4.8 mg/vial (4800 mcg/vial) recombinant human coagulation factor VIIa (rFVIIa); NovoSeven RT: 1 mg, 2 mg, 5, 8 mg powder for injection

Implementation
IV route (NovoSeven)
• Bring to room temperature; for 1.2-mg vial/2.2 ml sterile water for inj; 4.8-mg vial/8.5 ml sterile water for inj
• Remove caps from stopper, cleanse stopper with alcohol, allow to dry, draw back plunger of sterile syringe and allow air into syringe, insert needle of syringe into sterile water for inj, inject the air and withdraw amount required, insert syringe needle with diluent into product vial, aim to side so liquid runs down vial wall, gently swirl until dissolved, use within 3 hr, give by bol over 3-5 min
• Do not admix, keep refrigerated until ready to use, avoid sunlight

IV route (NovoSeven RT)
• May be stored in refrigerator or room temperature prior to reconstitution
• Reconstitute with hisitidine diluent 1.1 ml for 1-mg vial, 2.1 ml for 2-mg vial, 5.2 ml for 5-mg vial, 8.1 ml for 8-mg vial; allow diluent to run down side of vial; gently swirl until powder is dissolved (1 mg/ml)

ADVERSE EFFECTS
CNS: Fever, headache, **cerebral artery occlusion**
CV: Ischemic heart disease, MI, hypertension
INTEG: Pain, redness at inj site, pruritus, purpura, rash
SYST: Hemorrhage not otherwise specified, hemarthrosis, fibrinogen plasma decrease, hypertension, bradycardia, **DIC, coagulation disorder, thrombosis, acute renal failure**

Pharmacokinetics

Absorption	Unknown
Distribution	Unknown
Metabolism	Unknown
Excretion	Unknown
Half-life	2-3 hr

Pharmacodynamics

Unknown

INTERACTIONS

Individual drugs
Activated prothrombin complex concentrate, prothrombin complex concentrate: do not use together

NURSING CONSIDERATIONS

Assessment
• Assess VS, B/P, pulse, respirations, neurologic signs, temp at least q4hr, temp 104° F (40° C) or indicators of internal bleeding, cardiac rhythm
• Monitor pro-time, APTT, plasma FVII clotting
• Monitor for thrombosis; dose should be reduced or stopped

Nursing diagnoses

• Injury, risk for (uses, adverse reactions)

Evaluation
Positive therapeutic outcome

• Therapeutic response: hemostasis

⚠ HIGH ALERT

factor IX complex (human)
Alpha Nine SD, Bebulin VH, BeneFIX, Mononine, Profilnine SD
Func. class.: Hemostatic
Chem. class.: Factors II, VII, IX, X
Pregnancy category C

ACTION: Causes an increase in blood levels of clotting factors II, VII, IX, X; factor IX (human) has IX activity only

Therapeutic outcome: Replacement of factors II, VII, IX, X

USES: Hemophilia B (Christmas disease), factor IX deficiency, anticoagulant reversal, control of bleeding in patients with factor VIII inhibitors; reversal of overdose of anticoagulants in emergencies

CONTRAINDICATIONS:
Hypersensitivity to mouse/hamster protein, DIC, mild factor IX deficiency

Precautions: Pregnancy C, neonates, infants, elective surgery, hepatic disease

DOSAGE AND ROUTES

Bleeding in hemophilia A and inhibitors of factor VIII (Proplex T, Konyne 80)
Adult and child: 75 units/kg, repeat in 12 hr

Factor IX complex (human) bleeding in hemophilia B
Adult and child: IV Establish 25% of normal factor IX activity or 60-75 units/kg then 10-20 units/kg/day × 1-2 wk

Prophylaxis of bleeding in hemophilia B
Adult and child: IV 10-20 units/kg 1-2 ×/wk

Reversal of oral anticoagulant
Adult and child: 15 units/kg

Factor VII deficiency (use Proplex T only)
Adult and child: IV 0.5 units/kg × body weight (kg) × desired factor IX increase (in % of normal); repeat q4-6hr if needed

Factor IX (human) minor to moderate hemorrhage
Use only Alpha Nine, Alpha Nine SD
Adult and child: IV Dose to increase plasma factor IX level to 20%-30% in one dose

Serious hemorrhage
Adult and child: IV Dose to increase plasma factor IX level to 30%-50% given as daily INF

Minor hemorrhage (Mononine only)
Adult and child: IV dose to increase plasma factor IX level to 15%-25% (20-30 units/kg), may repeat in 24 hr if needed

Major hemorrhage
Adult and child: IV dose to increase plasma factor IX level to 25%-50% (75 units/kg) q18-30hr for up to 10 days

Available forms: Inj (number of units noted on label)

Implementation

IV route
• Give hepatitis B vaccine before administration
• Give **IV** after warming to room temperature 3 ml/min or less, with plastic syringe only; do not admix
• Give after dilution with provided diluent, 50 or 25 units/ml; max 10 ml/min; decrease rate if fever, headache, flushing, tingling occur
• Give after crossmatch is completed if patient has blood type A, B, AB, to determine incompatibility with factor
• Store reconstituted sol for 3 hr at room temperature or up to 2 yr if refrigerated (powder); check expiration date
• Incompatible with protein products

BeneFIX
• Allow vials of concentrate/diluent to warm to room temperature
• After removing flip-top cap from vial, wipe top of vial with alcohol swab; let dry
• Peel back cover from vial adapter package; do not remove
• Place vial adapter over vial; press firmly until it snaps; attach plunger rod to diluent syringe and break plastic tip cap from diluent syringe
• Lift the package away from the adapter and connect diluent syringe; depress plunger; swirl contents

ADVERSE EFFECTS
CNS: *Headache, dizziness,* malaise, paresthesia, *lethargy, chills, fever, flushing*
CV: *Hypotension,* tachycardia, **MI, venous thrombosis, pulmonary embolism**

GI: Nausea, vomiting, abdominal cramps, jaundice, **viral hepatitis**
HEMA: Thrombosis, hemolysis, AIDS, DIC
INTEG: Rash, flushing, *urticaria,* injection-site reactions
RESP: Bronchospasm

Pharmacokinetics

Absorption	40% (PO), complete (**IV**)
Distribution	Unknown
Metabolism	Rapidly cleared from plasma, liver 30%
Excretion	Kidneys—70% unchanged
Half-life	24 hr

Pharmacodynamics

Unknown

INTERACTIONS
Individual drugs
Aminocaproic acid: increased risk of thrombosis; do not use together
Warfarin: decreased effect of warfarin

Drug classifications
Incompatible with protein products

NURSING CONSIDERATIONS
Assesment
• Monitor blood studies (coagulation factor assays by % normal: 5% prevents spontaneous hemorrhage, 30%-50% for surgery, 80%-100% for severe hemorrhage); check for bleeding q15-30min, immobilize and apply ice to affected joints
• Monitor for increased B/P, pulse
• Monitor I&O; if urine becomes orange or red, notify prescriber
• **Assess for allergic or pyrogenic reaction:** fever, chills, rash, itching; slow inf rate if not severe
⚠ Assess for DIC: bleeding, ecchymosis, hypersensitivity, changes in coagulation tests

Nursing diagnoses
• Injury, risk for (uses)
• Knowledge, deficient (teaching)

Patient/family education
• Advise patient to report any signs of bleeding: gums, under skin, urine, stools, emesis; calf pain, joint pain, yellowing of eyes/skin
• Caution patient about risk of viral hepatitis, AIDS; that immunization for hepatitis B may be given first; to be tested q2-3mo for HIV, even though the risk is low

• Tell patient to carry/wear emergency ID identifying disease and treatment; avoid salicylates, NSAIDs; inform other health professionals about condition

Evaluation
Positive therapeutic outcome
• Prevention of hemorrhage

---

famciclovir (Rx)
(fam-sye-klo'vir)
Famvir, Sandoz Famciclovir ✦
Func. class.: Antiviral
Chem. class.: Guanosine nucleoside
Pregnancy category B

F

ACTION: Inhibits DNA polymerase and viral DNA synthesis by conversion of this guanosine nucleoside to penciclovir

Therapeutic outcome: Decreasing size and number of lesions

USES: Treatment of acute herpes zoster (shingles), genital herpes, recurrent mucocutaneous herpes simplex virus (HSV) in HIV patients, initial episodes of herpes genitalis, herpes labialis in the immunocompromised

CONTRAINDICATIONS:
Hypersensitivity to this product, penciclovir, acyclovir, ganciclovir, valacyclovir, or valganciclovir

Precautions: Pregnancy **B**, breastfeeding, renal disease

DOSAGE AND ROUTES
Herpes zoster
Adult: PO 500 mg q8hr × 7 days

Renal dose
Adult: PO CCr ≥ 60 ml/min 500 mg q8hr; 40-59 ml/min 500 mg q12hr; 20-39 ml/min 500 mg q24hr; CCr <20 ml/min 250 mg q24hr

Recurrent HSV
Adult: PO 125 mg q12hr × 5 days

Renal dose
Adult: PO CCr <39 ml/min 125 mg q24hr × 5 days

Suppression of recurrent HSV
Adult: PO 250 mg q12hr up to 1 yr

Renal dose
Adult: PO CCr 20-39 ml/min 125 mg q12hr × 5 days; CCr <20 ml/min 125 mg q24hr × 5 days

---

Genital herpes/herpes labialis (recurrent)
Adult: PO 125 mg bid × 5 days or 1000 mg bid for 1 day; begin treatment at first sign of recurrence

Suppression of recurrent genital herpes
Adult: PO 250 mg bid for up to a year

Herpes genitalis initial episodes
Adult: PO 250 mg tid × 7-10 days

Available forms: Tabs 125, 250, 500 mg

Implementation
• Give with or without meals; absorption does not appear to be lowered when taken with food
• Give within 72 hr of the appearance of rash in herpes zoster

ADVERSE EFFECTS
CNS: *Headache, fatigue, dizziness,* paresthesia, somnolence, fever
GI: Nausea, vomiting, diarrhea, constipation, abdominal pain, anorexia
GU: Decreased sperm count
INTEG: *Pruritus*
MS: Back pain, arthralgia
RESP: Pharyngitis, sinusitis

Pharmacokinetics

Absorption	Well absorbed, 77%
Distribution	Protein binding 20%
Metabolism	Intestinal tissue, blood, liver
Excretion	Breast milk, kidney, bile
Half-life	Terminal 2-3 hr

Pharmacodynamics

Onset	Unknown
Peak	1 hr
Duration	8 hr

INTERACTIONS
Individual drugs
Cimetidine: decreased metabolism
Digoxin, probenecid, theophylline: decreased renal excretion

NURSING CONSIDERATIONS
Assessment
• **Herpes zoster:** assess number and distribution of lesions; also burning, itching, or pain (early symptoms of herpes infection); neuralgia during, after treatment
• **Acute renal failure:** usually in high doses or in those >65 yr; monitor renal function

tests: urine CCr, BUN before, during treatment if patient has decreased renal function; dosage may need to be lowered
• Monitor bowel pattern before, during treatment; diarrhea may occur
• Assess for posttherapeutic neuralgia during and after treatment

Nursing diagnoses
• Infection, risk for (uses)
• Knowledge, deficient (teaching)

Patient/family education
• Teach patient how to recognize signs of beginning of infection
• Teach patient how to prevent the spread of infection to others
• Teach patient reason for medication and expected results
• Advise patient that this medication does not prevent spread of disease to others, that condoms should be used
• Advise women with genital herpes to have yearly Pap smears; cervical cancer is more likely

Evaluation
Positive therapeutic outcome
• Decreased size and spread of lesions
• Prevention of recurrence (genital herpes)
• Decreased time for healing

famotidine (Rx, OTC)
(fa-moe'ti-deen)
Apo-Famotidine ✦, **Equaline Heartburn Prevention, Gen-Famotidine** ✦, **Good Sense Acid Reducer, Heartburn Relief, Leader Acid Reducer, Nu-Famotidine** ✦, **Pepcid, Pepcid AC, Top Care Acid Reducer, Top Care Acid Reducer Maximum Strength, Walgreens Acid Controller**
Func. class.: H$_2$-histamine receptor antagonist, antiulcer agent
Pregnancy category B

ACTION: Inhibits histamine at H$_2$-receptor site in gastric parietal cells, which inhibits gastric acid secretion while pepsin remains at a stable level

Therapeutic outcome: Healing of duodenal ulcers or gastric ulcers; prevention of duodenal ulcers; decreases symptoms of gastroesophageal reflux disease or Zollinger-Ellison syndrome, heartburn

USES: Short-term treatment of active duodenal ulcer, maintenance therapy for duodenal ulcer, Zollinger-Ellison syndrome, multiple endocrine adenomas, gastric ulcers, heartburn, gastroesophageal reflux disease

Unlabeled uses: GI disorders in those taking NSAIDs, urticaria, prevention of stress ulcers, aspiration pneumonitis, inactivation of oral pancreatic enzymes in pancreatic disorders, prevention of paclitaxel hypersensitivity reactions

CONTRAINDICATIONS:
Hypersensitivity

Precautions: Pregnancy **B**, breastfeeding, children <12 yr, geriatric, severe renal/hepatic disease

DOSAGE AND ROUTES
Active ulcer
Adult: PO 40 mg/day at bedtime × 4-8 wk, then 20 mg/day at bedtime if needed (maintenance); **IV** 20 mg q12hr if unable to take PO
Child 1-16 yr: PO 0.5 mg/kg/day at bedtime or divided bid, max 40 mg/day

Hypersecretory conditions
Adult: PO 20 mg q6hr; may give 160 mg q6hr if needed; **IV** 20 mg q12hr if unable to take PO

Heartburn relief/prevention
Adult: PO 10 mg with water, 15 min-1 hr before eating

Renal dose
Adult: PO CCr <50 ml/min; give 50% of dose or extend interval to q36-48hr

Available forms: Tabs 10, 20, 40 mg; powder for oral susp 40 mg/5 ml; inj 10 mg/ml, 20 mg/50 ml 0.9% NaCl; orally disintegrating tabs (RPD) 20, 40 mg; chew tabs 10 mg; gel cap 10 mg

Implementation
PO route
• Give antacids 1 hr before or 2 hr after famotidine; may be given with foods or liquid
• Administer oral susp after shaking well; discard unused sol after 1 mo

Direct IV route
• Give **IV** direct after diluting 2 ml of product (10 mg/ml) in 0.9% NaCl to total volume of 5-10 ml; inject over 2 min to prevent hypotension

Intermittent IV infusion route
• Administer after diluting 20 mg of product in 100 ml of LR, 0.9% NaCl, D5W, D10W; run over 15-30 min

Continuous IV infusion route
• **Adults:** Dilute 40 mg/250 ml D5W or NS, infuse over 24 hr, run at 11 ml/hr, use infusion device
• Store in cool environment (oral); **IV** sol is stable for 48 hr at room temperature; do not use discolored sol

Y-site compatibilities: Acyclovir, allopurinol, amifostine, aminophylline, amphotericin, ampicillin, ampicillin/sulbactam, inamrinone, amsacrine, atropine, aztreonam, bretylium, calcium gluconate, ceFAZolin, cefoperazone, cefotaxime, cefotetan, cefoxitin, ceftazidime, ceftizoxime, cefTRIAXone, cefuroxime, cephalothin, cephapirin, chlorproMAZINE, CISplatin, cladribine, cyclophosphamide, cytarabine, dexamethasone, dextran 40, digoxin, diphenhydrAMINE, DOBUTamine, DOPamine, DOXOrubicin, droperidol, enalaprilat, EPINEPHrine, erythromycin lactobionate, esmolol, filgrastim, fluconazole, fludarabine, folic acid, gentamicin, granisetron, haloperidol, heparin, hydrocortisone, HYDROmorphone, hydrOXYzine, imipenem/cilastatin, regular insulin, isoproterenol, labetalol, lidocaine, LORazepam, magnesium sulfate, melphalan, meperidine, methotrexate, methylPREDNISolone, metoclopramide, mezlocillin, midazolam, morphine, nafcillin, nitroglycerin, nitroprusside, norepinephrine, ondansetron, oxacillin, paclitaxel, perphenazine, phenylephrine, phenytoin, phytonadione, piperacillin, potassium chloride, potassium phosphate, procainamide, propofol, sargramostim, sodium bicarbonate, teniposide, theophylline, thiamine, thiotepa, ticarcillin, ticarcillin-clavulanate, verapamil, vinorelbine

ADVERSE EFFECTS
CNS: *Headache, dizziness,* paresthesia, depression, anxiety, somnolence, insomnia, fever, **seizures in renal disease**
CV: **Dysrhythmias,** QT prolongation (impaired renal functioning)
EENT: Taste change, tinnitus, orbital edema
GI: *Constipation,* nausea, vomiting, anorexia, cramps, abnormal liver enzymes, diarrhea
HEMA: **Thrombocytopenia, aplastic anemia**
INTEG: Rash, **toxic epidermal necrolysis, Stevens-Johnson syndrome**
MS: Myalgia, arthralgia
RESP: **Pneumonia**

Pharmacokinetics

Absorption	50% absorbed (PO)
Distribution	Plasma, protein binding (15%-20%)
Metabolism	Liver (30% active metabolizing)
Excretion	Kidneys (70%)
Half-life	$2^{1}/_{2}$-$3^{1}/_{2}$ hr

Pharmacodynamics

	PO	IV
Onset	30-60 min	Immediate
Peak	1-3 hr	$^{1}/_{2}$-3 hr
Duration	6-12 hr	8-15 hr

INTERACTIONS

Individual drugs

Cefditoren, cefpodoxime, itraconazole, ketoconazole: decreased absorption of each specific product

Atazanivir, delavirdine: decreased effects of each specific product

Drug classifications

Antacids: decreased absorption of famotidine

NURSING CONSIDERATIONS

Assessment

• **Assess patient with ulcers or suspected ulcers:** epigastric, abdominal pain, hematemesis, occult blood in stools, blood in gastric aspirate before treatment; throughout treatment; monitor gastric pH (maintain at pH 5)

• Monitor I&O ratio, BUN, creatinine, CBC with differential monthly

Nursing diagnoses

• Knowledge, deficient (teaching)
• Pain, acute (uses)

Patient/family education

• Caution patient to avoid driving, other hazardous activities until stabilized on this medication; dizziness may occur

• Advise patient to avoid black pepper, caffeine, alcohol, harsh spices, extremes in temperature of food; tell patient to avoid OTC preparations: aspirin, cough/cold preparations; condition may worsen

• Advise patient to avoid taking OTC and prescription preparations of this product concurrently

• Tell patient that smoking decreases the effectiveness of the product; that smoking cessation should be considered

• Instruct patient that product must be continued for prescribed time to be effective and taken exactly as prescribed; doses are not to be doubled; take missed dose when remembered up to 1 hr before next dose

• Tell patient to report bruising, fatigue, malaise; blood dyscrasias may occur

• Tell patient to report diarrhea, black tarry stools, sore throat, rash, dizziness, confusion, or delirium to prescriber immediately

Evaluation

Positive therapeutic outcome

• Decreased pain in abdomen
• Healing of ulcers

---

fat emulsions (Rx)

(fat ee-mul'shuns)

Intralipid 10%, Intralipid 20%, Liposyn II 10%, Liposyn II 20%, Liposyn III 10%, Liposyn III 20%, Soyacal 20%

Func. class.: Caloric

Chem. class.: Fatty acid, long chain

Pregnancy category C

ACTION: Needed for energy, heat production; consists of neutral triglycerides, primarily unsaturated fatty acids

Therapeutic outcome: Increased available calories and fatty acids

USES: Increase calorie intake, prevent fatty acid deficiency

CONTRAINDICATIONS:
Hypersensitivity to this product, eggs, soybeans, or legumes; hyperlipemia; lipid necrosis; acute pancreatitis accompanied by hyperlipemia; hyperbilirubinemia of the newborn; renal insufficiency; hepatic damage

Precautions: Pregnancy **C**, term newborns, severe liver disease, diabetes mellitus, thrombocytopenia, gastric ulcers, sepsis

> **BLACK BOX WARNING:** Preterm infants

DOSAGE AND ROUTES

Deficiency

Adult and child: **IV** 8%-10% of required calorie intake (intralipid)

Adjunct to TPN

Adult: IV 1 ml/min over 15-30 min (10%) or 0.5 ml/min over 15-30 min (20%); may increase to 500 ml over 4-8 hr if no adverse reactions occur; max 2.5 g/kg

Child: IV 0.1 ml/min over 10-15 min (10%) or 0.05 ml/ min over 10-15 min (20%); may increase to 1 g/kg over 4 hr if no adverse reactions occur; max 4 g/kg

Prevention of deficiency

Adult: IV 500 ml 2 ×/wk (10%), given 1 ml/min for 30 min, max 500 ml over 6 hr
Child: IV 5-10 ml/kg/day (10%), given 0.1 ml/min for 30 min, max 100 ml/hr

Available forms: Inj 10% (50, 100, 200, 250, 500 ml), 20% (50, 100, 200, 250, 500 ml)

Implementation

Intermittent IV infusion route

• Administer using infusion pump at prescribed rate; do not use in-line filter sized for lipid emulsion; clogging will occur
• Do not use mixed sol that looks oily or is separated; discard unused sol
• Change **IV** tubing at each inf: infection may occur with old tubing
• Give by intermittent inf at a rate of 10% sol (1 ml/min); 20% sol (0.5 ml/min) initially for 15-30 min; may be increased to 10% sol (120 ml/hr) or 20% sol (62.5 ml/hr) if no adverse reactions occur; max 500 ml during the first day; children should be given 10% (0.1 mg/ml) or 20% (0.05 ml/min) initially for 15-30 min, may be increased 1 g/kg/4 hr, max 10% (100 ml/hr) or 20% (50 ml/hr)

ADVERSE EFFECTS

CNS: Dizziness, headache, drowsiness, **focal seizures**
CV: Shock
GI: Nausea, vomiting, **hepatomegaly**
HEMA: Hyperlipemia, hypercoagulation, thrombocytopenia, leukopenia, leukocytosis
RESP: Dyspnea, **fat in lung tissue**

Pharmacokinetics

Absorption	Completely absorbed
Distribution	Intravascular space
Metabolism	Conversion to triglycerides, then to free fatty acids
Excretion	Unknown
Half-life	Unknown

Pharmacodynamics

Unknown

NURSING CONSIDERATIONS

Assessment

• Monitor triglycerides, free fatty acid levels, platelet counts daily to prevent fat overload, thrombocytopenia
• Monitor liver function tests: AST, ALT, Hct, Hgb; notify prescriber if abnormal
• Assess nutritional status: calorie count by dietitian; monitor weight daily

Nursing diagnoses

• Knowledge, deficient (teaching)
• Nutrition: less than body requirements, imbalanced (uses)

Patient/family education

• Teach patient reason for use of lipids and expected results

Evaluation

Positive therapeutic outcome
• Increased weight
• Fatty acids at adequate levels

febuxostat (Rx)

(feb-ux'oh-stat)
Uloric
Func. class.: Antigout drug, antihyperuricemic
Chem. class.: Xanthine oxidase inhibitor
Pregnancy category C

ACTION: Inhibits the enzyme xanthine oxidase, reducing uric acid synthesis; more selective for xanthine oxidase than allopurinol

Therapeutic outcome: Decreased signs/symptoms of gout, hyperuricemia

USES: Chronic gout, hyperuricemia

CONTRAINDICATIONS: Hypersensitivity

Precautions: Pregnancy **C**, breastfeeding, children, renal/hepatic/cardiac/neoplastic disease, stroke, MI, organ transplant, Lesch-Nyhan syndrome

DOSAGE AND ROUTES

Adult: PO 40 mg daily, may increase to 80 mg daily if uric acid levels are >6 mg/dl after 2 wk of therapy

Available forms: Tabs 40, 80 mg

Implementation
PO route
- Give without regard to meals or antacid; may crush and add to foods or fluids
- Give a few days before antineoplastic therapy

ADVERSE EFFECTS
CNS: Weakness, flushing
CV: MI, atrial fibrillation, atrial flutter, AV block, bradycardia, hyper/hypotension, palpitations, **sinus tachycardia, stroke,** angina
EENT: Retinopathy, cataracts, epistaxis
GI: *Nausea, vomiting, anorexia,* constipation, diarrhea, dyspepsia, hematemesis, hepatitis, hepatomegaly, weight gain/loss, cholecystitis, cholelithiasis, melena
GU: Renal failure, urinary urgency/frequency/incontinence, nephrolithiasis, hematuria
HEMA: Thrombocytopenia, anemia, pancytopenia, leukopenia, bone marrow suppression
INTEG: Rash
MISC: Arthralgia, gout flare

Pharmacokinetics

Absorption	Unknown
Distribution	Protein binding 99.2%
Metabolism	Unknown
Excretion	Feces, urine
Half-life	5-8 hr

Pharmacodynamics

Onset	Unknown
Peak	1-1.5 hr
Duration	Unknown

INTERACTIONS
Individual drugs
AzaTHIOprine: increased toxicity
Rasburicase: increased xanthine nephropathy, calculi
Mercaptopurine, theophylline: increased myelosuppression

Drug classifications
Antineoplastics: increased xanthine nephropathy, calculi

NURSING CONSIDERATIONS
Assessment
- **Hyperuricemia:** Monitor uric acid levels q2wk; uric acid levels should be 6 mg/dl or less
- Monitor CBC, AST, BUN, creatinine before starting treatment, periodically

- **Renal disease:** Monitor I&O ratio; increase fluids to 2 L/day to prevent stone formation and toxicity
- Assess for rash, hypersensitivity reactions; discontinue
- **Assess for gout:** joint pain, swelling; may use with NSAIDs for acute gouty attacks and gout flare

Nursing diagnoses
- Pain, chronic (uses)
- Noncompliance (teaching)
- Knowledge, deficient (teaching)

Patient/family education
- Inform patient that tabs may be crushed
- Teach patient to take as prescribed; if dose is missed, take as soon as remembered; do not double dose
- Teach patient to increase fluid intake to 2 L/day unless contraindicated
- Advise patient to avoid alcohol, caffeine; will increase uric acid levels
- Advise patient to report cardiovascular events to prescriber, immediately

Evaluation
Positive therapeutic outcome
- Decreased pain in joints, decreased stone formation in kidneys, decreased uric acid levels

felodipine (Rx)
(feh-loh′dih-peen)
Plendil ❖, Renedil ❖, Sandoz Felodipine ❖
Func. class.: Calcium-channel blocker, antihypertensive, antianginal
Chem. class.: Dihydropyridine
Pregnancy category C

ACTION: Inhibits calcium ion influx across cell membrane, resulting in inhibition of excitation/contraction of vascular smooth muscle

Therapeutic outcome: Decreased B/P in hypertension

USES: Essential hypertension, alone or with other antihypertensives

CONTRAINDICATIONS:
Hypersensitivity to this product or dihydropyridines, sick sinus syndrome, 2nd- or 3rd-degree heart block, hypotension <90 mm Hg systolic

Precautions: Pregnancy **C**, breastfeeding, children, geriatric, CHF, hepatic injury, renal disease

DOSAGE AND ROUTES
Adult: PO 5 mg/day initially, usual range 2.5-10 mg/day; max 10 mg/day; do not adjust dosage at intervals of <2 wk
Geriatric: PO 2.5 mg/day

Hepatic dose
Adult: PO 2.5-5 mg/day, max 10 mg/day

Available forms: Ext rel tabs 2.5, 5, 10 mg

Implementation
• Do not break, crush, or chew ext rel tabs
• Give once a day with food for GI symptoms

ADVERSE EFFECTS
CNS: *Headache,* fatigue, drowsiness, dizziness, anxiety, depression, nervousness, insomnia, light-headedness, paresthesia, tinnitus, psychosis, somnolence
CV: **Dysrhythmias,** *edema,* **CHF,** hypotension, palpitations, **MI, pulmonary edema,** tachycardia, syncope, AV block, angina
GI: Nausea, vomiting, diarrhea, gastric upset, constipation, increased liver function studies, dry mouth
GU: Nocturia, polyuria
HEMA: Anemia
INTEG: Rash, pruritus
MISC: Flushing, sexual difficulties, cough, nasal congestion, shortness of breath, wheezing, epistaxis, respiratory infection, chest pain, **Angioedema,** gingival hyperplasia

Pharmacokinetics
Absorption	Well absorbed
Distribution	Unknown; protein binding >99%
Metabolism	Liver, extensively
Excretion	Kidneys
Half-life	11-16 hr

Pharmacodynamics
Onset	2-3 hr
Peak	$2^{1}/_{2}$-5 hr
Duration	<24 hr

INTERACTIONS
Individual drugs
Alcohol, carBAMazepine, cimetidine, clarithromycin, conivaptan, cycloSPORINE, dalfopristin, delavirdine, diltiazem, erythromycin, itraconazole, ketoconazole, miconazole, phenytoin, propranolol, quiNIDine, quinupristin, zileuton: increased hypotension
Digoxin, disopyramide, phenytoin: increased bradycardia, increased CHF

Drug classifications
β-Adrenergic blockers: increased bradycardia, CHF
Nitrates: increased hypotension
NSAIDs: decreased antihypertensive effects

Drug/herb
Ginkgo, ginseng, hawthorn: increased antihypertensive effect
Ephedra, St. John's wort: decreased antihypertensive effect

Drug/food
Grapefruit juice: increased felodipine level

NURSING CONSIDERATIONS
Assessment
• CHF: Assess fluid volume status: I&O ratio and record; weight; skin turgor; adequacy of pulses; moist mucous membranes; bilateral lung sounds; peripheral pitting edema; dehydration symptoms of decreasing output, thirst, hypotension, dry mouth, and mucous membranes should be reported; for CHF: weight gain, crackles, dyspnea, edema, jugular venous distention
• Monitor ALT, AST, bilirubin daily if these are elevated
• Monitor cardiac status: B/P, pulse, respiration, ECG, periodically
• **Assess for anginal pain:** duration; intensity; ameliorating, aggravating factors

Nursing diagnoses
• Cardiac output, decreased (uses)
• Knowledge, deficient (teaching)

Patient/family education
• Caution patient to avoid hazardous activities until stabilized on product and dizziness is no longer a problem
• Instruct patient to limit caffeine consumption; to avoid alcohol and OTC products unless directed by prescriber
• Urge patient to comply in all areas of medical regimen: diet, exercise, stress reduction, product therapy; to notify prescriber of irregular heartbeat, shortness of breath, swelling of feet and hands, pronounced dizziness, constipation, nausea, hypotension
• Advise patient to use protective clothing, sunscreen to prevent photosensitivity
• Teach patient to change positions slowly to prevent orthostatic hypotension
• Advise patient to obtain correct pulse; to contact prescriber if pulse is <50 bpm
• Teach patient to use as directed even if feeling better; may be taken with other CV products (nitrates, β-blockers); that capsules may appear in stools but are insignificant

Evaluation
Positive therapeutic outcome
- Decreased B/P
- Decreased anginal attacks
- Increase in activity tolerance

---

fenofibrate (Rx)
(fen-oh-fee′brate)
Antara, Apo-Fenofibrate ✦, Apo-Fero-Micro ✦, Fenoglide, Gen-Fenofibrate ✦, Lipidil Micro ✦, Lipidil Supracap, Lipofem, Lofibra, PMS-Fenofibrate ✦, Tricor, Triglide
Func. class.: Antilipemic
Chem. class.: Fibric acid derivative
Pregnancy category C

ACTION: Increases lipolysis and elimination of triglyceride-rich particles from plasma by activating lipoprotein lipase, resulting in triglyceride change in size and composition of LDL, leading to rapid breakdown of LDL; mobilizes triglycerides from tissue; increases excretion of neutral sterols

Therapeutic outcome: Decreasing cholesterol levels and low-density lipoproteins, decreased pruritus

USES: Hypercholesterolemia, patients with types IV, V hyperlipidemia who do not respond to other treatment and who are at risk for pancreatitis; Fredrickson type IIa or IIb hypertriglyceridemia

CONTRAINDICATIONS:
Hypersensitivity, severe renal/hepatic disease, primary biliary cirrhosis, preexisting gallbladder disease

Precautions: Pregnancy C, breastfeeding, geriatric, peptic ulcer, pancreatitis, renal/hepatic disease

DOSAGE AND ROUTES
Hypertriglyceridemia
Adult: PO (Antara) 43-130 mg/day; (Lofibra) 67-200 mg/day; (Tricor) 48-145 mg/day; (Triglide) 50-160 mg/day

Primary hypercholesterolemia/ mixed hyperlipidemia
Adult: PO (Antara) 130 mg/day; (Lofibra) 200 mg/day; (Tricor) 145 mg/day; (Triglide) 160 mg/day

Renal dose (geriatric)
Adult: PO (Tricor) CCr 30-80 ml/min 48 mg/day; CCr <30 ml/min contraindicated
Adult: PO (Triglide, Lipofem) CCr 11-49 ml/min 50 mg/day; (Antara) 43 mg/day; (Lofibra) 67 mg/day; (Antara, Lipofem, Lofibra, Triglide) CCr <10 ml/min, contraindicated

Available forms: Tabs (Triglide) 50, 160 mg; (Tricor) 48, 145 mg; micronized cap (Antara) 43, 130 mg; (Lofibra) 67, 134, 200 mg; cap (Lipofem) 50, 100, 150 mg; (Fenoglide) 40, 120 mg

Implementation
- Do not break, crush, or chew tabs
- Give with evening meal; if dose is increased, give with breakfast and evening meal
- Store in cool environment in tight, light-resistant container

ADVERSE EFFECTS
CNS: Fatigue, weakness, drowsiness, dizziness, insomnia, depression, vertigo
CV: Angina, **dysrhythmias,** hypertension
GI: Nausea, vomiting, dyspepsia, increased liver enzymes, flatulence, hepatomegaly, gastritis
GU: Dysuria, urinary frequency
HEMA: Anemia, **leukopenia, thrombosis, pulmonary embolism**
INTEG: *Rash,* urticaria, pruritus, photosensitivity
MISC: Polyphagia, weight gain, infection, flulike syndrome
MS: Myalgias, arthralgias, **myopathy, rhabdomyolysis**
RESP: Pharyngitis, bronchitis, cough

Pharmacokinetics
Absorption	Unknown
Distribution	Protein binding 99%
Metabolism	Liver
Excretion	Urine 60%
Half-life	20 hr

Pharmacodynamics
Onset	Unknown
Peak	6-8 hr
Duration	Unknown

INTERACTIONS
Individual drugs
CycloSPORINE: increased nephrotoxicity

Drug classifications
Anticoagulants (oral): increased effect of anticoagulants

Antidiabetics: increased effect of antidiabetics
Bile acid sequestrants: decreased absorption
HMG-CoA reductase inhibitors: do not use
together, rhabdomyolysis may occur

Drug/herb
Red yeast rice: increased effects

Drug/food
Increased absorption

Drug/lab test
Increase: ALT, AST, BUN, CK, creatinine
Decrease: WBC, uric acid, Hgb

NURSING CONSIDERATIONS

Assessment
• **Hypercholesterolemia:** Monitor lipid levels
(triglycerides, LDL, HDL, total cholesterol), fat
content
• Liver function tests, baseline and periodically
during treatment; CPK if muscle pain occurs,
CBC, Hct, Hgh, pro-time with anticoagulant
therapy
• **Assess for pancreatitis, cholelithiasis,
renal failure, rhabdomyolysis** (when
combined with HMG-CoA reductase inhibitors),
myositis; product should be discontinued
• Assess nutrition: fat, protein, carbohydrates,
nutritional analysis should be completed by
dietitian

Nursing diagnoses
• Knowledge, deficient (teaching)
• Noncompliance (teaching)

Patient/family education
• Inform patient that compliance is needed
• Teach patient that risk factors—high-fat diet,
smoking, alcohol consumption, absence of exercise—should be decreased
• Caution patient to notify prescriber if pregnancy is planned or suspected
• Teach patient to notify prescriber if the GI
symptoms of diarrhea, abdominal or epigastric
pain, nausea, or vomiting occur
• Instruct patient to report GU symptoms:
dysuria, proteinuria, oliguria, decreased libido,
impotence
• Advise patient to notify prescriber of muscle
pain, weakness, fever, fatigue, epigastric pain

Evaluation
Positive therapeutic outcome
• Decrease in cholesterol to desired level after
8 wk

fenofibric acid (Rx)
(fen-oh-fye-brick)
TriLipix, Fibricor
Func. class.: Antilipemic
Chem. class.: Fibric acid derivative
Pregnancy category C

ACTION: An active metabolite of fenofibrate; increases lipolysis and elimination
of triglyceride-rich particles from plasma by
activating lipoprotein lipase, resulting in triglyceride change in size and composition of LDL,
leading to rapid breakdown of LDL; mobilizes
triglycerides from tissue; increases excretion of
neutral sterols

Therapeutic outcome: Triglyceride level
returning to normal

USES: Hyperlipoproteinemia; hypertriglyceridemia

CONTRAINDICATIONS:
Hypersensitivity, severe renal/hepatic disease,
primary biliary cirrhosis, preexisting gallbladder
disease, breastfeeding

Precautions: Pregnancy **C**, geriatric, pancreatitis, thromboembolic disease

DOSAGE AND ROUTES

**Combination with HMG-CoA
reductase inhibitors to reduce
triglycerides and increase HDL-C in
those with mixed dyslipidemia or
coronary heart disease**
Adult: DEL REL cap PO 135 mg daily

Severe hypertriglyceridemia
Adult: DEL REL cap PO 45-135 daily; tabs
35-105 mg daily

Renal dose
Adult: PO CCr 30-80 ml/min 35 mg (Fibricor)
or 45 mg (TriLipix) q day, initially; CCr <30 ml/
min, do not use

Available forms: Tabs 35, 105 mg; cap
(Fibricor), gastro-resistant pellet 45, 135 mg
(TriLipix)

Implementation
• Give product with meals; may increase q4-
8wk

ADVERSE EFFECTS
CNS: Fatigue, weakness, drowsiness, dizziness, insomnia, depression, vertigo, asthenia,
headache

CV: Hypertension
EENT: Blurred vision
GI: *Nausea,* vomiting, dyspepsia, increased liver enzymes, abdominal pain, cholecystitis, cholelithiasis, constipation, diarrhea, hepatitis, jaundice, pancreatitis
GU: Impotence, decreased libido
HEMA: Anemia, leukopenia, **thrombosis/ pulmonary embolism, agranulocytosis, eosinophilia**
INTEG: *Rash,* urticaria, pruritus, **Stevens-Johnson syndrome**
MISC: Infection
MS: *Myalgias, arthralgias,* **myopathy,** back pain, MS pain, **rhabdomyolysis**
RESP: Pharyngitis, cough

Pharmacokinetics

Absorption	Unknown
Distribution	Protein binding 99%
Metabolism	Liver, converted to fenofibric acid
Excretion	Urine 60%
Half-life	20 hr

Pharmacodynamics

Onset	Unknown
Peak	4-5 hr (del rel cap), 2.5 hr (tab)
Duration	Unknown

INTERACTIONS

Individual drugs
CycloSPORINE: increased nephrotoxicity

Drug classifications
Monitor use with HMG-CoA reductase inhibitors; rhabdomyolysis may occur
Bile acid sequestrants: decreased absorption of fenofibrate
Oral anticoagulants: increased anticoagulant effect

Drug/herb
Glucomannan: increased effect
Gotu cola: decreased effect

Drug/food
Increase: absorption

NURSING CONSIDERATIONS

Assessment
• **Diet History:** monitor fat content, lipid levels (triglycerides, LDL, HDL, total cholesterol), LFTs baseline periodically during treatment, CBC with differential, CPK, serum bilirubin (direct/indirect)

• **Assess for pancreatitis, cholelithiasis renal failure, rhabdomyolysis** (when combined with HMG CoA reductase inhibitors), myositis; product should be discontinued

Nursing diagnosis
• Risk of injury (uses)
• Noncompliance (teaching)
• Knowledge, deficient (teaching)

Patient/family education
• Teach patient that compliance is needed
• Advise patient that risk factors should be decreased: high-fat diet, smoking, alcohol consumption, absence of exercise
• Advise patient to notify prescriber if pregnancy is suspected or planned
• Teach patient to report GU symptoms: decreased libido, impotence
• Advise patient to notify prescriber of muscle pain, weakness, fever, fatigue; epigastric pain

Evaluation:
Positive therapeutic outcome
• Decreased triglycerides

---

fenoldopam (Rx)
(fen-nahl′doh-pam)
Corlopam
Func. class.: Antihypertensive, vasodilator
Pregnancy category B

ACTION: Agonist at D_1-like dopamine receptors; binds to α_2-adrenoreceptors; increases renal blood flow

Therapeutic outcome: B/P, decreased

USES: Hypertensive crisis, malignant hypertension

Unlabeled uses: Prevention of contrast agent-associated nephrotoxicity

CONTRAINDICATIONS:
Hypersensitivity, sulfite sensitivity

Precautions: Pregnancy **B**, breastfeeding, children, tachycardia, intraocular pressure, hypokalemia, CVA, CAD, CHF, increased intraocular pressure

DOSAGE AND ROUTES
Adult: **IV** 0.1 mcg/kg/min, titrate upward or downward ≤15 min by 0.05-0.1 mcg/kg/min, max 0.8 mcg/kg/min

---

⚠ Nurse Alert

Child: CONT **IV** 0.2 mcg/kg/min with effects within 5 min; may increase dose to 0.3-0.5 mcg/kg/min q20-30min depending on response

Available forms: Inj 10 mg/ml

Implementation

IV route
• Give to patient in recumbent position; keep in that position for 1 hr after administration
• Diluted sol is stable in normal light/temperature for 24 hr

Adult
• Administer after diluting contents of ampules in 0.9% NaCl, or 5% dextrose inj (40 mcg/ml); then add 4 ml of conc (40 mg of product/1000 ml); 2 ml of conc (20 mg of product/500 ml); 1 ml of conc (10 mg of product/250 ml); do not admix

Child
• Use inf pump
• After dilution 3 ml (30 mg)/500 ml (60 mcg/ml); 1.5 ml (15 mg)/250 ml (60 mcg/ml); 0.6 ml (6 mg)/100 ml (60 mcg/ml)

Y-site compatibilities: Alfentanil, allopurinol, amifostine, aminocaproic acid, amiodarone, amphotericin B liposome, ampicillin-sulbactam, anidulafungin, argatroban, atenolol, atracurium, atropine, azithromycin, aztreonam, bivalirudin, bleomycin, buprenorphine, busulfan, butorphanol, calcium chloride/gluconate, CARBOplatin, carmustine, caspofungin, ceFAZolin, cefepime, cefoperazone, cefotaxime, cefotetan, ceftazidime, ceftizoxime, cefTRIAXone, cefuroxime, chloramphenicol, chlorproMAZINE, cimetidine, ciprofloxacin, cisatracurium, CISplatin, clindamycin, cyclophosphamide, cycloSPORINE, cytarabine, dacarbazine, DACTINomycin, DAPTOmycin, DAUNOrubicin, digoxin, diltiazem, diphenhydrAMINE, DOBUTamine, docetaxel, dolasetron, DOPamine, doxacurium, DOXOrubicin, doxycycline, droperidol, enalaprilat, ePHEDrine, EPINEPHrine, epirubicin, ertapenem, erythromycin, esmolol, etoposide, famotidine, fentaNYL, fluconazole, fludarabine, fluorouracil, foscarnet, gatifloxacin, gemcitabine, gentamicin, glycopyrrolate, granisetron hydrochloride, haloperidol, heparin, hydrALAZINE, hydrocortisone, HYDROmorphone, hydrOXYzine, IDArubicin, ifosfamide, imipenem-cilastatin, inamrinone, insulin (regular), irinotecan, isoproterenol, labetalol, leucovorin, levofloxacin, levorphanol, lidocaine, linezolid, LORazepam, magnesium sulfate, mannitol, mechlorethamine, meperidine, metaraminol, methotrexate, methyldopa, metoclopramide, metoprolol, metroNIDAZOLE, micafungin, midazolam, milrinone, minocycline, mitoxantrone, mivacurium, morphine, mycophenolate, nafcillin, nalbuphine, naloxone, niCARdipine, nitroglycerin, nitroprusside, norepinephrine, octreotide, ondansetron, oxaliplatin, oxytocin, paclitaxel, palonosetron, pamidronate, pancuronium, pemetrexed, pentamidine, pentazocine, PHENobarbital, phenylephrine, piperacillin, piperacillin-tazobactam, polymyxin B, potassium chloride/phosphates, procainamide, promethazine, propofol, propranolol, quiNIDine, quinupristin-dalfopristin, ranitidine, remifentanil, rocuronium, sodium acetate/phosphates, streptozocin, succinylcholine, SUFentanil, sulfamethoxazole-trimethoprim, tacrolimus, teniposide, theophylline, thiotepa, ticarcillin, ticarcillin-clavulanate, tigecycline, tirofiban, tobramycin, tolazoline, topotecan, trimethobenzamide, vancomycin, vasopressin, vecuronium, verapamil, vinBLAStine, vinCRIStine, vinorelbine, voriconazole, zidovudine, zoledronic acid

Y-site incompatibilities: Acyclovir, aminophylline, amphotericin B, ampicillin, bumetanide, cefoxitin, dexamethasone sodium phosphate, diazepam, fosphenytoin, furosemide, ganciclovir, ketorolac, meropenem, methohexital, methylPREDNISolone sodium succinate, pantoprazole, PENTobarbital, phenytoin, prochlorperazine, sodium bicarbonate, thiopental

ADVERSE EFFECTS
CNS: *Headache,* anxiety, dizziness, insomnia
CV: *Hypotension,* ST-T-wave changes, angina pectoris, palpitations, **MI, ischemic heart disease,** *flushing*
GI: Nausea, vomiting, constipation, diarrhea
HEMA: Leukocytosis, bleeding
INTEG: Sweating
META: Hypokalemia

Pharmacokinetics

Absorption	Unknown
Distribution	Steady state 20 min
Metabolism	Unknown
Excretion	Unknown
Half-life	5 min (elimination)

Pharmacodynamics
Unknown

INTERACTIONS

Individual drugs
Metoclopramide: decreased antihypertensive effects

Drug classifications
β-Adrenergic blockers: increased hypotension
Peripherally acting DOPamine antagonists: decreased antihypertensive effects

Drug/herb
Ephedra: decreased antihypertensive effect

NURSING CONSIDERATIONS

Assessment
• **Hypertensive crisis/malignant hypertension:** monitor B/P q5min until stabilized, then q1hr × 2 hr, then q4hr; pulse, jugular venous distention q4hr
• Monitor electrolytes, blood studies: K, Na, Cl, CO_2, CBC, serum glucose
• Assess skin turgor, dryness of mucous membranes for hydration status
• Assess **IV** site for extravasation, rate

Nursing diagnoses
• Knowledge, deficient (teaching)
• Noncompliance (teaching)

Patient/family education
• Teach patient reason for medication and expected results
• Instruct patient to report dyspnea, chest pain, bleeding

Evaluation
Positive therapeutic outcome
• Decreased B/P

⚠ HIGH ALERT

fentaNYL (Rx)
(fen′ta-nill)
ABSTRAL, Actiq, Fentora, Onsolis, RAN-Fentanyl ✤
fentaNYL transdermal (Rx)
Duragesic
Func. class.: Opioid analgesic
Chem. class.: Synthetic phenylpiperidine derivative
fentaNYL nasal spray (Rx)
Lazanda
fentaNYL SL spray (Rx)
Subsys
Pregnancy category C
Controlled substance schedule II

Do not confuse:
fentaNYL/Sufenta

ACTION: Inhibits ascending pain pathways in CNS, increases pain threshold, alters pain perception by binding to opiate receptors

Therapeutic outcome: Relief of pain, supplement to anesthesia

USES: Controls moderate to severe pain; preoperatively, postoperatively; adjunct to general anesthetic, adjunct to regional anesthesia; **FentaNYL:** for anesthesia as premedication, conscious sedation; **Actiq:** for breakthrough cancer pain

CONTRAINDICATIONS:
Hypersensitivity to opiates, myasthenia gravis

> **BLACK BOX WARNING:** headache, migraine (Actiq), Astral, Fentora, Lazanda, Onsolis, emergency dept use (Abstral, Lazanda), outpatient surgeries (Duragesic TD), opioid-naive patients

Precautions: Pregnancy **C,** breastfeeding, geriatric, increased ICP, seizure disorders, cardiac dysrhythmias, severe respiratory disorders

> **BLACK BOX WARNING:** Children, accidental exposure, ambient temperature increase, fever, skin abrasion (TD patch), substance abuse, respiratory disorders, depression, surgery

DOSAGE AND ROUTES
FentaNYL

Anesthetic
Adult: IV 25-100 mcg (0.7-2 mcg/kg) q2-3min prn

Anesthesia supplement
Adult and child >12 yr: IM/IV 2-20 mcg/kg **IV** INF 0.025-0.25 mcg/kg/min

Induction and maintenance
Adult: IV BOL 5-40 mcg/kg
Child 2-12 yr: IV 2-3 mcg/kg

Preoperatively
Adult and child >12 yr: IM/IV 0.05-0.1 mg q30-60min before surgery

Postoperatively
Adult and child >12 yr: IM/IV 0.05-0.1 mg q1-2hr prn

Sedation/analgesia
Adult and child >12 yr: IV 0.5-1 mcg/kg/dose; may repeat after 30-60 min

---

Child 1-12 yr: IV BOL 1-2 mcg/kg/dose; may repeat after 30-60 min intervals; CONT **IV** 1-5 mcg/kg/hr after **IV** BOL dose
Neonate: IV BOL 0.5-3 mcg/kg/dose; CONT **IV** 0.5-2 mcg/kg/hr after **IV** BOL

Actiq
Adult: Transmucosal 200 mcg, redose if needed 15 min after completion of 1st dose, max 2 doses during titration period

Fentora
Adult: BUCCAL 100 mcg placed above rear molar between upper cheek and gum

Onsolis
Adult: transmucosal 200 mcg, titrate, max 1200 mcg/dose or 4 doses/day

ABSTRAL
Adult: SL 100 mcg, another dose may be taken 30 min after first, max 2 doses per episode of breakthrough pain, ≥2 hr must elapse before treating again, titrate stepwise over consecutive episodes

FentaNYL transdermal
Adult: 25 mcg/hr; may increase until pain relief occurs; apply patch to flat surface on upper torso and wear for 72 hr; apply new patch to different site for continued relief

FentaNYL nasal spray
Adult: 100 mcg (1 spray in 1 nostril), may re-treat after ≥2 hr, titrate upward to adequate analgesia, treat a max of 4 episodes q day

FentaNYL SL spray
Adult: SL 100 mcg sprayed under the tongue; titrate stepwise carefully

Available forms: Inj 0.05 mg/ml; lozenges 100, 200, 300, 400 mcg; lozenges on a stick 200, 400, 600, 800, 1200, 1600 mcg; buccal tab 100, 200, 400, 600, 800 mcg; oral dissolving film (Onsolis) 120, 200, 400, 600, 800 mcg; transdermal patch 12, 25, 50, 75, 100 mcg/hr; SL tab (ABSTRAL) 100, 200, 300, 400, 600, 800 mcg; SL spray: 100, 200, 400, 600, 1200, 1600 mcg/spray

Implementation
• Store in light-resistant area at room temperature
Transmucosal route
• Remove foil just before administration; instruct patient to place between cheek and lower gum, moving it back and forth and sucking, not chewing (Actiq); place above rear molar (Fentora); place film on the inside of the cheek (Onsolis); all products not used or partially used should be flushed down the toilet

Transdermal route
• Apply patch to chest on a flat area with skin intact; for skin preparation, use clear water with no soap; clip hair, skin should be dry before applying patch; apply immediately after removing from package and press firmly in place with palm of hand; flush old patch down toilet immediately upon removal
Use pain dosing
• Dosage is titrated based on patient's report of pain; dosage is determined by calculating the previous 24-hr requirement and converting to equianalgesic morphine dose
• To convert to another opioid analgesic, remove transdermal patch and begin treatment with half the equal pain-controlling dose of the new analgesic in 12-18 hr
SL spray
• Open blister package with scissors immediately prior to use; spray contents under tongue; dispose of unit by placing it into disposable bags provided; seal bag, discard into trash container out of reach of children.

IV route
• Give by inj (IM, **IV**), only with resuscitative equipment available; give slowly to prevent rigidity
• Give **IV** undiluted by anesthesiologist or diluted with 5 ml or more sterile water or 0.9% NaCl given through Y-tube or 3-way stopcock given at 0.1 mg or less/ 1.2 min

Syringe compatibilities: Alprostadil, atracurium, atropine, bupivacaine/ketamine, butorphanol, chlorproMAZINE, cimetidine, cloNIDine/lidocaine, dimenhyDRINATE, diphenhydrAMINE, droperidol, heparin, HYDROmorphone, hydrOXYzine, lidocaine, meperidine, metoclopramide, midazolam, morphine, pentazocine, perphenazine, prochlorperazine, promazine, promethazine, ranitidine, scopolamine

Syringe incompatibilities: PENTobarbital

Y-site compatibilities: Abciximab, acyclovir, alfentanil, alprostadil, amikacin, aminocaproic acid, aminophylline, amiodarone, amphotericin B cholesteryl, amphotericin B lipid complex, amphotericin B liposome, anidulafungin, argatroban, ascorbic acid injection, atenolol, atracurium, atropine, azaTHIOprine, aztreonam, benztropine, bivalirudin, bleomycin, bumetanide, buprenorphine, butorphanol, calcium chloride/gluconate, CARBOplatin, caspofungin, cefamandole, ceFAZolin, cefmetazole, cefonicid, cefoperazone, cefotaxime, cefotetan,

*Adverse effects: italics = common; **bold** = life-threatening*

cefoxitin, ceftazidime, ceftizoxime, ceftobiprole, cefTRIAXone, cefuroxime, cephalothin, chloramphenicol, chlorproMAZINE, cimetidine, cisatracurium, CISplatin, clindamycin, cloNIDine, cyanocobalamin, cyclophosphamide, cycloSPORINE, cytarabine, DACTINomycin, DAPTOmycin, dexamethasone, dexmedetomidine, digoxin, diltiazem, diphenhydrAMINE, DOBUTamine, docetaxel, DOPamine, doripenem, doxacurium, doxapram, DOXOrubicin, doxycycline, enalaprilat, ePHEDrine, EPINEPHrine, epirubicin, epoetin alfa, eptifibatide, erythromycin, esmolol, etomidate, etoposide, famotidine, fenoldopam, fluconazole, fludarabine, fluorouracil, folic acid, furosemide, ganciclovir, gatifloxacin, gemcitabine, gentamicin, glycopyrrolate, granisetron, heparin, hydrocortisone, HYDROmorphone, hydrOXYzine, IDArubicin, ifosfamide, imipenem-cilastatin, inamrinone, insulin (regular), irinotecan, isoproterenol, ketorolac, labetalol, lansoprazole, levofloxacin, lidocaine, linezolid, LORazepam, LR, magnesium sulfate, mannitol, mechlorethamine, meperidine, metaraminol, methicillin, methotrexate, methotrimeprazine, methoxamine, methyldopate, methylPREDNISolone, metoclopramide, metoprolol, metroNIDAZOLE, mezlocillin, miconazole, midazolam, milrinone, minocycline, mitoxantrone, mivacurium, morphine, moxalactam, multiple vitamins injection, mycophenolate, nafcillin, nalbuphine, naloxone, nesiritide, netilmicin, niCARdipine, nitroglycerin, nitroprusside, norepinephrine, octreotide, ondansetron, oxacillin, oxaliplatin, oxytocin, paclitaxel, palonosetron, pamidronate, pancuronium, papaverine, pemetrexed, penicillin G potassium/sodium, pentamidine, pentazocine, PENTobarbital, PHENobarbital, phenylephrine, phytonadione, piperacillin, piperacillin-tazobactam, polymyxin B, potassium chloride, procainamide, prochlorperazine, promethazine, propofol, propranolol, protamine, pyridoxine, quiNIDine, quinupristin-dalfopristin, ranitidine, remifentanil, Ringer's, ritodrine, riTUXimab, rocuronium, sargramostim, scopolamine, sodium acetate/bicarbonate, succinylcholine, SUFentanil, tacrolimus, teniposide, theophylline, thiamine, thiopental, thiotepa, ticarcillin, ticarcillin-clavulanate, tigecycline, tirofiban, TNA, tobramycin, tolazoline, TPN, trastuzumab, trimetaphan, urokinase, vancomycin, vasopressin, vecuronium, verapamil, vinCRIStine, vinorelbine, vitamin B complex/C, voriconazole, zoledronic acid

Additive compatibilities: Bupivacaine, caffeine citrate, cloNIDine, droperidol, EPINEPHrine, ketamine, lidocaine, ziconotide

Additive incompatibilities: Methohexital, PENTobarbital, thiopental

Solution compatibilities: D_5W, 0.9% NaCl

ADVERSE EFFECTS
CNS: Dizziness, delirium, euphoria, sedation
CV: Bradycardia, cardiac arrest, hypo/hypertension
EENT: Blurred vision, miosis
GI: Nausea, vomiting, constipation
GU: Urinary retention
INTEG: Rash, diaphoresis
MS: Muscle rigidity
RESP: Respiratory depression, arrest, laryngospasm

Pharmacokinetics

Absorption	Well absorbed (IM), completely absorbed (**IV**)
Distribution	Unknown, crosses placenta
Metabolism	Extensively, liver; 80% bound to plasma proteins
Excretion	Kidneys, up to 25% unchanged; breast milk
Half-life	$1^1/_2$-6 hr; 17 hr after removal of patch (TD)

Pharmacodynamics

	IM	IV	TD
Onset	7-8 min	Rapid	6 hr
Peak	30 min	3-5 min	12-24 hr
Duration	1-2 hr	$^1/_2$-1 hr	72 hr

INTERACTIONS

Individual drugs
Alcohol: increased respiratory depression, hypotension, increased sedation

Drug classifications
Antipsychotics, opioids, skeletal muscle relaxants: effects increased
CNS depressants, sedative/hypnotics: increased respiratory depression, hypotension
CYP3A4 inducers (carBAMazepine, PHENobarbital, phenytoin, rifampin): decreased fentaNYL effect

Drug/herb
St. John's wort, valerian: increased fentaNYL action
Echinacea: decreased effect of fentaNYL

Drug/lab test
Increased: amylase, lipase

NURSING CONSIDERATIONS
Assessment
• Monitor VS after parenteral route (B/P, pulse, respiration); note muscle rigidity; take drug history before administering product; check renal/liver function tests; assess for respiratory dysfunction: respiratory depression, character, rate, rhythm; notify prescriber if respirations are <10/min
• Monitor CNS changes: dizziness, drowsiness, hallucinations, euphoria, LOC, pupil reaction
• Monitor allergic reactions: rash, urticaria; product should be discontinued
• **Assess for pain:** intensity, location, duration, type, before and 15 min after IM route or 3-5 min after **IV** route
Headache, migraine:
• Abstral, Actiq, Fentora, Lazanda, Onsolis are not to be used for this condition; Abstral, Lazanda is not to be used in the ED; Duragesic TD is not to be used for outpatient surgery patients
Apnea, respiratory arrest in opioid-naive patients:
• Do not use Abstral, Actiq, Duragesic, Fentora, Lazanda, Onsolis, opioid tolerant are those using ≥60 ml/day oral morphine, ≥30 mg/day oxyCODONE PO, 8 mg/day HYDROmorphone, 25 mcg tid fentaNYL/hr

Nursing diagnoses
• Breathing pattern, ineffective (adverse reactions)
• Knowledge, deficient (teaching)
• Pain, acute (uses)

Patient/family education
• Discuss the dangers of children or pets getting the product
• Advise patient to report any symptoms of CNS changes, allergic reactions
• Instruct patient to avoid CNS depressants: alcohol, sedative-hypnotics for at least 24 hr after taking this product
• Teach patient that dizziness, drowsiness, confusion are common, and to avoid getting up without assistance
• Discuss in detail with patient all aspects of the product
• Teach patient CNS changes: physical dependence; not to use with alcohol, other CNS depressants
Transdermal route
• **Ambient temperature increase:** Discuss with patient that excessive heat may increase absorption; excessive perspiration may alter adhesiveness; do not use with heating pads,

electric blankets, heat/tanning lamps, saunas, hot tubs, heated waterbeds, sunbathing
• Discuss with patient that hair may need to be clipped before applying
• Teach patient how to dispose of patch: place sticky sides together and flush in toilet

Evaluation
Positive therapeutic outcome
• Maintenance of anesthesia
• Decreased breakthrough cancer pain
• General pain relief

TREATMENT OF OVERDOSE:
Naloxone 0.2-0.8 **IV**, O₂, **IV** fluids, vasopressors

---

ferrous fumarate (Rx)
Ferretts, Ferrimin, Ferro-Sequels, Hemocyte, Palafer ✦, Walgreens Finest Iron
ferrous gluconate (Rx)
Apo-Ferrous Gluconate ✦, Ferate, Walgreens Gold Seal Ferrous Gluconate
ferrous sulfate (Rx)
Apo-Ferrous Sulfate ✦, Equaline Ferrous Sulfate, Leader Ferrous Sulfate, Slow Release Iron, Walgreens Gold Seal Ferrous Sulfate
ferrous sulfate, dried (Rx)
Slow Fe
carbonyl iron (OTC)
(kar'boh-nil)
ICAR Pediatric, Iron Chews
iron polysaccharide (OTC)
iFerex, Niferex, Nu-Iron
Func. class.: Hematinic
Chem. class.: Iron preparation
Pregnancy category B, C

ACTION: Replaces iron stores needed for red blood cell development, energy and O₂ transport, utilization; fumarate contains 33% elemental iron; gluconate, 12%; sulfate, 20%; iron, 30%; ferrous sulfate exsiccated

Therapeutic outcome: Prevention and correction of iron deficiency

USES: Iron deficiency anemia, prophylaxis for iron deficiency in pregnancy, nutritional supplementation

---

Adverse effects: *italics* = common; **bold** = life-threatening

CONTRAINDICATIONS:
Sideroblastic anemia, thalassemia, hemosiderosis/hemochromatosis

Precautions: Pregnancy **B** (ferric gluconate complex), **C** (iron dextran, oral products); anemia (long-term), peptic ulcer disease, hemolytic anemia, cirrhosis, ulcerative colitis/regional enteritis, sulfite sensitivity

> **BLACK BOX WARNING:** Accidental exposure

DOSAGE AND ROUTES
Fumarate
Adult: PO 50-100 mg tid
Child: PO 3 mg/kg/day (elemental iron) tid-qid
Infant: PO 10-25 mg/day (elemental iron) in 3-4 divided doses, max 15 mg/day

Gluconate
Adult: PO 60 mg bid-qid
Child 6-12 yr: PO 3 mg/kg/day divided

Sulfate
Adult: PO 0.750-1.5 g/day in divided doses tid
Child 6-12 yr: 600 mg/day in divided doses

Pregnancy
Adult: PO 300-600 mg/day in divided doses

Complex
Adult: IV INF (125 mg) 10 ml/100 ml of NaCl for inj given over 1 hr

Iron polysaccharide
Adult: 100-200 mg/day
Child: PO 4-6 mg/kg/day in 3 divided doses (severe iron deficiency)

Available forms: *Fumarate:* tabs 63, 195, 200, 324, 325 mg; chewable tabs 100 mg; controlled-release tabs 300 mg; oral susp 100 mg/5 ml, 45 mg/0.6 ml; *gluconate:* tabs 300, 320, 325 mg; caps 86, 325, 435 mg; film-coated tabs 300 mg; elix 300 mg/5 ml; *sulfate:* tabs 195, 300, 325 mg; enteric-coated tabs 325 mg; ext rel tabs, time-rel caps 525 mg; dried: tabs 200 mg; ext rel tabs 160 mg; ext rel caps 160 mg; *iron polysaccharide:* tabs 50 mg; caps 150 mg; sol 100 mg/5 ml

Implementation
• Swallow all tabs whole; do not break, crush, or chew
• Give between meals for best absorption; may give with juice; do not give with antacids or milk, delay at least 1 hr; if GI symptoms occur, give after meals even if absorption is decreased; eggs, milk products, chocolate, caffeine interfere with absorption; ferrous gluconate is less GI irritating than ferrous sulfate

• Give liquid preparations through plastic straw to avoid discoloration of tooth enamel; dilute thoroughly
• Give at least 1 hr before bedtime because corrosion may occur in stomach
• Give for <6 mo for anemia
• Store in airtight, light-resistant container

ADVERSE EFFECTS
GI: *Nausea, constipation, epigastric pain, black and red tarry stools,* vomiting, diarrhea
INTEG: Temporarily discolored tooth enamel and eyes
SYST: Hypersensitivity reactions (Ferrlecit)

Pharmacokinetics
Absorption	Up to 30%
Distribution	Bound to transferrin, crosses placenta
Metabolism	Recycled
Excretion	Feces, urine, skin, breast milk
Half-life	Unknown

Pharmacodynamics
Unknown

INTERACTIONS
Individual drugs
Chloramphenicol, vit C: increased absorption of iron products
Cholestyramine, L-thyroxine, levodopa, methyldopa, penicillamine, tetracycline, vitamin E: decreased absorption of each product
Drug classifications
Antacids, H_2 antagonists, proton pump inhibitors: decreased absorption of iron preparations
Fluoroquinolones: decreased absorption of fluoroquinolone
Drug/food
Caffeine, dairy products, eggs: decreased absorption
Drug/lab test
False positive: occult blood

NURSING CONSIDERATIONS
Assessment
• Monitor blood studies: Hct, Hgb, reticulocytes, bilirubin before treatment, at least monthly; iron studies (Fe, TIBC, ferritin)
• **Assess for toxicity:** nausea, vomiting, diarrhea (green, then tarry stools,) hematemesis, pallor, cyanosis, shock, coma

---

🅐 Nurse Alert

- Assess bowel elimination; if constipation occurs, increase water, bulk, activity before laxatives are required
- **Assess nutrition:** amount of iron in diet (meat, dark green leafy vegetables, dried beans, dried fruits, eggs); provide referral to dietitian if indicated
- Identify cause of iron loss or anemia, including salicylates, sulfonamides, antimalarials, quiNIDine

Nursing diagnoses
- Fatigue (uses)
- Knowledge, deficient (teaching)
- Nutrition, less than body requirements, imbalanced (uses)

Patient/family education
- Advise patient that iron will make stools black or dark green; that iron poisoning may occur if increased beyond recommended level
- Advise patient to keep out of reach of children, pets
- Caution patient not to substitute one iron salt for another; elemental iron content differs (e.g., 300 mg ferrous fumarate contains about 100 mg elemental iron, whereas 300 mg ferrous gluconate contains only about 30 mg elemental iron)
- Caution patient to avoid reclining position for 15-30 min after taking product to avoid esophageal corrosion; to follow diet high in iron
- Caution patient to avoid taking iron, dairy products, calcium supplements, vit C together; they compete for absorption

Evaluation
Positive therapeutic outcome
- Decreased fatigue, weakness
- Improvement in Hct, Hgb, reticulocytes

TREATMENT OF OVERDOSE:
Induce vomiting; give eggs, milk until lavage can be done

ferumoxytol (Rx)
(fer'ue-mox'i-tol)
Feraheme
Func. class.: Hematinic
Pregnancy category B

ACTION: Iron is carried by transferrin to the bone marrow, where it is incorporated into hemoglobin

USES: Iron deficiency anemia in chronic kidney disease

Therapeutic outcome: Resolution of iron deficiency anemia in chronic kidney disease

Unlabeled uses: MRI

CONTRAINDICATIONS:
Hypersensitivity, hemochromatosis

Precautions: Pregnancy **B,** breastfeeding, children, geriatric patients, all anemias excluding iron deficiency anemia, iron overload, dialysis, hepatic disease, hypotension, MRI, sideroblastic anemia, thalassemia

DOSAGE AND ROUTES
Adult: **IV** 510 mg of elemental iron followed by a second dose 3-8 days later; if giving during dialysis, give after B/P is stable and after 1 hr of hemodialysis

Available forms: 510 mg/17 ml solution for injection

Implementation
- Use only with epinephrine, Solu-Medrol available in case of anaphylactic reaction during dose

IV route
- Give directly in dialysis line by slow inj or inf, give by slow inj at 1 ml/min (5 min/vial); inf, dilute each vial exclusively in a max of 100 ml of 0.9% NaCl, give at rate of 100 mg of iron/15 min, discard unused portions

ADVERSE EFFECTS
CNS: Headache, dizziness
CV: Chest pain, hypo/hypertension, hypervolemia, edema
GI: *Nausea, vomiting, abdominal pain,* constipation, diarrhea
INTEG: Rash, pruritus, urticaria, fever
MISC: Anaphylaxis
MS: Back pain
RESP: Dyspnea, cough

Pharmacokinetics

Absorption	Unknown
Distribution	Unknown
Metabolism	Unknown
Excretion	Unknown
Half-life	15 hr

Pharmacodynamics
Unknown

INTERACTIONS
Oral iron; do not use: iron toxicity

NURSING CONSIDERATIONS
Assessment
• Monitor blood studies: Hct, Hgb, reticulocytes, transferrin, plasma iron concentrations, ferritin, total iron-binding, bilirubin before treatment, at least monthly
• **Assess for allergy: anaphylaxis,** rash, pruritus, fever, wheezing; notify prescriber immediately, keep emergency equipment available
• Assess cardiac status: hypo/hypertension, hypervolemia
• **Assess for toxicity:** nausea, vomiting, diarrhea, fever, abdominal pain (early symptoms), cyanotic-looking lips, nailbeds, seizures, CV collapse (late symptoms)

Nursing diagnoses
• Activity intolerance (uses)
• Knowledge deficient (teaching)

Perform/provide
• Store at room temperature in cool environment, do not freeze

Patient/family education
• Advise patient to report itching, rash, chest pain, headache, vertigo, nausea, vomiting, abdominal pain, joint/muscle pain, numbness, tingling
• Advise patient that iron poisoning may occur if increased beyond recommended level; not to take oral iron preparation
• Advise patient that product may alter MRI studies

Evaluation
Positive therapeutic outcome
• Increased serum iron levels, Hct, Hgb

TREATMENT OF OVERDOSE:
Discontinue product, treat allergic reaction, give diphenhydrAMINE or EPINEPHrine as needed, give iron-chelating product in acute poisoning

---

fesoterodine (Rx)
(fess′oh-ter-oh-deen)
Toviaz
Func. class.: Overactive bladder product
Chem. class.: Muscarinic receptor antagonist
Pregnancy category C

ACTION: Relaxes smooth muscles in urinary tract by inhibiting acetylcholine at postganglionic sites

Therapeutic outcome: Absence of urinary frequency, urgency, incontinence

USES: Overactive bladder (urinary frequency, urgency), urinary incontinence

CONTRAINDICATIONS:
GI obstruction, ileus, pyloric stenosis, urinary retention, gastric retention, hypersensitivity, closed-angle glaucoma

Precautions: Pregnancy **C**, breastfeeding, children, renal/hepatic disease, urinary tract obstruction, ambient temperature increase, autonomic neuropathy, constipation, contact lenses, hazardous activity, GERD, gastroparesis, myasthenia gravis, prostatic hypertrophy, toxic megacolon, ulcerative colitis, possible cross-sensitivity with tolterodine

DOSAGE AND ROUTES
Adult and geriatric: PO EXT REL 4 mg/day, may increase to 8 mg/day based on response, max 4 mg/day in those taking potent CYP3A4 inhibitors

Renal dose
Adult: PO EXT REL CCr <30 ml/min max 4 mg/day in severe renal impairment

Available forms: Ext rel tabs 4, 8 mg

Implementation
• Do not break, crush, or chew ext rel product
• Give without regard to meals
• Store at room temperature; protect from moisture

ADVERSE EFFECTS
CV: Chest pain, angina, **QT prolongation**
EENT: Xerophthalmia
GI: *Nausea, vomiting,* abdominal pain, constipation, dry mouth
GU: Dysuria, urinary retention
INTEG: Rash, angioedema
MISC: Peripheral edema, insomnia
MS: Back pain
RESP: Cough
SYST: Infection

Pharmacokinetics	
Absorption	Rapid
Distribution	Protein binding 50%
Metabolism	Unknown
Excretion	Urine, feces
Half-life	7 hr

Pharmacodynamics
Unknown

INTERACTIONS
Drug classifications
Anticholinergics, antimuscarinics: increased anticholinergic effect

Antiretroviral protease inhibitors, azole antifungals, macrolide antiinfectives: increased action of fesoterodine

Diuretics: increased urinary frequency

Drug/herb
Caffeine, green tea, guarana: decreased fesoterodine

Drug/food
Grapefruit juice: increased fesoterodine level
Cola, coffee, tea: decreased fesoterodine level

Drug/lab test
Increased: LFTs

NURSING CONSIDERATIONS
Assessment
• **Assess urinary patterns:** distention, nocturia, frequency, urgency, incontinence
• **Assess for allergic reactions:** rash, angioedema; if this occurs, product should be discontinued

Nursing diagnoses
• Knowledge, deficient (teaching)
• Incontinence, urge urinary (uses)
• Urinary elimination, impaired (uses)

Patient/family education
• Advise patient not to drink liquids before bedtime
• Instruct the patient on the importance of bladder maintenance

Evaluation
Positive therapeutic outcome
• Absence of urinary frequency, urgency, incontinence

fexofenadine (Rx, OTC)
(fex-oh-fin′a-deen)
Allegra, Allegra ODT
Func. class.: Histamine antagonist, 2nd generation
Chem. class.: Piperidine, peripherally selective
Pregnancy category C

Do not confuse:
Allegra/Viagra

ACTION: Acts on blood vessels, GI, respiratory system by competing with histamine for H_1-receptor site; decreases allergic response by blocking pharmacologic effects of histamine; less sedation rate than with other antihistamines

Therapeutic outcome: Absence of allergy symptoms and rhinitis

USES: Rhinitis, allergy symptoms, chronic idiopathic urticaria

CONTRAINDICATIONS:
Breastfeeding, newborn or premature infants, hypersensitivity, severe hepatic disease

Precautions: Pregnancy C, children, geriatric, respiratory disease, closed-angle glaucoma, prostatic hypertrophy, bladder neck obstruction, asthma

DOSAGE AND ROUTES
Adult and child >12 yr: PO Rx only 60 mg bid or 180 mg/day; PO OTC only 60 mg bid or 180 mg/day (self-treatment of allergic rhinitis)
Child 6-11 yr: PO 30 mg bid; Orally disintegrating tab 30 mg bid dissolved on tongue

Renal dose
Adult and child ≥12 yr: PO CCr <80 ml/min 60 mg/day
Child 2-11 yr: PO CCr <80 ml/min 30 mg q day
Child <2 yr: PO CCr <80 ml/min 15 mg q day

Available forms: Caps 60 mg; tabs 30, 60, 180 mg; oral susp 6 mg/ml; orally disintegrating tab 30 mg

Implementation
• Give without regard to meals; caps/tabs should not be given with or right before grapefruit, orange, or apple juice
• **Orally disintegrating tab:** allow to dissolve, swallow
• **Oral susp:** shake well, use calibrated measuring device
• Store in tight, light-resistant container

ADVERSE EFFECTS
CNS: Headache, stimulation, drowsiness, sedation, fatigue, confusion, blurred vision, tinnitus, restlessness, tremors, paradoxical excitation in children or geriatric
CV: Hypotension, palpitations, bradycardia, tachycardia, **dysrhythmias (rare)**
GI: Nausea, diarrhea, abdominal pain, vomiting, constipation
GU: Frequency, dysuria, urinary retention, impotence

HEMA: Hemolytic anemia, thrombocytopenia, leukopenia, agranulocytosis, pancytopenia
INTEG: Rash, eczema, photosensitivity, urticaria
RESP: Thickening of bronchial secretions; dry nose, throat

Pharmacokinetics

Absorption	Well absorbed
Distribution	Unknown
Metabolism	Liver
Excretion	Kidneys
Half-life	Unknown

Pharmacodynamics

Onset	1 hr
Peak	2-3 hr
Duration	12-24 hr

INTERACTIONS

Drug classifications
Aluminum, antacids, magnesium: decreased fexofenadine effect

Drug/food
Apple, orange, grapefruit juice: decreased absorption

Drug/lab test
False negative: skin allergy tests (discontinue antihistamine 3 days before testing)

NURSING CONSIDERATIONS

Assessment
• **Allergy:** assess for itchy, runny, watery eyes; congested nose; before and during treatment
• Assess respiratory status: rate, rhythm, increase in bronchial secretions, wheezing, chest tightness; provide fluids to 2 L/day to decrease secretion thickness
• Monitor I&O ratio: be alert for urinary retention, frequency, dysuria, especially geriatric; product should be discontinued if these occur

Nursing diagnoses
• Airway clearance, ineffective (uses)
• Injury, risk for (side effects)
• Knowledge, deficient (teaching)
• Noncompliance (teaching, overuse)

Patient/family education
• Teach all aspects of product uses; to notify prescriber if confusion, sedation, hypotension occur; to avoid driving or other hazardous activity if drowsiness occurs; to avoid alcohol or other CNS depressants that may potentiate effect
• Instruct patient to take 1 hr before or 2 hr after meals to facilitate absorption
• Instruct patient not to exceed recommended dose; dysrhythmias may occur
• Teach patient that hard candy, gum, frequent rinsing of mouth may be used for dryness

Evaluation
Positive therapeutic outcome
• Absence of running or congested nose, rashes

TREATMENT OF OVERDOSE:
Administer lavage, diazepam, vasopressors, **IV** phenytoin

fibrinogen, concentrate, human
Ria STAP
See Appendix A, Selected New Drugs

fidaxomicin (Rx)
(fye-dax-oh-mye'sin)
Dificid
Func. class.: Antiinfective-macrolide
Pregnancy category B

ACTION: Bactericidal against *Clostridium difficile*; is a fermentation product obtained from *Dactylosporangium aurantiacum*; inhibits RNA synthesis by inhibiting transcription of bacterial RNA polymerases; may act at the early stages of transcription

Therapeutic outcome: Resolution of *C. difficile* based on stool culture

USES: Pseudomembraneous colitis, *C. difficile*-associated diarrhea

CONTRAINDICATIONS:
Hypersensitivity

Precautions: Pregnancy B, breastfeeding, children

DOSAGE AND ROUTES
Adult: PO 200 mg bid × 10 days 1000 mg

Available forms: Tab 200 mg

Implementation:
• Give without regard to food

ADVERSE EFFECTS
GI: Nausea, vomiting, abdominal pain, **GI bleeding**
HEMA: Anemia, neutropenia

Pharmacokinetics

Absorption	Minimal
Distribution	GI tract
Metabolism	P-glucoprotein
Excretion	Feces 92%; parent drug
Half-life	6-16 hr

Pharmacodynamics

Onset	Unknown
Peak	2 hr
Duration	Unknown

INTERACTIONS

Individual drugs
CycloSPORINE: Increased fidaxomicin action

NURSING CONSIDERATIONS

Assessment
• **Pseudomembraneous colitis: Assess for diarrhea, abdominal pain, fever, fatigue, anorexia, possible anemia, elevated WBC and low serum albumin; this product may be used in place of vancomycin; monitor CBC with differential, and stool culture (*C. difficile*)**

Nursing diagnoses
• Risk for infection (uses)
• Diarrhea (uses)
• Knowledge deficit (teaching)

Patient/family education
• Advise patient to report GI bleeding, or severe abdominal pain
• Teach patient to report if pregnancy is planned or suspected or if breast feeding

Evaluation
Positive therapeutic outcome
• Resolution of *C. difficile*

---

filgrastim (Rx)
(fill-gras′stim)
G-CSF, granulocyte colony stimulator, Neupogen
Func. class.: Biological modifier
Chem. class.: Granulocyte colony-stimulating factor
Pregnancy category C

ACTION: Stimulates proliferation and differentiation of neutrophils; a glycoprotein

Therapeutic outcome: Absence of infection

USES: To decrease infection in patients receiving antineoplastics that are myelosuppressive; to increase WBC in patients with product-induced neutropenia; bone marrow depression

Unlabeled uses: Neutropenia in HIV infection, aplastic anemia, ganciclovir-induced neutropenia, zidovudine-induced neutropenia

CONTRAINDICATIONS:
Hypersensitivity to proteins of *Escherichia coli*

Precautions: Pregnancy **C**, breastfeeding, children, cardiac conditions, myeloid malignancies, radiation therapy, sepsis, sickle cell disease, chemotherapy, respiratory disease

DOSAGE AND ROUTES
After myelosuppressive chemotherapy
Adult and child: IV/SUBCUT 5 mcg/kg/day in a single dose × 14 days; may increase by 5 mcg/kg in each chemotherapy cycle

After bone marrow transplantation
Adult: IV/SUBCUT 10 mcg/kg as an INF (**IV**) over 4 or 24 hr, begin 24 hr after chemotherapy and 24 hr after bone marrow transplantation

Peripheral blood progenitor cell collection/therapy
Adult: 10 mcg/kg/day as a BOL or CONT INF × 4 days or more before leukapheresis, continue to last leukapheresis, may alter dose if WBC >100,000/mm^3

Severe neutropenia (chronic), idiopathic/cyclical
Adult: SUBCUT 5 mcg/kg daily

Available forms: Inj 300 mcg/ml, 480 mcg/1.6 ml, 480 mcg/0.8 ml, 3000 mcg/0.5 ml

Implementation
SUBCUT route
• May divide into 2 injections if dose is >1 ml

IV route
• Dilute in D$_5$W to a conc of 5-15 mcg/ml, vial is for one-time use; give over 15-30 min (chemotherapy); over 4-24 hr (bone marrow transplantation); do not use 0.9% NaCl to dilute product
• Use single-use vials; after dose is withdrawn, do not reenter vial
• Do not shake; discard any product left out for >24 hr
• Do not use earlier than 24 hr after antineoplastics, bone marrow infusion

---

• Give for 2 wk or until ANC $= 10,000/mm^3$ after the expected chemotherapy neutrophil nadir
• Store in refrigerator; do not freeze; may store at room temperature for up to 24 hr

Y-site compatibilities: Acyclovir, allopurinol, amikacin, aminophylline, ampicillin, ampicillin/sulbactam, aztreonam, bleomycin, bumetanide, buprenorphine, butorphanol, calcium gluconate, CARBOplatin, carmustine, ceFAZolin, cefotetan, ceftazidime, chlorproMAZINE, cimetidine, cisplatin, cyclophosphamide, cytarabine, dacarbazine, DAUNOrubicin, dexamethasone, diphenhydrAMINE, DOXOrubicin, doxycycline, droperidol, enalaprilat, famotidine, floxuridine, fluconazole, fludarabine, gallium, ganciclovir, granisetron, haloperidol, hydrocortisone, hydromorphone, hydrOXYzine, IDArubicin, ifosfamide, leucovorin, LORazepam, mechlorethamine, melphalan, meperidine, mesna, methotrexate, metoclopramide, miconazole, minocycline, mitoxantrone, morphine, nalbuphine, netilmicin, ondansetron, plicamycin, potassium chloride, promethazine, ranitidine, sodium bicarbonate, streptozocin, ticarcillin, ticarcillin/clavulanate, tobramycin, trimethoprim-sulfamethoxazole, vancomycin, vinBLAStine, vinCRIStine, vinorelbine, zidovudine

ADVERSE EFFECTS
CNS: Fever, headache
GI: Nausea, vomiting, diarrhea, mucositis, anorexia
HEMA: Thrombocytopenia, excessive leukocytosis
INTEG: Alopecia, exacerbation of skin conditions, urticaria, cutaneous vasculitis
MS: Osteoporosis, skeletal pain
OTHER: Chest pain, hypotension
RESP: Acute respiratory distress syndrome, wheezing, alveolar hemorrhage

Pharmacokinetics

Absorption	Well absorbed (SUBCUT), completely absorbed (**IV**)
Distribution	Unknown
Metabolism	Unknown
Excretion	Unknown
Half-life	Unknown

Pharmacodynamics

	IV	SUBCUT
Onset	5-60 min	5-60 min
Peak	24 hr	2-8 hr
Duration	up to 1 wk	up to 1 wk

INTERACTIONS
Individual drugs
Lithium: do not use concurrently

Drug classifications
Antineoplastics: increased neutrophils, do not use together 24 hr before or after antineoplastics

Drug/lab test
Increased: uric acid, lactate dehydrogenase, alkaline phosphatase

NURSING CONSIDERATIONS
Assessment
• Monitor blood studies: CBC, platelet count before treatment and twice weekly; neutrophil counts (ANC) may be increased for 2 days after therapy, but treatment should continue until ANC $>10,000/mm^3$
• Assess for bone pain: frequency, intensity, duration; analgesics may be given; opiates should not be used
• Check B/P, heart rate, respiration; baseline, during treatment

Nursing diagnoses
• Infection, risk for (uses)
• Knowledge, deficient (teaching)
• Pain, acute (adverse reaction)

Patient/family education
• Teach patient technique for self-administration: dose, side effects, disposal of containers and needles; provide instruction sheet

Evaluation
Positive therapeutic outcome
• Absence of infection

finasteride (Rx)
(fin-ass′te-ride)
Propecia, Proscar
Func. class.: Androgen hormone inhibitor, hair stimulant
Chem. class.: 5-α-Reductase inhibitor
Pregnancy category X

Do not confuse:
Proscar/ProSom/Prozac, finasteride/furosemide

ACTION: Inhibits 5-α-reductase and reduction in dihydrotestosterone (DHT); DHT induces androgenic effects by binding to androgen receptors in the cell nuclei of the prostate gland, liver, skin; prevents development of benign prostatic hypertrophy (BPH)

Therapeutic outcome: Reduced prostate size

USES: Symptomatic BPH; male-pattern baldness (Propecia)

CONTRAINDICATIONS:
Pregnancy **X**, breastfeeding, children, women who are pregnant or may become pregnant should not handle tabs, hypersensitivity

Precautions: Large residual urinary volume, severely diminished urinary flow, liver function abnormalities

DOSAGE AND ROUTES
BPH
Adult: PO 5 mg/day × 6-12 mo

Male-pattern baldness
Adult: PO 1 mg/day for 3 mo or more for results

Available forms: Tabs (Propecia) 1 mg, (Proscar) 5 mg

Implementation
• Administer without regard to meals; give for a minimum of 6 mo; not all patients will respond
• Store at temp <86° F (30° C); protect from light; keep container tightly closed

ADVERSE EFFECTS
GU: Impotence, decreased libido, decreased volume of ejaculate
INTEG: Rash
MISC: Breast tenderness, **secondary malignancy**

Pharmacokinetics

Absorption	63%, readily
Distribution	Plasma protein binding, crosses blood-brain barrier
Metabolism	Liver
Excretion	Kidneys, metabolites (39%); feces (57%)
Half-life	6-15 hr

Pharmacodynamics

Onset	Immediate
Peak	1-2 hr
Duration	14 days

INTERACTIONS
Drug classifications
Anticholinergics, bronchodilators (adrenergic), theophylline: decreased effect of finasteride

Drug/lab test
Decreased: PSA levels (finasteride)

NURSING CONSIDERATIONS
Assessment
• **BPH:** Assess urinary patterns, residual urinary volume, severely diminished urinary flow; PSA levels and digital rectal exam results before initiating therapy and periodically thereafter
• Monitor liver function tests before initiating treatment; extensively metabolized in liver

Nursing diagnoses
• Knowledge, deficient (teaching)
• Urinary elimination, impaired (uses)

Patient/family education
• Advise patient that pregnant women or women who may become pregnant should not touch crushed tab or come into contact with semen of a patient taking this product; may adversely affect development of male fetus
• Inform patient that volume of ejaculate may be decreased during treatment; impotence and decreased libido may also occur
• Inform patient that Propecia results may not occur for 3 mo
• Inform patient that Proscar results may not occur for 6-12 mo

Evaluation
Positive therapeutic outcome
• Decreased postvoiding dribbling, frequency, nocturia
• Increased urinary flow
• Regression of prostate size
• Hair growth within 3-6 mo

---

fingolimod (Rx)
(fin-gol'i-mod)
Gilenya
Func. class.: Biologic response modifier
Chem. class.: Sphingosine 1-phosphate receptor modulator
Pregnancy category C

ACTION: Binds with high affinity to sphingosine 1 phosphate receptors, blocks lymphocyte egress to lymph nodes, reducing the number of peripheral blood lymphocytes, may reduce lymphocyte migration into the CNS

Therapeutic outcome: Improved symptoms of multiple sclerosis and prevention of increasing disability

USES: To reduce frequency of exacerbation, to delay physical disability of relapsing forms of MS

CONTRAINDICATIONS:
Hypersensitivity

Precautions: AIDS, asthma, AV block, bradycardia, breastfeeding, dysrhythmias, cardiac disease, children, COPD, diabetes mellitus, heart failure, hepatic disease, HIV, hypertension, immunosuppression, infants, leukemia, lymphoma, neonates, pregnancy **C**, QT prolongation, respiratory insufficiency, sick sinus syndrome, syncope, uveitis

DOSAGE AND ROUTES
Adult: PO 0.5 mg q day

Hepatic dose
Adult: PO Child-Pugh C, total score >10: Closely monitor, fingolimod exposure is doubled

Available forms: Cap 0.5 mg

Implementation
PO route
• Watch patient for 6 hr after initial dose or if product is not given for >2 wk for development of bradycardia. Give without regard to food
• Store at room temperature, protect from moisture

ADVERSE EFFECTS
CNS: Asthenia, depression, fatigue, headache, dizziness, encephalopathy, migraine, paresthesias, **stroke**
CV: AV block, bradycardia, chest pain, hypertension, palpitations
EENT: Blurred vision, vision impairment, ocular pain, macular edema
GI: Abdominal pain, anorexia, diarrhea, jaundice, vomiting, weight loss
HEMA: Leukopenia, lymphopenia, neutropenia
INTEG: Alopecia, pruritus
MS: Back pain
RESP: Dyspnea, cough
SYST: Infection, influenza, **secondary malignancy**

Absorption	Protein binding (99.7%)
Distribution	Distributed to RBCs (86%)
Metabolism	Metabolized by CYP4F2 and CYP2D6 to a lesser extent
Excretion	Excreted in urine (81% inactive metabolites)
Half-life	Terminal half-life 6-9 days

Pharmacodynamics

Onset	Unknown
Peak	12-16 hrs
Duration	Steady state 1-2 mo

INTERACTIONS
Individual drugs
Ketoconazole: increased fingolimod effect

Drug classifications
Class Ia/III antidysrhythmics: increased risk of torsades de pointes
Antineoplastics, immunosuppressants, immune modulating therapies: increased immunosuppression
Inactive vaccines, toxoids: decreased effects
Live vaccines: increased infection risk

NURSING CONSIDERATIONS
Assessment
• **Multiple sclerosis:** Assess for improving paresthesia, muscle weakness, clonus, muscle spasms, difficulty in moving, difficulty in coordination in balance, speech, swallowing, vision problems, fatigue; prevention of increasing disability
• **Monitor laboratory values:** obtain before initial dose, CBC, LFTs, serum bilirubin, ophthalmologic exam, antibodies to VZ V if there is not a history of chickenpox or without vaccination, may give VZV vaccination of antibody-negative patient before giving product, postpone for 1 month after vaccination; obtain ECG for evidence of bradycardia, or AV block

Nursing diagnoses
• Activity intolerance (uses)

Patient/family education
• Provide med guide to patient and explain use of product and expected results
• Advise patient that continuing follow-up exams and laboratory tests will be required on a regular basis
• Instruct patient to report any side effects resulting from therapy
• Teach patient to protect from moisture

• Advise patient to report chest pain, palpitations, jaundice

Evaluation
Positive therapeutic outcome
• Improved symptoms of multiple sclerosis and prevention of increasing disability

flavocoxid (Rx)
(flav-uh-kox′id)
Limbrel
Func. class.: Oral nutritional supplement
Pregnancy category Unknown

ACTION: Exhibits antiinflammatory, analgesic properties, thought to be due to inhibition of prostaglandin synthesis via inhibition of cyclooxygenase

Therapeutic outcome: Decreased pain, inflammation in osteoarthritis

USES: For dietary management of osteoarthritis

CONTRAINDICATIONS:
Hypersensitivity

Precautions: Pregnancy **unknown,** breastfeeding, children <18 yr, history of stomach ulcers, angina, CAD, edema, geriatric patients, GI disease, rheumatoid arthritis, stroke, tachycardia/MI

DOSAGE AND ROUTES
Adult: PO 250-500 mg with or without 50 mg of citrated zinc bisglycinate 250/50 mg or 500/50 mg q12hr

Available forms: Caps 250 mg

Implementation
• Administer 1 hr before or after meals, food increases absorption

ADVERSE EFFECTS
MISC: Hypertension, increase in varicose veins, psoriasis
MS: Fluid accumulation in the knees

Pharmacokinetics

Absorption	Unknown
Distribution	Unknown
Metabolism	Primarily via glucuronidation and sulfation
Excretion	Unknown
Half-life	Unknown

Pharmacodynamics
Unknown

NURSING CONSIDERATIONS

Assessment
• **Assess for pain of rheumatoid arthritis, osteoarthritis;** check ROM, inflammation of joints, characteristics of pain
• Assess for history of GI ulcers, bleeding; use fecal occult blood test to determine GI bleeding

Nursing diagnoses
• Injury, risk for (uses)
• Knowledge, deficient (teaching)

Patient/family education
• Teach patient that product does not take the place of other products, including corticosteroids for osteoarthritis
• Advise patient to notify prescriber if pregnancy is planned or suspected

Evaluation
Positive therapeutic outcome
• Decreased pain, inflammation in arthritic conditions

flecainide (Rx)
(flek′a-nide)
Tambocor
Func. class.: Antidysrhythmic (Class IC)
Pregnancy category C

ACTION: Decreases conduction in all parts of the heart, with greatest effect on the His-Purkinje system, which stabilizes the cardiac membrane

Therapeutic outcome: Absence of dysrhythmias

USES: Life-threatening ventricular dysrhythmias, sustained ventricular tachycardia; supraventricular tachydysrhythmias, paroxysmal atrial fibrillation/flutter associated with disabling symptoms

Unlabeled uses: Atrial fibrillation, single dose

CONTRAINDICATIONS:
Hypersensitivity, severe heart block, cardiogenic shock, nonsustained ventricular dysrhythmias, frequent PVCs, non–life-threatening dysrhythmias

Precautions: Pregnancy **C,** breastfeeding, children, renal/hepatic disease, CHF, respiratory depression, myasthenia gravis, geriatric, electrolyte abnormalities, atrial fibrillation, sick sinus syndrome, torsades de pointes

> **BLACK BOX WARNING:** MI, cardiac arrhythmias

DOSAGE AND ROUTES
PSVT/PAT
Adult: PO 50 mg q12hr; may increase every 4 days by 50 mg q12hr to desired response; max 300 mg/day

Life-threatening ventricular dysrhythmias
Adult: PO 100 mg q12hr, may increase by 50 mg q12hr q4days; max 400 mg/day

Renal dose
Adult: PO CCr <35 ml/min dose 100 mg daily or 50 mg bid initially

Available forms: Tabs 50, 100, 150 mg

Implementation
• Give reduced dosage slowly with ECG monitoring; do not increase dose <4 days apart
• Give with meals if GI upset occurs

ADVERSE EFFECTS
CNS: *Headache, dizziness,* involuntary movement, confusion, psychosis, restlessness, irritability, paresthesias, ataxia, flushing, somnolence, depression, anxiety, malaise, fatigue, asthenia, tremors
CV: *Hypotension,* **bradycardia,** angina, PVCs, **heart block, cardiovascular collapse/arrest, dysrhythmias, CHF, fatal ventricular tachycardia,** palpitations, **QT prolongation, torsades de pointes**
EENT: Tinnitus, *blurred vision,* hearing loss, corneal deposits, dry eyes
GI: Nausea, vomiting, anorexia, constipation, abdominal pain, flatulence, change in taste, diarrhea
GU: Impotence, decreased libido, polyuria, urinary retention
HEMA: **Leukopenia, thrombocytopenia**
INTEG: Rash, urticaria, edema, swelling
RESP: Dyspnea, **respiratory depression**

Pharmacokinetics
Absorption	Well absorbed
Distribution	Widely distributed
Metabolism	Liver
Excretion	30% kidneys, unchanged
Half-life	14 hr

Pharmacodynamics
Onset	Unknown
Peak	3 hr
Duration	Unknown

INTERACTIONS
Individual drugs
Amiodarone, cimetidine, ritonavir: increased level of flecainide
Digoxin: increased digoxin levels
Disopyramide, verapamil: increased CV depressant action
Propanolol: increased effects of both products

Drug classifications
Acidifying agents, alkalizing agents: increased or decreased effect
β-Adrenergic blockers: increased CV depressant action

Drug/lab test
Increased: CPK

NURSING CONSIDERATIONS
Assessment
• **Dysrhythmias:** Monitor ECG continuously to determine product effectiveness; measure PR, QRS, QT intervals; check for PVCs, other dysrhythmias; monitor B/P continuously for hypo/hypertension and rebound hypertension (after 1-2 hr); check for dehydration or hypovolemia
• Monitor I&O ratio; electrolytes: potassium, sodium, chloride; check weight daily and for signs of CHF or pulmonary toxicity: dyspnea, fatigue, cough, fever, chest pain, jugular vein distention, crackles; if these occur, product should be discontinued
• Monitor liver function studies: AST, ALT, bilirubin, alkaline phosphatase
• Assess patient for CNS symptoms: confusion, psychosis, numbness, depression, involuntary movements; if these occur, product should be discontinued
• Monitor cardiac rate, respiration: rate, rhythm, character, chest pain; watch for ventricular tachycardia, supraventricular tachycardia, or fibrillation

Nursing diagnoses
• Cardiac output, decreased (uses)
• Knowledge, deficient (teaching)

Patient/family education
• Instruct patient to report side effects immediately to prescriber

• Instruct patient to complete follow-up appointment with health care provider, including pulmonary function tests, chest x-ray
• Teach patient to change position slowly from lying or sitting to standing to minimize orthostatic hypotension
• Advise patient not to skip or double doses
• Advise patient to carry/wear emergency ID with disorder, medications taken
• Advise patient to avoid hazardous activities that require alertness until response is known

Evaluation
Positive therapeutic outcome
• Absence of dysrhythmias

fluconazole (Rx)
(floo-kon'a-zole)
Apo-Fluconazole ✤, Diflucan, Gen-Fluconazole ✤
Func. class.: Antifungal
Chem. class.: Triazole
Pregnancy category C

Do not confuse:
Diflucan/Diprivan

ACTION: Inhibits ergosterol biosynthesis, causes direct damage to membrane phospholipids in the cell wall of fungi

Therapeutic outcome: Fungistatic fungicidal against the following susceptible organisms: *Candida, Cryptococcus neoformans*

USES: Oropharyngeal candidiasis; chronic mucocutaneous candidiasis; systemic, vaginal, urinary candidiasis; cryptococcal meningitis; prevention of candidiasis in bone marrow transplant in those who receive chemotherapy and/or radiation therapy, cystitis, fungal prophylaxis, peritonitis, pneumonia, pyelonephritis

CONTRAINDICATIONS:
Hypersensitivity to this product or azoles, pregnancy **D**

Precautions: Breastfeeding, renal/hepatic disease, torsades de pointes

DOSAGE AND ROUTES
Vaginal candidiasis
Adult: PO 150 mg as a single dose

Serious fungal infections
Adult: PO/IV 50-400 mg initially, then 200 mg once daily for 4 wk
Child: 6-12 mg/kg/day

Oropharyngeal candidiasis
Adult: PO/IV 200 mg initially, then 100 mg/day for at least 2 wk
Child: PO/IV 6 mg/kg initially, then 3 mg/kg/day for ≥2 wk

Prevention of candidiasis in bone marrow transplant
Adult: PO/IV 400 mg/day

Renal dose
Adult: PO CCr <50 ml/min after loading dose, give 50% of usual dose

Available forms: Tabs 50, 100, 150, 200 mg; inj 2 mg/ml; powder for oral susp 50, 200 mg/ml

Implementation
• Take with food to reduce GI effects
PO route
• Shake oral susp before each use

Intermittent IV infusion route
• Give after diluting according to package directions; run at 200 mg/hr or less; do not use plastic containers in connections
• Do not admix
• Administer **IV** using an in-line filter, using distal veins; check for extravasation and necrosis q2hr
• Give product only after C&S confirms organism, product needed to treat condition
• Store protected from moisture and light, diluted sol is stable for 24 hr

Y-site compatibilities: Acyclovir, aldesleukin, alfentanil, allopurinol, amifostine, amikacin, aminocaproic acid, aminophylline, amiodarone, anidulafungin, ascorbic acid injection, atenolol, atracurium, atropine, azaTHIOprine, aztreonam, benztropine, bivalirudin, bleomycin, bumetanide, buprenorphine, butorphanol, calcium chloride, CARBOplatin, caspofungin, cefamandole, ceFAZolin, cefepime, cefmetazole, cefonicid, cefoperazone, cefotetan, cefoxitin, cefpirome, ceftazidime, ceftizoxime, ceftobiprole, cephalothin, cephapirin, chlorproMAZINE, cimetidine, cisatracurium, CISplatin, codeine, cyanocobalamin, cyclophosphamide, cycloSPORINE, cytarabine, DACTINomycin, DAPTOmycin, dexamethasone, diltiazem, dimenhyDRINATE, diphenhydrAMINE, DOBUTamine, docetaxel, DOPamine, doripenem, doxacurium, DOXOrubicin, DOXOrubicin liposomal, doxycycline, droperidol, drotrecogin alfa, enalaprilat, ePHEDrine, EPINEPHrine, epirubicin, epoetin alfa, eptifibatide, ertapenem, erythromycin, esmolol, etoposide, famotidine, fenoldopam, fentaNYL, filgrastim, fludarabine,

Adverse effects: *italics* = common; **bold** = life-threatening

fluorouracil, folic acid, foscarnet, gallium, ganciclovir, gatifloxacin, gemcitabine, gentamicin, glycopyrrolate, granisetron, heparin, hydrocortisone, HYDROmorphone, IDArubicin, ifosfamide, IV immune globulin, inamrinone, indomethacin, insulin (regular), irinotecan, isoproterenol, ketorolac, labetalol, lansoprazole, leucovorin, levofloxacin, lidocaine, linezolid, LORazepam, LR, magnesium sulfate, mannitol, mechlorethamine, melphalan, meperidine, meropenem, metaraminol, methicillin, methotrexate, methoxamine, methyldopate, methylPREDNISolone, metoclopramide, metoprolol, metroNIDAZOLE, mezlocillin, miconazole, midazolam, milrinone, minocycline, mitoxantrone, morphine, moxalactam, multiple vitamins injection, mycophenolate, nafcillin, nalbuphine, naloxone, nesiritide, nitroglycerin, nitroprusside, norepinephrine, octreotide, ondansetron, oxacillin, oxaliplatin, oxytocin, paclitaxel, palonosetron, pamidronate, pancuronium, papaverine, pemetrexed, penicillin G potassium/sodium, pentazocine, PENTobarbital, PHENobarbital, phenylephrine, phenytoin, phytonadione, piperacillin-tazobactam, polymyxin B, potassium chloride, procainamide, prochlorperazine, promethazine, propofol, propranolol, protamine, pyridoxine, quiNIDine, quinupristin-dalfopristin, ranitidine, remifentanil, Ringer's, ritodrine, riTUXimab, rocuronium, sargramostim, sodium acetate/bicarbonate, succinylcholine, SUFentanil, tacrolimus, temocillin, teniposide, theophylline, thiotepa, ticarcillin-clavulanate, tigecycline, tirofiban, TNA, tobramycin, tolazoline, TPN, trastuzumab, trimetaphan, urokinase, vancomycin, vasopressin, vecuronium, verapamil, vinCRIStine, vinorelbine, voriconazole, zidovudine, zoledronic acid

Y-site incompatibilities: Amphotericin B, ampicillin, calcium gluconate, cefotaxime, cefTRIAXone, ceftazidime, cefuroxime, chloramphenicol, clindamycin, diazepam, digoxin, erythromycin lactobionate, furosemide, haloperidol, hydrOXYzine, imipenem/cilastatin, pentamidine, ticarcillin, trimethoprim/sulfamethoxazole

ADVERSE EFFECTS
CNS: Headache, **seizures**
CV: QT prolongation, torsades de pointes
GI: Nausea, vomiting, diarrhea, cramping, flatus, increased AST, ALT, **hepatotoxicity**
HEMA: Agranulocytosis, eosinophilia, leukopenia, neutropenia, thrombocytopenia
INTEG: Stevens-Johnson syndrome, angioedema, anaphylaxis, exfoliative dermatitis, toxic epidermal necrolysis

Pharmacokinetics
Absorption	Well absorbed (PO)
Distribution	Widely distributed (peritoneum, CSF)
Metabolism	<10%, liver
Excretion	80% kidneys (unchanged)
Half-life	30 hr, increased in renal disease

Pharmacodynamics
	PO	IV
Onset	Unknown	Immediate
Peak	2-4 hr	Infusion's end
Duration	Unknown	Unknown

INTERACTIONS
Individual drugs
Alfentanil, buprenorphine, ergot, fentaNYL, methadone, saquinavir, SUFentanil, zidovudine: increased effect of each specific drug
CycloSPORINE, phenytoin, rifabutin, sirolimus, tacrolimus, theophylline: increased plasma concentrations
Lovastatin, simvastatin: increased myopathy, rhabdomyolysis risk
Warfarin: increased anticoagulation

Drug classification
Contraceptives (oral), calcium-channel blockers: decreased effect
Oral antidiabetics: hypoglycemia

Drug/herb
Gossypol: increased nephrotoxicity

NURSING CONSIDERATIONS
Assessment
• **Assess for signs and symptoms of infection:** clearing of CSF culture during treatment, obtain C&S baseline and during treatment, product may be started as soon as culture is taken
• **Monitor for hepatotoxicity:** increased AST, ALT, alkaline phosphatase, bilirubin; discontinue product if hepatotoxicity occurs

Nursing diagnoses
• Infection, risk for (uses)
• Injury, risk for (adverse reactions)
• Knowledge, deficient (teaching)

Patient/family education
• Caution patient that long-term therapy may be needed to clear infection; to take entire course of medication; take in equal intervals (PO)

• **Teach patient the signs and symptoms of hepatotoxicity:** nausea, vomiting, clay-colored stools, dark urine, anorexia, fatigue, jaundice; prescriber should be notified immediately
• Inform patient that medication may be taken with food to reduce GI effects
• Advise patient to consider using alternative contraception if using oral contraceptives, pregnancy **D**

Evaluation
Positive therapeutic outcome
• Decreasing oral candidiasis, fever, malaise, rash
• Negative C&S for infecting organism

flumazenil (Rx)
(flu-maz'e-nil)
Anexate ✦, **Romazicon**
Func. class.: Antidote: Benzodiazepine receptor antagonist
Chem. class.: Imidazobenzodiazepine derivative
Pregnancy category C

ACTION: Antagonizes the actions of benzodiazepines on the CNS, competitively inhibits the activity at the benzodiazepine receptor complex

Therapeutic outcome: Reversed benzodiazepine toxic effects

USES: Reversal of the sedative effects of benzodiazepines

CONTRAINDICATIONS:
Hypersensitivity to this product or benzodiazepines, serious tricyclic overdose, patients given benzodiazepine for control of life-threatening condition

Precautions: Pregnancy **C**, breastfeeding, children, geriatric, ambulatory patients, renal/hepatic disease, status epilepticus, head injury, labor and delivery, hypoventilation, panic disorder, drug/alcohol dependency

> **BLACK BOX WARNING:** Benzodiazepine dependence, seizures

DOSAGE AND ROUTES
Reversal of conscious sedation or in general anesthesia
Adult: **IV** 0.2 mg (2 ml) given over 15 sec; wait 45 sec, then give 0.2 mg (2 ml) if consciousness

does not occur; may be repeated at 60-sec intervals as needed (max 3 mg/hr) or 1 mg/5 min
Child: **IV** 10 mcg (0.01 mg)/kg; cumulative dose of 1 mg or less

Management of suspected benzodiazepine overdose
Adult: **IV** 0.2 mg (2 ml) given over 30 sec; wait 30 sec, then give 0.3 mg (3 ml) over 30 sec if consciousness does not occur; further doses of 0.5 mg (5 ml) can be given over 30 sec at intervals of 1 min up to cumulative dose of 3 mg
Child: **IV** 10 mcg (0.01 mg/kg); cumulative dose of less than 1 mg

Available forms: Inj 0.1 mg/ml

Implementation
Direct IV route
• Give directly undiluted or diluted in 0.9% NaCl, D_5W, or LR; give over 15-30 sec into running **IV**
• Use large vein
• Check airway and **IV** access before administration
• Stable for 24 hr if drawn into a syringe or mixed with other solutions

ADVERSE EFFECTS
CNS: Dizziness, agitation, emotional lability, confusion, **seizures,** somnolence, panic attacks
CV: Hypertension, palpitations, cutaneous vasodilatation, **dysrhythmias,** bradycardia, tachycardia, chest pain
EENT: Abnormal vision, blurred vision, tinnitus
GI: Nausea, vomiting, hiccups
SYST: Headache, inj site pain, increased sweating, fatigue, rigors

Pharmacokinetics

Absorption	Complete
Distribution	Unknown
Metabolism	Liver
Excretion	Unknown
Half-life	41-79 min

Pharmacodynamics

Onset	1-2 min
Peak	10 min
Duration	Unknown

INTERACTIONS
Individual drugs
Zaleplon, zolpidem: antagonize action

Drug classifications
Benzodiazepines: antagonize action
Toxicity: mixed product overdosage

NURSING CONSIDERATIONS

Assessment
• Assess cardiac status using continuous monitoring
• Assess for seizures, protect patient from injury; most likely in those who usually experience withdrawal from sedatives
• Assess for GI symptoms: nausea, vomiting; place in side-lying position to prevent aspiration
• **Assess for allergic reactions:** flushing, rash, urticaria, pruritus
• **Seizures/benzodiazepine dependence:** Do not use in those who have used these products for interictal psychosis (IIP), or status epilepticus, use in ICU cautiously where there may be unrecognized benzodiazepine dependence

Nursing diagnoses
• Injury, risk for (uses)
• Poisoning, risk for (uses)

Patient/family education
• Caution patient that amnesia may continue
• Instruct patient to avoid any hazardous activities for 18-24 hr after discharge
• Caution patient not to take any alcohol or nonprescription products for 18-24 hr; serious reactions may occur

Evaluation
Positive therapeutic outcome
• Decreased sedation, respiratory depression
• Absence of toxicity

flunisolide nasal agent
See Appendix B

fluocinolone topical
See Appendix B

fluorometholone ophthalmic
See Appendix B

⚠ HIGH ALERT

fluorouracil (Rx)
(flure-oh-yoor'a-sil)
5-FU, Adrucil, Carac, Efudex
Func. class.: Antineoplastic, antimetabolite
Chem. class.: Pyrimidine antagonist
Pregnancy category X

Do not confuse:
fluorouracil/flucytosine

ACTION: Inhibits DNA, RNA synthesis; interferes with cell replication by competitively inhibiting thymidylate synthesis; cell cycle specific (S phase); a vesicant

Therapeutic outcome: Prevention of rapidly growing malignant cells

USES: *Systemic:* cancer of breast, colon, rectum, stomach, pancreas; *Topical:* superficial basal cell carcinoma; multiple actinic keratoses

CONTRAINDICATIONS:
Pregnancy **X**, breastfeeding, hypersensitivity, poor nutritional status, serious infections, major surgery within 1 mo

> **BLACK BOX WARNING:** Bone marrow suppression

Precautions: Children, renal/hepatic disease, angina

> **BLACK BOX WARNING:** GI bleeding

DOSAGE AND ROUTES
Doses vary widely, doses are based on actual body weight, unless obese, then based on lean body weight

Advanced colorectal cancer
Adult: IV 370 mg/m^2 given after leucovorin or 425 mg/m^2 given after leucovorin daily × 5 days; repeat q4-5wk

Other cancer
Adult: IV 12 mg/kg/day × 4 days, max 800 mg/day; may repeat with 6 mg/kg on day 6, 8, 10, 12; maintenance is 10-15 mg/kg/wk as a single dose, max 1 g/wk

Actinic/solar keratoses
Adult: TOP 1% cream/SOL 1-2 ×/day or 2%-5% SOL for hands

Superficial basal cell carcinoma
Adult: TOP 5% cream/SOL 2 ×/day × 3-12 wk

Available forms: Inj 50 mg/ml; cream 1%, 5%; SOL 1%, 2%, 5%

Implementation
• Avoid contact with skin (very irritating); wash completely to remove
• Give fluids **IV** or PO before chemotherapy to hydrate patient
• Give antiemetic 30-60 min before giving product to prevent vomiting, and prn for several days thereafter; antibiotics for prophylaxis of infection
• Provide liquid diet: carbonated beverages; gelatin may be added if patient is not nauseated or vomiting
• Rinse mouth tid-qid with water, club soda; brush teeth bid-qid with soft brush or cotton-tipped applicators for stomatitis; use unwaxed dental floss

Topical route
• Wear gloves when applying; may use with a loose dressing; use a plastic or wooden applicator

IV route
• Prepare in biological cabinet using gloves, gown, mask
• **IV** undiluted; may inject through Y-tube or 3-way stopcock; give over 1-3 min
• May be diluted in 0.9% NaCl, D$_5$W, given over 2-8 hr as an **IV** inf

Y-site compatibilities: Acyclovir, alfentanil, allopurinol, amifostine, amikacin, amphotericin B lipid complex, amphotericin B liposome, ampicillin, ampicillin-sulbactam, anidulafungin, atenolol, atracurium, azithromycin, aztreonam, bivalirudin, bleomycin, bumetanide, butorphanol, calcium gluconate, CARBOplatin, ceFAZolin, cefepime, cefoperazone, cefotaxime, cefotetan, cefoxitin, ceftazidime, ceftizoxime, cefTRIAXone, cefuroxime, cimetidine, cisatracurium, CISplatin, clindamycin, codeine, cyclophosphamide, cycloSPORINE, DAPTOmycin, dexamethasone, digoxin, docetaxel, DOPamine, doripenem, DOXOrubicin liposomal, enalaprilat, ePHEDrine, ertapenem, erythromycin, esmolol, etoposide phosphate, famotidine, fenoldopam, fentaNYL, fluconazole, fludarabine, foscarnet, fosphenytoin, furosemide, ganciclovir, gatifloxacin, gemcitabine, gentamicin, granisetron, heparin, hydrocortisone, HYDROmorphone, ifosfamide, imipenem-cilastatin, inamrinone, isoproterenol, ketorolac, labetalol, leucovorin, levorphanol, lidocaine, linezolid, magnesium sulfate, mannitol, melphalan, meperidine, meropenem, mesna, methohexital, methotrexate, methylPREDNISolone, metoprolol, metroNIDAZOLE, milrinone, mitomycin, mitoxantrone, morphine sulfate, nalbuphine, naloxone, nesiritide, nitroglycerin, nitroprusside, octreotide, ofloxacin, paclitaxel, palonosetron, pamidronate, pancuronium, pantoprazole, pemetrexed, PENTobarbital, PHENobarbital, phenylephrine, piperacillin, piperacillin-tazobactam, potassium chloride/phosphates, procainamide, propofol, propranolol, ranitidine, remifentanil, riTUXimab, sargramostim, sodium acetate/bicarbonate/phosphates, succinylcholine, SUFentanil, sulfamethoxazole-trimethoprim, teniposide, theophylline, thiopental, thiotepa, ticarcillin, ticarcillin-clavulanate, tigecycline, tirofiban, tobramycin, trastuzumab, vasopressin, vecuronium, vinBLAStine, vinCRIStine, vitamin B complex/C, voriconazole, zidovudine, zoledronic acid

Y-site incompatibilities: Droperidol, vinorelbine

ADVERSE EFFECTS

SYSTEMIC use
CNS: Lethargy, malaise, weakness, acute cerebellar dysfunction
CV: Myocardial ischemia, angina
EENT: Epistaxis, light intolerance, lacrimation
GI: *Anorexia, stomatitis,* diarrhea, nausea, vomiting, **hemorrhage,** enteritis, glossitis
HEMA: Thrombocytopenia, leukopenia, myelosuppression, anemia, agranulocytosis
INTEG: *Rash,* fever, photosensitivity

Pharmacokinetics

Absorption	Completely bioavailable (**IV**), minimal (topical)
Distribution	Widely distributed, concentration in tumor
Metabolism	Liver, converted to active metabolite
Excretion	Lungs (60%-80%), kidneys (up to 15%)
Half-life	20 hr terminal

Pharmacodynamics

Unknown	

INTERACTIONS

Individual drugs
Radiation: increased toxicity, bone marrow suppression

Adverse effects: *italics* = common; **bold** = life-threatening

Drug classifications
Antineoplastics: increased toxicity, bone marrow depression
Live virus vaccines: decreased antibody response

Drug/lab test
Increased: AST, ALT, LDH, serum bilirubin, Hct, Hgb, WBC, platelets, 5-HIAA
Decreased: albumin

NURSING CONSIDERATIONS

Assessment
• Monitor ECG; watch for ST-T wave changes, low QRS and T, possible dysrhythmias (sinus tachycardia, heart block, PVCs)
• Assess buccal cavity q8hr for dryness, sores or ulceration, white patches, oral pain, bleeding, dysphagia; obtain prescription for viscous lidocaine (Xylocaine)
• Assess tachypnea, ECG changes, dyspnea, edema, fatigue; identify dyspnea, crackles, unproductive cough, chest pain, tachypnea

> **BLACK BOX WARNING: Bone marrow suppression:** Monitor CBC, differential, platelet count daily (**IV**); withhold product if WBC is <4000/mm³ or platelet count is <100,000/mm³; notify prescriber of results if WBC <20,000/mm³, platelets <50,000/mm³; nadir of leukopenia within 2 wk, recovery 1 mo

• Monitor renal function studies: BUN, creatinine, serum uric acid, urine CCr before, during therapy; I&O ratio; report fall in urine output to <30 ml/hr
• Monitor temp q4hr (may indicate beginning of infection)
• Monitor liver function tests before, during therapy (bilirubin, AST, ALT, LDH) as needed or monthly; jaundice of skin, sclera, dark urine, clay-colored stools, itchy skin, abdominal pain, fever, diarrhea
• **Assess for bleeding:** hematuria, stool guaiac, bruising or petechiae, mucosa or orifices q8hr; inflammation of mucosa, breaks in skin

Nursing diagnoses
• Body image, disturbed (adverse reactions)
• Infection, risk for (adverse reactions)
• Injury, risk for (adverse reactions)
• Knowledge, deficient (teaching)

Patient/family education
• Caution patient that contraceptive measures are recommended during therapy, pregnancy X
• **Bleeding:** Teach patient to avoid using aspirin, NSAIDs, or ibuprofen-containing products, razors, commercial mouthwash because bleeding may occur; to report symptoms of bleeding (hematuria, tarry stools)
• **Instruct patient to report signs of anemia** (fatigue, headache, irritability, faintness, SOB)
• **Instruct patient to report signs of stomatitis** (bleeding, white spots, ulcerations in the mouth); tell patient to examine mouth daily, to report symptoms; viscous lidocaine (Xylocaine) may be used
• Teach patient to avoid crowds, persons with known infections
• Advise patient to avoid vaccinations during therapy, to use sunscreen or stay out of the sun to prevent burns; about hair loss; explore use of wigs or other products until hair regrowth occurs

Evaluation
Positive therapeutic outcome
• Prevention of rapid division of malignant cells

FLUoxetine (Rx)
(floo-ox'uh-teen)
Apo-Fluoxetine ✤, CO-Fluoxetine ✤, Gen-Fluoxetine ✤, Novo-Fluoxetine ✤, Nu-Fluoxetine ✤, PMS-Fluoxetine ✤, Prozac, Prozac Weekly, Sandoz Fluoxetine ✤, Sarafem, Selfemra
Func. class.: Antidepressant, selective serotonin reuptake inhibitor
Pregnancy category C

Do not confuse:
Prozac/Proscar/Prilosec/Prosom
Sarafem/Serophene

ACTION: Inhibits CNS neuron uptake of serotonin but not of norepinephrine

Therapeutic outcome: Decreased symptoms of depression after 2-3 wk

USES: Major depressive disorder, obsessive-compulsive disorder (OCD), bulimia nervosa; *Sarafem:* premenstrual dysphoric disorder (PMDD), panic disorder

Unlabeled uses: Alcoholism, anorexia nervosa, borderline personality disorder, obesity, posttraumatic stress disorder

CONTRAINDICATIONS:
Hypersensitivity

Precautions: Pregnancy **C,** breastfeeding, geriatric, diabetes mellitus, narrow-angle glaucoma, cardiac malformations in infants (exposed to fluoxetine in utero)

> **BLACK BOX WARNING:** Children, suicidal ideation

DOSAGE AND ROUTES
Depression/OCD
Adult: PO 20 mg/day AM; after 4 wk if no clinical improvement is noted, dosage may be increased to 20 mg bid in AM, afternoon; max 80 mg/day; PO 90 mg weekly
Geriatric: PO 5-10 mg/day, increase as needed
Child 5-18 yr: PO 5-10 mg/day, max 20 mg/day

Alcoholism (unlabeled)
Adult: PO 20-80 mg/day

Anorexia nervosa (unlabeled)
Adult: PO 10 mg every other day-20 mg/day

Borderline personality disorder (unlabeled)
Adult: PO 20 mg/day, max 80 mg/day

Kleptomania (unlabeled)
Adult: PO 60-80 mg/day

Posttraumatic stress disorder (unlabeled)
Adult: PO 10-80 mg/day

Premenstrual dysphoric disorder (Sarafem)
Adult: PO 20 mg/day, may be taken daily 14 days before menses

Available forms: Caps 10, 20, 40 mg; tabs 10, 20 mg; oral sol 20 mg/5 ml; del rel caps (Prozac Weekly) 90 mg; tab 10, 15, 20 mg (Sarafem)

Implementation
• Give without regard to meals
• Give dose at bedtime if oversedation occurs during day; may take entire dose at bedtime; geriatric may not tolerate once/day dosing, crush if patient unable to swallow whole (tabs only)
• **Prozac Weekly:** Give on same day each week, swallow whole, do not crush, cut, chew
• Store at room temperature; do not freeze

ADVERSE EFFECTS
CNS: *Headache, nervousness, insomnia, drowsiness, anxiety, tremor, dizziness, fatigue, sedation, poor concentration, abnormal dreams, agitation,* **seizures,** apathy, euphoria, hallucinations, delusions, psychosis, suicidal ideation, **neuroleptic malignant syndrome–like reactions,** serotonin syndrome
CV: *Hot flashes, palpitations,* **angina pectoris, hemorrhage,** hypertension, **tachycardia, 1st-degree AV block, bradycardia, MI, thrombophlebitis**
EENT: Visual changes, ear/eye pain, photophobia, tinnitus
GI: *Nausea, diarrhea, dry mouth, anorexia, dyspepsia, constipation, cramps, vomiting, taste changes, flatulence, decreased appetite*
GU: *Dysmenorrhea, decreased libido, urinary frequency, urinary tract infection,* amenorrhea, cystitis, impotence, urine retention
INTEG: *Sweating, rash, pruritus,* acne, alopecia, urticaria; **angioedema, exfoliative dermatitis, Stevens-Johnson syndrome, toxic epidermal necrolysis**
MS: *Pain,* arthritis, twitching
RESP: *Infection, pharyngitis, nasal congestion, sinus headache, sinusitis, cough, dyspnea, bronchitis,* asthma, hyperventilation, pneumonia
SYST: *Asthenia, viral infection, fever, allergy, chills*

Pharmacokinetics
Absorption	Well absorbed
Distribution	Crosses blood-brain barrier
Metabolism	Liver, extensively to norfluoxetine
Excretion	Kidneys, unchanged (12%), metabolite (7%); steady state 28-35 days, protein binding 94%
Half-life	1-3 days metabolite up to 1 wk

Pharmacodynamics
Onset	Unknown
Peak	6-8 hr
Duration	Unknown

INTERACTIONS
Individual drugs
Alcohol: increased CNS depression
Antidiabetics: increased levels or toxicity
Bosentan, budesonide, carBAMazepine, darifenacin, diazepam, digoxin, donepezil, lithium, paricalcitol, phenytoin, vinBLAStine, warfarin: increased toxicity
Cyproheptadine: decreased FLUoxetine effect

F

BusPIRone, haloperidol, loxapine, selegiline, thiothixene, tryptophan: increased serotonin syndrome, do not use concurrently

Drug classifications

Anticoagulants, NSAIDs, platelet inhibitors, salicylates, thrombolytics: increased bleeding risk

Antidepressants, opioids, sedative/hypnotics: increased CNS depression

MAOIs: hypertensive crisis, seizures; do not use with or 14 days prior to fluoxetine

SSRIs, SNRIs, serotonin-receptor agonists, tricyclics: increased serotonin syndrome, do not use concurrently

Drug/herb

Hops, kava, lavender, valerian: increased CNS effect

St. John's wort, SAM-e: do not use together; increased risk of serotonin syndrome

Drug/lab test

Increased: serum bilirubin, blood glucose, alkaline phosphatase, BUN, CK

NURSING CONSIDERATIONS

Assessment

• Monitor B/P (lying, standing), pulse q4hr; if systolic B/P drops 20 mm hg, hold product and notify prescriber; take VS q4hr in patients with CV disease

• Monitor blood studies: CBC, leukocytes, differential, cardiac enzymes if patient is receiving long-term therapy; check platelets, bleeding can occur; thyroid growth rate

• Monitor hepatic studies: AST, ALT, bilirubin

• Check weight qwk; appetite may increase with product

• Assess ECG for flattening of T-wave, bundle branch block, AV block, dysrhythmias in cardiac patients

> **BLACK BOX WARNING:** Assess mental status: mood, sensorium, affect, suicidal tendencies; increase in psychiatric symptoms: depression, panic; monitor for seizures; seizure potential is increased

• Monitor urinary retention, constipation; constipation is more likely to occur in children or geriatric

• Identify patient's alcohol consumption; if alcohol is consumed, hold dose until AM

• **Assess appetite in bulimia nervosa,** monitor weight daily, increase nutritious foods in diet, watch for bingeing and vomiting

• **Serious skin reactions:** angioedema, exfoliative dermatitis, **Stevens-Johnson syndrome,** toxic epidermal necrolysis

• Assess allergic reactions: itching, rash, urticaria, product should be discontinued; may need to give antihistamine

Nursing diagnoses

• Coping, ineffective (uses)
• Injury, risk for (side effects)
• Knowledge, deficient (teaching)
• Noncompliance (teaching)

Patient/family education

• Teach patient that therapeutic effects may take 1-4 wk

• Instruct patient to use caution in driving or other activities requiring alertness because of drowsiness, dizziness, blurred vision; to avoid rising quickly from sitting to standing, especially geriatric; to use sunscreen to prevent photosensitivity

• Caution patient to avoid alcohol ingestion, other CNS depressants

• Advise patient not to discontinue medication quickly after long-term use: may cause nausea, headache, malaise

• Instruct patient to increase fluids, bulk in diet if constipation, urinary retention occur, especially geriatric

• Advise patient to take gum, hard sugarless candy, or frequent sips of water for dry mouth

• Teach patient to avoid all OTC products unless approved by prescriber

• Advise patient to change positions slowly, orthostatic hypotension may occur

• Teach that suicidal thoughts, behavior may occur in young adults, children

Evaluation
Positive therapeutic outcome

• Decrease in depression
• Absence of suicidal thoughts
• Decreased symptoms of OCD

TREATMENT OF OVERDOSE:

Activated charcoal, supportive care

fluphenazine decanoate (Rx)

(floo-fen'ah-zeen)

Apo-Fluphenazine Decanoate ✤, **Modecate** ✤

fluphenazine hydrochloride (Rx)

Apo-Fluphenazine ✤

Func. class.: Antipsychotic/neuroleptic
Chem. class.: Phenothiazine, piperazine

Pregnancy category C

Do not confuse:
Prolixin/Proloid

ACTION: Depresses cerebral cortex, hypothalamus, limbic system, which control activity and aggression; blocks neurotransmission produced by dopamine at synapse; exhibits strong α-adrenergic and anticholinergic blocking action; mechanism for antipsychotic effects is unclear

Therapeutic outcome: Decreased signs and symptoms of psychosis

USES: Psychotic disorders, schizophrenia

CONTRAINDICATIONS:

Hypersensitivity, circulatory collapse, liver damage, cerebral arteriosclerosis, coronary disease, severe hypo/hypertension, blood dyscrasias, coma, brain damage, bone marrow depression, alcohol and barbiturate withdrawal, closed-angle glaucoma

Precautions: Pregnancy C, breastfeeding, children <12 yr, geriatric, seizure disorders, hypertension, hepatic/cardiac disease

> **BLACK BOX WARNING:** Dementia

DOSAGE AND ROUTES

Decanoate
Adult and child >16 yr: IM/SUBCUT 12.5-25 mg q1-3wk, may increase slowly
Child 12-16 yr: IM/SUBCUT 6.25-18.75 mg, then repeat q1-3wk, then increase slowly, max 25 mg
Child 5-12 yr: IM/SUBCUT 3.125-12.5 mg, then repeat q1-3wk, increase slowly

HCl
Adult: PO 2.5-10 mg, in divided doses q6-8hr, max 40 mg/day; IM initially 1.25 mg then 2.5-10 mg in divided doses q6-8hr

Child: PO 0.25-3.5 mg/day in divided doses q4-6hr, max 10 mg/day

Available forms: HCl: tabs 1, 2.5, 5, 10 mg; inj 2.5 mg/ml; decanoate: inj 25 mg/ml

Implementation
PO route
• **Oral solution:** Give product in liquid form mixed in glass of juice, milk, or water if hoarding is suspected; do not mix in caffeine drinks, tannics, or pectinates; decrease dose in geriatric patients
• Give PO with full glass of water, milk; or give with food to decrease GI upset
• Take antacids 2 hr before or after this product
• Store in tight, light-resistant container; oral sol in amber bottle
SUBCUT route
• May be given by this route; however, it is painful
IM route (HCl only)
• Inject in deep muscle mass, use a 21-G needle into dorsal gluteal site, keep patient recumbent for 30 min to prevent orthostatic hypotension

ADVERSE EFFECTS
CNS: *EPS, pseudoparkinsonism, akathisia, dystonia, tardive dyskinesia, drowsiness, headache,* **seizures, neuroleptic malignant syndrome**
CV: *Orthostatic hypotension,* hypertension, **cardiac arrest,** ECG changes, **tachycardia**
EENT: Blurred vision, glaucoma, dry eyes
GI: *Dry mouth, nausea, vomiting, anorexia, constipation,* diarrhea, jaundice, weight gain, **paralytic ileus, hepatitis,** cholecystic jaundice
GU: Urinary retention, urinary frequency, enuresis, impotence, amenorrhea, gynecomastia
HEMA: Anemia, **leukopenia, leukocytosis, agranulocytosis, aplastic anemia, thrombocytopenia**
INTEG: *Rash,* photosensitivity, dermatitis
RESP: **Laryngospasm,** dyspnea, **respiratory depression**

Pharmacokinetics

Absorption	Well absorbed (PO, IM)
Distribution	Widely absorbed, crosses blood-brain barrier, placenta
Metabolism	Liver, extensively, not dializable
Excretion	Kidneys (metabolites)
Half-life	HCl-4.7-15.3 hr, enanthate $3^{1}/_{2}$-4 days, decanoate 6.8-14.3 days

Pharmacodynamics

	PO/IM HCl	IM Enanthate	IM Decanoate
Onset	1 hr	1-2 days	1-3 days
Peak	1½-2 hr	2-3 days	1-2 days
Duration	6-8 hr	1-3 wk	>4 wk

INTERACTIONS

Individual drugs
Alcohol, haloperidol, metyrosine, risperidone: increased effects of both products, oversedation

Amiodarone, arsenic trioxide, astemizole, dasatinib, disopyramide, dofetilide, droperidol, erythromycin, flecainide, gatifloxacin, ibutilide, levomethadyl, ondansetron, paliperidone, palonosetron, pimozide, procainamide, probucol, ranolazine, quiNIDine, sotalol, sparfloxacin, saquinavir, sunitinib, vorinostat, ziprasidone: increased QT prolongation, torsades de pointes (at higher doses)

EPINEPHrine: increased toxicity

Levodopa: decreased antiparkinson activity

Lithium: decreased effects of lithium

Drug classifications
Anticholinergics: increased anticholinergic effects

Barbiturates: decreased effect of fluphenazine, oversedation

CNS depressants: oversedation

Smoking: decreased effects of fluphenazine

Drug/herb
Betel palm, kava: increased EPS

Cola tree, hops, kava, nettle, nutmeg: possible increased action

Henbane leaf: increased anticholinergic effect

Drug/lab test
Increased: liver function tests, cardiac enzymes, cholesterol, blood glucose, prolactin, bilirubin, cholinesterase

Decreased: hormones (blood and urine)

False positive: pregnancy tests, PKU, urinary steroids, 17-OHCS

NURSING CONSIDERATIONS

Assessment
• SSRIs, SNRIs, serotonin-receptor agonists: increased serotonin syndrome, malignant neuroleptic syndrome

• **Dementia:** deaths have occurred, not approved for this use

• **Serotonin syndrome, neuroleptic malignant syndrome:** severe EPS, increased CPK, altered mental state, sinus tachycardia, change in B/P; sweating often occurs in young men; heat stress, physical exhaustion, dehydration, organic brain disease

• **QT prolongation, torsades de pointes:** ECG for changes

• Assess mental status: orientation, mood, behavior, presence and type of hallucinations before initial administration and monthly; this product should significantly reduce psychotic behavior

• Check for swallowing of PO medication; check for hoarding or giving of medication to other patients

• Monitor I&O ratio, palpate bladder if low urinary output occurs, especially in geriatric; urinalysis recommended before, during prolonged therapy

• Monitor bilirubin, CBC, liver function tests monthly

• Assess affect, orientation, LOC, reflexes, gait, coordination, sleep pattern disturbances

• Monitor B/P with patient sitting, standing, and lying down; take pulse and respirations q4hr during initial treatment; establish baseline before starting treatment; report drops of 30 mm Hg; obtain baseline ECG, Q-wave and T-wave changes

• Check for dizziness, faintness, palpitations, tachycardia on rising; severe orthostatic hypotension is common

• **Assess for EPS** including akathisia (inability to sit still, no pattern to movements), tardive dyskinesia (bizarre movements of the jaw, mouth, tongue, extremities), pseudoparkinsonism (rigidity, tremors, pill rolling, shuffling gait); an antiparkinson product should be prescribed

• Assess for constipation, urinary retention daily; if these occur, increase bulk, water in diet

Nursing diagnoses
• Coping, ineffective (uses)
• Knowledge, deficient (teaching)
• Noncompliance (teaching)

Patient/family education
• Caution patient to avoid hazardous activities until product response is determined; dizziness, blurred vision may occur

• Inform patient that orthostatic hypotension occurs often and to rise from sitting or lying position gradually; tell patient to avoid hot tubs,

hot showers, tub baths because hypotension may occur; tell patient that in hot weather, heat stroke may occur; extra precautions are necessary to stay cool
• Instruct patient to avoid abrupt withdrawal of this product, or EPS may result; product should be withdrawn slowly
• Teach patient to avoid OTC preparations (cough, hay fever, cold) unless approved by physician because serious product interactions may occur; avoid use with alcohol, CNS depressants; increased drowsiness may occur
• Instruct patient to use a sunscreen and sunglasses to prevent burns
• Teach patient about EPS and necessity of meticulous oral hygiene because oral candidiasis may occur
• Instruct patient to take antacids 2 hr before or after this product
• Advise patient to report sore throat, malaise, fever, bleeding, mouth sores; if these occur, CBC should be performed and product discontinued

Evaluation
Positive therapeutic outcome
• Decrease in emotional excitement, hallucinations, delusions, paranoia
• Reorganization of patterns of thought, speech

TREATMENT OF OVERDOSE:
Lavage if orally ingested; provide airway; *do not induce vomiting or use epinephrine*

flurandrenolide topical
See Appendix B

flurazepam (Rx)
(flure-az'e-pam)
Apo-flurazepam ✦
Func. class.: Sedative-hypnotic
Chem. class.: Benzodiazepine, long-acting
Pregnancy category X
Controlled substance schedule IV (USA), Targeted (CDSA IV) (Canada)

Do not confuse:
flurazepam/temazepam

ACTION: Produces CNS depression at the limbic, thalamic, hypothalamic levels of CNS; may be mediated by neurotransmitter γ-aminobutyric acid (GABA); results are sedation, hypnosis, skeletal muscle relaxation, anticonvulsant activity, anxiolytic action

Therapeutic outcome: Ability to sleep, relaxation

USES: Insomnia, short term

CONTRAINDICATIONS:
Pregnancy **X**, breastfeeding

Precautions: Anemia, renal/hepatic disease, suicidal individuals, drug abuse, geriatric, psychosis, children <15 yr, angioedema, pulmonary disease, intermittent porphyria, uncontrolled pain, sleep apnea, hypersensitivity to this product or benzodiazepines

DOSAGE AND ROUTES
Adult: PO 15-30 mg at bedtime; may repeat dose once if needed
Geriatric: PO 15 mg at bedtime; may increase if needed

Hepatic dose
Dosage adjustment may be needed due to prolonged half-life

Available forms: Caps 15, 30 mg

Implementation
Give ¹/₂-1 hr before bedtime for sleeplessness; caps may be opened and mixed with food; give after meals to decrease GI symptoms if used for sedation
• Best to avoid in geriatric patients; long half-life
• Provide assistance with ambulation after giving dose
• Provide safety measures: night-light, call bell within easy reach
• Check to see if PO medication has been swallowed
• Store in tight container in cool environment

ADVERSE EFFECTS
CNS: *Lethargy, drowsiness, daytime sedation,* dizziness, confusion, light-headedness, headache, anxiety, irritability, complex sleep-related reactions (sleep driving, sleep eating)
CV: Chest pain, pulse changes, palpitations
GI: Nausea, vomiting, diarrhea, heartburn, abdominal pain, constipation
HEMA: Leukopenia, **granulocytopenia (rare)**
MISC: Physical, psychologic dependence, blurred vision, **apnea**

Pharmacokinetics

Absorption	Well absorbed
Distribution	Widely absorbed, crosses blood-brain barrier, crosses placenta, protein binding 97%
Metabolism	Liver to active, inactive metabolites
Excretion	Kidneys, breast milk
Half-life	$2^1/_2$ hr, 30-200 hr active metabolites

Pharmacodynamics

Onset	15-30 min
Peak	$^1/_2$-1 hr
Duration	7-8 hr

INTERACTIONS

Individual drugs

Alcohol: increased CNS depression
Cimetidine, disulfiram, fluoxetine, isoniazid, ketoconazole, propranolol, valproic acid: increased action of flurazepam
Probenecid: increased effects of flurazepam
Rifampin: decreased action of flurazepam
Theophylline: decreased effect of flurazepam

Drug classifications

Barbiturates: decreased effect of flurazepam
CNS depressants: increased CNS depression
CYP3A4 inhibitors, oral contraceptives: increased effect of flurazepam

Drug/herb

St. John's wort: decreased flurazepam effect

Drug/lab test

Increased: AST, ALT, serum bilirubin
Decreased: radioactive iodine uptake
False increase: urinary 17-OHCS

NURSING CONSIDERATIONS

Assessment

- Assess anxiety reaction: inability to sleep, apprehension, dread, foreboding, or uneasiness related to unidentified source of danger
- Assess for previous product dependence or tolerance; if product dependent or tolerant, amount of medication should be restricted
- Monitor B/P (lying, standing), pulse; if systolic B/P drops 20 mm Hg, hold product, notify prescriber; I&O, may indicate renal dysfunction
- Monitor blood studies: CBC during long-term therapy; blood dyscrasias have occurred rarely
- Monitor hepatic studies: AST, ALT, bilirubin, creatinine, LDH, alkaline phosphatase

- Monitor patient's mental status: mood, sensorium, affect, sleeping patterns, drowsiness, dizziness, suicidal tendencies
- Assess for withdrawal signs if discontinued abruptly
- Assess for excessive sedation, impaired coordination, especially in geriatric

Nursing diagnoses

- Knowledge, deficient (teaching)
- Noncompliance (teaching)
- Sleep pattern, disturbed (uses)

Patient/family education

- Inform patient that product may be taken with food; if dose is missed take as soon as remembered; do not double doses
- Advise patient to avoid OTC preparations unless approved by a physician, to avoid alcohol ingestion or other psychotropic medications unless approved by prescriber, that 1-2 wk of therapy may be required before therapeutic effects occur
- Caution patient to avoid driving, activities requiring alertness; drowsiness may occur; until medication response is known, tell patient that drowsiness may worsen at beginning of treatment
- Instruct patient not to discontinue medication abruptly after long-term use
- Caution patient to rise slowly or fainting may occur, especially in geriatric
- Inform patient that hangover is common in geriatric
- Teach patients to use contraceptives; pregnancy category **X**

Evaluation

Positive therapeutic outcome

- Increased well-being
- Decreased anxiety, restlessness, sleeplessness, dread

TREATMENT OF OVERDOSE:

Lavage, activated charcoal; monitor electrolytes, VS

flurbiprofen ophthalmic

See Appendix B

flutamide (Rx)

(floo'ta-mide)

Apo-Flutamide ✤, **Euflex** ✤

Func. class.: Antineoplastic hormone
Chem. class.: Antiandrogen

Pregnancy category D

ACTION: Interferes with androgen uptake in the nucleus or androgen activity in target tissues; arrests tumor growth in androgen-sensitive tissue (i.e., prostate gland)

Therapeutic outcome: Prevention of rapidly growing malignant cells

USES: Metastatic prostatic carcinoma, stage D_2 in combination with LHRH agonistic analogs (leuprolide), B_2-C in combination with goserelin and radiation

CONTRAINDICATIONS:

Pregnancy **D**, hypersensitivity

> **BLACK BOX WARNING:** Severe hepatic disease

Precautions: G6PD deficiency, hemoglobinopathy, lactase deficiency, polycystic ovary syndrome, tobacco smoking

DOSAGE AND ROUTES

Adult: PO 250 mg q8hr for a daily dose of 750 mg

Available forms: Caps 125, 250 ✤ mg

Implementation

• Used in combination with LHRH agonist (leuprolide)
• May be given with food or fluids

ADVERSE EFFECTS

CNS: *Hot flashes,* drowsiness, confusion, depression, anxiety, paresthesia
GI: *Diarrhea, nausea, vomiting,* increased liver function studies, **hepatitis,** anorexia, **hepatotoxicity,** abdominal pain, cholestasis, **hepatic necrosis/failure**
GU: *Decreased libido, impotence, gynecomastia*
HEMA: **Leukopenia, thrombocytopenia, hemolytic anemia**
INTEG: Irritation at site, rash, photosensitivity
MISC: Edema, neuromuscular and pulmonary symptoms, hypertension, **secondary malignancy**

Absorption	Well absorbed
Distribution	Unknown
Metabolism	Liver
Excretion	Unknown
Half-life	6 hr

Pharmacodynamics

Unknown

INTERACTIONS

Individual drugs

Leuprolide: decreased flutamide action
Warfarin: increased PT

NURSING CONSIDERATIONS

Assessment

• **Severe hepatic disease:** Monitor AST, ALT, alkaline phosphatase, which may be elevated; product may need to be discontinued; CBC, bilirubin, creatinine
• Identify CNS symptoms: drowsiness, confusion, depression, anxiety

Nursing diagnoses

• Body image, disturbed (adverse reactions)
• Infection, risk for (adverse reactions)
• Injury, risk for (adverse reactions)
• Knowledge, deficient (teaching)
• Sexual dysfunction (adverse reactions)

Patient/family education

• Tell the patient to report side effects: decreased libido, impotence, breast enlargement, hot flashes, diarrhea, which occur when the two products are given together; also nausea, vomiting; jaundice in eyes, skin; dark urine, clay-colored stools; hepatotoxicity may occur
• Inform patient that this product is taken with leuprolide for medical castration; do not change dosing
• Advise patient to use contraception during treatment, pregnancy **D**

Evaluation

Positive therapeutic outcome

• Prevention of rapid division of malignant cells

fluticasone (Rx)

(floo-tic'a-sone)
Flonase, Flovent HFA, Flovent Diskus ❧, Veramyst (nasal spray)
Func. class.: Corticosteroids, inhalation; antiasthmatic
Pregnancy category C

ACTION: Decreases inflammation by inhibiting mast cells, macrophages, and leukotrienes; antiinflammatory and vasoconstrictor properties

Therapeutic outcome: Decreased severity of asthma

USES: Prevention of chronic asthma during maintenance treatment in those requiring oral corticosteroids; nasal symptoms of seasonal/perennial and allergic/nonallergic rhinitis

CONTRAINDICATIONS:
Hypersensitivity to this product or milk protein, primary treatment in status asthmaticus

Precautions: Pregnancy C, breastfeeding, active infections, glaucoma, diabetes, immuno-compromised patients

DOSAGE AND ROUTES

Prevention of chronic asthma during maintenance treatment in those requiring oral corticosteroids

Flovent HFA
Adult and child ≥12 yr: INH 88-660 mcg bid (in those previously taking bronchodilators alone); INH 88-220 mcg bid, max 440 mcg bid (in those previously taking inhaled corticosteroids); INH 440 mcg bid, max 880 mcg bid (in those previously taking oral corticosteroids)
Child 4-11 yr: INH 88 mg bid

Flovent Diskus ❧
Adult and child ≥12 yr: INH 100 mcg bid, max 500 mcg (in those previously taking bronchodilators alone); INH 100-250 mcg bid, max 500 mcg bid (in those previously taking inhaled corticosteroids); INH 500-1000 mcg bid, max 1000 mcg bid (in those previously taking oral corticosteroids)
Child 4-11 yr: INH initially 50 mcg bid, max 100 mcg bid (in those previously taking bronchodilators alone or inhaled corticosteroids)

Nasal symptoms of seasonal/perennial rhinitis

Flonase
Adult: Nasal spray 2 sprays (100 mcg) in each nostril daily or 1 spray (50 mcg) in each nostril bid; when symptoms are controlled, decrease to 1 spray (50 mcg) in each nostril every day
Adolescent and child ≥4 yr: Nasal spray 1 spray (50 mcg) in each nostril daily; may increase to 2 sprays (100 mcg) in each nostril daily; max 2 sprays in each nostril daily

Available forms: Oral inh aerosol 44, 110, 220 mcg; oral inh powder 50, 100, 250 mcg

Implementation
• Give at 1 min intervals
• Decrease dose to lowest effective dose after desired effect; decrease dose at 2- to 4-wk intervals

ADVERSE EFFECTS
CNS: Fever, headache, nervousness, dizziness, migraines, numbness in fingers
EENT: *Pharyngitis,* sinusitis, rhinitis, laryngitis, hoarseness, dry eyes, cataracts, nasal discharge, epistaxis
GI: Diarrhea, abdominal pain, nausea, vomiting, *oral candidiasis,* gastroenteritis
GU: UTI
INTEG: Urticaria, dermatitis
META: Hyperglycemia, growth retardation in children, cushingoid features
MISC: Influenza, **eosinophilic conditions, angioedema, Churg-Strauss syndrome,** adrenal insufficiency (high doses), bone mineral density reduction
MS: Osteoporosis, muscle soreness, joint pain
RESP: *Upper respiratory infection,* dyspnea, cough, bronchitis, **bronchospasm**

Pharmacokinetics

Absorption	30% aerosol, 13.5% powder
Distribution	Protein binding 91%
Metabolism	In liver after absorption in lung
Excretion	<5% in urine and feces
Half-life	7.8 hr

Pharmacodynamics

Onset	12 hr	24 hr
Peak	Several days	Several days
Duration	1-2 wk	1-2 wk

INTERACTIONS

Individual drugs

Amprenavir, atazanavir, darunavir, delavirdine, fosamprenavir, nelfinavir, ritonavir, saquinavir: increased fluticasone levels

Mecasermin: decreased effects of mecasermin

Drug classifications

CYP3A4 inhibitors (ketoconazole, itraconazole): increased fluticasone levels

Growth hormones: decreased effects of growth hormones

Quinolones: increased tendinitis, tendon rupture

Drug/lab test

Increased: urine/serum glucose

NURSING CONSIDERATIONS

Assessment

• **Assess respiratory status:** lung sounds, pulmonary function tests during and several months after change from systemic to inhalation corticosteroids

• Assess for withdrawal symptoms from oral corticosteroids: depression, pain in joints, fatigue

⚠ Monitor adrenal insufficiency: nausea, weakness, fatigue, hypotension, hypoglycemia, anorexia; may occur when changing from systemic to inhalation corticosteroids; may be life-threatening

• Monitor growth rate in children; blood glucose, serum potassium in all patients

• Monitor adrenal function tests periodically: hypothalamic-pituitary-adrenal axis suppression in long-term treatment

Nursing diagnoses

• Airway clearance, ineffective (uses)
• Noncompliance (teaching)

Patient/family education

• Advise patient to use bronchodilator first before using inhalation, if taking both

• Caution patient not to use for acute asthmatic attack; acute asthma may require oral corticosteroids

• Advise patient to avoid smoking, smoke-filled rooms, those with URIs, those not immunized against chickenpox or measles

Evaluation

Positive therapeutic outcome

• Decreased severity of asthma

fluticasone nasal agent
See Appendix B

fluticasone topical
See Appendix B

fluvastatin (Rx)
(flu′vah-stay-tin)
Lescol, Lescol XL
Func. class.: Antilipidemic
Chem. class.: HMG-CoA reductase inhibitor
Pregnancy category X

F

ACTION: Inhibits HMG-CoA reductase enzyme, which reduces cholesterol synthesis

Therapeutic outcome: Decreased cholesterol levels and LDLs, increased HDLs

USES: As an adjunct in primary hypercholesterolemia (types Ia, Ib), coronary atherosclerosis in CAD; secondary prevention of coronary events in patients with CAD; adjunct to diet to reduce LDL, total cholesterol, apo B levels in heterozygous familial hypercholesterolemia (LDL-C ≥190 mg/dl) or LDL-C >160 mg/dl with history of premature CV disease

CONTRAINDICATIONS:

Pregnancy **X,** breastfeeding, hypersensitivity, active liver disease

Precautions: Past liver disease, alcoholism, severe acute infections, trauma, hypotension, uncontrolled seizure disorders, severe metabolic disorders, electrolyte imbalance, myopathy, rhabdomyolysis

DOSAGE AND ROUTES

Adult: PO 20-40 mg/day in PM initially, usual range 20-80 mg, max 80 mg; may be given in 2 doses (40 mg AM, 40 mg PM); dosage adjustments may be made in 4-wk intervals or more

Heterozygous familial hypercholesterolemia

Adolescents ≥1 yr postmenarche (10-16 yr): PO 20 mg daily at bedtime, may increase q6wk, max 40 mg bid (cap) or 80 mg (ext rel)

Available forms: Caps 20, 40 mg; ext rel tab 80 mg

Implementation

• Give with evening meal; if dosage is increased, give with breakfast and evening meal

• Store in cool environment in airtight, light-resistant container

ADVERSE EFFECTS
CNS: Headache, dizziness, insomnia
EENT: Lens opacities
GI: *Nausea, constipation, diarrhea, abdominal pain, cramps, dyspepsia, flatus,* liver dysfunction, **pancreatitis**
HEMA: Thrombocytopenia, hemolytic anemia, leukopenia
INTEG: Rash, pruritus
MISC: Fatigue, influenza, photosensitivity
MS: Myalgia, *arthritis, arthralgia,* myositis, **rhabdomyolysis**
RESP: Upper respiratory infection, rhinitis, cough, pharyngitis, sinusitis

Pharmacokinetics	
Absorption	Unknown
Distribution	Steady state 4-5 wk
Metabolism	Liver
Excretion	Feces, kidneys
Half-life	1-6 days

Pharmacodynamics
Unknown

INTERACTIONS
Individual drugs
Alcohol, cimetidine, ranitidine, omeprazole: increased fluvastatin effect
Cholestyramine: decreased fluvastatin effect
Colchicine, cycloSPORINE, niacin: increased myopathy
Digoxin, phenytoin, warfarin: increased action
Tramadol: increased serotonin syndrome

Drug classifications:
Fibric acid derivatives, protease inhibitors: increased myopathy

Drug/herb
Red yeast rice: increased adverse reactions
Gotu kola, St. John's wort: decreased effect

Drug/food
Grapefruit juice: possible increased fluvastatin toxicity

NURSING CONSIDERATIONS
Assessment
• **Hypercholesterolemia:** Assess nutrition: fat, protein, carbohydrates; nutritional analysis should be completed by dietitian before treatment
• Assess fasting lipid profile (cholesterol, LDL, HDL, triglycerides) q4-6wk, then q3-6mo when stable

• Monitor bowel pattern daily; diarrhea may be a problem
• **Hepatotoxicity/pancreatitis:** Monitor liver function studies q1-2mo during the first 1¹/₂ yr of treatment; AST, ALT, liver function test results may be increased
• Monitor renal studies in patients with compromised renal system: BUN, I&O ratio, creatinine
• Obtain ophth exam before, 1 mo after treatment begins, annually; lens opacities may occur
• **Myopathy, rhabdomyolysis:** Assess for muscle pain, tenderness; obtain baseline CPK, if elevated or if symptoms occur, product should be discontinued

Nursing diagnoses
• Diarrhea (adverse reactions)
• Knowledge, deficient (teaching)
• Noncompliance (teaching)

Patient/family education
• Inform patient that compliance is needed for positive results to occur, not to double doses
• Advise patient to notify prescriber if GI symptoms of diarrhea, abdominal or epigastric pain, nausea, vomiting, or if chills, fever, sore throat occur; also muscle pain, weakness, tenderness
• Advise patient that blood studies and eye exam will be necessary during treatment
• Instruct patient to report suspected pregnancy, not to use during pregnancy (**X**)
• Advise patient that previously prescribed regimen will continue, including diet, exercise, smoking cessation
• Instruct patient to notify all health care providers of products taken

Evaluation
Positive therapeutic outcome
• Decreased LDL, VLDL, total cholesterol levels
• Improved ratio of HDLs

folic acid (vitamin B₉) (PO, OTC; IM/IV, Ph)
(foe-lik a'sid)
Apo-Folic ✤, Equaline Folic Acid, Folacin, Vitamin B₉, Walgreens Gold Seal Folic Acid
Func. class.: Vitamin B-complex group, water-soluble vitamin
Chem. class.: Supplement
Pregnancy category A

ACTION: Needed for erythropoiesis; increases RBC, WBC, and platelet formation in megaloblastic anemias

Therapeutic outcome: Absence of macrocytic, megaloblastic anemias

USES: Megaloblastic or macrocytic anemia caused by folic acid deficiency; liver disease; alcoholism; hemolysis; intestinal obstruction; pregnancy; to reduce risk of neural tube defect

CONTRAINDICATIONS:
Hypersensitivity

Precautions: Pregnancy A, anemias other than megaloblastic/macrocytic anemia, vit B_{12} deficiency anemia, uncorrected pernicious anemia

DOSAGE AND ROUTES
RDA
Adult (pregnant/breastfeeding): PO 600 mcg/day
Adult and child ≥14 yr: PO 400 mcg
Child 9-13 yr: PO 300 mcg
Child 4-8 yr: PO 200 mcg
Child 1-3 yr: PO 150 mcg
Infant 6 mo-1 yr: PO 80 mcg
Neonate and infant <6 mo: PO 65 mcg

Megaloblastic/macrocytic anemia due to folic acid or nutritional deficiency
Pregnant/lactating: PO 800-1000 mcg

Therapeutic dose
Adult and child: PO/IM/SUBCUT/IV up to 1 mg/day

Maintenance dose
Adult and child >4 yr: PO/IM/IV/SUBCUT 0.4 mg/day
Child <4 yr: PO/IM/IV/SUBCUT up to 0.3 mg/day
Infant: PO/IM/IV/SUBCUT up to 0.1 mg/day
Pregnant/lactating: PO/IM/IV/SUBCUT 0.8-1 mg/day

Prevention of neural tube defects during pregnancy
Adult: PO 0.6 mg/day

Prevention of megaloblastic anemia during pregnancy
Adult: PO/IM/SUBCUT up to 1 mg/day during pregnancy

Tropical sprue
Adult: PO 3-15 mg/day

Available forms: Tabs 0.1, 0.4, 0.8, 1, 5 mg; inj 5, 10 mg/ml

Implementation
SUBCUT route
• Do not inject intradermally
IM route
• Inject deeply in large muscle mass, aspirate
Direct IV route
• Give **IV** directly, undiluted 5 mg or less over 1 min or more
Continuous IV route
• May be added to most **IV** sol or TPN
• Store in light-resistant container

ADVERSE EFFECTS
CNS: Confusion, depression, excitability, irritability
GI: Anorexia, nausea
INTEG: Flushing, pruritus, rash, erythema
RESP: Bronchospasm
SYST: Anaphylaxis (rare)

Pharmacokinetics
Absorption	Well absorbed
Distribution	Liver, crosses placenta
Metabolism	Liver (converted to active metabolite)
Excretion	Kidneys (unchanged)
Half-life	Unknown

Pharmacodynamics
Onset	Unknown
Peak	$1/2$-1 hr
Duration	Unknown

INTERACTIONS
Individual drugs
CarBAMazepine: increased need for folic acid
Fosphenytoin: decreased fosphenytoin levels, may increase seizures
Methotrexate, sulfasalazine, trimethoprim: decreased action of folic acid
Phenytoin: decreased phenytoin levels, may increase seizures

Drug classifications
Estrogens, glucocorticoids, hydantoins: increased need for folic acid
Sulfonamides: decreased action of folic acid

NURSING CONSIDERATIONS
Assessment
• **Megaloblastic anemia:** Assess patient for fatigue, dyspnea, weakness, activity intolerance (signs of megaloblastic anemia)

• Monitor Hgb, Hct, and reticulocyte count; folate levels: 6-15 mcg/ml baseline, throughout treatment
• Assess nutritional status: bran, yeast, dried beans, yeast, dried beans, nuts, fruits, fresh vegetables, asparagus; if high folic acid foods are missing from the diet, a referral to a dietitian may be indicated
• Identify products currently taken: alcohol, oral contraceptives, estrogens, glucocorticoids, carBAMazepine, hydantoins, trimethoprim; these products may cause increased folic acid use by the body and contribute to deficiency if taking other neurotoxic products

Nursing diagnoses
• Activity intolerance (uses)
• Fatigue (uses)
• Knowledge, deficient (teaching)
• Nutrition: less than body requirements, imbalanced (uses)

Patient/family education
• Advise patient to take product exactly as prescribed; not to double doses, toxicity may occur
• Instruct patient to notify prescriber of side effects; rash or fever may indicate hypersensitivity
• Advise patient that urine may become more yellow
• Instruct patient to increase intake of foods rich in folic acid in diet as recommended by dietitian or health care provider
• Advise patient to avoid breastfeeding

Evaluation
Positive therapeutic outcome
• Absence of fatigue, weakness, dyspnea
• Absence of symptoms of megaloblastic anemia
• Increase in reticulocyte count within 5 days
• Absence of neural tube defect

⚠ HIGH ALERT

fondaparinux (Rx)
(fon-dah-pair′ih-nux)
Arixtra
Func. class.: Anticoagulant, antithrombotic
Chem. class.: Synthetic, selective factor Xa inhibitor
Pregnancy category B

Do not confuse:
Arixtra/Anti-Xa

ACTION: Acts by antithrombin III (ATIII)-mediated selective inhibition of factor Xa; neutralization of factor Xa interrupts blood coagulation and inhibits thrombin formation; does not inactivate thrombin (activated factor II) or affect platelets

Therapeutic outcome: Prevention of deep vein thrombosis

USES: Prevention/treatment of deep vein thrombosis, pulmonary emboli in hip and knee replacement, hip fracture or abdominal surgery

CONTRAINDICATIONS:
Hypersensitivity to this product; hemophilia, leukemia with bleeding, peptic ulcer disease, hemorrhagic stroke, surgery, thrombocytopenic purpura, weight <50 kg, severe renal disease (CCr <30 ml/min), active major bleeding, bacterial endocarditis

Precautions: Pregnancy **B,** breastfeeding, children, geriatric, alcoholism, hepatic disease (severe), blood dyscrasias, heparin-induced thrombocytopenia, uncontrolled severe hypertension, subacute bacterial endocarditis, acute nephritis, mild to moderate renal disease

> **BLACK BOX WARNING:** Spinal/epidural anesthesia, lumbar puncture

DOSAGE AND ROUTES
Deep vein thrombosis/PE
Adult <50 kg: SUBCUT 5 mg/day × 5 days or more until INR is 2-3; may give warfarin within 72 hr of fondaparinux
Adult 50-100 kg: SUBCUT 7.5 mg/day × 5 days or more until INR is 2-3; may give warfarin within 72 hr of fondaparinux
Adult >100 kg: SUBCUT 10 mg/day × 5 days or more until INR is 2-3; may give warfarin within 72 hr of fondaparinux

Prevention of deep vein thrombosis
Adult: SUBCUT 2.5 mg/day, given 6 hr after surgery; continue for 5-9 days; hip surgery up to 32 days; abdominal surgery up to 24 days

Renal disease
Adult: Do not use if CCr <30 ml/min

Available forms: Inj 2.5 mg/0.5 ml, 5 mg/0.4 ml, 7.5 mg/0.6 ml, 10 mg/0.8 ml prefilled syringes

Implementation
• Do not mix with other products or solutions; cannot be used interchangeably (unit to unit) with other anticoagulants
• Administer for 5-9 days

- Give only after screening patient for bleeding disorders
- Store at 77° F (25° C); do not freeze

SUBCUT route
- Administer SUBCUT only; do not give IM
- Check for discolored sol or sol with particulate; if present, do not give
- Administer to recumbent patient, rotate inj sites (left/right anterolateral, left/right posterolateral abdominal wall), administer 6-8 hr after surgery
- Wipe surface of inj site with alcohol swab, twist plunger cap and remove, remove rigid needle guard by pulling straight off needle, do not aspirate, do not expel air bubble from surface
- Insert whole length of needle into skin fold held with thumb and forefinger
- When product is injected, a soft click may be felt or heard
- Give at same time each day to maintain steady blood levels
- Avoid all IM inj that may cause bleeding

A Administer only this product when ordered; not interchangeable with heparin

ADVERSE EFFECTS
CNS: *Fever,* confusion, headache, dizziness, *insomnia*
GI: *Nausea, vomiting,* diarrhea, dyspepsia, *constipation,* increased AST, ALT
GU: UTI, urinary retention
HEMA: *Anemia,* minor bleeding, purpura, hematoma, **thrombocytopenia, major bleeding (intracranial, cerebral, retroperitoneal hemorrhage), postoperative hemorrhage, heparin-induced thrombocytopenia**
INTEG: Local reaction—*rash,* pruritus, inj site bleeding, increased wound drainage, bullous eruption
META: Hypokalemia
MISC: Hypotension, pain, *edema*

Pharmacokinetics
Absorption	Rapidly, completely absorbed
Distribution	Blood; does not bind to plasma proteins except 94% to ATIII
Metabolism	Unknown
Excretion	Eliminated unchanged in 72 hr in normal renal function
Half-life	17-21 hr

Pharmacodynamics
Onset	Unknown
Peak	3 hr
Duration	Unknown

INTERACTIONS
Do not mix with other products or inf fluids
Individual drugs
Abciximab, clopidogrel, dipyridamole, eptifibatide, quiNIDine, tirofiban, valproic acid: increased risk of bleeding
Drug classifications
NSAIDs, salicylates: increased risk of bleeding
Drug/herb
Feverfew, garlic, ginger, ginkgo, ginseng, green tea, horse chestnut, kava: increased risk of bleeding

NURSING CONSIDERATIONS
Assessment

BLACK BOX WARNING: Monitor patients who have received epidural/spinal anesthesia or lumbar puncture for neurological impairment

- **Hemorrhage:** Assess for hemorrhage if coadministered with other products that may cause bleeding
- Assess blood studies (Hct, CBC, coagulation studies, platelets, occult blood in stools), anti-Xa; if platelets <100,000/mm³, treatment should be discontinued; renal studies: BUN, creatinine
- Assess for bleeding: gums, petechiae, ecchymosis, black tarry stools, hematuria; notify prescriber

Nursing diagnoses
- Injury, risk for (uses, adverse reactions)
- Knowledge, deficient (teaching)

Patient/family education
- Advise patient to use soft-bristle toothbrush to avoid bleeding gums, to use electric razor
- Advise patient to report any signs of bleeding: gums, under skin, urine, stools
- Caution patient to avoid OTC products containing aspirin

Evaluation
Positive therapeutic outcome
- Absence of deep vein thrombosis

formoterol (Rx)

(for-moh'ter-ahl)

**Foradil Aerolizer, Oxeze ✚,
Perforomist**

Func. class.: β-Adrenergic agonist

Chem. class.: Sympathomimetic catecholamine

Pregnancy category C

Do not confuse:

Foradil/Toradol

ACTION: Has β₁ and β₂ action; relaxes bronchial smooth muscle and dilates the trachea and main bronchi by increasing levels of cyclic AMP, which relaxes smooth muscles; causes increased contractility and heart rate by acting on β-receptors in the heart

Therapeutic outcome: Bronchodilation, increased heart rate and cardiac output from action on β-receptors in heart

USES: Maintenance, treatment of asthma, COPD, prevention of exercise-induced bronchospasm

CONTRAINDICATIONS:

Hypersensitivity to sympathomimetics, monotherapy for asthma

Precautions: Pregnancy C, geriatric, cardiac disorders, hyperthyroidism, diabetes mellitus, prostatic hypertrophy, hypertension, African descendants

> **BLACK BOX WARNING:** Asthma-related death

DOSAGE AND ROUTES

Maintenance, treatment of asthma

Adult and child ≥5 yr: INH AM and PM long-term, 1 cap (12 mcg) q12hr using aerolizer inhaler

Maintenance of COPD

Adult: INH 12 mcg q12hr

Prevention of exercise-induced bronchospasm

Adult and child ≥12 yr: INH prn 1 cap (12 mcg) at least 15 min before exercise, do not use additional doses for ≥12 hr

Available forms: INH powder in cap 12 mcg; nebulizer sol for inhalation 20 mcg/2 ml

Implementation

• Store at room temperature, protect from heat, moisture

Inhalation route

• Place cap in aerolizer inhaler; the cap is punctured; do not wash aerolizer inhaler

• Pull off cover, twist mouthpiece to open, push buttons in; make sure the four pins are visible; remove cap from blister pack, place cap in chamber; twist to close, press (a click will be heard), release; patient should exhale, place inhaler in mouth, inhale rapidly

ADVERSE EFFECTS

CNS: Tremors, *anxiety*, insomnia, headache, dizziness, stimulation

CV: Palpitations, tachycardia, hypertension, chest pain

GI: Nausea, vomiting, xerostomia

RESP: Bronchial irritation, dryness of oropharynx, **bronchospasms (overuse)**; infection, inflammatory reactions (child)

Pharmacokinetics

Absorption	Rapid (INH)
Distribution	Plasma protein binding 61%-64% at concentrations of 0.1-100 ng/mL; 31%-38% at concentrations of 5-500 ng/mL
Metabolism	Liver, lungs, GI tract
Excretion	Urine, feces
Half-life	10 hr mean terminal elimination half-life

Pharmacodynamics

Onset	Unknown
Peak	5 min (INH)
Duration	Unknown

INTERACTIONS

Amoxapine, arsenic trioxide, chloroquine, clarithromycin, dasatinib, dolasetron, droperidol, erythromycin, halofantrine, levomethadyl, ondansetron, paliperidone, palonosetron, pentamidine, probucol, ranolazine, sunitinib, vorinostat, pimozide, risperidone, ziprasidone: increased QT prolongation

Drug classifications

Class IA/III antidysrhythmics, phenothiazines, halogenated anesthetics, tricyclics, some quinolones: increase QT prolongation

β-blockers: decreased action of formoterol

MAOIs, antidepressants (tricyclics): serious dysrhythmias

Sympathomimetics, thyroid hormones, tricyclics, some quinolones: increased action of both products

Loop/thiazide diuretics: increased hypokalemia

NURSING CONSIDERATIONS

Assessment
• Assess respiratory function: B/P, pulse, lung sounds
• Assess I&O ratio; check for urinary retention, frequency, hesitancy
• Assess for paresthesias and coldness of extremities; peripheral blood flow may decrease

Nursing diagnoses
• Airway clearance, ineffective (uses)
• Gas exchange, impaired (uses)
• Knowledge, deficient (teaching)

Patient/family education
• Review package insert with patient and inform about all aspects of product
• Teach correct use of inhaler; not to swallow caps
• Teach use of spacer device in children or geriatric
• Advise patient to avoid getting aerosol in eyes
• Instruct patient to rinse mouth after use
• Advise patient to wash inhaler in warm water and dry daily
• Advise patient to avoid smoking, smoke-filled rooms, persons with respiratory infections
• Asthma-related death, severe asthma exacerbations: if wheezing worsens and cannot be relieved during an acute asthma attack, immediate medical attention should be sought

Evaluation
Positive therapeutic outcome
• Absence of dyspnea, wheezing
• Improved airway exchange
• Improved ABGs

TREATMENT OF OVERDOSE:
Administer β-blocker

fosamprenavir (Rx)
(fos-am-pren′a-veer)
Lexiva, Telzin ♣
Func. class.: Antiretroviral
Chem. class.: Protease inhibitor
Pregnancy category C

ACTION: Prodrug of amprenavir; inhibits human immunodeficiency virus (HIV) protease, which prevents maturation of the infectious virus

Therapeutic outcome: Decreasing symptoms of HIV

USES: HIV-1 infection in combination with antiretrovirals

CONTRAINDICATIONS:
Hypersensitivity to protease inhibitors

Precautions: Pregnancy C, breastfeeding, geriatric, liver disease, hemolytic anemia, diabetes, sulfa sensitivity

DOSAGE AND ROUTES
Therapy-naïve patients
Adult: PO 1400 mg bid without ritonavir, or fosamprenavir 1400 mg/day and ritonavir 200 mg/day, or fosamprenavir 700 mg bid and ritonavir 100 mg bid

Protease-experienced patients (PI)
Adult: PO 700 mg bid and ritonavir 100 mg bid

Combination with efavirenz
Adult: PO add another 100 mg/day of ritonavir for a total of 300 mg/day when all three products are given

Hepatic dose
Adult: PO (Child-Pugh 5-6) 700 mg bid without ritonavir (treatment-naive patients) or 700 mg bid with ritonavir 100 mg qd (treatment-naive or experienced patients); (Child-Pugh 7-9) 700 mg bid without ritonavir (treatment-naive patients) or 450 mg bid with ritonavir 100 mg qd (treatment-naive or experienced patients); (Child-Pugh 10-15) 350 mg bid without ritonavir (treatment-naive patients) or 300 mg bid with ritonavir 100 mg qd (treatment-naive or experienced patients)

Available forms: Tabs 700 mg (equivalent to 600 mg amprenavir); oral suspension 50 mg/ml

Implementation
• **Tabs:** Administer without regard to food
• **Oral susp:** *Adult:* give without food; *child:* give with food; if vomiting occurs within 30 min, readminister; shake oral susp vigorously prior to dosing, use calibrated device
• Patients receiving phosphodiesterase type 5 (PDE5) inhibitors may be at increased risk for PDE5 inhibitor adverse effects

ADVERSE EFFECTS
CNS: Headache, fatigue, depression, oral paresthesia
GI: *Nausea, diarrhea, vomiting, abdominal pain*

Adverse effects: *italics* = common; **bold** = life-threatening

INTEG: Rash, pruritus
MISC: Redistribution or accumulation of body fat, hyperglycemia, **Stevens-Johnson syndrome**

Pharmacokinetics

Absorption	Unknown
Distribution	90% protein binding
Metabolism	In the liver by CYP3A4
Excretion	Excretion of unchanged product is minimal
Half-life	Unknown

Pharmacodynamics

Onset	Unknown
Peak	$1^1/_2$-4 hr
Duration	Unknown

INTERACTIONS

Individual drugs

⚠ **Amiodarone, flecainide, lidocaine, midazolam, pimozide, propafenone, triazolam: serious life-threatening reactions**

CarBAMazepine, dexamethasone, efavirenz, lopinavir/ritonavir, nevirapine, phenytoin, ranitidine, saquinavir: decreased fosamprenavir levels, avoid concurrent use

Aripiprazole, itraconazole, ketoconazole, rifabutin, sildenafil, vardenafil: increased effect

Methadone: decreased effect

Warfarin: increased effect of warfarin

Drug classifications

Antacids: decreased fosamprenavir levels

⚠ **Barbiturates, proton-pump inhibitors, calcium channel blockers, ergots, H_2 receptor antagonists: serious life-threatening reactions**

Contraceptives (oral): decreased effect

Estrogens, H_2 receptor antagonists, oral contraceptives, proton-pump inhibitors: avoid use; may lose virologic response and possibly lead to resistance of fosamprenavir

HMG-CoA reductase inhibitors: increased toxicity

Drug/herb

Avoid use with St. John's wort, may lose virologic response and possibly lead to resistance of fosamprenavir

Drug/lab test

Increased: serum glucose, AST, ALT, triglycerides

NURSING CONSIDERATIONS

Assessment

• Assess bowel pattern before, during treatment; monitor hydration
• Assess skin eruptions, rash, urticaria, itching
• **HIV:** Monitor viral load, CD4 cell counts, plasma HIV RNA, serum cholesterol, lipid profile baseline, throughout treatment
• **Stevens-Johnson syndrome:** report immediately

Nursing diagnoses

• Infection, risk for (uses)
• Injury, risk for (adverse reactions)
• Knowledge, deficient (teaching)

Patient/family education

• Advise patient to avoid taking product with other medications unless directed by provider
• Teach patient that product does not cure, but does manage symptoms; that product does not prevent transmission of HIV to others
• Advise patient to use nonhormonal form of birth control while taking this product
• Instruct patient if dose is missed, take as soon as remembered up to 1 hr before next dose; do not double dose
• Instruct patient not to alter dose or stop therapy without talking to physician
• Advise physician if patient has a sulfa allergy
• Advise patient to report all medications, including herbal supplements, to prescriber

Evaluation

Positive therapeutic outcome
• Decreasing symptoms of HIV

---

fosaprepitant (Rx)

(phos-a-prep´ih-tant)
Emend
Func. class.: Antiemetic
Chem. class.: Miscellaneous
Pregnancy category B

ACTION: A selective antagonist of human substance P/neurokinin 1 (NK_1) receptors decreasing emetic reflex, prodrug of aprepitant

Therapeutic outcome: Absence of nausea, vomiting during cancer chemotherapy

USES: Prevention of nausea/vomiting associated with cancer chemotherapy (highly emetogenic/moderately emetogenic) including high-dose CISplatin, used in combination with other antiemetics; postoperative nausea/vomiting

---

⚠ Nurse Alert

CONTRAINDICATIONS:
Hypersensitivity to this product or polysorbate 80

Precautions: Pregnancy **B**, breastfeeding, children, hepatic disease, geriatric patients; continuous use for nausea and vomiting not recommended

DOSAGE AND ROUTES
Adult: **IV** INF 115 mg over 15 min, 30 min prior to chemotherapy as an alternate to the 1st dose of aprepitant on day 1 of the aprepitant-CINV regimen

Available forms: Powder for inj 115 mg

Implementation

IV INF route
- Give **IV** route
- Approved only as a substitute for the 1st dose of aprepitant in 3-day regimen
- Use aseptic technique for reconstitution; inject 5 ml of 0.9% NaCl into the vial, directing stream to wall of vial to prevent foam; swirl; do not shake
- Prepare inf bag with 110 ml of NS; do not dilute or reconstitute with any divalent cations such as calcium, magnesium, including LR, Hartmann's sol
- Withdraw the entire volume from vial and transfer to inf bag; total volume 115 ml (1 mg/ 1 ml)
- Gently invert bag 2-3 times; reconstituted sol is stable for 24 hr at lower room temp or <25°C
- Visually inspect for particulates and discoloration
- Infuse over 15 min

ADVERSE EFFECTS
CNS: *Headache, dizziness,* insomnia, anxiety, depression, confusion, peripheral neuropathy
CV: Bradycardia, tachycardia, DVT, hypo/ hypertension
GI: *Diarrhea, constipation,* abdominal pain, anorexia, gastritis, increased AST/ALT, *nausea,* vomiting, heartburn
GU: Increased BUN, serum creatine, proteinuria, dysuria
HEMA: Anemia, **thrombocytopenia, neutropenia**
INTEG: Pruritus, rash, urticaria, **anaphylaxis**
MISC: Asthenia, fatigue, dehydration, fever, hiccups, tinnitus

Pharmacokinetics

Absorption	Unknown
Distribution	Protein binding 95%
Metabolism	In liver by CYP3A4 enzymes to an active metabolite; rapidly converted to aprepitant (within 30 mins)
Excretion	Unknown
Half-life	13 hr

Pharmacodynamics
Unknown

INTERACTIONS

Individual drugs
Paroxetine: increased action of both products

Drug classifications
CYP2C9 substrates (warfarin, tolbutamide, phenytoin), oral contraceptives: decreased action
CYP3A4 inducers (rifampin, carBAMazepine, phenytoin): decreased aprepitant action
CYP3A4 inhibitors (ketoconazole, itraconazole, nefazodone, troleandomycin, clarithromycin, ritonavir, nelfinavir, diltiazem): increased aprepitant action
CYP3A4 substrates (pimozide, cisapride, dexamethasone, astemizole, methylPREDNISolone, midazolam, alprazolam, triazolam, docetaxel, paclitaxel, etoposide, irinotecan, imatinib, ifosfamide, vinorelbine, vinBLAStine, vinCRIStine): increased action

Drug/food
Grapefruit juice: decreased effect

NURSING CONSIDERATIONS

Assessment
- Assess CV status: hyper/hypotension, bradycardia, tachycardia, DVT
- Assess for absence of nausea, vomiting during chemotherapy
- Monitor LFTs

Nursing diagnoses
- Knowledge, deficient (teaching)
- Nausea (uses)

Patient/family education
- Instruct patient to report diarrhea, constipation
- Instruct patient to report all medications and herbals to prescriber prior to taking this medication
- Advise patient to use nonhormonal form of contraception while taking this agent; oral contraceptive effect may be decreased

---

• Advise patient on warfarin to have clotting monitored closely during 2-wk period following administration of aprepitant
• Instruct patient to avoid breastfeeding

Evaluation
Positive therapeutic outcome
• Absence of nausea, vomiting during cancer chemotherapy

---

foscarnet (Rx)
(foss-kar′net)
Foscavir
Func. class.: Antiviral
Chem. class.: Inorganic pyrophosphate organic analog
Pregnancy category C

ACTION: Antiviral activity is produced by selective inhibition at the pyrophosphate binding site on virus-specific DNA polymerases and reverse transcriptases at concentrations that do not affect cellular DNA polymerases

Therapeutic outcome: Virostatic agents against CMV retinitis

USES: Treatment of CMV, retinitis, herpes simplex virus (HSV) infections; used with ganciclovir for relapsing patients

CONTRAINDICATIONS:
Hypersensitivity, CCr <0.4 ml/min/kg

Precautions: Pregnancy C, breastfeeding, children, geriatric, seizure disorders, severe anemia

> **BLACK BOX WARNING:** Renal disease, electrolyte/mineral imbalances

DOSAGE AND ROUTES
CMV retinitis
Adult: IV INF 60 mg/kg given over at least 1 hr or 120 mg/kg over 2 hr, q8hr × 2-3 wk initially, or 90 mg/kg q12hr, usually given with at least 750-1000 ml of 0.9% NaCl daily

HSV
Adult: IV 40 mg/kg q8-12hr × 2-3 wk

Renal dose
Adult: IV
Male:

$$\frac{\text{weight (kg)} \times 140 - \text{age}}{72 \times \text{serum creatinine (mg/dl)}} = \text{CCr}$$

Female: 0.85 × male value; dose based on table provided in package insert

Available forms: Inj 6000 mg/250 ml, 12,000 mg/500 ml (24 mg/ml)

Implementation
Intermittent IV infusion route
• Administer increased fluids before, during product administration to induce diuresis and minimize renal toxicity
• Administer via inf pump, at no more than 1 mg/kg/min; do not give by rapid or bolus **IV;** give by central venous line or peripheral vein; standard 24 mg/ml sol may be used without dilution if using by central line; dilute the 24 mg/ml sol to 12 mg/ml with D_5W or 0.9% NaCl if using peripheral vein
• Monitor patient closely during therapy; if tingling, numbness, paresthesias occur, stop inf and obtain lab sample for electrolytes

Y-site incompatibilities: Manufacturer recommends that product not be given with other medications in syringe or admixed

ADVERSE EFFECTS
CNS: *Fever,* dizziness, *headache,* **seizures,** *fatigue,* neuropathy, asthenia, encephalopathy, malaise, meningitis, *paresthesia,* depression, *confusion, anxiety*
CV: ECG abnormalities, 1st-degree AV block, nonspecific ST-T segment changes, cerebrovascular disorder, cardiomyopathy, **cardiac arrest,** atrial fibrillation, CHF, sinus tachycardia
GI: *Nausea, vomiting, diarrhea, anorexia,* abdominal pain, **pancreatitis**
GU: **Acute renal failure,** decreased CCr and increased serum creatinine, azotemia, diabetes mellitus
HEMA: Anemia, **granulocytopenia, leukopenia, thrombocytopenia, thrombosis,** lymphadenopathy, neutropenia
INTEG: *Rash,* sweating, pruritus, skin discoloration
RESP: *Coughing, dyspnea,* pneumonia, **pulmonary infiltration, pneumothorax, hemoptysis**
SYST: *Hypokalemia, hypocalcemia, hypomagnesemia,* hypophosphatemia

Pharmacokinetics

Absorption	Complete (**IV**)
Distribution	14%-17% plasma protein binding
Metabolism	Not metabolized
Excretion	Kidneys (79%-92%) unchanged, breast milk
Half-life	18-88 hr; increased in renal disease

Pharmacodynamics

Onset	48 hr
Peak	2 wk
Duration	Unknown

INTERACTIONS

Individual drugs
Acyclovir, cidofovir, CISplatin, penicillamine, tacrolimus, tenofovir, vancomycin, amphotericin B, cycloSPORINE, lithium: increased nephrotoxicity

Pentamidine: increased hypocalcemia

Drug classifications
Aminoglycosides, gold compounds, NSAIDs: increased nephrotoxicity

NURSING CONSIDERATIONS

Assessment
• **General** culture should be done before treatment with foscarnet is begun; cultures of blood, urine, and throat may all be taken; CMV is not confirmed by this method; the diagnosis is made by an ophth exam

• **Renal tubular disorders:** Assess kidney: BUN, serum creatinine, creatinine clearance, if CCr <0.4 ml/min/kg, discontinue product

• Blood counts should be done q2wk; watch for decreasing granulocytes, Hgb; if low, therapy may have to be discontinued and restarted after hematologic recovery; blood transfusions may be required

• Assess for GI symptoms: severe nausea, vomiting, diarrhea; severe symptoms may necessitate discontinuing product

• Monitor electrolytes and minerals: calcium, phosphorous, magnesium, sodium, potassium; watch closely for tetany during first administration

⚠ Assess for symptoms of blood dyscrasias (anemia, granulocytopenia); bruising, fatigue, bleeding, poor healing

• **Assess for symptoms of allergic reactions:** flushing, rash, urticaria, pruritus

CMV retinitis
• Culture should be done prior to treatment (blood, urine, throat); a negative culture does not rule out CMV; ophthalmic exam should confirm diagnosis

Nursing diagnoses
• Infection, risk for (uses)
• Injury, risk for (adverse reactions)
• Knowledge, deficient (teaching)

Patient/family education
• Advise patient to notify prescriber if sore throat, swollen lymph nodes, malaise, fever occur; may indicate presence of other infections

• Advise patient to report perioral tingling, numbness in extremities, and paresthesias; inf should be stopped and electrolytes should be requested

• Caution patient that serious product interactions may occur if OTC products are ingested; check first with prescriber

• Inform patient that product is not a cure but will control symptoms

• Advise patient that ophth exams must be continued

Evaluation
Positive therapeutic outcome
• Improvement in CMV retinitis

---

fosinopril (Rx)
(foss-in-o'pril)
Monopril
Func. class.: Antihypertensive
Chem. class.: Angiotensin-converting enzyme (ACE) inhibitor
Pregnancy category D

Do not confuse:
Monopril/minoxidil/Accupril/Monoket

ACTION: Selectively suppresses renin-angiotensin-aldosterone system; inhibits ACE; prevents conversion of angiotensin I to angiotensin II; results in dilatation of arterial, venous vessels

Therapeutic outcome: Decreased B/P in hypertension

USES: Hypertension, alone or in combination with thiazide diuretics, systolic CHF

CONTRAINDICATIONS:
Breastfeeding, children, hypersensitivity to ACE inhibitors, history of ACE inhibitor–induced angioedema

BLACK BOX WARNING: Pregnancy **D**

Precautions: Geriatric, impaired liver function, hypovolemia, blood dyscrasias, CHF, COPD, asthma, angioedema, hyperkalemia, renal artery stenosis, renal disease

DOSAGE AND ROUTES
Hypertension
Adult: PO 10 mg/day initially, then 20-40 mg/day divided bid or daily, max 80 mg/day

CHF
Adult: PO 10 mg/day, then up to 40 mg/day, increased over several weeks; use lower dose in those undergoing diuresis before fosinopril

Available forms: Tabs 10, 20, 40 mg

Implementation
• Store in airtight container at 86° F (30° C) or less
• Severe hypotension may occur after 1st dose of this medication; hypotension may be prevented by reducing or discontinuing diuretic therapy 3 days before beginning benzapril therapy

ADVERSE EFFECTS
CNS: *Headache, dizziness,* fatigue
CV: *Hypotension,* orthostatic hypotension, tachycardia
GI: *Nausea,* constipation, vomiting, diarrhea, **hepatotoxicity, cholestatic jaundice, fulminant hepatic necrosis, hepatic failure, death**
GU: Increased BUN, creatinine, azotemia, **renal artery stenosis**
HEMA: Decreased Hct, Hgb, **eosinophilia, leukopenia, neutropenia**
META: Hyperkalemia
RESP: Cough
SYST: **Anaphylaxis, angioedema**

Pharmacokinetics

Absorption	30%
Distribution	Crosses placenta
Metabolism	Liver, converted to fosinoprilat
Excretion	50% kidneys (metabolites), 50% feces
Half-life	12 hr: fosinoprilat

Pharmacodynamics

Onset	1 hr
Peak	2-6 hr
Duration	24 hr

INTERACTIONS
Individual drugs
Alcohol (acute ingestion): increased hypotension (large amounts)
Digoxin, hydralazine, lithium, prazosin: increased toxicity

Drug classifications
Adrenergic blockers, antihypertensives, diuretics, ganglionic blockers, nitrates: increased hypotension
Antacids: decreased absorption
Diuretics (potassium-sparing), sympathomimetics, NSAIDs, vasodilators: increased toxicity
Salicylates: decreased antihypertensive effect

Drug/herb
Hawthorn: increased antihypertensive effect
Ephedra: decreased antihypertensive effect

Drug/lab test
Increased: AST, ALT, alkaline phosphatase, glucose, bilirubin, uric acid
Positive: ANA titer
False positive: urine acetone

NURSING CONSIDERATIONS
Assessment
• **Hypertension:** Monitor B/P, check for orthostatic hypotension, syncope; if changes occur, dosage change may be required
• **Collagen vascular disease:** Monitor blood studies: neutrophils, decreased platelets; obtain WBC with differential at baseline and qmo × 6 mo, then q2-3mo × 1 yr; if neutrophils <1000/mm^3, discontinue
• Monitor renal studies: protein, BUN, creatinine; watch for increased levels that may indicate nephrotic syndrome and renal failure; monitor urine daily for protein; monitor renal symptoms: polyuria, oliguria, frequency, dysuria
• Establish baselines in renal, liver function tests before therapy begins
• Check potassium levels throughout treatment although hyperkalemia rarely occurs
• **CHF:** Check for edema in feet, legs daily, monitor weight daily
• **Assess for allergic reactions:** rash, fever, pruritus, urticaria; product should be discontinued if antihistamines fail to help

Nursing diagnoses
• Cardiac output, decreased (uses)
• Injury, risk for (side effects)
• Knowledge, deficient (teaching)
• Noncompliance (teaching)

Patient/family education

• Advise patient not to discontinue product abruptly; warn patient to tell all persons associated with his or her care
• Teach patient not to use OTC products (cough, cold, allergy) unless directed by prescriber because serious side effects can occur; xanthines such as coffee, tea, chocolate, cola can prevent action of product
• Teach patient the importance of complying with dosage schedule, even if feeling better; to continue with medical regimen to decrease B/P: exercise, smoking cessation, decreasing stress, diet modifications
• Emphasize the need to rise slowly to sitting or standing position to minimize orthostatic hypotension; not to exercise in hot weather or increased hypotension can occur
• Advise patient to notify prescriber of mouth sores, sore throat, fever, swelling of hands or feet, irregular heartbeat, chest pain, coughing, shortness of breath
• Instruct patient to report excessive perspiration, dehydration, vomiting, diarrhea; may lead to fall in B/P
• Caution patient that product may cause dizziness, fainting, light-headedness; may occur during 1st few days of therapy; to avoid activities that may be hazardous
• Teach patient how to take B/P, normal readings for age-group

> **BLACK BOX WARNING:** Advise patient to notify prescriber if pregnancy is planned or suspected, pregnancy **D**

Evaluation
Positive therapeutic outcome
• Decreased B/P in hypertension

TREATMENT OF OVERDOSE:
0.9% NaCl **IV** inf, hemodialysis

fosphenytoin (Rx)
(foss-fen′i-toy-in)
Func. class.: Anticonvulsant
Chem. class.: Hydantoin, phosphate phenytoin ester
Pregnancy category D

ACTION: Inhibits spread of seizure activity in motor cortex by altering ion transport; increases AV conduction; prodrug of phenytoin

Therapeutic outcome: Decreased seizures, absence of dysrhythmias

USES: Generalized tonic-clonic seizures, status epilepticus, partial seizures

CONTRAINDICATIONS:
Pregnancy **D**, hypersensitivity, psychiatric conditions, bradycardia, SA and AV block, Stokes-Adams syndrome, absence seizures

Precautions: Breastfeeding, allergies, renal/hepatic disease, myocardial insufficiency, hypoalbuminemia, hypothyroidism, Asian patients positive for HLA-B 1502

> **BLACK BOX WARNING:** Rapid IV infusion

DOSAGE AND ROUTES
All doses in PE (phenytoin sodium equivalent)

Status epilepticus
Adult and adolescent: IV 15-20 mg PE/kg

Nonemergency/maintenance dosing
Adult and adolescent >16 yr: IM/IV 10-20 mg PE/kg 10 mg dose; 4-6 mg PE/kg/day (maintenance); start maintenance 12 hr after loading dose; give in 2-3 divided doses

Available forms: Inj 150 mg (100 mg PE), 750 mg (500 mg PE), 50 mg/ml vials

Implementation
Direct IV route
• Dilute with D_5W or 0.9% NaCl to 1.5-25 mg PE/ml
• Give at a rate of <150 mg PE/min (adult) or <3 mg PE/kg/min (child)

Y-site compatibilities: Aminocaproic acid, amphotericin B lipid complex, amphotericin B liposome, anidulafungin, atenolol, bivalirudin, bleomycin, CARBOplatin, CISplatin, cyclophosphamide, cytarabine, DACTINomycin, DAPTOmycin, dexmedetomidine, diltiazem, docetaxel, doxacurium, eptifibatide, ertapenem, etoposide, fludarabine, fluorouracil, gatifloxacin, gemcitabine, gemtuzumab, granisetron, ifosfamide, levofloxacin, linezolid, LORazepam, mechlorethamine, meperidine, methotrexate, metroNIDAZOLE, nesiritide, octreotide, oxaliplatin, oxytocin, paclitaxel, palonosetron, pamidronate, pantoprazole, pemetrexed, PHENobarbital, piperacillin-tazobactam, rocuronium, sodium acetate, tacrolimus, teniposide, thiotepa, tigecycline, tirofiban, vinCRIStine, vinorelbine, voriconazole, zoledronic acid

Y-site incompatibilities: Caspofungin, DOXOrubicin, epirubicin, fenoldopam, IDArubicin, midazolam, mitoxantrone, mycophenolate, quinupristin-dalfopristin

Adverse effects: *italics* = common; **bold** = life-threatening

ADVERSE EFFECTS

CNS: Drowsiness, dizziness, insomnia, paresthesias, depression, **suicidal tendencies,** aggression, headache, confusion, paresthesia

CV: Hypotension, **ventricular fibrillation,** hypertension, **CHF, shock**

EENT: Nystagmus, diplopia, blurred vision

GI: Nausea, vomiting, diarrhea, constipation, anorexia, weight loss, **hepatitis,** jaundice, gingival hyperplasia

HEMA: Agranulocytosis, leukopenia, aplastic anemia, thrombocytopenia, megaloblastic anemia

INTEG: Rash, lupus erythematosus, **Stevens-Johnson syndrome,** hirsutism, hypersensitivity, pruritus

SYST: Hyperglycemia, hypokalemia, **toxic epidermal necrolysis (Asian patients positive for HLA-B 1502)**

Pharmacokinetics

Absorption	Unknown
Distribution	Protein binding 99%
Metabolism	Liver: converted to phenytoin
Excretion	Kidneys
Half-life	Unknown

Pharmacodynamics

Unknown

INTERACTIONS

Individual drugs

Alcohol: decreased effects of fosphenytoin (chronic use)

Amiodarone, chloramphenicol, cimetidine: increased fosphenytoin level

CarBAMazepine, folic acid, rifampin, theophylline, tramadol: decreased effects of fosphenytoin

Drug classifications

Antacids, antihistamines, antineoplastics, CYP1A2 inducers: decreased effects of fosphenytoin

Antidepressants (tricyclics), CYP1A2 inhibitors, estrogens, H_2-receptor antagonists, phenothiazines, salicylates, sulfonamides: increased fosphenytoin level

Drug/herb

Ginseng, valerian: decreased anticonvulsant effect

Ginkgo: increased anticonvulsant effect

Drug/lab test

Increased: glucose, alkaline phosphatase

Decreased: dexamethasone, metyrapone test serum, PBI, urinary steroids

NURSING CONSIDERATIONS

Assessment

• Assess drug level: target level 10-20 mcg/ml; toxic level 30-50 mcg/ml, wait at least 2 hr after dose before testing, 4 hr after IM dose

• **Assess seizure activity** including type, location, duration, and character; provide seizure precaution

• Assess renal studies: urinalysis, BUN, urine creatinine

• Monitor hepatic studies: ALT, AST, bilirubin, creatinine

• Assess allergic reaction: red raised rash; if this occurs, product should be discontinued

• **Monitor for toxicity:** bone marrow depression, nausea, vomiting, ataxia, diplopia, cardiovascular collapse, slurred speech, confusion

• Assess product level: toxic level 30-50 mcg/ml

⚠ **Assess for rash, discontinue as soon as rash develops, serious adverse reactions such as Stevens-Johnson syndrome can occur**

⚠ **Assess mental status: mood, sensorium, affect, memory (long, short), especially geriatric; suicidal thoughts/behaviors**

• **Assess for blood dyscrasias:** fever, sore throat, bruising, rash, jaundice, epistaxis (long-term treatment only)

• Monitor blood studies: RBC, Hct, Hgb, reticulocyte counts weekly for 4 wk, then monthly; also check thyroid function tests, serum calcium, albumin, phosphorus

Nursing diagnoses

• Injury, risk for (uses, adverse reactions)
• Knowledge, deficient (teaching)
• Noncompliance (teaching)

Patient/family education

• Teach patient the reason for and expected outcome of treatment

• Instruct patient not to use machinery or engage in hazardous activity; drowsiness, dizziness may occur

• Advise patient to carry/wear emergency ID identifying product used, name of prescriber

• Advise patient to notify prescriber of rash, bleeding, bruising, slurred speech, jaundice of skin or eyes, joint pain, nausea, vomiting, severe headache

• Advise patient to keep all medical appointments, including lab work, physical assessment

• Advise patient to notify prescriber if pregnancy is planned or suspected; to use contraception with this product

Evaluation
Positive therapeutic outcome
• Decreased seizure activity

> **⚠ HIGH ALERT**

fospropofol (Rx)
(fos-proe′poe-fol)
Lusedra
Func. class.: General anesthetic
Pregnancy category B

ACTION: Prodrug of propofol; produces dose-dependent CNS depression by activation of GABA receptor inhibition of NMDA subtype of glutamate receptors by channel-gating modulation

Therapeutic outcome: Anesthesia

USES: Induction or maintenance of anesthesia as part of balanced anesthetic technique; sedation in mechanically ventilated patients

CONTRAINDICATIONS:
Hypersensitivity to product

Precautions: Pregnancy **B,** breastfeeding, children, geriatric patients, respiratory depression, severe respiratory disorders, cardiac dysrhythmias, labor and delivery, renal disease, hyperlipidemia

DOSAGE AND ROUTES
Induction/maintenance
Adult <65 (healthy): *>90 kg,* initially 577.5 mg **IV** bolus, as needed give supplemental doses up to a max of 140 mg **IV**/dose to achieve desired level of sedation, give no more frequently than q4min; *61-89 kg,* initially 6.5 mg/kg (max 577.5 mg) **IV** bolus, as needed give supplemental doses up to 1.6 mg/kg/dose (max 140 mg/dose) **IV** to achieve desired level of sedation, give no more frequently than q4min; *≤60 kg,* initially 385 mg **IV** bolus, as needed give supplemental doses up to a max of 105 mg **IV**/dose to achieve desired level of sedation, give no more frequently than q4min

Adult <65 yr (severe systemic disease): *≥90 kg,* initially 437.5 mg **IV** bolus, as needed give supplemental doses up to a max of 105 mg **IV**/dose to achieve desired level of sedation, give no more frequently than q4min; *61-89 kg,* initially give 75% of standard dosing regimen, which is 4.875 mg/kg (max 437.5 mg) **IV** bolus, as needed give supplemental doses that are 75%

of standard dosing regimen (up to 1.2 mg/kg/dose **IV**, max 105 mg/dose **IV**), give doses to achieve desired level of sedation, give no more frequently than q4min; *≤60 kg,* initially 297.5 mg **IV** bolus, as needed give supplemental doses up to a max of 70 mg **IV**/dose to achieve desired level of sedation, give no more frequently than q4min

Geriatric: *≥90 kg,* initially 437.5 mg **IV** bolus, as needed give supplemental doses up to a max 105 mg **IV**/dose to achieve desired level of sedation, give no more frequently than q4min; *61-89 kg,* initially give 75% of standard dosing regimen, which is 4.875 mg/kg (max 105 mg 1 dose) **IV** bolus, as needed give supplemental doses that are 75% of standard dosing regimen; give doses to achieve desired level of sedation; give no more frequently than q4min

Available forms: Inj 1050 mg/30 ml

Implementation
IV bolus route
• Visually inspect for particulate matter and discoloration
• Each vial is single patient/single use
• Draw from vial, discard unused portion
• Do not mix with other drugs prior to use
• Give by **IV** bolus in free-flowing peripheral **IV** line of D₅W, 5% dextrose/0.2% NaCl, 5% dextrose/0.45% NaCl D₅LR, LR, 0.45% NaCl, NS, 5% dextrose/0.45% NaCl/20 mEq KCl; do not mix with other fluids; flush line with NS before and after administration
• No filtration needed
• Give only with resuscitative equipment available
• Give only by qualified persons trained in anesthesia
• Store unopened vials at room temperature

ADVERSE EFFECTS
CNS: Involuntary movement, headache, jerking, fever, dizziness, shivering, tremor, confusion, somnolence, paresthesia, agitation, abnormal dreams, euphoria, fatigue, **increased intracranial pressure, impaired cerebral flow, seizures**
CV: *Bradycardia, hypotension,* hypertension, PVC, PAC, tachycardia, abnormal ECG, ST segment depression, **asystole, bradydysrhythmias**
EENT: Blurred vision, tinnitus, eye pain, strange taste, diplopia
GI: *Nausea, vomiting, abdominal cramping,* dry mouth, swallowing, hypersalivation, **pancreatitis**

GU: Urine retention, green urine, cloudy urine, oliguria
INTEG: *Flushing, phlebitis, hives, burning/ stinging at inj site,* rash, pain of extremities
MS: Myalgia
RESP: Apnea, *cough, hiccups,* dyspnea, hypoventilation, sneezing, wheezing, tachypnea, hypoxia, respiratory acidosis

Pharmacokinetics

Absorption	Unknown
Distribution	Rapid, 98% protein binding
Metabolism	Liver conjugated to inactive metabolites
Excretion	Urine 7%
Half-life	1-8 min; terminal 0.81-0.88 hr

Pharmacodynamics

Onset	15-30 sec
Peak	Unknown
Duration	Unknown

INTERACTIONS

Individual drugs
Alcohol: increased CNS depression

Drug classifications
• Alcohol, opioids, sedative/hypnotics, antipsychotics, skeletal muscle relaxants, inhalational anesthetics: increased CNS depression
• MAOIs: do not use within 10 days

Drug/herb
St. John's wort: increased fospropofol effect

NURSING CONSIDERATIONS

Assessment
• Assess inj site: phlebitis, burning, stinging
• **Monitor ECG** for changes: PVC, PAC, ST segment changes; monitor VS
• Assess CNS changes: movement, jerking, tremors, dizziness, LOC, pupil reaction
• Assess for allergic reactions: hives
• **Assess for respiratory depression,** character, rate, rhythm; notify prescriber if respirations are <10/min, hypoxemia is detectable by pulse oximetry

Nursing diagnoses
• Injury, risk for (adverse reactions)

Teach patient/family
• Teach patient that this medication will cause dizziness, drowsiness, sedation

Evaluation
Positive therapeutic outcome
• Induction of anesthesia

TREATMENT OF OVERDOSE:
Discontinue product; administer vasopressor agents or anticholinergics, artificial ventilation

---

frovatriptan (Rx)
(froh-vah-trip′tan)
Frova
Func. class.: Antimigraine agent
Chem. class.: 5-HT$_1$ receptor agonist
Pregnancy category C

ACTION: Binds selectively to the vascular 5-HT$_{1B}$, 5-HT$_{1D}$ receptor subtypes, exerts antimigraine effect; binds to benzodiazepine receptor sites, causes vasoconstriction in cranium

Therapeutic outcome: Absence of migraines

USES: Acute treatment of migraine with or without aura

CONTRAINDICATIONS:
Angina pectoris, history of MI, documented silent ischemia, Prinzmetal's angina, ischemic heart disease, concurrent ergotamine-containing preparations, uncontrolled hypertension, hypersensitivity, basilar or hemiplegic migraine; ischemic bowel disease; peripheral vascular disease, severe hepatic disease, prophylactic migraine treatment

Precautions: Pregnancy C, breastfeeding, children, geriatric, postmenopausal women, men >40 yr, risk factors for CAD, hypercholesterolemia, obesity, diabetes, impaired hepatic function, seizure disorder

DOSAGE AND ROUTES
Adult: PO 2.5 mg; a 2nd dose may be taken after ≥2 hr; max 3 tabs/day (7.5 mg)

Available forms: Tabs 2.5 mg

Implementation
• Ensure that tablets are swallowed whole
• Provide quiet, calm environment with decreased stimulation from noise, bright light, excessive talking

ADVERSE EFFECTS
CNS: *Hot sensation,* paresthesia, *dizziness,* headache, fatigue, cold sensation, insomnia, anxiety, somnolence, **seizures**

⚠ Nurse Alert

CV: *Flushing,* chest pain, palpitation
GI: Dry mouth, dyspepsia, abdominal pain, diarrhea, vomiting, nausea
MS: Skeletal pain

Pharmacokinetics

Absorption	Absolute bioavailability of PO dose ~20% in males, 30% in females
Distribution	Protein binding 15%; reversibly bound to blood cells at equilibrium 60%
Metabolism	Liver, by CYP1A2
Excretion	Urine (32%), feces (62%)
Half-life	25-29 hr

Pharmacodynamics

Onset	10 min-2 hr
Peak	2-4 hr
Duration	Unknown

INTERACTIONS

Individual drugs
Estrogen, propranolol: increased effects of frovatriptan

Drug classifications
CYP1A2 inhibitors (cimetidine, ciprofloxacin, erythromycin), oral contraceptives: increased frovatriptan levels
Selective serotonin reuptake inhibitors, other serotonin agonists (dextromethorphan, tramadol, antidepressants): increased toxicity

NURSING CONSIDERATIONS

Assessment
• **Migraine:** aura, alleviating/exacerbating factor, diet, character
• Assess for ingestion of tyramine-containing foods (pickled products, beer, wine, aged cheese), food additives, preservatives, colorings, artificial sweeteners, chocolate, caffeine, which may precipitate these types of headaches
• Assess B/P; signs/symptoms of coronary vasospasms
• Assess for stress level, activity, recreation, coping mechanisms
• Assess neurologic status: LOC, paresthesia, hot/cold sensations, dizziness, headache, fatigue

Nursing diagnoses
• Knowledge, deficient (teaching)
• Pain, acute (uses)

Patient/family education
• Instruct patient to report any side effects to prescriber

• Advise patient to use contraception while taking product
• Advise patient that photosensitivity may occur, to use sunscreen and wear protective clothing when outdoors
• Advise patient to have dark, quiet environment available

Evaluation
Positive therapeutic outcome
• Decrease in frequency, severity of migraine

TREATMENT OF OVERDOSE:
No specific antidote; monitor patient closely for ≥48 hr, treat any symptoms as necessary

fulvestrant (Rx)
(full-ves'trant)
Faslodex
Func. class.: Antineoplastic
Pregnancy category D

ACTION: Inhibits cell division by binding to cytoplasmic estrogen receptors; resembles normal cell complex but inhibits DNA synthesis and estrogen response of target tissue

Therapeutic outcome: Decreased tumor size, spread of malignancy

USES: Advanced breast carcinoma in estrogen-receptor–positive patients (usually postmenopausal)

CONTRAINDICATIONS:
Pregnancy **D,** breastfeeding, children, hypersensitivity

Precautions: Hepatic disease

DOSAGE AND ROUTES
Adult: IM 500 mg as 5-ml inj on days 1, 15, 29 and q mo thereafter

Available forms: Inj 50 mg/ml

Implementation
• Give IM 5 ml as a single inj or 2, 2.5 ml inj; give slowly in buttock
• Give antacid before oral agent; give product after evening meal, before bedtime
• Give antiemetic 30-60 min before giving product to prevent vomiting
• Provide liquid diet, if needed, including cola, Jell-O; dry toast or crackers may be added if patient is not nauseated or vomiting
• Increase fluids to 2 L/day unless contraindicated
• Store in refrigerator

ADVERSE EFFECTS

CNS: *Headache,* depression, dizziness, insomnia, paresthesia, anxiety
GI: *Nausea, vomiting,* anorexia, constipation, diarrhea, abdominal pain
HEMA: Anemia
INTEG: *Rash,* sweating, hot flashes, inj site pain
MS: Bone pain, arthritis, back pain
RESP: Pharyngitis, dyspnea, cough
SYST: Angioedema

Pharmacokinetics

Absorption	Unknown
Distribution	Unknown
Metabolism	CYP3A4
Excretion	Feces 90%
Half-life	40 days

Pharmacodynamics

Unknown

NURSING CONSIDERATIONS

Assessment
• Monitor for side effects, report to prescriber

Nursing diagnoses
• Infection, risk for (adverse reactions)
• Knowledge, deficient (teaching)
• Nutrition: less than body requirements, imbalanced (adverse reactions)

Patient/family education
• Advise patient to report any complaints, side effects to prescriber
• Teach patient to increase fluids to 2 L/day unless contraindicated
• Advise patient to report vaginal bleeding immediately
• Teach patient that tumor flare—increase in size of tumor, increased bone pain—may occur and will subside rapidly; may take analgesics for pain
• Teach patient to use contraception, pregnancy **D**

Evaluation
Positive therapeutic outcome
• Decreased tumor size, decreased spread of malignancy

furosemide (Rx)

(fur-oh′se-mide)
Apo-Furosemide ✦, Lasix
Func. class.: Loop diuretic
Chem. class.: Sulfonamide derivative
Pregnancy category C

Do not confuse:
furosemide/torsemide,
Lasix/Lanoxin/Lomotil/Luvox

ACTION: Acts on the ascending loop of Henle in the kidney, inhibiting reabsorption of electrolytes sodium and chloride, causing excretion of sodium, calcium, magnesium, chloride, water, and some potassium; decreases reabsorption of sodium and chloride and increases excretion of potassium in the distal tubule of the kidney; responsible for slight antihypertensive effect and peripheral vasodilatation

Therapeutic outcome: Decreased edema in lung tissue, peripherally; decreased B/P

USES: Pulmonary edema, edema in CHF, nephrotic syndrome, ascites, hepatic disease, hypertension

Unlabeled uses: Hypercalcemia in malignancy

CONTRAINDICATIONS:
Anuria, hypovolemia, breastfeeding, infants, electrolyte depletion

Precautions: Pregnancy C, diabetes mellitus, dehydration, severe renal disease, cirrhosis, ascites, hypersensitivity to sulfonamides

DOSAGE AND ROUTES
Adult: PO 20-80 mg/day in AM, may give another dose in 6 hr, up to 600 mg/day; IM/IV 20-40 mg, increased by 20 mg q2hr until desired response
Child: PO/IM/IV 2 mg/kg, may increase by 1-2 mg/kg/q6-8hr up to 6 mg/kg

Acute pulmonary edema
Adult: IV 40 mg given over several min, repeated in 1 hr; increase to 80 mg if needed
Child: IV/IM 1-2 mg/kg q6-12hr, max 6 mg/kg/dose
Premature neonates >32 wk postconception age: IV/IM 1-2 mg/kg q12-24hr
Premature neonates ≤32 wk postconception age: IV/IM max 1 mg/kg initially

Antihypercalcemia
Adult: IM/IV 80-100 mg q1-4hr or PO 120 mg/day or divided bid
Child: IM/IV 25-50 mg, repeat q4hr if needed

Acute/chronic renal failure
Adult: PO 80 mg q day, increase by 80-120 mg/day to desired response; **IV** 100-200 mg, max 600-800 mg

Available forms: Tabs 20, 40, 80 mg; oral sol 8 mg/ml, 10 mg/ml; inj IM, **IV** 10 mg/ml

Implementation
- Give in AM to avoid interference with sleep
- Potassium replacement if potassium level is <3.0 mg/dl; product may be crushed if patient is unable to swallow

PO route
- With food or milk or use oral sol if nausea occurs; absorption may be reduced slightly

IV route
- Do not use sol that is yellow, has a precipitate or crystals

IV, direct route
- Give undiluted through Y-tube on 3-way stopcock; give 20 mg or less/min

Intermittent IV inf route
- May be added to 0.9% NaCl, D₅W, use within 24 hr to ensure compatibility; give through Y-tube or 3-way stopcock; give at 4 mg/min or less, use inf pump

Y-site compatibilities: Acyclovir, alfentanil, allopurinol, alprostadil, amifostine, amikacin, aminocaproic acid, aminophylline, amphotericin B cholesteryl/lipid complex/liposome, anidulafungin, argatroban, ascorbic acid, atenolol, atropine, azaTHIOprine, aztreonam, bivalirudin, bleomycin, bumetanide, calcium chloride/gluconate, CARBOplatin, cefamandole, ceFAZolin, cefepime, cefmetazole, cefonicid, cefoperazone, cefotaxime, cefotetan, cefoxitin, ceftazIdime, ceftizoxime, ceftobiprole, cefTRIAXone, cefuroxime, cephalothin, cephapirin, chloramphenicol, CISplatin, cladribine, clindamycin, cyanocobalamin, cyclophosphamide, cycloSPORINE, cytarabine, DACTINomycin, DAPTOmycin, dexamethasone, dexmedetomidine, digoxin, docetaxel, doripenem, doxacurium, DOXOrubicin liposome, enalaprilat, ePHEDrine, EPINEPHrine, etoposide, fentaNYL, fludarabine, fluorouracil, folic acid, foscarnet, gallium nitrate, ganciclovir, granisetron, heparin, hydrocortisone, HYDROmorphone, ifosfamide, imipenem-cilastatin, indomethacin, insulin (regular), isosorbide, kanamycin, leucovorin, lidocaine, linezolid, LORazepam, LR, mannitol, mechlorethamine, melphalan, meropenem, methicillin, methotrexate, methylPREDNISolone, metoprolol, metroNIDAZOLE, mezlocillin, micafungin, miconazole, mitomycin, moxalactam, multiple vitamins injection, nafcillin, naloxone, nitroprusside, octreotide, oxacillin, oxaliplatin, oxytocin, paclitaxel, palonosetron, pamidronate, pantoprazole, pemetrexed, penicillin G, PENTobarbital, PHENobarbital, phytonadione, piperacillin, piperacillin-tazobactam, potassium chloride, procainamide, propofol, propranolol, ranitidine, remifentanil, Ringer's, ritodrine, sargramostim, sodium acetate/bicarbonate, succinylcholine, SUFentanil, temocillin, teniposide, theophylline, thiopental, thiotepa, ticarcillin, ticarcillin-clavulanate, tigecycline, tirofiban, TNA, tobramycin, urokinase, vit B/C, voriconazole, zoledronic acid

Y-site incompatibilities: Amsacrine, bleomycin, DOXOrubicin, droperidol, esmolol, fluconazole, gentamicin, IDArubicin, metoclopramide, milrinone, netilmicin, ondansetron, quiNIDine, vinBLAStine, vinCRIStine

ADVERSE EFFECTS
CNS: Headache, fatigue, weakness, vertigo, paresthesias
CV: Orthostatic hypotension, chest pain, ECG changes, **circulatory collapse**
EENT: *Loss of hearing,* ear pain, tinnitus, blurred vision
ELECT: *Hypokalemia, hypochloremic alkalosis, hypomagnesemia, hyperuricemia, hypocalcemia, hyponatremia,* metabolic alkalosis
ENDO: *Hyperglycemia*
GI: *Nausea,* diarrhea, dry mouth, vomiting, anorexia, cramps, oral or gastric irritations, pancreatitis
GU: *Polyuria,* renal failure, *glycosuria*
HEMA: **Thrombocytopenia, agranulocytosis, leukopenia, neutropenia,** anemia
INTEG: *Rash, pruritus, purpura,* **Stevens-Johnson syndrome,** sweating, photosensitivity, urticaria
MS: Cramps, stiffness

Pharmacokinetics

	PO
Absorption	GI tract (60%-70%)
	PO/IM/IV
Distribution	Crosses placenta
Metabolism	Liver (30%-40%)
Excretion	Breast milk, urine, feces
Half-life	½-1 hr

Adverse effects: *italics* = common; **bold** = life-threatening

Pharmacodynamics

	PO	IM	IV
Onset	1 hr	$1/2$ hr	5 min
Peak	1-2 hr	Unknown	$1/2$ hr
Duration	6-8 hr	4-8 hr	2 hr

INTERACTIONS

Individual drugs

CISplatin, vancomycin: increased risk of ototoxicity

Digoxin: increased toxicity

Lithium: decreased renal clearance, causing increased toxicity

Probenecid: decreased furosemide effect

Drug classifications

Aminoglycosides: increased ototoxicity

Anticoagulants, salicylates: increased effects

Antihypertensives: increased antihypertensive effect

Nitrates: increased hypotensive action

Nondepolarizing skeletal muscle relaxants: increased toxicity

Drug/lab test

Interference: GTT

Increase: LDL

NURSING CONSIDERATIONS

Assessment

• **Ototoxicity:** Assess patient for tinnitus, hearing loss, ear pain; periodic testing of hearing is needed when high doses of this product are given by **IV** route

• **Hypokalemia:** acidic urine, reduced urine osmolality, nocturia, polyuria and polydipsia; hypotension, broad T-wave, U-wave, ectopy, tachycardia, weak pulse; muscle weakness, altered LOC, drowsiness, apathy, lethargy, confusion, depression; anorexia, nausea, cramps, constipation, distention, paralytic ileus; hypoventilation, respiratory muscle weakness

• Monitor for CV, GI, neurologic manifestations of hyponatremia: increased B/P, cold, clammy skin, hypovolemia or hypervolemia; anorexia, nausea, vomiting, diarrhea, abdominal cramps; lethargy, increased ICP, confusion, headache, seizures, coma, fatigue, tremors, hyperreflexia

• Monitor for neurologic, respiratory manifestations of hyperchloremia: weakness, lethargy, coma; deep rapid breathing

• **CHF:** Assess fluid volume status: I&O ratios and record, count or weigh diapers as appropriate, weight, distended red veins, crackles in lung, color, quality, and specific gravity of urine, skin turgor, adequacy of pulses, moist mucous membranes, bilateral lung sounds, peripheral pitting edema; dehydration symptoms of decreasing output, thirst, hypotension, dry mouth and mucous membranes should be reported

• Monitor electrolytes: potassium, sodium, chloride, magnesium; also include BUN, blood pH, ABGs, uric acid, CBC, blood glucose

• **Hypertension:** Assess B/P before and during therapy lying, standing, and sitting as appropriate; orthostatic hypotension can occur rapidly

Nursing diagnoses

• Fluid volume, deficient (side effects)
• Fluid volume, excess (uses)
• Knowledge, deficient (teaching)

Patient/family education

• Teach patient to take the medication early in the day to prevent nocturia

• Instruct the patient to take with food or milk if GI symptoms of nausea and anorexia occur

• Teach patient to maintain a record of weight on a weekly basis and notify physician of weight loss of >5 lb

• Caution the patient that this product causes a loss of potassium, that food rich in potassium should be added to the diet; refer to a dietitian for assistance in planning

• Caution the patient to rise slowly from sitting or reclining positions, not to exercise in hot weather or stand for prolonged periods because orthostatic hypotension will be enhanced; lie down if dizziness occurs

• Advise patient to wear protective clothing and sunscreen to prevent photosensitivity

• Caution patient not to use alcohol or any OTC medications without physician's approval; serious product reactions may occur

• Emphasize the need to contact physician immediately if muscle cramps, weakness, nausea, dizziness, or numbness occurs

• Teach patient to take and record own B/P and pulse

• Advise patient to continue taking medication even if feeling better; this product controls symptoms but does not cure the condition

• Advise the patient with hypertension to continue other medical treatment (exercise, weight loss, relaxation techniques, cessation of smoking)

Evaluation

Positive therapeutic outcome

• Decreased edema
• Decreased B/P
• Lowered calcium level in malignancy
• Increased diuresis

gabapentin (Rx)

(gab'a-pen-tin)

Apo-Gabapentin ✦, CO
Gabapentin ✦, Gen-Gabapentin,
Gralise, Horizant, Neurontin, Novo-
Gabapentin ✦, PMS-Gabapentin ✦,
ratio-Gabapentin

Func. class.: Anticonvulsant

Pregnancy category C

Do not confuse:
Neurontin/Noroxin/Neoral

ACTION: Mechanism unknown; may increase seizure threshold; structurally similar to GABA; gabapentin binding sites in neocortex, hippocampus

Therapeutic outcome: Decreased seizure activity

USES: Adjunct treatment of partial seizures, with or without generalization in patients >12 yr; adjunct in partial seizures in children 3-12 yr, postherpetic neuralgia, primary restless leg syndrome (RLS) in adults

Unlabeled uses: Tremors in multiple sclerosis, neuropathic pain, bipolar disorder, migraine prophylaxis, diabetic neuropathy

CONTRAINDICATIONS:
Hypersensitivity to this product

Precautions: Pregnancy C, breastfeeding, children <3 yr, geriatric, renal disease, hemodialysis, suicidal thoughts, depression

DOSAGE AND ROUTES
Adult and child >12 yr: PO 900-1800 mg/day in 3 divided doses; may titrate by giving 300 mg on the first day, 300 mg bid on second day, 300 mg tid on third day; may increase to 1800 mg/day by adding 300 mg on subsequent days
Child 3-12 yr: PO 10-15 mg/kg/day in 3 divided doses, initially titrate dose upward over approximately 3 days; 25-35 mg/kg/day; all given in 3 divided doses

Postherpetic neuralgia
Adult: PO 300 mg on day 1, 600 mg/day divided bid on day 2, 900 mg/day divided tid, may titrate to 1800-3600 mg divided tid if needed; ext rel tab (Gralise only) 300 mg on day 1, then 600 mg on day 2, 900 mg on days 3-6, 1200 mg on days 7-10, 1500 mg on days 11-14, 1800 mg on day 15 and thereafter

Moderate to severe RLS (Horizant only)
Adult: PO ext rel tab 600 mg qd with food at about 5 PM; if dose is missed, take next day at 5 PM

Renal dose
Adult and child >12 yr: CCr 30-59 ml/min 200-700 mg bid; CCr 15-29 ml/min 200-700 mg/day; CCr <15 ml/min 100-300 mg/day

Available forms: Caps 100, 300, 400 mg; tabs 600, 800 mg; oral sol 250 mg/5 ml; Horizant: ext rel tab 600 mg

Implementation
• Do not break, crush, or chew caps, ext rel tabs; cap may be opened and contents put in applesauce or dissolved in juice; scored tab may be cut in half
• Give at least 2 hr apart when giving antacids; give without regard to meals
• Store at room temperature away from heat and light
• Provide assistance with ambulation during early part of treatment; dizziness occurs
• **Provide seizure precautions:** padded side rails, move objects that may harm patient
• **Oral sol:** measure with calibrated device
• **Ext release:** give with food at about 5 pm, bioavailability is increased with food; do not interchange Gralise with Horizant

ADVERSE EFFECTS
CNS: *Drowsiness, confusion,* dizziness, fatigue, anxiety, somnolence, ataxia, amnesia, abnormal thinking, unsteady gait, depression; 3-12 yr old: emotional lability, aggression, thought disorder, hyperkinesia, hostility, **seizures, suicidal ideation**
CV: Vasodilatation, peripheral edema, hypotension
EENT: Dry mouth, blurred vision, diplopia, nystagmus
GI: Constipation, increased appetite, dental abnormalities, nausea, vomiting
GU: Impotence, bleeding, *UTI*
HEMA: Leukopenia, decreased WBC
INTEG: Pruritus, abrasion, **Stevens-Johnson syndrome**
MS: Myalgia
RESP: Rhinitis, pharyngitis, coughing

Pharmacokinetics

Pharmacokinetics	
Absorption	Unknown
Distribution	Unknown
Metabolism	None
Excretion	Urine unchanged
Half-life	5-7 hr, 130 hr in ESRD

Pharmacodynamics

Unknown

INTERACTIONS

Individual drugs
Alcohol: increased CNS depression
Cimetidine, sevelamer: decreased gabapentin levels
Morphine: increased gabapentin levels
HYDROcodone: decreased effect of HYDROcodone

Drug classifications
Antacids: decreased gabapentin levels
Antihistamines, sedatives, all other CNS depressants: increased CNS depression

Drug/lab test
False positive: urinary protein using Ames N-multistix SG

NURSING CONSIDERATIONS

Assessment
• **Assess seizures:** aura, location, duration, activity at onset
• Assess renal studies: urinalysis, BUN, urine creatinine q3mo
⚠ **Assess mental status: mood, sensorium, affect, behavioral changes, suicidal thoughts/behaviors; if mental status changes, notify prescriber**
• Assess eye problems, need for ophth exam before, during, after treatment (slit lamp, fundoscopy, tonometry)

Nursing diagnoses
• Knowledge, deficient (teaching)
• Noncompliance (teaching)

Patient/family education
• Advise patient to carry/wear emergency ID stating patient's name, products taken, condition, prescriber's name and phone number
• Advise patient to avoid driving, other activities that require alertness
• Teach patient not to discontinue medication quickly after long-term use, withdrawal-precipitated seizures may occur, not to double dose; if dose is missed, take if 2 hr or more before next dose

• Teach patient to gradually withdraw over 7 days; abrupt withdrawal may precipitate seizures
• Teach patient to use hard candy, gum, and frequent rinsing of mouth for dry mouth
• Teach patient to increase fluids, bulk in diet for constipation
• Advise patient to notify prescriber if pregnancy is planned or suspected, avoid breastfeeding

Evaluation
Positive therapeutic outcome
• Decreased seizure activity; document on patient's chart

TREATMENT OF OVERDOSE:
Lavage, VS

galantamine (Rx)
(gah-lan'tah-meen)
Razadyne, Razadyne ER, Reminyl ✦
Func. class.: Anti-Alzheimer's agent
Chem. class.: Cholinesterase inhibitor
Pregnancy category B

ACTION: Enhances cholinergic functioning by increasing acetylcholine

Therapeutic outcome: Decreased signs and symptoms of Alzheimer's dementia

USES: Mild to moderate dementia of Alzheimer's disease, vascular dementia

CONTRAINDICATIONS:
Hypersensitivity to this product, breastfeeding, children, GI bleeding, jaundice, renal failure

Precautions: Pregnancy **B**, respiratory/renal/hepatic/cardiac disease, seizure disorder, peptic ulcer, asthma, bradycardia, heart block, geriatric patients, surgery, urinary tract obstruction

DOSAGE AND ROUTES
Adult: PO 4 mg bid with morning and evening meals; after 4 wk or more may increase to 8 mg bid; after another 4 wk may increase to 12 mg bid; usual dose 16-24 mg/day in 2 divided doses; EXT REL 8 mg/day in AM; may increase to 16 mg/day after 4 wk, and 24 mg/day after another 4 wk

Hepatic dose
Adult: (Child-Pugh 7-9) PO max 16 mg/day
Adult: (Child-Pugh 10-15) avoid PO use

Renal dose
Adult: PO CCr 10-70 ml/min; max 16 mg/day; CCr <9 ml/min: PO avoid use

Available forms: Tabs 4, 8, 12 mg; ext rel tabs 8, 16, 24 mg; oral sol 4 mg/ml

Implementation
• Give with meals, morning and evening, ext rel product can be opened and sprinkled on food; do not crush/chew
• Dose increase after minimum of 4 wk at prior dose; if dose is interrupted for several days, restart at lower dose, titrate to current dose
• Provide assistance with ambulation during beginning therapy
• Perform complete suicide assessment

ADVERSE EFFECTS
CNS: *Tremors, insomnia,* depression, dizziness, headache, somnolence, fatigue
CV: Bradycardia, chest pain
GI: *Nausea, vomiting, anorexia, abdominal distress, flatulence,* diarrhea
GU: Urinary incontinence, bladder outflow obstruction, hematuria
HEMA: Anemia
META: Weight decrease
MS: Asthenia
RESP: URI, rhinitis

Pharmacokinetics
Absorption	Rapidly and completely absorbed
Distribution	18% protein binding
Metabolism	Liver
Excretion	Kidneys; clearance decreased in geriatric, hepatic/renal disease, females (20% lower)
Half-life	Elimination 7 hr

Pharmacodynamics
Unknown

INTERACTIONS
Drug classifications
Cholinesterase inhibitors, cholinomimetics: synergistic effect
CYP3A4/CYP2D6 inducers (bosentan, carBAMazepine, fosphenytoin, nevirapine, oxcarbazepine, phenytoin, rifabutin, rifampin, rifapentine, troglitazone): decreased galantamine effect
CYP3A4/CYP2D6 inhibitors (antiretroviral protease inhibitors, clarithromycin, conivaptan, delavirdine, diltiazem, efavirenz, erythro-

mycin, fluconazole, fluvoxamine, imatinib, itraconazole, ketoconazole, nefazodone, niCARdipine, troleandomycin, verapamil, voriconazole, zafirlukast): increased galantamine effect
NSAIDs: increased GI effects

Drug/herb
St. John's wort: decreased galantamine effect

NURSING CONSIDERATIONS
Assessment
• **Alzheimer's disease:** Assess mental status: affect, mood, behavioral changes, depression, memory, attention, confusion, cognitive functioning
• Assess liver function enzymes: AST, ALT, alkaline phosphatase, LDH, bilirubin, CBC
• Assess for severe GI effects: nausea, vomiting, anorexia, weight loss
• Assess B/P, heart rate, respiration during initial treatment

Nursing diagnoses
• Knowledge, deficient (teaching)

Patient/family education
• Teach patient or caregiver correct procedure for giving oral sol, using instruction sheet provided
• Instruct patient or caregiver to notify prescriber of severe GI effects
• Instruct patient or caregiver to report hypo/hypertension, slow heart rate

Evaluation
Positive therapeutic outcome
• Decreased symptoms of dementia
• Increased coherence
• Improved cognitive performance (memory, orientation, attention, reasoning, language, praxis)

TREATMENT OF OVERDOSE:
Administer **IV** atropine titrated to effect at an initial dose of 0.5-1 mg, with subsequent doses based on clinical response; provide general supportive measures

---

ganciclovir (Rx)
(gan-sye′kloe-vir)
Cytovene, Vitrasert
Func. class.: Antiviral
Chem. class.: Synthetic nucleoside analog
Pregnancy category C

Do not confuse:
Cytovene/Cytosar

ACTION: Inhibits replication of herpes viruses in vitro; competitively inhibits human cytomegalovirus (CMV) DNA polymerase and is incorporated, resulting in termination of DNA elongation

Therapeutic outcome: Decreased proliferation of virus responsible for CMV retinitis

USES: Cytomegalovirus (CMV) retinitis in immunocompromised persons, including those with AIDS, after indirect ophthalmoscopy confirms diagnosis; prophylaxis of CMV in transplantation

Unlabeled uses: CMV pneumonia in organ transplant patients, CMV gastroenteritis in patients with irritable bowel syndrome, CMV pneumonitis

CONTRAINDICATIONS:
Hypersensitivity to acyclovir, famciclovir, penciclovir, valacyclovir, valganciclovir, or ganciclovir

BLACK BOX WARNING: ANC <500/mm^3, platelet count <25,000/mm^3 (intravitreal)

Precautions: Pregnancy C, breastfeeding, children <6 mo, geriatric, preexisting cytopenias, renal function impairment, radiation therapy

BLACK BOX WARNING: Secondary malignancy, bone marrow suppression, anemia, infertility, neutropenia

DOSAGE AND ROUTES
Induction treatment
Adult: IV 5 mg/kg/dose given over 1 hr q12hr × 2-3 wk

Maintenance treatment
Adult: IV INF 5 mg/kg/day given over 1 hr, daily × 7 days/wk; or 6 mg/kg/day × 5 days/wk; PO 1000 mg tid with food or 500 mg q3hr while awake; Intravitreal 4.5-mg implant

Prevention of CMV infection
Adult: IV 5 mg/kg/dose over 1 hr q12hr × 1-2 wk, then 5 mg/kg/day × 7 days/wk, then 6 mg/kg/day × 5 days/wk; PO 1000 mg tid, starting 10 days posttransplant × 14 days

Renal dose
Adult: IV CCr 50-69 ml/min, reduce to 2.5 mg/kg q12hr (induction), 2.5 mg/kg q24hr (maintenance); **PO** 1500 mg q day or 500 mg tid; **IV** CCr 25-49 ml/min reduce to 2.5 mg q24hr (induction); 1.25 mg/kg q24hr (maintenance); **PO** 1000 mg q day or 500 mg bid; **IV** CCr 10-24 ml/

min reduce to 1.25 mg/kg q24hr (induction); 0.625 mg/kg q24hr (maintenance); **PO** 500 mg q day; **IV** CCr <10 ml/min reduce to 1.25 mg/kg 3×/wk after hemodialysis (induction); 0.625 mg/kg 3×/wk after hemodialysis (maintenance); **PO** 500 mg 3×/wk after hemodialysis

Available forms: Powder for inj 500 mg/vial, caps 250, 500 mg; implant, intravitreal 4.5 mg

Implementation
PO route
• Give with food, do not open or crush caps

IV route
• Product should be mixed under strict aseptic conditions using gloves, gown, and mask and using precautions for antineoplastics

Intermittent IV inf route
• Administer **IV** after reconstituting 500 mg/10 ml of sterile water for inj (50 mg/ml); shake; further dilute in 100 ml of D$_5$W, 0.9% NaCl, LR, Ringer's and run over 1 hr; use inf pump, in-line filter
• Do not give by BOL **IV**, IM, SUBCUT inj
• Use reconstituted sol within 12 hr, do not refrigerate or freeze; do not use sol with particulate matter or discoloration, fludarabine, sargramostim

Y-site compatibilities: Allopurinol, CISplatin, cyclophosphamide, enalaprilat, etoposide, filgrastim, fluconazole, gatifloxacin, granisetron, linezolid, melphalan, methotrexate, paclitaxel, propofol, tacrolimus, teniposide, thiotepa

Y-site incompatibilities: Amsacrine, fludarabine, foscarnet, ondansetron, sargramostim, vinorelbine

Intravitreal implant route
• Implanted by surgeon only
• Handle carefully to prevent damage to coating

ADVERSE EFFECTS
CNS: *Fever,* chills, **coma,** *confusion,* abnormal thoughts, dizziness, bizarre dreams, *headache,* psychosis, tremors, somnolence, *paresthesia, weakness,* **seizures,** peripheral neuropathy
CV: Dysrhythmia, hypo/hypertension
EENT: Retinal detachment in CMV retinitis, cataracts, ocular hypertension, ocular pain, conjunctival scarring
GI: *Abnormal liver function tests, nausea, vomiting, anorexia, diarrhea, abdominal pain,* hemorrhage, **perforation, pancreatitis**
GU: Hematuria, *increased creatinine,* BUN

HEMA: Granulocytopenia, thrombocytopenia, irreversible neutropenia, anemia, eosinophilia, pancytopenia
INTEG: *Rash,* alopecia, *pruritus,* urticaria, pain at inj site, phlebitis
RESP: Dyspnea

Pharmacokinetics

Absorption	Completely absorbed, increased bioavailability with fatty foods
Distribution	Crosses blood-brain barrier, CSF
Metabolism	Not metabolized
Excretion	Kidneys (90%) unchanged, breast milk
Half-life	3 hr

Pharmacodynamics

Unknown

INTERACTIONS

Individual drugs

Adriamycin, amphotericin B, cycloSPORINE, dapsone, DOXOrubicin, flucytosine, mycophenolate, pentamidine, probenecid, tacrolimus, trimethoprim/sulfa combinations, vinBLAStine, vinCRIStine: increased ganciclovir toxicity

Didanosine: increased didanosine effect

Imipenem with cilastatin: increased risk for seizures

Probenecid: decreased renal clearance of ganciclovir

Radiation, zidovudine: severe granulocytopenia; do not give together

Tenofovir: increased effect

Drug classifications

Antineoplastics: severe granulocytopenia; do not give together

Nucleoside analogs, NSAIDs: increased toxicity

NURSING CONSIDERATIONS

Assessment

• **CMV retinitis:** Culture should be done before treatment with ganciclovir is initiated; cultures of blood, urine, and throat may all be taken; CMV is not confirmed by this method; the diagnosis is made by an ophthalmic exam

• Assess kidney, liver function; increases in hemopoietic studies: BUN, serum creatinine, AST creatinine clearance, ALT, A:G ratio, baseline, and drip treatment; blood counts should be done q2wk; watch for decreasing granulocytes, Hgb; if low, therapy may have to be discontinued

and restarted after hematologic recovery; blood transfusions may be required

• Assess for GI symptoms: severe nausea, vomiting, diarrhea; severe symptoms may necessitate discontinuing product

• Monitor electrolytes and minerals: calcium, phosphorus, magnesium, sodium, potassium; watch closely for tetany during 1st administration

• Assess for symptoms of allergic reactions: flushing, rash, urticaria, pruritus

• **Monitor for leukopenia/neutropenia/thrombocytopenia:** WBCs, platelets q2day during 2 ×/day dosing and qwk thereafter; check for leukopenia with daily WBC count in patients with prior leukopenia with other nucleoside analogs or for whom leukopenia counts are <1000 cells/mm^3 at start of treatment; bruising, fatigue, bleeding, poor healing

• Assess for seizures, dysrhythmias

Nursing diagnoses

• Infection, risk for (uses)
• Injury, risk for (uses, adverse reactions)
• Knowledge, deficient (teaching)

Patient/family education

• Advise patient to notify prescriber if sore throat, swollen lymph nodes, malaise, fever occur; may indicate other infections

• Advise patient to report perioral tingling, numbness in extremities, and paresthesias

• Caution patient that serious product interactions may occur if OTC products are ingested; check first with prescriber

• Inform patient that product is not a cure, but will control symptoms

• Advise patient that regular blood tests, ophth exams must be continued

• Inform patient that major toxicities may necessitate discontinuing product

• **Instruct patient to use contraception during treatment and that infertility may occur; men should use barrier contraception for 90 days after treatment**

• Teach patient to take PO with food

• **Teach patient to report infection:** fever, chills, sore throat; blood dyscrasias: bruising, bleeding, petechiae

• Tell patient to avoid crowds, persons with respiratory infection

• Advise patient to use sunscreen to prevent burns

Evaluation

Positive therapeutic outcome

• Decreased symptoms of CMV infection

G

ganciclovir ophthalmic
See Appendix B

ganirelix (Rx)
(gan-i-rell'-ex)
Orgalutran ✦
Func. class.: Gonadotropin-releasing hormone antagonist
Chem. class.: Synthetic decapeptide
Pregnancy category X

ACTION: Inhibitor of pituitary gonadotropin secretion; initially increases LH and FSH, induces a rapid suppression of gonadotropin secretion

Therapeutic outcome: Pregnancy

USES: For inhibition of premature LH surges in women undergoing controlled ovarian hyperstimulation

CONTRAINDICATIONS:
Pregnancy **X,** breastfeeding, hypersensitivity, latex allergy

DOSAGE AND ROUTES
Adult: Give FSH on day 2 or 3 of cycle, then SUBCUT 250 mcg/day during mid to late portion of follicular phase; continue until day of hCG administration

Available forms: Inj 250 mcg/0.5 ml

Implementation
• Administer SUBCUT using abdomen, around navel, or upper thigh, swab inj area with disinfectant, clean a 2-in circle and allow to dry, pinch up area between thumb and finger, insert needle at 45-90 degrees to surface; if positioned correctly, no blood will be drawn back into syringe; if blood is drawn into syringe, reposition needle without removing it, inject slowly
• Protect from light

ADVERSE EFFECTS
CNS: Headache
ENDO: Ovarian hyperstimulation syndrome, abdominal pain (gynecologic)
GI: Nausea
GU: *Spotting, breakthrough bleeding,* decreased urine, **fetal death**
INTEG: Pain on inj
SYST: Fetal death

Pharmacokinetics
Absorption	Unknown
Distribution	Unknown
Metabolism	To metabolites
Excretion	Unknown
Half-life	13-16 hr

Pharmacodynamics
Onset	Unknown
Peak	Unknown
Duration	Treatment length

NURSING CONSIDERATIONS
Assessment
• Monitor reproductive tests: serum progesterone, LH, estradiol, ovarian ultrasound, pelvic exam, baseline, during treatment
• Assess for suspected pregnancy; product should not be used (pregnancy **X**)
• Assess for latex allergy; product should not be used

Nursing diagnoses
• Knowledge, deficient (teaching)
• Sexual dysfunction (uses)

Patient/family education
• Teach patient to report abdominal pain, vaginal bleeding

Evaluation
Positive therapeutic outcome
• Pregnancy

gatifloxacin ophthalmic
See Appendix B

gefitinib (Rx)
(ge-fi'tye-nib)
Iressa
Func. class.: Antineoplastic, miscellaneous
Chem. class.: Epidermal growth factor receptor inhibitor
Pregnancy category D

ACTION: Not fully understood; inhibits intracellular phosphorylation of cell surface receptors associated with epidermal growth factor receptors

Therapeutic outcome: Decreased growth and spread of malignant cells

USES: Advanced/metastatic non–small cell lung cancer (NSCLC) in those who have not responded to platinum or docetaxel products

CONTRAINDICATIONS:
Pregnancy **D**, breastfeeding, children, hypersensitivity

Precautions: Renal/hepatic/ocular/pulmonary disorders, geriatric

DOSAGE AND ROUTES
Adult: PO 250 mg/day

CYP3A4 inducers concurrently (such as rifampin or phenytoin)
Adult: PO 500 mg/day

Available forms: Tabs 250 mg

Implementation
• Give without regard to food

ADVERSE EFFECTS
EENT: Amblyopia, conjunctivitis, eye pain, corneal erosion/ulcer
GI: Nausea, diarrhea, vomiting, anorexia, **pancreatitis**, mouth ulceration, **hepatotoxicity**
INTEG: Rash, pruritus, acne, dry skin, **toxic epidermal neurolysis, angioedema**
MISC: Peripheral edema, hemorrhage
RESP: **Interstitial lung disease,** cough, dyspnea, pneumonia

Pharmacokinetics

Absorption	Slowly
Distribution	Unknown
Metabolism	Unknown
Excretion	In feces (86%), urine (<4%)
Half-life	Unknown

Pharmacodynamics

Onset	Unknown
Peak	3-7 hr
Duration	Unknown

INTERACTIONS

Individual drugs
Cimetidine, phenytoin, ranitidine, rifampin, sodium bicarbonate: decreased levels
Clarithromycin, erythromycin, itraconazole, ketoconazole: increased concentration
Clozapine: increased bone marrow suppression
Metoprolol, warfarin: increased plasma concentration

Drug/herb
St. John's wort: decreased gefitinib levels

NURSING CONSIDERATIONS
Assessment
⚠ **Assess pulmonary changes: lung sounds, cough, dyspnea; interstitial lung disease may occur, may be fatal; discontinue therapy if confirmed**
• Assess ocular changes: eye irritation, corneal erosion/ulcer, aberrant eyelash growth
⚠ **Assess for pancreatitis: abdominal pain, levels of amylase, lipase**
⚠ **Assess for toxic epidermal necrosis, angioedema**
• Monitor GI symptoms: frequency of stools; if diarrhea is poorly tolerated, therapy may be discontinued for up to 14 days

Nursing diagnoses
• Body image, disturbed (adverse reactions)
• Infection, risk for (adverse reactions)
• Injury, risk for (adverse reactions)
• Knowledge, deficient (teaching)

Patient/family education
• Teach to report adverse reactions immediately: SOB, severe abdominal pain, occular changes, skin eruptions
• Advise of reason for treatment, expected results
• Advise to use contraception during treatment

Evaluation
Positive therapeutic outcome
• Decreased non–small cell lung cancer cells

---

gemcitabine (Rx)
(gem-sit'a-been)
Gemzar
Func. class.: Antineoplastic—miscellaneous
Chem. class.: Nucleoside analog
Pregnancy category D

Do not confuse:
Gemzar/Zinecard

ACTION: Exhibits antitumor activity by killing cells undergoing DNA synthesis (S phase) and blocking G_1/S-phase boundary

Therapeutic outcome: Prevention of growth of tumor

USES: Adenocarcinoma of the pancreas (nonresectable stage II, III, or metastatic stage IV); in combination with CISplatin for inoperable, advanced, or metastatic non–small cell lung cancer; advanced breast cancer in combination with paclitaxel; with CARBOplatin for ovarian cancer, biliary tract cancer

CONTRAINDICATIONS:
Pregnancy **D**, breastfeeding, hypersensitivity

Precautions: Children, geriatric, myelosuppression, radiation therapy, renal/hepatic disease

DOSAGE AND ROUTES

Pancreatic carcinoma (nonresectable stage II, III, IV)
Adult: IV 1000 mg/m² given over ½ hr qwk × 7 wk, then 1 wk rest period; subsequent cycles should be infused once qwk × 3 wk out of every 4 wk depending on hematologic toxicity

Non–small cell lung cancer

4 wk schedule
Adult: IV 1000 mg/m² given over ½ hr on days 1, 8, 15 of each 28-day cycle; give CISplatin IV 100 mg/m² on day 1 after gemcitabine

3 wk schedule
Adult: IV 1250 mg/m² given over ½ hr on days 1, 8 of each 21-day cycle; give CISplatin 100 mg/m² after the INF of gemcitabine on day 1

Advanced breast cancer
Adult: IV 1250 mg/m² over ½ hr on days 1 and 8 of a 21-day cycle; give with paclitaxel on day 1, 175 mg/m² over 3 hr prior to gemcitabine

Available forms: Lyophilized powder for inj 20 mg/ml

Implementation
• Give increased fluid intake to 2-3 L/day to prevent dehydration, unless contraindicated
• Provide antiemetic agents before and after treatment

IV route
• Prepare in biological cabinet using gown, mask, gloves
• After reconstituting with 0.9% NaCl 5 ml/200 mg vial of product or 25 ml/1 g of product, shake (38 mg/ml); may be further diluted with 0.9% NaCl to concentrate as low as 0.1 mg/ml; discard unused portion, give over ½ hr, do not admix

Y-site compatibilities: Amifostine, amikacin, aminophylline, ampicillin, aztreonam, bleomycin, bumetanide, butorphanol, calcium gluconate, cefoxitin, ceftazidime, ceftizoxime, cefTRIAXone, chlorproMAZINE, cimetidine, ciprofloxacin, CISplatin, clindamycin, cyclophosphamide, cytarabine, DACTINomycin, DAU-NOrubicin, diphenhydrAMINE, DOBUTamine, docetaxel, DOPamine, DOXOrubicin, droperidol, enalaprilat, etoposide, famotidine, floxuridine, fluconazole, fludarabine, fluorouracil, gentamicin, granisetron, haloperidol, heparin, hydrocortisone, HYDROmorphone, IDArubicin, ifosfamide, leucovorin, linezolid, LORazepam, mannitol, meperidine, mesna, metoclopramide, metroNIDAZOLE, minocycline, mitoxantrone, morphine, nalbuphine, ondansetron, paclitaxel, promethazine, ranitidine, streptozocin, teniposide, thiotepa, ticarcillin, tobramycin, topotecan, trimethoprim/sulfamethoxazole, vancomycin, vinBLAStine, vinCRIStine, vinorelbine, zidovudine, zoledronic acid

Y-site incompatibilities: Acyclovir, amphotericin B colloidal, amphotericin B lipid complex, amphotericin B liposome, cefepime, cefoperazone, cefotaxime, chloramphenicol, dantrolene, DAPTOmycin, diazepam, furosemide, ganciclovir, imipenem-cilastatin, irinotecan, ketorolac, lansoprazole, methotrexate, methylPREDNISolone, mitomycin, nafcillin, pantoprazole, pemetrexed, phenytoin, piperacillin, prochlorperazine, thiopental

ADVERSE EFFECTS
GI: Diarrhea, nausea, vomiting, anorexia, constipation, stomatitis
GU: Proteinuria, hematuria
HEMA: Leukopenia, anemia, neutropenia, thrombocytopenia
INTEG: Irritation at site, rash, alopecia
MISC: Dyspnea, fever, hemorrhage, infection, flulike syndrome, paresthesia, peripheral edema, myalgia

Pharmacokinetics
Absorption	Unknown
Distribution	Crosses placenta
Metabolism	Unknown
Excretion	Unknown
Half-life	42-379 min

Pharmacodynamics
Unknown

INTERACTIONS

Individual drug
Alcohol: increased bleeding

Drug classifications
Anticoagulants, NSAIDs, salicylates: increased bleeding
Antineoplastics, radiation: increased myelosuppression, diarrhea
Live virus vaccines: decreased antibody response

Drug/lab test
Increased: BUN, AST, ALT, alkaline phosphatase, bilirubin, creatinine

NURSING CONSIDERATIONS
Assessment
• **Bone marrow depression:** monitor CBC, differential, platelet count before each dose; single agent: absolute granulocyte count >1000, and platelets >100,000, give complete dose; absolute granulocyte count 500-999, platelets 50,000-99,999, give 75%; absolute granulocyte count <500 or platelets <50,000, do not give; combination with paclitaxel in breast cancer: absolute granulocyte count >1200 and platelets >75,000, give complete dose; absolute granulocyte count 1000-1199 or platelets 50,000-75,000, give 75%; absolute granulocyte 700-999 or platelets ≥50,000, give 50%; granulocyte count <700 or platelets <50,000, do not give; combination with CARBOplatin in ovarian cancer: absolute granulocyte count >1500 and platelet count >100,000, give complete dose; absolute granulocyte count 1000-1499 or platelets 75,000-99,999, give 75%; absolute granulocyte count <1000 or platelets <75,000, do not give
• **Assess for blood dyscrasias:** bruising, bleeding, petechiae
• Monitor I&O, nutritional intake
• Monitor renal/hepatic studies before, during treatment; may increase AST, ALT, alkaline phosphatase, bilirubin, BUN, creatinine
• Assess food preferences: list likes, dislikes
• Assess buccal cavity for dryness, sores or ulceration, white patches, oral pain, bleeding, dysphagia
• Assess GI symptoms: frequency of stools; cramping
• Assess signs of dehydration: rapid respirations, poor skin turgor, decreased urine output, dry skin, restlessness, weakness

Nursing diagnoses
• Infection, risk for (adverse reactions)
• Nutrition: less than body requirements, imbalanced (adverse reaction)

Patient/family education
• Teach patient to rinse mouth tid-qid with water, club soda; brush teeth bid-tid with soft brush or cotton-tipped applicator for stomatitis; use unwaxed dental floss
• Advise patient to avoid foods with citric acid or hot or rough texture if stomatitis is present; to drink adequate fluids

• Advise patient to report stomatitis; any bleeding, white spots, ulcerations in mouth; tell patient to examine mouth daily, report symptoms
• Advise patient to report signs of anemia: fatigue, headache, faintness, shortness of breath, irritability; hematuria, dysuria
• Advise patient to use contraception during therapy and for 4 mo after (pregnancy **D**)
• Instruct patient to avoid use with NSAIDs, salicylates, alcohol; not to receive vaccinations during treatment
• Teach about possible hair loss and what can be done
• Advise to report flulike symptoms, swelling of feet/legs, bruising; bleeding of gums, blood in urine, stools, emesis
• Teach to avoid crowds, persons with known upper respiratory infections
• Advise patient to use electric razor

Evaluation
Positive therapeutic outcome
• Decrease in tumor size, decrease in spread of cancer, symptom relief

TREATMENT OF OVERDOSE:
Induce vomiting, provide supportive care

gemfibrozil (Rx)
(gem-fye'broe-zil)
Apo-Gemfibrozil ✦, **gemfibrozil, Gen-Gemfibrozil** ✦, **Lopid, PMS-Gemfibrozil** ✦
Func. class.: Antilipemic
Chem. class.: Fibric acid derivative
Pregnancy category C

Do not confuse:
Lopid/Levbid/Slo-bid

ACTION: Inhibits biosynthesis of VLDL, decreases triglycerides, increases HDLs

Therapeutic outcome: Decreased hepatic triglyceride production, VLDL; accelerates removal of cholesterol from liver

USES: Type IIb, IV, V hyperlipidemia as adjunct with diet therapy, hypertriglyceridemia

CONTRAINDICATIONS:
Severe renal/hepatic disease, preexisting gallbladder disease, primary biliary cirrhosis, hypersensitivity

Precautions: Pregnancy **C**, breastfeeding, monitor hematologic and hepatic function

DOSAGE AND ROUTES

Adult: PO 1200 mg in divided doses bid 30 min before meals

Hepatic/renal dose
Avoid use

Available forms: Tabs 600 mg; caps 300 mg ✿

Implementation
• Give 30 min before AM and PM meals

ADVERSE EFFECTS

CNS: Fatigue, vertigo, headache, paresthesia, dizziness, somnolence
GI: Nausea, vomiting, *dyspepsia, diarrhea, abdominal pain*
HEMA: Leukopenia, anemia, eosinophilia, thrombocytopenia
INTEG: Rash, urticaria, pruritus
MISC: Task perversion
MS: Myopathy, rhabdomyolysis
SYST: Angioedema, exfoliative dermatitis

Pharmacokinetics

Absorption	Well absorbed
Distribution	Unknown, plasma protein binding >90%
Metabolism	Liver, minimal
Excretion	Kidney, unchanged (70%), feces (6%)
Half-life	$1^1/_2$ hr

Pharmacodynamics

Onset	1-2 hr
Peak	1-2 hr
Duration	2-4 months

INTERACTIONS

Individual drugs
CycloSPORINE: decreased cycloSPORINE effect
Repaglinide: increased hypoglycemic effect
Warfarin: increased anticoagulant properties

Drug classifications
Bile acid sequestrants: decreased effect of gemfibrozil, separate by >2 hr
HMG-CoA reductase inhibitors: increased risk of myositis, myalgia
Sulfonylureas: increased hypoglycemic effect

Drug/lab test
Increased: liver function tests, CK
Decreased: Hgb, Hct, WBC, potassium

NURSING CONSIDERATIONS

Assessment
• **Hypercholesteremia:** Assess nutrition: fat, protein, carbohydrates; nutritional analysis should be performed by dietitian before treatment is initiated; monitor triglycerides, cholesterol, lipids baseline, during treatment; LDL and VLDL should be watched closely and if increased, product should be discontinued
• Assess renal, liver function tests, CBC, blood glucose if patient is on long-term therapy; if liver function test results increase, product should be discontinued
• Monitor bowel pattern daily; diarrhea may be a problem
• **Myopathy, rhabdomyolysis:** Assess for muscle pain, tenderness; obtain baseline CPK: if elevated or if these occur, product should be discontinued

Nursing diagnoses
• Diarrhea (adverse reactions)
• Knowledge, deficient (teaching)
• Noncompliance (teaching)

Patient/family education
• Inform patient that compliance is needed for positive results to occur; not to double doses; that product may be discontinued if no improvement in 3 mo
• Caution patient to decrease risk factors: high-fat diet, smoking, alcohol consumption, lack of exercise
• Advise patient to notify prescriber if GI symptoms of diarrhea, abdominal or epigastric pain, nausea, vomiting occur; or if chills, fever, sore throat occur; also occurrence of muscle cramps, abdominal cramps, severe flatulence

Evaluation
Positive therapeutic outcome
• Decreased cholesterol levels, serum triglyceride and improved ratio with HDLs

gemifloxacin (Rx)
(gem-ah-flox′a-sin)
Factive
Func. class.: Antiinfective
Chem. class.: Fluoroquinolone
Pregnancy category C

ACTION: Inhibits DNA gyrase, which is an enzyme involved in replication, transcription, and repair of bacterial DNA

Therapeutic outcome: Negative C&S, decreasing symptoms of infection

⚠ Nurse Alert

USES: Acute bacterial exacerbation of chronic bronchitis caused by *Streptococcus pneumoniae, Haemophilus influenzae, Haemophilus parainfluenzae, Moraxella catarrhalis;* community-acquired pneumonia caused by *Streptococcus pneumoniae* including multiproduct-resistant strains, *H. influenzae, M. catarrhalis, Mycoplasma pneumoniae, Chlamydia pneumoniae, Klebsiella pneumoniae*

CONTRAINDICATIONS:
Hypersensitivity to quinolones

Precautions: Pregnancy **C,** breastfeeding, children, geriatric, hypokalemia, hypomagnesemia, renal disease, seizure disorders, excessive exposure to sunlight, psychosis, increased intracranial pressure, history of QT interval prolongation, dysrhythmias, myasthenia gravis, torsades de pointes

> **BLACK BOX WARNING:** Tendon pain/rupture, tendinitis

DOSAGE AND ROUTES
Adult: PO 320 mg/day × 5-10 days depending on type of infection

Renal dose
Adult: PO CCr ≤40 ml/min 160 mg q24hr

Available forms: Tabs 320 mg

Implementation
- Give with or without food
- Theophylline should not be used with this product; toxicity may result
- Administer 2 hr before or 3 hr after antacids, iron, zinc, or buffered products; 2 hr before sucralfate

ADVERSE EFFECTS
CNS: *Dizziness, headache,* somnolence, depression, insomnia, nervousness, confusion, agitation, **seizures**
CV: QT prolongation, vasodilatation
EENT: Visual disturbances
GI: Diarrhea, *nausea,* vomiting, anorexia, flatulence, heartburn, dry mouth; increased AST, ALT; constipation, abdominal pain, oral thrush, glossitis, stomatitis, **pseudomembranous colitis**
GU: Crystalluria (rare)
HEMA: Thrombocytopenia, neutropenia
INTEG: Rash, pruritus, urticaria, *photosensitivity*
SYST: Anaphylaxis, Stevens-Johnson syndrome

Pharmacokinetics
Absorption	Rapidly, bioavailability 71%
Distribution	Unknown
Metabolism	Unknown
Excretion	In urine as active product, metabolites
Half-life	4-12 hr

Pharmacodynamics
Onset	Unknown
Peak	1-2 hr
Duration	Unknown

INTERACTIONS
Individual drugs
Amoxapine, chloroquine, clozapine, dasatinib, dolasetron, dronedarone, droperidol, erythromycin, flecainide, haloperidol, lapatinib, maprotiline, methadone, octreotide, ondansetron, palonosetron, pentamidine, pimozide, propafenone, ranolazine, risperidone, sertindole, sunitinib, tacrolimus, telithromycin, troleandomycin, vardenafil, vorinostat, ziprasidone: increased QT prolongation
Probenecid: may increase toxicity
Theophylline: toxicity; do not use concurrently

Drug classifications
Antacids containing aluminum, iron, magnesium, sucralfate, zinc: decreased absorption; give 2 hr before or 3 hr after meals
Antiarrhythmics (amiodarone, disopyramide, procainamide, quinidine, sotalol), antidepressants (tricyclics), β-blockers, halogenated/local anesthetics: may decrease effect, resulting in life-threatening dysrhythmias, QT prolongation
Drugs that increase QT prolongation: increased QT prolongation
NSAIDs: increased CNS stimulation

NURSING CONSIDERATIONS
Assessment
- Monitor renal, liver function tests: BUN, creatinine, AST, ALT
- Monitor I&O ratio; urine pH, <5.5 is ideal
- Assess CNS symptoms: insomnia, vertigo, headache, agitation, confusion
⚠ Assess allergic reactions and anaphylaxis: rash, flushing, urticaria, pruritus, chills, fever, joint pain; may occur a few days after therapy begins; epinephrine and resuscitation equipment should be available for anaphylactic reaction

• **Pseudomembranous colitis:** Monitor bowel pattern daily; if severe diarrhea, fever, abdominal pain occurs, product should be discontinued
• **Assess for overgrowth of infection:** perineal itching, fever, malaise, redness, pain, swelling, drainage, rash, diarrhea, change in cough, sputum

Nursing diagnoses
• Infection, risk for (uses)
• Knowledge, deficient (teaching)
• Noncompliance (teaching)

Patient/family education
• Advise patient that fluids must be increased to 2 L/day to avoid crystallization in kidneys
• Instruct patient that if dizziness or light-headedness occurs, to ambulate, perform activities with assistance
• Instruct patient to complete full course of product therapy
• Teach patient to contact prescriber if adverse reactions occur
• Teach patient to avoid iron- or mineral-containing supplements or aluminum/magnesium antacids within 2 hr before or 3 hr after dosing
• Advise patient that photosensitivity may occur and sunscreen should be used
• Advise patient to use frequent rinsing of mouth, sugarless candy or gum for dry mouth
• Teach patient to avoid other medication unless approved by prescriber

Evaluation
Positive therapeutic outcome
• Negative C&S, absence of signs/symptoms of infection

⚠ HIGH ALERT

gemtuzumab (Rx)
(gem-tue-zue'mab)
Mylotarg
Func. class.: Antineoplastic—miscellaneous
Chem. class.: Monoclonal antibody
Pregnancy category D

ACTION: Composed of recombinant humanized IgG4κ antibody, binds to CD33 antigen that is released in myeloid cells

Therapeutic outcome: Decreasing signs/symptoms of leukemia

USES: Acute myeloid leukemia (AML) in patients with first relapse who are 60 yr or older

CONTRAINDICATIONS:
Pregnancy **D**, breastfeeding

> **BLACK BOX WARNING:** Hypersensitivity to this product or murine protein, severe myelosuppression

Precautions: Children, severe renal disease

> **BLACK BOX WARNING:** Hepatic disease, pulmonary disease, infusion-related reactions

DOSAGE AND ROUTES
Adult: **IV** 9 m/m^2 as a 2 hr INF; before giving INF, give diphenhydrAMINE 50 mg PO, acetaminophen 650-1000 mg PO 1 hr; then use acetaminophen 650-1000 mg q4hr for additional 2 doses prn

Available forms: Powder for inj, lyophilized 5 mg

Implementation
• Do not give **IV** push or bolus
• Protect from light, use biological safety hood, allow to come to room temperature
• Reconstitute each vial with 5 ml of sterile water for inj using sterile syringes, swirl each vial, check for discoloration or particulate matter, give over 2 hr, use a separate line with 1.2-micron terminal filter
• May be premedicated with methylPREDNISolone and antiemetics
• Store reconstituted sol for ≤8 hr in refrigerator

ADVERSE EFFECTS
CNS: *Dizziness,* insomnia, depression, headache
CV: Hypertension, **hemorrhage,** tachycardia, hypotension
HEMA: Prolonged neutropenia, thrombocytopenia
INTEG: *Rash,* herpes simplex, local reaction, petechiae, pruritus
GI: Anorexia, diarrhea, constipation, nausea, stomatitis, vomiting, **fatal liver toxicity**
GU: Hematuria, **vaginal hemorrhage**
META: Hypokalemia, hypomagnesemia
MISC: *Fever, myalgias, headache, chills,* peripheral edema
RESP: Cough, pneumonia, epistaxis, rhinitis, dyspnea

Pharmacokinetics

Absorption	Unknown
Distribution	Unknown
Metabolism	Unknown
Excretion	Unknown
Half-life	Biphasic; 45, 100 hr, respectively

Pharmacodynamics

Unknown

INTERACTIONS

Drug classifications

Antineoplastics, other, radiation: increased bone marrow suppression

NURSING CONSIDERATIONS

Assessment

• Assess for pulmonary symptoms: cough, dyspnea

• Monitor blood studies: BUN, creatinine, AST, ALT, electrolytes, bilirubin, CBC, uric acid

• Assess for symptoms of infection; chills, fever, headache may be masked by product

• Assess CNS reaction: LOC, mental status, dizziness, confusion

• Assess cardiac status: lung sounds; ECG before, during treatment, especially in those with cardiac disease

• Assess bone marrow depression: bruising, bleeding, blood in stools, urine, sputum, emesis

Nursing diagnoses

• Infection, risk for (adverse reactions)

• Nutrition: less than body requirements, imbalanced (adverse reactions)

• Oral mucous membrane, impaired (adverse reactions)

Patient/family education

• Advise patient to take acetaminophen for fever

• Instruct patient to avoid hazardous tasks, since confusion, dizziness may occur; avoid prolonged sunlight, use sunscreen

• Instruct patient to report signs of infection: sore throat, fever, diarrhea, vomiting

• Teach patient to avoid immunizations, crowds, people with known infections

• Caution patient that product is very toxic

Evaluation

Positive therapeutic outcome

• Improvement in blood counts

gentamicin (Rx)

(jen-ta-mye'sin)

Func. class.: Antiinfective

Chem. class.: Aminoglycoside

Pregnancy category C

Do not confuse:

Garamycin/kanamycin

ACTION: Interferes with protein synthesis in bacterial cell by binding to ribosomal subunit, causing misreading of genetic code; inaccurate peptide sequence forms in protein chain, causing bacterial death

Therapeutic outcome: Bactericidal effects for the following organisms: *Pseudomonas aeruginosa, Proteus, Klebsiella, Serratia, Escherichia coli, Enterobacter, Citrobacter, Staphylococcus, Shigella, Salmonella, Acinetobacter, Bacillus anthracis*

USES: Severe systemic infections of CNS; respiratory, GI, and urinary tracts; bone; skin; soft tissues; acute PID caused by susceptible strains

CONTRAINDICATIONS:

Hypersensitivity to this or other aminoglycosides, fungal/viral/mycobacterial infection

BLACK BOX WARNING: Severe renal disease, pregnancy **D**

Precautions: Breastfeeding, geriatric, neonates

BLACK BOX WARNING: Mild renal disease, hearing deficits, myasthenia gravis, Parkinson's disease, infant botulism

DOSAGE AND ROUTES

Severe systemic infections

Adult: IV INF 3-6 mg/kg/day in 3 divided doses q8hr; dilute in 50-200 ml 0.9% NaCl or D_5W given over 30 min-1 hr; IM 3 mg/kg/day in divided doses q8hr

Child: IV/IM 2-2.5 mg/kg q8hr

Neonate and infant: IV/IM 2.5 mg/kg q8-12hr

Neonate <1 wk: 2.5 mg/kg q12-24hr

Renal dose

Adult: IM/IV CCr 70-100 ml/min reduce dose by multiplying maintenance dose by 0.85, give q8-12hr; CCr 50-69 ml/min reduce dose as above, give q12hr; CCr 25-49 ml/min reduce as above, give q24hr; CCr <25 ml/min reduce as above, give based on serum concentrations

Available forms: Inj 10, 40 mg/ml; premixed inj 40, 60, 70, 80, 100 mg/50 ml

Implementation

Intermittent IV infusion route
• Give inj deeply in large muscle mass; rotate sites

Topical route
• Wash hands, wear gloves, clean skin before applying

IV route
• Give in even doses around the clock; product must be given for 10-14 days to ensure organism death and prevent superinfection
• Give by intermittent inf over ½-1 hr, flush with 0.9% NaCl or D₅W after inf
• Separate aminoglycosides and penicillins by ≥1 hr
• Store in tight container

Syringe compatibilities: Clindamycin, methicillin, penicillin G sodium

Y-site compatibilities: Amifostine, amiodarone, amsacrine, atracurium, aztreonam, cefpirome, ciprofloxacin, cyclophosphamide, cytarabine, diltiazem, enalaprilat, esmolol, famotidine, fluconazole, fludarabine, foscarnet, granisetron, hydromorphone, IL-2, insulin, labetalol, LORazepam, magnesium sulfate, melphalan, meperidine, meropenem, midazolam, morphine, multivitamins, ondansetron, paclitaxel, pancuronium, perphenazine, sargramostim, tacrolimus, teniposide, theophylline, thiotepa, tolazine, vecuronium, vinorelbine, vit B with C, zidovudine

Y-site incompatibilities: IDArubicin, indomethacin

ADVERSE EFFECTS

CNS: Confusion, depression, numbness, tremors, **seizures,** muscle twitching, **neurotoxicity,** dizziness, vertigo
CV: Hypotension, hypertension, palpitations, edema
EENT: Ototoxicity, deafness, visual disturbances, tinnitus
GI: *Nausea, vomiting, anorexia,* increased ALT, AST, bilirubin, hepatomegaly, **hepatic necrosis,** splenomegaly
GU: Oliguria, hematuria, renal damage, azotemia, **renal failure, nephrotoxicity,** proteinuria

HEMA: Agranulocytosis, thrombocytopenia, leukopenia, eosinophilia, anemia
INTEG: *Rash,* burning, urticaria, dermatitis, alopecia, photosensitivity

Pharmacokinetics

Absorption	Well absorbed (IM)
Distribution	Distributed in extracellular fluids, poorly distributed in CSF; crosses placenta
Metabolism	Liver, minimal
Excretion	Mostly unchanged (79%) kidneys
Half-life	1-2 hr; infants 6-7 hr; increased in renal disease

Pharmacodynamics

	IM	IV
Onset	Rapid	Rapid
Peak	½-1½ hr	Infusion's end
Duration	Unknown	Unknown

INTERACTIONS

Individual drugs
Acyclovir, amphotericin B, cidofovir, cisplatin, ethacrynic acid, furosemide, mannitol, methoxyflurane, polymyxin, vancomycin: increased ototoxicity, neurotoxicity, nephrotoxicity

Drug classifications
Aminoglycosides, cephalosporins, penicillins: increased ototoxicity, neurotoxicity, nephrotoxicity
Nondepolarizing neuromuscular blockers: increased neuromuscular blockade, respiratory depression
Penicillins: Do not use at the same time as or physically mix with penicillins

Drug/lab test
Increase: LDH, AST, ALT, bilirubin, BUN, creatinine, eosinophils
Decrease: Hgb, WBC, platelets, granulocytes

NURSING CONSIDERATIONS

Assessment
• Assess patient for previous sensitivity reaction
• **Assess patient for signs and symptoms of infection** including characteristics of wounds, sputum, urine, stool, WBC >10,000/mm³, fever; obtain baseline during treatment
• **Neuromuscular disease (myasthenia gravis, Parkinson's disease, infant botulism):** Assess for paresthesias, tetany, Chvostek's/Trousseau's signs, confusion (adults)

tetany, muscle weakness (infants); correct electrolyte imbalance

• Complete C&S before beginning product therapy; this will ensure that correct treatment has been initiated

• **Assess for allergic reactions:** rash, urticaria, pruritus, chills, fever, joint pain may occur a few days after therapy begins

> **BLACK BOX WARNING: Renal disease:** Identify urine output; if decreasing, notify prescriber (may indicate nephrotoxicity); also, increased BUN, creatinine, urine CCr <80 ml/min; monitor I&O ratio; urinalysis daily for proteinuria, cells, casts; report sudden change in urine output; assess urine pH if product is used for UTI; urine should be kept alkaline

• Monitor blood studies: AST, ALT, CBC, Hct, bilirubin, LDH, alkaline phosphatase, Coombs' test monthly if patient is on long-term therapy

• Monitor electrolytes: potassium, sodium, chloride, magnesium monthly if patient is on long-term therapy

• Monitor for bleeding: ecchymosis, bleeding gums, hematuria; assess stool guaiac daily if on long-term therapy

• **Assess for overgrowth of infection:** perineal itching, fever, malaise, redness, pain, swelling, drainage, rash, diarrhea, change in cough, sputum

• Obtain weight before treatment; calculation of dosage is usually based on ideal body weight but may be calculated on actual body weight

• Monitor VS during inf, watch for hypotension, change in pulse

• Assess **IV** site for thrombophlebitis including pain, redness, swelling q30min, change site if needed; apply warm compresses to discontinued site

• Obtain serum peak, measured at 30-60 min after **IV** inf or 60 min after IM inj, trough level measured just before next dose; blood level should be 2-4 times bacteriostatic level

> **BLACK BOX WARNING: Assess for deafness** by audiometric testing, ringing, roaring in ears, vertigo; assess hearing before, during, after treatment

• Assess for dehydration: high specific gravity, decrease in skin turgor, dry mucous membranes, dark urine

Nursing diagnoses
• Diarrhea (side effects)
• Infection, risk for (uses)
• Injury, risk for (side effects)

• Knowledge, deficient (teaching)
• Noncompliance (teaching)

Patient/family education
• Teach patient to report sore throat, bruising, bleeding, joint pain; may indicate blood dyscrasias (rare)

• Advise patient to contact prescriber if vaginal itching, loose foul-smelling stools, furry tongue occur; may indicate superimposed infection

Evaluation
Positive therapeutic outcome
• Absence of signs/symptoms of infection (WBC <10,000/mm^3, temp WNL, absence of red, draining wounds)
• Reported improvement in symptoms of infection

TREATMENT OF OVERDOSE:
Withdraw product, hemodialysis

> ### gentamicin ophthalmic
> *See Appendix B*

> ### gentamicin topical
> *See Appendix B*

> ### glatiramer (Rx)
> (glah-teer'a-mer)
> **Copaxone**
> *Func. class.:* Multiple sclerosis agent
> **Pregnancy category B**

ACTION: Unknown; may modify the immune responses responsible for multiple sclerosis (MS)

Therapeutic outcome: Decreased symptoms of MS

USES: Reduction of the frequency of relapses in patients with relapsing-remitting MS after first clinical episode with MRI results consistent with MS

CONTRAINDICATIONS:
Hypersensitivity to this product or mannitol

Precautions: Pregnancy **B**, breastfeeding, children <18 yr, immune disorders, renal disease

DOSAGE AND ROUTES
Adult: SUBCUT 20 mg/day

Available forms: Inj premixed 20 mg/ml

Implementation
SUBCUT route
• Use a sterile syringe/needle to transfer the supplied diluent into the vial, rotate vial gently, do not shake; withdraw medication using a syringe with 27-G needle; administer SUBCUT into hip, thigh, arm; discard unused portion
• Use SUBCUT route only; do not give IM or **IV**
• Do not use sol that contains precipitate or is discolored

ADVERSE EFFECTS
CNS: Anxiety, hypertonia, tremor, vertigo, speech disorder, agitation, confusion, flushing
CV: Migraine, syncope, tachycardia, vasodilatation, chest pain, hypertension
EENT: Ear pain, blurred vision
GI: Nausea, vomiting, diarrhea, anorexia, gastroenteritis
GU: Urgency, dysmenorrhea, vaginal moniliasis
HEMA: Ecchymosis, lymphadenopathy
INTEG: Pruritus, rash, sweating, urticaria, erythema, injection site reaction
META: Edema, weight gain
MS: Arthralgia, back pain, neck pain, increased muscle tone
RESP: Bronchitis, dyspnea, laryngismus, rhinitis

Pharmacokinetics
Unknown

Pharmacodynamics
Unknown

NURSING CONSIDERATIONS
Assessment
• Monitor blood, renal, liver function tests before treatment
• Assess for CNS symptoms: anxiety, confusion, vertigo
• Assess GI status: diarrhea, vomiting, abdominal pain, gastroenteritis
• Assess cardiac status: tachycardia, palpitations, vasodilatation, chest pain

Nursing diagnoses
• Knowledge, deficient (teaching)
• Noncompliance (teaching)

Patient/family education
• Give written, detailed instructions about the product; provide initial and return demonstrations on inj procedure; give information on use and disposal of product
• Advise patient that blurred vision, sweating may occur

• Advise patient that irregular menses, dysmenorrhea, or metorrhagia as well as breast pain may occur; use contraception during treatment
• Advise patient to notify prescriber if pregnancy is suspected or if nursing
• Advise patient not to change dosing or to stop taking product without advice of prescriber

Evaluation
Positive therapeutic outcome
• Decreased symptoms of multiple sclerosis

---

glimepiride (Rx)
(gly-meh′pih-ride)
Amaryl, CO Glimepiride ✤, ratio-Glimepiride ✤, Sandoz Glimepiride ✤
glipiZIDE (Rx)
(glip-i′zide)
Glucotrol, Glucotrol XL
Func. class.: Antidiabetic
Chem. class.: Sulfonylurea (2nd generation)
Pregnancy category C

Do not confuse:
glipiZIDE/glucotrol/glyBURIDE

ACTION: Causes functioning β cells in pancreas to release insulin, leading to drop in blood glucose levels; may improve insulin binding to insulin receptors or increase the number of insulin receptors with prolonged administration; may also reduce basal hepatic glucose secretion; not effective if patient lacks functioning β cells

Therapeutic outcome: Decrease in polyuria, polydipsia, polyphagia, clear sensorium, absence of dizziness, stable gait

USES: Type 2 diabetes mellitus

CONTRAINDICATIONS:
Hypersensitivity to sulfonylureas, type 1 diabetes, diabetic ketoacidosis

Precautions: Pregnancy **C**, geriatric, cardiac disease, severe renal/hepatic disease, G6PD deficiency

DOSAGE AND ROUTES
Glimepiride
Adult: PO 1-2 mg/day with breakfast, then increase by ≤2 mg/day at q1-2wk, max 8 mg/day
Geriatric: PO 1 mg/day, may increase if needed

⚠ Nurse Alert

Renal dose
Adult: PO 1 mg/day with breakfast, may titrate upward as needed

GlipiZIDE
Adult: PO 5 mg initially before breakfast, then increase by 2.5-5 mg after several days, to desired response; max 40 mg/day in divided doses or 15 mg/dose; (XL) PO 5 mg/day with breakfast, may increase to 10 mg/day; max 20 mg/day
Geriatric: PO 2.5 mg/day, may increase if needed

Hepatic dose
Adult: PO 2.5 mg initially, then increase to desired response; max 40 mg/day in divided doses or 15 mg/dose

Available forms: Glimepiride: tabs 1, 2, 4 mg; glipiZIDE: tabs 5, 10 mg scored; EXT REL tabs 2.5, 5, 10 mg

Implementation
• Do not break, crush, or chew ext rel tabs
• Convert from other oral hypoglycemic agents or insulin dosage of <40 units/day; change may be made without gradual dosage change
• Patients taking >40 units/day of insulin convert gradually by receiving oral hypoglycemic agents and 50% of previous insulin dosage for 3-5 days
• Monitor serum or urine glucose and ketones 3 ×/day during conversion
• **Glipizide:** 30 min before meals (regular release); with breakfast (ext rel)
• **Glimepiride:** with breakfast; if patient is NPO, may need to hold dose to prevent hypoglycemia
• Give tab crushed and mixed with meal or fluids for patients with difficulty swallowing
• For severe hypoglycemia give **IV** D$_{50}$W, then **IV** dextrose solution
• Store in tight container in cool environment

ADVERSE EFFECTS
CNS: *Headache, weakness, dizziness, drowsiness,* tinnitus, fatigue, vertigo
ENDO: Hypoglycemia
GI: Hepatotoxicity, cholestatic jaundice, nausea, vomiting, diarrhea, heartburn
HEMA: Leukopenia, thrombocytopenia, agranulocytosis, aplastic anemia, increased AST, ALT, alkaline phosphatase, **pancytopenia, hemolytic anemia**
INTEG: Rash, allergic reactions, pruritus, urticaria, eczema, photosensitivity, erythema, allergic vasculitis

Pharmacokinetics
Absorption	Completely absorbed, GI tract
Distribution	Unknown
Metabolism	Liver
Excretion	Via kidneys
Half-life	2-4 hr; 5 hr glimepiride

Pharmacodynamics
	Glipizide	Glimepiride
Onset	1-1½ hr	
Peak	1-3 hr	2-3 hr
Duration	10-24 hr	

G

INTERACTIONS
Individual drugs
Charcoal, cholestyramine, diazoxide, isoniazid, rifampin: possible decreased action of glipiZIDE
Chloramphenicol, cimetidine, clarithromycin, clofibrate, fenfluramine, fluconazole, gemfibrozil, guanethidine, insulin, methyldopa, phenylbutazone, probenecid, sulfinpyrizine, voriconazole: increased hypoglycemia
Digoxin: increased action of digoxin

Drug classifications
Androgens, anticoagulants, fibric acid derivatives, H$_2$-antagonists, magnesium salts, MAOIs, NSAIDs, salicylates, sulfonamides, tricyclics, urinary acidifiers: increased hypoglycemia
β-Blockers: may mask symptoms of hypoglycemia
Diuretics (thiazide), corticosteroids, hydantoins, urinary alkalinizers: possible decreased action of glipiZIDE
Glycosides: increased action of glycosides

Drug/herb
Garlic, horse chestnut: increased antidiabetic effect
Chromium: decreased antidiabetic effect
Chromium, coenzyme Q10, fenugreek, ginseng: increased or decreased hypoglycemic effect
Green tea: decreased hypoglycemic effect

Drug/lab test
Increase: AST, ALT, LDH, BUN, creatinine

NURSING CONSIDERATIONS
Assessment
• **Assess for hypoglycemic/hyperglycemic reactions** that can occur soon after meals; hypoglycemic reactions (sweating, weakness, dizziness, anxiety, tremors, hunger); hypergly-

cemic reactions; A1c (baseline, q3mo) during treatment
• **Blood dyscrasias:** Monitor CBC

Nursing diagnoses
• Injury, risk for (adverse reactions)
• Knowledge, deficient (teaching)
• Noncompliance (teaching)
• Nutrition: less than body requirements, imbalanced (adverse reactions)
• Nutrition: more than body requirements, imbalanced (uses)

Patient/family education
• **Teach patient to check for symptoms of cholestatic jaundice:** dark urine, pruritus, yellow sclera; if these occur, prescriber should be notified
• Teach patient to use capillary blood glucose test
• Teach patient to report bleeding, bruising, weight gain, edema, SOB, weakness, sore throat
• Teach patient symptoms of hypo/hyperglycemia, what to do about each
• Instruct patient that product must be continued on daily basis; explain consequence of discontinuing product abruptly
• Caution patient to avoid OTC medications unless approved by a prescriber
• Teach patient that diabetes is a lifelong illness; that this product is not a cure
• Teach patient to avoid alcohol; inform about disulfiram reaction (nausea, headache, cramps, flushing, hypoglycemia)
• Instruct patient that all food included in diet plan must be eaten to prevent hypoglycemia
• Advise patient to use sunscreen or stay out of the sun to prevent burns
• Advise patient to carry/wear emergency ID and carry a glucagon emergency kit for emergency purposes; also prescriber name, phone number, and medications taken
• Teach patient ext rel tab may appear in stool

Evaluation
Positive therapeutic outcome
• Decrease in polyuria, polydipsia, polyphagia; clear sensorium; absence of dizziness; stable gait
• Improved serum glucose, A1c

glyBURIDE (Rx)
(glye´byoor-ide)
Apo-Glyburide ✚, **DiaBeta** ✚, **Glynase PresTab, Novo-Glyburide** ✚, **Nu-Glyburide** ✚, **PMS-Glyburide** ✚, **ratio-Glyburide** ✚, **Sandoz Glyburide** ✚
Func. class.: Antidiabetic
Chem. class.: Sulfonylurea (2nd generation)
Pregnancy category C

Do not confuse:
glyBURIDE/Glucotrol/glipiZIDE, DiaBeta/Zebeta

ACTION: Causes functioning β cells in pancreas to release insulin, leading to drop in blood glucose levels; may improve insulin binding to insulin receptors and increase number of insulin receptors with prolonged administration; may also reduce basal hepatic glucose secretion; not effective if patient lacks functioning β cells

Therapeutic outcome: Decrease in polyuria, polydipsia, polyphagia, clear sensorium, absence of dizziness, stable gait

USES: Type 2 diabetes mellitus

CONTRAINDICATIONS:
Hypersensitivity to sulfonylureas, type 1 diabetes, diabetic ketoacidosis, renal failure

Precautions: Pregnancy **C**, geriatric, cardiac/thyroid disease, severe renal/hepatic disease, severe hypoglycemic reactions, sulfonamide/sulfonylurea hypersensitivity, G6PD deficiency

DOSAGE AND ROUTES
DiaBeta
Adult: PO 1.25-5 mg initially, then increased to desired response at weekly intervals up to 20 mg/day; may be given as a single or divided dose
Geriatric: PO 1.25 mg initially, then increased to desired response; max 20 mg/day, maintenance 1.25-20 mg/day

Glynase PresTab (micronized)
Adult: PO 1.5-3 mg/day initially, may increase by 1.5 mg/wk, max 12 mg/day
Geriatric: PO 0.75-3 mg/day, may increase by 1.5 mg/wk

Available forms: Tabs (DiaBeta) 1.25, 2.5, 5 mg; tabs micronized (Glynase PresTab) 1.5, 3, 6 mg

Implementation
• Conversion from other oral hypoglycemic agents or insulin dosage of <40 units/day; change may be made without gradual dosage change
• Patients taking >40 units/day of insulin convert gradually by receiving oral hypoglycemic agents and 50% of previous insulin dosage for 3-5 days
• Monitor serum or urine glucose and ketones 3 ×/day during conversion
• Give product 30 min before breakfast; if large dose is required, may be divided into two; give with meals to decrease GI upset and provide best absorption; if patient is NPO, may need to hold dose to avoid hypoglycemia, take at same time each day
• Give tab crushed and mixed with meal or fluids for patients with difficulty swallowing
• For severe hypoglycemia, give **IV** D$_{50}$W, then **IV** dextrose sol
• Store in tight container in cool environment

ADVERSE EFFECTS
CNS: *Headache, weakness,* paresthesia, tinnitus, fatigue, vertigo
EENT: Blurred vision
ENDO: Hypoglycemia
GI: Nausea, fullness, heartburn, **hepatoxicity, cholestatic jaundice,** vomiting, diarrhea, **hepatic failure** (rare)
HEMA: **Leukopenia, thrombocytopenia, agranulocytosis, aplastic anemia,** increased AST, ALT, alkaline phosphatase
INTEG: Rash, allergic reactions, pruritus, urticaria, eczema, photosensitivity, erythema
MS: Joint pains

Pharmacokinetics
Absorption	Completely absorbed GI tract
Distribution	99% plasma protein binding
Metabolism	Liver
Excretion	Urine, feces (metabolites), crosses placenta
Half-life	10 hr

Pharmacodynamics
Onset	2 hr
Peak	2-4 hr
Duration	24 hr

INTERACTIONS
Individual drugs
Bosentan: increased LFTs, avoid concurrent use
Charcoal, cholestyramine, isoniazid, rifampin thyroid, voriconazole: decreased action of glyBURIDE
Clarithromycin, chloramphenicol, fenfluramine, fluconazole, gemfibrozil, guanethidine, insulin, methyldopa, phenylbutazone, probenecid, sulfinpyrazone: increased hypoglycemia
Colesevelam: increased triglyceride levels
CycloSPORINE: increased action of cycloSPORINE
Diazoxide: both products may have action decreased
Digoxin: increased level

Drug classifications
Androgens, anticoagulants, antidepressants (tricyclics), β-blockers, H$_2$-antagonists, magnesium salts, MAOIs, NSAIDs, salicylates, sulfonamides, urinary acidifiers: increased hypoglycemia
β-Adrenergic blockers: increased masking of symptoms of hypoglycemia
Diuretics (thiazide), hydantoins, urinary alkalinizers, corticosteroids, phenothiazines, oral contraceptives, estrogens: decreased action of glyBURIDE

Drug/herb
Garlic, horse chestnut: increased antidiabetic effect
Green tea: decreased hypoglycemic effect

Drug/lab test
Increased: AST, ALT, LDH, BUN, creatinine

NURSING CONSIDERATIONS
Assessment
• Assess for hypo/hyperglycemic reactions that can occur soon after meals; hypoglycemic reactions (sweating, weakness, dizziness, anxiety, tremors, hunger); hyperglycemic reactions; A1c (baseline, q3mo) during treatment
• **Blood dyscrasias:** Monitor CBC, check liver function tests periodically, AST, LDH, and renal studies: BUN, creatinine during treatment

Nursing diagnoses
• Injury, risk for (adverse reactions)
• Knowledge, deficient (teaching)
• Noncompliance (teaching)
• Nutrition: less than body requirements, imbalanced (adverse reactions)
• Nutrition: more than body requirements, imbalanced (uses)

Patient/family education

• **Teach patient to check for symptoms of cholestatic jaundice:** dark urine, pruritus, yellow sclera; if these occur, prescriber should be notified

• Teach patient to use capillary blood glucose test

• **Teach patient symptoms of hypo/hyperglycemia,** what to do about each

• Instruct patient that product must be continued on daily basis; explain consequence of discontinuing product abruptly

• Teach patient to report bleeding, bruising, weight gain, edema, shortness of breath, weakness, sore throat

• Teach patient to take product in AM to prevent hypoglycemic reactions at night

• Caution patient to avoid OTC medications unless approved by a prescriber

• Teach patient that diabetes is a lifelong illness; that this product is not a cure

• Instruct patient that all food included in diet plan must be eaten to prevent hypoglycemia

• Advise patient to carry/wear emergency ID and carry a glucagon emergency kit for emergency purposes: have sugar packets available; also prescriber name, phone number, and medications

• Advise patient to use sunscreen or stay out of the sun to prevent burns

Evaluation

Positive therapeutic outcome

• Decrease in polyuria, polydipsia, polyphagia; clear sensorium; absence of dizziness; stable gait

• Improved serum glucose, A1c

glycopyrrolate (Rx)

(glye-koe-pye′roe-late)
Cuvposa, Robinul, Robinul-Forte
Func. class.: Cholinergic blocker, antispasmodic
Chem. class.: Quaternary ammonium compound
Pregnancy category B

ACTION: Inhibits action of acetylcholine at receptor sites in autonomic nervous system, which controls secretions, free acids in stomach

Therapeutic outcome: Decreased secretions in the respiratory tract, GI system

USES: Decreased secretions before surgery, reversal of neuromuscular blockade, peptic ulcer disease, irritable bowel syndrome, bradycardia, drooling

CONTRAINDICATIONS:

Children <3 yr, hypersensitivity, closed-angle glaucoma, myasthenia gravis, GI/GU obstruction, tachycardia, myocardial ischemia, hepatic disease, ulcerative colitis, toxic megacolon, prostatic hypertrophy

Precautions: Pregnancy **B,** breastfeeding, geriatric, pulmonary/renal disease, CHF, hyperthyroidism, CAD, Down syndrome, hiatal hernia, hypertension

DOSAGE AND ROUTES

Preoperatively
Adult: IM 4.4 mcg/kg $^1/_2$-1 hr before surgery, max 0.1 mg
Child >2 yr (unlabeled): IM 4 mcg/kg 30-60 min before surgery
Child <2 yr (unlabeled): IM 4-9 mcg/kg

Intraoperative
Adult: IV 0.1 mg; may repeat 2-3 min prn
Child: IM/IV 4 mcg/kg q2-3min prn; max 0.1 mg/dose

Reversal of neuromuscular blockage
Adult and child: IV 200 mcg for each 1 mg of neostigmine or 5 mg IV of pyridostigmine simultaneously

GI disorders
Adult: PO 1-2 mg bid-tid; max 6 mg/day; IM/IV 100-200 mcg tid-qid, titrated to patient response

Antidysrhythmic
Adult: IV 100 mcg, may repeat q2min
Child: IV 4.4 mcg/kg, may repeat q2min, max 100 mcg

Secretion control
Child: PO 40-100 mcg/kg/dose tid-qid; IM/IV 4-10 mcg/kg/dose q3-4hr; max 0.2 mg/dose or 0.8 mg/24hr

Chronic drooling
Children/adolescents (3-16 yr): PO (oral solution) 0.02 mg/kg tid, titrate by 0.02 mg/kg/dose q5-7days, max 0.1 mg/kg/dose tid or 13-17 kg 1.5 mg/dose, 18-22 kg 2 mg, 23-27 kg 2.5 mg dose, ≥28 kg 3 mg/dose

Available forms: Tabs 1, 2 mg; inj 200 mcg 0.2 mg/ml; oral sol 1 mg/5 ml

Implementation
PO route
• Give PO with or after meals to prevent GI upset; may give with fluids other than water
IM route
• Give IM inj deeply in large muscle mass
Direct IV route
• Administer **IV** undiluted, give at a rate of 0.2 mg or less over 5-15 min through Y-tube or 3-way stopcock; do not add to **IV** sol
• Administer parenteral dose with patient recumbent to prevent postural hypotension

Syringe compatibilities: Atropine, benzquinamide, chlorproMAZINE, cimetidine, codeine, diphenhydrAMINE, droperidol, droperidol/fentaNYL, hydromorphone, hydrOXYzine, levorphanol, lidocaine, meperidine, meperidine/promethazine, midazolam, morphine, nalbuphine, neostigmine, oxymorphone, procaine, prochlorperazine, promazine, promethazine, pyridostigmine, ranitidine, scopolamine, triflupromazine, trimethobenzamide

Y-site compatibilities: Propofol

Solution compatibilities: D₅W, 0.9% NaCl, Ringer's D₅/0.45% NaCl

ADVERSE EFFECTS
CNS: Confusion, anxiety, restlessness, irritability, delusions, hallucinations, headache, sedation, depression, incoherence, dizziness, lethargy, flushing, weakness, **seizures**
CV: Palpitations, tachycardia, postural hypotension, paradoxical bradycardia
EENT: Blurred vision, photophobia, dilated pupils, difficulty swallowing, increased intraocular pressure, mydriasis, cycloplegia
GI: *Dryness of mouth, constipation,* nausea, vomiting, abdominal distress, paralytic ileus, altered taste perception
GU: Hesitancy, retention, impotence
INTEG: Urticaria, allergic reactions
MISC: Suppression of breastfeeding, nasal congestion, decreased sweating, **malignant hyperthermia**
SYST: Anaphylaxis

Pharmacokinetics

Absorption	Well absorbed (PO, SUBCUT, IM)
Distribution	Unknown
Metabolism	Not metabolized
Excretion	Unchanged in feces
Half-life	2 hr

Pharmacodynamics

	PO	IM	IV
Onset	Unknown	15-30 min	Immediate
Peak	1 hr	30-45 min	10-15 min
Duration	8-12 hr	2-7 hr	2-7 hr

INTERACTIONS
Individual drugs
Alcohol, amantadine: increased anticholinergic effect

Drug classifications
Antacids: decreased absorption of glycopyrrolate
Antidepressants (tricyclic), antihistamines, phenothiazines: increased anticholinergic effect
Antidiarrheals: decreased absorption of glycopyrrolate

NURSING CONSIDERATIONS
Assessment
• Monitor I&O ratio; retention commonly causes decreased urinary output; check for urinary hesitation; palpate bladder if retention occurs
• Monitor ECG for ectopic ventricular beats, PVC, tachycardia
• Monitor for bowel sounds; check for constipation; increase fluids, bulk, exercise if constipation occurs
• Assess mental status: affect, mood, CNS depression, worsening of psychiatric symptoms during early therapy

Nursing diagnoses
• Knowledge, deficient (teaching)

Patient/family education
• Caution patient not to operate machinery or engage in hazardous activities if drowsiness, blurred vision occurs
• Advise patient not to take OTC products, cough, cold preparations with alcohol, antihistamines without approval of prescriber
• Teach patient to avoid hot temperature: sweating is decreased, so heat stroke is possible
• Advise patient to notify prescriber of eye pain, blurred vision, light sensitivity
• Caution patient not to discontinue this product abruptly; tapering should be done over 1 wk

Evaluation
Positive therapeutic outcome
• Decreased secretions, bronchial, GI
• Decreased pain in GI disorders
• Reversal of neuromuscular blockade

G

golimumab (Rx)

(goal-lim'yu-mab)
Simponi
Func. class.: Antirheumatic agent (disease modifying), immunomodulator
Chem. class.: Monoclonal antibody, DMARDS, tumor necrosis factor (TNF) modifier
Pregnancy category B

ACTION: Monoclonal antibody specific for human tumor necrosis factor (TNF); elevated levels of TNF are found in patients with rheumatoid arthritis

Therapeutic outcome: Decreased pain, decreased inflammation in joints, better ROM

USES: Rheumatoid arthritis, ankylosing spondylitis, psoriatic arthritis

CONTRAINDICATIONS:

Hypersensitivity active infections

Precautions: Pregnancy **B**, breastfeeding, children, geriatric patients, CNS demyelinating disease, Guillain-Barré syndrome, CHF, hepatitis B carriers, blood dyscrasias, surgery, MS, neurological disease, diabetes, immunosuppression

> **BLACK BOX WARNING:** Infection

DOSAGE AND ROUTES

Adult: SUBCUT 50 mg qmo; for RA give with methotrexate

Available forms: Inj 50 mg/0.5 ml prefilled syringe, SmartJect Auto Injector

Implementation
SUBCUT route
• Visually inspect solution for particulate or discoloration, solution should be clear to slightly opalescent and colorless to slightly yellow; there may be tiny white particles; do not shake
• *SmartJect autoinjector:* Allow to reach room temperature for 30 min prior to use, remove cap, inject within 5 min of removing cap, do not put cap back on, place the open end against the inj site at a 90-degree angle, without pushing button, push the injector firmly against the skin, press the button once and release, listen for the first click, wait for the second click or 15 sec, and remove the injector; do not rub site
• *Prefilled syringe:* Allow to warm to room temperature for 30 min, remove needle cover by pulling straight off, do not twist or recap,

inject within 5 min of needle cover removal, hold the syringe in one hand like a pencil and use the other to pinch the skin, inject needle at a 45-degree angle, push plunger down as far as it will go, keep pressure on the plunger head and remove needle from skin, remove pressure from the plunger head, the needle guard will cover the needle, do not rub site

ADVERSE EFFECTS

CNS: Dizziness, paresthesia, **CNS demyelinating disorder,** weakness
CV: Hypertension, **CHF**
GI: Hepatitis
HEMA: Agranulocytosis, aplastic anemia, leukopenia, polycythemia, thromocytopenia, pancytopenia
INTEG: Psoriasis
MISC: Increased risk of cancer, antibody development to this drug, **risk of infection (TB, invasive fungal infections, other opportunistic infections); may be fatal,** inj site reactions

Pharmacokinetics

Absorption	Unknown
Distribution	Unknown
Metabolism	Unknown
Excretion	Unknown
Half-life	Terminal 2 wk

Pharmacodynamics

Unknown

INTERACTIONS

Individual drugs
Abatacept, adalimumab, anakinra, etanercept, immunosuppressants, infliximab, rilonacept, riuximab: increased infection
Warfarin, cycloSPORINE, theophylline: dosage change may be needed

Drug classifications
Vaccines: do not give concurrently; immunization should be brought up to date before treatment

NURSING CONSIDERATIONS

Assessment
• **Assess for pain,** stiffness, ROM, swelling of joints during treatment
• Check for inj site pain, swelling; usually occur after 2 inj (4-5 days)

BLACK BOX WARNING: Check for infections (fever, flulike symptoms, dyspnea, change in urination, redness/swelling around any wounds), stop treatment if present; some serious infections including sepsis may occur, may be fatal; patients with active infections should not be started on this product

• **Blood dyscrasias:** CBC, differential before and periodically during treatment

Nursing diagnoses
• Activity intolerance (uses)
• Knowledge, deficient (teaching)
• Mobility, impaired physical (uses)
• Pain, chronic (uses)

Patient/family education
• Teach patient about self-administration if appropriate: inj should be made in thigh, abdomen, upper arm; rotate sites at least 1 inch from old site; do not inject in areas that are bruised, red, hard
• Advise patient that if medication is not taken when due, inject next dose as soon as remembered and inject next dose as scheduled

Evaluation
Positive therapeutic outcome
• Decreased inflammation, pain in joints

goserelin (Rx)
(goe′se-rel-lin)
Zoladex
Func. class.: Gonadotropin-releasing hormone, antineoplastic
Chem. class.: Synthetic decapeptide analog of LHRH
Pregnancy category D, X

ACTION: Inhibitor of pituitary gonadotropin secretion; initially increases LH and FSH, with increases in testosterone, reduction in sex steroid levels (substitute serum testosterone levels)

Therapeutic outcome: Decrease in tumor size and spread of malignant cells

USES: Advanced prostate cancer Stage B2-C (10.8 mg); endometriosis, advanced breast cancer, endometrial thinning (3.6 mg)

CONTRAINDICATIONS:
Pregnancy **D** (breast cancer), **X** (endometriosis), breastfeeding, nondiagnosed vaginal bleeding, children, 10.8 mg dose in women, hypersensitivity to LHRH, LHRH-agonist analogs

Precautions: Spinal cord decompression, renal disease, bone mineral density loss

DOSAGE AND ROUTES
Adult: SUBCUT 3.6 mg q4wk (implant) or 10.8 mg q12wk

Endometrial thinning
Adult: SUBCUT 1-2 depot inj; usually 1 depot, surgery performed at 4 wk; if 2 depots, surgery performed 2-4 wk after 2nd depot

Available forms: Depot inj 3.6, 10.8 mg

Implementation
Depot
• Give SUBCUT using implant, inserted by qualified person into upper subcutaneous tissue in abdominal wall q28days or q12wk (10.8 mg), do not attempt to remove air bubbles from syringe

ADVERSE EFFECTS
CNS: Headaches, **spinal cord compression,** anxiety, depression, dizziness, insomnia, lethargy, hot flashes, emotional lability
CV: Dysrhythmia, cerebrovascular accident, hypertension, **MI,** chest pain, **CHF; sudden cardiac death, stroke (men)**
ENDO: Gynecomastia, breast tenderness, hot flashes; hyperglycemia, diabetes (men)
GI: Nausea, vomiting, constipation, diarrhea, ulcer
GU: *Spotting, breakthrough bleeding, decreased libido,* renal insufficiency, urinary obstruction, urinary tract infection, impotence
INTEG: Rash, pain on inj, diaphoresis
MS: Osteoneuralgia
RESP: *COPD, URI*

Pharmacokinetics

Absorption	Well absorbed
Distribution	Unknown
Metabolism	Unknown
Excretion	Unknown
Half-life	$4^{1}/_{2}$ hr

Pharmacodynamics

Onset	Unknown
Peak	14-28 days
Duration	Treatment length

INTERACTIONS

Drug/lab test
Increased: alkaline phosphatase, estradiol, FSH, LH
Decreased: progesterone

NURSING CONSIDERATIONS

Assessment

• Reproductive studies: monitor pelvic ultrasound, pelvic exam, PSA, serum estradiol/testosterone, pregnancy test prior to therapy
• Monitor I&O ratios; palpate bladder for distention in urinary obstruction
• Cancer metastases: monitor for relief of bone pain (back pain), change in motor function
• Blood studies: monitor acid phosphatase; calcium in breast/prostate cancer, hypercalcemia may occur

Nursing diagnoses

• Knowledge, deficient (teaching)
• Sexual dysfunction (uses)

Patient/family education

• Caution patient that gynecomastia and postmenopausal symptoms may occur but will decrease after treatment is discontinued; that bone pain may increase, then decrease
• Teach patient to contact prescriber for difficulty urinating, hot flashes occur during treatment
• Advise patient not to breastfeed while taking product; use effective nonhormonal contraception

Evaluation

Positive therapeutic outcome

• More normal levels of PSA, acid phosphatase, alkaline phosphatase; testosterone level of <25 mg/dl

---

granisetron (Rx)

(grane-iss'e-tron)
Granisol, Kytril, Sancuso
Func. class.: Antiemetic
Chem. class.: 5-HT₃ receptor antagonist
Pregnancy category B

ACTION: Prevents nausea, vomiting by blocking serotonin peripherally, centrally, and in the small intestine

Therapeutic outcome: Absence of nausea and vomiting

USES: Prevention of nausea, vomiting associated with cancer chemotherapy including high-dose CISplatin, radiation

Unlabeled uses: Acute nausea, vomiting after surgery

CONTRAINDICATIONS:

Hypersensitivity to this product or benzyl alcohol

Precautions: Pregnancy **B**, breastfeeding, children, geriatric, ondansetron/palonosetron/dolasetron hypersensitivity, cardiac dysrhythmias, cardiac/hepatic disease, electrolyte imbalances

DOSAGE AND ROUTES

Nausea, vomiting in chemotherapy

Adult and child ≥2 yr: **IV** 10 mcg/kg over 5 min, 30 min before the start of cancer chemotherapy, TD apply 1 patch (3.1 mg/24 hr) to upper arm 24-48 hr before chemotherapy; patch may be worn up to 7 days
Adult: PO 1 mg bid, give 1st dose 1 hr before chemotherapy and next dose 12 hr after 1st or 2 mg as a single dose anytime within 1 hr prior to chemotherapy

Nausea, vomiting in radiation therapy

Adult: PO 2 mg/day 1 hr prior to radiation

Available forms: Inj 1 mg/ml; tabs 1 mg, oral sol 2 mg/10 ml; patch TD 3.1 mg/24 hr

Implementation

IV route
• May give undiluted over 30 sec via Y-site
IV intermittent infusion route
• Dilute in 0.9% NaCl for inj or D₅W (20-50 ml), give over 5-15 min, ½ hr prior to chemotherapy
• Store at room temp for 24-hr dilution

Y-site compatibilities: Acyclovir, allopurinol, amifostine, amikacin, aminophylline, amphotericin B cholesteryl, ampicillin, ampicillin/sulbactam, amsacrine, aztreonam, bleomycin, bumetanide, buprenorphine, butorphanol, calcium gluconate, CARBOplatin, carmustine, ceFAZolin, cefepime, cefonicid, cefoperazone, cefotaxime, cefotetan, cefoxitin, ceftazidime, ceftizoxime, cefTRIAXone, cefuroxime, chlorproMAZINE, cimetidine, ciprofloxacin, CISplatin, cladribine, clindamycin, cyclophosphamide, cytarabine, dacarbazine, DACTINomycin, DAUNOrubicin, dexamethasone, diphenhydrAMINE, DOBUTamine, DOPamine, DOXOrubicin, DOXOrubicin liposome, doxycycline, droperidol, enalaprilat, etoposide, famotidine, filgrastim, floxuridine, fluconazole, fluorouracil, fludarabine, furosemide, gallium, ganciclovir, gentamicin, haloperidol, heparin, hydrocortisone, HYDROmorphone, hydrOXYzine, IDArubicin, ifosfamide, imipenem-cilastatin, leucovorin, LORazepam, magnesium sulfate, melphalan, meperidine, mesna, methotrexate, methylPREDNISolone, metoclopramide, metroNIDAZOLE, mezlocillin, miconazole, minocycline, mito-mycin, mitoxantrone, morphine, nalbuphine, netilmicin, ofloxacin, paclitaxel, piperacillin, piperacillin/tazobactam, plicamycin, potassium chloride, prochlorperazine, promethazine, propofol, ranitidine, sargramostim, sodium bicarbonate, streptozocin, teniposide, thiotepa, ticarcillin, ticarcillin/clavulanate, tobramycin, trimethoprim/sulfamethoxazole, vancomycin, vinBLAStine, vinCRIStine, vinorelbine, zidovudine

Y-site incompatibilities: Amphotericin B coloidal, diazepam, phenytoin

Additive compatibilities: Dexamethasone, methylPREDNISolone

Solution compatibilities: D$_5$W, 0.9% NaCl

Transdermal route
• Apply to dry, clean, intact skin of upper, outer arm 24 hr prior to chemotherapy; firmly press on skin; keep on during chemotherapy; can bathe; avoid swimming, whirlpool; remove ≥24 hr after chemotherapy

ADVERSE EFFECTS
CNS: *Headache, asthenia,* anxiety, dizziness
CV: Hypertension, QT prolongation
GI: Diarrhea, *constipation,* increased AST, ALT, *nausea*
HEMA: **Leukopenia,** anemia, **thrombocytopenia**
MISC: Rash, **bronchospasm**

Pharmacokinetics

Absorption	Unknown
Distribution	Unknown
Metabolism	Liver
Excretion	Unknown
Half-life	10-12 hr

Pharmacodynamics
Unknown

INTERACTIONS
Individual drugs
Amoxapine, chloroquine, clozapine, dasatinib, dolasetron, dronedarone, droperidol, erythromycin, flecainide, haloperidol, lapatinib, maprotiline, methadone, octreotide, ondansetron, palonosetron, pentamidine, pimozide, propafenone, ranolazine, risperidone, sertindole, sunitinib, tacrolimus, telithromycin, troleandomycin, vardenafil, vorinostat, ziprasidone: increased QT prolongation

Drug classifications
Antipsychotics: increased EPS
β-blockers, class I, III antidysrhythmics, halogenated/local anesthetics, phenothiazines, tricyclics: increased QT prolongation

NURSING CONSIDERATIONS
Assessment
• Assess patient for absence of nausea, vomiting during chemotherapy
• **Assess patient for hypersensitive reaction:** rash, bronchospasm

Nursing diagnoses
• Fluid volume, deficient (uses)
• Knowledge, deficient (teaching)

Patient/family education
• Advise patient to report diarrhea, constipation, rash, or changes in respirations

Evaluation
Positive therapeutic outcome
• Absence of nausea, vomiting during cancer chemotherapy

---

guaiFENesin (Rx, OTC)
(gwye-fen'e-sin)
Alfen, Altarussin, Balminil ✦, Bidex, Diabetic Tussin, Elix Sure EX, Equaline Non-Drowsy Tussin, Equate Tussin Cough, Ganidin NR, Good Sense Mucus Relief, Good Sense Tussin Chest Congestion, Guaifenesin NR, Guiatuss, Humibid, Iophen NR, Liquibid, Miltuss EX, Mucinex, Mucinex Children's Mucus Relief, Mucinex Junior Strength, Naldecon Senior EX, Organ-1 NR, Organidin NR, Q-Tussin, Robafen, Robitussin Guaifenesin ✦, Scot-Tussin Expectorant, Siltussin DAS, Siltussin SA, Top Care Children's Mucus Relief, Top Care Tussin Chest Congestion Solution, Wal-Tussin Expectorant, XPect
Func. class.: Expectorant
Pregnancy category C

ACTION: Increases the volume and reduces the viscosity of secretions in the trachea and bronchi to facilitate secretion removal

Therapeutic outcome: Decreased cough

USES: Productive and nonproductive cough

CONTRAINDICATIONS:
Hypersensitivity, chronic persistent cough

Precautions: Pregnancy **C**, breastfeeding, CHF, asthma, emphysema, fever

DOSAGE AND ROUTES
Adult and child ≥12 yr: PO 200-400 mg q4hr, or EXT REL 600-1200 mg q12hr; max 2.4 g/day
Child 6-11 yr: PO 100-200 mg q4hr or EXT REL 600 mg q12hr; max 1.2 g/day
Child 2-5 yr: PO: 50-100 mg q4hr; max 600 mg/day, EXT REL 300 mg q12hr, max 600 mg/day

Available forms: Tabs 200, 400 mg; ext rel tabs 600, 1200 mg; syr 100 mg/5 ml; oral sol 100 mg/5 ml; oral granules 50, 100 mg/packet

Implementation
• Store at room temperature; provide room humidification to assist with liquefying secretions
• Avoid fluids for 1/2 hr after administration

ADVERSE EFFECTS
CNS: Drowsiness, headache, dizziness
GI: Nausea, anorexia, vomiting, diarrhea

Pharmacokinetics

Absorption	Well absorbed
Distribution	Unknown
Metabolism	Unknown
Excretion	Unknown
Half-life	1 hr

Pharmacodynamics

	PO	PO–EXT REL
Onset	1/2 hr	Unknown
Peak	Unknown	Unknown
Duration	4-6 hr	12 hr

NURSING CONSIDERATIONS
Assessment
• **Assess cough:** type, frequency, character, including characteristics of sputum; lung sounds bilaterally; fluids should be increased to 2 L/day to decrease secretion viscosity (thickness)

Nursing diagnoses
• Airway clearance, ineffective (uses)
• Knowledge, deficient (teaching)

Patient/family education
• Caution patient to avoid driving, other hazardous activities if drowsiness occurs (rare)

• Advise patient to avoid smoking, smoke-filled rooms, perfumes, dust, environmental pollutants, cleansers
• Instruct patient to notify prescriber if dry, nonproductive cough lasts over 7 days

Evaluation
Positive therapeutic outcome
• Absence of dry cough
• Thinner, more productive cough that raises secretions

---

halcinonide topical
See Appendix B

haloperidol (Rx)
(hal-oh-pehr'ih-dol)
Apo-Haloperidol ✤
haloperidol decanoate (Rx)
Haldol Decanoate
haloperidol lactate (Rx)
Haldol
Func. class.: Antipsychotic/neuroleptic
Chem. class.: Butyrophenone
Pregnancy category C

Do not confuse:
haloperidol/Halotestin, **Haldol**/Stadol

ACTION: Depresses cerebral cortex, hypothalamus, limbic system, which control activity and aggression; blocks neurotransmission produced by dopamine at synapse; exhibits strong α-adrenergic, anticholinergic blocking action; mechanism for antipsychotic effects unclear

Therapeutic outcome: Decreased signs and symptoms of psychosis

USES: Psychotic disorders, control of tics, vocal utterances in Tourette's syndrome, short-term treatment of hyperactive children showing excessive motor activity, prolonged parenteral therapy in chronic schizophrenia, organic mental syndrome with psychotic features, hiccups (short-term), emergency sedation of severely agitated or delirious patients, ADHD

Unlabeled uses: Nausea, vomiting in surgery, autism, migraine headache

CONTRAINDICATIONS:
Children <3 yr, hypersensitivity, blood dyscrasias, coma, brain damage, bone marrow depression, alcohol and barbiturate withdrawal states,

---

Parkinson's disease, angina, epilepsy, urinary retention, closed-angle glaucoma

Precautions: Pregnancy **C**, breastfeeding, geriatric, seizure disorders, hypertension, hepatic/cardiac/pulmonary disease

> **BLACK BOX WARNING:** Dementia

DOSAGE AND ROUTES

Acute psychosis
Adult: IM/IV (lactate) 2-10 mg, may repeat q1hr, convert to **PO** as soon as possible, **PO** should be 150% of total parenteral dose required
Child 6-12 yr: IM/IV (lactate) (unlabeled) 1-3 mg q4-8hr, max 0.15 mg/kg/day, switch to **PO** as soon as possible

Chronic schizophrenia
Adult: IM (decanoate) 50-100 mg q4wk, max 100 mg for 1st inj
Child 3-12 yr: PO/IM 0.05-0.15 mg/kg/day

Tourette's syndrome
Adult and adolescent: PO 0.5-2 mg bid-tid, increased until desired response occurs
Child 3-12 yr or weighing 15-40 kg: PO 0.25-0.5 mg/day in 2-3 divided doses, increase by 0.25-0.5 mg q5-7days, max 0.15 mg/kg/day

ADHD
Child 3-12 yr: PO 0.25-0.5 mg/day in 2-3 divided doses, may increase by 0.025-0.5 mg q5-7days; maintenance 0.01-0.03 mg/kg/day as a single dose

Autism (unlabeled)
Child: PO 0.04 mg/kg/day or 1-3 mg/day, max 4 mg/day

Migraine (unlabeled)
Adult: PO/IM (lactate) 5 mg at onset, may repeat once

Available forms: Tabs 0.5, 1, 2, 5, 10, 20 mg, *lactate:* oral sol 2 mg/ml; inj 5 mg/ml; *decanoate:* 50 mg/ml, 100 mg/ml

Implementation
PO route
• Give product in liquid form mixed in glass of juice or caffeine-free cola if hoarding is suspected; do not mix in caffeine drinks, tannics, pectins
• Give decreased dosage in geriatric because of slower metabolism
• Give PO with full glass of water, milk; or give with food to decrease GI upset
• Give antacids 2 hr before or after this product

• Store in tight, light-resistant container; oral sol in amber bottle
IM route
• Inject in deep muscle mass, do not give SUBCUT; use 21-gauge 2-in needle; do not administer sol with a precipitate; give <3 ml per inj site; give slowly, may be painful
• Patient should remain lying down after IM inj for at least 30 min
IV route (lactate)
• Give undiluted for psychotic episode at 5 mg/min
Intermittent IV infusion route
• Give after dilution in 30-50 ml of D_5W, run over $^1/_2$ hr

Y-site compatibilities: Amifostine, amsacrine, aztreonam, cimetidine, cisatracurium, cladribine, DOBUTamine, DOPamine, DOXOrubicin liposome, famotidine, filgrastim, fludarabine, granisetron, lidocaine, LORazepam, melphalan, midazolam, nitroglycerin, norepinephrine, ondansetron, paclitaxel, phenylephrine, propofol, remifentanil, SUFentanil, tacrolimus, teniposide, theophylline, thiotepa, vinorelbine

Y-site incompatibilities: Fluconazole, foscarnet, heparin, sargramostim

ADVERSE EFFECTS
CNS: *EPS, pseudoparkinsonism, akathisia, dystonia, tardive dyskinesia, drowsiness, headache,* **seizures, neuroleptic malignant syndrome,** confusion
CV: *Orthostatic hypotension,* hypertension, **cardiac arrest,** ECG changes, **tachycardia, QT prolongation, sudden death**
EENT: Blurred vision, glaucoma, dry eyes
GI: *Dry mouth, nausea, vomiting, anorexia, constipation,* diarrhea, jaundice, weight gain, **ileus, hepatitis**
GU: Urinary retention, urinary frequency, dysuria, enuresis, impotence, amenorrhea, gynecomastia
INTEG: *Rash,* photosensitivity, dermatitis
RESP: **Laryngospasm,** dyspnea, **respiratory depression**
SYST: Risk of death (dementia)

H

Pharmacokinetics

Absorption	Well absorbed (PO, IM); decanoate (IM) absorbed slowly
Distribution	High concentrations in liver, crosses placenta, protein binding 92%
Metabolism	Liver, extensively
Excretion	Kidneys, breast milk
Half-life	Terminal half-life 12-36 hr (metabolized)

Pharmacodynamics

	PO	IM	IM (decanoate)
Onset	Erratic	$^1/_2$ hr	3-9 days
Peak	2-6 hr	30-45 min	4-11 days
Duration	8-12 hr	4-8 hr	3 wk

INTERACTIONS

Individual drugs

Alcohol: increased effects of both products, oversedation

Amoxapine, chloroquine, clozapine, dasatinib, dolasetron, dronedarone, droperidol, erythromycin, flecainide, lapatinib, maprotiline, methadone, octreotide, ondansetron, palonosetron, pentamidine, pimozide, propafenone, ranolazine, risperidone, sertindole, sunitinib, tacrolimus, telithromycin, troleandomycin, vardenafil, vorinostat, ziprasidone: increased QT prolongation

CarBAMazepine: decreased effects of haloperidol

EPINEPHrine: increased toxicity

Levodopa: decreased effects of levodopa

Lithium: increased toxicity; decreased effects of lithium

PHENobarbital: decreased effects of haloperidol

Drug classifications

Anticholinergics: increased anticholinergic effects

Barbiturate anesthetics: oversedation

β-Adrenergic blockers: increased effects of both products

Class IA, III antidysrhythmics, halogenated/local anesthetics, phenothiazines, tricyclics, β-blockers: increased QT prolongation

CNS depressants: oversedation

SSRIs, SNRIs: increased serotonin syndrome, increased neuroleptic malignant syndrome

Drug/lab test

Increased: liver function tests, cardiac enzymes, cholesterol, blood glucose, prolactin, bilirubin, PBI, cholinesterase, alkaline phosphatase

Decreased: hormones (blood and urine), protime

False positive: pregnancy tests, PKU

False negative: urinary steroids

NURSING CONSIDERATIONS

Assessment

> **BLACK BOX WARNING:** Assess for dementia, affect, orientation, LOC, reflexes, gait, coordination, sleep pattern disturbances

• Assess mental status: orientation, mood, behavior, presence and type of hallucinations before initial administration and monthly; this product should significantly reduce psychotic behavior

• Check for swallowing of PO medication; check for hoarding and for giving medication to other patients

• Monitor I&O ratio; palpate bladder if low urinary output occurs, especially in geriatric; urinalysis is recommended before, during prolonged therapy

• Monitor bilirubin, CBC, liver function tests monthly

• Assess affect, orientation, LOC, reflexes, gait, coordination, sleep pattern disturbances

• Monitor B/P with patient sitting, standing, and lying; take pulse and respirations q4hr during initial treatment; establish baseline before starting treatment; report drops of ≥30 mm Hg; obtain baseline ECG, Q-wave and T-wave changes

• Check for dizziness, faintness, palpitations, tachycardia on rising; severe orthostatic hypotension is common

• **Assess for neuroleptic malignant syndrome:** hyperpyrexia, muscle rigidity, increased CPK, altered mental status; product should be discontinued immediately; if seizures, hypo/hypertension, tachycardia occur, notify prescriber immediately

• **Assess for EPS** including akathisia (inability to sit still, no pattern to movements), tardive dyskinesia (bizarre movements of the jaw, mouth, tongue, extremities), pseudoparkinsonism (ragged tremors, pill rolling, shuffling gait); an antiparkinsonian product should be prescribed

• Assess for constipation and urinary retention daily; if these occur, increase bulk, water in diet

Nursing diagnoses
* Coping, ineffective (uses)
* Knowledge, deficient (teaching)
* Noncompliance (teaching)

Patient/family education
* Teach patient to use good oral hygiene; use frequent rinsing of mouth, sugarless gum for dry mouth; oral candidiasis may occur
* Advise patient to avoid hazardous activities until product response is determined; dizziness, blurred vision are common
* Inform patient that orthostatic hypotension occurs often and to rise from sitting or lying position gradually; tell patient to avoid hot tubs, hot showers, tub baths, since hypotension may occur; tell patient that in hot weather heat stroke may occur; take extra precautions to stay cool
* Instruct patient to avoid abrupt withdrawal of this product, or EPS may result; product should be withdrawn slowly
* Caution patient to avoid OTC preparations (cough, hay fever, cold) unless approved by prescriber, since serious product interactions may occur; avoid use with alcohol, CNS depressants since increased drowsiness may occur
* Advise patient to use a sunscreen and sunglasses to prevent burns
* Tell patient to report impaired vision, jaundice, muscle twitching

Evaluation
Positive therapeutic outcome
* Decrease in emotional excitement, hallucinations, delusions, paranoia, reorganization of patterns of thought, speech; improvement in specific behaviors

TREATMENT OF OVERDOSE:
Lavage if orally ingested; provide airway; *do not induce vomiting*

> **⚠ HIGH ALERT**

heparin (Rx)
(hep'a-rin)
Hepalean ✢, Heparin Leo ✢, Hep-Lock, Hep-Lock U/P, Monoject Prefill
Func. class.: Anticoagulant, antithrombotic
Pregnancy category C

Do not confuse:
heparin/Hespan

ACTION: Prevents conversion of fibrinogen to fibrin and prothrombin to thrombin by enhancing inhibitory effects of antithrombin III

Therapeutic outcome: Prevention of thrombi

USES: Prevention of deep vein thrombosis (DVT) and pulmonary emboli (PE) (treatment and prevention), MI, open heart surgery, disseminated intravascular clotting syndrome, atrial fibrillation with embolization; as an anticoagulant in transfusion and dialysis procedures; to maintain patency of indwelling venipuncture devices; diagnosis, treatment of disseminated intravascular coagulation (DIC)

CONTRAINDICATIONS:
Hypersensitivity, hemophilia, leukemia with bleeding, peptic ulcer disease, severe thrombocytopenic purpura, renal/hepatic disease (severe), blood dyscrasias, severe hypertension, subacute bacterial endocarditis, acute nephritis; benzyl alcohol products in neonates, infants, pregnancy, lactation

Precautions: Pregnancy C, children, geriatric, alcoholism, hyperlipidemia, diabetes, renal disease

DOSAGE AND ROUTES
Deep vein thrombosis/pulmonary embolism
Adult: **IV BOL** 80 international units/kg, then maintenance **IV INF** 18 international units/kg/hr; if aPTT <35 (1.2×normal), increase **IV INF** rate by 4 international units/kg/hr and rebolus with 80 international units/kg; if aPTT 35-45 (1.2-1.5 × normal), increase **IV INF** by 2 international units/kg/hr and rebolus with 40 international units/kg; if aPTT 46-70 (1.5-2.3 × normal), maintain **IV INF;** if aPTT 71-90 (2.3-3 × normal), decrease **IV INF** by 2 international units/kg/hr; if aPTT >90 (>3 × normal), hold **IV INF** for 1 hr, then decrease rate 3 international units/kg/hr
Child/infant/neonate: **IV** loading dose 75 international units/kg
Child >1 yr: 20 international units/kg/hr, **infant, neonates <1 yr:** 28 international units/kg/hr as initial maintenance dose

Thrombosis prophylaxis (open heart/CV surgery)
Adult: **IV** ≥150 international units/kg, procedures <60 min up to 300 international units/kg, procedures >60 min up to 400 international units/kg, based on ACT

Thrombosis prophylaxis (PCI, not receiving abciximab)
Adult: IV BOL weight-adjusted with 60-100 international units/kg, maintain ACT within 250-300 sec (HemoTec) or 300-350 sec (Hemochron)
Child/infant/neonate: IV BOL 100-150 international units/kg

Prophylaxis for DVT/PE
Adult: SUBCUT 5000 units q8-12hr

IV catheter occlusion prophylaxis
Adult and child: IV 10-100 units/ml
Infant <10 kg: IV 10 units/ml

Available forms: Sol for inj 10, 100, 1000, 5000, 7500, 10,000, 20,000, 40,000 units/ml; premixed 1000 units/500 ml, 2000 units/1000 ml, 12,500 units/250 ml, 25,000 units/250 ml, 25,000 units/500 ml; lock flush preparations 10 units/ml

Implementation
• Give at same time each day to maintain steady blood levels
• Cannot be used interchangeably (unit for unit) with LMWHs or heparinoids
SUBCUT route
• Give SUBCUT with at least 25-G ³/₈-in needle; do not massage area or aspirate fluid when giving SUBCUT inj; give in abdomen between pelvic bones, rotate sites; leave in for 10 sec; apply gentle pressure for 1 min
• Changing needles is not recommended
Heparin lock route
• **Do not mistake heparin sodium injection 10,000 units/ml and Hep-Lock U/P 10 units/ml; they have similar blue labeling; deaths in pediatric patients have occurred when heparin sodium injection vials were confused with heparin flush vials**
• Inject 10-100 units/0.5-1 ml after each inf or q8-12hr

Direct IV route
• Give loading dose undiluted over ≥1 min; use before continuous infusion
Continuous IV infusion route
• Dilute 25,000 units/250-500 ml 0.9% NaCl or D₅W (50-100 units/ml); some solutions are premixed and ready for use
• When product is added to inf sol for cont **IV**, invert container at least 6 × to ensure adequate mixing

Y-site compatibilities: Acyclovir, aldesleukin, allopurinol, amifostine, aminophylline, ampicillin, ampicillin/sulbactam, atracurium, atropine, aztreonam, betamethasone, bleomycin, calcium gluconate, ceFAZolin, cefotetan, ceftazidime, cefTRIAXone, cephalothin, cephapirin, chlordiazepoxide, chlorproMAZINE, cimetidine, CISplatin, cladribine, clindamycin, conjugated estrogens, cyanocobalamin, cyclophosphamide, cytarabine, dexamethasone, digoxin, diphenhydrAMINE, DOPamine, DOXOrubicin liposome, edrophonium, enalaprilat, EPINEPHrine, erythromycin, esmolol, ethacrynate, famotidine, fentaNYL, fluconazole, fludarabine, fluorouracil, foscarnet, furosemide, gallium, granisetron, hydrALAZINE, hydrocortisone, HYDROmorphone, regular insulin, isoproterenol, kanamycin, leucovorin, lidocaine, LORazepam, magnesium sulfate, melphalan, menadiol sodium, meperidine, meropenem, methicillin, methotrexate, methoxamine, methyldopate, methylergonovine, metoclopramide, metroNIDAZOLE, midazolam, milrinone, minocycline, mitomycin, morphine, nafcillin, neostigmine, nitroglycerin, nitroprusside, norepinephrine, ondansetron, oxacillin, oxytocin, paclitaxel, pancuronium, penicillin G potassium, pentazocine, phytonadione, piperacillin, piperacillin/tazobactam, propofol, potassium chloride, prednisoLONE, procainamide, prochlorperazine, propofol, propranolol, pyridostigmine, ranitidine, remifentanil, sargramostim, scopolamine, sodium bicarbonate, streptokinase, succinylcholine, tacrolimus, teniposide, theophylline, thiopental, thiotepa, ticarcillin, ticarcillin/clavulanate, trimethobenzamide, vecuronium, vinBLAStine, vinorelbine, warfarin, zidovudine

Y-site incompatibilities: Alteplase, ciprofloxacin, dacarbazine, diazepam, DOBUTamine, DOXOrubicin, ergotamine, gentamicin, haloperidol, IDArubicin, methotrimeprazine, phenytoin, promethazine, tobramycin, triflupromazine

Additive compatibilities: Aminophylline, amphotericin, ascorbic acid, bleomycin, calcium gluconate, cefepime, cephapirin, chloramphenicol, clindamycin, colistimethate, dimenhyDRINATE, doxacillin, DOPamine, enalaprilat, erythromycin, esmolol, floxacillin, fluconazole, flumazenil, furosemide, hydrocortisone, isoproterenol, lidocaine, lincomycin, magnesium sulfate, meropenem, methyldopate, methylPREDNISolone, metronidazole/sodium bicarbonate, nafcillin, norepinephrine, octreotide, penicillin G, potassium chloride, prednisoLONE, promazine, ranitidine, sodium bicarbonate, verapamil, vit B complex, vit B complex with C

Additive incompatibilities: Amikacin, erythromycin lactobionate, gentamicin, kanamycin, meperidine, methadone, morphine, polymyxin B, streptomycin

ADVERSE EFFECTS

CNS: *Fever,* chills, headache
GU: Hematuria
HEMA: Hemorrhage, thrombocytopenia, anemia
INTEG: *Rash,* dermatitis, urticaria, pruritus, delayed transient alopecia, hematoma, cutaneous necrosis (SUBCUT)
SYST: Anaphylaxis

Pharmacokinetics

Absorption	Well absorbed (SUBCUT)
Distribution	Unknown
Metabolism	Partially in kidney, liver
Excretion	Lymph, spleen, in urine (<50% unchanged)
Half-life	1½ hr

Pharmacodynamics

	SUBCUT	IV
Onset	½-1 hr	5 min
Peak	2 hr	10 min
Duration	8-12 hr	2-6 hr

INTERACTIONS

Individual drugs
Dextran, dipyridole, ticlopidine, clopidogrel, presgrel: increased action of heparin
Digoxin: decreased action of heparin
Nicotine: decreased action of heparin

Drug classifications
Anticoagulants (oral), cephalosporins, NSAIDs, penicillins, platelet inhibitors, salicylates, antineoplastics, SSRIs, SNRIs: increased action of heparin
Antihistamines, tetracyclines, cardiac glycosides: decreased action of heparin
Corticosteroids, decreased action of corticosteroids

Drug/lab test
Increased: ALT, AST, INR, pro-time, PTT, potassium
Decreased: platelets, triglycerides, cholesterol, plasma free fatty acids

NURSING CONSIDERATIONS

Assessment
• Assess for blood studies (Hct, occult blood in stools) q3mo if patient is on long-term therapy
• Monitor PPT, which should be 1½-2 × control, PTT; often done daily, APTT, ACT

• Monitor platelet count q2-3day; thrombocytopenia may occur on fourth day of treatment and resolve, or continue to eighth day of treatment
⚠ **Bleeding, hemorrhage: Assess for bleeding gums, petechiae, ecchymosis, black tarry stools, hematuria, epistaxis, decrease in Hct, B/P; notify prescriber immediately; HIT may occur after product discontinuation**
• **Monitor for hypersensitivity:** fever, skin rash, urticaria; notify prescriber immediately

Nursing diagnoses
• Injury, risk for (uses, adverse reactions)
• Knowledge, deficient (teaching)

Patient/family education
• Advise patient to avoid OTC preparations that may cause serious product interactions unless directed by prescriber; may contain aspirin or other anticoagulants
• Tell patient that product may be withheld during active bleeding (menstruation), depending on condition
• Caution patient to use soft-bristle toothbrush to avoid bleeding gums; avoid contact sports; use electric razor; avoid IM inj
• Instruct patient to carry/wear emergency ID or other identification identifying product taken and condition treated
• Advise patient to report any signs of bleeding: gums, under skin, urine, stools; or unusual bruising even after discontinuing product

Evaluation
Positive therapeutic outcome
• Decrease of DVT
• PTT of 1.5-2.5 × control
• Free-flowing **IV**

TREATMENT OF OVERDOSE:
Withdraw product, give protamine sulfate 1 mg protamine/100 units heparin

hepatitis B immune globulin (Rx)
(hep-a-tite'iss)
HepaGam B, Hyper HEP B S/D, Nabi-HB
Func. class.: Immune globulin
Pregnancy category C

ACTION: Provides passive immunity to hepatitis B

Therapeutic outcome: Passive immunity to hepatitis B

USES: Prevention of hepatitis B virus in exposed patients, including passive immunity in neonates born to HBsAg-positive mothers, prevention of hepatitis B recurrence after liver transplant in HBsAg-positive patients

CONTRAINDICATIONS:
Hypersensitivity to immune globulins, coagulation disorders

Precautions: Pregnancy **C**, breastfeeding, children, geriatric, hemophilia, active infection, IgA deficiency

DOSAGE AND ROUTES
Adult and child: IM 0.06 ml/kg (usual 3-5 ml) within 7 days of exposure; repeat 28 days after exposure, if patient wishes not to receive the hepatitis B vaccine

Prevention of hepatitis B infection recurrence after liver transplant
Adult: IV (HepaGam B only) 20,000 international units concurrent with grafting transplanted liver, then 20,000 international units/day on days 1-7, then 20,000 international units q2wk starting on day 14, then 20,000 international units q mo, starting on month 4

Neonates born to hepatitis B surface antigen–positive mothers: IM 0.5 ml within 12 hr of birth

Available forms: Inj 1-, 4-, 5-ml vials; neonatal syringe 0.5 ml; HepaGam B sol for inj 312 units/ml; Hyper HEP B S/D 217 units/ml

Implementation
IM route
• After rotating vial, do not shake
• Only with EPINEPHrine 1:1000 on unit to treat laryngospasm
• In deltoid for better absorption (adult)

IV route (Hepa Gam B only)
• Calculate volume needed for each 20,000 international units dose by using measured potency of each lot, potency is stamped on label
• Promptly use after vial is entered, discard unused product
• Give at 2 ml/min through separate IV line, use inf pump, decrease to 1 ml/min, if infusion-related event occurs, patient becomes uncomfortable

ADVERSE EFFECTS
CNS: Headache, dizziness, fever
GI: Nausea, vomiting
INTEG: Soreness at inj site, urticaria, erythema, swelling

SYST: Induration, **anaphylaxis, angio-edema**

Pharmacokinetics
Absorption	Slowly absorbed
Distribution	Unknown
Metabolism	Unknown
Excretion	Unknown
Half-life	3 wk

Pharmacodynamics
Onset	1-7 days
Peak	3-10 days
Duration	2-6 mo

INTERACTIONS
Drug classifications
MMR, rotavirus vaccines, varicella: do not use within 3 mo of hepatitis B immune globulin

NURSING CONSIDERATIONS
Assessment
• Assess for history of allergies, skin conditions (eczema, psoriasis, dermatitis), reactions to vaccinations
• Assess for skin reactions: rash, induration, urticaria
• Assess for sneezing, pruritus, angioedema, dysphagia, vomiting, abdominal pain
⚠ Assess for anaphylaxis: inability to breathe, bronchospasm, hypotension, wheezing, diaphoresis, fever, flushing; epinephrine and emergency equipment should be available

Nursing diagnoses
• Infection, risk for (uses)
• Knowledge, deficient (teaching)

Patient/family education
• Teach patient purpose of product and expected results
• Give patient a list of adverse reactions that need to be reported immediately: wheezing, vomiting, sneezing, abdominal pain, sweating, tightness in chest
• Advise patient that pain, rash, swelling at inj site can be expected
• Give patient written record of immunization

Evaluation
Positive therapeutic outcome
• Prevention of hepatitis B

homatropine ophthalmic
See Appendix B

⚠ Nurse Alert

hydrALAZINE (Rx)
(hye-dral'a-zeen)
Apresoline, Apo-HydrALAZINE
Func. class.: Antihypertensive, direct-acting peripheral vasodilator
Chem. class.: Phthalazine
Pregnancy category C

Do not confuse:
hydrALAZINE/hydrOXYzine,
Apresoline/allopurinol

ACTION: Vasodilates arterioles in smooth muscle by direct relaxation; reduces B/P with reflex increases in heart rate, stroke volume, cardiac output

Therapeutic outcome: Decreased B/P in hypertension, decreased afterload in CHF

USES: Essential hypertension, severe essential hypertension

Unlabeled uses: CHF

CONTRAINDICATIONS:
Hypersensitivity to hydrALAZINEs, mitral valvular rheumatic heart disease, CAD

Precautions: Pregnancy **C**, breastfeeding, geriatric, CVA, advanced renal disease, liver disease, SLE, dissecting aortic aneurysm

DOSAGE AND ROUTES
Hypertension
Adult: PO 10 mg qid 2-4 days, then 25 mg for rest of 1st wk, then 50 mg qid individualized to desired response; max 300 mg/day
Child: PO 0.75-1 mg/kg/day in 2-4 divided doses; max 25 mg/dose, increase over 3-4 wk to max 7.5 mg/kg/day or 200 mg, whichever is less

Hypertensive crisis
Adult: IV BOL 10-20 mg q4-6hr; administer PO as soon as possible; IM 10-50 mg q4-6hr
Child: IV BOL 0.1-0.6 mg/kg q4hr; IM 0.1-0.6 mg/kg q4-6hr, max 1.7-3.5 mg/kg/day

CHF
Adult: PO 10-25 mg bid, max 75 mg tid

Available forms: Inj 20 mg/ml; tabs 10, 25, 50, 100 mg

Implementation
PO route
• Give with meals to enhance absorption
• Store protected from light and heat

Direct IV route
• Give by **IV** undiluted through Y-tube or 3-way stopcock, give each 10 mg over 1 min or more
• Administer with patient in recumbent position; keep in that position for 1 hr after administration

Y-site compatibilities: Heparin, hydrocortisone, potassium chloride, verapamil, vit B/C

Y-site incompatibilities: Aminophylline, ampicillin, diazoxide, furosemide, paclitaxel

ADVERSE EFFECTS
CNS: *Headache, tremors, dizziness, anxiety,* peripheral neuritis, depression, fever, chills
CV: *Palpitations, reflex tachycardia, angina,* **shock,** rebound hypertension, orthostatic hypotension
GI: *Nausea, vomiting, anorexia, diarrhea,* constipation, paralytic ileus
GU: Urinary retention, glomerulonephritis, hematuria
HEMA: Leukopenia, **agranulocytosis,** anemia, **thrombocytopenia**
INTEG: Rash, pruritus, urticaria
MISC: Nasal congestion, muscle cramps, *lupuslike symptoms,* flushing, edema, dyspnea

Pharmacokinetics

Absorption	Rapidly absorbed (PO); well absorbed (IM); completely absorbed (**IV**)
Distribution	Widely distributed; crosses placenta
Metabolism	GI mucosa, liver extensively
Excretion	Kidneys, urine (12%-14%)
Half-life	2-8 hr

Pharmacodynamics

	PO	IM	IV
Onset	½ hr	10-30 min	5-20 min
Peak	1-2 hr	1 hr	10-80 min
Duration	6-12 hr	4-6 hr	4-6 hr

INTERACTIONS
Individual drugs
Alcohol, levodopa: increased hypotension
Indomethacin: decreased effects of hydrALAZINE

Drug classifications
β-Adrenergic blockers: increased effects
MAOIs: severe hypotension
Other antihypertensives, thiazide diuretics: increased hypotension

Adverse effects: *italics* = common; **bold** = life-threatening

Sympathomimetics (EPINEPHrine, norepineph-rine): increased tachycardia, angina
NSAIDs, estrogens: decreased hydrALAZINE effects

NURSING CONSIDERATIONS

Assessment
• Assess cardiac status: B/P q5min for 2 hr, then qhr for 2 hr, then q4hr; pulse, jugular venous distention q4hr
• Monitor electrolytes, blood studies: potassium, sodium, chloride, carbon dioxide, CBC, serum glucose; LE prep, ANA titer before starting treatment
• Monitor weight daily, I&O; check for edema in feet, legs daily; check skin turgor, dryness of mucous membranes for hydration status
• Assess for crackles, dyspnea, orthopnea; peripheral edema, fatigue, weight gain, jugular vein distention (CHF)
• For fever, joint pain, rash, sore throat (lupus-like symptoms), notify prescriber

Nursing diagnoses
• Cardiac output, decreased (adverse reactions)
• Injury, risk for (side effects)
• Knowledge, deficient (teaching)

Patient/family education
• Teach patient to take with food to increase bioavailability (PO)
• Teach patient to avoid OTC preparations unless directed by prescriber
• Advise patient to notify prescriber if chest pain, severe fatigue, fever, muscle or joint pain occur
• Advise patient to rise slowly to prevent orthostatic hypertension
• Advise patient to notify prescriber if pregnancy is suspected

Evaluation
Positive therapeutic outcome
• Decreased B/P in hypertension

TREATMENT OF OVERDOSE:
Administer vasopressors, volume expanders for shock; if PO, lavage or give activated charcoal, digitalization

hydrochlorothiazide (Rx)
(hye-droe-klor-oh-thye'a-zide)
Apo-Hydro ✳, Diovan HCT ✳, Ezide, Neo-Codema ✳, PMS-Hydrochlorothiazide
Func. class.: Diuretic, antihypertensive
Chem. class.: Thiazide, sulfonamide derivative
Pregnancy category B

ACTION: Acts on the distal tubule in the kidney, increasing excretion of sodium, water, chloride, and potassium

Therapeutic outcome: Decreased B/P, decreased edema in lung tissues peripherally

USES: Edema, hypertension, diuresis, CHF; edema in corticosteroid, estrogen, NSAID therapy; idiopathic lower extremity edema therapy

CONTRAINDICATIONS:
Hypersensitivity to thiazides or sulfonamides, anuria, renal decompensation, hypomagnesemia

Precautions: Pregnancy **B**, breastfeeding, hypokalemia, renal/hepatic disease, gout, COPD, lupus erythematosus, diabetes mellitus, hyperlipidemia, CCr <30 ml/min

DOSAGE AND ROUTES
Adult: PO 12.5-25 mg/day, may increase to 50 mg/day in 1-2 divided doses
Child >6 mo: PO 1-2 mg/kg/day in divided doses
Child <6 mo: PO up to 2-3.3 mg/kg/day in divided doses

Available forms: Tabs 12.5, 25, 50 mg; caps 12.5 mg

Implementation
• Give in AM to avoid interference with sleep
• Provide potassium replacement if potassium level is ≤3.0 mg/dl; give whole tab or use oral sol lightly; product may be crushed if patient is unable to swallow
• Administer with food; if nausea occurs, absorption may be increased

ADVERSE EFFECTS
CNS: Drowsiness, paresthesia, depression, headache, *dizziness, fatigue, weakness,* fever
CV: Irregular pulse, orthostatic hypotension, palpitations, volume depletion, allergic myocarditis
EENT: Blurred vision

ELECT: *Hypokalemia,* hypercalcemia, hypo-natremia, hypochloremia, hypomagnesemia
GI: *Nausea, vomiting, anorexia,* constipation, diarrhea, cramps, pancreatitis, GI irritation, **hepatitis**
GU: *Frequency,* polyuria, **uremia,** glucosuria, hyperuricemia
HEMA: Aplastic anemia, hemolytic anemia, leukopenia, agranulocytosis, thrombocytopenia, neutropenia
INTEG: *Rash,* urticaria, purpura, photosensi-tivity, alopecia, erythema multiforme
META: *Hyperglycemia, hyperuricemia,* increased creatinine, BUN

Pharmacokinetics

Absorption	Variable
Distribution	Extracellular spaces; crosses placenta
Metabolism	Excreted unchanged in urine
Excretion	Breast milk
Half-life	6-15 hr

Pharmacodynamics

Onset	2 hr
Peak	4 hr
Duration	6-12 hr

INTERACTIONS

Individual drugs
Amphotericin B: increased hypokalemia
Cholestyramine, colestipol: decreased absorp-tion of hydrochlorothiazide
Diazoxide: increased hyperglycemia, hyperurice-mia, hypotension
Lithium: increased toxicity

Drug classifications
Antidiabetics: decreased effect of antidiabetic agent
Cardiac glycosides, nondepolarizing skeletal muscle relaxants: increased toxicity
Diuretics (loop): increased effects of diuretic
Glucocorticoids: increased hypokalemia
NSAIDs: increased risk of renal failure

Drug/lab test
Increased: amylase, parathyroid test

NURSING CONSIDERATIONS

Assessment
• Monitor glucose in urine if patient is diabetic
• Assess improvement in CVP q8hr
• Check for rashes, temp elevation daily
• Assess for confusion, especially in geriatric patients; take safety precautions if needed

• Monitor for acidic urine, reduced urine, osmolality, nocturia; hypotension, broad T-wave, U-wave, ectopy, tachycardia, weak pulse; muscle weakness, altered LOC, drowsiness, apathy, leth-argy, confusion, depression; anorexia, nausea, cramps, constipation, distention, paralytic ileus; hypoventilation, respiratory muscle weakness
• Assess fluid volume status: I&O ratios, record, count, or weigh diapers as appropriate; weight; distended red veins; crackles in lungs; color, quality, and specific gravity of urine; skin turgor; adequacy of pulses; moist mucous membranes; bilateral lung sounds; peripheral pitting edema; assess for dehydration: symptoms of decreas-ing output, thirst, hypotension; dry mouth and mucous membranes should be reported
• Monitor electrolytes: potassium, sodium, calcium, magnesium; also include BUN, blood pH, ABGs, uric acid, CBC, blood glucose, renal function
• Assess B/P before, during therapy with patient lying, standing, and sitting as appropriate; ortho-static hypotension can occur rapidly

Nursing diagnoses
• Fluid volume, deficient (side effects)
• Fluid volume, excess (uses)
• Knowledge, deficient (teaching)
• Urinary elimination, impaired (side effects)

Patient/family education
• Teach patient to take the medication early in the day to prevent nocturia
• Instruct patient to take with food or milk if GI symptoms of nausea and anorexia occur
• Teach patient to maintain a weekly record of weight and notify prescriber of weight loss >5 lb
• Caution patient that this product causes a loss of potassium and that food rich in potassium should be added to the diet; refer to a dietitian for assistance in planning
• Caution patient to rise slowly from sitting or reclining positions, not to exercise in hot weather or stand for prolonged periods since orthostatic hypotension will be enhanced; lie down if dizziness occurs
• Teach patient not to use alcohol or any OTC medications without prescriber's approval; seri-ous product reactions may occur
• Emphasize the need to contact prescriber im-mediately if muscle cramps, weakness, nausea, dizziness, or numbness occurs
• Teach patient to take own B/P and pulse and record findings
• Teach patient to continue taking medication even if feeling better; this product controls symptoms but does not cure the condition

• Advise patient with hypertension to continue other medical treatment (exercise, weight loss, relaxation techniques, cessation of smoking)

Evaluation

Positive therapeutic outcome

• Decreased edema
• Decreased B/P
• Increased diuresis

TREATMENT OF OVERDOSE:

Lavage if taken orally, monitor electrolytes, administer dextrose in saline, monitor hydration, CV, renal status

HYDROcodone (Rx)

(hye-droe-koe'done)

Hycodan ✤, Tussigon

HYDROcodone/acetamino-phen (Rx)

Co-Gesic, Dolorex Forte, Duocet, Hycet, Hydrocet, Hydrogesic, Liquicet, Lorcet, Lortab, Margesic H, Maxidone, NorCo, Panlor, Polygesic, Stagesic, T-Gesic, Vanacet, Vicodin, Vicodin ES, Vicodin HP, Xodol, Zamicet, Zydone

HYDROcodone/ibuprofen (Rx)

Ibudone, Reprexain, Vicoprofen

Func. class.: Antitussive opioid analgesic/nonopioid analgesic

Pregnancy category C

Controlled substance schedule III

Do not confuse:

HYDROcodone/hydrocortisone, Hycodan/Vicodin

ACTION: Acts directly on cough center in medulla to suppress cough; binds to opiate receptors in the CNS to reduce pain

Therapeutic outcome: Pain relief, decreased cough, decreased diarrhea

USES: Hyperactive and nonproductive cough, mild to moderate pain

CONTRAINDICATIONS:

Acne rosacea/vulgaris, Cushing's, measles, perioral dermatitis, varicella, abrupt discontinuation, hypersensitivity to this product or benzyl

Precautions: Pregnancy C, breastfeeding, neonates, addictive personality, increased ICP,

MI (acute), severe heart disease, respiratory depression, renal/hepatic disease, bowel impaction, urinary retention, viral infection, ulcerative colitis, seizures, sulfite hypersensitivity, psychosis, hypertension, hyperthyroidism

DOSAGES AND ROUTES

Analgesic

Adult: PO 2.5-10 mg q3-6hr prn, max 60 mg/day

Antitussive

Adult: PO 5 mg q4-6hr prn, max 30 mg/24 hr

Available forms: HYDROcodone: bulk powder; **HYDROcodone/acetaminophen:** 5 mg HYDROcodone/500 mg acetaminophen (Co-Gesic, Lorcet, Lortab 5/500, Stagesic, Vicodin); 7.5 mg HYDROcodone/400 mg acetaminophen (Zydone), 7.5 mg HYDROcodone/500 mg acetaminophen (Lortab 7.5/500), 7.5 mg HYDROcodone/750 mg acetaminophen (Vicodin ES), 5 mg HYDROcodone/325 acetaminophen, 10 mg HYDROcodone/325 acetaminophen (Norco), 10 mg HYDROcodone/500 mg acetaminophen (Lortab 10/500), 10 mg HYDROcodone/650 mg acetaminophen (Lorcet 10/650, Vicodin HP), 10 mg HYDROcodone/660 acetaminophen (Vicodin HP); caps 5 mg HYDROcodone/500 mg acetaminophen (Stagesic, Zydone); **HYDROcodone/ibuprofen:** tabs 7.5 mg HYDROcodone/200 mg ibuprofen (Vico-profen)

Implementation

• Do not break, crush, or chew tabs; only scored tabs may be broken
• Give with antiemetic if nausea, vomiting occur
• Give when pain is beginning to return; determine dosage interval by patient response; continuous dosing of medication is more effective than given prn
• Medication should be slowly withdrawn after long-term use to prevent withdrawal symptoms
• Max 4 g acetaminophen with combination product
• Store in light-resistant container at room temperature
• May be given with food or milk to lessen GI upset

ADVERSE EFFECTS

CNS: *Drowsiness,* dizziness, light-headedness, confusion, headache, sedation, euphoria, dysphoria, weakness, hallucinations, disorientation, mood changes, dependence, **seizures**

CV: Palpitations, tachycardia, bradycardia, change in B/P, **circulatory depression,** syncope, **cardiac arrest (child)**

⚠ Nurse Alert

EENT: Tinnitus, blurred vision, miosis, diplopia
GI: *Nausea, vomiting, anorexia, constipation,* cramps, dry mouth, ulcers
GU: Increased urinary output, dysuria, urinary retention
INTEG: Rash, urticaria, flushing, pruritus
RESP: Respiratory depression, pulmonary edema, bronchopneumonia, respiratory arrest (child)

Pharmacokinetics

Absorption	Well absorbed
Distribution	Unknown; crosses placenta
Metabolism	Liver, extensively
Excretion	Kidneys
Half-life	$3^{1}/_{2}$-$4^{1}/_{2}$ hr

Pharmacodynamics

	PO (analgesic)	PO (antitussive)
Onset	10-20 min	Unknown
Peak	30-60 min	Unknown
Duration	4-6 hr	4-6 hr

INTERACTIONS
Individual drugs
Alcohol: increased CNS depression

Drug classifications
Antidepressants (tricyclics), CNS depressants, general anesthetics, opioids, phenothiazines, sedative/hypnotics, skeletal muscle relaxants: increased CNS depression
MAOIs: increased severe reactions

Drug/herb
Lavender, valerian: increased CNS depression

Drug/lab test
Increased: amylase, lipase

NURSING CONSIDERATIONS
Assessment
• **Assess pain:** intensity, type, location, duration, precipitating factor before and 1 hr after giving product, titrate upward by 25%; assess need for pain medication, physical dependency
• Monitor VS after parenteral route; note muscle rigidity; product history; liver; renal function tests; cough; and respiratory dysfunction: respiratory depression, character, rate, rhythm; notify prescriber if respirations are <10/min
• **Monitor CNS changes:** dizziness, drowsiness, hallucinations, euphoria, LOC, pupil reaction

• Monitor allergic reactions: rash, urticaria
• Obtain history of ulcers if using ibuprofen combination product
• **Bowel status:** constipation; provide fluids, fiber in diet, may need stimulant laxative

Nursing diagnoses
• Breathing pattern, ineffective (adverse reactions)
• Knowledge, deficient (teaching)
• Pain, acute (uses)

Patient/family education
• Instruct patient to report any symptoms of CNS changes, allergic reactions; to avoid CNS depressants: alcohol, sedative/hypnotics for at least 24 hr after taking this product
• Teach patient that dizziness, drowsiness, and confusion are common and to avoid getting up without assistance, driving, or other hazardous activities
• Discuss in detail all aspects of the product

Evaluation
Positive therapeutic outcome
• Decreased pain
• Decreased cough

TREATMENT OF OVERDOSE:
Naloxone HCl (Narcan) 0.2-0.8 **IV**, O_2, **IV** fluids, vasopressors

hydrocortisone (Rx)
(hy-droh-kor'tih-sone)
Cortef, Colocort, Cortena
hydrocortisone acetate (Rx)
Anucort, Anusol, Cortifoam, Hemril, Protocort, Rectasol
hydrocortisone sodium succinate (Rx)
A-hydroCort, Solu-Cortef
Func. class.: Short-acting glucocorticoid
Chem. class.: Natural nonfluorinated, group IV potency (valerate), group VI potency (acetate and plain)
Pregnancy category C

Do not confuse:
hydrocortisone/HYDROcodone,
predniSONE/predinsoLONE

ACTION: Decreases inflammation by suppressing migration of polymorphonuclear leukocytes and fibroblasts and reversing increased capillary permeability and lysosomal stabilization (systemic); antipruritic, antiinflammatory (topical)

Therapeutic outcome: Decreased inflammation

USES: Severe inflammation, septic shock, adrenal insufficiency, ulcerative colitis, collagen disorders

CONTRAINDICATIONS:
Children <2 yr, psychosis, hypersensitivity, idiopathic thrombocytopenia (IM), acute glomerulonephritis, amebiasis, fungal infections, nonasthmatic bronchial disease, AIDS, TB, recent MI (associated with left-ventricular rupture)

Precautions: Pregnancy **C**, breastfeeding, diabetes mellitus, glaucoma, osteoporosis, seizure disorders, ulcerative colitis, CHF, myasthenia gravis, renal disease, esophagitis, peptic ulcer, metastatic carcinoma

DOSAGE AND ROUTES
Adrenal insufficiency/inflammation
Adult: PO 20-240 mg daily; IM/IV 100-500 mg (succinate), then 50-100 mg IM as needed

Shock prevention
Adult: IM/IV 50 mg/kg repeated q4hr; repeat q24hr as needed (succinate)
Child: IM/IV 0.16-1 mg/kg or 6-30 mg/m² given daily or bid (succinate)

Colitis
Adult: PO 20-240 mg (base)/day in 2-4 divided doses; enema 100 mg nightly for 21 days
Child: PO 2-8 mg (base)/kg/day or 60-240 mg (base)/m²/day in 3-4 divided doses

Topical route
Adult and child >2 yr: Apply to affected area daily-qid

Available forms: Tabs 5, 10, 20 mg; inj 25, 50 mg/ml; enema 100 mg/60 ml; **acetate:** inj 25 ✷, 50 mg/ml ✷, rectal 10% aerosol foam, supp 25, 30 mg; **succinate:** inj 100 mg, 250 mg, 500 mg, 1000 mg/vial

Implementation
PO route
• Give with food or milk to decrease GI symptoms
Rectal route
• Use applicator provided
• Clean applicator after each use
• Retain for 1 hr if possible

Topical route
• Apply only to affected areas; do not get in eyes
• Cleanse and dry area before applying medication, then cover with occlusive dressing (only if prescribed); seal to normal skin; change q12hr; systemic absorption may occur; use only on dermatoses; do not use on weeping, denuded, or infected area
• Use for a few days after area has cleared
• Store at room temperature
Nasal route
• Patient should clear nasal passages before administration; use decongestant if needed; shake inhaler, invert, tilt head backward, insert nozzle into nostril, away from septum; hold other nostril closed and depress activator, inhale through nose, exhale through mouth

IM route
• Give deeply in large muscle mass; rotate sites; avoid deltoid; use 21-gauge needle

IV route
• **Succinate: IV** in mix-o-vial or reconstitute 250 mg or less/2 ml bacteriostatic water for injection, mix gently; give direct IV over 1 min or more; may be further diluted in 100, 250, 500, or 1000 ml of D₅W, D₅/0.9% NaCl, 0.9% NaCl given over ordered rate

Sodium succinate preparations

Y-site compatibilities: Acyclovir, allopurinol, amifostine, aminophylline, ampicillin, amphotericin B cholesteryl, inamrinone, amsacrine, atracurium, atropine, aztreonam, betamethasone, calcium gluconate, cefepime, cefmetazole, cephalothin, cephapirin, chlordiazepoxide, chlorproMAZINE, cisatracurium, cladribine, cyanocobalamin, cytarabine, dexamethasone, digoxin, diphenhydrAMINE, DOPamine, DOXOrubicin liposome, droperidol, edrophonium, enalaprilat, EPINEPHrine, esmolol, conjugated estrogens, ethacrynate, famotidine, fentaNYL, fentaNYL/droperidol, filgrastim, fludarabine, fluorouracil, foscarnet, furosemide, gallium, granisetron, heparin, hydrALAZINE, regular insulin, isoproterenol, kanamycin, lidocaine, LORazepam, magnesium sulfate, melphalan, menadiol, meperidine, methicillin, methoxamine, methylergonovine, minocycline, morphine, neostigmine, norepinephrine, ondansetron, oxacillin, oxytocin, paclitaxel, pancuronium, penicillin G potassium, pentazocine, phytonadione, piperacillin/tazobactam, prednisoLONE, procainamide, prochlorperazine, propofol, propranolol, pyridostigmine, remifentanil, scopolamine, sodium bicarbonate, succinylcholine, tacrolimus, teniposide, theoph-

ylline, thiotepa, trimethaphan, trimethobenzamide, vecuronium, vinorelbine

Y-site incompatibilities: Diazepam,
ergotamine tartrate, IDArubicin, phenytoin,
sargramostim

ADVERSE EFFECTS

CNS: Depression, flushing, sweating, headache, mood changes, **pseudotumor cerebri**
CV: Hypertension, **circulatory collapse,
thrombophlebitis, embolism,** tachycardia,
edema
EENT: Fungal infections, increased intraocular
pressure, blurred vision
GI: Diarrhea, nausea, abdominal distention, **GI
hemorrhage,** increased appetite, **pancreatitis**
HEMA: Thrombocytopenia
INTEG: Acne, poor wound healing, ecchymosis, petechiae
MS: Fractures, osteoporosis, weakness

Pharmacokinetics

Absorption	Well absorbed (PO); systemic (topical)
Distribution	Crosses placenta
Metabolism	Liver, extensively
Excretion	Kidney
Half-life	3-5 hr, adrenal suppression 3-4 days

Pharmacodynamics

	PO	IM	IV	TOPICAL
Onset	1-2 hr	20 min	Rapid	Min to hr
Peak	1 hr	4-8 hr	Unkn	Hr to days
Duration	1½ days	1½ days	1½ days	Hr to days

INTERACTIONS

Individual drugs
Alcohol, amphotericin B, cycloSPORINE,
digoxin: increased side effects
Bosentan, cholestyramine, colestipol, ePHED-
rine, phenytoin, rifampin, theophylline:
decreased action of hydrocortisone

Drug classifications
Anticoagulants, calcium supplements, toxoids,
vaccines: decreased action of each specific
drug
Anticonvulsants: decreased effects of anticonvulsant
Antidiabetics: decreased effects of antidiabetics
Barbiturates: decreased action of hydrocortisone

Diuretics: increased side effects
NSAIDs, salicylates: increased risk of GI bleeding

Drug/lab test
Increased: cholesterol, sodium, blood glucose,
uric acid, calcium, urine glucose
Decreased: calcium, potassium, T_4, T_3, thyroid
^{131}I uptake test, urine 17-OHCS, 17-KS
False negative: skin allergy tests

NURSING CONSIDERATIONS

Assessment
• **Adrenal insufficiency (cushingoid
symptoms):** nausea, anorexia, shortness of
breath, moon face, fatigue, dizziness, weakness,
joint pain before and during treatment; monitor
plasma cortisol levels during long-term therapy
(normal level is 138-635 nmol/L when obtained
at 8 AM); check adrenal function periodically for
hypothalamic-pituitary-adrenal axis suppression
• Monitor potassium, blood glucose, urine
glucose while patient is on long-term therapy;
hypokalemia and hyperglycemia may occur
• Monitor I&O ratio; be alert for decreasing
urinary output and increasing edema; weigh
daily; notify prescriber of weekly gain >5 lb or
edema, hypertension, cardiac symptoms
• **Assess for infection:** increased temp, WBC
even after withdrawal of medication; product
masks infection symptoms; if fever develops,
product should be discontinued
• Check for potassium depletion: paresthesias,
fatigue, nausea, vomiting, depression, polyuria,
dysrhythmias, weakness
• Assess mental status: affect, mood, behavioral
changes, aggression
• Check nasal passages during long-term treatment for changes in mucus (nasal)
• Assess for systemic absorption: increased
temp, inflammation, irritation (topical)
• GI effects: nausea, vomiting, anorexia or
appetite stimulation, diarrhea, constipation, abdominal pain, hiccups, gastritis, pancreatitis, GI
bleeding/perforation with long-term treatment

Nursing diagnoses
• Infection, risk for (adverse reactions)
• Knowledge, deficient (teaching)
• Noncompliance (teaching) (topical/nasal
preparation)

Patient/family education
• Teach patient all aspects of product use,
including cushingoid symptoms
• Advise patient to carry/wear emergency ID as
corticosteroid user; not to discontinue abruptly;
adrenal crisis can result

H

Adverse effects: *italics* = common; **bold** = life-threatening

• Instruct patient to notify prescriber if therapeutic response decreases; dosage adjustment may be needed
• Instruct patient to notify prescriber of signs of infection
• Teach patient that product can mask infections and cause hypoglycemia (diabetic)
• Teach patient to avoid live-virus vaccines if using steroids long term
• Caution patient to avoid OTC products unless directed by prescriber: salicylates, alcohol in cough products, cold preparations
• **Teach patient symptoms of adrenal insufficiency:** nausea, anorexia, fatigue, dizziness, dyspnea, weakness, joint pain; and when to notify prescriber
• Advise patient that long-term therapy may be needed to resolve infection (1-2 mo depending on type of infection)
• Teach patient to report immediately abdominal pain, black tarry stools, as GI bleeding/perforation can occur
• Advise patient not to discontinue abruptly or adrenal crisis can result; product should be tapered
Nasal route
• Instruct patient to clear nasal passages if sneezing attack occurs, then repeat dose; to continue using product even if mild nasal bleeding occurs; bleeding is usually transient
• Teach method of instillation after providing written instruction from manufacturer on instillation

Evaluation
Positive therapeutic outcome
• Decrease in runny nose (nasal)
• Decreased inflammation
• Absence of severe itching, patches on skin, flaking (top)
• Decreased GI symptoms

hydrocortisone topical
See Appendix B

⚠ HIGH ALERT

HYDROmorphone (Rx)
(hye-droe-mor′fone)
Dilaudid, Dilaudid-HP, Exalgo, Hydromorph Contin ✤, PMS Hydromorphone
Func. class.: Antitussive, opioid analgesic agonist
Chem. class.: Phenanthrene derivative, guaifenesin
Pregnancy category C
Controlled substance schedule II

Do not confuse:
HYDROmorphone/meperidine/morphine, Dilaudid/Demerol

ACTION: Inhibits ascending pain pathways in CNS, increases pain threshold, alters pain perception

Therapeutic outcome: Decreased cough, decreased pain

USES: As an antitussive to suppress cough; moderate to severe pain

CONTRAINDICATIONS: Hypersensitivity

> **BLACK BOX WARNING:** Respiratory depression, opioid-naive patients, substance abuse

Precautions: Pregnancy C, breastfeeding, children <18 yr, increased ICP, addictive personality, renal/hepatic disease, MI (acute), severe heart disease, bowel impaction, abrupt discontinuation, COPD

DOSAGE AND ROUTES
Analgesic
Adult: PO (oral solution) 2.5-10 mg q3-6hr or (tabs) 2-4 mg q4-6hr; **EXT REL** (Exalgo): Convert to **EXT REL** by giving total daily dose of immediate release q day, titrate if needed **EXT REL** q3-4days until adequate pain relief; use 25%-50% increase for each titration step, if more than 2 doses of rescue medication is needed in 24 hr consider titration; **IM/SUBCUT/IV** 1-2 mg q4-6hr prn, may be increased; **RECT** 3 mg q6-8hr prn
Geriatric: PO 1-2 mg q4-6hr

Available forms: Inj 1, 2, 4, 10 mg/ml; tabs 2, 4, 8 mg; oral sol 5 mg/5 ml; supp 3 mg, ext rel tab 8, 12, 16 mg

Implementation

- Give with antiemetic if nausea, vomiting occur
- Give when pain is beginning to return; determine dosage interval by patient response; continuous dosing of medication is more effective given prn; explain analgesic effect
- Withdraw medication slowly after long-term use to prevent withdrawal symptoms
- Store in light-resistant container at room temperature

PO route

- May be given with food or milk to lessen GI upset

Extended release

> **BLACK BOX WARNING:** Do not use extended-release products in opioid-naive patients

- **Converting from oral opioids;** conversion ratios are approximate; initiate ext rel tabs at 50% of calculated total daily equivalent dose of ext rel, give q24hr; max increase q2-3days, consider titration increases of 25%-50% in each step
- **Converting from transdermal patch (fentaNYL)** initiate ext rel tabs 18 hr after removal of patch; for each 25 mcg/hr dose of transdermal fentaNYL the dose is 12 mg q24hr, start dose at 50% of calculated HYDROmorphone ext rel dose q24hr; titrate no more often than q3-4days, consider dose increases of 25%-50% with each step; if more than 2 rescue doses are required in 24 hr, consider titration

SUBCUT route

- Do not give if sol is cloudy or a precipitate has formed; rotate inj sites
- Use short 30-G needle, make sure not to inject intradermally

Direct IV route

- Give after diluting with 5 ml or more of sterile water or 0.9% NaCl for inj
- Give slowly at 2 mg over 3-5 min or less through Y-connector or 3-way stopcock

IV infusion route

- Dilute each 0.1-1 mg/ml in 0.9% NaCl, deliver by opioid syringe infusion; may be diluted in D5W, D5/NaCl, 0.45% NaCl or 0.9% NaCl for larger amounts and through an infusion pump

Syringe compatibilities: Atropine, bupivacaine, ceftazidime, chlorproMAZINE, cimetidine, dimenhyDRINATE, diphenhydrAMINE, fentaNYL, glycopyrrolate, haloperidol, hydrOXYzine, LORazepam, midazolam, pentazocine, PENTobarbital, prochlorperazine, promethazine, ranitidine, scopolamine, tetracaine, thiethylperazine, trimethobenzamide

Y-site compatibilities: Acyclovir, allopurinol, amifostine, amikacin, amsacrine, aztreonam, cefamandole, cefepime, cefmetazole, cefoperazone, cefotaxime, cefoxitin, ceftazidime, ceftizoxime, cefuroxime, cephalothin, cephapirin, chloramphenicol, CISplatin, cladribine, clindamycin, cyclophosphamide, cytarabine, diltiazem, DOBUTamine, DOPamine, DOXOrubicin, doxycycline, EPINEPHrine, erythromycin lactobionate, famotidine, fentaNYL, filgrastim, fludarabine, foscarnet, furosemide, gentamicin, granisetron, heparin, kanamycin, labetalol, LORazepam, magnesium sulfate, melphalan, methotrexate, metroNIDAZOLE, mezlocillin, midazolam, milrinone, morphine, moxalactam, nafcillin, niCARdipine, nitroglycerin, norepinephrine, ondansetron, oxacillin, paclitaxel, penicillin G potassium, piperacillin, piperacillin/tazobactam, propofol, ranitidine, teniposide, thiotepa, ticarcillin, tobramycin, trimethoprim/sulfamethoxazole, vancomycin, vecuronium, vinorelbine

Y-site incompatibilities: Ampicillin, diazepam, minocycline, PHENobarbital, phenytoin, sargramostim

Additive compatibilities: Bupivacaine, cloNIDine, fluorouracil, heparin, midazolam, ondansetron, potassium chloride, promethazine, verapamil, ziconotide

Additive incompatibilities: Sodium bicarbonate, thiopental

Solution compatibilities: D5W, D5/0.45% NaCl, D5/0.9% NaCl, D5/LR, D5/Ringer's, 0.45% NaCl, 0.9% NaCl, Ringer's, LR

ADVERSE EFFECTS

CNS: Dizziness, drowsiness, *sedation, confusion,* headache, euphoria, mood changes, **seizures**

CV: *Hypotension, bradycardia,* palpitations, change in B/P, tachycardia, peripheral vasodilatation

EENT: Miosis, diplopia, blurred vision, tinnitus

GI: *Nausea, constipation, vomiting, anorexia,* dry mouth, cramps, paralytic ileus

GU: Increased urinary output, dysuria, urinary retention

INTEG: Urticaria, rash, flushing, bruising, diaphoresis, pruritus

RESP: Respiratory depression, dyspnea

H

Pharmacokinetics

Absorption	Well absorbed (PO), complete (**IV**)	
Distribution	Unknown; crosses placenta	
Metabolism	Liver, extensively	
Excretion	Kidneys	
Half-life	2-3 hr	

Pharmacodynamics

	PO/IM/ SUBCUT	IV	RECT
Onset	15-30 min	10-15 min	15-30 min
Peak	30-60 min	15-30 min	30-90 min
Duration	4-5 hr	2-3 hr	4-5 hr

INTERACTIONS

Individual drugs
Alcohol: increased respiratory depression, hypotension, sedation

Drug classifications
Antipsychotics, opiates, sedative/hypnotics, skeletal muscle relaxants: increased effects
MAOIs: increased severe reactions
Opiate antagonists: decreased HYDROmorphone effects

Drug/herb
Chamomile, hops, kava, lavender, St. John's wort, valerian: increased action

Drug/lab test
Increased: amylase

NURSING CONSIDERATIONS

Assessment
• **Assess pain control,** sedation by scoring on 0-10 scale; around-the-clock dosing is best for pain control
• Monitor VS after parenteral route; note muscle rigidity; product history

> **BLACK BOX WARNING:** Respiratory dysfunction; respiratory depression; monitor character, rate, rhythm; notify prescriber if respirations are <10/min

• Monitor CNS changes: dizziness, drowsiness, hallucinations, euphoria, LOC, pupil reaction
• Monitor allergic reactions: rash, urticaria; bowel function, constipation

Nursing diagnoses
• Breathing pattern, ineffective (adverse reactions)

• Knowledge, deficient (teaching)
• Pain, acute (uses)

Patient/family education
• Instruct patient to report any symptoms of CNS changes, allergic reactions; to avoid CNS depressants: alcohol, sedative-hypnotics for at least 24 hr after taking this product
• Advise patient that dizziness, drowsiness, and confusion are common and to avoid getting up without assistance, driving, or other hazardous activities
• Discuss in detail all aspects of the product

Evaluation
Positive therapeutic outcome
• Decreased pain
• Decreased cough

TREATMENT OF OVERDOSE:
Naloxone HCl (Narcan) 0.2-0.8 **IV**, O_2, **IV** fluids, vasopressors

hydroxychloroquine (Rx)
(hye-drox-ee-klor'oh-kwin)
Apo-Hydroxyquine ❖, **Gen-Hydroxyquine** ❖, **Plaquenil**
Func. class.: Antimalarial, antirheumatic (DMARDs)
Chem. class.: 4-Aminoquinoline derivative
Pregnancy category C

ACTION: Impairs complement-dependent antigen-antibody reactions

Therapeutic outcome: Resolution of infection

USES: Malaria caused by *Plasmodium vivax, P. malariae, P. ovale, P. falciparum* (some strains); LE, rheumatoid arthritis

CONTRAINDICATIONS:
Hypersensitivity to this product or chloroquine, retinal field changes

> **BLACK BOX WARNING:** Children (long-term), ocular disease

Precautions: Pregnancy **C**, breastfeeding, blood dyscrasias, severe GI disease, neurologic disease, alcoholism, hepatic disease, G6PD deficiency, psoriasis, eczema

DOSAGE AND ROUTES

Malaria

Adult: PO suppression or prevention 400 mg qwk, begin 1-2 wk before travel, continue 4 wk after returning; treatment 800 mg, then 400 mg after 6-8 hr, then 400 mg q day on 2nd and 3rd day, total dose 2 g

Child: PO suppression or prevention 6.4 mg/kg (5 mg/kg base) qwk, begin 1-2 wk before travel, continue 4 wk after returning; treatment 10 mg/kg, 6.4 mg/kg (5 mg/kg base), at 6, 24, 48 hr after 1st dose

Lupus erythematosus

Adult: PO 400 mg (310 mg base) daily-bid; length depends on patient response; maintenance 200-400 mg/day

Rheumatoid arthritis

Adult: PO 400-600 mg/day for 4-12 wk; then 200-300 mg/day after good response

Available forms: Tabs 200 mg

Implementation

• Give before or after meals with milk, at same time each day to maintain product level
• Tabs may be crushed and mixed with food, fluids
• Malaria prophylaxis should be started 2 wk prior to exposure and 4-6 wk after leaving exposure area
• Store in tight, light-resistant container at room temperature

ADVERSE EFFECTS

CNS: Headache, stimulation, fatigue, irritability, **seizures**, bad dreams, dizziness, confusion, psychosis, decreased reflexes
CV: Hypotension, heart block, **asystole with syncope**
EENT: *Blurred vision, corneal changes, retinal changes, difficulty focusing,* tinnitus, vertigo, deafness, photophobia, corneal edema
GI: *Nausea, vomiting, anorexia,* diarrhea, cramps
HEMA: **Thrombocytopenia, agranulocytosis, leukopenia, aplastic anemia**
INTEG: Pruritus, pigmentation changes, skin eruptions, lichen planus–like eruptions, eczema, **exfoliative dermatitis,** alopecia, **Stevens-Johnson syndrome,** photosensitivity

Pharmacokinetics

Absorption	Well absorbed
Distribution	Widely distributed, crosses placenta
Metabolism	Liver
Excretion	Urine/feces
Half-life	3-5 day

Pharmacodynamics

Onset	Rapid
Peak	1-2 hr
Duration	Days-weeks

INTERACTIONS

Individual products

Magnesium, aluminum products: decreased malarial action
Digoxin: increased levels
Methotrexate: decreased levels
Rabies vaccine: increased antibody titer

Drug classifications

Live-virus vaccines, botulinum toxoids: decreased effects

NURSING CONSIDERATIONS

Assessment

• **Assess for lupus erythematosus, malaria symptoms** before treatment and daily
• **Assess for rheumatoid arthritis:** pain, swelling, ROM, temp of joints
• Assess ophthalmic exam baseline, q6mo if long-term treatment or product dosage >150 mg/day
• Assess hepatic studies qwk: AST, ALT, bilirubin
• **Blood dyscrasias:** Assess blood studies: CBC, platelets; WBC, RBC, platelets may be decreased; if severe, product should be discontinued; malaise, fever, bruising, bleeding (rare)
• Assess for decreased reflexes: knee, ankle
• Assess ECG during therapy
• Assess for depression of T-waves, widening of QRS complex
• **Assess allergic reactions:** pruritus, rash, urticaria
• **Assess for ototoxicity** (tinnitus, vertigo, change in hearing); audiometric testing should be done before, after treatment
⚠ **Assess for toxicity: blurring vision, difficulty focusing, headache, dizziness, knee, ankle reflexes; product should be discontinued immediately**

Nursing diagnoses
- Infection, risk for (uses)
- Knowledge, deficient (teaching)
- Pain, chronic (uses)

Patient/family education
- Teach patient to use sunglasses in bright sunlight to decrease photophobia
- Teach patient that urine may turn rust or brown
- Teach patient to report hearing, vision problems; fever, fatigue, bruising, bleeding, which may indicate blood dyscrasias

Evaluation
Positive therapeutic outcome
- Decreased symptoms of malaria, LE, rheumatoid arthritis

TREATMENT OF OVERDOSE:
Induce vomiting; gastric lavage; administer barbiturate (ultra–short-acting), vasopressor, ammonium chloride; tracheostomy may be necessary

---

hydroxyurea (Rx)
(hye-drox-ee-yoo-ree′ah)
Apo-Hydroxyurea, Droxia, Hydrea
Func. class.: Antineoplastic, antimetabolite
Chem. class.: Synthetic urea analog
Pregnancy category D

ACTION: Acts by inhibiting DNA synthesis without interfering with RNA or protein synthesis; incorporates thymidine into DNA, causing direct damage to DNA strands; cell cycle specific (S phase)

Therapeutic outcome: Prevention of rapidly growing malignant cells

USES: Melanoma, chronic myelogenous leukemia, recurrent or metastatic ovarian cancer, squamous cell carcinoma of the head and neck, sickle cell anemia

CONTRAINDICATIONS:
Pregnancy **D**, breastfeeding, hypersensitivity

> **BLACK BOX WARNING:** Leukopenia (<2500/mm³), thrombocytopenia (<100,000/mm³), anemia (severe)

Precautions: Renal disease (severe)

DOSAGE AND ROUTES

Ovarian cancer, malignant melanoma
Adult: PO 80 mg/kg as a single dose q3day or 20-30 mg/kg as a single dose daily

Ovarian cancer in combination with radiation
Adult: PO 80 mg/kg as a single dose q3day; should be started 7 days before irradiation

Sickle cell anemia
Adult: PO 15 mg/kg/day, may increase by 5 mg/kg/day q12wk; max 35 mg/kg/day

Renal/hepatic disease
Reduce dose

Available forms: Caps 200, 300, 400, 500 mg

Implementation
- Do not crush or chew caps; for difficulty swallowing, caps may be opened and contents mixed with water
- Avoid contact with skin, very irritating; wash completely to remove
- Give fluids **IV** or PO before chemotherapy to hydrate patient
- Give antiemetic 30-60 min before giving product and prn to prevent vomiting; antibiotics for prophylaxis of infection
- Provide liquid diet: carbonated beverages; gelatin may be added if patient is not nauseated or vomiting

ADVERSE EFFECTS
CNS: Headache, confusion, hallucinations, dizziness, **seizures**
CV: Angina, ischemia
GI: Nausea, vomiting, anorexia, diarrhea, stomatitis, constipation, **hepatotoxicity**
GU: Increased BUN, uric acid, creatinine, temporary renal function impairment
HEMA: Leukopenia, anemia, thrombocytopenia, megaloblastic erythropoiesis
INTEG: *Rash,* urticaria, pruritus, dry skin, facial erythema
MISC: Fever, chills, malaise, secondary cancers, tumor lysis syndrome
META: Hyperphosphatemia, hyperuricemia, hypocalcemia

Pharmacokinetics

Absorption	Well absorbed
Distribution	Crosses blood-brain barrier
Metabolism	Liver (50%)
Excretion	Kidneys, unchanged (50%), eliminated as CO_2
Half-life	Terminal 3.5-4.5 hr

Pharmacodynamics

Onset	Unknown
Peak	1-4 hr
Duration	Unknown

INTERACTIONS

Individual drugs
Didanosine, stavudine: increased pancreatitis
Radiation: increased toxicity

Drug classifications
Anticoagulants, NSAIDs, thrombolytics, salicylates, platelet inhibitors: increased bleeding
Antineoplastics: increased toxicity
Hematopoietic progenitor cells (sargramostim, filgrastim): do not use within 24 hr before or after antineoplastic
Live-virus vaccines: do not use together

Drug/lab test
Increased: renal function tests

NURSING CONSIDERATIONS

Assessment
• Assess buccal cavity q8hr for dryness, sores or ulceration, white patches, oral pain, bleeding, dysphagia; obtain prescription for viscous lidocaine (Xylocaine)
• Assess symptoms indicating severe allergic reaction: rash, pruritus, urticaria, purpuric skin lesions, itching, flushing
• **Bone marrow suppression:** Monitor CBC, differential, platelet count weekly; withhold product if WBC is <2500/mm³ or platelet count is <100,000/mm³; notify prescriber of results if WBC <20,000/mm³, platelets <150,000/mm³
• Assess for increased uric acid levels, swelling, joint pain primarily in extremities; patient should be well hydrated to prevent urate deposits
• Monitor renal function studies: BUN, creatinine, serum uric acid, urine CCr before, during therapy; I&O ratio; report fall in urine output to <30 ml/hr
• Monitor temp (may indicate beginning of infection)

• Monitor liver function tests before, during therapy (bilirubin, AST, ALT, LDH) as needed or monthly
• **Assess for bleeding:** hematuria, stool guaiac, bruising or petechiae, mucosa or orifices q8hr; check for inflammation of mucosa, breaks in skin
⚠ Assess for tumor lysis syndrome: hyperkalemia, hyperphosphatemia, hyperuricemia, hypocalcemia, uric acid nephropathy, acute renal failure; metabolic acidosis can occur, aggressive alkalinization of urine and allopurinol can prevent this
⚠ Severe allergic reaction: assess for rash, urticaria, itching, flushing
⚠ Neurotoxicity: assess for headaches, hallucinations, seizures, dizziness

Nursing diagnoses
• Body image, disturbed (adverse reactions)
• Infection, risk for (adverse reactions)
• Injury, risk for (adverse reactions)
• Knowledge, deficient (teaching)

Patient/family education
• Advise patient that contraceptive measures are recommended during therapy (pregnancy **D**)
• Teach patient to avoid use of products containing aspirin or ibuprofen, razors, commercial mouthwash, since bleeding may occur; instruct patient to report symptoms of bleeding (hematuria, tarry stools)
• Teach patient to rinse mouth tid-qid with water, club soda; brush teeth bid-qid with soft brush or cotton-tipped applicators for stomatitis; use unwaxed dental floss
• Instruct patient to report signs of anemia (fatigue, headache, irritability, faintness, shortness of breath)
• Advise patient to report any changes in breathing or coughing even several mo after treatment; to avoid crowds and persons with respiratory tract or other infections
• Caution patient not to have any vaccinations without the advice of the prescriber; serious reactions can occur

Evaluation
Positive therapeutic outcome
• Prevention of rapid division of malignant cells

H

Adverse effects: *italics* = common; **bold** = life-threatening

hydrOXYzine (Rx)

(hye-drox'i-zeen)

ANX, Apo-hydroxyzine ✹, Vistaril

Func. class.: Antianxiety, sedative, hypnotic, antihistamine, antiemetic

Chem. class.: Piperazine derivative

Pregnancy category C

Do not confuse:

hydrOXYzine/hydrALAZINE, Vistaril/Versed

ACTION: Depresses subcortical levels of CNS, including limbic system, reticular formation; anticholinergic, antiemetic, antihistaminic responses; competes with H_1-receptor sites

Therapeutic outcome: Absence of allergy symptoms, rhinitis, pruritus, absence of nausea/vomiting, sedation, absence of anxiety

USES: Anxiety preoperatively; postoperatively to prevent nausea, vomiting; to potentiate opioid analgesics; sedation; pruritus; prevention of alcohol withdrawal

CONTRAINDICATIONS:

Pregnancy (1st trimester), breastfeeding, acute asthma, hypersensitivity to this product or cetirizine

Precautions: Pregnancy C (2nd/3rd trimesters), geriatric, debilitated patients, renal/hepatic disease, closed-angle glaucoma, COPD, prostatic hypertrophy, asthma

DOSAGE AND ROUTES

Anxiety

Adult: PO 25-100 mg tid-qid, max 600 mg/day; IM 50-100 mg q4-6hr

Geriatric: PO max 50 mg/day

Child >6 yr: PO 50-100 mg/day in divided doses

Child <6 yr: PO 50 mg/day in divided doses

Alcohol withdrawal

Adult: IM 50-100 mg, then q4-6hr

Preoperatively/postoperatively (nausea/vomiting)

Adult: IM 25-100 mg q4-6hr

Child: IM 0.5-1.1 mg/kg as a single dose

Pruritus

Adult: PO 25 mg tid-qid; IM 50-100 mg, then q4-6hr prn, switch to PO as soon as feasible

Child ≥6 yr: PO 50-100 mg/day in divided doses; IM 0.5-1 mg/kg/dose q4-6hr prn, use PO when possible

Child <6 yr: PO 50 mg/day in divided doses

Renal dose

Adult: PO CCr <50 ml/min reduce dose by 50%

Available forms: Tabs 10, 25, 50 mg; caps 25, 50, 100 mg; oral sol 10 mg/5 ml; oral susp 25 mg/5 ml; inj 25, 50 mg/ml

Implementation

PO route

• Take 1 hr after or 2 hr before meals to facilitate absorption

• May crush tab if patient is unable to swallow whole

• Give with meals if GI symptoms occur; absorption may be slightly decreased

• Caps may be opened and product mixed with food/fluids for patients with swallowing difficulties

IM route

• Give IM inj in large muscle mass; aspirate to prevent IV administration; use Z-track method; severe necrosis can result with improper technique; never give IV/SUBCUT

Syringe compatibilities: Atropine, atropine/meperidine, benzquinamide, bupivacaine, butorphanol, chlorproMAZINE, cimetidine, codeine, diphenhydrAMINE, doxapram, droperidol, fentaNYL, fluphenazine, glycopyrrolate, HYDROmorphone, lidocaine, meperidine, meperidine/atropine, methotrimeprazine, metoclopramide, midazolam, morphine, nalbuphine, oxymorphone, pentazocine, perphenazine, procaine, prochlorperazine, promazine, promethazine, remifentanil, scopolamine, SUFentanil, thiothixene

Syringe incompatibilities: Aminophylline, chloramphenicol, dimenhyDRINATE, heparin, penicillin G potassium, PENTobarbital, PHENobarbital, phenytoin

Additive compatibilities: CISplatin, cyclophosphamide, cytarabine, dimenhyDRINATE, etoposide, lidocaine, mesna, methotrexate, nafcillin

ADVERSE EFFECTS

CNS: *Dizziness, drowsiness,* confusion, headache, tremors, fatigue, depression, **seizures**

CV: Hypotension

GI: Dry mouth, nausea, diarrhea, increased appetite, weight gain

---

⚠ Nurse Alert

Pharmacokinetics

Absorption	Well absorbed
Distribution	Not known
Metabolism	Liver, completely
Excretion	Feces, urine, bile
Half-life	3 hr

Pharmacodynamics

	PO/IM
Onset	15-60 min
Peak	2-4 hr
Duration	4-6 hr

INTERACTIONS

Individual drugs
Alcohol: increased CNS depression
Atropine, disopyramide, haloperidol, quiNIDine: increased anticholinergic reactions

Drug classifications
Analgesics, barbiturates, CNS depressants, opiates, sedative/hypnotics: increased CNS depression
Antidepressants, antihistamines, MAOIs, phenothiazines: increased anticholinergic reactions

NURSING CONSIDERATIONS

Assessment
• Assess mental status: mood, sensorium, affect, behavior, increased sedation
• Assess respiratory status: rate, rhythm, increase in bronchial secretions, wheezing, chest tightness; provide fluids to 2 L/day to decrease secretion thickness
• Monitor I&O ratio: be alert for urinary retention, frequency, dysuria, especially in geriatric; product should be discontinued if these occur
• Observe for drowsiness, dizziness
• Assess cough characteristics including type, frequency, thickness of secretions; evaluate response to this medication if using for cough

Nursing diagnoses
• Anxiety (uses)
• Injury, risk for (side effects)
• Knowledge, deficient (teaching)

Patient/family education
• Caution patient to avoid hazardous activities and activities requiring alertness, since dizziness may occur; instruct patient to request assistance with ambulation
• Advise patient to avoid alcohol, other CNS depressants including cough, cold preparations; CNS depression may occur

• Teach all aspects of product use; to notify prescriber if confusion, sedation, hypotension occur; to avoid driving and other hazardous activity if drowsiness occurs
• Caution patient not to exceed recommended dosage; dysrhythmias may occur
• Tell patient hard candy, gum, frequent rinsing of mouth may be used for dryness

Evaluation
Positive therapeutic outcome
• Absence of nausea, vomiting
• Decreased anxiety

TREATMENT OF OVERDOSE:
Lavage if orally ingested, VS, supportive care, **IV** norepinephrine for hypotension

Hylan G-F 20
Synvisc, Synvisc One
See Appendix A, Selected New Drugs

hyoscyamine (Rx)
(hye-oh-sye′a-meen)
Anaspaz, Colidrops, Colytrol Pediatric, Cystospaz-M, ED-SPAZ, HydroMax-DT, HydroMax-FT, HydroMax-SR, HyoMax, HyoMax SL, Hyosyne, Levbid, Levsin, Medispax, NuLev, Spacol, Spasdel, Symax
Func. class.: Anticholinergic/antispasmodics
Chem. class.: Belladonna alkaloid
Pregnancy category C

ACTION: Inhibits muscarinic actions of acetylcholine at postganglionic parasympathetic neuroeffector sites, reduces rigidity, tremors, hyperhidrosis of parkinsonism

Therapeutic outcome: Absence of peptic ulcer after treatment

USES: Treatment of peptic ulcer disease in combination with other products; other GI disorders, other spastic disorders, IBS, urinary incontinence

CONTRAINDICATIONS:
Hypersensitivity to anticholinergics, closed-angle glaucoma, GI obstruction, myasthenia gravis, paralytic ileus, GI atony, toxic megacolon, prostatic hypertrophy, urinary tract obstruction

Precautions: Pregnancy **C**, geriatric, hyperthyroidism, CAD, dysrhythmias, CHF, ulcerative colitis, hypertension, hiatal hernia, renal/hepatic disease, urinary retention

DOSAGE AND ROUTES
Adult/adolescent/child ≥12 yr: PO/SL 0.125-0.25 mg q4hr; EXT REL 0.375-0.75 mg q12hr
Adult: IM/SUBCUT/IV 0.25-0.5 mg single dose or 2-4×/day q6hr
Geriatric: Max 1.5 mg/day in divided doses or max 4 biphasic tabs
Child 2-12 yr: PO SL 0.0625-0.125 q4hr

Available forms: Tabs 0.125, 0.15 mg; ext rel caps 0.375 mg; time rel tabs 0.375 ml; sol 0.125 mg/ml; elix 0.125 mg/ml; inj 0.5 mg/ml, SL tab 0.125 mg, tab biphasic 0.125, 0.375 mg; orally disintegrating tab 0.125 mg

Implementation
• Do not break, crush, or chew time rel caps
• Give ½ hour before meals for better absorption
• Give decreased dose to geriatric patients; metabolism may be slowed
• Store in tight container protected from light

ADVERSE EFFECTS
CNS: *Confusion, stimulation in geriatric,* headache, insomnia, dizziness, drowsiness, anxiety, weakness, hallucination
CV: *Palpitations,* tachycardia
EENT: *Blurred vision,* photophobia, mydriasis, cycloplegia, increased ocular tension
GI: *Dry mouth, constipation, paralytic ileus,* heartburn, nausea, vomiting, dysphagia, absence of taste
GU: *Urinary hesitancy, retention,* impotence
INTEG: Urticaria, rash, pruritus, anhidrosis, fever, allergic reactions

Pharmacokinetics

Absorption	Well
Distribution	Cross blood-brain barrier, placenta
Metabolism	Liver
Excretion	Urine
Half-life	$3\frac{1}{2}$ hr

Pharmacodynamics

	PO	IM/IV/SUBCUT
Onset	30 min	2-3 min
Peak	Unknown	Unknown
Duration	4-6 hr	4-6 hr

INTERACTIONS
Individual drugs
Amantidine: increased anticholinergic effect
Ketoconazole, levodopa: decreased effects

Drug classifications
Antacids: decreased hyoscyamine effect
Antidepressants (tricyclics), antihistamines, H_1, MAOIs: increased anticholinergic effect
Phenothiazines: decreased effect of phenothiazines

NURSING CONSIDERATIONS
Assessment
• Monitor VS, cardiac status: checking for dysrhythmias, increased rate, palpitations
• Monitor I/O ratio; check for urinary retention or hesitancy
• Monitor GI complaints: pain, bleeding (frank or occult), nausea, vomiting, anorexia

Nursing diagnoses
• Constipation (adverse reactions)
• Injury, risk for (adverse reactions)
• Knowledge, deficient (teaching)

Patient/family education
• Teach patient to avoid driving, other hazardous activities until stabilized on medication
• Teach patient to avoid alcohol or other CNS depressants; will enhance sedating properties of this product
• Teach patient to avoid hot environments; heat stroke may occur; product suppresses perspiration
• Teach patient to use sunglasses when outside to prevent photophobia; may cause blurred vision
• Teach patient to use gum, hard candy, frequent rinsing of mouth for dryness of oral cavity
• Teach patient to increase fluids, bulk, exercise to decrease constipation

Evaluation
Positive therapeutic outcome
• Absence of epigastric pain, bleeding, nausea, vomiting

ibandronate (Rx)

(eye-ban'dro-nate)
Boniva
Func. class.: Bone-resorption inhibitor, electrolyte modifier
Chem. class.: Bisphosphonate
Pregnancy category C

ACTION: Inhibits bone resorption, apparently without inhibiting bone formation and mineralization; absorbs calcium phosphate crystals in bone and may directly block dissolution of hydroxyapatite crystals of bone; more potent than other products

Therapeutic outcome: Increased bone mineral density

USES: Osteoporosis and prophylaxis

Unlabeled uses: Hypercalcemia, osteolytic metastases, Paget's disease

CONTRAINDICATIONS:

Achalasia, esophageal stricture, hypocalcemia, intraarterial administration, renal failure, hypersensitivity to bisphosphonates

Precautions: Pregnancy C, breastfeeding, children, geriatric, anemia, chemotherapy, coagulopathy, dental disease, diabetes mellitus, dysphagia, GI/renal disease, GERD, hypertension, infection, multiple myeloma, phosphate hypersensitivity, vitamin D deficiency

DOSAGE AND ROUTES

Postmenopausal osteoporosis
Adult: PO 2.5 mg/day or 150 mg qmo; **IV** BOL 3 mg q3mo

Prophylaxis
Adult: PO 2.5 mg/day or 150 mg qmo

Paget's disease (unlabeled)
Adult: **IV** 2 mg as a single dose

Osteolytic metastases (unlabeled)
Adult: **IV** 6 mg over 1 hr × 3 days, repeat q4wk

Hypercalcemia (unlabeled)
Adult: **IV** INF 2 mg over 2 hr

Renal dose
Adult: PO CCr <30 ml/min, avoid use

Available forms: Tabs 2.5, 150 mg; sol for inj 3 mg/ml

Implementation
PO route
• Give early AM with a glass of water; if qmo, give on same day of each month

Direct IV route
• Use single-dose prefilled syringe; discard unused portion; give over 15-30 sec
• Store at room temperature

ADVERSE EFFECTS
CNS: Fever, insomnia, dizziness, headache
CV: Hypertension, **atrial fibrillation**
EENT: Ocular pain/inflammation, uveitis
GI: Constipation, nausea, vomiting, diarrhea, dyspepsia
INTEG: Rash, inj site reaction
META: *Hypomagnesemia, hypophosphatemia, hypocalcemia,* hypercholesterolemia
MS: Bone pain, myalgia, osteonecrosis of the jaw

Pharmacokinetics

Absorption	Poor
Distribution	Taken up primarily by bones, 86%-99% protein binding
Metabolism	Unknown
Excretion	Primarily by kidneys
Half-life	5-60 hr

Pharmacodynamics

Onset	Unknown
Peak	0.5-2 hr
Duration	Up to 1 mo

INTERACTIONS

Individual drugs
Calcium, vitamin D, iron, aluminum, magnesium salts: decreased ibandronate effect, separate by 1 hr
CycloSPORINE, tacrolimus: possible increased neurotoxicity

Drug classifications
Aminoglycosides, NSAIDs, radiopaque contrast agents: possible increased neurotoxicity
Loop diuretics: increased hypocalcemia

Drug/food
• Do not take with food, calcium

Drug/lab test
Decrease: Alk phos

NURSING CONSIDERATIONS

Assessment
- **Osteoporosis:** before and during treatment; monitor DEXA scan for bone mineral density
- Assess for blood studies: electrolytes, Ca, P, Mg; creatinine/BUN
- Assess for atrial fibrillation
- **Assess dental health;** before dental extraction, give antiinfectives
- Assess for bone pain; use analgesics

Nursing diagnoses
- Injury, risk for (uses)
- Knowledge, deficient (teaching)

Patient/family education
- **Teach patient to report hypercalcemic relapse:** nausea, vomiting, bone pain, thirst; unusual muscle twitching, muscle spasms, severe diarrhea, constipation
- Advise patient to continue with dietary recommendations, including calcium and vit D
- Instruct patient to obtain an analgesic from provider for bone pain
- Advise patient that if nausea/vomiting occur, small, frequent meals may help
- Teach patient to report vision symptoms: blurred vision, edema, inflammation; report to prescriber
- Teach to report if pregnancy is planned or suspected or if planning to breastfeed
- Encourage to exercise regularly, to stop smoking, and decrease alcohol
- Advise to take in AM at least 60 min before other meds, food, beverages
- Teach to sit upright ≥60 min after PO dose

Evaluation
Positive therapeutic outcome
- Increased bone mineral density

ibritumomab (Rx)
(ee-brit-u-moe'mab)
Zevalin
Func. class.: Radiopharmaceutical
Pregnancy category D

ACTION: High affinity for indium-111, yttrium-90; induces CD20⁺ B-cell lines

Therapeutic outcome: Decrease in tumor size, spread of malignancy

USES: Non-Hodgkin's lymphoma, B-cell NHL

CONTRAINDICATIONS:
Pregnancy **D**, hypersensitivity to murine proteins, prior murine antibody exposure

> **BLACK BOX WARNING:** Hypersensitivity to this agent, neutropenia, thrombocytopenia

Precautions: Breastfeeding, children, geriatric, cardiac conditions, immunizations after therapy

> **BLACK BOX WARNING:** Altered biodistribution, infusion-related reaction

DOSAGE AND ROUTES
Adult:
Step 1: IV RiTUXimab 250 mg/m² given first; premedicate with acetaminophen 650 mg and diphenhydrAMINE 50 mg

Adult (baseline platelets ≥150,000/mm³)
Step 2: 7-9 days after step 1, give a second dose of riTUXimab 250 mg/m² IV; within 4 hr of completing the riTUXimab infusion, give Y-90 ibritumomab tiuxetan 0.4 mCi/kg (14.8 MBq/kg) IV over 10 min; the dose given should be within 10% of the actual prescribed dose of Y-90 ibritumomab tiuxetan, the total dose given max 32 mCi (1184 MBq) regardless of the patient's weight

Adults (baseline platelets 100,000-149,000/mm³)
Step 2: 7-9 days after step 1, give a second dose of riTUXimab 250 mg/m² IV; within 4 hr of completing the riTUXimab infusion, give Y-90 ibritumomab tiuxetan 0.3 mCi/kg (11.1 MBq/kg) IV over 10 min; the dose given should be within 10% of the actual prescribed dose of Y-90 ibritumomab tiuxetan; the total dose given max 32 mCi (1184 MBq) regardless of the patient's weight

Adults (baseline platelets <100,000/mm³)
Do not use

Available forms: Inj 3.2 mg/2 ml

Implementation
- Do not use as BOL or IV direct
- Provide increased fluid intake to 2-3 L/day to prevent dehydration, unless contraindicated

IV infusion route
- See manufacturer's product labeling for preparation
- Have emergency equipment nearby with EPINEPHrine, antihistamines, corticosteroids

---

⚠ Nurse Alert

ADVERSE EFFECTS

CV: Cardiac dysrhythmias
GI: *Nausea, vomiting, anorexia,* abdominal pain, diarrhea
GU: Renal failure
HEMA: Leukopenia, neutropenia, thrombocytopenia, anemia
INTEG: *Irritation at site, rash,* fatal mucocutaneous infections (rare)
OTHER: Fever, chills, asthenia, headache, angioedema, hypotension, myalgia, bronchospasm, hemorrhage, infections, cough, dyspnea, dizziness, anxiety
SYST: Stevens-Johnson syndrome, secondary malignancies (AML, MDS), fatal infections

Pharmacokinetics

Absorption	Unknown
Distribution	Unknown
Metabolism	Unknown
Excretion	Unknown
Half-life	30 hr

Pharmacodynamics

Unknown

NURSING CONSIDERATIONS

Assessment

• Assess for infection, murine antibody titers

> **BLACK BOX WARNING: Assess for signs of fatal infusion reaction:** hypoxia, pulmonary infiltrates, ARDS, MI, ventricular fibrillation, cardiogenic shock; most fatal infusion reactions occur with first infusion; potentially fatal

• Assess biodistribution: first image 2-24 hr, second image 48-72 hr, third image 90-120 hr (optimal)
• **Assess for signs of severe mucocutaneous reactions:** Stevens-Johnson syndrome, lichenoid dermatitis, toxic epidermal lysis; occur 1-13 wk after product was given
⚠ **Assess for tumor lysis syndrome: acute renal failure requiring hemodialysis, hyperkalemia, hypocalcemia, hyperuricemia, hyperphosphatemia**

> **BLACK BOX WARNING: Bone marrow depression:** Monitor CBC, differential, platelet count weekly; withhold product if WBC is <3500/mm^3 or platelet count <150,000/mm^3; notify prescriber of these results

• Monitor GI symptoms: frequency of stools
• Assess for signs of dehydration: rapid respirations, poor skin turgor, decreased urine output, dry skin, restlessness, weakness

Nursing diagnoses

• Infection, risk for (adverse reactions)
• Knowledge, deficient (teaching)
• Nutrition: less than body requirements, imbalanced (adverse reactions)

Patient/family education

• Teach patient radiation safety precautions, disposal of body fluids
• Teach patient symptoms of infection
• Teach patient decreased blood count precautions
• Advise patient to report adverse reactions
• Advise patient to use contraception during and for 12 mo after therapy, pregnancy **D**
• Teach patient neutropenia and bleeding precautions

Evaluation

Positive therapeutic outcome

• Improvement in blood counts
• Decreased evidence of disease

---

ibuprofen (OTC, Rx)

(eye-byoo-proe'fen)

Advil, Advil Children's, Advil Infant's Concentrated, Advil Junior Strength, Apo-Ibuprofen ✦, Caldolor, ElixSure IB, Equaline Ibuprofen, Genpril, GoodSense Ibuprofen Junior Strength, Ibren, IBU, Infants Leader Ibu-drops, Leader Ibuprofen Jr, Midol Cramps and Body Aches Formula, Motrin ✦, Motrin IB, Motrin Infant's, Motrin Junior Strength, Pamprin IB ✦, Samson-8 Select Brand, Top Care Infant, Walgreens Ibuprofen, Wal-Profen

ibuprofen lysine (Rx)

NeoProfen

Do not confuse:

Nuprin/Lupron

ACTION: Inhibits COX-1, COX-2 by blocking arachidonate; analgesic, antiinflammatory, antipyretic

Therapeutic outcome: Decreased pain, inflammation, fever

USES: Rheumatoid arthritis, osteoarthritis, primary dysmenorrhea, gout, dental pain, musculoskeletal disorders, fever, migraine

CONTRAINDICATIONS:

Avoid in 3rd trimester of pregnancy (**D**), hypersensitivity to this product, NSAIDs, salicylates, asthma, severe renal/hepatic disease

> **BLACK BOX WARNING:** Perioperative pain in CABG

Precautions: Pregnancy **B** (1st and 2nd trimester), breastfeeding, children, geriatric, bleeding disorders, GI disorders, cardiac disorders, hypersensitivity to other antiinflammatory agents, CHF, CCr <25 ml/min

> **BLACK BOX WARNING:** GI bleeding, MI, stroke

DOSAGE AND ROUTES

Self-treatment of minor aches/pain
Adult/adolescent: PO (OTC product) 200 mg q4-6hr, may increase to 400 mg q4-6hr; max 1200 mg/day

Analgesia
Adult: PO 200-400 mg q4-6hr; max 3.2 g/day; OTC use max 1200 mg/day
Child: PO 4-10 mg/kg/dose q6-8hr

Moderate to severe pain (hospitalized patients) (Caldolor)
Adult: IV 400-800 mg q6hr as an adjunct to opiate agonist therapy

Dysmenorrhea
Adult: PO 400 mg q4hr; max 1200 mg/day

Antipyretic
Child 6 mo-12 yr: PO 5 mg/kg (temp <102.5° F or 39.2° C), 10 mg/kg (temp >102.5° F), may repeat q6-8hr; max 40 mg/kg/day

Antiinflammatory
Adult: PO 400-800 mg tid-qid; max 3.2 g/day
Child: PO 30-40 mg/kg/day in 3-4 divided doses; max 50 mg/kg/day

Patent ductus arteriosus (PDA) (Neoprofen)
Premature neonate ≤32 wk gestation who weighs 500-1500 g: IV 10 mg/kg initially, then if needed, 2 doses 5 mg/kg at 24 hr intervals; if oliguria occurs, hold dose

Available forms: Tabs 100, 200, 300, 400, 600, 800 mg; liqui-gel caps 200 mg; oral susp 100 mg/5 ml; liquid 100 mg/5 ml; chew tabs 50, 100 mg; drops 50 mg/1.25 ml; inj 10 mg/ml (NeoProfen); inj (Caldolor) 100 mg/ml

Implementation
PO route
- Administer to patient crushed or whole; 800-mg tab may be dissolved in water
- Give with food or milk to decrease gastric symptoms; give 2 hr before or 30 min after meals; absorption may be slowed
- Shake susp well before use

IV route
- Must be well hydrated prior to administration
- Dilute to ≤4 mg/ml (0.9% NaCl, LR, D_5); infuse over ≥30 min
- Discard unused portion

Intermittent IV infusion route
- Visually inspect for particulate
- Ibuprofen lysine: dilute with dextrose or saline to appropriate volume (10 mg/kg of ibuprofen is recommended) given within 30 min of preparation: give via port that is nearest insertion site; give over 15 min
- Check for extravasation; do not give in same line with TPN, interrupt TPN for 15 min before and after product administration

ADVERSE EFFECTS
CNS: *Headache,* dizziness, drowsiness, fatigue, tremors, confusion, insomnia, anxiety, depression
CV: Tachycardia, peripheral edema, palpitations, dysrhythmias, **CV thrombotic events, MI, stroke**
EENT: Tinnitus, hearing loss, blurred vision
GI: *Nausea, anorexia,* vomiting, diarrhea, jaundice, **hepatitis,** constipation, flatulence, cramps, dry mouth, peptic ulcer, **GI bleeding, ulceration, necrotizing enterocolitis, GI perforation**
GU: Nephrotoxicity, dysuria, hematuria, oliguria, azotemia
HEMA: Blood dyscrasias, increased bleeding time
INTEG: Purpura, rash, pruritus, sweating, urticaria, **necrotizing fasciitis**
SYST: Anaphylaxis, Stevens-Johnson syndrome

Pharmacokinetics

Absorption	Well absorbed
Distribution	Not known; crosses placenta
Metabolism	Liver, extensively
Excretion	Kidneys, unchanged (10%)
Half-life	1.8-2 hr

Pharmacodynamics

Onset	1/2 hr
Peak	1-2 hr
Duration	4-6 hr

INTERACTIONS

Individual drugs
Alcohol, aspirin: increased GI reactions
Aspirin: decreased ibuprofen action
CycloSPORINE, lithium, methotrexate: increased toxicity
Furosemide: decreased effect of furosemide
Radiation: increased risk of blood dyscrasias
Valproic acid, warfarin: increased risk of bleeding

Drug classifications
Anticoagulants, antiplatelet agents, salicylates, thrombolytics: increased risk of bleeding
Anticoagulants (oral): increased toxicity
Antidiabetics (oral): increased hypoglycemia
Antihypertensives: decreased effect of antihypertensives
Antineoplastics: increased risk of blood dyscrasias
Corticosteroids, NSAIDs: increased GI reactions
Diuretics: decreased effectiveness of diuretics (thiazides)

Drug/herb
Feverfew, garlic, ginger, ginkgo, ginseng *(Panax):* increased risk of bleeding

NURSING CONSIDERATIONS

Assessment
• **Assess for infection;** may mask symptoms
• **Assess pain:** location, duration, type, intensity before dose, 1 hr after
• Assess musculoskeletal status: ROM before dose, 1 hr after
• Monitor liver function tests: AST, ALT, bilirubin, creatinine if patient is on long-term therapy
• **Nephrotoxicity:** Monitor renal function tests: BUN, urine creatinine if patient is on long-term therapy
• Assess cardiac status: edema (peripheral), tachycardia, palpitations; monitor B/P, pulse for character, quality, rhythm
• Monitor blood studies: CBC, Hct, Hgb, protime if patient is on long-term therapy
• Check I&O ratio; decreasing output may indicate renal failure if patient is on long-term therapy
• Assess for history of peptic ulcer disorder; asthma, aspirin, hypersensitivity, check closely for hypersensitivity reactions
• **Assess for allergic reactions:** rash, urticaria; if these occur, product may have to be discontinued
• Assess for vision changes: blurring, halos; may indicate corneal, retinal damage
• Identify prior product history; there are many product interactions
• Identify fever: length of time in evidence and related symptoms

Nursing diagnoses
• Injury, risk for (side effects)
• Knowledge, deficient (teaching)
• Mobility, impaired physical (uses)
• Pain, acute (uses)
• Pain, chronic (uses)

Patient/family education
• Advise patient to read label on other OTC products
• Inform patient that the therapeutic response takes 1 mo (arthritis)
• Caution patient to avoid alcohol ingestion, salicylates, NSAIDs; GI bleeding may occur
• Advise patient with allergies that allergic reactions may develop
• Advise patient to use sunscreen to prevent photosensitivity
• Advise patient to report use of this product to all health care providers
• **Nephrotoxicity:** advise to report change in urinary pattern, weight increase, edema, increased pain in joints, fever, blood in urine

Evaluation
Positive therapeutic outcome
• Decreased pain
• Decreased inflammation
• Decreased fever
• Increased mobility

TREATMENT OF OVERDOSE:
Lavage, activated charcoal, induce diuresis

⚠ HIGH ALERT
ibutilide (Rx)
(eye-byoo′te-lide)
Corvert
Func. class.: Antidysrhythmic (Class III)
Pregnancy category C

ACTION: Prolongs duration of action potential and effective refractory period

USES: For rapid conversion of atrial fibrillation/flutter occurring within 1 wk of coronary artery bypass or valve surgery

CONTRAINDICATIONS:
Hypersensitivity

Precautions: Pregnancy C, breastfeeding, children <18 yr; geriatric, sinus node dysfuntion, 2nd- or 3rd-degree AV block, electrolyte imbalances, bradycardia, renal/hepatic disease, CHF

> **BLACK BOX WARNING:** QT prolongation, torsades de pointes, ventricular arrhythmias, ventricular tachycardia, cardiac dysrhythmias

DOSAGE AND ROUTES
Atrial fibrillation/flutter
Adult: IV INF (≥60 kg) 1 vial (1 mg) given over 10 min, may repeat same dose in 10 min; IV INF (<60 kg) 0.01 mg/kg given over 10 min, may repeat same dose in 10 min

Available forms: Inj 0.1 mg/ml

Implementation
IV route
• Give reduced dosage slowly with ECG monitoring only
• Give undiluted or diluted in 50 ml of 0.9% NaCl or D5W (0.017 mg/ml), give over 10 min
• Solution is stable for 48 hr refrigerated or 24 hr at room temperature
• Do not admix with other solution, products

ADVERSE EFFECTS
CNS: *Headache*
CV: *Hypotension, bradycardia,* **sinus arrest, CHF, dysrhythmias,** hypertension, extrasystoles, ventricular tachycardia, bundle branch block, AV block, palpitations, supraventricular extrasystoles, syncope, **prolonged QT interval, torsades de pointes**
GI: Nausea

Pharmacokinetics
Absorption	Unknown
Distribution	Unknown
Metabolism	Liver
Excretion	Kidney
Half-life	6 hr

Pharmacodynamics
Unknown

INTERACTIONS
Individual drugs
Digoxin: masking of cardiotoxicity

Drug classifications
Antidepressants (tricyclics/tetracyclics): prodysrhythmia
Antihistamines, H2-receptor antagonists, antidepressants, tetracyclines, tricyclics, phenothiazines: increased prodysrhythmia
Class Ia antidysrhythmics (disopyramide, quinidine, procainamide), class III agents (amiodarone, sotalol): do not use within 5 hr of ibutilide

NURSING CONSIDERATIONS
Assessment
• Monitor I&O ratio; monitor electrolytes: potassium, sodium, chloride
• Monitor liver function tests: AST, ALT, bilirubin, alkaline phosphatase
• Monitor ECG continuously to determine product effectiveness; measure PR, QRS, QT intervals; check for PVCs, other dysrhythmias; monitor B/P continuously for hypo/hypertension; check for rebound hypertension after 1-2 hr; discontinue product when atrial fibrillation/flutter ceases
• Monitor for dehydration or hypovolemia
• Assess for CNS symptoms: confusion, psychosis, numbness, depression, involuntary movements; if these occur product should be discontinued
• Monitor cardiac rate, respiration; rate, rhythm, character, chest pain, ventricular tachycardia, supraventricular tachycardia or fibrillation

Nursing diagnoses
• Cardiac output, decreased (uses)
• Gas exchange, impaired (adverse reactions)
• Knowledge, deficient (teaching)

Patient/family education
• Instruct patient to report side effects immediately to prescriber

---

⚠ *Nurse Alert*

Evaluation
Positive therapeutic outcome
• Decrease in atrial fibrillation/flutter

⚠ HIGH ALERT

IDArubicin (Rx)
(eye-da-roo'bi-sin)
Idamycin PFS
Func. class.: Antineoplastic, antibiotic
Chem. class.: Anthracycline glycoside
Pregnancy category D

Do not confuse:
IDArubicin/DOXOrubicin/DAUNOrubicin/
epirubicin, **Idamycin**/Adriamycin

ACTION: Not cell cycle specific; topo-isomerase II inhibitor, a vesicant

Therapeutic outcome: Prevention of rapidly growing malignant cells

USES: Used in combination with other antineoplastics for acute myelocytic leukemia in adults

Unlabeled uses: Breast cancer, liquid tumors

CONTRAINDICATIONS:
Pregnancy **D**, breastfeeding, hypersensitivity

> **BLACK BOX WARNING:** Myelosuppression, bilirubin >5 mg/dl

Precautions: Children, gout, bone marrow depression, preexisting CV disease

> **BLACK BOX WARNING:** Renal/hepatic disease, heart failure

DOSAGE AND ROUTES
Adult: IV 8-12 mg/m²/day × 3 days in combination with cytarabine (induction)

Renal/hepatic dose
Adult: IV if bilirubin is 2.5-5 mg/dl, give 50% of dose; if bilirubin >5 mg/dl, do not use; if CCr >2.5 mg/dl, reduce dose

Available forms: Inj 1 mg/ml

Implementation
IV route
• Avoid contact with skin; very irritating; wash completely to remove

• Administer antiemetic 30-60 min before giving product and prn to prevent vomiting; administer antibiotics for prophylaxis of infection

Intermittent IV infusion route
• Product should be prepared by experienced personnel using proper precautions (biological cabinet, wearing gown, gloves, mask)
• Do not give IM/subcut
• Give after reconstituting 5-mg vial with 5 ml of 0.9% NaCl (1 mg/1 ml); give over 10-15 min through Y-tube or 3-way stopcock of inf of D₅ or 0.9% NaCl; discard unused portion
• Apply ice compress after stopping infusion (extravasation)
• Store at room temperature for 3 days after reconstituting or 7 days refrigerated

Y-site compatibilities: Amifostine, amikacin, aztreonam, cimetidine, cladribine, cyclophosphamide, cytarabine, diphenhydrAMINE, droperidol, erythromycin, filgrastim, granisetron, imipenem/cilastatin, magnesium sulfate, mannitol, melphalan, metoclopromide, potassium chloride, ranitidine, sargramostim, thiotepa, vinorelbine

Y-site incompatibilities: Acyclovir, ampicillin/sulbactam, ceFAZolin, ceftazidine, clindamycin, dexamethasone, etoposide, furosemide, gentamicin, hydrocortisone, LORazepam, meperidine, methotrexate, mezlocillin, sargramostim, sodium bicarbonate, vancomycin, vinCRIStine

ADVERSE EFFECTS
CNS: Fever, chills, headache, **seizures**
CV: Dysrhythmias, CHF, pericarditis, myocarditis, peripheral edema, angina, **MI, myocardial toxicity**
GI: Nausea, vomiting, abdominal pain, mucositis, diarrhea, **hepatotoxicity**
GU: Nephrotoxicity, red urine
HEMA: Thrombocytopenia, leukopenia, anemia
INTEG: Rash, **extravasation,** dermatitis, reversible alopecia, urticaria, thrombophlebitis, tissue necrosis at inj site, radiation recall
SYST: Infection, tumor lysis syndrome

Pharmacokinetics	
Absorption	Complete bioavailability
Distribution	Rapidly distributed, protein binding 97%
Metabolism	Liver, extensively
Excretion	Bile
Half-life	22 hr

Adverse effects: *italics* = common; **bold** = life-threatening

Pharmacodynamics
Unknown

INTERACTIONS
Individual drugs
Radiation: increased toxicity

Drug classifications
Antineoplastics: increased toxicity
Live virus vaccines: decreased antibody response

Drug/lab test
Increased: uric acid

NURSING CONSIDERATIONS
Assessment
• **Assess for tumor lysis syndrome:** hyperkalemia, hyperphosphatemia, hyperuricemia, hypocalcemia
• **Assess symptoms indicating severe allergic reaction:** rash, pruritus, urticaria, purpuric skin lesions, itching, flushing; product should be discontinued
• Assess for tachypnea, dyspnea, edema, fatigue

> BLACK BOX WARNING: **Assess for cardiac toxicity:** CHF, dysrhythmias, cardiomyopathy; cardiac studies should be done before and periodically during treatment; ECG, chest x-ray, MUGA

• Monitor CBC, differential, platelet count weekly; withhold product if WBC is <4000/mm³ or platelet count is <100,000/mm³; notify prescriber of results if WBC <20,000/mm³, platelets <150,000/mm³
• Monitor renal function studies: BUN, uric acid, urine CCr, electrolytes, before, during therapy
• Monitor temp (may indicate beginning of infection)
• Monitor liver function tests before, during therapy (bilirubin, AST, ALT, LDH) as needed or monthly; note jaundice of skin and sclera, dark urine, clay-colored stools, itchy skin, abdominal pain, fever, diarrhea; hepatotoxicity can be severe
• Assess for bleeding: hematuria, stool guaiac, bruising or petechiae, mucosa or orifices, assess for inflammation of mucosa, breaks in skin
• Identify effects of alopecia on body image; discuss feelings about body changes
⚠ **Assess for local irritation, pain, burning at injection site, extravasation, a vesicant**

Nursing diagnoses
• Body image, disturbed (adverse reactions)
• Cardiac output, decreased (adverse reactions)
• Infection, risk for (adverse reactions)
• Injury, risk for (adverse reactions)
• Knowledge, deficient (teaching)

Patient/family education
• Teach patient to avoid use of products containing aspirin or ibuprofen, razors, commercial mouthwash, since bleeding may occur; to report symptoms of bleeding (hematuria, tarry stools)
• Instruct patient to report signs of anemia (fatigue, headache, irritability, faintness, shortness of breath)
• Advise patient that hair may be lost during treatment; a wig or hairpiece may make patient feel better; new hair may be different in color, texture
• Teach patient to rinse mouth tid-qid with water, club soda; brush teeth bid-qid with soft brush or cotton-tipped applicators for stomatitis; use unwaxed dental floss
• Tell patient not to have any vaccinations without the advice of the prescriber; serious reactions can occur
• Advise patient that contraception is needed during treatment and for several mo after the completion of therapy
• Teach patient to report signs of CHF, cardiac toxicity, beginning infection
• Advise patient to avoid crowds, those with upper respiratory illness
• Advise that all body fluids change color

Evaluation
Positive therapeutic outcome
• Prevention of rapid division of malignant cells

⚠ HIGH ALERT

ifosfamide (Rx)
(i-foss′fa-mide)
Ifex
Func. class.: Antineoplastic alkylating agent
Chem. class.: Nitrogen mustard
Pregnancy category D

Do not confuse:
ifosfamide/cyclophosphamide

ACTION: Alkylates DNA, RNA; inhibits enzymes that allow synthesis of amino acids in proteins; also responsible for cross-linking DNA strands; activity is not cell cycle stage specific

Therapeutic outcome: Prevention of rapidly growing malignant cells

---

⚠ Nurse Alert

USES: Testicular cancer

Unlabeled uses: Soft-tissue sarcoma, Ewing's sarcoma, non-Hodgkin's lymphoma, lung/pancreatic cancer, sarcoma

CONTRAINDICATIONS:
Pregnancy **D**, hypersensitivity

> **BLACK BOX WARNING:** Bone marrow suppression

Precautions: Renal/hepatic disease, breastfeeding, children

> **BLACK BOX WARNING:** Coma, hemorrhagic cystitis

DOSAGE AND ROUTES
Adult: IV 1.2-2 g/m^2/day × 5 days; repeat course q3wk; give with mesna

Renal dose
Adult: IV CCr 31-60 ml/min give 75% of dose; CCr 10-30 ml/min give 50% of dose; CCr <10 ml/min, do not give

Available forms: Inj 1, 3 g vials

Implementation

IV route
• Always give with mesna and increase fluids to 3 L/day to prevent ifosfamide-induced hemorrhagic cystitis
• Give ≥3 L/day fluids IV or PO before and after chemotherapy to hydrate patient to prevent hemorrhagic cystitis
• Give antiemetic 30-60 min before giving product and prn to prevent vomiting

Intermittent IV infusion route
• Dilute 1 g/20 ml or 3 g/60 ml of sterile or bacteriostatic water for inj with parabens or benzyl only; shake
• Give by intermittent inf after further diluting with D$_5$W, LR, 0.9% NaCl, sterile water for inj (1 g/20 ml = 50 mg/ml; 1 g/50 ml = 20 mg/ml; 1 g/200 ml = 5 mg/ml); give over ≥30 min; may also give as a cont inf over 72 hr
• Store powder at room temperature

Y-site compatibilities: Allopurinol, amifostine, aztreonam, filgrastim, fludarabine, gallium, granisetron, melphalan, ondansetron, paclitaxel, piperacillin/tazobactam, propofol, sargramostim, teniposide, thiotepa, vinorelbine

Additive compatibilities: CARBOplatin, CISplatin, etoposide, fluorouracil, mesna

ADVERSE EFFECTS
CNS: Facial paresthesia, fever, malaise, somnolence, confusion, depression, hallucinations, dizziness, disorientation, **seizures**, **coma**, cranial nerve dysfunction
GI: Nausea, vomiting, anorexia, **hepatotoxicity**, stomatitis, constipation, diarrhea
GU: Hematuria, **nephrotoxicity**, **hemorrhagic cystitis**, dysuria, urinary frequency
HEMA: **Thrombocytopenia, leukopenia, anemia**
INTEG: Dermatitis, alopecia, pain at inj site, hyperpigmentation
META: Metabolic acidosis

Pharmacokinetics
Absorption	Complete bioavailability
Distribution	Saturation at high dosages
Metabolism	Liver
Excretion	Breast milk
Half-life	15 hr, depends on dose

Pharmacodynamics
Unknown

INTERACTIONS

Individual drugs
Allopurinol: increased toxicity
Radiation: increased bone marrow suppression

Drug classifications
Anticoagulants, NSAIDs, salicylates, thrombolytics: increased bleeding risk
Antineoplastics: increased bone marrow suppression
CYP3A4 inducers, barbiturates: increased toxicity
CYP3A4 inhibitors: decreased ifosfamide effect
Live virus vaccines: decreased antibody response

NURSING CONSIDERATIONS

Assessment
⚠ Monitor CBC, differential, platelet count weekly; withhold product if WBC is <2000 or platelet count is <50,000; notify prescriber of results if WBC <10,000/mm^3, platelets <100,000/mm^3, severe myelosuppression
• Monitor renal function studies: BUN, serum uric acid, urine CCr before, during therapy; I&O ratio; report fall in urine output of 30 ml/hr
• Monitor for cold, fever, sore throat (may indicate beginning of infection); identify edema in feet and joints, stomach pain, shaking; prescriber should be notified

Adverse effects: *italics* = common; **bold** = life-threatening

• Assess for bleeding: hematuria, guaiac, bruising or petechiae, mucosa or orifices; no rect temp
• Monitor liver function tests before, during therapy (ALT, AST, LDH); jaundice of skin, sclera, dark urine, clay-colored stools, itching, abdominal pain, fever, diarrhea that may indicate liver involvement

Nursing diagnoses
• Body image, disturbed (adverse reactions)
• Infection, risk for (adverse reactions)
• Injury, risk for (adverse reactions)
• Knowledge, deficient (teaching)

Patient/family education
• Teach patient to avoid use of products containing aspirin or NSAIDs, razors, commercial mouthwash, since bleeding may occur; to report symptoms of bleeding (hematuria, tarry stools)
• Instruct patient to report signs of anemia (fatigue, headache, irritability, faintness, shortness of breath)
• Advise patient to report any changes in breathing or coughing even several mo after treatment; to avoid crowds and persons with respiratory tract or other infections
• Teach patient that hair loss is common; discuss the use of wigs or hairpieces; that hair may be a different texture when regrowth occurs
• Caution patient not to have any vaccinations without the advice of the prescriber; serious reactions can occur
• Advise patient that contraception is needed during treatment and for several mo after completion of therapy
• Advise patient to report confusion, hallucinations, extreme drowsiness, numbness, tingling; avoid use of alcohol for ≥4 months after treatment

Evaluation
Positive therapeutic outcome
• Prevention of rapid division of malignant cells
• Absence of swelling at night
• Increased appetite, increased weight

iloperidone (Rx)
(ill-o-pehr′ih-dohn)
Fanapt
Func. class.: Antipsychotic
Chem. class.: Benzisoxazole derivative
Pregnancy category C

ACTION: Unknown; may be mediated through both dopamine type 2 (D_2) and serotonin type 2 (5-HT_2) antagonism

Therapeutic outcome: Decreased signs/symptoms of schizophrenia

USES: Schizophrenia

CONTRAINDICATIONS:
Breastfeeding, hypersensitivity

Precautions: Pregnancy C, children, geriatric patients, renal/hepatic disease, breast cancer, Parkinson's disease, dementia with Lewy bodies, seizure disorder, QT prolongation, bundle branch block, acute MI, ambient temperature increase, AV block, stroke, substance abuse, suicidal ideation, tardive dyskinesia, torsades de pointes, blood dyscrasias

> **BLACK BOX WARNING:** Dementia

DOSAGE AND ROUTES
Adult: PO 1 mg bid, day 1; 2 mg bid, day 2, 4 mg bid, day 3; 6 mg bid, day 4; 8 mg bid, day 5; 10 mg bid, day 6; 12 mg bid, day 7; max 24 mg/day in two divided doses; reduce dose by 50% in poor metabolizer of CYP2D6 or when used with strong CYP2D6/CYP3A4 inhibitors

Available forms: Tabs 1, 2, 4, 6, 8, 10, 12 mg; titration pack

Implementation
• Give reduced dose in geriatric patients
• Give anticholinergic agent on order from prescriber, to be used for EPS
• Avoid use with CNS depressants
• Provide decreased stimulus by dimming lights, avoiding loud noises
• Provide supervised ambulation until patient is stabilized on medication; do not involve in strenuous exercise program because fainting is possible; patient should not stand still for a long time
• Give increased fluids to prevent constipation
• Provide sips of water, candy, gum for dry mouth
• Store in tight, light-resistant container (PO); unopened vials in refrigerator; protect from light; do not freeze

ADVERSE EFFECTS
CNS: *EPS, pseudoparkinsonism, akathisia, dystonia, tardive dyskinesia; drowsiness,* **seizures, neuroleptic malignant syndrome,** dizziness, delirium, depression, paranoia, fatigue, hostility, lethargy, restlessness, vertigo, tremor
CV: Orthostatic hypotension, **heart failure, AV block, QT prolongation,** tachycardia

EENT: Blurred vision, cataracts, nystagmus, tinnitus
GI: *Nausea,* vomiting, *anorexia, constipation,* jaundice, weight gain/loss, abdominal pain, stomatitis
GU: Hyperprolactinemia, urinary retention/incontinence, testicular pain, **renal failure**
MISC: **Renal artery occlusion**
HEMA: **Agranulocytosis, leukopenia, neutropenia**

Pharmacokinetics

Absorption	Unknown
Distribution	Unknown
Metabolism	Extensively, liver (major metabolite) CYP2D6, CYP3A4
Excretion	Urine
Half-life	Terminal 18 hr extensive metabolizers; 33 hr poor metabolizers

Pharmacodynamics

Onset	Unknown
Peak	2-4 hr
Duration	Unknown

INTERACTIONS

Individual drugs
Alcohol: increased sedation
Chloroquine, clarithromycin, droperidol, erythromycin, haloperidol, methadone, pentamidine: increased QT prolongation

Drug classifications
CYP2D6, CYP3A4 inducers (carBAMazepine, barbiturates, phenytoins, rifampin): decreased iloperidone action
CYP2D6, CYP3A4 inhibitors (delavirdine, indinavir, itraconazole, dalfopristin, ritonavir, tipranavir): increased iloperidone effect, decreased clearance
Class IA/ III antidysrhythmics, some phenothiazines, β-agonists, local anesthetics, tricyclics: increased QT prolongation
Other CNS depressants: increased sedation
SSRIs, SNRIs, serotonin-agonists: increased serotonin syndrome, neuroleptic malignant syndrome

Drug/lab test
Increase: prolactin levels

NURSING CONSIDERATIONS

Assessment
• Assess mental status before initial administration

• Monitor swallowing of PO medication; check for hoarding and for giving medication to other patients
• Monitor I&O ratio; palpate bladder if urinary output is low
• Monitor bilirubin, CBC, hepatic studies qmo
• Monitor urinalysis before, during prolonged therapy
• Assess affect, orientation, LOC, reflexes, gait, coordination, sleep pattern disturbances
• Monitor B/P standing and lying; also pulse, respirations; take these q4hr during initial treatment; establish baseline before starting treatment; report drops of 30 mm Hg; watch for ECG changes; QT prolongation may occur
• Assess for dizziness, faintness, palpitations, tachycardia on rising
• **Assess for EPS,** including akathisia, tardive dyskinesia (bizarre movements of the jaw, mouth, tongue, extremities), pseudoparkinsonism (rigidity, tremors, pill rolling, shuffling gait)

> **BLACK BOX WARNING:** Assess for serious reactions in the geriatric patient: fatal pneumonia, heart failure, sudden death

• **Assess for neuroleptic malignant syndrome:** hyperthermia, increased CPK, altered mental status, muscle rigidity
• Assess for constipation, urinary retention daily; if these occur, increase bulk and water in diet
• Monitor weight gain, hyperglycemia, metabolic changes in diabetes

Nursing Diagnoses
• Coping, ineffective (uses)
• Noncompliance (teaching)
• Knowledge, deficient (teaching)

Patient/family education
• Teach that orthostatic hypotension may occur and to rise from sitting or lying position gradually
• Advise to avoid hot tubs, hot showers, tub baths; hypotension may occur
• Teach to avoid abrupt withdrawal of this product; EPS may result; product should be withdrawn slowly
• Teach to avoid OTC preparations (cough, hay fever, cold) unless approved by prescriber; serious product interactions may occur; avoid use of alcohol; increased drowsiness may occur
• Advise to avoid hazardous activities if drowsy or dizzy
• Teach compliance with product regimen
• Teach to report impaired vision, tremors, muscle twitching

• Teach that heat stroke may occur in hot weather; take extra precautions to stay cool
• Advise to use contraception; inform prescriber if pregnancy is planned or suspected

Evaluation
Positive therapeutic outcome
• Decrease in emotional excitement, hallucinations, delusions, paranoia; reorganization of patterns of thought, speech

TREATMENT OF OVERDOSE:
Lavage if orally ingested; provide airway; *do not induce vomiting*

---

imatinib (Rx)
(im-ah-tin'ib)
Gleevec
Func. class.: Antineoplastic—miscellaneous
Chem. class.: Protein-tyrosine kinase inhibitor
Pregnancy category D

ACTION: Inhibits Bcr-Abl tyrosine kinase created in chronic myeloid leukemia (CML)

Therapeutic outcome: Decreased tumor size, prevention of spread of cancer

USES: Treatment of chronic myeloid leukemia (CML), Philadelphia chromosome positive in blast cell crisis or chronic failure after treatment failure with interferon alfa; gastrointestinal stromal tumors (GIST), positive for KIT; chronic eosinophilic leukemia, acute lymphocytic leukemia, dermatofibrosarcoma protuberans, myelodysplastic syndrome, systemic mastocytosis

CONTRAINDICATIONS:
Pregnancy **D**, hypersensitivity

Precautions: Breastfeeding, children, geriatric, cardiac/renal/hepatic/dental disease, GI bleeding, bone marrow suppression, infection, thrombocytopenia, neutropenia, immunosuppression

DOSAGE AND ROUTES

Acute lymphocytic leukemia (ALL)
Adult: PO 600 mg q day

CML, chronic phase
Adult: PO 400-600 mg/day
Adolescent/child ≥2 yr: PO 340 mg/m²/day, max 600 mg/day

CML, accelerated phase/blast crisis
Adult: PO 600-800 mg/day

GIST
Adult: PO 400-600 mg/day

Hepatic dose
Adult: PO total bilirubin 1.5-3 × ULN and any AST, decrease initial dose to 400 mg/day; total bilirubin >3 × ULN and any AST, decrease initial dose to 300 mg/day

Renal dose
Adult: PO CCr 40-59 ml/min, max 600 mg/day; CCr 20-39 ml/min decrease initial dose by 50%, max 400 mg/day; CCr <20 ml/min use with caution 100 mg/day

Available forms: Tabs 100, 400 mg

Implementation
PO route
• Give with meal and large glass of water to decrease GI symptoms, doses of 800 mg should be given 400 mg bid
• Tab may be dispersed in a glass of water or apple juice, use 50 ml of liquid for 100 mg tab, 200 ml/400 mg
• Store at 25° C (77° F)

ADVERSE EFFECTS
CNS: CNS hemorrhage, headache, dizziness, insomnia
CV: Hemorrhage, heart failure, cardiac tamponade, hypereosinophilia, cardiac toxicity
EENT: Blurred vision, conjunctivitis
GI: *Nausea,* **hepatotoxicity,** *vomiting, dyspepsia,* **GI hemorrhage,** *anorexia,* abdominal pain, GI perforation, diarrhea
HEMA: Neutropenia, thrombocytopenia, bleeding
INTEG: *Rash, pruritus,* alopecia, photosensitivity
META: Edema, fluid retention, hypokalemia
MISC: Fatigue, epistaxis, pyrexia, night sweats, increased weight, flulike symptoms, hypothyroidism
MS: Cramps, pain, arthralgia, myalgia
RESP: Cough, dyspnea, nasopharyngitis, pneumonia, URI, pleural effusion, edema

Pharmacokinetics

Absorption	Well absorbed; bound to plasma protein (98%)
Distribution	Unknown
Metabolism	Liver (metabolites)
Excretion	Feces, primarily (metabolites)
Half-life	18-40 hr

Pharmacodynamics

Onset	Unknown
Peak	2-4 hr
Duration	24 hr (imatinib), 40 hr (metabolite)

INTERACTIONS

Individual drugs

Acetaminophen: increased hepatotoxicity

Simvastatin: increased plasma concentrations

Warfarin: increased plasma concentration of warfarin; avoid coadministration; use low-molecular-weight anticoagulants instead

Drug classifications

Calcium channel blockers, ergots: increased plasma concentrations

CYP3A4 inducers (carBAMazepine, dexamethasone, PHENobarbital, phenytoin, rifampin): decreased imatinib concentrations

CYP3A4 inhibitors (clarithromycin, erythromycin, ketoconazole, itraconazole): increased imatinib concentrations

Drug/food

Grapefruit juice: increased imatinib effect, avoid while taking this product

Drug/herb

St. John's wort: decreased imatinib concentration

NURSING CONSIDERATIONS

Assessment

• **Bone marrow suppression:** Assess ANC and platelets; in chronic phase if ANC $<1 \times 10^9$/L and/or platelets $<50 \times 10^9$/L, stop until ANC $>1.5 \times 10^9$/L and platelets $>75 \times 10^9$/L; in accelerated phase/blast crisis if ANC $<0.5 \times 10^9$/L and/or platelets $<10 \times 10^9$/L, determine whether cytopenia is related to biopsy/aspirate; if not, reduce dose by 200 mg; if cytopenia continues, reduce dose by another 100 mg; if cytopenia continues for 4 wk, stop product until ANC $\geq 1 \times 10^9$/L

• **Assess for hepatotoxicity:** monitor liver function tests before treatment, qmo if line transaminases are $>5 \times$ IULN, withhold imatinib until transaminase levels return to $<2.5 \times$ IULN

• **Renal toxicity:** monitor bilirubin, if $>3 \times$ IULN, withhold imatinib until bilirubin levels return to $<1.5 \times$ IULN

• Assess GI symptoms: frequency of stools

• Assess signs of fluid retention, edema: weigh, monitor lung sounds, 50-ml fluid retention is dose dependent

Nursing diagnoses

• Injury, risk for (side effects)

• Knowledge, deficient (teaching)

Patient/family education

• Instruct patient to report adverse reactions immediately: shortness of breath, swelling of extremities, bleeding

• Teach patient reason for treatment, expected result

• Instruct patient to eat a nutritious diet with iron, vit supplement, low fiber, few dairy products

Evaluation

Positive therapeutic outcome

• Decrease in leukemic cells, size of tumors

---

imipenem/cilastatin (Rx)

(i-me-pen'em sye-la-stat'in)

Primaxin IM, Primaxin IV

Func. class.: Antiinfective, miscellaneous penicillin

Chem. class.: Carbapenem

Pregnancy category C

Do not confuse:

imipenem/Omnipen, **Primaxin**/Premarin

ACTION: Interferes with cell wall replication of susceptible organisms; osmotically unstable cell wall swells and bursts from osmotic pressure; addition of cilastatin prevents renal inactivation that occurs with high urinary concentrations of imipenem

Therapeutic outcome: Bactericidal action against the following: *Streptococcus pneumoniae,* group A β-hemolytic streptococci, *Staphylococcus aureus,* enterococcus; gram-negative organisms: *Klebsiella, Proteus, Escherichia coli, Acinetobacter, Serratia, Pseudomonas aeruginosu; Salmonella, Shigella, Haemophilus influenzae, Listeria* spp.

USES: Serious infections caused by gram-positive or gram-negative organisms

CONTRAINDICATIONS: Hypersensitivity, IM hypersensitivity to local anesthetics of the amide type, or carbapenems, AV block, shock (IM)

Precautions: Pregnancy **C**, breastfeeding, children, geriatric, hypersensitivity to cephalosporins, penicillins, seizure disorders, renal disease, head trauma, pseudomembranous colitis, ulcerative colitis

---

DOSAGE AND ROUTES

Adult: IV 250-500 mg q6-8hr; severe infections may require 1 g q8hr; may give IM q12hr (total daily IM dose >1500 mg not recommended); mild to moderate infections

Child: IV 60-100 mg/kg/day in divided doses, max 4 g/day; IM 10-15 mg/kg q6hr

Renal dose

Adult ≥70 kg (reduce normal dose of 1 g/day to): IV CCr 41-70 ml/min 250 mg q8hr; CCr 6-40 ml/min 250 mg q12hr; **(reduce normal dose of 1.5 g/day to):** CCr 41-70 ml/min 250 mg q6hr; CCr 21-40 ml/min 250 mg q8hr; CCr 6-20 ml/min 250 mg q12hr; **(reduce normal dose of 2 g/day to):** CCr 41-70 ml/min 500 mg q8hr; CCr 21-40 ml/min 250 mg q6hr; CCr 6-20 250 mg q12hr

Available forms: Powder for sol inj 250, 500; powder for susp 500 mg

Implementation

IM route

• Reconstitute 500 mg/2 ml lidocaine without epiNEPHrine; shake well, withdraw and administer entire vial; give inj deep in large muscle mass, aspirate, product for IM is not for IV use

Intermittent IV infusion route

• Reconstitute each 250 or 500 mg/10 ml of compatible diluent; shake well; transfer the resulting susp to ≥100 ml of compatible diluent; add 10 ml to each previously reconstituted vial and shake to ensure all medication is used; transfer the remaining contents of the vial to the inf container; do not administer susp by direct inj

• Give each 250- or 500-mg dose over 20-30 min, and each 1-g dose over 40-60 min; administer over 15-20 min for pediatric patients; do not administer direct **IV**; do not admix with other antibiotics

Y-site compatibilities: Acyclovir, amifostine, aztreonam, cefepime, diltiazem, famotidine, fludarabine, foscarnet, granisetron, IDArubicin, regular insulin, melphalan, methotrexate, ondansetron, propofol, tacrolimus, teniposide, thiotepa, vinorelbine, zidovudine

Y-site incompatibilities: Fluconazole, meperidine, sargramostim

ADVERSE EFFECTS

CNS: Fever, somnolence, **seizures,** confusion, dizziness, weakness, myoclonus

CV: Hypotension, palpitations, tachycardia

GI: *Diarrhea, nausea, vomiting,* **pseudomembranous colitis, hepatitis,** glossitis

GU: Renal toxicity/failure

HEMA: Eosinophilia, neutropenia, decreased Hgb, Hct

INTEG: Rash, urticaria, pruritus, pain at inj site, phlebitis, erythema at inj site

RESP: Chest discomfort, dyspnea, hyperventilation

SYST: Anaphylaxis, Stevens-Johnson syndrome

Pharmacokinetics

Absorption	Complete bioavailability (**IV**)
Distribution	Widely distributed; crosses placenta
Metabolism	Liver
Excretion	Kidneys, unchanged (70%-80%); breast milk
Half-life	1 hr; increased in renal disease

Pharmacodynamics

	IM	IV
Onset	Unknown	Rapid
Peak	Unknown	$1/2$-1 hr

INTERACTIONS

Individual drugs

Aminophylline, cycloSPORINE, ganciclovir, theophylline: increased risk of seizures

Probenecid: increased imipenem plasma levels

Valproic acid: decreased effect of valproic acid

Drug classifications

β-Lactam antibiotics: increased antagonistic effect

Drug/lab test

Increased: AST, ALT, LDH, BUN, alkaline phosphatase, bilirubin, creatinine

False positive: direct Coombs' test

NURSING CONSIDERATIONS

Assessment

• Assess patient for previous penicillin sensitivity reaction, may have sensitivity to this product

• **Assess patient for signs and symptoms of infection,** including characteristics of wounds, sputum, urine, stool, WBC >10,000/mm³, fever; obtain baseline information before, during treatment

• Complete C&S tests before beginning product therapy to identify if correct treatment has been initiated

• **Assess for allergic reactions, anaphylaxis:** rash, urticaria, pruritus, chills, wheezing, laryngeal edema, fever, joint pain; angioedema may occur a few days after therapy begins; epiNEPHrine, resuscitation equipment should be available for anaphylactic reaction

• Identify urine output; if decreasing, notify prescriber (may indicate nephrotoxicity); also check for increased BUN, creatinine

• Monitor blood studies: AST, ALT, CBC, Hct, bilirubin, LDH, alkaline phosphatase, Coombs' test monthly if patient is on long-term therapy

• Monitor electrolytes: potassium, sodium, chloride monthly if patient is on long-term therapy

• Assess bowel pattern daily; if severe diarrhea occurs, product should be discontinued; may indicate pseudomembranous colitis

• **Monitor for bleeding:** ecchymosis, bleeding gums, hematuria, stool guaiac daily if patient is on long-term therapy

• Assess for overgrowth of infection: perineal itching, fever, malaise, redness, pain, swelling, drainage, rash, diarrhea, change in cough, sputum

Nursing diagnoses
• Diarrhea (adverse reactions)
• Infection, risk for (uses)
• Injury, risk for (adverse reactions)
• Knowledge, deficient (teaching)
• Noncompliance (teaching)

Patient/family education
• Advise patient to report sore throat, bruising, bleeding, joint pain; may indicate blood dyscrasias (rare)

• Advise patient to contact prescriber if vaginal itching, loose foul-smelling stools, furry tongue occur; may indicate superinfection

• Advise patient to notify prescriber of diarrhea with blood or pus; may indicate pseudomembranous colitis

Evaluation
Positive therapeutic outcome
• Absence of signs/symptoms of infection (WBC <10,000/mm³, temp WNL, absence of red, draining wounds)

• Reported improvement in symptoms of infection

TREATMENT OF ANAPHY-LAXIS: EPINEPHrine, antihistamines, resuscitate if needed

imipramine (Rx)
(im-ip'ra-meen)
Apo-Imipramine ✦, Tofranil, Tofranil PM
Func. class.: Antidepressant, tricyclic
Chem. class.: Dibenzazepine, tertiary amine
Pregnancy category D

Do not confuse:
imipramine/desipramine

ACTION: Blocks reuptake of norepinephrine and serotonin into nerve endings, increasing action of norepinephrine and serotonin in nerve cells; has anticholinergic effects

Therapeutic outcome: Decreased symptoms of depression after 2-3 wk; decreased bedwetting in children

USES: Depression, enuresis in children

Unlabeled uses: Chronic pain, migraine headaches, cluster headaches as adjunct, incontinence

CONTRAINDICATIONS:
Pregnancy **D**, hypersensitivity to tricyclics, AV block, bundle-branch block, ileus, QT prolongation, acute MI

Precautions: Suicidal patients, severe depression, increased intraocular pressure, closed-angle glaucoma, urinary retention, cardiac/hepatic disease, hyperthyroidism, electroshock therapy, elective surgery, breast-feeding, geriatric, seizure disorders, prostatic hypertrophy, MI

BLACK BOX WARNING: Children other than for enuresis; suicidal ideation

DOSAGE AND ROUTES
Adult: PO 75-100 mg/day in divided doses; may increase by 25-50 mg up to 200 mg, 200 mg/day (outpatients), 300 mg/day (inpatients); may give daily dose at bedtime
Geriatric: PO 25-50 mg at bedtime, may increase to 100 mg/day in divided doses
Child ≥6 yr (unlabeled): PO 1.5 mg/kg/day in divided doses; max 2.5 mg/kg/day

Enuresis
Child 6-12 yr: PO 10-25 mg at bedtime, max 50 mg

Available forms: Tabs 10, 25, 50 mg; caps 75, 100, 125, 150 mg

Implementation
PO route
- Do not break, crush, or chew caps
- Give with food or milk
- Store at room temperature; do not freeze

ADVERSE EFFECTS
CNS: *Dizziness, drowsiness,* confusion, headache, anxiety, tremors, stimulation, weakness, insomnia, nightmares, EPS (geriatric), increased psychiatric symptoms, paresthesia, **seizures**

CV: *Orthostatic hypotension, ECG changes, tachycardia,* hypertension, palpitations, **dysrhythmias**

EENT: Blurred vision, tinnitus, mydriasis

GI: *Diarrhea, dry mouth,* nausea, vomiting, **paralytic ileus,** increased appetite, cramps, epigastric distress, jaundice, **hepatitis,** stomatitis, constipation, taste change

GU: *Retention,* **acute renal failure**

HEMA: **Agranulocytosis, thrombocytopenia, eosinophilia, leukopenia**

INTEG: Rash, urticaria, sweating, pruritus, photosensitivity, hyperpigmentation (rare)

Pharmacokinetics

Absorption	Well absorbed
Distribution	Widely distributed; crosses placenta
Metabolism	Liver, extensively
Excretion	Kidneys, breast milk
Half-life	6-20 hr

Pharmacodynamics

	PO
Onset	1 hr
Peak	Unknown
Duration	Unknown

INTERACTIONS
Individual drugs
Alcohol: increased effects

CloNIDine: hyperpyretic crisis, seizures, hypertensive episode

CloNIDine, guanethidine: decreased effects

Gatifloxacin, levofloxacin, moxifloxacin, ziprasidone: increased QT interval

Drug classifications
MAOIs: hyperpyretic crisis, hypertensive episode, seizures

SSRIs, SNRIs, serotonin-receptor agonists: increased serotonin syndrome, increased neuroleptic malignant syndrome; avoid concurrent use

Sympathomimetics (direct acting [EPINEPHrine]), barbiturates, benzodiazepines, CNS depressants: increased effects

Sympathomimetics (indirect acting [ePHEDrine]): decreased effects

Tricyclic antidepressants, class IA/III antidysrhythmics: increased QT interval

Drug/herb
St. John's wort: serotonin syndrome

Drug/lab test
Increased: serum bilirubin, blood glucose, alkaline phosphatase

Decreased: VMA, 5-HIAA, urinary catecholamines

NURSING CONSIDERATIONS
Assessment
- Monitor B/P (with patient lying, standing), pulse q4hr; if systolic B/P drops 20 mm Hg, hold product, notify prescriber; take vital signs q4hr in patients with CV disease
- Monitor blood studies: CBC, leukocytes, differential, cardiac enzymes if patient is receiving long-term therapy
- Monitor hepatic studies: AST, ALT, bilirubin
- Check weight weekly; appetite may increase with product
- **QT prolongation:** Assess ECG for flattening of T wave, bundle branch block, AV block, dysrhythmias in cardiac patients
- Assess for EPS primarily in geriatric: rigidity, dystonia, akathisia
- Assess mental status: mood, sensorium, affect, suicidal tendencies; increase in psychiatric symptoms: depression, panic
- Monitor urinary retention, constipation; constipation is more likely to occur in children or geriatric
- **⚠ Assess for withdrawal symptoms: headache, nausea, vomiting, muscle pain, weakness, diarrhea, insomnia, restlessness; do not usually occur unless product was discontinued abruptly**
- Identify alcohol consumption; if alcohol is consumed, hold dose until AM

Nursing diagnoses
- Coping, ineffective (uses)
- Injury, risk for (side effects)
- Knowledge, deficient (teaching)
- Noncompliance (teaching)

Patient/family education
- Teach patient that therapeutic effects may take 2-3 wk

⚠ Nurse Alert

- Teach patient to use caution in driving and other activities requiring alertness because of drowsiness, dizziness, blurred vision; to avoid rising quickly from sitting position, especially geriatric; orthostatic hypotension may occur
- Teach patient to avoid alcohol ingestion, other CNS depressants during treatment
- Teach patient not to discontinue medication quickly after long-term use: may cause nausea, headache, malaise
- Teach patient to wear sunscreen or large hat, since photosensitivity occurs
- Teach patient to increase fluids, bulk in diet if constipation, urinary retention occur, especially geriatric
- Teach patient to take gum, hard sugarless candy, frequent sips of water for dry mouth

Evaluation
Positive therapeutic outcome
- Decreased depression
- Absence of suicidal thoughts
- Decreased enuresis in children
- Decreased pain

TREATMENT OF OVERDOSE:
ECG monitoring, lavage, activated charcoal, administer anticonvulsant

immune globulin IM (IMIg, IgIM) (Rx)
Bay Gam 15%, Flebogamma 5%, Flebogamma DIF 5%, Gamunex 10%, Privigen 10%, Vivaglobin 10%
immune globulin IV (IGIV, IVIG) (Rx)
Bay Gam 15%, Carimune DF, Flebogamma 5%, Flebogamma 10% DIF, Gammaked, Gammaplex, Gammar-P IV, Gammagard S/D, Gamunex, Iveegram EN, Polygam S/D, Privigen, Vivaglobin
immune globulin SC (SCIG, IGSC) (Rx)
Bay Gam 15%, Flebogamma 5%, Flebogamma DIF 5%, Gammagard Liquid 10%, Gammaked, Gammaplex, Gamunex 10%, Privigen 10%, Vivaglobin

Func. class.: Immune serum
Chem. class.: IgG
Pregnancy category C

Do not confuse:
Iveegam/Invega

ACTION: Provides passive immunity to hepatitis A, measles, varicella, rubella, immune globulin deficiency; contains γ-globulin antibodies (IgG)

Therapeutic outcome: Absence of infection

USES: Immunodeficiency syndrome, B-cell chronic lymphocytic leukemia, Kawasaki's syndrome, bone marrow transplantation, pediatric HIV infection, agammaglobulinemia, hepatitis A, B exposure, measles exposure, measles vaccine complications, purpura, rubella exposure, chickenpox exposure, chronic inflammatory demyelinating polyneuropathy

Unlabeled uses: IV posttransfusion purpura, Guillain-Barré syndrome

CONTRAINDICATIONS:
Coagulopathy, hemophilia, IgA deficiency, thrombocytopenia

Precautions: Pregnancy C, breastfeeding, children, agammaglobulinemia, bleeding, hypogammaglobulinemia, infection, IV, viral infection

DOSAGE AND ROUTES
Immune globulin IM (IMIg, IgIM)

Hepatitis A prophylaxis
Adult, geriatric, adolescent, children, infant (unlabeled): IM 0.02 ml/kg for those who have not received Hepatitis A vaccine and have been exposed in the last 2 wk

Measles prophylaxis (exposed in last 6 days)
Adult: IM 0.25 ml/kg (immunocompetent)
Child (unlabeled): IM 0.5 ml/kg as a single dose, max 15 ml (immunocompromised)

Varicella prophylaxis
Adult: IM 0.6-1.2 ml/kg as soon as possible and if varicella-zoster immune globulin is not available

Rubella prophylaxis in exposed/ susceptible who will not consider a therapeutic abortion
Adult: Pregnant women IM 0.55 ml/kg

Immunoglobulin deficiency
Adult: 1.32 ml/kg, then 0.66 ml/kg (at least 100 mg/kg) q3-4wk

Immune globulin IV (IVIG, IGIV)

Primary immunodeficiency

Gammagard S/D
Adult/adolescent/child: IV 300-600 mg/kg q3-4wk

Polygam S/D
Adult/adolescent/child: IV 100 mg/kg qmo; initially 200-400 mg/kg may be used

Gammar-P IV
Adult: IV 200-400 mg/kg q3-4wk
Adolescent/child: IV 200 mg/kg q3-4wk

Gamunex
Adult/adolescent/child: IV INF 300-600 mg/kg (3-6 ml/kg) q3-4wk; initial infusion rate 1 mg/kg/min (max 8 mg/kg/min)

Iveegam EN
Adult/adolescent/child: IV 200 mg/kg qmo; max 800 mg/kg qmo

Panglobulin NF/Carimune NF
Adult/adolescent/child: IV 200 mg/kg qmo

Gammagard Liquid/Flebogamma 5%
Adult/adolescent/child: IV 300-600 mg/kg q3-4wk

Privigen
Adult/adolescent/child ≥3 yr: IV 200-800 mg q3-4wk

Idiopathic thrombocytopenic purpura (ITP)

Panglobulin NF/Carimune NF
Adult/child: IV 400 mg/kg qd × 2-5 days; in acute ITP of childhood, only 2 of the 5 days are needed if initial platelets are 30,000-50,000 mcl after 2 doses

Gammagard S/D/Polygam S/D
Adult/adolescent/child: IV 1000 mg/kg as a single dose; may give on alternate days for up to 3 doses

Gamunex
Adult/adolescent/child: IV INF total dose of 2000 mg/kg, divided as 1000 mg/kg (10 ml/kg) given on 2 consecutive days; initial rate is 1 mg/kg/min (max 8 mg/kg/min), if after 1st dose adequate platelets are observed after 24 hr, may withhold 2nd dose

Privigen
Adult/adolescent ≥15 yr: 1 g/kg/day × 2 days

Kawasaki's disease

Iveegam EN
Child: IV 400 mg/kg qd × 4 consecutive days or a single dose of 2000 mg/kg over 10 hr; give with aspirin 100 mg/kg/day through 14th day of illness, then 3-5 mg/kg each day thereafter for 5 wk

Gammagard S/D/Polygam S/D
Infant/child: IV 1000 mg/kg (single dose) or 400 mg/kg/day × 4 days beginning within 7 days of fever onset, with aspirin 80-100 mg/kg/day × 4 divided doses

Immune globulin SC (SCIG/IgSC)
Adult/child >2 yr: SC infusion 100-200 mg/kg qwk; **Vivaglobin** brand of SGIG 160 mg IgG/ml, SC inj; max 15 ml for injection, given at max of 20 ml/hr

Available forms: IM (Bay Gam) inj 2, 10 ml vial; IV (Gamimune N) 5%, 10% sol; powder for inj (Carimune NF) 1-, 3-, 6-, 12-g vials; (Gammagard S/D) 50 mg protein/ml in 2.5-, 5-, 10-g vials; (Gammar-P IV) 1-, 2.5-, 5-, 10-g vials; (Iveegam) 500 mg, 1-, 2.5-, 5-g vials; (Panglobulin) 6-, 12-g vials; (Polygam S/D) 2.5-, 5-, 10-g vials; sol for inj (Gamunex) 1-, 2.5-, 5-, 10-, 20-g vials; human sol for inj: Flebogamma 5%, 10% DIF

Implementation
IM route
• Give IM (IGIM) inj in deltoid or anterolateral thigh in adults or anterolateral thigh in young children; if large amounts are given, several injections may be needed
• Do not give the IM preparation IV, SUBCUT, or intradermally
• Sol should be transparent and clear or slightly colored

IV route
• Warm to room temperature before administration (diluent, powder for inj)
• A transfer device is provided by manufacturer; this product should not be agitated or shaken
• Do not give the IV preparation SUBCUT, IM, or intradermally
• Check for adverse reaction during inf; stop inf if adverse reactions occur

Y-site compatibilities: Fluconazole, sargramostim
Gamimune N: Dilute IV with D_5; give 0.01 ml/kg/min; may increase to 0.02-0.04 ml/kg/min if no adverse reactions occur; may increase to 0.08 ml/kg/hr; sol should be refrigerated; do not freeze

Gammagard S/D: Reconstitute with sterile water for inj (50 mg protein/ml); give within 2 hr of reconstitution; give 0.5 ml/kg/hr; may increase to 4 ml/kg/hr if no adverse reactions occur; use inf set provided

Gammar-P IV: Give 0.01 ml/kg/min (50 mg/ml sol) over 15-30 min; may increase to 0.02 ml/kg/min; if adverse reactions are not present, may increase to 0.03-0.06 ml/kg/min; do not freeze; store at room temperature

Iveegam (5%): Give 1-2 ml/min; refrigerate, do not freeze

ADVERSE EFFECTS

CNS: Headache, fatigue, malaise
GI: Abdominal pain
HEMA: Thromboembolism (Vivaglobin)
INTEG: Pain at inj site, rash, pruritus, chills
MS: Arthralgia, chest pain
SYST: Lymphadenopathy, **anaphylaxis**

Pharmacokinetics

Absorption	Well absorbed (IM); completely absorbed (**IV**)
Distribution	Rapidly
Metabolism	Liver, catabolism
Excretion	Kidneys
Half-life	3-4 wk

Pharmacodynamics

	IM	IV
Onset	Unknown	Rapid
Peak	Unknown	Unknown
Duration	Unknown	Unknown

INTERACTIONS

Drug classifications
Live virus vaccines: do not give within 3 mo

Drug/lab test
Interference: glucose testing system

NURSING CONSIDERATIONS

Assessment
• Assess for exposure date: this product should be given within 6 days of measles, 1 wk of hepatitis B, 14 days of hepatitis A; if the date of exposure is outside these limits, immune globulin will not be effective
• Monitor blood studies in leukemia, idiopathic thrombocytopenic purpura: WBCs (leukemia), platelets
• Identify the number of inj of this product patient has received; multiple inj may lead to sensitization (diaphoresis, fever, chills, malaise)

• Assess for anaphylaxis in patient receiving **IV** immune globulin: diaphoresis, flushing, nausea, vomiting, wheezing, difficulty breathing, hypotension, chest tightness, fever, weakness, sneezing, abdominal pain; VS should be monitored during inf and 1 hr after beginning inf; emergency equipment should be available with epinephrine and antihistamines to treat anaphylaxis

Nursing diagnoses
• Infection, risk for (uses)
• Knowledge, deficient (teaching)

Patient/family education
• Advise patient that passive immunity is temporary; explain reason for and expected results of this product
• Advise patient that pain and tenderness may occur at inj site

Evaluation
Positive therapeutic outcome
• Prevention of infection
• Increased platelets

TREATMENT OF ANAPHYLAXIS: EPINEPHrine, diphenhydrAMINE, O_2, vasopressors, corticosteroids

⚠ HIGH ALERT

inamrinone (Rx)
(in-am'rih-nohn)
Func. class.: Inotropic agent
Chem. class.: Bipyrimidine derivative
Pregnancy category C

Do not confuse:
inamrinone/amiodarone

ACTION: Positive inotropic agent with vasodilator properties; reduces preload and afterload by direct **Discontinued** vascular smooth muscle; increases myocardial contractility

Therapeutic outcome: Increased inotropic effect resulting in increased cardiac output

USES: Short-term management of CHF that has not responded to other medication (diuretics, other vasodilators); can be used with digoxin

CONTRAINDICATIONS: Hypersensitivity to this product or bisulfites, severe aortic disease, severe pulmonic valvular disease, acute MI

Adverse effects: *italics* = common; **bold** = life-threatening

Precautions: Pregnancy C, breastfeeding, children, geriatric, renal/hepatic disease, atrial flutter/fibrillation, asthma

DOSAGE AND ROUTES
Adult and child: IV BOL 0.75 mg/kg given over 2-3 min; start INF of 5-10 mcg/kg/min; may give another BOL 30 min after start of therapy, max 10 mg/kg total daily dose

Renal dose
Adult: IV CCr >10 ml/min 100% of dose; CCr <10 ml/min 50%-75% of dose

Available forms: Inj 5 mg/ml

Implementation
• Patients with low potassium levels (hypokalemia) should receive potassium supplements before inamrinone administration
• Administer potassium supplements if ordered for potassium levels <3.0 mg/dl; correct before using inamrinone

IV route
• Do not mix directly with dextrose sol; chemical reaction occurs over 24 hr; precipitate forms if inamrinone and furosemide come in contact

IV, direct route
• May inject into running dextrose inf through Y-connector or directly; **Discontinued** may give undiluted over 2-3 min or dilute with 0.9%, 0.45% NaCl to concentration of 1-3 mg/ml; run at prescribed rate by cont inf; another loading dose may be given in 30 min

Continuous IV route
• Give after diluting with 0.9% or 0.45% NaCl (1-3 mg/ml); do not dilute with dextrose sol; decomposition of product will occur; use inf pump; use sol within 24 hr of dilution; titrate to patient response

Syringe compatibilities: Propranolol, verapamil

Y-site compatibilities: Alfentanil, aminocaproic acid, anidulafungin, atracurium, atropine, benztropine, bivalirudin, bleomycin, buprenorphine, calcium chloride, CARBOplatin, caspofungin, cisatracurium, CISplatin, cyclophosphamide, cytarabine, DACTINomycin, DAPTOmycin, dexmedetomidine, diltiazem, docetaxel, doxacurium, DOXOrubicin, ePHEDrine, epirubicin, eptifibatide, ertapenem, etoposide, fenoldopam, fentaNYL, fluconazole, fludarabine, fluorouracil, gatifloxacin, glycopyrrolate, granisetron, hydrOXYzine, IDArubicin, ifosfamide, irinotecan, labetalol, lidocaine, linezolid, mechlorethamine, metaraminol,

metroNIDAZOLE, midazolam, minocycline, mitoxantrone, mycophenolate, naloxone, nitroprusside, oxaliplatin, paclitaxel, palonosetron, pamidronate, pantoprazole, propofol, propranolol, protamine, remifentanil, tacrolimus, teniposide, thiotepa, tolazoline, trimetaphan, vasopressin, verapamil, vinCRIStine, vinorelbine, voriconazole

Y-site incompatibilities: Furosemide, inamrinone, sodium bicarbonate

ADVERSE EFFECTS
CV: Dysrhythmias, *hypotension*, chest pain
GI: *Nausea, vomiting, anorexia*, abdominal pain, hepatotoxicity (rare), ascites, jaundice, hiccups
HEMA: Thrombocytopenia
INTEG: Allergic reactions, burning at inj site
RESP: Pleuritis, pulmonary densities, hypoxemia

Pharmacokinetics
Absorption	Complete bioavailability
Distribution	Protein binding 40%
Metabolism	Liver, 50%
Excretion	Kidney, metabolites (10%-40%)
Half-life	4-6 hr, increased in CHF **Discontinued**

Pharmacodynamics
Onset	2-5 min
Peak	10 min
Duration	0.5-2 hr

INTERACTIONS
Individual drugs
Disopyramide: excessive hypotension

Drug classifications
Antihypertensives: excessive hypotension
Cardiac glycosides: increased additive effect

Drug/lab test
Increased: hepatic enzymes
Decreased: potassium

NURSING CONSIDERATIONS
Assessment
• Monitor manifestations of hypokalemia: *RENAL:* acidic urine, reduced urine, osmolality, nocturia; *CV:* hypotension, broad T-wave, U-wave, ectopy, tachycardia, weak pulse; *NEURO:* muscle weakness, altered LOC, drowsiness, apathy, lethargy, confusion, depression; *GI:* anorexia, nausea, cramps, constipation, distention, paralytic ileus; *RESP:* hypoventilation, respiratory muscle weakness

• Assess fluid volume status: CVP in geriatric, I&O ratio and record, weight, distended red veins, crackles in lung, color, quality, and specific gravity of urine, skin turgor, adequacy of pulses, moist mucous membranes, bilateral lung sounds, peripheral pitting edema; dehydration symptoms of decreasing output, thirst, hypotension, dry mouth, and mucous membranes should be reported
• Monitor electrolytes: potassium, sodium, calcium, magnesium; also include BUN, blood pH, ABGs
• Monitor B/P and pulse, PCWP, CVP, index, often during inf; if B/P drops 30 mm Hg, stop inf and call prescriber
• Monitor ALT, AST, bilirubin daily; if these are elevated, hepatotoxicity is suspected
⚠ If platelets are <150,000/mm³, product is usually discontinued and another product started
• Assess for extravasation: change site q48hr

Nursing diagnosis **Discontinued**
• Cardiac output, decreased (uses)
• Fluid volume, excess (uses)
• Knowledge, deficient (teaching)

Patient/family education
• Teach patient reason for medication and expected results
• Instruct patient to make position changes slowly; orthostatic hypotension may occur
• Teach patient signs and symptoms of hypersensitivity reactions and hypokalemia
• Advise patient that burning may occur at **IV** site

Evaluation
Positive therapeutic outcome
• Increased cardiac output
• Decreased PCWP, adequate CVP
• Decreased dyspnea, fatigue, edema, ECG

TREATMENT OF OVERDOSE:
Discontinue product, support circulation

indacaterol
(in-da-kat′er-ol)
Arcapta Neohaler
Func. class.: β₂-agonist, long-acting
Pregnancy category C

ACTION: An agonist at β_2-receptors. These receptors are present in large numbers in the lungs and are located on bronchiolar smooth muscle. Stimulation of β_2-receptors in the lung causes relaxation of bronchial smooth muscle, which produces bronchodilation and an increase in bronchial airflow. These effects may be mediated, in part, by increased activity of adenyl cyclase, an intracellular enzyme responsible for the formation of cyclic-3′,5′-adenosine monophosphate (cAMP); has >24 times greater agonist activity at β_2-receptors (primarily in the lung) than at β_1-receptors (primarily in the heart)

USES: Bronchitis, chronic obstructive pulmonary disease (COPD), emphysema

CONTRAINDICATIONS:
Acute bronchospasm, acute asthma attack, status asthmaticus, acute respiratory insufficiency, monotherapy of asthma

Precautions: Cardiac arrhythmias, congenital long QT syndrome, diabetes mellitus, hypertension, hyperthyroidism (thyrotoxicosis, thyroid disease), hypokalemia, ischemic cardiac disease (coronary artery disease), milk protein hypersensitivity, pheochromocytoma, QT prolongation, seizure disorder, severe hepatic disease, tachycardia, torsades de pointes history, unusual responsiveness to other sympathomimetic amines; not indicated for neonates, infants, children, or adolescents under the age of 18 years, pregnancy C, breastfeeding

DOSAGE AND ROUTES
Adult: INH 75 mcg (contents of 1 capsule) inhaled once daily; administer at the same time every day, max 1 dose in 24 hours

Available forms:
Powder for inhalation: 75 mcg

Implementation
Inhalation route
• For oral inhalation use only; instruct patients *not* to swallow the capsules; always use the Neohaler inhaler to administer capsules; this inhaler should not be used with any other medication; do *not* use with a spacer
• To administer, use dry hands to remove a capsule from the blister pack immediately before use and place into the capsule chamber of the Neohaler inhaler; click the inhaler closed; do not place capsule into the mouthpiece; then, holding the inhaler upright, depress buttons fully one time to pierce capsule; a click will be heard; have patient breathe out fully away from inhaler; place inhaler in the mouth with lips closed around the mouthpiece and buttons positioned to the left and right (not up and down), then breathe deeply, rapidly, steadily in through

the inhaler. A whirring sound should be heard; if no sound is heard, check the chamber—capsule may be stuck. Gently tap the base of the device to loosen capsule if necessary. After inhalation, the patient should hold breath as long as comfortable while removing inhaler from the mouth; check the chamber to see if any powder remains in the capsule; repeat inhalation steps until no powder remains. Most patients can empty the capsule in one or two inhalations. After administration, open the chamber and discard the empty capsule

• Occasionally the gelatin capsule might break into very small pieces, which can pass through the inhaler screen and reach the mouth. Accidental inhalation or ingestion of these pieces is harmless; piercing the capsule more than once increases the risk of shattering capsule; do not wash inhaler; keep it dry. Cleaning is not necessary, but if desired, a clean, dry, lint-free cloth may be used to wipe out the inhaler

• Use the new inhaler provided with each new prescription

• To avoid the spread of infection, do not share the inhaler

ADVERSE EFFECTS

CNS: Headache, tremor
CV: Sinus tachycardia, hypertension, **QT prolongation and ST-T wave changes, prolonged QTc (an increase of >60 ms from baseline), nonsustained ventricular tachycardia, supraventricular tachycardia (SVT) episodes, intermittent ectopic atrial rhythm**
ENDO: Hyperglycemia
GI: Nausea, dry mouth (xerostomia)
META: Hypokalemia
MS: Muscle cramps/spasm, musculoskeletal pain
RESP: Paradoxical bronchospasm, cough, dyspnea, sputum purulence or volume, wheezing, nasopharyngitis, pneumonia, sinusitis and upper respiratory tract infection

Pharmacokinetics

Absorption	Unknown
Distribution	Steady state 12-15 days protein binding 94-96%
Metabolism	By CYP3A4, CYP1A1, CYP2D6, UTG1A1
Excretion	Renal 2-6%, fecally >90%
Half-life	Terminal 45.5-126 hrs

Pharmacodynamics

Onset	5 min
Peak	15 min
Duration	Unknown

INTERACTIONS

Individual drugs
Amoxapine, some antipsychotics (phenothiazines, pimozide, haloperidol risperidone, sertindole ziprasidone), arsenic trioxide, astemizole, bepridil, cisapride, citalopram, chloroquine, clarithromycin, dasatinib, dolasetron, dronedarone, droperidol, erythromycin, flecainide, halofantrine, levomethadyl, maprotiline, methadone, ondansetron, paliperidone, palonosetron, pentamidine, probucol, propafenone, some quinolones (ofloxacin, gatifloxacin, gemifloxacin, grepafloxacin, levofloxacin, moxifloxacin, sparfloxacin), ranolazine, sunitinib, terfenadine, thioridazine, troleandomycin, vorinostat, tetrabenazine: increased QT prolongation
Aminophylline, theophylline: increased hypokalemia
Furazolidone, procarbazine, rasagiline: increased cardiovascular reactions

Drug classifications
Class IA/III antiarrhythmics, halogenated anesthetics, tricyclic antidepressants: increased QT prolongation
Corticosteroids: increased hypokalemia
MAOIs: increased cardiovascular reactions

NURSING CONSIDERATIONS

Assessment
• **COPD, emphysema, bronchospasm:** Monitor pulmonary function tests
• **QT prolongation: Monitor ECG, ejection fraction for QT prolongation**
• **Paradoxical bronchospasm: If paradoxical bronchospasm occurs, discontinue this medication immediately, use a short-acting beta-agonist for rescue therapy, as appropriate**

Patient/Family Education
• Teach patient/family to report dyspnea, wheezing, bronchospasm
• Teach patient/family not to use with other products unless approved by prescriber; there are many interactions

indapamide (Rx)
(in-dap′a-mide)
Lozide ✦
Func. class.: Diuretic, thiazide-like, antihypertensive
Chem. class.: Thiazide-like sulfonamide derivative
Pregnancy category D

ACTION: Acts on proximal section of distal renal tubule by inhibiting reabsorption of sodium, may act by direct vasodilatation caused by blocking of calcium channels

Therapeutic outcome: Decreased B/P; decreased edema in lung tissues, peripherally

USES: Edema of CHF, hypertension, diuresis

CONTRAINDICATIONS:
Hypersensitivity to this product or sulfonamides, anuria, hepatic coma, pregnancy (**D**)

Precautions: Breastfeeding, hypokalemia, severe renal disease, hepatic disease, ascites, dehydration, CCr <30 ml/min (not effective), diabetes mellitus, gout

DOSAGE AND ROUTES
Edema
Adult: PO 2.5 mg/day in AM; may be increased to 5 mg/day if needed after 1 wk

Antihypertensive
Adult: PO 1.25-5 mg/day; may increase to 5 mg/day over 8 wk

Available forms: Tabs 1.25, 2.5 mg

Implementation
• Give in AM to avoid interference with sleep
• Provide potassium replacement if potassium level is <3.0 mg/dl; give whole
• Give with food and milk if nausea occurs, absorption may be increased

ADVERSE EFFECTS
CNS: Depression, *headache, dizziness, fatigue, weakness, nervousness, agitation,* extremity numbness
CV: Orthostatic hypotension, palpitations, volume depletion, PVCs, dysrhythmias, vaculitis
EENT: Blurred vision, nasal congestion, increased intraocular pressure
ELECT: *Hypokalemia, hypercalcemia, hyponatremia, hypochloremic alkalosis, hypomagnesemia,* hyperuricemia, hyperglycemia

GI: *Nausea,* vomiting, anorexia, constipation, diarrhea, cramps, abdominal pain, dry mouth
GU: *Frequency, polyuria, nocturia,* impotence
INTEG: Rash, *pruritus*
MS: Cramps

Pharmacokinetics
Absorption	Well absorbed
Distribution	Widely distributed
Metabolism	Liver, 7%
Excretion	Unchanged (urine)
Half-life	14-18 hr

Pharmacodynamics
Onset	1-2 hr
Peak	2 hr
Duration	Up to 36 hr

INTERACTIONS
Individual drugs
Amphotericin B: decreased potassium
Cholestyramine, colestipol: decreased absorption
Diazoxide: hyperglycemia
Digoxin, lithium: increased toxicity
Indomethacin: decreased hypotensive effect

Drug classifications
Anticoagulants, antidiabetics, antigout agents: decreased effects
Diuretics (other), steroids: decreased potassium
Muscle relaxants, steroids: increased toxicity
NSAIDs: decreased hypotensive effects

Drug/herb
St. John's wort: severe photosensitivity

Drug/lab test
Increased: calcium, parathyroid test, glucose, uric acid

NURSING CONSIDERATIONS
Assessment
• Check for rashes, temp elevation daily
• Monitor patients that receive cardiac glycosides for increased hypokalemia, toxicity
• Monitor for hypokalemia: acidic or reduced urine, osmolality, nocturia; hypotension, broad T-wave, U-wave, ectopy, tachycardia, weak pulse; muscle weakness, altered LOC, drowsiness, apathy, lethargy, confusion, depression; anorexia, nausea, cramps, constipation, distention, paralytic ileus; hypoventilation, respiratory muscle weakness
• Monitor for hypomagnesemia: agitation, muscle twitching, paresthesias, hyperactive

reflexes, positive Babinski reflex, dysphagia, nystagmus, seizures, tetany; nausea, vomiting, diarrhea, anorexia, abdominal distention; ectopy, tachycardia, broad, flat- or inverted T-waves, depressed ST segment, prolonged QT interval, decreased cardiac output, hypotension

• Monitor for hyponatremia: increased B/P, cold, clammy skin, hypo/hypervolemia; anorexia, nausea, vomiting, diarrhea, abdominal cramps; lethargy, increased ICP, confusion, headache, seizures, coma, fatigue, tremors, hyperreflexia

• Monitor for manifestations of hyperchloremia: weakness, lethargy, coma, deep rapid breathing

• Assess fluid volume status: I&O ratios and record, weight, distended red veins, crackles in lung, color, quality and specific gravity of urine, skin turgor, adequacy of pulses, moist mucous membranes, bilateral lung sounds, peripheral pitting edema; dehydration symptoms of decreasing output, thirst, hypotension, dry mouth and mucous membranes should be reported

• Monitor electrolytes: potassium, sodium, calcium, magnesium; also include BUN, blood pH, ABGs, uric acid, CBC, blood glucose

• Assess B/P before, during therapy with patient lying, standing, and sitting as appropriate; orthostatic hypotension can occur rapidly

Nursing diagnoses
• Fluid volume, deficient (side effects)
• Fluid volume, excess (uses)
• Knowledge, deficient (teaching)
• Urinary elimination, impaired (side effect)

Patient/family education
• Teach patient to take the medication early in the day to prevent nocturia
• Instruct the patient to take with food or milk if GI symptoms of nausea and anorexia occur
• Teach patient to maintain weekly record of weight and notify prescriber of weight loss >5 lb
• Caution the patient that this product causes a loss of potassium, so food rich in potassium should be added to the diet; refer to a dietitian for assistance in planning
• Caution the patient to rise slowly from sitting or reclining positions, not to exercise in hot weather or stand for prolonged periods, since orthostatic hypotension will be enhanced; lie down if dizziness occurs
• Teach patient not to use alcohol or any OTC medications without prescriber's approval; serious product reactions may occur
• Emphasize the need to contact prescriber immediately if muscle cramps, weakness, nausea, dizziness, or numbness occur

• Teach patient to take own B/P and pulse and record findings
• Instruct patient to continue taking medication even if feeling better; this product controls symptoms but does not cure the condition
• Advise the patient with hypertension to continue other medical treatment (exercise, weight loss, relaxation techniques, cessation of smoking)

Evaluation
Positive therapeutic outcome
• Decreased edema
• Decreased B/P
• Increased diuresis

TREATMENT OF OVERDOSE:
Lavage, monitor electrolytes, administer **IV** fluids, monitor hydration, CV, renal status

---

indinavir (Rx)
(en-den′a-veer)
Crixivan
Func. class.: Antiretroviral
Chem. class.: Protease inhibitor
Pregnancy category C

Do not confuse:
indinavir/Denavir

ACTION: Inhibits HIV-1 protease; this prevents maturation of the infectious virus

Therapeutic outcome: Decreased signs/symptoms of HIV-1 infection

USES: HIV-1 in combination with at least 2 other antiretrovirals

Unlabeled uses: Prevention of HIV-1 after exposure

CONTRAINDICATIONS:
Hypersensitivity, breastfeeding

Precautions: Pregnancy **C,** children, renal/hepatic disease, history of renal stones, diabetes, hypercholesterolemia, hemophilia

DOSAGE AND ROUTES
Adult: PO 800 mg q8hr; 400 mg bid with ritonavir 400 mg bid; or 800 mg bid with ritonavir 100-200 mg bid; decrease dose to 600 mg bid when given with lopinavir, ritonavir

Hepatic dose
Adult: PO 600 mg q8hr

Available forms: Caps 100, 200, 333, 400 mg

Implementation
• Do not break, crush, or chew caps
• Give with water 1 hr before or 2 hr after meals; may be given with other liquids or small meal; do not give with high-fat, high-protein meals
• Give in equal intervals around the clock
• Dosage adjustment will need to be considered when given with efavirenz
• Give water to 1.5 L/day minimum, to prevent nephrolithiasis

ADVERSE EFFECTS
CNS: *Headache, insomnia,* dizziness, somnolence
GI: *Diarrhea, abdominal pain, nausea, vomiting,* anorexia, dry mouth
GU: Nephrolithiasis
INTEG: Rash
MISC: Asthenia, **insulin-resistant hyperglycemia,** hyperlipidemia, **ketoacidosis,** lipodystrophy
MS: Pain

Pharmacokinetics

Absorption	Unknown
Distribution	Unknown
Metabolism	60% protein binding; liver
Excretion	<20% unchanged, urine; 83% feces
Half-life	Terminal 2 hr

Pharmacodynamics
Unknown

INTERACTIONS
Individual drugs
Amiodarone, alfuzosin, pimozide: life-threatening dysrhythmias
Clarithromycin, zidovudine: increased levels of both products
Isoniazid: increased isoniazid level
Midazolam, rifampin, triazolam: increased life-threatening dysrhythmias

Drug classifications
Anticonvulsants: decreased effect of both products
CYP3A4 inducers (barbiturates, carBAMazepine, efavirenz, fluconazole, modafinil, nevirapine, nonnucleoside reverse transcriptase inhibitors, phenytoin, rifamycins): decreased indinavir levels
CYP3A4 inhibitors (aprepitant, azole antifungals, delavirdine, itraconazole, ketoconazole, nefazodone, protease inhibitors, verapamil); phosphotriesterases: increased indinavir levels
CYP3A4 substrates (azole antifungals, benzodiazepines, calcium channel blockers, immunosuppressants, macrolides, sildenafil, SSRIs, statins, tadalafil, vardenafil): decreased effect of these substrates
Ergots: increased life-threatening dysrhythmias
Oral contraceptives: increased levels of oral contraceptives
Statins (atorvastatin, lovastatin, simvastatin): increased myopathy

Drug/herb
St. John's wort: decreased indinavir level, avoid use

Drug/food
High fat, high protein, grapefruit juice: decreased absorption

Drug/lab test
Increased: AST, ALT, amylase, total bilirubin

NURSING CONSIDERATIONS
Assessment
• Assess for lower back, flank pain: indicates kidney stones
• Monitor signs of infection, anemia
• Monitor liver studies: ALT, AST; total bilirubin, amylase; all may be elevated
• Determine the presence of other STDs
• Assess bowel pattern before, during treatment; if severe abdominal pain with bleeding occurs, product should be discontinued; monitor hydration
• Assess skin eruptions: rash, urticaria, itching
• Assess allergies before treatment, reaction to each medication; place allergies on chart
• Monitor viral load CD4 during treatment

Nursing diagnoses
• Infection, risk for (uses)
• Knowledge, deficient (teaching)

Patient/family education
• Advise to take as prescribed; if dose is missed, take as soon as remembered up to 1 hr before next dose; do not double dose
• Advise that product must be taken in equal intervals around the clock to maintain blood levels for duration of therapy
• Instruct patient to increase fluids to prevent kidney stones; if stone formation occurs, treatment may need to be interrupted

- Inform patient that product does not cure AIDS, controls symptoms only; not to donate blood
- Advise patient that hyperglycemia may occur; watch for symptoms (thirst, hunger, dry, itchy skin); notify prescriber

Evaluation
Positive therapeutic outcome
- Decreased signs/symptoms of infection, HIV

indomethacin (Rx)
(in-doe-meth′a-sin)
Indocin, Nu-Indo 🍁
Func. class.: NSAID (nonsteroidal antiinflammatory), antirheumatic
Chem. class.: Propionic acid derivative
Pregnancy category B (1st trimester), D (2nd/3rd trimesters)

Do not confuse:
Indocin/Endocet, minocin/Vicodin

ACTION: Inhibits prostaglandin synthesis by decreasing enzyme needed for biosynthesis; analgesic, antiinflammatory, antipyretic

Therapeutic outcome: Decreased pain, inflammation; closure of patent ductus arteriosus (premature infants)

USES: Rheumatoid arthritis, ankylosing spondylitis, osteoarthritis, bursitis, tendinitis, acute gouty arthritis; closure of patent ductus arteriosus in premature infants (**IV**)

CONTRAINDICATIONS:
Pregnancy **D** (3rd trimester) hypersensitivity, asthma, ulcer disease, neonates, aortic coarctation, bleeding, salicylate/NSAID hypersensitivity

> **BLACK BOX WARNING:** Perioperative pain in CABG

Precautions: Pregnancy **B** (1st trimester), breastfeeding, children, bleeding disorders, GI disorders, cardiac disorders, asthma, diabetes, acute bronchospasm, ulcerative colitis, seizures, Parkinson's disease, renal/hepatic disease, depression

> **BLACK BOX WARNING:** Stroke, GI bleeding, MI

DOSAGE AND ROUTES
Arthritis/antiinflammatory
Adult: PO 25-50 mg bid-tid, max 200 mg/day; SUS REL 75 mg daily; may increase to 75 mg bid

Acute gouty arthritis
Adult: PO 50 mg tid; use only for acute attack, then reduce dosage

Patent ductus arteriosus
Longer or repeated treatment courses may be necessary for very premature infants
Infant <2 days: **IV** 0.2 mg/kg, then 0.1 mg/kg × 2 doses after 12, 24 hr
Infant 2-7 days: **IV** 0.2 mg/kg, then 0.2 mg/kg × 2 doses after 12, 24 hr
Infant >7 days: **IV** 0.2 mg/kg, then 0.25 mg/kg × 2 doses after 12, 24 hr

Available forms: Caps 25, 50 mg; sus rel caps 75 mg; oral susp 5 mg/ml; inj 1-mg vials; supp 50 mg

Implementation
PO route
- Swallow sus rel cap whole; do not break, crush, or chew sus rel cap
- Give with food or milk to decrease gastric symptoms and prevent ulceration
- Shake susp; do not mix with other liquids
Rectal route
- Have patient retain rect supp for 1 hr after insertion

IV route
- Give after diluting 1-2 mg/ml or more normal saline or sterile water for inj without preservative; give over 5-10 sec to avoid dramatic shift in cerebral blood flow; avoid extravasation

Y-site compatibilities: Furosemide, insulin (regular), potassium chloride, sodium bicarbonate, sodium nitroprusside

ADVERSE EFFECTS
CNS: Dizziness, drowsiness, fatigue, tremors, confusion, insomnia, anxiety, depression, *headache*
CV: Tachycardia, peripheral edema, palpitations, dysrhythmias, hypertension, **CV thrombotic events, MI, stroke**
EENT: Tinnitus, hearing loss, blurred vision
GI: *Nausea,* anorexia, *vomiting,* diarrhea, jaundice, **cholestatic hepatitis,** *constipation,* flatulence, cramps, dry mouth, peptic ulcer, **ulceration, perforation, GI bleeding**
GU: Nephrotoxicity (dysuria, hematuria, oliguria, azotemia)

HEMA: Blood dyscrasias, prolonged bleeding
INTEG: Purpura, rash, pruritus, sweating

Pharmacokinetics

Absorption	Well absorbed (PO); erratic (RECT); complete (**IV**)
Distribution	Crosses blood-brain barrier; placenta, 99% plasma protein binding
Metabolism	Liver, extensively
Excretion	Breast milk; urine 60%, feces 33%
Half-life	1 hr first pass, 2.6-11.2 hr second pass

Pharmacodynamics

	PO	PO–ext rel	IV
Onset	1-2 hr	$1/2$ hr	2 day
Peak	3 hr	Unknown	Unknown
Duration	4-6 hr	4-6 hr	Unknown

INTERACTIONS

Individual drugs
Abciximab, aspirin, cefamandole, cefoperazone, cefotetan, clopidogrel, eptifibatide, plicamycin, ticlopidine, tirofiban, valproic acid: increased bleeding risk
CycloSPORINE, lithium, methotrexate, probenecid, zidovudine: increased toxicity
Digoxin, penicillamine, phenyton: increased effect of each specific product

Drug classifications
Aminoglycosides: increased effects of aminoglycosides
Anticoagulants, SNRIs, SSRIs, thrombolytics: increased risk of bleeding
Antihypertensives: decreased effect of antihypertensives
Diuretics (potassium sparing): increased hyperkalemia

NURSING CONSIDERATIONS

Assessment
• Assess for patent ductus arteriosus: respiratory rate, character, heart sounds
• Assess for joint pain (duration, intensity, ROM), baseline and during treatment
• Assess for confusion, mood changes, hallucinations, especially in geriatric
• Assess renal, liver, blood studies: BUN, creatinine, AST, ALT, Hgb before treatment, periodi-

cally thereafter; if renal function decreases, do not give subsequent doses

> **BLACK BOX WARNING:** Assess for cardiac disease, CV, thrombotic events (MI, stroke) prior to administration

Nursing diagnoses
• Knowledge, deficient (teaching)
• Mobility, impaired physical (uses)
• Pain, acute (uses)
• Pain, chronic (uses)

Patient/family education
• Advise patient to report change in vision, blurring, rash, tinnitus, black stools
• Tell patient not to use for any other condition than prescribed
• Advise patient to avoid use with OTC medications for pain unless approved by prescriber, to report use to all providers
• Advise patient to avoid hazardous activities, since dizziness or drowsiness can occur
• Instruct patient to use sunscreen to prevent photosensitivity

Evaluation
Positive therapeutic outcome
• Decreased stiffness
• Increased joint mobility
• Decreased pain

inFLIXimab (Rx)
(in-fliks'ih-mab)
Remicade
Func. class.: Monoclonal antibody
Chem. class.: Tumor necrosis factor modifiers
Pregnancy category B

ACTION: Monoclonal antibody that neutralizes the activity of tumor necrosis factor α (TNFα) that has been found in Crohn's disease; decreased infiltration of inflammatory cells

Therapeutic outcome: Decreased cramping and blood in stools

USES: Crohn's disease, fistulizing, moderate to severe; rheumatoid arthritis given with methotrexate, plaque psoriasis, ankylosing spondylitis, ulcerative colitis, psoriatic arthritis, psoriasis

Unlabeled uses: Behçet's syndrome, uveitis, juvenile arthritis

CONTRAINDICATIONS:

Hypersensitivity to murines, moderate to severe CHF (NYHA class III/IV)

Precautions: Pregnancy **B,** breastfeeding, children, geriatric, COPD, hepatotoxicity, hematologic abnormalities, hepatitis B, Guillain-Barré syndrome, seizures, multiple sclerosis

> **BLACK BOX WARNING:** Infection, neoplastic disease, TB

DOSAGE AND ROUTES

Crohn's disease (moderate to severe/fistulizing)

Adult/adolescent/child ≥6 yr: **IV** INF 5 mg/kg initially, then repeat dose 2, 6 wk, q8wk thereafter, may increase to 10 mg/kg if needed (adults)

Rheumatoid arthritis

Adult: **IV** 3 mg/kg initially, and 2, 6 wk and q8wk thereafter, max 10 mg/kg/dose

Available forms: Powder for inj 100 mg

Implementation

Intermittent IV infusion route

• Administer immediately after reconstitution; reconstitute each vial with 10 ml of sterile water for inj, further dilute total dose/250 ml of 0.9% NaCl inj to a total conc of between 0.4 and 4 mg/ml; use 21-G or smaller needle for reconstitution, direct sterile water at glass wall of vial, gently swirl, do not shake, may foam; allow to stand for 5 min, give within 3 hr
• Give over ≥2 hr, use polyethylene-lined inf with in-line, sterile, low-protein-bind filter
• Do not admix
• Provide refrigerated storage, do not freeze

ADVERSE EFFECTS

CNS: *Headache, dizziness, depression, vertigo, fatigue, anxiety, fever,* **seizures,** *chills, flulike symptoms,* demyelinating disease
CV: Chest pain, hypo/hypertension, tachycardia, **CHF, acute coronary syndrome**
GI: *Nausea, vomiting, abdominal pain, stomatitis, constipation, dyspepsia, flatulence*
GU: Dysuria, frequency
HEMA: Anemia, leukopenia, thrombocytopenia, pancytopenia
INTEG: *Rash, dermatitis, urticaria,* dry skin, sweating, flushing, hematoma, pruritus, keratoderma blennorrhagicum
MS: Myalgia, back pain, arthralgia
RESP: URI, pharyngitis, bronchitis, cough, dyspnea, sinusitis

SYST: Anaphylaxis, fatal infections, sepsis, malignancies, immunogenicity, Stevens-Johnson syndrome, toxic epidermal necrosis

Pharmacokinetics

Absorption	Unknown
Distribution	Vascular compartment
Metabolism	Unknown
Excretion	Unknown
Half-life	$9\frac{1}{2}$ days

Pharmacodynamics

Unknown

INTERACTIONS

Drug classifications

Live virus vaccines: do not administer live vaccines concurrently

NURSING CONSIDERATIONS

Assessment

• Assess GI symptoms: nausea, vomiting, abdominal pain
• Take periodic blood counts: CBC
• Assess CV status: B/P, pulse, chest pain
⚠ Assess for allergic reaction, anaphylaxis: rash, dermatitis, urticaria, fever, chills, dyspnea, hypotension; discontinue if severe; administer epinephrine, corticosteroids, antihistamines; assess for allergy to murine proteins before starting therapy

> **BLACK BOX WARNING:** Fatal infections: discontinue if infection occurs, do not administer to patients with active infections; identify TB before beginning treatment, a TB test should be obtained; if present, TB should be treated before giving infliximab; exercise caution when switching one DMARD to another

• Report suspected adverse reactions to the FDA (1-800-FDA-1088)

> **BLACK BOX WARNING:** Assess for neoplastic disease in those <18 yr, including heptosplenic T-cell lymphoma

Nursing diagnoses

• Diarrhea (uses)
• Injury, risk for (uses)
• Knowledge, deficient (teaching)

Patient/family education

• Advise patient not to breastfeed while taking this product

⚠ Nurse Alert

- Advise patient to notify prescriber of GI symptoms, hypersensitivity reactions
- Advise patient not to operate machinery or drive if dizziness, vertigo occurs

Evaluation
Positive therapeutic outcome
- Absence of blood in stool
- Reported improvement in comfort
- Weight gain

⚠ HIGH ALERT

INSULINS

RAPID ACTING
insulin glulisine (Rx)
Apidra, Apidra SoloStar
insulin aspart (Rx)
Novolog, Novolog Flexpen, Novolog PenFill, NovoMix 30 ✿, NovoRapid ✿
insulin lispro (Rx)
Humalog

SHORT ACTING
insulin, regular (OTC)
Humulin R ✿, Novolin R, ReliOn R
insulin, regular concentrated (Rx)
Humulin RU-500

INTERMEDIATE ACTING
insulin, isophane suspension (NPH) (OTC)
Humulin N, Novolin ge NPH ✿, Novolin N, Novolin N Prefilled, ReliOn N

LONG ACTING
insulin detemir (Rx)
Levemir
insulin glargine (Rx)
Lantus

MIXTURES
insulin, isophane suspension and regular insulin (Rx)
Humulin 70/30, Humalin 30/70 ✿, Novolin 70/30, Novolin 70/30 Prefilled, ReliOn 70/30

isophane insulin suspension (NPH) and insulin mixtures (Rx)
Humulin 50/50
insulin lispro mixture (Rx)
Humalog KwikPen Mix 50/50, Humalog Mix 25 ✿, Humalog Mix 50 ✿, Humalog Mix 75/25, Humalog Mix 50/50
insulin aspart mixture (Rx)
Novolog 70/30, Novolog Mix Flexpen Prefilled Syringe 70/30
Func. class.: Antidiabetic, pancreatic hormone
Chem. class.: Modified structures of endogenous human insulin
Pregnancy category B, C

Do not confuse:
Lantus/lente, Novolin 70/30 PenFill/Novolin 70/30 Prefilled

ACTION: Decreases blood glucose; by transport of glucose into cells and the conversion of glucose to glycogen, indirectly increases blood pyruvate and lactate, decreases phosphate and potassium; insulin may be human (processed by recombinant DNA technologies)

Therapeutic outcome: Decreased blood glucose levels in diabetes mellitus

USES: Type 1 diabetes mellitus, type 2 diabetes mellitus, gestational diabetes, insulin lispro may be used in combination with sulfonylureas in children >3 yr

CONTRAINDICATIONS: Hypersensitivity to protamine; creosol (aspart)

Precautions: Pregnancy **B** (lispro, aspart, regular), **C** (all others)

DOSAGE AND ROUTES
Insulin glulisine
Adult/adolescent/child ≥4 yr: SUBCUT dosage individualized, give within 15 min before or 20 min after starting a meal
Adult: IV dilute to 1 unit/ml in INF systems with 0.9% NaCl, using PVC Viaflex INF bags and PVC tubing, use dedicated line

Insulin aspart
Adult/adolescent/child ≥6 yr: Intermittent SUBCUT total daily dose is given as 2-4 inj/day

---

Adverse effects: *italics* = common; **bold** = life-threatening

just prior to beginning of a meal; in general, 50%-70% of total daily insulin may be given as insulin aspart, the remainder should be intermediate or long-acting insulin; CONTINU-OUS SUBCUT used with external insulin pump via cont SUBCUT insulin INF (CSII), the insulin dose should be based on the insulin dose from the previous regimen

Insulin lispro
Adult/adolescent/child ≥3 yr: SUBCUT 15 min before meals; **continuous subcut infusion (external insulin pump)** the total daily dose should be based on the insulin dose in previous regimen, 50% of total dose can be given as meal-related boluses and the remainder as basal infusion

Human regular
Adult: SUBCUT $^{1}/_{2}$-1 hr before meals

Insulin, isophane suspension
Adult: SUBCUT dosage individualized by blood, urine glucose; usual dose 7-26 units; may increase by 2-10 units/day if needed

Insulin detemir
Adult: SUBCUT 1 or 2 times/day; if 1 time, give with evening meal

Insulin glargine
Adult and child ≥6 yr: SUBCUT 10 international units/day, range 2-100 international units/day

Regular insulin (ketoacidosis)
Adult: **IV** 5-10 units, then 5-10 units/hr until desired response, then switch to SUBCUT dose; **IV/INF** 2-12 units (50 units/500 ml of normal saline)
Child: **IV** 0.1 units/kg

Replacement
Adult and child: SUBCUT 0.5-1 units/kg/day qid given 30 min before meals
Adolescent: SUBCUT 0.8-1.2 mg/kg/day; this dosage is used during rapid growth

Available forms: NPH inj 100 units/ml; **regular** inj 100 units/ml, cartridges 100 units/ml; **insulin analog** inj 100 units/ml; **isophane insulin** inj 100 units/ml, cartridges 100 units/ml; **insulin lispro** 100 units/ml, 1.5-ml cartridges; insulin lispro Humalog Pen sol for inj 100 units/ml; **insulin glulisine** inj 100 units/ml; **insulin glargine** inj 100 units/ml; **insulin detemir** inj 100 units/ml in 10 vials, 3-ml cartridges; **insulin aspart** inj 100 mg/ml (Flexpen, PenFill)

Implementation
• Store at room temperature for <1 mo (some insulins); keep away from heat and sunlight; refrigerate all other supply; NPH, premixed insulins are cloudy; regular, rapid-acting analogs, long-acting analogs are clear; do not freeze—**IV** route, regular only

SUBCUT route
• Give after warming to room temperature by rotating in palms to prevent injecting cold insulin; use only insulin syringes with markings or syringe matching units/ml; rotate inj sites within one area: abdomen, upper back, thighs, upper arm, buttocks; keep record of sites
• Give increased dosages if tolerance occurs
• Premixed insulins and NPH are cloudy suspensions
• Regular human insulin, rapid-acting analogs, and long-acting analogs are clear; do not use if cloudy, thick, or discolored

CONT SUBCUT route (insulin infusion CSII)
• Do not mix with other insulins when using a pump
• Insulin lispro 3 ml cartridges are to be used in Disetronic H-TRON plus V100 pump using Disetronic rapid inf sets; the inf set and the cartridge adapter should be changed q3day; replace 3 ml cartridge q6days

IV route (insulin glulisine only)
• Dilute to 1 international unit/ml in infusion systems with 0.9% NaCl using PVC viaflex inf bags and PVC tubing; use dedicated line; do not admix

IV route (regular only)
⚠ When regular insulin is administered IV, monitor glucose, potassium often to prevent fatal hypoglycemia, hypokalemia
• **IV** direct, undiluted via vein, Y-site, 3-way stopcock; give at 50 units/min or less
• Give by cont inf after diluting with **IV** sol and run at prescribed rate; use **IV** inf pump for correct dosing; give reduced dose at serum glucose level of 250 mg/100 ml

Additive compatibilities: Bretylium, cimetidine, lidocaine, meropenem, ranitidine, verapamil

Additive incompatibilities: Aminophylline, amobarbital, chlorothiazide, cytarabine, DOBUTamine, PENTobarbital, PHENobarbital, phenytoin, secobarbital, sodium bicarbonate, thiopental

Y-site compatibilities: Amiodarone, ampicillin, ampicillin/sulbactam, aztreonam, ceFAZolin, cefotetan, DOBUTamine, esmolol, famotidine, gentamicin, heparin, heparin/hydrocortisone, imipenem/cilastatin, indomethacin, magnesium sulfate, meperidine, meropenem, midazolam, morphine, nitroglycerin, oxytocin, PENTobarbital, potassium chloride, propofol, ritodrine, sodium bicarbonate, sodium nitroprusside, tacrolimus, terbutaline, ticarcillin, ticarcillin/clavulanate, tobramycin, vancomycin, vit B/C

Y-site incompatibilities: Nafcillin

ADVERSE EFFECTS
EENT: Blurred vision, dry mouth
INTEG: Flushing, rash, urticaria, warmth, *lipodystrophy,* lipohypertrophy, swelling, redness
META: *Hypoglycemia,* rebound hyperglycemia (Somogyi effect 12-72 hr or longer)
MISC: Peripheral edema
SYST: Anaphylaxis

Pharmacokinetics

Absorption	Rapidly absorbed (SUBCUT)
Distribution	Widely distributed
Metabolism	Liver, muscle, kidney
Excretion	Kidneys
Half-life	Regular 3-5 min; NPH 10 min

INTERACTIONS
Individual drugs
Alcohol: increased hypoglycemia
DOBUTamine: increased insulin need
EPINEPHrine: decreased hypoglycemia
Fenfluramine, guanethedine, phenylbutazone, sulfinpyrazone, tetracycline: decreased insulin need

Drug classifications
Anabolic steroids, β-adrenergic blockers, hypoglycemics (oral), salicylates: increased hypoglycemia
Contraceptives (oral), corticosteroids, diuretics (thiazide), thyroid hormones: decreased hypoglycemia
Estrogens: increased insulin need
MAOIs: decreased insulin need

Drug/lab test
Increased: VMA
Decreased: potassium, calcium
Interference: liver, thyroid function tests

NURSING CONSIDERATIONS
Assessment
• Fasting blood glucose, also Hgb A1c may be tested to identify treatment effectiveness q3mo

Pharmacodynamics

Rapid acting

Insulin glulisine	Onset 15-30 min, peak $^1/_2$-$1^1/_2$ hr, duration 3-4 hr
Insulin aspart	Onset 10-20 min, peak 1-3 hr, duration 3-5 hr
Insulin lispro	Onset 15-30 min, peak $^1/_2$-$1^1/_2$ hr, duration 3-4 hr

Short acting

Insulin regular	Onset 30 min, peak 2.5-5 hr, duration up to 6 hr

Intermediate acting

Insulin, isophane suspension (NPH)	Onset 1.5-4 hr, peak 4-12 hr, duration up to 24 hr

Long acting

Insulin detemir	Onset 0.8-2 hr, peak unknown, duration up to 24 hr (concentration dependent)
Insulin glargine	Onset 1.5 hr, no peak identified, duration ≥ 24 hr

Mixtures

Insulin, isophane suspension and regular insulin (70/30)	Onset 10-20 hr, peak 2.4 hr, duration up to 24 hr
Isophane insulin suspension (NPH) and insulin mixtures (50/50)	Onset $^1/_2$-1 hr, peak dual, duration 10-16 hr

• Urine ketones during illness; insulin requirements may increase during stress, illness, surgery
• For hypoglycemic reaction that can occur during peak time (sweating, weakness, dizziness, chills, confusion, headache, nausea, rapid weak pulse, fatigue, tachycardia, memory lapses, slurred speech, staggering gait, anxiety, tremors, hunger)
• For hyperglycemia: acetone breath, polyuria, fatigue, polydipsia, flushed, dry skin, lethargy

Nursing diagnoses
• Injury, risk for (adverse reactions)
• Knowledge, deficient (teaching)
• Noncompliance (teaching)

Patient/family education
• Advise patient that blurred vision occurs; not to change corrective lens until vision is stabilized 1-2 mo
• Advise patient to keep insulin, equipment available at all times; carry a glucagon kit, candy, or lump sugar to treat hypoglycemia
• Inform patient that product does not cure diabetes but controls symptoms
• Advise patient to carry emergency ID as diabetic
• Instruct patient to recognize hypoglycemia reaction: headache, tremors, fatigue, weakness
• Instruct patient to recognize hyperglycemia reaction: frequent urination, thirst, fatigue, hunger
• Teach patient the dosage, route, mixing instructions, any diet restrictions, disease process
• Teach patient the symptoms of ketoacidosis: nausea, thirst, polyuria, dry mouth, decreased B/P, dry, flushed skin, acetone breath, drowsiness, Kussmaul respirations
• Advise patient that a plan is necessary for diet, exercise; all food on diet should be eaten; exercise routine should not vary
• Teach patient about blood glucose testing; make sure patient is able to determine glucose level
• Advise patient to avoid OTC products unless directed by prescriber

Evaluation
Positive therapeutic outcome
• Decrease in polyuria, polydipsia, polyphagia; clear sensorium; absence of dizziness; stable gait
• Blood glucose level under control

TREATMENT OF OVERDOSE:
Glucose 25 g **IV,** via dextrose 50% sol, 50 ml, or glucagon 1 mg

---

interferon alfa-2a (recombinant) (Rx)
(in-ter-feer′on)
Roferon-A
interferon alfa-2b (recombinant) (Rx)
Intron-A
Func. class.: Antineoplastic, miscellaneous
Chem. class.: Protein product
Pregnancy category C

Do not confuse:
Roferon-A/Imferon

ACTION: Antiviral action inhibits viral replication by reprogramming virus; antitumor action suppresses cell proliferation; immuno-modulating action phagocytizes target cells; may also inhibit virus replication in virus-infested cells

Therapeutic outcome: Prevention of rapid growth of malignant cells; treatment of hepatitis non-A, non-B (liver function improvement)

USES: Hairy cell leukemia in persons >18 yr; condylomata acuminata (alfa 2b); chronic hepatitis C (alfa 2b); 2a only chronic myelogenous leukemia; 2b only hepatitis B, malignant melanoma

Unlabeled uses: Bladder tumors, carcinoid tumors, non-Hodgkin's lymphoma, essential thrombocytopenia, cytomegaloviruses, herpes simplex, human papilloma virus–associated diseases

CONTRAINDICATIONS:
Hypersensitivity

Precautions: Pregnancy **C,** breastfeeding, children, severe hypotension, dysrhythmia, tachycardia, severe renal/hepatic disease, seizure disorder, optic neuritis, ocular disease, thyroid/pulmonary disease

BLACK BOX WARNING: Autoimmune disorders, cardiac disease, infection, depression

DOSAGE AND ROUTES
Hairy cell leukemia (2a)
Adult: SUBCUT/IM 3 million international units/day × 16-24 wk, then 3 million international units 3 ×/wk maintenance

---

Condylomata acuminata (2a)
Adult: Intralesional 1 million international units/lesion 3 ×/wk × 3 wk

Alfa-2b hairy-cell leukemia
Adult: SUBCUT/IM 2 million international units/m² 3 ×/wk × up to 6 mo

Condylomata acuminata
Adult: Intralesional 1 million international units (0.1 ml) injected into each lesion 3 ×/wk on alternating days for 3 wk; treat ≤5 warts per course

Chronic hepatitis B
Adult: SUBCUT/IM 30-35 million international units/wk × 16 wk given 5 million international units/day or 10 million international units 3 ×/wk

Available forms: Alfa-2a: inj 3, 6, 36 million international units/ml; alfa-2b: inj 3, 5, 10, 18, 25 million international units/vial, powder for inj 5, 10, 18, 25, 50 million international units/vial

Implementation
• Sol should be prepared by qualified personnel only under controlled conditions in biological cabinet using gown, gloves, and mask
• Use Luer-Lok tubing to prevent leakage; do not let sol come in contact with skin; if contact occurs, wash well with soap and water
• Give at bedtime to minimize side effects
• Give acetaminophen as ordered to alleviate fever and headache

Alfa-2a
• Give **SUBCUT/IM** after reconstituting 18 million units/3 ml of diluent provided (6 million units/ml)
• 36 million units/ml is used for Kaposi's sarcoma only
• Store reconstituted sol; must be used within 24 hr

Alfa-2b
• Give by **IM/SUBCUT** after reconstituting 3-5 million international units/1 ml, 10 million international units/2 ml, 25 million international units/5 ml, of diluent provided; mix gently, do not shake; each brand has different dilution directions; check package insert

Intralesional route (2b)
• Give by intralesional route after reconstituting 10 million international units/1 ml of bacteriostatic water for inj; no more than 5 lesions can safely be treated at a time; using a 25-G needle inject 0.1 ml into base at center

ADVERSE EFFECTS
CNS: *Dizziness, confusion, numbness, paresthesia,* hallucinations, **seizures, coma,** amnesia, anxiety, mood changes, depression, somnolence, paranoia, irritability, hostility, encephalopathy
CV: *Edema, hypotension,* hypertension, chest pain, palpitations, dysrhythmias, **CHF, MI, CVA,** tachycardia, syncope
GI: *Weight loss, taste changes,* nausea, anorexia, diarrhea, xerostomia
GU: *Impotence*
HEMA: Neutropenia, thrombocytopenia
INTEG: *Rash, dry skin, itching, alopecia,* flushing, photosensitivity, **serious skin infection**
MISC: *Flulike symptoms: fever, fatigue, myalgias, headache, chills,* optic neuritis, **anaphylaxis, angioedema**

Pharmacokinetics
Absorption	80%-90% (SUBCUT/IM)
Distribution	Unknown
Metabolism	Renal tubules (degraded)
Excretion	Kidneys
Half-life	3.7-8.5 hr (2a); 2-7 hr (2b)

Pharmacodynamics
Onset	Unknown
Peak	3-8 hr
Duration	Unknown

INTERACTIONS
Individual drugs
Aminophylline: increased toxicity, blood levels
Clozapine, warfarin, zidovudine: increased neutropenia

Drug/lab test
Interference: AST, ALT, LDH, alkaline phosphatase, WBC, platelets, granulocytes, creatinine

NURSING CONSIDERATIONS
Assessment
• Assess cardiac status: lung sounds, ECG before, during treatment, especially in those with cardiac disease, hypo/hypertension—MI, CHF, CVA may occur
• Assess bone marrow depression: bruising, bleeding, blood in stools, urine, sputum, emesis
• Assess mental status: depression, suicidal thoughts, hallucinations, amnesia
• Assess for symptoms of infection; may be masked by drug fever; fever, chills, headache,

sore throat may occur 6 hr after dose; give acetaminophen for symptoms
• Assess liver, thyroid function tests
• In AIDS patients with Kaposi's sarcoma, assess characteristics of lesions during therapy; symptoms should decrease
• Assess for bleeding: hematuria, stool guaiac, bruising or petechiae, mucosa or orifices q8hr; check for inflammation of mucosa, breaks in skin; avoid IM inj, rectal temp, or any other procedures that break the skin
• Assess for CNS reaction: LOC, mental status, dizziness, confusion, poor coordination, difficulty speaking, behavior changes; notify prescriber (alfa-2b)

Nursing diagnoses
• Body image, disturbed (adverse reactions)
• Infection, risk for (adverse reactions)
• Injury, risk for (adverse reactions)
• Knowledge, deficient (teaching)

Patient/family education
• Caution patient to avoid hazardous tasks, since confusion, dizziness may occur; fatigue is common; activity may have to be altered; to take at bedtime to minimize flulike symptoms; to take acetaminophen for fever; avoid prolonged sunlight
• Advise patient that brands of this product should not be changed; each form is different, with different dosages
• Caution patient not to become pregnant while taking product; possible mutagenic effects; impotence may occur during treatment but is temporary
• Advise patient to report signs of infection: sore throat, fever, diarrhea, vomiting; sores or white patches in mouth
⚠ Advise patient that suicidal ideation is common; notify prescriber if severe or incapacitating

Evaluation
Positive therapeutic outcome
• Improved leukocytes, Hgb, platelets
• Decreased amount of genital warts

---

interferon alfacon-1 (Rx)
(in-ter-feer'on al'fa-kon)
Infergen
Func. class.: Recombinant type 1 interferon
Pregnancy category C

ACTION: Induces biologic responses and has antiviral, antiproliferative, and immunomodulatory effects

Therapeutic outcome: Decreased signs/symptoms of hepatitis C

USES: Chronic hepatitis C infections in those 18 yr and older with compensated liver disease who have anti-HCV antibodies or HCV RNA, may use in combination with ribavirin

Unlabeled uses: Hairy cell leukemia when used with G-CSF

CONTRAINDICATIONS:
Hypersensitivity to α-interferons, or products from *Escherichia coli,* uncompensated hepatic disease, autoimmune hepatitis

Precautions: Pregnancy C, breastfeeding, children <18 yr, thyroid disorders, myelosuppression, hepatic disease, alcoholism, geriatric patients, seizure disorder, hepatitis

> **BLACK BOX WARNING:** Cardiac disease, autoimmune disorder, infection, depression

DOSAGE AND ROUTES
Adult: Monotherapy: SUBCUT 9 mcg as a single inj 3 ×/wk × 24 wk; leave at least 48 hr between injections; those who did not respond or relapsed after discontinuation, give 15 mcg 3×/wk × 48 wk; **combination:** subcut 15 mcg q day with ribavirin 1000 mg/day PO (<75 kg), 1200 mg/day PO (≥75 kg) give in 2 divided doses for up to 48 wks, use stepwise dose reduction in the interferon dose from 15 mcg to 9 mcg to 6 mcg for serious adverse reactions

Available forms: Inj 9 mcg/0.3 ml, 15 mcg/0.5 ml

ADVERSE EFFECTS
CNS: Headache, fatigue, fever, rigors, insomnia, dizziness, agitation, nervousness, anxiety, lability, abnormal thinking, depression
CV: Hypertension, palpitation, tachycardia
EENT: Tinnitus, earache, conjunctivitis, eye pain
GI: Abdominal pain, nausea, diarrhea, anorexia, dyspepsia, vomiting, constipation, flatulence, hemorrhoids, decreased salivation
GU: Dysmenorrhea, vaginitis, menstrual disorders
HEMA: Granulocytopenia, thrombocytopenia, leukopenia, ecchymosis, aplastic anemia
INTEG: Alopecia, pruritus, rash, erythema, dry skin
MISC: Anaphylaxis, angioedema, flulike illness

⚠ Nurse Alert

MS: Back, limb, neck, skeletal pain, rigors
RESP: Pharyngitis, upper respiratory infection, cough, sinusitis, rhinitis, respiratory tract congestion, epistaxis, dyspnea, bronchitis

Pharmacokinetics	
Unknown	

Pharmacodynamics	
Onset	Unknown
Peak	24-36 hr
Duration	Unknown

NURSING CONSIDERATIONS

Assessment
• Assess CBC, liver function tests, ECG, platelet counts, heme concentration, ANC, serum creatinine concentration, albumin, bilirubin, TSH, T₄
• Assess for myelosuppression, low dose if neutrophil count is <500 × 10-6/L or if platelets are <50 × 10-9/L
• Assess for hypersensitivity; discontinue immediately if hypersensitivity occurs

Nursing diagnoses
• Infection, risk for (uses)
• Knowledge, deficient (teaching)

Patient/family education
• Provide patient or family member with written, detailed instructions about the product
• Caution patient to use contraception during treatment

Evaluation
Positive therapeutic outcome
• Decreased hepatitis C signs/symptoms

---

interferon beta-1a (Rx)
(in-ter-feer′on)
Avonex, Rebif
interferon beta-1b (Rx)
Betaseron, Extavia
Func. class.: Multiple sclerosis agent, immune modifier
Chem. class.: Interferon, *Escherichia coli* derivative
Pregnancy category C

ACTION: Antiviral, immunoregulatory; action not clearly understood; biologic response-modifying properties mediated through specific receptors on cells, inducing expression of interferon-induced gene products

Therapeutic outcome: Decreased symptoms of multiple sclerosis

USES: Ambulatory patients with relapsing or remitting multiple sclerosis

Unlabeled uses: May be useful in treatment of AIDS, AIDS-related Kaposi's sarcoma, malignant melanoma, metastatic renal cell carcinoma, cutaneous T-cell lymphoma, acute non-A/non-B hepatitis

CONTRAINDICATIONS:
Hypersensitivity to natural or recombinant interferon-beta or human albumin, hamster protein, rotavirus vaccine

Precautions: Pregnancy **C**, breastfeeding, children <18 yr, chronic progressive multiple sclerosis, depression, mental disorders, seizure disorders, latex allergy, autoimmune disorders, bone marrow suppression, hepatotoxicity, cardiac disease, alcoholism, chickenpox, herpes zoster

DOSAGE AND ROUTES
Interferon beta-1a
Remitting-relapsing multiple sclerosis
Adult: IM (Avonex) 30 mcg qwk; SUBCUT (Rebif) 22 or 44 mcg 3 ×/wk with each dose 48 hr apart, titrate to full dose over 4-wk period

Interferon beta-1b
Relapsing/remitting multiple sclerosis
Adult: SUBCUT 0.0625 mg every other day for wk 1 and 2; then 0.125 mg every other day for wk 3 and 4; then 0.1875 mg every other day for wk 5 and 6; then 0.25 mg every other day thereafter; higher doses should not be used

Available forms: Beta-1a (Avonex): 33 mcg (6.6 million international units/vial); (Rebif) 22 mcg, 44 mcg/0.5 ml; beta-1b: powder for Inj 0.3 mg (9.6 m international units)

Implementation
• Reconstitute 0.3 mg (9.6 million international units)/1.2 ml of supplied diluent (0.2 mg or 8 million international units concentration); rotate vial gently, do not shake; withdraw 1 ml using a syringe with 27-G needle; administer SUBCUT only into hip, thigh, arm; discard unused portion
• Products are not interchangeable
Interferon beta-1a
• Reconstitute with 1.1 ml of diluent, swirl, give within 6 hr

---

Adverse effects: *italics* = common; **bold** = life-threatening

Interferon beta-1b
- Reconstitute by injecting diluent provided (1.2 ml) into vial, swirl (8 milli-international units/ml), use 27-G needle for inj
- Give acetaminophen for fever, headache; use SUBCUT route only; do not give IM or **IV**
- Store reconstituted sol in refrigerator; do not freeze; do not use sol that contains precipitate or is discolored

ADVERSE EFFECTS

CNS: *Headache, fever, pain, chills, mental changes,* depression, hypertonia, **suicide attempts, seizures**
CV: *Migraine, palpitations, hypertension,* tachycardia, peripheral vascular disorders
EENT: Conjunctivitis, blurred vision
GI: *Diarrhea, constipation, vomiting, abdominal pain*
GU: *Dysmenorrhea, irregular menses, metrorrhagia,* cystitis, breast pain
HEMA: **Decreased lymphocytes,** ANC, **WBC,** *lymphadenopathy,* anemia
INTEG: *Sweating, inj site reaction*
MS: *Myalgia,* **myasthenia**
RESP: *Sinusitis,* dyspnea

Pharmacokinetics

Absorption	50% is absorbed
Distribution	Unknown
Metabolism	Unknown
Excretion	Unknown
Half-life	8 min-4½ hr (beta-1b), 8.6 hr (beta-1a)

Pharmacodynamics

	Beta-1a	Beta-1b
Onset	Up to 12 hr	Rapid
Peak	48 hr	2-8 hr
Duration	4 days	Unknown

INTERACTIONS

Individual drugs
Zidovudine: decreased clearance

Drug classifications
Antiretrovirals (NNRTIs, NRTIs, protease inhibitors: increased hepatic damage
Antineoplastics: increased myelosuppression

Drug/herb
Astragalus, echinacea, melatonin: change in immunomodulation

Drug/lab test
Increased: liver function tests
Interference: vaccines, toxoids; avoid concurrent use

NURSING CONSIDERATIONS

Assessment
- Monitor blood, renal, liver function tests: CBC, differential, platelet counts, BUN, creatinine, ALT, urinalysis; if neutrophil count is <750/mm^3, or if AST, ALT is 10 × greater than ULN, or if bilirubin is 5 × greater than ULN, discontinue product; when neutrophil count exceeds 750/mm^3 and liver function or renal studies return to normal, treatment may resume at 50% original dosage
- Assess for CNS symptoms: headache, fatigue, depression; if depression occurs and is severe, product should be discontinued
- Assess for multiple sclerosis symptoms
- Assess mental status: depression, depersonalization, suicidal thoughts, insomnia
- Monitor GI status: diarrhea or constipation, vomiting, abdominal pain
- Monitor cardiac status: increased B/P, tachycardia

Nursing diagnoses
- Knowledge, deficient (teaching)
- Mobility, impaired physical (uses)

Patient/family education
- Provide patient or family member with written, detailed instructions about the product; provide initial and return demonstrations on inj procedure; give information on use and disposal of product
- Inform patient that blurred vision, sweating may occur
- Advise female patients that irregular menses, dysmenorrhea, or metrorrhagia as well as breast pain may occur; use contraception during treatment; product may cause spontaneous abortion
- Teach patient to use sunscreen to prevent photosensitivity
- Instruct patient to notify prescriber if pregnancy is suspected
- Teach patient inj technique and care of equipment
- Instruct patient to notify prescriber of increased temp, chills, muscle soreness, fatigue

Evaluation
Positive therapeutic outcome
- Decreased symptoms of multiple sclerosis

interferon gamma-1b (Rx)
(in-ter-feer′on)
Actimmune
Func. class.: Biologic response modifier
Chem. class.: Lymphokine, interleukin type
Pregnancy category C

ACTION: Species-specific protein synthesized in response to viruses; potent phagocyte-activating effects; capable of mediating the killing of *Staphylococcus aureus, Toxoplasma gondii, Leishmania donovani, Listeria monocytogenes, Mycobacterium avium-intracellulare;* enhances oxidative metabolism of macrophages; enhances antibody-dependent cellular cytotoxicity

Therapeutic outcome: Decreased signs/symptoms of infection (serious) in chronic granulomatous disease

USES: Serious infections associated with chronic granulomatous disease, osteopetrosis

Unlabeled uses: Osteoporosis, *Mycobacterium avium* complex (MAC), ovarian cancer, pulmonary fibrosis

CONTRAINDICATIONS:
Hypersensitivity to interferon γ, *Escherichia coli*–derived products

Precautions: Pregnancy C, breastfeeding, children <1 yr, cardiac disease, seizure/CNS disorders, myelosuppression

DOSAGE AND ROUTES
Adult: SUBCUT 50 mcg/m^2 (1.5 million units/m^2) for patient with a surface area of >0.5 m^2; 1.5 mcg/kg/dose for patient with a surface area of <0.5/m^2; give on Monday, Wednesday, Friday for 3 ×/wk dosing

Available forms: Inj 100 mcg (2 million units)/single-dose vial

Implementation
• Give at bedtime to minimize adverse reactions; administer acetaminophen for fever, headache; use 50% of the dosage prescribed if severe reactions occur or discontinue treatment until reactions subside
• Give in right or left deltoid and anterior thigh; warm to room temperature before use; do not leave at room temperature >12 hr (unopened vial); does not contain preservatives
• Store in refrigerator upon receipt; do not freeze; do not shake

ADVERSE EFFECTS
CNS: *Headache, fatigue,* depression, fever, chills
GI: *Nausea, anorexia,* abdominal pain, weight loss, diarrhea, vomiting, colitis
HEMA: **Leukopenia, thrombocytopenia,** neutropenia
INTEG: Rash, pain at inj site, **Stevens-Johnson syndrome**
MS: Myalgia, arthralgia

Pharmacokinetics
Absorption	Slowly absorbed 89%
Distribution	Unknown
Metabolism	Unknown
Excretion	Unknown
Half-life	5.9 hr

Pharmacodynamics
Onset	Unknown
Peak	7 hr
Duration	Unknown

INTERACTIONS
Individual drugs
Aminophylline, theophylline: increased levels

Drug classifications
Myelosuppressive agents: increased myelosuppression
Protease inhibitors, nucleoside reverse transcriptase inhibitors (NRTIs), nonnucleoside reverse transcriptase inhibitors (NNRTIs): increased liver toxicity

NURSING CONSIDERATIONS
Assessment
• Monitor blood, renal, hepatic studies: CBC with differential, platelet count, BUN, creatinine, ALT, urinalysis before, q3mo during treatment
• Assess for infection: headache, fever, chills, fatigue; these are common adverse reactions
• Monitor CNS symptoms: headache, fatigue, depression

Nursing diagnoses
• Infection, risk for (uses)
• Knowledge, deficient (teaching)

Patient/family education
• Provide patient or family member with written, detailed instructions about the product; provide initial and return demonstrations on inj procedure; give information on use and disposal of product
• Caution patient to use contraception during treatment

Evaluation
Positive therapeutic outcome
- Decreased serious infections
- Improvement in existing infections and inflammatory conditions

ipilimumab
(ip-i-lim'ue-mab)
Yervoy
Func. class.: Antineoplastic; biologic response modifier
Pregnancy category C

ACTION: A recombinant, human monoclonal antibody that binds to the cytotoxic T-lymphocyte-associated antigen 4 (CTLA-4); action is indirect, possibly through T-cell mediated antitumor immune responses

Therapeutic outcome: Decreased spread of malignant cells

USES: Treatment of unresectable or metastatic malignant melanoma

CONTRAINDICATIONS:
Hypersensitivity

Precautions: Pregnancy, breastfeeding, Crohn's disease, hepatitis, immunosuppression, inflammatory bowel disease, iritis, ocular disease, organ transplant, pancreatitis, renal disease, rheumatoid arthritis, sarcoidosis, systemic lupus erythematosus, thyroid disease, ulcerative colitis, uveitis

DOSAGE AND ROUTES
Adult and geriatric: **IV** 3 mg/kg over 90 min q3wk × 4 doses. Permanently discontinue if the full treatment course is not completed within 16 wk from first dose or for severe or life-threatening adverse reactions; withhold a dose for any moderate endocrine or immune-mediated adverse reactions; if the moderate adverse reaction completely or partially resolves (Grade 0-1) and if the patient is receiving less than 7.5 mg predniSONE or equivalent per day, resume at a dose of 3 mg/kg IV every 3 wk until all 4 planned doses or 16 wk from first dose, whichever occurs earlier; if moderate adverse reactions are persistent or if the corticosteroid dose cannot be reduced to 7.5 mg predniSONE or equivalent per day, permanently discontinue

Available forms: Solution for inj 50 mg/10 ml, 200 mg/40 ml

Implementation
Intermittent IV Infusion route
- Visually inspect parenteral products for particulate matter and discoloration before using whenever solution and container permit; solution may have a pale yellow color and have translucent-to-white, amorphous particles; discard the vial if the solution is cloudy, if there is pronounced discoloration, or if particulate matter is present
- Allow vials to stand at room temperature for 5 min before infusion preparation; withdraw the required volume and transfer into an IV bag. Discard partially used vials or empty vials; dilute with 0.9% sodium chloride injection, or 5% dextrose injection, to a final concentration (1-2 mg/ml); mix diluted solution by gentle inversion; do not admix
- Give infusion over 90 min through an IV line with a low-protein binding in-line filter, do not give with other products; after each infusion, flush the line with 0.9% sodium chloride Injection, or 0.5% dextrose injection
- Store once diluted, store for no more than 24 hr refrigerated or at room temperature

ADVERSE EFFECTS
CNS: **Severe and fatal immune-mediated neuropathies,** fatigue, fever, headache
EENT: Episcleritis, iritis, Uveitis
ENDO: **Severe and fatal immune-mediated endocrinopathies**
GI: **Severe and fatal immune-mediated enterocolitis, hepatitis;** pancreatitis, abdominal pain, colitis, constipation, decreased appetite, diarrhea, nausea, vomiting
INTEG: **Severe and fatal immune-mediated dermatitis,** pruritus, rash, urticaria
MISC: **Anemia, cough, dyspnea, eosinophilia, nephritis**
SYST: Antibody formation, **Stevens-Johnson syndrome, toxic epidermal necrolysis**

> **BLACK BOX WARNING:** Adrenal insufficiency, diarrhea, Guillain-Barré syndrome, hepatic disease, myasthenia gravis, hyperhypothyroidism, hypopituitarism, peripheral neuropathy, serious rash

Pharmacokinetics

Absorption	Unknown
Distribution	Steady state (end of 3rd dose)
Metabolism	Unknown
Excretion	Unknown
Half-life	Terminal 14.7 days

Pharmacodynamics

Onset	Unknown
Peak	Unknown
Duration	Unknown

NURSING CONSIDERATIONS

Assessment

• **Serious skin disorders: Stevens-Johnson syndrome, toxic epidermal necrolysis:** permanently discontinue in these or rash complicated by full thickness dermal ulceration or necrotic, bullous, or hemorrhagic manifestations like bullous rash; give systemic corticosteroids at a dose of 1-2 mg/kg/day of predniSONE or equivalent; when dermatitis is controlled, taper corticosteroids over a period of at least 1 month. Withhold in those with moderate to severe reactions; for mild to moderate dermatitis (localized rash and pruritus), give topical or systemic corticosteroids

• **Hepatotoxicity:** Monitor liver function tests baseline and before each dose; rule out infectious or malignant causes and increase the frequency of liver function test monitoring until resolution; permanently discontinue in those with Grade 3-5 give systemic corticosteroids at a dose of 1-2 mg/kg/day of prednisone or equivalent

• **Neuropathy:** Monitor for motor or sensory neuropathy (unilateral or bilateral weakness, sensory alterations, or paresthesias) before each dose; permanently discontinue if severe neuropathy (interfering with daily activities) such as Guillain-Barré-like syndromes occur

• **Endocrinopathy:** Monitor thyroid function tests at baseline and before each dose; monitor hypophysitis, adrenal insufficiency, adrenal crisis, hyperthyroidism, hypothyroidism (fatigue, headache, mental status changes, abdominal pain, unusual bowel habits, hypotension, or nonspecific symptoms that may resemble other causes)

Nursing diagnoses

• Risk for injury (uses, adverse reactions)

Patient/family education

• Instruct patient/family to report immediately allergic reaction, skin rash, severe abdominal pain, yellowing of skin, eyes; tingling of extremities, change in bowel habits

• Discuss reason for treatment and expected results

Evaluation
Positive therapeutic outcome
• Decreasing spread of malignant melanoma

ipratropium (Rx)
(i-pra-troe′pee-um)
Atrovent HFA
Func. class.: Anticholinergic, bronchodilator
Chem. class.: Synthetic quaternary ammonium compound
Pregnancy category B

Do not confuse:
Atrovent/Alupent

ACTION: Inhibits interaction of acetylcholine at receptor sites on the bronchial smooth muscle, resulting in decreased cyclic guanosine monophosphate (cyclic GMP) and bronchodilatation

Therapeutic outcome: Bronchodilatation

USES: COPD; rhinorrhea (nasal spray)

CONTRAINDICATIONS:
Hypersensitivity to this product, atropine, bromide, soybean, or peanut products

Precautions: Pregnancy **B,** breastfeeding, children <12 yr, angioedema, heart failure, surgery, acute bronchospasm, closed-angle glaucoma, prostatic hypertrophy, bladder neck obstruction, urinary retention

DOSAGE AND ROUTES
Adult: INH 2 sprays (17 mcg/spray) 3-4×/day, max 12 INH/24 hr, SOL 500 mcg (1 unit dose) given 3-4×/day by nebulizer; nasal spray: 2 sprays (42 mcg/spray) 3-4×/day
Child 5-12 yr: NASAL 2 sprays in each nostril 3×/day

Available forms: Aerosol 17 mcg/actuation; nasal spray 0.03%, 0.06%; sol for inh 0.0125% ✤, 0.02%

Implementation
• Give after shaking container; have patient exhale, place mouthpiece in mouth, inhale slowly, hold breath, remove, exhale slowly; allow at least 1 min between inhalations
• Give this medication before other medications and allow at least 5 min between each

Nebulizer route
• Use solution in nebulizer with a mouthpiece rather than a face mask
Nasal route
• Prime pump, initially requires 7 actuations of the pump, priming again is not necessary if used regularly
• Store in light-resistant container; do not expose to temperature over 86° F (30° C)

ADVERSE EFFECTS

CNS: *Anxiety, dizziness, headache,* nervousness
CV: Palpitations
EENT: Dry mouth, blurred vision, nasal congestion
GI: *Nausea, vomiting, cramps*
INTEG: Rash
RESP: *Cough, worsening of symptoms,* bronchospasm

Pharmacokinetics

Absorption	Minimal
Distribution	Does not cross blood-brain barrier
Metabolism	Liver, minimal
Excretion	Unknown
Half-life	2 hr

Pharmacodynamics

Onset	5-15 min
Peak	$1-1\frac{1}{2}$ hr
Duration	3-6 hr

INTERACTIONS

Individual drugs
Disopyramide: increased anticholinergic action

Drug classifications
Antihistamines, phenothiazines: increased anticholinergic action
Bronchodilators (other): increased toxicity

Drug/herb
Belladonna: increased anticholinergic effect
Green tea (large amounts), guarana: increased bronchodilator effect

NURSING CONSIDERATIONS

Assessment
• Monitor respiratory function: vital capacity, FEV, ABGs, lung sounds, heart rate, rhythm (baseline, during treatment); if severe bronchospasm is present, a more rapid medication is required
• Monitor for evidence of allergic reactions, paradoxical bronchospasm; withhold dose and notify prescriber; identify if patient is allergic to belladonna products or atropine; allergy to this product may occur

Nursing diagnoses
• Gas exchange, impaired (uses)
• Knowledge, deficient (teaching)

Patient/family education
• Advise patient not to use OTC medications unless approved by prescriber; extra stimulation may occur; to use this medication before other medications and allow at least 5 min between each to prevent overstimulation
• Teach patient that compliance is necessary with number of inhalations/24 hr, or overdose may occur
• Instruct geriatric patients to use spacer device
• Teach patient the proper use of the inhaler; review package insert with patient; to avoid getting aerosol in eyes: blurring may result; to wash inhaler in warm water daily and dry; to avoid smoking, smoke-filled rooms, persons with respiratory tract infections
• Teach patient if paradoxical bronchospasm occurs to stop product immediately and notify prescriber; to limit caffeine products such as chocolate, coffee, tea, and colas
• Instruct patient on administration of dose, not to use more than prescribed; serious side effects may occur; if dose is missed, take when remembered; space other doses on new time schedule; do not double doses

Evaluation
Positive therapeutic outcome
• Absence of dyspnea, wheezing after 1 hr
• Improved airway exchange
• Improved ABGs

---

irbesartan (Rx)
(er-be-sar'tan)
Avapro
Func. class.: Antihypertensive
Chem. class.: Angiotensin II receptor (type AT_1)
Pregnancy category C (1st trimester), D (2nd/3rd trimesters)

Do not confuse:
Avapro/Anaprox

ACTION: Blocks the vasoconstrictor and aldosterone-secreting effects of angiotensin II;

---

selectively blocks the binding of angiotensin II to the AT_1 receptor found in tissues

Therapeutic outcome: Decreased B/P

USES: Hypertension, alone or in combination, nephropathy in patients with type 2 diabetes mellitus; proteinuria

Unlabeled uses: Heart failure

CONTRAINDICATIONS:
Hypersensitivity

> **BLACK BOX WARNING:** Pregnancy **D** (2nd/3rd trimesters)

Precautions: Pregnancy **C** (1st trimester), breastfeeding, children <6 yr, geriatric, renal/hepatic disease, renal artery stenosis, hypersensitivity to ACE inhibitors

DOSAGE AND ROUTES

Hypertension
Adult: PO 150 mg/day; may be increased to 300 mg/day; volume-depleted patients: start with 75 mg/day

Nephropathy in patients with type 2 diabetes mellitus
Adult: PO maintenance dose 300 mg/day, start 75 mg/day

Available forms: Tabs 75, 150, 300 mg

Implementation
• Administer without regard to meals

ADVERSE EFFECTS
CNS: Dizziness, anxiety, headache, fatigue
CV: Hypotension
GI: *Diarrhea, dyspepsia*
MISC: Edema, chest pain, rash, tachycardia, UTI, **angioedema**, hyperkalemia
RESP: *Cough, upper respiratory infection,* rhinitis, pharyngitis, sinus disorder

Pharmacokinetics

Absorption	Well absorbed
Distribution	Bound to plasma proteins (90%)
Metabolism	Liver (minimal)
Excretion	Feces, urine
Half-life	11-15 hr

Pharmacodynamics
Unknown

INTERACTIONS

Drug classifications
CYP2C9 inhibitors (amiodarone, delavirdine, fluconazole, fluoxetine, fluvastatin, fluvoxamine, imatinib, sulfonamides, sulfinpyrazone, voriconazole, zafirlukast): increased irbesartan level

Diuretics (potassium sparing), ACE inhibitors, potassium salt substitutes: increased hyperkalemia

NSAIDs: decreased antihypertensive effect

Drug/herb
Astragalus, cola tree: increased or decreased antihypertensive effect

Black cohosh, goldenseal, hawthorn, kelp: increased antihypertensive effect

Guarana, khat, licorice, yohimbe: decreased antihypertensive effect

NURSING CONSIDERATIONS

Assessment
• Assess B/P, pulse q4hr; note rate, rhythm, quality
• Monitor electrolytes: potassium, sodium, chloride
• Obtain baselines for renal, liver function tests before therapy begins
• Monitor for edema in feet, legs daily
• Assess for skin turgor, dryness of mucous membranes for hydration status

Nursing diagnoses
• Fluid volume, deficient (side effects)
• Knowledge, deficient (teaching)
• Noncompliance (teaching)

Patient/family education
• Advise patient to comply with dosage schedule, even if feeling better
• Inform patient that product may cause dizziness, fainting, light-headedness
• Caution patient to rise slowly to sitting or standing position to minimize orthostatic hypotension
• Advise patient to notify prescriber if pregnancy is suspected

Evaluation
Positive therapeutic outcome
• Decreased B/P

⚠ HIGH ALERT

irinotecan (Rx)
(ear-een-oh-tee′kan)
Camptosar
Func. class.: Antineoplastic hormone
Chem. class.: Topoisomerase inhibitor
Pregnancy category D

ACTION: Cytotoxic by producing damage to single-strand DNA during DNA synthesis, binds to topoisomerase I

Therapeutic outcome: Prevention in growth of tumor

USES: Metastatic carcinoma of colon or rectum, or 1st-line treatment in combination with fluorouracil (5-FU) and leucovorin for metastatic carcinoma of colon or rectum

CONTRAINDICATIONS:
Pregnancy **D**, hypersensitivity

Precautions: Breastfeeding, children, geriatric, irradiation, hepatic disease

> **BLACK BOX WARNING:** Myelosuppression, diarrhea

DOSAGE AND ROUTES
Single agent
Adult: IV 125 mg/m^2 given over 1^1/$_2$ hr qwk × 4 wk, q6wk

Combination dosage schedule

Regimen 1: Irinotecan 75-125 mg/m^2, leucovorin 20 mg/m^2, 5-FU 300-500 mg/m^2, depending on dosing levels

Regimen 2: Irinotecan 120-180 mg/m^2, leucovorin 200 mg/m^2, 5-FU-BOL 240-400 mg/m^2, 5-FU INF 360-600 mg/m^2

Available forms: Inj 20 mg/ml

Implementation
• Give antiemetics and dexamethasone 10 mg at least ^{1}/$_2$ hr before antineoplastics
• Give after preparing in biological cabinet using gloves, mask, gown

Intermittent IV infusion route
• Give by intermittent inf after diluting with 0.9% NaCl or D$_5$W (0.12-2.8 mg/ml); give over 1^1/$_2$ hr
• Do not admix with other solutions or medications
• Stable for 24 hr at room temperature, 48 hr if refrigerated

ADVERSE EFFECTS
CNS: Fever, headache, chills, dizziness
CV: Vasodilatation, edema, **thromboembolism**
GI: Severe diarrhea, *nausea, vomiting,* anorexia, constipation, cramps, flatus, stomatitis, dyspepsia, **hepatotoxicity**
HEMA: Leukopenia, anemia, **neutropenia**
INTEG: Irritation at site, rash, sweating, alopecia
MISC: Asthenia, weight loss, back pain
RESP: Dyspnea, increased cough, rhinitis

Pharmacokinetics

Absorption	Complete
Distribution	Widely, 30%-68% bound to plasma proteins, increased risk of toxicity in those homozygous for UGT1A128
Metabolism	Unknown
Excretion	Urine/bile
Half-life	6-12 hr

Pharmacodynamics

Unknown

INTERACTIONS
Individual products
CarBAMazepine, PHENobarbital, phenytoin: decreased irinotecan levels
Dexamethasone: increased lymphocytopenia, hyperglycemia
Fluorouracil: increased toxicity
Prochlorperazine: increased akathisia
Radiation: increased myelosuppression, diarrhea

Drug classifications
Anticoagulants, NSAIDs: increased bleeding risk
Antineoplastics: increased myelosuppression, diarrhea
CYP3A4 inhibitors (ketoconazole): increased irinotecan levels
CYP3A4 inducers (phenytoin, carBAMazepine, PENTobarbital): decreased irinotecan levels
Diuretics: increased dehydration

Drug/herb
St. John's wort: decreased product level; avoid concurrent use

Drug/lab test
Increased: ALK phos, AST

NURSING CONSIDERATIONS
Assessment
• Assess for CNS symptoms: fever, headache, chills, dizziness

---

BLACK BOX WARNING: Assess CBC, differential, platelet count weekly; use colony-stimulating factor if WBC is <2000/mm³, platelet count is <100,000/mm³, Hgb ≤9 g/dl, neutrophils ≤1000/mm³; notify prescriber of these results, product should be discontinued and colony-stimulating factor given

• Assess buccal cavity for dryness, sores or ulceration, white patches, oral pain, bleeding, dysphagia

BLACK BOX WARNING: Assess GI symptoms: frequency of stools; cramping; severe life-threatening diarrhea may occur with fluid and electrolyte imbalances

• Assess early diarrhea and other cholinergic symptoms, treat with atropine; late diarrhea can be life threatening, must be treated promptly with loperimide
• Assess signs of dehydration: rapid respirations, poor skin turgor, decreased urine output; dry skin, restlessness, weakness
• Assess for bone marrow depression: bruising, bleeding, blood in stools, urine, sputum, emesis

Nursing diagnoses
• Infection, risk for (adverse reactions)
• Knowledge, deficient (teaching)

Patient/family education
• Advise patient to avoid foods with citric acid or hot or rough texture if stomatitis is present; to drink adequate fluids
• Advise patient to report stomatitis; any bleeding, white spots, ulcerations in mouth; tell patient to examine mouth daily, report symptoms
• Advise patient to report signs of anemia: fatigue, headache, faintness, shortness of breath, irritability
• Advise patient to use contraception during therapy
• Advise patient to avoid vaccinations while taking this product
• Instruct patient to report diarrhea that occurs 24 hr after administration; severe dehydration can occur rapidly
• Teach patient to avoid salicylates, NSAIDs, alcohol; bleeding may occur

Evaluation
Positive therapeutic outcome
• Decrease in tumor size, decrease in spread of cancer

TREATMENT OF OVERDOSE:
Induce vomiting, provide supportive care, prevent dehydration

iron, carbonyl
See ferrous fumarate

iron dextran (Rx)
DexFerrum, InFed
Func. class.: Hematinic
Chem. class.: Ferric hydroxide complex with dextran
Pregnancy category C

Do not confuse:
Imferon/Imuran/Roferon-A/Interferon

ACTION: Iron is carried by transferrin to the bone marrow, where it is incorporated into hemoglobin

Therapeutic outcome: Prevention and resolution of iron-deficiency anemia

USES: Iron-deficiency anemia

CONTRAINDICATIONS:

BLACK BOX WARNING: Hypersensitivity

Precautions: Pregnancy **C**, breastfeeding, infants <4 mo, children, acute renal disease, asthma, rheumatoid arthritis (**IV**), all anemias excluding iron-deficiency anemia, hepatic/cardiac/renal disease, neonates, ankylosing spondylitis, lupus, hypotension

DOSAGE AND ROUTES
Adult and child: IM 0.5 ml as a test dose by Z-track, then no more than the following per day:
Adult <50 kg: IM 100 mg
Adult >50 kg: IM 250 mg
Child 5-9 kg: IM 50 mg
Infant <5 kg: IM 25 mg
Adult: **IV** 0.5 ml (25 mg) test dose, then 100 mg/day after 2-3 days; give 25 mg test dose, wait 5 min, then INF over 6-12 hr or follow equation:

$$\frac{0.3 \times weight\ (lb) \times \frac{100\ Hgb\ (g/dl) \times 100}{14.8}} = mg\ iron$$

Patients <30 lb (66 kg) should be given 80% of above formula dose

Available forms: Inj IM/IV 50 mg/ml (2 ml, 10 ml vials)

Implementation
IM route
• Discontinue oral iron before parenteral; give only after test dose of 25 mg by preferred route;

Adverse effects: *italics* = common; **bold** = life-threatening

wait at least 1 hr before giving remaining portion
• Give IM inj deep in large muscle mass; use Z-track method and 19-G, 20-G 2-, 3-inch needle; ensure needle is long enough to place product deep in muscle; change needles after withdrawing medication and injecting to prevent skin and tissue staining

IV route
• Give **IV** after flushing tubing with 10 ml of 0.9% NaCl; give undiluted; give 1 ml (50 mg) or less over 1 min or more; flush line after use with 10 ml of 0.9% NaCl; patient should remain recumbent for 30-60 min to prevent orthostatic hypotension
• **IV** inj requires single-dose vial without preservative; verify on label **IV** use is approved
• Give by cont inf after diluting in 50-250 ml of 0.9% NaCl for inf; administer over 4-5 hr
• Give only with epinephrine available in case of anaphylactic reaction during dose
• Store at room temperature in cool environment

ADVERSE EFFECTS
CNS: Headache, paresthesia, dizziness, shivering, weakness, **seizures**
CV: Chest pain, **shock,** hypotension, tachycardia
GI: *Nausea,* vomiting, metallic taste, abdominal pain
HEMA: Leukocytosis
INTEG: Rash, pruritus, urticaria, fever, sweating, chills, brown skin discoloration, pain at inj site, necrosis, sterile abscesses, phlebitis
MISC: Anaphylaxis
RESP: Dyspnea

Pharmacokinetics

Absorption	Well absorbed; lymphatics over wk or mo
Distribution	Crosses placenta
Metabolism	Slow; blood loss, desquamation
Excretion	Breast milk, feces, urine, bile
Half-life	6 hr

Pharmacodynamics
Unknown

INTERACTIONS
Individual drugs
Chloramphenicol: decreased reticulocyte response
Oral iron: do not use together, increased toxicity

Drug/lab test
False increase: serum bilirubin
False decrease: serum calcium
False positive: ^{99m}Tc diphosphate bone scan, iron test (large doses >2 ml)

NURSING CONSIDERATIONS
Assessment
• Observe for 1 hr after test dose
• Monitor blood studies: Hct, Hgb, reticulocytes, transferrin, plasma iron concentrations, ferritin, total iron-binding bilirubin before treatment, at least monthly

> **BLACK BOX WARNING:** Assess for allergic reaction and anaphylaxis; rash, pruritus, fever, chills, wheezing; notify prescriber immediately, keep emergency equipment available

• Assess cardiac status: anginal pain, hypotension, tachycardia
• Assess for nutrition: amount of iron in diet (meat, dark green leafy vegetables, dried fruits, eggs); cause of iron loss or anemia, including salicylates, sulfonamides
• Monitor pulse, B/P during **IV** administration
• Assess for toxicity: nausea, vomiting, diarrhea, fever, abdominal pain (early symptoms); cyanotic lips, nailbeds, seizures, CV collapse (late symptoms)

Nursing diagnoses
• Activity intolerance (uses)
• Fatigue (uses)
• Knowledge, deficient (teaching)

Patient/family education
• Caution patient that iron poisoning may occur if increased beyond recommended level; to not take oral iron preparation or vitamins containing iron unless approved by prescriber
• Advise patient that delayed reaction may occur 1-2 days after administration and last 3-4 days (**IV**) or 3-7 days (IM); report fever, chills, malaise, muscle/joint aches, nausea, vomiting, backache
• Advise patient to avoid breastfeeding
• Advise patient that stools may become dark

Evaluation
Positive therapeutic outcome
• Increased serum iron levels, Hct, Hgb

TREATMENT OF OVERDOSE:
Discontinue product, treat allergic reaction, give diphenhydrAMINE or EPINEPHrine as needed for anaphylaxis; give iron-chelating product in acute poisoning

iron polysaccharide
See ferrous fumarate

iron sucrose (Rx)
Venofer
Func. class.: Hematinic
Chem. class.: Ferric hydroxide complex with dextran
Pregnancy category B

ACTION: Iron is carried by transferrin to the bone marrow, where it is incorporated into hemoglobin

Therapeutic outcome: Improved signs/symptoms of iron deficiency anemia; iron levels improved

USES: Iron deficiency anemia

Unlabeled uses: Dystrophic epidermolysis bullosa (DEB)

CONTRAINDICATIONS:
Hypersensitivity, all anemias excluding iron deficiency anemia, iron overload

Precautions: Pregnancy **B**, breastfeeding (**IV**), children, geriatric, abdominal pain, anaphylactic shock, arthralgia, chest pain, cough, diarrhea, dizziness, dyspnea, edema, increased LFTs, fever, headache, heart failure, hyper/hypotension, infection, MS pain, nausea/vomiting, seizures, weakness

DOSAGE AND ROUTES
Adult: **IV** 5 ml (100 mg of elemental iron) given during dialysis, most will need 1000 mg of elemental iron over 10 sequential dialysis sessions

Available forms: Inj 20 mg/ml

Implementation
⚠ **Give only with epinephrine, solu-medrol in case of anaphylactic reaction during dose**

IV route
• Give directly in dialysis line by slow inj or inf; give by slow inj at 1 ml/min (5 min/vial); inf dilute each vial exclusively in a maximum of 100 ml of 0.9% NaCl, give at rate of 100 mg of iron/15 min, discard unused portions
• Store at room temperature in cool environment, do not freeze

ADVERSE EFFECTS
CNS: Headache, dizziness
CV: Chest pain, hypo/hypertension, hypervolemia
GI: *Nausea, vomiting, abdominal pain*
INTEG: Rash, pruritus, urticaria, fever, sweating, chills
MISC: Anaphylaxis
RESP: Dyspnea, pneumonia, cough

Pharmacokinetics

Absorption	Unknown
Distribution	Unknown
Metabolism	Unknown
Excretion	Urine
Half-life	6 hr

Pharmacodynamics
Unknown

INTERACTIONS
Individual drugs
Chloramphenicol: decreased iron sucrose
Dimercaprol, iron (oral): increased toxicity; do not use together

NURSING CONSIDERATIONS
Assessment
• Monitor blood studies: Hct, Hgb, reticulocytes, transferrin, plasma iron concentrations, ferritin, total iron binding, bilirubin before treatment, at least monthly
• Assess for allergy: anaphylaxis, rash, pruritus, fever, chills, wheezing; notify prescriber immediately, keep emergency equipment available
• Assess cardiac status: hypotension, hypertension, hypervolemia
• Assess for toxicity: nausea, vomiting, diarrhea, fever, abdominal pain (early symptoms), cyanotic-looking lips and nailbeds, seizures, CV collapse (late symptoms)

Nursing diagnoses
• Knowledge, deficient (teaching)
• Nutrition, less than body requirements, imbalanced (uses)

Patient/family education
• Teach patient that iron poisoning may occur if increased beyond recommended level; not to take oral iron preparations
• Teach patient to report itching, rash, chest pain, headache, vertigo, nausea, vomiting, abdominal pain, joint/muscle pain, numbness, tingling

---

Evaluation
Positive therapeutic outcome
• Increased serum iron levels, Hct, Hgb

TREATMENT OF OVERDOSE:
Discontinue product, treat allergic reaction, give diphenhydrAMINE or epinephrine as needed, give iron-chelating product in acute poisoning

isoflurophate ophthalmic
See Appendix B

isoniazid (Rx)
(eye-soe-nye′a-zid)
Isotamine ✦
Func. class.: Antitubercular
Chem. class.: Isonicotinic acid hydrazide
Pregnancy category C

ACTION: Bactericidal interference with lipid, nucleic acid biosynthesis

Therapeutic outcome: Resolution of TB infection

USES: Treatment, prevention of TB

CONTRAINDICATIONS:
Hypersensitivity

> **BLACK BOX WARNING:** Acute liver disease

Precautions: Pregnancy **C**, diabetic retinopathy, cataracts, ocular defects, renal disease, **IV** drug users, people >35 yr, postpartum period, HIV, neuropathy

> **BLACK BOX WARNING:** Female (African descent, Hispanic), alcoholism

DOSAGE AND ROUTES
Treatment
Adult/adolescent with or without HIV: PO/IM 5 mg/kg/day up to 300 mg/day or 15 mg/kg 2-3 ×/week, max 900 mg 2-3 ×/wk
Child and infant HIV positive: PO/IM 10-15 mg/kg/day; max 300 mg/day

Available forms: Tabs 100, 300 mg; inj 100 mg/ml

Implementation
• Give antiemetic for vomiting
• Provide a list of foods to avoid while taking this product

PO route
• Give with meals to decrease GI symptoms; absorption is better when taken on empty stomach, 1 hr before or 2 hr after meals
IM route
• Give inj deep in large muscle mass, massage; rotate inj sites, warm inj to room temperature to dissolve crystals

ADVERSE EFFECTS

Hypersensitivity: Fever, skin eruptions, lymphadenopathy, vasculitis
CNS: *Peripheral neuropathy, dizziness,* memory impairment, **toxic encephalopathy, seizures**, psychosis, slurred speech
EENT: Blurred vision, optic neuritis
GI: *Nausea, vomiting,* epigastric distress, **jaundice, fatal hepatitis**
HEMA: **Agranulocytosis, hemolytic anemia, aplastic anemia, thrombocytopenia, eosinophilia, methemoglobinemia**
MISC: Dyspnea, vit B_6 deficiency, pellagra, hyperglycemia, metabolic acidosis, gynecomastia, rheumatic syndrome, systemic lupus erythematosus–like syndrome

Pharmacokinetics
Absorption	Well absorbed
Distribution	Widely
Metabolism	Liver
Excretion	Kidneys
Half-life	1-4 hr

Pharmacodynamics
	PO	IM
Onset	Rapid	Rapid
Peak	1-2 hr	45-60 min
Duration	6-8 hr	6-8 hr

INTERACTIONS

Individual drugs
Alcohol, carBAMazepine, cycloSERINE, ethionamide, meperidine, phenytoin, rifampin, warfarin: increased toxicity
BCG vaccine, ketoconazole: decreased effectiveness

Drug classifications
Antacids, aluminum: decreased absorption
Benzodiazepines: increased toxicity
SSRIs, SNRIs: increased serotonin syndrome

Drug/food
Tyramine foods: increased toxicity

⚠ Nurse Alert

NURSING CONSIDERATIONS

Assessment

• Obtain C&S tests, including sputum tests, before treatment; monitor every mo to detect resistance

> **BLACK BOX WARNING:** Monitor liver function tests weekly: ALT, AST, bilirubin, increased results may indicate hepatitis; renal studies during treatment, monthly: BUN, creatinine, output, specific gravity, urinalysis, uric acid

• Assess mental status often: affect, mood, behavioral changes; psychosis may occur with hallucinations, confusion
• Assess hepatic status: decreased appetite, jaundice, dark urine, fatigue
• Assess for visual disturbance that may indicate optic neuritis: blurred vision, change in color perception; may lead to blindness

Nursing diagnoses

• Diarrhea (adverse reactions)
• Infection, risk for (uses)
• Injury, risk for (adverse reactions)
• Knowledge, deficient (teaching)
• Noncompliance (teaching)

Patient/family education

• Instruct patient that compliance with dosage schedule for duration is necessary; not to skip or double doses; that scheduled appointments must be kept or relapse may occur
• Caution patient to avoid alcohol while taking product or hepatoxicity may result; to avoid ingestion of aged cheeses, fish or hypertensive crisis may result; give patient written directions on which foods to avoid while taking this medication
• Tell patient to report peripheral neuritis: weakness, tingling/numbness of hands/feet, fatigue; hepatoxicity: loss of appetite, nausea, vomiting, jaundice of skin or eyes

Evaluation

Positive therapeutic outcome

• Decreased symptoms of TB
• Culture negative for TB

TREATMENT OF OVERDOSE:

Pyridoxine

isosorbide dinitrate (Rx)

(eye-soe-sor'bide)
Apo-ISDN ❖, Dilatrate-SR, Isochren, IsoDitrate, Isordil

isosorbide mononitrate (Rx)

Apo-ISMN ❖, Imdur, Monoket
Func. class.: Antianginal, vasodilator
Chem. class.: Nitrate
Pregnancy category C

Do not confuse:

Imdur/Imuran/Inderal/K-Dur, Monoket/Monopril

ACTION: Relaxation of vascular smooth muscle, which leads to decreased preload, afterload, thus decreasing left ventricular end-diastolic pressure, and systemic vascular resistance and reducing cardiac O_2 demand

Therapeutic outcome: Relief and prevention of angina pectoris

USES: Treatment, prevention of chronic stable angina pectoris

CONTRAINDICATIONS:

Hypersensitivity to this product or nitrates, severe anemia, increased ICP, cerebral hemorrhage, acute MI

Precautions: Pregnancy **C**, breastfeeding, children, postural hypotension, MI, CHF, severe renal/hepatic disease

DOSAGE AND ROUTES

Dinitrate
Adult: PO 5-20 mg bid-tid, initially, maintenance 10-40 mg bid-tid; SL buccal tab 2.5-5 mg; may repeat q5-10min × 3 doses; EXT REL 40-80 mg q8-12hr, max 160 mg/day

Mononitrate
Adult: PO (Monoket) 10-20 mg bid, 7 hr apart; (Imdur) initiate at 30-60 mg/day as a single dose, increase q3day as needed; may increase to 120 mg/day; max 240 mg/day

Available forms: Dinitrate: sus rel caps 40 mg; SR tabs 40 mg; tabs 5, 10, 20, 30, 40 mg; SL tabs 2.5, 5 mg; chew tabs 5, 10 mg; mononitrate: tabs (Monoket) 10, 20 mg; ext rel tabs (Imdur) 30, 60, 120 mg

Implementation
PO route
• Swallow sus rel cap and ext rel tab whole; do not break, crush, or chew
• Do not swallow SL tab; tab should be dissolved under tongue
• Chew tab should be chewed thoroughly
• Give 1 hr before or 2 hr after meals with 8 oz of water
SL route
• Hold SL tab under tongue until dissolved (a few min); do not take anything PO when SL tab is in place

ADVERSE EFFECTS
CNS: *Vascular headache, flushing, dizziness,* weakness, faintness
CV: *Postural hypotension,* tachycardia, **collapse,** syncope, palpitations
GI: Nausea, vomiting, diarrhea
INTEG: Pallor, sweating, rash
MISC: Twitching, hemolytic anemia, **methemoglobinemia,** tolerance

Pharmacokinetics

Absorption	Well absorbed
Distribution	Unknown
Metabolism	Liver
Excretion	Urine, metabolites
Half-life	Dinitrate 1 hr, mononitrate 5 hr

Pharmacodynamics

	Sus rel	SL	PO
Onset	Up to 4 hr	2-5 min	15-30 min
Peak	Unknown	Unknown	Unknown
Duration	6-8 hr	1-4 hr	4-6 hr

INTERACTIONS
Individual drugs
Alcohol: increased hypotension
⚠ **Sildenafil, tadalafil, vardenafil: fatal hypotension**

Drug classifications
Antihypertensives, β-adrenergic blockers, calcium channel blockers, diuretics, phenothiazines: increased hypotension

NURSING CONSIDERATIONS
Assessment
• **Assess for pain:** duration, time started, activity being performed, character, intensity

• Monitor for orthostatic B/P, pulse at baseline, during treatment

Nursing diagnoses
• Cardiac output, decreased (uses)
• Knowledge, deficient (teaching)

Patient/family education
• Instruct patient to not skip or double doses; if dose is missed take when remembered if 2 hr before next dose (dinitrate), 6 hr before next dose (sus rel), or 8 hr before next dose (mononitrate)
• Caution patient to avoid alcohol and OTC medications unless approved by prescriber
• Inform patient that product may be taken before stressful activity: exercise, sexual activity
• Advise patient that SL tab may sting mucous membranes
• Caution patient to avoid driving and hazardous activities if dizziness occurs
• Advise patient to comply with complete medical regimen
• Caution patient to make position changes slowly to prevent orthostatic hypotension

Evaluation
Positive therapeutic outcome
• Decrease in, prevention of anginal pain

---

isradipine (Rx)
(is-ra′di-peen)
DynaCirc CR
Func. class.: Calcium channel blocker, antihypertensive, antianginal
Chem. class.: Dihydropyridine
Pregnancy category C

Do not confuse:
DynaCirc/Dynabac/Dynacin

ACTION: Inhibits calcium ion influx across cell membrane during cardiac depolarization; produces relaxation of coronary vascular smooth muscle and peripheral vascular smooth muscle; dilates coronary vascular arteries

Therapeutic outcome: Decreased B/P

USES: Essential hypertension

CONTRAINDICATIONS:
Hypersensitivity to this product or dihydropyridines

Precautions: Pregnancy C, breastfeeding, children, geriatric, CHF, hypotension, renal/hepatic disease, acute MI, bradycardia, cardiogenic shock, GERD, hiatal hernia, ventricular dysfunction

DOSAGE AND ROUTES
Adult: PO 2.5 mg bid; increase at 2-4 wk intervals up to 5 mg bid or 10 mg/day; CONT REL 5 mg/day, may be increased q2-4wk, max 20 mg/day

Available forms: Caps 2.5, 5 mg; cont rel tabs (CR) 5, 10 mg

Implementation
• Do not break, crush, or chew caps, cont rel tabs
• Give once a day with full glass of water; with food for GI symptoms

ADVERSE EFFECTS
CNS: Headache, fatigue, dizziness, fainting, sleep disturbances, weakness, depression, drowsiness
CV: Peripheral edema, tachycardia, hypotension, chest pain, **dysrhythmias,** syncope
GI: Nausea, vomiting, diarrhea, gastric upset, constipation, **hepatitis,** abdominal pain, distention, dry mouth
GU: Nocturia, urinary frequency
HEMA: Leukopenia
INTEG: Rash, pruritus, urticaria, **angioedema**
MISC: Flushing

Pharmacokinetics
Absorption	Well absorbed
Distribution	High plasma protein binding (95%)
Metabolism	Liver, extensively and rapidly
Excretion	Kidney
Half-life	Biphasic 1-1$^{1}/_{2}$ hr, 8 hr

Pharmacodynamics
Onset	1-2 hr
Peak	1.5 hr (immediate rel), 7-18 hr (cont rel)
Duration	12 hr

INTERACTIONS
Individual drugs
Cimetidine, ranitidine: decreased serum concentration of isradipine
Disopyramide: increased bradycardia, conduction effects
FentaNYL: increased hypotension
Lovastatin: decreased lovastatin concentration

Rifampin: increased serum concentration of isradipine

Drug classifications
Antihypertensives, nitrates: increased hypotension
β-Adrenergic blockers: increased synergistic effect
CYP3A4 inducers: decreased serum concentration of isradipine
CYP3A4 inhibitors: increased serum concentration of isradipine
NSAIDs, salicylates: decreased antihypertensive action

Drug/herb
Black cohosh, ginkgo, ginseng, goldenseal, hawthorn: increased antihypertensive effect
St. John's wort: decreased antihypertensive effect

NURSING CONSIDERATIONS
Assessment
• Assess fluid volume status: I&O ratio and record, weight, distended red veins, crackles in lung, color, quality, and specific gravity of urine, skin turgor, adequacy of pulses, moist mucous membranes, bilateral lung sounds, peripheral pitting edema; dehydration symptoms of decreasing output, thirst, hypotension, dry mouth and mucous membranes should be reported
• Monitor ALT, AST, bilirubin; if these are elevated, hepatotoxicity is suspected
• Assess renal, hepatic status, electrolytes before, during treatment
• Monitor cardiac status: B/P, pulse, respiration, ECG; assess anginal pain, precipitating, ameliorating factors

Nursing diagnoses
• Cardiac output, decreased (uses)
• Knowledge, deficient (teaching)

Patient/family education
• Instruct patient to avoid hazardous activities until stabilized on product and dizziness is no longer a problem
• Instruct patient to limit caffeine consumption; to avoid alcohol and OTC products unless directed by prescriber
• Advise patient to comply in all areas of medical regimen: diet, exercise, stress reduction, product therapy; to notify prescriber of irregular heartbeat, shortness of breath, swelling of feet and hands, pronounced dizziness, constipation, nausea, hypotension
• Instruct patient to use as directed even if feeling better
• Teach patient to take with a full glass of water

Evaluation
Positive therapeutic outcome
• Decreased B/P

TREATMENT OF OVERDOSE:
Defibrillation, atropine for AV block, vasopressor for hypotension

itraconazole (Rx)
(it-tra-kon′a-zol)
Sporanox
Func. class.: Antifungal (systemic)
Chem. class.: Triazole derivative
Pregnancy category C

ACTION: Alters cell membranes and inhibits several fungal enzymes

Therapeutic outcome: Fungistatic against *Histoplasma capsulatum, Blastomyces dermatitis, Cryptococcus neoformans, Aspergillus fumigatus, Candida*

USES: Histoplasmosis, blastomycosis (pulmonary and extrapulmonary), aspergillosis onychomycosis of toenail/fingernail

Unlabeled uses: Dermatomycosis, chromoblastomycosis, coccidioidomycosis, pityriasis versicolor, sebopsoriasis, vaginal candidiasis, cryptococcal, subcutaneous mycoses, dimorphic infections, fungal keratitis, alternariosis, zygomycosis

CONTRAINDICATIONS:
Hypersensitivity, fungal meningitis, onychomycosis, or dermatomycosis in cardiac dysfunction, females

> **BLACK BOX WARNING:** Heart failure, ventricular dysfunction, coadministration with other drugs

Precautions: Pregnancy **C**, breastfeeding, children, cardiac/renal/hepatic disease, achlorhydria or hypochlorhydria (product-induced), dialysis

DOSAGE AND ROUTES
Dose varies with type of infection
Adult: PO 200 mg/day with food; may increase to 400 mg/day if needed; life-threatening infections may require a loading dose of 200 mg tid × 3 days; **IV** 200 mg bid × 4 doses, then 200 mg/day; give each dose over 1 hr, maintenance PO 200-400 mg/day
Child: PO 3-5 mg/kg/day

Available forms: Caps 100 mg; oral sol 10 mg/ml; inj 10 mg/ml

Implementation
PO route
• Swallow caps whole; do not break, crush, or chew
• Give caps after full meal to ensure absorption
• Give with food or milk to prevent nausea and vomiting
• Take 2 hr before administration of other products that increase gastric pH
• Store in tight container at room temperature
• *Oral sol and caps are not interchangeable on a mg/mg basis*
• **Oral sol:** patient should swish in mouth vigorously

IV route
• **IV** after adding full contents 25 ml to 50 ml bag of NaCl, mix gently, use flow control device, give at a rate of 1 ml/min; use separate line, flush after use

ADVERSE EFFECTS
CNS: Headache, dizziness, insomnia, somnolence, depression
CV: Hypertension
GI: Nausea, vomiting, anorexia, diarrhea, cramps, abdominal pain, flatulence, **GI bleeding, hepatotoxicity**
GU: Gynecomastia, impotence, decreased libido
INTEG: Pruritus, fever, rash, **toxic epidermal necrolysis**
MISC: Edema, fatigue, malaise, hypokalemia, tinnitus, **rhabdomyolysis**

Pharmacokinetics
Absorption	Variable
Distribution	Tissue, plasma, CSF, 99.8% protein bound
Metabolism	Liver, extensively, inhibits CYP4503A enzyme
Excretion	Feces, breast milk
Half-life	IV 35.4 hr; terminal 29.4 hr; PO 64 hr; pediatric 35.8 hr

Pharmacodynamics
Onset	Unknown
Peak	4 hr
Duration	Unknown

INTERACTIONS

Individual drugs

BusPIRone: increased busPIRone levels, toxicity

Busulfan, clarithromycin, cycloSPORINE, atorvastatin, carBAMazepine, disopyramide, quetiapine, diazepam, digoxin, felodipine, fentaNYL, indinavir, isradipine, niCARdipine, NIFEdipine, nimoldipine, phenytoin, ritonavir, saquinavir, tacrolimus, warfarin: increased toxicity

CarBAMazepine, isoniazid: decreased itraconazole action

Didanosine: decreased antifungal action

Dofetilide, levomethadyl, pimozide, quiNIDine: life-threatening CV reaction

Alprazolam, clorazepam, diazepam, estazolam, flurazepam, midazolam (oral), triazolam: increased sedation

QuiNIDine: increased tinnitus, hearing loss, increased toxicity

Rifamycins: decreased action of itraconazole

Drug classifications

Antacids, H_2-receptor antagonists: decreased action of itraconazole

Calcium channel blockers: increased edema

Contraceptives (oral): decreased effect

Proton pump inhibitors: decreased itraconazole action

Hepatotoxic products: hepatotoxicity

Oral hypoglycemics: increased effects of oral hypoglycemics

Drug/food

Increased: absorption

NURSING CONSIDERATIONS

Assessment

• Assess for infection: WBC, sputum baseline, periodically, may start treatment before obtaining results

⚠ Monitor for hepatotoxicity: increasing AST, ALT, alkaline phosphatase, bilirubin

• Monitor for allergic reaction: dermatitis, rash; product should be discontinued, antihistamines (mild reaction) or epinephrine (severe reaction) administered; check inj site for thrombophlebitis

• Monitor for hypokalemia, check potassium level: anorexia, drowsiness, weakness, decreased reflexes, dizziness, increased urinary output, increased thirst, paresthesias; if these occur, product should be decreased or discontinued and potassium administered

Nursing diagnoses

• Infection, risk for (uses)

• Injury, risk for (adverse reaction)

• Knowledge, deficient (teaching)

Patient/family education

• Advise patient that long-term therapy may be needed to clear infection (1 wk-6 mo depending on type of infection)

• Teach patient side effects and when to notify prescriber

• Instruct patient to avoid hazardous activities if dizziness occurs

• Instruct patient to take 2 hr before administration of other products that increase gastric pH (antacids, H_2-blockers, omeprazole, sucralfate, anticholinergics)

• Teach patient importance of compliance with product regimen

• Instruct patient to notify prescriber of GI symptoms, signs of liver dysfunction (fatigue, nausea, anorexia, vomiting, dark urine, pale stools)

Evaluation

Positive therapeutic outcome

• Decreased fever, malaise, rash

• Negative C&S for infectious organism

---

ixabepilone (Rx)

(ix-ab-ep′i-lone)

Ixempra

Func. class.: Antineoplastic—miscellaneous

Chem. class.: Epothilone

Pregnancy category D

ACTION: Microtubule stabilizing agent; microtubles are needed for cell division

Therapeutic outcome: Decreased tumor size, decreased spread of malignancy

USES: Breast cancer

CONTRAINDICATIONS:

Pregnancy **D**, hypersensitivity to products with polyoxyethylated castor oil, breastfeeding, neutropenia <1500/mm^3, thrombocytopenia <100,000/mm^3

BLACK BOX WARNING: Hepatic disease

Precautions: Children, geriatric, alcoholism, bone marrow suppression, cardiac dysrhythmias, cardiac/renal disease, diabetes mellitus, peripheral neuropathy, ventricular dysfunction

---

DOSAGE AND ROUTES

Breast cancer, metastatic or locally advanced given with capecitabine, and resistant to anthracycline, taxane

Adult: IV INF 40 mg/m² over 3 hr q3wk plus capecitabine PO 2000 mg/m²/day in 2 divided doses on days 1-14 q21day; in those with BSA >2.2 m², dose should be calculated for a BSA of 2.2 m²

Breast cancer, metastatic or locally advanced resistant/refractory to anthracyclines, taxanes, capecitabine

Adult: IV INF 40 mg/m² over 3 hr q3wk; in those with BSA >2.2 m², dose should be calculated for a BSA of 2.2 m²

Dosage reduction in those taking a strong CYP3A4 inhibitor

Adult: IV INF 20 mg/m² over 3 hr q3wk

Available forms: Powder for inj 15, 45 mg

Implementation

• Give antiemetic 30-60 min before giving product and prn

IV route
• Let kit stand at room temperature for 30 min; to reconstitute, withdraw supplied diluent (8 ml for 15 mg vials, 23.5 ml for 45 mg vials); slowly inject solution into vial; gently swirl and invert to mix, final conc 2 mg/ml; further dilute in LR in DEHP-free bags; final conc should be 0.2-0.6 mg/ml; after added, mix by manual rotation
• Diluted sol is stable for 6 hr at room temperature; inf must be completed within 6 hr
• Use in-line filter 0.2-1.2 mcm
• Give over 3 hr

ADVERSE EFFECTS

CNS: *Peripheral neuropathy,* chills, fatigue, fever, flushing, headache, insomnia, impaired cognition, asthenia
CV: Bradycardia, *hypotension,* abnormal ECG, angina, atrial flutter, cardiomyopathy, chest pain, edema, MI, vasculitis
GI: *Nausea, vomiting, diarrhea,* abdominal pain, anorexia, colitis, constipation, gastritis, jaundice, GERD, **hepatic failure,** trismus
GU: Renal failure
HEMA: Neutropenia, thrombocytopenia, anemia, infections, coagulopathy
INTEG: *Alopecia,* rash, hot flashes
META: Hypokalemia, metabolic acidosis
MS: *Arthralgia, myalgia*
RESP: Bronchospasm, cough, dyspnea

SYST: *Hypersensitivity reactions,* anaphylaxis, dehydration, **radiation recall reaction**

Pharmacokinetics

Absorption	Unknown
Distribution	Unknown
Metabolism	Liver by CYP3A4
Excretion	Feces 65%, urine 21%
Half-life	Terminal 52 hr

Pharmacodynamics
Unknown

INTERACTIONS

Drug classifications

CYP3A4 inducers (aminoglutethimide, barbiturates, bexarotene, bosentan, carBAMazepine, dexamethasone, efavirenz, griseofulvin, modafinil, nafcillin, nevirapine, oxcarbazepine, phenytoin, rifamycin, topiramate): decreased ixabepilone levels

CYP3A4 inhibitors (amiodarone, amprenavir, aprepitant, atazanavir, chloramphenicol, clarithromycin, conivaptan, cycloSPORINE, danazol, darunavir, dalforpristan, delavirdine, diltiazem, erythromycin, estradiol, fluconazole, fluvoxamine, fosamprenavir, imatinib, indinavir, isoniazid, itraconazole, ketoconazole, lopinavir, miconazole, nefazodone, nelfinavir, propoxyphene, ritonavir, RU-486, saquinavir, tamoxifen, telithromycin, troleandomycin, verapamil, voriconazole, zafirlukast): increased ixabepilone level

Drug/herb
St. John's wort: avoid use

Drug/food
Grapefruit products: avoid use

NURSING CONSIDERATIONS

Assessment

• Monitor CBC, differential, platelet count prior to therapy, qwk; withhold product if WBC is <1500/mm³ or platelet count is <100,000/mm³, notify prescriber
• Monitor temp q4hr (may indicate beginning infection)

> **BLACK BOX WARNING:** Monitor liver function tests before, during therapy (bilirubin, AST, ALT, LDH) prn or qmo; check for jaundiced skin and sclera, dark urine, clay-colored stools, itchy skin, abdominal pain, fever, diarrhea

• Monitor VS during 1st hr of inf; check IV site for signs of infiltration

⚠ Assess for hypersensitive reactions, anaphylaxis including hypotension, dyspnea, angioedema, generalized urticaria; discontinue inf immediately; keep emergency equipment available

• Assess effects of alopecia on body image; discuss feelings about body changes

Nursing diagnoses
• Injury, risk for (uses, adverse reactions)
• Knowledge, deficient (teaching)

Patient/family education
• Teach patient to report signs of infection: fever, sore throat, flulike symptoms
• Teach patient to report signs of anemia: fatigue, headache, faintness, shortness of breath
• Teach patient to report any complaints or side effects to nurse or prescriber
• Caution patient that hair may be lost during treatment; a wig or hairpiece may make patient feel better; new hair may be different in color, texture
• Advise patient that pain in muscles and joints 2-5 days after inf is common
• Advise patient to use nonhormonal type of contraception
• Instruct patient to avoid receiving vaccinations while on this product

Evaluation
Positive therapeutic outcome
• Decreased tumor size, decreased spread of malignancy

---

ketoconazole (Rx)
(kee-toe-koe′na-zole)
Func. class.: Antifungal
Chem. class.: Imidazole derivative
Pregnancy category C

ACTION: Alters cell membrane and inhibits several fungal enzymes leading to cell death

Therapeutic outcome: Fungistatic/fungicidal against susceptible organisms: *Blastomycoses, Candida, Coccidioides, Cryptococcus, Histoplasma;* topical route: tinea cruris, tinea corporis, tinea versicolor, *Pityrosporum ovale*

USES: Systemic candidiasis, chronic mucocandidiasis, oral thrush, candiduria, coccidioidomycosis, histoplasmosis, chromomycosis, paracoccidioidomycosis, blastomycosis, tinea cruris, tinea corporis, tinea versicolor, *Pityrosporum ovale*

Unlabeled uses: Cushing's syndrome, advanced prostatic cancer

CONTRAINDICATIONS:
Breastfeeding, hypersensitivity, fungal meningitis

> **BLACK BOX WARNING:** Coadministration with other drugs

Precautions: Pregnancy C, children <2 yr, renal disease, achlorhydria (product induced)

> **BLACK BOX WARNING:** Hepatic disease

DOSAGE AND ROUTES
Adult: PO 200-400 mg once/day for 1-2 wk (candidiasis), 6 wk (other infections); 400 mg tid (prostate cancer, unlabeled)
Children >2 yr: 3.3-6.6 mg/kg/day as single daily dose

Available forms: Tabs 200 mg; oral susp ✦ 100 mg/5 ml topical (see Appendix B)

Implementation
PO route
• Give in the presence of acid products only; do not use alkaline products, proton pump inhibitors, H₂-antagonists, or antacids within 2 hr of product; may give coffee, tea, acidic fruit juices, cola; give with food to decrease GI symptoms; dissolve tab/4 ml of aqueous sol 0.2 N HCl, use straw to avoid contact, rinse with water afterward and swallow
• Give with HCl if achlorhydria is present
• Store in tight container at room temperature
Topical route
• Use enough medication to cover fungally infected and surrounding area; rub in; do not use occlusive dressing; do not get in eyes
Shampoo
• Hair should be wet; apply shampoo, lather, rub gently into scalp and hair for 1 min; rinse; reapply × 3 min; continue treatment 2 ×/wk for 1 mo, no more than once q3day

ADVERSE EFFECTS
CNS: Headache, dizziness, somnolence
GI: Nausea, vomiting, anorexia, diarrhea, abdominal pain, **hepatotoxicity**
GU: Gynecomastia, impotence
HEMA: Thrombocytopenia, leukopenia, hemolytic anemia
INTEG: Pruritus, fever, chills, photophobia, rash, dermatitis, purpura, urticaria
SYST: Anaphylaxis

K

Adverse effects: *italics* = common; **bold** = life-threatening

Pharmacokinetics

Absorption	pH dependent; decreased pH, increased absorption
Distribution	Widely distributed; crosses placenta
Metabolism	Liver, partially
Excretion	Feces, bile, breast milk
Half-life	Biphasic: 2 hr, 8 hr

Pharmacodynamics

Onset	Unknown
Peak	1-3 hr
Duration	Unknown

INTERACTIONS

Individual drugs

Alcohol: increased hepatotoxicity

Alfentanil, alprazolam, amprenavir, aripiprazole, atorvastatin, carBAMazepine, cerivastatin, clarithromycin, cyclophosphamide, cyclo-SPORINE, donepezil, eletriptan, erythromycin, fentaNYL, ifosfamide, indinavir, lovastatin, midazolam, nelfinavir, nisoldipine, quiNIDine, ritonavir, saquinavir, sildenafil, simvastatin, SUFentanil, tamoxifen, triazolam, vinBLAStine, vinCRIStine, zolpidem: increased toxicity, inhibition of CYP3A4 pathway

ddI, isoniazid, phenytoin, rifampin: decreased effect of ketoconazole

Paclitaxel: inhibited metabolism

Theophylline: decreased effectiveness

Warfarin: increased effects of warfarin

Drug classifications

Antacids, anticholinergics, gastric acid pump inhibitors, H_2-receptor agonists: decreased ketoconazole action

Anticoagulants (oral): increased effects of oral anticoagulants

Calcium channel blockers, corticosteroids, vinca alkaloids: increased toxicity, decreased CYP3A4 pathway

Contraceptives (oral): decreased effect of oral contraceptives

Hepatotoxic agents: increased hepatotoxicity

NURSING CONSIDERATIONS

Assessment

• Assess for signs and symptoms of infection: drainage, sore throat, urinary pain, hematuria, fever

• Obtain cultures for C&S before beginning treatment; therapy may be started after culture is taken

---

> **BLACK BOX WARNING: Monitor for hepatotoxicity:** increased AST, ALT, alkaline phosphatase, bilirubin; discontinue product if hepatotoxicity occurs; nausea, vomiting, jaundice, clay-colored stools, fatigue

Nursing diagnoses

• Infection, risk for (uses)
• Injury, risk for (adverse reactions)
• Knowledge, deficient (teaching)

Patient/family education

• Advise patient that long-term therapy may be needed to clear infection (1 wk-6 mo depending on infection)

• Advise patient to avoid hazardous activities if dizziness occurs

• Instruct patient to take 2 hr before administration of other products that increase gastric pH (antacids, H_2-blockers, omeprazole, sucralfate, anticholinergics)

• Stress the importance of compliance with product regimen

> **BLACK BOX WARNING:** Advise patient to notify prescriber of GI symptoms, signs of liver dysfunction (fatigue, nausea, anorexia, vomiting, dark urine, pale stools)

• Teach patient proper hygiene: hand washing, nail care, use of concomitant topical agents if prescribed

• Caution patient to avoid alcohol, since nausea, vomiting, hypertension may occur

• Advise patient to use sunscreen or avoid direct sunlight to prevent photosensitivity

• Advise patient to notify prescriber of sore throat, fever, skin rash, which may indicate superinfection

• Advise patient to use sunglasses to prevent photophobia

Evaluation

Positive therapeutic outcome

• Decreased oral candidiasis, fever, malaise, rash

• Negative C&S for infectious organism

• Absence of dandruff, scaling

---

ketoconazole topical

See Appendix B

---

ketoprofen (OTC, Rx)
(ke-to-proe'fen)
Apo-Keto ♣
Func. class.: NSAID; nonopioid analgesic, antirheumatic
Chem. class.: Propionic acid derivative
Pregnancy category B (1st trimester), D (2nd/3rd trimesters)

ACTION: Inhibits COX-1, COX-2; analgesic, antiinflammatory, antipyretic

Therapeutic outcome: Decreased pain, inflammation

USES: Mild to moderate pain; osteoarthritis; rheumatoid arthritis; dysmenorrhea; OTC relief of minor aches, pains

CONTRAINDICATIONS:
Pregnancy **D**, 2nd/3rd trimesters; hypersensitivity to this product, NSAIDs, salicylates, asthma, severe renal/hepatic disease, ulcer disease

> **BLACK BOX WARNING:** Perioperative pain in CABG

Precautions: Pregnancy **B** (1st trimester), breastfeeding, children, geriatric, bleeding/GI/cardiac disorders, hypersensitivity to other antiinflammatory agents

> **BLACK BOX WARNING:** GI bleeding, MI, stroke

DOSAGE AND ROUTES
Antiinflammatory
Adult: PO 50 mg qid or 75 mg tid, max 300 mg/day or EXT REL 200 mg/day

Analgesic
Adult: PO 25-50 mg q6-8hr, max 300 mg/day

Available forms: Caps 50, 75 mg; ext rel caps 200 mg

Implementation
• Swallow whole; do not break, crush, chew, or open ext rel cap
• Give with 8 oz of water and sit upright for 30 min after dose to prevent ulceration
• Give with food or milk to decrease gastric symptoms; give 30 min before or 2 hr after meals; absorption may be slowed

ADVERSE EFFECTS
CNS: Dizziness, drowsiness, fatigue, tremors, confusion, insomnia, anxiety, depression, headache
CV: Tachycardia, peripheral edema, palpitations, dysrhythmias, hypertension, **CV thrombotic events, MI, stroke**
EENT: Tinnitus, hearing loss, blurred vision
GI: *Nausea, anorexia, vomiting, diarrhea,* jaundice, **hepatitis,** constipation, flatulence, cramps, dry mouth, peptic ulcer, **GI bleeding**
GU: Nephrotoxicity: dysuria, hematuria, oliguria, azotemia
HEMA: Blood dyscrasias
INTEG: Purpura, rash, pruritus, sweating
SYST: Anaphylaxis

Pharmacokinetics
Absorption	Well absorbed
Distribution	Not known
Metabolism	Liver
Excretion	Kidneys
Half-life	2-4 hr; 5.4 hr (ext rel)

Pharmacodynamics
Onset	Unknown
Peak	1.2 hr; 6.8 hr (ext rel)
Duration	Unknown

INTERACTIONS
Individual drugs
Alcohol: increased adverse GI reactions, toxicity
Aspirin: increased ketoprofen levels, increased adverse GI reactions
Clopidogrel, eptifibatide, plicamycin, ticlopidine, tirofiban, valproic acid: increased risk of bleeding
CycloSPORINE, lithium, methotrexate, phenytoin: increased ketoprofen levels, increased toxicity
Insulin: increased hypoglycemia
Probenecid: increased ketoconazole levels
Radiation: increased risk of hematologic toxicity

Drug classifications
Anticoagulants, thrombolytics: increased risk of bleeding
Antihypertensives: decreased effect of antihypertensives
Antineoplastics: increased hematologic toxicity
Corticosteroids: increased adverse GI reactions
Diuretics: decreased effectiveness of diuretics
NSAIDs: increased adverse GI reactions
Sulfonylureas: increased hypoglycemia
SSRIs, SNRIs: increased serotonin syndrome

Drug/herb
Feverfew, garlic, ginger, ginkgo, ginseng *(Panax):* increased risk of bleeding

Drug/lab test
Increased: bleeding time, potassium, BUN, alkaline phosphatase, AST, ALT, creatinine, LDH
Decreased: blood glucose, Hct, Hgb, CCr, platelets, leukocytes
Interference: urine albumin, 17 KS, 17 hydroxycorticosteroids, bilirubin

NURSING CONSIDERATIONS

Assessment
• **Assess for pain:** type, location, intensity; ROM before and 1-2 hr after treatment
• Monitor renal, liver function tests: AST, ALT, bilirubin, creatinine, BUN, urine creatinine, CBC Hct, Hgb, pro-time if patient is on long-term therapy
• Check I&O ratio; decreasing output may indicate renal failure (long-term therapy)
• **Assess hepatotoxicity:** dark urine, clay-colored stools, jaundice of skin and sclera, itching, abdominal pain, fever, diarrhea if patient is on long-term therapy
• Assess for allergic reactions: rash, urticaria; if these occur, product may have to be discontinued
• Assess for ototoxicity: tinnitus, ringing, roaring in ears; audiometric testing needed before, after long-term therapy
• Assess for vision changes: blurring, halos; may indicate corneal, retinal damage
• Check edema in feet, ankles, legs
• Identify prior product history; there are many product interactions

> **BLACK BOX WARNING:** Assess for CV thrombotic events: MI, stroke

> **BLACK BOX WARNING:** For GI bleeding: blood in sputum, emesis, stools

Nursing diagnoses
• Injury, risk for (adverse reactions)
• Knowledge, deficient (teaching)
• Mobility, physical impaired (uses)
• Pain, acute (uses)
• Pain, chronic (uses)

Patient/family education
• Teach patient to report any symptoms of hepatotoxicity, renal toxicity, vision changes, ototoxicity, allergic reactions, bleeding (long-term therapy)

• Advise patient to take with 8 oz of water and sit upright for 30 min after dose to prevent ulceration
• Caution patient not to exceed recommended dosage, acute poisoning may result; to take as prescribed; do not double dose
• Advise patient to read label on other OTC products; many contain other antiinflammatories
• Advise patient to use sunscreen to prevent photosensitivity
• Inform patient that the therapeutic response takes 2 wk (arthritis)
• Teach patient to report tinnitus, confusion, diarrhea, sweating, hyperventilation, blurred vision, fever, joint aches
• Caution patient to avoid alcohol ingestion; GI bleeding may occur
• Teach patient to report use to all providers

Evaluation
Positive therapeutic outcome
• Decreased pain
• Decreased inflammation
• Increased mobility
• Decreased fever

ketorolac (Rx)
(kee′toe-role-ak)
Acular, Toradol 🍁
Func. class.: Nonsteroidal antiinflammatory (NSAID), nonopioid analgesic
Chem. class.: Acetic acid
Pregnancy category C; D (third trimester)

ACTION: Inhibits prostaglandin synthesis by decreasing an enzyme needed for biosynthesis; analgesic, antiinflammatory, antipyretic effects

Therapeutic outcome: Decreased pain, inflammation, ocular itching

USES: Mild to moderate pain (short term); decreased ocular itching in seasonal allergic conjunctivitis (ophthalmic)

CONTRAINDICATIONS:
Pregnancy **D** (3rd trimester), hypersensitivity, asthma, hepatic disease, peptic ulcer disease, CV bleeding

BLACK BOX WARNING: Breastfeeding, severe renal disease, labor and delivery, perioperative pain in CABG, prior to major surgery, epidural/intrathecal administration, GI bleeding, hypovolemia

Precautions: Pregnancy **C**, GI/cardiac disorders, hypersensitivity to other antiinflammatory agents, CCr <25 ml/min

BLACK BOX WARNING: Children, geriatric, bleeding, MI, stroke

DOSAGE AND ROUTES
Adult/adolescent >17 yr and ≥50 kg: PO continuation from **IM/IV** only 20 mg, then 10 mg q4-6hr prn, max 40 mg/day
Adult/adolescent >17 yr and <50 kg: IM (single dose) 30-60 mg, **IV** 15-30 mg; **IM/IV** (multiple dosing) 15-30 mg q6hr, max 60 mg/day × 5 day combined either **PO/IM/IV**

Ophthalmic route
Adult: 1 gtt (0.25 mg) qid × 7 days
Child: IV 1 mg/kg, then 0.5 mg/kg q6hr

Available forms: Inj 15, 30 mg/ml (prefilled syringes); ophth 0.5% sol; tabs 10 mg

Implementation
PO route
• Administer to patient crushed or whole
• Max 5 days
• Give with full glass of water; give with food or milk to decrease gastric symptoms; give 30 min before or 2 hr after meals; absorption may be slowed

IM/IV route
• IV give undiluted ≥15 sec
• Give IM inj deeply into large muscle mass
• Store at room temperature, protect from light

Y-site compatibilities: Cisatracurium, remifentanil, SUFentanil

Syringe incompatibilities: Morphine, meperidine, promethazine, hydrOXYzine

Solution compatibilities: D$_5$W, 0.9% NaCl, LR, D$_5$, plasmalate

ADVERSE EFFECTS
CNS: Dizziness, *drowsiness,* tremors, **seizures**
CV: Hypertension, flushing, syncope, pallor, edema, vasodilatation, **CV thrombotic events, MI, stroke**
EENT: Tinnitus, hearing loss, blurred vision

GI: Nausea, anorexia, vomiting, diarrhea, constipation, flatulence, cramps, dry mouth, peptic ulcer, **GI bleeding, perforation,** taste change, **hepatitis, hepatic failure**
GU: Nephrotoxicity: dysuria, hematuria, oliguria, azotemia
HEMA: Blood dyscrasias, prolonged bleeding
INTEG: Purpura, rash, pruritus, sweating, **angioedema, Stevens-Johnson syndrome, toxic epidermal necrolysis**

Pharmacokinetics

Absorption	Rapidly, completely absorbed
Distribution	Bound to plasma proteins (99%)
Metabolism	Liver (<50%)
Excretion	Kidney, metabolites (92%); breast milk (6%); feces
Half-life	6 hr (IM); increased in renal disease

Pharmacodynamics

	IM	Ophth/PO
Onset	Up to 10 min	Unknown
Peak	50 min IM; 2-3 hr PO	Unknown
Duration	4-6 hr PO	Unknown

INTERACTIONS
Individual drugs
Alcohol, aspirin: increased GI effects
Aspirin: increased ketorolac levels, contraindicated
Cefamandole, cefoperazone, cefotetan, clopidogrel, eptifibatide, plicamycin, ticlopidine, tirofiban, valproic acid: increased risk of bleeding
CycloSPORINE, lithium, methotrexate, pentoxifylline, probenecid: increased toxicity

Drug classifications
ACE inhibitors: increased renal impairment
Anticoagulants: increased effects
Antihypertensives: decreased antihypertensive effect
Salicylates, SNRIs, SSRIs, thrombolytics: increased risk of bleeding
Corticosteroids, NSAIDs, potassium products, steroids: increased GI effects
Diuretics: decreased diuretic effect
NSAIDs (other): increased ketorolac levels; contraindicated

K

Drug/lab test
Increased: AST, ALT, LDH, alkaline phosphatase, bleeding time, BUN, creatinine, potassium
Decreased: blood glucose, Hct/Hgb, platelets

NURSING CONSIDERATIONS

Assessment

> **BLACK BOX WARNING:** Monitor renal, hepatic, blood studies: BUN, creatinine, AST, ALT, Hgb before treatment, periodically thereafter, check for dehydration

• Monitor for aspirin sensitivity, asthma; these patients may be more likely to develop hypersensitivity to NSAIDs
• Assess patient's eyes: redness, swelling, tearing, itching
• **Monitor for pain:** type, location, intensity, ROM before and 1 hr after treatment

> **BLACK BOX WARNING:** Assess for GI bleeding: blood in sputum, emesis, stools

> **BLACK BOX WARNING:** Assess for CV thrombotic events: MI, stroke

Nursing diagnoses
• Injury, risk for (adverse reactions)
• Knowledge, deficient (teaching)
• Mobility, impaired physical (uses)
• Pain, acute (uses)

Patient/family education
• Teach patient that product must be continued for prescribed time to be effective; to avoid aspirin, alcoholic beverages, other NSAIDs, acetaminophen
• Caution patient to report bleeding, bruising, fatigue, malaise, since blood dyscrasias do occur
• Instruct patient to use caution when driving; drowsiness, dizziness may occur
• Instruct patient to take with a full glass of water to enhance absorption
• Caution patient that this product may cause eye redness, burning if soft contact lenses are worn
• Advise to report use to all health care providers
• Instruct patient to report change in urine pattern, weight increase, edema; pain in joints, fever, blood in urine (indicates nephrotoxicity); bruising, black tarry stools (indicates bleeding)
• Caution patient not to breastfeed

Evaluation
Positive therapeutic outcome
• Decreased pain
• Decreased inflammatory response
• Increased mobility
• Decreased ocular itching

ketorolac ophthalmic
See Appendix B

ketotifen ophthalmic
See Appendix B

labetalol (Rx)
(la-bet'a-lole)
Trandate
Func. class.: Antihypertensive, antianginal
Chem. class.: α- and β-blocker
Pregnancy category C

Do not confuse:
Trandate/Tridate

ACTION: Produces decreases in B/P without reflex tachycardia or significant reduction in heart rate through mixture of α-blocking, β-blocking effects; elevated plasma resins are reduced

Therapeutic outcome: Decreased B/P

USES: Mild to moderate hypertension; treatment of severe hypertension (**IV**)

Unlabeled uses: Hypertension in patients with pheochromocytoma, hypertension in clonidine withdrawal

CONTRAINDICATIONS:
Hypersensitivity to β-blockers, cardiogenic shock, heart block (2nd or 3rd degree), sinus bradycardia, CHF, bronchial asthma

Precautions: Pregnancy C, breastfeeding, geriatric, major surgery, diabetes mellitus, thyroid/renal/hepatic disease, COPD, well-compensated heart failure, CAD, nonallergic bronchospasm, peripheral vascular disease

> **BLACK BOX WARNING:** Abrupt discontinuation

DOSAGE AND ROUTES

Hypertension
Adult: PO 100 mg bid; may be given with a diuretic; may increase to 200 mg bid after 2

days; may continue to increase q1-3days; max 2400 mg/day in divided doses

Hypertensive crisis

Adult: **IV** INF 200 mg/160 ml D$_5$W, run at 2 mg/min or 1.6 ml/min; stop INF after desired response obtained; repeat q6-8hr as needed; **IV** BOL 20 mg over 2 min; may repeat 20-80 mg q10min, max 300 mg

Available forms: Tabs 100, 200, 300 mg; inj 5 mg/ml in 20-ml ampules

Implementation

PO route

• Give before meals, at bedtime; tab may be crushed or swallowed whole; give with food to prevent GI upset, increase absorption; reduce dosage in renal dysfunction
• Do not discontinue prior to surgery
• Store protected from light, moisture; place in cool environment

Direct IV route

• Give undiluted (5 mg/ml) over 2 min

Continuous IV infusion route

• Give after diluting in LR, D$_5$W, D$_5$ in 0.2%, 0.9%, 0.33% NaCl or Ringer's; infusion is titrated to patient's response; 200 mg of product/160 ml sol (1 mg/ml); 300 mg of product/240 ml sol (1 mg/ml); 200 mg of product/250 ml sol (2 mg/3 ml); use inf pump
• Keep patient recumbent during and for 3 hr after inf, monitor VS q5-15min

Y-site compatibilities: Amikacin, aminophylline, amiodarone, ampicillin, butorphanol, calcium gluconate, ceftazidime, ceftizoxime, cimetidine, diltiazem, DOBUTamine, DOPamine, enalaprilat, EPINEPHrine, erythromycin, esmolol, famotidine, fentaNYL, gentamicin, HYDROmorphone, lidocaine, LORazepam, magnesium sulfate, meperidine, metroNIDAZOLE, midazolam, milrinone, morphine, niCARdipine, nitroglycerin, nitroprusside, norepinephrine, oxacillin, potassium chloride, potassium phosphate, propofol, ranitidine, sodium acetate, tobramycin, vancomycin, vecuronium

Y-site incompatibilities: Cefoperazone, nafcillin

ADVERSE EFFECTS

CNS: Dizziness, mental changes, drowsiness, fatigue, headache, catatonia, depression, anxiety, nightmares, paresthesias, lethargy
CV: *Orthostatic hypotension*, **bradycardia**, **CHF**, chest pain, **ventricular dysrhythmias**, AV block, scalp tingling

EENT: *Tinnitus*, vision changes, sore throat, double vision, dry burning eyes, floppy iris syndrome
GI: *Nausea, vomiting, diarrhea*, dyspepsia, taste distortion
GU: Impotence, dysuria, ejaculatory failure
HEMA: **Agranulocytosis, thrombocytopenia, purpura** (rare)
INTEG: Rash, alopecia, urticaria, pruritus, fever, **exfoliative dermatitis**
RESP: **Bronchospasm**, dyspnea, wheezing

Pharmacokinetics

Absorption	Bioavailability 25% (PO); complete (**IV**)
Distribution	Crosses placenta, CNS
Metabolism	Liver, extensively
Excretion	Breast milk, kidneys, bile
Half-life	6-8 hr

Pharmacodynamics

	PO	IV
Onset	30 min	5 min
Peak	2-4 hr	15 min
Duration	8-12 hr	2-4 hr

INTERACTIONS

Individual drugs

Alcohol (large amounts), cimetidine, nitroglycerin: increased hypotension
Lidocaine: decreased effect
Verapamil: increased myocardial depression

Drug classifications

Antidepressants, tricyclics: increased tremor
Antidiabetics: increased or decreased effect
Antihypertensives: increased hypotension
β-Blockers, bronchodilators, sympathomimetics, xanthines: decreased effects
Diuretics: increased hypotension
General anesthetics, hydantoins, class IC antidysrhythmics: increased myocardial depression
MAOIs: do not use within 2 wk
NSAIDs, salicylates: decreased antihypertensive effect
Theophyllines: decreased bronchodilatation

Drug/herb

Hawthorn: increased antihypertensive effect
Ephedra: decreased antihypertensive effect

Drug/lab test

Increased: ANA titer, blood glucose, alkaline phosphatase, LDH, AST, ALT, BUN, potassium, triglycerides, uric acid, serum lipoprotein
False increase: urinary catecholamines

L

NURSING CONSIDERATIONS
Assessment
- **Hypertension:** monitor B/P at beginning of treatment, periodically thereafter; pulse q4hr; note rate, rhythm, quality: apical/radial pulse before administration; notify prescriber of any significant changes (pulse <50 bpm)
- Check for baselines in renal, liver function tests before therapy begins
- **CHF:** assess for edema in feet, legs daily, monitor I&O, daily weight; check for jugular vein distention, crackles bilaterally, dyspnea

> **BLACK BOX WARNING:** Abrupt discontinuation: Product should be tapered to prevent adverse reactions

Nursing diagnoses
- Cardiac output, decreased (uses)
- Injury, risk for (side effects)
- Knowledge, deficient (teaching)
- Noncompliance (teaching)

Patient/family education

> **BLACK BOX WARNING:** Teach patient not to discontinue product abruptly, precipitate angina might occur; taper over 2 wk

- Teach patient not to use OTC products containing α-adrenergic stimulants (such as nasal decongestants, cold preparations); to avoid alcohol, smoking; to limit sodium intake as prescribed
- Teach patient how to take pulse and B/P at home; advise when to notify prescriber
- Instruct patient to comply with weight control, dietary adjustments, modified exercise program
- Advise patient to carry/wear emergency ID to identify products being taken, allergies; that product controls symptoms but does not cure the condition
- **Teach patient to report symptoms of CHF:** difficulty breathing, especially on exertion or when lying down, night cough, swelling of extremities, bradycardia, dizziness, confusion, depression, fever
- Teach patient to take product as prescribed, not to double or skip doses; take any missed doses as soon as remembered if at least 4 hr until next dose
- Advise patient to avoid driving or other hazardous activities until response is known; dizziness, drowsiness occurs
- Teach patient to take product at bedtime to prevent orthostatic hypotension, to rise slowly

Evaluation
Positive therapeutic outcome
- Decreased B/P in hypertension (after 1-2 wk)
- Absence of dysrhythmias

TREATMENT OF OVERDOSE:
Lavage, **IV** glucagon or atropine for bradycardia, **IV** theophylline for bronchospasm, digoxin, O_2, diuretic for cardiac failure, hemodialysis, **IV** glucose for hyperglycemia, **IV** diazepam (or phenytoin) for seizures

---

lacosamide (Rx)
(la-koe′sa-mide)
Vimpat
Func. class.: Anticonvulsant
Chem. class.: Functionalized amino acid
Pregnancy category C

ACTION: May act through action at sodium channels; exact action is unknown

Therapeutic outcome: Decrease in severity of seizures

USES: Adjunctive therapy of partial seizures

CONTRAINDICATIONS:
Hypersensitivity

Precautions: Pregnancy **C,** breastfeeding, allergies, renal/hepatic disease, geriatric patients, child <17 yr, acute MI, atrial fibrillation/flutter, AV block, bradycardia, cardiac disease, congenital heart disease, dehydration, depression, dialysis, hazardous activity, electrolyte imbalance, heart failure, labor, PR prolongation, sick sinus syndrome, substance abuse, suicidal ideation, syncope, torsades de pointes

DOSAGE AND ROUTES
Adult and child ≥17 yr: PO 50 mg bid, may increase qwk by 100 mg bid to 200-400 mg/day; **IV** 50 mg 2 ×/day, infuse over 30-60 min, may be increased 100 mg/day weekly, up to 200-400 mg/day maintenance

Renal/hepatic dose
Adult: PO/**IV** max 300 mg/day in mild to moderate hepatic disease or CCr ≤30 ml/min

Available forms: Film-coated tabs 50, 100, 150, 200 mg; **IV** 20 ml single use vials (200 mg/20 ml), oral sol 10 mg/ml

Implementation
- Store PO products/**IV** vials at room temperature; solution is stable for 24 hr when mixed

---

with compatible diluents in glass or PVC bags at room temperature

PO route
• **Tablet:** give without regard to meals
• **Oral sol:** measure with calibrated measuring device

IV route
• May give undiluted or mixed in 0.9% NaCl, D_5, or LR
• Infuse over 30-60 min
• Do not use if discolored or particulates are present; discard unused portions

ADVERSE EFFECTS

CNS: Dizziness, syncope, tremor, vertigo, ataxia, drowsiness, fever, hypoesthesia, paresthesias, depression, fatigue, headache, confusion, irritability, psychological dependence, **suicidal ideation**
CV: *Atrial fibrillation/flutter,* **AV block,** bradycardia, myocarditis, orthostatic hypotension, palpitations, **PR prolongation**
EENT: Diplopia, blurred vision, nystagmus, tinnitus
GI: Nausea, constipation, vomiting, **hepatitis,** diarrhea, dyspepsia
HEMA: **Anemia, neutropenia**
INTEG: Rash, erythemia, inj site reaction, pruritus, xerostomia
MS: Asthenia, dysarthria
SYST: **Drug reaction with eosinophilia and systemic symptoms (DRESS)**

Pharmacokinetics

Absorption	Unknown
Distribution	Protein binding <15%
Metabolism	Liver
Excretion	Kidneys (95%)
Half-life	13 hr (PO), elimination half-life 15-23 hr

Pharmacodynamics

	PO	IV
Onset	Unknown	Unknown
Peak	1-4 hr (PO)	30-60 min
Duration	Unknown	Unknown

INTERACTIONS

Individual drugs
Atazanavir, dronedarone, digoxin, lopinavir, ritonavir: increase PR prolongation

Drug classifications
β-blockers, calcium-channel blockers: increase PR prolongation

CYP2C19 inhibitors (fluconazole, isoniazid, miconazole): increase lacosamide effect

Drug/lab test
Increased: LFTs

NURSING CONSIDERATIONS

Assessment
• **Assess for seizures:** duration, type, intensity, precipitating factors
• Monitor for renal function: albumin concentration
• Assess CV status: orthostatic hypotension, PR prolongation; monitor cardiac status throughout treatment
• Assess mental status: mood, sensorium, affect, memory (long, short), depression, suicidal ideation, psychological dependence
• Assess for rash, hypersensitivity reactions

Nursing diagnoses
• Injury, risk for (uses)
• Knowledge, deficient (teaching)

Patient/family education
• Caution patient not to discontinue product abruptly, taper over 1 wk; seizures may occur
• Advise patient to avoid hazardous activities until stabilized on product
• Instruct patient to carry emergency ID stating product use
• Advise patient to notify prescriber of suicidal thoughts or actions, syncope, cardiac changes
• Instruct patient to notify prescriber if pregnancy is planned or suspected
• Teach patient that interactions with other medications may occur
• Give patient MediGuide for proper use and risks

Evaluation
Positive therapeutic outcome
• Decrease in severity of seizures

---

lactulose (Rx)

(lak′tyoo-lose)
Constulose, Enulose, Generlac, Kristalose
Func. class.: Laxative (hyperosmotic/ammonia detoxicant)
Chem. class.: Lactose synthetic derivative
Pregnancy category B

ACTION: Prevents absorption of ammonia in colon by acidifying stool; increases water, softens stool

Therapeutic outcome: Decreased constipation, decreased blood ammonia level

USES: Chronic constipation, portal-systemic encephalopathy in patients with hepatic disease

CONTRAINDICATIONS:
Hypersensitivity, low-galactose diet

Precautions: Pregnancy **B**, breastfeeding, geriatric and debilitated patient, diabetes mellitus

DOSAGE AND ROUTES
Constipation
Adult: PO 15-30 ml/day (10-20 g), may increase to 60 ml/day prn
Child (unlabeled): PO 7.5 ml/day

Hepatic encephalopathy
Adult: PO 30-45 ml (20-30 g) tid or qid until stools are soft; retention enema 300 ml diluted
Infant: PO 2.5-10 ml/day in divided doses
Child: PO 40-90 ml/day in divided doses given 3-4 ×/day

Available forms: Oral sol (encephalopathy) 10 g/15 ml; oral sol (constipation) 10 g/15 ml

Implementation
PO route
• Give with full glass of fruit juice, water, milk to increase palatability of oral form; for rapid effect, give on empty stomach; increase fluids by 2 L/day; do not give with other laxatives; if diarrhea occurs, reduce dosage
• Kristalose: dissolve contents of packet in 4 oz of water
Rectal route
• **Administer retention enema** by diluting 300 ml of lactulose/700 ml of water or of 0.9% NaCl; administer by rect balloon catheter; retain for 30-60 min; repeat if evacuated too quickly

ADVERSE EFFECTS
GI: *Nausea, vomiting, anorexia, abdominal cramps, diarrhea,* flatulence, *distention, belching*
META: Hypernatremia

Pharmacokinetics

Absorption	Poorly absorbed
Distribution	Not known
Metabolism	Colonic bacteria to acids
Excretion	Kidneys, unchanged
Half-life	Unknown

Pharmacodynamics
Unknown

INTERACTIONS
Individual drugs
Neomycin: decreased lactulose effect
NIFEdipine extended release tab: increased GI obstruction

Drug classifications
Antiinfectives (oral), antacids: decreased lactulose effect
Laxatives: do not use together (hepatic encephalopathy)

Drug/herb
Flax, senna: increased laxative effect

Drug/lab test
Blood glucose (diabetic patients): increase
Blood ammonia: decrease

NURSING CONSIDERATIONS
Assessment
• **Stool:** Assess for amount, color, consistency
• Monitor glucose levels in diabetic patients (increases)
• **Cause of constipation:** Determine whether fluids, bulk, or exercise is missing from lifestyle
• Monitor blood, urine, electrolytes if used often by patient; may cause diarrhea, hypokalemia, hypernatremia; check I&O ratio to identify fluid loss
• Assess cramping, rectal bleeding, nausea, vomiting; if these symptoms occur, product should be discontinued; identify cause of constipation: identify whether fluids, bulk, or exercise is missing from lifestyle
• **Hepatic encephalopathy:** Monitor blood ammonia level (30-70 mg/100 ml); monitor for clearing of confusion, lethargy, restlessness, irritability (hepatic encephalopathy); may decrease ammonia level by 50%

Nursing diagnoses
• Constipation (uses)
• Diarrhea (adverse reactions)
• Knowledge, deficient (teaching)
• Noncompliance (teaching)

Patient/family education
• Discuss with patient that adequate fluid consumption is necessary
• Teach patient that normal bowel movements do not always occur daily
• Teach patient not to use in presence of abdominal pain, nausea, vomiting; tell patient to notify prescriber of unrelieved constipation

---

⚠ Nurse Alert

or if symptoms of electrolyte imbalance occur:
muscle cramps, pain, weakness, dizziness,
excessive thirst
• Teach patient not to use laxatives for long-
term therapy; bowel tone will be lost
• Do not give at bedtime as a laxative; may
interfere with sleep
• Notify prescriber if diarrhea occurs; may
indicate overdosage

Evaluation
Positive therapeutic outcome
• Decreased constipation
• Decreased blood ammonia level
• Clearing of mental state

lamiVUDine (3TC) (Rx)
(lam-i'vue-dine)
Epivir, Epivir-HBV, Heptovir ❧
Func. class.: Antiretroviral
Chem. class.: Nucleoside reverse tran-
scriptase inhibitor (NRTI)
Pregnancy category C

Do not confuse:
lamiVUDine/LamoTRIgine

ACTION: Inhibits replication of HIV virus
by incorporating into cellular DNA by viral
reverse transcriptase, thereby terminating the
cellular DNA chain

Therapeutic outcome: Improved symptoms of HIV infection

USES: HIV infection in combination with at
least 2 other antiretrovirals; chronic hepatitis B
(Epivir-HBV)

Unlabeled uses: Prophylaxis of HIV postexposure with indinavir and zidovudine

CONTRAINDICATIONS:
Hypersensitivity

> **BLACK BOX WARNING:** Lactic acidosis

Precautions: Pregnancy **C**, breastfeeding,
children, geriatric, granulocyte count <1000/
mm³ or Hgb <9.5 g/dl, renal disease, pancreatitis, peripheral neuropathy

> **BLACK BOX WARNING:** Severe hepatic
> dysfunction

DOSAGE AND ROUTES
HIV infection
Adult and adolescent >16 yr: PO 150 mg bid
or 300 mg/day
Child 3 mo-16 yr: PO 4 mg/kg bid; max 150
mg bid

Renal dose
Adult: PO CCr 30-49 ml/min: Epivir 150 mg
q day; Epivir HBV 100 mg 1st dose, then 50
mg q day; CCr 15-29 ml/min: Epivir 150 mg 1st
dose, then 100 mg q day; Epivir HBV 100 mg
1st dose, then 25 mg q day; CCr 5-14 ml/min:
Epivir 150 mg 1st dose, then 50 mg q day;
Epivir HBV 35 mg 1st dose, then 15 mg q day;
CCr <5 ml/min: Epivir 50 mg 1st dose, then
25 mg q day; Epivir HBV 35 mg 1st dose, then
10 mg q day

Chronic hepatitis B
Adult: PO 100 mg/day
Child/adolescent 2-17 yr: PO 3 mg/kg/day,
max 100 mg

Available forms: Oral sol **(Epivir)** 10 mg/
ml, tabs 150, 300/mg; oral sol **(Epivir-HBV)** 5
mg/ml, tabs 100 mg

Implementation
• Epivir and Epivir-HBV are not interchangeable
• Administer PO daily, bid without regard to
meals
• Give with other antiretrovirals only
• Store in cool environment; protect from light

ADVERSE EFFECTS
CNS: *Fever, headache, malaise, dizziness,
insomnia, depression, fatigue, chills,* **sei-
zures,** peripheral neuropathy, paresthesia
EENT: Taste change, hearing loss, photopho-
bia
GI: *Nausea, vomiting, diarrhea,* anorexia,
cramps, dyspepsia, **hepatomegaly with
steatosis, pancreatitis**
HEMA: **Neutropenia,** anemia, **thrombocy-
topenia**
INTEG: *Rash*
MS: *Myalgia, arthralgia, pain*
RESP: *Cough*
SYST: **Lactic acidosis, anaphylaxis,
Stevens-Johnson syndrome**

Pharmacokinetics	
Absorption	Rapidly absorbed
Distribution	Extravascular space
Metabolism	Protein binding <36%
Excretion	Unchanged in urine
Half-life	Terminal half-life 5-7 hr

Pharmacodynamics
Unknown

INTERACTIONS
Individual drugs
Amiloride, dofetilide, entecavir, metformin, memantine, procainamide, trospium, trimethoprim/sulfamethoxazole: increased level of lamiVUDine

Emtricitabine: do not combine, duplication

Zalcitabine: decreased both products, avoid concurrent use

Drug classifications
Interferons: decrease lamiVUDine

Drug/lab test
Increased: ALT, bilirubin

Decreased: Hgb, neutrophil, platelet count

NURSING CONSIDERATIONS
Assessment
• **HIV:** Monitor blood counts q2wk; watch for neutropenia, thrombocytopenia, Hgb, CD4, viral load, lipase, triglycerides periodically during treatment; if low, therapy may have to be discontinued and restarted after hematologic recovery; blood transfusions may be required; assess for lessening of symptoms

• **Hepatitis B:** Assess for fatigue, anorexia, pruritus, jaundice during and for several months after discontinuation; monitor liver function tests: AST, ALT, bilirubin; amylase; bilirubin, triglycerides, lipase

• **Monitor children for pancreatitis:** abdominal pain, nausea, vomiting, neuropathy

> BLACK BOX WARNING: **Assess for lactic acidosis, severe hepatomegaly with steatosis:** obtain baseline liver function tests; if elevated, discontinue treatment; discontinue even if liver function tests are normal and symptoms of lactic acidosis, severe hepatomegaly develops; may be fatal

Nursing diagnoses
• Infection, risk for (uses)
• Injury, risk for (adverse reactions)
• Knowledge, deficient (teaching)

Patient/family education
• Teach patient that GI complaints and insomnia resolve after 3-4 wk of treatment
• Tell patient that product is not a cure for AIDS but will control symptoms; compliance is needed, take as directed, to complete full course of treatment even if feeling better

• Teach patient to notify prescriber of sore throat, swollen lymph nodes, malaise, fever, peripheral neuropathy; other infections may occur
• Teach patient that virus is still infective, may pass AIDS virus to others
• Encourage patient to continue follow-up visits since serious toxicity may occur; blood counts must be done q2wk
• Tell patient that other products may be necessary to prevent other infections
• Teach patient that product may cause fainting or dizziness

Evaluation
Positive therapeutic outcome
• Absence of infection, symptoms of HIV infection

---

lamoTRIgine (Rx)
(lam-o-trye′geen)
Lamictal, Lamictal CD, Lamictal ODT, Lamictal XR
Func. class.: Anticonvulsant— miscellaneous
Chem. class.: Phenyltriazine
Pregnancy category C

Do not confuse:
lamoTRIgine/lamiVUDine,
LaMICtal/LamISIL/Lomotil

ACTION: May inhibit voltage-sensitive sodium channels, decreasing seizures

Therapeutic outcome: Decrease in intensity and number of seizures

USES: Adjunct in the treatment of partial, tonic-clonic seizures, children with Lennox-Gastaut syndrome, bipolar disorder

Unlabeled uses: Absence seizures

CONTRAINDICATIONS:
Hypersensitivity

Precautions: Pregnancy **C** (cleft lip/palate in 1st trimester), breastfeeding, geriatric, renal/hepatic/cardiac disease, severe depression, suicidal ideation, blood dyscrasias

> BLACK BOX WARNING: Children <16 yr

DOSAGE AND ROUTES

Seizures: monotherapy

Adult and adolescent ≥16 yr: PO 50 mg/day for wk 1 and 2, then increase to 100 mg divided bid for wk 3 and 4; maintenance 300-500 mg/day; receiving enzyme inducing AEDs (carBAMazepine, PHENobarbital, phenytoin, primidone but not valproic acid); EXT REL 50 mg/day × 1-2 wks, then 100 mg/day during wk 3-4, then 200 mg/day during wk 5, then 300 mg/day during wk 6, then 400 mg/day during wk 7; after wk 7 range is 400-600 mg/day

Adolescent <16 yr and child: PO 0.3 mg/kg/day wk 1 and 2, then 0.6 mg/kg/day wk 3 and 4; depends on use of AED; usual dosage 4.5-7.5 mg/kg/day, max 300 mg/day

Monotherapy for patients taking valproate

Adult/adolescent ≥16 yr: receiving lamoTRIgine and valproate, without enzyme-inducing drug PO (immediate-release) stabilize on valproate and target dose of 200 mg/day lamoTRIgine; if patient is not taking lamoTRIgine 200 mg/day, increase dose by 25-50 mg/day q1-2wk to reach 200 mg/day; while maintaining lamoTRIgine 200 mg/day, decrease valproate to 500 mg/day by ≤500 mg/day/wk, maintain valproate at 500 mg/day × 1 wk, then increase lamoTRIgine to 300 mg/day, while decreasing valproate 250 mg/day × 1 wk, then discontinue valproate and increase lamoTRIgine by 100 mg/day q wk to maintenance dosage of 500 mg/day

Seizures: multiple therapy with valproate

Adult and adolescent ≥16 yr: PO 25 mg every other day, then 25 mg/day wk 3-4, increase by 25-50 mg q1-2wk; maintenance 100-400 mg/day

Adolescent <16 yr and child: PO 0.1-0.2 mg/kg/day initially, then increase q2wk as needed to 1.5 mg/kg/day or 200 mg/day

Bipolar disorder (Escalation regimen in those not taking carBAMazepine, or other enzyme-inducing drugs or valproate)

Adult and adolescent ≥16 yr: PO wk 1-2 25 mg/day; wk 3-4 50 mg/day; wk 5 100 mg/day; wk 6-7 200 mg/day; for patients taking valproic acid: wk 1-2 25 mg every other day; wk 3-4 25 mg/day; wk 5 50 mg/day; wk 6 100 mg/day; wk 7 100 mg/day

Hepatic dose

Adult (moderate hepatic impairment or severe without ascites): PO reduce by 25%

Adult (severe hepatic impairment with ascites): PO reduce by 50%

Available forms: Tabs 25, 100, 150, 200 mg; chew tabs 5, 25 mg; oral disintegrating tab 25, 50, 100, 200 mg; oral disintegrating 25-50, 50-100, 25-50-100 mg titration kit; PO ext rel 25-50-100, 50-100-200 mg titration kit; PO 25-100 mg starter kit, ext rel 25, 50, 100, 250 mg

Implementation

PO route

• Discontinue all products gradually ≥2 wk, abrupt discontinuation can increase seizures

• **Chewable dispersible tab:** may be swallowed whole, chewed, mixed in water or fruit juice; to mix add to small amount of liquid in a glass or spoon, tabs will dissolve in 1 min, then mix in more liquid and swirl and swallow immediately

• **Orally disintegrating tabs:** place on tongue, move around in mouth, when disintegrated, swallow; examine blister pack before use, do not use if blisters are torn or missing

• **Extended-release tabs:** swallow whole, do not cut, break, chew

• Give correct starter kit, errors have occurred

• Give in divided doses with or after meals to decrease adverse effects

ADVERSE EFFECTS

CNS: Fever, insomnia, tremor, depression, anxiety, *dizziness,* ataxia, *headache,* **suicidal ideation**

EENT: Nystagmus, *diplopia, blurred vision*

GI: *Nausea, vomiting, anorexia,* abdominal pain, **hepatotoxicity**

GU: *Dysmenorrhea*

HEMA: Anemia, **DIC, leukopenia, thrombocytopenia**

INTEG: **Rash (potentially life-threatening),** alopecia, photosensitivity

SYST: **Stevens-Johnson syndrome, angioedema, toxic epidermal necrolysis**

Pharmacokinetics

Absorption	Well absorbed, rapid
Distribution	Protein binding 55%, crosses placenta
Metabolism	Glucuronic acid conjunction
Excretion	Excreted in breast milk
Half-life	Terminal 24 hr; 15 hr with enzyme inducers

Pharmacodynamics

Onset	Unknown
Peak	1.4-2.3 hr
Duration	Unknown

INTERACTIONS

Individual drugs
Acetaminophen, carBAMazepine, OXcarbazepine, PHENobarbital, phenytoin, primidone: decreased lamoTRIgine serum concentration
Valproic acid: decreased metabolic clearance of lamoTRIgine

Drug classifications
CYP3A4 inhibitors: decreased metabolic clearance of lamoTRIgine
Contraceptives (oral), estrogens, succinimides, rifamycins: decreased lamoTRIgine serum concentration

Drug/herb
Ginkgo: increased anticonvulsant effect
Ginseng, santonica: decreased anticonvulsant effect

NURSING CONSIDERATIONS

Assessment
⚠ Assess for rash (Stevens-Johnson syndrome or toxic epidermal necrolysis) in pediatric patients; product should be discontinued at first sign of rash
• Assess for seizure activity: duration, type, intensity, halo before seizure
• Assess for hypersensitive reactions
⚠ Bipolar disorder: suicidal thoughts/behaviors

Nursing diagnoses
• Injury, risk for (uses)
• Knowledge, deficient (teaching)

Patient/family education
• Caution patient not to discontinue product abruptly; seizures may occur
• Caution patient to avoid hazardous activities until stabilized on product
• Advise patient to notify prescriber of skin rash or increased seizure activity
• Instruct patient to report to prescriber if pregnancy is suspected or planned
• Teach patient to use sunscreen and protective clothing; photosensitivity occurs
• Advise patient to carry/wear emergency ID stating product use
• Advise patient to notify prescriber immediately of suicidal thoughts, behaviors

Evaluation
Positive therapeutic outcome
• Decrease in severity of seizures or severity of bipolar symptoms

lansoprazole (Rx, OTC)
(lan-soe′prah-zole)
Prevacid, Prevacid SoluTab
Func. class.: Anti-ulcer proton-pump inhibitor
Chem. class.: Benzimidazole
Pregnancy category B

Do not confuse:
Prevacid/Pravachol/Prinivil

ACTION: Suppresses gastric secretion by inhibiting hydrogen/potassium ATPase enzyme system in gastric parietal cell; characterized as gastric acid pump inhibitor since it blocks final step of acid production

Therapeutic outcome: Reduction in gastric pain, swelling, fullness

USES: Gastroesophageal reflux disease (GERD), severe erosive esophagitis, poorly responsive systemic GERD, pathologic hypersecretory conditions (Zollinger-Ellison syndrome, systemic mastocytosis, multiple endocrine adenomas); possibly effective for treatment of duodenal, gastric ulcers, maintenance of healed duodenal ulcers

CONTRAINDICATIONS:
Hypersensitivity

Precautions: Pregnancy B, breastfeeding, children

DOSAGE AND ROUTES

Frequent heartburn
Adult: PO 15 mg qd up to 14 days

Duodenal ulcer
Adult: PO 15 mg/day before meals for 4 wk, then 15 mg/day to maintain healing of ulcers; ulcers associated with *Helicobacter pylori*: 30 mg lansoprazole, 500 mg clarithromycin, 1 g amoxicillin bid × 14 days or 30 mg lansoprazole, 1 g amoxicillin tid × 14 days

Pathologic hypersecretory conditions
Adult: PO 60 mg/day, may give up to 90 mg bid, administer >120 mg/day in divided doses

GERD/esophagitis
Adult/adolescent: PO 15-30 mg/day × 8 wk
Child 1-11 yr (>30 kg): PO 30 mg/day ≤12 wk
Child 1-11 yr (≤30 kg): 15 mg/day ≤12 wk

Stress gastric prophylaxis
Adult: NG use 30 mg oral cap or 300 mg disintegrating tab

Available forms: del rel caps 15, 30 mg; orally disintegrating tabs 15, 30 mg

Implementation
PO route
• Swallow del rel cap whole; do not break, crush, chew, or open
• Administer before eating
NG route
• **Oral cap:** Open cap and pour ¹/₄ of granules into NG feeding syringe with plunger removed, slowly add water and depress plunger, repeat until all granules are used, flush tube with 15 ml water
• **Oral disintegrating tab:** Mix 30 mg tab in 10 ml water give via NG tube, flush tube with 10 ml sterile water and clamp for 60 min

ADVERSE EFFECTS
CNS: Headache, dizziness, confusion, agitation, amnesia, depression
CV: Chest pain, angina, tachycardia, bradycardia, palpitations, **CVA**, hypo/hypertension, **MI, shock,** vasodilatation
EENT: Tinnitus, taste perversion, deafness, eye pain, otitis media
GI: Diarrhea, abdominal pain, vomiting, nausea, constipation, flatulence, acid regurgitation, anorexia, irritable colon, microscopic colitis
GU: **Hematuria,** glycosuria, impotence, kidney calculus, breast enlargement
HEMA: **Hemolysis,** anemia
INTEG: Rash, urticaria, pruritus, alopecia
META: Weight gain/loss, gout
RESP: Upper respiratory infections, cough, epistaxis, asthma, bronchitis, dyspnea, **pneumonia**

Pharmacokinetics

Absorption	Rapid after granules leave stomach
Distribution	Protein binding 97%
Metabolism	Liver extensively
Excretion	Urine, feces; clearance decreased in geriatric, renal/hepatic disease
Half-life	Plasma 1.5 hr

Pharmacodynamics
Unknown

INTERACTIONS
Individual products
Octreotide, misoprostol: decreased lansoprazole effect
Extended release amphetamine/dextroamphetamine: decreased release of extended-release product
Calcium carbonate, iron salts, itraconazole, ketoconazole, atazanavir, ampicillin: decreased absorption of each specific product
Fluvoxamine, voriconazole: increased lansoprazole toxicity
Sucralfate: delayed absorption of lansoprazole
Clopidogrel: decreased antiplatelet effect

Drug/lab test
Increase: AST, ALT, alk phos, creatinine, LDH, gastrin, bilirubin

Drug/herb
• Avoid use with red yeast rice

Drug classifications
Loop/thiazide diuretics: increase hypomagnesemia
Antimuscarinics, H_2 blockers: decrease lansoprazole effect

NURSING CONSIDERATIONS
Assessment
• Assess GI system; bowel sounds q8hr, abdomen for pain, swelling, anorexia, blood in stool, emesis
• Monitor liver enzymes (AST, ALT, alkaline phosphatase) during treatment
• Monitor INR and pro-time when taking warfarin

Nursing diagnoses
• Knowledge, deficient (teaching)
• Pain, chronic (uses)

Patient/family education
• Instruct patient to report severe diarrhea; product may have to be discontinued
• Inform diabetic patient that hypoglycemia may occur
• Encourage patient to avoid hazardous activities; dizziness may occur
• Tell patient to avoid alcohol, salicylates, ibuprofen; may cause GI irritation

Evaluation
Positive therapeutic outcome
• Absence of gastric pain, swelling, fullness

⚠ HIGH ALERT

lapatinib (Rx)

(la-pa'tin-ib)

Tykerb

Func. class.: Antineoplastic—miscellaneous

Chem. class.: Biologic response modifier, signal transduction inhibitor (STIs)

Pregnancy category D

ACTION: Reverses tyrosine kinase of both the epidermal growth factor receptor (ERbB1) and human epidermal receptor type 2 (HER2) (ERbB2)

Therapeutic outcome: Decrease in breast cancer progression

USES: Advanced/metastatic breast cancer patients with tumor that overexpresses HER2 protein and who have received previous chemotherapy; those for whom hormonal therapy is indicated

CONTRAINDICATIONS:

Pregnancy **D**, hypersensitivity, breastfeeding, torsades de pointes

Precautions: Geriatric, cardiac disease, bradycardia, hypertension, hypokalemia, hypomagnesemia, QT prolongation

> **BLACK BOX WARNING:** Hepatic disease

DOSAGE AND ROUTES

Advanced/metastatic breast cancer with HER2 overexpression who have received previous therapy

Adult: PO 1250 mg (5 tabs)/day 1 hr before or after food on days 1-21 plus capecitabine 2000 mg/m^2/day in 2 divided doses on days 1-14 in a repeating 21-day cycle; continue until therapeutic response or toxicity occurs

Metastatic breast cancer with HER2 overexpression for whom hormonal therapy is indicated

Adult: PO 1500 mg (6 tabs) 1 hr before food with letrozole 2.5 q/day

Hepatic dose

Adult (Child-Pugh C): PO 750 mg/day (with capecitabine); 1000 mg/day (with letrozole)

Available forms: Tabs 250 mg

Implementation

- Give once a day with water on an empty stomach, 1 hr before or after food
- Do not use with grapefruit products
- Store at room temperature away from heat

ADVERSE EFFECTS

CNS: Fatigue, insomnia, palmar-plantar erythrodysesthesia (hand/foot syndrome)

CV: Heart failure, palpitations, QT prolongation

GI: Anorexia, diarrhea, dyspepsia, mouth ulcerations, nausea, vomiting, xerosis

HEMA: Anemia, neutropenia, thrombocytopenia

INTEG: Rash

RESP: Dyspnea, pneumonitis

Pharmacokinetics

Absorption	Incomplete
Distribution	Steady state 6-7 days
Metabolism	Liver, extensively, by CYP3A4, CYP3A5; >99% protein bound
Excretion	Unknown
Half-life	Elimination 24 hr; increased in hepatic disease

Pharmacodynamics

Onset	Unknown
Peak	4 hr
Duration	Unknown

INTERACTIONS

Individual drugs

Arsenic trioxide, bepridil, chlorpromazine, chloroquine, grepafloxacin, halofantrine, haloperidol, levomethadyl, mesoridazine, pentamine, probucol, sparfloxacin, thioridazine: increased QT prolongation

Drug classifications

CYP3A4 inhibitors (amiodarone, amprenavir, aprepitant, atazanavir, chloramphenicol, clarithromycin, conivaptan, dalfopristin, danazol, darunavir, delavirdine, diltiazem, efavirenz, erythromycin, estradiol, fluconazole, fluvoxamine, imatinib, indinavir, isoniazid, itraconazole, ketoconazole, miconazole, mifepristone, nefazodone, nelfinavir, propoxyphene, quinupristin, ritonavir, RU-486, saquinavir, telithromycin, troleandomycin, verapamil, voriconazole, zafirlukast): increased effect of lapatinib; avoid concurrent use

CYP3A4 inhibitors (amiodarone, clarithromycin, erythromycin, telithromycin, troleandomycin), class IA, III antidysrhythmics: increased QT prolongation

CYP3A4 substrates (methadone, pimozide, quetiapine, quiNIDine, risperidone, terfenadine, ziprasidone): increased effect of these products, QT prolongation

NURSING CONSIDERATIONS

Assessment

• Assess cardiac status: EEG for QT prolongation, ejection fraction; chest pain, palpitations, dyspnea

• Assess hepatic status: liver function tests; jaundice of sclera, skin; dose should be reduced in hepatic disease

• Assess for skin toxicities NCI CTC grade 2 or greater; discontinue use in those with decreased left ventricular ejection fraction (LVEF) or for LVEF that drops below the institution's lower limit of normal; the product may be restarted after 2 wk if the LVEF recovers to normal at 1000 mg/day; restart at 1250 mg/day when toxicity improves to grade 1 or better

Nursing diagnoses

• Injury, risk for (uses, adverse reactions)
• Knowledge, deficient (teaching)

Patient/family education

• Instruct patient to take with a full glass of water, once a day, 1 hr before or after food; do not take with food or grapefruit products

• Advise patient to take as directed only; if a dose is missed, take as soon as remembered; if it is close to the next dose, take only that dose; do not double

• Teach patient to report to prescriber: chest pain, difficulty breathing, fever, chills, sore throat, bleeding, bruising, yellow skin or eyes, severe fatigue, dizziness, palpitations

• Advise patient of other side effects that can occur but do not need to be reported: nausea, diarrhea, heartburn, mouth sores, rash, numbness/pain in hands/feet

• Advise patient to use adequate contraception because this drug is teratogenic, pregnancy **D**

Evaluation
Positive therapeutic outcome
• Decrease in breast cancer progression

latanoprost ophthalmic
See Appendix B

leflunomide (Rx)
(leh-floo′noh-mide)
Arava
Func. class.: Antirheumatic (DMARDs)
Chem. class.: Immune modulator, pyrimidine synthesis inhibitor
Pregnancy category X

ACTION: Inhibits an enzyme involved in pyrimidine synthesis and has antiproliferative, antiinflammatory effect

Therapeutic outcome: Decreased pain, joint swelling, increased mobility

USES: Rheumatoid arthritis, to reduce disease process as well as symptoms

Unlabeled uses: Juvenile rheumatoid arthritis

CONTRAINDICATIONS:
Breastfeeding, hypersensitivity, jaundice, lactase deficiency, hepatic disease

> **BLACK BOX WARNING:** Pregnancy **X**

Precautions: Children, renal disorders, vaccinations, infection, alcoholism, immunosuppression

DOSAGE AND ROUTES
Adult: PO loading dose 100 mg/day × 3 days, maintenance 20 mg/day; may be decreased to 10 mg/day if not well tolerated

Juvenile rheumatoid arthritis (unlabeled)
Adolescent and child >40 kg: PO 20 mg
Adolescent and child 20-40 kg: PO 15 mg
Adolescent and child 10-19.9 kg: PO 10 mg

Available forms: Tabs 10, 20, 100 mg

Implementation
• Give a loading dose of 100 mg/day × 3 days, then 200 mg/day, decrease to 100 mg/day if poorly tolerated
• Give with full glass of water to enhance absorption
• Give PO with food, milk, or antacids for GI upset
• **Drug elimination:** to eliminate product give cholestyramine 8 g tid × 11 days, check levels

ADVERSE EFFECTS
CNS: Dizziness, insomnia, depression, paresthesia, anxiety, migraine, neuralgia, headache

CV: Palpitations, hypertension, chest pain, angina pectoris, peripheral edema
EENT: Pharyngitis, oral candidiasis, stomatitis, dry mouth, blurred vision
GI: *Nausea, anorexia, vomiting, constipation, flatulence, diarrhea, increased liver function tests,* **hepatotoxicity**
HEMA: Anemia, ecchymosis, hyperlipidemia
INTEG: Rash, pruritus, alopecia, acne, hematoma, herpes infections
RESP: Pharyngitis, rhinitis, bronchitis, cough, respiratory infection, pneumonia, sinusitis, **interstitial lung disease**
SYST: Opportunistic/fatal infections

Pharmacokinetics

Absorption	Unknown
Distribution	Unknown
Metabolism	Liver
Excretion	Kidneys
Half-life	Unknown

Pharmacodynamics
Unknown

INTERACTIONS

Individual drugs
Activated charcoal, cholestyramine: decreased effect of leflunomide
Methotrexate: increased leflunomide side effects
Rifampin: increased rifampin levels

Drug classifications
Hepatotoxic agents: increased side effects of leflunomide
Live virus vaccines: decreased antibody reaction
NSAIDs: increased NSAID effect

NURSING CONSIDERATIONS

Assessment
• Screen for latent TB before starting treatment; if TB is present, treat before using this product
• **Interstitial lung disease:** assess for worsening cough, dyspnea, fever; may need to be discontinued
• Monitor liver function tests: if ALT elevations are >2 times baseline, reduce dosage to 10 mg/day
• Obtain CBC with differential q6mo, then q6-8mo thereafter, pregnancy test, electrolytes
• **Assess arthritic symptoms:** ROM, mobility, swelling of joints, baseline, during treatment
• **Assess for infection:** fatal opportunistic infections can occur

Nursing diagnoses
• Knowledge, deficient (teaching)
• Mobility, impaired physical (uses)
• Pain, chronic (uses)

Patient/family education
• Teach patient that product must be continued for prescribed time to be effective
• Instruct patient to take with food, milk, or antacids to avoid GI upset, take at same time of day
• Advise patient to use caution when driving; drowsiness, dizziness may occur
• Advise patient to take with a full glass of water to enhance absorption
• Advise patient not to become pregnant (**X**) while taking this product
• Inform patient that hair may be lost, review alternatives
• Advise patient to avoid live virus vaccinations during treatment

Evaluation
Positive therapeutic outcome
• Increased joint mobility without pain
• Decreased joint swelling

TREATMENT OF OVERDOSE:
Give cholestyramine tid × 24 hr, or activated charcoal

lenalidomide (Rx)
(len-a-lid'o-mide)
Revlimid
Func. class.: Antianemic, biologic response modifier, hormone
Chem. class.: Thalidomide derivative/TNF modifier
Pregnancy category X

ACTION: Decreases secretion of inflammatory cytokines and increases secretion of antiinflammatory cytokines, also inhibits COX-2

Therapeutic outcome: Increase in reticulocyte count

USES: Transfusion-dependent anemia due to low- or intermediate-1–risk myelodysplastic syndrome (MDS); multiple myeloma in combination with dexamethasone

CONTRAINDICATIONS:
Breastfeeding, hypersensitivity

BLACK BOX WARNING: Pregnancy X, females

Precautions: Accidental exposure, bone marrow suppression, children, dental disease, uterine bleeding, geriatric, fungal/viral infections, smoking

> **BLACK BOX WARNING:** Neutropenia/thrombocytopenia, thromboembolic disease

DOSAGE AND ROUTES

Transfusion-dependent anemia due to low- or intermediate-1–risk MDS associated with a deletion 5q cytogenetic abnormality with or without additional cytogenetic abnormalities

Adult: PO 10 mg/day; continue/adjust based on clinical toxicity/lab findings

Multiple myeloma in combination with dexamethasone in patients who have failed to respond to at least one prior therapy

Adult: PO 25 mg/day on days 1-21 with dexamethasone 40 mg/day PO on days 1-4, 9-12, 17-20 of each 28-day cycle for the first 4 therapy cycles; starting with cycle 5, the lenalidomide dose stays the same, but only give dexamethasone 40 mg/day PO on days 1-4 q28day; continue/adjust dosing based on clinical and laboratory findings

Dosage adjustments for hematologic toxicities associated with MDS

Thrombocytopenia or neutropenia within 4 wk of starting at 10 mg/ day PO: Reduce dose from 10 mg/day PO to 5 mg/day PO; withhold lenalidomide if platelet count $<50,000/mm^3$ from a baseline of at least $100,000/mm^3$, if platelet count falls to 50% of the baseline value, if the baseline is $<100,000/mm^3$, if absolute neutrophil count (ANC) $<750/mm^3$ from a baseline of at least $1000/mm^3$, or if $<500/mm^3$ from a baseline of $<1000/mm^3$; the new dose of 5 mg/day PO may begin once the platelet count is at least $50,000/mm^3$ ($30,000/mm^3$ if the baseline $<60,000/mm^3$), and the ANC returns to at least $1000/mm^3$ or $500/mm^3$ for patients with a baseline $<1000/mm^3$

Thrombocytopenia or neutropenia after 4 wk of starting at 10 mg/day PO: Reduce dose from 10 mg/day PO to 5 mg/day PO; withhold lenalidomide if platelet count $<30,000/mm^3$, if platelet count $<50,000/mm^3$ and a platelet transfusion, if neutrophils $<500/mm^3$ for at least 7 days, or if $<500/mm^3$ and

a temp of at least 38.5° C are present; the new dose of 5 mg/day PO may begin once the platelet count is at least $30,000/mm^3$ without hemostatic failure and the ANC is at least $500/mm^3$

Thrombocytopenia or neutropenia that develops while taking 5 mg/ day PO:

Reduce dose from 5 mg/day PO to 5 mg PO every other day; withhold lenalidomide if platelet count $<30,000/mm^3$, platelet count $<50,000/mm^3$ and a platelet transfusion, neutrophils $<500/mm^3$ for at least 7 days, or if $<500/mm^3$ and a temp of at least 38.5° C are present; the new dose of 5 mg PO every other day may begin once the platelet count is at least $30,000/mm^3$ without hemostatic failure, and the ANC is at least $500/mm^3$

Dosage adjustments for toxicities (multiple myeloma)

Thrombocytopenia: Reduce dose from 25 mg/day PO to 15 mg/day PO; withhold lenalidomide if platelet count $<30,000/mm^3$; check CBC qwk; the new dose of 15 mg/day PO may begin once the platelet count is at least $30,000/mm^3$; withhold lenalidomide each time the platelet count is $<30,000/mm^3$; a new dose of 5 mg less than the previous dose should be started once the platelet count is at least $30,000/mm^3$; do not dose below 5 mg/day PO

Neutropenia without other toxicity: Hold dose; withhold lenalidomide and add G-CSF if neutrophils $<1000/mm^3$; check CBC weekly; resume lenalidomide at 25 mg/day PO once neutrophils are at least $1000/mm^3$, and neutropenia is the only toxicity

Neutropenia with other toxicity: Reduce dose from 25 mg/day PO to 15 mg/day PO; withhold lenalidomide and add G-CSF if neutrophils $<1000/mm^3$; check CBC qwk; resume lenalidomide at 15 mg/day PO once neutrophils are at least $1000/mm^3$; withhold lenalidomide and add G-CSF each time the neutrophils are $<1000/mm^3$; if other toxicity is present, a new dose of 5 mg less than the previous dose should be started once the neutrophils are at least $1000/mm^3$; do not dose below 5 mg/day PO

Other grade 3 or 4 toxicity related to lenalidomide: Reduce dosage from 25 mg/day PO to 15 mg/day PO; withhold lenalidomide and resume lenalidomide at 15 mg/day PO once the toxicity has resolved to grade 2 or less; withhold lenalidomide each time a grade 3 or 4 toxicity occurs; a new dose of 5 mg less than the previous dose should be started once the toxicity has resolved to grade 2 or less; do not dose below 5 mg/day PO

Renal dose

Adult: PO CCr 30-59 ml/min, 5 mg q24hr (MDS), 10 mg q24hr (multiple myeloma); CCr <30 ml/min (not requiring dialysis), 5 mg q48hr (MDS), 15 mg q48hr (multiple myeloma)

Available forms: Caps 5, 10, 15, 25 mg

Implementation

• Give PO, with dexamethasone for multiple myeloma
• Do not crush or open caps
• All persons involved must comply with the condition of rev assist program

ADVERSE EFFECTS

CNS: Depression, dizziness, fatigue, fever, headache, sweating, peripheral enuropathy
CV: Chest pain, hypotension, palpitations
GI: Abdominal pain, anorexia, constipation, diarrhea, nausea/vomiting, dysgeusia, xerosis
HEMA: Anemia, leukopenia, pancytopenia, thrombocytopenia, neutropenia
META: Hypokalemia, hypomagnesemia
MS: Arthralgia, back pain, myalgia
RESP: Cough, dyspnea, **pulmonary embolism**, epistaxis, rhinitis
SYST: Angioedema, secondary malignancy

Pharmacokinetics

Absorption	Rapid
Distribution	Unknown
Metabolism	Unknown
Excretion	Unknown
Half-life	Elimination 3 hr

Pharmacodynamics

Unknown

INTERACTIONS

Drug classifications

Anticoagulants, NSAIDs, platelet inhibitors, salicylates, thrombolytics: increased bleeding risk
Toxoids, vaccines: decreased immune response

NURSING CONSIDERATIONS

Assessment

> **BLACK BOX WARNING:** Monitor blood tests: HCT, Hgb, electrolytes

• Monitor B/P for hypotension
• Assess blood dyscrasias

> **BLACK BOX WARNING:** Assess for hypersensitivity reactions: skin rashes, urticaria (rare)

> **BLACK BOX WARNING:** Assess for pregnancy before use, pregnancy **X**

Nursing diagnoses

• Activity intolerance (uses)
• Knowledge, deficient (teaching)

Patient/family education

• Advise patient to avoid driving or hazardous activity during beginning of treatment

Evaluation

Positive therapeutic outcome
• Increase in reticulocyte count

⚠ HIGH ALERT

lepirudin (Rx)

(lep-ih-roo′din)
Refludan
Func. class.: Anticoagulant
Chem. class.: Thrombin inhibitor, hirudin
Pregnancy category B

ACTION: Direct inhibitor of thrombin that is highly specific

Therapeutic outcome: Absence of thrombocytopenia, stroke, MI, or other thromboembolic conditions

USES: Anticoagulation in those with heparin-induced thrombocytopenia (HIT) and other thromboembolic conditions

Unlabeled uses: Adjunct therapy in unstable angina, acute MI without ST elevation, prevention of DVT, PCI

CONTRAINDICATIONS: Hypersensitivity to hirudins

Precautions: Pregnancy **B,** breastfeeding, children, women, geriatric, intracranial bleeding, hepatic disease, recent major surgery, hemorrhagic diathesis, bacterial endocarditis, severe uncontrolled hypertension, advanced renal disease, recent active peptic ulcer, recent CVA, stroke, intracerebral surgery

---

DOSAGE AND ROUTES

Heparin-induced thrombocytopenia (not receiving concurrent thrombolytic therapy)
Adult: IV BOL 0.4 mg/kg over 15-20 sec; then 0.15 mg/kg as a CONT INF for 2-10 days or longer

Concomitant use with thrombolytic therapy
Adult: IV BOL 0.2 mg/kg initially, then CONT IV INF 0.1 mg/kg/hr

Renal dose
Adult: IV BOL 0.2 mg/kg over 15-20 sec; CCr 45-60 ml/min 0.075 mg/kg/hr; CCr 30-44 ml/min 0.045 mg/kg/hr; CCr 15-29 ml/min 0.0225 mg/kg/hr

Available forms: Powder for inj 50 mg

Implementation
• Administer after reconstitution and further dilution under sterile conditions; use water for inj or 0.9% NaCl; for further dilution 0.9% NaCl or D₅; for rapid and complete reconstitution, inject 1 ml of diluent into vial and shake gently, use immediately, warm to room temperature before use
• Avoid all IM inj that may cause bleeding

Direct IV route
• Use sol with conc of 5 mg/ml, reconstitute 5 mg (1 vial)/1 ml of water for inj or 0.9% NaCl, use body weight for correct weight calculation, shake gently; transfer contents of vial into a 10-ml syringe and dilute to a volume of 10 ml with sterile water for inj D₅W, or 0.9% NaCl

Continuous IV infusion route
• Use sol with a conc of 0.2 or 0.4 mg/ml; reconstitute 100 mg (2 vials) with 1 ml each (2 ml) water for inj or 0.9% NaCl, transfer to inf bag with either 500 or 250 ml of 0.9% NaCl or D₅W

Y-site compatibilities: Amiodarone

ADVERSE EFFECTS
CNS: *Fever*, **intracranial bleeding**
CV: **Heart failure, pericardial effusion, ventricular fibrillation**
GI: GI bleeding, abnormal LFTs
GU: **Hematuria**, abnormal kidney function, vaginal bleeding
HEMA: **Hemorrhage, thrombocytopenia, anemia**
INTEG: Allergic skin reactions
RESP: Pneumonia, stridor, dyspnea, **bronchospasm**

SYST: **Multiorgan failure, sepsis, anaphylaxis**

Pharmacokinetics
Absorption	Unknown
Distribution	Distributed to extracellular fluids
Metabolism	By the release of amino acids during catabolism
Excretion	50% unchanged in urine
Half-life	Unknown

Pharmacodynamics
Unknown

INTERACTIONS
Individual drugs
Aspirin, cefamandole, cefoperazone, cefotetan, clopidogrel, dipyridamole, eptifibatide, plicamycin, ticlopidine, tirofiban, valproic acid: increased bleeding risk

Drug classifications
NSAIDs, thrombolytics, warfarin derivatives: increased bleeding risk

NURSING CONSIDERATIONS
Assessment
• **Anticoagulation:** obtain baseline aPTT before treatment: do not start treatment if aPTT ratio is ≥2.5; then aPTT 4 hr after initiation of treatment and at least daily thereafter; if aPTT is above target, stop infusion for 2 hr, then restart at 50%, take aPTT in 4 hr; if below target, increase inf rate by 20%, take aPTT in 4 hr, max inf rate 0.21 mg/kg/hr without checking for coagulation abnormalities
• Monitor aPTT, which should be 1.5-2.5 × control
⚠ **Bleeding/hemorrhage: Assess bleeding gums, petechiae, ecchymosis, black tarry stools, hematuria/epistaxis, B/P, vaginal bleeding, puncture sites; may indicate bleeding and possible hemorrhage**
• Assess fever, skin rash, urticaria
• Monitor Hgb, Hct, platelets, serum creatinine, urinalysis, stool guaiac

Nursing diagnoses
• Injury, risk for (side effects)
• Knowledge, deficient (teaching)

Patient/family education
• Teach patient to use soft-bristle toothbrush to prevent bleeding gums, avoid contact sports, use electric razor, avoid IM inj
• Teach patient to report any signs of bleeding: gums, under skin, urine, stools

Evaluation
Positive therapeutic outcome
• Anticoagulation, aPTT 1.5-2.5, absence of bleeding

letrozole (Rx)
(let'tro-zohl)
Femara
Func. class.: Antineoplastic, nonsteroidal aromatase inhibitor
Pregnancy category D

ACTION: Binds to the heme group of aromatase; inhibits conversion of androgens to estrogens to reduce plasma estrogen levels

Therapeutic outcome: Decreased spread of malignancy

USES: Early, advanced, or metastatic breast cancer in postmenopausal women

CONTRAINDICATIONS:
Pregnancy **D**, hypersensitivity, premenopausal females

Precautions: Hepatic disease, respiratory disease, osteoporosis

DOSAGE AND ROUTES
Adult: PO 2.5 mg/day

Available forms: Tabs 2.5 mg

Implementation
• May administer bisphosphates to increase bone density
• Give with food or fluids for GI upset
• Give in equal intervals q6hr

ADVERSE EFFECTS
CNS: Somnolence, dizziness, depression, anxiety, *headache, lethargy*
CV: Angina, **MI, CVA, thromboembolic events,** peripheral edema, hypertension
GI: *Nausea, vomiting, anorexia,* constipation, heartburn, diarrhea
GU: Endometrial cancer, vaginal bleeding, endometrial proliferation disorder
INTEG: *Rash, pruritus,* alopecia, sweating
MISC: Hot flashes, night sweats, **second malignancies, anaphylaxis, angioedema**
MS: Arthralgia, arthritis, bone fracture, myalgia, osteoporosis
RESP: Dyspnea, cough

Pharmacokinetics
Absorption	Well absorbed
Distribution	Widely distributed, steady state 2-6 wk
Metabolism	Liver
Excretion	Kidneys
Half-life	Terminal 48 hr

Pharmacodynamics
Onset	Unknown
Peak	2 days
Duration	Unknown

INTERACTIONS
Drug classifications
Estrogens, oral contraceptives: decreased letrozole effect

NURSING CONSIDERATIONS
Assessment
• Monitor temperature q4hr; may indicate beginning of infection
• Monitor LFTs before, during therapy (bilirubin, AST, ALT, LDH) as needed or monthly

Nursing diagnoses
• Body image, disturbed (adverse reactions)
• Infection, risk for (adverse reactions)
• Injury, risk for (adverse reactions)
• Knowledge, deficient (teaching)

Patient/family education
• Advise patient to avoid use of alcohol, which potentiates this product
• Tell patient that product may be taken without regard to meals
• Teach patient to report vaginal bleeding, diarrhea, chest/bone pain
• Advise patient to use adequate contraception in perimenopausal, recently menopausal women, pregnancy **D**

Evaluation
Positive therapeutic outcome
• Prevention of rapid division of malignant cells, postmenopausal cancer, prostate cancer

TREATMENT OF OVERDOSE:
Induce vomiting, provide supportive care

leucovorin (Rx)

(loo-koe-vor'in)
Func. class.: Vitamin/folic acid antagonist antidote
Chem. class.: Tetrahydrofolic acid derivative
Pregnancy category C

Do not confuse:
leucovorin/Leukeran/Leukine,
folinic acid/folic acid

ACTION: Needed for normal growth patterns; prevents toxicity during antineoplastic therapy by protecting normal cells

Therapeutic outcome: Reversal of severe toxic effects of folic acid antagonists

USES: Megaloblastic or macrocytic anemia caused by folic acid deficiency, overdose of folic acid antagonist, methotrexate toxicity, toxicity caused by pyrimethamine/trimethoprim/trimetrexate, pneumocystosis, toxoplasmosis

CONTRAINDICATIONS:
Hypersensitivity to this product or folic acid, benzyl alcohol, anemias other than megaloblastic not associated with vit B_{12} deficiency

Precautions: Pregnancy **C**, seizures, geriatric, neonates, stomatitis, vomiting, breastfeeding

DOSAGE AND ROUTES

Megaloblastic anemia caused by enzyme deficiency
Adult and child: PO/IM/IV up to 6 mg/day

Megaloblastic anemia caused by deficiency of folate
Adult and child: IM 1 mg or less/day until adequate response

Advanced colorectal cancer
Adult: IV 200 mg/m², then 5-fluorouracil 370 mg/m²; or leucovorin 20 mg/m², then 5-fluorouracil 425 mg/m²; give daily × 5 days q4-5wk

Methotrexate toxicity—leucovorin rescue
Adult and child: PO/IM/IV **(normal elimination)** given 6 hr after dose of methotrexate 10 mg/m² until methotrexate is <5 × 10⁻⁸ m, CCr has increased 50% above prior level, or methotrexate level is 5 × 10⁻⁸ m at 24 hr or at 48 hr level is >9 × 10⁻⁸ m; give leucovorin 100 mg/m² q3hr until level drops to <10⁻⁸ m

Pyrimethamine/trimethoprim toxicity
Adult and child: PO/IM 5-15 mg/day

Available forms: Tabs 5, 10, 15, 25 mg; inj 3, 5 mg/ml; powder for inj 10 mg/ml

Implementation
• Instruct patient about leucovorin rescue; have patient drink 3 L of fluid each day of rescue
• Do not give concurrently with systemic methotrexate

PO route
• Use PO route only if patient is not vomiting
• Within 1 hr of folic acid antagonist, do not give concurrently with systemic methotrexate

IM route
• Treatment of megaloblastic anemia uses IM dosing
• Give within 1 hr of folic acid antagonist, no reconstitution needed
• Give increased fluid intake if used to treat folic acid inhibitor overdose
• Provide protection from light and heat when storing ampules

IV route
• Reconstitute 50 mg/5 ml of bacteriostatic water or sterile water for inj (10 mg/ml) or 100 mg/10 ml; use immediately if sterile water for inj is used to reconstitute

Direct IV route
• Give over 160 mg/min or less (16 ml of 10 mg/ml sol/min)

Intermittent IV infusion route
• Give after diluting in 100-500 ml of 0.9% NaCl, D₅W, D₁₀W, LR, Ringer's

Syringe compatibilities: Bleomycin, CISplatin, cyclophosphamide, DOXOrubicin, fluorouracil, furosemide, heparin, methotrexate, metoclopramide, mitomycin, vinBLAStine, vinCRIStine

Y-site compatibilities: Amifostine, aztreonam, bleomycin, cefepime, CISplatin, cladribine, cyclophosphamide, DOXOrubicin, filgrastim, fluconazole, fluorouracil, furosemide, granisetron, heparin, methotrexate, metoclopramide, mitomycin, piperacillin/tazobactam, tacrolimus, teniposide, thiotepa, vinBLAStine, vinCRIStine

Additive compatibilities: CISplatin, CISplatin/floxuridine, floxuridine

ADVERSE EFFECTS
HEMA: Thrombocytosis (intraarterial)
INTEG: Rash, pruritus, erythema, urticaria
RESP: Wheezing

Pharmacokinetics

Absorption	Rapidly absorbed (PO); completely absorbed (**IV**)
Distribution	Widely distributed
Metabolism	Liver
Excretion	Kidney
Half-life	$3^1/_2$ hr

Pharmacodynamics

	PO/IM/IV
Onset	Up to 5 min
Peak	Unknown
Duration	4-6 hr

INTERACTIONS

Individual drugs

Sulfamethoxazole-trimethoprim: decreased effect

Capecitabine, floxuridine, fluorouracil: increased toxicity

Drug classifications

Barbiturates: increased metabolism of barbiturates

Hydantoins: increased metabolism of hydantoins

NURSING CONSIDERATIONS

Assessment

• Obtain CCr before leucovorin rescue and daily to detect nephrotoxicity, methotrexate level
• Monitor I&O, urine pH q6hr; maintain at >7 to prevent neurotoxicity; watch for nausea and vomiting; if vomiting occurs IM or **IV** route may be necessary
• Assess products currently taken: alcohol, hydantoins, trimethoprim may cause increased folic acid use by body
• Assess for allergic reactions: rash, dyspnea, wheezing
• Assess neurologic status (rescue), weakness, fatigue
• Monitor calcium levels
• Assess for megaloblastic anemia, plasma lactic acid, reticulocyte count, Hct, Hgb

Nursing diagnoses

• Injury, risk for (uses)
• Knowledge, deficient (teaching)
• Nutrition: less than body requirements, imbalanced (uses)

Patient/family education

• **For leucovorin rescue:** Drink 3 L fluid day of rescue

• Advise patient to take product exactly as prescribed; to notify prescriber of side effects immediately
• Advise patient to report signs of hypersensitivity reaction immediately
• **Advise patient with folic acid deficiency** to eat folic acid–rich foods: bran, yeast, dried beans, nuts, fruits, fresh green leafy vegetables, asparagus
• Advise patient to avoid breastfeeding

Evaluation

Positive therapeutic outcome
• Increased weight
• Improved orientation, well-being
• Absence of fatigue
• Reversal of toxicity: methotrexate, folic acid antagonist overdose

---

⚠ HIGH ALERT

leuprolide (Rx)

(loo-proe'lide)

Eligard, Lupron Depo, Viadur
Func. class.: Antineoplastic hormone
Chem. class.: Gonadotropin-releasing hormone
Pregnancy category X

Do not confuse:
Lupron/Lopurin/Nuprin

ACTION: Causes initial increase in circulating levels of LH, FSH; continuous administration results in decreased LH, FSH; in men testosterone is reduced to castration levels; in premenopausal women estrogen is reduced to menopausal levels

Therapeutic outcome: Prevention of rapidly growing malignant cells in prostate cancer, decreased pain in endometriosis, resolution of central precocious puberty (CPP)

USES: Metastatic prostate cancer (inj implant), management of endometriosis (depot), CPP, uterine leiomyomata (fibroids)

CONTRAINDICATIONS:
Pregnancy **X,** breastfeeding, hypersensitivity to GnRH or analogs, thromboembolic disorders, undiagnosed vaginal bleeding; Viadur implant or Eligard should not be used in women or children

Precautions: Edema, hepatic disease, CVA, MI, seizures, hypertension, diabetes mellitus,

---

⚠ Nurse Alert

CHF, depression, osteoporosis, spinal cord compression, urinary tract obstruction

DOSAGE AND ROUTES

Prostate cancer
Adult: SUBCUT 1 mg/day; IM 7.5 mg/dose qmo; Viadur implant (72 mg) qyr; or IM 22.5 mg q3mo; or IM 30 mg q4mo; or IM 45 mg q6mo

Endometriosis/fibroids
Adult: IM 3.75 mg qmo for 6 mo, 11.25 mg q3mo for 6 mo, or IM 30 mg q4mo

Central precocious puberty
Child: SUBCUT 50 mcg/kg/day; increase as needed by 10 mcg/kg/day
Child >37.5 kg: IM 15 mg q4wk
Child 25-37.5 kg: IM 11.25 mg q4wk
Child ≤25 kg: 7.5 mg q4wk

Available forms: Powder for inj depot 1 mo 3.75 mg, depot 3 mo/1.25 mg, 22.5 mg; depot 4 mo 30 mg; depot-ped 7.5, 11.25, 15 mg; sol for inj 1 mg/0.2 ml; susp for inj 7.5, 22.5, 30, 45 mg; implant (Viadur) 65 mg

Implementation
• Use depot only IM; never give SUBCUT
• Unused vials may be stored at room temperature

Subcut route
• No dilution needed; if patient is self-administering make sure patient uses syringes provided by manufacturer
• **Viadur Duros implant:** Insert in inner aspect of arm, remove after 12 mo
• **Eligard subcut:** Bring to room temp, once mixed give within 30 min; prepare the 2 syringes for mixing, join the 2 syringes by pushing in and twisting until secure; mix the product by pushing the contents of both syringes back and forth between syringes until uniform, should be light tan to tan; hold syringes vertically with syringe B on the bottom, draw entire mixed product into syringe B (short, wide syringe) by depressing the syringe A plunger and slightly withdrawing syringe B plunger, uncouple syringe A while pushing down on syringe A plunger, small air bubbles will remain; hold syringe B upright, remove pink cap, attach needle cartridge to the end of syringe B, remove needle cover, give by subcut route

IM route
• **Give monthly:** reconstitute single-use vial with 1 ml of diluent; if multiple vials are used, withdraw 0.5 ml and inject into each vial (1 ml), withdraw all and inject

• **Give 3 month:** reconstitute microspheres using 1.5 ml of diluent and inject in vial, shake, withdraw and inject
• **12-month:** inserted into upper arm; at the end of 12 months, implant must be removed
• Use syringe and product packaged together; give deep in large muscle mass; rotate sites

ADVERSE EFFECTS
CNS: Memory impairment, depression, **seizures**
CV: MI, pulmonary emboli, dysrhythmias, peripheral edema
GI: Anorexia, diarrhea, **GI bleeding,** nausea, vomiting
GU: Edema, hot flashes, impotence, decreased libido, amenorrhea, vaginal dryness, gynecomastia, **profuse vaginal bleeding**
INTEG: Alopecia
MS: Bone pain
Prostate cancer: increased bone pain for the first 4 wk of treatment, those with metastases in spinal column might have severe back pain

Pharmacokinetics
Absorption	Rapidly absorbed (SUBCUT); slowly absorbed (IM depot)
Distribution	Unknown
Metabolism	Unknown
Excretion	Unknown
Half-life	3-4 hr

Pharmacodynamics
Unknown

INTERACTIONS

Individual drugs
Flutamide, megestrol: increased antineoplastic action

NURSING CONSIDERATIONS

Assessment
• **Assess for symptoms of endometriosis/ fibroids** including lower abdominal pain, excessive vaginal bleeding, bloating if product is given for the diagnosis of endometriosis
• **For central precocious puberty (CPP):** the diagnosis should have been confirmed by development of secondary sex characteristics in children <9 yr; also included to confirm the diagnosis of CPP is estradiol/testosterone, GnRH test, tomography of head, adrenal steroid, chorionic gonadotropin, wrist x-ray, height, weight; patients with CPP display the signs of testicular

growth, facial, body hair (boys), breast development, menses (girls)
• Monitor liver function tests before, during therapy (bilirubin, AST, ALT, LDH) as needed or monthly; prostate-specific antigen in prostate cancer; calcium, testosterone, bone mineral density, blood glucose, HbA1c
• Monitor pituitary gonadotropic and gonadal function during therapy and 4-8 wk after therapy is decreased; check LH, FSH, acid phosphate at beginning of treatment
• **Tumor flare:** monitor worsening of signs and symptoms (normal during beginning therapy): fatigue, increased pulse, pallor, lethargy, edema in feet, joints, stomach pain, shaking
• Monitor renal status: I&O ratio, check for bladder distention daily during beginning therapy (renal obstruction)
• **Severe allergic reaction:** rash, pruritus, urticaria, purpuric skin lesions, itching, flushing

Nursing diagnoses
• Injury, risk for (adverse reactions)
• Knowledge, deficient (teaching)
• Sexual dysfunction (adverse reactions)

Patient/family education
• Advise patient to notify prescriber if menstruation continues (menstruation should stop); to use a nonhormonal method of contraception during therapy
• Instruct patient to report any complaints, side effects to nurse or prescriber; hot flashes may occur; record weight, report gain of 2 lb/day
• Teach patient how to prepare, administer; to rotate sites for SUBCUT inj; to keep accurate records of dosing (prostate cancer)
• Instruct patient that tumor flare may occur: increase in size of tumor, increased bone pain; tell patient that bone pain disappears after 1 wk; may take analgesics for pain; premenopausal women must use mechanical birth control; ovulation may be induced
• Advise the patient not to breastfeed while taking this product
• Inform patient that voiding problems may increase in beginning of therapy, but will decrease in several weeks

Evaluation
Positive therapeutic outcome
• Decreased size, spread of malignancy
• Decreased pain in endometriosis, fibroids
• Decreased signs of CPP
• Increased follicle maturation

levalbuterol (Rx)
(lev-al-bute′er-ole)
Xopenex, Xopenex HFA
Func. class.: Bronchodilator
Chem. class.: Adrenergic β_2-agonist
Pregnancy category C

ACTION: Causes bronchodilatation by action on β_2 (pulmonary) receptors by increasing levels of cyclic adenosine monophosphate (AMP), which relaxes smooth muscle; produces bronchodilatation; CNS, cardiac stimulation, increased diuresis, and increased gastric acid secretion

Therapeutic outcome: Increased ability to breathe because of bronchodilatation

USES: Treatment or prevention of bronchospasm (reversible obstructive airway disease)

CONTRAINDICATIONS:
Hypersensitivity to sympathomimetics, this product, or albuterol

Precautions: Pregnancy C, breastfeeding, hyperthyroidism, diabetes mellitus, hypertension, prostatic hypertrophy, closed-angle glaucoma, seizures, renal disease, QT prolongation, tachydysrhythmias, severe cardiac disease, hypokalemia

DOSAGE AND ROUTES
Adult and child ≥12 yr: INH 0.63 mg tid, q6-8hr by nebulization; may increase to 1.25 mg q8hr
Adult/adolescent/child >4 yr: (HFA, metered dose) 90 mcg (2 INH) q4-6hr
Child 6-11 yr: INH 0.31 mg tid via nebulization, max 0.63 mg tid

Available forms: Inh pediatric 0.31 mg/3 ml; sol 0.63, 1.25 mg/3 ml; 45 mcg per actuation (HFA)

Implementation
• Give by nebulization q6-8hr; wait at least 1 min between inhalation of aerosols
• Use this medication before other medications and allow 5 min between each to prevent overstimulation

ADVERSE EFFECTS
CNS: *Tremors, anxiety,* insomnia, headache, dizziness, stimulation, *restlessness,* weakness, irritability
CV: Palpitations, tachycardia, hypertension, angina, hypotension, dysrhythmias, **QT prolongation**

EENT: Dry nose, irritation of nose and throat
GI: Heartburn, nausea, vomiting, diarrhea, rhinitis
INTEG: Rash
META: Hypokalemia, hyperglycemia
MS: Muscle cramps
RESP: Cough
SYST: Anaphylaxis, angioedema

Pharmacokinetics

Absorption	Unknown
Distribution	Unknown
Metabolism	Liver extensively, tissues
Excretion	Unknown, breast milk
Half-life	Unknown

Pharmacodynamics

	INH SOL	INH AEROSOL
Onset	5-15 min	4.5-10.2 min
Peak	1½ hr	76-78 min
Duration	5-6 hr	6 hr

INTERACTIONS

Individual drugs
Haloperidol, chloroquine, droperidol, pentamidine, arsenic trioxide, levomethadyl: increased QT prolongation

Drug classifications
Adrenergics: increased levalbuterol action
β-Adrenergic blockers: decreased levabuterol action
Bronchodilators (aerosol): increased action of bronchodilator
Class IA/III antidysrhythmics, some phenothiazines, beta agonists, local anesthetics, tricyclics, CYP3A4 inhibitors (amiodarone, clarithromycin, erythromycin, telithromycin, troleandomycin), CYP3A4 substrates (methadone, pimozide, quetiapine, quiNIDine, risperidone, ziprasidone): increased QT prolongation
MAOIs: increased levalbuterol action

Drug/herb
Cola nut, guarana, tea (black/green), coffee, yerba maté: increased stimulation

NURSING CONSIDERATIONS

Assessment
• Assess cardiac status: palpitations, increased or decreased B/P, dysrhythmias
• **QT prolongation:** Monitor ECG for QT prolongation, ejection fraction; assess for chest pain, palpitations, dyspnea

• **Assess respiratory function:** vital capacity, forced expiratory volume, ABGs, lung sounds, heart rate, rhythm (baseline, during therapy); character of sputum: color, consistency, amount
• Determine that patient has not received theophylline therapy before giving dose, to prevent additive effect; client's ability to self-medicate
• **Monitor for evidence of allergic reactions;** paradoxic bronchospasm, anaphylaxis, angioedema; withhold dose; notify prescriber

Nursing diagnoses
• Gas exchange, impaired (uses)
• Knowledge, deficient (teaching)

Patient/family education
• Tell patient not to use OTC medications before consulting prescriber; extra stimulation may occur; instruct patient to use this medication before other medications and allow at least 5 min between each to prevent overstimulation; to limit caffeine products such as chocolate, coffee, tea, and cola or herbs such as cola nut, guarana, yerba maté
⚠ Teach patient that if paradoxical bronchospasm occurs to stop product immediately and notify prescriber
• Teach patient to use this product first, if using other inhalers, wait 5 min or more between products; rinse mouth with water after each dose to prevent dry mouth

Evaluation
Positive therapeutic outcome
• Absence of dyspnea and wheezing after 1 hr
• Improved airway exchange
• Improved ABGs

TREATMENT OF OVERDOSE:
Administer a β₁-adrenergic blocker

---

levetiracetam (Rx)
(lev-ee-tye′ra-see-tam)
Keppra, Keppra XR
Func. class.: Anticonvulsant
Pregnancy category C

ACTION: Unknown; may inhibit nerve impulses by limiting influx of sodium ions across cell membrane in motor cortex

Therapeutic outcome: Absence of seizures

USES: Adjunctive therapy in partial-onset seizures, primary generalized tonic-clonic seizures

Adverse effects: *italics* = common; **bold** = life-threatening

CONTRAINDICATIONS:
Hypersensitivity, breastfeeding

Precautions: Pregnancy **C**, children, geriatric, cardiac/renal disease, psychosis

DOSAGE AND ROUTES
Adjunctive treatment of partial seizures
Adult and adolescent ≥16 yr: **IV** 500 mg bid, may titrate by 1000 mg/day q2wk; max 3000 mg/day in divided doses; EXT REL 1000 mg/day, may increase q2wk, max 3000 mg/day
Adolescent <16 yr/child/infant: PO 10 mg/kg bid, increase the daily dose q2wk, by 20 mg/kg to 30 mg/kg bid; if unable to tolerate, may reduce dose

Myoclonic seizures/tonic-clonic seizures/partial seizures
Adult and adolescent >16 yr: PO/IV 500 mg bid, may increase by 1000 mg/day q2wk; max 3000 mg/day

Renal dose
Adult: PO CCr 50-80 ml/min, 500-1000 mg q12hr, EXT REL 1000-2000 q24hr, max 2000 mg/day; CCr 30-49 ml/min, 250-750 mg q12hr, EXT REL 500-1500 mg q24hr, max 1500 mg/day; CCr <30 ml/min 250-500 mg q12hr, EXT REL 500-1000 mg q24hr, max 1000 mg/day

Available forms: Tabs 250, 500, 750, 1000; oral sol 100 mg/ml; SOL for inj 100 mg/ml, ext rel tab 500, 750 mg

Implementation
PO route
• Give with food, milk to decrease GI symptoms (rare)
• **Child <20 kg:** give oral sol, use calibrated device
• Store at room temperature (PO); diluted preparation stable for 24 hr at room temperature in polyvinyl bags

Intermittent IV route
• Single-use vials: dilute in 100 mg of 0.9% NaCl, D₅, LR; give over 15 min, discard unused vial contents, do not use product with particulates or discoloration

Additive compatibilities: diazepam, LORazepam, valproate

ADVERSE EFFECTS
CNS: Dizziness, somnolence, asthenia, psychosis, **suicidal ideation**
HEMA: Decreased Hct, Hgb, RBC, infection
MISC: Abdominal pain, pharyngitis, infection

Pharmacokinetics
Absorption	Rapidly absorbed
Distribution	Widely distributed, not protein bound
Metabolism	Liver, small amount
Excretion	Kidneys, 66% unchanged
Half-life	6-8 hr, longer in renal disease/geriatric

Pharmacodynamics
Unknown

INTERACTIONS
Individual drugs
Alcohol: avoid using
CarBAMazepine: increased carBAMazepine toxicity
Sevelamer: decreased levetiracetam absorption; separate by 1 hr before, 3 hr after sevelamer

NURSING CONSIDERATIONS
Assessment
• Monitor urine function tests (BUN, urine protein) periodically during treatments
⚠ **Assess seizure activity including type, location, duration, and character; provide seizure precautions**
• Assess blood studies: RBC, Hct, Hgb
⚠ **Assess mental status: mood, sensorium, affect, behavioral changes, suicidal thoughts/behaviors**

Nursing diagnoses
• Injury, risk for (side effects)
• Knowledge, deficient (teaching)

Patient/family education
• Teach patient to carry/wear emergency ID stating patient's name, products taken, condition, prescriber's name, phone number
• Caution patient to avoid driving, other activities that require alertness until stabilized on medication
• Teach patient not to discontinue medication quickly after long-term use
• Teach patient to use a nonhormonal type of contraception to prevent harm to the fetus
• Teach patient to take exactly as prescribed, do not double or omit doses
• Advise not to breastfeed, excreted in breast milk

Evaluation
Positive therapeutic outcome
• Decreased seizure activity

⚠ Nurse Alert

levobetaxolol ophthalmic
See Appendix B

levobunolol ophthalmic
See Appendix B

levocabastine ophthalmic
See Appendix B

levocetirizine (Rx)
(lee-voh-she-teer'ah-zeen)
Xyzal
Func. class.: Antihistamine, low sedating
Chem. class.: H$_1$-histamine blocker
Pregnancy category B

ACTION: Acts on blood vessels, GI, respiratory system by competing with histamine for H$_1$-receptor site; decreases allergic response by blocking pharmacologic effects of histamine; minimal anticholinergic action

Therapeutic outcome: Absence of running or congested nose or rashes

USES: Perennial or seasonal rhinitis, allergy symptoms, chronic idiopathic urticaria

CONTRAINDICATIONS:
Breastfeeding; end-stage renal disease; dialysis; child 6-11 yr with renal disease; hypersensitivity to this product, cetrizine, hydroxyzine

Precautions: Pregnancy **B,** driving, renal disease

DOSAGE AND ROUTES
Adult and child ≥12 yr: PO 2.5-5 mg/day in the evening
Child 6-11 yr: PO (oral SOL) 2.5 mg/day in the evening
Child 2-5 yr: PO (oral SOL) 1.25 mg/day in the evening
Geriatric: PO 2.5-5 mg/day in the evening

Renal dose
Adult: PO CCr 50-80 ml/min 2.5 mg/day; CCr 30-50 ml/min 2.5 mg every other day; CCr 10-30 ml/min 2.5 mg 2 ×/wk; CCr <10 ml/min, do not use

Available forms: Tabs 5 mg; oral sol 2.5 mg/5 ml

Implementation
• Give without regard to meals in the evening; tabs are scored and may be broken in half
• Store in tight, light-resistant container

ADVERSE EFFECTS
CNS: *Drowsiness, fatigue,* asthenia, dizziness, depression, **seizures, suicidal ideation,** insomnia, hallucinations, orofacial dyskinesia (rare)
CV: Hypotension, palpitations, sinus tachycardia
GI: Dry mouth, increased liver function tests, **hepatitis**
HEMA: Hemolytic anemia, thrombocytopenia (rare)
INTEG: Rash, transient, **anaphylaxis, angioedema,** fixed drug eruption, pruritus
RESP: Pneumonia, cough
OTHER: Stillbirth (rare)

Pharmacokinetics

Absorption	Rapid
Distribution	Unknown
Metabolism	Protein binding 91%-92%
Excretion	Urine 85.4%, feces 12.9%
Half-life	8 hr

Pharmacodynamics

Onset	Unknown
Peak	0.9 hr
Duration	Unknown

INTERACTIONS
Individual drugs
Alcohol: increased CNS depression
Ritonavir: increased half-life; decreased clearance of levocetirizine

Drug classifications
MAOIs, phenothiazines, tricyclics: increased anticholinergic/sedative effect
Other CNS depressants: increased CNS depression

Drug/lab test
False negative: skin allergy tests

NURSING CONSIDERATIONS
Assessment
• Allergy symptoms: pruritus, urticaria, watering eyes, baseline, during treatment
• Respiratory status: rate, rhythm, increase in bronchial secretions, wheezing, chest tightness
• Liver function tests, serum creatinine, BUN

Nursing diagnoses
• Knowledge, deficient (teaching)
• Noncompliance (teaching)

L

Patient/family education
• Teach patient all aspects of product use; to notify prescriber if confusion, sedation, hypotension occur
• Advise patient to avoid driving, other hazardous activities if drowsiness occurs
• Advise patient to avoid alcohol, other CNS depressants
• Inform patient that product is not recommended during breastfeeding

Evaluation
Positive therapeutic outcome
• Absence of running or congested nose or rashes

TREATMENT OF OVERDOSE:
Administer diazepam, vasopressors, IV phenytoin

levofloxacin (Rx)
(lev-o-floks′a-sin)
Levaquin
Func. class.: Antiinfective
Chem. class.: Fluoroquinolone antibacterial
Pregnancy category C

ACTION: Interferes with conversion of intermediate DNA fragments into high molecular weight DNA in bacteria; DNA gyrase inhibitor; inhibits topoisomerase IV

Therapeutic outcome: Bacteriocidal action against the following: *Streptococcus pneumoniae, Haemophilus influenzae, Haemophilus parainfluenzae, Moraxella catarrhalis, Klebsiella pneumoniae, Mycoplasma pneumoniae, Escherichia coli, Serratia marcescens, Chlamydia pneumoniae, Legionella pneumophilia, Enterococcus faecalis, Staphylococcus epidermidis, Staphylococcus pyogenes*

USES: Acute sinusitis, acute chronic bronchitis, community-acquired pneumonia, uncomplicated skin infections, complicated UTI, cellulitis, PID, prostatitis, inhalational anthrax (postexposure), acute pyelonephritis, inhalation anthrax in children

Unlabeled uses: Gonococcal infections, disseminated

CONTRAINDICATIONS:
Hypersensitivity to quinolones

Precautions: Pregnancy **C**, breastfeeding, children; photosensitivity, acute MI, atrial fibrillation, colitis, dehydration, diabetes, QT prolongation, myasthenia gravis, renal disease, seizure disorder, syphilis

> **BLACK BOX WARNING:** Tendon pain/rupture, tendinitis

DOSAGE AND ROUTES
Acute bacterial exacerbation of chronic bronchitis
Adult: PO/IV 500 mg q24hr × 7 days

Acute bacterial sinusitis
Adult: PO 500 mg q24hr × 10-14 days or 750 mg q24hr × 5 days

Acute pyelonephritis
Adult: PO 250 mg q24hr × 10 days or 750 mg q24hr × 5 days

Chronic bacterial prostatitis
Adult: PO 500 mg q24hr × 28 days

Postexposure inhalational anthrax
Adult/adolescent/child >50 kg: PO/IV 500 mg q24hr × 60 days
Infant >6 mo and child <50 kg: IV 8 mg/kg q12hr × 60 days, max 250 mg/dose

Pneumonia, community acquired
Adult: PO/IV 500 mg q24hr × 7-14 days or 750 mg q24hr × 5 days

Pneumonia, nosocomial
Adult: PO/IV 750 mg q24hr × 7-14 days

SSSI, complicated
Adult: PO/IV 750 mg q24hr × 7-14 days

SSSI, uncomplicated
Adult: PO 500 mg q24hr × 7-10 days

UTI, complicated
Adult: PO/IV 250 mg q24hr × 10 days

UTI, uncomplicated
Adult: PO 250 mg q24hr × 3 days

Gonococcal infection, disseminated (unlabeled)
Adult: IV 250 mg q24hr × 24-48 hr, then PO 500 mg/day × 7 days

PID
Adult: IV 500 mg q24hr × 14 days

Renal disease
Adult: PO/IV CCr 20-49 ml/min initial 500 mg, then 250 mg q24hr; CCr 10-19 ml/min 250 or 500 mg, depending on condition, then 250 mg q48hr

Available forms: Single-use vials (500, 750 mg), premixed flexible container; 250 mg/50 ml D₅W, 500 mg/100 ml D₅W, 750 mg/150 ml D₅W; tabs 250, 500, 750 mg; oral sol 25 mg/ml

Implementation
• Give PO 4 hr before or 2 hr after antacids, iron, calcium, zinc
• Check for irritation, extravasation, phlebitis daily

Intermittent IV infusion route
• Discard any unused sol in the single-dose vial
• Dilute with 0.9% NaCl, D₅W, to 5 mg/ml, give 250 mg over 60 min or 750 mg over 90 min
• Using premix, tear outer wrap at notch and remove sol container; check for leaks; close control clamps; remove cover from port at bottom of container; insert pin into port with a twist; suspend container from hanger; squeeze and release drip chamber to proper fluid level; open flow control to expel air, close clamp; regulate rate with flow control clamps

Y-site compatibilities: Alfentanil, amifostine, amikacin, aminocaproic acid, aminophylline, ampicillin, anidulafungin, atenolol, atracurium, aztreonam, bivalirudin, bleomycin, bumetanide, buprenorphine, busulfan, butorphanol, caffeine citrate, calcium gluconate, CARBOplatin, carmustine, caspofungin, cefepime, cefotetan, ceftazidime, ceftizoxime, cefTRIAXone, cefuroxime, chlorproMAZINE, cimetidine, cisatracurium, CISplatin, clindamycin, cyclophosphamide, cycloSPORINE, cytarabine, DACTINomycin, DAPTOmycin, dexamethasone, dexrazoxane, digoxin, diltiazem, diphenhydrAMINE, DOBUTamine, docetaxel, dolasetron, DOPamine, doripenem, doxacurium, doxycycline, droperidol, enalaprilat, ePHEDrine, EPINEPHrine, epirubicin, ertapenem, erythromycin, esmolol, etoposide, famotidine, fenoldopam, fentaNYL, filgrastim, floxuridine, fluconazole, fludarabine, fosphenytoin, gemcitabine, gentamicin, granisetron, haloperidol, hydrocortisone, HYDROmorphone, IDArubicin, ifosfamide, imipenem-cilastatin, isoproterenol, labetalol, leucovorin, levorphanol, lidocaine, linezolid, magnesium sulfate, mannitol, mechlorethamine, meperidine, mesna, methylPREDNISolone, metoclopramide, metroNIDAZOLE, midazolam, milrinone, mitomycin, mitoxantrone, morphine, nalbuphine, naloxone, nesiritide, octreotide, ondansetron, oxacillin, oxaliplatin, oxytocin, paclitaxel, palonosetron, pancuronium, pemetrexed, penicillin G sodium, pentamidine, phenylephrine, plicamycin, potassium chloride, promethazine, propranolol, ranitidine, remifentanil, rocuronium, sargramostim, succinylcholine, SUFentanil, tacrolimus, teniposide, theophylline, thiotepa, tirofiban, tobramycin, trimethoprim-sulfamethoxazole, vancomycin, vasopressin, vecuronium, verapamil, vinBLAStine, vinCRIStine, vinorelbine, voriconazole, zidovudine

Solution compatibilities: 0.9% NaCl, D₅W, D₅/0.9% NaCl, D₅LR, D₅/0.45% NaCl, sodium lactate, plasma-lyte 56/D₅W

ADVERSE EFFECTS:
CNS: *Headache*, dizziness, *insomnia*, anxiety, **seizures**, encephalopathy, paresthesia
CV: Chest pain, palpitations, vasodilatation, QT prolongation
EENT: Dry mouth, visual impairment
GI: *Nausea*, flatulence, *vomiting*, diarrhea, abdominal pain, **pseudomembranous colitis, hepatotoxicity**
GU: Vaginitis, crystalluria
HEMA: Eosinophilia, **hemolytic anemia,** lymphophemia
INTEG: Rash, pruritus, photosensitivity, **epidermal necrolysis**
MISC: Hypoglycemia, hypersensitivity, tendon rupture
RESP: Pneumonitis
SYST: **Anaphylaxis, multisystem organ failure, Stevens-Johnson syndrome**

Pharmacokinetics
Absorption	Unknown
Distribution	Unknown
Metabolism	Liver
Excretion	Kidneys unchanged
Half-life	6-8 hr

Pharmacodynamics
Onset	Immediate
Peak	Infusion's end
Duration	Unknown

INTERACTIONS
Individual drugs
Calcium, iron, sucralfate, zinc: decreased absorption of levofloxacin
Foscarnet: increased CNS stimulation, seizures
Haloperidol, chloroquine, droperidol, pentamidine, arsenic trioxide, levomethadyl: increased QT prolongation
Magnesium: decreased levofloxacin absorption; do not use in same **IV** line
Probenecid: increased levofloxacin levels

Adverse effects: *italics* = common; **bold** = life-threatening

Theophylline: decreased theophylline clearance; toxicity may result

Warfarin: increased bleeding

Drug classifications

Antacids (magnesium, aluminum): decreased absorption of levofloxacin

Class IA/III antidysrhythmics, some phenothiazines, beta agonists, local anesthetics, tricyclics, CYP3A4 inhibitors (amiodarone, clarithromycin, erythromycin, telithromycin, troleandomycin), CYP3A4 substrates (methadone, pimozide, QUEtiapine, quiNIDine, risperidone, ziprasidone): increased QT prolongation

NSAIDs: increased CNS stimulation, seizures

Drug/lab test

Decreased: glucose, lymphocytes

NURSING CONSIDERATIONS

Assessment

• Assess patient for previous sensitivity reaction

• **Assess patient for signs and symptoms of infection,** including characteristics of wounds, sputum, urine, stool, WBC >10,000/mm³, fever; baseline, during treatment

• Obtain C&S before beginning product therapy to identify if correct treatment has been initiated

• **QT prolongation:** Monitor for QT prolongation, ejection fraction; assess for chest pain, palpitations, dyspnea

• **Pseudomembranous colitis:** Assess for diarrhea, abdominal pain, fever, fatigue, anorexia; possible anemia, elevated WBC and low serum albumin; stop product and give usually either vancomycin or IV metroNIDAZOLE

• **Assess for allergic reactions and anaphylaxis:** rash, urticaria, pruritus, chills, fever, joint pain; may occur a few days after therapy begins; epinephrine and resuscitation equipment should be available for anaphylactic reaction

• Determine urine output; if decreasing, notify prescriber (may indicate nephrotoxicity); also check for increased BUN, creatinine

• Monitor blood tests: AST, ALT, CBC, Hct, bilirubin, LDH, alkaline phosphatase, Coombs' test monthly if patient is on long-term therapy

• Monitor electrolytes: potassium, sodium, chloride monthly if patient is on long-term therapy

• Monitor for bleeding: ecchymosis, bleeding gums, hematuria, stool guaiac daily if on long-term therapy

• **Assess for overgrowth of infection:** perineal itching, fever, malaise, redness, pain, swelling, drainage, rash, diarrhea, change in cough, sputum

Nursing diagnoses

• Diarrhea (side effects)

• Infection, risk for (uses)

• Injury, risk for (side effects)

• Knowledge, deficient (teaching)

• Noncompliance (teaching)

Patient/family education

• Teach patient to report sore throat, bruising, bleeding, joint pain; may indicate **blood dyscrasias (rare)**

• Advise patient to contact prescriber if vaginal itching, loose foul-smelling stools, furry tongue occur, may indicate superinfection; report itching, rash, pruritus, urticaria

• Instruct patient to take all medication prescribed for the length of time ordered; product must be taken around the clock to maintain blood levels; do not give medication to others

• Advise patient to notify prescriber of diarrhea with blood or pus

• Instruct patient to take 4 hr before antacids, iron, calcium, zinc products

• Tell patient to complete full course of therapy; to increase fluid intake to 2 L/day to prevent crystalluria

• Advise patient to avoid hazardous activities until response to product is known

• Instruct patient to rinse mouth frequently and use sugarless candy or gum for dry mouth

• Instruct patient to avoid taking other medications unless approved by prescriber

• Advise patient to avoid sun exposure or use sunscreen to prevent phototoxicity

Evaluation

Positive therapeutic outcome

• Absence of signs/symptoms of infection (WBC <10,000/mm³, temp WNL)

• Reported improvement in symptoms of infection

levofloxacin ophthalmic

See Appendix B

levoleucovorin (Rx)

(lee-voe-loo-koe-voe′rin)

Fusilev

Func. class.: Chemotherapy protectant

Chem. class.: Tetrahydrofolic acid derivative

Pregnancy category C

ACTION: Acts as a replacement to rescue cells from the effects of folate antagonists

Therapeutic outcome: Prevention of methotrexate toxicity

USES: For methotrexate toxicity prophylaxis, colorectal cancer (to potentiate fluorouracil therapy)

CONTRAINDICATIONS:
Hypersensitivity to this agent or folic acid, mannitol; intrathecal administration

Precautions: Pregnancy **C**, breastfeeding, children <6 yr, megaloblastic/pernicious anemia, seizure disorder, vitamin B_{12} deficiency

DOSAGE AND ROUTES

For levoleucovorin rescue following high-dose methotrexate treatment for osteosarcoma
Adult and child >6 yr: **IV** 7.5 mg (approximately 5 mg/m²) q6hr × 10 doses starting 24 hr after the beginning of methotrexate INF; max >16 ml (160 mg) of the reconstituted SOL/min

For inadvertent overdose of methotrexate
Adult and child >6 yr: **IV** 7.5 mg q6hr until serum methotrexate conc <0.01 micromolar; max >16 ml (160 mg) of the reconstituted SOL/min

Colorectal cancer
Adult: **IV** 100 mg/m² over ≥3 min, then fluorouracil 370 mg/m² **IV** each day × 5 days or levoleucovorin 10 mg/m² **IV,** then fluorouracil 425 mg/m² **IV** each day × 5 days; the course may be repeated q28days × 2, then repeated at 28-35 day intervals if complete recovery from toxic effects has occurred

Available forms: Powder for inj 50 mg

Implementation
• Give within 1 hr of folic acid antagonist
• Do not give concurrently with systemic methotrexate
• Increase fluid intake if used to treat folic acid inhibitor overdose
• Protect from light and heat

IV route
• For **IV** reconstitute 50 mg vial/5.3 ml of normal saline (10 mg/ml)

Intermittent IV route
• Further dilute to a final concentration of 0.5-5 mg/ml
• Give ≤160 mg/min

ADVERSE EFFECTS
CNS: **Seizures,** syncope
GI: Nausea, vomiting, stomatitis
GU: Abnormal renal function
INTEG: *Rash, pruritus,* anaphylaxis, *urticaria*
RESP: Dyspnea

INTERACTIONS

Individual drugs
Capecitabine, floxuridine, fluorouracil: increased toxicity
Methotrexate, pyrimethamine, trimethoprim, trimetrexate: decreased effect of these products

Drug classifications
Barbiturates, hydantoins: increased metabolism

NURSING CONSIDERATIONS

Assessment
• Monitor CCr, creatinine before levoleucovorin rescue and daily to detect methotrexate level
• Monitor CBC with differential
• Assess other products taken: hydantoins, trimethoprim may cause increased folic acid use by body
• **Assess neurologic status** (rescue): weakness, fatigue
• **Anaphylaxis:** dyspnea, rash, temperature change, pruritus when given with a methotrexate regimen

Nursing diagnoses
• Injury, risk for (uses)
• Knowledge, deficient (teaching)

Patient/family education
• Teach patient to eat folic acid–rich foods for folic acid deficiency: bran, yeast, dried beans, nuts, fresh green leafy vegetables
• Advise patient to notify prescriber of side effects
• Instruct patient to report signs of hyposensitivity reaction immediately
• Inform patient to avoid breastfeeding

Evaluation
Positive therapeutic outcome
• Prevention of methotrexate toxicity

levothyroxine (Rx)
(lee-voe-thye-rox′een)
Eltroxin ✦, Levothroid, Levoxyl, Synthroid, Tirosint, Unithroid
Func. class.: Thyroid hormone
Chem. class.: Levoisomer of thyroxine
Pregnancy category A

Do not confuse:
Synthroid/Symmetrel

ACTION: Controls protein synthesis; increases metabolic rate, cardiac output, renal blood flow, O_2 consumption, body temp, blood volume, growth, development at cellular level via action on thyroid hormone receptors

Therapeutic outcome: Correction of lack of thyroid hormone

USES: Hypothyroidism, myxedema coma, thyroid hormone replacement, thyrotoxicosis, congenital hypothyroidism, some types of thyroid cancer, pituitary TSH suppression

CONTRAINDICATIONS:
Adrenal insufficiency, recent MI, thyrotoxicosis, hypersensitivity to beef, alcohol intolerance (inj only)

> **BLACK BOX WARNING:** Obesity treatment

Precautions: Pregnancy **A**, breastfeeding, geriatric, angina pectoris, hypertension, ischemia, cardiac disease, diabetes

DOSAGE AND ROUTES
Severe hypothyroidism
Adult ≤50 yr: PO 1.7 mcg/kg/day, 6-8 wk, average dose 100-200 mcg/day, max 200 mcg/day; IM/IV 50-100 mcg/day as a single dose or 50% of usual oral dosage
Adult >50 yr without heart disease or <50 yr with heart disease: PO 25-50 mcg/day, titrate q6-8wk
Adult >50 yr with heart disease: PO 12.5-25 mcg/day, titrate by 12.5-25 mcg q6-8wk
Child >12 yr: PO 2-3 mcg/kg/day given as a single dose AM
Child 6-12 yr: PO 4-5 mcg/kg/day given as a single dose AM
Child 1-5 yr: PO 5-6 mcg/kg/day given as a single dose AM
Child 6-12 mo: PO 6-8 mcg/kg/day given as a single dose AM

Child <6 mo: PO 8-10 mcg/kg/day given as a single dose AM

Myxedema coma
Adult: IV 200-500 mcg; may increase by 100-300 mcg after 24 hr; give oral medication as soon as possible

Subclinical hypothyroidism
Adult: PO 1 mcg/kg/day may be sufficient

Available forms: Powder for inj 200, 500 mcg/vial; tabs 25, 50, 88, 100, 112, 125, 137, 150, 175, 200, 300; cap (liquid filled) 13, 25, 50, 75, 88, 100, 112, 125, 137, 150 mcg

Implementation
PO route
• Give in AM if possible as a single dose to decrease sleeplessness; give at same time each day to maintain product level
• Give crushed and mixed with water, nonsoy formula, or breast milk for infants/children
• Give only for hormone imbalances; not to be used for obesity, male infertility, menstrual conditions, lethargy; give lowest dosage that relieves symptoms; lower dosage for geriatric and in cardiac disease
• Store in tight, light-resistant container
• Remove medication 4 wk before RAIU test
• Separate antacids, iron, calcium products by 4 hr

Direct IV route
• Give **IV** after diluting with provided diluent (0.9% NaCl), 500 mcg/5 ml, 200 mcg/2 ml; shake well; give through Y-tube or 3-way stopcock; give 100 mcg or less over 1 min; do not add to **IV** infusion; considered incompatible in syringe with all other products

ADVERSE EFFECTS
CNS: *Anxiety, insomnia, tremors,* headache, **thyroid storm,** excitability
CV: *Tachycardia, palpitations, angina, dysrhythmias,* hypertension, **cardiac arrest**
GI: Nausea, diarrhea, increased or decreased appetite, cramps
MISC: Menstrual irregularities, weight loss, sweating, heat intolerance, fever, alopecia, decreased bone mineral density

Pharmacokinetics

Absorption	Erratic (PO); complete (IV)
Distribution	Widely distributed
Metabolism	Liver; enterohepatic recirculation
Excretion	Feces via bile; breast milk (small amounts)
Half-life	6-7 days

Pharmacodynamics

	PO	IV
Onset	3-5 days	6-8 hr
Peak	12-48 hr	12-48 hr
Duration	Unknown	Unknown

INTERACTIONS

Individual drugs
Aluminum, calcium, iron, magnesium, sucralfate, rifampin, rifabutin: decreased levothyroxine effects

Orlistat, ferrous sulfate: decreased absorption of levothyroxine

Drug classifications
Antacids: decreased levothyroxine effects

Anticoagulants (oral): increased anticoagulant effect

Antidepressants (tricyclics): increased tricyclic effect

Bile acid sequestrants: decreased levothyroxine absorption

EPINEPHrine products: increased cardiac insufficiency risk

Estrogens: decreased thyroid hormone effects

Selective serotonin reuptake inhibitors: decreased levothyroxine effects

Sympathomimetics: increased sympathomimetic effect

Drug/herb
Soy: decreased thyroid hormone effect

Drug/lab test
Increased: CPK, LDH, AST, blood glucose
Decreased: thyroid function tests

NURSING CONSIDERATIONS

Assessment
• Determine if the patient is taking anticoagulants, antidiabetic agents; document on chart
• Take B/P, pulse before each dose; monitor I&O ratio and weight every day in same clothing, using same scale, at same time of day
• Monitor height, weight, psychomotor development, and growth rate if given to a child

• Monitor T_3, T_4, which are decreased; radioimmunoassay of TSH, which is increased; radioactive iodine uptake (RAIU), which is increased if patient's dosage of medication is too low
• Monitor pro-time (may require decreased anticoagulant); check for bleeding, bruising
• Assess for increased nervousness, excitability, irritability, which may indicate a too-high dosage of medication, usually after 1-3 wk of treatment
• Assess cardiac status: angina, palpitations, chest pain, change in VS; the geriatric patient may have undetected cardiac problems and baseline ECG should be completed before treatment

Nursing diagnoses
• Knowledge, deficient (teaching)
• Noncompliance (teaching)

Patient/family education
• Teach patient that product is not a cure but controls symptoms and that treatment is long term
• Instruct patient to report excitability, irritability, anxiety, sweating, heat intolerance, chest pain, palpitations, which indicate overdose
• Advise patient not to switch brands unless approved by prescriber; bioavailability may differ; do not take with food; absorption will be decreased
• Teach patient that product may be discontinued after giving birth; thyroid panel will be evaluated after 1-2 mo
• Teach patient or parent that hyperthyroid child will show almost immediate behavior/personality change; that hair loss will occur in child but is temporary
• Caution patient that product is not to be taken to reduce weight
• Caution patient to avoid OTC preparations with iodine; read labels; other medications should not be used unless approved by prescriber
• Teach patient to avoid iodine-rich food: iodized salt, soybeans, tofu, turnips, high-iodine seafood, some bread

Evaluation
Positive therapeutic outcome
• Absence of depression
• Weight loss, increased diuresis, pulse, appetite
• Absence of constipation, peripheral edema, cold intolerance, pale, cool dry skin, brittle nails, alopecia, coarse hair, menorrhagia, night blindness, paresthesias, syncope, stupor, coma, rosy cheeks

• Improved levels of T_3, T_4 by laboratory tests
• Child: age-appropriate weight, height, and psychomotor development

TREATMENT OF OVERDOSE:
Withhold dose for up to 1 wk; acute overdose: gastric lavage or induced emesis, activated charcoal; provide supportive treatment to control symptoms

---

⚠ HIGH ALERT

lidocaine, parenteral (Rx)
(lye′doe-kane)
LidoPen Auto-Injector, Xylocaine, Xylocard ✦
Func. class.: Antidysrhythmic (class IB)
Chem. class.: Aminoacyl amide
Pregnancy category B

ACTION: Increases electrical stimulation threshold of ventricle and His-Purkinje system, which stabilizes cardiac membrane and decreases automaticity

Therapeutic outcome: Decreased ventricular dysrhythmia

USES: Ventricular tachycardia, ventricular dysrhythmias during cardiac surgery, MI, digoxin toxicity, cardiac catheterization

CONTRAINDICATIONS:
Hypersensitivity to amides, severe heart block, supraventricular dysrhythmias, Adams-Stokes syndrome, Wolff-Parkinson-White syndrome

Precautions: Pregnancy **B,** breastfeeding, children, geriatric, renal/hepatic disease, CHF, respiratory depression, malignant hyperthermia, myasthenia gravis, weight <50 kg

DOSAGE AND ROUTES
Adult: IV BOL 50-100 mg (1-1.5 mg/kg) 25-50 mg/min, repeat q3-5min, max 300 mg in 1 hr; begin **IV** INF 1-4 mg/min (20-50 mcg/kg/min); IM 200-300 mg (4.3 mg/kg) in deltoid muscle, may repeat in 1-1½ hr if needed

Available forms: IV inf 0.2% (2 mg/ml), 0.4% (4 mg/ml), 0.8% (8 mg/ml); IV admixture 4% (40 mg/ml), 10% (100 mg/ml), 20% (200 mg/ml); **IV direct** 1% (10 mg/ml), 2% (20 mg/ml); **IM** 10% (300 mg/3 ml)

Implementation
IM route
• Administer in deltoid, aspirate to prevent **IV** administration
• Check site daily for extravasation

Direct IV route
• Give undiluted (1%, 2% only); give 6 mg or less over 1 min; if using an **IV** line, use port near insertion site, flush with 0.9% NaCl (50 ml)
• Store at room temperature; sol should be clear

Continuous IV infusion route
• Give after adding 1 g/250-1000 ml of D₅W; give 1-4 mg/min; use infusion pump for correct dosage; pediatric inf is 120 mg of lidocaine/100 ml of D₅W; 1-2.5 ml/kg/hr = 20-50 mcg/kg/min; use only 1%, 2% sol

Solution compatibilities: D₅W, D₅/0.9% NaCl, D₅/0.45% NaCl, D₅/LR, LR, 0.9% NaCl, 0.45% NaCl

Y-site compatibilities: Alemtuzumab, alteplase, amikacin, aminophylline, amiodarone, argatroban, atropine, aztreonam, bivalirudin, bumetanide, calcium chloride/gluconate, ceFAZolin, cefotaxime, cefoxitin, ceftazidime, ceftizoxime, cefTRIAXone, cefuroxime, chloramphenicol, cimetidine, ciprofloxacin, cisatracurium, clindamycin, cycloSPORINE, DAPTOmycin, dexamethasone, dexmedetomidine, digoxin, diltiazem, diphenhydrAMINE, DOBUTamine, DOPamine, doxycycline, enalaprilat, EPINEPHrine, eptifibatide, ertapenem, erythromycin, esmolol, etomidate, famotidine, fenoldopam, fentaNYL, fluconazole, furosemide, gentamicin, granisetron, haloperidol, heparin, hydrocortisone, imipenem/cilastatin, inamrinone, insulin, isoproterenol, ketorolac, labetalol, levofloxacin, linezolid, LORazepam, magnesium sulfate, meperidine, methylPREDNISolone, metoclopramide, metoprolol, metroNIDAZOLE, micafungin, midazolam, morphine, nafcillin, niCARdipine, nitroglycerin, nitroprusside, norepinephrine, ondansetron, palonosetron, penicillin G potassium, phenylephrine, phytonadione, piperacillin/tazobactam, potassium chloride, procainamide, prochlorperazine, promethazine, propofol, propranolol, protamine, quinupristin/dalfopristin, ranitidine, remifentanil, sodium bicarbonate, tacrolimus, theophylline, ticarcillin/clavulanate, tigecycline, tirofiban, tobramycin, vancomycin, vasopressin, verapamil, vitamin B complex with C, voriconazole, warfarin

Y-site incompatibilities: Acyclovir, amphotericin B cholesteryl sulfate complex/colloidal, azaTHIOprine, caspofungin, diazepam, ganciclovir, lansoprazole, pantoprazole, phenytoin, thiopental, trimethoprim/sulfamethoxazole

ADVERSE EFFECTS

CNS: *Headache, dizziness,* involuntary movement, confusion, tremor, *drowsiness,* euphoria, **seizures,** shivering
CV: *Hypotension, bradycardia,* **heart block, cardiovascular collapse, arrest**
EENT: Tinnitus, blurred vision
GI: Nausea, vomiting, anorexia
HEMA: Methemoglobinemia
INTEG: Rash, urticaria, edema, swelling, petechiae, pruritus
MISC: Febrile response, phlebitis at inj site
RESP: Dyspnea, **respiratory depression**

Pharmacokinetics

Absorption	Complete bioavailability (**IV**)
Distribution	Erythrocytes, cardiovascular endothelium
Metabolism	Liver
Excretion	Kidneys
Half-life	Biphasic 8 min, 1-2 hr

Pharmacodynamics

	IV	IM
Onset	2 min	5-15 min
Peak	Unknown	$^1/_2$ hr
Duration	20 min	$1^1/_2$ hr

INTERACTIONS

Individual drugs

Amiodarone, phenytoin, procainamide, propranolol: increase cardiac depression, toxicity
Cimetidine, metoprolol, phenytoin: increased lidocaine effects
CycloSPORINE: decreased effect of cycloSPORINE
Tubocurarine: increased neuromuscular blockade

Drug classifications

Antihypertensives, MAOIs: increased hypotensive effects
β-blockers, protease inhibitors: increased lidocaine effects
Barbiturates: decreased lidocaine effects
Neuromuscular blockers: increased neuromuscular blockade

Drug/lab test

Increased: CPK

NURSING CONSIDERATIONS

Assessment

• Assess for oxygenation or perfusion deficit: decreased B/P, chest pain, dizziness, loss of consciousness
• Assess respiratory status: auscultate lung fields for bibasilar crackles in patients with advanced CHF
• Assess for urinary retention: check for pain, abdominal absorption, palpate bladder; check males with benign prostatic hypertrophy; anticholinergic reaction may cause retention
• Monitor I&O ratio, electrolytes (potassium, sodium, chloride); watch for decreasing urinary output, possible retention
• Monitor liver function tests: AST, ALT, bilirubin, alk phos
• Monitor ECG continuously to determine product effectiveness, measure PR, QRS, QT intervals, check for PVCs, other dysrhythmias; monitor B/P continuously for hypo/hypertension; check for rebound hypertension after 1-2 hr, prolonged PR/QT intervals, QRS complex; if QT or QRS increases by 50% or more, withhold next dose, notify prescriber
• Monitor for CNS symptoms: confusion, numbness, depression, involuntary movements; if these occur, product should be discontinued
• Monitor blood levels (therapeutic level 1.5-5 mcg/ml), notify prescriber of abnormal results

Nursing diagnoses

• Cardiac output, decreased (uses)
• Gas exchange, impaired (adverse reactions)
• Knowledge, deficient (teaching)

Patient/family education

• Teach patient or family reason for use of medication and expected results
⚠ Instruct patient in at-home use of Lidopen Auto-Injector; patient should call prescriber before use if heart attack is imminent

Evaluation

Positive therapeutic outcome
• Decreased B/P, dysrhythmias
• Decreased heart rate
• Normal sinus rhythm

TREATMENT OF OVERDOSE:

Oxygen, artificial ventilation, ECG, administer DOPamine for circulatory depression, diazepam or thiopental for seizures; decreased product or discontinuation may be required

lidocaine topical
See Appendix B

Adverse effects: *italics* = common; **bold** = life-threatening

linagliptin

(lin-a-glip'tin)
Tradjenta
Func. class.: Antidiabetic
Chem. class.: Dipeptidyl peptidase-4
inhibitor
Pregnancy category B

ACTION: Slows the inactivation of incretin hormones. Concentrations of the active, intact hormones are increased by linagliptin, thereby increasing and prolonging the action of these hormones. Incretin hormones are released by the intestine throughout the day, and levels are increased in response to a meal.

Therapeutic outcome: Decreasing blood glucose level, A1c; decreasing polydipsia, polyphagia

USES: Type 2 diabetes mellitus

CONTRAINDICATIONS:
Hypersensitivity to linagliptin, type 1 diabetes mellitus, diabetic ketoacidosis (DKA)

Precautions: Pregnancy category B, breast-feeding, adolescents or children <18 years old, debilitated physical condition, malnutrition, uncontrolled adrenal insufficiency, pituitary insufficiency, hypothyroidism, diarrhea, gastroparesis, GI obstruction, ileus, female hormonal changes, high fever, severe psychological stress, uncontrolled hypercortisolism, hyperthyroidism

DOSAGE AND ROUTES
Adult: PO 5 mg q day; when used with a sulfonylurea, a lower dose of the sulfonylurea may be necessary to minimize the risk of hypoglycemia
Available forms: Tab 5 mg

Implementation:
• Given once daily; may give without regard to food
• Store at room temperature

ADVERSE EFFECTS
CNS: Headache
EENT: Nasopharyngitis
ENDO: Hyperuricemia, hypoglycemia
GI: Body weight loss, **pancreatitis**
INTEG: Angioedema, exfoliative dermatitis, hypersensitivity reactions, urticaria
MISC: Arthralgia, back pain
RESP: Bronchial hyperreactivity (with **bronchospasm**), cough, nasopharyngitis

Pharmacokinetics
Absorption	Rapidly, bioavailability 30%
Distribution	Extensive, tissues; protein binding concentration dependent
Metabolism	Weak CYP3A4 inhibitor
Excretion	90% unchanged, 80% enterohepatic, urine 5%
Half-life	Terminal >100 hr, effective 12 hr

Pharmacodynamics
Onset	Unknown
Peak	Unknown
Duration	Unknown

INTERACTIONS
Individual drugs
Alcohol, cisapride, lithium, metoclopramide, tegaserod: Increased need for dosing change
Bumetanide, dextrothyroxine, ethacrynic acid, ethotoin, fosphenytoin, furosemide, glucagon, niacin (nicotinic acid), phenothiazine, phenytoin, torsemide, triamterene: Decreased hypoglycemic effect
CloNIDine, dexfenfluramine, disopyramide, fenfluramine, fluoxetine, guanethidine, octreotide: Increased or prolonged hypoglycemia
Reserpine: Increased masking the signs and symptoms of hypoglycemia

Drug classifications
Beta blockers, ACE inhibitors, angiotensin II receptor antagonists, fibric acid derivatives, monoamine oxidase inhibitors (MAOIs), salicylates, sulfonylureas: Increased or prolonged hypoglycemia
Atypical antipsychotics (aripiprazole, clozapine, OLANZapine, quetiapine, risperidone, and ziprasidone), carbonic anhydrase inhibitors, estrogens, glucocorticoids, oral contraceptives, progestins, thiazide diuretics, thyroid hormones: Decreased hypoglycemic effect
Androgens, quinolones: Increased need for dosing change
CYP3A4 inducers (topiramate, rifabutin, pioglitazone, OXcarbazepine, carBAMazepine, nevirapine, modafinil, metyrapone, etravirine, efavirenz, bosentan, barbiturates, aprepitant, fosaprepitant): Decreased effect of linagliptin

NURSING CONSIDERATIONS
Assessment
• Hypoglycemia/hypoglycemia: Monitor reactions that may occur after meals; for severe hypoglycemia use IV Dextrose

• Monitor blood glucose, A1c, during treatment to determine diabetes control
• Monitor CBC baseline and periodically during treatment, report decreased blood counts

Nursing diagnoses
• Nutrition, more than body requirements, imbalanced (uses)
• Nutrition, less than body requirements, imbalanced (adverse reactions)
• Injury, risk for injury (adverse reactions)
• Knowledge deficit (teaching)
• Noncompliance (teaching)

Patient/family education
• Teach patient the symptoms of hypo/hyperglycemia and what to do about each; to have glucagon emergency kit available, carry sugar packets
• Advise patient that product must be continued on a daily basis, explain consequences of discontinuing product abruptly; to take only as directed
• Direct patient to avoid OTC products unless approved by prescriber
• Teach patient that diabetes is a life-long illness, product will not cure diabetes
• Teach patient that all food in diet plan must be eaten to prevent hypoglycemia
• Advise patient to carry emergency ID with prescriber, condition and medications taken
• Report immediately, skin disorders, swelling, difficulty breathing, or severe abdominal pain

Evaluation
• Improving blood glucose level, A1c; decreasing polydipsia, polyphagia, polyuria, clear sensorium, absence of dizziness

---

lindane (OTC)
(lin-dane)
Hexit ✤, **PMS-Lindane** ✤
Func. class.: Scabicide/pediculicide
Chem. class.: Chlorinated hydrocarbon (synthetic)
Pregnancy category C

ACTION: Stimulates nervous system of arthropods, resulting in seizures, death of organism

Therapeutic outcome: Resolution of infestation

USES: Scabies, lice (head/pubic/body), nits in those intolerant to or who do not respond to other agents

CONTRAINDICATIONS:
Hypersensitivity; patients with known seizure disorders; Norwegian (crusted) scabies

> **BLACK BOX WARNING:** Premature neonate; inflammation of skin, abrasions, or breaks in skin; seizure disorder

Precautions: Pregnancy **C**, breastfeeding, infants, children <10 yr; avoid contact with eyes

DOSAGE AND ROUTES
Lice
Adult and child: Shampoo using 30 ml, work into lather, rub for 5 min, rinse, dry with towel; use fine-toothed comb to remove nits; most require 1 oz, max 2 oz

Scabies
Adult and child: TOP cream/lotion wash area with soap and water, remove visible crusts; apply to skin surfaces; remove with soap, water 8-12 hr after application; may reapply in 1 wk if needed; TOP apply 1% cream/lotion to skin from neck to bottom of feet, toes; repeat in 1 wk if necessary; most require 1 oz, max 2 oz

Available forms: Lotion, shampoo, cream (1%)

Implementation
• Apply to body areas, scalp only; do not apply to face, lips, mouth, eyes, any mucous membrane, anus, or meatus
• Give topical corticosteroids as ordered to decrease contact dermatitis; provide antihistamines
• Apply menthol or phenol lotions to control itching
• Give topical antibiotics for infection
• Provide isolation until areas on skin, scalp have cleared and treatment is completed
• Remove nits by using a fine-toothed comb rinsed in vinegar after treatment; use gloves
• Caregivers applying these products to another person should wear gloves less permeable to lindane, thoroughly clean hands after application, avoid natural latex gloves
Cream/ointment/lotion
• Use for scabies only; skin should be clean without other products on it, wait 1 hr after bathing or showering before application, shake well, apply under fingernails after trimming, a toothbrush can be used to apply; after application wrap toothbrush in paper and discard, use only a single application, apply as a thin layer over all skin from neck down, close bottle with leftover and discard

---

• Do not cover, wash off after 8-12 hr using warm (not hot) water, do not leave on >12 hr
Shampoo
• For lice only, do not use other hair products before use, shake well, hair should be completely dry, use only enough shampoo to lightly wet the hair and scalp, work into hair, do not use water, allow to remain only 4 min, rinse and lather away, towel briskly

ADVERSE EFFECTS
CNS: Tremors, **seizures,** stimulation, dizziness (chronic inhalation of vapors), anxiety, **CNS toxicity**
CV: Ventricular fibrillation (chronic inhalation of vapors)
GI: *Nausea, vomiting, diarrhea,* liver damage (inhalation of vapors)
GU: Kidney damage (chronic inhalation of vapors)
HEMA: Aplastic anemia (chronic inhalation of vapors), myelosuppression
INTEG: *Pruritus, rash, irritation, contact dermatitis*

Pharmacokinetics
Absorption	20%
Distribution	Fat
Metabolism	Liver
Excretion	Kidneys
Half-life	18 hr

Pharmacodynamics
Onset	Rapid
Peak	Rapid
Duration	3 hr

INTERACTIONS
Oil-based hair dressing: increased absorption; wash, rinse, and dry hair before using lindane

NURSING CONSIDERATIONS
Assessment

> **BLACK BOX WARNING:** Skin with abrasions, breaks, inflammation; do not use on these areas

• **Infestation:** Assess head, hair for lice and nits before, after treatment; if scabies are present, check all skin surfaces
• Identify source of infection: school, family members, sexual contacts

Nursing diagnoses
• Knowledge, deficient (teaching)
• Skin integrity, impaired (uses)

Patient/family education
• Advise patient to wash all inhabitants' clothing, using insecticide; preventive treatment may be required for all persons living in same house, using lotion or shampoo to decrease spread of infection; use rubber gloves when applying product
• Instruct patient that itching may continue for 4-6 wk; that product must be reapplied if accidently washed off, or treatment will be ineffective; remove after specified time to prevent toxicity
• Advise patient not to apply to face; if contact with eyes occurs, flush with water
• Advise patient that sexual contacts should be treated simultaneously
• Inform the patient of CNS toxicity: dizziness, cramps, anxiety, nausea, vomiting, seizures

Evaluation
Positive therapeutic outcome
• Decreased crusts, nits, brownish trails on skin, itching papules in skinfolds
• Decreased itching after several wk

TREATMENT OF INGESTION:
Gastric lavage, saline laxatives, **IV** diazepam (Valium) for seizures (if taken orally)

linezolid (Rx)
(lih-nee′zoh-lid)
Zyvox
Func. class.: Broad-spectrum antiinfective
Chem. class.: Oxazolidinone
Pregnancy category C

Do not confuse:
Zyvox/Ziox/Zosyn

ACTION: Inhibits protein synthesis by interfering with translation; binds to bacterial 23S ribosomal RNA of the 50S subunit, preventing formation of the bacterial translation process in primarily gram-positive organisms

Therapeutic outcome: Negative blood cultures, absence of signs/symptoms of infection

USES: Vancomycin-resistant *Enterococcus faecium* infections, nosocomial pneumonia, uncomplicated or complicated skin and skin structure infections, community-acquired pneumonia

CONTRAINDICATIONS:
Hypersensitivity

Precautions: Pregnancy **C**, breastfeeding, children, thrombocytopenia, bone marrow suppression, hypertension, hyperthyroidism, pheochromocytoma, seizure disorder, ulcerative colitis, MI, PKU, renal/GI disease

DOSAGE AND ROUTES

Vancomycin-resistant *E. faecium* infections
Adult/adolescent/child ≥12 yr: IV/PO 600 mg q12hr × 14-28 days; max 1200 mg/day
Child <12 yr/infant/term neonate: IV/PO 10 mg/kg q8hr × 14-28 days

Nosocomial pneumonia/complicated skin infections/community-acquired pneumonia/concurrent bacterial infection
Adult: IV/PO 600 mg q12hr × 10-14 days; max 1200 mg/day
Child birth-11 yr: PO 10 mg/kg q8hr × 10-14 days

Uncomplicated skin infections
Adult: IV/PO 400 mg q12hr × 10-14 days; max 1200 mg/day
Adolescent: PO 600 mg q12hr × 10-14 days, max 1200 mg/day
Infant, preterm <7 days old: PO 10 mg/kg q12hr × 10-14 days

Available forms: Tabs 600 mg; oral susp 100 mg/5 ml; inj 2 mg/ml

Implementation
PO route
• Store reconstituted oral susp at room temperature, use within 3 wk
• Give over 30-120 min; do not use **IV** inf bag in series connections, do not use with additives in sol, do not use with another product, administer separately, flush line before and after use

Intermittent IV infusion route
• Premixed solutions are ready to use (2 mg/ml)

Y-site compatibilities: Acyclovir, alfentanil, amikacin, aminophylline, ampicillin, aztreonam, bretylium, buprenorphine, butorphanol, calcium gluconate, CARBOplatin, ceFAZolin, cefoperazone, cefotetan, cefoxitin, ceftazidime, ceftizoxime, cefTRIAXone, cefuroxime, cimetidine, ciprofloxacin, cisatracurium, cisplatin, clindamycin, cyclophosphamide, cycloSPORINE, cytarabine, HYDROmorphone, ifosfamide, labetalol, leucovorin, levofloxacin, lidocaine, LORazepam, magnesium sulfate, mannitol, meperidine, meropenem, mesna, methotrexate, methylPREDNISolone, metoclopramide, metroNIDAZOLE, midazolam, minocycline, mitoxantrone, morphine, nalbuphine, naloxone, nitroglycerin, ofloxacin, ondansetron, paclitaxel, PENTobarbital, piperacillin, potassium chloride, prochlorperazine, promethazine, propranolol, ranitidine, remifentanil, theophylline, ticarcillin, tobramycin, vancomycin, vecuronium, verapamil, vinCRIStine, zidovudine

Solution compatibilities: D₅, 0.9% NaCl, LR

ADVERSE EFFECTS
CNS: *Headache,* dizziness, insomnia
GI: *Nausea, diarrhea,* increased ALT, AST, *vomiting,* taste change, tongue color change, **pseudomembranous colitis**
HEMA: Myelosuppression
MISC: Vaginal moniliasis, fungal infection, oral moniliasis, **lactic acidosis,** anaphylaxis, angioedema, **Stevens-Johnson syndrome**

Pharmacokinetics

Absorption	Rapid, excessive
Distribution	Protein binding 31%
Metabolism	Oxidation of the morpholine ring
Excretion	Unknown
Half-life	Unknown

Pharmacodynamics
Unknown

INTERACTIONS

Individual drugs
Amoxapine, cyclobenzaprine, maprotiline, methyldopa, mirtazapine, trazodone: increased hypertensive crisis, seizures, coma

Drug classifications
Adrenergic blockers: increased effects of adrenergics
Antidepressants (tricyclics): increased hypertensive crisis, seizures, coma
MAOIs or those that possess MAOI-like action (flurazolidone, isoniazid, procarbazine): do not use together; hypertensive crisis may occur
SSRIs, SNRIs: increased serotonin syndrome
Serotoninergic agents: increased effect

Drug/herb
Green tea, valerian, ginseng, yohimbe, kava: avoid use

Drug/food
Tyramine foods: avoid; increased pressor response

Adverse effects: *italics* = common; **bold** = life-threatening

NURSING CONSIDERATIONS

Assessment
- Assess CNS symptoms: headache, dizziness
- Monitor liver function tests: AST, ALT
- Monitor allergic reactions: fever, flushing, rash, urticaria, pruritus
- Monitor CBC weekly, assess for myelosuppression (anemia, leukopenia, pancytopenia, thrombocytopenia)
- **Pseudomembranous colitis:** Assess for diarrhea, abdominal pain, fever, fatigue, anorexia; possible anemia, elevated WBC, and low serum albumin; stop product and usually give either vancomycin or IV metroNIDAZOLE
- **Serotonin syndrome:** at least 2 wk should elapse between continuing linezolid and start of serotonergic agents; assess for increased heart rate, shivering, sweating, dilated pupils, tremor, high B/P, hyperthermia, headache, confusion; if these occur stop linezolid; administer a serotonin antagonist if needed
- **Lactic acidosis:** repeated nausea/vomiting, unexplained acidosis, low bicarbonate level: notify prescriber immediately
- **Anaphylaxis/angioedema/Stevens-Johnson syndrome:** rash, pruritus, difficulty breathing, fever: have emergency equipment nearby

Nursing diagnoses
- Infection, risk for (uses)
- Knowledge, deficient (teaching)

Patient/family education
- Advise patient if dizziness occurs, to ambulate and perform activities with assistance
- Advise patient to complete full course of product therapy
- Advise patient to contact prescriber if adverse reaction occurs
- Advise patient to avoid large amounts of tyramine-containing foods (give list)

Evaluation
Positive therapeutic outcome
- Decreased symptoms of infection, blood cultures negative

---

liothyronine (T₃) (Rx)
(lye-oh-thye'roe-neen)
Cytomel, ʟ-Triiodothyronine, Triostat
Func. class.: Thyroid hormone
Chem. class.: Synthetic T₃
Pregnancy category A

ACTION: Increases metabolic rates, cardiac output, O_2 consumption, body temp, blood volume, growth, development at cellular level; exact mechanism unknown

Therapeutic outcome: Correction of lack of thyroid hormone

USES: Hypothyroidism, myxedema coma, thyroid hormone replacement, nontoxic goiter, T₃ suppression test, congenital hypothyroidism

CONTRAINDICATIONS:
Adrenal insufficiency, MI, thyrotoxicosis, untreated hypertension

BLACK BOX WARNING: Obesity treatment

Precautions: Pregnancy **A**, breastfeeding, geriatric, angina pectoris, hypertension, ischemia, cardiac disease, diabetes

DOSAGE AND ROUTES
Adult: PO 25 mcg/day, increase by 12.5-25 mcg q1-2wk until desired response; maintenance dose 25-75 mcg/day; max 100 mcg/day
Geriatric: PO 5 mcg/day, increase by 5 mcg/day q1-2wk, maintenance 25-75 mcg/day

Congenital hypothyroidism
Child >3 yr: PO 50-100 mcg/day
Child <3 yr: PO 5 mcg/day, increase by 5 mcg q3-4day titrated to response; infant maintenance 20 mcg/day; 1-3 yr 50 mcg/day

Myxedema, severe hypothyroidism
Adult: PO 25-50 mcg, then may increase by 5-10 mcg q1-2wk; maintenance dose 50-100 mcg/day

Myxedema coma/precoma
Adult: IV 25-50 mcg initially; 5 mcg in geriatric; 10-20 mcg in cardiac disease; give doses q4-12hr

Nontoxic goiter
Adult: PO 5 mcg/day, increase by 12.5-25 mcg q1-2wk; maintenance dose 75 mcg/day

Suppression test (T₃)
Adult: PO 75-100 mcg daily × 1 wk; ¹³¹I is given before and after 1st wk dose

Available forms: Tabs 5, 25, 50 mcg; inj 10 mcg/ml

Implementation
PO route
- Give in ᴀᴍ if possible as a single dose to decrease sleeplessness; give at same time each day to maintain product level
- Do not take with food or absorption will be decreased

• Give only for hormone imbalances; not to be used for obesity, male infertility, menstrual conditions, lethargy; give lowest dose that relieves symptoms; give lower dose to geriatric and those with cardiac disease
• Store in airtight, light-resistant container

IV route
• Administer **IV** for myxedema coma and precoma; do not give IM or SUBCUT; give q4-12hr; use PO dose as soon as feasible

ADVERSE EFFECTS

CNS: *Insomnia, tremors,* headache, **thyroid storm**
CV: *Tachycardia, palpitations, angina, dysrhythmias,* hypertension, **cardiac arrest**
GI: Nausea, diarrhea, increased or decreased appetite, cramps
MISC: Menstrual irregularities, weight loss, sweating, heat intolerance, fever, alopecia

Pharmacokinetics

Absorption	Well (PO); complete (**IV**)
Distribution	Widely distributed; does not cross placenta
Metabolism	Liver
Excretion	Feces via bile, breast milk
Half-life	1-2 days

Pharmacodynamics

	PO/IV
Onset	Unknown
Peak	12-24 hr
Duration	72 hr

INTERACTIONS

Individual drugs
Cholestyramine, colestipol: decreased absorption of thyroid hormone

Drug classifications
Amphetamines, anticoagulants (oral), antidepressants (tricyclics), decongestants, sympathomimetics, vasopressors: increased effect of each specific product
Calcium, iron, aluminum, magnesium products: decreased absorption of liothyronine
Estrogens: decreased effects of liothyronine

Drug/herb
Soy: decreased thyroid hormone effect

Drug/lab test
Increased: CPK, LDH, AST, PBI, blood glucose
Decreased: thyroid function tests

NURSING CONSIDERATIONS

Assessment
• Determine if the patient is taking anticoagulants, antidiabetic agents; document on patient record
• Take B/P, pulse before each dose; monitor I&O ratio and weight every day in same clothing, using same scale, at same time of day
• Monitor height, weight, psychomotor development, and growth rate of child
• Monitor T₃, T₄, FTIs, which are decreased; radioimmunoassay of TSH, which is increased; radioactive iodine uptake, which is increased if medication dose is too low
• Monitor pro-time; may require decreased anticoagulant; check for bleeding, bruising
• Assess for increased nervousness, excitability, irritability, which may indicate a too-high dose, usually after 1-3 wk of treatment
• Assess cardiac status: angina, palpitations, chest pain, change in VS; geriatric may have undetected cardiac problems, and baseline ECG should be completed before treatment

Nursing diagnoses
• Knowledge, deficient (teaching)
• Noncompliance (teaching)

Patient/family education
• Teach patient that product is not a cure but controls symptoms, treatment is long term
• Instruct patient to report excitability, irritability, anxiety, sweating, heat intolerance, chest pain, palpitations, which indicate overdose
• Advise patient not to switch brands unless approved by prescriber; bioavailability may differ
• Teach patient that product might be discontinued after giving birth; thyroid panel will be evaluated after 1-2 mo
• Teach patient that hyperthyroid child will show almost immediate behavior/personality change; that hair loss will occur in child but is temporary
• Caution patient that product is not to be taken to reduce weight
• Caution patient to avoid OTC preparations with iodine; read labels; other medications should not be used unless approved by prescriber
• Teach patient to avoid iodine-rich food: iodized salt, soybeans, tofu, turnips, high-iodine seafood, some bread

Evaluation
Positive therapeutic outcome
• Absence of depression
• Weight loss
• Increased diuresis, pulse, appetite

• Absence of constipation, peripheral edema, cold intolerance, pale cool dry skin, brittle nails, alopecia, coarse hair, menorrhagia, night blindness, paresthesias, syncope, stupor, coma, rosy cheeks
• Improved levels of T_3, T_4 by laboratory tests
• Child: age-appropriate weight, height, and psychomotor development

TREATMENT OF OVERDOSE:
Withhold dose for up to 1 wk; for acute overdose: gastric lavage or induce emesis, then activated charcoal; provide supportive treatment to control symptoms

liotrix (Rx)
(lye'oh-trix)
T_3/T_4, Thyrolar
Func. class.: Thyroid hormone
Chem. class.: Levothyroxine/liothyronine (synthetic T_4, T_3)
Pregnancy category A

Do not confuse:
Thyrolar/Thyrar

ACTION: Increases metabolic rates, cardiac output, O_2 consumption, body temp, blood volume, growth, development at cellular level; exact mechanism unknown

Therapeutic outcome: Correction of lack of thyroid hormone

USES: Hypothyroidism, thyroid hormone replacement

CONTRAINDICATIONS:
Adrenal insufficiency, MI, thyrotoxicosis

BLACK BOX WARNING: Obesity treatment

Precautions: Pregnancy A, breastfeeding, geriatric, angina pectoris, hypertension, ischemia, cardiac disease, diabetes mellitus

DOSAGE AND ROUTES
Adult: PO a single dose of Thyrolar $1/4$ or $1/2$ adult dose, adjust as needed at 2-wk intervals
Geriatric: PO $1/4$ tab initially, adjust q6-8wk

Available forms: Tabs levothyroxine 12.5 mcg/liothyronine 3.1 mcg; levothyroxine 25 mcg/liothyronine 6.25 mcg (Thyrolar-$1/2$); levothyroxine 50 mcg/liothyronine 12.5 mcg (Thyrolar-1); levothyroxine 100 mcg/liothyronine 25 mcg (Thyrolar-2); levothyroxine 150 mcg/liothyronine 37.5 mcg (Thyrolar-3)

Implementation
• Give in AM if possible as a single dose to decrease sleeplessness; give at same time each day to maintain product level
• Do not give with food or absorption will be decreased
• Give only for hormone imbalances; not to be used for obesity, male infertility, menstrual conditions, lethargy; give lowest dose that relieves symptoms; give lower dose to the geriatric and those with cardiac disease
• Store in airtight, light-resistant container
• Remove medication 4 wk before RAIU test

ADVERSE EFFECTS
CNS: *Insomnia, tremors,* headache, **thyroid storm**, nervousness
CV: *Tachycardia, palpitations, angina, dysrhythmias,* hypertension, **cardiac arrest**
GI: Nausea, diarrhea, increased or decreased appetite, cramps, vomiting
MISC: Menstrual irregularities, weight loss, sweating, heat intolerance, fever

Pharmacokinetics
Absorption	50%-80% (T_4); 95% (T_3)
Distribution	Widely distributed; does not cross placenta
Metabolism	Liver, tissues
Excretion	Feces via bile; breast milk
Half-life	6-7 days (T_4); 2 days (T_3)

Pharmacodynamics
	PO (T_4)	PO (T_3)
Onset	Unknown	Unknown
Peak	Unknown	24-72 hr
Duration	Unknown	72 hr

INTERACTIONS
Individual drugs
CarBAMazepine, phenytoin, rifampin: decreased effects of liotrix
Cholestyramine: decreased absorption of thyroid hormone
Colestipol: decreased absorption of liotrix

Drug classifications
Amphetamines, decongestants, vasopressors: increased effect of each specific product
Anticoagulants (oral): increased effect of anticoagulants
Antidepressants (tricyclics): increased tricyclic effect
Catecholamines: increased catecholamine effect
Estrogens: decreased liotrix effect

⚠ Nurse Alert

Sympathomimetics: increased sympathomimetic effect

Drug/herb
Soy: decreased thyroid hormone effect

Drug/lab test
Increased: CPK, LDH, AST, PBI, blood glucose
Decreased: thyroid function tests

NURSING CONSIDERATIONS
Assessment
• Determine if the patient is taking anticoagulants, antidiabetic agents; document on chart
• Take B/P, pulse before each dose; monitor I&O ratio and weight every day in same clothing, using same scale, at same time of day
• Monitor height, weight, psychomotor development, and growth rate if given to a child
• Monitor T_3, T_4, FTIs, which are decreased; radioimmunoassay of TSH, which is increased; radioactive iodine uptake (RA international units), which is increased if medication dose is too low
• Monitor pro-time; may require decreased anticoagulant; check for bleeding, bruising
• Assess for increased nervousness, excitability, irritability, which may indicate a too-high dose of medication, usually after 1-3 wk of treatment
• Assess cardiac status: angina, palpitations, chest pain, change in VS; the geriatric patient may have undetected cardiac problems, and baseline ECG should be completed before treatment

Nursing diagnoses
• Knowledge, deficient (teaching)
• Noncompliance (teaching)

Patient/family education
• Teach patient that product is not a cure but controls symptoms, treatment is long term
• Instruct patient to report excitability, irritability, anxiety, sweating, heat intolerance, chest pain, palpitations, which indicate overdose
• Advise patient not to switch brands unless approved by prescriber; bioavailability may differ
• Teach patient that product might be discontinued after giving birth; thyroid panel will be evaluated after 1-2 mo
• Teach patient that hyperthyroid child will show almost immediate behavior/personality change; that hair loss will occur in child but is temporary
• Caution patient that product is not to be taken to reduce weight
• Caution patient to avoid OTC preparations with iodine; read labels; other medications should not be used unless approved by prescriber
• Teach patient to avoid iodine-rich food: iodized salt, soybeans, tofu, turnips, high iodine seafood, some bread

Evaluation
Positive therapeutic outcome
• Absence of depression
• Weight loss
• Increased diuresis, pulse, appetite
• Absence of constipation, peripheral edema, cold intolerance, pale cool dry skin, brittle nails, alopecia, coarse hair, menorrhagia, night blindness, paresthesias, syncope, stupor, coma, rosy cheeks
• Improved levels of T_3, T_4 by laboratory tests
• Child: age-appropriate weight, height, and psychomotor development

TREATMENT OF OVERDOSE:
Withhold dose for up to 1 wk; acute overdose: gastric lavage or induce emesis, then activated charcoal; provide supportive treatment to control symptoms

liraglutide (Rx)
(lir′a-gloo′tide)
Victoza
Func. class.: Antidiabetic agent
Chem. class.: Incretin mimetics
Pregnancy category C

ACTION: Improved glycemic control and potential weight loss via activation of the glucagon-like peptide-1 (GLP-1) receptor

Therapeutic outcome: Stable and improved serum glucose, HbA1C, weight loss

USES: Type 2 diabetes mellitus in combination with diet and exercise

CONTRAINDICATIONS:
Hypersensitivity

Precautions: Alcoholism, breastfeeding, burns, children, cholelithiasis, type 1 diabetes mellitus, ketoacidosis, diarrhea, elderly, fever, gastroparesis, hepatic disease, hypoglycemia, infection, pancreatitis, renal disease, surgery, thyroid disease, trauma, vomiting, pregnancy **C**

BLACK BOX WARNING: Medullary thyroid carcinoma (MTC), multiple endocrine neoplasia syndrome type 2 (MEN 2), thyroid cancer

Adverse effects: *italics* = common; **bold** = life-threatening

DOSAGE AND ROUTES

Adult: Subcut 0.6 mg q day × 1 wk, then increase to 1.2 mg q day, max 1.8 mg/day

Available forms: Solution for injection 18mg/3 ml prefilled pen

Implementation
SUBCUT route

• Give by subcut only, inspect for particulate matter or discoloration, do not use if unusually viscous, cloudy, discolored, or if particles are present; give daily at any time without regard to meals; pen needles must be purchased separately, use Novo Nordisk needles, prime before first use, see manual for directions; give in thigh, abdomen, or upper arm; lightly pinch fold of skin, insert needle at 90-degree angle or 45-degree angle if thin, release skin, aspiration is not needed, give over 6 seconds, rotate injection sites

• Storage: do not store pen with needle attached; avoid direct heat and sunlight, discard 30 days after first use, after first use may be stored at room temperature or refrigerated, do not freeze

ADVERSE EFFECTS

CNS: Dizziness, headache
CV: Hypertension
ENDO: Hypoglycemia
EENT: Sinusitis
GI: Abdominal pain, anorexia, constipation, diarrhea, dyspepsia, nausea, vomiting, **pancreatitis**
INTEG: **Angioedema,** erythema, injection site reaction, urticaria
MS: Back pain
SYST: Antibody formation, infection, influenza, **secondary thyroid malignancy**

Pharmacokinetics

Absorption	Protein binding (98%)
Distribution	Binds to albumin, then released into circulation
Metabolism	Unknown
Excretion	Unknown
Half-life	12-13 hr

Pharmacodynamics

Onset	Unknown
Peak	Peak 8-12 hr
Duration	Unknown

INTERACTIONS
Individual drugs

Dexfenfluramine, fenfluramine, disopyramide, fluoxetine, mecasermin, octreotide, pegvisomant, salicylates: increased hypoglycemic reactions

Baclofen, cycloSPORINE, tacrolimus, dextrothyroxine, diazoxide, phenytoin, fosphenytoin, ethotoin, isoniazid, niacin, nicotine: increased hyperglycemic reactions

Bortezomib, cloNIDine, alcohol, lithium, pentamidine: increased or decreased hypoglycemic reactions

Atorvastatin, acetaminophen, griseofulvin: increased or decreased effects of each specific drug

Drug classifications

Angiotensin II receptor antagonists, ACE inhibitors, other antidiabetics, β-blockers, fibric acid derivatives, MAOIs, salicylates: increased hypoglycemic reactions

Protease inhibitors, phenothiazines, atypical antipsychotics, corticosteroids, carbonic anhydrase inhibitors, estrogens, progestins, oral contraceptives, growth hormones, sympathomimetics: increased hyperglycemic reactions

Androgens, quinolones: increased or decreased hypoglycemic reactions

NURSING CONSIDERATIONS

> **BLACK BOX WARNING:** Thyroid C-cell tumors: monitor during treatment

Assessment

• Watch for hypoglycemic reactions that can occur soon after meals: hunger, sweating, weakness, dizziness, tremors, restlessness, tachycardia
• Assess for hypersensitivity to this product
• Monitor serum glucose, A1c, CBC during treatment
• **Assess for stress:** diabetic patients exposed to stress, surgery, fever, infections may require insulin administration temporarily
• **Assess for serious skin reactions:** angioedema, pancreatitis, secondary thyroid malignancy

Nursing diagnoses

• Imbalanced nutrition: more than body requirements (uses)
• Noncompliance (teaching)

Patient/family education

• Teach patient the symptoms of hypo/hyper-glycemia and what to do about each, to have glucagon emergency kit available, carry a carbohydrate source at all times

• Teach patient about side effects associated with therapy such as nausea and vomiting; upward dose titration can be delayed or ignored depending on tolerance

• Teach patient that diabetes is a life-long illness, product does not cure disease and must be continued on a daily basis

• Instruct patient to carry emergency ID with prescriber's phone number and medications taken

• Advise patient to continue with other recommendations: diet, exercise, hygiene

• Teach patient to test blood glucose using a blood glucose meter

• Advise patient to avoid other medications, herbs, supplements unless approved by prescriber

• Advise patient to report serious skin effects, abdominal pain with nausea/vomiting

• Provide patient with written instructions if self-administration is ordered

Evaluation

Positive therapeutic outcome

• Stable and improved serum glucose, A1C, weight loss

lisdexamfetamine (Rx)

(lis-dex'am-fet'a-meen)

Vyvanse

Func. class.: CNS stimulant
Chem. class.: Amphetamine

Pregnancy category C
Controlled substance schedule II

ACTION: Increases release of norepinephrine, dopamine in cerebral cortex to reticular activating system

Therapeutic outcome: Ability to focus, decreased hyperactivity

USES: Attention-deficit disorder with hyperactivity (ADHD)

CONTRAINDICATIONS:

Hyperthyroidism, hypertension, glaucoma, severe arteriosclerosis, CV disease, anxiety, breastfeeding, hypersensitivity to sympathomimetic amines

---

BLACK BOX WARNING: Substance abuse

Precautions: Pregnancy **C**, children <6 yr, Tourette's syndrome, depression, anorexia nervosa, psychosis, seizure disorder, suicidal ideation, MI, heart failure, alcoholism, aortic stenosis, bipolar disorder

DOSAGE AND ROUTES

Child 6-12 yr: PO 30 mg/day in the AM, may increase by 20 mg/day at weekly intervals; max 70 mg/day

Available forms: Caps 30, 50, 70 mg

Implementation

• Provide gum, hard candy, frequent sips of water for dry mouth

BLACK BOX WARNING: Before giving this product, identify substance abuse; there is a high potential for abuse

ADVERSE EFFECTS

CNS: *Hyperactivity, insomnia, restlessness, talkativeness,* dizziness, headache, dysphoria, irritability, aggressiveness, CNS tumor, dependence, addiction, mild euphoria, somnolence, lability, psychosis, mania, hallucinations, aggression

CV: *Palpitations, tachycardia,* hypertension, decrease in heart rate, **dysrhythmias,** MI, **cardiomyopathy**

EENT: Blurred vision, mydriasis, diplopia

ENDO: Growth inhibition

GI: *Anorexia,* dry mouth, diarrhea, weight loss

GU: Impotence, change in libido

INTEG: Urticaria, **angioedema, Stevens-Johnson syndrome, toxic epidermal necrolysis**

Pharmacokinetics

Absorption	Unknown
Distribution	Crosses placenta, breast milk
Metabolism	Liver
Excretion	Urine pH dependent
Half-life	<1 hr

Pharmacodynamics

Unknown

INTERACTIONS

Individual drugs

AcetaZOLAMIDE, sodium bicarbonate: increased lisdexamfetamine effect

---

Ascorbic acid, ammonium chloride: decreased lisdexamfetamine effect

Haloperidol, meperidine, modafinil, PHENobarbital, phenytoin: increased CNS effect

Melatonin: increased CNS stimulation

Phenytoin: decreased absorption

Drug classifications

Adrenergic blockers, antidiabetics: decreased effect

Antacids: increased lisdexamfetamine effect

⚠ MAOIs or within 14 days of MAOIs: hypertensive crisis

Phenothiazines, tricyclics: increased CNS effect

Urinary acidifiers: decreased lisdexamfetamine effect

Urinary alkalinizers: increased lisdexamfetamine effect

Drug/herb

Eucalyptus: decreased stimulant effect

Green tea, guarana, khat, melatonin: increased stimulant effect

St. John's wort: serotonin syndrome

Drug/food

Caffeine: increased amine effect

NURSING CONSIDERATIONS

Assessment

• Monitor VS, B/P; this product may reverse antihypertensives; check patients with cardiac disease often

• Monitor CBC, urinalysis; in diabetes: blood glucose; insulin changes may be required, since eating may decrease

• **Serotonin syndrome, neuroleptic malignant syndrome:** Assess for increased heart rate, shivering, sweating, dilated pupils, tremors, high B/P, hyperthermia, headache, confusion; if these occur, stop product, administer a serotonin antagonist if needed; at lease 2 wk should elapse between discontinuation of serotonergic agents and start of this product

• Monitor height, growth rate in children; growth rate may be decreased

• Assess mental status: mood, sensorium, affect, stimulation, insomnia, irritability

• Assess for tolerance or dependency: an increased amount may be used to get same effect; will develop after long-term use

• Assess for overdose: pain, fever, dehydration, insomnia, hyperactivity

Nursing diagnoses

• Knowledge, deficient (teaching)

• Noncompliance (teaching)

Patient/family education

• Advise patient to decrease caffeine consumption (coffee, tea, cola, chocolate); may increase irritability, stimulation

• Advise patient to avoid OTC preparations unless approved by prescriber

• Teach patient to taper product over several weeks; depression, increased sleeping, lethargy

• Advise to take every day in AM

• Give without regard to meals

• Caps: may take whole or opened with contents dissolved in water and taken

• Avoid breastfeeding

• Advise to use as part of a comprehensive treatment program

• Caution patient to avoid alcohol ingestion

• Advise patient to avoid hazardous activities until stabilized on medication

• Instruct patient to get needed rest; patient will feel more tired at end of day

Evaluation

Positive therapeutic outcome

• Ability to stay on task, decreased hyperactivity

TREATMENT OF OVERDOSE:

Administer fluids, antihypertensive for increased B/P, ammonium chloride for increased excretion, chlorproMAZINE to antagonize CNS effect

lisinopril (Rx)

(lyse-in'oh-pril)

Zestril

Func. class.: Antihypertensive, angiotensin converting enzyme (ACE) I inhibitor

Chem. class.: Enalaprilat lysine analog

Pregnancy category D

Do not confuse:

lisinopril/Risperdal,
Prinivil/Plendil/Prilosec/Proventil

ACTION: Selectively suppresses renin-angiotensin-aldosterone system; inhibits ACE; prevents conversion of angiotensin I to angiotensin II

Therapeutic outcome: Decreased B/P in hypertension, decreased preload, afterload in CHF

USES: Mild to moderate hypertension, adjunctive therapy of systolic CHF, acute MI

CONTRAINDICATIONS:

Hypersensitivity, angioedema

⚠ Nurse Alert

BLACK BOX WARNING: Pregnancy **D** (2nd/3rd trimesters)

Precautions: Pregnancy **C** (1st trimester), breastfeeding, renal disease, hyperkalemia, renal artery stenosis, CHF

DOSAGE AND ROUTES

Hypertension
Adult: PO 10-40 mg/day; may increase to 80 mg/day if required
Child ≥6 yr: PO 0.7 mg/kg q day, up to 5 mg/day; titrate q1-2wk up to 0.6 mg/kg/day or 40 mg/day
Geriatric: PO 2.5-5 mg/day, increase q7day

CHF
Adult: PO 5 mg initially with diuretics/digoxin, range 5-40 mg

Acute myocardial infarction
Adults who are hemodynamically stable: PO give 5 mg within 24 hr of onset of symptoms, then 5 mg after 24 hr, 10 mg after 48 hr, then 10 mg q day

Renal dose
Adult: PO CCr <30 ml/min reduce dose by 50%, initially 5 mg/day, max 40 mg/day; CCr <10 ml/min 2.5 mg/day, max 40 mg/day

Available forms: Tabs 2.5, 5, 10, 20, 30 40 mg

Implementation
• Store in airtight container at 86° F (30° C) or less
• Severe hypotension may occur after 1st dose of this medication; may be prevented by reducing or discontinuing diuretic therapy 3 days before beginning lisinopril therapy

ADVERSE EFFECTS
CNS: *Vertigo,* depression, **stroke,** insomnia, paresthesias, *headache,* fatigue, asthenia, dizziness
CV: Chest pain, hypotension, sinus tachycardia
EENT: Blurred vision, nasal congestion
GI: Nausea, vomiting, anorexia, constipation, flatulence, GI irritation, diarrhea, **hepatic failure, hepatic necrosis**
GU: **Proteinuria, renal insufficiency,** sexual dysfunction, impotence
INTEG: Rash, pruritus
MISC: Muscle cramps, hyperkalemia
RESP: Dry cough, dyspnea
SYST: **Angioedema, anaphylaxis, toxic epidermal necrolysis**

Pharmacokinetics
Absorption	Variable
Distribution	Unknown
Metabolism	Not metabolized
Excretion	Kidneys, unchanged
Half-life	12 hr

Pharmacodynamics
Onset	1 hr
Peak	6-8 hr
Duration	24 hr

INTERACTIONS

Individual drugs
Alcohol (large amounts), probenecid: increased hypotension
Allopurinol: increased hypersensitivity
Aspirin: decreased lisinopril effect
CycloSPORINE: increased hyperkalemia
Indomethacin: decreased antihypertensive effect
Lithium: increased levels of lithium, toxicity

Drug classifications
Antihypertensives, diuretics, nitrates, phenothiazines: increased hypotension
Diuretics, potassium-sparing, potassium salt substitutes, potassium supplements: increased hyperkalemia
NSAIDs: decreased lisinopril effect

Drug/food
High-potassium diet (bananas, orange juice, avocados, broccoli, nuts, spinach) should be avoided; hyperkalemia may occur

Drug/lab test
Interference: glucose/insulin tolerance tests, ANA titer

NURSING CONSIDERATIONS

Assessment
• Assess blood studies: platelets, WBC with differential: baseline, q3mo; if neutrophils are <1000/mm^3, discontinue treatment
• **Hypertension:** monitor B/P, check for orthostatic hypotension, syncope; if changes occur, dosage change may be required
• Establish baselines in renal/liver function tests before therapy begins
• Monitor renal/liver function tests: protein, BUN, creatinine; watch for increased levels that may indicate nephrotic syndrome and renal failure; monitor renal symptoms: polyuria, oliguria, frequency, dysuria
• Check potassium levels throughout treatment, although hyperkalemia rarely occurs

• **CHF:** check for edema in feet, legs daily, weight daily, dyspnea, wet crackles
• Assess for anaphylaxis, toxic epidermal necrolysis, angioedema, allergic reactions: rash, fever, pruritus, urticaria; facial swelling, dyspnea, tongue swelling (rare); product should be discontinued if antihistamines fail to help

Nursing diagnoses
• Cardiac output, decreased (uses)
• Injury, risk for (side effects)
• Knowledge, deficient (teaching)
• Noncompliance (teaching)

Patient/family education
• Caution patient not to discontinue product abruptly; advise patient to inform all health care providers about taking this product
• Teach patient not to use OTC products (cough, cold, allergy) unless directed by prescriber; serious side effects can occur
• Teach patient the importance of complying with dosage schedule, even if feeling better; to continue with medical regimen to decrease B/P: exercise, cessation of smoking, decreasing stress, diet modifications
• Teach patient to notify prescriber of mouth sores, sore throat, fever, swelling of hands or feet, irregular heartbeat, chest pain, coughing, shortness of breath
• Caution patient to report excessive perspiration, dehydration, vomiting, diarrhea; may lead to fall in B/P
• Emphasize the need to rise slowly to sitting or standing position to minimize orthostatic hypotension; not to exercise in hot weather or increased hypotension can occur
• Caution patient that product may cause dizziness, fainting, light-headedness; may occur during 1st few days of therapy; to avoid activities that may be hazardous
• Teach patient how to take B/P, and normal readings for age-group; advise patient to take B/P regularly
• Instruct patient to avoid increasing potassium in the diet

> **BLACK BOX WARNING:** Advise patient to report if pregnancy is planned or suspected (pregnancy **D**), 2nd/3rd trimesters

Evaluation
Positive therapeutic outcome
• Decreased B/P in hypertension
• Decreased CHF symptoms

TREATMENT OF OVERDOSE:
0.9% NaCl **IV** inf, hemodialysis

lithium (Rx)
(li'thee-um)
Carbolith ✦, Duralith ✦, Lithobid
Func. class.: Antimanic, antipsychotic
Chem. class.: Alkali metal ion salt
Pregnancy category D

ACTION: May alter sodium, potassium ion transport across cell membrane in nerve, muscle cells; may balance biogenic amines of norepinephrine, serotonin in CNS areas involved in emotional responses

Therapeutic outcome: Stable mood

USES: Bipolar disorder (manic phase), prevention of bipolar manic-depressive psychosis

CONTRAINDICATIONS:
Pregnancy **D**, breastfeeding, children <12 yr, hepatic disease, brain trauma, organic brain syndrome, schizophrenia, severe cardiac/renal disease, severe dehydration

Precautions: Geriatric, thyroid disease, seizure disorders, diabetes mellitus, systemic infection, urinary retention

> **BLACK BOX WARNING:** Lithium level >1.5 mmol/L

DOSAGE AND ROUTES
Adult: PO 300-600 mg tid; maintenance 300 mg tid or qid; SLOW REL Tab 300 mg bid; dosage should be individualized to maintain blood levels at 0.5-1.5 mEq/L
Geriatric: PO 300 mg bid, increase q7day by 300 mg to desired dose
Child: PO 15-20 mg/kg/day in 3-4 divided doses; increase as needed; do not exceed adult doses; maintain blood levels at 0.4-0.5 mEq/L

Renal dose
Adult: PO CCr 10-50 ml/min 50%-75% of dose; CCr <10 ml/min 25%-50% of dose

Available forms: Caps 150, 300, 600 mg; tabs 300 mg; ext rel tabs 300, 450 mg; syr 300 mg/5 ml (8 mEq/5 ml); slow rel caps 150, 300 mg ✦

Implementation
• Do not break, crush, or chew caps and slow rel caps
• Administer reduced dosage to geriatric; give with meals to avoid GI upset

- Provide adequate fluids (2-3 L/day) to prevent dehydration during initial treatment, 1-2 L/day during maintenance
- Give list of products that interact with lithium

ADVERSE EFFECTS

CNS: *Headache, drowsiness, dizziness, tremors,* twitching, ataxia, **seizures,** slurred speech, restlessness, *confusion,* stupor, memory loss, clonic movements, *fatigue*
CV: *Hypotension,* ECG changes, **dysrhythmias, circulatory collapse, edema**
EENT: Tinnitus, blurred vision
ENDO: Hypothyroidism, goiter, hyperglycemia, hyperthyroidism, hyponatremia
GI: *Dry mouth, anorexia, nausea, vomiting, diarrhea,* incontinence, abdominal pain, metallic taste
GU: **Polyuria, glycosuria, proteinuria, albuminuria,** urinary incontinence, polydipsia
HEMA: Leukocytosis
INTEG: Drying of hair, alopecia, rash, pruritus, hyperkeratosis, *acneiform rash, folliculitis*
MS: *Muscle weakness*

Pharmacokinetics

Absorption	Completely absorbed
Distribution	Reabsorbed by renal tubules (80%); crosses blood-brain barrier; crosses placenta
Metabolism	Unknown
Excretion	Urine, unchanged
Half-life	18-36 hr depending on age

Pharmacodynamics

Onset	Rapid
Peak	$1/2$-12 hr
Duration	Unknown

INTERACTIONS

Individual drugs
AcetaZOLAMIDE, aminophylline, mannitol, sodium bicarbonate: increased renal clearance
Calcium iodide, iodinated glycerol, potassium iodide: increased hypothyroid effect
CarBAMazepine, fluoxetine, methyldopa, probenecid: increased lithium effect/toxicity
Haloperidol: increased neurotoxicity
Indomethacin, losartan: increased toxicity
Thioridazine: brain damage
Urea: decreased lithium effect

Drug classifications
Antithyroid agents: increased hypothyroid effects
β-Blockers used for lithium tremor: increase masking of lithium toxicity

Neuromuscular blocking agents: increased effect of neuromuscular blocking effects
NSAIDs, thiazides: increased lithium toxicity
Phenothiazines: increased effect of phenothiazines
Theophyllines, urinary alkalinizers: decreased effect of lithium

Drug/herb
Guarana, tea (black/green): decreased lithium effect
- Avoid use with kava, St. John's wort, valerian

Drug/food
Significant changes in sodium intake will alter lithium excretion

Drug/lab test
Increased: potassium excretion, urine glucose, blood glucose, protein, BUN
Decreased: VMA, T_3, T_4, PBI, ^{131}I

NURSING CONSIDERATIONS

Assessment
- **Bipolar disorder:** manic symptoms, mood, behavior before and during treatment
- **Assess for lithium toxicity:** Vomiting, diarrhea, poor coordination, fine motor tremors, weakness, lassitude; major toxicity: coarse tremors, severe thirst, tinnitus, dilute urine
- Assess weight daily; check for edema in legs, ankles, wrists; report if present; check skin turgor at least daily
- Monitor sodium intake; decreased sodium intake with decreased fluid intake may lead to lithium retention; increased sodium and fluids may decrease lithium retention
- Monitor urine for albuminuria, glycosuria, uric acid during beginning treatment, q2mo thereafter
- Assess neurologic status: LOC, gait, motor reflexes, hand tremors

BLACK BOX WARNING: Monitor serum lithium levels weekly initially, then q2mo (therapeutic level: 0.5-1.5 mEq/L); toxic level >1.5 mcg/L; toxicity and therapeutic levels are very close; toxicity may occur rapidly; blood levels are measured before the AM dose

Nursing diagnoses
- Coping, ineffective (uses)
- Knowledge, deficient (teaching)
- Noncompliance (teaching)

Patient/family education
- Provide patient with written information on symptoms of **minor toxicity:** vomiting, diarrhea, poor coordination, fine motor tremors,

weakness, lassitude; **major toxicity:** coarse tremors, severe thirst, tinnitus, dilute urine
• Advise patient to monitor urine specific gravity; emphasize need for follow-up care to determine lithium effects
• Advise patient that contraception is necessary, since lithium may harm fetus, pregnancy **D**
• Caution patient not to operate machinery until lithium levels are stable and response determined; that beneficial effects may take 1-3 wk
• Provide to the patient a list of products that interact with lithium and discuss need for adequate, stable intake of salt and fluid
• Advise to have lithium levels monitored to ensure effectiveness

Evaluation
Positive therapeutic outcome
• Decrease in excitement, poor judgment, insomnia (manic phase)
• Decreased mood swings and lability

TREATMENT OF OVERDOSE:
Induce emesis or lavage, maintain airway, respiratory function; dialysis for severe intoxication

Iodoxamide ophthalmic
See Appendix B

loperamide (OTC, Rx)
(loe-per'a-mide)
Anti-Diarrheal, Equaline Anti-Diarrheal ✿, Good Sense Anti-Diarrheal, Imodium, Imodium A-D, Rx Choice Loperamide, Select Brand Anti-Diarrheal, Top Care Anti-Diarrheal, Walgreens Anti-Diarrheal
Func. class.: Antidiarrheal
Chem. class.: Piperidine derivative
Pregnancy category C

Do not confuse:
Imodium/Indocin, Loperimide/furosemide

ACTION: Direct action on intestinal muscles to decrease GI peristalsis; reduces volume, increases bulk; electrolytes are not lost

Therapeutic outcome: Absence of diarrhea

USES: Diarrhea (cause undetermined), chronic diarrhea, to decrease amount of ileostomy discharge, traveler's diarrhea

CONTRAINDICATIONS:
Hypersensitivity, pseudomembranous colitis, constipation, dysentery, GI bleeding/obstruction/perforation, ileus, vomiting

Precautions: Pregnancy **C**, breastfeeding, children <2 yr, hepatic disease, gastroenteritis, toxic megacolon, geriatric patients, dehydration, bacterial disease, AIDS, severe ulcerative colitis

DOSAGE AND ROUTES
Adult: PO 4 mg, then 2 mg after each loose stool, max 16 mg/24 hr
Child 9-11 yr: PO 2 mg, then 1 mg after each loose stool, max 6 mg/24 hr
Child 6-8 yr: PO 2 mg, then 0.1 mg/kg after each loose stool, max 4 mg/day
Child 2-5 yr: PO 1 mg, then 0.1 mg/kg after each loose stool, max 4 mg/24 hr

Available forms: Caps 2 mg; liquid 1 mg/5 ml; tabs 2 mg

Implementation
• Do not break, crush, or chew caps
• Store in airtight containers
• Do not mix oral sol with other sol

ADVERSE EFFECTS
CNS: Dizziness, drowsiness, fatigue
GI: *Nausea, dry mouth, vomiting, constipation,* abdominal pain, anorexia, **toxic megacolon,** bacterial enterocolitis, flatulence
INTEG: Rash
MISC: Hyperglycemia
SYST: Anaphylaxis, angioedema, toxic epidermal necrolysis

Pharmacokinetics

Absorption	Poor
Distribution	Unknown
Metabolism	Liver
Excretion	Feces, unchanged; small amount in urine
Half-life	9-14 hr

Pharmacodynamics

Onset	$^{1}/_{2}$-1 hr
Peak	Unknown
Duration	4-5 hr

INTERACTIONS
Individual drugs
Alcohol: increased CNS depression

Drug classifications
Antihistamines, analgesics (opioids), sedative/hypnotics: increased CNS depression

⚠ Nurse Alert

Drug/herb
Chamomile, hops, kava, skullcap, valerian: increased CNS depression
Nutmeg: increased antidiarrheal effect

NURSING CONSIDERATIONS

Assessment
• Monitor electrolytes (potassium, sodium, chloride) if patient is on long-term therapy; check fluid status, skin turgor
• **Stools:** Assess bowel pattern before, during treatment; check for rebound constipation after termination of medication; check bowel sounds
• Check response after 48 hr; if no response, product should be discontinued and other treatment initiated
• Assess for abdominal distention, toxic megacolon, which may occur in ulcerative colitis
• Assess for dehydration, CNS symptoms in children or those with hepatic disease

Nursing diagnoses
• Constipation (adverse reactions)
• Diarrhea (uses)
• Knowledge, deficient (teaching)
• Noncompliance (teaching)

Patient/family education
• Caution patient to avoid alcohol and OTC products unless directed by prescriber; may cause increased CNS depression
• Advise patient not to exceed recommended dosage; product may be habit forming; ileostomy patient may take this product for extended time
• Advise patient that product may cause drowsiness and to avoid hazardous activities until response to product is determined
• Teach patient that dry mouth can be decreased by frequent sips of water, hard candy, sugarless gum

Evaluation
Positive therapeutic outcome
• Decreased diarrhea

loratadine (Rx, OTC)
(lor-a′ti-deen)
Alavert, Claritin, Children's Claritin RediTabs, Dimetapp, Equaline Non-Drowsy, Equate Allergy Relief, Good Sense Non-Drowsy, Leader Allergy Relief, Leader Loratadine, Tavist ND, Walgreens Loratadine, Wal-itin Aller-Melts, Wal-vert
Func. class.: Antihistamine (2nd generation)
Chem. class.: Selective histamine (H_1) receptor antagonist
Pregnancy category B

Do not confuse:
loratadine/lovastatin/LORazepam/losartan

ACTION: Binds to peripheral histamine receptors, which provides antihistamine action without sedation

Therapeutic outcome: Decreased nasal stuffiness, itching, swollen eyes

USES: Seasonal rhinitis, chronic idiopathic urticaria for those ≥2 yr

CONTRAINDICATIONS: Hypersensitivity, acute asthma attacks, lower respiratory tract disease

Precautions: Pregnancy **B,** increased intraocular pressure, bronchial asthma, breastfeeding, hepatic/renal disease

DOSAGE AND ROUTES
Adult and child ≥6 yr: PO 10 mg/day
Child 2-5 yr: PO 5 mg/day

Renal dose
Adult: PO CCr <30 ml/min 10 mg every other day

Hepatic dose
Adult: PO 10 mg every other day

Available forms: Tabs 10 mg; rapid-disintegrating tabs 10 mg; orally disintegrating tabs 10 mg; syr 1 mg/ml; susp 5 mg/ml

Implementation
• Give on an empty stomach, 1 hr before or 2 hr after meals to facilitate absorption
• **Rapid-disintegrating tabs:** Place rapidly disintegrating tabs on tongue, then swallow after disintegrated with or without water

L

- Use within 6 mo of opening pouch; immediately after opening blister pack
- Store in airtight, light-resistant container

ADVERSE EFFECTS

CNS: Sedation (more common with increased dosages), headache, fatigue, restlessness
CV: Sinus tachycardia
RESP: Wheezing

Pharmacokinetics

Absorption	Well absorbed
Distribution	Unknown
Metabolism	Liver, extensively, to active metabolite desloratadine
Excretion	Kidneys
Half-life	17-28 hr

Pharmacodynamics

Onset	1-3 hr
Peak	8-12 hr
Duration	>24 hr

INTERACTIONS

Individual drugs
Alcohol: increased CNS depression
Cimetidine, ketoconazole: increased loratadine level

Drug classifications
Antidepressants, antihistamines (other), sedative-hypnotics: increased CNS depression
Macrolides (clarithromycin, erythromycin): increased loratadine level
MAOIs: increased antihistamine effects

Drug/lab test
False negative: skin allergy tests (discontinue antihistamine 3 days before testing)

NURSING CONSIDERATIONS

Assessment
- **Assess allergy:** hives, rash, rhinitis
- Assess respiratory status: rate, rhythm, increase in bronchial secretions, wheezing, chest tightness; provide fluids to 2 L/day to decrease secretion thickness
- Monitor LFTs, serum creatinine/BUN

Nursing diagnoses
- Knowledge, deficient (teaching)
- Noncompliance (teaching, overuse)

Patient/family education
- Teach all aspects of product uses; to notify prescriber if confusion, sedation, hypotension occur; to avoid driving and other hazardous activity if drowsiness occurs; to avoid alcohol and other CNS depressants that may potentiate effect
- Teach patient to take 1 hr before or 2 hr after meals to facilitate absorption
- Advise patient to use sunscreen or stay out of the sun to prevent burns
- Caution patient not to exceed recommended dosage; dysrhythmias may occur
- Teach patient that hard candy, gum, frequent rinsing of mouth may be used for dryness

Evaluation
Positive therapeutic outcome
- Absence of runny or congested nose, other allergy symptoms

LORazepam (Rx)
(lor-az′e-pam)
Ativan
Func. class.: Sedative-hypnotic, antianxiety agent
Chem. class.: Benzodiazepine, short acting
Pregnancy category D
Controlled substance schedule IV

Do not confuse:
LORazepam/ALPRAZolam/clonazePAM

ACTION: Potentiates the actions of GABA, an inhibitory neurotransmitter, especially in the limbic system and reticular formation, which depresses the CNS

Therapeutic outcome: Decreased anxiety, relaxation

USES: Anxiety, irritability in psychiatric or organic disorders, preoperatively; adjunct in endoscopic procedures, status epilepticus

Unlabeled uses: Antiemetic before chemotherapy, rectal use, insomnia

CONTRAINDICATIONS:
Pregnancy **D**, breastfeeding, hypersensitivity to benzodiazepines/benzyl alcohol, closed-angle glaucoma, psychosis, history of drug abuse, COPD, sleep apnea

Precautions: Geriatric, debilitated patients, children <12 yr, renal/hepatic disease, addiction, suicidal ideation, abrupt discontinuation

DOSAGE AND ROUTES
Anxiety
Adult/adolescent: PO 2-3 mg/day in divided doses, max 10 mg/day
Geriatric: PO 1-2 mg/day in divided doses, or 0.5-1 mg at bedtime

Insomnia (unlabeled)
Adult: PO 2-4 mg at bedtime; only minimally effective after 2 wk continuous therapy
Geriatric: PO 0.5-1 mg initially

Preoperatively
Adult: IM 50 mcg/kg 2 hr before surgery; **IV** 44 mcg/kg 15-20 min before surgery, max 2 mg 15-20 min before surgery
Child ≥12 yr: **IV** 0.05 mg/kg

Status epilepticus
Neonate: IV 0.05 mg/kg
Child: IV 0.1 mg/kg up to 4 mg/dose; RECT (unlabeled) 0.05-0.1 mg × 2; wait 7 min before giving 2nd dose

Available forms: Tabs 0.5, 1, 2 mg; inj 2, 4 mg/ml; conc sol 2 mg/ml

Implementation
PO route
• Give largest dose before bedtime if giving in divided dose
• Concentrate: use calibrated dropper; add to food/drink, consume immediately
• Give with food or milk for GI symptoms; crush tab if patient is unable to swallow medication whole; provide sugarless gum, hard candy, frequent sips of water for dry mouth
SUBCUT route
• Use by SUBCUT route for rapid response (investigational use)
IM route
• Give deep in muscle mass; if using for preoperative sedation, give 2 hr or more before surgical procedure
Direct IV route
• Prepare immediately before use; short stability time
• Dilute with sterile water for inj, 0.9% NaCl, or D₅W just before using; give by Y-site or 3-way stopcock at 2 mg/min
• Do not use sol that is discolored or contains a precipitate

Y-site compatibilities: Acyclovir, albumin, allopurinol, amifostine, amikacin, amoxicillin, amoxicillin/clavulanate, amphotericin B cholesteryl, amsacrine, atenolol, atracurium, bivalirudin, bleomycin, bumetanide, butorphanol, calcium chloride/gluconate, CARBOplatin, ceFAZolin, cefepime, cefotaxime, cefotetan, cefoxitin, ceftazidime, ceftizoxime, ceftobiprole, cefTRIAXone, cefuroxime, chloramphenicol, chlorproMAZINE, cimetidine, ciprofloxacin, cisatracurium, CISplatin, cladribine, clindamycin, cloNIDine, cyclophosphamide, cycloSPORINE, cytarabine, DACTINomycin, DAPTOmycin, dexamethasone, dexmedetomidine, diltiazem, DOBUTamine, docetaxel, DOPamine, doripenem, DOXOrubicin, DOXOrubicin liposomal, droperidol, enalaprilat, ePHEDrine, EPINEPHrine, epirubicin, eptifibatide, erythromycin, esmolol, etomidate, famotidine, fenoldopam, fentaNYL, filgrastim, fluconazole, fludarabine, fosphenytoin, furosemide, ganciclovir, gatifloxacin, gemcitabine, gentamicin, glycopyrrolate, granisetron, haloperidol, heparin, hydrocortisone, HYDROmorphone, hydrOXYzine, ifosfamide, inamrinone, insulin (regular), irinotecan, isoproterenol, ketorolac, labetalol, lidocaine, linezolid, magnesium sulfate, mannitol, mechlorethamine, melphalan, meropenem, metaraminol, methadone, methotrexate, methyldopate, methylPREDNISolone, metoclopramide, metoprolol, metroNIDAZOLE, micafungin, midazolam, milrinone, minocycline, mitoxantrone, morphine, mycophenolate, nafcillin, nalbuphine, naloxone, nesiritide, niCARdipine, nitroglycerin, nitroprusside, norepinephrine, octreotide, oxaliplatin, oxytocin, paclitaxel, palonosetron, pamidronate, pancuronium, pemetrexed, pentamidine, PENTobarbital, PHENobarbital, piperacillin, piperacillin-tazobactam, polymyxin B, potassium chloride, propofol, ranitidine, remifentanil, tacrolimus, teniposide, theophylline, thiotepa, ticarcillin, ticarcillin-clavulanate, tigecycline, tirofiban, tobramycin, TPN, trastuzumab, trimethobenzamide, trimethoprim-sulfamethoxazole, vancomycin, vasopressin, vecuronium, verapamil, vinCRIStine, vinorelbine, voriconazole, zidovudine

Y-site incompatibilities: IDArubicin, ondansetron, sargramostim

ADVERSE EFFECTS
CNS: *Dizziness, drowsiness,* confusion, headache, anxiety, tremors, stimulation, fatigue, depression, insomnia, hallucinations, weakness, unsteadiness
CV: *Orthostatic hypotension,* **ECG changes, tachycardia,** hypotension, **apnea, cardiac arrest (IV, rapid)**
EENT: *Blurred vision,* tinnitus, mydriasis
GI: Constipation, dry mouth, nausea, vomiting, anorexia, diarrhea
INTEG: Rash, dermatitis, itching
MISC: Acidosis

Pharmacokinetics

Absorption	Well absorbed (PO); completely absorbed (IM)
Distribution	Widely distributed; crosses placenta, blood-brain barrier
Metabolism	Liver, extensively
Excretion	Kidneys, breast milk
Half-life	14 hr

Pharmacodynamics

	PO	IM	IV
Onset	$1/2$ hr	15-30 min	5-15 min
Peak	1-3 hr	1-1$1/2$ hr	Unknown
Duration	12-24 hr	6-8 hr	6-8 hr

INTERACTIONS

Individual drugs
Alcohol: increased CNS depression
Disulfiram: increased LORazepam effects
Valproic acid: decreased LORazepam effects

Drug classifications
CNS depressants, oral contraceptives: increased LORazepam effects

Drug/herb
Chamomile, hops, kava, lavender, valerian: increased CNS depression

Drug/lab test
Increased: AST, ALT, serum bilirubin
Decreased: radioactive iodine uptake
False increase: 17-OHCS

NURSING CONSIDERATIONS

Assessment
• **Assess degree of anxiety;** what precipitates anxiety and whether product controls symptoms; other signs of anxiety: dilated pupils, inability to sleep, restlessness, inability to focus
• **Assess for alcohol withdrawal symptoms,** including hallucinations (visual, auditory), delirium, irritability, agitation, fine to coarse tremors
• Monitor B/P (with patient lying/standing), pulse; check respiratory rate; if systolic B/P drops 20 mm Hg, hold product, notify prescriber; respirations q5-15min if given **IV**
• Monitor CBC during long-term therapy; blood dyscrasias have occurred (rare)

• Monitor for seizure control; type, duration, and intensity of seizures; what precipitates seizures
• Monitor hepatic studies: AST, ALT, bilirubin, creatinine, LDH, alkaline phosphatase
• Assess mental status: mood, sensorium, affect, sleeping pattern, drowsiness, dizziness, suicidal tendencies, and ability of product to control these symptoms; check for tolerance, withdrawal symptoms: headache, nausea, vomiting, muscle pain, weakness after long-term use

Nursing diagnoses
• Coping, ineffective (uses)
• Knowledge, deficient (teaching)
• Noncompliance (teaching)
• Sleep deprivation (uses)

Patient/family education
• Advise patient that product may be taken with food; that product is not to be used for everyday stress or used longer than 4 mo unless directed by a prescriber; to take no more than prescribed amount; may be habit forming
• Caution patient to avoid OTC preparations unless approved by prescriber; to avoid alcohol, other psychotropic medications unless prescribed by physician; not to discontinue medication abruptly after long-term use
• Inform patient to avoid driving and activities that require alertness; drowsiness may occur; to rise slowly or fainting may occur, especially in geriatric
• Inform patient that drowsiness may worsen at beginning of treatment

Evaluation
Positive therapeutic outcome
• Decreased anxiety, restlessness, insomnia

TREATMENT OF OVERDOSE:
Lavage, VS, supportive care

Iosartan (Rx)
(low-sar'tan)
Cozaar
Func. class.: Antihypertensive
Chem. class.: Angiotensin II receptor (type AT$_1$)
Pregnancy category C (1st trimester), D (2nd/3rd trimesters)

Do not confuse:
Iosartan/valsartan, **Cozaar**/Zocor

ACTION: Blocks the vasoconstrictor and aldosterone-secreting effects of angiotensin II;

selectively blocks the binding of angiotensin II to the AT_1 receptor found in tissues

Therapeutic outcome: Decreased B/P

USES: Hypertension, alone or in combination; nephropathy in type 2 diabetes, proteinuria, stroke prophylaxis in hypertensive patients with left ventricular hypertrophy

CONTRAINDICATIONS:
Hypersensitivity

> **BLACK BOX WARNING:** Pregnancy **D** (2nd/3rd trimesters)

Precautions: Pregnancy **C** (1st trimester), breastfeeding, children, geriatric, hypersensitivity to ACE inhibitors, hepatic disease, angioedema, renal artery stenosis, those of African descent

DOSAGE AND ROUTES
Hypertension
Adult: PO 50 mg/day alone or 25 mg/day when used in combination with diuretic; maintenance 25-100 mg/day
Child ≥6 yr: PO 0.7 mg/kg q day, max 50 mg/day

Hepatic dose
Adult: PO 25 mg/day as starting dose

Hypertension with left ventricular hypertrophy (benefit does not apply to those of African descent)
Adult: PO 50 mg/day, add hydrochlorothiazide 12.5 mg/day and/or increase losartan to 100 mg/day, then increase hydrochlorothiazide to 25 mg/day

Nephropathy in type 2 diabetes patients
Adult: PO 50 mg/day, may increase to 100 mg/day

Available forms: Tabs 25, 50, 100 mg

Implementation
• Administer without regard to meals

ADVERSE EFFECTS
CNS: *Dizziness, insomnia,* anxiety, confusion, abnormal dreams, migraine, tremor, vertigo, headache, malaise, depression
CV: Angina pectoris, 2nd-degree AV block, **CVA**, hypotension, **MI, dysrhythmias**
EENT: Blurred vision, burning eyes, conjunctivitis

GI: *Diarrhea, dyspepsia,* anorexia, constipation, dry mouth, flatulence, gastritis, vomiting
GU: Impotence, nocturia, urinary frequency, urinary tract infection, **renal failure**
HEMA: Anemia, **thrombocytopenia**
INTEG: Alopecia, dermatitis, dry skin, flushing, photosensitivity, rash, pruritus, sweating **angioedema**
META: Gout
MS: Cramps, myalgia, pain, stiffness
RESP: *Cough, upper respiratory infection,* congestion, dyspnea, bronchitis

Pharmacokinetics
Absorption	Well absorbed
Distribution	Bound to plasma proteins
Metabolism	Extensive
Excretion	Feces, urine
Half-life	Biphasic, 2 hr, 6-9 hr

Pharmacodynamics
Unknown

INTERACTIONS
Individual drugs
Fluconazole: increased antihypertensive effect
Lithium: increased toxicity
PHENobarbital, rifamycin: decreased antihypertensive effect

Drug classifications
ACE inhibitors, diuretics (potassium-sparing), potassium supplements: increased hyperkalemia
NSAIDs, salicylates: decreased antihypertensive effect

NURSING CONSIDERATIONS
Assessment
• Assess B/P with position changes, pulse q4hr; note rate, rhythm, quality
• Monitor electrolytes: potassium, sodium, chloride
• Obtain baselines for renal, liver function tests before therapy begins
• **CHF:** assess for jugular vein distention, weight daily, edema in feet, legs daily
• **Angioedema:** facial swelling, dyspnea, wheezing, may occur rapidly, tongue swelling (rare)
• **Blood dyscrasias:** thrombocytopenia, anemia (rare)

Nursing diagnoses
• Fluid volume, deficient (side effects)
• Noncompliance (teaching)
• Knowledge, deficient (teaching)

Patient/family education
• Teach patient to avoid sunlight or wear sunscreen if in sunlight; photosensitivity may occur
• Advise patient to comply with dosage schedule, even if feeling better
• Teach patient to notify prescriber of mouth sores, fever, swelling of hands or feet, irregular heartbeat, chest pain
• Advise patient that excessive perspiration, dehydration, vomiting, diarrhea may lead to fall in blood pressure, consult prescriber if these occur
• Inform patient that product may cause dizziness, fainting; light-headedness may occur
• Caution patient to rise slowly to sitting or standing position to minimize orthostatic hypotension

> **BLACK BOX WARNING:** Advise patient to use contraception while taking this product, pregnancy **D** 2nd/3rd trimesters

Evaluation
Positive therapeutic outcome
• Decreased B/P

loteprednol ophthalmic
See Appendix B

lovastatin (Rx)
(loe′va-sta-tin)
Altoprev, Mevacor
Func. class.: Antilipemic
Chem. class.: HMG-CoA reductase inhibitor
Pregnancy category X

Do not confuse:
lovastatin/Lotensin/Leustatin,
Mevacor/mivacron

ACTION: By inhibiting HMG-CoA reductase, which reduces cholesterol synthesis

Therapeutic outcome: Decreased cholesterol levels and LDL, increased HDL

USES: As an adjunct in primary hypercholesterolemia (types IIa, IIb), atherosclerosis, heterozygous familial hypercholesterolemia (adolescents)

CONTRAINDICATIONS:
Pregnancy **X**, breastfeeding, hypersensitivity, active liver disease

Precautions: Past liver disease, alcoholism, severe acute infections, trauma, hypotension, uncontrolled seizure disorders, severe metabolic disorders, electrolyte imbalances, visual condition, children

DOSAGE AND ROUTES
Adult: PO 20 mg/day with evening meal; may increase to 20-40 mg/day in single or divided doses; max 40 mg/day; EXT REL 20-60 mg/day at bedtime; max 40 mg/day

Heterozygous familial hypercholesterolemia
Adolescent 10-17 yr: PO 10-40 mg with evening meal

Renal dose
Adult: PO CCr <30 mg/min max 20 mg/day unless titrated

Available forms: Tabs 10, 20, 40 mg; ext rel tab (Altocor) 10, 20, 40, 60 mg

Implementation
• Give with evening meal; if dosage is increased, take with breakfast and evening meal
• Altroprev is not equivalent to Mevacor
• Store in cool environment in airtight, light-resistant container

ADVERSE EFFECTS
CNS: Dizziness, headache, tremor, insomnia, paresthesia
EENT: Blurred vision, lens opacities
GI: Nausea, constipation, diarrhea, dyspepsia, *flatus,* abdominal pain, heartburn, **liver dysfunction,** vomiting, acid regurgitation, dry mouth, dysgeusia
HEMA: Thrombocytopenia, hemolytic anemia, leukopenia
INTEG: Rash, pruritus, photosensitivity
MS: Muscle cramps, myalgia, **myositis, rhabdomyolysis;** leg, shoulder, or localized pain

Pharmacokinetics

Absorption	Poorly absorbed, erratic
Distribution	Crosses placenta, blood-brain barrier
Metabolism	Liver, extensively
Excretion	Feces (83%); kidneys, urine (10%)
Half-life	3-4 hr

Pharmacodynamics

Onset	Unknown
Peak	2-4 hr
Duration	Unknown

INTERACTIONS

Individual drugs

Bosentan, exonatide: decreased action of
lovastatin

Clarithromycin, clofibrate, cycloSPORINE,
dalfopristin, danazol, diltiazem, erythromycin,
gemfibrozil, niacin, quinupristin, telithromycin, verapamil: increased myalgia, myositis,
rhabdomyolysis

Diltiazem: increased lovastatin effects

Warfarin: increased bleeding

Drug classifications

Azole antifungals, protease inhibitors: increased
myositis, myalgia, rhabdomyolysis

Bile acid sequestrants: decreased lovastatin
effects

Drug/herb

Pectin, St. John's wort: decreased effect

Red yeast rice: increased adverse reactions

Drug/food

Increased levels of lovastatin with food, must be
taken with food

Grapefruit juice: increased toxicity

Oat bran: decreased absorption

Drug/lab test

Increased: CPK, liver function tests

NURSING CONSIDERATIONS

Assessment

• Assess nutrition: fat, protein, carbohydrates;
nutritional analysis should be completed by
dietitian before treatment

• Monitor bowel pattern daily; diarrhea may be
a problem

• Monitor triglycerides, fasting cholesterol LDL,
HDL at baseline, throughout treatment; watch
LDL and VLDL closely; if increased, product
should be discontinued

• Assess for muscle pain, tenderness, obtain
CPK; if these occur, product may need to be
discontinued

• **Rhabdomyolysis:** muscle pain, increased
CPK, weakness, swelling of affected muscles; if
these occur and if confirmed by CPK, product
should be discontinued

Nursing diagnoses

• Diarrhea (adverse reactions)

• Knowledge, deficient (teaching)

• Noncompliance (teaching)

Patient/family education

• Inform patient that compliance is needed for
positive results to occur; not to double doses

• Inform patient that blood work and ophthalmic exam will be necessary during treatment

• Teach patient that risk factors should be
decreased: high-fat diet, smoking, alcohol
consumption, absence of exercise

• Advise patient to report if pregnancy is suspected, pregnancy **X**, do not breastfeed

• Advise patient to notify prescriber if the GI
symptoms of diarrhea, abdominal or epigastric
pain, nausea, vomiting occur; or if chills, fever,
sore throat, blurred vision, dizziness, headache,
muscle pain, weakness occur

• Advise patient to stay out of the sun or use
sunscreen to prevent burns

Evaluation

Positive therapeutic outcome

• Decreased cholesterol, serum triglyceride
levels

• Improved level of HDL

loxapine (Rx)

(lox′a-peen)

Loxapac � , Loxitane

Func. class.: Antipsychotic/neuroleptic

Chem. class.: Dibenzoxazepine

Pregnancy category C

Do not confuse:
Loxitane/Soriatane

ACTION: Depresses cerebral cortex,
hypothalamus, limbic system, which control
activity and aggression; blocks neurotransmission produced by DOPamine at synapse; exhibits
strong α-adrenergic, anticholinergic blocking
action; mechanism for antipsychotic effects is
unclear

Therapeutic outcome: Decreased
psychotic behavior

USES: Psychotic disorders, nonpsychotic
symptoms associated with dementia

Unlabeled uses: Depression, anxiety

CONTRAINDICATIONS:
Hypersensitivity, blood dyscrasias, coma, severe
CNS depression, brain damage, bone marrow
depression, alcohol and barbiturate withdrawal
states, closed-angle glaucoma

Precautions: Pregnancy **C**, breastfeeding,
children <16 yr, geriatric, seizure disorders,
cardiac/renal/hepatic disease, prostatic hypertrophy, cardiac conditions

BLACK BOX WARNING: Dementia

DOSAGE AND ROUTES
Adult: PO 10 mg bid-qid initially; may be rapidly increased depending on severity of condition; maintenance 60-100 mg/day
Geriatric: PO 5-10 mg/day bid, increase q4-7day by 5-10 mg, max 250 mg/day

Available forms: Caps 5, 10, 25, 50 mg; conc 25 mg/ml; tabs 5, 10, 25, 50 mg

Implementation
PO route
• Administer product in liquid form mixed in glass of juice or soft drink if hoarding is suspected; do not mix in caffeine drinks, tannics, pectins
• Administer lowered dose in geriatric, since metabolism is slowed
• Administer with full glass of water or milk; or give with food to decrease GI upset
• Give antacids 2 hr before or after taking this product
• Store in airtight, light-resistant container, oral sol in amber bottle

ADVERSE EFFECTS
CNS: *EPS: pseudoparkinsonism, akathisia, dystonia, tardive dyskinesia, drowsiness, headache,* **seizures,** confusion, **neuroleptic malignant syndrome**
CV: *Orthostatic hypotension,* **cardiac arrest,** ECG changes, tachycardia
EENT: Blurred vision, glaucoma
GI: *Dry mouth, nausea, vomiting, anorexia, constipation,* diarrhea, jaundice, weight gain
GU: Urinary retention, urinary frequency, enuresis, impotence, amenorrhea, gynecomastia
HEMA: **Anemia, leukopenia, leukocytosis, agranulocytosis**
INTEG: *Rash,* photosensitivity, dermatitis
RESP: **Laryngospasm,** dyspnea, **respiratory depression**

Pharmacokinetics

Absorption	Well absorbed (PO)
Distribution	Unknown
Metabolism	Liver, extensively
Excretion	Kidneys
Half-life	Biphasic 5 hr, 19 hr

Pharmacodynamics

	PO
Onset	$1/2$ hr
Peak	2-4 hr
Duration	12 hr

INTERACTIONS
Individual drugs
Alcohol: increased CNS depression
EPINEPHrine: increased toxicity
Guanadrel, guanethidine, levodopa: decreased effects

Drug classifications
Antidepressants, MAOIs: increased CNS depression
Antipsychotics: increased EPS

NURSING CONSIDERATIONS
Assessment
• Assess mental status: orientation, mood, behavior, presence and type of hallucinations before initial administration, monthly; this product should significantly reduce psychotic behavior
• Check for swallowing of PO medication; check for hoarding or giving medication to other patients
• Monitor I&O ratio; palpate bladder if low urinary output occurs, especially in geriatric; urinalysis recommended before, during prolonged therapy, urinary retention may be cause
• Monitor bilirubin, CBC, LFTs monthly
• Assess affect, orientation, LOC, reflexes, gait, coordination, sleep pattern disturbances
• Monitor B/P with patient sitting, standing, and lying; take pulse and respirations q4hr during initial treatment; establish baseline before starting treatment; report drops of 30 mm Hg
• Check for dizziness, faintness, palpitations, tachycardia on rising; severe orthostatic hypotension is common
⚠ **Identify neuroleptic malignant syndrome: hyperpyrexia, muscle rigidity, increased CPK, altered mental status; product should be discontinued**
• **Assess for EPS,** including akathisia (inability to sit still, no pattern to movements), tardive dyskinesia (bizarre movements of the jaw, mouth, tongue, extremities), pseudoparkinsonism (ragged tremors, pill rolling, shuffling gait); an antiparkinsonian product should be prescribed
• Assess for constipation, urinary retention daily; if these occur, increase bulk, water in diet

Nursing diagnoses
• Coping, ineffective (uses)
• Knowledge, deficient (teaching)
• Noncompliance (teaching)

Patient/family education
• Teach patient to use good oral hygiene; suggest frequent rinsing of mouth, sugarless gum for dry mouth; oral candidiasis can occur
• Caution patient to avoid hazardous activities until product response is determined; dizziness, blurred vision may occur
• Inform patient that orthostatic hypotension occurs often and to rise from sitting or lying position gradually; caution patient to avoid hot tubs, hot showers, tub baths, since hypotension may occur; tell patient that in hot weather heat stroke may occur; take extra precautions to stay cool
• Advise patient to avoid abrupt withdrawal of this product, or EPS may result; product should be withdrawn slowly
• Advise patient to avoid use with alcohol, CNS depressants; increased drowsiness may occur
• Advise patient to use a sunscreen and sunglasses to prevent burns
• Teach patient to take antacids 2 hr before or after taking this product
• Instruct patient to report sore throat, malaise, fever, bleeding, mouth sores; if these occur, CBC should be performed and product discontinued

Evaluation
Positive therapeutic outcome
• Decrease in emotional excitement, hallucinations, delusions, paranoia
• Reorganization of patterns of thought, speech

TREATMENT OF OVERDOSE:
Lavage; barbiturates; provide airway, **IV** fluids; do not use EPINEPHrine, which may increase hypotension

---

lubiprostone (Rx)
(loo-bee-pros'-tone)
Amitiza
Func. class.: Miscellaneous gastrointestinal agent
Pregnancy category C

ACTION: Locally acting chloride channel activator, enhances a chloride-rich intestinal fluid secretion without altering other electrolytes; increases motility in the intestine, increasing softening and passage of stool

Therapeutic outcome: Decreased constipation

USES: Chronic idiopathic constipation, constipation-predominant irritable bowel syndrome in women >18 yr

CONTRAINDICATIONS:
Hypersensitivity, GI obstruction

Precautions: Pregnancy **C**, breastfeeding, children, diarrhea, IBD, abdominal pain, cholelithiasis, fecal inpaction, GI/hepatic disease

DOSAGE AND ROUTES

Chronic idiopathic constipation
Adult: PO 24 mcg bid with food/water

IBS with constipation (women)
Adult and adolescent ≥18 yr: PO 8 mcg bid with food and water

Hepatic dosage
Adult: For chronic constipation 16 mcg bid (Child-Pugh B); 8 mcg bid (Child-Pugh C); **for irritable bowel:** 8 mcg daily (Child-Pugh C), may be increased if tolerated

Available forms: Caps 8, 24 mcg

Implementation
• Give with food bid
• Store at room temperature

ADVERSE EFFECTS
CNS: *Headache,* dizziness, depression, fatigue, insomnia
CV: Hypertension, chest pain
GI: *Nausea, abdominal pain, eructation,* abdominal distention, constipation, diarrhea, dry mouth, dyspepsia, flatulence, viral gastroenteritis, gastroesophageal reflux disease, vomiting, fecal incontinence, fecal urgency
GU: UTI
MISC: Chest pain, peripheral edema, influenza, pyrexia, viral infection
MS: Back pain, arthralgia, muscle cramps, pain in extremities
RESP: Bronchitis; cough, dyspnea, nasopharyngitis, sinusitis, URI

Pharmacokinetics
Absorption	Unknown
Distribution	Protein binding 94%
Metabolism	Rapid in stomach, jejunum
Excretion	Unknown
Half-life	0.9-1.4 hr

Pharmacodynamics
Onset	Unknown
Peak	1.14 hr
Duration	Unknown

INTERACTIONS

Individual drugs
• Anticholinergics, antidiarrheals: decreased effects of lubiprostone
• Do not use with sodium phosphate monobasic monohydra, sodium phosphate dibasic anhydrous, with other laxative, purgatives, when evacuating the bowel before radiologic exam or surgery
• Possible GI obstruction with NIFEdipine extended rel tab

NURSING CONSIDERATIONS

Assessment
• Assess GI symptoms: nausea, abdominal pain
• Assess periodically for need for continued treatment

Nursing diagnoses
• Constipation (uses)
• Knowledge, deficient (teaching)

Patient/family education
• Teach patient to notify prescriber of GI symptoms, diarrhea, hypersensitivity reactions

Evaluation
Positive therapeutic outcome
• Decreased constipation

---

lurasidone (Rx)
(loo-ras'i-done)
Latuda
Func. class.: Atypical antipsychotic
Chem. class.: Benzoisothiazol derivative
Pregnancy category B

ACTION: May modulate central dopaminergic and serotoninergic activity, high affinity for dopamine-D_2 receptors, serotonin 5-HT_{2A} receptors, and partial agonist at serotonin 5-HT_{1A} receptor

Therapeutic outcome: Decreasing hallucinations, delusions, agitation, social withdrawal

USES: Schizophrenia

CONTRAINDICATIONS:
Hypersensitivity

Precautions: Abrupt discontinuation, ambient temperature increase, breast cancer, breastfeeding, cardiac disease, children, dehydration, diabetes, ketoacidosis, driving/operating machinery, dysphagia, geriatrics, heart failure, hematological/hepatic/renal disease, hypotension, hypovolemia, MI, infertility, obesity, Parkinson's disease, pregnancy **B,** seizures, strenuous exercise, stroke, substance abuse, suicidal ideation, syncope, tardive dyskinesia

> **BLACK BOX WARNING:** Dementia: antipsychotics, such as lurasidone, are not approved for the treatment of dementia-related psychosis in geriatric patients and may increase the risk of death in this population

DOSAGE AND ROUTES
Adult: PO 40 mg q day, range 40-80 mg/day, those receiving CYP3A4 inhibitors (max 40 mg/day), do not use with strong CYP3A4 inducers/inhibitors

Hepatic/renal dose
Adult: PO Child-Pugh class B/C , CCr $\geq$10 ml/min-<50 ml/min max 40 mg/day

Available forms: 40 mg and 80 mg tabs

Implementation
• Give with a meal of at least 350 calories
• Store at room temperature, protect from moisture

ADVERSE EFFECTS
CNS: Agitation, akathisia, anxiety, dizziness, drowsiness, fatigue, hyperthermia, insomnia, dystonic reactions; **neuroleptic malignant syndrome (rare)**, pseudoparkinsonism, restlessness, **seizures, suicidal ideation,** syncope, tardive dyskinesia, vertigo
CV: Angina, **AV block, bradycardia,** hypertension, orthostatic hypotension, **sinus tachycardia, stroke**
EENT: Blurred vision
ENDO: Diabetes mellitus, ketoacidosis, hyperglycemia, hyperprolactimemia
GI: Abdominal pain, diarrhea, dyspepsia, nausea, vomiting, gastritis, weight gain/loss
GU: Amenorrhea, breast enlargement, dysmenorrhea, impotence, dysuria, renal failure
HEMA: Agranulocytosis, anemia, leucopenia, neutropenia
INTEG: Pruritus, rash
MS: Back pain, dysarthria; **rhabdomyolysis (rare)**
SYST: Angioedema

Pharmacokinetics	
Absorption	9-19%
Distribution	99% protein binding
Metabolism	Unknown
Excretion	80% feces, 9% urine
Half-life	18 hr

⚠ Nurse Alert

Pharmacodynamics

Onset	Unknown
Peak	1-3 hr
Duration	Steady state 7 days

INTERACTIONS

Drug classifications
Strong CYP3A4 inhibitors: increased lurasidone effect, do not use concurrently

SSRIs, SNRIs: increased serotonin syndrome, neuroleptic malignant syndrome

NURSING CONSIDERATIONS

Assessment
• **Assess for schizophrenia:** hallucinations, delusions, agitation, social withdrawal; monitor orientation, behavior, mood prior to and periodically during therapy

• **Assess for neuroleptic malignant syndrome (rare):** fever, dyspnea, tachycardia, seizures, sweating, hyper-hypotension, muscle stiffness, pallor, report immediately

• **Monitor for blood dyscrasias:** CBC periodically, blood dyscrasias may occur

• **Monitor for serious cardiac symptoms:** AV block, stroke, bradycardia may occur

• **Assess for EPS:** restlessness, difficulty speaking, loss of balance, pill rolling, mask-like face, shuffling gait, rigidity, tremors, muscle spasms; monitor prior to and periodically during therapy; report tardive dyskinesia immediately

Nursing diagnoses
• Ineffective coping (uses)
• Noncompliance (teaching)

Patient/family education
• Explain reason for treatment and expected results
• Teach patient to report EPS, blood dyscrasias: sore throat, fever, unusual bleeding/bruising

Evaluation
Positive therapeutic outcome
• Decreasing hallucinations, delusions, agitation, social withdrawal

lymphocyte immune globulin (antithymocyte) (Rx)
Atgam

Func. class.: Immune globulin immunosuppressant

Pregnancy category C

ACTION: Produces immunosuppression by inhibiting the function of T-lymphocytes

Therapeutic outcome: Absence of transplant rejection; hematologic remission (aplastic anemia)

USES: Organ transplants to prevent rejection, aplastic anemia

Unlabeled uses: Multiple sclerosis, myasthenia gravis, immunosuppressant in liver, bone marrow, heart and other organ transplants, pure red cell aplasia, scleroderma

CONTRAINDICATIONS:
Hypersensitivity to this product or equine/porcine protein, acute viral illness

Precautions: Pregnancy C, breastfeeding, children, severe renal/hepatic disease, leukopenia, thrombocytopenia

> **BLACK BOX WARNING:** Infection, neoplastic disease

DOSAGE AND ROUTES

Renal allograft
Adult/child: IV 10-30 mg/kg/day × 14 days

Delay of renal allograft rejection
Adult: IV 15 mg/kg/day × 7-14 days, then every other day × 14 days for a total of 21 doses in 28 days

Aplastic anemia
Adult: IV 10-20 mg/kg/day × 8-14 days, then every other day for up to 21 total doses

Available forms: Inj 50 mg horse gamma globulin/ml

Implementation
IV route
• Do not infuse <4 hr
• Keep emergency equipment nearby for severe allergic reactions
• **Aplastic anemia:** Skin testing must be completed before treatment; use intradermal inj of 0.1 ml of a 1:1000 dilution (5 mcg of horse

Adverse effects: *italics* = common; **bold** = life-threatening

IgG) in 0.9% NaCl; if a wheal or rash or both >10 mm, use caution during inf
• Dilute in saline sol before inf; invert **IV** bag, so undiluted product does not contact the air inside; concentration should not be >1 mg/ml

ADVERSE EFFECTS

Renal transplant
CNS: Fever, chills, headache, dizziness, weakness, faintness, **seizures**
CV: Chest pain, hypo/hypertension, tachycardia
GI: Diarrhea, nausea, vomiting, epigastric pain, **GI bleeding**
INTEG: Rash, pruritus, urticaria, wheal
SYST: Anaphylaxis

Aplastic anemia
CNS: Fever, chills, headache, **seizures**, lightheadedness, encephalitis, postviral encephalopathy
CV: Bradycardia, myocarditis, irregularity
GI: Nausea, liver function test abnormality
HEMA: Thrombocytopenia

Pharmacokinetics
Absorption	Unknown
Distribution	Unknown
Metabolism	Unknown
Excretion	Unknown
Half-life	5.7 days

Pharmacodynamics
Onset	Rapid
Peak	Unknown
Duration	Unknown

NURSING CONSIDERATIONS

Assessment
• Assess for infection; if infection occurs, evaluation will be needed to continue treatment
• Monitor renal function tests: BUN, creatinine at least monthly during treatment, 3 mo after treatment
• Monitor liver function tests: alkaline phosphatase, AST, ALT, bilirubin

Nursing diagnoses
• Infection, risk for (uses)
• Knowledge, deficient (teaching)
• Mobility, impaired physical (uses)

Patient/family education
• Advise patient to report fever, rash, chills, sore throat, fatigue, since serious infections may occur

• Caution patient to use contraceptive measures during treatment and for 12 wk after ending therapy; product is teratogenic
• Caution patient to avoid crowds and persons with known infections to reduce risk of infection

Evaluation
Positive therapeutic outcome
• Absence of graft rejection
• Hematologic recovery (aplastic anemia)

---

mafenide topical
See Appendix B

magaldrate (OTC)
(mag'al-drate)
Isopan, Losapan ✤, Riopan, Riopan Extra Strength ✤
Func. class.: Antacid
Chem. class.: Aluminum/magnesium hydroxide
Pregnancy category C

ACTION: Neutralizes gastric acidity; product is dissolved in gastric contents; this product is a combination of aluminum and magnesium

Therapeutic outcome: Decreased pain of ulcers

USES: Antacid, hiatal hernia, indigestion/heartburn, hyperacidity

Unlabeled uses: Duodenal and gastric ulcers, peptic ulcer disease (adjunct), reflex esophagitis

CONTRAINDICATIONS:
Hypersensitivity to this product or benzyl alcohol

Precautions: Pregnancy **C,** geriatric, fluid restriction, decreased GI motility, GI obstruction, dehydration, renal disease, sodium-restricted diets, bone disease, hypertension, appendicitis, diverticulitis, ulcerative colitis, neonates/infants, hypermagnesemia, hypophosphatemia

DOSAGE AND ROUTES
Adult/child/geriatric: SUSP 5-10 ml (480-1080 mg) with water between meals, at bedtime

Available forms: Susp 540 mg/5 ml

Implementation
• Take antacids 2 hr before or 2 hr after taking enteric-coated products
• Give laxatives or stool softeners if constipation occurs

- Give susp after shaking; give between meals and at bedtime
- Give when stomach is empty after meals and at bedtime

ADVERSE EFFECTS
GI: Constipation, diarrhea, anorexia
META: Hypermagnesemia, hypophosphatemia

Pharmacokinetics

Absorption	Not absorbed
Distribution	Not distributed
Metabolism	Not metabolized
Excretion	Kidneys
Half-life	Unknown

Pharmacodynamics

Onset	Unknown
Peak	$^{1}/_{2}$ hr
Duration	1 hr

INTERACTIONS
Individual drugs
ChlordiazePOXIDE, cimetidine, isoniazid, ketoconazole, phenytoin, tetracycline: decreased absorption of each specific product
Flecainide, quiNIDine: increased action when taken in large amounts

Drug classifications
Amphetamines: increased action when taken in large amounts
Anticholinergics, corticosteroids, fluoroquinolones, iron salts, phenothiazines, salicylates: decreased absorption of each specific product
Salicylates: decreased action when taken in large amounts

NURSING CONSIDERATIONS
Assessment
- **Antacid:** location of pain, intensity, characteristics, what aggravates, ameliorates pain; heartburn/indigestion; hematemesis
- Monitor serum magnesium, calcium, phosphate, potassium if using long term or with impaired renal function
- Assess for constipation: increase bulk in diet if needed or obtain order for stool softener

Nursing diagnoses
- Knowledge, deficient (teaching)
- Pain, acute (uses)

Patient/family education
- Advise patient to separate ingestion of enteric-coated products and antacid by 2 hr
- Advise patient to use product 2 wk or less; product should not be used for long periods
- Teach patient to notify prescriber immediately if coffee-ground emesis, emesis with frank blood, or black tarry stools occur

Evaluation
Positive therapeutic outcome
- Absence of abdominal pain
- Decreased acidity

magnesium salts
(mag-neez'ee-um)
magnesium chloride (Rx)
Mag-64
magnesium citrate (OTC)
Walgreens Magnesium Citrate
magnesium gluconate (OTC)
Mag-G, Magtrate
magnesium hydroxide (OTC)
Ex-Lax Milk of Magnesia, Freelax, Good Sense Milk of Magnesia, Leader Milk of Magnesia, Phillips Milk of Magnesia, MOM, Top Care Milk of Magnesia, Walgreens Milk of Magnesia
magnesium oxide (OTC)
Mag-Ox 400, Uro-Mag
magnesium sulfate (OTC, Rx)
epsom salt, magnesium sulfate (IV)— HIGH ALERT
Func. class.: Electrolyte; anticonvulsant, laxative, saline; antacid
Pregnancy category A, B

ACTION: Increases osmotic pressure, draws fluid into colon, neutralizes HCl

Therapeutic outcome: Magnesium levels WNL, absence of constipation

USES: Constipation, bowel preparation before surgery or exam, electrolyte, anticonvulsant, in preeclampsia, eclampsia (magnesium sulfate)

CONTRAINDICATIONS:
Hypersensitivity, abdominal pain, nausea/vomiting, obstruction, acute surgical abdomen, rectal bleeding, heart block, myocardial damage

Precautions: Pregnancy **A, B** (magnesium sulfate), renal disease/cardiac disease

DOSAGE AND ROUTES

Laxative
Adult: PO 15-60 ml at bedtime (Milk of Magnesia)
Adult and child >12 yr: PO 15 g in 8 oz of H_2O (magnesium sulfate); PO 5-30 ml (Concentrated Milk of Magnesia); PO 5-10 oz at bedtime (magnesium citrate)
Child 2-6 yr: 5-15 ml/day (Milk of Magnesia)

Prevention of magnesium deficiency
Adult and child ≥10 yr: PO (male): 350-400 mg/day; (female): 280-300 mg/day; (breastfeeding): 335-350 mg/day; (pregnancy): 320 mg/day
Child 8-10 yr: PO 170 mg/day
Child 4-7 yr: PO 120 mg/day

Magnesium sulfate deficiency
Adult: PO 200-400 mg in divided doses tid-qid; IM 1 g q6hr × 4 doses; **IV** 5 g (severe)
Child 6-12 yr: 3-6 mg/kg/day in divided doses tid-qid

Preeclampsia/eclampsia magnesium sulfate
Adult: **IM/IV** INF 4-5 g; with 5 g IM in each gluteus, then 5 g q4hr or 4 g **IV** INF, then 1-2 g/hr cont INF, max 40 g/day or 20 g/48 hr in severe renal disease

Available forms: Chloride: sus rel tabs 535 mg (64 mg Mg); enteric tabs 833 mg (100 mg Mg); hydroxide: liquid 400 mg/5 ml (164 mg Mg/5 ml); conc liquid 800 mg/5 ml (328 mg Mg/5 ml); chew tabs 300, 600 mg; oxide: tabs 400 mg (241.3 mg Mg); caps 140 mg (84.5 mg Mg); sulfate: powder for oral; bulk packages; (epsom salts) bulk packages; inj 10, 12.5, 25, 50%; citrate: oral sol 240, 296, 300 ml bottles (77 mEq/100 ml)

Implementation
PO route
• Administer with 8 oz of water
• Refrigerate magnesium citrate before administration
• Shake susp before using
• Administer to patient crushed or whole; chewable tablets may be chewed
• Administer with food or milk to decrease gastric symptoms; give 30 min before or 2 hr after antacids

• Tablets should be chewed thoroughly before swallowing, give 4 oz of water afterward
• **Laxative:** give on empty stomach

IM route (magnesium sulfate)
• Give deeply in gluteal site

IV route (magnesium sulfate)
• Only when calcium gluconate available for magnesium toxicity

Direct IV route
• Dilute 50% solution to 20% or less give at ≤150 mg/min

Continuous IV INF route
• May dilute to 20% sol, infuse over 3 hr
• IV at less than 125 mg/kg/hr; circulatory collapse may occur; use inf pump

Y-site compatibilities: Acyclovir, aldesleukin, amifostine, amikacin, ampicillin, aztreonam, cefamandole, ceFAZolin, cefmetazole, cefoperazone, cefotaxime, cefoxitin, cephalothin, cephapirin, chloramphenicol, cisatracurium, DOBUTamine, doxycycline, DOXOrubicin liposome, enalaprilat, erythromycin, esmolol, famotidine, fludarabine, gallium, gentamicin, granisetron, heparin, HYDROmorphone, IDArubicin, insulin, kanamycin, labetalol, meperidine, metronidazole, minocycline, morphine, moxalactam, nafcillin, ondansetron, oxacillin, paclitaxel, penicillin G potassium, piperacillin, piperacillin/tazobactam, potassium chloride, propofol, remifentanil, sargramostim, thiotepa, ticarcillin, tobramycin, trimethoprim/sulfamethoxazole, vancomycin, vit B complex/C

ADVERSE EFFECTS

CNS: Muscle weakness, flushing, sweating, confusion, sedation, depressed reflexes, **flaccid paralysis, hypothermia**
CV: Hypotension, heart block, **circulatory collapse,** vasodilatation
GI: *Nausea, vomiting, anorexia, cramps,* diarrhea
HEMA: Prolonged bleeding time
META: Electrolyte, fluid imbalances
RESP: Respiratory depression/paralysis

Pharmacokinetics

Absorption	Unknown
Distribution	Unknown
Metabolism	Unknown
Excretion	Kidneys
Half-life	Unknown effective anticonvulsant levels 2.5-7.5 mEq/L

⚠ Nurse Alert

Pharmacodynamics

	PO	IM	IV
Onset	3-6 hr	1 hr	Unknown
Peak	Unknown	Unknown	Unknown
Duration	Unknown	4 hr	$\frac{1}{2}$ hr

INTERACTIONS

Individual products
Digoxin: decreased effect of digoxin
Nitrofurantoin: decreased absorption

Drug classifications
Antihypertensives: increased hypotension
Antiinfectives (fluoroquinolones), tetracyclines: decreased absorption
Neuromuscular blockers: increased effect

NURSING CONSIDERATIONS

Assessment
• Assess I&O ratio; check for decrease in urinary output
• **Laxative:** assess cause of constipation; lack of fluids, bulk, exercise
• Assess cramping, rectal bleeding, nausea, vomiting; product should be discontinued
⚠ **Assess magnesium toxicity: thirst, confusion, decrease in reflexes**
• Assess visual changes: blurring, halos, corneal and retinal damage
• Assess edema in feet, ankles, legs
• Assess prior product history; there are many product interactions
• Eclampsia: seizure precautions, BP, ECG (magnesium sulfate)

Nursing diagnoses
• Constipation (uses)
• Injury, risk for
• Knowledge, deficient (teaching)

Patient/family education
• Teach not to use laxatives for long-term therapy; bowel tone will be lost
• Teach that chilling helps the taste of magnesium citrate
• Teach to shake suspension well
• Teach to not use at bedtime as a laxative; may interfere with sleep
• Teach to give citrus fruit after administering to counteract unpleasant taste
• Teach reason for product, expected result

Evaluation
• Positive therapeutic response; decreased constipation; absence of seizures (eclampsia), normal serum calcium levels

---

mannitol (Rx)
(man′i-tole)
Osmitrol, Resectisol
Func. class.: Diuretic-osmotic
Chem. class.: Hexahydric alcohol
Pregnancy category C

ACTION: Increases osmolarity of glomerular filtrate, which raises osmotic pressure of fluid in renal tubules; there is a decrease in reabsorption of water, electrolytes; increases in urinary output, sodium, chloride, potassium, calcium, phosphorus, uric acid, urea, magnesium

USES: Edema; promote systemic diuresis in cerebral edema, decrease intraocular pressure, improve renal function in acute renal failure, chemical poisoning

CONTRAINDICATIONS:
Active intracranial bleeding, hypersensitivity, anuria, severe pulmonary congestion, edema, severe dehydration, progressive heart disease, renal failure

Precautions: Pregnancy C, breastfeeding, geriatric, dehydration, severe renal disease, CHF, electrolyte imbalances

DOSAGE AND ROUTES

Oliguria, prevention
Adult: IV after initial test dose and if urine output is 30-50 mg/hr × 2 hr, give 20-100 g of a 15% or 20% SOL in a 24-hr period

Oliguria, treatment
Adult: IV after initial test dose, give balance of 50 g of a 20% SOL over 1 hr, then 5% via CONT IV INF to maintain output at 50 ml/hr
Child (unlabeled): IV 0.5-2 g/kg as a 15%-20% SOL, run over 30-60 min; maintenance 0.25-0.5 g/kg q4-6hr

Intraocular pressure
Adult: IV 1.5-2 g/kg of a 15%-25% SOL over 30-60 min

ICP
Adult: IV 1-2 g/kg, then 0.25-1 g/kg q4hr

Diuresis in product intoxication
Adult and child >12 yr: 5%-10% SOL continuously up to 200 g IV, while maintaining 100-500 ml urine output/hr

Available forms: Inj 5%, 10%, 15%, 20%, 25%; GU irrigation 5%

M

Adverse effects: *italics* = common; **bold** = life-threatening

Implementation
Irrigation
• Use 100 ml of 25%/900 ml of sterile water for inj (2.5% sol)
• Administer potassium replacement if potassium level is <3 mg/ml

IV route
• Use an in-line filter for 15%, 20%, 25%; give with inf pump; check **IV** patency at inf site before, during administration; do not use sol that is yellow or has a precipitate or crystals; to redissolve, run bottle under hot water and shake vigorously; cool to body temp before giving
• Run at 30-50 ml/hr in oliguria; run over 30-60 min in increased ICP; run over 30 min for intraocular pressure; 60-90 min after surgery
• **Test dose** with severe oliguria, 0.2 g/kg over 3-5 mins; if continued oliguria give 2nd test dose; if no response, reassess patient

Y-site compatibilities: Acyclovir, alemtuzumab, amifostine, amikacin, ampicillin, atropine, aztreonam, bivalirudin, bumetanide, calcium gluconate, caspofungin, ceFAZolin, cefotaxime, cefoxitin, ceftazidime, ceftizoxime, chloramphenicol, cimetidine, cisatracurium, clindamycin, DAPTOmycin, dexmedetomidine, digoxin, diltiazem, diphenhydrAMINE, DOBUTamine, DOPamine, DOXOrubicin liposome, doxycycline, enalaprilat, EPINEPHrine, ertapenem, esmolol, famotidine, fenoldopam, fentaNYL, fluconazole, fludarabine, gentamicin, granisetron, heparin, HYDROmorphone, hydrOXYzine, IDArubicin, imipenem/cilastatin, insulin, isoproterenol, ketorolac, labetalol, levofloxacin, lidocaine, linezolid, LORazepam, meperidine, metoclopramide, metoprolol, metroNIDAZOLE, micafungin, midazolam, milrinone, morphine, nafcillin, niCARdipine, nitroglycerin, nitroprusside, norepinephrine, ondansetron, oxaliplatin, paclitaxel, palonosetron, pantoprazole, penicillin G potassium, phenylephrine, piperacillin/tazobactam, potassium chloride, procainamide, prochlorperazine, promethazine, propofol, propranolol, protamine, quinupristin/dalfopristin, ranitidine, remifentanil, sargramostim, sodium bicarbonate, tacrolimus, thiotepa, ticarcillin/clavulanate, tirofiban, tobramycin, trimethoprim/sulfamethoxazole, vancomycin, vasopressin, verapamil, vitamin B complex with C, voriconazole

Y-site incompatibilities: Aminophylline, amphotericin B cholesteryl sulfate complex, calcium chloride, cefepime, cefTRIAXone, cefuroxime, ciprofloxacin, dexamethasone sodium phosphate, diazepam, drotrecogin, haloperidol, lansoprazole, methylPREDNISolone sodium succinate, phenytoin, phytonadione

ADVERSE EFFECTS
CNS: Dizziness, headache, **seizures, rebound increased ICP,** confusion
CV: Edema, hypotension, hypertension, **tachycardia, CHF,** thrombophlebitis, angina-like chest pains, fever, chills, **circulatory overload**
EENT: Loss of hearing, blurred vision, nasal congestion, decreased intraocular pressure
ELECT: Fluid, electrolyte imbalances, **acidosis,** electrolyte loss, dehydration, hyper/hypokalemia
GI: *Nausea, vomiting,* dry mouth, diarrhea
GU: Marked diuresis, urinary retention, thirst
RESP: Pulmonary congestion

Pharmacokinetics
Absorption	Complete
Distribution	Extracellular spaces
Metabolism	Minimal
Excretion	Renal
Half-life	100 min

Pharmacodynamics
Onset	$1/2$-1 hr
Peak	1 hr
Duration	6-8 hr

INTERACTIONS
Individual drugs
Lithium: increased elimination of mannitol
Imipramine: increased excretion of imipramine
Arsenic trioxide, levomethadyl: increased hypokalemia

Drug classifications
Salicylates, barbiturates, bromides: increased excretion of each specific product

Drug/food
Potassium foods: increased hyperkalemia

Drug/lab test
Interference: inorganic phosphorus, ethylene glycol

NURSING CONSIDERATIONS
Assessment
• Assess neurologic status: LOC, ICP reading, pupil size and reaction when product is given for increased ICP
• Assess for vision changes or eye discomfort or pain before, during treatment (increases intraocular pressure); neurologic checks, ICP during treatment (increased ICP)
• Assess patient for tinnitus, hearing loss, ear pain; periodic testing of hearing is needed when high doses of this product are given by **IV** route

⚠ Nurse Alert

• Assess fluid volume status: check I&O ratios and record hourly urine values, CVP, breath sounds, weight, distended red veins, crackles in lungs, color, quality, and specific gravity of urine, skin turgor, adequacy of pulses, moist mucous membranes, bilateral lung sounds, peripheral pitting edema

• Assess for dehydration; symptoms of decreasing output, thirst, hypotension, dry mouth and mucous membranes should be reported

• Monitor electrolytes: potassium, sodium, calcium, magnesium; also include BUN, ABGs, CVP, PAP, CBC; regularly monitor serum and urine levels of sodium and potassium

• Assess B/P before, during therapy with patient lying, standing, and sitting as appropriate; orthostatic hypotension can occur rapidly

• Monitor for rebound ICP: headache, confusion

Nursing diagnoses
• Fluid volume, deficient (adverse reactions)
• Fluid volume, excess (uses)
• Knowledge, deficient (teaching)
• Urinary elimination, impaired (adverse reactions)

Patient/family education
• Teach patient reason for and method of treatment

Evaluation
Positive therapeutic outcome
• Decreased intraocular pressure
• Prevention of hypokalemia (diuretic use)
• Decreased edema
• Decreased ICP
• Increased diuresis of >30 ml/hr
• Increased excretion of toxic substances

TREATMENT OF OVERDOSE:
Discontinue infusion; correct fluid, electrolyte imbalances; hemodialysis; monitor hydration, CV, renal function

---

maraviroc (Rx)
(mah-rav′er-rock)
Selzentry
Func. class.: Antiretroviral
Chem. class.: Fusion inhibitor, CCR5-receptor antagonist
Pregnancy category B

ACTION: Interferes with entry into HIV-1 by inhibiting the fusion of the virus and cell membrane

Therapeutic outcome: Improvement in CD4, viral load, T-cell count

USES: CCR5-tropic HIV in combination with other antiretroviral agents in treating experienced patients

CONTRAINDICATIONS:
Hypersensitivity

Precautions: Pregnancy **B**, breastfeeding, Asian patients, renal/hepatic/cardiac disease, electrolyte imbalance, dehydration, immune reconstitution syndrome, infection, MI, orthostatic hypotension, children, geriatric

BLACK BOX WARNING: Hepatitis

DOSAGE AND ROUTES
Those not taking CYP3A inducers/inhibitors
Adult: PO 300 mg bid

Those taking CYP3A4 inhibitors with/without a CYP3A inducer
Adult: PO 150 mg bid

Those taking CYP3A4 inducers without a strong CYP3A inhibitor
Adult: PO 600 mg bid

Available forms: Tabs 150, 300 mg

Implementation
• May give without regard to meals, with 8 oz of water
• Store at room temperature

ADVERSE EFFECTS
CNS: Dizziness, depression, **viral meningitis,** disturbances in consciousness, peripheral neuropathy, paresthesia, dysesthesia, fever
CV: MI, cardiac ischemia, orthostatic hypotension
EENT: Gingival hyperplasia
GI: Diarrhea, constipation, dyspepsia, **pseudomembranous colitis, hepatotoxicity**
INTEG: Rash, urticaria, pruritus, folliculitis
MS: Joint pain, leg pain, muscle cramps
RESP: Cough, URI, sinusitis, bronchitis, pneumonia, **bronchospasm, obstruction**
SYST: Herpes virus

M

Pharmacokinetics

Absorption	Unknown
Distribution	Unknown
Metabolism	By P450 system, CYP3A metabolism
Excretion	Urine 20%, feces 76%
Half-life	Unknown

Pharmacodynamics

Unknown

INTERACTIONS

Drug classifications

CYP3A inhibitors (amiodarone, aprepitant, chloramphenicol, clarithromycin, conivaptan, cycloSPORINE, dalfopristin, danazol, diltiazem, erythromycin, estradiol, fluconazole, fluvoxamine, imatinib, isoniazid, itraconazole, ketoconazole, miconazole, nefazodone, niCARdipine, propoxyphene, RU-486, tamoxifen, telithromycin, troleandomycin, verapamil, voriconazole, zafirlukast): increased maraviroc levels

CYP3A4 inducers (aminoglutethimide, barbiturates, bexaroten, bosentan, carBAMazepine, dexamethasone, efavirenz, fosphenytoin, griseofulvin, modafinil, nafcillin, OXcarbazepine, phenytoin, rifabutin, rifamipin, rifapentine, topiramate, tipranavir): decreased maraviroc effect

Drug/food

High-fat meal: decreased absorption 33%

Drug/herb

St. John's wort: decreased maraviroc effect

NURSING CONSIDERATIONS

Assessment

• **HIV:** CD_4, T-cell count, plasma HIV RNA, CCR5-tropic HIV-1; assess for change in symptoms, other infections during treatment
• Monitor renal tests: serum creatinine
• Assess bowel pattern before, during treatment
• **Allergies:** skin eruptions: rash, urticaria, itching; assess allergies before treatment and before each dose

> **BLACK BOX WARNING: Hepatitis:** assess for dark urine, abdominal pain, vomiting, yellowing of skin/eyes, hepatomegaly: if present, discontinue product; monitor LFTs

Nursing diagnoses

• Injury, risk for (uses, adverse reactions)
• Knowledge, deficient (teaching)

Patient/family education

• Advise patient to take as prescribed; if dose is missed, take as soon as remembered up to 1 hr before next dose; do not double dose
• Teach patient that product does not cure infection, just controls symptoms, and does not prevent infecting others
⚠ **Teach patient to report sore throat, fever, fatigue; may indicate superinfection; yellow skin/eyes, abdominal pain, vomiting (hepatitis); itching, dyspnea (allergic reaction)**
• Advise patient that product must be taken in equal intervals around the clock to maintain blood levels for duration of therapy
• Instruct patient to notify prescriber of side effects
• Advise patient to avoid driving or other hazardous activities until reaction is known; dizziness may occur
• Teach patient to make position changes slowly to prevent postural hypotension
• Inform patient to notify prescriber if pregnancy is planned or suspected

Evaluation

Positive therapeutic outcome

• Improvement in CD4, viral load, T-cell count

mecasermin (Rx)

(mec-a′sir-men)
Increlex
Func. class.: Biologic response modifier; insulin-like growth factor
Pregnancy category C

ACTION: Stimulates growth; IGF-1 is the principal hormonal mediator of statural growth; GH binds to its receptor in the liver and other tissues

Therapeutic outcome: Increased height

USES: Growth failure in children with severe primary insulin-like growth factor-1 (IGF-1) deficiency (primary IGFD) or with growth hormone (GH) gene deletion who have developed neutralizing antibodies to GH

Unlabeled uses: ALS

CONTRAINDICATIONS:

Hypersensitivity, benzyl alcohol, closed epiphyses, active/suspected neoplasia, **IV** use

Precautions: Pregnancy **C,** breastfeeding, children <2 yr, diabetes mellitus, hypothyroidism, lymphoid tissue hypertrophy, increased ICP, malnutrition, scoliosis, sleep apnea

DOSAGE AND ROUTES
Child: SUBCUT 0.04-0.08 mg/kg (40-80 mcg/kg) bid; if well tolerated for 1 wk, may increase by 0.04 mg/kg/dose, max 0.12 mg/kg bid

Available forms: Inj 10 mg/ml

Implementation
SUBCUT route
• Give within 20 min of a meal or snack
• Rotate inj site; use sterile, disposable syringe/needles; use small-volume syringe for accurate measurement
• Store in refrigerator before opening, avoid freezing; after opening, stable for 30 days after initial vial entry, store in refrigerator, do not use if particulate matter is present, avoid direct light, do not use after expiration date

ADVERSE EFFECTS
CNS: Headache, **seizures,** dizziness, cardiac valvulopathy, increased intracranial pressure
CV: Cardiac murmur
EENT: Ear pain, otitis media, abnormal tympanometry, papilledema, visual impairment, tonsillar hypertrophy
ENDO: Hypoglycemia, ketosis, hypothyroidism, hypercholesterolemia, hypertriglyceridemia
GI: Vomiting, nausea
HEMA: Thymus hypertrophy
INTEG: Pruritus, urticaria, **anaphylaxis, angioedema**
MISC: Bruising, lipohypertrophy, hypersensitivity reactions, inj site reaction
MS: Arthralgia, joint pain, slipped upper femoral epiphysis
RESP: Snoring, **apnea**
SYST: Antibodies to growth hormone, secondary malignancy

Pharmacokinetics
Absorption	Near 100%
Distribution	Unknown
Metabolism	Liver/kidneys
Excretion	Unknown
Half-life	5.8 hr

Pharmacodynamics
Unknown

INTERACTIONS
Drug classifications
Antidiabetics, corticosteroids: increased hypoglycemia
Psychostimulants: decrease in growth suppression possible

NURSING CONSIDERATIONS
Assessment
• Monitor preprandial glucose at beginning of treatment and until well tolerated
• Monitor by funduscopic exam at beginning, periodically during treatment
• Assess for allergic reactions; if present, interrupt treatment and notify prescriber
• Assess growth rate of child at intervals during treatment
• Serious skin disorders: angioedema; anaphylaxis

Nursing diagnoses
• Knowledge, deficient (teaching)

Patient/family education
• Teach patient that treatment may continue for years; regular assessments are required
• Advise patient to avoid hazardous activities, driving within 2-3 hr of dosing
• Teach patient correct administration and needle disposal

Evaluation
Positive therapeutic outcome
• Growth in children

meclizine (OTC, Rx)
(mek′li-zeen)
Antivert, Bonamine ✦, Bonine, Dramamine Less Drowsy Formula, Medivert, Travel Sickness, Wal-Dram II
Func. class.: Antiemetic, antihistamine, anticholinergic
Chem. class.: H₁-receptor antagonist, piperazine derivative
Pregnancy category B

ACTION: Acts centrally by blocking chemoreceptor trigger zone, which in turn acts on vomiting center

Therapeutic outcome: Decreased nausea in motion sickness; decreased vertigo

USES: Vertigo, motion sickness

CONTRAINDICATIONS:
Hypersensitivity to cyclizines, shock

Precautions: Pregnancy **B,** breastfeeding, children, geriatric, closed-angle glaucoma, glaucoma, urinary retention, prostatic hypertrophy, CV disease, hypertension, seizure disorder

DOSAGE AND ROUTES

Vertigo
Adult/adolescent: PO 25-100 mg/day in divided doses

Motion sickness
Adult/adolescent: PO 25-50 mg 1 hr before traveling; repeat dose q24hr prn

Available forms: Tabs 12.5, 25, 50 mg; chew tabs 25 mg; caps 25, 30 mg

Implementation
• Tabs may be swallowed whole, chewed, or allowed to dissolve; give with food to decrease GI upset
• Give lowest possible dose in geriatric, anticholinergic effects

ADVERSE EFFECTS
CNS: *Drowsiness,* fatigue, restlessness, headache, insomnia
CV: Hypotension
EENT: Dry mouth, blurred vision
GI: Nausea, anorexia, constipation, increased appetite
GU: Urinary retention

Pharmacokinetics

Absorption	Well absorbed
Distribution	Unknown
Metabolism	Unknown
Excretion	Unknown
Half-life	6 hr

Pharmacodynamics

Onset	1 hr
Peak	Unknown
Duration	8-24 hr

INTERACTIONS

Individual drugs
Alcohol: increased effects
Atropine: increased anticholinergic effects

Drug classifications
Antihistamines, antidepressants, phenothiazines: increased anticholinergic effect
CNS depressants, opioids: increased CNS depression

Drug/herb
Hops, valerian, kava: increased sedative effect

Drug/lab test
False negative: allergy skin testing (allergen extracts)

NURSING CONSIDERATIONS

Assessment
• **Vertigo/motion sickness:** nausea, vomiting after 1 hr, assess vertigo periodically
• Monitor VS, B/P
⚠ **Assess for signs of toxicity of other products or masking of symptoms of disease: brain tumor, intestinal obstruction**
• Observe for drowsiness, dizziness, LOC

Nursing diagnoses
• Injury, risk for (adverse reactions)
• Knowledge, deficient (teaching)

Patient/family education
• Teach patient that a false-negative result may occur with skin testing for allergies; these procedures should not be scheduled for 4 days after discontinuing use
• Teach patient to avoid hazardous activities, activities requiring alertness; dizziness may occur; instruct patient to request assistance with ambulation
• Teach patient to avoid alcohol, other depressants, breastfeeding

Evaluation
Positive therapeutic outcome
• Absence of dizziness, vomiting

medroxyPROGESTERone (Rx)
(me-drox-ee-proe-jess'te-rone)
Depo-Provera, Gen-Medroxy ✦, Provera
Func. class.: Hormone: progestogen, contraceptive, antineoplastic
Chem. class.: Progesterone derivative
Pregnancy category X

Do not confuse:
medroxyPROGESTERone/methylPREDNISolone, **Amen**/Ambien, **Provera**/Premarin/Covera

ACTION: Inhibits secretion of pituitary gonadotropins, which prevents follicular maturation and ovulation; stimulates growth of mammary tissue; antineoplastic action against endometrial cancer

Therapeutic outcome: Decreased abnormal uterine bleeding, absence of amenorrhea

USES: Uterine bleeding (abnormal), secondary amenorrhea, contraceptive, prevention of endometrial changes associated with estrogen replacement therapy (ERT), inoperable, recurrent, metastatic endometrial/renal cancer

CONTRAINDICATIONS:
Pregnancy **X,** hypersensitivity, reproductive cancer, genital bleeding (abnormal, undiagnosed), missed abortion

> **BLACK BOX WARNING:** Breast cancer, MI, stroke, thromboembolic disease, thrombophlebitis

Precautions: Breastfeeding, hypertension, asthma, blood dyscrasias, gallbladder disease, CHF, diabetes mellitus, bone disease, depression, migraine headache, seizure disorders, renal/hepatic disease, family history of cancer of breast or reproductive tract, bone mineral density loss, ocular disorders

> **BLACK BOX WARNING:** Use of this product has been shown to increase dementia in women ≥65 yr old; use may increase osteoporosis in long-term treatment, those at greater risk also smoke, adequate calcium and vitamin D should be taken

DOSAGE AND ROUTES
Secondary amenorrhea
Adult: PO 5-10 mg/day × 5-10 days

Uterine bleeding
Adult: PO 5-10 mg/day × 5-10 days starting on 16th or 21st day of menstrual cycle

With ERT
Adult: PO 5-10 mg qd × 10-14 or more days/mo (sequential estrogen); 2.5-5 mg qd (continuous estrogen)

Contraceptive
Adult: IM 150 mg q12wk; SUBCUT (depot SUBCUT Provera 104 inj) 104 mg q 3 mo

Endometrial/renal cancer
Adult: IM 400 mg-1 g (using 400 mg/ml depot inj susp) q wk

Available forms: Tabs 2.5, 5, 10 mg; inj susp 50, 150, 400 mg/ml; depot SUBCUT inj: 104 mg/0.65 ml

Implementation
PO route
• Give with food or milk to decrease GI symptoms
IM route
• Store in dark area
• Give titrated dosage; use lowest effective dosage; give oil sol deep in large muscle mass

(IM); rotate sites; use after warming to dissolve crystals

ADVERSE EFFECTS
CNS: Dizziness, headache, migraine, depression, fatigue, nervousness
CV: Hypotension, thrombophlebitis, edema, **thromboembolism, stroke, pulmonary embolism, MI**
EENT: Diplopia
GI: *Nausea,* vomiting, anorexia, cramps, increased weight, **cholestatic jaundice,** abdominal pain
GU: Amenorrhea, cervical erosion, breakthrough bleeding, dysmenorrhea, vaginal candidiasis, breast changes, *gynecomastia, testicular atrophy, impotence,* endometriosis, **spontaneous abortion**
INTEG: Rash, urticaria, acne, hirsutism, alopecia, oily skin, seborrhea, purpura, melasma, photosensitivity
META: Hyperglycemia
MS: Decreased bone density
SYST: Angioedema, anaphylaxis

Pharmacokinetics		
Unknown		

Pharmacodynamics		
	PO	IM
Onset	Unknown	Unknown
Peak	Unknown	Unknown
Duration	2-4 hr	Unknown

INTERACTIONS
Individual drugs
Aminoglutethimide: decreased contraceptive effect

Drug/lab test
Increased: alk phos, pregnanediol, amino acids, sodium
Decreased: GTT, HDL

NURSING CONSIDERATIONS
Assessment
• **Assess for symptoms indicating severe allergic reaction, angioedema;** have EPINEPHrine and resuscitative equipment available
• Monitor B/P at beginning of treatment and periodically; check weight daily; notify prescriber of weekly weight gain >5 lb; bone mineral density
• Monitor I&O ratio: be alert for decreasing urinary output, increasing edema, hypertension
• Assess liver function tests: ALT, AST, bilirubin, periodically during long-term therapy

M

- Assess for edema, hypertension, cardiac symptoms, jaundice
- Assess mental status: affect, mood, behavioral changes, depression

Nursing diagnoses
- Injury, risk for (adverse reactions)
- Knowledge, deficient (teaching)
- Sexual dysfunction (uses)

Patient/family education
- Advise patients to avoid sunlight or use sunscreen; photosensitivity and melasma (brown patches on the face) can occur
- Teach patient about cushingoid symptoms: weight gain, moon face, buffalo hump, acne
- Teach women patients to report breast lumps, vaginal bleeding, edema, jaundice, dark urine, clay-colored stools, dyspnea, headache, blurred vision, abdominal pain, sudden changes in speech/coordination, numbness or stiffness in legs, chest pain; teach men to report impotence or gynecomastia
- Teach patient to report suspected pregnancy (X) immediately; fertility returns in 6-12 mo after discontinuing

> **BLACK BOX WARNING:** Long-term use decreases bone density; exercise, calcium supplements can help lessen osteoporosis

Evaluation
Positive therapeutic outcome
- Decreased abnormal uterine bleeding
- Absence of amenorrhea
- Prevention of pregnancy
- Arrested spread of malignant cells

medrysone ophthalmic
See Appendix B

megestrol (Rx)
(me-jess′trole)
Megace, Megace ES
Func. class.: Antineoplastic hormone
Chem. class.: Progestin
Pregnancy category D (tabs), X (susp)

Do not confuse:
Megace/Reglan

ACTION: Affects endometrium by antiluteinizing effect; this is thought to bring about cell death

Therapeutic outcome: Prevention of rapidly growing malignant cells; weight gain, increased appetite in AIDS

USES: Breast, endometrial, renal cell cancer; increased weight, decreased cachexia and anorexia associated with AIDS

Unlabeled uses: Hot flashes, prostate cancer

CONTRAINDICATIONS:
Pregnancy **X** (susp), **D** (tabs), hypersensitivity

Precautions: Diabetes, thrombosis, adrenal insufficiency

DOSAGE AND ROUTES
Endometrial/ovarian carcinoma
Adult: PO 40-320 mg/day in divided doses

Breast carcinoma
Adult: PO 40 mg qid or 160 mg/day

Anorexia (AIDS)
Adult: PO 800 mg/day (oral SUSP) or 625 mg/day (ES)

Hot flashes (unlabeled)
Adult: PO 20 mg bid

Available forms: Tabs 20, 40 mg; oral susp 40, 125 mg/ml

Implementation
- Administer with meals for GI symptoms
- Oral susp is usually used for AIDS patients; shake well
- Give tablets for carcinoma

ADVERSE EFFECTS
CNS: Mood swings, insomnia
CV: Thrombophlebitis, thromboembolism, hypertension
ENDO: Adrenal insufficiency
GI: Nausea, vomiting, diarrhea, abdominal cramps, weight gain, flatus, indigestion
GU: Gynecomastia, fluid retention, hypercalcemia, vaginal bleeding, discharge, impotence, decreased libido
INTEG: Alopecia, rash, pruritus, purpura, itching, sweating
META: Hyperglycemia

⚠ Nurse Alert

Pharmacokinetics

Absorption	Well absorbed; food increases oral sol
Distribution	Unknown
Metabolism	Liver, completely
Excretion	Unknown
Half-life	1 hr

Pharmacodynamics

Onset	Several wk to mo
Peak	Unknown
Duration	1-3 days

INTERACTIONS

Individual drugs
Dofetilide: do not use with megestrol

Drug/lab test
Increased: alkaline phosphatase, urinary pregnanediol, plasma amino acids, urinary sodium
Decreased: HDL, GTT
False positive: urine glucose

NURSING CONSIDERATIONS

Assessment
• PSA levels in men (prostate cancer); blood glucose, liver function studies, serum calcium, weight
• Monitor effects of alopecia on body image; discuss feelings about body changes
• In AIDS patients monitor calorie counts, weight, appetite
• **Assess for thrombophlebitis:** Homan's sign, pain, redness, swelling in calf, thigh; notify prescriber immediately if these occur

Nursing diagnoses
• Knowledge, deficient (teaching)

Patient/family education
• Teach patient to report any complaints or side effects to prescriber
• Advise patient that contraceptive measures must be used during and 4 mo after treatment; product is teratogenic: pregnancy **D** tabs, pregnancy **X** susp
• Explore with patient the need for wig or a hairpiece for hair loss
• Caution patient to report vaginal bleeding to prescriber
• Review with patient the need to comply with dosage schedule, not to miss or double doses; missed doses may be taken up to 1 hr before next dose

• Teach patient how to recognize signs of fluid retention, thromboembolism and report immediately
• Teach that gynecomastia and alopecia can occur; reversible after discontinuing treatment
• Advise to monitor blood glucose if diabetic

Evaluation
Positive therapeutic outcome
• Decreased spread of malignant cells
• Weight gain, increased appetite in AIDS patients
• Resolved dysfunctional uterine bleeding

meloxicam (Rx)

(mel-ox'i-kam)
Mobic, Mobicox ✚
Func. class.: Nonsteroidal antiinflammatory/nonopioid analgesic (NSAIDs)
Chem. class.: Oxicam
Pregnancy category C (1st trimester), D (2nd/3rd trimesters)

ACTION: Inhibits COX-1, COX-2 by blocking arachidonate; analgesic, antiinflammatory, antipyretic effects

Therapeutic outcome: Decreased pain, swelling of joints; improved mobility

USES: Osteoarthritis, rheumatoid arthritis, juvenile arthritis

CONTRAINDICATIONS:
Pregnancy **D** (after 30 wk), labor and delivery, breastfeeding, hypersensitivity, asthma, severe renal/hepatic disease, peptic ulcer disease, CV bleeding

BLACK BOX WARNING: Perioperative pain in CABG surgery

Precautions: Pregnancy **C** (before 30 wk), children, geriatric, bleeding/GI/cardiac disorders, hypersensitivity to other antiinflammatory agents, CCr <25 ml/min

BLACK BOX WARNING: GI bleeding, MI, stroke

DOSAGE AND ROUTES
Adult: PO 7.5 mg/day, may increase to 15 mg/day; max 15 mg/day

Juvenile rheumatoid arthritis
Child ≥2 yr: PO 0.125 mg/kg, max 7.5 mg q day

Available forms: Tabs 7.5, 15 mg; susp 7.5 mg/5 ml

Implementation
- May take without regard to meals; take with food for GI upset
- Take with full glass of water and sit upright for $^1/_2$ hr
- Store at room temperature

ADVERSE EFFECTS
CNS: Dizziness, drowsiness, tremors, headache, nervousness, malaise, fatigue, insomnia, depression, **seizures**
CV: Hypertension, angina, **cardiac failure, MI,** hypotension, palpitations, **dysrhythmias,** tachycardia, stroke
EENT: Tinnitus, hearing loss, blurred vision
GI: Pancreatitis, nausea, colitis, GERD, vomiting, diarrhea, constipation, flatulence, cramps, dry mouth, peptic ulcer, **GI bleeding, perforation,** jaundice
GU: Nephrotoxicity: dysuria, hematuria, oliguria, azotemia
HEMA: Blood dyscrasias, anemia, prolonged bleeding
INTEG: Rash, urticaria, photosensitivity
SYST: Angioedema, anaphylaxis, Stevens-Johnson syndrome, toxic epidermal necrolysis

Pharmacokinetics

Absorption	Unknown
Distribution	Protein binding 99.4%
Metabolism	Liver <50%
Excretion	Breast milk, kidneys, feces
Half-life	15-20 hr

Pharmacodynamics

	PO	IM
Onset	Unknown	Unknown
Peak	4-5 hr	50 min
Duration	Unknown	Unknown

INTERACTIONS
Individual drugs
Cholestyramine: decreased action of meloxicam
CycloSPORINE, tacrolimus: increased nephrotoxicity
Lithium, methotrexate: increased action of each of these

Drug classifications
Aminoglycosides, anticoagulants, diuretics: increased action of each specific product

β-Adrenergic blockers, ACE inhibitors, thiazides, other antihypertensives: decreased action of β-blockers
Salicylates, sulfonamides: increased action of meloxicam

Drug/herb
Feverfew, ginko: decreased meloxicam effect
Garlic: increased bleeding risk

NURSING CONSIDERATIONS
Assessment
- Monitor renal, liver, blood tests: BUN, creatinine, AST, ALT, Hgb before treatment, periodically thereafter

> **BLACK BOX WARNING:** Check for GI bleeding, perforation, stool guaiac

⚠ Assess for anaphylaxis and angioedema; emergency equipment should be nearby
⚠ Fatal fulminant hepatitis, hepatic necrosis, hepatic failure: Assess for jaundice, yellow sclera and skin, clay-colored stools; monitor for liver function studies, hepatic reactions are more common in those with liver disease
- Assess for audiometric, ophth exam before, during, after treatment

> **BLACK BOX WARNING:** Assess for hypertension, MI, stroke, cardiac conditions

Nursing diagnoses
- Knowledge, deficient (teaching)
- Mobility, impaired physical (uses)
- Pain, chronic (uses)

Patient/family education
- Advise patient to report blurred vision or ringing, roaring in ears (may indicate toxicity)
- Advise patient to avoid driving, other hazardous activities if dizziness or drowsiness occurs
- Teach patient to report change in urine pattern, weight increase, edema, pain increase in joints, fever, blood in urine (indicates nephrotoxicity); to report rash, black stools, or continuing headache
- Teach patient to not use alcohol, aspirin, acetaminophen without consulting prescriber
- Advise to report use to all health care providers

Evaluation
Positive therapeutic outcome
- Decreased pain, stiffness, swelling in joints, able to move more easily

---

⚠ Nurse Alert

⚠ HIGH ALERT

melphalan (Rx)

(mel'fa-lan)

Alkeran

Func. class.: Antineoplastic, alkylating agent

Chem. class.: Nitrogen mustard

Pregnancy category D

Do not confuse:
melphalan/myleran

ACTION: Responsible for cross-linking DNA strands leading to cell death; activity is not cell cycle phase specific

Therapeutic outcome: Prevention of rapidly growing malignant cells

USES: Multiple myeloma, malignant melanoma, advanced ovarian cancer

Unlabeled uses: Breast, testicular, prostate carcinoma; osteogenic sarcoma, chronic myelogenous leukemia, non-Hodgkin's lymphoma

CONTRAINDICATIONS:

Pregnancy **D,** breastfeeding, or other nitrogen mustards

> **BLACK BOX WARNING:** Hypersensitivity to this product

Precautions: Children, radiation therapy, infection, renal disease

> **BLACK BOX WARNING:** Bone marrow depression, secondary malignancy

DOSAGE AND ROUTES

Multiple myeloma

Adult: PO 6 mg qd × 2-3 wk, adjust dose based on blood counts or 10 mg qd × 7-10 days and 2 mg qd once WBC >4000 cells/mm³, platelets >100,000 cells/mm³, then 2-4 mg/day or 7 mg/m² × 5 days q5-6 wk

Adult: IV INF 16 mg/m²; reduce in renal insufficiency; give over 15-20 min; give at 2-wk intervals × 4 doses, then at 4-wk intervals

Ovarian carcinoma

Adult: PO 200 mcg/kg/day × 5 days q4-5wk

Available forms: Tabs 2 mg; powder for inj 50 mg

Implementation

• Give fluids **IV** or PO before chemotherapy to hydrate patient

• Give antacid before oral agent; give product after evening meal, before bedtime; provide antiemetic 30-60 min before giving product and prn to prevent vomiting; give antibiotics for prophylaxis of infection

• Give in AM so product can be eliminated before bedtime

• Use a liquid diet: carbonated beverages; gelatin may be added if patient is not nauseated or vomiting

PO route

• Give 1 hr before or 2 hr after meals to prevent nausea/vomiting

Intermittent IV INF route

• Use gloves during administration; if skin exposure occurs, wash immediately with soap and water

• Reconstitute with provided diluent (10 ml) to 5 mg/ml; shake until clear; further dilute with 0.9% NaCl to <0.45 mg/ml; give over ≥15 min, give within 1 hr

Y-site compatibilities: Acyclovir, amikacin, aminophylline, ampicillin, aztreonam, bleomycin, bumetanide, buprenorphine, butorphanol, calcium gluconate, CARBOplatin, carmustine, ceFAZolin, cefepime, cefoperazone, cefotaxime, cefotetan, ceftazidime, ceftizoxime, cefTRIAXone, cefuroxime, cimetidine, CISplatin, clindamycin, cyclophosphamide, cytarabine, dacarbazine, DACTINomycin, DAUNOrubicin, dexamethasone, diphenhydrAMINE, DOXOrubicin, doxycycline, droperidol, enalaprilat, etoposide, famotidine, floxuridine, fluconazole, fludarabine, fluorouracil, furosemide, gallium, ganciclovir, gentamicin, granisetron, haloperidol, heparin, hydrocortisone sodium phosphate, hydromorphone, hydrOXYzine, IDArubicin, ifosfamide, imipenem-cilastatin, LORazepam, mannitol, mechlorethamine, meperidine, mesna, methylPREDNISolone, metoclopramide, methotrexate, metroNIDAZOLE, miconazole, minocycline, mitomycin, mitoxantrone, morphine, nalbuphine, netilmicin, ondansetron, pentostatin, piperacillin, plicamycin, potassium chloride, prochlorperazine, promethazine, ranitidine, sodium bicarbonate, streptozocin, teniposide, thiotepa, ticarcillin, ticarcillin/clavulanate, tobramycin, trimethoprim/sulfamethoxazole, vancomycin, vinBLAStine, vinCRIStine, vinorelbine, zidovudine

M

ADVERSE EFFECTS

GI: *Nausea, vomiting,* stomatitis, diarrhea, **hepatitis**
GU: Amenorrhea, hyperuricemia, gonadal suppression
HEMA: Thrombocytopenia, neutropenia, leukopenia, anemia
INTEG: Rash, urticaria, alopecia, pruritus
RESP: Fibrosis, dysplasia, dyspnea, pneumonitis
SYST: Anaphylaxis, allergic reaction, **secondary malignancies,** edema

Pharmacokinetics

Absorption	Variable; incompletely absorbed
Distribution	Rapidly distributed, protein binding 80%-90%
Metabolism	Bloodstream
Excretion	Kidneys, unchanged (10%)
Half-life	$1^1/_2$ hr

Pharmacodynamics

Unknown

INTERACTIONS

Individual drugs

Sargramostim, GM-CSF, filgrastim, G-CSF: avoid administration 14 hr before or 24 hr after this product
Carmustine: increased pulmonary toxicity
CycloSPORINE: increased renal failure risk
Nalidixic acid: increased enterocolitis risk
Radiation: increased toxicity

Drug classifications

Anticoagulants, NSAIDs, salicylates, thrombolytics, platelet inhibitors: increased bleeding risk
Antineoplastics: increased toxicity
Live virus vaccines: increased adverse reactions; decreased antibody reaction

NURSING CONSIDERATIONS

Assessment

> **BLACK BOX WARNING:** Monitor CBC, differential, platelet count weekly; withhold product if WBC is <3000/mm³ or platelet count is <100,000/mm³; notify prescriber; recovery usually occurs in 6 wk

• **Hyperuricemia:** assess for increased uric acid levels, swelling, joint pain primarily in extremities; patient should be well hydrated to prevent urate deposits
• **Infection:** monitor for cold, fever, chills, sore throat

• **Assess for bleeding:** hematuria, guaiac, bruising or petechiae, from mucosa or orifices q8hr; no rectal temp
• **Assess for symptoms indicating severe allergic reaction:** rash, pruritus, urticaria, purpuric skin lesions, itching, flushing; assess allergy to chlorambucil; cross-sensitivity may occur

Nursing diagnoses

• Body image, disturbed (adverse reactions)
• Infection, risk for (adverse reactions)
• Injury, risk for (adverse reactions)
• Knowledge, deficient (teaching)

Patient/family education

• Teach patient to avoid use of products containing aspirin or ibuprofen, razors, commercial mouthwash, since bleeding may occur; to report symptoms of bleeding (hematuria, tarry stools)
• Instruct patient to report signs of anemia (fatigue, headache, irritability, faintness, shortness of breath)
• Instruct patient to report any changes in breathing or coughing even several mo after treatment; to avoid crowds and persons with respiratory tract or other infections
• Tell patient hair loss is common; discuss the use of wigs or hairpieces
• Caution patient not to have any vaccinations without the advice of the prescriber, serious reactions can occur
• Advise patient that contraception is needed during treatment and for several mo after the completion of therapy, pregnancy **D**
• Teach patient to rinse mouth tid-qid with water, club soda; brush teeth bid-qid with soft brush or cotton-tipped applicators for stomatitis; use unwaxed dental floss

Evaluation

Positive therapeutic outcome
• Decreased size of tumor
• Decreased spread of malignancy

---

memantine (Rx)
(me-man'teen)
Ebixa ✦, Namenda, Namenda XR
Func. class.: Anti–Alzheimer's disease agent
Chem. class.: NMDA receptor antagonist
Pregnancy category B

ACTION: Antagonist action of CNS NMDA receptors that may contribute to the symptoms of Alzheimer's disease

---

⚠ Nurse Alert

Therapeutic outcome: Improved mood, orientation, decreasing confusion

USES: Moderate to severe dementia in Alzheimer's disease

Unlabeled uses: Vascular dementia

CONTRAINDICATIONS:
Hypersensitivity, children

Precautions: Pregnancy **B**, breastfeeding, renal disease, seizures, severe hepatic disease, GU conditions that raise urine pH, renal failure

DOSAGE AND ROUTES
Adult: PO 5 mg/day, may increase dose in 5-mg increments ≥1-wk intervals; recommended target dose 20 mg/day as 10 mg bid

Available forms: Tabs 5, 10 mg; tab titration pak 5, 10 mg; oral sol 2 mg/ml, 10 mg/5 ml

Implementation
• Can be taken without regard to meals
• Give twice a day if dose >5 mg
• Dosage is adjusted to response no more than q1wk
• Provide assistance with ambulation during beginning therapy; dizziness may occur
• **Extended Release Caps:** Do not crush, chew, divide; swallow whole or open and sprinkle on applesauce

ADVERSE EFFECTS
CNS: *Dizziness, confusion,* somnolence, headache, hallucinations
CV: Hypertension
GI: Vomiting, constipation
INTEG: Rash
MISC: Back pain, fatigue, pain
RESP: Coughing, dyspnea

Pharmacokinetics

Absorption	Rapidly absorbed PO
Distribution	44% protein binding
Metabolism	Very little
Excretion	57%-82% excreted unchanged in urine
Half-life	Terminal elimination half-life 60-80 hr

Pharmacodynamics
Unknown

INTERACTIONS
Individual drugs
Cimetidine, hydrochlorothiazide, nicotine, quiNIDine, ranitidine, triamterene: may alter levels of both products
Ergot, levodopa: increased effect of each

Drug classifications
Drugs that make the urine alkaline (sodium bicarbonate, carbonic anhydrase inhibitors): decreased clearance

NURSING CONSIDERATIONS
Assessment
• Alzheimer's dementia: affect, mood, behavioral changes; hallucinations, confusion, attention, orientation, memory

Nursing diagnoses
• Injury, risk for (uses)
• Knowledge, deficient (teaching)
• Noncompliance (teaching)

Patient/family education
• Advise to report side effects: restlessness, psychosis, visual hallucinations, stupor, loss of consciousness; indicate overdose
• Advise to use product exactly as prescribed; product is not a cure

Evaluation
Positive therapeutic outcome
• Decrease in confusion, improved mood or ability to maintain function, even with no improvement in symptoms

M

menotropins (Rx)
(men-oh-troe'pinz)
Menopur, Repronex
Func. class.: Gonadotropin
Chem. class.: Exogenous gonadotropin
Pregnancy category X

ACTION: In women, increases follicular growth, maturation; in men, when given with hCG, stimulates spermatogenesis

Therapeutic outcome: Pregnancy, ovulation

USES: Infertility, anovulation in women; stimulates spermatogenesis in men; usually used with hCG

CONTRAINDICATIONS:
Pregnancy **X**, primary ovarian failure, abnormal bleeding, thyroid/adrenal dysfunction, organic

intracranial lesion, ovarian cysts, primary testicular failure, high FSH, neoplastic disease

Precautions: Ascites, children, geriatric patients, endometriosis, polycystic ovary syndrome, thromboembolic disease; uterine leiomyomata, smoking

DOSAGE AND ROUTES

Infertility
Adult (men): IM 1 ampule 3 ×/wk with hCG 2000 units 2 ×/wk × 4 mo
Adult (women): IM 75 international units of FSH, LH daily × 9-12 days, then 10,000 units of hCG 1 day after these products; repeat × 2 menstrual cycles, then increase to 150 international units of FSH, LH daily × 9-12 days, then 10,000 units of hCG 1 day after these products × 2 menstrual cycles

Anovulation
Adult (women): IM (Humegon) 75 international units FSH, LH daily × 7-12 days, then 10,000 units hCG 1 day after last dose of these products: repeat × 1-3 menstrual cycles; IM/SUBCUT (Repronex only) 75 international units FSH/LH activity daily × 5 days, adjust dose by no more than 75-150 international units/day q2days

Available forms: Powder for inj lyophilized 75, 150 international units FSH, LH activity

Implementation
• Give after reconstituting with 1-2 ml of sterile saline inj; use immediately

ADVERSE EFFECTS
CNS: Fever, hot flashes, dizziness
CV: Hypovolemia, tachycardia
GI: *Nausea,* vomiting, diarrhea, anorexia
GU: Ovarian hyperstimulation syndrome (OHSS), multiple births, abdominal distention, pain, sudden ovarian enlargement, ascites with or without pain, ectopic pregnancy, gynecomastia in men
HEMA: Hemoperitoneum, arterial thromboembolism
INTEG: Rash, swelling of inj site
OTHER: Anaphylaxis
RESP: ARDS, pulmonary embolism, pulmonary infarction, pleural effusion, atelectasis, dyspnea, tachypnea

Pharmacokinetics

Absorption	Well absorbed
Distribution	Unknown
Metabolism	Unknown
Excretion	Kidneys, unchanged (8%)
Half-life	70 hr (FSH); 4 hr (LH)

Pharmacodynamics

Unknown

NURSING CONSIDERATIONS

Assessment
• Monitor weight daily; notify prescriber if weight gain increases rapidly
• Monitor estrogen excretion level; if >100 mcg/24 hr, product is withheld; serum progesterone, LH, estradiol level, pelvic exam, ovarian ultrasound; hyperstimulation syndrome may occur
• Monitor I&O ratio; be alert for decreasing urinary output
• Assess for ovarian enlargement, abdominal distention/pain; report symptoms immediately

Nursing diagnoses
• Knowledge, deficient (teaching)
• Sexual dysfunction (uses)

Patient/family education
• Advise patient that multiple births are possible; if pregnancy occurs, it is usually 4-6 wk after start of treatment
• Instruct patient to keep daily appointment

Evaluation
Positive therapeutic outcome
• Pregnancy

⚠ HIGH ALERT

meperidine (Rx)
(me-per'i-deen)
Demerol, Meperitab
Func. class.: Opioid analgesic
Chem. class.: Phenylpiperidine derivative
Pregnancy category C
Controlled substance schedule II

Do not confuse:
meperidine/HYDROmorphone/meprobamate/morphine,
Demerol/Dilaudid/Desyrel/Demulen

ACTION: Depresses pain impulse transmission at the spinal cord level by interacting with opioid receptors

Therapeutic outcome: Relief of pain

USES: Moderate to severe pain, preoperatively, postoperatively

CONTRAINDICATIONS:
Hypersensitivity

Precautions: Pregnancy **C**, breastfeeding, child <18 yr, geriatric, addictive personality, increased ICP, MI (acute), severe heart disease, respiratory depression, renal/hepatic disease, seizure disorder, abrupt discontinuation, chronic pain

DOSAGE AND ROUTES
Moderate to severe pain
Adult: PO/SUBCUT/IM 50-150 mg q3-4hr prn; IV 15-35 mg/hr as a CONT INF; PCA 10 mg, then 1-5 mg incremental dose; lockout interval 6-10 min
Child: PO/SUBCUT/IM 1-1.8 mg/kg q3-4hr prn, max 100 mg q4hr

Preoperatively
Adult: IM/SUBCUT 50-100 mg 30-90 min before surgery
Child: IM/SUBCUT 1-2 mg/kg 30-90 min before surgery, max 100 mg

Labor analgesia
Adult: SUBCUT/IM 50-100 mg given when contractions are regulary spaced, repeat q1-3hr prn

Available forms: Inj 10, 25, 50, 75, 100 mg/ml; tabs 50, 100 mg; syr 50 mg/5 ml

Implementation
• Give with antiemetic if nausea, vomiting occur
• Administer when pain is beginning to return; determine dosage interval by patient response; continuous dosing of medication is more effective given prn
• Medication should be slowly withdrawn after long-term use to prevent withdrawal symptoms
• Store in light-resistant container at room temperature
PO route
• May be given with food or milk to lessen GI upset
• Syr should be mixed with 4 oz of water
IM/SUBCUT route
• Do not give if cloudy or a precipitate has formed
• Patient should remain recumbent for 1 hr after administration
• Inject IM into a large muscle mass; IM is preferred route for multiple injections

Direct IV route
• Give after diluting to 10 mg/ml with sterile water, 0.9% NaCl for inj; give slowly at ≤25 mg/min; rapid administration may cause respiratory depression, hypotension, circulatory collapse
• Have emergency equipment and opiate antagonist on hand
Continuous IV infusion route
• Give after diluting to 1 mg/ml with D_5W, $D_{10}W$, dextrose/saline combinations, dextrose/Ringer's, inj combinations, 0.45% NaCl, 0.9% NaCl, Ringer's, LR; give by inf pump; titrate according to response

Syringe compatibilities: Butorphanol, chlorproMAZINE, cimetidine, dimenhyDRINATE, diphenhydrAMINE, droperidol, fentanyl, glycopyrrolate, hydrOXYzine, ketamine, metoclopramide, midazolam, pentazocine, perphenazine, prochlorperazine, promazine, promethazine, ranitidine, scopolamine

Syringe incompatibilities: Heparin, morphine, pentobarbital

Y-site compatibilities: Amifostine, amikacin, ampicillin, atenolol, aztreonam, bumetanide, cefamandole, ceFAZolin, cefmetazole, cefotaxime, cefotetan, cefoxitin, ceftazidime, ceftizoxime, cefTRIAXone, cefuroxime, cephalothin, cephapirin, chloramphenicol, cladribine, clindamycin, dexamethasone, diltiazem, diphenhydrAMINE, DOBUTamine, DOPamine, doxycycline, droperidol, erythromycin lactobionate, famotidine, filgrastim, fluconazole, fludarabine, gallium, gentamicin, granisetron, heparin, hydrocortisone, regular insulin, kanamycin, labetalol, lidocaine, magnesium sulfate, melphalan, methyldopate, methylPREDNISolone, metoclopramide, metoprolol, metroNIDAZOLE, moxalactam, ondansetron, oxacillin, oxytocin, paclitaxel, penicillin G potassium, piperacillin, potassium chloride, propofol, propranolol, ranitidine, sargramostim, teniposide, thiotepa, ticarcillin, ticarcillin/clavulanate, tobramycin, trimethoprim/sulfamethoxazole, vancomycin, verapamil, vinorelbine

Y-site incompatibilities: Cefoperazone, IDArubicin, imipenem/cilastatin, mezlocillin, minocycline
Continuous intrathecal infusion route
• Use controlled-infusion device, an implantable controlled-microinfusion device is used for highly concentrated infusion, monitor for several days after implantation
• Infusion reservoir should only be filled by those fully qualified

M

• To prevent pain, depletion of reservoir should be avoided

ADVERSE EFFECTS

CNS: Drowsiness, dizziness, confusion, headache, sedation, euphoria, **increased ICP, seizures,** serotonin syndrome
CV: Palpitations, bradycardia, hypotension, change in B/P, tachycardia (**IV**)
EENT: Tinnitus, blurred vision, miosis, diplopia, depressed corneal reflex
GI: Nausea, vomiting, anorexia, constipation, cramps, biliary spasm, paralytic ileus
GU: Urinary retention, dysuria
INTEG: Rash, urticaria, bruising, flushing, diaphoresis, pruritus
RESP: Respiratory depression
SYST: Anaphylaxis

Pharmacokinetics

Absorption	Well absorbed (IM, SUBCUT); 50% (PO)
Distribution	Widely distributed; crosses placenta; protein binding 65%-75%; toxic by-product accumulation can result from regular use or in renal disease
Metabolism	Liver, extensively to active/inactive metabolites
Excretion	Kidneys; breast milk
Half-life	3-4 hr

Pharmacodynamics

	PO	IM/SUBCUT	IV
Onset	15 min	10 min	5 min
Peak	$1/2$-1 hr	$1/2$-1 hr	5-7 min
Duration	2-4 hr	2-4 hr	2 hr

INTERACTIONS

Individual drugs

Alcohol: increased respiratory depression, hypotension, sedation
Phenytoin: decreased meperidine effect
Procarbazine: fatal reaction, do not use together

Drug classifications

CNS depressants, opioids, sedative/hypnotics, antipsychotics, skeletal muscle relaxants: increased effects
SSRIs, SNRIs, serotonin-receptor agonists: increased serotonin syndrome, increased neuroleptic malignant syndrome
MAOIs: do not use for 2 wk before taking meperidine; may cause fatal reaction

Protease inhibitor antiretrovirals: increased adverse reactions

Drug/herb

St. John's wort: increased CNS depression

Drug/lab test

Increased: amylase, lipase

NURSING CONSIDERATIONS

Assessment

• **Assess pain:** location, duration, intensity before and 1 hr (IM, SUBCUT, PO), 5-10 min (**IV**) after administration
• Assess renal function before initiating therapy; poor renal function can lead to accumulation of toxic metabolite and seizures
• Monitor VS after parenteral route; note muscle rigidity, product history, liver, kidney function tests, respiratory dysfunction: respiratory depression, character, rate, rhythm; notify prescriber if respirations are <10/min
• Monitor CNS changes: dizziness, drowsiness, hallucinations, euphoria, LOC, pupil reaction; these are due to metabolite produced; CNS stimulation occurs with chronic or high doses
• Monitor allergic reactions: rash, urticaria
• Assess for constipation; increase fluids, bulk in diet; give stimulant laxatives if needed

Nursing diagnoses

• Breathing pattern, ineffective (adverse reactions)
• Injury, risk for (adverse reactions)
• Knowledge, deficient (teaching)
• Pain, acute (uses)
• Sensory perception, disturbed: visual, auditory (adverse reactions)

Patient/family education

• Advise patients to avoid CNS depressants (alcohol, sedative/hypnotics) for at least 24 hr after taking this product
• Discuss with patient that dizziness, drowsiness, and confusion are common; to avoid getting up without assistance
• Discuss in detail with patient all aspects of the product, including its purpose and what to expect
• Caution patient to make position changes carefully to lessen orthostatic hypotension

Evaluation

Positive therapeutic outcome
• Decreased pain

TREATMENT OF OVERDOSE:

Naloxone 0.2-0.8 mg **IV,** O_2, **IV** fluids, vasopressors

mercaptopurine (6-MP) (Rx)

(mer-kap-toe-pyoor'een)

Purinethol

Func. class.: Antineoplastic, antimetabolite

Chem. class.: Purine analog

Pregnancy category D

ACTION: Inhibits purine metabolism at multiple sites, which inhibits DNA and RNA synthesis S phase of cell cycle

Therapeutic outcome: Prevention of rapidly growing malignant cells

USES: Chronic myelocytic leukemia, acute lymphoblastic leukemia in children

Unlabeled uses: Polycythemia vera, psoriatic arthritis, colitis, lymphoma, acute myelogenous leukemia

CONTRAINDICATIONS:

Pregnancy **D**, breastfeeding, patients with prior product resistance, leukopenia, thrombocytopenia, anemia

Precautions: Renal/hepatic disease, tumor lysis syndrome, dental disease, herpes, radiation therapy

DOSAGE AND ROUTES

Acute lymphocytic leukemia

Adult: PO 2.5-5 mg/kg/day or 80-100 mg/m²/day, maintenance 1.5-2.5 mg/kg/day

Child: PO 2.5-5 mg/kg/day, maintenance 1.5-2.5 mg/kg/day or 70-100 mg/m²/day

Available forms: Tabs 50 mg

Implementation

• Give fluids **IV** or PO before chemotherapy to hydrate patient
• Give antiemetic 30-60 min before giving product and prn to prevent vomiting
• Give in PM on empty stomach
• Give entire dose at one time
• Provide liquid diet: carbonated beverages; gelatin may be added if patient is not nauseated or vomiting
• Tab may be crushed and added to fluids or food to facilitate swallowing

ADVERSE EFFECTS

CNS: Weakness

GI: *Nausea, vomiting, anorexia, diarrhea, stomatitis,* **hepatotoxicity** (with high doses), jaundice, gastritis, **pancreatitis**

GU: **Renal failure,** hyperuricemia, **oliguria,** crystalluria, **hematuria**

HEMA: Thrombocytopenia, leukopenia, myelosuppression, anemia

INTEG: *Rash,* dry skin, urticaria, alopecia

Pharmacokinetics

Absorption	Variable
Distribution	Widely, body water
Metabolism	Liver, extensively
Excretion	Kidneys unchanged (small amounts)
Half-life	Terminal 1-1.5 hr

Pharmacodynamics

Onset	Unknown
Peak	1-2 hr
Duration	Unknown

INTERACTIONS

Individual products

Allopurinol, sulfamethoxazole-trimethoprim: increased bone marrow depression

Radiation: increased effects

Warfarin: increased effect of warfarin

Drug classifications

Anticoagulants, NSAIDs, platelet inhibitors, salicylates, thrombolytics: increased bleeding risk

Antineoplastics, immunosuppressants: increased effects

Live virus vaccines: decreased antibodies

NURSING CONSIDERATIONS

Assessment

• Assess buccal cavity for dryness, sores or ulceration, white patches, oral pain, bleeding, dysphagia; obtain prescription for viscous lidocaine (Xylocaine)

⚠ Assess symptoms indicating severe allergic reaction: rash, pruritus, urticaria, purpuric skin lesions, itching, flushing, laryngeal edema

• **Bone marrow suppression:** monitor CBC, differential, platelet count weekly; withhold product if WBC is <4000/mm³ or platelet count is <100,000/mm³; notify prescriber of results if WBC <20,000/mm³, platelets <150,000/mm³

• Assess for increased uric acid levels, swelling, joint pain primarily in extremities; patient should be well hydrated to prevent urate deposits

• Monitor renal function tests: BUN, creatinine, serum uric acid, urine CCr before, during

M

therapy; check I&O ratio; report fall in urine output to <30 ml/hr
• Monitor temp q4hr (may indicate beginning of infection)
• Monitor liver function tests before, during therapy (bilirubin, AST, ALT, LDH) as needed or monthly; check for yellowing of skin or sclera, dark urine, clay-colored stools, itchy skin, abdominal pain, fever, diarrhea
• **Assess for bleeding:** hematuria, stool guaiac, bruising or petechiae, mucosa or orifices q8hr; check for inflammation of mucosa, breaks in skin

Nursing diagnoses
• Body image, disturbed (adverse reactions)
• Infection, risk for (adverse reactions)
• Injury, risk for (adverse reactions)
• Knowledge, deficient (teaching)

Patient/family education
• Encourage patient to rinse mouth tid-qid with water, club soda; brush teeth bid-qid with soft brush or cotton-tipped applicators for stomatitis; use unwaxed dental floss
• Advise patient that contraceptive measures are recommended during therapy; serious teratogenic effects may occur, to avoid breast-feeding
• Teach patient to avoid use of products containing aspirin or NSAIDs, razors, commercial mouthwash, since bleeding may occur; to report symptoms of bleeding (hematuria, tarry stools)
• Instruct patient to report signs of anemia (fatigue, headache, irritability, faintness, shortness of breath)
• Instruct patient to report any changes in breathing or coughing even several mo after treatment; to avoid crowds and persons with respiratory tract or other infections
• Caution patient not to have any vaccinations without the advice of the prescriber; serious reactions can occur
• Advise patient to take entire dose at one time

Evaluation
Positive therapeutic outcome
• Prevention of rapid division of malignant cells

meropenem (Rx)
(mer-oh-pen'em)
Merrem IV
Func. class.: Antiinfective—miscellaneous
Pregnancy category B

ACTION: Interferes with cell wall replication of susceptible organisms; osmotically unstable cell wall swells and bursts from osmotic pressure

Therapeutic outcome: Bactericidal action against the following: *Streptococcus pneumoniae,* group A β-hemolytic streptococci, *viridans* group streptococci, enterococcus; gram-negative organisms *Klebsiella, Proteus, Escherichia coli, Pseudomonas aeruginosa, Bacteroides fragilis, Bacteroides thetaiotamicron,* bacterial meningitis (>3 mo old)

USES: Serious infections caused by gram-positive or gram-negative organisms (appendicitis, peritonitis)

Unlabeled uses: Febrile neutropenic, community-acquired pneumonia

CONTRAINDICATIONS:
Hypersensitivity to meropenem, carbapenems, cephalosporins, penicillins

Precautions: Pregnancy **B**, breastfeeding, geriatric, renal disease, seizure disorder

DOSAGE AND ROUTES
Adult: IV 1 g q8hr, given over 15-30 min or as an IV BOL 5-20 ml given over 3-5 min
Adolescent < 50 kg/Child ≥ 3 mo: IV 20-40 mg/kg q8hr (max 2 g q8hr meningitis)
Child >50 kg: IV 1 g q8hr (intraabdominal infection) or 2 g q8hr (meningitis) given over 15-30 min or as an IV BOL 5-20 ml over 3-5 min; max 2 g q8hr

Renal dose
Adult: IV CCr 26-50 ml/min give dose q12hr; CCr 10-25 ml/min give $^1/_2$ dose q12hr; CCr <10 ml/min give $^1/_2$ dose q24hr

Available forms: Powder for inj 500 mg, 1 g

Implementation
Direct IV route
• Reconstitute 500 mg or 1 g vials with 10, 20 ml of sterile water for inj respectively, shake to dissolve and let stand until clear (average conc 50 mg/ml) reconstituted sol may be stored for 2 hr at room temperature or 12 hr refrigerated, inject up to 1 g in 5-20 ml over 3-5 min
Intermittent IV infusion route
• Vials may be directly constituted with compatible inf fluid (NS, D_5W) to 2.5-50 mg/ml vials; vials with 0.9% NaCl can be stored up to 2 hr at room temperature, or 18 hr refrigerated, D_5W may be stored up to 1 hr at room temperature or up to 8 hr refrigerated, infuse over 15-30 min

Y-site compatibilities: Aminophylline, atenolol, atropine, cimetidine, dexamethasone, digoxin, diphenhydrAMINE, enalaprilat, fluconazole, furosemide, gentamicin, heparin, insulin (regular), metoclopramide, morphine, norepinephrine, PHENobarbital, vancomycin

Additive compatibilities: Aminophylline, atropine, cimetidine, dexamethasone, DOBUTamine, DOPamine, enalaprilat, fluconazole, furosemide, gentamicin, heparin, insulin (regular), magnesium sulfate, metoclopramide, morphine, norepinephrine, PHENobarbital, ranitidine, vancomycin

ADVERSE EFFECTS

CNS: Fever, somnolence, *seizures,* dizziness, weakness, *headache,* myoclonia, confusion
CV: Hypotension, palpitations, tachycardia
GI: Diarrhea, nausea, vomiting, **pseudomembranous colitis, hepatitis,** glossitis
HEMA: Eosinophilia, **neutropenia,** decreased Hgb, Hct, **agranulocytosis**
INTEG: *Rash,* urticaria, *pruritus,* pain at inj site, phlebitis, erythema at inj site
RESP: Chest discomfort, dyspnea, hyperventilation, **pulmonary embolism**
SYST: **Anaphylaxis, Stevens-Johnson syndrome, angioedema**

Pharmacokinetics

Absorption	Complete bioavailability
Distribution	Widely distributed
Metabolism	Liver
Excretion	Kidneys
Half-life	1 hr; increased in renal disease

Pharmacodynamics

Onset	Rapid
Peak	Dose dependent
Duration	Unknown

INTERACTIONS

Individual drugs
Probenecid: increased meropenem levels
Valproic acid: decreased effect of valproic acid

Drug/herb
Do not use acidophilus with antiinfectives; separate by several hours

Drug/lab test
Increased: AST, ALT, LDH, BUN, alkaline phosphatase, bilirubin, creatinine
False positive: direct Coombs' test

NURSING CONSIDERATIONS

Assessment
• Assess patient for previous sensitivity reaction to carbapenem antiinfectives, penicillins
• **Assess patient for signs and symptoms of infection,** including characteristics of wounds, sputum, urine, stool, WBC >10,000/100 mm³, fever; obtain baseline information before, during treatment
• Complete C&S tests before beginning product therapy to identify if correct treatment has been initiated
• **Assess for allergic reactions, anaphylaxis:** rash, urticaria, pruritus, chills, fever, joint pain; angioedema may occur a few days after therapy begins; epinephrine and resuscitation equipment should be available for anaphylactic reaction
• Identify urine output; if decreasing, notify prescriber (may indicate nephrotoxicity); also check for increased BUN, creatinine
• Monitor blood studies: AST, ALT, CBC, Hct, bilirubin, LDH, alkaline phosphatase, Coombs' test monthly if patient is on long-term therapy
• Monitor electrolytes: potassium, sodium, chloride monthly if patient is on long-term therapy
• Assess bowel pattern daily; if severe diarrhea occurs, product should be discontinued; **may indicate pseudomembranous colitis**
• Monitor for bleeding: ecchymosis, bleeding gums, hematuria, stool guaiac daily if on long-term therapy
• **Assess for overgrowth of infection:** perineal itching, fever, malaise, redness, pain, swelling, drainage, rash, diarrhea, change in cough, sputum

Nursing diagnoses
• Diarrhea (adverse reactions)
• Infection, risk for (uses)
• Injury, risk for (adverse reactions)
• Knowledge, deficient (teaching)
• Noncompliance (teaching)

Patient/family education
• Teach patient to report sore throat, bruising, bleeding, joint pain; may indicate blood dyscrasias (rare)
• Advise patient to contact prescriber if vaginal itching, loose foul-smelling stools, furry tongue occur; may indicate superinfection
• Advise patient to avoid breastfeeding; product is excreted in breast milk
• Advise patient to notify prescriber of diarrhea with blood or pus; may indicate **pseudomembranous colitis**

Evaluation
Positive therapeutic outcome
• Absence of signs/symptoms of infection (WBC <10,000/mm^3, temp WNL, absence of red draining wounds)
• Reported improvement in symptoms of infection

TREATMENT OF ANAPHYLAXIS: EPINEPHrine, antihistamines, resuscitate if needed

mesalamine, 5-ASA (Rx)
(mez-al'a-meen)
Apriso, Asacol, Asacol HD, Canasa, Lialda, Pentasa, Rowasa, sf Rowasa, Salofalk ♣
Func class.: GI antiinflammatory
Chem. class.: 5-Aminosalicylic acid
Pregnancy category B

Do not confuse:
Asacol/Ansaid/Os-Cal

ACTION: May diminish inflammation by blocking cyclooxygenase, inhibiting prostaglandin production in colon, local action only

Therapeutic outcome: Decreased cramping, pain in GI conditions

USES: Mild to moderate active distal ulcerative colitis, proctosigmoiditis, proctitis

Unlabeled uses: Crohn's disease

CONTRAINDICATIONS:
Hypersensitivity to this product or salicylates, 5-aminosalicylates

Precautions: Pregnancy **B**, breastfeeding, children, geriatric, renal disease, sulfite sensitivity, pyloric stenosis

DOSAGE AND ROUTES
Treatment of ulcerative colitis
Adult: RECT 60 ml (4 g) at bedtime, retained for 8 hr × 3-6 wk; DEL REL tab (Lialda) 2.4-4.8 g/day × 8 wk; DEL REL tab (Asacol) 800 mg tid × 6 wk; CONT REL cap (Pentasa) 1 g qid up to 8 wk; EXT REL cap (Apriso) 1500 mg (4 caps) qd AM up to 6 mo; RECT SUPP 500 mg bid retained for 1-3 hr × 3-6 wk until remission, may increase to tid if needed

Maintenance of remission
Adult: PO (delayed release tabs: Asacol) 800 mg bid or 400 mg qid; (delayed release caps:

Apriso) 1500 mg (4 caps) each AM; (delayed release tabs: Lialda) 2.4 g (2 tab) q day with a meal

Available forms: Enema 4 g/60 ml (Rowasa, ss Rowasa); del rel tabs 400 mg (Asacol); 800 mg (Asacol HD); ext rel tab 500 mg; ext rel cap 250 mg, 500 mg (Pentasa); del rel tab (Lialda) 1.2 g; 0.375 g (Apriso); rect supp 1000 mg

Implementation
PO route
• Do not break, crush, or chew del rel tabs
• **Lialda:** take with a meal
• **Apriso caps:** without regard to meals in AM
Rectal route (susp)
• Give at bedtime, retained until AM; empty bowel before insertion
• Store at room temperature
• Usual course of therapy is 3-6 wk
• Give after shaking bottle well

ADVERSE EFFECTS
CNS: *Headache, fever, dizziness,* insomnia, asthenia, weakness, fatigue
CV: Pericarditis, myocarditis, chest pain, palpitations
EENT: Sore throat, cough, pharyngitis, rhinitis
GI: *Cramps, gas, nausea, diarrhea,* rectal pain, constipation
INTEG: *Rash, itching,* acne
SYST: *Flulike symptoms, malaise,* back pain, peripheral edema, leg and joint pain, arthralgia, dysmenorrhea, **anaphylaxis,** acute intolerance syndrome

Pharmacokinetics
Absorption	20%-30% (PO), 10%-25% (RECT)
Distribution	Unknown
Metabolism	Unknown
Excretion	Feces
Half-life	1 hr; metabolite 5-10 hr

Pharmacodynamics
Unknown

INTERACTIONS
Individual drugs
Azathioprine: increased azathioprine action
Digoxin: decreased digoxin level
Lactulose: decreased mesalamine absorption
Omeprazole: increased mesalamine absorption
Warfarin: decreased effect of warfarin

Drug classifications
H₂ blockers: do not give with Apriso
NSAIDs: increased nephrotoxicity
Antacids: decreased mesalamine absorption

Drug/lab test
Increased: AST, ALT, alkaline phosphatase, LDH, GGTP, amylase, lipase

NURSING CONSIDERATIONS
Assessment
• Assess for GI symptoms: cramping, gas, nausea, diarrhea, rectal pain, abdominal pain; if severe, the product should be discontinued
• Assess for allergy to salicylates, sulfonamides; if allergic reactions occur, discontinue product
• Assess renal function before, during treatment: BUN, creatinine
• Monitor I&O ratios, increase fluids to 1500 ml daily to prevent crystalluria

Nursing diagnoses
• Diarrhea (uses)
• Knowledge, deficient (teaching)
• Pain, chronic (uses)

Patient/family education
• Advise patient to notify prescriber if abdominal pain, cramping, diarrhea with blood, headache, fever, rash, chest pain occur; product should be discontinued
• Teach correct administration for PO or enema

Evaluation
Positive therapeutic outcome
• Absence of pain, bleeding from GI tract

---

metformin (Rx)
(met-for′min)
Fortamet, Glucophage, Glucophage XR, Glumetza, Riomet
Func. class.: Antidiabetic, oral
Chem. class.: Biguanide
Pregnancy category B

ACTION: Inhibits hepatic glucose production and increases sensitivity of peripheral tissue to insulin

Therapeutic outcome: Blood glucose at normal levels

USES: Type 2 diabetes mellitus

CONTRAINDICATIONS:
Hypersensitivity; hepatic disease; creatinine >1.5 mg/ml (males), ≥1.4 (females); alcohol-ism; cardiopulmonary disease; acidemia; acute MI; cardiogenic shock; diabetic ketoacidosis; metabolic acidosis

BLACK BOX WARNING: History of lactic acidosis

Precautions: Pregnancy B, breastfeeding, geriatric, thyroid disease, previous hypersensitivity, CHF

DOSAGE AND ROUTES
Type 2 diabetes mellitus
Adult: PO 500 mg bid or 850 mg q day initially, then 500 mg weekly or 850 mg q2wk up to 2000 mg/day in divided doses; dosage adjustment q2-3wk or 850 mg/day with morning meal with dosage increased every other week, max 2550 mg/day; EXT REL (Glucophage XR) 500 mg qd with evening meal; may increase by 500 mg qwk, max 2000 mg/day; (Glumetza) 1000 mg qd with food, preferably with the PM meal, may increase by 500 mg qwk, max 2000 mg/day; (Fortamet) 500-1000 mg qd with PM meal, may increase by 500 mg qwk, max 2550 mg/day
Geriatric: PO use lowest effective dose

Available forms: Tabs 500, 850, 1000 mg; ext rel tabs 500, 750, 1000 mg; oral sol (Riomet) 500 mg/5 ml

Implementation
• Conversion from other oral hypoglycemic agents; change may be made without gradual dosage change; monitor serum or urine glucose and ketones tid during conversion
• **Immediate rel:** give twice a day with meals to decrease GI upset and provide best absorption
• Give immediate rel tabs crushed and mixed with meal or fluids for patients with difficulty swallowing
• **Extended release product:** may also be taken as a single dose; titrate slowly to therapeutic response, side-effect tolerance
• Do not break, crush, or chew ext rel tabs
• Give in AM to prevent hypoglycemic reactions in PM
• Store in tight container in cool environment

ADVERSE EFFECTS:
CNS: *Headache, weakness, dizziness, drowsiness,* tinnitus, fatigue, vertigo, *agitation*
CV: **Heart failure**
ENDO: **Lactic acidosis,** hypoglycemia
GI: Nausea, vomiting, diarrhea, heartburn, anorexia, metallic taste

M

HEMA: Thrombocytopenia, decreased vit B_{12} levels
INTEG: Rash

Pharmacokinetics

Absorption	Unknown
Distribution	Unknown
Metabolism	Unknown
Excretion	Kidneys, unchanged (35%-50%)
Half-life	$1^{1}/_{2}$-5 hr, terminal 6-20 hr

Pharmacodynamics

Onset	Unknown
Peak	1-3 hr
Duration	Unknown

INTERACTIONS

Individual drugs

Cimetidine, digoxin, morphine, procainamide, quiNIDine, ranitidine, triamterone, vancomycin: increased metformin level

Cimetidine, phenytoin: increased hypoglycemia

Dofetilide: increased lactic acidosis, do not use together

Radiologic contrast media: do not give together; may cause renal failure

Drug classifications

Calcium channel blockers, contraceptives (oral), corticosteroids, diuretics, estrogens, phenothiazines, sympathomimetics: increased hypoglycemia

Drug/herb

Garlic, green tea: increased hypoglycemia
Glucosamine: increased hyperglycemia

NURSING CONSIDERATIONS

Assessment

• Assess for hypoglycemic reactions (sweating, weakness, dizziness, anxiety, tremors, hunger), hyperglycemic reactions soon after meals; these occur rarely with this product

• Monitor CBC (baseline, q3mo) during treatment; check liver function tests (AST, LDH) and renal tests (BUN, creatinine) periodically during treatment; glucose, A1c; folic acid, vitamin B_{12} q1-2 yr

> **BLACK BOX WARNING:** Monitor for lactic acidosis: malaise, myalgia, abdominal distress; risk increases with age, poor renal function; monitor electrolytes, lactate, pyruvate, blood pH, ketones, glucose

Nursing diagnoses

• Knowledge, deficient (teaching)

Patient/family education

• Teach patient to regularly self-monitor blood glucose using blood glucose meter

• Teach patient symptoms of hypo/hyperglycemia, what to do about each (rare)

• Advise patient that product must be continued on daily basis; explain consequence of discontinuing product abruptly

• Advise patient to take product in morning to prevent hypoglycemic reactions at night

• Advise patient to avoid OTC medications, alcohol unless approved by the prescriber

• Teach patient that diabetes is a lifelong illness; that this product controls symptoms, but does not cure the condition

> **BLACK BOX WARNING: Teach patient symptoms of lactic acidosis**—hyperventilation, fatigue, malaise, myalgia, chills, somnolence—and to notify prescriber immediately

• Teach patient to carry/wear emergency ID and glucagon emergency kit for emergencies

• Advise patient that glucophage XR tab may appear in stool

• Advise patient to take with meals

Evaluation

Positive therapeutic outcome

• Decrease in polyuria, polydipsia, polyphagia; clear sensorium; absence of dizziness; stable gait; blood glucose, A1c at normal level

---

⚠ HIGH ALERT

methadone (Rx)

(meth'a-done)
Dolophine, Metadol ✦, Methadose
Func. class.: Opioid analgesic
Chem. class.: Synthetic diphenylheptane derivative
Pregnancy category C
Controlled substance schedule II

Do not confuse:
methadone/methylphenidate

ACTION: Depresses pain impulse transmission at the spinal cord level by interacting with opioid receptors; produces CNS depression

Therapeutic outcome: Relief of pain; successful opioid withdrawal

USES: Severe pain, opiate withdrawal

CONTRAINDICATIONS:
Hypersensitivity to this product, or hypersensitivity to chlorobutanol (inj route), asthma, ileus

> **BLACK BOX WARNING:** Respiratory depression

Precautions: Pregnancy **C,** breastfeeding, children <18 yr, geriatric, addictive personality, increased ICP, MI (acute), severe heart disease, respiratory depression, renal/hepatic disease, respiratory insufficiency, torsades de pointes, pulmonary disease, COPD

> **BLACK BOX WARNING:** QT prolongation, pain

DOSAGE AND ROUTES
Severe pain
Adult: PO/SUBCUT/IM 2.5-10 mg q8-12hr prn

Opiate withdrawal
Adult including pregnant women: PO 20-30 mg initially, unless low opioid tolerance is expected, additional 5-10 mg q2-4hr as needed after initial dose, if symptoms continue may give for up to 5 days

Renal dose
Adult: PO may need to be modified

Available forms: Inj 10 mg/ml; tabs 5, 10 mg; oral sol 5, 10 mg/5 ml, 10 mg/ml

Implementation
• Medication should be slowly withdrawn after long-term use to prevent withdrawal symptoms
PO route
• May be given with food or milk to lessen GI upset
• Store in light-resistant container at room temperature
IM/SUBCUT route
• Do not give if cloudy or a precipitate has formed
• Give deeply in large muscle mass (IM); rotate inj sites

ADVERSE EFFECTS
CNS: *Drowsiness, dizziness, confusion, headache, sedation,* euphoria, **seizures**
CV: Palpitations, bradycardia, change in B/P, **cardiac arrest, shock,** hypotension, **torsades de pointes, QT prolongation**
EENT: Tinnitus, blurred vision, miosis, diplopia
GI: *Nausea, vomiting, anorexia, constipation, cramps,* biliary tract spasm

GU: Increased urinary output, dysuria, urinary retention, impotence
INTEG: *Rash,* urticaria, bruising, flushing, diaphoresis, pruritus
RESP: **Respiratory depression, respiratory arrest**

Pharmacokinetics
Absorption	Well absorbed (PO, SUBCUT, IM)
Distribution	Widely distributed; crosses placenta, half as active PO, as inj
Metabolism	Liver, extensively
Excretion	Kidneys, breast milk
Half-life	8-59 hr; extended interval with continued dosing

Pharmacodynamics
	PO	IM/SUBCUT
Onset	$^{1}/_{2}$-1 hr	20 min
Peak	1-1.5 hr	$1^{1}/_{2}$-2 hr
Duration	4-12 hr	4-6 hr

INTERACTIONS
Individual drugs
Alcohol: increased respiratory depression, hypotension, sedation
Nalbuphine, pentazine, phenytoin, rifampin: decreased analgesia
Selegiline: do not use within 2 wk of methadone

Drug classifications
Antipsychotics, opiates, sedative/hypnotics, skeletal muscle relaxants: increased respiratory depression, hypotension
Class IA antiarrhythmics (disopyramide, procainamide, quiNIDine), class III antiarrhythmics (amiodarone, bretylium, dofetilide, ibutilide, sotalol), astemizole, arsenic trioxide, bepridil, cisapride, chloroquine, clarithromycin, levomethadyl, pentamidine, some phenothiazines, pimozide, probucol, sparfloxacin, terfenadine: increased QT prolongation
CYP3A4 inducers (barbiturates, bosentan, carBAMazepine, efavirenz, phenytoins, nevirapine, rifabutin, rifampin): decreased methadone effect
CYP3A4 inhibitors (aprepitant, antiretroviral protease inhibitors, clarithromycin, danazol, delavirdine, diltiazem, erythromycin, fluconazole, fluoxetine, fluvoxamine, imatinib, ketoconazole, mibefradil, nefazodone, telithromycin, voriconazole): increased toxicity

M

MAOIs: do not use for 2 wk before taking methadone: unpredictable reactions

Drug/herb
Chamomile, hops, kava, valerian: increased CNS depression

St. John's wort: avoid use, withdrawal may result

Drug/lab test
Increased: amylase, lipase

NURSING CONSIDERATIONS

Assessment
• **Assess for pain:** type, location, intensity, grimacing before and $1^1/_2$-2 hr after administration; use pain scoring
• Monitor VS after parenteral route; note muscle rigidity, product history, liver, kidney function tests
• Monitor CNS changes: dizziness, drowsiness, hallucinations, euphoria, LOC, pupil reaction
• Monitor allergic reactions: rash, urticaria
• Monitor opioid detoxification: no analgesia occurs, only prevention of withdrawal symptoms

> **BLACK BOX WARNING:** Monitor B/P, pulse, ECG: QT prolongation, hypotension, palpitations may occur

• Monitor bowel changes; bulk, fluids, laxatives should be used for constipation

> **BLACK BOX WARNING:** Respiratory dysfunction: respiratory depression, character, rate, rhythm; notify prescriber if respirations <10/min

Nursing diagnoses
• Breathing pattern, ineffective (adverse reactions)
• Knowledge, deficient (teaching)
• Pain, acute (uses)

Patient/family education
• Instruct patient to report any symptoms of CNS changes, allergic reactions; to avoid CNS depressants (alcohol, sedative-hypnotics) for at least 24 hr after taking this product
• Discuss with patient that dizziness, drowsiness, and confusion are common; to avoid getting up without assistance
• Discuss in detail with patient all aspects of the product
• Caution patient to make position changes slowly to prevent orthostatic hypotension
• Teach patient withdrawal symptoms may occur: nausea, vomiting, cramps, fever, faintness, anorexia

• Advise patient to maintain proper hydration, avoid alcohol use

Evaluation
Positive therapeutic outcome
• Decreased pain
• Successful opioid withdrawal

TREATMENT OF OVERDOSE:
Naloxone (Narcan) 0.2-0.8 mg **IV**, O_2, **IV** fluids, vasopressors

---

methimazole (Rx)
(meth-im′a-zole)
Tapazole
Func. class.: Thyroid hormone antagonist (antithyroid)
Chem. class.: Thioamide
Pregnancy category D

Do not confuse:
methimazole/metoprolol/minoxidil

ACTION: Inhibits synthesis of thyroid hormones by decreasing iodine use in the manufacture of thyroglobin and iodothyronine; does not affect already formed hormones, does not affect circulatory T_4, T_3

Therapeutic outcome: Decreased T_4 levels, hyperthyroid symptoms

USES: Hyperthyroidism, preparation for thyroidectomy, thyrotoxic crisis, thyroid storm when PTU is contraindicated

CONTRAINDICATIONS:
Pregnancy **D**, breastfeeding, hypersensitivity

Precautions: Infection, bone marrow depression, hepatic disease, bleeding disorders

DOSAGE AND ROUTES
Hyperthyroidism
Adult: PO 15 mg/day (mild hyperthyroidism); 30-40 mg/day (moderate-severe); 60 mg/day (severe); maintenance dosage 5-15 mg/day, may be divided
Child: PO 0.4 mg/kg/day in divided doses q8hr; continue until euthyroid; maintenance dosage 0.2 mg/kg/day in divided doses q8hr, max 30 mg/24 hr, may be divided

Preparation for thyroidectomy
Adult and child: PO same as above; iodine may be added for 10 days before surgery

---

Thyrotoxic crisis
Adult and child: PO same as hyperthyroidism with iodine and propranolol

Available forms: Tabs 5, 10, 15, 20 mg

Implementation
• Give with meals to decrease GI upset; give at same time each day to maintain product level
• Give lowest dosage that relieves symptoms
• Store in light-resistant container
• Increase fluids to 3-4 L/day, unless contraindicated

ADVERSE EFFECTS
CNS: *Drowsiness, headache, vertigo, fever,* paresthesias, neuritis
ENDO: *Enlarged thyroid*
GI: *Nausea, diarrhea, vomiting, jaundice,* **hepatitis,** loss of taste
GU: **Nephritis**
HEMA: **Agranulocytosis, leukopenia, thrombocytopenia, hypothrombinemia, lymphadenopathy,** bleeding, vasculitis
INTEG: *Rash, urticaria, pruritus, alopecia, hyperpigmentation,* lupuslike syndrome
MS: Myalgia, arthralgia, nocturnal muscle cramps

Pharmacokinetics
Absorption	Rapidly absorbed
Distribution	Crosses placenta
Metabolism	Liver, extensively
Excretion	Kidneys, unchanged; breast milk
Half-life	5-13 hr

Pharmacodynamics
Onset	$1/2$ hr
Peak	Unknown
Duration	2-4 hr

INTERACTIONS
Individual drugs
Amiodarone, potassium iodide: decreased effectiveness
Digoxin: increased response
Radiation: increased bone marrow depression
Warfarin: decreased anticoagulant effect

Drug classifications
Antineoplastics: increased bone marrow depression
Phenothiazines: increased agranulocytosis

Drug/lab test
Increased: pro-time, AST, ALT, alkaline phosphatase

NURSING CONSIDERATIONS
Assessment
• **Hyperthyroidism:** palpitations, nervousness/loss of hair, insomnia, heat intolerance, weight loss, diarrhea
• **Hypothyroidism:** constipation, dry skin, weakness, fatigue, headache, intolerance to cold, weight gain; adjustment may be needed
• Monitor pulse, B/P, temp; check I&O ratio; check for edema (puffy hands, feet, periorbitis); indicates hypothyroidism
• Check weight daily; same clothing, scale, time of day
• Monitor T_3, T_4, which are increased; serum TSH, which is decreased; free thyroxine index, which is increased if dosage is too low; discontinue product 3-4 wk before radioactive iodine uptake
⚠ **Monitor blood studies: CBC for blood dyscrasias (leukopenia, thrombocytopenia, agranulocytosis); if these occur, product should be discontinued and other treatment initiated; LFTs**
• **Assess for hypersensitivity** (rash, enlarged cervical lymph nodes); product may have to be discontinued
• **Assess for hypoprothrombinemia** (bleeding, petechiae, ecchymosis)
• Monitor clinical response: after 3 wk should include increased weight, pulse, decreased T_4
⚠ **Assess for bone marrow depression: sore throat, fever, fatigue**

Nursing diagnoses
• Knowledge, deficient (teaching)
• Noncompliance (teaching)

Patient/family education
• Advise patient to abstain from breastfeeding after delivery; product appears in breast milk
• Instruct patient to take pulse daily; to keep graph of weight, pulse, mood
• Advise patient to report redness, swelling, sore throat, mouth lesions, which indicate blood dyscrasias
• Caution patient to avoid OTC products that contain iodine; that seafood and other iodine-containing products may be restricted by prescriber
• Caution patient not to discontinue this medication abruptly; thyroid crisis may occur; stress patient compliance
• Advise patient that response may take several mo if thyroid is large
• **Teach patient symptoms/signs of overdose:** periorbital edema, cold intolerance, mental depression; notify prescriber at once

• **Teach patient symptoms of inadequate dosage**: tachycardia, diarrhea, fever, irritability; prescriber should be notified to adjust
• Teach patient to take medication exactly as prescribed, not to skip or double doses; missed doses should be taken when remembered up to 1 hr before next dose
• Instruct patient to carry ID describing medication taken and condition being treated

Evaluation
Positive therapeutic outcome
• Decreased weight gain
• Decreased pulse
• Decreased T_4
• Decreased B/P

methocarbamol (Rx)
(meth-oh-kar′ba-mole)
Robaxin
Func. class.: Skeletal muscle relaxant, central acting
Chem. class.: Carbamate derivative
Pregnancy category C

Do not confuse:
Relaxin/Reglan/Relafen/Rolephin

ACTION: Depresses multisynaptic pathways in the spinal cord, causing skeletal muscle relaxation

Therapeutic outcome: Decreased pain, spasm, resolution of tetanic spasms

USES: Adjunct for relief of spasm and pain in musculoskeletal conditions, tetanus

CONTRAINDICATIONS:
Hypersensitivity to this product or PEG300 (inj), children <12 yr, intermittent porphyria, renal disease (IM/**IV**)

Precautions: Pregnancy **C**, renal/hepatic disease, addictive personalities, myasthenia gravis, epilepsy

DOSAGE AND ROUTES
Muscle spasm
Adult: PO 1.5 g qid × 2-3 days; then 1 g qid; IM 500 mg in each gluteal region; may repeat q8hr; **IV** BOL 1-3 g/day max at 3 ml/min; **IV** INF 1 g/250 ml D_5W or 0.9% NaCl, max 3 g/day
Geriatric: PO 500 mg qid, titrate to needed dose

Tetanus management
Adult: **IV** DIRECT 1-2 g or **IV** INF 1-3 g q6hr, max 3 g
Child: **IV** 15 mg/kg q6hr prn, max 1-8 g/m^2/day for 3 consecutive days, max 3 ml/min **IV**

Available forms: Tabs 500, 750 mg; inj 100 mg/ml

Implementation
• Methocarbamol incompatible with any product in sol or syringe
PO route
• Give with meals if GI symptoms occur
• Store in airtight container at room temperature
IM route
• Give inj deep in large muscle mass; rotate sites
• Do not give SUBCUT
Direct IV route
• Give undiluted over 1 min or more; give 300 mg or less 1 min or longer
Intermittent IV infusion route
• May be diluted in 250 ml or less D_5 or isotonic NaCl sol for slow **IV** inf
• Give by slow **IV** to prevent phlebitis; keep recumbent during and for 15 min after to prevent orthostatic hypotension; check for extravasation

ADVERSE EFFECTS
CNS: *Dizziness, weakness, drowsiness,* syncope, flushing, headache, tremor, depression, insomnia, **seizures** (**IV,** IM only)
CV: Postural hypotension, *bradycardia*
EENT: Diplopia, temporary loss of vision, conjunctivitis, nasal congestion, blurred vision, nystagmus
GI: *Nausea,* vomiting, hiccups, anorexia, metallic taste, dyspepsia, jaundice
GU: Brown, black, green urine
HEMA: Hemolysis, increased hemoglobin, **leukopenia** (**IV** only)
INTEG: Rash, pruritus, fever, facial flushing, urticaria, phlebitis, extravasation
MISC: Anaphylaxis, angioneurotic edema (IM, **IV**)

Pharmacokinetics
Absorption	Rapidly absorbed (PO)
Distribution	Widely distributed; crosses placenta
Metabolism	Liver, partially
Excretion	Kidney, unchanged
Half-life	1-2 hr

Pharmacodynamics

	PO	IM	IV
Onset	$1/2$ hr	Rapid	Rapid
Peak	1-2 hr	Unknown	Inf end
Duration	>8 hr	Unknown	Unknown

INTERACTIONS

Individual drugs
Alcohol: increased CNS depression

Drug classifications
Antidepressants (tricyclic), barbiturates, opioids, sedative-hypnotics: increased CNS depression

Drug/herb
Chamomile, hops, kava, skullcap, St. John's wort, valerian: increased CNS depression

Drug/lab test
False increase: VMA, urinary 5-HIAA

NURSING CONSIDERATIONS

Assessment
• Assess for pain and spasm: location, duration, intensity, range of motion
• Assess blood studies: CBC, WBC differential; blood dyscrasias may occur
• Assess hepatic studies: AST, ALT, alk phos; hepatitis may occur; renal studies: BUN, creatinine with **IV** use
• Monitor during and after inj: CNS effects, rash, conjunctivitis, and nasal congestion may occur
• Monitor EEG in epileptic patients; poor seizure control has occurred in patients taking this product
• Assess allergic reactions: rash, fever, respiratory distress; check for severe weakness, numbness in extremities
• Assess for tolerance: increased need for medication, more frequent requests for medication, increased pain
• Assess for CNS depression: dizziness, drowsiness, psychiatric symptoms

Nursing diagnoses
• Injury, risk for (adverse reactions)
• Knowledge, deficient (teaching)
• Mobility, impaired physical (uses)

Patient/family education
• Advise patient not to discontinue medication quickly; insomnia, nausea, headache, spasticity, tachycardia will occur; product should be tapered off over 1-2 wk
• Inform patient that urine may turn green, black, or brown
• Caution patient not to take with alcohol, other CNS depressants; increased CNS depression can occur
• Advise patient to avoid altering activities while taking this product
• Caution patient to avoid hazardous activities if drowsiness, dizziness occur; driving should be avoided until product response is known
• Advise patient to avoid using OTC medications that are CNS depressants (cough preparations, antihistamines) unless directed by prescriber; CNS depression can occur

Evaluation
Positive therapeutic outcome
• Decreased pain, spasticity

TREATMENT OF OVERDOSE:
Activated charcoal, dialysis; have EPINEPHrine, antihistamines, and corticosteroids available, enhance elimination with osmotic diureses, **IV** fluids for hypotension

---

▲ HIGH ALERT

methotrexate (Rx)
(meth-oh-trex'ate)
Rheumatrex, Trexall
Func. class.: Antineoplastic, antimetabolite
Chem. class.: Folic acid antagonist
Pregnancy category X

Do not confuse:
methotrexate/metolazone/mitoxantrone

ACTION: Inhibits an enzyme that reduces folic acid, which is needed for nucleic acid synthesis in all cells; cell cycle specific (S phase); immunosuppressive

Therapeutic outcome: Prevention of rapidly growing malignant cells; immunosuppression

USES: Acute lymphocytic leukemia, in combination for breast, lung, head, neck carcinoma, lymphosarcoma, gestational choriocarcinoma, hydatidiform mole, psoriasis, rheumatoid arthritis, mycosis fungoides, osteosarcoma

CONTRAINDICATIONS:
Hypersensitivity, leukopenia (<3500/mm³), thrombocytopenia (<100,000/mm³), anemia, psoriatic patients with severe renal disease, alcoholism, HIV infection

M

> **BLACK BOX WARNING:** Pregnancy **X**, hepatic disease

Precautions: Breastfeeding, children

> **BLACK BOX WARNING:** Renal disease, ascites, diarrhea, exfoliative dermatitis, infection, intrathecal administration, lymphoma, pleural effusion, pulmonary disease, radiation therapy, stomatitis, tumor lysis syndrome

DOSAGE AND ROUTES

Acute lymphocytic leukemia
Adult and child: PO/IM/**IV** 3.3 mg/m^2/day × 4-6 wk until remission, then 20-30 mg/m^2 PO/IM qwk in 2 divided doses or 2.5 mg/kg **IV** × 2 wk

Burkitt's lymphoma (stages I, II, III) (unlabeled)
Adult: PO 10-25 mg/day × 4-8 days with 7-day rest period

Lymphosarcoma (stage III)
Adult: PO/IM/**IV** 0.625-2.5 mg/kg/day

Meningeal leukemia
Adult and child: 12 mg/m^2 IT q2-5days until CSF is normal, then one additional dose, max 15 mg

Choriocarcinoma
Adult and child: PO/IM 15-30 mg/kg/day × 5 days, then off 1 wk; may repeat

Breast cancer
Adult: **IV** 40-60 mg/m^2 on day 1 of every 21-28 days with other antineoplastics

Rheumatoid arthritis
Adult: PO 7.5 mg/wk or divided doses of 2.5 mg q12hr × 3 given qwk, max 20 mg/wk

Polyarticular-course juvenile RA
Child: PO/IM 10 mg/m^2 qwk

Osteosarcoma
Adult and child: **IV** 12 g/m^2 given over 4 hr, then leucovorin rescue is given

Mycosis fungoides
Adult: PO 2.5-10 mg/day until cleared (may be many mo); IM 50 mg qwk or 15-37.5 mg 2 ×/wk

Psoriasis
Adult: PO/IM/**IV** 10-25 mg qwk or 2.5 mg PO q12hr × 3 doses qwk; may increase to 25 mg qwk

Available forms: Tabs 2.5, 5, 7.5, 10, 15 mg; inj 25 mg/ml; powder for inj 20 mg, 1 g

Implementation
• Avoid contact with skin, since product is very irritating; wash completely to remove
⚠ Leucovorin rescue: Administer leucovorin calcium within 24 hr of giving this product to prevent tissue damage; check agency policy; continue until methotrexate level <10^{-8} m
• Give antiemetic 30-60 min before giving product and prn to prevent vomiting; administer antibiotics for infection prophylaxis
• Give in AM so product can be eliminated before bedtime
• Provide liquid diet: carbonated beverages; gelatin may be added if patient is not nauseated or vomiting

PO route
• Give 1 hr before or 2 hr after meals to prevent vomiting
• Make sure product is taken weekly in RA, JRA

IM route
• Give deeply in large muscle mass

Direct IV route
• Give **IV** after diluting 5 mg/2 ml of sterile water for inj; give through Y-tube or 3-way stopcock

Intermittent/continuous IV route
• Further dilute in D$_5$W, D$_5$/0.9% NaCl, 0.9% NaCl; prior to infusion check patency of vein, flush with 5-10 ml of D$_5$W, 0.9% NaCl, infuse at 4-20 mg/hr or prescribed rate

IV infusion
• Intermediate or high dose: 500 mg/m^2 over <4 hr or >1 g/m^2 over >4 hr; confirm WBC >15 mm^3, neutrophils >200 mm^3, platelets > 75,000/mm^3, serum bilirubin <1.2 mg/dl, serum creatinine WNL, SGPT <450 U, creatinine clearance >60 ml/min
⚠ Give sodium bicarbonate tabs or IV fluids to prevent precipitation of product at high doses; urine pH should be >7; may need to reduce dose if BUN is 20-30 mg/dl or creatinine is 1.2-2 mg/dl; stop product if BUN >30 mg/dl or creatitine is >2 mg/dl

Syringe compatibilities: Bleomycin, CISplatin, cyclophosphamide, doxapram, DOXOrubicin, fluorouracil, furosemide, heparin, leucovorin, mitomycin, vinBLAStine, vinCRIStine

Syringe incompatibilities: Droperidol, ranitidine

Y-site compatibilities: Allopurinol, amifostine, asparaginase, aztreonam, bleomycin, cefepime, cefTRIAXone, cimetidine, CISplatin, cyclophosphamide, cytarabine, DAUNOrubicin, dexchlorpheniramine, diphenhydrAMINE,

---

DOXOrubicin, etoposide, famotidine, filgrastim, fludarabine, fluorouracil, furosemide, gallium, ganciclovir, granisetron, heparin, HYDROmorphone, imipenem-cilastatin, leucovorin, LORazepam, melphalan, mesna, methylPREDNISolone, metoclopramide, mitomycin, morphine, ondansetron, oxacillin, paclitaxel, piperacillin/tazobactam, prochlorperazine, ranitidine, sargramostim, teniposide, thiotepa, vinBLAStine, vinCRIStine, vinorelbine

Y-site incompatibilities: Droperidol, IDArubicin

Additive compatibilities: Cephalothin, cyclophosphamide, cytarabine, fluorouracil, hydrOXYzine, mercaptopurine, ondansetron, sodium bicarbonate, vinCRIStine

Additive incompatibilities: Bleomycin, prednisoLONE

Solution compatibilities: Amino acids, 4.25%/D$_{25}$, D$_5$W, sodium bicarbonate 0.05 mol/L, 0.9% NaCl
Intrathecal route
• Use preservative-free solutions, reconstitute with normal saline, the dose should be drawn into a 5-10 ml syringe after lumbar puncture, the volume of CSF should be withdrawn equal to volume of methotrexate, allow CSF to flow into syringe and mix, inject over 15-30 sec with bevel of needle upward

ADVERSE EFFECTS
CNS: Dizziness, **seizures,** headache, confusion, hemiparesis, malaise, fatigue, chills, fever, **leukoencephalopathy; arachnoiditis** (intrathecal)
EENT: Blurred vision, optic neuropathy
GI: *Nausea, vomiting, anorexia, diarrhea, ulcerative stomatitis,* **hepatotoxicity,** cramps, ulcer, gastritis, **GI hemorrhage,** abdominal pain, hematemesis, **hepatic fibrosis, acute toxicity**
GU: Urinary retention, **renal failure,** menstrual irregularities, defective spermatogenesis, **hematuria, azotemia, uric acid nephropathy**
HEMA: **Leukopenia, thrombocytopenia, myelosuppression, anemia**
INTEG: *Rash, alopecia,* dry skin, urticaria, photosensitivity, folliculitis, vasculitis, petechiae, ecchymosis, acne, alopecia, **severe fatal skin reactions**
RESP: **Methotrexate-induced lung disease**
SYST: **Sudden death,** *Pneumocystis jiroveci* **pneumonia, tumor lysis syndrome**

Pharmacokinetics
Absorption	Well absorbed (GI)
Distribution	Widely distributed; crosses placenta
Metabolism	Not metabolized
Excretion	Kidneys, unchanged; breast milk (minimal)
Half-life	Terminal 10-12 hr; increased in renal disease

Pharmacodynamics
	PO	IM/IV	IT
Onset	Unknown	Unknown	Unknown
Peak	1-4 hr	$^1/_2$-2 hr	Unknown
Duration	Unknown	Unknown	Unknown

INTERACTIONS
Individual drugs
Alcohol, phenylbutazone, probenecid, radiation, theophylline: increased toxicity
Digoxin (PO), fosphenytoin, phenytoin: decreased effect of each specific product
Folic acid: decreased effect of methotrexate
Radiation: increased bone marrow suppression

Drug classifications
Anticoagulants (oral): increased hypoprothrombinemia
Antineoplastics, NSAIDs, penicillins, salicylates, sulfa products: increased toxicity
Live virus vaccines: decreased antibodies

NURSING CONSIDERATIONS
Assessment
• Assess buccal cavity q8hr for dryness, sores or ulceration, white patches, oral pain, bleeding, dysphagia; obtain prescription for viscous lidocaine (Xylocaine)
• **Assess symptoms indicating severe allergic reaction:** rash, pruritus, urticaria, purpuric skin lesions, itching, flushing
• Assess tachypnea, ECG changes, dyspnea, edema, fatigue; identify dyspnea, crackles, unproductive cough, chest pain, tachypnea
• Monitor CBC, differential, platelet count weekly; withhold product if WBC is <3500/mm^3 or platelet count is <100,000/mm^3; notify prescriber of results if WBC <20,000/mm^3, platelets <150,000/mm^3; WBC, platelet nadirs occur on day 7
• Assess for increased uric acid levels, swelling, joint pain primarily in extremities; patient should be well hydrated to prevent urate deposits

> **BLACK BOX WARNING:** Renal disease: avoid use in renal failure; monitor renal function studies: BUN, creatinine, serum uric acid, urine CCr before, during therapy; check I&O ratio; report fall in urine output to <30 ml/hr

• Monitor temp (may indicate beginning of infection)
• **Hepatotoxicity:** monitor liver function tests before, during therapy (bilirubin, AST, ALT, LDH) as needed or monthly; check for jaundice of skin and sclera, dark urine, clay-colored stools, itchy skin, abdominal pain, fever, diarrhea (hepatotoxicity)
• Assess for bleeding: hematuria, stool guaiac, bruising or petechiae, mucosa or orifices; check for inflammation of mucosa, breaks in skin
• Identify effects of alopecia on body image; discuss feelings about body changes
• Identify edema in feet, joint and stomach pain, shaking; prescriber should be notified
• Monitor methotrexate levels, adjust leucovorin dose based on the level

> **BLACK BOX WARNING:** Pulmonary toxicity: those with ascites or pleural effusions are at greater risk for toxicity, fluid should be removed before treatment, monitor plasma methotrexate level

> **BLACK BOX WARNING:** Tumor lysis syndrome: hyperkalemia, hyperphosphatemia, hyperuricemia, hypocalcemia, decreased urine output; use aggressive hydration and allopurinol to correct severe electrolyte imbalances, renal toxicity

• **Rheumatoid arthritis:** ROM, pain, joint swelling, prior to and during treatment
• **Psoriasis:** assess skin lesions prior to and during treatment

Nursing diagnoses
• Body image, disturbed (adverse reactions)
• Infection, risk for (adverse reactions)
• Injury, risk for (adverse reactions)
• Knowledge, deficient (teaching)

Patient/family education
• Encourage patient to rinse mouth tid-qid with water, club soda; brush teeth bid-qid with soft brush or cotton-tipped applicators for stomatitis; use unwaxed dental floss
• Advise patient that contraceptive measures are recommended during therapy; product is teratogenic; contraception should be used for 3 mo (male) and 4-6 wk (female); to discontinue breastfeeding; toxicity to infant may occur (X)

• Teach patient to avoid use of products containing aspirin or NSAIDs, razors, commercial mouthwash, since bleeding may occur; to report symptoms of bleeding (hematuria, tarry stools)
• Caution patient to report signs of anemia (fatigue, headache, irritability, faintness, shortness of breath); seizures
• Advise patient to report any changes in breathing or coughing even several mo after treatment; to avoid crowds and persons with respiratory tract or other infections
• Advise patient to report stomatitis: any bleeding, white spots, ulcerations in mouth to prescriber; tell patient to examine mouth daily, report symptoms, use good oral hygiene
• Teach patient that hair may be lost during treatment; a wig or hairpiece may make patient feel better; new hair may be different in color, texture
• Caution patient not to have any vaccinations without the advice of the prescriber; serious reactions can occur
• Advise patient to use sunblock or protective clothing to prevent burns

Evaluation
Positive therapeutic outcome
• Prevention of rapid division of malignant cells
• Decreased joint inflammation in RA

methoxy polyethylene glycol-epoetin beta (Rx)
(meth-ox′ee pol′ee-eth′i-leen glye′kol-e-poe′e-tin bay′ta)
Mircera
Func. class.: Antianemic, biological modifier, hormone
Chem. class.: Amino acid polypeptide
Pregnancy category C

ACTION: Erythropoietin is one factor controlling rate of red cell production; product is developed by recombinant DNA technology

Therapeutic outcome: Increase in reticulocyte count in 2-6 wk, Hgb/Hct; increased appetite, enhanced sense of well-being

USES: Anemia caused by reduced endogenous erythropoietin production, primarily end-stage renal disease; to correct hemostatic defect in uremia on all dosages

CONTRAINDICATIONS: Red cell aplasia, neoplastic disease, hypersensitivity to mannitol, uncontrolled hypertension

⚠ Nurse Alert

BLACK BOX WARNING: Hgb >12 g/dl

Precautions: Pregnancy **C**, seizure disorder, porphyria, children <1 mo, breastfeeding, multidose preserved formulation contains benzyl alcohol and should not be used in premature infants, CV disease, hemodialysis, latex allergy, surgery, hypertension, history of CABG

BLACK BOX WARNING: Neoplastic disease

DOSAGE AND ROUTES
For all dosages
Adult and geriatric: Reduce by 25% if Hgb >1 g/dl in any 2-wk period or if Hgb is close to 12 g/dl; if Hgb continues to rise after decrease, hold until Hgb starts to decrease

Treatment of anemia in chronic renal failure (dialysis dependent/ independent)—not currently using ESA
Adult and geriatric: IV/SUBCUT 0.6 mcg q2wk

Using >80 mcg/wk darbepoetin or >16000 units/wk epoetin
Adult and geriatric: IV/SUBCUT 180 mcg q2wk or 360 mcg q4wk

Using 40-80 mcg/wk darbepoetin or 8000-16,000 units/wk epoetin
Adult and geriatric: IV/SUBCUT 100 mcg q2wk

Using <40 mcg/wk darbepoetin or <8000 units/wk epoetin
Adult and geriatric: IV/SUBCUT 60 mcg q2wk or 120 mcg q4wk

Implementation
• Do not shake vial
• Give iron supplements as needed; adequate iron stores are needed for this agent to work properly
SUBCUT route
• Inject into outer aspect of upper arms, abdomen (except for 2 inches around navel) or front aspect of middle thigh; do not inject in areas that have stretch marks or are scarred or bruised
• Rotate inj sites
Direct IV route
• Give additional heparin to lower chance of clots
• Give by direct inj or bolus into venous line at end of dialysis

Solution compatibilities: Do not dilute or administer with other sol

ADVERSE EFFECTS
CNS: Seizures, encephalopathy, headache
CV: *Hypertension,* edema, heart failure, hypotension, sinus tachycardia, stroke, myocardial infarction
GI: Diarrhea
HEMA: Anemia, red cell aplasia, thrombocytopenia, thromboembolism, thrombosis
INTEG: Pruritus, rash, erythema, inj site reaction
MS: Muscle spasms, back pain
SYST: Antibody formation

Pharmacokinetics
Absorption	Unknown
Distribution	Unknown
Metabolism	Unknown
Excretion	Unknown
Half-life	Half-life 139 ± 67 hr rise in reticulocytes on day 7, rise in Hgb in 7-14 days (SUBCUT); Half-life 134 ± 65 hr (**IV**)

Pharmacodynamics
Unknown

INTERACTIONS
Drug classifications
Androgens: increased action of methoxy polyethylene gycol-epoetin
Other erythropoiesis stimulating agents (ESA) (epoetin, darbepoetin): adverse reactions; do not give concurrently

NURSING CONSIDERATIONS
Assessment
• Monitor renal studies: urinalysis, protein, blood, BUN, creatinine; I&O, report drop in output <50 ml/hr

BLACK BOX WARNING: Assess CBC, blood studies: ferritin, transferrin monthly; transferrin ≥20%, ferritin ≥100 ng/ml; Hct 2 ×/wk until stabilized in target range (30%-36%) then at regular intervals; those with endogenous erythropoietin levels of <500 units/L respond to this agent; monitor Hct 2 ×/wk in chronic renal failure; cancer patients and patients treated with zidovudine should be monitored weekly, then periodically after stabilization; death may occur in Hgb >12g/dl

M

- Monitor B/P; check for rising B/P as Hct rises, antihypertensives may be needed; hypertension may occur rapidly, leading to hypertensive encephalopathy
- Assess CNS symptoms: for seizures if Hct is increased within 2 wk by 4 points
- Assess for hypersensitivity reactions: skin rashes, urticaria (rare), antibody development
⚠ **For pure cell aplasia (PRCA) in absence of other causes, evaluate by testing serum for recombinant erythropoetin antibodies; any loss of response to epoetin should be evaluated**
- Assess dialysis patients: thrill, bruit of shunts, monitor for circulation impairment
- **Hypersensitivity reactions:** assess for skin reactions, rash, urticaria (rare), antibody development

Nursing diagnoses
- Injury, risk for (uses)
- Knowledge, deficient (teaching)
- Urinary elimination, impaired (uses)

Patient/family education
- Caution patient to avoid driving or hazardous activities during beginning of treatment
- Instruct patient to monitor B/P
- Instruct patient to take iron supplements, vitamin B_{12}, folic acid as directed

Evaluation
Positive therapeutic outcome
- Increase in reticulocyte count in 2-6 wk, Hgb/Hct; increased appetite, enhanced sense of well-being

methyldopa/methyldopate (Rx)
(meth-ill-doe′pa)
Apo-methyldopa ✶
Func. class.: Antihypertensive
Chem. class.: Centrally acting α-adrenergic inhibitor
Pregnancy category B (PO) C (IV)

Do not confuse:
methyldopa/L-dopa (levodopa)

ACTION: Stimulates central inhibitory $α_2$-adrenergic receptors or acts as false transmitter, resulting in reduction of arterial pressure

Therapeutic outcome: Decreased B/P in hypertension

USES: Hypertension, hypertensive crisis

CONTRAINDICATIONS:
Active hepatic disease, hypersensitivity

Precautions: Pregnancy **B**, geriatric patients, cardiac disease, autoimmune disease, depression, dialysis, hemolytic anemia, Parkinson's disease, pheochromocytoma, sulfite hypersensitivity

DOSAGE AND ROUTES
Adult: PO 250-500 mg bid or tid, then adjusted q2day prn, 0.5-2 g/day in 2-4 divided doses (maintenance), max 3 g/day; **IV** 250-500 mg in 100 ml D_5W q6hr, run over 30-60 min, max 1 g q6hr, switch to PO as soon as possible
Geriatric: PO 125 mg bid/tid, increase q2day as needed, max 3 g/day
Child: PO 10 mg/kg/day in 2-4 divided doses, max 65 mg/kg or 3 g/day, whichever is less; **IV** 20-40 mg/kg/day in 4 divided doses, max 65 mg/kg or 3 g, whichever is less

Available forms: Methyldopa: tabs 250, 500 mg; methydopate: inj 50 mg/ml (250 mg/5 ml)

Implementation
PO route
- Give before meals
- Shake susp before using
- Store in airtight container at room temperature

Intermittent IV infusion route
- Give after diluting in 100 ml of 0.9% NaCl, D_5W, D_5/0.9% NaCl, 5% sodium bicarbonate, Ringer's; administer over 30-60 min

Y-site compatibilities: Alfentanil, amikacin, aminophylline, anidulafungin, ascorbic acid, atenolol, atracurium, atropine, aztreonam, benztropine, bivalirudin, bleomycin, bumetanide, buprenorphine, butorphanol, calcium chloride/gluconate, caspofungin, cefamandole, ceFAZolin, cefmetazole, cefonicid, cefotaxime, cefotetan, cefoxitin, ceftazidime, ceftizoxime, cefTRIAXone, cefuroxime, cephalothin, chlorproMAZINE, cimetidine, clindamycin, cyanocobalamin, cycloSPORINE, DACTINomycin, DAPTOmycin, dexamethasone, digoxin, diltiazem, diphenhydrAMINE, docetaxel, DOPamine, doxycycline, enalaprilat, ePHEDrine, EPINEPHrine, epoetin alfa, ertapenem, erythromycin, esmolol, etoposide, etoposide phosphate, famotidine, fenoldopam, fentaNYL, fluconazole, fludarabine, gatifloxacin, gemcitabine, gentamicin, glycopyrrolate, granisetron, heparin, hydrocortisone, HYDROmorphone, hydrOXYzine, IDArubicin, insulin(regular), irinotecan, isoproterenol, labetalol, lidocaine, linezolid,

LORazepam, magnesium sulfate, mannitol, mechlorethamine, meperidine, metaraminol, methicillin, methoxamine, methylPREDNISolone, metoclopramide, metoprolol, metroNIDAZOLE, mezlocillin, miconazole, midazolam, milrinone, minocycline, mitoxantrone, morphine, moxalactam, multiple vitamins, mycophenolate mofetil, nafcillin, nalbuphine, naloxone, netilmicin, nitroglycerin, nitroprusside, norepinephrine, octreotide, ondansetron, oxacillin, oxaliplatin, oxytocin, paclitaxel, palonosetron, pamidronate, pancuronium, pantoprazole, papaverine, pemetrexed, penicillin G potassium/sodium, pentazocine, phentolamine, phenylephrine, phytonadione, piperacillin, polymyxin B, potassium chloride, procainamide, prochlorperazine, promethazine, propranolol, protamine, pyridoxine, quiNIDine, ranitidine, ritodrine, sodium bicarbonate, succinylcholine, SUFentanil, tacrolimus, teniposide, theophylline, thiamine, thiotepa, ticarcillin, ticarcillin-clavulanate, tigecycline, tirofiban, tobramycin, tolazoline, trimetaphan, urokinase, vancomycin, vasopressin, vecuronium, verapamil, vinorelbine, voriconazole, zoledronic acid

Additive compatibilities: Aminophylline, ascorbic acid, chloramphenicol, diphenhydrAMINE, heparin, magnesium sulfate, multivitamins, netilmicin, potassium chloride, promazine, sodium bicarbonate, succinylcholine, verapamil, vit B/C

Additive incompatibilities: Amphotericin B, barbiturates, methohexital, sulfonamides

Solution compatibilities: D_5W, $D_5/0.9\%$ NaCl, Ringer's, sodium bicarbonate 5%, 0.9% NaCl, amino acids 4.25%/D_{25}, Dextran$_6$/0.9% NaCl, Normosol R, Normosol M/D_5W

ADVERSE EFFECTS
CNS: *Drowsiness, weakness, dizziness, sedation, headache,* depression, psychosis, paresthesias, parkinsonism, Bell's palsy, nightmares
CV: Bradycardia, **myocarditis,** orthostatic hypotension, angina, edema, weight gain, **CHF,** paradoxical pressor response (**IV** use)
EENT: Nasal congestion
ENDO: Breast enlargement, gynecomastia, amenorrhea
GI: Nausea, vomiting, diarrhea, constipation, **hepatic dysfunction,** sore or "black" tongue, **pancreatitis,** colitis, flatulence
GU: Impotence, failure to ejaculate
HEMA: Leukopenia, thrombocytopenia, hemolytic anemia, granulocytopenia, positive Coombs' test

INTEG: Lupus-like syndrome, rash, **toxic epidural necrolysis**

Pharmacokinetics
Absorption	50% (PO)
Distribution	Crosses placenta, blood-brain barrier
Metabolism	Liver, moderately
Excretion	Kidneys, unchanged (partially)
Half-life	$1^1/_2$ hr

Pharmacodynamics
	PO	IV
Onset	Unknown	Unknown
Peak	2-4 hr	2 hr
Duration	12-24 hr	10-16 hr

INTERACTIONS
Individual drugs
Alcohol: CNS depression
Haloperidol: increased psychosis
Iron: decreased methyldopa absorption
Levodopa: increased CNS toxicity, hypotension
Lithium: increased lithium toxicity
TOLBUTamide: increased hypoglycemia

Drug classifications
Amphetamines, antidepressants (tricyclics), barbiturates, NSAIDs, phenothiazines: decreased antihypertensive effect
Analgesics, antidepressants, antihistamines, sedative/hypnotics: increased CNS depression
Antihypertensives, diuretics: increased hypotension
β-Adrenergic blockers: increased B/P
MAOIs: increased pressor effect, do not use concurrently
Sympathomimetic amines: increased pressor effect

Drug/lab test
Interference: urinary uric acid, serum creatinine, AST
False increase: urinary catecholamines

NURSING CONSIDERATIONS
Assessment
• Monitor blood tests: neutrophils, decreased platelets; direct Coombs' test before, after 6, 12 mo of therapy
• Monitor renal studies: protein, BUN, creatinine; watch for increased levels that may indicate nephrotic syndrome: polyuria, oliguria, frequency; report weight gain >5 lb

M

• Obtain baselines in renal, liver function tests before therapy begins; check potassium levels, although hyperkalemia rarely occurs
• Monitor B/P, pulse if the product is being used for hypertension; notify prescriber of changes
• Monitor edema in feet, legs daily; monitor I&O; check weight for decreasing output
• Assess for allergic reaction: rash, fever, pruritus, urticaria; product should be discontinued if antihistamines fail to help
• Monitor CNS symptoms, especially in the geriatric; depression; change in mental status

Nursing diagnoses
• Cardiac output, decreased (uses)
• Injury, risk for (side effects)
• Knowledge, deficient (teaching)
• Noncompliance (teaching)

Patient/family education
• Instruct patient not to discontinue product abruptly, or withdrawal symptoms may occur: anxiety, increased B/P, headache, insomnia, increased pulse, tremors, nausea, sweating
• Caution patient not to use OTC (cough, cold, or allergy) products unless directed by prescriber
• Teach patient to comply with dosage schedule even if feeling better; product controls symptoms, does not cure
• Caution patient to change position slowly, to rise slowly to sitting or standing position to minimize orthostatic hypotension, especially geriatric
• Teach patient about excessive perspiration, dehydration, vomiting, diarrhea; may lead to fall in B/P; consult prescriber if these occur
• Advise patient that product may cause dizziness, fainting; light-headedness may occur during 1st few days of therapy; that product may cause dry mouth, use hard candy, saliva product, or frequent rinsing of mouth
• Caution patient that compliance is necessary; not to skip or stop product unless directed by prescriber
• Teach patient that product may cause skin rash
• Teach patient to avoid hazardous activities, since product may cause drowsiness, dizziness

Evaluation
Positive therapeutic outcome
• Decreased B/P

TREATMENT OF OVERDOSE:
Gastric evacuation, sympathomimetics may be indicated if severe; hemodialysis

methylergonovine (Rx)
(meth-ill-er-goe-noe′veen)
Methergine
Func. class.: Oxytocic
Chem. class.: Ergot alkaloid
Pregnancy category C

ACTION: Stimulates uterine and vascular smooth muscle, causing contractions, decreased bleeding, arterial vasoconstriction

Therapeutic outcome: Absence of hemorrhage

USES: Treatment of hemorrhage postpartum or after abortion, uterine contractions

CONTRAINDICATIONS:
Pregnancy (4th stage of labor), hypersensitivity to ergot preparations, angina, arteriosclerosis, CAD, dysfunctional uterine bleeding, eclampsia, MI, neonates, Raynaud's disease, sepsis, stroke, Buerger's disease, thrombophlebitis, hypertension, PID, respiratory disease, cardiac disease, peripheral vascular disease

Precautions: Pregnancy C, severe renal/hepatic disease, jaundice, diabetes mellitus, seizure disorders, sepsis, CAD

DOSAGE AND ROUTES
Adult: PO 200 mcg tid-qid up to 7 days; IM/IV 200 mcg q2-4hr for 1-5 doses

Available forms: Inj 200 mcg/ml; tabs 200 mcg

Implementation
PO route
• PO is the preferred route
IM route
• Give inj deeply in large muscle mass

Direct IV route
• Give by this route for severe, life-threatening hemorrhage
• Give directly undiluted or diluted with 5 ml of 0.9% NaCl given through Y-site or 3-way stopcock; give 0.2 mg/min; use clear, colorless sol
• Store up to 2 mo if unused

Y-site compatibilities: Heparin, hydrocortisone sodium succinate, potassium chloride, vit B/C

ADVERSE EFFECTS
CNS: *Headache, dizziness,* seizures
CV: Hypotension, chest pain, palpitations, *hypertension,* **dysrhythmias; CVA (IV)**

EENT: Tinnitus
GI: *Nausea, vomiting*
GU: Cramping
INTEG: Sweating, rash, allergic reactions
RESP: *Dyspnea*

Pharmacokinetics

Absorption	Well absorbed (PO, IM)
Distribution	Unknown
Metabolism	Liver, possibly
Excretion	Unknown
Half-life	$1/2$-2 hr

Pharmacodynamics

	PO	IM	IV
Onset	5-15 min	5 min	Immediate
Peak	Unknown	Unknown	Unknown
Duration	3 hr	3 hr	Unknown

INTERACTIONS

Individual drugs
Smoking: increased vasoconstriction

Drug classifications
Vasopressors: increased vasoconstriction

NURSING CONSIDERATIONS

Assessment
• Monitor B/P, pulse; watch for change that may indicate hemorrhage
• Assess fundal tone, nonphasic contractions; check for relaxation or severe cramping
• **Assess for ergotism or overdose:** nausea, vomiting, weakness, muscular pain, insensitivity to cold, paresthesia of extremities; product should be decreased or infusion discontinued
• Before administering ergonovine, check calcium levels; if hypocalcemia is present, correction should be made to increase effectiveness of this product
• Monitor prolactin levels and for decreased breast milk production

Nursing diagnoses
• Injury, risk for (adverse reactions)
• Knowledge, deficient (teaching)
• Tissue perfusion, ineffective (uses)

Patient/family education
• Advise patient to stop smoking, since increased vasoconstriction will result
• Inform patient that abdominal cramps are a side effect of this medication
• Instruct patient to notify prescriber if chest pain, nausea, vomiting, headache, muscle pain, weakness, or cold, numb extremities occur

Evaluation
Positive therapeutic outcome
• Prevention of hemorrhage

---

methylnaltrexone (Rx)
(meth-il-nal-trex'one)
Relistor
Func. class.: Opioid antagonist
Pregnancy category B

ACTION: Peripheral mu-opioid receptor antagonist that reduces constipation associated with opiate agonists

Therapeutic outcome: Decreased constipation

USES: Treatment of opioid-induced constipation in patients with advanced illness who are receiving palliative care when response to laxative therapy has been insufficient

CONTRAINDICATIONS: Hypersensitivity, GI obstruction, **IV** route

Precautions: Pregnancy **B**, breastfeeding, renal disease, children, diarrhea, driving, operating machinery, geriatric patients, neoplastic disease, Crohn's disease, peptic ulcer, ulcerative colitis

DOSAGE AND ROUTES

Opiate-agonist induced constipation
Adult >114 kg: SUBCUT 0.15 mg/kg every other day prn
Adult 62-114 kg: SUBCUT 12 mg every other day prn
Adult 38-62 kg: SUBCUT 8 mg every other day prn
Adult <38 kg: SUBCUT 0.15 mg/kg every other day prn

Renal dose
Adult: SUBCUT CCr <30 ml/min, reduce normal adult dose by 50%

Available forms: Solution for inj 12 mg/0.6 ml

Implementation
• Give SUBCUT only; oral dose is investigational and not currently available
• Do not give **IV**; IV dosing for urinary retention is investigational
• Store at 15°-30° C (59°-86° F); do not freeze
• Store away from light

M

SUBCUT route

• Inspect the solution before use; it should be a clear, colorless to pale yellow aqueous solution; do not use if particulate matter or discoloration are present

• Withdraw the needed amount of solution into a sterile syringe; if immediate administration is impossible, the syringe may be kept at room temperature for up to 24 hr; the syringe does not need to be kept away from light during the 24-hr period; immediately discard any unused portion in the vial; no preservatives are present

• Administer into the upper arm, abdomen, or thigh no more than 1 ×/24 hr; rotate inj sites; do not inject the same spot each time; do not inject into areas where skin is tender, bruised, red, or hard; avoid areas with scars or stretch marks

• If using with retractable needle, slowly push down on the plunger past the resistance point until the syringe is empty and a click is heard

ADVERSE EFFECTS

CNS: Dizziness
GI: Nausea, vomiting, diarrhea, flatulence, abdominal pain
INTEG: Hyperhidrosis

Pharmacokinetics

Absorption	Unknown
Distribution	Protein binding 11%-15.3%
Metabolism	Unknown
Excretion	Unknown
Half-life	Terminal 8 hr

Pharmacodynamics

Onset	Unknown
Peak	30 min (SUBCUT)
Duration	Unknown

NURSING CONSIDERATIONS

Assessment

• Monitor serum creatinine
• Assess for stool characteristics: amount, consistency; bowel sounds during treatment

Nursing diagnoses

• Constipation (uses)
• Knowledge, deficient (teaching)

Patient/family education

• Caution patient not to drive or operate machinery until effect is known
• Teach patient that after 30 min, toilet facilities should be nearby, bowel relaxation occurs
• Advise patient to notify prescriber of abdominal pain, continuous or severe diarrhea, nausea or vomiting

Evaluation

Positive therapeutic outcome
• Decreased constipation

---

methylphenidate (Rx)

(meth-ill-fen'i-date)
**Apo-Methylphenidate ✦,
Biphentin ✦, Concerta, Daytrana,
Metadate CD, Methidate, Methylin,
PMS-Methylphenidate ✦, Ritalin,
Ritalin LA, Ritalin SR**
Func. class.: Cerebral stimulant
Chem. class.: Piperidine derivative
Pregnancy category C
Controlled substance schedule II

Do not confuse:
methylphenidate/methadone

ACTION: Increases release of norepinephrine and dopamine in cerebral cortex to reticular activating system; exact action not known

Therapeutic outcome: Increased alertness, decreased fatigue, ability to stay awake (narcolepsy), increased attention span, decreased hyperactivity (ADHD)

USES: Attention deficit disorder with hyperactivity (ADHD), narcolepsy (except Concerta, Metadate CD, Ritalin LA), attention deficit disorder (ADD)

CONTRAINDICATIONS:
Hypersensitivity, anxiety, history of Tourette's syndrome, children <6 yr, glaucoma, anorexia nervosa, tartrazine dye hypersensitivity, glaucoma

Precautions: Pregnancy **C,** breastfeeding, hypertension, depression, seizures

> **BLACK BOX WARNING:** Substance abuse

DOSAGE AND ROUTES

Attention-deficit/hyperactivity disorder (ADHD) initial treatment (not currently on methylphenidate)

Regular release: Ritalin, Methylin, Methylin oral sol, Methylin chew tabs
Adult: PO 20-30 mg/day, range 10-60 mg/day in 2-3 divided doses, 30-45 min before meals
Child ≥6 yr: PO 5 mg bid initially, increase 5-10 mg/day q wk, usual dose 0.3-2 mg/kg/day, max 60 mg/day

---

⚠ Nurse Alert

Extended release: Ritalin SR, Metadate ER, Methylin ER
Adult/adolescent/child ≥6 yr: **PO** max 20-30 mg tid

Extended-release once-daily tabs: Concerta
Adult: **PO** 18-36 mg/day initially, then adjust by 18 mg q wk, max 72 mg/day
Adolescent: **PO** 18 mg/day initially, then adjust by 18 mg q wk, max 72 mg/day
Child ≥6 yr: **PO** 18 mg/day initially, then adjust by 18 mg q wk, max 54 mg/day

Extended-release once-daily capsules: Ritalin LA
Adult/adolescent/child ≥6 yr: **PO** 20 mg q day in AM initially, adjust by 10 mg q wk, max 60 mg/day

Extended-release once-daily capsules: Metadate CD
Adult/adolescent/child ≥6 yr: **PO** 20 mg q day in AM, adjust by 20 mg q wk, max 60 mg/day

Transdermal: Daytrana
Adolescent/child ≥6 yr: **TD** wk 1: 10 mg q day (9-mg patch); wk 2: 15 mg q day (9-mg patch); wk 3: 20 mg q day (9-mg patch); wk 4: 30 mg q day (9-mg patch)

Conversion to once-daily from other forms for ADHD
Extended-release once-daily capsules: Metadate CD
Adult/adolescent/child ≥6 yr: **PO** give no more than total daily dose of other forms, may adjust by 20 mg q wk, max 60 mg/day

Extended-release once-daily capsules: Ritalin LA
Adult/adolescent/child ≥6 yr: **PO** give no more than total daily dose of other forms, may adjust by 10 mg q wk, max 60 mg/day

Extended-release once-daily tablets: Concerta
Adult/adolescent/child ≥6 yr (currently receiving 10-15 mg/day): **PO** 18 mg q AM initially, adjust by 18 mg q wk, max 72 mg/day (adult); max 72 mg/day, 2 mg/kg/day (adolescent); 54 mg/day (child)
Adult/adolescent/child ≥6 yr (currently receiving 20-30 mg/day): **PO** 36 mg q AM, adjust by 18 mg q wk, max 72 mg/day (adult); 72 mg/day, 2 mg/kg/day (adolescent); 54 mg/day (child)
Adult/adolescent/child ≥6 yr (currently receiving 30-45 mg/day): **PO** 54 mg q AM, adjust by 18 mg q wk, max 72 mg/day (adult); 72 mg/day, 2 mg/kg/day (adolescent); 54 mg/day (child)

Adult/adolescent/child ≥6 yr (currently receiving 40-60 mg/day): **PO** 72 mg q AM, 72 mg/day

Transdermal: Daytrana
Adolescent and child ≥6 yr: **TD** wk 1: 10 mg q day (9-mg patch); wk 2: 15 mg q day (9-mg patch); wk 3: 20 mg q day (9-mg patch); wk 4: 30 mg q day (9-mg patch)

Narcolepsy

Immediate release: Ritalin, Methylin oral sol, Methylin chew tabs
Adult: **PO** 20-30 mg/day, range 10-60 mg/day in 2-3 divided doses
Child ≥6 yr: **PO** 5 mg bid, may increase by 5-10 mg q wk, max 60 mg/day

Extended-release tabs: Ritalin SR, Metadate ER
Adult/adolescent/child ≥6 yr: **PO** max 20 mg tid

Poststroke depression; major depression (unlabeled)
Adult and geriatric: **PO** (immediate rel tabs) 2.5 mg bid, may increase by 2.5-5 mg q2-3days

Available forms: Tabs 5, 10, 20 mg; ext rel tabs 10, 20, mg; ext rel tabs (Concerta) 18, 27, 36, 54 mg; ext rel caps 10, 20, 30, 40 mg; oral sol 5 mg, 10 mg/ml; chew tabs (Methylin) 2.5, 5, 10 mg; transdermal patch 12.5 cm² (10 mg), 18.75 cm² (15 mg), 25 cm² (20 mg), 37.5 cm² (30 mg)

Implementation
PO route
• Do not chew, crush time rel tabs; caps may be opened and beads sprinkled over spoonful of applesauce
• Give at least 6 hr before bedtime (regular release); at least 10 hr (ext rel) to avoid sleeplessness; titrate to patient's response; lowest dosage should be used to control symptoms
• Give gum, hard candy, frequent sips of water for dry mouth at beginning of treatment; these symptoms tend to lessen with time
• Avoid Metadate CD on day of surgery
Transdermal route
• Place on clean, dry area of the hip; avoid waist; removal is 9 hr after application; fold after removal and flush down toilet
• If patch falls off, apply a new patch to a different site; total wear time should be 9 hr

ADVERSE EFFECTS
CNS: *Hyperactivity, insomnia, restlessness, talkativeness,* dizziness, headache, akathisia, dyskinesia, masking or worsening of Tourette's

syndrome, **seizures,** drowsiness, toxic psychosis, hallucinations, **neuroleptic malignant syndrome, aggression, cerebral vasculitis, hemorrhage, stroke (rare)**
CV: *Palpitations, tachycardia,* B/P changes, angina, **dysrhythmias**
ENDO: Growth retardation
GI: Nausea, anorexia, dry mouth, weight loss, abdominal pain
HEMA: Leukopenia, anemia, thrombocytopenic purpura
INTEG: Exfoliative dermatitis, urticaria, rash, erythema multiforme, **hypersensitivity reactions**
MISC: Fever, arthralgia, scalp hair loss

Pharmacokinetics

Absorption	Well absorbed (PO); delayed (ext rel)
Distribution	Widely distributed; crosses placenta
Metabolism	Liver
Excretion	Kidneys
Half-life	1-3 hr

Pharmacodynamics

	PO	PO–ext rel
Onset	$^1/_2$-1 hr	2 hr
Peak	1-3 hr	4 hr
Duration	4-6 hr	6-8 hr

INTERACTIONS

Individual drugs
Guanethidine: decreased effect of guanethidine

Drug classifications
Anticonvulsants, antidepressants (tricyclics), SNRIs, CNS stimulants, selective serotonin reuptake inhibitors (SSRIs): increased effects
MAOIs (or within 14 days of MAOIs), vasopressors: hypertensive crisis
Antihypertensives: decreased effects of antihypertensives

Drug/herb
Cola nut, guarana, horsetail, yerba maté, yohimbe: increased CNS stimulation
Melatonin: synergistic effect

Drug/food
Caffeine: increased stimulation

NURSING CONSIDERATIONS

Assessment
• **ADHD:** In children or adults with ADHD, monitor for improved organizational skills, attention span, attending to tasks, impulse control, socialization, and ability to get along better with others
• Monitor VS, B/P, since this product may reverse antihypertensives; check patients with cardiac disease more often for increased B/P
• Perform CBC, urinalysis; for diabetic patients monitor blood glucose, urine glucose; insulin changes may be required, since eating will decrease
• Monitor height and weight q3mo since growth rate in children may be decreased; appetite is suppressed, weight loss is common during the first few mo of treatment
• Monitor mental status: mood, sensorium, affect, stimulation, insomnia; aggressiveness may occur; depression with crying spells may occur after product has worn off
• Assess for tolerance; should not be used for extended time except in ADHD; dosage should be discontinued gradually to prevent withdrawal symptoms
• **Assess for narcoleptic symptoms** before medication and after; ability to stay awake should increase significantly
⚠ Assess for withdrawal symptoms: headache, nausea, vomiting, muscle pain, weakness; product tolerance will develop after long-term use; dosage should not be increased if tolerance develops
• Assess appetite, sleep, speech patterns

Nursing diagnoses
• Coping, ineffective (uses)
• Knowledge, deficient (teaching)

Patient/family education
• Teach patient to decrease caffeine consumption (coffee, tea, cola, chocolate); not to use guarana, cola nut, yerba maté, which may increase irritability and stimulation; to avoid OTC preparations unless approved by prescriber; to avoid alcohol ingestion; these may cause serious product interactions
• Advise patient to taper off product over several wk, or depression, increased sleeping, lethargy may occur
• Caution patient to avoid hazardous activities until stabilized on medication
• Instruct patient not to double doses if medication is missed; prescriber may suggest product holidays (ADHD) during the school year to assess progress and determine continued product necessity
• Instruct patient/family to notify prescriber if significant side effects occur: tremors, insomnia, palpitations, restlessness; product changes may be needed

⚠ Nurse Alert

- Inform patient that if dry mouth occurs to use frequent sips of water, sugarless gum, hard candy during beginning therapy; dry mouth lessens with continued treatment
- Encourage patient to get needed rest; patient will feel more tired at end of day; to take last dose at least 6 hr before bedtime to avoid insomnia
- Advise patient that shell of Concerta tab may appear in stools

Evaluation
Positive therapeutic outcome
- Decreased hyperactivity in ADHD
- Improved attention span in ADHD
- Absence of sleeping during day in narcolepsy

TREATMENT OF OVERDOSE:
Administer fluids, hemodialysis, peritoneal dialysis, antihypertensives for increased B/P; administer short-acting barbiturate before lavage

methylPREDNISolone (Rx)
(meth-ill-pred-niss′oh-lone)
A-Methapred, Depo-Medrol, Medrol, Solu-Medrol
Func. class.: Corticosteroid, synthetic
Chem. class.: Glucocorticoid, immediate acting
Pregnancy category C

Do not confuse:
methylPREDNISolone/medroxyPROGESTERone, **predniSONE**/methylTESTOSTERone

ACTION: Decreases inflammation by suppression of migration of polymorphonuclear leukocytes, fibroblasts; reverses increased capillary permeability and lysosomal stabilization

Therapeutic outcome: Decreased inflammation

USES: Severe inflammation, shock, adrenal insufficiency, collagen disorders, management of acute spinal cord injury, multiple sclerosis

CONTRAINDICATIONS:
Hypersensitivity, Cushing's syndrome, measles, varicella, fungal infections

Precautions: Pregnancy C, breastfeeding, diabetes mellitus, glaucoma, osteoporosis, seizure disorders, ulcerative colitis, CHF, myasthenia gravis, renal disease, esophagitis, peptic ulcer, tartrazine, benzyl alcohol, corticosteroid hypersensitivity, viral infection, TB, traumatic brain injury

DOSAGE AND ROUTES
Adrenal insufficiency/inflammation
Adult: PO 4-48 mg in 4 divided doses; IM 10-80 mg (acetate); IM/**IV** 10-250 mg (succinate); intraarticular 4-80 mg (acetate)
Child: **IV** 0.5-1.7 mg/kg in 3-4 divided doses (succinate)

Shock
Adult: **IV** 100-250 mg q2-6hr or 30 mg/kg, then q4-6hr prn × 2-3 days (succinate)

Multiple sclerosis
Adult: PO 160 mg/day × 1 wk, then 64 mg every other day × 30 days

Available forms: Tabs 2, 4, 6, 8, 16, 24, 32 mg; inj 20, 40, 80 mg/ml acetate; inj 40, 125, 500, 1000, 2000 mg/vial succinate

Implementation
PO route
- Give with food or milk to decrease GI symptoms
IM route
- Give IM inj deep in large muscle mass; rotate sites; avoid deltoid; use 21-G needle
- Give in one dose in AM to prevent adrenal suppression; avoid SUBCUT administration; may damage tissue

IV route
- Use only methylPREDNISolone sodium succinate (Solu-Medrol) **IV**, never use methylPREDNISolone acetate suspension **IV**
- Give after diluting with provided diluent, agitate slowly; give 500 mg or less over 1 min or longer

Intermittent/continuous IV infusion route
- Dilute further in D₅W, 0.9% NaCl, D₅NS, haze may form, give over 15-60 min, large doses (≥500 mg) give over 30-60 min
- Give after shaking susp (parenteral)
- Give titrated dosage; use lowest effective dosage

Syringe compatibilities: Granisetron, metoclopramide

Y-site compatibilities: Acyclovir, amifostine, aztreonam, cefepime, CISplatin, cladribine, cyclophosphamide, cytarabine, DOPamine, DOXOrubicin, enalaprilat, famotidine, fludarabine, granisetron, heparin, inamrinone, melphalan, meperidine, methotrexate, metronidazole, midazolam, morphine, piperacillin/tazobactam,

M

sodium bicarbonate, tacrolimus, teniposide, theophylline, thiotepa, vit B with C

Y-site incompatibilities: Ondansetron, paclitaxel, sargramostim, vinorelbine

Inhalation route
• Give inh with water to decrease possibility of fungal infections
• Give titrated dosage; use lowest effective dosage
• Clean aerosol topically daily with warm water; dry thoroughly
• Store in cool environment; do not puncture or incinerate container

Topical route
• Cleanse area before applying product
• Apply only to affected areas; do not get in eyes
• Apply medication, then cover with occlusive dressing (only if prescribed); seal to normal skin; change q12hr; systemic absorption may occur
• Apply only to dermatoses; do not use on weeping, denuded, or infected area
• Apply treatment for a few days after area has cleared
• Store at room temperature

ADVERSE EFFECTS

CNS: Depression, flushing, sweating, headache, mood changes
CV: Hypertension, **circulatory collapse, thrombophlebitis, embolism,** tachycardia
EENT: Fungal infections, increased intraocular pressure, blurred vision, cataracts
GI: Diarrhea, nausea, abdominal distention, **GI hemorrhage,** increased appetite, **pancreatitis**
HEMA: Thrombocytopenia
INTEG: Acne, poor wound healing, ecchymosis, petechiae
MS: Fractures, osteoporosis, weakness

Pharmacokinetics

Absorption	Well absorbed (PO); systemic (topical)
Distribution	Crosses placenta
Metabolism	Liver, extensively
Excretion	Kidney
Half-life	3-5 hr (plasma) 18-36 hr (tissue); adrenal suppression 3-4 days

Pharmacodynamics

	PO	IM	IV	Topical
Onset	Unknown	Unknown	Rapid	Min to hr
Peak	2 hr	4-8 days	Unknown	Hr to days
Duration	$1\frac{1}{2}$ days	1-4 wk	Unknown	Hr to days

INTERACTIONS

Individual drugs
Amphotericin B: increased side effects
Insulin: increased need for insulin
Phenytoin, rifampin: decreased action; increased metabolism
Somatrem: decreased effect

Drug classifications
Contraceptives, oral: increased methylPREDNISolone action
CYP3A4 inducers (barbiturates, bosentan, carBAMazepine, efavirenz, phenytoins, nevirapine, rifabutin, rifampin): decreased methylPREDNISolone effect
CYP3A4 inhibitors (aprepitant, antiretroviral protease inhibitors, clarithromycin, danazol, delavirdine, diltiazem, erythromycin, fluconazole, fluoxetine, fluvoxamine, imatinib, ketoconazole, mibefradil, nefazodone, telithromycin, voriconazole): increased adrenal suppression
Diuretics: increased side effects
Hypoglycemic agents: increased need for hypoglycemic agents
Vaccines: decreased effects of vaccines

Drug/herb
St. John's wort: avoid use

Drug/food
Grapefruit juice: increased methylPREDNISolone level; do not use concurrently

Drug/lab test
Increased: cholesterol, sodium, blood glucose, uric acid, calcium, urine glucose
Decreased: calcium, potassium, T_4, T_3, thyroid radioactive iodine uptake test, urine 17-OHCS, 17-KS
False negative: skin allergy tests

NURSING CONSIDERATIONS

Assessment
• **Adrenal insufficiency:** assess for weight loss, nausea, vomiting, confusion, anxiety, hypotension, weakness

• Monitor plasma cortisol levels during long-term therapy (normal level 138-635 nmol/L when drawn at 8 AM)

• Monitor potassium, blood glucose, urine glucose while patient is on long-term therapy; hypokalemia and hyperglycemia

• Monitor weight daily; notify prescriber of weekly gain >5 lb

• Monitor B/P q4hr, pulse; notify prescriber if chest pain occurs

• Monitor I&O ratio; be alert for decreasing urinary output and increasing edema

• Monitor adrenal function periodically for hypothalamic-pituitary-adrenal axis suppression

• **Assess for infection:** increased temp, WBC even after withdrawal of medication; product masks infection symptoms

• Assess for potassium depletion: paresthesias, fatigue, nausea, vomiting, depression, polyuria, dysrhythmias, weakness

• Assess for edema, hypertension, cardiac symptoms

• Assess mental status: affect, mood, behavioral changes, aggression

• Check temp; if fever develops, product should be discontinued

• Assess for systemic absorption: increased temp, inflammation, irritation (topical)

Nursing diagnoses

• Infection, risk for (adverse reactions)
• Knowledge, deficient (teaching)
• Noncompliance (teaching)

Patient/family education

• Teach patient that emergency ID as corticosteroid user should be carried/worn

• Advise patient to notify prescriber if therapeutic response decreases; dosage adjustment may be needed

⚠ Caution patient not to discontinue abruptly; adrenal crisis can result

• Caution patient to avoid OTC products: salicylates, alcohol in cough products, cold preparations unless directed by prescriber

• Teach patient all aspects of product use including cushingoid symptoms

• Teach patient symptoms of adrenal insufficiency: nausea, anorexia, fatigue, dizziness, dyspnea, weakness, joint pain

• Inform patient that long-term therapy may be needed to clear infection (1-2 mo depending on type of infection)

Nasal route

• Advise patient to clear nasal passages if sneezing attack occurs; repeat dose

• Advise patient to continue using product even if mild nasal bleeding occurs; is usually transient

• Teach patient method of instillation after providing written instructions from manufacturer

Topical route

• Advise patient to avoid sunlight on affected area; burns may occur

Evaluation

Positive therapeutic outcome

• Ease of respirations, decreased inflammation
• Absence of severe itching, patches on skin, flaking (top)

metipranolol ophthalmic
See Appendix B

metoclopramide (Rx)
(met-oh-kloe-pra′mide)
Apo-Metoclop ✦, Metozolv ODT, Nu-Metoclopramide ✦, Reglan
Func. class.: Cholinergic, antiemetic
Chem. class.: Central dopamine receptor antagonist
Pregnancy category B

Do not confuse:
metoclopramide/metolazone,
Reglan/Megace/Renagel

ACTION: Enhances response to acetylcholine of tissue in upper GI tract, which causes contraction of gastric muscle, relaxes pyloric, duodenal segments, increases peristalsis without stimulating secretions, blocks dopamine in chemoreceptor trigger zone of CNS

Therapeutic outcome: Decreased symptoms of delayed gastric emptying, decreased nausea, vomiting

USES: Prevention of nausea, vomiting induced by chemotherapy, radiation; delayed gastric emptying, gastroesophageal reflux

CONTRAINDICATIONS: Hypersensitivity to this product or procaine or procainamide, seizure disorder, pheochromocytoma, breast cancer (prolactin dependent), GI obstruction

Precautions: Pregnancy **B**, breastfeeding, GI hemorrhage, CHF, Parkinson's disease

BLACK BOX WARNING: Tardive dyskinesia

M

DOSAGE AND ROUTES

Nausea/vomiting (chemotherapy)
Adult: IV 1-2 mg/kg 30 min before administration of chemotherapy, then q2hr × 2 doses, then q3hr × 3 doses
Child (unlabeled): IV 1-2 mg/kg/dose

Facilitation of small bowel intubation in radiologic exams
Adult and child >14 yr: IV 10 mg over 1-2 min
Child 6-14 yr: IV 2.5-5 mg
Child <6 yr: IV 0.1 mg/kg

Diabetic gastroparesis
Adult: PO 10 mg 30 min before meals, at bedtime × 2-8 wk
Geriatric: PO 5 mg $\frac{1}{2}$ hr before meals, at bedtime, increase to 10 mg if needed

Gastroesophageal reflux
Adult: PO 10-15 mg qid 30 min before meals and at bedtime
Child: PO 0.4-0.8 mg/kg/day divided in 4 doses

Renal dose
Adult: IV CCr <40 ml/min 50% of dose

Available forms: Tabs 5, 10 mg; syr 5 mg/5 ml; inj 5 mg/ml, conc sol 10 mg/ml, orally disintegrating tab 5, 10 mg

Implementation
PO route
• Use gum, hard candy, frequent rinsing of mouth for dryness of oral cavity
• Give $\frac{1}{2}$-1 hr before meals for better absorption
• **Oral disintegrating:** place on tongue, allow to dissolve, swallow, remove from bottle immediately before use
IM route
• Give for postop nausea and vomiting before end of surgery
Direct IV route
• Give **IV** undiluted if dose is ≤10 mg; give over 2 min
• Give diphenhydrAMINE **IV** for EPS
• Discard open ampules
Intermittent IV infusion route
• Dilute more than 10 mg in 50 ml or more D_5W, NaCl, Ringer's, LR and give over 15 min or more

Y-site compatibilities: Acyclovir, aldesleukin, alfentanil, amifostine, amikacin, aminophylline, ascorbic acid, atracurium, atropine, azaTHIOprine, aztreonam, bivalirudin, bleomycin, bumetanide, buprenorphine, butorphanol, calcium chloride/gluconate, CARBOplatin, caspofungin, ceFAZolin, cefonicid, cefoperazone, cefotaxime, cefotetan, cefoxitin, ceftazidime, ceftizoxime, cefTRIAXone, cefuroxime, chloramphenicol, chlorproMAZINE, cimetidine, ciprofloxacin, cisatracurium, CISplatin, cladribine, clindamycin, cyanocobalamin, cyclophosphamide, cycloSPORINE, cytarabine, DACTINomycin, DAPTOmycin, dexamethasone, dexmedetomidine, digoxin, diltiazem, diphenhydrAMINE, DOBUTamine, docetaxel, DOPamine, doripenem, doxapram, DOXOrubicin hydrochloride, doxycycline, droperidol, enalaprilat, ePHEDrine, EPINEPHrine, epirubicin, epoetin alfa, ertapenem, erythromycin, esmolol, etoposide, etoposide phosphate, famotidine, fenoldopam, fentaNYL, filgrastim, fluconazole, fludarabine, folic acid, foscarnet, gallium nitrate, gemcitabine, gentamicin, glycopyrrolate, granisetron, heparin, hydrocortisone, HYDROmorphone, IDArubicin, ifosfamide, imipenem/cilastatin, indomethacin, insulin, isoproterenol, ketorolac, labetalol, leucovorin, levofloxacin, lidocaine, linezolid, LORazepam, magnesium sulfate, mannitol, mechlorethamine, melphalan, meperidine, meropenem, metaraminol, methadone, methotrexate, methoxamine, methyldopate, methylPREDNISolone, metoprolol, metroNIDAZOLE, miconazole, midazolam, milrinone, minocycline, mitomycin, morphine, moxalactam, multiple vitamins, nafcillin, nalbuphine, naloxone, nesiritide, nitroglycerin, nitroprusside, norepinephrine, octreotide, ondansetron, oxaliplatin, oxytocin, paclitaxel, palonosetron, pantoprazole, papaverine, pemetrexed, penicillin G, pentamidine, pentazocine, PENTobarbital, PHENobarbital, phentolamine, phenylephrine, phytonadione, piperacillin/tazobactam, potassium chloride, procainamide, prochlorperazine, promethazine, propranolol, protamine, pyridoxine, quinupristin/dalfopristin, ranitidine, remifentanil, riTUXimab, rocuronium, sargramostim, sodium acetate/bicarbonate, succinylcholine, SUFentanil, tacrolimus, teniposide, theophylline, thiamine, thiotepa, ticarcillin/clavulanate, tigecycline, tirofiban, tobramycin, tolazoline, topotecan, trastuzumab, trimethaphan, urokinase, vancomycin, vasopressin, vecuronium, verapamil, vinBLAStine, vinCRIStine, vinorelbine, voriconazole, zidovudine

Y-site incompatibilities: Amphotericin B cholesteryl/colloidal, amphotericin B liposome, amsacrine, cefepime, dantrolene, diazepam, diazoxide, DOXOrubicin liposome, ganciclovir, inamrinone, phenytoin, propofol, trimethoprim/sulfamethoxazole

ADVERSE EFFECTS

CNS: *Sedation, fatigue, restlessness, headache, sleeplessness, dystonia,* dizziness, drowsiness, **suicidal ideation, seizures,** EPS, **neuroleptic malignant syndrome; tardive dyskinesia** (>3 mo, high doses)
CV: Hypotension, **supraventricular tachycardia**
GI: Dry mouth, constipation, nausea, anorexia, vomiting, diarrhea
GU: Decreased libido, prolactin secretion, amenorrhea, galactorrhea
HEMA: Neutropenia, leukopenia, agranulocytosis
INTEG: Urticaria, rash

Pharmacokinetics

Absorption	Well absorbed (PO)
Distribution	Widely distributed; crosses blood-brain barrier, placenta
Metabolism	Liver, minimally
Excretion	Kidneys, breast milk
Half-life	4 hr

Pharmacodynamics

	PO	IM	IV
Onset	¹/₂-1 hr	10-15 min	1-3 min
Peak	Unknown	Unknown	Unknown
Duration	1-2 hr	1-2 hr	1-2 hr

INTERACTIONS

Individual drugs
Alcohol: increased sedation
Haloperidol: increased extrapyramidal reaction

Drug classifications
Anticholinergics, opiates: decreased action of metoclopramide
CNS depressants: increased sedation
MAOIs: avoid use
Phenothiazines: increased extrapyramidal reaction

Drug/lab test
Increased: prolactin, aldosterone, thyrotropin

NURSING CONSIDERATIONS

Assessment
• Assess GI complaints: nausea, vomiting, anorexia, constipation, abdominal distention before, after administration

> **BLACK BOX WARNING:** Assess for EPS and tardive dyskinesia (more likely to occur in geriatric): rigidity, grimacing, shuffling gait, tremors, rhythmic involuntary movements of tongue, mouth, jaw, feet, hands; these side effects should be reported to prescriber immediately; some effects may be irreversible

• Assess mental status: depression, anxiety, irritability during treatment
• **Neuroleptic malignant syndrome:** assess for hyperthermia, change in B/P, pulse, tachycardia, sweating, rigidity, altered consciousness

Nursing diagnoses
• Injury, risk for (adverse reactions)
• Knowledge, deficient (teaching)

Patient/family education
• Instruct patient to avoid driving, other hazardous activities until stabilized on this medication
• Advise patient to avoid alcohol and other CNS depressants that enhance sedating properties of this product
• Advise patient to notify prescriber if involuntary movements occur

Evaluation
Positive therapeutic outcome
• Absence of nausea, vomiting, anorexia, fullness

metolazone (Rx)
(me-tole′a-zone)
Zaroxolyn
Func. class.: Diuretic, antihypertensive
Chem. class.: Thiazide-like quinazoline derivative
Pregnancy category B

Do not confuse:
metolazone/methotrexate/metoclopramide

ACTION: Acts on the distal tubule and cortical thick ascending limb of the loop of Henle in the kidney, increasing excretion of sodium, water, chloride, magnesium, potassium, and bicarbonate

Therapeutic outcome: Decreased B/P, decreased edema in lung tissue and peripherally

USES: Edema, hypertension

CONTRAINDICATIONS:
Hypersensitivity to thiazides or sulfonamides, anuria, coma

M

BLACK BOX WARNING: Hepatic encephalopathy

Precautions: Pregnancy **B**, breastfeeding, geriatric, hypokalemia, renal/hepatic disease, gout, COPD, lupus erythematosus, diabetes mellitus, hypotension, history of pancreatitis, hypersensitivity to sulfonamides, thiazides, electrolyte imbalance

DOSAGE AND ROUTES

Edema
Adult: PO 5-10 mg/day; max 20 mg/day

Hypertension
Adult: PO 2.5-5 mg/day

Available forms: Tabs 2.5, 5, 10 mg

Implementation
- Give in AM to avoid interference with sleep
- Provide potassium replacement if potassium level is 3.0; product may be crushed if patient is unable to swallow
- Give with food; if nausea occurs, absorption may be increased; extended-release product is Zaroxolyn; prompt action product is Mykrox; the two formulations are not equivalent

ADVERSE EFFECTS

CNS: Anxiety, depression, headache, *dizziness, fatigue, weakness*
CV: Orthostatic hypotension, palpitations, volume depletion, chest pain, hypotension
EENT: Blurred vision
ELECT: *Hypokalemia,* hypercalcemia, hyponatremia
GI: *Nausea, vomiting, anorexia,* constipation, diarrhea, cramps, **pancreatitis,** GI irritation, dry mouth, jaundice
GU: *Frequency,* polyuria, **uremia,** glucosuria, nocturia, impotence
HEMA: Aplastic anemia, hemolytic anemia, leukopenia, agranulocytosis, neutropenia
INTEG: *Rash,* urticaria, purpura, photosensitivity, fever, dry skin
META: *Hyperglycemia,* increased creatinine, BUN
MS: Muscle cramps, joint pain, swelling

Pharmacokinetics
Absorption	GI tract (10%-20%)
Distribution	Crosses placenta
Metabolism	Urine, unchanged
Excretion	Breast milk
Half-life	8 hr (extended); 14 hr (prompt)

Pharmacodynamics
Onset	1 hr
Peak	2 hr
Duration	12-24 hr

INTERACTIONS

Individual drugs
Alcohol: increased hypotension (large amounts)
Amphotericin B, digoxin, mezlocillin, piperacillin: increased hypokalemia
Lithium: increased toxicity

Drug classifications
Antihypertensives: increased antihypertensive effect
Barbiturates, nitrates, opioids: increased hypotension
Diuretics (loop): increased metolazone effect
Glucocorticoids, laxatives (stimulant): increased hypokalemia
NSAIDs, salicylates: decreased action of metolazone

NURSING CONSIDERATIONS

Assessment
- **Hypertension:** assess B/P before, during therapy with patient lying, standing, and sitting as appropriate; orthostatic hypotension can occur rapidly
- Monitor blood glucose if patient is diabetic
- **CHF:** assess for improvement in feet, legs, sacral area daily if medication is being used
- Check for rashes, temp elevation daily
- Monitor patients receiving cardiac glycosides for increased hypokalemia
- **Hypokalemia:** assess for postural hypotension, malaise, fatigue, tachycardia, leg cramps, weakness

---

BLACK BOX WARNING: Hepatic encephalopathy: do not use in hepatic coma or precoma, fluctuations in electrolytes can occur rapidly and precipitate hepatic coma, use caution in those with impaired hepatic function

---

- Assess and record fluid volume status: I&O ratios; monitor weight, distended red veins, crackles in lung, color, quality, and specific

gravity of urine; skin turgor, adequacy of pulses, moist mucous membranes, bilateral lung sounds, peripheral pitting edema; dehydration symptoms of decreasing output, thirst, hypotension, dry mouth and mucous membranes should be reported
• Monitor electrolytes: potassium, sodium, calcium, magnesium; also include BUN, blood pH, ABGs, uric acid, CBC, blood glucose

Nursing diagnoses
• Fluid volume, deficient (adverse reactions)
• Fluid volume, excess (uses)
• Knowledge, deficient (teaching)
• Urinary elimination, impaired (adverse reactions)

Patient/family education
• Teach patient to take the medication early in the day to prevent nocturia
• Instruct patient to take with food or milk if GI symptoms of nausea and anorexia occur
• Teach patient to maintain a weekly record of weight and notify prescriber of weight loss >5 lb
• Caution patient that this product causes a loss of potassium, so foods rich in potassium should be added to the diet; refer to a dietitian for assistance in planning
• Caution the patient to rise slowly from sitting or reclining positions, not to exercise in hot weather or stand for prolonged periods, since orthostatic hypotension will be enhanced; lie down if dizziness occurs
• Teach patient not to use alcohol or any OTC medications without prescriber's approval; serious product reactions may occur
• Emphasize the need to contact prescriber immediately if muscle cramps, weakness, nausea, dizziness, or numbness occur
• Teach patient to take own B/P and pulse and record
• Advise patient to use sunscreen to prevent burns
• Teach patient to continue taking medication even if feeling better; this product controls symptoms but does not cure the condition
• Advise patient with hypertension to continue other medical regimen (exercise, weight loss, relaxation techniques, smoking cessation)

Evaluation
Positive therapeutic outcome
• Decreased edema
• Decreased B/P

TREATMENT OF OVERDOSE:
Lavage if taken orally, monitor electrolytes; administer dextrose in saline; monitor hydration, CV, renal status

metoprolol (Rx)
(met-oh-proe'lole)
Betaloc ✦, Lopressor, Nu-Metop ✦, Toprol-XL
Func. class.: Antihypertensive, antianginal
Chem. class.: β₁-Adrenergic blocker
Pregnancy category C

Do not confuse:
metoprolol/misoprostol

ACTION: Lowers B/P by β-blocking effects; reduces elevated renin plasma levels; blocks β₂-adrenergic receptors in bronchial, vascular smooth muscle only at high doses, negative chronotropic effect

Therapeutic outcome: Decreased B/P, heart rate, AV conduction

USES: Mild to moderate hypertension, acute MI to reduce cardiovascular mortality, angina pectoris, New York Heart Association class II, III heart failure

CONTRAINDICATIONS:
Hypersensitivity to β-blockers, cardiogenic shock, heart block (2nd and 3rd degree), sinus bradycardia, pheochromocytoma, sick sinus syndrome

Precautions: Pregnancy C, breastfeeding, geriatric, major surgery, diabetes mellitus, thyroid/renal/hepatic disease, COPD, CAD, nonallergic bronchospasm, CHF, bronchial asthma, CVA, children, depression, vasospastic angina

BLACK BOX WARNING: Abrupt discontinuation

DOSAGE AND ROUTES
Hypertension
Adult: PO 50 mg bid, or 100 mg/day; may give 200-450 mg in divided doses; EXT REL 25-100 mg qd, titrate at weekly intervals, max 400 mg/day
Child/adolescent 6-16 yr: PO EXT REL 1 mg/kg up to 50 mg qd
Geriatric: PO 25 mg/day initially, increase weekly as needed

Myocardial infarction
Adult: IV BOL (early treatment) 5 mg q2 min × 3 doses, then 50 mg PO 15 min after last dose and q6hr × 48 hr (late treatment); PO maintenance 50-100 mg bid for 1-3 yr

Heart failure (NYHA class II/III)
Adult: PO EXT REL 25 mg qd × 2 wk (class II); 12.5 mg qd (class III)

Angina
Adult: PO 100 mg/day as a single dose or in 2 divided doses, increase qwk as needed, or 100 mg EXT REL tab daily, max 400 mg/day ext rel

Migraine prevention (unlabeled)
Adult: PO 25-100 mg bid-qid; 50-200 mg daily (XL)

Available forms: Tabs 50, 100 mg; inj 1 mg/ml; ext rel tabs (tartrate) 100 mg; EXT REL tabs (succinate) (XL) 25, 50, 100, 200 mg

Implementation
PO route
• Do not break, crush, or chew ext rel tabs
• Give regular release tab before meals, at bedtime; tab may be crushed or swallowed whole; give with food to prevent GI upset; reduced dosage in renal dysfunction; give at same time each day
• Store protected from light, moisture; place in cool environment

Direct IV route
• Give 5 mg/2 min or more × 3 doses at 2 min intervals, start PO 15 min after last **IV** dose

Y-site compatibilities: Abciximab, acyclovir, alemtuzumab, alfentanil, alteplase, amikacin, aminophylline, amiodarone, amphotericin B liposome, anidulafungin, argatroban, ascorbic acid, atracurium, atropine, azaTHIOprine, aztreonam, benztropine, bivalirudin, bleomycin, bumetanide, buprenorphine, butorphanol, calcium chloride/gluconate, CARBOplatin, caspofungin, ceFAZolin, cefonicid, cefoperazone, cefotaxime, cefotetan, cefoxitin, ceftazidime, ceftizoxime, cefTRIAXone, cefuroxime, chloramphenicol, chlorproMAZINE, cimetidine, CISplatin, clindamycin, cyanocobalamin, cyclophosphamide, cycloSPORINE, cytarabine, DACTINomycin, DAPTOmycin, dexamethasone, dexmedetomidine, digoxin, diltiazem, diphenhydrAMINE, DOBUTamine, docetaxel, DOPamine, doxacurium, DOXOrubicin, doxycycline, enalaprilat, ePHEDrine, EPINEPHrine, epirubicin, epoetin alfa, eptifibatide, esmolol, etoposide, etoposide phosphate, famotidine, fenoldopam, fentaNYL, fluconazole, fludarabine, fluorouracil, folic acid, furosemide, ganciclovir, gemcitabine, gentamicin, glycopyrrolate, granisetron, heparin, hydrocortisone, HYDROmorphone, IDArubicin, ifosfamide, imipenem/cilastatin, indomethacin, insulin, isoproterenol, ketorolac, labetalol, linezolid, LORazepam, magnesium sulfate, mannitol, mechlorethamine, meperidine, metaraminol, methotrexate, methoxamine, methyldopate, methylPREDNISolone, metoclopramide, metroNIDAZOLE, midazolam, milrinone, mitoxantrone, morphine, multivitamins, nafcillin, nalbuphine, naloxone, nitroprusside, norepinephrine, octreotide, ondansetron, oxacillin, oxaliplatin, oxytocin, paclitaxel, palonosetron, pancuronium, papaverine, pemetrexed, penicillin G, pentamidine, pentazocine, PENTobarbital, PHENobarbital, phentolamine, phenylephrine, phytonadione, piperacillin/tazobactam, potassium chloride, procainamide, prochlorperazine, promethazine, propranolol, protamine, pyridoxine, quinupristin/dalfopristin, ranitidine, rocuronium, sodium bicarbonate, succinylcholine, SUFentanil, tacrolimus, teniposide, theophylline, thiamine, thiotepa, ticarcillin/clavulanate, tigecycline, tirofiban, tobramycin, tolazoline, trimetaphan, urokinase, vancomycin, vasopressin, vecuronium, verapamil, vinCRIStine, vinorelbine, voriconazole

Y-site incompatibilities: Allopurinol, amphotericin B cholesteryl/colloidal/lipid complex, dantrolene, diazepam, diazoxide, lepirudin, pantoprazole, phenytoin, trimethoprim/sulfamethoxazole

ADVERSE EFFECTS
CNS: *Insomnia, dizziness,* mental changes, hallucinations, depression, anxiety, headaches, nightmares, confusion, fatigue
CV: CHF, *palpitations,* dysrhythmias, **cardiac arrest, AV block,** *hypotension,* **bradycardia, pulmonary/peripheral edema, chest pain**
EENT: Sore throat, dry burning eyes
GI: *Nausea, vomiting,* colitis, cramps, *diarrhea,* constipation, flatulence, dry mouth, *hiccups*
GU: Impotence
HEMA: Agranulocytosis, eosinophilia, thrombocytopenic purpura
INTEG: Rash, purpura, alopecia, dry skin, urticaria, pruritus
RESP: Bronchospasm, dyspnea, wheezing

Pharmacokinetics

Absorption	Well absorbed (PO); completely absorbed (**IV**)
Distribution	Crosses blood-brain barrier, placenta
Metabolism	Liver, extensively
Excretion	Kidneys, breast milk
Half-life	3-4 hr

Pharmacodynamics

	PO	IV
Onset	15 min	Immediate
Peak	2-4 hr	20 min
Duration	6-19 hr	5-8 hr

INTERACTIONS

Individual drugs
Cimetidine: increased metoprolol level
EPINEPHrine, hydrALAZINE, methyldopa prazosin, reserpine: increased hypotension, bradycardia
Insulin: increased hypoglycemia

Drug classifications
Antidiabetics (oral): increased hypoglycemia
Amphetamines, calcium channel blockers, histamine H_2 antagonists: increased hypotension, bradycardia
Barbiturates: decreased metoprolol level
MAOIs: do not use together
NSAIDs, salicylates: decreased antihypertensive effect
Xanthines: decreased effects of xanthines

Drug/food
Increased: absorption with food

Drug/lab test
Increased: BUN, potassium, ANA titer, serum lipoprotein, triglycerides, uric acid, alkaline phosphatase, LDH, AST, ALT

NURSING CONSIDERATIONS

Assessment
• Monitor ECG directly when giving IV during initial treatment
• Monitor B/P during beginning treatment, periodically thereafter; pulse q4hr; note rate, rhythm, quality; check apical/radial pulse before administration; notify prescriber of any significant changes (pulse <50 bpm)
• Check for baselines in renal, liver function tests before therapy begins and periodically thereafter

• Assess for edema in feet, legs daily; monitor I&O, daily weight; check for jugular vein distention, crackles bilaterally, dyspnea (CHF)
• Monitor skin turgor, dryness of mucous membranes for hydration status, especially geriatric

Nursing diagnoses
• Cardiac output, decreased (uses)
• Injury, risk for (adverse reactions)
• Knowledge, deficient (teaching)
• Noncompliance (teaching)

Patient/family education

> **BLACK BOX WARNING:** Teach patient not to discontinue product abruptly; taper over 2 wk; may cause precipitate angina if stopped abruptly

• Teach patient not to use OTC products containing α-adrenergic stimulants (such as nasal decongestants, cold preparations); to avoid alcohol, smoking and to limit sodium intake as prescribed
• Teach patient how to take pulse and B/P at home; advise when to notify prescriber
• Instruct patient to comply with weight control, dietary adjustments, modified exercise program
• Tell patient to carry/wear emergency ID to identify product being taken, allergies; tell patient product controls symptoms but does not cure
• Caution patient to avoid hazardous activities if dizziness, drowsiness is present, to avoid driving until product response is known
• Teach patient to report symptoms of CHF; difficult breathing, especially with exertion or when lying down, night cough, swelling of extremities or bradycardia, dizziness, confusion, depression, fever, decreased vision
• Teach patient to take product as prescribed, not to double doses or skip doses; take any missed doses as soon as remembered if at least 4 hr until next dose
• Advise to monitor blood glucose closely if diabetic
• Advise to report Raynaud's symptoms

Evaluation
Positive therapeutic outcome
• Decreased B/P in hypertension (after 1-2 wk)
• Absence of dysrhythmias
• Decreased anginal pain

TREATMENT OF OVERDOSE:
Lavage, **IV** atropine for bradycardia, **IV** theophylline for bronchospasm, digoxin, O_2, diuretic for cardiac failure, hemodialysis, **IV** glucose for

M

Adverse effects: *italics* = common; **bold** = life-threatening

hyperglycemia, **IV** diazepam (or phenytoin) for seizures

metroNIDAZOLE (Rx)

(me-troe-ni'da-zole)

Flagyl, Flagyl 375, Flagyl ER, Flagyl IV, Flagyl IV RTU, Florazone ER ✿, Novonidazole ✿

Func. class.: Antiinfective, miscellaneous
Chem. class.: Nitroimidazole derivative

Pregnancy category B (2nd, 3rd trimesters)

ACTION: Direct-acting amebicide/trichomonacide; binds, degrades DNA structure, inhibiting bacterial nucleic acid synthesis

Therapeutic outcome: Trichomonacidal, amebicidal, bactericidal for the following susceptible organisms: *Bacteroides, Clostridium, Trichomonas vaginalis, Giardia lamblia, Entamoeba histolytica*

USES: Intestinal amebiasis, amebic abscess, trichomoniasis, refractory trichomoniasis, bacterial anaerobic infections, giardiasis; septicemia, endocarditis, bone, joint, and lower respiratory tract infections, rosacea

Unlabeled uses: Crohn's disease

CONTRAINDICATIONS:

Pregnancy (1st trimester), breastfeeding, hypersensitivity to this product

Precautions: Pregnancy **B** (2nd/3rd trimesters), candidal infections, heart failure, fungal infection, geriatric, dental disease, bone marrow suppression, hematologic disease, renal/hepatic/GI disease, contracted visual or color fields, blood dyscrasias, CNS disorders

> **BLACK BOX WARNING:** Secondary malignancy

DOSAGE AND ROUTES

Trichomoniasis

Adult: PO 500 mg bid × 7 days or 2 g in single dose; do not repeat treatment for 4-6 wk
Child (unlabeled): PO 15 mg/kg/day divided in 3 doses × 7-10 days

Refractory trichomoniasis

Adult: PO 250 mg bid × 10 days

Amebic hepatic abscess

Adult: PO 500-750 mg tid × 5-10 days

Child: PO 35-50 mg/kg/day in 3 divided doses × 10 days

Intestinal amebiasis

Adult: PO 750 mg tid × 5-10 days
Child: PO 35-50 mg/kg/day in 3 divided doses × 10 days; then oral iodoquinol

Anaerobic bacterial infections

Adult: **IV** INF 15 mg/kg/over 1 hr, then 7.5 mg/kg **IV** or PO q6hr, max 4 g/day; first maintenance dose should be administered 6 hr after loading dose

Bacterial vaginosis

Adult: PO REG REL 500 mg bid or 250 mg tid × 7 days; EXT REL 750 mg/day × 7 days

Giardiasis (unlabeled)

Adult: PO 250 mg tid × 5-7 days
Child: PO 5 mg/kg divided tid × 5 days

Antibiotic-associated pseudomembranous colitis

Adult (unlabeled): PO 250-500 mg 3-4 ×/day × 7-14 days
Child: PO 20 mg/kg/day (max 2 g) divided q6hr

Available forms: Tabs 250, 500 mg; ext rel tabs 750 mg; caps 375 mg; inj 500 mg/100 ml; powder for inj 500 mg single dose

Implementation

PO route

• Give with or after a meal to avoid GI symptoms, metallic taste; crush tab if needed
• Store in light-resistant container; do not refrigerate

Topical route

• A thin coating should be applied to affected area after cleaning with soap and water and patting dry

IV route

• Give intermittent **IV** prediluted; for Flagyl **IV** dilute with 4.4 ml of sterile water or 0.9% NaCl; must be diluted further with 8 mg/ml or more 0.9% NaCl, D_5W, or LR; must neutralize with 5 mEq of $NaCO_3$/500 mg; CO_2 gas will be generated and may require venting; run over 1 hr or more; primary **IV** must be discontinued; may be given as cont inf; do not use aluminum products; **IV** may require venting

Y-site compatibilities: Acyclovir, alemtuzumab, alfentanil, allopurinol, amifostene, amikacin, aminophylline, amiodarone, ampicillin, ampicillin/sulbactam, anidulafungin, atracurium, bivalirudin, bumetanide, buprenorphine, busulfan, butorphanol, calcium acetate/chloride/gluconate, CARBOplatin, ceFAZolin, cefepime, cefoperazone, cefotetan, cefotaxime, cefTRIAXone, cefuroxime, chloramphenicol, chlorproMAZINE, cimetidine, ciprofloxacin, cisatracurium, CISplatin, clindamycin, codeine, cyclophosphamide, cycloSPORINE, cytarabine, DACTINomycin, dexamethasone, dexmedetomidine, dexrazoxane, digoxin, diltiazem, dimenhyDRINATE, diphenhydrAMINE, DOBUTamine, docetaxel, DOPamine, doripenem, doxacurium, doxapram, DOXOrubicin, DOXOrubicin liposome, doxycycline, droperidol, enalaprilat, ePHEDrine, EPINEPHrine, epirubicin, eptifibatide, ertapenem, erythromycin, esmolol, etoposide, etoposide phosphate, famotidine, fenoldopam, fentaNYL, fluconazole, fludarabine, fluorouracil, foscarnet, fosphenytoin, furosemide, gemcitabine, gentamicin, glycopyrrolate, granisetron, haloperidol, heparin, hydrALAZINE, hydrocortisone, HYDROmorphone, IDArubicin, ifosfamide, imipenem/cilastatin, inamrinone, insulin, isoproterenol, ketorolac, labetalol, leucovorin, levofloxacin, lidocaine, linezolid, LORazepam, magnesium sulfate, mannitol, mechlorethamine, melphalan, meperidine, meropenem, mesna, metaraminol, methotrexate, methyldopate, methylPREDNISolone, metoclopramide, metoprolol, midazolam, milrinone, mitoxantrone, morphine, nafcillin, nalbuphine, naloxone, nesiritide, niCARdipine, nitroglycerin, nitroprusside, norepinephrine, octreotide, ondansetron, oxaliplatin, oxytocin, paclitaxel, palonosetron, pancuronium, pentamidine, pentazocine, PENTobarbital, perphenazine, PHENobarbital, phentolamine, phenylephrine, piperacillin/tazobactam, potassium chloride/phosphates, prochlorperazine, promethazine, propranolol, ranitidine, remifentanil, riTUXimab, rocuronium, sargramostim, sodium acetate/bicarbonate/phosphates, streptozocin, succinylcholine, SUFentanil, tacrolimus, teniposide, theophylline, thiopental, thiotepa, ticarcillin/clavulanate, tigecycline, tirofiban, tobramycin, trastuzumab, trimethobenzamide, trimethoprim/sulfamethoxazole, vancomycin, vasopressin, vecuronium, verapamil, vinCRIStine, vinorelbine, voriconazole, zidovudine, zoledronic acid

Y-site incompatibilities: Amphotericin B cholesteryl/colloidal/liposome, aztreonam, dantrolene, DAPTOmycin, diazepam, drotrecogin, filgrastim, ganciclovir, pantoprazole, pemetrexed, phenytoin, procainamide, quinupristin/dalfopristin

ADVERSE EFFECTS

CNS: *Headache, dizziness,* confusion, irritability, restlessness, ataxia, depression, fatigue, drowsiness, insomnia, paresthesia, peripheral neuropathy, **seizures,** incoordination, depression, encephalopathy, **aseptic meningitis**

CV: Flat T-waves

EENT: Blurred vision, sore throat, retinal edema, dry mouth, metallic taste, furry tongue, glossitis, stomatitis, photophobia, optic neuritis

GI: *Nausea, vomiting, diarrhea,* epigastric distress, *anorexia,* constipation, *abdominal cramps,* **pseudomembranous colitis**

GU: Darkened urine, vaginal dryness, polyuria, **albuminuria,** dysuria, cystitis, decreased libido, **nephrotoxicity,** incontinence, dyspareunia, candidiasis

HEMA: Leukopenia, bone marrow depression, aplasia, thrombocytopenia

INTEG: Rash, pruritus, urticaria, flushing

Pharmacokinetics

Absorption	80% (PO)
Distribution	Widely distributed, crosses placenta
Metabolism	Liver
Excretion	Urine, unchanged; feces
Half-life	6-11 hr

Pharmacodynamics

	PO	IV
Onset	Rapid	Immediate
Peak	1-2 hr	Infusion's end
Duration	Unknown	Unknown

INTERACTIONS

Individual drugs

Alcohol: increased disulfiram-like reaction

AzaTHIOprine, fluorouracil: increased leukopenia

Amprenavir: do not use bortezomib; norfloxacin, zalcitabine: avoid use

Busulfan: increased busulfan toxicity, avoid concurrent use

Cholestyramine: decreased metroNIDAZOLE

Fosphenytoin, lithium, phenytoin, warfarin: increased action of these drugs

Drug classifications

Barbiturates: decreased metroNIDAZOLE half-life

CYP3A4 substrates: increased levels

Drug/lab test

Altered: AST, ALT, LDH

Decrease: WBC, neutrophils

False decrease: triglycerides

M

Adverse effects: *italics* = common; **bold** = life-threatening

NURSING CONSIDERATIONS
Assessment
• **Assess patient for signs and symptoms of infection** including characteristics of wounds, WBC >10,000/mm^3, vaginal secretions, fever; obtain baseline information and during treatment
• Obtain C&S before beginning product therapy to identify if correct treatment has been initiated
• **Assess for allergic reactions:** rash, urticaria, pruritus
• Identify urine output; if decreasing, notify prescriber **(may indicate nephrotoxicity)**; also check for increased BUN, creatinine
• Assess bowel pattern daily; if severe diarrhea occurs, product should be discontinued
• Assess for overgrowth of infection: perineal itching, fever, malaise, redness, pain, swelling, drainage, rash, diarrhea, change in cough, sputum

> **BLACK BOX WARNING: Secondary malignancy:** use only when indicated, avoid unnecessary use

Nursing diagnoses
• Diarrhea (adverse reactions)
• Infection, risk for (uses)
• Injury, risk for (adverse reactions)
• Knowledge, deficient (teaching)
• Noncompliance (teaching)

Patient/family education
• Teach patient to report sore throat, bruising, bleeding, joint pain; may indicate blood dyscrasias (rare)
• Advise patient to contact prescriber if vaginal itching, loose foul-smelling stools, furry tongue occur; may indicate superinfection
• Advise patient to notify physician of numbness or tingling of extremities
• Teach trichomoniasis patient that both partners need to be treated; condoms should be used during intercourse to prevent reinfection
• Advise patient of disulfiram-like reaction to alcohol ingestion; alcohol should not be used within 48 hr of this product
• Inform patient product has a metallic taste and urine may turn dark
• Advise patient to contact prescriber if pregnancy is suspected
• Advise patient to use sips of water, sugarless gum, candy for dry mouth

Evaluation
Positive therapeutic outcome
• Decreased symptoms of infection

metroNIDAZOLE topical
See Appendix B

micafungin (Rx)
(my-ca-fun'gin)
Mycamine
Func. class.: Antifungal, systemic
Chem. class.: Echinocandin
Pregnancy category C

ACTION: Inhibits an essential component in fungal cell walls; causes direct damage to fungal cell wall

Therapeutic outcome: Prevention of *Candida* infection in hematopoietic stem cell transplantation (HSCT); or decreased symptoms of *Candida* infection, negative culture

USES: Treatment of esophageal candidiasis; prophylaxis of *Candida* infections in patients undergoing HSCT; susceptible *Candida* species: *C. albicans, C. glabrata, C. krusei, C. parapsilosis, C. tropicalis*

CONTRAINDICATIONS:
Hypersensitivity to this product or other echinocandins

Precautions: Pregnancy **C,** breastfeeding, children, geriatric, severe hepatic disease

DOSAGE AND ROUTES
Candidemia/acute disseminated candidiasis, abscess, peritonitis
Adult: IV 100 mg q day over 1 hr
Esophageal candidiasis
Adult: IV 150 mg/day, given over 1 hr
Prophylaxis of *Candida* infections
Adult: IV 50 mg/day, given over 1 hr

Available forms: Powder for injection 50 mg, in single-dose vials; 50, 100 mg vial

Implementation
• Do not use if cloudy or precipitated; do not admix product
• Flush line before, after administration with 0.9% NaCl

IV route
• **For *Candida* prevention:** reconstitute with provided diluent 0.9% NaCl without bacteriostatic product; 50 mg vial/5 ml (10 mg/ml), swirl to dissolve, do not shake; further dilute with 100 ml 0.9% NaCl, only; run over 1 hr

• For *Candida* infection: reconstitute with provided diluent 50 mg/5 ml (10 mg/ml); further dilute 3 reconstituted vials in 100 ml of 0.9% NaCl, run over 1 hr
• Store at room temperature, away from light; do not freeze; discard unused solution

Y-site compatibilities: Aminophylline, bumetanide, calcium chloride/gluconate, cycloSPORINE, DOPamine, eptifibatide, esmolol, fenoldopam, furosemide, heparin, HYDRO-morphone, lidocaine, LORazepam, magnesium sulfate, milrinone, nitroglycerin, nitroprusside, norepinephrine, phenylephrine, potassium chloride, potassium phosphate, tacrolimus, vasopressin

Y-site incompatibilities: Albumin, amiodarone, cisatracurium, diltiazem, DOBUTamine, EPINEPHrine, insulin, labetalol, meperidine, midazolam, morphine, mycophenolate mofetil, nesiritide, niCARdipine, octreotide, ondansetron, phenytoin, telavancin, vecuronium

ADVERSE EFFECTS
CNS: **Convulsions,** dizziness, *headache, somnolence,* fever, anxiety
CV: Flushing, hypertension, phlebitis, tachycardia
GI: Abdominal pain, *nausea, anorexia, vomiting, diarrhea, increased AST, ALT, alkaline phosphatase, blood dehydrogenase, hyperbilirubinemia*
HEMA: **Neutropenia, thrombocytopenia, leukopenia, coagulopathy, anemia, hemolytic anemia**
INTEG: *Rash, pruritus, inj site pain*
META: Hypokalemia, hypocalcemia, hypomagnesemia
MS: *Rigors*

Pharmacokinetics

Absorption	Unknown
Distribution	Protein binding 99%
Metabolism	Liver
Excretion	Feces, urine
Half-life	Terminal 14-17.2 hr

Pharmacodynamics
Unknown

INTERACTIONS
Individual drugs
Itraconazole, sirolimus, NIFEdipine: increased plasma concentrations; may need dosage reduction

NURSING CONSIDERATIONS
Assessment
• Assess for signs and symptoms of infection, clearing of cultures during treatment; obtain culture baseline, throughout; product may be started as soon as culture is taken (esophageal candidiasis); monitor cultures during HSCT, for prevention of *Candida* infections
• Monitor CBC (RBC, Hct, Hgb), differential, platelet count periodically; notify prescriber of results
• Monitor renal studies: BUN, urine CCr, electrolytes before, during therapy
• Monitor hepatic studies before, during treatment: bilirubin, AST, ALT, alkaline phosphatase, as needed
• Assess for bleeding: hematuria, heme-positive stools, bruising or petechiae of mucosa or orifices; blood dyscrasias can occur
• Assess for hypersensitivity: rash, pruritus, facial swelling; also for phlebitis
• Assess for hemolytic anemia
• Assess GI symptoms: frequency of stools, cramping; if severe diarrhea occurs, electrolytes may need to be given

Nursing diagnoses
• Infection, risk for (uses)
• Injury, risk for (adverse reactions)
• Knowledge, deficient (teaching)

Patient/family education
• Advise patient to notify prescriber if pregnancy is suspected or planned; use nonhormonal form of contraception while taking this product
• Teach patient to avoid breastfeeding while taking this product
• Teach patient to inform prescriber of renal or hepatic disease
• Teach patient to report bleeding, facial swelling, wheezing, difficulty breathing, itching, rash, hives, increasing warmth, flushing
• Instruct patient to report signs of infection: increased temp, sore throat, flulike symptoms
• Advise patient to notify prescriber of nausea, vomiting, diarrhea, jaundice, anorexia, clay-colored stools, dark urine; hepatotoxicity may occur

Evaluation
Positive therapeutic outcome
• Prevention of *Candida* infection in HSCT; decreased symptoms of *Candida* infection, negative culture

M

miconazole (Rx, OTC)

(mi-kon'a-zole)
Femizole-M, Monistat, Monistat 3, Monistat 7, Monistat-Derm, Monistat Dual-Pak, M-Zole 7 Dual Pack, topical: Micatin, Micatin Liquid, miconazole nitrate
Func. class.: Antifungal
Chem. class.: Imidazole
Pregnancy category C

ACTION: Alters cell membranes, inhibits fungal enzymes, inhibits sterols so intracellular contents are lost, prevents biosynthesis of phospholipids/triglycerides

Therapeutic outcome: Fungistatic/fungicidal against *Aspergillus, Coccidioides, Cryptococcus, Candida, Dermatophytes, Histoplasma*

USES: Coccidioidomycosis, candidiasis, cryptococcosis, paracoccidioidomycosis, chronic mucocutaneous candidiasis, fungal meningitis; **IV** used for severe infections only; topical for tinea pedis, tinea cruris, tinea corporis, tinea versicolor, vaginal or vulva candidal infections

CONTRAINDICATIONS: Hypersensitivity

Precautions: Pregnancy **C**, renal/hepatic disease

DOSAGE AND ROUTES

Adult: **IV** INF 200-3600 mg/day; may be divided in 3 INF at 200-1200 mg/INF; may have to repeat course; IT 20 mg given simultaneously with **IV** for fungal meningitis q1-2day
Child: **IV** 20-40 mg/kg/day, max 15 mg/kg/day
Adult and child: TOP apply to affected area bid × 2-4 wk
Adult: Intravaginal 200 mg SUPP at bedtime × 3 days or 100 mg SUPP × 1 wk

Available forms: Inj 10 mg/ml; aerosol 2%; cream 2%; lotion 2%; powder 2%; spray 2%; vag cream 2%; vag supp 100, 200 mg

Implementation

• Have adrenalin, suction, tracheostomy set, endotracheal intubation equipment available
Topical route
• Apply after cleansing area with soap and water before each application; use enough medication to cover lesions completely; dry well
• Store at room temperature in dry place

Vaginal route
• Administer 1 applicator full every night high into the vagina
• Store at room temperature in dry place
IV route
• Give 200 mg initially to prevent severe hypersensitive reaction
• Give **IV** after diluting in ≤1 g/10 ml of sterile water, D₅W, or 0.45% NaCl over 3-5 min
• Give by intermittent **IV** after diluting in 200 ml or more D₅W or 0.9% NaCl; give over 30-60 min
• Store at room temperature; reconstituted sol is stable for 24 hr refrigerated

Y-site compatibilities: Allopurinol, filgrastim, foscarnet, granisetron, melphalan, ondansetron, propofol, sargramostim, teniposide, thiotepa, vinorelbine

Y-site incompatibilities: Fludarabine

ADVERSE EFFECTS

CNS: Drowsiness, headache, lethargy
CV: Tachycardia, **dysrhythmias** (rapid **IV**)
GI: Nausea, vomiting, anorexia, diarrhea, cramps
GU: Vulvovaginal burning, itching, hyponatremia, pelvic cramps (topical forms)
HEMA: Decreased Hct, thrombocytopenia, hyperlipidemia
INTEG: Pruritus, rash, fever, flushing, hives
SYST: Anaphylaxis

Pharmacokinetics

Absorption	Poorly absorbed (PO)
Distribution	Widely distributed (**IV**); bound to serum proteins (90%)
Metabolism	Liver, extensively
Excretion	Unknown
Half-life	Triphasic: 0.4, 2.1, 24 hr

Pharmacodynamics

	IV	Topical	Vag
Onset	Rapid	Unknown	Unknown
Peak	Infusion's end	Unknown	Unknown
Duration	Unknown	Unknown	Unknown

INTERACTIONS

Individual drugs

Amphotericin B: decreased effect of amphotericin B
Amphotericin B, isoniazid, rifampin: decreased effect of miconazole

Phenytoin: increased effect
Warfarin: increased anticoagulant effect

Drug classifications
Sulfonylureas: increased effect

Drug/lab test
False positive: urine glucose, urine protein

NURSING CONSIDERATIONS

Assessment
• Assess for signs and symptoms of infection: drainage, sore throat, urinary pain, hematuria, fever
• Obtain C&S before beginning treatment; therapy may be started after culture is taken; monitor signs of infection before, throughout treatment
• Monitor bowel pattern before, during treatment; diarrhea may occur
• Monitor cardiac system: B/P, pulse; watch for increasing pulse, cardiac dysrhythmias; product should be discontinued
• Monitor blood studies: WBC, RBC, Hgb, Hct, bleeding time; patients taking anticoagulants may need a decreased dosage; monitor liver and renal studies periodically for patients on long-term therapy
• Monitor I&O ratio; watch for decreasing urinary output, change in specific gravity; discontinue product to prevent renal damage; patients with renal disease may require lowered dose
• Monitor **IV** site for thrombophlebitis; site should be changed q48-72hr
• Monitor for allergies before initiation of treatment and reaction to each medication; highlight allergies on chart; check for allergic reaction: burning, stinging, swelling, redness (topical); observe for skin eruptions after administration of product to 1 wk after discontinuing product

Nursing diagnoses
• Infection, risk for (uses)
• Injury, risk for (adverse reactions)
• Knowledge, deficient (teaching)
• Skin integrity, impaired (uses)

Patient/family education
• Inform patient that culture may be performed after completed course of medication
• Advise patient to notify nurse of diarrhea, symptoms of candidal vaginitis
Topical route
• Teach patient to use medical asepsis (hand washing) before, after each application; to apply with glove to prevent further infection; to avoid contact with eyes; not to use occlusive dressings

• Caution patient to avoid use of OTC creams, ointments, lotions unless directed by prescriber
• Instruct patient to notify prescriber if condition does not improve in 4 wk or if symptoms return in 2 mo; pregnancy or a serious medical condition may be the cause
• Teach patient to use for full prescribed treatment time, or reinfection may occur
Vaginal route
• Instruct patient in asepsis (hand washing) before, after each application
• Teach patient to apply with applicator only; to avoid use of any other vaginal product unless directed by prescriber; sanitary napkin may prevent soiling of undergarments; to abstain from sexual intercourse until treatment is completed or reinfection and irritation may occur
• Instruct patient to notify prescriber if symptoms persist

Evaluation
Positive therapeutic outcome
• Decreasing oral candidiasis, fever, malaise, rash
• Negative C&S for infectious organism
• Decrease in size, number of lesions
• Decrease in itching or white discharge (vaginal)

TREATMENT OF OVERDOSE:
Withdraw product; maintain airway; administer EPINEPHrine, aminophylline, O_2, **IV** corticosteroids for anaphylaxis

miconazole topical
See Appendix B

miconazole vaginal antifungal
See Appendix B

midazolam (Rx)
(mid'ay-zoe-lam)
Func. class.: Sedative/hypnotic, antianxiety
Chem. class.: Benzodiazepine, short-acting
Pregnancy category D
Controlled substance schedule IV

ACTION: Depresses subcortical levels in CNS; may act on limbic system, reticular formation; may potentiate GABA by binding to specific benzodiazepine receptors

Therapeutic outcome: Sedation for anesthesia induction and procedures

USES: Preoperative sedation, general anesthesia induction, sedation for diagnostic endoscopic procedures, intubation, anxiety

Unlabeled uses: Refractory status epilepticus

CONTRAINDICATIONS:

Pregnancy **D**, hypersensitivity to benzodiazepines, acute closed-angle glaucoma, status asthmaticus

Precautions: Breastfeeding, children, geriatric, COPD, CHF, chronic renal failure, chills, debilitated, hepatic disease, shock, coma, alcohol intoxication

> **BLACK BOX WARNING:** Neonates (contains benzyl alcohol), **IV** administration, respiratory depression/insufficiency

DOSAGE AND ROUTES

Preoperative sedation
Adult and child ≥12 yr: IM 0.07-0.08 mg/kg 30-60 min before general anesthesia
Child 1-6 mo: IM 0.1-0.15 mg/kg, may give up to 0.5 mg/kg if needed, max 10 mg
Child 6 mo-5 yr: IV 0.05-0.1 mg/kg, a total dose of 0.6 mg/kg may be needed
Child 6-11 yr: IV 0.025-0.05 mg/kg, a total dose of 0.4 mg/kg may be needed

Induction of general anesthesia
Adult >55 yr: (ASA I/II) IV 150-300 mcg/kg over 30 sec; (ASA III/IV) limit dose to 250 mcg/kg (nonpremedicated) or 150 mcg/kg (premedicated)
Adult <55 yr: IV 200-350 mcg/kg over 20-30 sec; if patient has not received premedication, may repeat by giving 20% of original dose; if patient has received premedication reduce dosage by 50 mcg/kg
Child: No safe and effective dosage is established; however, doses of 50-200 mcg/kg IV have been used

Continuous infusion for intubation (critical care)
Adult: IV 0.01-0.05 mg/kg over several min; repeat at 10-15 min intervals until adequate sedation, then 0.02-0.10 mg/kg/hr maintenance; adjust as needed
Child: IV 0.05-0.2 mg/kg over 2-3 min, then 0.06-0.12 mg/kg/hr by CONT INF; adjust as needed
Neonates: IV 0.03-0.06 mg/kg/hr titrate using lowest dose

Available forms: Inj 1, 5 mg/ml; syr 2 mg/ml

Implementation
PO route
• Remove cap of press-in bottle adaptor and push adaptor into neck of bottle; close with cap, remove cap, and insert tip of dispenser and insert into adaptor; turn upside-down and withdraw correct dose; place in mouth
IM route
• Give inj deep into large muscle mass
• Store at room temperature; protect from light
IV route
• Give **IV** undiluted or after diluting with D₅W or 0.9% NaCl to a conc of 0.25 mg/ml; give over 2 min (conscious sedation) or over 30 sec (anesthesia induction)
• Ensure immediate availability of resuscitation equipment, O₂ to support airway; do not give by rapid bol

Syrinxe compatibilities: Alfentanil, atracurium, atropine, benzquinamide, buprenorphine, butorphanol, chlorproMAZINE, cimetadine, cisatracurium, diphenhyDRAMINE, droperidol, fentaNYL, glycopyrrolate, hydromorphine, hydrOXYzine, ketamine, meperidine, metoclopramide, morphine, nalbuphine, promazine, promethazine, remifentanil, scopolamine, SUFentanil, thiethylperazine, trimethobenzamide

Syringe incompatibilities: DimenhyDRINATE, PENTobarbital, perphenazine, prochlorperazine, ranitidine

Y-site compatibilities: Abciximab, alfentamil, amikacin, amiodarone, argatroban, atracurium, atropine, aztreonam, benzotropine, calcium gluconate, ceFAZolin, cefotaxime, cefoxitine, cefTRIAXone, cimetidine, ciprofloxacin, CISplatin, clindamycin, clonidine, cyanocobalamin, cycloSPORINE, DACTINomycin, digoxin, diltiazem, diphenhydrAMINE, docetaxal, DOPamine, doxycycline, enalaprilat, EPINEPHrine, erythromycin, esmolol, etomidate, etoposide, famotidine, fentaNYL, fluconazole, folic acid, gatifloxacin, gemcitabine, gentamicin, glycopyrrolate, granisetron, heparin, hetastarch, HYDROmorphone, hydrOXYzine, inamrinone, isoproterenol, labetalol, lactated Ringer's, levofloxacin, lidocaine, linezolid, LORazepam, magnesium, mannitol, meperidine, methadone, methyldopa, methylPREDNISolone, metoclopramide, metomolol, metroNIDAZOLE, milrinone, morphine, nalbuphine, naloxone, niCARdipine, nitroglycerin, nitroprusside, norepinephrine, ondansetron, oxacillin, oxytocin, paclitaxel,

---

⚠ Nurse Alert

palonosetron, pancuronium, papaverin, phentolamine, phytonadione, piperacillin, potassium chloride, propanolol, protamine, pyridoxine, ranitidine, remifentanil, sodium nitroprusside, streptokinase, succinylcholine, SUFentanil, teniposide, theophylline, thiotepa, ticarcillin, tobramycin, vancomycin, vasopressin, vecuronium, verapamil, voriconazole

Y-site incompatibilities: Foscarnet

ADVERSE EFFECTS

CNS: Retrograde amnesia, euphoria, confusion, headache, anxiety, insomnia, slurred speech, paresthesia, tremors, weakness, chills, agitation, paradoxical reactions
CV: Hypotension, PVCs, tachycardia, bigeminy, nodal rhythm, **cardiac arrest**
EENT: Blurred vision, nystagmus, diplopia, loss of balance
GI: *Nausea, vomiting,* increased salivation, hiccups
INTEG: Urticaria, pain at injection site, swelling at inj site, rash, pruritus at injection site
RESP: Coughing, **apnea, bronchospasm, laryngospasm,** dyspnea, **respiratory depression**

Pharmacokinetics

Absorption	Well absorbed
Distribution	Crosses placenta, blood-brain barrier; protein binding 97%
Metabolism	Liver
Excretion	Kidneys, breast milk
Half-life	1.8-6.4 hr

Pharmacodynamics

	PO	IM	IV
Onset	20-30 min	15 min	3-5 min
Peak	Unknown	½-1 hr	Unknown
Duration	Unknown	2-3 hr	<2 hr

INTERACTIONS

Individual drugs
Alcohol: increased respiratory depression
Cimetidine, erythromycin, ranitidine, theophylline: decreased midazolam metabolism
Fluvoxamine, indinavir, ritonavir, verapamil: increased respiratory depression

Drug classifications
Antihypertensives, nitrates, opiates: increase in hypotension
Barbiturates, opiate analgesics, other CNS depressants: increased respiratory depression

CYP3A4 inducers (azole antifungals, theophylline): increased half-life of midazolam
CYP3A4 inhibitors: increased levels of midazolam

Drug/herb
Kava, valerian: increased sedation
St. John's wort: decreased midazolam

Drug/food
Grapefruit juice: increased midazolam effect (PO)

NURSING CONSIDERATIONS

Assessment
• Monitor B/P, pulse, respiration during **IV**; O_2 and emergency equipment should be nearby
• Monitor inj site for redness, pain, swelling
• Assess degree of amnesia in geriatric; may be increased
• Assess anterograde amnesia
• Assess vital signs for recovery period in obese patient, since half-life may be extended
• **Respiratory depression/insufficiency:** assess for apnea, respiratory depression, which may be increased in the geriatric

Nursing diagnoses
• Knowledge, deficient (teaching)

Patient/family education
• Inform patient that amnesia occurs; events might not be remembered
• Caution patient to avoid CNS depressants including alcohol for 24 hr after taking this product

Evaluation
Positive therapeutic outcome
• Induction of sedation, amnesia

TREATMENT OF OVERDOSE:
O_2, flumazenil

mifepristone (Rx)
(mif-ee-press'tone)
Mifeprex
Func. class.: Abortifacient
Chem. class.: Antiprogestational
Pregnancy category C

ACTION: Stimulates uterine contractions, causing complete abortion

Therapeutic outcome: Termination of pregnancy

USES: Abortion through 49 days of gestation

M

Unlabeled uses: Postcoital contraception/contragestation, intrauterine fetal death, endometriosis, Cushing's syndrome, unresectable meningioma

CONTRAINDICATIONS:

Hypersensitivity to this product, misoprostol, or prostaglandins; severe renal/hepatic disease, PID, respiratory/cardiac disease, IUD, ectopic pregnancy, chronic adrenal failure, bleeding disorder, inherited porphyrias

Precautions: Pregnancy **C,** women >35 yr/ smoking ≥10 cigarettes/day, asthma, anemia, jaundice, diabetes mellitus, seizure disorders, past uterine surgery

> **BLACK BOX WARNING:** Infection, sepsis, vaginal bleeding

DOSAGE AND ROUTES

Coadministration of mifepristone/ misoprostol

Adult: Day 1: PO single dose 600 mg mifepristone, 400 mcg misoprostol day 3 if needed (unless complete termination is confirmed)

Available forms: Tabs 200 mg

Implementation

• Provide emotional support before and after abortion

ADVERSE EFFECTS

CNS: Dizziness, insomnia, anxiety, syncope, fainting, headache
GI: *Nausea, vomiting, diarrhea,* dyspepsia
GU: Uterine cramping, uterine hemorrhage, vaginitis, pelvic pain
MISC: Fatigue, back pain, fever, viral infections, chills, sinusitis

Pharmacokinetics

Absorption	Rapidly
Distribution	98% protein binding, albumin, glycoprotein
Metabolism	Unknown
Excretion	Feces, urine
Half-life	Unknown

Pharmacodynamics

Onset	Unknown
Peak	90 min
Duration	Unknown

INTERACTIONS

Individual drugs

Erythromycin, itraconazole, ketoconazole: decreased metabolism of each specific product

Drug classifications

Anticoagulants, long-term corticosteroids: do not use together

Drug/herb

St. John's wort: decreased mifepristone action

Drug/food

Grapefruit juice: decreased metabolism of mifepristone

NURSING CONSIDERATIONS

Assessment

• Monitor B/P, pulse; watch for change that may indicate hemorrhage
• Monitor respiratory rate, rhythm, depth; notify prescriber of abnormalities
• Assess for length, duration of contraction; notify prescriber of contractions lasting > 1 min or absence of contractions
• **Assess for incomplete abortion;** pregnancy must be terminated by another method; product is teratogenic

Nursing diagnoses

• Knowledge, deficient (teaching)
• Pain, acute (adverse reactions)

Patient/family education

• **Sepsis:** advise patient to report increased blood loss, abdominal cramps, increased temp, foul-smelling lochia
• Teach patient some methods of comfort control and pain control
• Advise patient to continue with follow-up
• Advise patient that cramping and vaginal bleeding will occur

Evaluation

Positive therapeutic outcome
• Expulsion of fetus

---

miglitol (Rx)

(mig′le-tol)
Glyset
Func. class.: Oral hypoglycemic
Chem. class.: α-Glucosidase inhibitor
Pregnancy category B

ACTION: Delays the digestion/absorption of ingested carbohydrates, results in a smaller rise in blood glucose after meals; does not increase insulin production

Therapeutic outcome: Decreased blood glucose levels in diabetes mellitus

USES: Type 2 diabetes mellitus

CONTRAINDICATIONS:
Hypersensitivity, diabetic ketoacidosis, cirrhosis, IBD, colonic ulceration, partial intestinal obstruction, chronic intestinal disease, ileus

Precautions: Pregnancy **B,** breastfeeding, children, renal/hepatic disease

DOSAGE AND ROUTES
Initial dose
Adult: PO 25 mg tid initially, with first bite of meal

Maintenance dose
Adult: PO may be increased to 50 mg tid; may increase to 100 mg tid if needed with dosage adjustment at 4-8 wk intervals

Available forms: Tabs 25, 50, 100 mg

Implementation
• Give tid with first bite of each meal
• Provide storage in airtight container at room temperature

ADVERSE EFFECTS
GI: *Abdominal pain, diarrhea, flatulence,* **hepatotoxicity**
HEMA: Low iron
INTEG: Rash

Pharmacokinetics

Absorption	Unknown
Distribution	Unknown
Metabolism	Not metabolized
Excretion	Kidneys, unchanged product
Half-life	2 hr

Pharmacodynamics

Onset	Unknown
Peak	2-3 hr
Duration	Unknown

INTERACTIONS
Individual drugs
Digoxin: decreased levels of digoxin
Propranolol: decreased levels of propranolol
Ranitidine: decreased levels of ranitidine

Drug classifications
Adsorbents (intestinal), enzymes (digestive): decreased miglitol levels; do not use together

Drug/food
Carbohydrates: increased diarrhea

NURSING CONSIDERATIONS
Assessment
• Assess for hypo/hyperglycemia; even though this product does not cause hypoglycemia, if taking a sulfonylurea or insulin, hypoglycemia may be additive (rare)
• Monitor blood glucose levels, A1c, liver function tests; if hypoglycemia occurs with monotherapy, treat with glucose

Nursing diagnoses
• Knowledge, deficient (teaching)
• Noncompliance (teaching)
• Nutrition: less than body requirements, imbalanced (adverse reactions)
• Nutrition: more than body requirements, imbalanced (uses)

Patient/family education
• Teach patient the symptoms of hypo/hyperglycemia and what to do about each
• Instruct that medication must be taken as prescribed; explain consequences of discontinuing the medication abruptly; that during periods of stress, infection, surgery, insulin may be required
• Tell patient to avoid OTC medications unless approved by prescriber
• Teach patient that diabetes is a lifelong illness; product will not cure condition
• Instruct patient to carry/wear emergency ID as diabetic
• Teach patient that diet and exercise regimen must be followed
• Teach patient GI side effects and what to do about them

Evaluation
Positive therapeutic outcome
• Decreased signs, symptoms of diabetes mellitus (polyuria, polydipsia, polyphagia, clear sensorium, absence of dizziness, stable gait)
• Improved blood glucose, A1c

M

⚠ HIGH ALERT

milrinone (Rx)
(mill-re'none)
Func. class.: Inotropic/vasodilator agent
with phosphodiesterase activity
Chem. class.: Bipyridine derivative
Pregnancy category C

ACTION: Positive inotropic agent with
vasodilator properties; increases contractility of
cardiac muscle; reduces preload and afterload
by direct relaxation of vascular smooth muscle;
increases myocardial contractility

Therapeutic outcome: Increased inotropic effect resulting in increased cardiac output

USES: Short-term management of advanced
CHF that has not responded to other medication

CONTRAINDICATIONS:
Hypersensitivity to this product, severe aortic
disease, severe pulmonic valvular disease, acute
MI

Precautions: Pregnancy **C**, breastfeeding,
children, geriatric, renal/hepatic disease, atrial
flutter/fibrillation

DOSAGE AND ROUTES
Adult: IV BOL 50 mcg/kg given over 10 min;
start INF of 0.375-0.75 mcg/kg/min; reduce dosage in renal impairment

Renal dose
Adult: IV CCr 41-50 ml/min 0.43 mcg/kg/min,
titrate up; CCr 31-40 ml/min 0.38 mcg/kg/min,
titrate up; CCr 21-30 ml/min 0.33 mcg/kg/min,
titrate up; CCr 11-20 ml/min 0.08 mcg/kg/min;
CCr 6-10 ml/min 0.23 mcg/kg/min; CCr <6 ml/
min 0.20 mcg/kg/min; max all dosages 0.75
mcg/kg/min

Available forms: Inj 1 mg/ml; premixed
inj 200 mcg/ml in D_5W

Implementation
Direct IV route
• Give **IV** loading dose undiluted over 10 min;
use controlled-rate device
• Administer by direct **IV** into inf through
Y-connector or directly into tubing
Continuous IV infusion route
• Dilute 20 mg vial with 80, 112, 180 ml of
0.45% NaCl, 0.9% NaCl, or D_5W to a concentra-
tion of 200, 150, 100 mcg/ml respectively
• Do not mix directly with glucose sol (chemi-
cal reaction occurs over 24 hr) precipitate

forms if milrinone and furosemide come into
contact
• Titrate rate based on hemodynamic and clinical response, use controlled device
• Administer potassium supplements if ordered
for potassium levels <3.0 mg/dl

Y-site compatibilities: Acyclovir,
alfentanil, allopurinol, amifostine, amikacin,
aminocaproic acid, aminophylline, amiodarone,
amphotericin B liposome, ampicillin, ampicillin-
sulbactam, anidulafungin, argatroban, atenolol,
atracurium, aztreonam, bivalirudin, bleomycin, bumetanide, buprenorphine, busulfan,
butorphanol, calcium chloride/gluconate,
CARBOplatin, caspofungin, ceFAZolin, cefepime,
cefotaxime, cefotetan, cefoxitin, ceftazidime,
ceftizoxime, cefTRIAXone, cefuroxime, chloramphenicol, chlorproMAZINE, cimetidine, ciprofloxacin, cisatracurium, CISplatin, clindamycin,
cyclophosphamide, cycloSPORINE, cytarabine,
DACTINomycin, DAPTOmycin, dexamethasone,
digoxin, diltiazem, DOBUTamine, docetaxel, DO-
Pamine, doripenem, doxacurium, DOXOrubicin,
doxycycline, droperidol, enalaprilat, ePHED-
rine, EPINEPHrine, epirubicin, eptifibatide,
ertapenem, erythromycin, etoposide, famotidine,
fenoldopam, fentaNYL, fluconazole, fludarabine,
fluorouracil, gallium, ganciclovir, gatifloxacin, gemcitabine, gentamicin, glycopyrrolate,
granisetron, haloperidol, heparin, hydrALAZINE,
hydrocortisone, HYDROmorphone, IDArubicin, ifosfamide, insulin (regular), irinotecan,
isoproterenol, ketorolac, labetalol, levofloxacin,
linezolid, LORazepam, magnesium sulfate,
mannitol, mechlorethamine, melphalan, meperidine, meropenem, methohexital, methotrexate,
methyldopate, methylPREDNISolone, metoclopramide, metoprolol, metroNIDAZOLE, micafungin, midazolam, mitoxantrone, morphine,
mycophenolate, nafcillin, nalbuphine, naloxone,
nesiritide, norepinephrine, octreotide, oxacillin,
oxaliplatin, oxytocin, paclitaxel, palonosetron,
pamidronate, pancuronium, pemetrexed,
pentamidine, pentazocine, PENTobarbital,
PHENobarbital, phenylephrine, piperacillin,
piperacillin-tazobactam, polymyxin B, potassium
chloride/phosphates, prochlorperazine, promethazine, propofol, propranolol, quiNIDine,
quinupristin-dalfopristin, ranitidine, remifentanil, rocuronium, sodium acetate/bicarbonate/
phosphates, streptozocin, succinylcholine,
SUFentanil, sulfamethoxazole-trimethoprim,
tacrolimus, teniposide, theophylline, thiopental,
thiotepa, ticarcillin, ticarcillin-clavulanate,
tigecycline, tirofiban, tobramycin, torsemide,
vancomycin, vasopressin, vecuronium, verap-

amil, vinCRIStine, vinorelbine, voriconazole, zidovudine, zoledronic acid

ADVERSE EFFECTS

CV: Dysrhythmias, hypotension, chest pain, PVCs
GI: Nausea, vomiting, anorexia, abdominal pain, **hepatotoxicity,** jaundice
HEMA: Thrombocytopenia
MISC: Headache, hypokalemia, tremor, injection site reactions

Pharmacokinetics

Absorption	Completely absorbed
Distribution	Unknown
Metabolism	Liver (50%)
Excretion	Kidney, unchanged (83%), metabolites (12%)
Half-life	2.4 hr; increased in CHF

Pharmacodynamics

Onset	2-5 min
Peak	10 min
Duration	Variable

INTERACTIONS

Drug classifications
Antihypertensives, diuretics: increased effects

NURSING CONSIDERATIONS

Assessment
• Monitor for hypokalemia: acidic urine, reduced urine, osmolality, nocturia; hypotension, broad T-wave, U-wave, ectopy, tachycardia, weak pulse; muscle weakness, altered LOC, drowsiness, apathy, lethargy, confusion, depression; anorexia, nausea, cramps, constipation, distention, paralytic ileus; hypoventilation, respiratory muscle weakness
• Assess fluid volume status: complete I&O ratio and record; note weight, distended red veins, crackles in lung; color, quality, and specific gravity of urine; skin turgor, adequacy of pulses, moist mucous membranes, bilateral lung sounds, peripheral pitting edema; dehydration symptoms of decreasing output, thirst, hypotension, dry mouth and mucous membranes should be reported
• Monitor electrolytes: potassium, sodium, calcium, magnesium; also include BUN, blood pH, ABGs
⚠ Monitor B/P and pulse, ECG continuously during IV; ventricular dysrhythmia can occur; PCWP, CVP, index often during

inf; if B/P drops 30 mm Hg, stop inf and call prescriber
• Monitor ALT, AST, bilirubin daily; if these are elevated, hepatotoxicity is suspected
• Monitor platelets; if <150,000/mm³, product is usually discontinued and another product started
• Assess for extravasation: change site q48hr

Nursing diagnoses
• Cardiac output, decreased (uses)
• Fluid volume, excess (uses)
• Knowledge, deficient (teaching)

Patient/family education
• Teach patient reason for medication and expected results
• Instruct patient to make position changes slowly; orthostatic hypotension may occur
• Teach patient signs and symptoms of hypersensitivity reactions and hypokalemia

Evaluation
Positive therapeutic outcome
• Increased cardiac output
• Decreased PCWP, adequate CVP
• Decreased dyspnea, fatigue, edema, ECG

TREATMENT OF OVERDOSE:
Discontinue product, support circulation

minocycline (Rx)
(min-oh-sye′kleen)
Arestin, Dynacin, Minocin, Solodyn
Func. class.: Broad-spectrum antiinfective
Chem. class.: Tetracycline
Pregnancy category D

ACTION: Inhibits protein synthesis and phosphorylation in microorganisms by binding to 30S ribosomal subunits and reversibly binding to 50S ribosomal subunits; bacteriostatic

Therapeutic outcome: Bactericidal action against susceptible organisms, including *Neisseria meningitidis, Neisseria gonorrhoeae, Treponema pallidum, Chlamydia trachomatis, Ureaplasma urealyticum, Mycoplasma pneumoniae, Nocardia, Rickettsia*

USES: Syphilis, chlamydial infection, gonorrhea, lymphogranuloma venereum, rickettsial infections, inflammatory acne, meningitis carriers, periodontitis, methicillin-resistant *Staphylococcus aureus* (MRSA) infections, nonnodular moderate to severe acne vulgaris

Unlabeled uses: Rheumatoid arthritis

CONTRAINDICATIONS:

Pregnancy **D,** hypersensitivity to tetracyclines, children <8 yr

Precautions: Breastfeeding, hepatic disease

DOSAGE AND ROUTES

Adult: PO/**IV** 200 mg, then 100 mg q12hr, max 400 mg/24 hr **IV;** subgingival insert into periodontal pocket

Child >8 yr: PO/**IV** 4 mg/kg then 4 mg/kg/day PO in divided doses q12hr

Gonorrhea

Adult: PO 200 mg, then 100 mg q12hr × 4 days or more

C. trachomatis infection

Adult: PO 100 mg bid × 7 days

Syphilis

Adult: PO 200 mg, then 100 mg q12hr × 10-15 days

Uncomplicated gonococcal urethritis in men

Adult: PO 100 mg q12hr × 5 days

Rheumatoid arthritis (unlabeled)

Adult: PO 100 mg bid for ≤48 wk

Acne vulgaris (solodyn only)

Adults/adolescents/children ≥12 yr: EXT REL 1 mg/kg/day × 12 wk or those weighing 126-136 kg: 135 mg/day; 111-125 kg: 115 mg/day; 97-110 kg: 105 mg/day; 85-96 kg: 90 mg/day; 72-84 kg: 80 mg/day; 60-71 kg: 65 mg/day; 50-59 kg: 55 mg/day

Acne vulgaris (all except solodyn)

Adults/adolescents/children ≥12 yr: EXT REL 1 mg/kg × 12 wk or 91-136 kg/35 mg/day; 60-90 kg 90 mg/day; 45-59 kg 45 mg/day

Available forms: Caps 50, 75, 100 mg; oral susp 50 mg/5 ml; powder for inj 100 mg; pellet-filled caps 50, 100 mg; tabs 50, 75, 100 mg; ext rel tabs 45, 65, 90, 115, 135 mg

Implementation

PO route

• Give around the clock to maintain proper blood levels; give with food to increase absorption of product; do not give within 3 hr of other agents; product interactions may occur

• Give with 8 oz of water 1 hr before bedtime to prevent ulceration

• Shake liquid preparation well before giving; use calibrated device for proper dosing

• Do not give with iron, calcium, magnesium products, or antacids, which decrease absorption and form insoluble chelate

IV route

• Check for irritation, extravasation, phlebitis daily; change site q72hr

• For intermittent inf, dilute each 100 mg/10 ml of 0.9% NaCl, sterile water for inj; further dilute in 500-1000 ml of 0.9% NaCl, D$_5$W, Ringer's, LR, D$_5$/LR; give over 6 hr

Y-site compatibilities: Alfentanil, amikacin, atracurium, benztropine, bretylium, buprenorphine, butorphanol, calcium chloride, CARBOplatin, caspofungin, cefonicid, chlorproMAZINE, cimetidine, codeine, cyclophosphamide, cycloSPORINE, cytarabine, DACTINomycin, dexmedetomidine, diltiazem, diphenhydrAMINE, DOBUTamine, docetaxel, doxacurium, doxycycline, enalaprilat, ePHEDrine, EPINEPHrine, eptifibatide, etoposide, fenoldopam, fentaNYL, fludarabine, gatifloxacin, gemcitabine, gentamicin, glycopyrrolate, granisetron, heparin, hetastarch, IDArubicin, ifosfamide, inamrinone, isoproterenol, labetalol, levofloxacin, lidocaine, linezolid, LORazepam, magnesium sulfate, mannitol, melphalan, metaraminol, methotrexate, methyldopa, metoclopramide, metoprolol, midazolam, mitoxantrone, nalbuphine, naloxone, perphenazine, potassium chloride, sargramostim, sodium succinate, vinorelbine, vit B/C

Y-site incompatibilities: Aztreonam, filgrastim, HYDROmorphone, meperidine, morphine, teniposide

ADVERSE EFFECTS

CNS: *Dizziness,* fever, light-headedness, vertigo, seizures, **increased intracranial pressure**

CV: Pericarditis

EENT: Dysphagia, glossitis, decreased calcification, permanent discoloration of teeth, oral candidiasis

GI: *Nausea,* abdominal pain, *vomiting, diarrhea,* anorexia, enterocolitis, **hepatotoxicity,** flatulence, abdominal cramps, epigastric burning, stomatitis, **pseudomembranous colitis**

GU: Increased BUN, polyuria, polydipsia, **renal failure, nephrotoxicity**

HEMA: Eosinophilia, neutropenia, **thrombocytopenia, hemolytic anemia,** pancytopenia

INTEG: *Rash, urticaria, photosensitivity, increased pigmentation,* **exfoliative dermatitis,** pruritus, blue-gray color of skin and mucous membranes

MS: Myalgia, arthritis, bone discoloration, joint stiffness

SYST: Angioedema, Stevens-Johnson syndrome

Pharmacokinetics

Absorption	Well absorbed (PO)
Distribution	Widely distributed (70%-75% protein bound); some distribution in CSF, crosses placenta
Metabolism	Liver, some
Excretion	Kidneys, unchanged (20%), bile, feces
Half-life	11-17 hr

Pharmacodynamics

	PO	IV
Onset	Rapid	Rapid
Peak	2-3 hr	Infusion's end
Duration	Unknown	Unknown

INTERACTIONS

Individual drugs
Calcium: forms chelates, decreased absorption
CarBAMazepine, phenytoin: decreased effect
Digoxin: increased effect
Insulin: increased effect
Kaolin/pectin, sodium bicarbonate, cimetidine, quinapril, sucralfate, iron: decreased minocycline effect
Theophylline: increased effect
Warfarin: increased effect

Drug classifications
Alkali products, antacids: decreased minocycline effect
Anticoagulants (oral neuromuscular blockers): increased effect
Barbiturates, penicillins: decreased effect
Oral contraceptives: decreased effect of oral contraception
Retinoids: increased chance of pseudomotor cerebri, do not use concurrently

Drug/lab test
False negative: urine glucose with Clinistix, Tes-Tape

NURSING CONSIDERATIONS

Assessment
• Assess patient for previous sensitivity reaction
• **Assess patient for signs and symptoms of infection** including characteristics of wounds, sputum, urine, stool, WBC >10,000/mm³, fever; obtain baseline information before, during treatment

• Obtain C&S before beginning product therapy to identify if correct treatment has been initiated
• **Assess for allergic reactions:** rash, urticaria, pruritus, angioedema
• Monitor blood studies: AST, ALT, CBC, Hct, bilirubin, alkaline phosphatase, amylase monthly if patient is on long-term therapy
• **Pseudomembranous colitis:** assess bowel pattern daily; if severe diarrhea occurs, product should be discontinued
• Monitor for bleeding: ecchymosis, bleeding gums, hematuria, stool guaiac daily if on long-term therapy; blood dyscrasias may occur
• **Assess for overgrowth of infection:** perineal itching, fever, malaise, redness, pain, swelling, drainage, rash, diarrhea, change in cough, sputum; black, furry tongue

Nursing diagnoses
• Diarrhea (adverse reactions)
• Infection, risk for (uses)
• Knowledge, deficient (teaching)
• Noncompliance (teaching)

Patient/family education
• Teach patient to use sunscreen when outdoors to decrease photosensitivity reaction
• Teach patient to report sore throat, bruising, bleeding, joint pain; may indicate blood dyscrasias (rare)
• Advise patient to contact prescriber if vaginal itching, loose foul-smelling stools, furry tongue occur; may indicate superinfection; report itching, rash, pruritus, urticaria
• Instruct patient to take all medication prescribed for the length of time ordered; product must be taken around the clock to maintain blood levels; do not give medication to others; take with a full glass of water; may take with food; not to use outdated product, Fanconi's syndrome may occur
• Advise patient to use a form of contraception other than hormonal

Evaluation
Positive therapeutic outcome
• Absence of signs/symptoms of infection (WBC <10,000/mm³, temp WNL, absence of red, draining wounds)
• Reported improvement in symptoms of infection

minoxidil (Rx, OTC)
(mi-nox'i-dill)
Loniten, Rogaine (TOP)
Func. class.: Antihypertensive, hair growth stimulant
Chem. class.: Vasodilator, peripheral
Pregnancy category C

Do not confuse:
Loniten/Lipitor
minoxidil/Monopril

ACTION: Directly relaxes arteriolar smooth muscle, causing vasodilatation; reduces peripheral vascular resistance, decreases B/P; increased cutaneous blood flow; stimulation of hair follicles

Therapeutic outcome: Decreased B/P in hypertension; hair growth

USES: Severe hypertension unresponsive to other therapy (use with diuretic and β-blocker); topically to treat alopecia

CONTRAINDICATIONS:
Dissecting aortic aneurysm, hypersensitivity, pheochromocytoma

> **BLACK BOX WARNING:** Acute MI

Precautions: Pregnancy **C**, breastfeeding, children, geriatric, renal disease, CVD

> **BLACK BOX WARNING:** CAD, CHF, cardiac disease, cardiac tamponade, edema, hypotension, orthostatic hypotension, pericardial effusion

DOSAGE AND ROUTES
Severe hypertension
Adult: PO 2.5-5 mg/day in 1-2 divided doses, max 100 mg/day; usual range 10-40 mg/day in single doses
Geriatric: PO 2.5 mg/day, may be increased gradually
Child <12 yr: PO initial 0.1-0.2 mg/kg/day; effective range, 0.25-1 mg/kg/day; max, 50 mg/day

Alopecia
Adult: TOP 1 ml bid, rub into scalp daily, max 2 ml/day

Available forms: Tabs 2.5, 10 mg; topical 2%, 5% sol, topical foam 5%

Implementation
PO route
- Give with meals to decrease GI symptoms
- Give with β-blockers and/or diuretic for hypertension
- Store protected from light and heat

Topical route
- Administer 1 ml dose no matter how much balding has occurred; increasing dose does not speed hair growth
- Treatment must continue long term or new hair will be lost again

ADVERSE EFFECTS
Systemic
CNS: Headache, fatigue
CV: *Severe rebound hypertension (on withdrawal in children),* tachycardia, angina, increased T-wave, **CHF, pulmonary edema, pericardial effusion,** edema, sodium retention, water retention, hypotension
GI: Nausea, vomiting
GU: Breast tenderness
HEMA: Hct, Hgb, erythrocyte count may decrease initially
INTEG: Pruritus, **Stevens-Johnson syndrome,** rash, hirsutism

Pharmacokinetics

Absorption	Well absorbed (PO); minimally absorbed (topical)
Distribution	Widely distributed, protein binding minimal
Metabolism	Liver
Excretion	Kidneys, breast milk
Half-life	4.2 hr

Pharmacodynamics

	PO	Topical
Onset	$1/2$ hr	4 mo
Peak	2-3 hr	Unknown
Duration	75 hr	4 mo

INTERACTIONS
Individual
Guanethidine, nitroprusside: increased hypotension

Drug classifications
Antihypertensives, MAOIs, nitrates: increased hypotension
Estrogens, NSAIDs, salicylates: decreased antihypertensive effect

Drug/herb
Hawthorn: increased antihypertensive effect

Drug/lab test
Increased: renal function tests
Decreased: Hgb, Hct, RBC

NURSING CONSIDERATIONS
Assessment
⚠ Monitor closely; usually given with β-blocker to prevent tachycardia and increased myocardial workload; usually given with diuretic to prevent serious fluid accumulation; patient should be hospitalized during beginning treatment
• Monitor B/P, pulse, jugular venous distention periodically throughout treatment
• Monitor electrolytes, blood studies: potassium, sodium, chloride, CBC, serum glucose
⚠ Monitor weight daily, I&O; assess edema in feet, legs daily; check skin turgor, dryness of mucous membranes for hydration status
• Assess for crackles, dyspnea, orthopnea, peripheral edema, fatigue, weight gain, jugular vein distention (CHF)
• Assess for signs of hyperglycemia: acetone breath, increased urinary output, severe thirst, lethargy, dizziness

Nursing diagnoses
• Cardiac output, decreased (adverse reactions)
• Injury, risk for (side effects)
• Knowledge, deficient (teaching)

Patient/family education
Topical route
• Teach patient that new hair will be soft and hardly visible
• Caution patient not to use on other parts of the body; product is to be used on the scalp only
• Instruct patient that hair should be clean before applying medication; do not get on clothing
• Caution patient not to get medication near mucous membranes (mouth, nose, eyes) and to contact prescriber if burning, stinging, or rash occurs

Evaluation
Positive therapeutic outcome
• Decreased B/P in hypertension
• Hair growth (TOP)

mirtazapine (Rx)
(mer-ta′za-peen)
CO Mirtazapine ✱, Gen-Mirtazapine ✱, Novo-Mirtazapine ✱, PMS-Mirtazapine ✱, ratio-Mirtazapine ✱, Remeron, Remeron Soltab, Sandoz Mirtazapine ✱
Func. class.: Antidepressant
Chem. class.: Tetracyclic
Pregnancy category C

ACTION: Blocks reuptake of norepinephrine, serotonin into nerve endings, increasing action of norepinephrine, serotonin in nerve cells; antagonist of central α_2-receptors, blocks histamine receptors; has anticholinergic action

Therapeutic outcome: Decreased symptoms of depression after 2-3 wk

USES: Depression, dysthymic disorder, bipolar disorder: depression, agitated depression

CONTRAINDICATIONS: Hypersensitivity to tricyclics, recovery phase of MI, agranulocytosis, jaundice

Precautions: Pregnancy C, geriatric, suicidal patients, severe depression, increased intraocular pressure, closed-angle glaucoma, urinary retention, cardiac/renal/hepatic disease, hypo/hyperthyroidism, electroshock therapy, elective surgery, seizure disorder, bone marrow suppression, thrombocytopenia

BLACK BOX WARNING: Suicidal ideation, children

DOSAGE AND ROUTES
Adult: PO 15 mg/day at bedtime, maintenance to continue for 6 mo, titrate up to 45 mg/day; orally disintegrating tabs open blister pack, place tab on tongue, allow to disintegrate, swallow
Geriatric: PO 7.5 mg nightly, increase by 7.5 mg q1-2wk to desired dose, max 45 mg/day

Available forms: Tabs 15, 30, 45 mg; orally disintegrating tabs (Soltab) 15, 30, 45 mg

Implementation
• Give with food or milk for GI symptoms; crush if patient is unable to swallow medication whole
• Give dose at bedtime if oversedation occurs during day; may take entire dose at bedtime; geriatric may not tolerate once/day dosing
• Store at room temperature; do not freeze

• Allow orally disintegrating tablets to dissolve on tongue; no water needed; do not split

• **Serotonin syndrome, neuroleptic malignant syndrome:** assess for increased heart rate, shivering, sweating, dilated pupils, tremors, high B/P, hyperthermia, headache, confusion; if these occur, stop product, administer a serotonin antagonist if needed; at least 2 wk should elapse between discontinuation of serotoninergic agents and start of this product

ADVERSE EFFECTS

CNS: *Dizziness, drowsiness,* confusion, headache, anxiety, tremors, stimulation, weakness, nightmares, EPS (geriatric), increased psychiatric symptoms, **seizures**
CV: *Orthostatic hypotension, ECG changes, tachycardia, hypertension,* palpitations
EENT: *Blurred vision,* tinnitus, mydriasis
GI: *Diarrhea, dry mouth,* nausea, vomiting, **paralytic ileus,** increased appetite, cramps, epigastric distress, **jaundice, hepatitis,** stomatitis, constipation, weight gain
GU: *Retention,* **acute renal failure**
HEMA: **Agranulocytosis, thrombocytopenia, eosinophilia, leukopenia**
INTEG: Rash, urticaria, sweating, pruritus, photosensitivity
SYST: Flulike symptoms, increased cholesterol levels

Pharmacokinetics

Absorption	Slow, complete
Distribution	Widely distributed; crosses placenta
Metabolism	Liver, extensively
Excretion	Feces; breast milk
Half-life	20-40 hr

Pharmacodynamics

Onset	Unknown
Peak	2 hr
Duration	Unknown

INTERACTIONS

Individual drugs
Alcohol: increased CNS depression
CloNIDine: decreased effects
Fenfluramine, dexfenfluramine, sibutramine, nefazodone: increased serotonin syndrome

Drug classifications
Barbiturates, benzodiazepines, CNS depressants (other): increased effects
MAOIs: hypertensive episode, seizures, hyperpyretic crisis

Sympathomimetics, indirect acting (ePHEDrine): decreased effects
SSRIs, SNRIs, serotonin-receptor agonists: increased serotonin syndrome

Drug/herb
Kava: increased CNS depression
St. John's wort, SAM-e: serotonin syndrome

Drug/lab test
Increased: serum bilirubin, blood glucose, alkaline phosphatase
Decreased: VMA, 5-HIAA
False increase: urinary catecholamines

NURSING CONSIDERATIONS

Assessment
• Monitor B/P (with patient lying, standing), pulse q4hr during beginning treatment; if systolic B/P drops 20 mm Hg, hold product, notify prescriber; take VS q4hr in patients with CV disease
• Monitor blood studies: CBC, leukocytes, differential, cardiac enzymes if patient is receiving long-term therapy
• Monitor liver function tests: AST, ALT, bilirubin
• Check weight weekly; product may increase appetite
• Assess ECG for flattening of T-wave, bundle branch block, AV block, dysrhythmias in cardiac patients
• Assess for EPS primarily in geriatric: rigidity, dystonia, akathisia
• Assess mental status: mood, sensorium, affect, suicidal tendencies; assess increase in psychiatric symptoms: depression, panic
• Identify alcohol consumption; if alcohol is consumed, hold dose until AM

Nursing diagnoses
• Coping, ineffective (uses)
• Injury, risk for (side effects)
• Knowledge, deficient (teaching)
• Noncompliance (teaching)

Patient/family education
• Inform patient that therapeutic effects may take 2-3 wk; take at bedtime
• Advise patient to use caution in driving and other activities requiring alertness because of drowsiness, dizziness, blurred vision; to avoid rising quickly from sitting to standing, especially geriatric
• Caution patient to avoid alcohol ingestion, other CNS depressants
• Teach patient to increase fluids, bulk in diet if constipation, urinary retention occur, especially geriatric

⚠ Nurse Alert

- Teach patient to use gum, hard sugarless candy, or frequent sips of water for dry mouth
- Teach patient to report immediately urinary retention, worsening of depression, suicidal thoughts/behavior
- Advise not to use within 14 days of MAOIs

Evaluation
Positive therapeutic outcome
- Decrease in depression
- Absence of suicidal thoughts

TREATMENT OF OVERDOSE:
ECG monitoring, lavage, activated charcoal, administer anticonvulsant

misoprostol (Rx)
(mye-soe-prost'ole)
Apo-Misoprostol ✦, Cytotec
Func. class.: Gastric mucosa protectant; antiulcer
Chem. class.: Prostaglandin E₁ analog
Pregnancy category X

Do not confuse:
misoprostol/metoprolol, **Cytotec**/Cytoxan

ACTION: Inhibits gastric acid secretion; may protect gastric mucosa; can increase bicarbonate, mucus production

Therapeutic outcome: Prevention of gastric ulcers

USES: Prevention of NSAID-induced gastric ulcers

CONTRAINDICATIONS:
Hypersensitivity to this product or prostaglandins

> **BLACK BOX WARNING:** Pregnancy **X**, females

Precautions: Breastfeeding, children, geriatric, renal disease, CV disease, abnormal fetal position, cardiac/renal/inflammatory bowel disease, C-section, dehydration, diarrhea, fever, ectopic pregnancy, fetal distress, sepsis, vaginal bleeding

DOSAGE AND ROUTES
Adult: PO 200 mcg qid with food for duration of NSAID therapy with last dose at bedtime; if 200 mcg is not tolerated, 100 mcg may be given

Available forms: Tabs 100, 200 mcg

Implementation
- Give with meals for prolonged product effect; avoid use of magnesium antacids

ADVERSE EFFECTS
GI: *Diarrhea,* nausea, vomiting, flatulence, constipation, dyspepsia, abdominal pain
GU: Spotting, cramps, hypermenorrhea, menstrual disorders

Pharmacokinetics
Absorption	Well absorbed
Distribution	Unknown
Metabolism	Liver
Excretion	Kidneys
Half-life	$^1/_2$-1 hr

Pharmacodynamics
Onset	$^1/_2$ hr
Peak	Unknown
Duration	3 hr

INTERACTIONS
Drug/food
Maximum concentrations when taken with food

NURSING CONSIDERATIONS
Assessment
- Assess patient for GI symptoms: hematemesis, occult or frank blood in stools, also severe abdominal pain, cramping, severe diarrhea
- Obtain a negative pregnancy test in women of childbearing age before starting medication; miscarriages are common

Nursing diagnoses
- Knowledge, deficient (teaching)
- Pain, chronic (uses)

Patient/family education
- Advise patient to avoid black pepper, caffeine, alcohol, harsh spices, extremes in temperature of food, which may aggravate condition
- Caution patient to avoid OTC preparations: aspirin, cough, cold preparations; condition may worsen
- Teach patient that product must be continued for prescribed time to be effective and taken exactly as prescribed; doses are not to be doubled
- Instruct patient to report to prescriber diarrhea, black tarry stools, abdominal pain, cramping, menstrual disorders

> **BLACK BOX WARNING:** Caution patient to prevent pregnancy while taking this product; spontaneous abortion may occur, pregnancy **X**

M

Adverse effects: *italics* = common; **bold** = life-threatening

Evaluation
Positive therapeutic outcome
• Prevention of ulcers

⚠ HIGH ALERT

mitomycin (Rx)
(mye-toe-mye′sin)
mitomycin
Func. class.: Antineoplastic, antibiotic
Pregnancy category D

Do not confuse:
mitomycin/mithramycin/mitotane/mitoxantrone

ACTION: Inhibits DNA synthesis, primarily; derived from *Streptomyces caespitosus;* appears to cause cross-linking of DNA; a vesicant

Therapeutic outcome: Prevention of rapidly growing malignant cells

USES: Pancreas, stomach, colorectal, bladder cancer

CONTRAINDICATIONS:
Pregnancy **D** (1st trimester), breastfeeding, hypersensitivity, as a single agent, coagulation disorders

BLACK BOX WARNING: Thrombocytopenia

Precautions: Accidental exposure, acute bronchospasm, anemia, children, dental disease/work, extravasation, females, hemolytic-uremic syndrome, infection, radiation therapy, surgery, vaccines, renal/respiratory disease

BLACK BOX WARNING: Bone marrow suppression, hemolytic uremic syndrome

DOSAGE AND ROUTES
Adult: **IV** 10-20 mg/m^2 q6-8wk

Available forms: Inj 5, 20, 40 mg/vial

Implementation
Direct IV route
• Use cytotoxic handling procedures
• Give antiemetic 30-60 min before product to prevent vomiting
• Use port if possible, product is very irritating to tissues
• Reconstitute 5 mg/10 ml; 20 mg/40 ml; 40 mg/80 ml of sterile water for injection (0.5 mg/ml); shake to dissolve, let stand until completely dissolved; stable for 1 wk at room temperature,

2 wk refrigerated, can be further diluted to 20-40 mcg/ml
• Inject reconstituted injection slowly over 5-10 min **IV** push into free-flowing **IV** infusion of 0.9% NaCl or D$_5$W

Syringe compatibilities: Bleomycin, CISplatin, cyclophosphamide, DOXOrubicin, droperidol, fluorouracil, furosemide, heparin, leucovorin, methotrexate, metoclopramide, vinBLAStine, vinCRIStine

Y-site compatibilities: Allopurinol, amifostine, bleomycin, CISplatin, cyclophosphamide, DOXOrubicin, droperidol, fluorouracil, furosemide, granisetron, heparin, leucovorin, melphalan, methotrexate, metoclopramide, ondansetron, teniposide, thiotepa, vinBLAStine, vinCRIStine

Y-site incompatibilities: Sargramostim, vinorelbine

ADVERSE EFFECTS
CNS: Fever, headache, confusion, drowsiness, syncope, fatigue
EENT: Blurred vision
GI: *Nausea, vomiting, anorexia, stomatitis,* **hepatotoxicity,** diarrhea
GU: Urinary retention, **renal failure,** edema
HEMA: **Thrombocytopenia, leukopenia, anemia**
INTEG: *Rash,* alopecia, **extravasation,** nail discoloration
MISC: **Hemolytic uremic syndrome, CHF**
RESP: **Fibrosis, pulmonary infiltrate,** dyspnea

Pharmacokinetics

Absorption	Complete bioavailability
Distribution	Widely distributed; concentrates in tumor
Metabolism	Liver, extensively
Excretion	Kidneys, unchanged
Half-life	1 hr

Pharmacodynamics
Unknown

INTERACTIONS
Individual drugs
Radiation: increased toxicity

Drug classifications
Anticoagulants, NSAIDs: increased bleeding risk
Antineoplastics: increased toxicity

Drug/herb
Black cohosh: avoid use

NURSING CONSIDERATIONS
Assessment

> **BLACK BOX WARNING:** Assess for fatal hemolytic uremic syndrome: hypertension, thrombocytopenia, microangiopathic hemolytic anemia; occurs during long-term therapy

- Assess buccal cavity q8hr for dryness, sores or ulceration, white patches, oral pain, bleeding, dysphagia; obtain prescription for viscous lidocaine (Xylocaine)
- Assess symptoms indicating severe allergic reaction: rash, pruritus, urticaria, purpuric skin lesions, itching, flushing

> **BLACK BOX WARNING:** Bone marrow suppression: Monitor CBC, differential, platelet count weekly; withhold product if WBC is <2000/mm³ or platelet count is <100,000/mm³ or granulocyte count is <1000/mm³; notify prescriber; bleeding: hematuria, guaiac, bruising, petechiae, mucosa, or orifices

- Monitor renal function tests: BUN, creatinine, serum uric acid, urine CCr before, during therapy; check I&O ratio; report fall in urine output to <30 ml/hr; adjust dose based on renal function
- ⚠ Assess for pulmonary fibrosis, bronchospasm, dyspnea, crackles, unproductive cough, chest pain, tachypnea, fatigue, increased pulse, pallor, lethargy
- Monitor temp q4hr (may indicate beginning of infection)
- Monitor liver function tests before, during therapy (bilirubin, AST, ALT, LDH) as needed or monthly; check for jaundiced skin and sclera, dark urine, clay-colored stools, itchy skin, abdominal pain, fever, diarrhea
- Assess for bleeding: hematuria, stool guaiac, bruising or petechiae, mucosa or orifices q8hr; inflammation of mucosa, breaks in skin
- Identify effects of alopecia on body image; discuss feelings about body changes
- Identify edema in feet, joint pain, stomach pain, shaking; check for inflammation of mucosa, breaks in skin

Nursing diagnoses
- Body image, disturbed (adverse reactions)
- Infection, risk for (adverse reactions)
- Injury, risk for (adverse reactions)
- Knowledge, deficient (teaching)

Patient/family education
- Advise patient to get adequate fluids 2-3 L/day unless contraindicated

- Encourage patient to rinse mouth tid-qid with water, club soda, brush teeth bid-qid with soft brush or cotton-tipped applicators for stomatitis, use unwaxed dental floss
- Teach patient to avoid use of products containing aspirin or ibuprofen, razors, commercial mouthwash, since bleeding may occur; to report symptoms of bleeding (hematuria, tarry stools)
- Caution patient to report signs of anemia (fatigue, headache, irritability, faintness, shortness of breath)
- Advise patient to report any changes in breathing or coughing even several mo after treatment; to avoid crowds and persons with respiratory tract or other infections
- Inform patient that hair may be lost during treatment; a wig or hairpiece may make patient feel better; new hair may be different in color, texture
- Advise patient not to have any vaccinations without the advice of the prescriber; serious reactions can occur
- Teach patient that contraception is needed during treatment and for several mo after completion of therapy
- Teach patient to report immediately urine retention, absence of urine, dyspnea, bleeding, jaundice

Evaluation
Positive therapeutic outcome
- Prevention of rapid division of malignant cells

⚠ HIGH ALERT

mitoxantrone (Rx)
(mye-toe-zan′trone)
Novantrone
Func. class.: Antineoplastic-antibiotic, immunomodulator
Chem. class.: Synthetic anthraquinone
Pregnancy category D

Do not confuse:
mitoxantrone/mitomycin/mithramycin/mitotane

ACTION: DNA reactive agent; cytocidal effect on both proliferating and nonproliferating cells; topoisomerase II inhibitor; a vesicant

Therapeutic outcome: Prevention of rapidly growing malignant cells

USES: Acute myelogenous leukemia (adult), relapsed leukemia, multiple sclerosis; used with steroids to treat bone pain (advanced prostate cancer); multiple sclerosis

Unlabeled uses: Liver malignancies, non-Hodgkin's lymphoma, breast cancer, ALL

CONTRAINDICATIONS:
Pregnancy **D**, hypersensitivity

Precautions: Breastfeeding, children, myelosuppression, cardiac/renal/hepatic disease, gout

> **BLACK BOX WARNING:** Secondary malignancy, neutropenia, intrathecal administration, extravasation, heart failure

DOSAGE AND ROUTES

Acute nonlymphatic leukemia/induction
Adult: **IV** INF 12 mg/m^2/day on days 1-3, and 100 mg/m^2 cytosine arabinoside $\times$ 7 days as a CONT 24-hr INF

Consolidation
Adult: **IV** INF 12 mg/m^2 given as a short 5-15 min INF

Advanced prostate cancer
Adult: **IV** 12-14 mg/m^2 as a single dose or short INF q21day

Multiple sclerosis, relapsing
Adult: **IV** INF 12 mg/m^2 as a 5-15 min INF q3mo

Available forms: Inj 2, 10, 12.5, 15 mg/ml

Implementation
⚠ Do not mix with any other product
• Avoid contact with skin, since medication is very irritating; wash completely to remove
• Give fluids **IV** or PO before chemotherapy to hydrate patient
• Give antacid before oral agent; give product after evening meal, before bedtime; provide antiemetic 30-60 min before giving product and prn to prevent vomiting; administer antibiotics for prophylaxis of infection
• Give topical or systemic analgesics for pain
• Liquid diet: carbonated beverages; gelatin may be added if patient is not nauseated or vomiting
• Sol should be prepared by qualified personnel only under controlled conditions in a biological cabinet using mask, gloves, gown
• Use Luer-Lok tubing to prevent leakage; do not let sol come in contact with skin; if contact occurs, wash well with soap and water

Direct IV route
• Give after diluting with 50 ml or more of 0.9% NaCl or D$_5$W; give over 3-5 min into running **IV** of D$_5$W or 0.9% NaCl

Intermittent IV infusion route
• May be diluted further in D$_5$W, 0.9% NaCl and run over 15-30 min; check for extravasation

Continuous IV infusion route
• Give over 24 hr

Y-site compatibilities: Allopurinol, amifostine, cladribine, filgrastim, fludarabine, granisetron, melphalan, ondansetron, sargramostim, teniposide, thiotepa, vinorelbine

Y-site incompatibilities: Paclitaxel

Additive compatibilities: Cyclophosphamide, cytarabine, fluorouracil, hydrocortisone, potassium chloride

Additive incompatibilities: Heparin

Solution compatibilities: D$_5$/0.9 NaCl, D$_5$W, 0.9% NaCl

ADVERSE EFFECTS
CNS: Headache, **seizures,** fatigue
CV: CHF, cardiomyopathy, dysrhythmias
EENT: Conjunctivitis, blue-green sclera, blurred vision
GI: *Nausea, vomiting, diarrhea, anorexia, mucositis,* **hepatoxicity**
GU: Amenorrhea, menstrual disorders
HEMA: Thrombocytopenia, leukopenia, myelosuppression, anemia, secondary leukemia
INTEG: *Rash, necrosis at inj site,* alopecia, dermatitis, thrombophlebitis at inj site
MISC: Fever
RESP: Cough, dyspnea

Pharmacokinetics
Absorption	Completely absorbed
Distribution	Widely distributed, protein binding 78%
Metabolism	Liver
Excretion	Bile; kidneys, unchanged ($<$10%)
Half-life	23-215 hr

Pharmacodynamics
Unknown

INTERACTIONS

Individual drugs
Heparin: do not mix; precipitate will form
Radiation: increased toxicity, bone marrow suppression

Drug classifications
Do not mix with any other product
Anticoagulants, NSAIDs: increased bleeding risk

Antineoplastics: increased toxicity, bone marrow suppression
Live virus vaccines: increased adverse reactions

Drug/herb
Black cohosh, dong quai: avoid use

NURSING CONSIDERATIONS
Assessment
• **Multiple sclerosis:** obtain baseline multigated angiogram, left ventricular ejection fraction (LVEF) if symptoms of CHF occur, repeat LVEF or if cumulative dose is >100 mg/m²; do not administer to patients who have received a lifetime dose of ≥140 mg/m² or if LVEF is <50% or significant decrease in LVEF
• Do not administer in multiple sclerosis if neutrophils <1500/mm³
• Obtain pregnancy test in all women of childbearing age

> **BLACK BOX WARNING:** Monitor ECG; watch for ST-T wave changes, low QRS and T, possible dysrhythmias (sinus tachycardia, heart block, PVCs); also monitor ECHO, MUGA, chest x-ray, RAI angiography to assess ejection fraction before, during treatment; product is cardiotoxic: may develop during treatment or months to years after treatment

• Assess buccal cavity q8hr for dryness, sores or ulceration, white patches, oral pain, bleeding, dysphagia; obtain prescription for viscous lidocaine (Xylocaine)
• **Assess symptoms indicating severe allergic reaction:** rash, pruritus, urticaria, purpuric skin lesions, itching, flushing
• Assess tachypnea, ECG changes, dyspnea, edema, fatigue
• Monitor CBC, differential, platelet count weekly; withhold product if WBC is <4000/mm³ or platelet count is <75,000/mm³, notify prescriber of results if WBC is <20,000/mm³, platelets are <150,000/mm³; neutrophil count or ANC
• Assess for increased uric acid levels, swelling, joint pain primarily in extremities; patient should be well hydrated to prevent urate deposits
• Monitor renal function tests: BUN, creatinine, urine CCr before, during therapy; determine I&O ratio
• Monitor temp q4hr: may indicate beginning of infection
• Monitor liver function tests before, during therapy (bilirubin, AST, ALT, LDH) as needed or monthly; dose reduction needed in hepatic dis-

ease; check for jaundiced skin and sclera, dark urine, clay-colored stools, itchy skin, abdominal pain, fever, diarrhea
• **Assess for bleeding:** hematuria, stool guaiac, bruising or petechiae, mucosa or orifices q8hr; check for inflammation of mucosa, breaks in skin
• Identify effects of alopecia on body image; discuss feelings about body changes
⚠ **Assess for MS:** obtain MUGA, LVEF baselines; repeat LVEF if symptoms of CHF occur or if cumulative dose is >100 mg/m²; do not give to patients who have received a lifetime dose of ≥140 mg/m² or if LVEF is <50% or significant LVEF

> **BLACK BOX WARNING:** Assess for secondary acute myelogenous leukemia (AML), which can develop after taking this product

Nursing diagnoses
• Body image, disturbed (adverse reactions)
• Infection, risk for (adverse reactions)
• Injury, risk for (adverse reactions)
• Knowledge, deficient (teaching)

Patient/family education
• Encourage patient to rinse mouth tid-qid with water, club soda; brush teeth bid-qid with soft brush or cotton-tipped applicators for stomatitis; use unwaxed dental floss
• Teach patient to avoid use of products containing aspirin or NSAIDs, razors, commercial mouthwash, since bleeding may occur; to report symptoms of bleeding (hematuria, tarry stools)
• Caution patient to report signs of anemia (fatigue, headache, irritability, faintness, shortness of breath)
• Inform patient that hair may be lost during treatment; a wig or hairpiece may make patient feel better; new hair may be different in color, texture
• Caution patient not to have any vaccinations without the advice of the prescriber; serious reactions can occur
• Advise patient that contraception is needed during treatment and for several mo after completion of therapy
• Advise patient that sclera, urine may turn blue or green
• Advise patient to increase fluids to 2-3 L/day unless contraindicated
• Teach patient to avoid crowds, persons with infections
• Teach patient to report immediately bleeding, dyspnea, possible infections, seizure, jaundice

Evaluation
Positive therapeutic outcome
• Prevention of rapid division of malignant cells

modafinil (Rx)
(mo-daf'i-nil)
Alertec ✦, Provigil
Func. class.: CNS stimulant
Chem. class.: Racemic compound
Pregnancy category C
Controlled substance IV

ACTION: Similar action as sympathomimetics; does not alter release of dopamine, norepinephrine

Therapeutic outcome: Ability to stay awake

USES: Narcolepsy, shift work sleep disturbance, obstructive sleep apnea

CONTRAINDICATIONS:
Hypersensitivity, ischemic heart disease, left ventricular hypertrophy, chest pain, dysrhythmias

Precautions: Pregnancy C, breastfeeding, child <16 yr, geriatric, unstable angina, history of MI, severe hepatic disease

DOSAGE AND ROUTES
Adult/adolescent ≥16 yr: PO 200 mg qd

Hepatic dose (severe hepatic disease)
Adult: PO 100 mg qd

Available forms: Tabs 100, 200 mg

Implementation
• Give 1 hr before start of shift work, or in the AM for those with narcolepsy or sleep apnea
• Store at room temperature

ADVERSE EFFECTS
CNS: *Headache,* anxiety, cataplexy, depression, dizziness, insomnia, amnesia, confusion, ataxia, tremors, paresthesia, dyskinesia, **suicidal ideation**
CV: Dysrhythmias, hyper/hypotension, chest pain, vasodilation
EENT: Change in vision, *rhinitis,* pharyngitis, epistaxis
GI: Nausea, vomiting, changes in LFTs, anorexia, diarrhea, thirst, mouth ulcers
GU: Ejaculation disorder, urinary retention, albuminuria
HEMA: Eosinophilia

INTEG: Rash, dry skin, herpes simplex, **Stevens-Johnson syndrome**
MISC: Infection, hyperglycemia, neck pain
RESP: *Dyspnea,* lung changes

Pharmacokinetics

Absorption	Rapid
Distribution	60% protein binding
Metabolism	Liver (90%)
Excretion	Unknown
Half-life	15 hr

Pharmacodynamics

Onset	Unknown
Peak	2-4 hr
Duration	Unknown

INTERACTIONS

Individual drugs
Diazepam, phenytoin, propranolol, warfarin: increased effects of these drugs
CycloSPORINE, theophylline: decreased effects of these drugs

Drug classifications
Antidepressants (tricyclics): increased effects
Hormonal contraceptives: decreased effects

Drug/herb
Coffee, cola nut, guarana, mate, tea: increased stimulation

Drug/lab test
Increased: eosinophils, glucose, LFTs

NURSING CONSIDERATIONS

Assessment
• For narcolepsy, shift work, history of sleep apnea
• For depression, suicidal ideation
• Monitor B/P in those with hypertension

Nursing diagnosis
• Sleep pattern disturbance (uses)

Patient/family education
• Advise patient to take only as directed; may be taken with or without food
• Advise patient to use other form of contraception during and at least 30 days after discontinuing medication, if using hormonal birth control; advise patient to notify prescriber if pregnancy is planned or suspected or if breastfeeding
• Advise patient to notify prescriber of allergic reaction, tremors, confusion
• Teach patient to avoid all OTC medications unless approved by prescriber

- Teach patient to avoid hazardous activities until drug effect is known

Evaluation
- Ability to stay awake

moexipril (Rx)

(moe-ex′i-pril)
Univasc
Func. class.: Antihypertensive
Chem. class.: Angiotensin-converting enzyme (ACE) inhibitor
Pregnancy category D

ACTION: Selectively suppresses renin-angiotensin-aldosterone system; inhibits ACE; prevents conversion of angiotensin I to angiotensin II; results in dilatation of arterial, venous vessels

Therapeutic outcome: Decreased B/P in hypertension

USES: Hypertension, alone or in combination with thiazide diuretics

CONTRAINDICATIONS:

Breastfeeding, hypersensitivity, children, heart block, bilateral renal stenosis, history of angioedema

BLACK BOX WARNING: Pregnancy **D**

Precautions: Dialysis patients, hypovolemia, leukemia, scleroderma, lupus erythematosus, blood dyscrasias, CHF, diabetes mellitus, renal/thyroid disease, COPD, asthma, potassium-sparing diuretics

DOSAGE AND ROUTES

Initial treatment
Adult: PO 7.5 mg 1 hr before meals initially, may be increased or divided depending on B/P response

Maintenance
Adult: PO 7.5-30 mg/day in 1-2 divided doses 1 hr before meals

Renal dose
Adult: PO CCr <40 ml/min 3.75 mg/day titrate to desired dose, max 15 mg/day

Available forms: Tabs 7.5, 15 mg

Implementation
- Give PO 1 hr before meals
- Store in airtight container at 86° F or less

ADVERSE EFFECTS

CNS: Fever, chills, headache, fatigue
CV: Hypotension, postural hypotension
GI: Loss of taste, hepatic failure/necrosis, hepatitis
GU: Impotence, dysuria, nocturia, proteinuria, nephrotic syndrome, acute reversible renal failure, polyuria, oliguria, frequency
HEMA: Neutropenia
INTEG: Rash, photosensitivity
META: Hypokalemia, hyperkalemia, hyponatremia
RESP: Bronchospasm, dyspnea, dry cough, pneumonitis
SYST: Angioedema, anaphylaxis

Pharmacokinetics

Absorption	Unknown
Distribution	Unknown
Metabolism	Liver to metabolites
Excretion	Feces (52%), kidneys, crosses placenta, excreted in breast milk
Half-life	Unknown

Pharmacodynamics

Unknown

INTERACTIONS

Individual drugs
AzaTHIOprine: increased myelosuppression
CycloSPORINE: increased hyperkalemia
Digoxin, lithium: increased toxicity

Drug classification
Adrenergic blockers, antihypertensives, diuretics, ganglionic blockers, phenothiazines: increased hypotension
Diuretics (potassium-sparing), potassium supplements, sympathomimetics: do not use together
Diuretics (potassium-sparing): increased hyperkalemia
NSAIDs: decreased antihypertensive effect

Drug/herb
Hawthorn: increased antihypertensive effect
Yohimbe: decreased antihypertensive effect

Drug/lab test
False positive: urine acetone

NURSING CONSIDERATIONS

Assessment
- Monitor blood studies: neutrophils, decreased platelets
- Monitor B/P

M

• Monitor renal function tests: protein, BUN, creatinine; watch for increased levels that may indicate **nephrotic syndrome**
• Monitor baselines in renal, liver function tests before therapy begins
• Monitor potassium levels, although hyperkalemia rarely occurs
• Assess edema in feet, legs daily
• **Assess allergic reaction:** rash, fever, pruritus, urticaria; product should be discontinued if antihistamines fail to help
• **Assess for symptoms of CHF:** edema, dyspnea, wet crackles, B/P
• Monitor for renal symptoms: polyuria, oliguria, frequency

Nursing diagnoses
• Knowledge, deficient (teaching)

Patient/family education
• Instruct patient not to discontinue product abruptly
• Tell patient not to use OTC (cough, cold, allergy) products unless directed by prescriber
• Teach patient to comply with dosage schedule, even if feeling better
• Encourage patient to rise slowly to sitting or standing position to minimize orthostatic hypotension
• Teach patient to notify prescriber of mouth sores, sore throat, fever, swelling of hands or feet, irregular heartbeat, chest pain, signs of angioedema
• Tell patient that excessive perspiration, dehydration, vomiting, diarrhea may lead to fall in B/P; consult prescriber if this occurs
• Teach patient that dizziness, fainting, lightheadedness may occur during first few days of therapy
• Tell patient that rash or impaired perspiration may occur

> **BLACK BOX WARNING:** Advise patient to notify prescriber if pregnancy is planned or suspected

• Teach patient how to take B/P

Evaluation
Positive therapeutic outcome
• Decreased B/P in hypertension

TREATMENT OF OVERDOSE:
0.9% NaCl **IV** inf, hemodialysis

montelukast (Rx)
(mon-teh-loo'kast)
Singulair
Func. class.: Bronchodilator
Chem. class.: Leukotriene antagonist, cysteinyl
Pregnancy category B

ACTION: Inhibits leukotriene (LTD_4) formation; leukotrienes exert their effects by increasing neutrophil, eosinophil migration; aggregation of neutrophils, monocytes; smooth muscle contraction, capillary permeability; these actions further lead to bronchoconstriction, inflammation, edema

Therapeutic outcome: Ability to breathe with ease

USES: Chronic asthma in adults and children, seasonal allergic rhinitis, bronchospasm prophylaxis

Unlabeled uses: Chronic urticaria

CONTRAINDICATIONS:
Hypersensitivity

Precautions: Pregnancy **B**, breastfeeding, children <6 yr, acute attacks of asthma, alcohol consumption, severe hepatic disease, corticosteroid withdrawal, phenylketonuria

DOSAGE AND ROUTES
Asthma
Adult and child ≥15 yr: PO 10 mg/day PM
Child 6-14 yr: PO 5 mg chew tabs/day PM
Child 2-5 yr: PO (chew tabs, granules) 4 mg/day
Child 12-23 mo: PO 1 packet of granules taken PM

Exercise-induced bronchoconstriction
Adult and adolescent ≥15 yr: PO 10 mg 2 hr prior to exercise; do not take another dose within 24 hr

Available forms: Tabs 10 mg; chewable tabs 4, 5 mg; oral granules 4 mg/packet

Implementation
PO route
• Give PO in PM daily for all uses except exercise-induced bronchoconstriction; then take 2 hr prior to exercise
• Do not open packet until ready to use; mix whole dose, give within 15 min

---

⚠ Nurse Alert

- Granules may be given directly in mouth or mixed with a spoonful of soft food (carrots, applesauce, ice cream, rice)

ADVERSE EFFECTS
CNS: Dizziness, fatigue, headache, behavior changes, **suicidal ideation, suicide, seizures,** agitation, anxiety, depression, fever, hallucinations, drowsiness
GI: Abdominal pain, dyspepsia, nausea, vomiting, diarrhea, **pancreatitis**
HEMA: Thrombocytopenia
INTEG: Rash, pruritus, erythema
MS: Asthenia, myalgia, muscle cramps
RESP: Influenza, cough, nasal congestion
SYST: Anaphylaxis, angioedema, Churg-Strauss syndrome

Pharmacokinetics

Absorption	Rapidly absorbed
Distribution	Protein binding 99%
Metabolism	Liver
Excretion	Bile
Half-life	2.7-5.5 hr

Pharmacodynamics

Onset	Unknown
Peak	3-4 hr
Duration	Unknown

INTERACTIONS
Individual drugs
Rifabutin, rifapentine, carBAMazepine, fosphenytoin, phenytoin, rifampin: decreased montelukast levels

Drug classifications
Barbiturates: decreased montelukast levels

Drug/herb
Tea (green, black), guarana: increased stimulation

Drug/lab test
Increased: ALT, AST

NURSING CONSIDERATIONS
Assessment
⚠ Assess adult patients carefully for symptoms of Churg-Strauss syndrome (rare), including eosinophilia, vasculitic rash, worsening pulmonary symptoms, cardiac complications and/or neuropathy
- Monitor CBC, blood chemistry during treatment

- Assess respiratory rate, rhythm, depth; auscultate lung fields bilaterally; notify prescriber of abnormalities
- Assess allergic reactions: rash, urticaria; product should be discontinued
- Assess for behavior changes and suicidal ideation, other neuropsychiatric reactions

Nursing diagnoses
- Activity intolerance (uses)
- Knowledge, deficient (teaching)

Patient/family education
- Advise patient to avoid hazardous activities; dizziness may occur
- Teach patient that product is not to be used for acute asthma attacks
- Advise patient to avoid NSAIDs if sensitive to aspirin
- Advise patient to continue to use inhaled β-agonists if exercise-induced asthma occurs

Evaluation
Positive therapeutic outcome
- Increased ease of breathing
- Decreased bronchospasm

M

⚠ HIGH ALERT

morphine (Rx)
(mor′feen)
Astramorph PF, Avinza, Depo Dur, Infumorph PF, Kadian, M.O.S. ✽, MS Contin, MSIR ✽, Oramorph SR
Func. class.: Opioid analgesic
Chem. class.: Alkaloid
Pregnancy category C
Controlled substance schedule II

Do not confuse:
morphine/HYDROmorphone,
MS Contin/oxyCONTIN

ACTION: Depresses pain impulse transmission at the spinal cord level by interacting with opioid receptors

Therapeutic outcome: Decreased pain

USES: Moderate to severe pain

CONTRAINDICATIONS:
Hypersensitivity, addiction (opioid), hemorrhage, bronchial asthma, increased ICP, paralytic ileus, hypovolemic shock

> **BLACK BOX WARNING:** Respiratory depression

Precautions: Pregnancy **C**, breastfeeding, children <18 yr, geriatric, addictive personality, acute MI, severe heart disease, renal/hepatic disease, bowel impaction

> **BLACK BOX WARNING:** Abrupt discontinuation, accidental exposure, epidural/intrathecal administration, opioid-naive patients, substance abuse

DOSAGE AND ROUTES

Adult: 5-10 mg q4hr (opiate naïve) 5-20 mg q4hr (prior opiate use); PO 10-30 mg q4hr prn; EXT REL 15-30 mg q8-12hr; RECT 10-20 mg q4hr prn; **IV** 2.5-15 mg diluted in 4-5 ml of water for inj, over 5 min; SUS REL cap (Kadian), EXT REL cap (Avinza) give total daily dose q24hr; for those with no tolerance to opioids, 30 mg/day, may adjust by no more than 30 mg q4day; MS Contin may be given in divided doses
Child: SUBCUT/IV 0.05-0.2 mg/kg, max 15 mg; PO 0.2-0.5 mg/kg q4-6hr (regular REL), q12hr (SUS REL)

Available forms: Inj 0.5, 1, 2, 3, 4, 5, 8, 10, 15, 25, 50 mg/ml; oral sol 10, 20 mg/5 ml, 10 mg/0.5 ml; oral tabs 15, 30 mg; rect supp 5, 10, 20, 30 mg; ext rel tabs 15, 30, 60, 100, 200 mg; caps 15, 30 mg; syr 1, 5 mg/ml; cont rel cap pellets (Kadian) 10, 20, 30, 50, 60, 100, 200 mg; ext rel caps (Avinza) 30, 60, 90, 120 mg

Implementation

• Give with antiemetic if nausea, vomiting occur
• Administer when pain is beginning to return; determine dosage interval by patient response; continuous dosing of medication is more effective than giving prn
• Withdraw medication slowly after long-term use to prevent withdrawal symptoms
• Store in light-resistant container at room temperature
• Kadian is not bioequivalent to other controlled-release forms
• 20 mg/ml concentrated oral sol for opioid-tolerant patient only

PO route

• Swallow ext rel tabs whole; do not break, crush, or chew
⚠ **Kadian tabs may be opened and sprinkled on applesauce immediately before use; do not break, crush, chew, or dissolve pellets in Kadian cap, which may lead to an overdose; adjustments may need**

to be made when converting from another form of morphine
• 20 mg/ml concentrated oral sol for opioid-tolerant patient only
• May be given with food or milk to lessen GI upset; other forms may be crushed and mixed with food or fluids

IM/SUBCUT route

• Do not give if cloudy or a precipitate has formed

Direct IV route

• Give direct **IV** after diluting with ≥5 ml of sterile water or 0.9% NaCl for inj; give 2.5-15 mg/4-5 min; rapid administration may lead to increased respiratory depression, death

Continuous IV infusion route

• Give by adding to 5% dextrose
• Give by inf pump to deliver correct dosage; titrate to provide adequate pain relief without serious sedation, respiratory depression, hypotension

Patient-controlled anesthesia (PCA)

• May be given by patient-controlled analgesia (PCA) pump in terminal illnesses; patient is able to control amount of morphine, dilute solution to a concentration of 1 or 10 mg/ml for ease in calculation and programming PCA pump
• Administer epidurally with caution in the geriatric

Syringe compatibilities: Atropine, benzquinamide, bupivacaine, butorphanol, cimetidine, dimenhyDRINATE, diphenhydrAMINE, droperidol, fentaNYL, glycopyrrolate, hydrOXYzine, ketamine, metoclopramide, midazolam, milrinone, pentazocine, perphenazine, promazine, ranitidine, scopolamine

Syringe incompatibilities: Meperidine, thiopental

Y-site compatibilities: Allopurinol, amifostine, amikacin, aminophylline, amiodarone, ampicillin, ampicillin/sulbactam, amsacrine, atenolol, atracurium, aztreonam, bumetanide, calcium chloride, cefamandole, ceFAZolin, cefmetazole, cefoperazone, cefotaxime, cefotetan, cefoxitin, ceftazidime, ceftizoxime, cefTRIAXone, cefuroxime, cephalothin, cephapirin, chloramphenicol, CISplatin, cladribine, clindamycin, cyclophosphamide, cytarabine, dexamethasone, digoxin, diltiazem, DOBUTamine, DOPamine, doxycycline, enalaprilat, EPINEPHrine, erythromycin, esmolol, etomidate, famotidine, fentaNYL, filgrastim, fluconazole, fludarabine, foscarnet, gentamicin, granisetron, heparin, hydrocortisone, HYDROmorphone, IL-2, insulin (regular), kanamycin, labetalol, lidocaine,

LORazepam, magnesium sulfate, melphalan, meropenem, methotrexate, methyldopate, methylPREDNISolone, metoclopramide, metoprolol, metroNIDAZOLE, mezlocillin, midazolam, milrinone, moxalactam, nafcillin, niCARdipine, nitroglycerin, norepinephrine, ondansetron, oxacillin, oxytocin, paclitaxel, pancuronium, penicillin G potassium, piperacillin, piperacillin/tazobactam, potassium chloride, propofol, propranolol, ranitidine, sodium bicarbonate, sodium nitroprusside, teniposide, thiotepa, ticarcillin, ticarcillin/clavulanate, tobramycin, trimethoprim/sulfamethoxazole, vancomycin, vecuronium, vinorelbine, vit B/C, warfarin, zidovudine

Y-site incompatibilities: Furosemide, minocycline, tetracycline

ADVERSE EFFECTS

CNS: Drowsiness, dizziness, *confusion,* headache, *sedation,* euphoria, insomnia, **seizures**
CV: Palpitations, **bradycardia,** change in B/P, **shock, cardiac arrest,** chest pain, hyper/hypotension, edema, **tachycardia**
EENT: Tinnitus, blurred vision, miosis, diplopia
GI: Nausea, vomiting, anorexia, *constipation,* cramps, biliary tract pressure
GU: Urinary retention
HEMA: Thrombocytopenia
INTEG: Rash, urticaria, bruising, flushing, diaphoresis, pruritus
RESP: Respiratory depression, respiratory arrest, apnea

Pharmacokinetics

Absorption	Variably absorbed (PO); well absorbed (IM, SUBCUT, RECT); completely absorbed (**IV**)
Distribution	Widely distributed; crosses placenta
Metabolism	Liver, extensively
Excretion	Kidneys
Half-life	$1^1/_2$-2 hr

INTERACTIONS

Individual drugs
Alcohol: increased effects with other CNS depressants
Rifampin: decreased analgesic action

Drug classifications
Antipsychotics, opiates, sedative-hypnotics, skeletal muscle relaxants: increased effects with other CNS depressants
MAOIs: unpredictable reaction may occur; avoid use

Drug/herb
Chamomile, hops, kava, St. John's wort, valerian: increased CNS depression
Corkwood: increased anticholinergic effect

Drug/food
Cranberry juice (excessive amounts), oats: decreased morphine effect

Drug/lab test
Increased: amylase

NURSING CONSIDERATIONS

Assessment
• Assess pain: location, type, character, intensity; give dose before pain becomes extreme
• Monitor I&O ratio; check for decreasing output; may indicate urinary retention; check for constipation; increase fluids, bulk in diet if needed, or stimulant laxatives may be prescribed

> **BLACK BOX WARNING:** Abrupt discontinuation: gradually taper to prevent withdrawal symptoms; decrease by 50% q1-2 days, avoid use of narcotic antagonist

• Monitor CNS changes: dizziness, drowsiness, hallucinations, euphoria, LOC, pupil reactions
• Monitor allergic reactions: rash, urticaria

> **BLACK BOX WARNING:** Accidental exposure: if Duramorph or Infamorph gets on skin, remove contaminated clothing and rinse affected area with water

Pharmacodynamics

	PO	PO EXT REL	IM	SUBCUT	RECT	IV	IT
Onset	Variable	Unknown	10-30 min	20 min	Unknown	Rapid	Rapid
Peak	1 hr	Unknown	50-90 min	1-$1^1/_2$ hr	$^1/_2$-1 hr	20 min	Unknown
Duration	4-5 hr	8-12 hr	3-7 hr	4-5 hr	4-5 hr	4-5 hr	Ext

Adverse effects: *italics* = common; **bold** = life-threatening

BLACK BOX WARNING: Assess respiratory dysfunction: depression, character, rate, rhythm; notify prescriber if respirations are <12/min; accidental overdose has occurred with high-potency oral sol

Nursing diagnoses
• Breathing pattern, ineffective (adverse reactions)
• Knowledge, deficient (teaching)
• Pain, acute (uses)

Patient/family education
• Advise patient to report any symptoms of CNS changes, allergic reactions
• Caution patients to avoid CNS depressants (alcohol, sedative/hypnotics) for at least 24 hr after taking this product
• Discuss with patient that dizziness, drowsiness, and confusion are common; to avoid getting up without assistance
• Discuss in detail all aspects of the product and expected response

Evaluation
Positive therapeutic outcome
• Decreased pain

TREATMENT OF OVERDOSE:
Naloxone (Narcan) 0.2-0.8 **IV**, O_2, **IV** fluids, vasopressors

moxifloxacin (Rx)
(mox-i-floks′a-sin)
Avelox, Avelox IV
Func. class.: Antiinfective
Chem. class.: Fluoroquinolone
Pregnancy category C

ACTION: Interferes with conversion of intermediate DNA fragments into high molecular weight DNA in bacteria; DNA gyrase inhibitor

Therapeutic outcome: Bactericidal action against the following: *Staphylococcus aureus, Streptococcus pneumoniae, Haemophilus influenzae, Haemophilus parainfluenzae, Moraxella catarrhalis, Klebsiella pneumoniae, Mycoplasma pneumoniae, Chlamydia pneumoniae; Streptococcus pyogenes, Escherichia coli, Bacteroides fragilis, Streptococcus arginosus, Streptococcus constellatus, Enterococcus faecalis, Proteus mirabilis, Clostridium perfringens, Bacteroides thetalomicron, Peptostreptococcus, Enterobacter cloacae*

USES: Acute bacterial sinusitis, acute bacterial exacerbation of chronic bronchitis, community-acquired pneumonia (mild to moderate), uncomplicated skin/skin structure infections, complicated intraabdominal infections including polymicrobial infections, complicated skin/skin structure infections

CONTRAINDICATIONS:
Hypersensitivity to quinolones

Precautions: Pregnancy **C**, breastfeeding, children, renal/hepatic/cardiac disease, epilepsy, uncorrected hypokalemia, prolonged QT interval, patients receiving class IA, III antidysrhythmics, GI disease, seizure disorder

BLACK BOX WARNING: Tendon pain/rupture, tendinitis

DOSAGE AND ROUTES
Acute bacterial sinusitis
Adult: PO/**IV** 400 mg q24hr × 10 days

Acute bacterial exacerbation of chronic bronchitis
Adult: PO/**IV** 400 mg q24hr × 5 days

Community-acquired pneumonia
Adult: PO/**IV** 400 mg q24hr × 7-14 days

Uncomplicated skin/skin structure infections
Adult: PO/**IV** 400 mg q24hr × 7 days

Complicated intraabdominal infections
Adult: **IV** 400 mg/day × 5-14 days

Complicated skin/skin structure infections
Adult: PO/**IV** 400 mg/day × 7-21 days

Available forms: Tabs 400 mg; inj premix 400 mg/250 ml

Implementation
• Do not use theophylline with this product; may cause toxicity
PO route
• Give once a day for 5-10 days depending on condition

IV route
• Discontinue primary **IV** while administering moxifloxacin, give over 60 min
• Do not give SUBCUT, IM
• Available as premixed sol, may be diluted at ratios from 1:10 to 10:1, do not refrigerate, give by direct infusion or through Y-type infusion set, do not add other medications to sol or infuse through same IV line at same time

Solution compatibilities: 0.9% NaCl, D_5, D_{10}, LR, sterile water for inj

ADVERSE EFFECTS

CNS: Headache, dizziness, fatigue, insomnia, depression, restlessness, **seizures,** confusion, **increased intracranial pressure,** peripheral neuropathy
CV: Prolonged QT interval, dysrhythmias, torsades de pointes, tachycardia
EENT: Blurred vision, tinnitus, taste changes
GI: Nausea, increased ALT, AST, flatulence, heartburn, vomiting, diarrhea, oral candidiasis, dysphagia, **pseudomembranous colitis**
INTEG: Rash, pruritus, urticaria, photosensitivity, flushing, fever, chills
MS: Tremor, arthralgia, **tendon rupture,** myalgia
SYST: Anaphylaxis, Stevens-Johnson syndrome

Pharmacokinetics

Absorption	Well absorbed (75%) (PO)
Distribution	Widely distributed
Metabolism	Liver
Excretion	Kidneys
Half-life	Increased in renal disease

Pharmacodynamics

	PO
Onset	Rapid
Peak	1 hr
Duration	Unknown

INTERACTIONS

Individual drugs
Aluminum hydroxide, calcium, didanosine, iron, sucralfate, zinc sulfate: decreased absorption of moxifloxacin
CycloSPORINE: increased cycloSPORINE effect
Haloperidol, chloroquine, droperidol, pentamidine; arsenic trioxide, levomethadyl: increased QT prolongation
Probenecid: increased blood levels
Warfarin: increased warfarin effect

Drug classifications
Antacids (magnesium), iron salts: decreased absorption of moxifloxacin
Class IA/III antidysrhythmics, some phenothiazines, β-agonists, local anesthetics, tricyclics, CYP3A4 inhibitors (amiodarone, clarithromycin, erythromycin, telithromycin, troleandomycin), CYP3A4 substrates (methadone, pimozide, quetiapine, quiNIDine,

risperidone, ziprasidone): increased QT prolongation
NSAIDs: increased seizure risk
Corticosteroids: increased tendon rupture

Drug/food
Enteral feeding: decreased absorption of moxifloxacin

NURSING CONSIDERATIONS

Assessment
• Assess patient for previous sensitivity reaction
• Assess patient for signs and symptoms of infection including characteristics of wounds, sputum, urine, stool, WBC $>10,000/mm^3$, fever baseline, during treatment
• Obtain C&S before beginning product therapy to identify if correct treatment has been initiated
• **Assess for allergic reactions, Stevens-Johnson syndrome, toxic epidermal necrolysis, and anaphylaxis:** rash, urticaria, pruritus, chills, fever, joint pain; may occur a few days after therapy begins; epinephrine and resuscitation equipment should be available for anaphylactic reaction
• Assess for CNS symptoms: headache, dizziness, fatigue, insomnia, depression, **seizures**
• Identify urine output; if decreasing, notify prescriber (may indicate nephrotoxicity); also check for increased BUN, creatinine
• Monitor blood tests: AST, ALT, CBC, Hct, bilirubin, LDH, alkaline phosphatase, Coombs' test monthly if patient is on long-term therapy
• Monitor electrolytes: potassium, sodium chloride monthly if patient is on long-term therapy
• **Pseudomembranous colitis:** assess for diarrhea, abdominal pain, fever, fatigue, anorexia; possible anemia, elevated WBC and low serum albumin; stop product and usually give either vancomycin or IV metroNIDAZOLE
• Monitor for bleeding: ecchymosis, bleeding gums, hematuria, stool guaiac daily if on long-term therapy
• Assess for overgrowth of infection: perineal itching, fever, malaise, redness, pain, swelling, drainage, rash, diarrhea, change in cough, sputum

BLACK BOX WARNING: Assess for tendon pain, rupture, tendinitis; if tendon becomes inflamed, drug should be discontinued

⚠ **QT prolongation:** Monitor ECG for QT prolongation, ejection fraction; assess for chest pain, palpitations, dyspnea

M

Adverse effects: *italics* = common; **bold** = life-threatening

Nursing diagnoses
- Diarrhea (side effects)
- Infection, risk for (uses)
- Injury, risk for (side effects)
- Knowledge, deficient (teaching)
- Noncompliance (teaching)

Patient/family education
- Teach patient to report sore throat, bruising, bleeding, joint pain; may indicate blood dyscrasias (rare)
- Advise patient to contact prescriber if vaginal itching, loose foul-smelling stools, furry tongue occur; may indicate superinfection; report itching, rash, pruritus, urticaria
- Instruct patient to take all medication prescribed for the length of time ordered; not to give medication to others
- Advise patient to notify prescriber of diarrhea with blood or pus
- Advise patient to rinse mouth frequently, use sugarless candy or gum for dry mouth
- Advise patient to take as prescribed, not to double or miss doses

Evaluation
Positive therapeutic outcome
- Absence of signs/symptoms of infection (WBC <10,000/mm³, temp WNL)
- Reported improvement in symptoms of infection

moxifloxacin ophthalmic
See Appendix B

multivitamins (PO, OTC, IV, Rx)
Many brands available
Func. class.: Vitamins, multiple
Pregnancy category A

Do not confuse:
Theragran/Phenergan

ACTION: Needed for adequate metabolism

Therapeutic outcome: Prevention and treatment of vitamin deficiencies

USES: Prevention and treatment of vitamin deficiencies

Precautions: Pregnancy A

DOSAGE AND ROUTES
Adult and child: PO/IV—depends on brand

Available forms: Many forms available

Implementation
PO route
- Liquid multivitamins can be diluted or dropped into patient's mouth using dropper provided with some brands
- Chew tabs should be chewed and not swallowed whole

IV route
- Give by cont inf only after diluting 5-10 ml (multivitamins)/500-1000 ml of D$_5$W, D$_{10}$W, D$_{20}$W, LR, D$_5$/LR, D$_5$/0.9% NaCl, 0.9% NaCl, 3% NaCl
- Do not use sol with crystals, precipitate, or color other than bright yellow

Y-site compatibilities: Acyclovir, ampicillin, ceFAZolin, cephalothin, cephapirin, diltiazem, erythromycin, fludarabine, gentamicin, tacrolimus, tetracycline

Additive compatibilities: Cefoxitin, isoproterenol, methyldopa, metoclopramide, metroNIDAZOLE, netilmicin, norepinephrine, sodium bicarbonate, verapamil

Additive incompatibilities: Penicillin G, erythromycin, tetracycline, kanamycin, streptomycin, doxycycline, lincomycin should not be admixed

ADVERSE EFFECTS
Rare at recommended dosage

Pharmacokinetics

Absorption	Well absorbed (PO)
Distribution	Widely distributed; crosses placenta
Metabolism	Widely metabolized
Excretion	Kidney, unchanged (water soluble)
Half-life	Unknown

Pharmacodynamics

Unknown

NURSING CONSIDERATIONS
Assessment
- Assess patient for vitamin deficiency; usually more than one vitamin deficiency is present

Nursing diagnoses
- Knowledge, deficient (teaching)
- Nutrition: less than body requirements, imbalanced (uses)

Patient/family education
- Advise patient that adequate nutrition must be maintained to prevent further deficiencies; to comply with treatment regimen

• Advise patient to avoid treating flavored multivitamins as candy; child may overdose
• Caution patient to store vitamins out of children's reach

Evaluation
Positive therapeutic outcome
• Check each individual vitamin for guidelines
• Absence of vitamin deficiencies

mupirocin topical
See Appendix B

muromonab-CD3 (Rx)
(mur-oe-mone'ab)
Orthoclone OKT3
Func. class.: Immunosuppressive
Chem. class.: Murine monoclonal antibody
Pregnancy category C

ACTION: Recognizes and reacts with the T$_3$ antigens on T lymphocytes, leads to cytokine release, blocks T-cell function

Therapeutic outcome: Prevention of graft rejection

USES: Acute allograft rejection in renal, cardiac, hepatic transplant patients

CONTRAINDICATIONS:
Hypersensitivity to murine origin, CHF, uncontrolled hypertension, breastfeeding, pregnancy **C**

> **BLACK BOX WARNING:** Fluid overload, seizures

Precautions: Pregnancy **C**, children <2 yr, fever, cerebral edema, thrombus, CV/vascular disease, MI, seizure disorder, lymphoma, human anti-murine antibody (HAMA), pulmonary edema, infection

> **BLACK BOX WARNING:** Angioedema, immunosuppressants

DOSAGE AND ROUTES
Adult: **IV** BOL 5 mg/day × 10-14 days
Child ≤30 kg: **IV** 2.5 mg qd × 10-14 days

Cardiac/hepatic allograft rejection, steroid resistant
Adult: **IV** BOL 5 mg/day × 10-14 days; begin when it is known that rejection has not been reversed by steroids

Available forms: Inj 5 mg/5 ml

Implementation
• Give by direct **IV** undiluted; withdraw with a 0.2-0.22 low–protein binding μm filter; discard and use new needle for administration; give over 1 min
• Give for several days before transplant surgery

ADVERSE EFFECTS
CNS: *Pyrexia, chills, tremors,* **aseptic meningitis,** fever, headache, **encephalopathy, seizures**
CV: *Chest pain,* sinus tachycardia, hypertension, angina
EENT: Vision impairment, irreversible blindness
GI: *Vomiting, nausea, diarrhea*
MISC: **Infection, cytokine release syndrome, anaphylaxis,** malaise, **secondary malignancy**
RESP: *Dyspnea, wheezing,* **pulmonary edema**

Pharmacokinetics
Absorption	Completely absorbed
Distribution	Unknown
Metabolism	Unknown
Excretion	Unknown
Half-life	Unknown

Pharmacodynamics
Unknown

INTERACTIONS
Individual drugs
AzaTHIOprine, cycloSPORINE: increased risk of infection
Indomethacin: increased CNS symptoms

Drug classifications
Corticosteroids: increased risk of infection
Immunosuppressants: increased immunosuppression
Live virus vaccines: decreased antibody response

Drug/herb
Astragalus, echinacea, melatonin: interference with immunosuppression
Ginseng, St. John's wort: decreased effect

NURSING CONSIDERATIONS
Assessment
⚠ Assess for cytosine release syndrome (CRS): nausea, vomiting, chills, fever, joint pain, weakness, dizziness, diarrhea, tremors, abdominal pain; occurs 30-60 min after first dose; methylPREDNISolone sodium

M

succinate may be prescribed to lessen this reaction

• **Assess for hypersensitivity reaction, anaphylaxis:** dyspnea, bronchospasm, urticaria, tachycardia, hypotension, angioedema; discontinue product; emergency equipment must be nearby

• Assess for headache, photophobia, fever, rigidity: indicate **aseptic meningitis** has developed

• Assess for sore throat, fever, chills, rash, dysuria, which may indicate infection; therapy may be discontinued

• Assess for fluid overload: edema, pulmonary edema, increasing weight

• Monitor blood studies: CBC with differential, platelets, BUN, creatinine, alkaline phosphatase, bilirubin during treatment monthly

• Monitor AST, ALT, BUN, creatinine, alkaline phosphatase, bilirubin

• Obtain human-mouse antibody; if titer is >1:1000, this product should not be used

• Monitor T-cells with CD3, CD4, CD8 antigen daily; report should be CD3 positive and T-cells <25/mm^3

• **Hepatotoxicity:** assess for dark urine, jaundice, itching, light-colored stools; product should be discontinued

• **Fluid overload:** monitor for increased weight, I&O, edema, crackles, B/P

Nursing diagnoses
• Infection, risk for (uses)
• Knowledge, deficient (teaching)

Patient/family education
• Instruct patient to report fever, chills, sore throat, fatigue, since serious infections may occur; rash, rapid heartbeat

• Advise patient to use contraceptive measures during treatment and several months after, do not breastfeed

• Advise patient to avoid crowds and persons with known infections to reduce risk of infection

• Advise patient to report symptoms of cytokine release syndrome, aseptic meningitis, give list of symptoms

• Instruct patient to avoid vaccinations during treatment

Evaluation
Positive therapeutic outcome
• Absence of graft rejection

mycophenolate (Rx)
(mie-koe-feen′oh-late)
Mycophenolate Mofetil CellCept, Myfortic (Rx)
Func. class.: Immunosuppressant
Pregnancy category C

ACTION: Inhibits inflammatory responses that are mediated by the immune system; prolongs survival of allogenic transplants

Therapeutic outcome: Absence of graft rejection

USES: Organ transplants to prevent rejection (renal); prophylaxis of rejection in allogenic cardiac, hepatic, renal transplants

Unlabeled uses: Refractory uveitis, 2nd-line therapy for Churg-Strauss syndrome, diffuse proliferative lupus nephritis (in combination), rheumatoid arthritis, psoriasis

CONTRAINDICATIONS:
Hypersensitivity to this product or mycophenolic acid

> **BLACK BOX WARNING:** Pregnancy **D**

Precautions: Breastfeeding, lymphomas, neutropenia, renal disease, accidental exposure, anemia

> **BLACK BOX WARNING:** Infection, neoplastic disease

DOSAGE AND ROUTES
Renal transplant
Adult: PO 1 g or 720 mg bid given to renal transplant patients in combination with corticosteroids and cycloSPORINE; mycophenolate mofetil or 720 mg mycophenolate sodium
Child: PO-ER 400 mg/m^2 bid, max 720 mg bid

Renal dose
Adult: PO/IV GFR <25 ml/min, max 2 g/day

Cardiac transplant
Adult: PO/IV 1.5 g bid, **IV** can be started ≤24 hr after transplant, switch to PO when able

Hepatic transplant
Adult: PO 1.5 g bid, IV 1 g over ≥2 hr

Available forms: Caps 250 mg; tabs 500 mg; inj (powder) 500 mg/20 ml vial; powder for oral susp 200 mg/ml; ext rel tab (Myfortic) 180, 360 mg

Implementation
- May be given in combination with corticosteroids and cycloSPORINE

PO route
- Do not crush, chew tabs; do not open caps; avoid inhalation or direct contact with skin, mucous membranes; tetratogenic in animals
- Give alone for better absorption
- Delayed rel tabs and caps; oral susp and tab are not interchangeable

Intermittent IV infusion route
- Reconstitute each vial with 14 ml D_5W, shake gently, further dilute to 6 mg/ml, dilute 1-g doses in 140 ml D_5W, and 1.5-g doses in 210 ml D_5W, give by slow **IV** infusion ≥2 hr, never give by bolus or rapid **IV** injection
- Do not give with other medications or solutions

Y-site compatibilities: Alemtuzumab, alfentanil, amikacin, anidulafungin, argatroban, bivalirudin, caspofungin, cefepime, DAPTOmycin, DOPamine, norepinephrine, octreotide, oxytocin, tacrolimus, tigecycline, tirofiban, vancomycin

Y-site incompatibilities: Acyclovir, allopurinol, amifostine, aminocaproic acid, aminophylline, amphotericin B, colloidal/lipid complex/liposome, ampicillin, atenolol, azithromycin, aztreonam

ADVERSE EFFECTS
CNS: *Tremor, dizziness, insomnia, headache, fever,* **progressive multifocal leukoencephalopathy,** anxiety, pain
CV: *Hypertension, chest pain,* hypotension
GI: *Nausea, vomiting,* stomatitis, *diarrhea, constipation,* **GI bleeding,** abdominal pain, anorexia, dyspepsia
GU: *UTI, hematuria,* **renal tubular necrosis, polyomavirus-associated nephropathy**
HEMA: Leukopenia, thrombocytopenia, anemia, pancytopenia, pure red cell aplasia
INTEG: *Rash*
META: *Peripheral edema, hypercholesterolemia, hypophosphatemia, edema, hypo/hyperkalemia, hyperglycemia,* hypocalcemia, hypomagnesemia
MS: Arthralgia, muscle wasting, back pain, weakness
RESP: *Dyspnea, respiratory infection, increased cough, pharyngitis, bronchitis, pneumonia*
SYST: Lymphoma, nonmelanoma skin carcinoma, sepsis

Absorption	Rapid and complete
Distribution	Unknown
Metabolism	To active metabolite (MPA)
Excretion	Urine, feces
Half-life	Unknown

Pharmacodynamics
Unknown

INTERACTIONS
Individual drugs
Acyclovir, ganciclovir: increased concentration of both products
AzaTHIOprine: avoid use
Cholestyramine, colestopol: decreased levels of mycophenolate
Phenytoin: increased effects; decreased protein binding of phenytoin
Probenecid: increased levels of mycophenolate
Theophylline: increased effects; decreased protein binding of theophylline

Drug classifications
Antacids (magnesium, aluminum): decreased levels of mycophenolate
Contraceptives (oral), live attenuated vaccines: decreased effects
Anticoagulants, NSAIDs, thrombolytics, salicylates: increased risk of bleeding

Drug/herb
Astragalus, echinacea, melatonin: interferes with immunosuppression

Drug/food
Decreased absorption if taken with food

Drug/lab test
- Increase: serum creatinine, BUN, abnormal LFTs

NURSING CONSIDERATIONS
Assessment
- **Progressive multifocal leukoencephalopathy; may be fatal:** ataxia, confusion, apathy, hemiparesis, visual problems, weakness; side effects should be reported to the FDA
- Monitor blood tests: CBC monthly during treatment
- Monitor liver function tests: alkaline phosphatase, AST, ALT, bilirubin
- Monitor renal studies: BUN, CCr, electrolytes
- Obtain pregnancy test within 1 wk prior to initiation of treatment; confirm negative pregnancy test

M

Nursing diagnoses
- Infection, risk for (uses)
- Knowledge, deficient (teaching)

Patient/family education
- Teach patient to report fever, rash, severe diarrhea, chills, sore throat, fatigue, since serious infections may occur
- Instruct patient to avoid crowds to reduce risk of infection
- Advise patient that repeated lab tests are necessary
- Advise patient to limit exposure to sunlight/UV light
- Instruct patient to use two forms of contraception before, during, and 6 wk after therapy

Evaluation
Positive therapeutic outcome
- Absence of graft rejection

---

nabumetone (Rx)
(na-byoo′me-tone)
Apo-Nabumetone ✦,
Gen-Nabumetone ✦
Func. class.: Nonsteroidal antiinflammatory
Chem. class.: Acetic acid derivative
Pregnancy category C

ACTION: Metabolite inhibits COX-1, COX-2 by blocking arachidonate; analgesic, antiinflammatory, antipyretic

Therapeutic outcome: Decreased pain, swelling of joints

USES: Osteoarthritis, rheumatoid arthritis, acute or chronic treatment

CONTRAINDICATIONS:
Pregnancy **D** (3rd trimester), hypersensitivity to this product or aspirin, iodides, NSAIDs

> **BLACK BOX WARNING:** Perioperative pain in CABG surgery

Precautions: Pregnancy **C**, breastfeeding, children, geriatric, bleeding disorders, GI/cardiac/renal disorders, hepatic dysfunction, asthma, bone marrow suppression, lupus (SLE), ulcerative colitis, blood dyscrasias

> **BLACK BOX WARNING:** MI, stroke, GI bleeding

DOSAGE AND ROUTES
Adult: PO 1 g as a single dose or divided bid; may increase to 2 g/day if needed; max 2 g/day if needed (as a divided dose)

Available forms: Tabs 500, 750 mg

Implementation
- Administer tab to patient crushed or whole
- Give with food or milk to decrease gastric symptoms
- Patient should take with a full glass of water and sit upright

ADVERSE EFFECTS
CNS: Dizziness, headache, drowsiness, fatigue, tremors, confusion, insomnia, anxiety, depression, nervousness
CV: Tachycardia, peripheral edema, palpitations, **dysrhythmias, CHF, MI, stroke**
EENT: Tinnitus
GI: Nausea, anorexia, vomiting, diarrhea, jaundice, cholestatic hepatitis, constipation, flatulence, cramps, dry mouth, peptic ulcer, gastritis, **ulceration, perforation,** bleeding
GU: Nephrotoxicity, dysuria, hematuria, oliguria, azotemia, cystitis
HEMA: Blood dyscrasias
INTEG: Purpura, rash, pruritus, sweating, photosensitivity
RESP: Dyspnea, pharyngitis, **bronchospasm**
SYST: Anaphylaxis, angioneurotic edema

Pharmacokinetics
Absorption	Well absorbed
Distribution	Protein binding >99%
Metabolism	Liver, extensively, to inactive metabolite
Excretion	Unknown
Half-life	24 hr

Pharmacodynamics
Onset	Unknown
Peak	$2^1/_2$-4 hr
Duration	Unknown

INTERACTIONS
Individual drugs
Alcohol, potassium: increased GI reactions
Cefamandole, cefoperazone, cefotetan, clopidogrel, eptifibatide, plicamycin, ticlopidine, valproic acid: increased risk of bleeding
Lithium, methotrexate: increased effect of each
Radiation: increased risk of hematologic reactions

Drug classifications
Anticoagulants, thrombolytics, SSRIs, SNRIs: increased risk of bleeding
Antihypertensives: decreased effect of antihypertensives
Antineoplastics: increased risk of hematologic reactions
Corticosteroids, NSAIDs, potassium supplements, salicylates: increased GI reactions
Diuretics: decreased effectiveness of diuretics

Drug/herb
Arginine, gossypol: increased gastric irritation
Bearberry, bilberry: increased NSAID effect
Garlic, ginger, ginkgo: increased bleeding risk

Drug/lab test
Increased: bleeding time, K, BUN, AST, ALT, LDH, alkaline phosphatase, creatinine
Decreased: CCr, blood glucose, Hct, Hgb

NURSING CONSIDERATIONS
Assessment

> **BLACK BOX WARNING: Cardiac status:** CV thrombic events, MI, stroke; may be fatal, not to be used in perioperative pain after CABG

> **BLACK BOX WARNING: GI status:** ulceration, bleeding, perforation; may be fatal

• **Assess for pain:** frequency, characteristics, location, duration, intensity, relief of pain after medication; and for inflammation of joints, ROM
• Monitor blood counts during therapy; watch for decreasing platelets; if low, therapy may need to be discontinued, restarted after hematologic recovery; check for blood dyscrasias (thrombocytopenia): bruising, fatigue, bleeding, poor healing; monitor liver function tests: AST, ALT, alkaline phosphatase; LDH, blood glucose, WBC, CCr
• Assess for asthma, aspirin sensitivity, nasal polyps; increased hypersensitivity reactions

Nursing diagnoses
• Injury, risk for (adverse reactions)
• Knowledge, deficient (teaching)
• Mobility, impaired physical (uses)
• Pain, acute (uses)
• Pain, chronic

Patient/family education
• Tell patient that product must be continued for prescribed time to be effective; to avoid aspirin, alcoholic beverages, NSAIDs, and OTC medications unless approved by prescriber

• Caution patient to report bleeding, bruising, fatigue, malaise, since blood dyscrasias do occur
• Instruct patient to use caution when driving; drowsiness, dizziness may occur
• Advise patient to use sunscreen, hat, and other protective clothing to prevent burns
• Advise patient to report dark stools, a change in urine pattern, increased weight, edema, increased pain in joints, fever, blood in urine, blurred vision, ringing or roaring in ears
• Advise to report use to all health care providers

Evaluation
Positive therapeutic outcome
• Decreased pain
• Decreased inflammation
• Increased mobility

nadolol (Rx)
(nay-doe′lole)
Apo-Nadolol ✦, Corgard
Func. class.: Antihypertensive, antianginal
Chem. class.: β-Adrenergic receptor blocker
Pregnancy category C

Do not confuse:
Corgard/Cognex/Coreg/nadolol/mandol

ACTION: Long-acting, nonselective β-adrenergic receptor blocking agent, blocks β_1 in the heart and β_2 in the lungs, uterus, and circulatory system; mechanism is similar to that of propranolol

Therapeutic outcome: Decreased B/P, heart rate

USES: Chronic stable angina pectoris, mild to moderate hypertension

Unlabeled uses: Tachydysrhythmias, anxiety, tremors, esophageal varices (rebleeding only), prophylaxis of migraine headaches

CONTRAINDICATIONS:
Hypersensitivity to this product, cardiac failure, cardiogenic shock, 2nd- or 3rd-degree heart block, bronchospastic disease, sinus bradycardia, CHF, COPD

Precautions: Pregnancy C, breastfeeding, diabetes mellitus, renal disease, hyperthyroidism, peripheral vascular disease, myasthenia gravis, major surgery, nonallergic bronchospasm

---

> **BLACK BOX WARNING:** Abrupt discontinuation

DOSAGE AND ROUTES
Adult: PO 40 mg/day; increase by 40-80 mg q3-7day; maintenance 40-240 mg/day for angina, 40-320 mg/day for hypertension
Geriatric: PO 20 mg/day, may increase by 20 mg until desired dose

Renal dose
Adult: PO CCr 31-50 ml/min give q24-36hr; CCr 10-30 ml/min give q24-48hr; CCr <10 ml/min give q40-60hr

Migraine Prevention (unlabeled)
Adult: PO 80-240 mg q day × 2-18 mo

Available forms: Tabs 20, 40, 80 mg

Implementation
• Give before meals, at bedtime; tab may be crushed or swallowed whole; give with food to prevent GI upset; give reduced dosage in renal dysfunction; check apical pulse prior to use, if <60 bpm, withhold dose and contact prescriber
• Store protected from light, moisture; place in cool environment

ADVERSE EFFECTS
CNS: Depression, dizziness, fatigue, lethargy, paresthesia, headache, *weakness,* insomnia, memory loss, nightmares
CV: Bradycardia, *hypotension,* **CHF,** palpitations, AV block, chest pain, peripheral ischemia, flushing, edema, vasodilatation, conduction disturbances
EENT: Blurred vision, dry eyes, nasal congestion
ENDO: Hyperglycemia, hypoglycemia
GI: Nausea, vomiting, diarrhea, colitis, constipation, cramps, dry mouth, flatulence, hepatomegaly, **pancreatitis,** taste distortion
GU: *Impotence,* decreased libido
HEMA: Agranulocytosis, thrombocytopenia
INTEG: Rash, pruritus, fever, alopecia
RESP: Dyspnea, respiratory dysfunction, **bronchospasm,** cough, wheezing, pharyngitis, **laryngospasm, pulmonary edema**

Pharmacokinetics
Absorption	Variably absorbed
Distribution	Crosses placenta; minimal concentration in CNS, protein binding 30%
Metabolism	Unknown
Excretion	Kidneys, unchanged
Half-life	10-24 hr; increased in renal disease

Pharmacodynamics
Onset	Variable
Peak	3-4 hr
Duration	20-24 hr

INTERACTIONS
Individual drugs
CloNIDine, EPINEPHrine: increased hypotension, bradycardia
Digoxin: increased bradycardia
Thyroid: decreased β-blocking effect

Drug classifications
Antihypertensives: increased hypotension
Ergots: peripheral ischemia
MAOIs: increased bradycardia; do not use together
NSAIDs: decreased antihypertensive effect
Phenothiazines: increased hypotensive effects

Drug/lab test
Increased: serum potassium, serum uric acid, ALT, AST, alkaline phosphatase, LDH, blood glucose, cholesterol, ANA, triglycerides

NURSING CONSIDERATIONS
Assessment
• **Pain:** assess for duration, time started, activity being performed, location, character
• Monitor B/P at beginning of treatment, periodically thereafter; note rate, rhythm, quality of apical/radial pulse before administration; notify prescriber of any significant changes (pulse <60 bpm), orthostatic hypotension
• Check for baselines in renal, liver function tests before therapy begins
• Assess for edema in feet, legs daily; monitor I&O, daily weight; check for jugular vein distention and crackles bilaterally, dyspnea **(CHF)**
• Headache, light-headedness, decreased B/P; may indicate a need for decreased dosage

---

⚠ Nurse Alert

BLACK BOX WARNING: Abrupt discontinuation: can result in MI, myocardial ischemia, ventricular dysrhythmias, severe hypertension, withdraw slowly by tapering over 2 wk

Nursing diagnoses
• Cardiac output, decreased (uses)
• Injury, risk for (adverse reactions)
• Knowledge, deficient (teaching)
• Noncompliance (teaching)

Patient/family education
• Teach patient not to discontinue product abruptly; taper over 2 wk; may cause precipitate angina, serious dysrhythmias if stopped abruptly
• Teach patient not to use OTC products containing α-adrenergic stimulants (such as nasal decongestants, cold preparations); to avoid alcohol and smoking and to limit sodium intake as prescribed
• Teach patient how to take pulse and B/P at home; to hold dose if pulse is ≤50 bpm, systolic B/P <90 mm Hg; advise when to notify prescriber
• **Hypertension:** instruct patient to comply with weight control, dietary adjustments, modified exercise program; to report weight gain >5 lb, swelling, unusual bruising, bleeding
• Advise patient to carry/wear emergency ID to identify product being taken, allergies; teach patient product controls symptoms but does not cure condition
• Caution patient to avoid hazardous activities if dizziness, drowsiness are present; to rise slowly to prevent orthostatic hypotension
• **Teach patient to report symptoms of CHF:** difficult breathing, especially on exertion or when lying down, night cough, swelling of extremities or bradycardia, dizziness, confusion, depression, fever
• Teach patient to take product as prescribed, not to double doses, skip doses; take any missed doses as soon as remembered if at least 4 hr until next dose

Evaluation
Positive therapeutic outcome
• Decreased B/P in hypertension

nafcillin (Rx)
(naf-sill′in)
Func. class.: Antiinfective, broad-spectrum
Chem. class.: Penicillinase-resistant penicillin
Pregnancy category B

ACTION: Interferes with cell wall replication of susceptible organisms; osmotically unstable cell wall swells, bursts from osmotic pressure

Therapeutic outcome: Bactericidal effects for gram-positive cocci *Staphylococcus aureus, Streptococcus viridans, Streptococcus pneumoniae* and infections caused by penicillinase-producing *Staphylococcus*

USES: Infections caused by penicillinase-producing staphylococci, streptococci; respiratory tract, skin, skin structure, urinary tract, bone, joint infections; sinusitis; endocarditis; septicemia; meningitis

CONTRAINDICATIONS:
Hypersensitivity to penicillins or corn

Precautions: Pregnancy **B**, breastfeeding, neonates, GI disease, asthma, hypersensitivity to cephalosporins or carbapenems

DOSAGE AND ROUTES
Adult: IV 500-2000 mg q4hr
Infant and child >1 mo: IV 50-200 mg/kg/day in divided doses q4-6hr
Neonate >7 days (weight >2 kg): IV 25 mg/kg q6hr
Neonate ≤7 days (weight ≤2 kg): IV 25 mg/kg q8hr

Meningitis
Adult: IV 100-200 mg/kg/day divided q4-6hr, max 12 g/day
Neonate >7 days (weight >2 kg): IV 50 mg/kg q6hr
Neonate ≤7 days (weight <2 kg): IV 50 mg/kg q12hr

Available forms: Powder for inj 1, 2, premixed or Add-Vantage vials

Implementation
IM route
• Give deep in large muscle mass

IV route
• Reconstitute vials: add 1.7 (1.8 nafcil), 3, 4, or 6.4 ml (6.6 ml NaCl) sterile water for inj, 0.9% NaCl, bacteriostatic water for inj with

benzyl alcohol or parabens to vials with 500 mg, 1 g, 2 g of nafcillin, respectively (250 mg/ml)
- **Nallpen piggyback units:** reconstitute 1 or 2 g with 50-100 ml or 99 ml, respectively, of sterile water for inj, 0.45% NaCl, 0.9% NaCl
- **Unipen piggyback units:** reconstitute according to manufacturer

Direct intermittent IV INJ route
- Further dilute the reconstituted sol in 15-30 ml of sterile water for inj, 0.45% NaCl, 0.9% NaCl; inj slowly over 5-10 min into the tubing of a free-flowing compatible IV solution

Intermittent IV infusion route
- Vials, further dilute reconstituted solution to 2-40 mg/ml, for peripheral vein inf ≤20 mg/ml (preferred); piggyback unit no further dilution needed; infuse ≥30-60 min, make sure entire dose is given before 10% or more of solution is inactivated

Y-site compatibilities: Acyclovir, atropine, cyclophosphamide, diazepam, enalaprilat, esmolol, famotidine, fentaNYL, fluconazole, foscarnet, HYDROmorphone, magnesium sulfate, morphine, perphenazine, propofol, theophylline, zidovudine

Y-site incompatibilities: Droperidol, fentaNYL/droperidol, labetalol, nalbuphine, pentazocine, regular insulin, verapamil

ADVERSE EFFECTS

CNS: Lethargy, hallucinations, anxiety, depression, muscle twitching, **coma, seizures**
GI: *Nausea, vomiting, diarrhea,* increased AST, ALT, abdominal pain, glossitis, **pseudomembranous colitis**
GU: Oliguria, **proteinuria, hematuria,** vaginitis, moniliasis, **glomerulonephritis, interstitial nephritis**
HEMA: Anemia, increased bleeding time, **bone marrow depression, neutropenia**
SYST: Anaphylaxis, serum sickness, Stevens-Johnson syndrome

Pharmacokinetics

Absorption	Well absorbed (IM); erratic (PO)
Distribution	Widely distributed; crosses placenta
Metabolism	Not metabolized
Excretion	Kidneys, unchanged; breast milk
Half-life	1 hr; increased in renal disease

Pharmacodynamics

	PO	IM	IV
Onset	$^{1}/_{2}$ hr	$^{1}/_{2}$ hr	Immediate
Peak	1-2 hr	1-2 hr	Infusion end
Duration	Unknown	Unknown	Unknown

INTERACTIONS

Individual drugs
CycloSPORINE: decreased effect of cycloSPORINE
NDR: decrease: effect of cycloSPORINE: warfarin
Probenecid: increased nafcillin levels

Drug classifications
Tetracyclines: avoid use

Drug/food
Food, carbonated drinks, citrus fruit juices: decreased absorption

Drug/lab test
False positive: urine glucose, urine protein

NURSING CONSIDERATIONS

Assessment
- Assess patient for previous sensitivity reaction to penicillins or other cephalosporins; cross-sensitivity between penicillins and cephalosporins is common
- Assess patient for signs and symptoms of infection including characteristics of wounds, sputum, urine, stool, WBC >10,000/mm^3, earache, fever; obtain information baseline, during treatment
- Obtain C&S before beginning product therapy to identify if correct treatment has been initiated
- **Assess for allergic reactions, anaphylaxis:** rash, urticaria, pruritus, chills, fever, dyspnea, laryngeal edema, joint pain; angioedema may occur a few days after therapy begins; EPINEPHrine, resuscitation equipment should be available for anaphylactic reaction
- Assess renal function tests: urinalysis, protein, blood, BUN, creatinine; abnormal urinalysis may indicate nephrotoxicity
- ⚠ **Identify urine output; if decreasing, notify prescriber (may indicate nephrotoxicity)**
- Monitor blood studies: AST, ALT, CBC, Hct, bilirubin, LDH, alkaline phosphatase, Coombs' test monthly if patient is on long-term therapy
- Monitor electrolytes: potassium, sodium, chloride monthly if patient is on long-term therapy

⚠ Nurse Alert

- **Pseudomembranous colitis:** assess for diarrhea, abdominal pain, fever, fatigue, anorexia; possible anemia, elevated WBC and low serum albumin; stop product and usually give either vancomycin or IV metroNIDAZOLE
- Monitor for bleeding: ecchymosis, bleeding gums, hematuria, stool guaiac daily if on long-term therapy
- Assess for overgrowth of infection: perineal itching, fever, malaise, redness, pain, swelling, drainage, rash, diarrhea, change in cough, sputum

Nursing diagnoses
- Diarrhea (adverse reactions)
- Infection, risk for (uses)
- Injury, risk for (adverse reactions)
- Knowledge, deficient (teaching)
- Noncompliance (teaching)

Patient/family education
- Teach patient to report sore throat, bruising, bleeding, joint pain; may indicate blood dyscrasias (rare)
- Advise patient to contact prescriber if vaginal itching, loose foul-smelling stools, furry tongue occur; may indicate superinfection
- Instruct patient to take all medication prescribed for the length of time ordered
- Advise patient to notify prescriber of diarrhea with blood or pus, which may indicate pseudomembranous colitis
- Advise patient to carry/wear emergency ID if allergic to penicillins

Evaluation
Positive therapeutic outcome
- Absence of signs/symptoms of infection (WBC <10,000/mm³, temp WNL, absence of red, draining wounds, earache)
- Reported improvement in symptoms of infection

TREATMENT OF ANAPHYLAXIS: Withdraw product, maintain airway, administer epinephrine, aminophylline, O₂, **IV** corticosteroids

⚠ HIGH ALERT

nalbuphine (Rx)
(nal'byoo-feen)
Func. class.: Opioid analgesic
Chem. class.: Synthetic opioid agonist/antagonist
Pregnancy category C

ACTION: Depresses pain impulse transmission at the spinal cord level by interacting with opioid receptors

Therapeutic outcome: Relief of pain

USES: Moderate to severe pain

CONTRAINDICATIONS:
Hypersensitivity, addiction (opioid)

Precautions: Pregnancy **C**, breastfeeding, addictive personality, increased ICP, MI (acute), severe heart disease, respiratory depression, renal/hepatic disease, bowel impaction

DOSAGE AND ROUTES
Analgesic
Adult: SUBCUT/IM/**IV** 10 mg q3-6hr prn, max 160 mg/day

Balanced anesthesia adjunct
Adult: IV 0.3-3 mg/kg given over 10-15 min; may give 0.25-0.5 mg/kg as needed (maintenance)

Available forms: Inj 10, 20 mg/ml

Implementation
- Give by inj (IM, **IV**), only with resuscitative equipment available; give slowly to prevent rigidity
- Store in light-resistant area at room temperature
IM route
- Give inj deeply in large muscle mass; rotate inj sites; protect vial from light
Direct IV route
- Give direct **IV** undiluted 10 mg or less over 3-5 min or more into free-flowing IV line of D₅W, NS, LR

Syringe compatibilities: Atropine, cimetidine, diphenhydrAMINE, droperidol, glycopyrrolate, hydrOXYzine, lidocaine, midazolam, prochlorperazine, promethazine, ranitidine, scopolamine, trimethobenzamide

Syringe incompatibilities: Diazepam, PENTobarbital

Y-site compatibilities: Amifostine, aztreonam, cefmetazole, cladribine, filgrastim, fludarabine, granisetron, melphalan, paclitaxel, propofol, teniposide, thiotepa, vinorelbine

Y-site incompatibilities: Nafcillin, sargramostim

ADVERSE EFFECTS

CNS: *Drowsiness, dizziness, confusion, headache, sedation, euphoria,* dysphoria (high doses), hallucinations, increased dreaming, tolerance, physical and psychological dependency
CV: Palpitations, bradycardia, change in B/P, orthostatic hypotension, **cardiac arrest**
EENT: Tinnitus, blurred vision, miosis, diplopia
GI: *Nausea, vomiting, anorexia, constipation, cramps,* abdominal pain, dyspepsia, xerostomia, bitter taste
GU: Increased urinary output, dysuria, urinary retention, urgency
INTEG: *Rash,* urticaria, bruising, flushing, *diaphoresis,* pruritus
RESP: Respiratory depression, pulmonary edema

Pharmacokinetics

Absorption	Well absorbed (SUBCUT, IM); completely absorbed (**IV**)
Distribution	Crosses placenta
Metabolism	Liver, extensively
Excretion	Feces, kidneys, unchanged (small amounts); breast milk
Half-life	3-6 hr

Pharmacodynamics

	IM	SUBCUT	IV
Onset	Up to 15 min	Up to 15 min	Rapid
Peak	1 hr	Unknown	$1/2$ hr
Duration	3-6 hr	3-6 hr	3-6 hr

INTERACTIONS

Individual drugs
Alcohol: increased respiratory depression, hypotension, sedation

Drug classifications
Antipsychotics, CNS depressants, sedative/hypnotics, skeletal muscle relaxants: increased respiratory depression, hypotension
MAOIs: avoid use, results are unpredictable
Opiates: increased effects with other CNS depressants

Drug/lab test
Increased: amylase

NURSING CONSIDERATIONS

Assessment
• **Assess pain characteristics** (location, intensity, type) before medication administration, 30-60 min after treatment, titrate upward by 25%-50% until pain is reduced by 50%
• Assess bowel status; constipation is common
• Monitor VS after parenteral route; note muscle rigidity, product history, liver, kidney function tests; **respiratory dysfunction: respiratory depression, character, rate, rhythm; notify prescriber if respirations are <10/min**
• **Monitor CNS changes:** dizziness, drowsiness, hallucinations, euphoria, LOC, pupil reaction
• Monitor allergic reactions: rash, urticaria

Nursing diagnoses
• Breathing pattern, ineffective (adverse reactions)
• Knowledge, deficient (teaching)
• Pain, acute (uses)
• Sensory perception, disturbed: visual, auditory (adverse reactions)

Patient/family education
• Instruct patient to report any symptoms of CNS changes, allergic reactions
• Teach patient that physical dependency can result from long-term use, although there is a low potential for dependency
• Caution patients to avoid CNS depressants: alcohol, sedative/hypnotics for at least 24 hr after taking this product
• Discuss with patient that dizziness, drowsiness, confusion are common; to avoid getting up without assistance
• Discuss in detail all aspects of the product: reason for taking product and expected results
• Instruct patient to change position slowly to prevent orthostatic hypotension

Evaluation
Positive therapeutic outcome
• Relief of pain without respiratory depression

TREATMENT OF OVERDOSE:
Naloxone (Narcan) 0.2-0.8 **IV**, O_2, **IV** fluids, vasopressors

⚠ Nurse Alert

naloxone (Rx)

(nal-oks'one)
naloxone HCl
Func. class.: Opioid antagonist, antidote
Chem. class.: Thebaine derivative
Pregnancy category C

ACTION: Competes with opioids at opioid-receptor sites

Therapeutic outcome: Absence of opioid overdose

USES: Respiratory depression induced by opioids, pentazocine, propoxyphene; refractory circulatory shock, asphyxia neonatorum, coma, hypotension

Unlabeled uses: IBS, opiate agonist dependence, opiate agonist-induced constipation, pruritus

CONTRAINDICATIONS:
Hypersensitivity

Precautions: Pregnancy **C,** breastfeeding, neonates, children, CV disease, opioid dependency, seizure disorder, drug dependency

DOSAGE AND ROUTES
Opioid-induced respiratory depression
Adult: IV/SUBCUT/IM 0.4-2 mg; repeat q2-3min if needed, max 10 mg
Child <5 yr or ≤20 kg: IV/SUBCUT/IM 0.01 mg/kg slowly followed by 0.1 mg/kg if needed or as an INF titrated to response

Postoperative opioid-induced respiratory depression
Adult: IV 0.1-0.2 mg q2-3min prn
Child: IV/IM/SUBCUT 0.005-0.01 mg/kg q2-3min prn

Opioid overdose
Adult: IV/SUBCUT/IM 0.4 mg (10 mcg/kg) (not opioid dependent), may repeat q2-3min; 0.1-0.2 mg q2-3min (opioid dependent)

Available forms: Inj 0.02, 0.4 mg/ml

Implementation
Direct IV route
• Give undiluted; give 0.4 mg or less over 15 sec or titrate inf to response
Continuous IV infusion route
• Dilute 2 mg/500 ml 0.9% NaCl or D₅W (4 mcg/ml), titrate to response

• Give only with resuscitative equipment, O₂ nearby
• Use only sol prepared within 24 hr
• Store at room temperature in darkness

Y-site compatibilities: Acyclovir, alfentanil, amikacin, aminocaproic acid, aminophylline, anidulafungin, ascorbic acid, atenolol, atracurium, atropine, azaTHIOprine, aztreonam, benztropine, bivalirudin, bleomycin, bumetanide, buprenorphine, butorphanol, calcium chloride/gluconate, CARBOplatin, caspofungin, cefamandole, ceFAZolin, cefmetazole, cefonicid, cefoperazone, cefotaxime, cefotetan, cefoxitin, ceftazidime, ceftizoxime, cefTRIAXone, cefuroxime, cephalothin, cephapirin, chloramphenicol, chlorproMAZINE, cimetidine, CISplatin, clindamycin, cyanocobalamin, cyclophosphamide, cycloSPORINE, cytarabine, DACTINomycin, DAPTOmycin, dexamethasone, digoxin, diltiazem, diphenhydrAMINE, DOBUTamine, docetaxel, DOPamine, doxacurium, DOXOrubicin, doxycycline, enalaprilat, ePHEDrine, EPINEPHrine, epirubicin, epoetin alfa, eptifibatide, ertapenem, erythromycin, esmolol, etoposide, etoposide phosphate, famotidine, fenoldopam, fentaNYL, fluconazole, fludarabine, fluorouracil, folic acid, furosemide, ganciclovir, gatifloxacin, gemcitabine, gentamicin, glycopyrrolate, granisetron, heparin, hydrocortisone, hydrOXYzine, IDArubicin, ifosfamide, imipenem-cilastatin, inamrinone, indomethacin, insulin (regular), irinotecan, isoproterenol, ketorolac, labetalol, levofloxacin, lidocaine, linezolid, LORazepam, mannitol, mechlorethamine, meperidine, metaraminol, methicillin, methotrexate, methoxamine, methyldopate, methylPREDNISolone, metoclopramide, metoprolol, metroNIDAZOLE, mezlocillin, miconazole, midazolam, milrinone, minocycline, mitoxantrone, morphine, moxalactam, multiple vitamins, mycophenolate, nafcillin, nalbuphine, nesiritide, netilmicin, nitroglycerin, nitroprusside, norepinephrine, octreotide, ondansetron, oxacillin, oxaliplatin, oxytocin, paclitaxel, palonosetron, pamidronate, pancuronium, papaverine, pemetrexed, penicillin G potassium/sodium, pentamidine, pentazocine, PENTobarbital, PHENobarbital, phentolamine, phenylephrine, phytonadione, piperacillin, piperacillin-tazobactam, polymyxin B, potassium chloride, procainamide, prochlorperazine, promethazine, propofol, propranolol, protamine, pyridoxine, quiNIDine, quinupristin-dalfopristin, ranitidine, ritodrine, rocuronium, sodium acetate/bicarbonate, succinylcholine, SUFentanil, tacrolimus, teniposide, theophylline, thiamine, ticarcillin, ticarcillin-clavulanate, tigecycline, tirofiban,

N

    Adverse effects: *italics* = common; **bold** = life-threatening

tobramycin, tolazoline, trimetaphan, urokinase, vancomycin, vasopressin, vecuronium, verapamil, vinCRIStine, vinorelbine, voriconazole, zoledronic acid

ADVERSE EFFECTS

CNS: Drowsiness, nervousness, **seizures,** tremor
CV: Rapid pulse, **ventricular tachycardia, fibrillation,** increased systolic B/P (high doses), hypo/hypertension, **cardiac arrest, sinus tachycardia**
GI: Nausea, vomiting, **hepatotoxicity**
RESP: Hyperpnea, **pulmonary edema**

Pharmacokinetics

Absorption	Well absorbed (SUBCUT, IM); completely absorbed (**IV**)
Distribution	Rapidly distributed; crosses placenta
Metabolism	Liver
Excretion	Kidneys
Half-life	1 hr; up to 3 hr (neonates)

Pharmacodynamics

	IV	IM/SUBCUT
Onset	1 min	2-5 min
Peak	Unknown	Unknown
Duration	45 min	30-81 min

INTERACTIONS

Individual drugs
Tramadol: increased seizures

Drug classifications
Analgesics (opioids): decreased effects of opioid analgesics

Drug/lab test
Interference: urine VMA, 5-HIAA, urine glucose

NURSING CONSIDERATIONS

Assessment
• **Assess for signs of opioid withdrawal** in drug-dependent individuals: cramping, hypertension, anxiety, vomiting; may occur up to 2 hr after administration
• Monitor VS q3-5min; ABGs including Po_2, Pco_2
• Assess cardiac status: tachycardia, hypertension; monitor ECG
• **Assess for pain:** duration, intensity, location before, after administration; may be used for respiratory depression
• **Assess for respiratory dysfunction:** respiratory depression, character, rate, rhythm;

if respirations are <10/min, probably due to opioid overdose, administer naloxone; monitor LOC

Nursing diagnoses
• Breathing pattern, ineffective (uses)
• Coping, ineffective (uses)
• Knowledge, deficient (teaching)
• Pain, acute (adverse reactions)

Patient/family education
• Explain reason for and expected results of medication when patient is alert

Evaluation
Positive therapeutic outcome
• Reversal of respiratory depression
• LOC: alert

naphazoline nasal
See Appendix B

naphazoline ophthalmic
See Appendix B

naproxen
(na-prox′en)
Aleve, Anaprox, Anaprox DS, Apo-Napro-Na ✹, Apo-Naproxen ✹, EC-Naprosyn, Equaline All Day Relief, Gen-Naproxen EC ✹, Good Sense All Day Pain Relief, Leader Naproxen, Midol Extended Relief, Novo-Naprox ✹, Novo-Naprox Sodium ✹, Nu-Naprox ✹, Select Brand Naproxen, Top Care All Day Pain Relief, Wal-Proxen
Func. class.: Nonsteroidal antiinflammatory, nonopioid analgesic
Chem. class.: Propionic acid derivative
Pregnancy category B (1st trimester), D (2nd/3rd trimesters)

Do not confuse:
Naprosyn/Natacyn/Naprelan

ACTION: Completely inhibits COX-1, COX-2 by blocking arachidonate; analgesic, antiinflammatory, antipyretic

Therapeutic outcome: Decreased pain, inflammation

USES: Mild to moderate pain, osteoarthritis, rheumatoid arthritis, gouty arthritis, primary dysmenorrhea, tendinitis, ankylosing spondylitis, bursitis, myalgia, dental pain

CONTRAINDICATIONS:

Pregnancy **D** (2nd/3rd trimesters), hypersensitivity to NSAIDs, salicylates, asthma, severe renal/hepatic/ulcer disease

> **BLACK BOX WARNING:** Perioperative pain in CABG surgery

Precautions: Pregnancy **C** (1st trimester), breastfeeding, children <2 yr, geriatric, bleeding disorders, GI/cardiac disorders, hypersensitivity to other antiinflammatory agents, CCr <30 ml/min

> **BLACK BOX WARNING:** MI, GI bleeding, stroke

DOSAGE AND ROUTES

200 mg base = 220 mg naproxen sodium

Antiinflammatory/analgesic/ antidysmenorrheal

Adult: PO 250-500 mg bid, max 1250 mg/day; DEL REL TAB 375-500 mg bid
Child ≥2 yr: PO 5-7 mg/kg/q 8-12 hr

Antigout
Adult: PO 750 mg, then 250 mg q8hr

OTC use
Adult: PO 220 mg q8-12hr or 440 mg, then 220 mg q12hr, max 660 mg/24 hr, taken no longer than 10 days
Geriatric >65 yr: PO max 220 mg q12hr

Available forms: Naproxen: tabs: 250, 375, 500 mg; del rel tabs (EC-Naprosyn, Naprosyn-E) 250♣, 375, 500 mg; oral susp 125 mg/5 ml; ext rel tabs (CR) 375, 500, 750 mg♣; **naproxen sodium;** tabs 220, 275, 550 mg; ext rel tab 220 mg

Implementation

• Administer to patient crushed or whole **(regular release)**; do not crush, break, or chew **extended rel tab**
• Give OTC for 10 days or less unless approved by prescriber
• Give with food or milk to decrease gastric symptoms; give ½ hr before or 2 hr after meals for better absorption
• Patient should take with 8 oz of water and sit upright for 30 min after dose to prevent ulceration

ADVERSE EFFECTS

CNS: Dizziness, drowsiness, fatigue, tremors, confusion, insomnia, anxiety, depression
CV: Tachycardia, peripheral edema, palpitations, **dysrhythmias, MI, stroke**
EENT: Tinnitus, hearing loss, blurred vision
GI: Nausea, anorexia, vomiting, diarrhea, jaundice, **hepatitis,** constipation, flatulence, cramps, peptic ulcer, **GI ulceration, bleeding, perforation**
GU: Nephrotoxicity: dysuria, hematuria, oliguria, azotemia
HEMA: Blood dyscrasias
INTEG: Purpura, rash, pruritus, sweating
SYST: Anaphylaxis

Pharmacokinetics

Absorption	Completely absorbed
Distribution	Crosses placenta, 99% protein binding
Metabolism	Liver, extensively
Excretion	Breast milk
Half-life	10-20 hr

Pharmacodynamics

Onset	1 hr
Peak	2-4 hr
Duration	<7 hr

INTERACTIONS

Individual drugs
Alcohol, aspirin: increased risk of GI side effects
Cefamandole, cefoperazone, cefotetan, clopidogrel, eptifibatide, plicamycin, ticlopidine, tirofiban, valproic acid: increased bleeding risk
Lithium, methotrexate, probenecid, radiation: increased toxicity
Cholestyramine, sucralfate: decreased/delayed absorption of naproxen

Drug classifications
ACE inhibitors: possible renal impairment
Antacids: decreased/delayed absorption of naproxen
Anticoagulants, SSRIs, SNRIs, thrombolytics, tricyclics: increased risk of bleeding
Antihypertensives: decreased effect of antihypertensives
Antineoplastics: increased risk of hematologic toxicity
Corticosteroids, NSAIDs: increased risk of GI adverse reactions
Diuretics: decreased effectiveness of diuretics

Drug/herb
Fenugreek, feverfew, garlic, ginger, ginkgo, ginseng *(Panax),* licorice: increased bleeding risk

Drug/lab test
Increased: BUN, alkaline phosphatase
False: increased 5-HIAA, 17KS

N

NURSING CONSIDERATIONS
Assessment

> **BLACK BOX WARNING: Cardiac status:** CV thrombotic events, MI, stroke; may be fatal; not to be used in CABG

> **BLACK BOX WARNING: GI status:** ulceration, bleeding, perforation; may be fatal

- Monitor liver function, renal function, other blood tests: AST, ALT, bilirubin, creatinine, BUN, CBC, Hct, Hgb, pro-time, LDH, blood glucose, WBC, platelets; if patient is on long-term therapy
- Check I&O ratio; decreasing output may indicate renal failure (long-term therapy)
- **Assess hepatotoxicity:** dark urine, clay-colored stools, yellowing of the skin and sclera, itching, abdominal pain, fever, diarrhea if patient is on long-term therapy
- Assess for allergic reactions: rash, urticaria; if these occur, product may have to be discontinued
- **Assess for ototoxicity:** tinnitus, ringing, roaring in ears; audiometric testing needed before, after long-term therapy
- Assess for vision changes: blurring, halos; may indicate corneal, retinal damage
- Check for edema in feet, ankles, legs
- Identify prior product history; there are many product interactions
- **Monitor pain:** location, frequency, duration, characteristics, type, intensity before dose and 1 hour after
- **Arthritis:** Assess ROM, pain, swelling before and 1-2 hr after use
- **Fever:** Assess before use and 1 hr after use
- Assess for asthma, aspirin hypersensitivity, or nasal polyps, increased risk of hypersensitivity

Nursing diagnoses
- Injury, risk for (adverse reactions)
- Knowledge, deficient (teaching)
- Mobility, impaired physical (uses)
- Pain, acute (uses)
- Pain, chronic

Patient/family education
- Teach patient to report any symptoms of renal/hepatic toxicity, vision changes, ototoxicity, allergic reactions, bleeding (long-term therapy); to report use to all health care providers
- Caution patient not to exceed recommended dosage; acute poisoning may result; to take as prescribed, do not double dose
- Advise patient to use sunscreen to prevent photosensitivity reactions
- Teach patient to read label on other OTC products; many contain other antiinflammatories; caution patient to avoid alcohol ingestion; GI bleeding may occur
- Inform patient that the therapeutic response takes 2 wk (arthritis)
- Teach patient to report tinnitus, confusion, diarrhea, sweating, hyperventilation, blurred vision, fever, joint aches, black stools, flulike symptoms

Evaluation
Positive therapeutic outcome
- Decreased pain
- Decreased inflammation
- Increased mobility

naratriptan (Rx)
(nair′ah-trip-tan)
Amerge
Func. class.: Antimigraine agent
Chem. class.: 5-HT₁-like receptor agonist
Pregnancy category C

ACTION: Binds selectively to the vascular 5-HT₁ receptor subtype, exerts antimigraine effect; causes vasoconstriction in cranial arteries

Therapeutic outcome: Decreased intensity and incidence of migraines

USES: Acute treatment of migraine with or without aura

CONTRAINDICATIONS: Angina pectoris, history of MI, documented silent ischemia, ischemic heart disease, concurrent ergotamine-containing preparations, uncontrolled hypertension, hypersensitivity, severe renal disease (CCr <15 ml/min), severe hepatic disease (Child-Pugh grade C), CV syndromes, hemiplegic or basilar migraines

Precautions: Pregnancy **C,** breastfeeding, children, geriatric, postmenopausal women, men >40 yr, risk factors for CAD, hypercholesterolemia, obesity, diabetes, impaired renal/hepatic function, peripheral vascular disease

DOSAGE AND ROUTES
Adult: PO 1 or 2.5 mg with fluids; if headache returns, repeat once after 4 hr, max 5 mg/24 hr

Renal/hepatic dose
Adult: PO CCr 15-39 ml/min
Max 2.5 mg/24 hr

Available forms: Tabs 1, 2.5 mg

Implementation
• Do not use product if another 5-HT$_1$ agonist or an ergot preparation has been used in past 24 hr
• Give with fluids as soon as symptoms appear; may take another dose after 4 hr; max 5 mg in any 24-hr period
• Provide a quiet, calm environment with decreased stimulation, including noise, bright light, excessive talking

ADVERSE EFFECTS
CNS: Dizziness, sedation, fatigue
CV: Increased B/P, palpitations, **tachydys-rhythmias, PR and QT$_C$ prolongation, ST/T wave changes, PVCs, atrial flutter, fibrillation, coronary vasospasm**
EENT: EENT infections, photophobia
GI: *Nausea, vomiting*
MISC: Temp change sensations, tightness, pressure sensations
MS: *Weakness, neck stiffness,* myalgia

Pharmacokinetics
Absorption	Unknown
Distribution	28%-31% protein binding
Metabolism	Liver (metabolite)
Excretion	Urine/feces
Half-life	6 hr

Pharmacodynamics
Onset	Unknown
Peak	2-3 hr
Duration	Unknown

INTERACTIONS
Individual drugs
Sibutramine: increased serotonin syndrome risk

Drug classifications
5-HT$_1$ agonists, ergot derivatives: increased vasospastic effect
MAOIs: increased risk of adverse reactions, do not use together
SSRIs (fluoxetine, fluvoxamine, PARoxetine, sertraline), SNRIs, serotonin receptor agonists, sibutramine: increased serotonin syndrome, **neuroleptic malignant syndrome**

Drug/herb
SAMe, St. John's wort: increased serotonin syndrome

NURSING CONSIDERATIONS
Assessment
• **Serotonin syndrome, neuroleptic malignant syndrome:** assess for increased heart rate, shivering, sweating, dilated pupils, tremors, high B/P, hyperthermia, headache, confusion; if these occur, stop product, administer a serotonin antagonist if needed; at least 2 wk should elapse between discontinuing serotoninergic agents and starting this product
• **Migraines:** assess for aura, duration, effect of lifestyle, aggravating/alleviating factors
• Cardiac status: ECG, increased B/P, dysrhythmias
• Assess for stress level, activity, recreation, coping mechanisms
• Assess neurologic status: LOC, blurred vision, nausea, tics preceding headache

Nursing diagnoses
• Knowledge, deficient (teaching)
• Noncompliance (teaching)
• Pain, acute (uses)

Patient/family education
• Teach patient to report pain, tightness in chest, neck, throat, or jaw; notify prescriber immediately if sudden, severe abdominal pain occurs
• Teach patient to use contraception while taking product, to notify prescriber if pregnancy is planned or suspected
• Teach patient not to use if another 5-HT$_1$ agonist or an ergot preparation has been used in the past 24 hr; avoid using >2 days/wk, rebound headache may occur

Evaluation
Positive therapeutic outcome
• Absence of migraine headaches

---

natalizumab (Rx)
(na-ta-liz'u-mab)
Tysabri
Func. class.: Biological response modifier, immunoglobulins, monoclonal antibody
Pregnancy category C

ACTION: Biological response modifying properties mediated through specific receptors on cells, may be secondary to blockade of the interaction by inflammatory cells on vascular endothelial cells

Therapeutic outcome: Decreased symptoms of multiple sclerosis

USES: Ambulatory patients with relapsing-remitting multiple sclerosis who have not responded to other treatment, moderate to severe Crohn's disease

N

CONTRAINDICATIONS:
Hypersensitivity, immunocompromised individuals (HIV, AIDS, leukemia, lymphoma, transplants), PML, murine (mouse) protein allergy

> **BLACK BOX WARNING:** Progressive multifocal leukoencephalopathy

Precautions: Pregnancy **C**, breastfeeding, geriatric, chronic progressive multiple sclerosis, depression, mental disorders, diabetes, TB, active infections, hepatotoxicity

DOSAGE AND ROUTES
Adult: IV INF 300 mg q4wk, give over 1 hr, observe during and for 1 hr after inf

Available forms: Single-use vial, 300 mg/100 ml 0.9% NaCl

Implementation
• Give acetaminophen for fever, headache
• Give only after being enrolled in the TOUCH Prescribing Program

Intermittent IV INF route
• Use only clear, colorless solution, without particulates
• Withdraw 15 ml from the vial using aseptic technique: inject conc into 100 ml 0.9% NaCl; do not use other diluents; mix completely; do not shake; infuse immediately or refrigerate for up to 8 hr; warm to room temperature before using; flush with 0.9% NaCl before, after inf; do not admix or use in same line with other agents
• Withhold product at first sign of PML
• Store solution in refrigerator; do not freeze or shake; protect from light; use within 8 hr of preparation

ADVERSE EFFECTS
CNS: *Headache, fatigue,* rigors, syncope, tremors, *depression,* **PML (progressive multifocal leukoencephalopathy), suicidal ideation,** anxiety
CV: Chest discomfort, hyper/hypotension, tachycardia
GI: *Abdominal discomfort,* abnormal liver function tests, gastroenteritis, **severe hepatic injury**
GU: Amenorrhea, *UTI, irregular menses,* vaginitis, urinary frequency
INTEG: *Rash,* dermatitis, pruritus, **skin melanoma,** infusion-related reactions
MS: *Arthralgia,* myalgia
RESP: *Lower respiratory tract infection,* dyspnea
SYST: **Anaphylaxis, angioedema**

Pharmacokinetics
Absorption	Unknown
Distribution	Unknown
Metabolism	Unknown
Excretion	Unknown
Half-life	Approximately 11 days

Pharmacodynamics
Unknown

INTERACTIONS
Drug classifications
Do not use with vaccines
Immunosuppressants, antineoplastics, immunomodulators: increased infection

NURSING CONSIDERATIONS
Assessment

> **BLACK BOX WARNING:** Assess for progressive multifocal leukoencephalopathy (weakness, paralysis, vision loss, impaired speech, cognitive deterioration), notify prescriber immediately

• Monitor blood, renal, hepatic tests: CBC, differential, platelet counts, BUN, creatinine, ALT, urinalysis, for hypersensitivity reactions
• Assess CNS symptoms: headache, fatigue, depression, rigors, tremors
• Assess GI status: abdominal discomfort
• Assess mental status: depression, depersonalization, suicidal thoughts, insomnia
• **Assess for multiple sclerosis symptoms;** this product should only be used in patients who have not responded to other treatments
⚠ **Assess for anaphylaxis: shortness of breath, hives; swelling, tightness in throat, chest pain; usually within 2 hr of inf**
• Monitor using gadolinium-enhanced MRI scan of the brain, possibly CSF for JC viral DNA

Nursing diagnoses
• Injury, risk for (uses, adverse reactions)
• Knowledge, deficient (teaching)
• Mobility, impaired physical (uses)

Patient/family education
• Provide patient or family member with written, detailed information about the product
• Teach female patients they may experience irregular menses, amenorrhea
• Instruct patient to notify prescriber if pregnancy is suspected
• Instruct patient to avoid breastfeeding while taking this product

• Instruct patient to notify prescriber of possible infection: sore throat, cough, increased temp

Evaluation
Positive therapeutic outcome
• Decreased symptoms of multiple sclerosis

natamycin ophthalmic
See Appendix B

nebivolol (Rx)
(ne-biv'oh-lol)
Bystolic
Func. class.: Antihypertensive
Chem. class.: β_1-Blocker
Pregnancy category C

ACTION: Competitively blocks stimulation of β-adrenergic receptors within vascular smooth muscle; decreases rate of SA node discharge, increases recovery time, slows conduction of AV node resulting in decreased heart rate (negative chronotropic effect), which decreases O_2 consumption in myocardium due to β_1-receptor antagonism; also decreases renin-aldosterone-angiotensin system at high doses, inhibits β_2-receptors in bronchial system (high doses)

Therapeutic outcome: Decreased B/P after 1-2 wk

USES: Hypertension alone or in combination

Unlabeled uses: Heart failure

CONTRAINDICATIONS:
Cardiogenic shock, sick sinus syndrome, AV heart block, hypersensitivity to this agent or β-blockers, heart failure, severe hepatic disease, severe bradycardia

Precautions: Pregnancy C, breastfeeding, children, major surgery, peripheral vascular disease, diabetes mellitus, thyrotoxicosis, COPD, asthma, well-compensated heart failure, renal/hepatic disease, abrupt discontinuation, acute bronchospasm

DOSAGE AND ROUTES
Hypertension
Adult: PO 5 mg/day, may be increased to desired response q2wk; max 40 mg/day
Geriatric: PO max 40 mg/day

Renal dose
Adult: PO CCr <30 ml/min, 2.5 mg/day; may increase cautiously

Hepatic dose
Adult: PO (Child-Pugh class B) 2.5 mg qd; use dose escalation cautiously

Heart failure (unlabeled)
Adult: PO 1.25 mg titrated to max 10 mg/day

Available forms: Tabs 2.5, 5, 10, 20 mg

Implementation
PO route
• Give without regard for meals; tab may be crushed or swallowed whole; give with food to prevent GI upset
• Store protected from light, moisture; place in cool environment

ADVERSE EFFECTS
CNS: *Insomnia, fatigue, dizziness, mental changes,* drowsiness, headache
CV: Bradycardia, MI, AV heart block, edema
GI: *Nausea, diarrhea,* vomiting, abdominal pain
GU: *Impotence*
HEMA: Thrombocytopenia
INTEG: Rash, pruritus, vasculitis, urticaria, psoriasis, **angioedema**
MISC: Renal failure, pulmonary edema, hyperuricemia, hypercholesterolemia
RESP: Bronchospasm, dyspnea

Pharmacokinetics

Absorption	Unknown
Distribution	Unknown
Metabolism	In liver by CYP2D6
Excretion	38% excreted in urine, 44% in feces
Half-life	12 hr

Pharmacodynamics

Onset	Unknown
Peak	1.5-4 hr
Duration	Unknown

INTERACTIONS
Individual drugs
Cimetidine: increased nebivolol action
Mefloquine: do not give
Sildenafil: decreased nebivolol action

Drug classifications
β-blockers, others: do not use concurrently
Calcium channel blockers (nondihydropyridine), CYP2D6 inhibitors (amiodarone,

N

buPROPion, chloroquine, chlorpheniramine, chlorproMAZINE, cinacalcet, diphenhydrA-MINE, duloxetine, fluoxetine, haloperidol, imatinib, paroxetine, promethazine, propoxyphene, quiNIDine, quiNINE, ritonavir, terbinafine, thioridazine): increased nebivolol action

CYP2D6 inducers (rifampin): decreased nebivolol action

Drug/herb
Hawthorn: may increase nebivolol effect
Ephedra: decreased nebivolol effect

Drug/lab test
Increased: serum lipoprotein levels, BUN, potassium, triglyceride, uric acid, LDH, AST, ALT, blood glucose, alkaline phosphatase
Positive: ANA titer

NURSING CONSIDERATIONS

Assessment
• **Hypertension:** monitor B/P during beginning treatment, periodically thereafter; assess apical/radial pulse before administration; notify prescriber of any significant changes (pulse <50 bpm); **signs of CHF** (dyspnea, crackles, weight gain, jugular vein distention)
• Assess baselines in renal/hepatic studies before therapy begins and periodically
• Monitor I&O, edema in feet, legs daily
• Monitor skin turgor, dryness of mucous membranes for hydration status, especially geriatric patients

Nursing diagnoses
• Cardiac output, decreased (uses)
• Knowledge, deficient (teaching)
• Noncompliance (teaching)

Patient/family education
⚠ **Caution patient not to discontinue product abruptly; severe cardiac reactions may occur; taper over 2 wk; do not double dose; if a dose is missed, take as soon as remembered up to 4 hr before next dose**
• Inform patient product may mask signs of hypoglycemia or alter blood glucose levels
• Advise patient not to use OTC products containing α-adrenergic stimulants (such as nasal decongestants, OTC cold preparations) unless directed by prescriber
• Instruct patient to report low pulse, dizziness, confusion, depression, fever
• Teach patient to take pulse, B/P at home; advise when to notify prescriber
• Advise patient to comply with weight control, dietary adjustments, modified exercise program

• Instruct patient to carry emergency ID to identify product, allergies
• Caution patient to avoid hazardous activities if dizziness, drowsiness are present
• **Instruct patient to report symptoms of CHF:** difficulty breathing, especially on exertion or when lying down, night cough, swelling of extremities
• Teach patient to continue with required lifestyle changes (exercise, diet, weight loss, stress reduction)

Evaluation
Positive therapeutic outcome
• Decreased B/P after 1-2 wk
• Decreased dysrhythmias

TREATMENT OF OVERDOSE:
Lavage, **IV** atropine for bradycardia, **IV** theophylline for bronchospasm, digoxin, O$_2$, diuretic for cardiac failure, **IV** glucose for hypoglycemia, **IV** diazepam (or phenytoin) for seizures, **IV** fluids, **IV** pressors

---

⚠ HIGH ALERT

nelarabine (Rx)
(nella-ra′ben)
Arranon, Atriance ✤
Func. class.: Antineoplastic
Chem. class.: Purine analog
Pregnancy category D

ACTION: Leukemic blasts allow incorporation into DNA, thus interfering with cell replication, leading to cell death

Therapeutic outcome: Decreased growth of malignant cells

USES: T-cell lymphoblastic leukemia, T-cell lymphoblastic lymphoma after relapse or treatment failure with at least two chemotherapeutic agents

CONTRAINDICATIONS:
Pregnancy **D**, hypersensitivity

Precautions: Breastfeeding, children, geriatric, renal/hepatic disease

BLACK BOX WARNING: Seizure disorder, IM administration, neurological disease, peripheral neuropathy

---

DOSAGE AND ROUTES

Adult: IV 1500 mg/m² over 2 hr on days 1, 3, 5 repeated q21day

Infant ≥2 mo, child, adolescent: IV 650 mg/m² over 1 hr/day × 5 days, repeated q21day

Available forms: Sol for inj 5 mg/ml (50 ml)

Implementation

Intermittent IV infusion route
• Visually inspect for particulate or discoloration whenever possible
• Do not dilute before use; transfer needed amount to PVC infusion bag or glass container; stable up to 8 hr in these containers; infuse over 2 hr (adult), 1 hr (child)
• Provide **IV** hydration and allopurinol in risk of hyperuricemia
• Use procedures for proper handling/disposal of anticancer products
• Rinse mouth tid-qid with water, club soda; brush teeth bid-tid with soft brush or cotton-tipped applicators for stomatitis; use unwaxed dental floss
• Store at room temperature

ADVERSE EFFECTS

CNS: Dizziness, *fatigue*, insomnia, rigors, **seizures,** peripheral neuropathy, **paralysis,** confusion, headache, **Guillain-Barré syndrome,** depression, drowsiness, encephalopathy
CV: Edema
GI: *Nausea, vomiting, anorexia, diarrhea, stomatitis, constipation*
HEMA: **Neutropenia,** leukopenia, **thrombocytopenia,** anemia
META: Decreased potassium, calcium, magnesium, albumin, bilirubin, AST, ALT, hyperuricemia; increased glucose
MS: Myalgia, arthralgia, back pain, weakness
RESP: **Pleural effusion,** cough, dyspnea, wheezing, epistaxis
SYST: **Tumor lysis syndrome (TLS)**

Pharmacokinetics

Absorption	Unknown
Distribution	Unknown
Metabolism	Liver
Excretion	Kidneys
Half-life	30 min-3 hr

Pharmacodynamics
Unknown

INTERACTIONS

Drug classifications
Anticoagulants, NSAIDs, platelet inhibitors, salicylates: increased bleeding risk
Toxoids, vaccinations (live virus): do not use

NURSING CONSIDERATIONS

Assessment
• **Tumor lysis syndrome:** assess for hyperkalemia, hyperphosphatemia, hyperuricemia, hypocalcemia
• Monitor CBC (RBC, Hct, Hgb), differential platelet count weekly; withhold products if WBC is <4000/mm³, platelet count is <75,000/mm³, or RBC, Hct, Hgb low; notify prescriber of these results
• Monitor renal function tests: BUN, serum uric acid, urine CCr, electrolytes before, during therapy
• Monitor temp; fever may indicate beginning infection; no rectal temps
• Monitor liver function tests before, during therapy: bilirubin, ALT, AST, alk phos as needed or monthly
• Assess for bleeding: hematuria, heme-positive stools, bruising or petechiae, mucosa or orifices

> **BLACK BOX WARNING: Assess for neurotoxicity:** somnolence, confusion, seizures, ataxia, paresthesias, hypoesthesia, coma, status epilepticus, craniospinal demyelination; contact prescriber immediately, those with NCI common toxicity criteria ≥ grade 2, product should be discontinued

• Assess for dyspnea, crackles, unproductive cough, chest pain, tachypnea, fatigue, increased pulse, pallor, lethargy, personality changes
• Assess buccal cavity q8hr for dryness, sores or ulceration, white patches, oral pain, bleeding, dysphagia
• **Assess for GI symptoms:** frequency of stools, cramping; if severe diarrhea occurs, fluid and electrolytes may need to be given

Nursing diagnoses
• Injury, risk for (uses, adverse reactions)

Patient/family education
• Advise patient to avoid foods with citric acid, hot or rough texture if stomatitis is present; OTC products
• Advise patient to use contraception while taking this product, pregnancy **D**
• Advise patient to avoid using while breastfeeding

• **Teach patient to report signs of infection:** increased temp, sore throat, flulike symptoms
• Teach patient to report signs of anemia: fatigue, headache, faintness, shortness of breath, irritability
• Teach patient to report bleeding; to avoid use of razors, commercial mouthwash
• Advise patient that seizures may occur; not to operate machinery or drive until effects are known; to report numbness, paresthesias, weakness
• Advise patient not to receive vaccinations while taking this product

Evaluation
Positive therapeutic outcome
• Decreased spread of malignancy

nelfinavir (Rx)
(nell-fin′a-veer)
Viracept
Func. class.: Antiretroviral
Chem. class.: Protease inhibitor
Pregnancy category B

ACTION: Inhibits HIV-1 protease, which prevents maturation of the infectious virus

USES: HIV-1 in combination with other antiretrovirals

CONTRAINDICATIONS:
Hypersensitivity to protease inhibitors

Precautions: Pregnancy **B**, breastfeeding, hemophilia, PKU, renal/hepatic disease, pancreatitis, diabetes, infection

DOSAGE AND ROUTES
HIV infection
Adult and child >13 yr: PO 750 mg tid or 1250 mg bid
Child 2-13 yr: PO 25-30 mg/kg tid, max 2500 mg/day

Prevention of HIV infection after exposure (unlabeled)
Adult: PO 1250 mg bid with two other antiretroviral agents × 4 wk

Available forms: Tabs 250, 625 mg; oral powder 50 mg/g/scoop

Implementation
• Administer with food
• Oral powder can be mixed with fluids; do not mix with juice or acidic fluids; stable mixed for 6 hr; do not mix with water in original bottle

ADVERSE EFFECTS
CNS: Headache, asthenia, poor concentration, **seizures, suicidal ideation**
CV: Bleeding
ENDO: Hyperglycemia, hyperlipidemia
GI: Diarrhea, nausea, anorexia, dyspepsia, *flatulence,* **hepatitis, pancreatitis**
HEMA: Anemia, leukopenia, thrombocytopenia, Hgb abnormalities
INTEG: Rash, dermatitis, **anaphylaxis**
MS: Pain, arthralgia, myalgia, myopathy
OTHER: Hypoglycemia, redistribution/accumulation of body fat, **immune reconstitution syndrome**

Pharmacokinetics
Absorption	Unknown
Distribution	98% protein binding
Metabolism	Liver (minimal)
Excretion	Feces/urine
Half-life	$3^{1}/_{2}$-5 hr

Pharmacodynamics
Onset	Unknown
Peak	2-4 hr
Duration	Unknown

INTERACTIONS
Individual drugs
Amiodarone, lovastatin, midazolam, pimozide, quiNIDine, salmeterol, simvastatin, triazolam: increased serious dysrhythmias
Alfentanil, alosetron, atorvastatin, azithromycin, bortezomib, buprenorphine, busPIRone, cilostazol, cycloSPORINE, disopyramide, docetaxel, dofetilide, donepezil, ethosuximide, fentaNYL, galantamine, gefitinib, halofantrine, indinavir, levomethadyl, systemic lidocaine, paclitaxel, rifabutin, saquinavir, sibutramine, sildenafil, sirolimus, SUFentanil, tacrolimus, trazadone, ziprasidone, zonisamide: increased effect of each product
CarBAMazepine, nevirapine, PHENobarbital, phenytoin, rifamycin: decreased nelfinavir levels
Delavirdine: increased protease inhibitor levels
Didanosine, methadone, phenytoin: decreased effect
Indinavir, ketoconazole, ritonavir: increased nelfinavir levels

Drug classifications
Calcium channel blockers, tricyclic antidepressants, vinca alkaloids: increased effects
Contraceptives (oral): decreased effect
Ergots: increased serious dysrhythmias

HIV protease inhibitors: increased protease inhibitor levels

Drug/herb
St. John's wort: decreased antiretroviral effect, do not use concurrently

Drug/food
Increased: absorption with food

Drug/lab test
Increased: AST, ALT, alkaline phosphatase, total bilirubin, CPK, LDH

NURSING CONSIDERATIONS
Assessment
• Assess resistance testing at initiation and failure of treatment
• Assess signs of infection, anemia
• Monitor liver function tests: ALT, AST
• Assess bowel pattern before, during treatment; if severe abdominal pain with bleeding occurs, product should be discontinued; monitor hydration
• **Anaphylaxis, hypersensitivity reaction:** assess for wheezing, flushing, swelling of lips, tongue, throat, skin eruptions, rash, urticaria, itching
• **HIV:** Monitor blood studies: serum lipid profile, plasma HIV RNA, blood glucose, viral load, CD_4 cell counts baseline, throughout treatment
• **Immune reconstitution syndrome:** occurs with combination therapy; includes MAC, CMV, PCP, TB that require treatment

Nursing diagnoses
• Infection, risk for (uses)
• Knowledge, deficient (teaching)

Patient/family education
• Advise patient to take with meal or snack; if dose is missed, take as soon as remembered up to 1 hr before next dose; do not double dose
• Advise patient to avoid taking with other medications, unless directed by prescriber
• Teach patient that product does not cure, but manages symptoms; does not prevent transmission of HIV to others
• Teach patient to use nonhormonal form of contraception while taking this product
• Teach to report symptoms of hyperglycemia

Evaluation
Positive therapeutic outcome
• Decreasing symptoms of HIV
• Improving viral load and CD4 cell counts

neomycin topical
See Appendix B

nepafenac ophthalmic
See Appendix B

⚠ HIGH ALERT

nesiritide (Rx)
(nes-eer'ih-tide)
Natrecor
Func. class.: Vasodilator
Chem. class.: Human B-type natriuretic peptide
Pregnancy category C

ACTION: Uses DNA technology; human B-type natriuretic peptide binds to the receptor in vascular smooth muscle and endothelial cells, leading to smooth muscle relaxation

Therapeutic outcome: Improvement in symptoms of CHF

USES: Acutely decompensated CHF

CONTRAINDICATIONS:
Hypersensitivity to this product or *E. coli* protein, cardiogenic shock or B/P <90 mm Hg as primary therapy

Precautions: Pregnancy **C,** breastfeeding, children, mitral stenosis; significant valvular stenosis, restriction, or obstructive cardiomyopathy, or any condition that depends on venous return; renal disease, constrictive pericarditis

DOSAGE AND ROUTES
Adult: BOL **IV** 2 mcg/kg, then CONT **IV** INF 0.01 mcg/kg/min

Available forms: Powder for inj, 1.5 mg single-use vial

Implementation
IV route
• Do not administer nesiritide through a central heparin-coated catheter; heparin should be administered through a separate catheter
• Reconstitute one 1.5 mg vial/5 ml of diluent from prefilled 250 ml plastic **IV** bag with diluent of choice (D_5, 0.9% NaCl, D_5/0.9% NaCl, D_5/0.2% NaCl); do not shake vial, roll gently; use only clear sol
• Withdraw all contents of reconstituted vial and add to the 250-ml plastic **IV** bag (6 mcg/ml); invert bag several times
• Use within 24 hr of reconstituting

N

Adverse effects: *italics* = common; **bold** = life-threatening

Direct IV route
- Prime tubing with 5 ml of inf sol, calculate dose based on patients' weight, $0.33 \times$ patient weight (kg) = bolus vol (ml) (6 mcg/ml), withdraw prescribed bolus dose (volume) from prepared inf bag; give over 1 min through IV port

Intermittent IV INF route
- After bolus dose, use inf, give at 0.1 ml/kg/hr (0.01 mcg/kg/min)

Y-site compatibilities: Acyclovir, alfentanil, allopurinol, amifostine, aminocaproic acid, aminophylline, amiodarone, amphotericin B colloidal, amphotericin B lipid complex, amphotericin B liposome, anidulafungin, argatroban, atenolol, atracurium, azithromycin, aztreonam, bivalirudin, bleomycin, buprenorphine, busulfan, butorphanol, calcium acetate/chloride/gluconate, CARBOplatin, carmustine, ceFAZolin, cefotaxime, cefotetan, cefoxitin, ceftazidime, ceftizoxime, cefTRIAXone, cefuroxime, chloramphenicol, cimetidine, ciprofloxacin, cisatracurium, CISplatin, clindamycin, cyclophosphamide, cycloSPORINE, cytarabine, dacarbazine, DACTINomycin, DAUNOrubicin, digoxin, diltiazem, diphenhydrAMINE, docetaxel, dolasetron, doxacurium, DOXOrubicin, doxycycline, droperidol, ePHEDrine, epirubicin, ertapenem, erythromycin, esmolol, etoposide, etoposide phosphate, famotidine, fenoldopam, fentaNYL, filgrastim, fluconazole, fludarabine, fluorouracil, foscarnet, fosphenytoin, ganciclovir, gatifloxacin, gemcitabine, gemtuzumab, glycopyrrolate, granisetron, haloperidol, hydrocortisone, HYDROmorphone, hydrOXYzine, IDArubicin, ifosfamide, imipenem-cilastatin, irinotecan, ketorolac, leucovorin, levofloxacin, lidocaine, linezolid, LORazepam, magnesium sulfate, mannitol, mechlorethamine, melphalan, meropenem, mesna, metaraminol, methohexital, methotrexate, methylPREDNISolone, metoclopramide, metroNIDAZOLE, midazolam, milrinone, minocycline, mitomycin, mitoxantrone, mivacurium, moxifloxacin, mycophenolate, nalbuphine, naloxone, niCARdipine, nitroglycerin, nitroprusside, octreotide, ondansetron, oxaliplatin, oxytocin, paclitaxel, palonosetron, pamidronate, pancuronium, pemetrexed, pentamidine, PENTobarbital, PHENobarbital, phentolamine, phenylephrine, polymyxin B sulfate, potassium chloride/phosphates, prochlorperazine, propranolol, quiNIDine, quinupristin-dalfopristin, ranitidine, remifentanil, rocuronium, sodium acetate/bicarbonate/phosphates, streptozocin, succinylcholine, SUFentanil, tacrolimus, teniposide, theophylline, thiotepa, ticarcillin, tigecycline, tirofiban, tolazoline, topotecan, torsemide, trimethobenzamide, vancomycin, vasopressin, vecuronium, verapamil, vinBLAStine, vinCRIStine, vinorelbine, zidovudine, zoledronic acid

ADVERSE EFFECTS

CNS: Headache, insomnia, dizziness, anxiety, confusion, paresthesia, tremor
CV: *Hypotension,* **tachycardia,** dysrhythmias, bradycardia, ventricular tachycardia, ventricular extrasystoles, **atrial fibrillation**
GI: Vomiting, nausea
INTEG: Rash, sweating, pruritus, inj site reaction
MISC: Back pain, abdominal pain
RESP: Increased cough, hemoptysis, **apnea**

Pharmacokinetics

Absorption	Vascular smooth muscle and endothelial cells
Distribution	Unknown
Metabolism	Unknown
Excretion	Bound to cell surfaces, internalized, and proteolyzed; cleaved by endopeptidases on vascular lumenal surface; renal filtration
Half-life	18 min

Pharmacodynamics

Onset	15 min
Peak	1 hr
Duration	Unknown

INTERACTIONS

Drug classifications
ACE inhibitors, antihypertensives, inotropes, **IV** nitrates: increased symptomatic hypotension

NURSING CONSIDERATIONS

Assessment
- Assess PCWP, RAP, cardiac index, MPAP, B/P, pulse during treatment until stable
- Monitor I&O, daily weight, serum creatinine, BUN
- **Assess for CHF:** weight gain, dyspnea, crackles, I&O ratios, peripheral edema

Nursing diagnoses
- Knowledge, deficient (teaching)
- Tissue perfusion, ineffective (uses)

Patient/family education
- Explain purpose of medication and expected results

⚠ Nurse Alert

• Instruct patient to report pain at IV site

Evaluation
Positive therapeutic outcome
• Improvement in CHF with improved PCWP, RAP, MPAP

nevirapine (Rx)
(ne-veer′a-peen)
Viramune, Viramune XR
Func. class.: Antiretroviral
Chem. class.: Non-nucleoside reverse transcriptase inhibitor (NNRTI)
Pregnancy category B

Do not confuse:
nevirapine/nelfinavir, **Viramune**/Viracept

ACTION: Binds directly to reverse transcriptase and blocks RNA, DNA, causing a disruption of the enzyme's site

Therapeutic outcome: Improvement of HIV-1 infection

USES: HIV-1 in combination with other highly active antiretroviral treatments (HAART)

CONTRAINDICATIONS:

> **BLACK BOX WARNING:** Hypersensitivity, hepatic disease

Precautions: Pregnancy **B**, breastfeeding, children, renal disease, Hispanic patients

> **BLACK BOX WARNING:** Females, hepatitis

DOSAGE AND ROUTES
Treatment of HIV infection in combination with other antiretrovirals
Adult and adolescent: PO 200 mg/day × 2 wk, then 200 mg bid in combination; ext rel tab (adults not currently taking immediate release nevirapine) 200 mg/day (immediate rel tab) × 14 days with other antiretrovirals; if rash develops during lead-in period and persists beyond 14 days, do not use ext rel tab; if no consistent rash is present then give 400 mg q day ext rel tab with other antiretrovirals; if interrupted > 7 days, restart 14-day lead-in dosing; adults switched from immediate-release tab, 400 mg q day ext rel tab
Neonate ≥15 days old/infant/child: PO 150 mg/m²/day × 14 days, then 150 mg/m² bid; max 400 mg/day

Perinatal transmission prophylaxis (unlabeled)
Females with no previous antiretroviral therapy: PO 200 mg as a single dose at onset of labor with zidovudine 2 mg/kg over 1 hr followed by zidovudine 1 mg/kg/hr until delivery
Neonate ≥34 wk gestation: PO nevirapine 2 mg/kg as a single dose at age 48-72 hr and PO zidovudine 2 mg/kg q6hr for 6 wk

Hepatic dose
Adult: PO do not use in Child-Pugh B or C

Available forms: Tabs 200 mg; oral susp 50 mg/5 ml; ext rel tabs: 400 mg

Implementation
• Do not initiate treatment in females when CD4 counts >250 cells/mm³, or in males when >400 cells/mm³ unless benefit outweighs risks
• Give without regard to meals
• Give at equal intervals around the clock to maintain blood levels

ADVERSE EFFECTS
CNS: *Paresthesia, headache, fever, peripheral neuropathy*
GI: *Diarrhea,* abdominal pain, *nausea, stomatitis,* **hepatotoxicity, hepatic failure**
HEMA: **Neutropenia, anemia, thrombocytopenia**
INTEG: *Rash,* **toxic epidermal necrolysis**
MISC: **Stevens-Johnson syndrome, anaphylaxis**
MS: Pain, myalgia, **rhabdomyolysis**

Pharmacokinetics
Absorption	Rapid
Distribution	Protein binding 60%
Metabolism	Liver, by P450 enzyme system
Excretion	91% urine
Half-life	25-30 hr 50% removed by peritoneal dialysis; slower clearance rate in Hispanics, African Americans

Pharmacodynamics
Onset	Unknown
Peak	4 hr
Duration	Unknown

INTERACTIONS
Individual drugs
Cimetidine: increased nevirapine levels
ClonazePAM, diazepam, warfarin: decreased nevirapine level

Adverse effects: *italics* = common; **bold** = life-threatening

Itraconazole: decreased effect of itraconazole
Ketoconazole: decreased effect of ketoconazole
Methadone: decreased effect of methadone

Drug classifications
Anticonvulsants, rifamycins: decreased nevirapine levels
Antiinfectives, macrolides: increased nevirapine levels
Oral contraceptives, protease inhibitors: decreased action

Drug/herb
St. John's wort: decreased nevirapine levels, do not use together

Drug/lab test
Increased: ALT, AST, GGT, bilirubin, Hgb
Decreased: neutrophil count

NURSING CONSIDERATIONS

Assessment
• Use resistance testing before starting and when therapy fails
• **Assess signs of infection,** anemia, hepatotoxicity, immune reconstitution syndrome
• **HIV:** Assess liver, renal, blood tests: ALT, AST, viral load, CD4, plasma HIV RNA, glucose levels in diabetic patients; if liver function tests are elevated significantly, product should be withheld
• Assess bowel pattern before, during treatment; if severe abdominal pain with bleeding occurs, product should be discontinued; monitor hydration
⚠ **Assess skin eruptions; rash, urticaria, itching; if rash is severe or systemic symptoms occur, discontinue immediately**
• Assess allergies before treatment, reaction to each medication
• **Rhabdomyolysis:** assess for pain, tenderness, weakness, edema; product should be discontinued
⚠ **Stevens-Johnson syndrome, toxic epidermal necrolysis, assess for allergies before treatment, reaction to each medication; skin eruptions; rash, urticaria, itching; if rash is severe or systemic symptoms occur, discontinue immediately**

Nursing diagnoses
• Diarrhea (side effects)
• Infection, risk for (uses)
• Knowledge, deficient (teaching)

Patient/family education
• Instruct patient to report immediately any right quadrant pain, yellowing of eyes/skin, dark urine, nausea, anorexia, muscle pain/tenderness, rash

• Inform patient that product may be taken with food, antacids
• Advise patient to take as prescribed; if dose is missed, take as soon as remembered up to 1 hr before next dose; do not double dose
• Advise patient that product must be taken in equal intervals around the clock to maintain blood levels for duration of therapy
• Advise patient that product is not a cure, controls symptoms of HIV, does not prevent transmission
• Instruct patient to avoid OTC agents unless approved by prescriber
• Advise patient to use a nonhormonal form of contraception during treatment

Evaluation
Positive therapeutic outcome
• Improving viral load and CD4 cell counts
• Absence of AIDS-defining symptoms
• Improvement in quality of life

---

niacin (Rx, OTC)
(nye′a-sin)
Equaline Niacin, Niaspan, Ni-Odan ✦, Slo-Niacin
niacinamide (Rx, OTC)
(nye-a-sin′a-mide)
Func. class.: Vitamin B₃ lipid-lowering product
Chem. class.: Water-soluble vitamin
Pregnancy category C

ACTION: Needed for conversion of fats, protein, carbohydrates by oxidation-reduction; acts directly on vascular smooth muscle, causing vasodilatation; reduces LDL, VLDL, total cholesterol, triglycerides, increases HDL

Therapeutic outcome: Decreasing cholesterol and LDL levels, B₃ supplementation

USES: Pellagra, hyperlipidemias (types IV, V), peripheral vascular disease that presents a risk for pancreatitis

CONTRAINDICATIONS: Breastfeeding, hypersensitivity, peptic ulcer, hepatic disease, hemorrhage, severe hypotension

Precautions: Pregnancy **C**, breastfeeding, glaucoma, CV disease, CAD, diabetes mellitus, gout, schizophrenia

---

⚠ Nurse Alert

DOSAGE AND ROUTES

Niacin deficiency
Adult: PO 100-500 mg/day in divided doses; IM/SUBCUT 5-100 mg 5 or more times a day; **IV** 25-100 mg bid or tid
Child: PO up to 300 mg/day in divided doses

Adjunct in hyperlipidemia
Adult: 250 mg after evening meal, may increase dosage at 1-4 wk intervals to 1-2 g tid, max 6 g/day; EXT REL 500 mg at bedtime, ×4 wk, then 1000 mg at bedtime for wk 5-8, do not increase by more than 500 mg q4wk, max 2000 mg/day

Pellagra
Adult: PO 300-500 mg/day in divided doses, IM 50-100 mg 5 ×/day or IV 25-100 mg bid by slow IV INF
Child: PO 100-300 mg/day in divided doses; IV up to 300 mg/day by slow IV/INF

Peripheral vascular disease (unlabeled)
Adult: PO 250-800 mg/day in 3-5 divided doses

Available forms: Niacin: tabs 50, 100, 250, 500 mg; ext rel caps 250, 500 mg; ext rel tabs 250, 500, 750, 1000 mg; niacinamide: tabs 100, 500 mg

Implementation
PO route
• Do not break, crush, or chew ext rel products
• Give with meals or milk for GI symptoms, with 81-325 mg of aspirin or NSAIDs $\frac{1}{2}$ hr before dose to decrease flushing

ADVERSE EFFECTS
CNS: Paresthesias, headache, dizziness, anxiety
CV: Postural hypotension, vasovagal attacks, dysrhythmias, vasodilatation
EENT: Blurred vision, ptosis
GI: Nausea, vomiting, anorexia, *jaundice,* diarrhea, peptic ulcer, **hepatotoxicity,** dyspepsia, **hepatitis**
GU: Hyperuricemia, **glycosuria, hypoalbuminemia**
INTEG: Flushing, dry skin, rash, pruritus, itching, tingling

Pharmacokinetics

Absorption	Well absorbed (PO)
Distribution	Widely distributed
Metabolism	Converted to niacinamide
Excretion	Urine, unchanged (30%); breast milk
Half-life	45 min

Pharmacodynamics

	PO	IV
Onset	Unknown	Unknown
Peak	30-70 min	Unknown
Duration	Unknown	Unknown

INTERACTIONS

Individual drugs
Alcohol: increased flushing, pruritus, avoid use

Drug classifications
Ganglionic blockers: increased postural hypotension
HMG-CoA reductase inhibitors: increased myopathy, rhabdomyolysis

Drug/herb
Red yeast rice: increased myopathy, rhabdomyolysis

Drug/lab test
Increased: bilirubin, alkaline phosphatase, liver enzymes, LDH, uric acid, glucose
Decreased: cholesterol
False increase: urinary catecholamines
False positive: urine glucose

NURSING CONSIDERATIONS

Assessment
• **Assess for niacin deficiency (pellagra):** nausea, vomiting, stomatitis, confusion, hallucinations before, throughout treatment
• **Hyperlipidemia:** assess for lipid, triglyceride, cholesterol level, if using for hyperlipidemia
• Assess nutrition: fat, protein, carbohydrates, nutritional analysis should be completed by dietitian
• **Hepatotoxicity:** monitor liver function tests: AST, ALT, bilirubin, uric acid, alkaline phosphatase; blood glucose before, during treatment; liver dysfunction: clay-colored stools, itching, dark urine, jaundice
• Monitor niacin levels during administration of this product
• Monitor cardiac status: rate, rhythm, quality; postural hypotension, dysrhythmias
• Monitor nutritional status: liver, yeast, legumes, organ meat, lean poultry; high-level niacin products should be included in the diet
• Assess for CNS symptoms: headache, paresthesias, blurred vision

Nursing diagnoses
• Knowledge, deficient (teaching)
• Noncompliance (teaching)
• Nutrition: less than body requirements, imbalanced (uses)

N

Patient/family education
• Advise patient that flushing and increase in feelings of warmth will occur several hr after taking product (PO); after 2 wk of therapy these side effects diminish
• Instruct patient to remain recumbent if postural hypotension occurs; to rise slowly from sitting or recumbency
• Caution patient to abstain from alcohol if product is prescribed for hyperlipidemia
• Caution patient to avoid sunlight if skin lesions are present
• **Hepatotoxicity:** Advise patient to report clay-colored stools, anorexia, yellow eyes/skin, dark urine

Evaluation
Positive therapeutic outcome
• Decreased lipid levels
• Warm extremities
• Absence of numbness in extremities

niCARdipine (Rx)
(nye-card'i-peen)
Cardene IV, Cardene SR
Func. class.: Calcium channel blocker, antianginal, antihypertensive
Chem. class.: Dihydropyridine
Pregnancy category C

Do not confuse:
niCARdipine/NIFEdipine, **Cardene**/Cardizem, **Cardene SR**/Cardizem SR

ACTION: Inhibits calcium ion influx across cell membrane during cardiac depolarization, produces relaxation of coronary vascular smooth muscle and peripheral vascular smooth muscle, dilates coronary arteries, increases myocardial oxygen delivery in patients with vasospastic angina

Therapeutic outcome: Decreased angina pectoris, decreased B/P in hypertension

USES: Chronic stable angina pectoris, hypertension

CONTRAINDICATIONS:
Sick sinus syndrome, 2nd- or 3rd-degree heart block, hypersensitivity to this product or dihydropyridine, advanced aortic stenosis

Precautions: Pregnancy C, breastfeeding, children, geriatric, CHF, hypotension, hepatic injury, renal disease

DOSAGE AND ROUTES
Hypertension
Adult: PO 20 mg tid initially; may increase after 3 days (range 20-40 mg tid) or SUS REL 30 mg bid; may increase to 60 mg bid **IV** 5 mg/hr; may increase by 2.5 mg/hr q15min; max 15 mg/hr

Angina
Adult: PO 20 mg tid, may be adjusted q3day, may use 20-40 mg tid

Renal dose
Adult: PO 20 mg tid or SUS REL 30 mg bid

Hepatic dose
Adult: PO 20 mg bid

Available forms: Caps 20, 30 mg; sus rel caps 30, 45, 60 mg; inj 2.5 mg/ml, premixed 20 mg/200 ml, 40 mg/200 ml

Implementation
PO route
• Do not break, crush, chew, or open sus rel caps
• Give without regard to meals
• Store in airtight container at room temperature

IV route
• Dilute each 25 mg/240 ml of compatible sol (0.1 mg/ml), give slowly, titrate to patient's response, stable for 24 hr at room temperature, change IV site q30 min

Solution compatibilities: D_5W, $D_5/0.45\%$ NaCl, $D_5/0.9\%$ NaCl

Y-site compatibilities: Alemtuzumab, amikacin, aminophylline, aztreonam, bivalirudin, butorphanol, calcium gluconate, CARBOplatin, caspofungin, ceFAZolin, ceftizoxime, chloramphenicol, cimetidine, CISplatin, clindamycin, cytarabine, DAPTOmycin, dexmedetomidine, diltiazem, DOBUTamine, docetaxel, DOPamine, DOXOrubicin hydrochloride, enalaprilat, EPINEPHrine, epirubicin, erythromycin, esmolol, famotidine, fenoldopam, fentaNYL, gentamicin, hydrocortisone, HYDROmorphone, labetalol, lidocaine, linezolid, LORazepam, magnesium sulfate, mechlorethamine, methylPREDNISolone, metroNIDAZOLE, midazolam, milrinone, morphine, nafcillin, nesiritide, nitroglycerin, nitroprusside, norepinephrine, octreotide, oxaliplatin, oxytocin, palonosetron, penicillin G potassium, potassium chloride/phosphate, quinupristin-dalfopristin, ranitidine, rocuronium, tacrolimus, tirofiban, tobramycin, trimethoprim/sulfamethoxazole, vancomycin, vasopressin, vecuronium, vinCRIStine, voriconazole, zoledronic acid

Y-site incompatibilities: Amphotericin B liposome/lipid complex, ampicillin,
ampicillin/sulbactam, cefepime, cefoperazone,
ertapenem, fluorouracil, furosemide, methotrexate, micafungin, pantoprazole, pemetrexed,
thiopental, thiotepa, tigecycline

ADVERSE EFFECTS
CNS: *Headache, dizziness,* anxiety, depression, confusion, paresthesia, somnolence,
flushing
CV: Edema, bradycardia, hypotension, palpitations, **pulmonary edema,** chest pain, tachycardia, increased angina, **arrhythmias, CHF**
GI: Nausea, vomiting, gastric upset, constipation, **hepatitis,** abdominal cramps, dry mouth,
sore throat
GU: Nocturia, polyuria
INTEG: Rash, infusion site discomfort,
Stevens-Johnson syndrome
MISC: Blurred vision, flushing, sweating, SOB,
impotence

Pharmacokinetics
Absorption	Well absorbed (PO); bioavailability poor
Distribution	Unknown
Metabolism	Liver, extensively
Excretion	Kidneys 60%, feces 35%
Half-life	2-5 hr

Pharmacodynamics
	PO	PO SUS REL
Onset	$1/2$ hr	Unknown
Peak	1-2 hr	2-6 hr
Duration	8 hr	10-12 hr

INTERACTIONS
Individual drugs
Alcohol: increased hypotension
CarBAMazepine, cycloSPORIINE, prazosin, pro-
pranolol, quiNIDine: increased risk of toxicity
Cimetidine: increased niCARdipine effects
Digoxin, quiNIDine, theophylline: increased
effects
Rifampin: decreased antihypertensive effect

Drug classifications
Antihypertensives, neuromuscular blocking
agents, nitrates: increased hypotension
NSAIDs: decreased antihypertensive effect

Drug/herb
Ginkgo, ginseng, hawthorn: increased effect
Ephedra, melatonin, St. John's wort, yohimbe:
decreased effect

Drug/food
Grapefruit juice: increased hypotensive effect

NURSING CONSIDERATIONS
Assessment
• Assess fluid volume status (I&O ratio) and
record weight, color, quality, and specific gravity
of urine, skin turgor, adequacy of pulses, moist
mucous membranes, bilateral lung sounds,
peripheral pitting edema; dehydration symptoms
of decreasing output, thirst, hypotension, dry
mouth, and mucous membranes should be
reported
• **Monitor for CHF:** weight gain, crackles,
jugular venous distention, dyspnea
• **Hypertension:** assess for decreasing B/P;
salt in diet, smoking, exercise, diet, weight
• **Assess anginal pain:** intensity, location,
duration, alleviating factors
• Monitor potassium, renal/liver function tests,
periodically

Nursing diagnoses
• Cardiac output, decreased (uses)
• Knowledge, deficient (teaching)

Patient/family education
• Advise patient to avoid hazardous activities
until stabilized on product and dizziness is no
longer a problem
• Instruct patient to limit caffeine consumption; to avoid alcohol and OTC products unless
directed by a prescriber
⚠ **Hypertension: instruct patient to comply
with all areas of medical regimen: diet,
exercise, stress reduction, product therapy**
• Instruct patient to notify prescriber of irregular heartbeat, shortness of breath, swelling of
feet and hands, pronounced dizziness, constipation, nausea, hypotension, change in severity/
pattern/incidence of angina
• Teach patient to use medication as directed
even if feeling better; may be taken with other
cardiovascular products (nitrates, β-blockers)
• Teach patient to take medication exactly as
prescribed
• Advise patient to contact prescriber if anginal
attacks continue or become worse

Evaluation
Positive therapeutic outcome
• Decreased angina attacks
• Decreased B/P

TREATMENT OF OVERDOSE:
Defibrillation, atropine for AV block, vasopressor for hypotension

Adverse effects: *italics* = common; **bold** = life-threatening

nicotinamide
See niacin

nicotine
(nik'o-teen)
nicotine chewing gum (OTC, Rx)
CVS Nicotine Polacrilex, Equate Nicotine, Good Sense Nicotine, Leader Nicotine Gum, GNP Nicotine, NICO-relief, Nicorette, Publix Stop Smoking Aid, TopCare Nicotine, Walgreens Nicotine
nicotine inhaler (OTC, Rx)
Nicotrol Inhaler
nicotine lozenge (OTC)
CVS Nicotine Polacrilex, GNP Nicotine Polacrilex, Good Sense Nicotine, Polacrilex Lozenge, TopCare Nicotine Polacrilex Lozenge, Walgreens Nicotine Polacrilex Lozenge
nicotine nasal spray (Rx)
Nicotrol NS
nicotine transdermal (OTC, Rx)
CVS Nicotine Transdermal System, Equate Nicotine Transdermal System, Habitrol ✿, Leader Nicotine Transdermal Patch, Nicoderm CQ, Sunmark Nicotine Transdermal System, Walgreens Nicotine Transdermal Patch

Func. class.: Smoking deterrent
Chem. class.: Ganglionic cholinergic agonist
Pregnancy category D (transdermal), C (gum)

ACTION: Agonist at nicotinic receptors in the peripheral and central nervous systems; acts at sympathetic ganglia, on chemoreceptors of the aorta and carotid bodies; also affects adrenalin-releasing catecholamines

Therapeutic outcome: Decreased withdrawal effects when smoking cessation is attempted

USES: Deter cigarette smoking

Unlabeled uses: Tourette's syndrome

CONTRAINDICATIONS:
Pregnancy **D** (transdermal, inhaler), hypersensitivity, immediate post-MI recovery period, severe angina pectoris

Precautions: Pregnancy **C** (gum), breastfeeding, vasospastic disease, dysrhythmias, diabetes mellitus, hyperthyroidism, pheochromocytoma, coronary disease, esophagitis, peptic ulcer, renal/hepatic disease; MRI (patch)

DOSAGE AND ROUTES
Nicotine chewing gum
Adult: If patient smokes ≤25 cigarettes/day, start with 2 mg gum; if >25 cigarettes/day, start with 4 mg gum; then 1 piece of gum q1-2hr × 6 wk, then 1 piece of gum q2-4hr × 2 wk, then 1 piece of gum q4-8hr × 2 wk, then discontinue; max 24/day

Nicotine inhaler
Adult: Inhale 6 cartridges/day for first 3-6 wk, max 16/day × 12 wk

Nicotine lozenge
Adult: If cigarette is desired >30 min after awakening, start with 1-2–mg lozenge; if <30 min after awakening, start with 4-mg lozenge; then 1 q1-2hr, max 20 lozenges/day or 5 lozenges/6 hr × 6 wk, then 1 lozenge q2-4hr × 2 wk, then 1 lozenge q4-8hr × 2 wk, then discontinue

Nicotine nasal spray
Adult: 1 spray in each nostril 1-2 ×/hr, max 5 ×/hr or 40 ×/day, max 3 mo

Nicotine transdermal/inhaler system
Habitrol ✿, NicoDerm
Adult: 21 mg/day × 4-8 wk; 14 mg/day × 2-4 wk; 7 mg/day × 2-4 wk

Nicotrol
Adult: 15 mg/day × 12 wk; 10 mg/day × 2 wk; 5 mg/day × 2 wk

Nicotrol inhaler
Adult: Delivers 30% of what a smoker receives from an actual cigarette

Tourette's syndrome (unlabeled)
Adult and child: Chewing gum 2 mg chewed × ¹/₂ hr bid × 1-6 mo; transdermal 7 or 10 mg patch daily × 2 days

Available forms: Gum: 2, 4 mg/piece; nicotine transdermal system (Habitrol ✿, NicoDerm, Nicotine Transdermal System); 7, 14, 21 mg/day delivered; (NicoDerm) 5, 10, 15 mg/day; nicotine inhaler: 4 mg delivered; nasal spray: 0.5 mg of nicotine/actuation; lozenge: 2 mg, 4 mg

Implementation

- Give only prescribed amount, or toxicity may occur
- **Gum:** chew gum slowly for 30 min to promote buccal absorption of the product; do not chew > 45 min
- Begin product withdrawal after 3 mo of use; do not exceed 6 mo
- **Transdermal patch:** apply once a day to a nonhairy, clean, dry area of skin on upper body or upper outer arm; rotate sites to prevent skin irritation
- **Inhaler:** puffing on mouthpiece delivers nicotine through the mouth

ADVERSE EFFECTS

CNS: Dizziness, vertigo, insomnia, headache, confusion, **seizures,** depression, euphoria, numbness, tinnitus, strange dreams
CV: Dysrhythmias, tachycardia, palpitations, edema, flushing, hypertension
EENT: Jaw ache, irritation in buccal cavity
GI: *Nausea, vomiting, anorexia, indigestion,* diarrhea, abdominal pain, constipation, eructation, irritation
RESP: Breathing difficulty, cough, hoarseness, sneezing, wheezing, bronchial spasm

Pharmacokinetics

Absorption	Slowly absorbed, buccal cavity
Distribution	Unknown
Metabolism	Liver; some by lungs, kidneys
Excretion	Kidneys, unchanged (20%); breast milk
Half-life	1-2 hr

Pharmacodynamics

Onset	Rapid
Peak	$1/2$ hr
Duration	Unknown

INTERACTIONS

Individual drugs

Bromocriptine, cabergoline: increased vasoconstriction
Adenosine: increased effects
BuPROPion: increased B/P
Insulin: decreased effect
Cimetidine: decreased nicotine clearance

Drug classifications

Ergots: increased vasoconstriction
α-Blockers: decreased effect

Drug/food

Acidic foods (colas, coffee): avoid use of gum with and for 15 min after

NURSING CONSIDERATIONS

Assessment

- **Assess for adverse reaction to gum:** irritation of buccal cavity, dislike of taste, jaw ache
- **Assess for withdrawal symptoms:** headache, fatigue, drowsiness, restlessness, irritability, severe cravings for nicotine products before, during, and after treatment
- **Smoking:** obtain a nicotine assessment: brand of cigarettes, chewing tobacco, cigars, number of each used per day; what increases need or activities performed when each is used
- Gum should not be used if temporomandibular condition exists
- **Assess for nicotine toxicity:** GI symptoms (nausea, vomiting, diarrhea), cardiopulmonary symptoms (decreased B/P, dyspnea, change in pulse), weakness, abdominal cramping, headache, blurred vision, tinnitus; product should be discontinued

Nursing diagnoses

- Coping, ineffective (uses)
- Knowledge, deficient (teaching)
- Noncompliance (teaching)

Patient/family education

- Advise patient to begin product withdrawal after 3 mo use; max 6 mo
- Teach patient all aspects of product; give package insert to patient and explain; caution patient not to exceed prescribed dose
- Caution patient not to use during pregnancy; birth defects may occur

Gum

- Advise patient to chew gum slowly for 30 min to promote buccal absorption of the product; do not chew over 45 min
- Inform patient that gum will not stick to dentures, dental appliances
- Caution patient that gum is as toxic as cigarettes; it is to be used only to deter smoking

Transdermal patch

- Caution patient that patch is as toxic as cigarettes; to be used only to deter smoking
- Caution patient not to use during pregnancy; birth defects may occur
- Instruct patient to keep used and unused system out of reach of children and pets

N

• Instruct patient to apply once a day to a non-hairy, clean, dry area of skin on upper body or upper outer arm; to rotate sites to prevent skin irritation
• Instruct patient to stop smoking immediately when beginning patch treatment
• Teach patient to apply promptly after removing from protective pouch; system may lose strength
• **Nasal spray:** tilt head back, do not swallow or inhale during administration; after smoking is stopped, use spray up to 8 wk, then discontinue over 6 wk by tapering
• **Lozenges:** allow to dissolve, avoid swallowing
• **Inhalation:** use the inhaler for 20 min
• Advise patient that puffing on mouthpiece delivers nicotine through the mouth lining

Evaluation
Positive therapeutic outcome
• Decrease in urge to smoke
• Decreased need for gum after 3-6 mo

NIFEdipine (Rx)
(nye-fed'i-peen)
Adalat CC, Afedtab CR, Apo-Nifed ✻, Apo-Nifed PA ✻, Nifediac CC, Nifedical XL, Procardia, Procardia XL
Func. class.: Calcium channel blocker, antianginal, antihypertensive
Chem. class.: Dihydropyridine
Pregnancy category C

Do not confuse:
NIFEdipine/niCARdipine/niMODipine

ACTION: Inhibits calcium ion influx across cell membrane during cardiac depolarization, produces relaxation of coronary vascular smooth muscle, dilates coronary vascular arteries, increases myocardial oxygen delivery in patients with vasospastic angina, dilates peripheral arteries

Therapeutic outcome: Decreased angina pectoris, decreased B/P in hypertension

USES: Chronic stable angina pectoris, vasospastic angina, hypertension

CONTRAINDICATIONS:
Hypersensitivity to this product or dihydropyridine, cardiogenic shock

Precautions: Pregnancy C, breastfeeding, children, CHF, hypotension, sick sinus

syndrome, 2nd- or 3rd-degree heart block, hypotension less than 90 mm Hg systolic, hepatic injury, renal disease, acute MI, aortic stenosis, GERD, heart failure

DOSAGE AND ROUTES
Adult: PO immediate release, 10 mg tid; increase in 10-mg increments q7-14day, max 180 mg/24 hr or single dose of 30 mg; SUS REL 30-60 mg/day; may increase q7-14day; doses >120 mg not recommended

Hypertension
Adult: PO EXT REL 30-60 mg qd, titrate upward as needed; max 90 mg/day (Adalat CC); 120 mg/day (Procardia XL)
Adolescent/child (unlabeled): PO EXT REL 0.25-0.5 mg/kg/day, max 3 mg/kg/day

Available forms: Caps 5 ✻, 10, 20 mg; ext rel tabs (CC, XL) 10 ✻, 20 ✻, 30, 60, 90 mg; tabs 10 mg ✻

Implementation
PO route
• Give without regard to meals
• Store in airtight container at room temperature
Sublingual route
• Using a sterile needle, puncture the cap and squeeze medication in buccal/sublingual area (not an FDA-approved use)

ADVERSE EFFECTS
CNS: *Headache,* fatigue, drowsiness, *dizziness,* anxiety, depression, weakness, insomnia, *light-headedness,* paresthesia, tinnitus, blurred vision, nervousness, tremor, flushing
CV: Dysrhythmias, edema, hypotension, palpitations, tachycardia
GI: *Nausea,* vomiting, diarrhea, gastric upset, constipation, increased LFTs, dry mouth, flatulence, gingival hyperplasia
GU: Nocturia, polyuria
HEMA: Bruising, bleeding, petechiae
INTEG: Rash, pruritus, *flushing,* hair loss, **Stevens-Johnson syndrome, toxic epidermal necrolysis, exfoliative dermatitis**
MISC: Sexual difficulties, cough, fever, chills

Pharmacokinetics

Absorption	Well absorbed (PO)
Distribution	Unknown
Metabolism	Liver, extensively
Excretion	Unknown
Half-life	2-5 hr

Pharmacodynamics

	PO	PO EXT REL
Onset	$^1/_2$ hr	Unknown
Peak	Unknown	Unknown
Duration	6-8 hr	24 hr

INTERACTIONS

Individual drugs
Cimetidine, ranitidine: increased risk of toxicity
CarBAMazepine, cycloSPORINE, phenytoin, prazosin, digoxin: increased levels of each product
QuiNIDine: decreased effects
Smoking: decreased NIFEdipine level

Drug classifications
Strong CYP3A4 inducers: use is contraindicated
Antihypertensives, β-adrenergic blockers: increased effects
NSAIDs: decreased antihypertensive effect

Drug/herb
Ginkgo biloba, ginseng, hawthorn: increased effect
Ephedra, melatonin, St. John's wort, yohimbe: decreased effect

Drug/food
Grapefruit juice: increased NIFEdipine level

Drug/lab test
Positive: ANA titer, direct Coombs' test
Increased: CPK, LDH, AST

NURSING CONSIDERATIONS

Assessment
• **Assess anginal pain:** location, intensity, duration, character, alleviating, aggravating factors
• Assess for bruising, petechiae, bleeding
• Monitor potassium, renal/liver function tests periodically during treatment
• **Serious skin disorders:** rash starts suddenly, assess for fever, cutaneous lesions, may have pustules; discontinue product
• Assess fluid volume status (I&O ratio) and record weight, distended red veins, crackles in lung, color, quality, and specific gravity of urine, skin turgor, adequacy of pulses, moist mucous membranes, bilateral lung sounds, peripheral pitting edema; dehydration symptoms of decreasing output, thirst, hypotension, dry mouth, and mucous membranes should be reported
• Monitor cardiac status: B/P, pulse, respirations, ECG

Nursing diagnoses
• Cardiac output, decreased (uses)
• Knowledge, deficient (teaching)
• Pain, acute (uses)

Patient/family education
• Advise patient to avoid hazardous activities until stabilized on product and dizziness is no longer a problem
• Instruct patient to limit caffeine consumption; to avoid alcohol and OTC products unless directed by prescriber
• Tell patient that ext rel tab has nonabsorbable shell, may appear in stools
• **Hypertension:** instruct patient to comply in all areas of medical regimen: diet, exercise, stress reduction, product therapy
• Tell patient to notify prescriber of irregular heartbeat, SOB, swelling of feet and hands, pronounced dizziness, constipation, nausea, hypotension, severe rash, changes in pattern/frequency/severity of angina
• Teach patient to use as directed even if feeling better; may be taken with other cardiovascular products (nitrates, β-blockers)
• Advise patient to increase fluid intake to prevent constipation
• Teach patient to check for gingival hyperplasia and report promptly
• Teach patient not to discontinue abruptly; gradually taper

Evaluation
Positive therapeutic outcome
• Decreased angina attacks
• Decreased B/P

TREATMENT OF OVERDOSE:
Defibrillation, atropine for AV block, vasopressor for hypotension

---

nilotinib (Rx)
(nye-loe'ti-nib)
Tasigna
Func. class.: Antineoplastic—miscellaneous
Chem. class.: Protein-tyrosine kinase inhibitor
Pregnancy category D

ACTION: Inhibits BCR-ABL tyrosine kinase created in chronic myeloid leukemia (CML)

Therapeutic outcome: Decrease in progression of disease

USES: Chronic phase/accelerated phase Philadelphia chromosome–positive chronic myelogenous leukemia that is resistant/intolerant to imatinib

N

Adverse effects: *italics* = common; **bold** = life-threatening

CONTRAINDICATIONS:
Pregnancy **D**, breastfeeding, hypersensitivity

> **BLACK BOX WARNING:** Hypokalemia, hypomagnesemia, QT prolongation

Precautions: Children, women, geriatric patients, active infections, anemia, cardiac disease, bone marrow suppression, cholestasis, diabetes, gelatin hypersensitivity, infertility, galactose-free diet, lactase deficiency, neutropenia, pancreatitis, thrombocytopenia

> **BLACK BOX WARNING:** Hepatic disease

DOSAGE AND ROUTES
Adult: PO 400 mg q12h; continue until disease progression or unacceptable toxicity

Escalation regimen for those taking a strong CYP3A4 inducer
Adult: PO increase dose as required

Adjustment following discontinuation of a strong CYP3A4 inducer
Adult: PO reduce to 400 mg/bid

For those taking a strong CYP3A4 inhibitor
Adult: PO reduce dose to 400 mg/day

QT prolongation
QTcF >480 msec: Withhold dose

ANC 1 × 10⁹/L or platelets <50 × 10⁹/L: Withhold dose

Myelosuppression
ANC 1×10^9/L or platelets $<50 \times 10^9$/L: Withhold dose

Hepatic Dose
Adult: PO (Child-Pugh classes A-C): newly diagnosed CML 200 mg bid, then escalation to 300 mg bid initially

Available forms: Caps 150, 200 mg

Implementation
• Do not break, crush, or chew caps; if a whole capsule cannot be swallowed, disperse capsule contents in 1 tsp of applesauce
• Give without regard to meals; separate doses by 12 hr; a make-up dose should not be taken if a dose is missed
• Store at 15°-30° C (59°-86° F)

ADVERSE EFFECTS
CNS: Headache, dizziness, fatigue, fever, flushing, paresthesia
CV: QT prolongation, palpitations, **torsades de pointes**
GI: *Nausea,* hepatotoxicity, vomiting, dyspepsia, *anorexia, abdominal pain,* constipation, **pancreatitis,** diarrhea

HEMA: Neutropenia, thrombocytopenia, anemia, pancytopenia
INTEG: *Rash,* alopecia, erythema
META: Hyperamylasemia, hyperbilirubinemia, hyperglycemia, hyperkalemia, hypocalcemia, hyponatremia, hypomagnesemia
MISC: Diaphoresis
MS: Arthralgia, myalgia, back/bone pain, muscle cramps
RESP: Cough, dyspnea
SYST: Bleeding

Pharmacokinetics
Absorption	Unknown
Distribution	Protein binding 98%, plasma levels 3 hr
Metabolism	By CYP3A4
Excretion	Unknown
Half-life	Elimination 17 hr

Pharmacodynamics
Unknown

INTERACTIONS
Individual drugs
• Product interactions are numerous
Acetaminophen: increased hepatotoxicity
CarBAMazepine, dexamethasone, PHENobarbital, phenytoin, rifampin: decreased concentrations
Clarithromycin, erythromycin, itraconazole, ketoconazole: increased concentrations
Haloperidol, chloroquine, droperidol, pentamidine, arsenic trioxide, levomethadyl: increased QT prolongation
Pimozide, ziprasidone: do not use concurrently
Simvastatin: increased plasma concentrations
Warfarin: increased plasma concentration; avoid use with warfarin, use low-molecular-weight anticoagulants instead

Drug classifications
Class IA/III antidysrhythmics, some phenothiazines, β-agonists, local anesthetics, tricyclics, CYP3A4 inhibitors (amiodarone, clarithromycin, erythromycin, telithromycin, troleandomycin), CYP3A4 substrates (methadone, pimozide, quetiapine, quiNIDine, risperidone, ziprasidone): increased QT prolongation
Calcium channel blockers: increased plasma concentrations
Phenothiazines: do not use concurrently

Drug/herb
St. John's wort: decreased concentration

⚠ Nurse Alert

Drug/food
Grapefruit juice: increased plasma concentrations

NURSING CONSIDERATIONS

Assessment
- Assess ANC and platelets; if ANC $<1 \times 10^9$/L and/or platelets $<50 \times 10^9$/L, stop until ANC $>1.5 \times 10^9$/L and platelets $>75 \times 10^9$/L
- Monitor CV status: hypertension, QT prolongation can occur; monitor left ventricular ejection fraction (LVEF) baseline periodically
- Assess for renal toxicity: if bilirubin $>3 \times$ IULN, withhold until bilirubin levels return to $<1.5 \times$ IULN
- **Assess for hepatotoxicity:** monitor hepatic function tests, before treatment and qmo; if liver transaminases $>5 \times$ IULN, withhold until transaminase levels return to $<2.5 \times$ IULN
- **Myelosuppression:** Monitor CBC, differential, platelet count weekly; withhold product if WBC is <3500/mm^3 or platelet count $<100,000$/mm^3; notify prescriber of these results; product should be discontinued
- Monitor for bleeding: epistaxis, rectal, gingival, upper GI, genital, and wound bleeding; tumor-related hemorrhage may occur rapidly
- **Monitor electrolytes:** calcium, potassium, magnesium, sodium; lipase, phosphate; hypokalemia, hypomagnesemia should be corrected prior to use
- **QT prolongation:** ECG for QT prolongation, ejection fraction; assess for chest pain, palpitations, dyspnea

Nursing diagnoses
- Knowledge, deficient (teaching)

Patient/family education
- Instruct patient to report adverse reactions immediately: SOB, bleeding
- Inform patient reason for treatment, expected result
- Advise patient that many adverse reactions may occur
- Teach patient to avoid persons with known upper respiratory infections; immunosuppression is common
- Instruct in signs/symptoms of low potassium or magnesium

Evaluation
Positive therapeutic outcome
- Decrease in progression of disease

niMODipine (Rx)
(ni-moe′dip-een)
Nimotop
Func. class.: Calcium channel blocker
Chem. class.: Dihydropyridine
Pregnancy category C

ACTION: Unknown, may have greater effect on cerebral arteries

Therapeutic outcome: Prevention of vascular spasm (subarachnoid hemorrhage)

USES: Prevention of cerebrovascular spasm in subarachnoid hemorrhage

CONTRAINDICATIONS:
Sick sinus syndrome, 2nd- or 3rd-degree heart block, hypotension less than 90 mm Hg systolic, hypersensitivity

Precautions: Pregnancy **C**, breastfeeding, children, geriatric, CHF, hypotension, hepatic injury, renal disease

DOSAGE AND ROUTES
Adult: PO begin therapy within 96 hr, 60 mg q4hr $\times$ 21 days

Available forms: Caps 30 mg

Implementation
- May puncture cap and dilute in water and give through nasogastric tube; flush tube with 0.9% NaCl
- Store in airtight container at room temperature

ADVERSE EFFECTS
CNS: Headache, fatigue, drowsiness, dizziness, anxiety, depression, weakness, insomnia, confusion, paresthesia, somnolence
CV: Dysrhythmia, edema, CHF, bradycardia, hypotension, palpitations, MI, **pulmonary edema**
GI: Nausea, vomiting, diarrhea, gastric upset, constipation, **hepatitis,** abdominal cramps
GU: Nocturia, polyuria, **acute renal failure**
INTEG: Rash, pruritus, urticaria, photosensitivity, hair loss
MISC: Blurred vision, flushing, nasal congestion, sweating, shortness of breath, gynecomastia, hyperglycemia, sexual difficulties

N

Adverse effects: *italics* = common; **bold** = life-threatening

Pharmacokinetics

Absorption	Well absorbed, poor bioavailability
Distribution	Crosses blood-brain barrier
Metabolism	Liver, extensively
Excretion	Kidneys
Half-life	1-2 hr

Pharmacodynamics

Onset	Unknown
Peak	1 hr
Duration	Unknown

INTERACTIONS

Individual drugs
Alcohol: increased hypotension
Digoxin: increased digoxin levels, bradycardia
PHENobarbital, phenytoin: decreased effectiveness
Propranolol: increased toxicity

Drug classifications
Antihypertensives: increased hypotension
β-Adrenergic blockers: increased bradycardia
Nitrates: increased nitrates

Drug/herb
Barberry, betel palm, burdock, goldenseal, khat, khella, lily of the valley, plantain: increased effect
Yohimbe: decreased effect

NURSING CONSIDERATIONS

Assessment
• Assess fluid volume status (I&O ratio) and record weight; distended red veins; crackles in lung; color, quality, and specific gravity of urine; skin turgor; adequacy of pulses; moist mucous membranes; bilateral lung sounds; peripheral pitting edema; dehydration symptoms of decreasing output, thirst, hypotension, dry mouth and mucous membranes should be reported
• Monitor B/P and pulse; if B/P drops 30 mm Hg, call prescriber
• Monitor ALT, AST, bilirubin daily; if these are elevated, hepatotoxicity is suspected

Nursing diagnoses
• Injury, risk for (uses)
• Knowledge, deficient (teaching)

Evaluation
Positive therapeutic outcome
• Prevention of neurologic damage from subarachnoid hemorrhage

nisoldipine (Rx)
(nye'sol-dye-peen)
Sular
Func. class.: Antihypertensive, calcium channel blocker
Chem. class.: Dihydropyridine
Pregnancy category C

ACTION: Inhibits calcium ion influx across cell membrane, resulting in dilatation of peripheral arteries

Therapeutic outcome: Decreased B/P in hypertension

USES: Essential hypertension, alone or with other antihypertensives

CONTRAINDICATIONS: Hypersensitivity to this product or dihydropyridines, sick sinus syndrome, 2nd- or 3rd-degree heart block, aortic stenosis

Precautions: Pregnancy **C,** breastfeeding, children, geriatric, CHF, hypotension <90 mm Hg systolic, hepatic injury, renal disease, acute MI, unstable angina, CAD, cardiogenic shock

DOSAGE AND ROUTES
Adult: PO 17 mg/day initially, may increase by 8.5 mg/wk, usual dose 17-34 mg/day, max 34 mg/day
Geriatric/hepatic dose: PO 8.5 mg/day, increase based on response

Hepatic Dose
Adult: PO 8.5 mg/day

Available forms: Ext rel tabs 8.5, 17, 20, 25.5, 30, 34, 40 mg

Implementation
PO route
• Give once a day, with food to decrease GI symptoms; avoid high-fat foods, grapefruit

ADVERSE EFFECTS
CNS: Headache, fatigue, drowsiness, dizziness, anxiety, depression, nervousness, insomnia, light-headedness, paresthesia, tinnitus, psychosis, somnolence, ataxia, confusion, malaise, migraine, flushing
CV: Dysrhythmias, edema, **CHF,** hypotension, palpitations, **MI, pulmonary edema,** tachycardia, syncope, AV block, angina, chest pain, ECG abnormalities
GI: Nausea, vomiting, diarrhea, gastric upset, constipation, elevated liver function tests, dry mouth, dyspepsia, dysphagia, flatulence

GU: Nocturia, hematuria, dysuria
HEMA: Anemia, leukopenia, petechiae
INTEG: Rash, pruritus
MISC: Sexual difficulties, gingival hyperplasia, chills, fever, gout, sweating, cough, nasal congestion, shortness of breath, wheezing, epistaxis, dyspnea

Pharmacokinetics	
Absorption	Well absorbed
Distribution	Highly protein bound
Metabolism	Liver
Excretion	Kidneys
Half-life	Unknown

Pharmacodynamics	
Onset	Unknown
Peak	6-12 hr
Duration	Unknown

INTERACTIONS
Individual drugs
Cimetidine, ranitidine: increased nisoldipine level
Digoxin: increased effects

Drug classifications
Antifungals (azole), CYP3A4 inhibitors: increased nisoldipine level
Antihypertensives: increased hypotension
β-Adrenergic blockers: increased effects
Hydantoins, CYP3A4 inducers: decreased nisoldipine effect

Drug/herb
Ephedra, melatonin: increased B/P
Hawthorn: decreased B/P
St. John's wort, ginseng, ginkgo biloba: decreased effect

Drug/food
Grapefruit juice: increased hypotension
High-fat foods: increased nisoldipine level

NURSING CONSIDERATIONS
Assessment
• Assess fluid volume status: I&O ratio and record; weight; skin turgor; adequacy of pulses; moist mucous membranes; bilateral lung sounds; peripheral pitting edema; dehydration symptoms of decreasing output, thirst, hypotension, dry mouth and mucous membranes should be reported
• Monitor ALT, AST, bilirubin daily if these are elevated and hepatotoxicity is suspected
• Monitor cardiac status: B/P, pulse, respiration, ECG

Nursing diagnoses
• Cardiac output, decreased (uses)
• Knowledge, deficient (teaching)

Patient/family education
• Caution patient to avoid hazardous activities until stabilized on product and dizziness is no longer a problem
• Instruct patient to limit caffeine consumption; to avoid alcohol and OTC products unless directed by prescriber
• Urge patient to comply in all areas of medical regimen: diet, exercise, stress reduction, product therapy; to notify prescriber of irregular heartbeat, SOB, swelling of feet and hands, pronounced dizziness, constipation, nausea, hypotension
• Teach patient to use as directed even if feeling better; may be taken with other cardiovascular products (nitrates, β-blockers)
• Advise patient to rise slowly to prevent orthostatic hypotension
• Teach patient to report nausea, dizziness, edema, SOB, palpitations

Evaluation
Positive therapeutic outcome
• Decreased B/P

N

nitazoxanide (Rx)
(nye-taz-ox′a-nide)
Alinia
Func. class.: Antiprotozoal
Pregnancy category B

ACTION: Interferes with DNA/RNA synthesis in protozoa

Therapeutic outcome: C&S negative for organism

USES: Diarrhea caused by *Cryptosporidium parvum* or *Giardia lamblia*

CONTRAINDICATIONS:
Hypersensitivity

Precautions: Pregnancy **B,** breastfeeding, children <1 yr or >11 yr, renal/hepatic disease, diabetes mellitus (contains sucrose), HIV, immunocompromised patients

DOSAGE AND ROUTES
Adult: PO 500 mg q12hr × 3 days
Child 4-11 yr: **PO** 10 ml (200 mg) q12hr × 3 days
Child 12-47 mo: **PO** 5 ml (100 mg) q12hr × 3 days

Available forms: Powder for oral susp 100 mg/5 ml; tab 500 mg

Implementation
PO route
- Give with food
- Shake oral susp before giving

ADVERSE EFFECTS
CNS: *Dizziness, fever, headache*
CV: Hypotension
GI: *Nausea,* anorexia, flatulence, increased appetite, enlarged salivary glands, abdominal pain, diarrhea, vomiting
HEMA: Anemia, **leukopenia,** neutropenia
INTEG: Pruritus, sweating
MISC: Increased creatinine, pale yellow eye discoloration, rhinitis, discolored urine, infection, malaise

Pharmacokinetics

Absorption	Unknown
Distribution	Metabolite protein binding >99%
Metabolism	Hydrolyzed to active metabolite, undergoes conjugation
Excretion	Urine, bile, feces
Half-life	Unknown

Pharmacodynamics
Unknown

INTERACTIONS
Drug classifications
Other highly protein-bound products (phenytoin, aspirin): competes for binding sites

Drug/lab test
Increase: creatinine, GPT

NURSING CONSIDERATIONS
Assessment
- Assess for signs of infection
- Assess bowel pattern before, during treatment

Nursing diagnoses
- Infection, risk for (uses)
- Knowledge, deficient (teaching)

Patient/family education
- Advise to take with food; shake susp well before each dose

Evaluation
Positive therapeutic outcome
- C&S negative for organism
- Decreased diarrhea

nitrofurantoin (Rx)
(nye-troe-fyoor′an-toyn)
Apo-Nitrofurantoin ✤, Furadantin, Macrobid, Macrodantin, Novo-Furantoin ✤
Func. class.: Urinary tract antiinfective
Chem. class.: Synthetic nitrofuran derivative
Pregnancy category B

ACTION: Inhibits bacterial acetyl-CoA from interfering with carbohydrate metabolism

Therapeutic outcome: Resolution of infection

USES: Urinary tract infections caused by *Escherichia coli, Klebsiella, Pseudomonas, Proteus vulgaris, Proteus morganii, Serratia, Citrobacter, Staphylococcus aureus, Staphylococcus epidermidis, Enterococcus, Salmonella, Shigella*

CONTRAINDICATIONS:
Infants <1 mo, hypersensitivity, anuria, severe renal disease, CCr <60 ml/min, at term pregnancy (38-42 wk), labor, delivery

Precautions: Pregnancy **B**, breastfeeding, geriatric, G6PD deficiency, GI disease, diabetes, cholestatic jaundice due to nitrofurantoin therapy

DOSAGE AND ROUTES
Active infections
Adult: PO 50-100 mg qid after meals or 50-100 mg at bedtime for long-term treatment
Child: PO 5-7 mg/kg/day in 4 divided doses; 1-2 mg/kg/day for long-term treatment; max 7 mg/kg/day

Chronic suppression
Adult: PO 50-100 mg qPM
Child: PO 2 mg/kg/day qPM or 0.5-1 mg/kg q12hr if dose is not well tolerated

Available forms: Caps 25, 50, 100 mg; susp 25 mg/ml; macrocrystal caps (Macrodantin) 25, 50, 100 mg; cap (Macrobid) 100 mg (25 macrocrystals, 75 monohydrate)

Implementation
- Do not break, crush, chew, or open tabs, caps
- Give after clean-catch urine for C&S
- Give two daily doses if urine output is high or if patient has diabetes

ADVERSE EFFECTS

CNS: *Dizziness, headache,* drowsiness, peripheral neuropathy, chills, confusion, vertigo
CV: Bundle branch block, chest pain
GI: *Nausea, vomiting, abdominal pain, diarrhea,* **cholestatic jaundice,** loss of appetite, **pseudomembranous colitis, hepatitis,** pancreatitis
HEMA: Anemia, agranulocytosis, hemolytic anemia, leukopenia, thrombocytopenia
INTEG: Pruritus, rash, urticaria, **angioedema,** alopecia, tooth staining, **exfoliative dermatitis**
MS: Arthralgia, myalgia, numbness, peripheral neuropathy
RESP: Cough, dyspnea, pneumonitis, pulmonary fibrosis/infiltrate
SYST: Stevens-Johnson syndrome, super-infection, SLE-like syndrome

Pharmacokinetics	
Absorption	Readily absorbed
Distribution	Crosses placenta, excreted in breast milk
Metabolism	Liver, partially
Excretion	Kidneys, 30%-50% unchanged
Half-life	20-60 min

Pharmacodynamics	
Onset	Unknown
Peak	30 min
Duration	6-12 hr

INTERACTIONS

Individual products
Magnesium trisilicate: decreased absorption
Norfloxacin: antagonist effect
Probenecid: increased nitrofurantoin levels

Drug/lab test
Increased: BUN, alkaline phosphatase, bilirubin, creatinine, blood glucose

NURSING CONSIDERATIONS

Assessment
• Monitor blood count during chronic therapy
• Assess CNS symptoms: insomnia, vertigo, headache, drowsiness, seizures
• Assess allergy: fever, flushing, rash, urticaria, pruritus
• **Urinary tract infection:** assess for burning, pain on urination, fever; cloudy, foul-smelling urine; I&O ratio; C&S before treatment, after completion; serum creatinine, BUN

• **Hepatotoxicity:** assess for yellowing of skin, eyes, dark urine, clay-colored stools; monitor AST, ALT
• **Pulmonary fibrosis, pneumonitis:** assess for dyspnea, tachypnea, persistent cough
• **Serious skin disorders:** assess for fever, flushing, rash, urticaria, pruritus
• **Peripheral neuropathy:** assess for paresthesias (more common in diabetes mellitus, electrolyte imbalances, vit B deficiency, debilitated patients)
• **Pseudomembranous colitis:** assess for diarrhea, abdominal pain, fever, fatigue, anorexia; possible anemia, elevated WBC and low serum albumin; stop product and usually give either vancomycin or IV metroNIDAZOLE

Nursing diagnoses
• Infection, risk for (uses)
• Knowledge, deficient (teaching)

Patient/family education
• Teach patient to take with food or milk; avoid alcohol
• Teach patient to protect susp from freezing and shake well before taking
• Teach patient that product may cause drowsiness; instruct client to seek aid in walking and other activities; advise patient not to drive or operate machinery while on medication
• Teach patient that diabetics should monitor blood glucose level
• Teach patient that product may turn urine rust-yellow to brown
⚠ **Teach patient to notify prescriber of symptoms of pseudomembranous colitis: fever, diarrhea with mucous, pus, or blood**

Evaluation
Positive therapeutic outcome
• Decreased dysuria, fever; negative C&S

nitrofurazone topical
See Appendix B

nitroglycerin (Rx)
(nye-troe-gli′ser-in)
extended release caps (Rx)
Nitro-Time
translingual spray (Rx)
Nitrolingual
sublingual (Rx)
Nitrostat
rectal ointment
Rectiv
topical ointment (Rx)
Nitro-Bid
transdermal (Rx)
Minitran, Nitro-Dur
Func. class.: Coronary vasodilator, antianginal
Chem. class.: Nitrate
Pregnancy category C

Do not confuse:
Nitro-Bid/Nicobid

ACTION: Decreases preload and afterload, which thus decreases left ventricular end-diastolic pressure and systemic vascular resistance; dilates coronary arteries and improves blood flow through coronary vasculature, dilates arterial, venous beds systemically

Therapeutic outcome: Prevention of anginal attack

USES: Chronic stable angina pectoris, prophylaxis of angina pain, CHF associated with acute MI, controlled hypotension in surgical procedures, anal fissures

CONTRAINDICATIONS:
Hypersensitivity to this product or nitrites, severe anemia, increased ICP, cerebral hemorrhage, closed-angle glaucoma, cardiac tamponade, cardiomyopathy, constrictive pericarditis

Precautions: Pregnancy **C**, breastfeeding, children, postural hypotension, severe renal/hepatic disease, acute MI, abrupt discontinuation, hyperthyroidism

DOSAGE AND ROUTES
Adult: SL dissolve tab under tongue when pain begins; may repeat q5min until relief occurs; take no more than 3 tab/15 min; use 1 tab prophylactically 5-10 min before activities; SUS REL cap q6-12hr on empty stomach; TOP 1-2 in q8hr; increase to 4 in q4hr as needed; **IV** 5 mcg/min, then increase by 5 mcg/min q3-5min; if no response after 20 mcg/min, increase by 10-20 mcg/min until desired response; transdermal apply a pad daily to a site free from hair; remove patch at bedtime to provide 10-12 hr nitrate-free interval to avoid tolerance
Child: **IV** initial 0.25-0.5 mcg/kg/min, titrate to patient response, usual dose 1-3 mcg/kg/min transmucosal

Anal fisures (Rectiv)
Adult: rectal apply 1 in of 0.4% ointment q12hr × 3 wk

Available forms: Translingual aerosol 0.4 mg/m spray; sus rel caps 2.5, 6.5, 9, 13 mg; sus rel tabs 2.6, 6.5, 9 mg; SL tabs 0.3, 0.4, 0.6 mg; topical joint 2%; trans syst 0.1, 0.2, 0.3, 0.4, 0.6, 0.8 mg/hr; inj 25 mg/250 ml, 50 mg/250 ml, 100 mg/250 ml, 50 mg/500 ml, 100 mg/500 ml, 200 mg/500 ml; rectal ointment 0.4% (Rectiv)

Implementation
PO route
• Swallow sus rel tabs whole; do not break, crush, or chew sus rel tabs
• Give 1 hr before or 2 hr after meals with 8 oz of water
SL route
• Should be dissolved under tongue, not swallowed
Aerosol route
• Sprayed under tongue (nitrolingual); not inhaled, prime before 1st-time use or if product has not been used in > 6 wk; press valve head with forefinger
Transmucosal route
• Tab should be placed between cheek and gum line
• Do not take anything PO when tab is in place
Topical ointment route
• Apply ointment using dose-measuring papers supplied; apply to an area without hair; ointment should cover 2-3–inch area; may apply an occlusive dressing as directed
Transdermal route
• Apply transdermal patches to area without hair; press hard to adhere; if patch becomes dislodged, apply a new one
SL route
• Keep tab in original container
• If 3 SL tab in 15 min do not relieve pain, consider diagnosis of MI
• SL tab should be held under tongue until dissolved (a few min); do not take anything by mouth when SL tab is in place

Rectal route
• Cover finger with plastic wrap, disposable glove or finget cot, lay finger alongside 1 inch dosing line on carton, squeeze tube until equal to 1 inch dosing line, insert covered finger no further than 1st finger joint gently into anal canal and on sides, wash hands thoroughly, if too painful, apply directly to outside of anus

Continuous IV infusion route
• Diluted in D_5, D_5W, 0.9% NaCl for inf to 200-400 mcg/ml depending on patient's fluid status, common dilution is 50 mg/250 ml, use controlled inf device; use glass inf bottles, non–polyvinyl chloride inf tubing; titrate to patient response; do not use filters

Y-site compatibilities: Acyclovir, alfentanil, amikacin, aminocaproic acid, aminophylline, amiodarone, amphotericin B lipid complex, amphotericin B liposome, anidulafungin, argatroban, ascorbic acid, atenolol, atracurium, atropine, azaTHIOprine, aztreonam, benztropine, bivalirudin, bleomycin, bumetanide, buprenorphine, butorphanol, calcium chloride/gluconate, CARBOplatin, caspofungin, cefamandole, ceFAZolin, cefmetazole, cefonicid, cefoperazone, cefotaxime, cefotetan, cefoxitin, ceftazidime, ceftizoxime, cefTRIAXone, cefuroxime, cephalothin, cephapirin, chloramphenicol, chlorproMAZINE, cimetidine, cisatracurium, CISplatin, clindamycin, cloNIDine, cyanocobalamin, cyclophosphamide, cycloSPORINE, cytarabine, DACTINomycin, dexamethasone, digoxin, diltiazem, diphenhydrAMINE, DOBUTamine, docetaxel, DOPamine, doxacurium, DOXOrubicin, doxycycline, drotrecogin alfa, enalaprilat, ePHEDrine, EPINEPHrinc, epirubicin, epoetin alfa, eptifibatide, ertapenem, erythromycin, esmolol, etoposide, famotidine, fenoldopam, fentaNYL, fluconazole, fludarabine, fluorouracil, folic acid, ganciclovir, gatifloxacin, gemcitabine, gemtuzumab, gentamicin, glycopyrrolate, granisetron, heparin, hydrocortisone, HYDROmorphone, hydrOXYzine, IDArubicin, ifosfamide, imipenem-cilastatin, indomethacin, insulin (regular), irinotecan, isoproterenol, ketorolac, labetalol, lidocaine, linezolid, LORazepam, magnesium sulfate, mannitol, mechlorethamine, meperidine, metaraminol, methicillin, methotrexate, methoxamine, methyldopate, methylPREDNISolone, metoclopramide, metroNIDAZOLE, mezlocillin, micafungin, miconazole, midazolam, milrinone, minocycline, mitoxantrone, morphine, moxalactam, mycophenolate, nafcillin, nalbuphine, naloxone, nesiritide, netilmicin, niCARdipine, nitroprusside, norepinephrine, octreotide, ondansetron, oxacillin, oxaliplatin, oxytocin, paclitaxel, palonosetron, pamidronate, pancuronium, pantoprazole, papaverine, pemetrexed, penicillin G potassium/sodium, pentamidine, pentazocine, PENTobarbital, PHENobarbital, phentolamine, phenylephrine, phytonadione, piperacillin, piperacillin-tazobactam, polymyxin B, potassium chloride, procainamide, prochlorperazine, promethazine, propofol, propranolol, protamine, pyridoxine, quiNIDine, quinupristin-dalfopristin, ranitidine, remifentanil, ritodrine, rocuronium, sodium bicarbonate, succinylcholine, SUFentanil, tacrolimus, teniposide, theophylline, thiamine, thiopental, thiotepa, ticarcillin, ticarcillin-clavulanate, tigecycline, tirofiban, tobramycin, tolazoline, trimetaphan, urokinase, vancomycin, vasopressin, vecuronium, verapamil, vinCRIStine, vinorelbine, voriconazole, warfarin, zoledronic acid

Y-site incompatibilities: Alteplase

ADVERSE EFFECTS
CNS: *Headache, flushing, dizziness*
CV: *Postural hypotension,* tachycardia, **collapse,** syncope, palpitations
GI: Nausea, vomiting
INTEG: Pallor, sweating, rash

Pharmacokinetics

Absorption	Well absorbed (PO, buccal, SL)
Distribution	Unknown
Metabolism	Liver, extensively
Excretion	Kidney
Half-life	1-4 min

Pharmacodynamics

	SUS REL	SL	TD	IV	TRANS-MUCOSAL	AEROSOL	TOPICAL OINT
Onset	20-45 min	1-3 min	$1/_2$-1 hr	1-2 min	1-2 min	2 min	$1/_2$-1 hr
Peak	Unknown	Unknown	Unknown	Unknown	Unknown	Unknown	Unknown
Duration	3-8 hr	$1/_2$ hr	12-24 hr	3-5 min	3-5 hr	$1/_2$-1 hr	2-12 hr

Adverse effects: *italics* = common; **bold** = life-threatening

INTERACTIONS

Individual drugs
Alcohol: increased hypotension, CV collapse
Aspirin: increased nitrate level
Heparin: decreased effects (with IV nitroglycerin)
Sildenafil, tadalafil, vardenafil: increased fatal hypotension, do not use together

Drug classifications
Antihypertensives, β-adrenergic blockers, calcium channel blockers, diuretics: increased hypotension

Drug/lab test
Increased: urine catecholamine, urine VMA
False increase: cholesterol

NURSING CONSIDERATIONS

Assessment
• Monitor orthostatic B/P, pulse
• **Assess pain:** duration, time started, activity being performed, character; check for tolerance if taken over long period
• Monitor for headache, light-headedness, decreased B/P; may indicate a need for decreased dosage

Nursing diagnoses
• Cardiac output, decreased (uses)
• Knowledge, deficient (teaching)
• Noncompliance (teaching)
• Poisoning, risk for (uses)
• Tissue perfusion, ineffective (uses)

Patient/family education
• Instruct patient to avoid alcohol
• Advise patient that product may cause headache; tolerance usually develops; use nonopioid analgesic
• Teach patient that product may be taken before stressful activity, exercise, sexual activity
• Inform patient that SL tab may sting when product comes in contact with mucous membranes
• Caution patient to avoid hazardous activities if dizziness occurs
• Instruct patient to comply with complete medical regimen
• Advise patient to make position changes slowly to prevent fainting
⚠ **Advise patient to never use erectile dysfunction products (sildenafil, tadalafil, vardenafil); may cause severe hypotension, death**

Evaluation
Positive therapeutic outcome
• Decreased, prevention of anginal pain

⚠ HIGH ALERT

nitroprusside (Rx)
(nye-troe-pruss'ide)
Nitropress
Func. class.: Antihypertensive, vasodilator
Pregnancy category C

ACTION: Directly relaxes arteriolar, venous smooth muscle, resulting in reduction in cardiac preload, afterload

Therapeutic outcome: Decreased B/P in hypertensive crisis, decreased preload, afterload

USES: Hypertensive crisis, to decrease bleeding by creating hypotension during surgery, acute CHF

CONTRAINDICATIONS:
Hypersensitivity, hypertension (compensatory) due to aortic coarctation or AV shunting, acute CHF associated with reduced peripheral vascular resistance, AV shunt, Leber's disease, toxic amblyopia

BLACK BOX WARNING: Cyanide toxicity

Precautions: Pregnancy C, breastfeeding, children, geriatric, fluid, electrolyte imbalances, renal/hepatic disease, hypothyroidism

BLACK BOX WARNING: Hypotension

DOSAGE AND ROUTES
Adult and child: IV INF 0.25-1.0 mcg/kg/min; max 10 mcg/kg/min

Renal dose
Adult: IV INF CCr <60 ml/min maintain doses <3 mcg/kg/min to reduce thiocyanate accumulation

Available forms: Inj 50 mg 12 ml

Implementation
Continuous IV infusion route
• Depending on B/P reading q15min
• Reconstitute 50 mg/2-3 ml of D₅W, further dilute in 250, 500, or 1000 ml of D₅W to 200, 100, 50 mcg/ml respectively; use an infusion pump only; wrap bottle with aluminum foil to protect from light; observe for color change in the inf; discard if highly discolored (blue, green, dark red); titrate to patient response

Y-site compatibilities: Alfentanil, alprostadil, amikacin, aminocaproic acid,

---

⚠ Nurse Alert

aminophylline, amphotericin B lipid complex, amphotericin B liposome, anidulafungin, argatroban, atenolol, atropine, aztreonam, benztropine, bivalirudin, bleomycin, bumetanide, buprenorphine, butorphanol, calcium chloride/gluconate, CARBOplatin, cefamandole, ceFAZolin, cefmetazole, cefonicid, cefoperazone, cefotaxime, cefotetan, cefoxitin, ceftazidime, ceftizoxime, cefTRIAXone, cefuroxime, cephalothin, chloramphenicol, cimetidine, CISplatin, clindamycin, cyanocobalamin, cyclophosphamide, cycloSPORINE, cytarabine, DACTINomycin, DAPTOmycin, dexamethasone, digoxin, diltiazem, docetaxel, DOPamine, doxacurium, DOXOrubicin, doxycycline, enalaprilat, ePHEDrine, EPINEPHrine, epirubicin, epoetin alfa, eptifibatide, fenoldopam, fentaNYL, fluconazole, fludarabine, fluorouracil, folic acid, furosemide, ganciclovir, gatifloxacin, gemcitabine, gemtuzumab, gentamicin, glycopyrrolate, granisetron, heparin, hydrocortisone, HYDROmorphone, IDArubicin, ifosfamide, inamrinone, indomethacin, insulin (regular), isoproterenol, ketorolac, labetalol, lidocaine, linezolid, LORazepam, magnesium sulfate, mannitol, mechlorethamine, meperidine, metaraminol, methicillin, methoxamine, methyldopate, methylPREDNISolone, metoclopramide, metoprolol, metroNIDAZOLE, mezlocillin, micafungin, miconazole, midazolam, milrinone, minocycline, morphine, moxalactam, multiple vitamins injection, nafcillin, nalbuphine, naloxone, nesiritide, netilmicin, niCARdipine, nitroglycerin, norepinephrine, octreotide, ondansetron, oxacillin, oxaliplatin, oxytocin, paclitaxel, palonosetron, pamidronate, pancuronium, pantoprazole, penicillin G potassium/sodium, pentamidine, PENTobarbital, PHENobarbital, phentolamine, phenylephrine, phytonadione, piperacillin, piperacillin-tazobactam, polymyxin B, potassium chloride/phosphates, procainamide, propofol, propranolol, protamine, pyridoxine, ranitidine, ritodrine, rocuronium, sodium acetate/bicarbonate, succinylcholine, SUFentanil, tacrolimus, teniposide, theophylline, thiamine, ticarcillin, ticarcillin-clavulanate, tigecycline, tirofiban, tobramycin, tolazoline, trimetaphan, urokinase, vancomycin, vasopressin, vecuronium, verapamil, vinCRIStine, zoledronic acid

ADVERSE EFFECTS

CNS: *Dizziness, headache,* agitation, twitching, decreased reflexes, restlessness
CV: Bradycardia, ECG changes, tachycardia, hypotension
GI: Nausea, vomiting, abdominal pain

INTEG: Pain, irritation at inj site, sweating
MISC: Cyanide, thiocyanate toxicity, flushing, hypothyroidism

Pharmacokinetics

Absorption	Complete bioavailability
Distribution	Not known
Metabolism	RBCs, tissues
Excretion	Kidneys
Half-life	3 days; circulating half-life 2 min

Pharmacodynamics

Onset	1-2 min
Peak	Rapid
Duration	1-10 min

INTERACTIONS

Individual drugs
Enflurane, halothane; severe hypotension

Drug classifications
Circulatory depressants, ganglionic blockers, volatile liquid anesthetics: severe hypotension

Drug/herb
Hawthorn: increased antihypertensive effect

NURSING CONSIDERATIONS

Assessment
• Monitor B/P q5min × 2 hr, then qhr × 2 hr; monitor pulse q4hr; monitor jugular venous distention q4hr; ECG should be monitored continuously; monitor PCWP; rebound hypertension may occur after nitroprusside is discontinued
• Monitor electrolytes, blood studies: potassium, sodium, chloride, CO_2, CBC, serum glucose, serum methemoglobin if pulmonary oxygen levels are decreased
• Check weight, I&O, edema in feet and legs daily; assess skin turgor, dryness of mucous membranes for hydration status
• Assess for signs of CHF: dyspnea, edema, wet crackles
⚠ Monitor for increased lactate, cyanide, thiocyanate levels if on long-term treatment; thiocyanate level should be ≤1 millimole/L
• Monitor for decrease in bicarbonate, Pco_2, and blood pH; acidosis may occur with this product

Nursing diagnoses
• Injury, risk for (adverse reactions)
• Knowledge, deficient (teaching)
• Tissue perfusion, ineffective (uses)

N

Patient/family education
• Teach patient to report headache, dizziness, loss of hearing, blurred vision, dyspnea, faintness; may indicate adverse reactions

Evaluation
Positive therapeutic outcome
• Decreased B/P in hypertension
• Absence of bleeding in surgery

TREATMENT OF OVERDOSE:
Administer amyl nitrate inh until 3% sodium nitrate sol can be prepared for **IV** administration, then inject sodium thiosulfate **IV**; correct drop in B/P with vasopressor

---

⚠ HIGH ALERT

norepinephrine
(nor-ep-i-nef′rin)
Levophed
Func. class.: Adrenergic
Chem. class.: Catecholamine
Pregnancy category C

Do not confuse:
norepinephrine/EPINEPHrine

ACTION: Causes increased contractility and heart rate by acting on β-receptors in heart; also acts on a-receptors, thereby causing vasoconstriction in blood vessels; B/P is elevated, coronary blood flow improves, and cardiac output increases

Therapeutic outcome: Increased B/P with stabilization; adequate tissue perfusion

USES: Acute hypotension, shock

CONTRAINDICATIONS:
Hypersensitivity to this product or cyclopropane/halothane anesthesia; ventricular fibrillation, tachydysrhythmias, pheochromocytoma, hypotension, hypovolemia

BLACK BOX WARNING: Extravasation

Precautions Pregnancy C, breastfeeding, geriatric patients, arterial embolism, peripheral vascular disease, hypertension, hyperthyroidism, cardiac disease

DOSAGE AND ROUTES
Adult: IV INF 0.5-1 mcg/min titrated to B/P; maintenance 2-4 mcg/min; max 30 mcg/min

Child: IV INF 0.1-0.2 mcg/kg/min titrated to B/P; max 2 mcg/kg/min

Available forms: Inj 1 mg/ml

Implementation
CONT IV INF route
• Dilute with 500-1000 ml D_5W or D_5/0.9% NaCl; average dilution 4 mg/1000 ml diluent (4 mcg base/ml); give as inf 2-3 ml/min; titrate to response

Y-site compatibilities: Alfentanil, amikacin, amiodarone, anidulafungin, argatroban, ascorbic acid, atenolol, atracurium, atropine, aztreonam, benztropine, bivalirudin, bleomycin, bumetanide, buprenorphine, butorphanol, calcium chloride/gluconate, CARBOplatin, caspofungin, cefamandole, ceFAZolin, cefmetazole, cefonicid, cefoperazone, cefotaxime, cefotetan, cefoxitin, ceftazidime, ceftizoxime, ceftobiprole, cefTRIAXone, cefuroxime, cephalothin, chloramphenicol, chlorproMAZINE, cimetidine, cisatracurium, CISplatin, clindamycin, cloNIDine, cyanocobalamin, cyclophosphamide, cycloSPORINE, cytarabine, DAPTOmycin, dexamethasone, digoxin, diltiazem, diphenhydrAMINE, DOBUTamine, docetaxel, DOPamine, doripenem, doxycycline, enalaprilat, ePHEDrine, EPINEPHrine, epirubicin, epoetin alfa, ertapenem, erythromycin, esmolol, etoposide, famotidine, fenoldopam, fentaNYL, fluconazole, fludarabine, gatifloxacin, gemcitabine, gentamicin, glycopyrrolate, granisetron, heparin, hydrocortisone, HYDROmorphone, hydrOXYzine, IDArubicin, ifosfamide, imipenem-cilastatin, irinotecan, isoproterenol, ketorolac, labetalol, lidocaine, linezolid, LORazepam, magnesium sulfate, mannitol, mechlorethamine, meperidine, meropenem, metaraminol, methicillin, methotrexate, methoxamine, methyldopate, methylPREDNISolone, metoclopramide, metoprolol, metroNIDAZOLE, mezlocillin, micafungin, miconazole, midazolam, milrinone, minocycline, mitoxantrone, morphine, moxalactam, multiple vitamins injection, mycophenolate, nafcillin, nalbuphine, naloxone, netilmicin, niCARdipine, nitroglycerin, nitroprusside, octreotide, ondansetron, oxacillin, oxaliplatin, oxytocin, paclitaxel, palonosetron, pamidronate, pancuronium, papaverine, pemetrexed, penicillin G potassium/sodium, pentamidine, pentazocine, phenylephrine, phytonadione, piperacillin, piperacillin-tazobactam, polymyxin B, potassium chloride, procainamide, prochlorperazine, promethazine, propofol, propranolol, protamine, pyridoxine, quiNIDine, ranitidine, remifentanil, ritodrine, succinylcholine, SUFentanil, tacrolimus, tenipo-

---

side, theophylline, thiamine, thiotepa, ticarcillin, ticarcillin-clavulanate, tigecycline, tirofiban, tobramycin, tolazoline, trimetaphan, urokinase, vancomycin, vasopressin, vecuronium, verapamil, vinCRIStine, vinorelbine, vitamin B complex with C, voriconazole, zoledronic acid

ADVERSE EFFECTS

CNS: *Headache,* anxiety, dizziness, insomnia, restlessness, tremor, **cerebral hemorrhage**
CV: *Palpitations, tachycardia, hypertension, ectopic beats, angina*
GI: *Nausea, vomiting*
GU: Decreased urine output
INTEG: Necrosis, tissue sloughing with extravasation, **gangrene**
RESP: Dyspnea
SYST: Anaphylaxis

Pharmacokinetics	
Absorption	Complete
Distribution	Crosses placenta
Metabolism	Liver
Excretion	Urine

Pharmacodynamics	
Onset	Immediate
Peak	Rapid
Duration	1 min

INTERACTIONS

Individual drugs
Bicarbonate, sodium: incompatible with alkaline solutions
⚠ **Guanethidine, methyldopa: do not use norepinephrine within 2 wk of using these drugs because hypertensive crisis may result**

Drug classifications
α-blockers: decreased norepinephrine action
⚠ **Antihistamines, ergots, MAOIs, oxytocics, tricyclics: do not use norepinephrine within 2 wk of using these drugs because hypertensive crisis may result**
Oxytocics: Increased B/P
MAOIs, tricyclics: increased pressor effect

NURSING CONSIDERATIONS

Assessment
• Assess I&O ratio; notify prescriber if output <30 ml/hr
• Assess B/P, pulse q2-3min after parenteral route, ECG during administration continuously; if B/P increases, product is decreased, CVP or PWP during inf if possible
• Assess paresthesias and coldness of extremities; peripheral blood flow may decrease

> **BLACK BOX WARNING: Extravasation:** inj site: tissue sloughing

• Assess for sulfite sensitivity, which may be life-threatening

Nursing diagnoses
• Potential for injury (uses, adverse reactions)

Patient/family education
• Teach patient about the reason for product administration
• Advise family to report dyspnea, dizziness, chest pain

Evaluation
Positive therapeutic outcome
• Increased B/P with stabilization
• Adequate tissue perfusion

TREATMENT OF OVERDOSE:
Administer fluids, electrolyte replacement

norfloxacin ophthalmic
See Appendix B

N

nortriptyline (Rx)
(nor-trip′ti-leen)
Apo-Nortriptyline ✷**, Arentyl** ✷**, Pamelor**
Func. class.: Antidepressant, tricyclic
Chem. class.: Dibenzocycloheptene, secondary amine
Pregnancy category D

Do not confuse:
nortriptyline/amitriptyline

ACTION: Blocks reuptake of norepinephrine, serotonin into nerve endings, increasing action of norepinephrine, serotonin in nerve cells; has anticholinergic effects

Therapeutic outcome: Decreased symptoms of depression after 2-3 wk

USES: Major depression

Unlabeled uses: Chronic pain management

CONTRAINDICATIONS:
Pregnancy **D,** hypersensitivity to tricyclics, recovery phase of MI, seizure disorders, prostatic hypertrophy

Precautions: Breastfeeding, suicidal ideation, severe depression, increased intraocular pressure, closed-angle glaucoma, urinary retention, cardiac/hepatic disease, hyperthyroidism, electroshock therapy, elective surgery

> **BLACK BOX WARNING:** Children, suicidal ideation

DOSAGE AND ROUTES
Adult: PO 25 mg tid or qid; may increase to 150 mg/day; may give daily dose at bedtime
Adolescent: PO 1-3 mg/kg/day in 3-4 divided doses or qd at bedtime; max 150 mg/day
Geriatric: PO 10-25 mg nightly, increase by 10-25 mg at weekly intervals to desired dose; usual maintenance 75 mg/day, max 150 mg/day

Available forms: Caps 10, 25, 50, 75 mg; sol 10 mg/5 ml

Implementation
• Give with food or milk to decrease GI symptoms; mix conc with water, milk, fruit juice to disguise taste
• Give dose at bedtime if oversedation occurs during day; may take entire dose at bedtime; geriatric may not tolerate once/day dosing
• Store at room temperature; do not freeze

ADVERSE EFFECTS
CNS: *Dizziness, drowsiness,* confusion, headache, anxiety, tremors, stimulation, weakness, insomnia, nightmares, EPS (geriatric), increased psychiatric symptoms, **seizures**
CV: *Orthostatic hypotension, ECG changes, tachycardia,* **hypertension,** palpitations, **dysrhythmias**
EENT: Blurred vision, tinnitus, mydriasis
GI: *Constipation, dry mouth,* nausea, vomiting, **paralytic ileus,** increased appetite, cramps, epigastric distress, jaundice, **hepatitis,** stomatitis
GU: *Retention,* **acute renal failure**
HEMA: **Agranulocytosis, thrombocytopenia, eosinophilia, leukopenia**
INTEG: Rash, urticaria, sweating, pruritus, photosensitivity

Pharmacokinetics

Absorption	Well absorbed
Distribution	Widely distributed; crosses placenta
Metabolism	Liver, extensively
Excretion	Kidneys, breast milk
Half-life	18-28 hr; steady state 4-19 days

Pharmacodynamics
Unknown

INTERACTIONS
Individual drugs
Alcohol: increased CNS depression
CloNIDine, guanethidine: decreased effects
Smoking (heavy): decreased product effect
Haloperidol, chloroquine, droperidol, pentamidine, arsenic trioxide, levomethadyl: increased QT prolongation

Drug classifications
Barbiturates, benzodiazepines, CNS depressants: increased effects
MAOIs: hypertensive episode, hyperpyretic crisis, seizures
SSRIs, SNRIs, serotonin-receptor agonists: increased serotonin syndrome, neuroleptic malignant syndrome
Class IA/III antidysrhythmics, some phenothiazines, β-agonists, local anesthetics, tricyclics, CYP3A4 inhibitors (amiodarone, clarithromycin, erythromycin, telithromycin, troleandomycin), CYP3A4 substrates (methadone, pimozide, quetiapine, quiNIDine, risperidone, ziprasidone): increased QT prolongation
Sympathomimetics (direct-acting), products increasing QT interval: increased effects
Sympathomimetics (indirect-acting): decreased effects

Drug/herb
Kava, valerian: increased CNS effect
St. John's wort: decreased nortriptyline level

Drug/lab test
Increased: serum bilirubin, blood glucose, alkaline phosphatase
Decreased: VMA, 5-HIAA
False increase: urinary catecholamines

NURSING CONSIDERATIONS
Assessment
• Monitor B/P (with patient lying, standing), pulse q4hr; if systolic B/P drops 20 mm Hg,

---

⚠ Nurse Alert

hold product, notify prescriber; take VS q4hr of patients with CV disease

• Monitor blood studies: CBC, leukocytes, differential, cardiac enzymes if patient is receiving long-term therapy

• Monitor liver function tests: AST, ALT, bilirubin

• Check weight weekly; appetite may increase

• **QT prolongation:** assess for chest pain, palpitations, dyspnea

• Assess ECG for flattening of T-wave, bundle branch block, AV block, dysrhythmias in cardiac patients

• Assess for EPS primarily in geriatric: rigidity, dystonia, akathisia

• Assess mental status: mood, sensorium, affect, suicidal tendencies; increase in psychiatric symptoms: depression, panic

• Monitor urinary retention, constipation; constipation is more likely to occur in children or geriatric

⚠ **Assess for withdrawal symptoms: headache, nausea, vomiting, muscle pain, weakness; do not usually occur unless product was discontinued abruptly**

• Identify alcohol consumption; if alcohol is consumed, hold dose until AM

• **Serotonin syndrome, neuroleptic malignant syndrome:** assess for increased heart rate, shivering, sweating, dilated pupils, tremors, high B/P, hyperthermia, headache, confusion; if these occur, stop product, administer a serotonin antagonist if needed (rare)

Nursing diagnoses
• Coping, ineffective (uses)
• Injury, risk for (adverse reactions)
• Knowledge, deficient (teaching)
• Noncompliance (teaching)

Patient/family education
• Teach patient that therapeutic effects may take 2-3 wk

• Teach patient to use caution in driving and other activities requiring alertness because of drowsiness, dizziness, blurred vision; to avoid rising quickly from sitting to standing, especially geriatric

• Teach patient to avoid alcohol ingestion, MAOIs within 14 days, other CNS depressants; teach patient not to discontinue medication quickly after long-term use; may cause nausea, headache, malaise

• Teach patient to wear sunscreen or large hat to avoid burns, because photosensitivity occurs

• Teach patient to increase fluids, bulk in diet if constipation, urinary retention occur, especially geriatric, worsening depression, suicidal thoughts/behavior

• Teach patient to take gum, hard sugarless candy, or frequent sips of water for dry mouth

Evaluation
Positive therapeutic outcome
• Decrease in depression
• Absence of suicidal thoughts

TREATMENT OF OVERDOSE:
ECG monitoring, lavage, activated charcoal, administer anticonvulsant

---

nystatin (Rx, OTC)
(nis'ta-tin)
Bio-Statin, Nystat, Nystop, Pedi-Dri, ratio-Nystatin �canada
Func. class.: Antifungal
Chem. class.: Amphoteric polyene
Pregnancy category C

ACTION: Interferes with fungal DNA replication; binds sterols in fungal cell membrane, which increases permeability, resulting in leaking of cell nutrients

Therapeutic outcome: Fungistatic/fungicidal against *Candida* organisms

USES: *Candida* species causing oral, vaginal, intestinal infections

CONTRAINDICATIONS:
Hypersensitivity

Precautions: Pregnancy C

DOSAGE AND ROUTES
Oral infection
Adult/adolescent/child: Susp 400,000-600,000 units qid, use ¹/₂ dose in each side of mouth, swish and swallow, use for at least 48 hr after symptoms are resolved
Infant: SUSP 200,000 units qid (100,000 units in each side of mouth)

Newborn and premature infant:
SUSP 100,000 units qid
Adult and child: Troches 200,000-400,000 units qid × up to 2 wk

GI infection
Adult: PO 500,000-1,000,000 units tid

Cutaneous candidiasis
Adult/child:
Top cream/ointment
Apply to affected area bid
Powder
Apply to affected area bid-tid

Available forms: Tabs 500,000, 1,000,000 units; powder 50, 150, 500 million units; susp 100,000 units/ml; oral caps 500,000, 1,000,000 units bulk powder

Implementation
PO route
• Give oral susp dose by placing ¹/₂ in each cheek, swish for several min, then swallow; shake susp before use
• Store oral susp in refrigerator, tab in airtight, light-resistant containers at room temperature
Topical route
• Administer by moistening lesions with a swab coated with cream or ointment; use enough medication to cover lesions completely; give after cleansing with soap, water before each application; dry well; very moist lesions are best treated with topical powder
Vaginal route
• Insert vag tab high into vagina with applicator provided; administer in gravid client 3-6 wk before term to decrease candidiasis in the newborn
• Store at room temperature in dry place; protect from light, air, heat

ADVERSE EFFECTS
GI: Nausea, vomiting, anorexia, diarrhea, cramps
INTEG: Rash, urticaria (rare)

Pharmacokinetics	
Absorption	Poorly absorbed
Distribution	Unknown
Metabolism	Not metabolized
Excretion	Feces, unchanged
Half-life	Unknown

Pharmacodynamics	
Onset	Rapid
Peak	Unknown
Duration	6-12 hr

NURSING CONSIDERATIONS
Assessment
• **Assess for allergic reaction:** rash, urticaria; product may have to be discontinued
• Assess for predisposing factors for candidal infection: antibiotic therapy, pregnancy, diabetes mellitus, sexual partner infection (vag infections), AIDS
• Obtain culture and histologic tests to confirm organism

Nursing diagnoses
• Infection, risk for (uses)
• Knowledge, deficient (teaching)
• Skin integrity, impaired (uses)

Patient/family education
• Instruct patient that long-term therapy may be needed to clear infection; to complete entire course of medication
• Teach patient proper hygiene: use no commercial mouthwashes for mouth infection
• Advise patient to avoid getting preparation on hands
• Instruct patient to wear light-day pad for vag preparations to avoid soiling clothing; to avoid sexual contact during treatment to minimize reinfection
• Instruct patient to notify prescriber if irritation occurs; product may have to be discontinued
• Inform patient that relief from itching may occur after 24-72 hr
Topical route
• Advise patient to discontinue use and notify prescriber if irritation occurs
• Teach patient to apply with glove to prevent further infection; product may stain
• Caution patient not to use occlusive dressings; to avoid use of OTC creams, ointments, lotions unless directed by prescriber

Evaluation
Positive therapeutic outcome
• Culture negative for *Candida*
• Decrease in size, number of lesions
• Decreased itching, white patches on vulva (vaginal)

nystatin topical
See Appendix B

nystatin vaginal antifungal
See Appendix B

octreotide (Rx)

(ok-tree´-o-tide)

Sandostatin, Sandostatin LAR Depot

Func. class.: Growth hormone, antidiarrheal

Chem. class.: Synthetic octapeptide

Pregnancy category B

ACTION: A potent growth hormone similar to somatostatin

Therapeutic outcome: Decreased diarrhea; decreased symptoms of acromegaly, carcinoid tumors, vasoactive intestinal peptide tumors (VIPomas)

USES: **Sandostatin:** acromegaly, carcinoid tumors, VIPomas; **LAR Depot:** long-term maintenance of acromegaly, carcinoid tumors, VIPomas, short bowel syndrome, insulinoma, hepatorenal syndrome

Unlabeled uses: GI fistula, variceal bleeding, diarrheal conditions, pancreatic fistula, IBS, dumping syndrome

CONTRAINDICATIONS:

Hypersensitivity

Precautions: Pregnancy **B,** breastfeeding, children, geriatric, diabetes mellitus, hypothyroidism, renal disease

DOSAGE AND ROUTES

Acromegaly

Adult: SUBCUT/**IV** 50-100 mcg bid-tid, adjust q2wk based on growth hormone levels (Sandostatin) or IM 20 mg q4wk × 3 mo, adjust by growth hormone levels (Sandostatin LAR)

VIPomas

Adult: SUBCUT/**IV** 200-300 mcg/day in 2-4 doses for 2 wk, max 450 mcg/day; (Sandostatin) or IM 20 mg q2wk × 2 mo, adjust dose (Sandostatin LAR)

Flushing/diarrhea in carcinoid tumors

Adult: SUBCUT/**IV** 100-600 mcg/day in 2-4 doses for 2 wk, titrated to patient response (Sandostatin) or IM 20 mg q4wk × 2 mo, adjust dose (Sandostatin LAR)

GI fistula

Adult: SUBCUT 50-200 mcg q8hr

Antidiarrheal in AIDS patients (unlabeled)

Adult: SUBCUT 50 mcg q8h PRN, increase to 500 mcg q8h

Irritable bowel syndrome (unlabeled)

Adult: SUBCUT 100 mcg single dose to 125 mcg bid

Dumping syndrome (unlabeled)

Adult: SUBCUT 50-150 mcg/day

Variceal bleeding (unlabeled)

Adult: **IV** 25-50 mcg/hr CONT **IV** INF for 18 hr-5 days

Available forms: Sandostatin: inj 0.05, 0.1, 0.2, 0.5, 1 mg/ml; LAR Depot: inj powder for susp 10 mg, 20, 30 mg/5 ml

Implementation

• Store unopened amps, vials in refrigerator; or room temperature for 2 wk, protect from light; do not use discolored or cloudy sol

IM route

• Reconstitute with diluent provided; give into gluteal

SUBCUT route

• Rotate inj sites; use hip, thigh, abdomen

• Avoid using medication that is cold; allow to reach room temperature; do not use LAR Depot

Direct IV route

• Give over 3 min; in an emergency carcinoid crisis, give rapid bolus

Intermittent IV INF route

• Dilute in 50-200 ml D_5W, 0.9% NaCl; give over 15-30 min

Y-site compatibilities: Acyclovir, alfentanil, allopurinol, amifostine, amikacin, aminocaproic acid, aminophylline, amiodarone, amphotericin B colloidal, amphotericin B lipid complex, amphotericin B liposome, ampicillin, ampicillin-sulbactam, anidulafungin, argatroban, arsenic trioxide, atenolol, atracurium, azithromycin, aztreonam, bivalirudin, bleomycin, bumetanide, buprenorphine, busulfan, butorphanol, calcium chloride/gluconate, capreomycin, CARBOplatin, carmustine, caspofungin, ceFAZolin, cefepime, cefotaxime, cefotetan, cefoxitin, ceftazidime, ceftizoxime, cefTRIAXone, cefuroxime, chloramphenicol, chlorproMAZINE, cimetidine, ciprofloxacin, cisatracurium, CISplatin, clindamycin, cyclophosphamide, cycloSPORINE, cytarabine, dacarbazine, DACTINomycin, DAPTOmycin, DAUNOrubicin, DAUNOrubicin liposome, dexamethasone, digoxin, diltiazem, diphenhydrAMINE, DOBUTamine, docetaxel,

O

dolasetron, DOPamine, DOXOrubicin, DOXO-rubicin liposomal, doxycycline, droperidol, enalaprilat, ePHEDrine, EPINEPHrine, epirubicin, eptifibatide, ertapenem, erythromycin, esmolol, etoposide, famotidine, fenoldopam, fentaNYL, fluconazole, fludarabine, fluorouracil, foscarnet, fosphenytoin, furosemide, gallium nitrate, ganciclovir, gatifloxacin, gemcitabine, gentamicin, glycopyrrolate, granisetron, haloperidol, heparin, hydrALAZINE, hydrocortisone, HYDROmorphone, hydrOXYzine, IDArubicin, ifosfamide, imipenem-cilastatin, insulin (regular), irinotecan, isoproterenol, ketorolac, labetalol, lansoprazole, leucovorin, levofloxacin, lidocaine, linezolid, LORazepam, magnesium sulfate, mannitol, mechlorethamine, melphalan, meperidine, meropenem, mesna, methohexital, methotrexate, methyldopate, methylPREDNISolone, metoclopramide, metoprolol, metroNIDAZOLE, midazolam, milrinone, minocycline, mitomycin, mitoxantrone, mivacurium, morphine, moxifloxacin, mycophenolate, nafcillin, nalbuphine, naloxone, nesiritide, niCARdipine, nitroglycerin, nitroprusside, norepinephrine, ondansetron, oxaliplatin, paclitaxel, palonosetron, pamidronate, pancuronium, pemetrexed, pentamidine, pentazocine, PENTobarbital, PHENobarbital, phenylephrine, piperacillin, piperacillin-tazobactam, polymyxin B, potassium acetate/chloride/phosphates, procainamide, prochlorperazine, promethazine, propranolol, quiNIDine, quinupristin-dalfopristin, ranitidine, remifentanil, rocuronium, sodium acetate/bicarbonate/phosphates, streptozocin, succinylcholine, SUFentanil, sulfamethoxazole-trimethoprim, tacrolimus, teniposide, thiopental, thiotepa, ticarcillin, ticarcillin-clavulanate, tigecycline, tirofiban, tobramycin, topotecan, vancomycin, vasopressin, vecuronium, verapamil, vinBLAStine, vinCRIStine, vinorelbine, voriconazole, zidovudine, zoledronic acid

ADVERSE EFFECTS

CNS: *Headache, dizziness, fatigue, weakness,* depression, anxiety, tremors, **seizures,** paranoia
CV: *Sinus bradycardia, conduction abnormalities,* **dysrhythmias,** chest pain, shortness of breath, thrombophlebitis, ischemia, **CHF,** hypertension, palpitations, **QT prolongation, ST-T wave changes**
ENDO: *Hypo/hyperglycemia, ketosis, hypothyroidism,* galactorrhea, diabetes insipidus
GI: *Diarrhea, nausea, abdominal pain, vomiting, flatulence, distension, constipation,* **hepatitis,** elevated liver function tests, **GI bleeding, pancreatitis,** cholelithiasis, ileus

GU: UTI
HEMA: Hematoma of inj site, bruise
INTEG: Rash, urticaria, pain, inflammation at inj site
MS: Joint and muscle pain

Pharmacokinetics

Absorption	Rapidly, completely absorbed
Distribution	Unknown
Metabolism	Little
Excretion	Urine, unchanged
Half-life	1.7 hr

Pharmacodynamics

	Subcut/IV	IM
Onset	Unknown	Unknown
Peak	$1/2$ hr	2-4 wk
Duration	12 hr	Unknown

INTERACTIONS

Individual drugs
Other products that prolong QT: increased QT prolongation
CycloSPORINE: decreased effect of cycloSPORINE
Haloperidol, chloroquine, droperidol, pentamidine, arsenic trioxide, levomethadyl: increased QT prolongation

Drug classifications
Class IA/III antidysrhythmics, some phenothiazines, β-agonists, local anesthetics, tricyclics, CYP3A4 inhibitors (amiodarone, clarithromycin, erythromycin, telithromycin, troleandomycin), CYP3A4 substrates (methadone, pimozide, quetiapine, quiNIDine, risperidone, ziprasidone): increased QT prolongation

Drug/food
Decreased: absorption of dietary fat, vit B_{12} levels

Drug/lab test
Decreased: T_4

NURSING CONSIDERATIONS

Assessment
• Identify growth hormone antibodies, IGF-1, 1-4 hr intervals for 8-12 hr after dose in acromegaly; 5-HIAA; blood glucose, serotonin levels (carcinoid tumors), plasma substance P, plasma vasoactive intestinal peptide (VIP) (VIPomas)
• Monitor for fecal fat, serum carotene
• Monitor thyroid function tests: T_3, T_4, T_7, TSH to identify hypothyroidism

- Assess for allergic reaction: rash, itching, fever, nausea, wheezing
- **Assess for cardiac status:** bradycardia, conduction abnormalities, dysrhythmias; monitor ECG for QT prolongation, low voltage, axis shifts, early repolarization, R/S transition, early wave progression
- **Allergic reaction:** assess for rash, itching, fever, nausea, wheezing

Nursing diagnoses
- Body image, disturbed (uses)
- Knowledge, deficient (teaching)

Patient/family education
- Explain reason for medication and expected results
- Advise patient that routine follow-up is needed
- Advise diabetic patients to monitor glucose
- Instruct parents on procedure for medication preparation and inj use; request demonstration, return demonstration; provide written instructions
- Advise patient that dizziness, drowsiness, weakness may occur; to avoid hazardous activities if these occur; to report abdominal pain immediately

Evaluation
Positive therapeutic outcome
- Decreased symptoms of acromegaly, carcinoid, VIPoma
- Decreased diarrhea in AIDS

---

ofloxacin (Rx)
(o-flox′a-sin)
Apo-Ofloxacin ✦
Func. class.: Antiinfective
Chem. class.: Fluoroquinolone
Pregnancy category C

ACTION: Interferes with conversion of intermediate DNA fragments into high molecular weight DNA in bacteria, inhibits DNA gyrase

Therapeutic outcome: Bactericidal action against gram-positive pathogens *Staphylococcus epidermidis,* methicillin-resistant strains of *Staphylococcus aureus, Streptococcus pyogenes, Streptococcus pneumoniae;* gramnegative pathogens *Escherichia coli, Klebsiella* species, *Enterobacter, Salmonella, Shigella, Proteus vulgaris, Proteus rettgeri, Providencia stuartii, Morganella morganii, Pseudomonas aeruginosa, Serratia, Haemophilus* species, *Acinetobacter, Neisseria gonorrhoeae, Neisseria meningitidis, Yersinia, Vibrio, Brucella, Campylobacter,* and *Aeromonas* species;

anaerobic pathogens *Bacteroides fragilis intermedius, Clostridium perfringens, Gardnerella vaginalis, Peptococcus niger, Peptostreptococcus* species; *Chlamydia pneumoniae, Chlamydia trachomatis, Legionella pneumoniae, Mycobacterium tuberculosis, Mycoplasma pneumoniae*

USES: Treatment of lower respiratory tract infections (pneumonia, bronchitis), genitourinary infections (prostatitis, UTIs), skin and skin structure infections, gonorrhea, otitis media, conjunctivitis (ophth)

CONTRAINDICATIONS:
Hypersensitivity to quinolones, QT prolongation

Precautions: Pregnancy **C**, breastfeeding, children, geriatric, renal disease, seizure disorders, excessive sunlight, hypokalemia

> **BLACK BOX WARNING:** Tendon pain/rupture, tendinitis, myasthenia gravis

DOSAGE AND ROUTES
Lower respiratory tract infection/ skin and skin structure infections
Adult: PO 400 mg q12hr × 10 days

Cervicitis, urethritis
Adult: PO 300 mg q12hr × 7 days (nongonococcal): 400 mg as a single dose (gonococcal)

Prostatitis from *E. Coli*
Adult: PO 300 mg q12hr × 6 wk

Urinary tract infection
Adult: PO 200 mg q12hr × 10 days

Pelvic inflammatory disease
Adult: PO 400 mg q12hr × 10-14 days

Renal dose
Adult: PO CCr 20-50 ml/min give q24hr; CCr <20 ml/min give ¹/₂ of dose q24hr

Hepatic dose
Adult (Child-Pugh class C): PO max 400 mg/ day

Available forms: Tabs 200, 300, 400 mg
Implementation
PO route
- Give in equal intervals q12hr around the clock to maintain proper blood levels; do not give within 2 hr of other agents, since product interactions are possible: give with 8 oz of water
- Do not give with iron, aluminum, zinc products or antacids, which decrease absorption and form insoluble chelate

---

Adverse effects: *italics* = common; **bold** = life-threatening

ADVERSE EFFECTS

CNS: Dizziness, headache, fatigue, somnolence, depression, insomnia, lethargy, malaise, **seizures,** vertigo
CV: QT prolongation, dysrhythmias, chest pain
EENT: Visual disturbances
GI: Diarrhea, nausea, vomiting, anorexia, flatulence, heartburn, dry mouth, increased AST, ALT, abdominal pain, constipation, **pseudomembranous colitis,** abnormal taste, xerostomia
HEMA: Blood dyscrasias
INTEG: Rash, pruritus, photosensitivity
MS: Tendinitis, **tendon rupture, rhabdomyolysis**
SYST: Anaphylaxis, Stevens-Johnson syndrome, toxic epidermal necrosis

Pharmacokinetics

Absorption	Well absorbed (PO)
Distribution	Widely distributed
Metabolism	Unknown
Excretion	Kidneys, unchanged; breast milk
Half-life	5-9 hr; increased in renal disease

Pharmacodynamics

	PO	Ophth
Onset	Rapid	Unknown
Peak	1-2 hr	Unknown
Duration	Unknown	Unknown

INTERACTIONS

Individual drugs

Chloroquine, clarithromycin, droperidol, erythromycin, haloperidol, methadone, pentamidine: increased QT prolongation
Sucralfate, zinc sulfate: decreased absorption of ofloxacin, separate by 2 hr
Theophylline: possible toxicity
Warfarin: increased anticoagulation

Drug classifications

Antacids with aluminum, iron salts, magnesium: decreased absorption of ofloxacin, separate by 2 hr
Antidiabetics: altered blood glucose levels
β-agonists, class IA/III antidysrhythmics, local anesthetics, some phenothiazines, tricyclics: increased QT prolongation

> **BLACK BOX WARNING: Corticosteroids:**
> Increased tendon rupture/tendinitis

NSAIDs: increased CNS stimulation, seizures

NURSING CONSIDERATIONS

Assessment

• Assess patient for previous sensitivity reaction
• Assess patient for signs and symptoms of infection including characteristics of wounds, sputum, urine, stool, WBC $>10,000/mm^3$, fever; obtain baselines and monitor during treatment
• Obtain C&S before beginning product therapy to identify if correct treatment has been initiated
• **QT prolongation:** assess ECG for QT prolongation, ejection fraction; assess for chest pain, palpitations, dyspnea
• **Pseudomembranous colitis:** assess for diarrhea, abdominal pain, fever, fatigue, anorexia; possible anemia, elevated WBC and low serum albumin; stop product and usually give either vancomycin or IV metroNIDAZOLE
• **Rhabdomyolysis:** assess muscle pain, increased CPK, weakness, swelling of affected muscles; if these occur and if confirmed by CPK, product should be discontinued
• Assess for allergic reactions: rash, urticaria, pruritus
• Monitor blood studies: AST, ALT, CBC, serum glucose monthly if patient is on long-term therapy
• Assess for overgrowth of infection: perineal itching, fever, malaise, redness, pain, swelling, drainage, rash, diarrhea, change in cough, sputum
• Assess for CNS symptoms: seizures, vertigo, drowsiness, agitation, confusion, tremors

Nursing diagnoses

• Diarrhea (adverse reactions)
• Infection, risk for (uses)
• Injury, risk for (adverse reactions)
• Knowledge, deficient (teaching)
• Noncompliance (teaching)

Patient/family education

• Instruct patient to take all medication prescribed for the length of time ordered; product must be taken around the clock to maintain blood levels; do not give medication to others
• Teach patient to use sunscreen when outdoors to decrease phototoxicity
• Advise patient to increase fluids to 2 L/day to prevent crystalluria
• Caution patient to avoid driving and other hazardous activities until response is known; dizziness, confusion, drowsiness may occur

Evaluation

Positive therapeutic outcome
• Absence of signs/symptoms of infection
• Reported improvement in symptoms of infection
• Absence of red or itching eyes (ophth)

ofloxacin ophthalmic
See Appendix B

OLANZapine (Rx)
(oh-lanz′a-peen)
Zyprexa, Zyprexa Intramuscular, Zyprexa Relprevv, Zyprexa Zydis
Func. class.: Antipsychotic/neuroleptic
Chem. class.: Thienobenzodiazepine
Pregnancy category C

Do not confuse:
OLANZapine/osalazlne,
zyprexa/Celexa/Zyrtec

ACTION: May mediate antipsychotic activity by both dopamine and serotonin type 2 (5-HT$_2$) antagonism; also, may antagonize muscarinic, histaminic (H$_1$), and α-adrenergic receptors

Therapeutic outcome: Decreased psychotic symptoms

USES: Schizophrenia, acute manic episodes in bipolar disorder, acute agitation

Unlabeled uses: Dementia related to Alzheimer's disease, OCD, acute psychosis

CONTRAINDICATIONS:
Hypersensitivity

Precautions: Pregnancy C, breastfeeding, geriatric, hypertension, cardiac/renal/hepatic disease, diabetes, agranulocytosis, abrupt discontinuation, Asian patients, closed-angle glaucoma, coma, leukopenia, QT prolongation, tardive dyskinesia, torsades de pointes

> **BLACK BOX WARNING:** Dementia, postinjection delirium/sedation syndrome

DOSAGE AND ROUTES
Schizophrenia
Adult: PO 5-10 mg/day initially, may increase dosage by 5 mg at ≥1 wk intervals; orally disintegrating tabs: open blister pack, place tab on tongue, let disintegrate, swallow; max 20 mg/day
Geriatric: PO 5 mg, may increase cautiously at 1 wk intervals, max 20 mg/day
Adolescent: PO 2.5 mg or 5 mg/day, target 10 mg/day

Bipolar mania
Adult: PO 10-15 mg/day, may increase dose after 24 hr by 5 mg

Adolescent: PO 2.5 or 5 mg/day, target 10 mg/day

Agitation associated with schizophrenia, bipolar I mania
Adult: IM 10 mg

Available forms: Tabs 2.5, 5, 7.5, 10, 15, 20 mg; **orally disintegrating tabs** 5, 10, 15, 20 mg (Zyprexa Zydis; **powder for injection** 10 mg

Implementation
• Give antiparkinsonian agent for EPS
• Give decreased dose in geriatric
PO route
• Give with full glass of water/milk or with food to decrease GI upset
• **Orally disintegrating tabs:** open blister pack; place tab on tongue until dissolved; swallow; no water needed
IM route (Zyprexa Intramuscular)
• Dissolve contents of vials with 2.1 ml sterile water for injection (5 mg/ml), use immediately
• Do not use IV or SUBCUT
• Inject slowly, deep into muscle mass
IM route (Zyprexa Relprevv)

> **BLACK BOX WARNING:** Available only through restricted distribution program due to postinjection delirium/sedation syndrome; give at a facility with emergency services

• Use deep IM gluteal inj only
• Use only diluent provided in kit; give q2-4wk using 19G 1.5-inch needle in kit, in obesity use 19G 2 inch or larger needle
• Provide supervised ambulation until stabilized on medication; do not involve in strenuous exercise program because fainting is possible; patients should not stand still for long periods
• Give increased fluids to prevent constipation
• Give sips of water, candy, gum for dry mouth
• Store in airtight, light-resistant container
• Give orally disintegrating tabs: open blister pack, place tab on tongue until dissolved, swallow; no water needed

ADVERSE EFFECTS
CNS: EPS (pseudoparkinsonism, akathisia, dystonia, tardive dyskinesia), **seizures,** headache, **neuroleptic malignant syndrome (rare),** agitation, nervousness, hostility, dizziness, hypertonia, tremor, euphoria, confusion, *drowsiness,* fatigue, *abnormal gait, insomnia, fever*
CV: Hypotension, tachycardia, chest pain, **heart failure, sudden death (geriatric, IM),** orthostatic hypotension

Adverse effects: *italics* = common; **bold** = life-threatening

ENDO: Increased prolactin levels, hypoglycemia
GI: Dry mouth, nausea, vomiting, anorexia, constipation, abdominal pain, weight gain, appetite, dyspepsia, jaundice, **hepatitis**
GU: Urinary retention, urinary frequency, enuresis, impotence, amenorrhea, gynecomastia, breast engorgement, premenstrual syndrome
HEMA: Neutropenia
INTEG: Rash
MISC: Peripheral edema, accidental injury, hypertonia, hyperlipidemia
MS: Joint pain, twitching
RESP: *Cough, pharyngitis,* **fatal pneumonia (geriatric, IM)**

Pharmacokinetics

Absorption	Well absorbed
Distribution	93% plasma protein binding
Metabolism	Liver
Excretion	Kidneys
Half-life	Unknown

Pharmacodynamics

Onset	Unknown
Peak	6 hr
Duration	Unknown

INTERACTIONS

Individual drugs
Alcohol: increased sedation, hypotension
Bromocriptine, levodopa: decreased antiparkinson activity
CarBAMazepine, omeprazole, rifampin: decreased levels of OLANZapine
Diazepam: increased hypotension
Fluvoxamine: increased OLANZapine levels

Drug classifications
SSRIs, SNRIs: increased serotonin syndrome, increased neuroleptic malignant syndrome
Anesthetics (barbiturates), antidepressants, antihistamines, CNS depressants, sedative/hypnotics: increased sedation
Anticholinergics: increased anticholinergic effects
Antihypertensives: increased hypotension
DOPamine agonists: decreased antiparkinson activity

Drug/lab test
Increased: liver function tests, prolactin, CPK

NURSING CONSIDERATIONS

Assessment

> **BLACK BOX WARNING:** Postinjection delirium/sedation syndrome (Zyprexa Relprevv): monitor continuously for ≥3 hr after injection; this patient must be accompanied when leaving: sedation, coma, delirium, EPS, slurred speech, altered gait, aggression, dizziness, weakness, hypertension, seizures; before leaving, confirm the patient is alert, oriented, and free of any other symptoms

• Assess mental status, orientation, mood, behavior, presence of hallucinations and type before initial administration and monthly
• Monitor I&O ratio; palpate bladder if low urinary output occurs, especially in geriatric
• Monitor bilirubin, CBC
• Monitor urinalysis; recommended before, during prolonged therapy
• Assess affect, orientation, LOC, reflexes, gait, coordination, sleep pattern disturbances
• Monitor B/P sitting, standing, lying; take pulse and respirations q4hr during initial treatment; establish baseline before starting treatment; report drops of 30 mm Hg; obtain baseline ECG
• **Serotonin syndrome:** assess for increased heart rate, shivering, sweating, dilated pupils, tremors, high B/P, hyperthermia, headache, confusion; if these occur, stop product, administer a serotonin antagonist if needed
• Assess dizziness, faintness, palpitations, tachycardia on rising
• **Assess for neuroleptic malignant syndrome:** hyperpyrexia, muscle rigidity, increased CPK, altered mental status, for acute dystonia (cheek chewing, swallowing, eyes, pill rolling)
• **EPS** including akathisia (inability to sit still, no pattern to movements), tardive dyskinesia (bizarre movements of the jaw, mouth, tongue, extremities), pseudoparkinsonism (rigidity, tremors, pill rolling, shuffling gait)
• Monitor constipation, urinary retention daily; increase bulk, water in diet

Nursing diagnoses
• Knowledge, deficient (teaching)
• Noncompliance (teaching)

Patient/family education

> **BLACK BOX WARNING:** Teach patient about postinjection delirium/sedation syndrome; teach about all symptoms

• Teach patient to use good oral hygiene; frequent rinsing of mouth, candy, ice chips, sugarless gum for dry mouth
• Advise patient to avoid hazardous activities until product response is determined
• Advise patient that orthostatic hypotension occurs often and to rise from sitting or lying position gradually
• Advise patient to avoid hot tubs, hot showers, tub baths, since hypotension may occur
• Advise patient to avoid abrupt withdrawal of this product, or EPS may result; product should be withdrawn slowly
• Advise patient to avoid OTC preparations (cough, hay fever, cold) unless approved by prescriber, since serious product interactions may occur; avoid use with alcohol, CNS depressants, increased drowsiness may occur
• Advise patient that in hot weather, heat stroke may occur; take extra precautions to stay cool

Evaluation
Positive therapeutic outcome
• Decrease in emotional excitement, hallucinations, delusions, paranoia, reorganization of patterns of thought, speech

TREATMENT OF OVERDOSE:
Lavage if orally ingested; provide airway; do not induce vomiting or use epinephrine

olmesartan (Rx)
(ol-meh-sar'tan)
Benicar
Func. class.: Antihypertensive
Chem. class.: Angiotensin II receptor (type AT_1) antagonist
Pregnancy category C (1st trimester), D (2nd/3rd trimesters)

ACTION: Blocks the vasoconstrictor and aldosterone-secreting effects of angiotensin II; selectively blocks the binding of angiotensin II to the AT_1 receptor found in tissues

Therapeutic outcome: Decreased B/P

USES: Hypertension, alone or in combination with other antihypertensives

CONTRAINDICATIONS:
Hypersensitivity
Pregnancy **D** (2nd/3rd trimesters)

Precautions: Pregnancy **C** (1st trimester), breastfeeding, children, geriatric, hepatic disease, CHF

DOSAGE AND ROUTES
Adult: PO single agent 20 mg/day initially in patients who are not volume depleted; may be increased to 40 mg/day if needed after 2 wk

Available forms: Tabs 5, 20, 40 mg

Implementation
• Give without regard to meals; refrigerate suspension and store for up to 1 month; shake suspension before use

ADVERSE EFFECTS
CNS: *Dizziness,* fatigue, headache, insomnia
CV: Chest pain, peripheral edema, tachycardia
EENT: Sinusitis, rhinitis, pharyngitis
GI: *Diarrhea,* abdominal pain
MS: Arthralgia, pain
RESP: *Upper respiratory infection,* bronchitis
SYST: **Angioedema**

Pharmacokinetics
Absorption	Unknown
Distribution	Unknown
Metabolism	Unknown
Excretion	Urine, feces
Half-life	Unknown

Pharmacodynamics
Onset	Unknown
Peak	1-2 hr
Duration	Unknown

INTERACTIONS
Individual drugs
Lithium: increased effect

Drug classifications
Antihypertensives (other), diuretics: increased antihypertensive effects
NSAIDs: decreased antihypertensive effect
Antioxidants: increased effects
Potassium supplements, potassium-sparing diuretics: increased hyperkalemia

Drug/herb
Aconite: increased toxicity, death
Astragalus, cola tree: increased or decreased antihypertensive effect
Hawthorn: increased antihypertensive effect
Ephedra: decreased antihypertensive effect

NURSING CONSIDERATIONS
Assessment
• **Assess for pregnancy;** this product can cause fetal death when given in pregnancy, 2nd/3rd trimester

O

- Assess response and adverse reactions, especially in renal disease
- Monitor B/P, pulse q4hr; note rate, rhythm, quality; electrolytes: K, Na, Cl; baselines in renal, liver function tests before therapy begins
- Assess skin turgor, dryness of mucous membranes for hydration status; for angioedema: facial swelling, dyspnea

Nursing diagnoses
- Cardiac output, decreased (uses)
- Knowledge, deficient (teaching)
- Noncompliance (teaching)
- Tissue perfusion, ineffective (uses)

Patient/family education
- Advise to comply with dosage schedule, even if feeling better
- Advise patient to notify prescriber of mouth sores, fever, swelling of hands or feet, irregular heartbeat, chest pain
- Teach that excessive perspiration, dehydration, vomiting, diarrhea may lead to fall in B/P; to consult prescriber if these occur
- Teach that product may cause dizziness, fainting; light-headedness may occur
- Advise to rise slowly to sitting or standing position to minimize orthostatic hypotension
- Teach to notify prescriber immediately if pregnant; not to use during breastfeeding
- Advise to avoid all OTC medications, unless approved by prescriber
- Advise to inform all health care providers of medication use
- Advise to use proper technique for obtaining B/P and acceptable parameters

Evaluation
Positive therapeutic outcome
- Decreased B/P

olopatadine ophthalmic
See Appendix B

olsalazine (Rx)
(ohl-sal′ah-zeen)
Dipentum
Func. class.: Antiinflammatory
Chem. class.: Salicylate derivative
Pregnancy category C

Do not confuse:
olsalazine/OLANZapine

ACTION: Bioconverted to 5-aminosalicylic acid, which decreases inflammation

Therapeutic outcome: Lessening of loose diarrhea stools and cramping

USES: Maintenance of remission of ulcerative colitis in patients intolerant to sulfasalazine

CONTRAINDICATIONS:
Hypersensitivity to this product or salicylates

Precautions: Pregnancy **C**, breastfeeding, children <14 yr, impaired renal/hepatic function, severe allergy, bronchial asthma

DOSAGE AND ROUTES
Adult: PO 500 mg bid, max 3 g/day

Available forms: Caps 250 mg

Implementation
- Give total daily dose evenly spaced to minimize GI intolerance, give with food
- Store in tight, light-resistant container at room temperature

ADVERSE EFFECTS
CNS: Headache, hallucinations, depression, vertigo, fatigue, dizziness
GI: Nausea, vomiting, abdominal pain, **hepatitis**, diarrhea, bloating, **pancreatitis**
HEMA: Leukopenia, neutropenia, thrombocytopenia, agranulocytosis, anemia
INTEG: Rash, dermatitis, urticaria

Pharmacokinetics	
Absorption	Colon 99% converted to mesalamine
Distribution	Colon
Metabolism	Liver
Excretion	Feces
Half-life	0.9 hr

Pharmacodynamics	
Onset	Unknown
Peak	1 hr
Duration	12 hr

INTERACTIONS

Individual drugs
AzaTHIOprine: increased toxicity
Mercaptopurine, thioguanine: increased myelosuppression
Warfarin: increased pro-time, INR

Drug/lab test
Increased: AST, ALT

NURSING CONSIDERATIONS
Assessment
⚠ **Assess for blood dyscrasias: skin rash, fever, sore throat, bruising, bleeding, fatigue, joint pain (rare)**
• **Assess for allergic reaction:** rash, dermatitis, urticaria, pruritus, dyspnea, bronchospasm
• **Colitis:** assess bowel pattern, number of stools, consistency, frequency, pain, mucus before treatment and periodically

Nursing diagnoses
• Diarrhea (uses)
• Knowledge, deficient (teaching)
• Pain, acute (uses)

Patient/family education
• Advise patient to take as prescribed, take missed dose as soon as remembered
• Inform patient not to operate machinery or drive until effects are known, may cause dizziness
• Advise patient to notify prescriber if symptoms do not improve or if allergic reaction or sore throat occurs
• Teach patient to report diarrhea, rash, bleeding, bruising, fever, hallucinations

Evaluation
Positive therapeutic outcome
• Absence of fever, mucus in stools

---

omalizumab (Rx)
(oh-mah-lye-zoo′mab)
Xolair
Func. class.: Antiasthmatic
Chem. class.: Monoclonal antibody
Pregnancy category B

ACTION: Recombinant DNA-derived humanized IgG murine monoclonal antibody that selectively binds to IgE to limit the release of mediators in the allergic response

Therapeutic outcome: Ability to breathe more easily

USES: Moderate to severe persistent asthma

Unlabeled uses: Seasonal allergic rhinitis, food allergy

CONTRAINDICATIONS:
Hypersensitivity to hamster protein

BLACK BOX WARNING: Hypersensitivity to this product

Precautions: Pregnancy **B**, breastfeeding, children <12 yr, acute attacks of asthma, lymphoma, nephrotic disease, bronchospasm, neoplastic disease, status asthmaticus

DOSAGE AND ROUTES
Adult/adolescent/child ≥12 yr: SUBCUT 150-375 mg × 2-4 wk, divide inj into 2 sites, if dose is >150 mg; dose is adjusted based on IgE levels and significant changes in body weight

Available forms: Powder for inj, lyophilized 202.5 mg (150 mg/1.2 ml after reconstitution)

Implementation
SUBCUT route
• Reconstitute using 1.4 ml sterile water for inj (150 mg/1.2 ml or 125 mg/ml); gently swirl to dissolve; allow vial to stand and q5min gently swirl for 5-10 sec to dissolve, some vials take ≥20 min, do not use if contents do not dissolve within 40 min, should be clear or slightly opalescent; use large-bore needle to withdraw medication; replace needle with small-bore needle
• Given q2-4wk; product is viscous; if >150 mg is given, divide into two sites; the inj may take 5-10 sec to administer
• Do not give more than 150 mg/inj site

ADVERSE EFFECTS
CV: **Heart failure,** cardiomyopathy, hypotension
HEMA: **Serious systemic eosinophilia**
INTEG: Pruritus, dermatitis, inj site reactions, rash
MISC: Earache, dizziness, fatigue, pain, **malignancies,** viral infections, **anaphylaxis, thrombocytopenia,** headache
MS: Arthralgia, fracture, leg, arm pain
RESP: Sinusitis, upper respiratory tract infections, pharyngitis, pulmonary hypertension, **bronchospasm**

Pharmacokinetics
Absorption	Slow
Distribution	Unknown
Metabolism	Degradation by liver
Excretion	In bile
Half-life	26 days

Pharmacodynamics
Onset	Unknown
Peak	7-8 days
Duration	Unknown

INTERACTIONS
Drug classifications
Vaccines (live virus): use cautiously

NURSING CONSIDERATIONS
Assessment
• Monitor respiratory rate, rhythm, depth; auscultate lung fields bilaterally; notify prescriber of abnormalities; monitor pulmonary function tests; serum IgE

> **BLACK BOX WARNING: Assess for anaphylaxis, allergic reactions:** rash, urticaria, inability to breathe, edema of throat; observe for 2 hr, reaction can occur up to 24 hr; have emergency equipment available; product should be discontinued

Nursing diagnoses
• Gas exchange, impaired (uses)
• Knowledge, deficient (teaching)

Patient/family education
• Advise patient that improvement will not be immediate
• Teach patient not to stop taking or decrease current asthma medications unless instructed by prescriber

> **BLACK BOX WARNING:** Instruct patient to report signs of allergic reaction

Evaluation
Positive therapeutic outcome
• Ability to breathe more easily

omeprazole (Rx, OTC)
(oh-mep′ra-zole)
Apo-Omeprazole ✤, Good Sense Omeprazole, Losec ✤, Prilosec, Prilosec OTC
Func. class.: Antiulcer, proton pump inhibitor
Chem. class.: Benzimidazole
Pregnancy category C

Do not confuse:
PriLOSEC/Prinivil/predniSONE/PROzac

ACTION: Suppresses gastric secretion by inhibiting hydrogen/potassium ATPase enzyme system in the gastric parietal cell; characterized as a gastric acid pump inhibitor, since it blocks the final step of acid production

Therapeutic outcome: Absence of duodenal ulcers; decreased gastroesophageal reflux

USES: Gastroesophageal reflux disease (GERD), severe erosive esophagitis, poorly responsive systemic GERD, pathologic hypersecretory conditions (Zollinger-Ellison syndrome, systemic mastocytosis, multiple endocrine adenomas); possibly effective for treatment of duodenal ulcers with or without antiinfectives for *Helicobacter pylori*

CONTRAINDICATIONS:
Hypersensitivity

Precautions: Pregnancy **C,** breastfeeding, children

DOSAGE AND ROUTES
Active duodenal ulcers
Adult: PO 20 mg/day × 4-8 wk; associated with *H. pylori* 40 mg qAM and clarithromycin 500 mg tid on days 1-14, then 20 mg/day days 15-28

Severe erosive esophagitis/poorly responsive GERD
Adult: PO (DEL REL cap/SUSP) 20 mg/day × 4-8 wk

Pathologic hypersecretory conditions
Adult: PO 60 mg/day; may increase to 120 mg tid; daily doses >80 mg should be divided

Gastric ulcer
Adult: PO 40 mg/day × 4-8 wk
Geriatric: PO max 20 mg/day

Heartburn (OTC)
Adult: PO 1 DEL REL tab (20 mg) daily before AM meal with glass of water

Available forms: Del rel caps 10, 20, 40 mg, del rel tabs (PriLOSEC OTC) 20 mg; granules for oral susp 2.5, 10 mg (del rel)

Implementation
• Swallow sus rel caps whole; do not break, crush, chew, or open
• Give before patient eats; may give with antacids

ADVERSE EFFECTS
CNS: *Headache, dizziness, asthenia*
CV: Chest pain, angina, tachycardia, bradycardia, palpitations, peripheral edema, **heart failure**
EENT: Tinnitus, taste perversion
GI: *Diarrhea, abdominal pain, vomiting, nausea, constipation, flatulence, acid regurgitation,* abdominal swelling, anorexia, irritable colon, esophageal candidiasis, dry mouth, **hepatic failure**

⚠ Nurse Alert

GU: UTI, frequency, increased creatinine, pro-
teinuria, **hematuria,** testicular pain, glycosuria
**HEMA: Pancytopenia, thrombocytopenia,
neutropenia, leukocytosis,** anemia
INTEG: Rash, dry skin, urticaria, pruritus,
alopecia
META: Hypoglycemia, increased hepatic
enzymes, weight gain, hypomagnesemia, hyponatremia, vit B$_{12}$ deficiency
MISC: *Back pain,* fever, fatigue, malaise
RESP: *Upper respiratory tract infections,
cough,* epistaxis, **pneumonia**
**SYST: Angioedema, exfoliative dermatitis,
Stevens-Johnson syndrome, toxic epider-
mal necrolysis**

Pharmacokinetics

Absorption	Rapidly absorbed
Distribution	Protein binding (95%); gastric parietal cells
Metabolism	Liver, extensively; by CYP450 enzyme system
Excretion	Kidneys, feces
Half-life	$^{1}/_{2}$-1 hr; increased in the geriatric, hepatic disease

Pharmacodynamics

Onset	1 hr
Peak	$^{1}/_{2}$-3$^{1}/_{2}$ hr
Duration	3-4 days

INTERACTIONS

Individual drugs
Ampicillin: decreased effect of ampicillin
Calcium carbonate: decreased absorption of
calcium carbonate
Cyanocobalamin: decreased absorption of
cyanocobalamin
CycloSPORINE: increased cycloSPORINE levels
Diazepam: increased serum levels of diazepam
Digoxin: increased serum levels, delayed
absorption of digoxin
Disulfiram: increased disulfiram levels
Flurazepam: increased flurazepam level
Gefitinib: decreased effect of gefitinib
Indinavir: decreased effect of indinavir
Iron salts: decreased absorption
Ketoconazole: decreased absorption of keto-
conazole
Phenytoin: increased serum levels of phenytoin
Triazolam: increased triazolam level
Warfarin: increased bleeding tendencies

Drug classifications
Iron products: decreased absorption of iron

Drug/lab test
Increased: alkaline phosphatase, AST, ALT,
bilirubin, gastrin

NURSING CONSIDERATIONS

Assessment
• **Electrolyte imbalances:** hyponatremia,
hypomagnesemia in those using this product 3
mo-1 yr; if hypomagnesemia occurs, use of magnesium supplement may be sufficient; if severe,
discontinue use
• **Serious skin reactions:** toxic epidermal
necrolysis, **Stevens-Johnson syndrome,**
angioedema, exfoliative dermatitis; assess for
fever, sore throat, fatigue, thin ulcers, lesions in
mouth, lips; discontinue product
• Assess GI system: bowel sounds q8hr, abdomen for pain and swelling, anorexia
• **Monitor hepatic enzymes:** AST, ALT,
increased alkaline phosphatase during treatment; blood studies; CBC, differential during
treatment, blood dyscrasias may occur; vitamin
B$_{12}$ in long-term treatment

Nursing diagnoses
• Knowledge, deficient (teaching)
• Pain, chronic (uses)

Patient/family education
• Advise patient to report severe diarrhea;
black, tarry stools; abdominal cramps/pain,
continuing headache; product may have to be
discontinued
• Caution patient to avoid driving and other
hazardous activities until response to product is
known
• Caution patient to avoid alcohol, salicylates,
ibuprofen; may cause GI irritation

Evaluation
Positive therapeutic outcome
• Absence of epigastric pain, swelling, fullness

ondansetron (Rx)
(on-dan′sa-tron)
Zofran, Zofran ODT, Zuplenz
Func. class.: Antiemetic
Chem. class.: 5-HT receptor antagonist
Pregnancy category B

Do not confuse:
Zofran/Zantac

ACTION: Prevents nausea, vomiting by
blocking serotonin (5-HT) peripherally, centrally, and in the small intestine

Therapeutic outcome: Control of nausea, vomiting

USES: Prevention of nausea, vomiting associated with cancer chemotherapy, radiotherapy, and prevention of postoperative nausea, vomiting

Unlabeled uses: Bulimia, pruritus (rectal use), alcoholism, hyperemesis gravidarum

CONTRAINDICATIONS:

Hypersensitivity; phenylketonuric hypersensitivity (oral disintegrating tab), torsades de pointes

Precautions: Pregnancy **B**, breastfeeding, children, geriatric, granisetron hypersensitivity

DOSAGE AND ROUTES

Prevention of nausea/vomiting (cancer chemotherapy)

Adult and child 4-18 yr: IV 0.15 mg/kg infused over 15 min, 30 min before start of cancer chemotherapy; 0.15 mg/kg is given 4 hr and 8 hr after first dose or 32 mg as a single dose; dilute in 50 ml of D₅ or 0.9% NaCl before giving; RECT (unlabeled) 16 mg daily 2 hr before chemotherapy; PO 8 mg ½ hr prior to chemotherapy, repeat 4, 8 hr after 1st dose
Child ≥4 yr: PO 4 mg ½ hr prior to chemotherapy

Prevention of nausea/vomiting (radiotherapy)

Adult: PO 8 mg tid, may repeat q8hr

Prevention of postoperative nausea/vomiting

Adult: IV/IM 4 mg undiluted over >30 sec prior to induction of anesthesia
Child 2-12 yr: IV 0.1 mg/kg (≤40 kg); 4 mg (≥40 kg), give ≥30 sec

Hepatic dose
Adult: PO/IM/**IV** max dose 8 mg daily

Hyperemesis gravidarum (unlabeled)
Adult: PO/IV 4-8 mg bid-tid

Pruritus (unlabeled)
Adult: PO 4 mg bid

Alcoholism (unlabeled)
Adult: PO 4 mcg/kg bid

Available forms: Inj 2 mg/ml, 32 mg/50 ml (premixed); tabs 4, 8 mg; oral sol 4 mg/5 ml; oral disintegrating tabs 4, 8 mg; oral dissolving film 4.8 mg

Implementation
PO route
• **Oral disintegrating tab:** do not push through foil; gently remove and immediately place on tongue to dissolve, swallow with saliva
• **Oral dissolving film:** fold pouch along dotted line to expose near notch; while folded, tear and remove film, place film on tongue until dissolved, swallow after dissolved; to reach desired dose, administer successive films, allowing each to dissolve before using another

Direct IV route
• Give **IV** after diluting a single dose in 50 ml of 0.9% NaCl or D₅W, 0.45% NaCl; give over 15 min
• Store at room temperature for 48 hr after dilution

Y-site compatibilities: Aldesleukin, amifostine, amikacin, aztreonam, bleomycin, carboplatin, carmustine, ceFAZolin, ceforanide, cefotazime, cefoxitin, ceftazidime, ceftizoxime, cefuroxime, chlorproMAZINE, cimetidine, cisatracurium, CISplatin, cladribine, clindamycin, cyclophosphamide, cytarabine, dacarbazine, DACTINomycin, DAUNOrubicin, dexamethasone, diphenhydrAMINE, DOXOrubicin, DOXOrubicin liposome, doxycycline, droperidol, etoposide, famotidine, filgrastim, floxuridine, fluconazole, fludarabine, gentamicin, haloperidol, heparin, hydrocortisone, HYDROmorphone, hydrOXYzine, ifosfamide, imipenem/cilastatin, magnesium sulfate, mannitol, mechlorethamine, melphalan, meperidine, mesna, methotrexate, metoclopramide, miconazole, mitomycin, mitoxantrone, morphine, paclitaxel, pentostatin, potassium chloride, prochlorperazine, ranitidine, remifentanil, streptozocin, teniposide, thiotepa, ticarcillin, ticarcillin/clavulanate, vancomycin, vinBLAStine, vinCRIStine, vinorelbine, zidovudine

Y-site incompatibilities: Acyclovir, aminophylline, amphotericin B, ampicillin, ampicillin/sulbactam, cefoperazone, furosemide, ganciclovir, LORazepam, methylPREDNISolone, mezlocillin, piperacillin, sargramostim, sodium bicarbonate

ADVERSE EFFECTS
CNS: *Headache*, dizziness, drowsiness, fatigue, EPS
GI: *Diarrhea, constipation, abdominal pain*, dry mouth
MISC: Rash, **bronchospasm** (rare), *musculoskeletal pain, wound problems, shivering, fever, hypoxia, urinary retention*

Pharmacokinetics

Absorption	Completely absorbed (**IV**)
Distribution	Unknown
Metabolism	Liver, extensively
Excretion	Kidneys
Half-life	3.5-4.7 hr

Pharmacodynamics

Unknown

INTERACTIONS

Individual drugs
CarBAMazepine, phenytoin, rifampin: decreased ondansetron effect

NURSING CONSIDERATIONS

Assessment
• Assess for absence of nausea, vomiting during chemotherapy
• Assess for hypersensitivity reaction: rash, bronchospasm
• **Assess for EPS** shuffling gait, tremors, grimacing, rigidity

Nursing diagnoses
• Knowledge, deficient (teaching)
• Noncompliance (teaching)

Patient/family education
• Instruct patient to report diarrhea, constipation, rash, changes in respirations, or discomfort at insertion site
• Teach patient reason for medication and expected results

Evaluation
Positive therapeutic outcome
• Absence of nausea, vomiting during cancer chemotherapy

orlistat (Rx, OTC)
(or-li'stat)
Alli, Xenical
Chem. class.: Weight control agent, lipase inhibitor
Pregnancy category B

ACTION: Inhibits the absorption of dietary fat

Therapeutic outcome: Decrease in weight

USES: Obesity management

CONTRAINDICATIONS:
Breastfeeding, hypersensitivity, chronic malabsorption syndrome, cholestasis

Precautions: Pregnancy **B**, children, hypothyroidism, other organic causes of obesity, anorexia nervosa, bulimia, nephrolithiasis, GI disease, diabetes, fat-soluble vitamin deficiency

DOSAGE AND ROUTES
Adult: PO 60 mg (Alli)-120 mg (Xenical) tid with each main meal containing fat, max 360 mg/day

Available forms: Caps 60 mg (Alli), 120 mg (Xenical)

Implementation
• Patient should be on a diet with 30% of calories from fat; omit dose of orlistat if a meal contains no fat

ADVERSE EFFECTS
CNS: *Insomnia,* dizziness, headache, depression, anxiety, fatigue
GI: *Oily spotting, flatus with discharge, fecal urgency, fatty/oily stool, oily evacuation, fecal incontinence,* frequent defecation, nausea, vomiting, abdominal pain, infectious diarrhea, rectal pain, tooth disorder, hypovitaminosis, **hepatic failure, hepatitis, pancreatitis**
GU: UTI, vaginitis, menstrual irregularity
INTEG: Dry skin, rash
MS: Back pain, arthritis, myalgia, tendinitis
RESP: Influenza, upper, lower respiratory tract infection, EENT symptoms

Pharmacokinetics

Absorption	Minimal
Distribution	99% protein binding
Metabolism	Unknown
Excretion	Feces
Half-life	1-2 hr

Pharmacodynamics

Onset	Unknown
Peak	8 hr
Duration	Unknown

INTERACTIONS

Individual drugs
CycloSPORINE: decreased absorption
Pravastatin: increased lipid-lowering effect
Warfarin: increased effects of warfarin

Drug classifications
Fat-soluble vitamins: decreased absorption

O

Adverse effects: *italics* = common; **bold** = life-threatening

NURSING CONSIDERATIONS

Assessment
• Monitor weight weekly, diabetic patients may need reduction in oral hypoglycemics
• Assess for misuse in certain populations (anorexia nervosa, bulimia)
• **Hepatotoxicity/pancreatitis:** assess for liver injury: jaundice, weakness, abdominal pain (rare)

Nursing diagnoses
• Knowledge, deficient (teaching)
• Noncompliance (teaching)

Patient/family education
• Advise patient that 60 mg cap can be obtained OTC; 60 mg tid is the highest OTC dose
• Warn patient that safety and effectiveness beyond 2 yr have not been determined
• Instruct patient to read patient's information sheet, discuss unpleasant GI side effects
• Advise patient to avoid hazardous activities until stabilized on medication
• Instruct patient to take a multivitamin containing fat-soluble vitamins, take 2 hr before or after orlistat; psyllium taken with each dose or at bedtime may decrease GI symptoms
• Instruct patient/family to notify prescriber if significant side effects occur
• Advise prescriber if pregnancy is planned or suspected
• **Hepatotoxicity/pancreatitis:** advise patient to report yellowing skin/eyes, dark urine, weakness, abdominal pain

Evaluation
Positive therapeutic outcome
• Decreased weight

---

oseltamivir (Rx)
(oh-sell-tam′ih-ver)
Tamiflu
Func. class.: Antiviral
Chem. class.: Neuramidase inhibitor
Pregnancy category C

ACTION: Inhibits influenza virus neuraminidase with possible alteration of virus particle aggregation and release

Therapeutic outcome: Decreased symptoms of influenza type A

USES: Prevention/treatment of influenza type A or B

Unlabeled uses: Avian influenzae (H5N1), swine flu (H1N1), encephalitis

CONTRAINDICATIONS:
Hypersensitivity

Precautions: Pregnancy **C**, geriatric, renal/hepatic/pulmonary/cardiac disease, infants, children, neonates, psychosis, viral infection, breastfeeding

DOSAGE AND ROUTES

Treatment
Adult and child >40 kg: PO 75 bid mg × 5 days, begin treatment within 2 days of onset of symptoms
Child 23-40 kg and ≥1 yr: PO 60 mg bid
Child 15-23 kg and ≥1 yr: PO 45 mg bid
Child ≤15 kg and ≥1 yr: PO 30 mg bid

Prevention
Adult and child ≥13 yr: PO 75 mg/day × ≥7 days; begin treatment within 2 days of contact, max use 6 wk

Renal dose
Adult: PO CCr 10-30 ml/min 75 mg/day × 5 days (treatment); 75 mg every other day or 30 mg/day (prophylaxis)

H1N1 influenzae A virus (unlabeled)
Adult/adolescent/child >40 kg: PO 75 mg bid × 5 days
Child/adolescent 24-40 kg: PO 60 mg bid × 5 days
Child >1 yr and 15-23 kg: PO 45 mg bid × 5 days
Child >1 yr and <15 kg: PO 30 mg bid × 5 days

Available forms: Caps 30, 45, 75 mg; powder for oral susp 6 mg/ml

Implementation
• Give within 2 days of symptoms of influenza; continue for 5 days
• Give at least 4 hr before bedtime to prevent insomnia
• 12 mg/ml concentration will be available for a limited time, new product is 6 mg/ml concentration, take care to give correct dose
• Give without regard to food, give with food for GI upset
• **Oral susp:** loosen powder from side of bottle 55 ml shake well (6 mg/ml); remove child-resistant cap and push bottle adapter into neck of bottle, close tightly with child-resistant cap to ensure sealing; use within 17 days of preparation when refrigerated or 10 days at room temperature, write expiration date on bottle, shake well before use, use oral syringe provided but

---

⚠ Nurse Alert

only with markings for 30, 45, 60 mg, confirm dosing instructions are in same units as syringe provided
• Store in airtight, dry container

ADVERSE EFFECTS
CNS: Headache, fatigue, insomnia, dizziness, delirium, **self-injury (children)**
ENDO: Hyperglycemia
GI: *Nausea, vomiting,* diarrhea, abdominal pain
INTEG: **Toxic epidermal necrolysis, Stevens-Johnson syndrome, erythema multiforme**
RESP: Cough

Pharmacokinetics
Absorption	Rapidly absorbed
Distribution	Protein binding 3%
Metabolism	Converted to oseltamivir carboxylate (active form)
Excretion	Eliminated by conversion, urine 99%
Half-life	1-3 hr (active form)

Pharmacodynamics
Unknown

INTERACTIONS
Avoid use with H1N1 virus vaccine, intranasal influenza vaccine

NURSING CONSIDERATIONS
Assessment
• **Influenza:** assess for symptoms of influenza A: increased temperature, malaise, aches and pains

Nursing diagnoses
• Infection, risk for (uses)
• Knowledge, deficient (teaching)

Patient/family education
• Teach patient about aspects of product therapy
• Teach patient to avoid hazardous activities if dizziness occurs
• Advise patient to take as soon as symptoms appear, to take full course, even if feeling better
• Advise patient to take missed dose as soon as remembered if within 2 hr of next dose
• Teach patient to stop product immediately and report to prescriber skin rash, delirium, psychosis, hallucinations (child)
• Advise patient that product is not a substitute for a flu shot

• Inform patient to avoid other products without approval of prescriber

Evaluation
Positive therapeutic outcome
• Absence of fever, malaise, cough, dyspnea in influenza A

⚠ HIGH ALERT

oxaliplatin (Rx)
(ox-al-i′plat-in)
Eloxitin
Func. class.: Antineoplastic
Chem. class.: 3rd generation platinum analog
Pregnancy category D

ACTION: Forms cross links, inhibiting DNA replication and transcription, cell-cycle nonspecific

Therapeutic outcome: Decreased size of tumor, spread of malignancy

USES: Metastatic carcinoma of the colon or rectum in combination with 5-FU/leucovorin

Unlabeled uses: Relapsed or refractory non-Hodgkin's lymphoma, advanced ovarian cancer

CONTRAINDICATIONS:
Pregnancy **D**, breastfeeding, radiation therapy or chemotherapy within 1 mo, thrombocytopenia, smallpox vaccination

BLACK BOX WARNING: Hypersensitivity to this product or other platinum products

Precautions: Children, geriatric, pneumococcus vaccination, renal disease

DOSAGE AND ROUTES
Colorectal cancer
Dosage protocols may vary
Adult: IV INF *Day 1:* oxaliplatin 85 mg/m² in 250-500 ml D₅W and leucovorin 200 mg/m² in D₅W, give both over 2 hr at the same time in separate bags using a Y-line, followed by 5-FU 400 mg/m² IV BOL over 2-4 min, then 5-FU 600 mg/m² IV INF in 500 ml D₅W as a 22-hr CONT INF; *Day 2:* leucovorin 200 mg/m² IV INF over 2 hr, then 5-FU 400 mg/m² IV BOL over 2-4 min, then 5-FU 600 mg/m² IV INF in 500 ml D₅W as a 22-hr CONT INF; repeat cycle q2wk

Available forms: Powder for inj 50, 100 mg single-use vials (5 mg/ml)

Implementation

Intermittent IV INF route

- Premedicate with antiemetics including 5-HT₃ blockers, with or without dexamethasone, prehydration is not needed
- Do not reconstitute or dilute with sodium chloride or any chloride-containing solutions, do not use aluminum equipment during any preparation or administration, will degrade platinum; do not refrigerate unopened powder or solution; do not freeze; protect from light
- Use cytotoxic handling procedures; prepare in biological cabinet using gown, gloves, mask; do not allow product to come in contact with skin; use soap and water if contact occurs
- EPINEPHrine, antihistamines, corticosteroids for hypersensitivity reaction
- **Lyophilized powder:** reconstitute vial 50 mg/10 ml, or 100 mg/20 ml sterile water for inj or D₅W, after reconstitution, solution may be stored for ≤24 hr in refrigerator, after dilution in 250-500 ml D₅W, may store ≤24 hr in refrigerator or 6 hr at room temp, infuse over 2 hr
- **Aqueous solution:** dilute in 250-500 ml of D₅W, after dilution may store ≤24 hr refrigerator, 6 hr at room temp, infuse over 2 hr

Y-site compatibilities: Alfentanil, amifostine, amikacin, aminocaproic acid, amiodarone, amphotericin B colloidal, amphotericin B lipid complex, amphotericin B liposome, ampicillin, ampicillin-sulbactam, anidulafungin, atenolol, atracurium, azithromycin, aztreonam, bivalirudin, bleomycin, bumetanide, buprenorphine, butorphanol, calcium chloride/gluconate, CARBOplatin, caspofungin, ceFAZolin, cefotaxime, cefotetan, cefoxitin, ceftazidime, ceftizoxime, cefTRIAXone, cefuroxime, chloramphenicol, chlorproMAZINE, cimetidine, ciprofloxacin, cisatracurium, CISplatin, clindamycin, cyclophosphamide, cycloSPORINE, cytarabine, dacarbazine, DACTINomycin, DAPTOmycin, DAUNOrubicin, dexamethasone, digoxin, diltiazem, diphenhydrAMINE, DOBUTamine, docetaxel, dolasetron, DOPamine, doxacurium, DOXOrubicin, doxycycline, droperidol, enalaprilat, ePHEDrine, EPINEPHrine, epirubicin, ertapenem, erythromycin, esmolol, etoposide, famotidine, fenoldopam, fentaNYL, fluconazole, fludarabine, foscarnet, fosphenytoin, furosemide, gatifloxacin, gemcitabine, gemtuzumab, gentamicin, glycopyrrolate, granisetron, haloperidol, heparin, hydrALAZINE, hydrocortisone, HYDROmorphone, hydrOXYzine, IDArubicin, ifosfamide, imipenem-cilastatin, inamrinone, insulin (regular), irinotecan, isoproterenol, ketorolac, labetalol, leucovorin, levofloxacin, levorphanol, lidocaine, linezolid, LORazepam, magnesium sulfate, mannitol, meperidine, meropenem, mesna, metaraminol, methyldopate, methylPREDNISolone, metoclopramide, metoprolol, metroNIDAZOLE, midazolam, milrinone, minocycline, mitomycin, mitoxantrone, mivacurium, morphine, nafcillin, nalbuphine, naloxone, nesiritide, niCARdipine, nitroglycerin, nitroprusside, norepinephrine, octreotide, ondansetron, paclitaxel, palonosetron, pancuronium, pemetrexed, pentamidine, pentazocine, phenylephrine, piperacillin, polymyxin B, potassium chloride/phosphates, procainamide, prochlorperazine, promethazine, propranolol, quiNIDine, quinupristin-dalfopristin, ranitidine, rocuronium, sodium acetate/phosphates, succinylcholine, SUFentanil, sulfamethoxazole-trimethoprim, tacrolimus, teniposide, theophylline, thiotepa, ticarcillin, ticarcillin-clavulanate, tigecycline, tirofiban, tobramycin, tolazoline, topotecan, trimethobenzamide, vancomycin, vasopressin, vecuronium, verapamil, vinBLAStine, vinCRIStine, vinorelbine, voriconazole, zidovudine, zoledronic acid

ADVERSE EFFECTS

CNS: Peripheral neuropathy, fatigue, headache, dizziness, insomnia
CV: Cardiac abnormalities, **thromboembolism**
EENT: *Decreased visual acuity, tinnitus, hearing loss*
GI: *Severe nausea, vomiting, diarrhea, weight loss,* stomatitis, anorexia, gastroesophageal reflux, constipation, dyspepsia, mucositis, flatulence
GU: Hematuria, dysuria, creatinine
HEMA: Thrombocytopenia, leukopenia, pancytopenia, neutropenia, anemia, hemolytic uremic syndrome
INTEG: *Alopecia,* rash, flushing, extravasation, redness, swelling, pain at inj site
META: Hypokalemia
RESP: Fibrosis, dyspnea, cough, rhinitis, URI, pharyngitis
SYST: Anaphylaxis, angioedema

Pharmacokinetics

Absorption	Unknown
Distribution	15% of platinum in systemic circulation; 85% is either in tissues or being eliminated in urine
Metabolism	Liver
Excretion	Urine
Half-life	40 days

Pharmacodynamics

Unknown

INTERACTIONS
Individual drugs
Alcohol, aspirin: increased risk of bleeding
Radiation: increased myelosuppression

Drug classifications
Aminoglycosides, diuretics (loop): increased nephrotoxicity
Anticoagulants, NSAIDs, platelet inhibitors, thrombolytics, salicylates: increased risk of bleeding
Live virus vaccines: decreased antibody response
Myelosuppressives: increased myelosuppression
Tannins: increased oxaliplatin toxicity

Drug/lab test
Increased: ALT, AST, bilirubin, creatinine
Decreased: potassium, neutrophils, WBC, platelets

NURSING CONSIDERATIONS
Assessment
• **Bone marrow depression:** monitor CBC, differential, platelet count weekly; withhold product if WBC is <4000 or platelet count is <100,000; notify prescriber of results
• Monitor renal function tests: BUN, creatinine, serum uric acid, urine CCr before, electrolytes during therapy; dose should not be given if BUN >19 mg/dl; creatinine <1.5 mg/dl; I&O ratio; report fall in urine output of <30 ml/hr

> **BLACK BOX WARNING: Assess for anaphylaxis:** wheezing, tachycardia, facial swelling, fainting; discontinue product and report to prescriber; resuscitation equipment should be nearby

• Monitor temp (may indicate beginning infection)
• Monitor liver function tests before, during therapy (bilirubin, AST, ALT, LDH) as needed or monthly

• **Assess for bleeding:** hematuria, guaiac, bruising or petechiae, mucosa or orifices q8hr; obtain prescription for viscous lidocaine (Xylocaine)
• Assess effects of alopecia on body image; discuss feelings about body changes
• Assess for jaundice of skin, sclera; dark urine; clay-colored stools; itchy skin; abdominal pain; fever; diarrhea
• Assess for edema in feet, joint pain, stomach pain, shaking
• **Pulmonary fibrosis:** assess for cough, crackles, dyspnea, pulmonary infiltrate; discontinue immediately; may be fatal

Nursing diagnoses
• Infection, risk for (adverse reactions)
• Knowledge, deficient (teaching)
• Nutrition: less than body requirements, imbalanced (adverse reactions)

Patient/family education
• **Advise patient to report signs of infection:** increased temp, sore throat, flulike symptoms
• **Advise patient to report signs of anemia:** fatigue, headache, faintness, shortness of breath, irritability
• **Advise patient to report bleeding;** avoid use of razors, commercial mouthwash
• Advise patient to avoid aspirin, ibuprofen, NSAIDs, alcohol; may cause GI bleeding
• Advise patient to report any changes in breathing, coughing
• Advise patient that hair may be lost during treatment; a wig or hairpiece may make patient feel better; new hair may be different in color, texture
• Advise patient to report numbness, tingling in face or extremities, poor hearing or joint pain, swelling
• Advise patient not to receive vaccines during treatment
• Advise patient to use contraception during treatment and 4 mo after; this product may cause infertility, pregnancy **D**
• Teach patient to avoid contact with cold (air, ice, liquid); causes acute dysesthesias

Evaluation
Positive therapeutic outcome
• Decreased tumor size, spread of malignancy

oxazepam (Rx)

(ox-az′e-pam)

Apo-Oxazepam ✦

Func. class.: Sedative-hypnotic; antianxiety

Chem. class.: Benzodiazepine, short-acting

Pregnancy category D

Controlled substance schedule IV

ACTION: Depresses subcortical levels of CNS, including limbic system, reticular formation; potentiates GABA

Therapeutic outcome: Decreased anxiety, successful alcohol withdrawal, relaxation

USES: Anxiety, alcohol withdrawal, insomnia

CONTRAINDICATIONS:

Pregnancy **D,** breastfeeding, children <12 yr, hypersensitivity to benzodiazepines, closed-angle glaucoma, psychosis

Precautions: Geriatric, debilitated, renal/hepatic disease, depression, suicidal ideation, dementia, sleep apnea, seizure disorder

DOSAGE AND ROUTES

Anxiety

Adult: PO 10-30 mg tid-qid, max 120 mg/day

Geriatric: PO 5 mg daily-bid initially, may increase, max 15 mg qid

Alcohol withdrawal

Adult: PO 15-30 mg tid-qid

Available forms: Caps 10, 15, 30 mg

Implementation

• Give with food or milk for GI symptoms; tab may be crushed if patient is unable to swallow medication whole

ADVERSE EFFECTS

CNS: *Dizziness, drowsiness,* confusion, headache, anxiety, tremors, fatigue, depression, insomnia, hallucinations, paradoxical excitement, transient amnesia

CV: *Orthostatic hypotension,* **ECG changes, tachycardia,** hypotension

EENT: *Blurred vision,* tinnitus, mydriasis

GI: Nausea, vomiting, anorexia

HEMA: Leukopenia

INTEG: Rash, dermatitis, itching

SYST: Dependence

Pharmacokinetics

Absorption	Well absorbed
Distribution	Widely distributed; crosses placenta, blood-brain barrier
Metabolism	Liver
Excretion	Kidneys, breast milk
Half-life	5-15 hr

Pharmacodynamics

Onset	$1/2$-$1^1/_2$ hr
Peak	Unknown
Duration	6-12 hr

INTERACTIONS

Individual drugs

Alcohol: increased CNS depression

Disulfiram: increased oxazepam effects

Levodopa: decreased effects of levodopa

Phenytoin, theophylline, valproic acid: decreased oxazepam effects

Drug classifications

CNS depressants: increased oxazepam effects

Oral contraceptives: increased or decreased oxazepam effect

Drug/herb

Kava, melatonin, valerian: increased CNS depression

Drug/lab test

Increased: AST, ALT, serum bilirubin

Decreased: radioactive iodine uptake

False increase: 17-OHCS

NURSING CONSIDERATIONS

Assessment

• Assess mental status: mood, sensorium, anxiety, affect, sleeping pattern, drowsiness, dizziness, **suicidal thoughts, behavior; physical dependency, withdrawal symptoms:** anxiety, panic attacks, agitation, seizures, headache, nausea, vomiting, muscle pain, weakness; suicidal thoughts, behavior; indications of increasing tolerance and abuse

• Monitor B/P with patient lying, standing; pulse; if systolic B/P drops 20 mm Hg, hold product, notify prescriber

Nursing diagnoses

• Anxiety (uses)

• Injury, risk for (adverse reactions)

• Knowledge, deficient (teaching)

⚠ Nurse Alert

Patient/family education
• Teach patient that product may be taken with food or fluids; tab may be crushed or swallowed whole
• Caution patient not to use for everyday stress or longer than 4 mo unless directed by prescriber; not to take more than prescribed amount; not to double doses or skip doses
• Advise patient to avoid OTC preparations unless approved by prescriber; alcohol and CNS depressants will increase CNS depression
• Caution patient to avoid driving and activities that require alertness, since drowsiness may occur; to avoid alcohol and other psychotropic medications; to rise slowly or fainting may occur, especially geriatric; that drowsiness may worsen at beginning of treatment
• Caution patient not to discontinue medication abruptly after long-term use; withdrawal symptoms include vomiting, cramping, tremors, seizures
• Advise patient to use sugarless gum, hard candy, frequent sips of water for dry mouth
• Teach patient that drowsiness may worsen at beginning of treatment

Evaluation
Positive therapeutic outcome
• Decreased anxiety, restlessness, sleeplessness (short-term treatment only)

TREATMENT OF OVERDOSE:
Lavage, VS, supportive care

OXcarbazepine (Rx)
(ox′kar-baz′uh-peen)
Trileptal
Func. class.: Anticonvulsant
Pregnancy category C

ACTION: May inhibit nerve impulses by limiting influx of sodium ions across cell membrane in motor cortex

Therapeutic outcome: Absence of seizures

USES: Partial seizures

Unlabeled uses: Trigeminal neuralgia, atypical panic disorder, bipolar disorder

CONTRAINDICATIONS:
Hypersensitivity

Precautions: Pregnancy C, breastfeeding, children <4 yr, hypersensitivity to carbamaze-pine, renal disease, fluid restriction, hyponatremia, abrupt discontinuation, suicidal ideation

DOSAGE AND ROUTES
Seizures adjunctive therapy
Adult: PO 300 mg bid, may be increased by 600 mg/day in divided doses bid at weekly intervals; maintenance 1200 mg/day
Child 4-16 yr: PO 8-10 mg/kg/day divided bid, dose is determined by weight, increase by 5 mg/kg/day q3 days, max doses are weight dependent

Conversion to monotherapy in partial seizures
Adult: PO 300 mg bid with reduction in other anticonvulsants, increase OXcarbazepine by 600 mg/day qwk over 2-4 wk; withdraw other anticonvulsants over 3-6 wk, max 2400 mg/day

Initiation of monotherapy in partial seizures
Adult: PO 300 mg bid, increase by 300 mg/day q3day to 1200 mg divided bid

Renal dose
Adult: PO CCr <30 ml/min 150 mg bid and increase slowly

Available forms: Film-coated tabs 150, 300, 600 mg; oral susp 300 mg/5 ml

Implementation
• Store product at room temperature
• Provide assistance with ambulation during early part of treatment; dizziness may occur
• Give product with food, milk to decrease GI symptoms
• **Oral susp:** shake well, use calibrated oral syringe provided, use or discard within 7 days of opening

ADVERSE EFFECTS
CNS: *Headache, dizziness, confusion, fatigue,* feeling abnormal, ataxia, abnormal gait, tremors, anxiety, agitation, **worsening of seizures, suicidal ideation/behavior**
CV: *Hypotension,* chest pain, edema
EENT: *Blurred vision, diplopia, nystagmus,* rhinitis, sinusitis
GI: *Nausea, constipation, diarrhea,* anorexia, vomiting, abdominal pain, gastritis
INTEG: Purpura, rash, acne
SYST: **Angioedema, anaphylaxis, Stevens-Johnson syndrome, toxic epidermal necrolysis, drug reaction with eosinophilia and systemic symptoms (DRESS)**

Absorption	Unknown
Distribution	Unknown
Metabolism	Liver
Excretion	Unknown
Half-life	Unknown

Pharmacodynamics

Onset	Unknown
Peak	4-6 hr
Duration	Unknown

INTERACTIONS

Individual products
Alcohol: increased CNS depression
CarBAMazepine: decreased carBAMazepine level, decreased OXcarbazepine levels
Felodipine: decreased effects of felodipine
Nisoldipine, ranolazine: do not use concurrently
PHENobarbital, valproic acid, verapamil: decreased OXcarbazepine level
Phenytoin: decreased OXcarbazepine level

Drug classifications
Contraceptives (oral): decreased oral contraceptive level
MAOIs: do not use concurrently

Drug/herb
Ginkgo: increased anticonvulsant effect
Ginseng, santonica: decreased anticonvulsant effect

NURSING CONSIDERATIONS

Assessment
• **Assess seizure activity,** including frequency, duration, and aura; provide seizure precautions
• Assess mental status including mood, sensorium, affect, behavioral changes, suicidal thoughts, behavior; if mental status changes, notify prescriber
• Assess eye problems: ophthalmic examinations (slit lamp, funduscopy, tonometry) are needed before, during, after treatment
• Assess patient for hypersensitivity to carBAMazepine
• **Assess for serious skin reactions:** angioedema, anaphylaxis, Stevens-Johnson syndrome

Nursing diagnoses
• Injury, risk for (side effects)
• Knowledge, deficient (teaching)

Patient/family education
• Caution patient to avoid driving, other activities that require alertness
• Advise patient not to discontinue medication quickly after long-term use
• Instruct patient to avoid use of alcohol while taking this medication
• Instruct patient to use alternative contraception if using hormonal method
• Instruct patient to inform prescriber if allergic to carBAMazepine; multisystem hypersensitivity may occur, to report fever, other allergic symptoms

Evaluation
Positive therapeutic outcome
• Decreased seizure activity

TREATMENT OF OVERDOSE:
Activated charcoal, give 0.9% NaCl (hypotensive state), atropine (bradycardia); use benzodiazepines, barbiturates for seizures

---

oxybutynin (Rx)
(ox-i-byoo'ti-nin)
Ditropan, Ditropan XL, Gelnique, Oxytrol ❧, Oxytrol Transdermal, Uromax ❧
Func. class.: Anticholinergic
Chem. class.: Synthetic tertiary amine
Pregnancy category B

Do not confuse:
Ditropan/diazepam

ACTION: Relaxes smooth muscles in urinary tract by inhibiting acetylcholine at postganglionic sites

Therapeutic outcome: Decreased symptoms of urgency, nocturia, incontinence

USES: Antispasmodic for neurogenic bladder, overactive bladder

CONTRAINDICATIONS:
Hypersensitivity, GI obstruction, urinary retention, glaucoma, severe colitis, myasthenia gravis, unstable CV, infants

Precautions: Pregnancy **B,** breastfeeding, children <12 yr, geriatric, suspected glaucoma, cardiac disease, dementia

DOSAGE AND ROUTES
Adult: PO 5 mg bid-tid, max 5 mg qid; EXT REL tabs 5-10 mg/day, may increase by 5 mg, max 30 mg/day; transdermal apply one patch to abdomen, hip, buttock 2 ×/wk (q3-4day); GEL apply contents of 1 packet to abdomen, upper arms, shoulders, thighs daily

---

⚠ Nurse Alert

Geriatric: PO 2.5-5 mg bid-tid, increase by 2.5 mg q several days
Child ≥6 yr: PO 5 mg bid, not to exceed 5 mg tid; EXT REL 5 mg/day, max 20 mg/day
Child 1-5 yr: PO 0.2 mg/kg/dose 2-3 ×/day

Available forms: Syr 5 mg/5 ml; tabs 5 mg; ext rel tabs 5, 10, 15 mg; transdermal 3.9 mg/day; top gel 10% (Gelnique)

Implementation
PO route
• Do not break, crush, or chew ext rel tabs
• May be given with meals or fluids or on an empty stomach
Topical route
• Wash hands, apply to clean, dry, intact skin on abdomen, upper arms/shoulders, thighs, avoid navel, rotate sites
• Squeeze contents in palm of hand or directly on this site, rub gently
• Do not bathe, exercise, swim for 1 hr after application
• Allow to dry before putting on clothing
• Do not be near flame, fire, or smoke until gel has dried
• Delivers 100 mg
Transdermal route
• Apply to clean, dry, intact skin on the abdomen, hip, buttock, use firm pressure, not affected by showering/bathing; rotate sites
• Delivers 3.9 mg/day

ADVERSE EFFECTS
CNS: *Anxiety, restlessness, dizziness,* somnolence, insomnia, nervousness, **seizures,** headache, drowsiness, confusion
CV: *Palpitations, sinus tachycardia,* hypertension, peripheral edema, **QT prolongation**
EENT: Blurred vision, increased intraocular tension; dry mouth, throat, dry eyes
GI: *Nausea, vomiting, anorexia,* abdominal pain, constipation, *dyspepsia,* diarrhea, taste perversion, GERD
GU: Dysuria, impotence, retention, hesitancy
MISC: **Hyperthermia, anaphylaxis, angioedema**

Pharmacokinetics
Absorption	Rapidly absorbed
Distribution	Unknown
Metabolism	Liver
Excretion	Unknown
Half-life	Unknown

Pharmacodynamics
Onset	$1/2$-1 hr
Peak	3-4 hr
Duration	6-10 hr

INTERACTIONS
Individual drugs
Acetaminophen: decreased levels of acetaminophen
Amantadine: increased anticholinergic effects
Atenolol: increased levels of atenolol
Digoxin: increased levels of digoxin
Haloperidol, chloroquine, droperidol, pentamidine, arsenic trioxide, levomethadyl: increased QT prolongation
Levodopa: decreased levels of levodopa
Nitrofurantoin: increased levels of nitrofurantoin

Drug classifications
Antihistamines, other anticholinergics: increased anticholinergic effects
Benzodiazepines, sedatives, hypnotics, opioids: increased CNS depression
Class IA/III antidysrhythmics, some phenothiazines, β-agonists, local anesthetics, tricyclics, CYP3A4 inhibitors (amiodarone, clarithromycin, erythromycin, telithromycin, troleandomycin), CYP3A4 substrates (methadone, pimozide, quetiapine, quiNIDine, risperidone, ziprasidone): increased QT prolongation

NURSING CONSIDERATIONS
Assessment
• **Assess for allergic reactions:** rash, urticaria; if these occur, product should be discontinued
• **Assess urinary patterns:** distention, nocturia, frequency, urgency, incontinence; catheterization may be required to remove residual urine
• **QT prolongation:** assess ECG for QT prolongation, ejection fraction; assess for chest pain, palpitations, dyspnea

Nursing diagnoses
• Knowledge, deficient (teaching)
• Pain, acute (uses)
• Urinary elimination, impaired (uses)

Patient/family education
• Advise patient to avoid hazardous activities until response to product is known; dizziness, blurred vision may occur
• Caution patient to avoid OTC medication with alcohol or other CNS depressants

O

- Teach patient to use frequent rinsing of mouth, sips of water for dry mouth
- Teach patient to stay cool; avoid hot weather, strenuous activity since overheating may occur; product decreases perspiration
- Advise patient to report CNS effects: confusion, anxiety, anticholinergic effect in the geriatric

Evaluation
Positive therapeutic outcome
- Absence of dysuria, frequency, nocturia, incontinence

⚠ HIGH ALERT

oxyCODONE (Rx)
(ox-i-koe'done)
ETH-Oxydose, Oxecta, OxyContin, Roxicodone, Supeudol ✦
oxyCODONE/acetaminophen (Rx)
Magnacet, Percocet, Primalev, Roxicet, Tylox, Xolox
oxyCODONE/aspirin (Rx)
Endodan ✦, Percodan
oxyCODONE/ibuprofen (Rx)
Func. class.: Opiate analgesic
Chem. class.: Semisynthetic derivative
Pregnancy category B
Controlled substance schedule II

Do not confuse:
Percodan/Decadron, **Roxicet**/Roxanol, **Tylox**/Trimox/Wymox/Xanax

ACTION: Inhibits ascending pain pathways in CNS, increases pain threshold, alters pain perception

Therapeutic outcome: Decreased pain

USES: Moderate to severe pain

Unlabeled uses: Postherpetic neuralgia (cont rel)

CONTRAINDICATIONS:
Hypersensitivity, addiction (opiate), asthma, ileus

BLACK BOX WARNING: Respiratory depression

Precautions: Pregnancy **B**, breastfeeding, children <18 yr, addictive personality,

increased ICP, MI (acute), severe heart disease, renal/hepatic disease, bowel impaction

BLACK BOX WARNING: Opioid-naïve patients, substance abuse

DOSAGE AND ROUTES
Adult: PO 10-30 mg q4hr (5 mg q6hr for Oxyl R, OxyFast); **OxyFast CONC SOL is extremely concentrated, do not use interchangeably;** CONT REL 10 mg q12hr in opiate-naïve patients

Available forms: OxyCODONE: cont rel tabs (OxyCONTIN) 10, 15, 20, 40, 80, 160 mg; immediate rel tabs 5, 15, 30 mg; immediate rel caps 5 mg; oral sol 5 mg/5 ml, 20 mg/ml; oxyCODONE with acetaminophen: tabs 2.5 mg/300 mg, 2.5 mg/325 mg, 5 mg/300 mg, 5 mg/325 mg; 7.5 mg/325 mg, 7.5 mg/500 mg, 10 mg/325 mg, 10 mg/400 mg, 10 mg/650 mg; caps 5 mg/500 mg; oral sol 5 mg/325 mg/5 ml; oxyCODONE with aspirin: 4.88 mg/325 mg oxyCODONE with ibuprofen: 5 mg/400 mg

Implementation
- Give with antiemetic if nausea, vomiting occur
- Give when pain is beginning to return; determine dosage interval by patient response; continuous dosing of medication is more effective than when given prn
- Medication should be slowly withdrawn after long-term use to prevent withdrawal symptoms
- Store in light-resistant container at room temperature
PO route
- Do not break, crush, or chew cont rel tabs; give q12hr, no more frequently
- May be given with food or milk to lessen GI upset
- Use 80, 160 mg cont rel tabs (oxyCONTIN) only in opioid-tolerant patients

ADVERSE EFFECTS
CNS: *Drowsiness, dizziness, confusion, headache, sedation, euphoria,* fatigue, abnormal dreams, thoughts, hallucinations
CV: Palpitations, bradycardia, change in B/P
EENT: Tinnitus, blurred vision, miosis, diplopia
GI: *Nausea, vomiting, anorexia, constipation, cramps,* gastritis, dyspepsia, biliary spasms
GU: Increased urinary output, dysuria, urinary retention
INTEG: *Rash,* urticaria, bruising, flushing, diaphoresis, pruritus
RESP: Respiratory depression

⚠ Nurse Alert

Pharmacokinetics

Absorption	Well absorbed
Distribution	Widely distributed; crosses placenta, protein binding 45%
Metabolism	Liver, extensively
Excretion	Kidneys, breast milk
Half-life	3-5 hr

Pharmacodynamics

	PO	RECT
Onset	15-30 min	Unknown
Peak	$1/2$-1 hr	Unknown
Duration	3-4 hr	4-6 hr

INTERACTIONS

Individual drugs
Alcohol: increased respiratory depression, hypotension, sedation
Cimetidine: increased toxicity

Drug classifications
Antipsychotics, CNS depressants, opioids, sedative/hypnotics, skeletal muscle relaxants: increased respiratory depression, hypotension
MAOIs: increased toxicity

Drug/herb
St. John's wort, valerian: increased sedative effect

Drug/lab test
Increased: amylase, lipase

NURSING CONSIDERATIONS

Assessment
• **Pain:** assess intensity, location, type, characteristics; need for pain medication by pain/sedation scoring; physical dependence
• Monitor I&O ratio; check for decreasing output; may indicate urinary retention
• **CNS changes:** assess for dizziness, drowsiness, hallucinations, euphoria, LOC, pupil reaction
• **Allergic reactions:** assess for rash, urticaria

BLACK BOX WARNING: Respiratory dysfunction: assess for respiratory depression, character, rate, rhythm; notify prescriber if respirations are <10/min; also B/P, pulse

• **Bowel status:** assess for constipation; stimulate laxative may be needed with fluids, fiber
• Monitor VS after parenteral route; note muscle rigidity, product history, renal, liver function tests, respiratory dysfunction: respiratory depression, character, rate, rhythm; notify prescriber if respirations are <10/min

Nursing diagnoses
• Injury, risk for (adverse reactions)
• Knowledge, deficient (teaching)
• Pain, acute (uses)
• Pain, chronic

Patient/family education
• Advise patients to avoid CNS depressants: alcohol, sedative/hypnotics
• Discuss with patient that dizziness, drowsiness, and confusion are common; to avoid getting up without assistance
• Discuss in detail all aspects of the product, including purpose and what to expect
• Advise patient to make position changes slowly to lessen orthostatic hypotension
• Advise patient to avoid CNS depressants, alcohol
• Advise patient to avoid operating machinery, driving if drowsiness occurs
• Teach patient that withdrawal symptoms may occur after long-term use: nausea, vomiting, cramps, fever, faintness, anorexia

Evaluation
Positive therapeutic outcome
• Decreased pain

TREATMENT OF OVERDOSE: Naloxone 0.2-0.8 **IV,** O_2, **IV** fluids, vasopressors

oxymetazoline nasal agent
See Appendix B

oxymetazoline ophthalmic
See Appendix B

⚠ HIGH ALERT

oxymorphone (Rx)
(ox-i-mor'fone)
Opana, Opana ER
Func. class.: Opiate analgesic
Chem. class.: Semisynthetic phenanthrene derivative
Pregnancy category B
Controlled substance schedule II

ACTION: Depresses pain impulse transmission at the spinal cord level by interacting with opioid receptors, increases pain threshold, alters pain perception

Therapeutic outcome: Decreased pain

USES: Moderate to severe pain

CONTRAINDICATIONS:
Hypersensitivity, addiction (opioid), asthma, hepatic disease, ileus, intrathecal use, surgery

> **BLACK BOX WARNING:** Respiratory depression

Precautions: Pregnancy **B** (short-term), breastfeeding, children <18 yr, addictive personality, increased ICP, MI (acute), severe heart disease, respiratory depression, renal/hepatic disease, bowel impaction

> **BLACK BOX WARNING:** Alcoholism, opioid-naïve patients, substance abuse

DOSAGE AND ROUTES
Adult: IM/SUBCUT 1-1.5 mg q4-6hr prn; **IV** 0.5 mg q4-6hr prn; PO (immediate release only) 5-20 mg q4-6hr prn; PO-ER 5 mg q12hr in those requiring around the clock dosing

Labor analgesia
Adult: IM 0.5-1 mg

Available forms: Inj 1, 1.5 mg/ml; supp 5 mg; ER tab 5, 10, 20, 40 mg; tabs 5, 10 mg

Implementation
• Give 1 hr before or 2 hr after food (PO)
• Give with antiemetic if nausea, vomiting occur
• Do not break, crush, chew ER product
• Give when pain is beginning to return; determine dosage interval by patient response; continuous dosing of medication is more effective than when given prn
• Medication should be slowly withdrawn after long-term use to prevent withdrawal symptoms
• Store in light-resistant container at room temperature

CONTROLLED REL
• **Opiate naive:** start with lowest dose, titrate upward in 5-10 mg q12hr q3-7days to therapeutic response
• When converting from immediate release to ext rel, give ½ daily dose of ER product q12hr

Direct IV route
• Give undiluted over 2-3 min

Syringe compatibilities: Glycopyrrolate, hydrOXYzine, ranitidine

ADVERSE EFFECTS
CNS: *Drowsiness, dizziness, confusion, headache, sedation, euphoria (geriatric),* seizures, hallucinations, **increased ICP**

CV: Palpitations, **bradycardia,** change in B/P, hypotension
EENT: Tinnitus, blurred vision, miosis, diplopia
GI: *Nausea, vomiting, anorexia, constipation, cramps*
GU: Dysuria, urinary retention
INTEG: *Rash,* urticaria, bruising, flushing, diaphoresis, pruritus
RESP: Respiratory depression

Pharmacokinetics

Absorption	Well absorbed (RECT, IM, SUBCUT); completely absorbed (**IV**)
Distribution	Widely distributed; crosses placenta
Metabolism	Liver, extensively
Excretion	Kidneys
Half-life	2½-4 hr

Pharmacodynamics

	IM/SUBCUT	IV	RECT
Onset	15 min	10 min	30 min
Peak	1-1½ hr	15-30 min	Unknown
Duration	3-6 hr	3-4 hr	3-6 hr

INTERACTIONS
Individual drugs
Alcohol: increased respiratory depression, hypotension, sedation

Drug classifications
CNS depressants, opiates, antipsychotics, skeletal muscle relaxants, sedative/hypnotics: increased respiratory depression, hypotension
MAOIs: do not use 2 wk before oxymorphone; unpredictable effects

Drug/herb
Kava, St. John's wort, valerian: increased sedative effect

Drug/lab test
Increased: amylase

NURSING CONSIDERATIONS
Assessment
• **Pain:** assess location, intensity, type, other characteristics, before and 1 hr after (IM) IV 30 min; need for pain medication, physical dependence, give 25%-50% until there is pain reduction of 50% on pain rating scale, repeat

oxytocin **803**

dose may be given at time of peak, if previous dose does not control pain, and respiratory depression has not occurred; give short-acting opioids for breakthrough pain if on controlled rel product

> **BLACK BOX WARNING: Respiratory dysfunction:** Assess for respiratory depression, character, rate, rhythm; notify prescriber if respirations are <10/min

• **Assess bowel/bladder status:** constipation, may need stimulant laxative; I&O ratio for decreasing output, may indicate urinary retention
• Monitor VS after parenteral route; note muscle rigidity, product history, liver, kidney function tests
• Monitor CNS changes: dizziness, drowsiness, hallucinations, euphoria, LOC, pupil reaction
• Monitor allergic reactions: rash, urticaria

Nursing diagnoses
• Injury, risk for (adverse reactions)
• Knowledge, deficient (teaching)
• Pain, acute (uses)

Patient/family education
• Advise patient not to use other CNS depressants: alcohol, sedative/hypnotics
• Discuss with patient that dizziness, drowsiness, and confusion are common; to avoid getting up without assistance
• Discuss in detail all aspects of the product, including purpose and what to expect
• Advise patient to make position changes slowly to lessen orthostatic hypotension
• Advise patient not to drive, operate machinery if drowsiness occurs

Evaluation
Positive therapeutic outcome
• Decreased pain

TREATMENT OF OVERDOSE:
Naloxone (Narcan) 0.2-0.8 mg **IV**, O₂, **IV** fluids, vasopressors

---

⚠ HIGH ALERT

oxytocin (Rx)
(ox-i-toe′sin)
Pitocin
Func. class.: Oxytocic hormone
Pregnancy category N/A

ACTION: Acts directly on myofibrils, producing uterine contraction; stimulates breast milk letdown, vasoactive antidiuretic effect

Therapeutic outcome: Stimulation of labor, control of bleeding; stimulation of milk letdown

USES: Stimulation, induction of labor; missed or incomplete abortion; postpartum bleeding

CONTRAINDICATIONS:
Hypersensitivity, serum toxemia, cephalopelvic disproportion, fetal distress, hypertonic uterus, prolapsed umbilical cord, active genital herpes

Precautions: Cervical/uterine surgery, uterine sepsis, primipara >35 yr, 1st/2nd stage of labor

> **BLACK BOX WARNING:** Elective induction of labor

DOSAGE AND ROUTES
Labor induction
Adult: IV 1-2 milliunit/min, increase by 1-2 milliunit q15-60min until regular contractions occur, then decrease dosage

Postpartum hemorrhage
Adult: IV 10-40 units in 1000 ml nonhydrating diluent infused at 20-40 milliunit/min
Adult: IM 3-10 units after placenta delivery

Incomplete abortion
Adult: IV INF 10 units/500 ml D₅W or 0.9% NaCl run at 10-20 milliunit/min; max 30 units/12 hr

Fetal stress test
Adult: IV 0.5 milliunit/min; increase q20min until 3 contractions occur at 10 min

Available forms: Inj 10 units/ml

Implementation
IV route
• Use an inf pump; rotate sol for mixing; have magnesium sulfate available
Labor induction
• Give after diluting 10 units/1000 ml of 0.9% NS or D₅ NS run at 1-2 mU/min at 15-30 min intervals to begin normal labor; dilute 10-40 mU/min; titrate to control postpartum bleeding; dilute 10 units/500 ml sol; run 10 units-20 mU/ml; administer by only 1 route at a time; use inf pump; rotate inf to provide mixing; do not shake
Control of postpartum bleeding
• Dilute 10-40 units/1000 ml of sol; run at 10-20 mU/min; adjust rate as needed
• Have crash cart available on unit (magnesium sulfate at bedside)

♦ Canada only   Adverse effects: *italics* = common; **bold** = life-threatening

Incomplete, inevitable, elective abortion
• Dilute 10 units/500 ml compatible IV solution

Y-site compatibilities: Heparin, hydrocortisone, insulin (regular), meperidine, morphine, potassium chloride, vit B/C, warfarin

ADVERSE EFFECTS
CNS: Seizures, tetanic contractions
CV: Hypo/hypertension, dysrhythmias, increased pulse, bradycardia, tachycardia, premature ventricular contractions
FETUS: Dysrhythmias, jaundice, hypoxia, **intracranial hemorrhage**
GI: Anorexia, nausea, vomiting, constipation
GU: Abruptio placentae, decreased uterine blood flow
HEMA: Increased hyperbilirubinemia
INTEG: Rash
RESP: Asphyxia
SYST: Water intoxication of mother

Pharmacokinetics

Absorption	Well absorbed (nasal); completely absorbed (**IV**)
Distribution	Widely distributed (extracellular fluid)
Metabolism	Liver, rapidly
Excretion	Kidneys
Half-life	3-12 min

Pharmacodynamics

	Nasal	IV	IM
Onset	5 min	Rapid	3-7 min
Peak	Unknown	Unknown	Unknown
Duration	20 min	1 hr	1 hr

INTERACTIONS
Drug classifications
Vasopressors: increased hypertension

Drug/herb
Ephedra: hypertension

NURSING CONSIDERATIONS
Assessment
• Assess labor contractions: fetal heart tones, frequency, duration, intensity of contractions; if fetal heart tones increase or decrease significantly or if contractions are longer than 1 min, notify prescriber; turn patient on left side to increase oxygen to fetus
⚠ **Assess for water intoxication: confusion, anuria, drowsiness, headache; notify prescriber**

• Watch for fetal distress, acceleration, deceleration, fetal presentation, pelvic dimensions
• Monitor B/P, pulse, respiratory rate, rhythm, depth
• Monitor I&O ratio
• Provide an environment conducive to letdown reflex

Nursing diagnoses
• Injury, risk for (uses)
• Knowledge, deficient (teaching)

Patient/family education
• Teach patient to report increased blood loss, abdominal cramps, increased temp or foul-smelling lochia
• Advise patient that contractions will be similar to menstrual cramps, gradually increasing in intensity

Evaluation
Positive therapeutic outcome
• Stimulation of milk letdown (nasal)
• Induction of labor
• Decreased postpartum bleeding

---

paclitaxel (Rx)
(pa-kli-tax'el)
Taxol
paclitaxel protein-bound particles (Rx)
Abraxane
Func. class.: Antineoplastic—miscellaneous
Chem. class.: Taxane
Pregnancy category D

Do not confuse:
paclitaxel/paroxetine/Paxil,
Taxol/Paxil/Taxotere

ACTION: Inhibits the reorganization of the microtubule network needed for interphase and mitotic cellular functions; also causes abnormal bundles of microtubules during cell cycle and multiple esters of microtubules during mitosis

Therapeutic outcome: Prevention of rapidly growing malignant cells

USES: Taxol: metastatic carcinoma of the ovary, breast carcinoma, AIDS-related Kaposi's sarcoma (second line), non–small cell lung cancer (first line), adjuvant treatment for node-positive breast cancer

Unlabeled uses: Advanced head, neck, small cell lung cancer; non-Hodgkin's lym-

---

⚠ Nurse Alert

phoma, adenocarcinoma of the upper GI tract, hormone-refractory prostate cancer

CONTRAINDICATIONS:

Pregnancy **D**, hypersensitivity to paclitaxel or other products with polyoxyethylated castor oil, albumin

> **BLACK BOX WARNING:** Neutropenia (neutrophils <1500/mm^3)

Precautions: Breastfeeding, children, CV/hepatic disease, CNS disorder, renal disease, bone marrow suppression, dental disease/work, extravasation, females, geriatric patients, herpes, infection, infertility, jaundice, ocular exposure, radiation therapy, thrombocytopenia, vaccination

> **BLACK BOX WARNING:** Taxane hypersensitivity

DOSAGE AND ROUTES

Paclitaxel

Ovarian carcinoma

Adult: IV INF 135 mg/m^2 given over 24 hr q3wk, then CISplatin 75 mg/m^2 or 175 mg/m^2 over 3 hr q3wk or 175 mg/m^2 over 3 hr

Advanced ovarian carcinoma

Adult: IV INF 175 mg/m^2 with CISplatin 75 mg/m^2 over 3 hr q3wk

Breast carcinoma

Adult: IV INF 175 mg/m^2 over 3 hr q3wk × 4 courses

AIDS-related Kaposi's sarcoma

Adult: IV INF 135 mg/m^2 over 3 hr q3wk or 100 mg/m^2 over 3 hr q2wk

1st line non–small cell lung cancer

Adult: IV INF 135 mg/m^2/24 hr with CISplatin 75 mg/m^2 × 3 wk

Paclitaxel protein-bound particles

Adult: IV 260 mg/m^2 q3wk

Available forms: Inj 30 mg/5-ml vial, 100 mg/16.7-ml vial, 150 mg/24-ml vial, 300 mg/5-ml vials; powder for inj, lyophilized 100 mg in single-use vials (Abraxane)

Implementation

Continuous IV INF route

• After premedicating with dexamethasone 20 mg PO 12 hr and 6 hr before paclitaxel, diphenhydrAMINE 50 mg IV ½-1 hr before paclitaxel

and cimetidine 300 mg or ranitidine 50 mg IV ½-1 hr before paclitaxel
• For extravasation if given by regular IV, not port

Paclitaxel

• After diluting in 0.9% NaCl, D$_5$, D$_5$ and 0.9% NaCl, D$_5$LR (0.3-1.2 mg/ml) chemo dispensing pin or similar devices with spikes should not be used in vials of Taxol, use in-line filter ≤0.22 micron, may be given as 3 hr or 24 hr inf
• Use only glass bottles, polypropylene, polyolefin bags and administration sets; do not use PVC inf bags or sets

Y-site compatibilities: Acyclovir, amikacin, aminophylline, ampicillin/sulbactam, bleomycin, butorphanol, calcium chloride, CARBOplatin, cefepime, cefotetan, ceftazidime, cefTRIAXone, cimetidine, CISplatin, cladribine, cyclophosphamide, cytarabine, dacarbazine, dexamethasone, diphenhydrAMINE, DOXOrubicin, droperidol, etoposide, famotidine, floxuridine, fluconazole, fluorouracil, furosemide, ganciclovir, gentamicin, granisetron, haloperidol, heparin, hydrocortisone, HYDROmorphone, ifosfamide, LORazepam, magnesium sulfate, mannitol, meperidine, mesna, methotrexate, metoclopramide, morphine, nalbuphine, ondansetron, pentostatin, potassium chloride, prochlorperazine, propofol, ranitidine, sodium bicarbonate, thiotepa, vancomycin, vinBLAStine, vinCRIStine, zidovudine

Abraxane

Intermittent IV INF route

• Reconstitute vial by injecting 20 ml of 0.9% NaCl; slowly inject the 20 ml of 0.9% NaCl over at least 1 min to direct the sol flow on wall of vial; do not inject 0.9% NaCl directly onto lyophilized cake (foaming will occur); allow vial to sit for at least 5 min to ensure proper wetting of lyophilized cake; gently swirl or invert vial slowly for at least 2 min until completely dissolved
• Calculate dosing by dosing vol/ml = total dose (mg) ÷ 5 (mg/ml)

ADVERSE EFFECTS

CNS: Peripheral neuropathy
CV: *Bradycardia, hypotension, abnormal ECG,* supraventricular tachycardia (SVT)
GI: *Nausea, vomiting, diarrhea, mucositis; increased bilirubin, alkaline phosphatase, AST*
HEMA: **Neutropenia, leukopenia, thrombocytopenia, anemia,** bleeding, infections
INTEG: Alopecia, tissue necrosis, generalized urticaria, flushing

P

MS: *Arthralgia, myalgia*
RESP: Pulmonary embolism, dyspnea
SYST: *Hypersensitivity reactions,* anaphy-laxis, Stevens-Johnson syndrome, toxic epidermal necrolysis, angioedema

Pharmacokinetics

Absorption	Completely absorbed
Distribution	89%-98% protein binding
Metabolism	Liver, extensively
Excretion	Unknown
Half-life	5-17 hr

Pharmacodynamics

Onset	Unknown
Peak	1-2 wk
Duration	3 wk

INTERACTIONS

Individual drugs

CycloSPORINE, dexamethasone, diazepam, eto-poside, quiNIDine, teniposide, testosterone, verapamil, vinCRIStine: decreased metabolism of paclitaxel
DOXOrubicin: increased levels of DOXOrubicin
Ketoconazole: increased toxicity, decreased metabolism; avoid concurrent use
Radiation: increased myelosuppression

Drug classifications

Anticoagulants, NSAIDs: increased bleeding risk
Antineoplastics: increased myelosuppression
CYP2C8, CYP2C9 inducers: decreased paclitaxel level
Vaccines (live virus): decreased immune response

NURSING CONSIDERATIONS

Assessment

• Assess CNS changes: confusion, paresthesias, psychosis, tremors, seizures, neuropathies; product should be discontinued
• Check buccal cavity q8hr for dryness, sores or ulceration, white patches, oral pain, bleed-ing, dysphagia; obtain prescription for viscous lidocaine (Xylocaine) to use in mouth
• Monitor CBC, differential, platelet count weekly; withhold product if WBC is <1500/mm³ or platelet count is <100,000/mm³, notify prescriber of results
• **Cardiovascular status:** monitor ECG continuously in CV conditions; monitor for hypotension, sinus bradycardia/tachycardia
• **Peripheral neuropathy:** assess for pares-thesias, numbness; during inf use ice packs on extremities to lessen continued neuropathy

• **Arthralgia, myalgia:** may begin 2-3 days after infusion and continue for 4-5 days, may use analgesics
• **Nausea, vomiting:** premedicate with anti-emetics, nausea and vomiting occur often
• Monitor renal function tests: BUN, creatinine, serum uric acid, urine CCr before, during therapy; check I&O ratio; report fall in urine output to <30 ml/hr
• Monitor temp q4hr (may indicate beginning of infection)
• Monitor liver function tests before, during therapy (bilirubin, AST, ALT, LDH) as needed or monthly; check for jaundice of skin and sclera, dark urine, clay-colored stools, itchy skin, abdominal pain, fever, diarrhea
• Assess for bleeding: hematuria, stool guaiac, bruising or petechiae, mucosa or orifices q8hr; check for inflammation of mucosa, breaks in skin
• Assess effects of alopecia on body image; discuss feelings about body changes
• VS during 1st hr of inf, check IV site for signs of infiltration
⚠ Hypersensitive reactions, anaphylaxis, hypotension, dyspnea, angioedema, gener-alized urticaria; discontinue inf immediate-ly; keep emergency equipment available, monitor continuously during first 30-60 min, then periodically
• **Taxol flush:** for mild to moderate flush, may continue diphenhydrAMINE for up to 48 hr
• Effects of alopecia on body image; discuss feelings about body changes

Nursing diagnoses

• Body image, disturbed (adverse reactions)
• Infection, risk for (adverse reactions)
• Injury, risk for (adverse reactions)
• Knowledge, deficient (teaching)

Patient/family education

• Inform patient that nonhormonal contracep-tive measures are recommended during therapy and >4 mo after; teratogenic effects are pos-sible
• Teach patient to avoid use of products con-taining aspirin or ibuprofen, razors, commercial mouthwash, since bleeding may occur; to report symptoms of bleeding (hematuria, tarry stools)
• Instruct patient to report signs of anemia (fa-tigue, headache, irritability, faintness, shortness of breath) and CNS reactions (confusion, psy-chosis, nightmares, seizures, severe headaches)
• Teach patient to rinse mouth tid-qid with water, club soda; brush teeth bid-qid with soft brush or cotton-tipped applicators for stomati-tis; use unwaxed dental floss

• Inform patient that hair may be lost during treatment; a wig or hairpiece may make patient feel better; new hair may be different in color, texture
• Inform patient that receiving vaccinations during therapy may cause serious reactions

Evaluation
Positive therapeutic outcome
• Prevention of rapid division of malignant cells

---

paliperidone (Rx)
(pal-ee-per′i-done)
Invega, Invega Sustenna
Func. class.: Antipsychotic
Chem. class.: Benzisoxazole derivative
Pregnancy category C

Do not confuse:
Invega/Iveegan, **paliperidone**/risperidone

ACTION: Mediated through both dopamine type 2 (D_2) and serotonin type 2 (5-HT_2) antagonism

Therapeutic outcome: Decrease in emotional excitement, hallucinations, delusions, paranoia; reorganization of patterns of thought, speech

USES: Schizophrenia

CONTRAINDICATIONS:
Breastfeeding, seizure disorders, AV block, geriatric, QT prolongation, torsades de pointes, hypersensitivity to this product or risperidone

Precautions: Pregnancy C, children, renal/hepatic disease, obesity, Parkinson's disease

> **BLACK BOX WARNING:** Dementia

DOSAGE AND ROUTES
Adult: PO 6 mg/day; max 12 mg/day; IM 234 mg on day 1, then 156 mg 1 wk later; after 2nd dose, give 117 mg qmo, range 39-234 mg
Child/adolescent ≥12 yr and ≥51 kg: PO 3 mg q day, may increase if needed by 3 mg/day in intervals >5 days up to max 12 mg/day; <51 kg max 6 mg/day

Renal dose
Adult: PO CCr 50-79 ml/min, 3 mg/day, max 6 mg/day; EXT REL IM 156 mg on day 1, 117 mg 1 wk later, then 78 mg each mo CCr 10-49 ml/min, 1.5 mg/day, max 3 mg/day

Available forms: Ext rel tabs 1.5, 3, 6, 9 mg; ext rel susp for inj 39 mg/0.25 ml, 78 mg/0.5 ml, 117 mg/0.75 ml, 156 mg/1 ml, 234 mg/1.5 ml

Implementation
PO route
• Do not break, crush, or chew ext rel tabs
• Give without regard for food
• Give a reduced dose to the geriatric patient
• Give antiparkinsonian agent on order from prescriber; to be used for EPS
• Avoid use with CNS depressants
• Supervise ambulation until patient is stabilized on medication; do not involve in strenuous exercise program, because fainting is possible; patient should not stand still for a long time
• Increase fluids to prevent constipation
• Decrease stimulus by dimming lights, avoiding loud noise
• Provide sips of water, candy, gum for dry mouth
• Store in airtight, light-resistant container
IM route
• Use for IM only, do not use IV or SUBCUT, injection kits contain a prefilled syringe and 2 safety needles, for single use only, shake for 10 secs
• **Deltoid injection:** ≥ 90 kg use 1.5 inch, 22 G needle; < 90 kg use 1 inch, 23 G needle, alternate injections between deltoid muscles
• **Gluteal injection:** use 1.5 inch, 22 G needle; while holding syringe upright, twist rubber tip clockwise to remove, peel safety needle pouch half way open, grasp needle sheath using plastic peel pouch, attach needle to luer connection in clockwise motion, pull needle sheath away using straight pull, bring syringe with attached needle upright to de-aerate, de-aerate, inject; after injection, use finger, thumb or flat surface to activate needle protection system, until click heard, use deltoid × 2 dosages

ADVERSE EFFECTS
CNS: *EPS, pseudoparkinsonism, akathisia, dystonia, tardive dyskinesia; drowsiness, insomnia, agitation, anxiety, headache,* **seizures, neuroleptic malignant syndrome,** dizziness
CV: Orthostatic hypotension, **tachycardia, heart failure, QT prolongation,** heart block, dysrhythmias
EENT: Blurred vision
ENDO: Insulin increase, hyperinsulinemia
GI: *Nausea,* vomiting, *anorexia, constipation,* weight gain in adolescents, xerostomia
HEMA: **Agranulocytosis**

P

Pharmacokinetics

Absorption	Unknown
Distribution	Unknown
Metabolism	Unknown
Excretion	80% urine, 11% feces
Half-life	Elimination 23 hr

Pharmacodynamics

Onset	Unknown
Peak	24 hr
Duration	Unknown

INTERACTIONS

Individual drugs

Abarelix, alfuzosin, amoxapine, apomorphine, chloroquine, dasatinib, dolasetron, droperidol, flecainide, pimozide: increased QT prolongation

Alcohol: increased sedation

Levodopa: decreased levodopa effect

Paliperidone: decreased effect

Drug classifications

Azole antifungals; β-blockers; class IA, III antidysrhythmics; halogenated anesthetics; some antipsychotics; some phenothiazines; tricyclics (high doses): increased QT prolongation

SSRIs, SNRIs: increased serotonin syndrome, increased neuroleptic malignant syndrome

Other antipsychotics: increased EPS

Other CNS depressants, sedatives/hypnotics, opiates: increased sedation

Drug/herb

Betel palm, kava: increased EPS

Cola tree, hops, nettle, nutmeg: increased action

Kava: increased CNS depression

Drug/lab test

Increased: prolactin levels

NURSING CONSIDERATIONS

Assessment

> **BLACK BOX WARNING:** Assess mental status; mood, behavior, confusion, orientation, suicidal thoughts/behaviors; dementia especially in geriatric patients before initial administration

• **QT prolongation:** monitor ECG for QT prolongation, ejection fraction; assess for chest pain, palpitations, dyspnea
• Monitor for swallowing of PO medication; check for hoarding or giving of medication to other patients

• Monitor I&O ratio; palpate bladder if urinary output is low
• Assess affect, orientation, LOC, reflexes, gait, coordination, sleep pattern disturbances
• Monitor B/P standing and lying; also pulse, respirations; take these q4hr during initial treatment; establish baseline before starting treatment; report drops of 30 mm Hg; watch for ECG changes
• Assess for dizziness, faintness, palpitations, tachycardia on rising
• **Hyperprolactinemia:** assess for sexual dysfunction, decreased menstruation, breast pain
• **Assess for EPS,** including akathisia, tardive dyskinesia (bizarre movements of the jaw, mouth, tongue, extremities), pseudoparkinsonism (rigidity, tremors, pill rolling, shuffling gait)
⚠ Assess for serious reactions in the geriatric patient
⚠ **Serotonin syndrome, neuroleptic malignant syndrome:** assess for increased heart rate, shivering, sweating, dilated pupils, tremors, high B/P, hyperthermia, headache, confusion; if these occur, stop product, administer a serotonin antagonist if needed
• Assess skin turgor daily
• Assess for constipation, urinary retention daily; if these occur, increase bulk and water in diet; monitor for weight gain in adolescents

Nursing diagnoses

• Knowledge, deficient (teaching)
• Noncompliance (teaching)

Patient/family education

• Advise patient that orthostatic hypotension may occur and to rise from sitting or lying position gradually
• Advise patient to avoid hot tubs, hot showers, tub baths; hypotension may occur
• Caution patient to avoid abrupt withdrawal of this product; EPS may result; product should be withdrawn slowly
• Teach patient to avoid OTC preparations (cough, hay fever, cold) unless approved by prescriber; serious product interactions may occur; avoid use of alcohol; increased drowsiness may occur
• Advise patient to avoid hazardous activities if drowsy or dizzy
• Teach patient compliance with product regimen; non-absorbable tab shell is expelled in stool
• Teach patient to report impaired vision, tremors, muscle twitching
• Caution patient that heat stroke may occur in hot weather; take extra precautions to stay cool

• Teach patient to use contraception, inform prescriber if pregnancy is planned or suspected

> **BLACK BOX WARNING:** Teach patient to notify prescriber of suicidal thoughts, behaviors, or other changes in behavior

Evaluation
Positive therapeutic outcome
• Decrease in emotional excitement, hallucinations, delusions, paranoia; reorganization of patterns of thought, speech

TREATMENT OF OVERDOSE:
Lavage if orally ingested; provide airway; *do not induce vomiting*

---

palonosetron (Rx)
(pa-lone-o′se-tron)
Aloxi
Func. class.: Antiemetic
Chem. class.: 5-HT$_3$ receptor antagonist
Pregnancy category B

ACTION: Prevents nausea, vomiting by blocking serotonin peripherally, centrally, and in the small intestine at the 5-HT$_3$ receptor

Therapeutic outcome: Decreased nausea, vomiting during chemotherapy

USES: Prevention of nausea, vomiting associated with cancer chemotherapy; postoperative nausea/vomiting

CONTRAINDICATIONS:
Hypersensitivity

Precautions: Pregnancy **B**, breastfeeding, children, geriatric, with hypokalemia, hypomagnesemia, patients taking diuretics

DOSAGE AND ROUTES
Adult: PO 0.5 mg as a single dose 1 hr prior to chemotherapy; **IV** 0.25 mg as a single dose over 30 sec, 30 min prior to chemotherapy, max 0.25 mg **IV** over q 7 days

Postoperative nausea/vomiting prophylaxis for up to 24 hr after surgery
Adult: **IV** 0.075 mg given over 10 sec immediately before induction

Available forms: Inj 0.25 mg/5 ml, caps 0.5 mg

Implementation
Direct IV route
• Do not mix with other products; flush **IV** line before, after administration
• Store at room temperature
• **Chemotherapy nausea/vomiting:** give as a single dose over 30 seconds
• **Postoperative nausea/vomiting:** give over 10 seconds immediately prior to anesthesia induction

Syringe compatibilities: Dexamethasone

Y-site compatibilities: Alemtuzumab, alfentanil, amikacin, aminocaproic acid, aminophylline, amiodarone, amphotericin B liposome, ampicillin, ampicillin/sulbactam, atracurium, atropine, azithromycin, aztreonam, bivalirudin, bleomycin, bumetanide, buprenorphine, busulfan, butorphanol, calcium acetate/chloride/gluconate, CARBOplatin, carmustine, caspofungin, ceFAZolin, cefepime, cefotaxime, cefotetan, cefoxitin, ceftazidime, ceftizoxime, cefTRIAXone, cefuroxime, chloramphenicol, chlorproMAZINE, cimetidine, ciprofloxacin, cisatracurium, CISplatin, clindamycin, cyclophosphamide, cycloSPORINE, cytarabine, dacarbazine, DACTINomycin, dantrolene, DAPTOmycin, DAUNOrubicin, dexamethasone, dexmedetomidine, dexrazoxane, digoxin, diltiazem, diphenhydrAMINE, DOBUTamine, docetaxel, DOPamine, doxacurium, DOXOrubicin hydrochloride, droperidol, enalaprilat, ePHEDrine, EPINEPHrine, epirubicin, eptifibatide, erythromycin, esmolol, etoposide, etoposide phosphate, famotidine, fenoldopam, fentaNYL, fluconazole, fludarabine, fluorouracil, foscarnet, fosphenytoin, furosemide, gemcitabine, gentamicin, glycopyrrolate, haloperidol, heparin, hydrALAZINE, hydrocortisone, HYDROmorphone, IDArubicin, ifosfamide, inamrinone, insulin, irinotecan, isoproterenol, ketorolac, labetalol, leucovorin, levofloxacin, lidocaine, linezolid, LORazepam, magnesium sulfate, mannitol, mechlorethamine, melphalan, meperidine, meropenem, mesna, metaraminol, methotrexate, methyldopate, metoclopramide, metoprolol, metroNIDAZOLE, midazolam, milrinone, mitomycin, mitoxantrone, mivacurium, morphine, nalbuphine, naloxone, neostigmine, nesiritide, niCARdipine, nitroglycerin, nitroprusside, norepinephrine, octreotide, oxaliplatin, oxytocin, paclitaxel, pamidronate, pancuronium, pentazocine, PHENobarbital, phentolamine, phenylephrine, piperacillin/tazobactam, potassium acetate/chloride/phosphates, procainamide, prochlorperazine, promethazine, propranolol, quinupristin/dalfopristin, ranitidine, remifentanil, rocuronium, sodium acetate/bicarbonate/phosphates, streptozocin, succinylcholine, SUFentanil, tacrolimus, teniposide, theophylline, thiotepa, ticarcillin/clavulanate, tigecycline, tirofiban, tobramycin, topotecan, trimethobenzamide, trimethoprim/sulfamethoxazole, vancomycin, vasopressin, vecuronium, verapamil, vinBLAStine, vinCRIStine, vinorelbine, zidovudine

Y-site incompatibilities: Acyclovir, allopurinol, amphotericin B colloidal, diazepam, doxycycline, ganciclovir, imipenem/cilastatin, methylPREDNISolone, minocycline, nafcillin, pantoprazole, pentamidine, PENTobarbital, phenytoin, thiopental

ADVERSE EFFECTS

CNS: *Headache, dizziness, drowsiness, fatigue, insomnia*
GI: *Diarrhea, constipation,* abdominal pain
MISC: Weakness, hyperkalemia, anxiety, rash, **bronchospasm** (rare), arthralgia, *fever, urinary retention*

Pharmacokinetics

Absorption	Unknown
Distribution	62% protein bound
Metabolism	Liver
Excretion	Unchanged product and metabolites excreted by kidney
Half-life	40 hr

Pharmacodynamics
Unknown

INTERACTIONS

Individual drugs
Chloroquine, clarithromycin, droperidol, erythromycin, grepafloxacin, halofantrine, haloperidol, levomethadyl, methadone, pentamidine: possible QT prolongation

Drug classifications
Class 1A antidysrhythmics (disopyramide, procainamide, quiNIDine), class III antidysrhythmics (amiodarone, dofetilide, ibutilide), diuretics (except potassium sparing), some phenothiazines: possible QT prolongation

NURSING CONSIDERATIONS

Assessment
• Monitor for absence of nausea, vomiting during chemotherapy

• Assess hypersensitivity reaction: rash, bronchospasm

Nursing diagnoses
• Knowledge, deficient (teaching)

Patient/family education
• Teach to report diarrhea, constipation, rash, or changes in respirations or discomfort at insertion site
• Advise patient to avoid alcohol, barbiturates

Evaluation
Positive therapeutic outcome
• Absence of nausea, vomiting during cancer chemotherapy

pamidronate (Rx)
(pam-i-drone′ate)
Aredia
Func. class.: Bone resorption inhibitor, electrolyte modifier
Chem. class.: Bisphosphonate
Pregnancy category D

Do not confuse:
Aredia/Adriamycin

ACTION: Inhibits bone resorption, apparently without inhibiting bone formation and mineralization; absorbs calcium phosphate crystals in bone and may directly block dissolution of hydroxyapatite crystals of bone

Therapeutic outcome: Serum calcium at normal level

USES: Moderate to severe Paget's disease, hypercalcemia, osteolytic bone metastases in breast cancer patients, multiple myeloma

Unlabeled uses: Postmenopausal osteoporosis, hyperparathyroidism

CONTRAINDICATIONS:
Pregnancy **D,** hypersensitivity to bisphosphonates

Precautions: Children, nursing mothers, renal dysfunction, poor dentition

DOSAGE AND ROUTES

Hypercalcemia of malignancy
Adult: IV INF 60-90 mg as a single dose in moderate hypercalcemia, 90 mg in severe hypercalcemia given over 2-24 hr; dose should be diluted in 1000 ml 0.45% NaCl, 0.9% NaCl, or D_5W; wait 7 days before 2nd course

Osteolytic lesions
Adult: IV 90 mg/500 ml of D_5W, 0.45% NaCl, or 0.9% NaCl given over 4 hr on a monthly basis (multiple myeloma) or over 2 hr q3-4wk (breast carcinoma)

Paget's disease
Adult: IV INF 30 mg/day given over 4 hr × 3 days

Available forms: Powder for inj 30, 90 mg/vial; inj 3, 6, 9 mg/ml

Implementation
IV route
• After reconstituting by adding 10 ml of sterile water for inj to each vial (30 mg/10 ml or 90 mg/10 ml depending on vial used); add to 1000 ml of sterile 0.45%, 0.9% NaCl, D_5W, run over 2-24 hr **(hypercalcemia)**; dilute reconstituted sol in 500 ml of 0.9% NaCl, 0.45% NaCl, or D_5W, give over 4 hr **(multiple myeloma, Paget's disease)**; dilute reconstituted sol in 250 ml of 0.9% NaCl, 0.45% NaCl or D_5W, give over 2 hr **(osteolytic bone metastases of breast cancer)**
• Store inf sol for up to 24 hr at room temperature
• Reconstituted sol with sterile water may be stored under refrigeration for up to 24 hr
• Do not mix with calcium-containing inf sol such as Ringer's sol

Y-site compatibilities: Acyclovir, alfentanil, allopurinol, amifostine, amikacin, aminocaproic acid, aminophylline, amphotericin B lipid complex, amphotericin B liposome, ampicillin, anidulafungin, atenolol, atracurium, azithromycin, aztreonam, bivalirudin, bleomycin, bumetanide, buprenorphine, butorphanol, CARBOplatin, carmustine, ceFAZolin, cefepime, cefoperazone, cefotaxime, cefotetan, cefoxitin, ceftazidime, ceftizoxime, cefTRIAXone, cefuroxime, chloramphenicol, chlorproMAZINE, cimetidine, ciprofloxacin, cisatracurium, CISplatin, clindamycin, cyclophosphamide, cycloSPORINE, cytarabine, dacarbazine, DAPTOmycin, dexamethasone, dexmedetomidine, dexrazoxane, digoxin, diltiazem, diphenhydrAMINE, DOBUTamine, docetaxel, dolasetron, DOPamine, doxacurium, DOXOrubicin, doxycycline, droperidol, enalaprilat, ePHEDrine, EPINEPHrine, epirubicin, ertapenem, erythromycin, esmolol, etoposide, famotidine, fenoldopam, fentaNYL, fluconazole, fludarabine, fluorouracil, foscarnet, fosphenytoin, furosemide, gallium, ganciclovir, gatifloxacin, gemcitabine, gentamicin, glycopyrrolate, granisetron, haloperidol, heparin, hetastarch 6%, hydrALAZINE, hydrocortisone, HYDROmorphone, hydrOXYzine, ifosfamide, imipenem-cilastatin, inamrinone, insulin (regular), isoproterenol, ketorolac, labetalol, levofloxacin, levorphanol, lidocaine, linezolid, LORazepam, magnesium sulfate, mannitol, mechlorethamine, melphalan, meperidine, meropenem, mesna, metaraminol, methotrexate, methyldopate, methylPREDNISolone, metoclopramide, metoprolol, metroNIDAZOLE, midazolam, milrinone, minocycline, mitoxantrone, mivacurium, morphine, mycophenolate, nafcillin, nalbuphine, naloxone, nesiritide, niCARDipine, nitroglycerin, nitroprusside, norepinephrine, octreotide, ondansetron, oxytocin, paclitaxel, palonosetron, pancuronium, pemetrexed, pentamidine, pentazocine, PENTobarbital, PHENobarbital, phenylephrine, piperacillin, polymyxin B, potassium chloride/phosphates, procainamide, prochlorperazine, promethazine, propranolol, quiNIDine, quinupristin-dalfopristin, ranitidine, remifentanil, rocuronium, sodium acetate/bicarbonate/phosphates, succinylcholine, SUFentanil, sulfamethoxazole-trimethoprim, teniposide, theophylline, thiopental, thiotepa, ticarcillin, ticarcillin-clavulanate, tigecycline, tirofiban, tobramycin, tolazoline, topotecan, trimethobenzamide, vancomycin, vasopressin, vecuronium, verapamil, vinBLAStine, vinCRIStine, vinorelbine, voriconazole, zidovudine

ADVERSE EFFECTS
CNS: Fatigue, fever
CV: *Hypertension,* **atrial fibrillation**
EENT: Ocular pain, inflammation, vision impairment
GI: *Abdominal pain, anorexia, constipation, nausea, vomiting,* dyspepsia
GU: Renal failure
INTEG: Redness, swelling, induration, pain on palpation at site of catheter insertion
META: Anemia, hypokalemia, hypomagnesemia, hypophosphatemia, hypocalcemia, hypothyroidism
MS: *Severe bone pain,* myalgia, **osteonecrosis of the jaw**
RESP: Coughing, dyspnea, URI
SYST: **Angioedema, anaphylaxis**

P

Absorption	Rapidly cleared from circulation
Distribution	Mainly to bones, primarily in areas of high bone turnover
Metabolism	Unknown
Excretion	Kidneys, unchanged (50%)
Half-life	Biphasic 27 hr; from bone to 300 days

Pharmacodynamics

Onset	1 day
Peak	1 wk
Duration	Unknown

INTERACTIONS

Individual drugs
Calcium, vitamin D: decreased pamidronate effect

CycloSPORINE, tacrolimus, vancomycin: increased nephrotoxicity

Entecavir: increased effect of entecavir

Drug classifications
Aminoglycosides, NSAIDs, radiopaque contrast agents: increased nephrotoxicity

Loop diuretics: increased hypokalemia

NURSING CONSIDERATIONS

Assessment
• **Dental health:** give antiinfectives for dental extractions

• **Hypocalcemia:** assess for nausea, vomiting, constipation, thirst, dysrhythmias, hypocalcemia, paresthesia, twitching, laryngospasm, Chvostek's, Trousseau's signs; **hypercalcemia:** thirst, nausea, vomiting, dysrhythmias

• Assess for atrial fibrillation

• Assess fluid volume status: check I&O ratio and record, assess for distended red veins, crackles in lung, color, quality, and specific gravity of urine, skin turgor, adequacy of pulses, moist mucous membranes, bilateral lung sounds, peripheral pitting edema

• Monitor electrolytes: phosphorus, potassium, sodium, calcium, magnesium; also include BUN, creatinine, CBC, platelets, hemoglobin

• Assess B/P before, during therapy

• Assess for pain: in joints or on exertion, duration and characteristics; analgesics may be ordered

• Assess for phlebitis at **IV** site: swelling, redness, pain, warmth

Nursing diagnoses
• Fluid volume, excess (side effects)
• Injury, risk for (uses, adverse reactions)
• Knowledge, deficient (teaching)

Patient/family education
• Advise patient to report hypercalcemic relapse: nausea, vomiting, bone pain, thirst; unusual muscle twitching, muscle spasms, severe diarrhea, constipation, ocular symptoms

• Advise patient to continue with dietary recommendations, including calcium and vit D

• To obtain an analgesic from provider for bone pain

• Advise patient that small, frequent meals may help nausea/vomiting

Evaluation
Positive therapeutic outcome
• Decreased calcium levels to normal

---

pancrelipase (Rx)
(pan-kre-li′pase)
Cotazym-65B ✷, Creon, Creon Minimicrospheres, DMH ✷, Dygase, Lipram, Lipram-CR, Lipram-CR5, Lipram-PN, Lipram-PN10, Lipram-UL, Lipram-UL20, Pancrease ✷, Pancreaze, Panrecarb MS, Ultrase, Ultrase MT, Viokase, Zenpep
Func. class.: Digestant
Chem. class.: Pancreatic enzyme (bovine/porcine)
Pregnancy category B

ACTION: Pancreatic enzyme needed for breakdown of substances released from the pancreas

Therapeutic outcome: Increases protein, fat, carbohydrate digestion

USES: Exocrine pancreatic secretion insufficiency, cystic fibrosis (digestive aid), steatorrhea, pancreatic enzyme deficiency

CONTRAINDICATIONS: Allergy to pork

Precautions: Pregnancy **B**, ileus, pancreatitis, Crohn's disease

DOSAGE AND ROUTES
Many products listed above are not interchangeable

Del rel caps—Creon caps, Zenpep caps, Pancreaze caps
Adult/adolescents/child ≥4 yr: PO 500 lipase units/kg/meal, titrate based on response, max 2500 lipase units/kg/meal
Child 1<4 yr: PO 1000 lipase units/kg/meal, titrate based on response, max 2500 lipase units/kg/meal

Available forms: Powder 16,800 units lipase/70,000 units protease and amylase; caps 8000 units lipase/30,000 units protease and amylase; del rel caps, 4000 units lipase/12,000 units protease and amylase, 4000 units lipase/25,000 units protease/20,000 units amylase, 5000 units lipase/20,000 units protease and amylase, 10,000 units lipase/30,000 units protease and amylase, 12,000 units lipase/24,000 units protease and amylase, 12,000 units lipase/39,000 units protease and amylase, 16,000 units lipase/48,000 units protease and amylase 20,000 units lipase/65,000 units protease and amylase, 24,000 units lipase/78,000 units protease and amylase; del rel cap 5000, 15,000 units

Implementation
• Avoid inhaling powder
• Give tab with 8 oz of water and sitting up only; do not let tab sit in mouth; give with meals
• Give after antacid or cimetidine; decreased pH inactivates product
• Give powder mixed in prepared fruit for infants, children
• Administer low-fat diet to decrease GI symptoms
• Provide adequate hydration
• Store in airtight container at room temperature

ADVERSE EFFECTS
GI: Anorexia, *nausea, vomiting, diarrhea,* cramping, bloating
GU: Hyperuricuria, hyperuricemia

Pharmacokinetics
Unknown

Pharmacodynamics
Unknown

INTERACTIONS
Individual drugs
Acarbose, miglitol: decreased effects of each specific drug
Cimetidine, iron (oral): decreased absorption of pancrelipase

Drug classifications
Antacids: decreased absorption of pancrelipase

NURSING CONSIDERATIONS
Assessment
• Monitor I&O ratio; watch for increasing urinary output
• Monitor fecal fat, nitrogen, pro-time during treatment
• Monitor for polyuria, polydipsia, polyphagia (may indicate diabetes mellitus)
• Assess for allergy to pork; patient may also be sensitive to this product
• Assess for appropriate weight, height, development; there may be a developmental lag
• Check stools for steatorrhea, which signifies undigested fat content

Nursing diagnoses
• Knowledge, deficient (teaching)
• Nutrition: less than body requirements, imbalanced (uses)

Patient/family education
• Teach patient to take tab with 8 oz or more water, not to let tab sit in mouth; have patient take tab sitting up only
• Advise patient to notify prescriber of allergic reactions, abdominal pain, cramping, or hematuria
• Teach patient not to inhale powder, very irritating to mucous membranes, some powder may irritate skin

Evaluation
Positive therapeutic outcome
• Absence of steatorrhea
• Improved digestion of carbohydrates, proteins, fat

⚠ HIGH ALERT

pancuronium (Rx)
(pan-cure-oh′nee-yum)
Func. class.: Neuromuscular blocker (nondepolarizing)
Chem. class.: Synthetic curariform
Pregnancy category C

ACTION: Inhibits transmission of nerve impulses by binding with cholinergic receptor sites, antagonizing action of acetylcholine

Therapeutic outcome: Paralysis of all skeletal muscles

P

USES: Facilitation of endotracheal intubation, skeletal muscle relaxation during mechanical ventilation, surgery, or general anesthesia

CONTRAINDICATIONS:
Hypersensitivity to bromide ion

Precautions: Pregnancy C, breastfeeding, children <2 yr, renal/hepatic/cardiac/neuromuscular disease, electrolyte imbalances, dehydration, previous anaphylactic reactions (other neuromuscular blockers)

> **BLACK BOX WARNING:** Respiratory insufficiency

DOSAGE AND ROUTES
Adult/child/infant >1 mo: IV 0.04-0.1 mg/kg initially or 0.05 mg/kg after initial dose of succinylcholine; maintenance 0.01 mg/kg 60-100 min after initial dose, then 0.01 mg/kg q25-60min as needed; in obese patients, use ideal body weight

Neonate <1 mo: IV test dose 0.02 mg/kg, then 0.03 mg/kg/dose initially, repeat 2 × as needed at 5-10 min intervals; maintenance 0.03-0.09 mg/kg/dose q30min-4hr as needed

Available forms: Inj 1, 2 mg/ml

Implementation
• Use peripheral nerve stimulator (anesthesiologist) to determine neuromuscular blockade; deep tendon reflexes should be monitored during extended periods

Direct IV route
• Give undiluted over 1-2 min (1 mg/ml [10 ml vial], 2 mg/ml [2, 5 ml vial])

Intermittent IV infusion route
• Add 100 mg of product to 250 ml D₅W, 0.9% NaCl, or LR (0.4 mg/ml)
• Store in light-resistant area
• Give anticholinesterase to reverse neuromuscular blockade

Y-site compatibilities: Aminophylline, ceFAZolin, cefuroxime, cimetidine, DOBUTamine, DOPamine, EPINEPHrine, esmolol, fentaNYL, fluconazole, gentamicin, heparin, hydrocortisone, isoproterenol, LORazepam, midazolam, morphine, nitroglycerin, nitroprusside, ranitidine, sulfamethoxazole/trimethoprim, vancomycin

Y-site incompatibilities: Diazepam

Additive compatibilities: Verapamil

Additive incompatibilities: Barbiturates

ADVERSE EFFECTS
CV: Bradycardia, tachycardia, increased, decreased B/P, ventricular extrasystoles, edema, hypotension
EENT: Increased secretions
INTEG: Rash, flushing, pruritus, urticaria, sweating, salivation
MS: Weakness to prolonged skeletal muscle relaxation
RESP: Prolonged apnea, bronchospasm, cyanosis, respiratory depression, dyspnea
SYST: Anaphylaxis

Pharmacokinetics
Absorption	Complete bioavailability
Distribution	Extracellular space; crosses placenta
Metabolism	Plasma
Excretion	Kidneys, unchanged
Half-life	2 hr

Pharmacodynamics
Onset	3-5 min, dose dependent
Peak	3-5 min
Duration	35-40 min

INTERACTIONS
Individual products
Clindamycin, enflurane, isoflurane, lincomycin, lithium, quiNIDine: increased neuromuscular blockade
Theophylline: dysrhythmias

Drug classifications
Aminoglycosides, anesthetics (local), analgesics (opioid), polymyxin antiinfectives, thiazides: increased neuromuscular blockade

Drug/lab test
Decreased: cholinesterase

NURSING CONSIDERATIONS
Assessment
• Monitor vital signs (B/P, pulse, respirations, airway) until fully recovered; note rate, depth, pattern of respirations, strength of hand grip; patient should be intubated before use
• Monitor for electrolyte imbalances (potassium, magnesium) before product is used; electrolyte imbalances may lead to increased action of this product
• **Monitor for recovery:** decreased paralysis of face, diaphragm, leg, arm, rest of body; residual weakness and respiratory problems may occur during recovery period

🔺 Nurse Alert

⚠ Assess for hypersensitive reactions, anaphylaxis: rash, fever, respiratory distress, pruritus; product should be discontinued

Nursing diagnoses
• Breathing pattern, ineffective (uses)
• Communication, impaired verbal (adverse reactions)
• Fear (adverse reactions)
• Knowledge, deficient (teaching)

Patient/family education
• Provide reassurance if communication is difficult during recovery from neuromuscular blockade
• Provide explanation to patients regarding all procedures or treatments; patient will remain conscious if anesthesia is not given also

Evaluation
Positive therapeutic outcome
• Paralysis of jaw, eyelid, head, neck, rest of body as evaluated by peripheral nerve stimulator

TREATMENT OF OVERDOSE:
Neostigmine, atropine; monitor VS; may require mechanical ventilation

---

panitumumab (Rx)
(pan-i-tue′moo-mab)
Vectibix
Func. class.: Antineoplastic—miscellaneous
Chem. class.: Multikinase inhibitor, signal transduction inhibitor
Pregnancy category C

ACTION: Decreases growth and survival of cancer cells by competitive inhibition of EGF receptor

Therapeutic outcome: Decrease in colon carcinoma progression

USES: EGFR expressing metastatic colorectal cancer, not beneficial in *KRAS* mutations in codon 12 or 13

CONTRAINDICATIONS:
Hypersensitivity

Precautions: Pregnancy **C**, breastfeeding, children, hepatic disease, acute bronchospasm, diarrhea, hamster protein allergy, hypomagnesemia, hypotension, pulmonary fibrosis, sepsis, *KRAS* mutations

---

BLACK BOX WARNING: Exfoliative dermatitis, infusion-related reactions

DOSAGE AND ROUTES
Adult: IV INF 6 mg/kg over 60 min q2wk; doses > 1000 mg over 90 min

Available forms: Sol for inj 20 mg/ml

Implementation
Intermittent IV infusion route
• Give in hospital or clinic setting with full resuscitation equipment
• Give only as IV inf using controlled IV inf pump; do not give **IV** push or bolus; use low-protein binding 0.2 or 0.22 micron in-line filter; flush line with 0.9% NaCl before, after administration
• Give over 60 min through a peripheral line or in-dwelling catheter; inf doses of >1000 mg over 90 min
• Dilute in 100 ml of 0.9% NaCl; dilute doses >1000 mg in 150 ml of 0.9% NaCl; mix by inverting; max 10 mg/ml; use within 6 hr if stored at room temperature; can be stored between 2°-8° C for up to 24 hr
• Store unopened vials in refrigerator; do not shake; protect from direct sunlight; do not freeze

ADVERSE EFFECTS

P

CNS: Fatigue
CV: Peripheral edema
EENT: Ocular irritation, **ocular toxicity**
GI: *Nausea, diarrhea, vomiting,* anorexia, mouth ulceration, abdominal pain, constipation
HEMA: Thrombophlebitis
INTEG: *Rash,* pruritus, **exfoliative dermatitis,** skin fissure, **angioedema, severe/fatal infusion reactions**
META: Hypocalcemia, hypomagnesemia, antibody formation
RESP: **Bronchospasm, cough,** dyspnea, **hypoxia, pulmonary fibrosis/embolism,** pneumonitis, wheezing

---

　　　Adverse effects: *italics* = common; **bold** = life-threatening

Absorption	38%-49%, high-fat meal decreases absorption
Distribution	Protein binding 99.5%
Metabolism	Liver, oxidative metabolism by CYP3A4, glucuronidation by UGT1A9, some Asian patients (15%-20%) are poor metabolizers
Excretion	Feces 77%
Half-life	Elimination 7.5 day

Pharmacodynamics

Onset	Unknown
Peak	3 hr
Duration	Unknown

INTERACTIONS

Drug classifications
Antineoplastics, other: do not use with other products

NURSING CONSIDERATIONS

Assessment
• **Pulmonary fibrosis:** assess for dyspnea, cough, wheezing, may need to discontinue

> **BLACK BOX WARNING: Serious skin disorders:** assess for fever, sore throat, fatigue, then lesions in mouth, lips; withhold product, notify prescriber

• Monitor serum electrolytes periodically (calcium, magnesium)
• Assess for signs of infection: increased temperature

> **BLACK BOX WARNING:** Assess for signs of infusion reactions: bronchospasm, fever, chills, hypotension; may require discontinuation; have emergency equipment available

• **Assess for signs of ocular toxicity:** ocular irritation, hyperemia

Nursing diagnoses
• Infection, risk for (uses)
• Knowledge, deficient (teaching)
• Nutrition: less than body requirements, imbalanced (adverse reactions)

Patient/family education
⚠ **Instruct patient to report adverse reactions immediately: difficulty breathing, mouth sores, skin rash, ocular toxicity**
• Teach patient reason for treatment, expected results, adverse reactions

• Teach males/females to use contraception while taking this product and for 6 mo after treatment; do not breastfeed for at least 2 mo after treatment
• Advise to use sunscreen while taking, 2 mo after

Evaluation
Positive therapeutic outcome
• Decrease in colon carcinoma progression

---

pantoprazole (Rx)
(pan-toe-pray′zole)
Panto ✦, Pantoloc ✦, Protonix, Protonix IV
Func. class.: Proton pump inhibitor
Chem. class.: Benzimidazole
Pregnancy category C

ACTION: Suppresses gastric secretion by inhibiting hydrogen/potassium ATPase enzyme system in gastric parietal cell; characterized as gastric acid pump inhibitor, since it blocks final step of acid production

Therapeutic outcome: Absence of epigastric fullness, pain, swelling

USES: Gastroesophageal reflux disease (GERD), severe erosive esophagitis, maintenance, long-term pathological hypersecretory conditions including Zollinger-Ellison syndrome

CONTRAINDICATIONS: Hypersensitivity to this product or benzimidazole

Precautions: Pregnancy **C**, breastfeeding, children, proton pump hypersensitivity

DOSAGE AND ROUTES
GERD
Adult: PO 40 mg/day × 8 wk, may repeat course

Erosive esophagitis
Adult: **IV** 40 mg/day × 7-10 days; PO 40 mg/day × 8 wk; may repeat PO course

Pathologic hypersecretory conditions
Adult: PO 40 mg bid; **IV** 80 mg q12hr; max 240 mg/day

Available forms: Del rel tabs 20, 40 mg; powder for inj 40 mg/vial; del rel granules for susp 40 mg

---

⚠ Nurse Alert

Implementation
- Swallow del rel tabs whole; do not break, crush, or chew
- May take with or without food

IV route
- Reconstitute with 10 ml 0.9% NaCl; give as **IV** push ≥2 min; further dilute with 80 ml LR, D₅W, 0.9% NaCl (0.8 mg/ml), give over 15 min (≤6 mg/min)

ADVERSE EFFECTS
CNS: *Headache,* insomnia
GI: *Diarrhea, abdominal pain,* flatulence, **pancreatitis**
INTEG: *Rash*
META: Hyperglycemia, weight gain/loss, hyponatremia, hypomagnesemia
MS: **Rhabdomyolysis,** myalgia
RESP: **Pneumonia**
SYST: **Stevens-Johnson syndrome, toxic epidermal necrolysis, anaphylaxis, angioedema**

Pharmacokinetics

Absorption	Unknown
Distribution	Protein binding 97%
Metabolism	Unknown
Excretion	Urine-metabolites, feces, decreased rate in geriatric
Half-life	1½ hr

Pharmacodynamics

Onset	Unknown
Peak	2.4 hr
Duration	>24 hr

INTERACTIONS
Individual drugs
Calcium carbonate, sucralfate, vit B₁₂, ketoconazole, itraconazole, atazanair, ampicillin, iron salts: decreased absorption of pantoprazole
Clarithromycin, diazepam, flurazepam, phenytoin, triazolam: increased levels of pantoprazole
Clopidogrel: decreased clopidogrel effect
Warfarin: increased risk of bleeding

NURSING CONSIDERATIONS
Assessment
- **Rhabdomyolysis:** muscle pain, increased CPK, weakness, swelling of affected muscles; if these occur and if confirmed by CPK, product should be discontinued
- Assess GI system: bowel sounds q8hr, abdomen for pain, swelling, anorexia

- Monitor hepatic enzymes: AST, ALT, alkaline phosphatase during treatment
- **Serious skin reactions:** assess for toxic epidermal necrolysis, **Stevens-Johnson syndrome,** exfoliative dermatitis; fever, sore throat, fatigue, thin ulcers, lesions in the mouth, lips
- **Electrolytic imbalances:** hyponatremia; hypomagnesemia in those using this product (3 mo-1 yr) if hypomagnesemia occurs, use of magnesium supplements may be sufficient; if severe, discontinuation of this product may be required

Nursing diagnoses
- Knowledge, deficient (teaching)

Patient/family education
- Advise patient to report severe diarrhea; product may have to be discontinued
- Advise patient with diabetes that hyperglycemia may occur
- Advise patient to avoid hazardous activities; dizziness may occur
- Advise patient to avoid alcohol, salicylates, ibuprofen; may cause GI irritation

Evaluation
Positive therapeutic outcome
- Absence of epigastric pain, swelling, fullness

PARoxetine (Rx)
(par-ox′e-teen)
Paxil, Paxil CR, Pexeva, PMS
Func. class.: Antidepressant, selective serotonin reuptake inhibitor (SSRI)
Chem. class.: Phenylpiperidine derivative
Pregnancy category D

P

Do not confuse:
PARoxetine/paclitaxel,
Paxil/paclitaxel/Taxol

ACTION: Inhibits CNS neuron reuptake of serotonin but not of norepinephrine or DOPamine

Therapeutic outcome: Relief of depression

USES: Major depressive disorder, obsessive-compulsive disorder, panic disorder, generalized anxiety disorder, posttraumatic stress disorder, premenstrual disorders, social anxiety disorder

Unlabeled uses: Premature ejaculation

CONTRAINDICATIONS:
Pregnancy **D,** hypersensitivity, MAOI use, alcohol use

Adverse effects: *italics* = common; **bold** = life-threatening

Precautions: Breastfeeding, geriatric, seizure history, patients with history of mania, renal/hepatic disease

> **BLACK BOX WARNING:** Children, suicidal ideation

DOSAGE AND ROUTES

Depression
Adult: PO 20 mg/day in AM; after 4 wk if no clinical improvement is noted, dosage may be increased by 10 mg/day weekly to desired response; max 50 mg/day; or CONT REL 25 mg/day, may increase by 12.5 mg/day weekly up to 62.5 mg/day
Geriatric: PO 10 mg/day, increase by 10 mg to desired dose, max 40 mg/day

Obsessive-compulsive disorder
Adult: PO 40 mg/day in AM; start with 20 mg/day, increase 10 mg/day increments, max 60 mg/day

Panic disorder
Adult: Start with 10 mg/day and increase in 10 mg/day increments to 40 mg/day, max 60 mg/day; or CONT REL 12.5 mg/day max 75 mg/day

Generalized anxiety disorder
Adult: PO 20 mg/day in AM, range 20-50 mg/day

Posttraumatic stress disorder
Adult: PO 20 mg/day, range 20-60 mg/day

Premenstrual disorders
Adult: CONT REL 12.5 mg/day in AM

Renal dose
Adult: PO CCr 30-60 ml/min lower doses may be needed, CCr <30 ml/min 10 mg/day in AM, may increase by 10 mg/day qwk, max 40 mg/day; or CONT REL 12.5 mg/day max 50 mg/day

Hepatic dose
Adult: PO 10 mg/day initially, max 40 mg **regular release, CONT REL** 12.5 mg/day initially, max 50 mg/day

Available forms: Tabs 10, 20, 30, 40 mg; oral susp 10 mg/5 ml; cont rel 12.5, 25, 37.5 mg

Implementation
• Give with food or milk for GI symptoms; store at room temperature; do not freeze
• Give crushed if patient is unable to swallow whole, regular release only
• Use gum, hard candy, frequent sips of water for dry mouth
• Avoid use with other CNS depressants

• **Oral susp:** shake, measure with oral syringe or calibrated measuring device
• **Cont rel tab:** do not cut, chew, crush; do not give concurrently with antacids

ADVERSE EFFECTS
CNS: *Headache, nervousness, insomnia, drowsiness, anxiety, tremor, dizziness, fatigue, sedation,* abnormal dreams, agitation, apathy, euphoria, hallucinations, delusions, psychosis, **seizures, malignant neuroleptic syndrome–like reactions,** restless legs syndrome
CV: Vasodilatation, postural hypotension, palpitations
EENT: Visual changes
GI: *Nausea, diarrhea, constipation, dry mouth, anorexia,* dyspepsia, vomiting, taste changes, flatulence, decreased appetite, cramps
GU: Dysmenorrhea, decreased libido, urinary frequency, UTI, amenorrhea, cystitis, impotence, decreased sperm quality, decreased fertility, *abnormal ejaculation* (male)
INTEG: *Sweating,* rash
MS: Pain, arthritis, myalgia, myopathy, myasthenia
RESP: Infection, pharyngitis, nasal congestion, sinus headache, sinusitis, cough, dyspnea, yawning
SYST: Asthenia, fever, abrupt withdrawal syndrome

Pharmacokinetics

Absorption	Well absorbed
Distribution	Widely distributed; crosses blood-brain barrier, protein-binding 95%
Metabolism	Liver, mostly by CYP2D6 enzyme system
Excretion	Kidneys, unchanged (2%); breast milk
Half-life	21 hr (reg rel); 15-20 hr (cont rel)

Pharmacodynamics

Onset	Unknown
Peak	5.2 hr
Duration	Unknown

INTERACTIONS

Individual drugs
Methylphenidate, tramadol: increased serotonin syndrome
Cimetidine: increased PARoxetine levels
Digoxin: decreased effect of digoxin
L-tryptophan: increased agitation

PHENobarbital: decreased PARoxetine levels
Phenytoin: decreased effect of PARoxetine
⚠ **Pimozide: potentially fatal reactions**
Theophylline: increased theophylline levels
⚠ **Thioridazine: do not use with PARox-**
etine; hypertensive crisis, seizures, poten-
tially fatal reactions can occur
Warfarin: increased bleeding

Drug classifications

CYP2D6 inhibitors (aprepitant, delavirdine,
  imatinib, nefazodone): increased toxicity
Highly protein-bound products: increased side
  effects
⚠ **MAOIs: hypertensive crisis, seizures; do**
not use together; potentially fatal reactions
can occur
SSRIs, SNRIs, atypical antipsychotics, serotonin-
  receptor agonists, tricyclics, amphetamines:
  increased serotonin syndrome
NSAIDs, thrombolytics, salicylates, platelet inhibitors, anticoagulants: increased bleeding

Drug/herb

Ephedra: hypertensive crisis
Kava: avoid use
St. John's wort: possible serotonin syndrome,
  avoid use

Drug/lab test

Increased: serum bilirubin, blood glucose,
  alkaline phosphatase
Decreased: VMA, 5-HIAA
False increase: urinary catecholamines

NURSING CONSIDERATIONS
Assessment

> **BLACK BOX WARNING: Depression/OCD/**
> **anxiety/panic attacks:** assess mental status:
> mood, sensorium, affect, suicidal tendencies
> (especially in child/young adult), increase in
> psychiatric symptoms, increasing obsessive
> thoughts, compulsive behaviors, restrict
> amount available

• **Postural hypotension:** monitor B/P (lying/
standing), pulse q4hr; if systolic B/P drops 20
mm Hg, hold product, notify prescriber; take
vital signs q4hr in patients with CV disease
• **Renal status:** monitor BUN, creatinine,
urinary retention
• **Withdrawal symptoms:** assess for headache, nausea, vomiting, muscle pain, weakness;
not usual unless product discontinued abruptly
⚠ **Serotonin, neuroleptic malignant**
syndrome: assess for hallucinations, coma,
headache, agitation, shivering/sweating,
tachycardia, diarrhea, tremor, hyperten-
sion, hyperthermia, rigidity, delirium, coma,
myoclonus, agitation, nausea, vomiting
• Monitor blood studies: CBC, leukocytes, differential, cardiac enzymes if patient is receiving
long-term therapy
• Monitor hepatic studies: AST, ALT, bilirubin
• Check weight weekly; appetite may increase
with product
• Assess ECG for flattening of T-wave, bundle
branch block, AV block, dysrhythmias in cardiac
patients
• Assess for EPS primarily in geriatric: rigidity,
dystonia, akathisia
• Monitor urinary retention, constipation;
constipation is more likely to occur in children
or geriatric
• Identify alcohol consumption; if alcohol is
consumed, hold dose until AM

Nursing diagnoses

• Coping, ineffective (uses)
• Injury, risk for (adverse reactions)
• Knowledge, deficient (teaching)
• Noncompliance (teaching)

Patient/family education

• Advise patient that therapeutic effects may
take 1-4 wk
• Teach patient to use caution in driving and
other activities requiring alertness because of
drowsiness, dizziness, blurred vision; to avoid
rising quickly from sitting to standing, especially
geriatric
• Caution patient to avoid alcohol ingestion,
other CNS depressants, and OTC medication
unless prescribed
• Caution patient not to discontinue medication
quickly after long-term use; may cause nausea,
anxiety, headache, malaise; do not double doses
if one is missed
• Advise patient to use gum, hard sugarless
candy, or frequent sips of water for dry mouth; if
dry mouth continues an artificial saliva product
may be used

> **BLACK BOX WARNING:** Advise patient that
> depression may worsen, suicidal thoughts/
> behavior may occur, to notify prescriber

• Advise patient to discuss sexual side effects:
impotence, possible male infertility while taking
this product

Evaluation
Positive therapeutic outcome

• Decrease in depression
• Absence of suicidal thoughts

TREATMENT OF OVERDOSE:
Activated charcoal, gastric lavage, maintain airway; for seizures give diazepam, symptomatic treatment

pegaptanib (Rx)
(peg-ap′ta-nib)
Macugen
Func. class: Ophthalmic agent—miscellaneous
Pregnancy category B

ACTION: Binds to vascular endothelial growth factor (VEGF), thereby inhibiting angiogenesis

Therapeutic outcome: Stabilization of vision in macular degeneration

USES: Treatment of neovascular (wet) age-related macular degeneration; may be used alone or with photodynamic therapy (PDT)

CONTRAINDICATIONS:
Hypersensitivity, ocular or periocular infections

Precautions: Pregnancy **B**, inflammatory eye disease, ocular hypertension

DOSAGE AND ROUTES
Adult: Intravitreal inj 0.3 mg inj q6wk

Available forms: Inj 0.3 mg, single glass syringes

Implementation
• Administer anesthesia and a broad-spectrum antiinfective prior to injection
• The inj should be done under aseptic conditions
• Remove all air bubbles prior to use
• Store at 36°-46° F, do not freeze or shake vigorously

ADVERSE EFFECTS
EENT: *Anterior chamber inflammation, blurred vision, conjunctival hemorrhage, corneal edema, cataract, eye discharge, eye pain, increased intraocular pressure, punctate keratitis, reduced visual acuity, vitreous floaters, vitreous opacities, blepharitis, conjunctivitis, photophobia,* retinal detachment, iatrogenic traumatic cataract

Pharmacokinetics
Absorption	Unknown
Distribution	Unknown
Metabolism	Unknown
Excretion	Unknown
Half-life	87-100 hr in vitreous humor of the monkey

Pharmacodynamics
Onset	Unknown
Peak	Unknown
Duration	May remain fully active in the eye for 7-28 days

NURSING CONSIDERATIONS
Assessment
• Test visual acuity periodically
• Assess treated eye for increased intraocular pressure, infection, endophthalmitis
• Monitor perfusion of the optic nerve head immediately after injection, tonometry $\frac{1}{2}$ hr after inj, biomicroscopy 2-7 days after inj

Nursing diagnoses
• Knowledge, deficient (teaching)

Patient/family education
• Instruct patient to report any inflammation, bleeding, eye discharge, opacities to prescriber
• Instruct patient to continue with follow-up care during treatment

Evaluation
Positive therapeutic outcome
• Macular degeneration stabilized

⚠ HIGH ALERT

pegaspargase (Rx)
(peg-as′per-gase)
Oncaspar, PEG-L-asparaginase
Func. class.: Antineoplastic
Chem. class.: *Escherichia coli* enzyme
Pregnancy category C

ACTION: Indirectly inhibits protein synthesis in tumor cells; without amino acid, DNA, RNA synthesis is halted; asparagine, protein synthesis is halted; G_1 phase of cell cycle specific; a nonvesicant; a modified version of L-asparaginase

Therapeutic outcome: Prevention of rapidly growing malignant cells

USES: Acute lymphocytic leukemia unresponsive to other agents in combination with other antineoplastics

CONTRAINDICATIONS:
Breastfeeding, infants, hypersensitivity, pancreatitis, acute bronchospasm, bleeding, coagulopathy, coronary thrombosis, DIC, hypotension

Precautions: Pregnancy **C**, renal/hepatic/CNS disease, *E. coli* protein hypersensitivity, hemophilia, tumor lysis syndrome, infection

DOSAGE AND ROUTES
In combination
Adult and child: IV/IM 2500 international units/m^2 q14day, run **IV** over 1-2 hr in 100 ml of 0.9% NaCl or D$_5$W through a running **inj**; IM should be no more than 2 ml in one inj site used in combination with other chemotherapeutics

Available forms: Inj 750 international units/ml in a phosphate-buffered saline sol

Implementation
• Preparation by trained personnel is required in controlled environment
• Provide antiemetic 30-60 min before giving product and prn to prevent vomiting; administer antibiotics for prophylaxis of infection
• Provide a liquid diet: carbonated beverages; gelatin may be added if patient is not nauseated or vomiting
IM route
• No dilution needed, inject in large muscle, do not give more than 2 ml in one injection site, aspirate; preferred route

Intermittent IV infusion route
• Dilute contents of vial 1100 ml 0.9% NaCl or D$_5$W, give over 1-2 hr through freely running IV solution, keep refrigerated, do not freeze
• Provide allopurinol or sodium bicarbonate to reduce uric acid levels, alkalinization of urine

ADVERSE EFFECTS
CNS: Neuritis, dizziness, headache, **coma,** depression, fatigue, confusion, hallucinations, **seizures, intracranial bleeding**
CV: Chest pain, **hypotension**
ENDO: Hyperglycemia
GI: *Nausea, vomiting, anorexia, cramps, stomatitis,* **hepatotoxicity, pancreatitis,** *diarrhea*
GU: Urinary retention, **renal failure,** glycosuria, polyuria, azotemia, uric acid neuropathy
HEMA: **Thrombocytopenia, leukopenia, myelosuppression, anemia, decreased clotting factors, pancytopenia, DIC**
INTEG: *Rash,* urticaria, chills, fever
RESP: **Fibrosis, pulmonary infiltrate, severe bronchospasm**

SYST: Anaphylaxis, hypersensitivity, angioedema

Pharmacokinetics
Absorption	Complete bioavailability
Distribution	Intravascular spaces
Metabolism	Unknown
Excretion	Reticuloendothelial system
Half-life	5^1/$_2$ days

Pharmacodynamics
Onset	Rapid
Peak	Unknown
Duration	2 wk

INTERACTIONS
Individual drugs
Aspirin, heparin, warfarin: coagulation factor imbalances
Methotrexate: decreased action of methotrexate

Drug classifications
Corticosteroids: increased hypoglycemia
NSAIDs, salicylates, platelet inhibitors, thrombolytics: increased bleeding risk
Live virus vaccines: decreased immune responses

NURSING CONSIDERATIONS
Assessment
⚠ Assess for signs and symptoms of pancreatitis (nausea, vomiting, severe abdominal pain), anaphylaxis (bronchospasm, dyspnea), cyanosis; monitor amylase, glucose
⚠ Assess symptoms indicating severe allergic reaction: rash, pruritus, urticaria, purpuric skin lesions, itching, flushing; monitor for joint pain, bronchospasm, hypotension; epinephrine and crash carts should be nearby
• Monitor for frequency of stools, characteristics: cramping, acidosis; signs of dehydration: rapid respirations, poor skin turgor, decreased urine output, dry skin, restlessness, weakness
• Monitor CBC, differential, platelet count weekly; withhold product if WBC is <4000/mm^3 or platelet count is <100,000/mm^3; notify physician of results; also assess pro-time, PTT, and thrombin time, which may be increased
• Monitor renal function tests: BUN, creatinine, serum uric acid, urine CCr before, during therapy; check I&O ratio; report fall in urine output to <30 ml/hr; patient should be well hydrated with 2-3 L/day to prevent urate deposits

• Monitor temp q4hr (may indicate beginning of infection)
• Monitor liver function tests before, during therapy (bilirubin, AST, ALT, LDH) as needed or monthly; check for jaundice of skin and sclera, dark urine, clay-colored stools, itchy skin, abdominal pain, fever, diarrhea; also monitor cholesterol, alkaline phosphatase
• Assess for bleeding: hematuria, stool guaiac, bruising or petechiae, mucosa or orifices q8hr; check for inflammation of mucosa, breaks in skin
• Identify edema in feet, joint pain, stomach pain, shaking

Nursing diagnoses
• Infection, risk for (adverse reactions)
• Injury, risk for (adverse reactions)
• Knowledge, deficient (teaching)

Patient/family education
• Advise patient that contraceptive measures are recommended during therapy; product is teratogenic
• Teach patient to avoid use of products containing aspirin or NSAIDs, razors, commercial mouthwash, since bleeding may occur; to report symptoms of bleeding (hematuria, tarry stools)
• Teach patient to report signs of anemia (fatigue, headache, irritability, faintness, shortness of breath)
• Tell patient to avoid crowds and persons with respiratory tract infections to prevent patient infection
• Advise patient to avoid vaccinations, since serious reactions can occur
• Teach patient to report nausea, vomiting, bruising, bleeding, stomatitis, severe diarrhea, jaundice, chest pain, abdominal pain, trouble breathing, rash

Evaluation
Positive therapeutic outcome
• Prevention of rapid division of malignant cells

pegfilgrastim (Rx)
(peg-fill-grass'stim)
Neulasta
Func. class.: Hematopoietic agent
Pregnancy category C

ACTION: Stimulates proliferation and differentiation of neutrophils

Therapeutic outcome: Absence of infection

USES: To decrease infection in patients receiving antineoplastics that are myelosuppressive; to increase WBC in patients with product-induced neutropenia

CONTRAINDICATIONS:
Hypersensitivity to proteins of *E. coli,* filgrastim

Precautions: Pregnancy **C,** breastfeeding, child <45 kg, adolescents, myeloid malignancies, sickle cell disease, leukocytosis, splenic rupture, allergic-type reactions, ARDS, peripheral blood stem cell mobilization (PBSC)

DOSAGE AND ROUTES
Adult: SUBCUT 6 mg give once per chemotherapy cycle

Available forms: Sol for inj 10 mg/0.6 ml

Implementation
SUBCUT route
• Give using single-use vials; after dose is withdrawn, do not reenter vial
• Do not use 6-mg fixed dose in infants, children, or others <45 kg
• Inspect sol for discoloration, particulates; if present, do not use
• Do not administer in the period 14 days before and 24 hr after cytotoxic chemotherapy
• Store in refrigerator; do not freeze; may store at room temp up to 6 hr, avoid shaking, protect from light

ADVERSE EFFECTS
CNS: Fever, fatigue, headache, dizziness, insomnia, peripheral edema
GI: *Nausea,* vomiting, diarrhea, mucositis, anorexia, constipation, dyspepsia, abdominal pain, stomatitis, **splenic rupture**
HEMA: Leukocytosis, granulocytopenia, sickle cell crisis, hemoglobin S disease with crisis
INTEG: Alopecia
MISC: Chest pain, hyperuricemia, **anaphylaxis, flulike syndrome, angioedema, antibody formation**
MS: Skeletal pain
RESP: Respiratory distress syndrome

Pharmacokinetics

Absorption	Unknown
Distribution	Unknown
Metabolism	Unknown
Excretion	Unknown
Half-life	15-80 hr; 20-38 hr (child)

Pharmacodynamics

Unknown

INTERACTIONS

Individual drug
Lithium: increased release of neutrophils

Drug classifications
Cytotoxic chemotherapy agents: do not use this product concomitantly or 2 wk before or 24 hr after administration of cytotoxics

Drug/lab test
Increased: uric acid, LDH, alkaline phosphatase

NURSING CONSIDERATIONS

Assessment
• **Assess for allergic reactions, anaphylaxis:** rash, urticaria; discontinue this product, have emergency equipment nearby
• Monitor blood studies: CBC, platelet count before treatment and twice weekly; neutrophil counts may be increased for 2 days after therapy
• **ARDS:** assess for dyspnea, fever, tachypnea, occasional confusion; obtain ABGs, chest x-ray, product may need to be discontinued
• Monitor B/P, respirations, pulse before, during therapy
• **Assess for bone pain,** give mild analgesics

Nursing diagnoses
• Infection, risk for (uses)
• Knowledge, deficient (teaching)

Patient/family education
• Teach the technique for self-administration: dose, side effects, disposal of containers and needles; provide instruction sheet

Evaluation
Positive therapeutic outcome
• Absence of infection

---

peginterferon alfa-2a (Rx)
(peg-in-ter-feer'on)
Pegasys
peginterferon alfa-2b (Rx)
PegIntron, Sylatron
Func. class.: Immunomodulator
Pregnancy category C

ACTION: Stimulates genes to modulate many biologic effects, including inhibition of viral replication; inhibits ion cell proliferation, immunomodulation, stimulates effector proteins, decreases leukocyte, platelet counts

Therapeutic outcome: Undetectable viral load; decreasing signs, symptoms of chronic hepatitis C

USES: Chronic hepatitis C infections in adults with compensated liver disease, chronic hepatitis B in adults with HBe Ag–positive, HBe Ag–negative; HCV patients coinfected with HIV, nonresponders, or relapsers with chronic hepatitis C

CONTRAINDICATIONS:
Hypersensitivity to interferons, benzyl alcohol, *Escherichia coli* protein, neonates, infants, sepsis

Precautions: Pregnancy **C**, breastfeeding, children <18 yr, geriatric, thyroid disorders, myelosuppression, renal/hepatic disease, suicidal/homicidal ideation, preexisting ophthalmologic disorders, pancreatitis, hemodialysis

> **BLACK BOX WARNING:** Cardiac/autoimmune disease, depression, infection, use with ribavirin

DOSAGE AND ROUTES

Pegasys
Adult: SUBCUT 180 mcg qwk × 48 wk; if poorly tolerated, reduce dose to 135 mcg qwk; in some cases reduction to 90 mcg may be needed

PegIntron
(chronic hepatitis C with compensated liver disease)
Adult >105 kg: SUBCUT 1.5 mcg/kg/wk plus ribavirin 600 mg in AM and 800 mg in PM plus a HCV NS3/4A protease inhibitor
Adult 86-105 kg: 150 mcg/0.5 ml (0.5 ml of 150 mcg vial or Redipen) per wk plus ribavirin 1200 mg/day in 2 divided doses plus a HCV NS3/4A protease inhibitor
Adult: 81-85 kg: 120 mcg/0.5 ml (0.5 ml of 120 mcg vial or Redipen) per wk plus ribavirin 1200 mg/day in 2 divided doses plus a HCV NS3/4A protease inhibitor
Adult 76-80 kg: 120 mcg/0.5 ml (0.5 ml of 120 mcg vial or Redipen) per wk plus ribavirin 400 mg in AM and 600 mg in PM plus a HCV NS3/4A protease inhibitor
Adult 66-75 kg: 96 mcg/0.4 ml (0.4 ml of 120 mcg vial or Redipen) per wk plus ribavirin 400 mg in AM and 600 mg in PM plus a HCV NS3/4A protease inhibitor
Adult 61-65 kg: 96 mcg/0.4 ml (0.4 ml of 120 mcg vial or Redipen) per wk plus ribavirin 800

P

mg/day in 2 divided doses plus a HCV NS3/4A protease inhibitor
Adult 51-60 kg: 80 mcg/0.5 ml (0.5 ml of 80 mcg vial or Redipen) per wk plus ribavirin 800 mg/day in 2 divided doses plus a HCV NS3/4A protease inhibitor
Adult 40-50 kg: 64 mcg/0.4 ml (0.4 ml of 80 mcg vial or Redipen) per wk plus ribavirin 800 mg/day in 2 divided doses plus a HCV NS3/4A protease inhibitor
Adult <40 kg: 50 mcg/0.5 ml (0.5 ml of 50 mcg vial or Redipen) per wk plus ribavirin 800 mg/day in 2 divided doses plus a HCV NS3/4A protease inhibitor

Malignant melanoma (Sylatron only)
Adult: SUBCUT 6 mcg/kg/wk × 8 wk then 3 mcg/kg/wk × up to 5 yr, premedicate with acetaminophen 500-1000 mg 30 min before first dose and prn for subsequent doses

Available forms: Pegasys: inj 180 mcg/0.5 ml, 180 mcg/ml; PegIntron inj 50, 80, 120, 150 mcg/0.5 ml; Sylatron 296, 444, 888 mcg powder for inj

Implementation
• Give in PM to reduce discomfort, sleep through side effects
• Continue pediatric dose in those who turn 18 yr

ADVERSE EFFECTS
CNS: *Headache, insomnia, dizziness,* anxiety, hostility, lability, nervousness, depression, fatigue, poor concentration, pyrexia, **suicidal ideation, homicidal ideation,** relapse of drug addiction, emotional lability, mania, psychosis
CV: Ischemic CV events
ENDO: Hypothyroidism, diabetes
GI: *Abdominal pain, nausea, diarrhea, anorexia, vomiting,* dry mouth, **fatal colitis, fatal pancreatitis**
HEMA: Thrombocytopenia, neutropenia, anemia, lymphopenia
INTEG: *Alopecia, pruritus, rash,* dermatitis
MISC: Blurred vision, inj site reaction, rigors
MS: *Back pain,* myalgia, arthralgia
RESP: Cough, dyspnea

Pharmacokinetics

Absorption	Large variability
Distribution	Large variability
Metabolism	Large variability
Excretion	Large variability
Half-life	15-80 hr

Pharmacodynamics
Unknown

INTERACTIONS
Individual drugs
Theophylline: use caution if giving together
Drug classifications
Myelosuppressives: use caution if giving together
Drug/lab test
Increased: triglycerides, ALT, neutrophils, platelets
Abnormal: thyroid function test

NURSING CONSIDERATIONS
Assessment
• **Neuropsychiatric symptoms:** severe depression with suicidal ideation; monitor q3wk, then q8wk, then q6 mo
• Monitor platelet counts, heme concentration, ANC, serum creatinine concentration, albumin, bilirubin, TSH, T_4, AFP
• Assess for myelosuppression, hold dose if neutrophil count is $<500 \times 10^6$/L or if platelets are $<50 \times 10^9$/L
• Monitor B/P, blood glucose, ophthalmic exam, pulmonary function
• Monitor ALT, HCV viral load; patients who show no reduction in ALT, HCV are unlikely to show benefit of treatment after 6 mo
• **Myelosuppression:** hold dose if neutrophil count is $<500 \times 10^6$/L or if platelets are $<50 \times 10^9$/L
• **Hypersensitivity:** discontinue immediately if hypersensitivity occurs
• **Infection:** monitor vital signs, increased WBCs, fever; product may need to be discontinued
• **Colitis/pancreatitis:** may be fatal; diarrhea, fever, nausea, vomiting, severe abdominal pain, if these occur discontinue product

Nursing diagnoses
• Infection, risk for (uses)
• Knowledge, deficient (teaching)

Patient/family education
• Provide patient or family member with written, detailed information about product
• Give instructions for home use if appropriate
• Advise to take in evening to reduce discomfort, sleep through some side effects

Evaluation
Positive therapeutic outcome
• Decreased chronic hepatitis C signs/symptoms, undetectable viral load

---

⚠ Nurse Alert

⚠ HIGH ALERT

pemetrexed (Rx)

(pem-ah-trex′ed)

Alimta

Func. class.: Antineoplastic-antimetabolite

Chem. class.: Folic acid antagonist

Pregnancy category D

ACTION: Inhibits multiple enzymes that reduce folic acid, which is needed for cell replication

Therapeutic outcome: Decreased spread of mesothelioma, decreased tumor size

USES: Malignant pleural mesothelioma in combination with CISplatin; non–small cell lung cancer as a single agent; non-squamous non–small cell lung cancer (first-line treatment)

CONTRAINDICATIONS:

Pregnancy **D**, hypersensitivity, ANC <1500 cells/mm^3, CCr <45 ml/min, thrombocytopenia (<100,000/mm^3), anemia

Precautions: Breastfeeding, children, renal/hepatic disease

DOSAGE AND ROUTES

Adult: IV INF 500-600 mg/m^2 given over 10 min on day 1 of a 21-day cycle with CISplatin 75 mg/m^2 INF over 2 hr beginning $^1/_2$ hr after end of pemetrexed INF

ANC <500/mm^3 and platelets = 50,000/mm^3 75% of previous dose

Renal dose

Adult: IV infusion CCr <45 ml/min, not recommended

Available forms: Inj, single-use vials, 500 mg

Implementation

• Administer vit B$_{12}$ and low-dose folic acid as a prophylactic measure to treat related hematologic, GI toxicity; at least 5 daily doses of folic acid must be taken in the 7 days preceding first dose

• Premedicate with a corticosteroid (dexamethasone) given PO bid the day before, day of, and day after administration of pemetrexed

• **Neurotoxicity:** assess for CTC grade 2: withhold until resolution to at least pretherapy value/condition, reduce CISplatin by 50%; CTC grade 3/4; immediately discontinue this product and CISplatin if given in combination

• **Mucositis:** assess for CTC 3-4; withhold until resolution to at least pretherapy value/condition, reduce dose by 50%, if grade 3-4 occurs after 2 dosage reductions, discontinue this product and CISplatin

• **Bleeding:** assess for bleeding time, coagulation time during treatment; bleeding; hematuria, guaiac, brusing or petechiae, mucosa or orifices q8hr

• Use a liquid diet: carbonated beverage, gelatin; dry toast, crackers may be added when patient is not nauseated or vomiting

• Assist patient with rinsing of mouth tid-qid with water, club soda; brushing of teeth bid-tid with soft brush or cotton-tipped applicators for stomatitis; use unwaxed dental floss

IV route

• Use cytotoxic handling procedures

• Reconstitute 500-mg vial/20 ml 0.9% NaCl inj (preservative free) = 25 mg/ml, swirl until dissolved, further dilute with 100 ml 0.9% NaCl inj (preservative free), give as IV inf over 10 min

• Use only 0.9% NaCl inj (preservative free) for reconstitution, dilution

• Store at 77° F, excursions permitted 59°-86°F, not light sensitive, discard unused portions

Y-site compatibilities: Acyclovir sodium, alfentanil, allopurinol, amifostine, amikacin, aminocaproic acid, aminophylline, amiodarone, amphotericin B lipid complex, amphotericin B liposome, ampicillin, ampicillin-sulbactam, atenolol, atracurium, azithromycin, aztreonam, bivalirudin, bleomycin, bumetanide, buprenorphine, butorphanol, CARBOplatin, carmustine, ceftizoxime, cefTRIAXone, cefuroxime, cimetidine, cisatracurium, CISplatin, clindamycin, cyclophosphamide, cycloSPORINE, cytarabine, DACTINomycin, DAPTOmycin, dexamethasone, digoxin, diltiazem, diphenhydrAMINE, docetaxel, dolasetron, DOPamine, doxacurium, enalaprilat, ePHEDrine, EPINEPHrine, eptifibatide, ertapenem, esmolol, etoposide, famotidine, fenoldopam, fentaNYL, fluconazole, fludarabine, fluorouracil, foscarnet, fosphenytoin, furosemide, ganciclovir, gatifloxacin, glycopyrrolate, granisetron, haloperidol, heparin, hydrocortisone, HYDROmorphone, hydrOXYzine, ifosfamide, imipenem-cilastatin, insulin (regular), isoproterenol, ketorolac, labetalol, leucovorin, levofloxacin, lidocaine, linezolid, LORazepam, magnesium, mannitol, meperidine, meropenem, mesna, methyldopate, methylPREDNISolone, metoclopramide, metoprolol, midazolam, milrinone, mitomycin, mivacurium, morphine, moxifloxacin, nafcillin, naloxone, nesiritide, nitroglycerin, norepinephrine,

P

*Adverse effects: italics = common; **bold** = life-threatening*

octreotide, oxaliplatin, paclitaxel, pamidronate, pancuronium, PENTobarbital, PHENobarbital, piperacillin-tazobactam, polymyxin B, potassium chloride/phosphates, procainamide, promethazine, propranolol, ranitidine, remifentanil, rocuronium, sodium acetate/bicarbonate/phosphates, succinylcholine, SUFentanil, sulfamethoxazole-trimethoprim, tacrolimus, theophylline, thiopental, thiotepa, ticarcillin, ticarcillin-clavulanate, tigecycline, tirofiban, trimethobenzamide, vancomycin, vecuronium, verapamil, vinBLAStine, vinCRIStine, vinorelbine, zidovudine, zoledronic acid

ADVERSE EFFECTS

CNS: *Fatigue, fever, mood alteration, neuropathy*
CV: Thrombosis/embolism, *chest pain*
GI: *Nausea, vomiting, anorexia, diarrhea, ulcerative stomatitis, constipation, dysphagia, dehydration*
GU: *Renal failure, creatinine elevation*
HEMA: Neutropenia, leukopenia, thrombocytopenia, myelosuppression, anemia
INTEG: *Rash, desquamation*
RESP: *Dyspnea*
SYST: Infection with/without neutropenia, radiation recall reaction

Pharmacokinetics

Absorption	Unknown
Distribution	81% protein binding
Metabolism	Not metabolized
Excretion	Excreted in urine (unchanged 70%-90%) Not known if it is excreted in breast milk
Half-life	3.5 hr

Pharmacodynamics

Unknown

INTERACTIONS

Drug classifications

Anticoagulants, NSAIDs, platelet inhibitors, salicylates, thrombolytics: increased bleeding risk
Nephrotoxic products (NSAIDs): decreased pemetrexed clearance

NURSING CONSIDERATIONS

Assessment

⚠ **Bone marrow depression: monitor CBC, differential, platelet count; monitor for nadir and recovery; a new cycle should not begin if ANC < 1500 cells/mm³, platelets are** < 100,000 cells/mm³, creatinine clearance < 45 ml/min
• Monitor renal tests: BUN, serum uric acid, urine CCr, electrolytes before, during therapy
• For previous radiation treatments; radiation recall reactions have occurred (erythema, exfoliative dermatitis, pain, burning)
• Monitor I&O ratio; report fall in urine output to <30 ml/hr
• Monitor temp q4hr; fever may indicate beginning infection; no rectal temps
• Assess bleeding time, coagulation time during treatment; bleeding: hematuria, guaiac, bruising or petechiae, mucosa or orifices q8hr
• Assess buccal cavity q8hr for dryness, sores, ulceration, white patches, oral pain, bleeding, dysphagia
⚠ **Assess for symptoms indicating severe allergic reaction: rash, urticaria, itching, flushing**
• **Neurotoxicity:** CTC grade 2: withhold until resolution to at least pretherapy value/condition; reduce CISplatin by 50%; CTC grade 3-4; immediately discontinue product and CISplatin if given in combination
• **Mucositis:** CTC grade 3-4: withhold until resolution to at least pretherapy value/condition; reduce dose by 50%; if grade 3-4 occurs after 2 dosage reductions, discontinue product and CISplatin

Nursing diagnoses

• Body image, disturbed (adverse reactions)
• Infection, risk for (adverse reactions)
• Injury, risk for (adverse reactions)
• Knowledge, deficient (teaching)

Patient/family education

• Instruct patient to report any complaints, side effects to nurse or prescriber: black tarry stools, chills, fever, sore throat, bleeding, bruising, cough, shortness of breath, dark or bloody urine
• Instruct patient to avoid foods with citric acid, hot or rough texture if stomatitis is present
• Instruct patient to report stomatitis: any bleeding, white spots, ulcerations in mouth to prescriber; tell patient to examine mouth daily, report symptoms to nurse, use good oral hygiene
• Advise patient that contraceptive measures are recommended during therapy and for at least 8 wk following cessation of therapy, to discontinue breastfeeding; toxicity to infant may occur
• Advise patient to avoid alcohol, salicylates, live vaccines
• Advise patient to avoid use of razors, commercial mouthwash

- Teach to eat foods high in folic acid and take supplements as prescribed

Evaluation
Positive therapeutic outcome
- Decreased spread of malignancy

penciclovir topical
See Appendix B

PENICILLINS

penicillin G benzathine (Rx)
(pen-i-sill′in)
Bicillin L-A
penicillin G (Rx)
Pfizerpen
penicillin G procaine (Rx)
penicillin V (Rx)
Apo-Pen-VK ✿, Penicillin VK
Func. class.: Broad-spectrum antiinfective
Chem. class.: Natural penicillin
Pregnancy category B

ACTION: Interferes with cell wall replication of susceptible organisms; osmotically unstable cell wall swells and bursts from osmotic pressure, resulting in cell death

Therapeutic outcome: Bactericidal effects on the gram-positive cocci *Staphylococcus, Streptococcus pyogenes, Streptococcus viridans, Streptococcus faecalis, Streptococcus bovis, Streptococcus pneumoniae;* gram-negative cocci *Neisseria gonorrhoeae;* gram-positive bacilli *Actinomyces, Bacillus anthracis, Clostridium perfringens, Clostridium tetani, Corynebacterium diphtheriae, Listeria monocytogenes;* gram-negative bacilli *Escherichia coli, Proteus mirabilis, Salmonella, Shigella, Enterobacter, Streptobacillus moniliformis;* spirochete *Treponema pallidum*

USES: Respiratory tract infections, scarlet fever, erysipelas, otitis media, pneumonia, skin and soft tissue infections, gonorrhea

CONTRAINDICATIONS:
Hypersensitivity to penicillins, corn

Precautions: Pregnancy **B,** breastfeeding, hypersensitivity to cephalosporins/carbapenem/sulfite, severe renal disease, GI disease, asthma

DOSAGE AND ROUTES
Penicillin G benzathine

Early syphilis
Adult: IM 2.4 million units in single dose

Congenital syphilis
Child <2 yr: IM 50,000 units/kg in single dose, max 2.4 million units as a single inj

Prophylaxis of rheumatic fever, glomerulonephritis
Adult and child: IM 1.2 million units in single dose

Upper respiratory tract infections (group A streptococcal)
Adult: IM 1.2 million units in single dose
Child >27 kg: IM 900,000 units in single dose
Child <27 kg: IM 300,000-600,000 units in single dose

Available forms: Inj 300,000 units/ml; 600,000 units/ml

Penicillin G

Pneumococcal/streptococcal infections (serious)
Adult: IM/IV 5-24 million units in divided doses q4-6hr
Child <12 yr: IV 150,000-300,000 units/kg/day in 4-6 divided doses; max 24 million units/day

Renal dose
CCr <10 ml/min, give full loading dose, then ½ of loading dose q8-10hr

Available forms: Inj 1, 2, 3 million units/50 ml; powder for inj 1, 5, 20 million units/vial

Penicillin G procaine

Moderate to severe pneumococcal infections
Adult and child: IM 600,000-1.2 million units in 1 or 2 doses/day for 10 days to 2 wk

Newborn: Avoid use in newborns

Pneumococcal pneumonia
Adult and child >12 yr: IM 600,000-1.2 million units/day × 7-10 days

Available forms: Inj 600,000, 1,200,000 units/dose

Moderately severe group A streptococcal/staphylococcal pneumonia
Adult, adolescent, child ≥60 lb: IM 600,000-1 million units/day

P

Adolescent and child <60 lb: IM 300,000 units/day

Penicillin V

Pneumococcal/staphylococcal infections
Adult: PO 250-500 mg q6hr
Child <12 yr/adolescent/child >12 yr: PO 25-50 mg/kg/day in divided doses q6-8hr, max 3 g/day

Streptococcal infections
Adult/adolescent/child >12 yr: PO 125 mg q6-8hr × 10 days
Child <12 yr and >27 kg: PO 500 mg q8hr or 12hr × 10 days
Child <12 yr and ≤27 kg: PO 250 mg q8hr or q12hr or 40 mg/kg/day in 3 divided doses × 10 days

Prevention of recurrence of rheumatic fever/chorea
Adult: PO 125-250 mg bid continuously

Vincent's gingivitis/pharyngitis
Adult: PO 250 mg q6-8hr

Renal dose
CCr <50 ml/min dosage reduction indicated based on clinical response, degree of impairment

Available forms: Tabs 250, 500 mg; powder for oral sol 125, 250 mg/5 ml

Implementation

Penicillin G benzathine
IM route
• No dilution needed, shake well, give deeply IM in large muscle mass, avoid intravascular inj; aspirate; do not give **IV**

Penicillin G
• Penicillin G sodium or potassium can be given IM or IV, vials containing 10 or 20 million units are not for IM use

Intermittent IV infusion route
• Vials/bulk packages; dilute according to manufacturer's directions
• Frozen bags: thaw at room temp, do not force thaw, no reconstitution needed
• Final conc (100,000-500,000 units/ml, adults; 50,000 units/ml, neonate/infant)
• Total daily dose divided q4-6hr and given over 1-2 hr (adult), 15 min (infant/neonate)

Penicillin G potassium
Y-site compatibilities: Acyclovir, amiodarone, cyclophosphamide, diltiazem, enalaprilat, esmolol, fluconazole, foscarnet, heparin, HYDROmorphone, labetalol, magnesium sulfate, meperidine, morphine, perphenazine, potassium chloride, tacrolimus, theophylline, verapamil, vit B/C

Penicillin G procaine
• No dilution needed, give deep IM inj; avoid intravascular inj; aspirate; do not give IV

Penicillin V
• Orally on empty stomach for best absorption
• Oral susp: tap bottle to loosen, add $^1/_2$ total amount of water, shake, add remaining water, shake; final conc (125 or 250); store in refrigerator after reconstitution, discard after 14 days

Penicillin G procaine
• Do not give **IV**
• Give deeply in large muscle mass
• Reconstitute with 0.9% NaCl, sterile water for inj, D_5W; refrigerate unused portion
• Shake medication before administering
• IM route may include procaine reactions: fear of death, depression, seizures, anxiety, confusion, hallucinations

Penicillin V
• Give in even doses around the clock; if GI upset occurs, give with food; product must be given for 10-14 days to ensure organism death and prevent superinfection; store in tight container
• Shake susp; store in refrigerator for 2 wk or for 1 wk at room temperature

ADVERSE EFFECTS
CNS: Lethargy, hallucinations, anxiety, depression, twitching, **coma**, **seizures**, hyperreflexia
GI: *Nausea, vomiting, diarrhea,* increased AST, ALT, abdominal pain, glossitis, colitis, **pseudomembranous colitis**
GU: Oliguria, proteinuria, hematuria, *vaginitis, moniliasis,* **glomerulonephritis,** renal tubular damage
HEMA: Anemia, increased bleeding time, **bone marrow depression, granulocytopenia,** hemolytic anemia
META: Hyperkalemia, hypokalemia, alkalosis, hypernatremia
MISC: Local pain, tenderness and fever with IM inj, **anaphylaxis serum sickness, Stevens-Johnson syndrome**

Penicillin G benzathine

Pharmacokinetics

Absorption	Delayed; prolonged drug levels
Distribution	Widely distributed; crosses placenta
Metabolism	Liver, minimally
Excretion	Kidneys, unchanged; breast milk
Half-life	$^1/_2$-1 hr

Pharmacodynamics

Onset	Slow
Peak	12-24 hr
Duration	1-4 wk

Penicillin G

Pharmacokinetics

Absorption	Variably absorbed (PO); well absorbed (IM)
Distribution	Widely distributed; crosses placenta
Metabolism	Liver, minimally
Excretion	Kidneys, unchanged; breast milk
Half-life	$^1/_2$-1 hr

Pharmacodynamics

	PO	IM	IV
Onset	Rapid	Rapid	Rapid
Peak	1 hr	$^1/_4$-$^1/_2$ hr	Immediate
Duration	Unknown	Unknown	Unknown

Penicillin G procaine

Pharmacokinetics

Absorption	Delayed; prolonged drug levels
Distribution	Widely distributed; crosses placenta
Metabolism	Liver, minimally
Excretion	Kidneys, unchanged; breast milk
Half-life	$^1/_2$-1 hr

Pharmacodynamics

Onset	Slow
Peak	1-4 hr
Duration	15 hr

Penicillin V

Pharmacokinetics

Absorption	Widely absorbed
Distribution	Widely distributed; crosses placenta
Metabolism	Liver, minimally
Excretion	Kidneys, unchanged; breast milk
Half-life	$^1/_2$-1 hr

Pharmacodynamics

Onset	Rapid
Peak	$^1/_2$ hr
Duration	Unknown

INTERACTIONS

Individual drugs
Aspirin, probenecid: increased penicillin levels
Heparin: increased effect of heparin
Methotrexate: increased effect of methotrexate
Typhoid vaccine: decreased effect of toxoid vaccine

Drug classifications
Contraceptives (oral): decreased contraceptive effectiveness
Tetracyclines: decreased antimicrobial effectiveness of penicillin

Drug/lab test
False positive: urine glucose, urine protein

NURSING CONSIDERATIONS

Assessment
• Assess patient for previous sensitivity reaction to penicillins or cephalosporins; cross-sensitivity between penicillins and cephalosporins is common
• **Assess patient for signs and symptoms of infection** including characteristics of wounds, sputum, urine, stool, WBC >10,000/mm^3, earache, fever; obtain information baseline, during treatment
• Obtain C&S before beginning drug therapy to identify if correct treatment has been initiated
• **Assess for allergic reactions:** rash, urticaria, pruritus, chills, fever, joint pain; angioedema may occur a few days after therapy begins; epinephrine, resuscitation equipment should be available for anaphylactic reaction
• **Pseudomembranous colitis:** Assess for diarrhea, abdominal pain, fever, fatigue, anorexia; possible anemia, elevated WBC and low serum albumin; stop product and usually give either vancomycin or IV metroNIDAZOLE

⚠ Identify urine output; if decreasing, notify prescriber (may indicate nephrotoxicity); also check for increased BUN, creatinine
• Monitor blood studies: AST, ALT, CBC, Hct, bilirubin, LDH, alkaline phosphatase, Coombs' test monthly if patient is on long-term therapy
• Monitor electrolytes: potassium, sodium, chloride monthly if patient is on long-term therapy
• Assess bowel pattern daily; if severe diarrhea occurs, product should be discontinued; may indicate pseudomembranous colitis
• Monitor for bleeding: ecchymosis, bleeding gums, hematuria, stool guaiac daily if on long-term therapy
• **Assess for overgrowth of infection:** perineal itching, fever, malaise, redness, pain, swelling, drainage, rash, diarrhea, change in cough, sputum

Nursing diagnoses
• Diarrhea (adverse reactions)
• Infection, risk for (uses)
• Injury, risk for (adverse reactions)
• Knowledge, deficient (teaching)
• Noncompliance (teaching)

Patient/family education
• Teach patient to report sore throat, bruising, bleeding, joint pain; may indicate **blood dyscrasias (rare)**
• Advise patient to contact prescriber if vaginal itching, loose foul-smelling stools, furry tongue occur; may indicate **superinfection**
• Instruct patient to take all medication prescribed for the length of time ordered
• Advise patient to notify prescriber of diarrhea with blood or pus, which may indicate **pseudomembranous colitis**

Evaluation
Positive therapeutic outcome
• Absence of signs/symptoms of infection (WBC <10,000/mm^3, temp WNL, absence of red, draining wounds, earache)
• Reported improvement in symptoms of infection

TREATMENT OF ANAPHYLAXIS: Withdraw product, maintain airway, administer EPINEPHrine, aminophylline, O$_2$, IV corticosteroids

pentamidine (Rx)
(pen-tam′i-deen)
Nebupent, Pentam 300
Func. class.: Antiprotozoal
Chem. class.: Aromatic diamide derivative
Pregnancy category C

ACTION: Interferes with DNA/RNA synthesis in protozoa; has direct effect on islet cells in the pancreas

Therapeutic outcome: Protozoa death

USES: Treatment/prevention of *Pneumocystis jiroveci* infections

Unlabeled uses: Leishmaniasis, African trypanosomiasis

CONTRAINDICATIONS:
Hypersensitivity

Precautions: Pregnancy **C**, breastfeeding, children, blood dyscrasias, cardiac/renal/hepatic disease, diabetes mellitus, hypocalcemia, hyper/hypotension, anemia

DOSAGE AND ROUTES
Adult and child ≥4 mo: **IV**/IM 4 mg/kg/day × 2-3 wk; NEB 300 mg via specific nebulizer given q4wk for prevention

Available forms: Inj; aerosol 300 mg/vial; sol for aerosol 60 mg/vial ✦

Implementation
Inhalation route
• Through nebulizer, using Raspirgard II jet nebulizer; mix contents in 6 ml of sterile water; do not use low pressure (<20 psi); flow rate should be 5-7 L/min (40-50 psi) air or O$_2$ source over 30-45 min until chamber is empty
IM route
• 300 mg diluted in 3 ml sterile water; give deep IM by Z-track; painful by this route, rotate inj site

Intermittent IV infusion route
• 300 mg/3-5 ml of sterile water for inj, D$_5$W; withdraw dose and further dilute in 50-250 ml of D$_5$W; diluted sol is stable for 48 hr; discard unused sol; give over 1 hr or more

Y-site compatibilities: Alfentanil, atracurium, atropine, benztropine, buprenorphine, calcium gluconate, CARBOplatin, caspofungin, chlorpromazine, cimetidine, CISplatin, cyclophosphamide, cycloSPORINE, cytarabine, DACTINomycin, diltiazem, gatifloxacin, zidovudine

Y-site incompatibilities: Foscarnet, fluconazole

ADVERSE EFFECTS
CNS: Disorientation, hallucinations, dizziness, confusion, drowsiness
CV: Hypotension, ventricular tachycardia, **QT prolongation, dysrhythmias**
GI: *Nausea, vomiting, anorexia,* increased AST, ALT, **acute pancreatitis,** metallic taste
GU: Acute renal failure, increased serum creatinine, renal toxicity, decreased urination
HEMA: Anemia, **leukopenia, thrombocytopenia**
INTEG: Sterile abscess, pain at inj site, pruritus, urticaria, rash
META: Hyperkalemia, hypocalcemia, *hypoglycemia,* hypomagnesemia
MISC: Fatigue, fever, chills, night sweats, **anaphylaxis, Stevens-Johnson syndrome**
RESP: Cough, shortness of breath, **bronchospasm** (with aerosol), sore throat

Pharmacokinetics

Absorption	Well absorbed (IM); minimally absorbed (INH); completely absorbed (**IV**)
Distribution	Widely distributed; does not appear in CSF
Metabolism	Not known
Excretion	Kidneys, unchanged (up to 30%)
Half-life	$6^{1}/_{2}$-$9^{1}/_{2}$ hr; increased in renal disease

Pharmacodynamics

	IM	IV	INH
Onset	Unknown	Unknown	Unknown
Peak	$^{1}/_{2}$-1 hr	Inf end	Unknown
Duration	Unknown	Unknown	Unknown

INTERACTIONS
Individual drugs
Amphotericin B, CISplatin, vancomycin: increased nephrotoxicity
⚠ **Erythromycin IV: fatal dysrhythmias**
Haloperidol, chloroquine, droperidol, pentamidine; arsenic trioxide, levomethadyl: increased QT prolongation
Radiation: bone marrow suppression

Drug classifications
Aminoglycosides NSAIDs: increased nephrotoxicity
Antineoplastics: increased bone marrow depression
Class IA/III antidysrhythmics, some phenothiazines, β-agonists, local anesthetics, tricyclics, CYP3A4 inhibitors (amiodarone, clarithromycin, erythromycin, telithromycin, troleandomycin), CYP3A4 substrates (methadone, pimozide, QUEtiapine, quiNIDine, risperidone, ziprasidone): increased QT prolongation

Drug/lab test
Decrease: WBC, platelets, Hbg, Hct
Increase: BUN, creatinine

NURSING CONSIDERATIONS
Assessment
⚠ **Assess any patient with compromised renal system: product is excreted slowly in poor renal system function; toxicity may occur rapidly**
• **QT prolongation:** ECG for QT prolongation, ejection fraction; assess for chest pain, palpitations, dyspnea
• **Assess patient for infection,** including increased temp, thick sputum, WBC >10,000/mm³; monitor these signs of infection throughout treatment; obtain C&S before beginning therapy; treatment may begin after culture is obtained
• Assess respiratory system including rate, rhythm, bilateral lung sounds, SOB, wheezing, dyspnea
• Monitor ECG for cardiac dysrhythmias; ECG and pulse should be checked frequently during treatment, since cardiotoxicity can occur
• Assess for hypoglycemia including nausea, tremors, anxiety, chills, diaphoresis, headache, hunger, cold, pale skin; this side effect can last for several mo after treatment is completed
• Monitor for hyperglycemia including flushed, dry skin, acetone breath, thirst, anorexia, drowsiness, polyuria; this side effect can last for several mo after treatment is completed
• Monitor renal function tests including BUN, urinalysis, creatinine; obtain at baseline and frequently during treatment; nephrotoxicity may occur; check I&O, report hematuria, oliguria
• Monitor blood studies including blood glucose, CBC, platelets; blood glucose fluctuations are common; anemia, leukopenia, thrombocytopenia can occur
• Monitor liver function studies including AST, ALT, alkaline phosphatase, bilirubin before

P

beginning treatment and every 3 days during therapy
• Monitor calcium and magnesium before beginning treatment and every 3 days during therapy; hypocalcemia may occur

Nursing diagnoses
• Infection, risk for (uses)
• Knowledge, deficient (teaching)

Patient/family education
• Teach patient to report sore throat, fever, fatigue; could indicate superinfection
• Advise patient not to drink alcohol or take aspirin, since gastric bleeding may occur
• Teach patient to make position changes slowly to prevent orthostatic hypotension
• Advise patient to maintain adequate fluid intake

Evaluation
Positive therapeutic outcome
• Decreased signs and symptoms of protozoan infections
• Decreased signs and symptoms of *P. jiroveci* pneumonia in HIV infections

---

⚠ HIGH ALERT

pentazocine (Rx)
(pen-taz′oh-seen)
Talwin, Talwin NX
Func. class.: Opiate analgesic
Chem. class.: Synthetic benzomorphan (agonist/antagonist)
Pregnancy category C
Controlled substance schedule IV

ACTION: Inhibits ascending pain pathways in limbic system, thalamus, midbrain, hypothalamus by binding to opiate receptor sites, altering pain perception and response

Therapeutic outcome: Relief of pain

USES: Moderate to severe pain

CONTRAINDICATIONS:
Hypersensitivity to this product or sulfites, addiction (opioid)

Precautions: Pregnancy **C**, breastfeeding, child <18 yr, addictive personality, increased ICP, MI (acute), severe heart disease, respiratory depression, renal/hepatic disease, seizure disorder, head trauma, bowel impaction, geriatric patients

DOSAGE AND ROUTES
Adult: PO 50-100 mg q3-4hr prn, max 600 mg/day; **IV/IM/SUBCUT** 30 mg q3-4hr prn, max 360 mg/day

Labor
Adult: IM 30 mg; **IV** 20 mg q2-3hr when contractions are regular

Renal dose
Adult: CCr 10-50 ml/min reduce dose by 25%; CCr <10 ml/min reduce dose by 50%

Available forms: Inj 30 mg/ml; tabs 50 mg

Implementation
• Give by inj (IM, **IV**), only when resuscitative equipment available; give slowly to prevent rigidity
• Store in light-resistant area at room temperature
PO route
• Tabs made in the United States contain naloxone 0.5 mg to prevent abuse if the PO preparation is used **IV**
• Give without regard to food
• PO tabs are intended for PO, lethal reactions have occurred from giving tabs by inj
IM/SUBCUT route
• Give IM inj deeply in large muscle mass; rotate inj sites; repeated SUBCUT inj may cause necrosis

Direct IV route
• Give after diluting 5 mg/ml of sterile water for inj; give 5 mg or less over 1 min

Syringe compatibilities: Atropine, benzquinamide, butorphanol, chlorproMAZINE, cimetidine, dimenhyDRINATE, diphenhydrAMINE, droperidol, fentaNYL, HYDROmorphone, hydrOXYzine, meperidine, metoclopramide, morphine, perphenazine, prochlorperazine, promazine, promethazine, propiomazine, ranitidine, scopolamine

Syringe incompatibilities: Glycopyrrolate, heparin, PENTobarbital, other barbiturates

Y-site compatibilities: Heparin, hydrocortisone, potassium chloride, vit B/C

Y-site incompatibilities: Nafcillin

Additive incompatibilities: Aminophylline, amobarbital, PENTobarbital, PHENobarbital, secobarbital, sodium bicarbonate

ADVERSE EFFECTS
CNS: *Drowsiness, dizziness, confusion, headache, sedation, euphoria, hallucinations,* dreaming, insomnia, light-headedness

---

⚠ Nurse Alert

CV: Palpitations, bradycardia, change in B/P, tachycardia, increased B/P (high doses), hypotension, syncope, flushing
EENT: Tinnitus, blurred vision, miosis, diplopia
GI: *Nausea,* vomiting, anorexia, constipation, cramps, dry mouth
GU: Urinary retention, increased urinary output, dysuria
HEMA: Eosinophilia, decreased WBC
INTEG: *Rash,* urticaria, bruising, flushing, diaphoresis, pruritus, severe irritation at inj sites, **Stevens-Johnson syndrome**
RESP: **Respiratory depression**

Pharmacokinetics

Absorption	Well absorbed (PO, SUBCUT, IM); completely absorbed (**IV**)
Distribution	Widely distributed; crosses placenta
Metabolism	Liver, extensively
Excretion	Kidneys, small amounts (unchanged)
Half-life	2-3 hr

Pharmacodynamics

	PO	SUB-CUT/IM	IV
Onset	15-30 min	15-30 min	Rapid
Peak	1-3 hr	1-2 hr	15 min
Duration	3 hr	2-4 hr	1 hr

INTERACTIONS

Individual drugs
Alcohol: increased effects

Drug classifications
Antipsychotics, CNS depressants, sedative-hypnotics, skeletal muscle relaxants: increased effects
MAOIs: use cautiously; results are unpredictable
Opiates: decreased effects

Drug/lab test
Increased: amylase

NURSING CONSIDERATIONS

Assessment
• **Assess pain:** location, intensity, type of pain before, after treatment
• Assess bowel status: constipation; may need stimulant laxative/stool softener

• Monitor VS after parenteral route; note muscle rigidity, product history, liver, kidney function tests, respiratory dysfunction: respiratory depression, character, rate, rhythm; notify prescriber if respirations <10/min
• Monitor CNS changes: dizziness, drowsiness, hallucinations, euphoria, LOC, pupil reaction
• **Monitor allergic reactions:** rash, urticaria
• Assess for withdrawal symptoms in opiate-dependent patients

Nursing diagnoses
• Breathing pattern, ineffective (adverse reactions)
• Knowledge, deficient (teaching)
• Pain, acute (uses)

Patient/family education
• Teach patient to report any symptoms of CNS changes, allergic reactions
• Advise patients to avoid CNS depressants: alcohol, sedative-hypnotics for at least 24 hr after taking this product
• Discuss with patient that dizziness, drowsiness, and confusion are common; to avoid getting up without assistance
• Discuss in detail all aspects of the product
• Instruct patient to change position slowly to prevent orthostatic hypotension
• Teach patient to turn, cough, breathe deeply after surgery to prevent atelectasis
• Teach patient to avoid operating machinery if drowsiness occurs

Evaluation
Positive therapeutic outcome
• Relief of pain

TREATMENT OF OVERDOSE:
Naloxone (Narcan) 0.2-0.8 mg **IV**, O$_2$, **IV** fluids, vasopressors

---

pentoxifylline (Rx)
(pen-tox-if'i-lin)
Apo-Pentoxifylline �це, ratio-**Pentoxifylline** ✦, **Trental**
Func. class.: Hemorheologic agent
Chem. class.: Dimethylxanthine derivative
Pregnancy category C

ACTION: Decreases blood viscosity, stimulates prostacyclin formation, increases blood flow by increasing flexibility of RBCs; decreases RBC hyperaggregation; reduces platelet aggregation, decreases fibrinogen concentration

Therapeutic outcome: Decreased claudication and improved blood flow

---

USES: Intermittent claudication related to chronic occlusive vascular disease

Unlabeled uses: Diabetic neuropathies, sickle cell anemia

CONTRAINDICATIONS:
Hypersensitivity to this product or xanthines, retinal/cerebral hemorrhage

Precautions: Pregnancy **C**, breastfeeding, children, angina pectoris, impaired renal function, recent surgery, peptic ulcer, cardiac/hepatic disease, bleeding disorders

DOSAGE AND ROUTES
Adult: PO 400 mg tid with meals, may decrease to bid if side effects occur, must be taken for ≥8 wk for maximal effect

Available forms: Cont rel tabs 400 mg; ext rel tabs 400 mg

Implementation
• Do not break, crush, or chew cont rel or ext rel tab
• Give with meals to prevent GI upset

ADVERSE EFFECTS
CNS: *Headache,* anxiety, *tremors,* confusion, *dizziness*
GI: *Dyspepsia, nausea, vomiting*

Pharmacokinetics	
Absorption	Well absorbed
Distribution	Unknown
Metabolism	Liver, degradation
Excretion	Kidneys
Half-life	$1/2$-1 hr

Pharmacodynamics	
Onset	Unknown
Peak	2-4 hr
Duration	Unknown

INTERACTIONS
Individual drugs
Abciximab, clopidogrel, eptifibatide, ticlopidine, tirofiban, warfarin: increased bleeding risk
Cimetidine, ciprofloxacin: increased pentoxifylline level
Theophylline: increased theophylline level

Drug classifications
Antihypertensives, nitrates: increased hypotension
Thrombin inhibitors: increased bleeding risk

NURSING CONSIDERATIONS
Assessment
• Monitor B/P, respirations in patient taking antihypertensives
• Assess for intermittent claudication baseline, during treatment
• Monitor blood tests: pro-time, Hgb, Hct in patients at risk for hemorrhage

Nursing diagnoses
• Activity intolerance (uses)
• Knowledge, deficient (teaching)
• Noncompliance (teaching)
• Pain, chronic (uses)

Patient/family education
• Teach patient that therapeutic response may take 2-4 wk
• Instruct patient to observe feet for arterial insufficiency
• Instruct patient to use cotton socks, well-fitted shoes; not to go barefoot
• Advise patient to watch for bleeding, bruises, petechiae, epistaxis
• Advise that there are many drug, herb interactions

Evaluation
Positive therapeutic outcome
• Decreased pain, cramping
• Increased ambulation

perindopril (Rx)
(per-in-doe-pril)
Aceon, Coversye ♣
Func. class.: Antihypertensive
Chem. class.: Angiotensin-converting enzyme (ACE) inhibitor
Pregnancy category D

ACTION: Selectively suppresses renin-angiotensin-aldosterone system; inhibits ACE; prevents conversion of angiotensin I to angiotensin II, resulting in dilatation of arterial and venous vessels

Therapeutic outcome: Decreased B/P in hypertension

USES: Hypertension alone or in combination, stable artery disease

CONTRAINDICATIONS:
Hypersensitivity, history of angioedema

BLACK BOX WARNING: Pregnancy **D**

Precautions: Breastfeeding, renal disease, hyperkalemia, hepatic failure, dehydration, bilateral renal artery stenosis, cough, angioedema, severe CHF

DOSAGE AND ROUTES

Hypertension
Adult: PO 4 mg/day, may increase or decrease to desired response; range 4-8 mg/day may give in 2 divided doses or as a single dose; max 16 mg/day

Patients taking diuretics
Adult: PO 2-4 mg/day in 1-2 divided doses, range 4-8 mg/day

Stable CAD
Adult: PO 4 mg/day × 2 wk, then increase as tolerated to 8 mg/day

Renal dose
Adult: PO CCr 16-29 ml/min, 2 mg every other day; CCr 30-59 ml/min 2 mg/day

Available forms: Tabs, scored 2, 4, 8 mg

Implementation
• Store in airtight container at 86° F (30° C) or less
• Severe hypotension may occur after 1st dose of this medication; decreased hypotension may be prevented by reducing or discontinuing diuretic therapy 3 days before beginning perindopril therapy
• Give by IV inf of 0.9% NaCl (as ordered) to expand fluid volume if severe hypotension occurs

ADVERSE EFFECTS

CNS: *Insomnia, dizziness,* paresthesias, headache, fatigue, anxiety, depression
CV: *Hypotension,* chest pain, tachycardia, dysrhythmias, syncope
EENT: *Tinnitus,* visual changes, sore throat, double vision, dry burning eyes
GI: Nausea, vomiting, colitis, cramps, diarrhea, constipation, flatulence, dry mouth, loss of taste
GU: Proteinuria, renal failure, increased frequency of polyuria or oliguria
HEMA: Agranulocytosis, neutropenia
INTEG: Rash, purpura, alopecia, hyperhidrosis
META: Hyperkalemia
RESP: Dyspnea, dry cough, crackles
SYST: Angioedema

Pharmacokinetics

Absorption	Well absorbed
Distribution	Unknown
Metabolism	Liver
Excretion	Kidneys
Half-life	Unknown

Pharmacodynamics
Unknown

INTERACTIONS

Individual drugs
Allopurinol: increased hypersensitivity
Lithium: increased serum levels

Drug classifications
Antihypertensives, diuretics: increased hypotension
Antihypertensives, neuromuscular blocking agents: increased effects
Diuretics (potassium-sparing), potassium supplements, salt substitutes: hyperkalemia
NSAIDs: decreased effects
NSAIDs, salicylates: decreased antihypertensive effect

Drug/herb
Hawthorn: increased antihypertensive effect
Ephedra: decreased antihypertensive effect

Drug/lab test
Interference: glucose/insulin tolerance tests

NURSING CONSIDERATIONS

Assessment
• **Hypertension:** monitor B/P, orthostatic hypotension, syncope; if changes occur dosage change may be required
• Monitor blood studies: neutrophils, decreased platelets
• **CHF:** Check for edema in feet, legs daily
• Monitor renal studies: protein, BUN, creatinine; increased levels may indicate nephrotic syndrome and renal failure
• Monitor renal symptoms: polyuria, oliguria, frequency, dysuria
• Establish baselines in renal, liver function tests before therapy begins
• Check potassium levels throughout treatment, although hyperkalemia rarely occurs
• **Assess for allergic reactions:** rash, fever, pruritus, urticaria; product should be discontinued if antihistamines fail to help; angioedema: facial swelling, urticaria, product should be discontinued, may be more common in African-Americans

Adverse effects: *italics* = common; **bold** = life-threatening

Nursing diagnoses
• Cardiac output, decreased (uses)
• Injury, risk for (adverse reactions)
• Knowledge, deficient (teaching)
• Noncompliance (teaching)

Patient/family education
• Advise patient not to discontinue product abruptly; advise patient to tell all persons associated with health care
• Teach patient not to use OTC products (cough, cold, allergy medications) unless directed by physician; serious side effects can occur; xanthines, such as coffee, tea, chocolate, cola can prevent action of product
• Instruct patient on the importance of complying with dosage schedule, even if feeling better; to continue with medical regimen to decrease B/P: exercise, cessation of smoking, decreasing stress, diet modifications
• Emphasize the need to rise slowly to sitting or standing position to minimize orthostatic hypotension; not to exercise in hot weather, which can cause increased hypotension
• Advise patient to notify prescriber of mouth sores, sore throat, fever, swelling of hands or feet, irregular heartbeat, chest pain, coughing, shortness of breath
• Caution patient to report excessive perspiration, dehydration, vomiting, diarrhea; may lead to fall in B/P
• Caution patient that product may cause dizziness, fainting, light-headedness; may occur during 1st few days of therapy; to avoid activities that may be hazardous
• Teach patient how to take B/P, normal readings for age-group

> **BLACK BOX WARNING:** Notify prescriber if pregnancy is planned or suspected, pregnancy category **D**

Evaluation
Positive therapeutic outcome
• Decreased B/P in hypertension

TREATMENT OF OVERDOSE:
Lavage, **IV** atropine for bradycardia, **IV** theophylline for bronchospasm, digoxin, O_2; diuretic for cardiac failure, hemodialysis

---

phenazopyridine (Rx, OTC)
(fen-az-o-peer′i-deen)
AZO-Gesic, AZO-Standard, Baridium, Geridium, Phenazo ✽, Prodium, Pyridiate, Pyridium, Urodine, Urogesic, UTI-Relief
Func. class.: Nonopioid analgesic, urinary
Chem. class.: Azodye
Pregnancy category B

ACTION: Exerts analgesic, anesthetic action on the urinary tract mucosa

Therapeutic outcome: Decreased pain, burning when urinating

USES: Urinary tract irritation, infection (for symptoms only of pain, burning, itching) used with urinary antiinfectives

CONTRAINDICATIONS:
Hypersensitivity, renal insufficiency, hepatic disease, uremia

Precautions: Pregnancy **B,** breastfeeding, children <12 yr, geriatric patient, contact lens use

DOSAGE AND ROUTES
Adult: PO 200 mg tid × 2 days or less when used with antibacterial for UTI
Child 6-12 yr: PO 4 mg/kg tid × 2 days

Renal dose
Adult: PO CCr 50-80 ml/min give dose 8-16 hr; CCr <50 ml/min do not use

Available forms: Tabs 95, 97.2, 100, 200 mg

Implementation
• Give to patient crushed or whole; chew tab should be chewed
• Give with food or milk to decrease gastric symptoms

ADVERSE EFFECTS
CNS: Headache, **aseptic meningitis**
GI: *Nausea,* **hepatic toxicity**
GU: Renal toxicity, *orange-red urine*
HEMA: Methemoglobinemia
INTEG: Rash, pruritus, skin pigmentation
SYST: Anaphylaxis

Pharmacokinetics

Absorption	Well absorbed
Distribution	Unknown; crosses placenta
Metabolism	Unknown
Excretion	Kidneys, unchanged
Half-life	Unknown

Pharmacodynamics

Onset	Unknown
Peak	5-6 hr
Duration	8 hr

INTERACTIONS

Drug/lab test
Interference: urinalysis

NURSING CONSIDERATIONS

Assessment
• Assess urinary status: burning, pain, itching, urgency, frequency, hematuria before, during, after completion of product therapy
• Monitor liver function tests: AST, ALT, bilirubin if patient is on long-term therapy
⚠ **Assess for hepatotoxicity: dark urine, clay-colored stools, yellowing of skin and sclera, itching, abdominal pain, fever, diarrhea if patient is on long-term therapy**
• **Assess for allergic reactions:** rash, urticaria; if these occur, product may have to be discontinued

Nursing diagnoses
• Knowledge, deficient (teaching)
• Pain, acute (uses)
• Urinary elimination, impaired (uses)

Patient/family education
• Advise patient to report any symptoms of hepatotoxicity
• Caution patient not to exceed recommended dosage and to take with meals; to read label on other OTC products
• Teach patient not to discontinue after pain is relieved but continue to take concurrent prescribed antiinfective until finished
• Inform patient urine may turn red-orange; body fluids may stain clothing or contact lenses

Evaluation
Positive therapeutic outcome
• Decrease in pain, burning, itching when urinating

TREATMENT OF OVERDOSE:
Methylene blue 1-2 mg/kg **IV** or vit C 100-200 mg PO

⚠ HIGH ALERT

PHENobarbital (Rx)
(fee-noe-bar'bit-tal)
Luminal, PMS-PHENobarbital
Func. class.: Anticonvulsant
Chem. class.: Barbiturate
Pregnancy category D
Controlled substance schedule IV

Do not confuse:
PHENobarbital/PENTobarbital

ACTION: Decreases impulse transmission, increases seizure threshold at cerebral cortex level

Therapeutic outcome: Sedation, anticonvulsant, improved energy

USES: All forms of epilepsy, status epilepticus, febrile seizures in children, sedation, insomnia

Unlabeled uses: Hyperbilirubinemia, chronic cholestasis

CONTRAINDICATIONS:
Pregnancy **D**, breastfeeding, geriatric, hypersensitivity to barbiturates, porphyria, hepatic/respiratory disease, nephritis, hyperthyroidism, diabetes mellitus

Precautions: Anemia, renal disease

DOSAGE AND ROUTES
Seizures
Adult: PO 1-3 mg/kg/day in divided doses bid-tid or total dose at bedtime
Child 5-12 yr: PO 3-6 mg/kg/day in 1-2 divided doses
Child 1-5 yr: PO 6-8 mg/kg/day in 1-2 divided doses
Infant: PO 5-6 mg/kg/day in 1-2 divided doses

Neonate: PO 3-4 mg/kg/day as a single dose

Status epilepticus
Adult: IV INF 10 mg/kg; run no faster than 50 mg/min; may give up to 30 mg/kg
Child: IV INF 5-10 mg/kg; may repeat q10-15min up to 20 mg/kg; run no faster than 50 mg/min

Insomnia
Adult: PO/IM/SUBCUT 100-200 mg
Child (unlabeled): PO/IM/SUBCUT 3-5 mg/kg

P

Adverse effects: *italics* = common; **bold** = life-threatening

Sedation
Adult: PO 30-120 mg/day in 2-3 divided doses
Child: PO 3-5 mg/kg/day in 3 divided doses

Preoperative sedation
Adult: IM 100-200 mg 1-1$\frac{1}{2}$ hr before surgery
Child: PO/IM/IV 1-3 mg/kg 1-1$\frac{1}{2}$ hr before surgery

Available forms: Caps 15 mg; elix 20 mg/5 ml; tabs 15, 30, 32, 60, 65, 100 mg; inj 30, 60, 65, 130 mg/ml

Implementation
• Give medication after removal of cigarettes to prevent fires
• Give medication after trying conservative measures for insomnia

PO route
• Tab may be crushed and mixed with food if swallowing is difficult; also may be mixed with other fluids 30-60 min before bedtime for expected sleeplessness; on empty stomach for best absorption
• **Oral sol:** use undiluted or mixed with water or other fluids, use calibrated measuring device

IM route
• Give inj in deep muscle mass (gluteal) to minimize irritation to tissues
• Split inj of >5 ml into two, since irritation to tissues may occur

Direct IV route
• Use large vein to prevent extravasation; if extravasation occurs, use moist heat to the area and 5% procaine sol injected into area; give at 65 mg or less/min; titrate to patient's response

Y-site compatibilities: Doxapram, enalaprilat, fentaNYL, fosphenytoin, levofloxacin, meropenem, methadone, morphine, propofol, SUFentanil

Y-site incompatibilities: HYDROmorphone

ADVERSE EFFECTS
CNS: Paradoxical excitement (geriatric), drowsiness, lethargy, *hangover headache,* flushing, hallucinations, **coma**
GI: Nausea, vomiting, diarrhea, constipation
HEMA: Agranulocytosis, megaloblastic anemia, thrombocytopenia, thrombophlebitis
INTEG: Rash, urticaria, **Stevens-Johnson syndrome, angioedema,** local pain, swelling, necrosis, scaling eczema

Absorption	Slow (70%-90%) (PO/IM/**IV**)	
Distribution	Not known; crosses placenta	
Metabolism	Liver (75%)	
Excretion	Kidneys (25% unchanged)	
Half-life	2-6 days	

Pharmacodynamics

	PO	IM	IV
Onset	30-60 min	10-30 min	5 min
Peak	Unknown	Unknown	30 min
Duration	6-8 hr	4-6 hr	4-6 hr

INTERACTIONS
Individual drugs
Alcohol: increased CNS depression
Chloramphenicol, disulfiram: increased effects
Doxycycline, metroNIDAZOLE, quiNIDine, theophylline: decreased effectiveness
Furosemide: increased orthostatic hypotension
Valproic acid: increased sedation

Drug classifications
Anticoagulants, glucocorticoids, estrogens, hormonal contraceptives: decreased effectiveness
CNS depressants: increased effects
MAOIs, skeletal muscle relaxants (nondepolarizing), sulfonamides: increased effects

Drug/herb
Chamomile, eucalyptus, hops, kava, valerian: increased CNS depression
St. John's wort: decreased barbiturate effect

NURSING CONSIDERATIONS
Assessment
• Assess mental status: mood, sensorium, affect, memory (long, short), especially geriatric; if using as a hypnotic, assess sleep patterns during therapy; product suppresses REM sleep with dreaming
• Withdrawal insomnia may occur after short-term use; do not start using product again; insomnia improves in 1-3 nights; may experience increased dreaming
• Assess respiratory dysfunction: respiratory depression, character, rate, rhythm when using **IV;** hold product if respirations are <10/min or if pupils are dilated; also check VS q30min after parenteral route for 2 hr
• **Assess for barbiturate toxicity:** hypotension, pulmonary constriction, cold, clammy skin, cyanosis of lips, CNS depression, nausea,

vomiting, hallucinations, delirium, weakness, coma, pupillary constriction; mild symptoms occur in 8-12 hr without product
• **Assess for pain** in postop patients; pain threshold is lowered in patients taking this medication
• **Assess for blood dyscrasias:** fever, sore throat, bruising, rash, jaundice, epistaxis (long-term treatment only)
• **Assess seizure activity** including type, location, duration, character; provide seizure precaution

Nursing diagnoses
• Injury, risk for (adverse reactions)
• Knowledge, deficient (teaching)
• Sleep deprivation (uses)

Patient/family education
• Teach patient that hangover is common
• Instruct patient that product is indicated only for short-term treatment of insomnia and is probably ineffective after 2 wk
• Inform patient that physical dependency may result when used for extended time (45-90 days depending on dosage)
• Teach patient to avoid driving and other activities requiring alertness
• Caution patient to avoid alcohol ingestion and CNS depressants; serious CNS depression may result
• Instruct patient not to discontinue medication quickly after long-term use; may cause seizures; product should be tapered over 1 wk; take exactly as prescribed
• Emphasize the need to tell all prescribers that a barbiturate is being taken
• Teach the patient to make position changes slowly; orthostatic hypotension may occur
• Teach patient that response may take 4 days to 2 wk
• Instruct patient to notify prescriber immediately if bruising, bleeding occur, which may indicate blood dyscrasias

Evaluation
Positive therapeutic outcome
• Improved sleeping patterns
• Decreased seizure activity
• Sedative preoperatively

TREATMENT OF OVERDOSE:
Lavage, activated charcoal, warming blanket, VS, hemodialysis, alkalinize urine, give **IV** volume expanders, **IV** fluids

phentolamine (Rx)
(fen-tole′a-meen)
Func. class.: Antihypertensive
Chem. class.: α-Adrenergic blocker
Pregnancy category C

Do not confuse:
phentolamine/phentermine

ACTION: α-Adrenergic blocker; binds to α-adrenergic receptors, dilating peripheral blood vessels, lowering peripheral resistance, lowering blood pressure

Therapeutic outcome: Decreased B/P, reversal of vasoconstriction (dermal necrosis)

USES: Hypertension; pheochromocytoma; prevention, treatment of dermal necrosis after extravasation of norepinephrine, DOPamine, EPINEPHrine

Unlabeled uses: Impotence, hypertensive crisis due to MAOIs

CONTRAINDICATIONS:
Hypersensitivity, MI, coronary insufficiency, angina

Precautions: Pregnancy **C,** breastfeeding, dysrhythmia

DOSAGE AND ROUTES

Treatment of hypertensive episodes in pheochromocytoma
Adult: IV/IM 5 mg; repeat if necessary
Child: IV 0.05-0.1 mg/kg; repeat if necessary, max 5 mg

Diagnosis of pheochromocytoma
Adult: IV 2.5 mg; if negative, repeat with 5 mg **IV**
Child: IV 0.05 mg/kg; if negative, repeat with 0.1 mg/kg **IV**

Treatment of necrosis
Adult: 5-10 mg/10 ml 0.9% NaCl injected into area of extravasation within 12 hr
Child: 0.1-0.2 mg/kg; max 5 mg

Prevention of dermal necrosis
Adult: **IV** 10 mg/L of norepinephrine-containing sol
Child: **IV** 0.1-0.2 mg/kg, max 5 mg

Available forms: Inj 5 mg/ml

Implementation
• Give with vasopressor nearby

IV route
• Give by direct **IV** after diluting 5 mg/1 ml of sterile water for inj or 0.9% NaCl; give 5 mg or less/min
• Give by cont inf by further diluting 5-10 mg/500 ml of D$_5$W, titrate to patient response
• Add 10 mg/L to norepinephrine in **IV** sol for prevention of dermal necrosis

Syringe compatibilities: Papaverine

Y-site compatibilities: Amiodarone

Additive compatibilities: DOBUTamine, verapamil

ADVERSE EFFECTS
CNS: *Dizziness,* flushing, weakness, **cerebro-vascular spasm**
CV: *Hypotension,* **tachycardia,** *angina,* **dysrhythmias, MI**
EENT: Nasal congestion
GI: *Dry mouth, nausea, vomiting, diarrhea, abdominal pain*

Pharmacokinetics

Absorption	Well absorbed (IM); completely absorbed (**IV**)
Distribution	Unknown
Metabolism	Unknown
Excretion	Kidneys, unchanged (10%)
Half-life	Unknown

Pharmacodynamics

	IM	IV
Onset	Unknown	Rapid
Peak	20 min	2 min
Duration	$^1/_2$-1 hr	$^1/_2$ hr

INTERACTIONS

Individual drugs
EPINEPHrine: increased effects of EPINEPHrine

Drug classifications
Antihypertensives: increased effects of antihypertensives

NURSING CONSIDERATIONS

Assessment
• Monitor B/P, orthostatic hypotension, syncope, pulse, ECG until stable

Nursing diagnoses
• Cardiac output, decreased (uses)
• Injury, risk for (adverse reactions)
• Knowledge, deficient (teaching)
• Noncompliance (teaching)

Patient/family education
• Caution patient not to discontinue product abruptly
• Teach patient not to use OTC products (cough, cold, allergy) unless directed by prescriber
• Teach patient the importance of complying with dosage schedule, even if feeling better
• Emphasize the need to rise slowly to sitting or standing position to minimize orthostatic hypotension
• Teach patient to notify prescriber of mouth sores, sore throat, fever, swelling of hands or feet, irregular heartbeat, chest pain
• Caution patient to report excessive perspiration, dehydration, vomiting, diarrhea; may lead to fall in B/P
• Caution patient that product may cause dizziness, fainting, light-headedness; may occur during 1st few days of therapy
• Teach patient how to take B/P, teach normal readings for age group

Evaluation
Positive therapeutic outcome
• Decreased B/P in hypertension
• Resolution of impotence
• Prevention of dermal necrosis

TREATMENT OF OVERDOSE:
Administer norepinephrine; discontinue product

---

phenylephrine (Rx)
(fen-ill-ef′rin)
Neo-Synephrine
Func. class.: Adrenergic, direct acting
Chem. class.: Direct sympathomimetic amine (α-agonist)
Pregnancy category C

ACTION: Powerful and selective receptor agonist causing contraction of blood vessels, vasoconstriction of eye arterioles; decreases eye engorgement by stimulation of α-adrenergic receptors

Therapeutic outcome: Increased B/P, decreased nasal congestion, decreased eye irritation

USES: Hypotension, paroxysmal supraventricular tachycardia, shock, B/P maintenance during spinal anesthesia, topical ocular vasoconstrictor in uveitis, open-angle glaucoma; preoperatively, diagnostic procedures, refraction without cycloplegia; nasal congestion

CONTRAINDICATIONS:
Hypersensitivity, closed-angle glaucoma, ventricular fibrillation, tachydysrhythmias, pheochromocytoma, severe hypertension

Precautions: Pregnancy **C**, breastfeeding, geriatric, hyperthyroidism, severe arteriosclerosis, arterial embolism, peripheral vascular disease, bradycardia, myocardial disease, partial heart block

BLACK BOX WARNING: Cardiac disease, extravasation

DOSAGE AND ROUTES
Hypotension
Adult: SUBCUT/IM 2-5 mg; may repeat q10-15min if needed, do not exceed initial dose; **IV** 0.1-0.5 mg; may repeat q10-15min if needed, do not exceed initial dose
Child: IM/SUBCUT 0.1 mg/kg/dose q1-2hr prn

Supraventricular tachycardia
Adult: **IV** max 0.5 mg given rapidly, max single dose 1 mg

Shock
Adult: **IV** INF 10 mg/500 ml of D$_5$W given 100-180 mcg/min (if 20 gtt/ml device is used), then maintenance of 40-60 mcg/min (if 20 gtt/ml device is used); use inf pump
Child: **IV** BOL 5-20 mcg/kg/dose q10-15min; **IV** INF 0.1-0.5 mg/kg/min

Available forms: Inj 1% (10 mg/ml)

Implementation
IV route
- Give plasma expanders for hypovolemia
- Give **IV** after diluting 1 mg/9 ml of sterile water for inj; give dose over 30-60 sec; may be diluted 10 mg/500 ml of D$_5$W or 0.9% NaCl; titrate to patient's response; low normal B/P; check for extravasation; check site for infiltration; use inf pump
- Store reconstituted sol in refrigerator for no longer than 24 hr
- Do not use discolored sol

Y-site compatibilities: Famotidine, haloperidol, inamrinone, zidovudine

Additive compatibilities: Chloramphenicol, DOBUTamine, lidocaine, potassium chloride, sodium bicarbonate

ADVERSE EFFECTS
CNS: *Headache, dizziness, anxiety, tremor, insomnia*

CV: Reflex bradycardia, **dysrhythmias,** *hypertension,* **tachycardia,** palpitations, ectopic beats, angina
GI: *Nausea, vomiting*
INTEG: Necrosis, tissue sloughing with extravasation, **gangrene**
MISC: **Anaphylaxis**

Pharmacokinetics
Absorption	Well absorbed (IM); completely absorbed (**IV**); minimally absorbed (nasal, ophth)
Distribution	Unknown
Metabolism	Liver
Excretion	Unknown
Half-life	Unknown

Pharmacodynamics
	SUBCUT/IM	IV
Onset	15 min	Rapid
Peak	Unknown	Unknown
Duration	45-60 min	20-30 min

INTERACTIONS
Individual drugs
Digoxin: increased dysrhythmias

Drug classifications
α-Blockers: decreased phenylephrine action
Antidepressants (tricyclics), β-adrenergic blockers, H$_1$ antihistamines: increased pressor effect
General anesthetics: increased dysrhythmias
MAOIs: do not use within 2 wk, hypertensive crisis may result
Oxytocics: increased B/P

NURSING CONSIDERATIONS
Assessment
- Monitor I&O ratio; notify prescriber if output <30 ml/hr
- Monitor ECG during administration continuously; if B/P increases, product is decreased
- Monitor B/P and pulse q5min after parenteral route; CVP or PWP during inf if possible
- Assess for paresthesias and coldness of extremities; peripheral blood flow may decrease

Nursing diagnoses
- Cardiac output, decreased (uses)
- Knowledge, deficient (teaching)
- Tissue perfusion, ineffective (uses)

Patient/family education
- Inform patient of reason for product administration and expected result

- Advise patient to report pain at inf site immediately
- Instruct patient to report change in vision, blurring, loss of sight; breathing trouble, sweating, flushing

Evaluation
Positive therapeutic outcome
- Increased B/P with stabilization

phenylephrine nasal agent
See Appendix B

phenylephrine ophthalmic
See Appendix B

phenytoin (Rx)
(fen′i-toyn)
Dilantin, Phenytek
Func. class.: Anticonvulsant/
antidysrhythmic (class IB)
Chem. class.: Hydantoin
Pregnancy category D

ACTION: Inhibits spread of seizure activity in motor cortex by altering ion transport; increases AV conduction to decrease dysrhythmias

Therapeutic outcome: Decreased seizures, absence of dysrhythmias

USES: Generalized tonic-clonic seizures, status epilepticus, nonepileptic seizures associated with Reye's syndrome or after head trauma, Bell's palsy, complex/partial seizures

CONTRAINDICATIONS:
Pregnancy **D**, hypersensitivity, psychiatric condition, bradycardia, SA and AV block, Stokes-Adams syndrome, hepatic failure, acute intermittent porphyria

Precautions: Geriatric, allergies, renal/hepatic disease, petit mal seizures, hypotension, myocardial insufficiency, Asian patients positive for HLA-B 1502

DOSAGE AND ROUTES
Seizures
Adult: PO 15-20 mg/kg (EXT REL) in 3-4 divided doses given q2hr or 400 mg, then 300 mg q2hr × 2 doses, maintenance 4-7 mg/kg/day; max 600 mg/day; **IV** 15-20 mg/kg, max 25-50 mg/min then 100 mg q6-8hr
Child: PO 5 mg/kg/day in 2-3 divided doses, maintenance 4-8 mg/kg/day in 2-3 divided

doses, max 300 mg/day; **IV** 15-20 mg/kg at 1-3 mg/kg/min

Status epilepticus
Adult: **IV** 15-20 mg/kg, max 25-50 mg/min; may give 100 mg q6-8hr thereafter
Child: **IV** 15-20 mg/kg, max in divided doses 1-3 mg/kg/min

Ventricular dysrhythmias
Adult: PO loading dose 1 g divided over 24 hr, then 500 mg/day × 2 days; **IV** 250 mg given over 5 min until dysrhythmias subside or 1 g is given, or 100 mg q15min until dysrhythmias subside or 1 g is given
Child: PO 3-8 mg/kg or 250 mg/m²/day as single dose or divided in 2 doses; **IV** 3-8 mg/kg given over several min, or 250 mg/m²/day as single dose or divided in 2 doses

Renal dose
Adult: Do not use loading dose if CCr <10 ml/min or hepatic failure

Available forms: Susp 25 mg/5 ml; chew tabs 50 mg; inj 50 mg/ml; ext rel caps 100, 200, 300 mg; prompt rel caps 100 mg

Implementation
PO route
- Do not interchange chewable product with caps, not equivalent; only ext rel caps are to be used for once-a-day dosing
- Give with meals to decrease GI upset
- Chew tab can be crushed or chewed; cap can be opened and mixed with foods or fluids; cap and tab are not interchangeable, only ext rel cap is to be used for once a day dosing
- Do not take antacids or antidiarrheals within 2-3 hr of taking phenytoin
- **Oral suspension:** shake well before each dose G tube/NG tube; dilute susp prior to administration; flush tube with 20 ml water after dose
- Allow 7-10 days between dosage changes
- Divided PO doses with or after meals to decrease adverse effects
- 2 hr before or after antacid, enteral feeding
- Shake oral susp well; use measuring device for correct dose

Direct IV route
- Give undiluted at ≤50 mg/min (adult) 1-3 mg/kg/min (neonates)

Intermittent IV INF route
- Dilute dose in NS to ≤6.7 mg/ml, complete inf within 1 hr of preparation, use 0.22 or 0.45 micron in-line particulate final filter between **IV** catheter and tubing, flush the **IV** line or catheter with NS before and after use, give at ≤50 mg/min (adult), 0.5-1 mg/kg/min (child, infant, neonate)

Additive compatibilities: Bleomycin, verapamil

Y-site compatibilities: Esmolol, famotidine, fluconazole, foscarnet, tacrolimus

Y-site incompatibilities: Enalaprilat, potassium chloride, vit B/C

ADVERSE EFFECTS

CNS: Drowsiness, dizziness, insomnia, paresthesias, depression, **suicidal tendencies,** aggression, headache, confusion, slurred speech, peripheral neuropathy

CV: Hypotension, **ventricular fibrillation**

EENT: Nystagmus, diplopia, blurred vision

ENDO: Diabetes insipidus

GI: Nausea, vomiting, constipation, anorexia, weight loss, **hepatitis,** jaundice, gingival hyperplasia

GU: Nephritis, urine discoloration

HEMA: Agranulocytosis, leukopenia, aplastic anemia, thrombocytopenia, megaloblastic anemia

INTEG: Rash, **lupus erythematosus, Stevens-Johnson syndrome,** hirsutism, **toxic epidermal necrolysis**

SYST: Hypocalcemia, **purple glove syndrome (IV)**

Pharmacokinetics

Absorption	Slowly absorbed from GI tract; erratic (IM)
Distribution	Crosses placenta, 90%-95% protein binding
Metabolism	Liver, extensively
Excretion	Kidneys, minimally; enters breast milk
Half-life	7-42 hr, dose dependent

Pharmacodynamics

	PO	PO-EXT REL	IM	IV
Onset	2-24 hr	2-24 hr	Erratic	1-2 hr
Peak	$1^{1}/_{2}$-3 hr	4-12 hr	Erratic	Unknown
Duration	6-12 hr	12-36 hr	12-24 hr	12-24 hr

INTERACTIONS

Individual drugs

Alcohol (chronic use), carBAMazepine, folic acid, rifampin: decreased effects of phenytoin

Chloramphenicol, cimetidine, cycloSERINE, disulfiram, alcohol, amiodarone, FLUoxetine, gabapentin, methylphenidate, felbamate, traZODone, diazepam, valproate: increased phenytoin effect

Drug classifications

Antacids, barbiturates: decreased effect of phenytoin

Antidepressants (tricyclics), benzodiazepines, sulfonamides, H_2 antagonists, azole antifungals, estrogens, succinimides, phenothiazines, salicylates: increased phenytoin level

Drug/food

Enteral tube feeding: may decrease absorption of oral product, do not use enteral feedings 2 hr before and after dose

Drug/lab test

Increased: glucose, alkaline phosphatase, BSP

Decreased: dexamethasone, metyrapone test serum, urinary steroids

NURSING CONSIDERATIONS

Assessment

• Assess product level: toxic level 30-50 mcg/ml; therapeutic level 7.5-20 mcg/ml, wait ≥1 wk to determine level

A Assess mental status: mood, sensorium, affect, memory (long, short), especially geriatric; suicidal thoughts/behaviors

A Phenytoin hypersensitivity syndrome: assess 3-12 wk after start of treatment: rash, temp, lymphadenopathy; may cause hepatotoxicity, renal failure, rhabdomyolysis

A Serious skin disorders: assess for beginning rash that may lead to Stevens-Johnson syndrome or toxic epidermal necrolysis; phenytoin should not be used again, may occur more often in Asian patients with HLA-B 1502

A Purple glove syndrome: with IV use

• Phenytoin level: toxic level 30-50 mcg/ml, therapeutic level: 7.5-20 mcg/ml, wait ≥1 wk to draw levels

• **Seizures:** assess for duration, type, intensity precipitating factors, obtain EEG periodically

• Blood studies: CBC, platelets q2wk until stabilized, then q mo × 12, then q3mo; discontinue product if neutrophils <1600/mm^3; renal function: albumin conc; folic acid levels

• **Blood dyscrasias:** assess fever, sore throat, bruising, rash, jaundice, epistaxis (long-term treatment only)

• Assess renal studies: urinalysis, BUN, urine creatinine

• Monitor blood studies: RBC, Hct, Hgb, reticulocyte counts weekly for 4 wk then monthly; also check thyroid function tests, serum calcium
• Monitor liver function tests for renal failure: ALT, AST, bilirubin, creatinine
• Assess for signs of physical withdrawal if medication suddenly discontinued
• Assess eye problems: need for ophth exam before, during, after treatment (slit lamp, funduscopy, tonometry)
• **Monitor for toxicity:** bone marrow depression, nausea, vomiting, ataxia, diplopia, CV collapse, slurred speech, confusion

Nursing diagnoses
• Injury, risk for (uses, adverse reactions)
• Knowledge, deficient (teaching)
• Noncompliance (teaching)

Patient/family education
• Teach patient to carry/wear emergency ID stating name, products taken, condition, prescriber's name and phone number
• Advise patient to avoid driving and other activities that require alertness until product response is known; dizziness, drowsiness can occur
• Advise patient to avoid alcohol ingestion and CNS depressants unless approved by prescriber; increased sedation may occur
• Teach patient not to discontinue medication quickly after long-term use; taper off over several wk
• Advise patient that urine may turn pink, red, or brown
• Caution patient to avoid antacids or antidiarrheals within 2-3 hr of taking phenytoin
• Instruct patient in proper oral hygiene to prevent gingival hyperplasia; to visit dentist routinely
• Teach patient to use nonhormonal contraception, to notify prescriber if pregnancy is planned or suspected, pregnancy **D**
• Teach patient to notify prescriber of unusual bleeding, bruising, petechiae (bleeding), clay-colored stools, abdominal pain, dark urine, yellowing of skin/eyes (hepatotoxicity); slurred speech, headache, drowsiness

Evaluation
Positive therapeutic outcome
• Decreased seizure activity
• Decreased dysrhythmias
• Relief of pain

physostigmine ophthalmic
See Appendix B

phytonadione (vit K₁) (Rx)
(fye-toe-na-dye´one)
Mephyton
Func. class.: Vitamin K₁, fat-soluble vitamin
Pregnancy category C

ACTION: Needed for adequate blood clotting (factors II, VII, IX, X)

Therapeutic outcome: Prevention of bleeding

USES: Vitamin K malabsorption, hypoprothrombinemia, prevention of hypoprothrombinemia caused by oral anticoagulants, prevention of hemorrhagic disease of the newborn

CONTRAINDICATIONS:
Hypersensitivity, severe hepatic disease, last few wk of pregnancy

Precautions: Pregnancy **C**, neonates, hepatic disease

> **BLACK BOX WARNING:** IV use

DOSAGE AND ROUTES
Hypoprothrombinemia caused by vitamin K malabsorption
Adult: PO/IM 2.5-25 mg; may repeat or increase to 50 mg
Child: PO 2.5-5 mg
Infant: PO/IM 2 mg

Prevention of hemorrhagic disease of the newborn

Neonate: IM 0.5-1 mg within 1 hr after birth; repeat in 2-3 wk if required

Hypoprothrombinemia caused by oral anticoagulants
Adult and child: PO/SUBCUT/IM 1-10 mg, may repeat 12-48 hr after PO dose or 6-8 hr after SUBCUT/IM dose, based on INR

Available forms: Tabs 5 mg; inj 10 mg/ml, 1 mg/0.5 ml

Implementation
Intermittent IV infusion route
• Give **IV** after diluting with D₅ NS 10 ml or more; give max 1 mg/min

- Give **IV** only when other routes not possible (deaths have occurred)
- Store in airtight, light-resistant container

Y-site compatibilities: Alfentanil, amikacin, aminophylline, ascorbic acid, atracurium, atropine, azaTHIOprine, aztreonam, bumetanide, buprenorphine, butorphanol, calcium chloride/gluconate, ceFAZolin, cefonicid, cefoperazone, cefotaxime, cefotetan, cefoxitin, ceftazidime, ceftizoxime, cefTRIAXone, cefuroxime, chloramphenicol, chlorproMAZINE, cimetidine, clindamycin, cyanocobalamin, cycloSPORINE, dexamethasone, digoxin, diphenhydrAMINE, DOPamine, doxycycline, enalaprilat, ePHEDrine, EPINEPHrine, epoetin alfa, erythromycin, esmolol, famotidine, fentaNYL, fluconazole, folic acid, furosemide, ganciclovir, gentamicin, glycopyrrolate, heparin, hydrocortisone, imipenem-cilastatin, indomethacin, insulin, isoproterenol, ketorolac, labetalol, lidocaine, mannitol, meperidine, metaraminol, methoxamine, methyldopa, metoclopramide, metoprolol, metroNIDAZOLE, midazolam, morphine, multivitamins, nafcillin, nalbuphine, naloxone, nitroglycerin, nitroprusside, norepinephrine, ondansetron, oxacillin, oxytocin, papaverine, penicillin G potassium, pentamidine, pentazocine, PENTobarbital, PHENobarbital, phentolamine, phenylephrine, potassium chloride, procainamide, prochlorperazine, propranolol, pyridoxime, ranitidine, sodium bicarbonate, succinylcholine, SUFentanil, theophylline, thiamine, ticarcillin/clavulanate, tobramycin, tolazoline, trimethaphan, urokinase, vancomycin, vasopressin, verapamil, vitamin B with C

Y-site incompatibilities: Dantrolene, diazepam, diazoxide, magnesium sulfate, phenytoin, trimethoprim/sulfamethoxazole

ADVERSE EFFECTS
CNS: Headache, **brain damage** (large doses)
GI: Nausea, decreased liver function tests
HEMA: Hemolytic anemia, **hemoglobinuria, hyperbilirubinemia**
INTEG: Rash, urticaria
RESP: **Bronchospasm**, dyspnea, chest constriction, **respiratory arrest**

Pharmacokinetics

Absorption	Well absorbed (PO, IM, SUBCUT)
Distribution	Crosses placenta
Metabolism	Liver, rapidly
Excretion	Breast milk
Half-life	Unknown

Pharmacodynamics

	PO	SUBCUT/IM
Onset	6-12 hr	1-2 hr
Peak	Unknown	6 hr
Duration	Unknown	14 hr

INTERACTIONS
Individual drugs
Sucralfate, mineral oil: decreased action of phytonadione
Warfarin: decreased action of warfarin (large dose of this product)

Drug classifications
Oral anticoagulants: decreased anticoagulant effect
Bile acid sequestrants, antiinfectives, salicylates: decreased action of phytonadione

Drug/food
Olestra: decreased vit K levels

NURSING CONSIDERATIONS
Assessment
- Monitor pro-time during treatment (2-sec deviation from control time, bleeding time, and clotting time)
- Monitor for bleeding, INR pulse, and B/P
- Assess nutritional status: liver (beef), spinach, tomatoes, coffee, asparagus, broccoli, cabbage, lettuce, greens
- Assess for bleeding or bruising: hematuria, black tarry stools, hematemesis

Nursing diagnoses
- Knowledge, deficient (teaching)
- Nutrition: less than body requirements, imbalanced (uses)
- Tissue perfusion, ineffective (uses)

Patient/family education
- Teach patient not to take other supplements unless directed by prescriber; to take this medication as directed
- Teach patient necessary foods high in vit K to be included in diet
- Advise patient to avoid IM inj, hard toothbrush, flossing; use electric razor until treatment is terminated
- Instruct patient to report symptoms of bleeding: bruising, nosebleeds, blood in urine, heavy menstruation, black tarry stools
- Caution patient not to use OTC medications unless approved by prescriber
- Stress the need for periodic lab tests to monitor coagulation levels

P

Adverse effects: *italics* = common; **bold** = life-threatening

• Stress the need for patient to carry/wear emergency ID with condition, treatment, and medications taken

Evaluation
Positive therapeutic outcome
• Decreased bleeding tendencies
• Decreased pro-time
• Decreased clotting time

pilocarpine ophthalmic
See Appendix B

pimecrolimus topical
See Appendix B

pioglitazone (Rx)
(pie-oh-glye′ta-zone)
Actos
Func. class.: Antidiabetic, oral
Chem. class.: Thiazolidinedione
Pregnancy category C

ACTION: Specifically targets insulin resistance, an insulin sensitizer; regulates the transcription of a number of insulin-responsive genes

Therapeutic outcome: Decreased symptoms of diabetes mellitus

USES: Type 2 diabetes mellitus

CONTRAINDICATIONS:
Breastfeeding, children, hypersensitivity to thiazolidinediones, diabetic ketoacidosis

> **BLACK BOX WARNING:** CHF

Precautions: Pregnancy C, thyroid/renal/hepatic disease, edema, geriatric patients with CV disease, polycystic ovary syndrome, bladder cancer, osteoporosis, pulmonary disease, secondary malignancy

DOSAGE AND ROUTES
Monotherapy
Adult: PO 15-30 mg/day, may increase to 45 mg/day; with strong CYP2C8 max 15 mg/day; those with NYHA class I/II heart failure max 15 mg/day

Combination therapy
Adult: PO 15-30 mg/day with a sulfonylurea, metformin, or insulin; decrease sulfonylurea dose if hypoglycemia occurs; decrease insulin dose by 10%-25% if hypoglycemia occurs or if plasma glucose is <100 mg/dl; max 45 mg/day

Hepatic dose
Do not use in active liver disease or if ALT >2.5 × ULN

Available forms: Tabs 15, 30, 45 mg

Implementation
• Convert from other oral hypoglycemic agents; change may be made with gradual dosage change; monitor serum glucose during conversion
• Give once a day without regard to meals
• Give tabs crushed and mixed with meal or fluids for patients with difficulty swallowing
• Store in airtight container in cool environment

ADVERSE EFFECTS
CNS: *Headache*
CV: MI, **heart failure, death** (geriatric patients)
ENDO: Hyper/hypoglycemia
MISC: *Myalgia, sinusitis, upper respiratory tract infection, pharyngitis,* **hepatotoxicity,** edema, weight gain, anemia, macular edema; **risk of bladder cancer (use >1 yr)**
MS: Fractures (females), **rhabdomyolysis,** myalgia

Pharmacokinetics

Absorption	Unknown
Distribution	Protein binding >99%
Metabolism	Unknown
Excretion	Kidneys
Half-life	3-7 hr, terminal 16-24 hr

Pharmacodynamics

Onset	Unknown
Peak	6-12 wk
Duration	Unknown

INTERACTIONS
Individual drugs
Fluconazole, itraconazole, ketoconazole, miconazole, voriconazole: decreased pioglitazone effect

Drug classifications
CYP2C8 inducers: decreased pioglitazone effect
Oral contraceptives: decreased effect, use an alternative contraceptive method

Drug/herb
Garlic, green tea, horse chestnut: increased hypoglycemia

Drug/lab test
Increase: CPK

NURSING CONSIDERATIONS
Assessment

> **BLACK BOX WARNING:** For CHF: excessive/rapid weight gain > 5 lb, dyspnea, edema; may need to be reduced or discontinued

• **Hypoglycemic reactions:** assess for hypoglycemic reactions (sweating, weakness, dizziness, anxiety, tremors, hunger), hyperglycemic reactions soon after meals (rare)
• **Rhabdomyolysis:** muscle pain, increased CPK, weakness, swelling of affected muscles; if these occur and if confirmed by CPK, product should be discontinued
• Check LFTs periodically: AST, LDH; do not start treatment in active heart disease or if ALT >2.5× upper limit of normal; if treatment has already begun, follow closely with continuing ALT levels; if ALT increases to >3× upper limit of normal, recheck ALT as soon as possible, if ALT remains >3× upper limit of normal, discontinue
• Monitor FBS, glycosylated HbA1c, plasma lipids/lipoproteins, B/P, body weight during treatment
• Monitor CBC with differential prior to and during therapy, more necessary in those with anemia

Nursing diagnoses
• Knowledge, deficient (teaching)
• Nutrition: more than body requirements, imbalanced (uses)

Patient/family education
• Teach patient to self-monitor using a blood glucose meter
• Teach patient symptoms of hypo/hyperglycemia, what to do about each (rare)
• Advise patient that product must be continued on daily basis; explain consequence of discontinuing product abruptly
• Advise patient to avoid OTC medications or herbal preparations unless approved by prescriber; to report weight gain, edema
• Advise patient that diabetes is life-long illness; that this product is not a cure, only controls symptoms
• Instruct patient to notify prescriber if oral contraceptives are used
• Teach patient not to use if breastfeeding

Evaluation
Positive therapeutic outcome
• Decrease in polyuria, polydipsia, polyphagia; clear sensorium; absence of dizziness; stable gait; blood glucose, A1c improvement

piperacillin/tazobactam (Rx)
Zosyn
Func. class.: Broad-spectrum antiinfective
Chem. class.: Extended-spectrum penicillin
Pregnancy category B

ACTION: Interferes with cell wall replication of susceptible organisms; osmotically unstable cell wall swells and bursts from osmotic pressure; tazobactam is a β-lactamase inhibitor, protects piperacillin from enzymatic degradation

Therapeutic outcome: Bactericidal effects for piperacillin-resistant β-lactamase, *Escherichia coli, Staphylococcus aureus, Bacteroides fragilis, Bacteroides ovatus, Bacteroides thetaiotaomicron, Bacteroides vulgatus, Haemophilus influenzae*

USES: Moderate to severe infections: piperacillin-resistant, β-lactamase strains causing infections in respiratory tract, skin, skin structure, urinary tract, bone, and joint; gonorrhea, pneumonia, infections from penicillinase-producing staphylococci, streptococci

CONTRAINDICATIONS: Hypersensitivity to penicillins; neonates, carbapenem allergy

Precautions: Pregnancy **B,** breastfeeding, CHF, seizures, hypersensitivity to cephalosporins, renal insufficiency in children, GI disease, electrolyte imbalances

DOSAGE AND ROUTES
Nosocomial pneumonia
Adult: IV 4.5 g q6hr or 3.375 g q4hr with an aminoglycoside or antipseudomonal fluoroquinolone × 1-2 wk; continue aminoglycoside only if *Pseudomonas aeruginosa* is isolated

Other infections
Adult: IV INF 6-12 g/day, given 2.25 g q8hr to 3.375 g q6hr over 30 min × 7-10 days

Renal dose
Adult: IV CCr 20-40 ml/min give 3.375 g q6hr (nosocomial pneumonia); give 2.25 g q6hr (all

other indications); CCr <20 ml/min, give 2.25 g q6hr (nosocomial pneumonia); give 2.25 g q8hr (all other indications)

Available forms: Powder for inj 2 g piperacillin/0.25 g tazobactam, 3 g piperacillin/0.375 g tazobactam, 4 g piperacillin/0.5 g tazobactam, 36 g piperacillin/4.5 g tazobactam

Implementation

• Separate aminoglycoside from piperacillin to avoid inactivation
• Product after C&S is complete

Intermittent IV infusion route
• Reconstitute each 1 g of product/5 ml 0.9% NaCl for inj or sterile water for inj, dextrose 5%; shake well; further dilute in at least 50 ml compatible IV sol and run as int inf over at least 30 min

Y-site compatibilities: Alfentanil, allopurinol, amifostine, amikacin, aminocaproic acid, aminophylline, amphotericin B lipid complex, amphotericin B liposome, anidulafungin, atenolol, aztreonam, bivalirudin, bleomycin, bumetanide, buprenorphine, busulfan, butorphanol, calcium acetate/chloride/gluconate, CARBOplatin, carmustine, cefepime, chloramphenicol, cimetidine, clindamycin, cyclophosphamide, cycloSPORINE, cytarabine, DACTINomycin, DAPTOmycin, dexamethasone, dexrazoxane, diazepam, digoxin, diphenhydrAMINE, docetaxel, DOPamine, doxacurium, enalaprilat, ePHEDrine, EPINEPHrine, eptifibatide, erythromycin, esmolol, etoposide, fenoldopam, fentaNYL, floxuridine, fluconazole, fludarabine, fluorouracil, foscarnet, fosphenytoin, furosemide, gallium, granisetron, heparin, hydrocortisone, HYDROmorphone, ifosfamide, isoproterenol, ketorolac, lansoprazole, leucovorin, lidocaine, linezolid, LORazepam, magnesium sulfate, mannitol, mechlorethamine, melphalan, meperidine, mesna, metaraminol, methotrexate, methylPREDNISolone, metoclopramide, metoprolol, metroNIDAZOLE, milrinone, morphine, naloxone, nitroglycerin, nitroprusside, norepinephrine, octreotide, ondansetron, oxytocin, paclitaxel, palonosetron, pamidronate, pancuronium, pantoprazole, pemetrexed, PENTobarbital, PHENobarbital, phenylephrine, plicamycin, potassium chloride/phosphates, procainamide, ranitidine, remifentanil, riTUXimab, sargramostim, sodium acetate/bicarbonate/phosphates, succinylcholine, SUFentanil, sulfamethoxazole-trimethoprim, tacrolimus, teniposide, theophylline, thiotepa, tigecycline, tirofiban, trimethobenzamide, vasopressin, vinBLAStine, vinCRIStine, voriconazole, zidovudine, zoledronic acid

Y-site incompatibilities: Fluconazole, ondansetron, sargramostim, vinorelbine

ADVERSE EFFECTS

CNS: Headache, insomnia, dizziness, fever, lethargy, hallucinations, anxiety, depression, twitching, **seizures,** vertigo
CV: Cardiac toxicity
GI: *Nausea, vomiting, diarrhea,* increased AST, ALT, abdominal pain, glossitis, constipation, **pseudomembranous colitis**
GU: Oliguria, proteinuria, hematuria, *vaginitis, moniliasis,* **glomerulonephritis, renal failure**
HEMA: Anemia, increased bleeding time, **bone marrow depression, agranulocytosis,** hemolytic anemia
INTEG: Rash, pruritus, **exfoliative dermatitis**
META: Hypokalemia, hypernatremia
SYST: Serum sickness, anaphylaxis, Stevens-Johnson syndrome

Pharmacokinetics

Absorption	Well absorbed (80%)
Distribution	Widely distributed; crosses placenta
Metabolism	Not metabolized
Excretion	Kidneys, unchanged (90%); bile (10%); breast milk
Half-life	0.7-1.3 hr

Pharmacodynamics

Onset	Rapid
Peak	Inf end
Duration	Unknown

INTERACTIONS

Individual drugs
Aspirin, probenecid: increased piperacillin levels
Methotrexate: increased effect of methotrexate

Drug classifications
Aminoglycosides (**IV**): decreased piperacillin effect
Anticoagulants (oral): increased effect of anticoagulants
Contraceptives (oral): decreased contraceptive effectiveness
Neuromuscular blockers: increased effects
Tetracyclines: decreased antimicrobial effectiveness of piperacillin

Drug/lab test
Increased: platelet count, eosinophilia, neutropenia, leucopenia, serum creatinine, PTT, AST, ALT, alkaline phosphatase, bilirubin, BUN, electrolytes
Decreased: Hct, Hgb, electrolytes
False positive: urine glucose, urine protein, Coombs' test

NURSING CONSIDERATIONS

Assessment
• Assess patient for previous sensitivity reaction to penicillins or other cephalosporins; cross-sensitivity between penicillins and cephalosporins is common
• Assess patient for signs and symptoms of infection, including characteristics of wounds, sputum, urine, stool, WBC $>10,000/mm^3$, fever; obtain information baseline, during treatment
• Obtain C&S before beginning product therapy to identify if correct treatment has been initiated
• **Assess for allergic reactions:** rash, urticaria, pruritus, chills, fever, joint pain; angioedema may occur a few days after therapy begins; epinephrine, resuscitation equipment should be available for anaphylactic reaction
⚠ Identify urine output; if decreasing, notify prescriber (may indicate nephrotoxicity); also check for increased BUN, creatinine
• Monitor blood studies: AST, ALT, CBC, Hct, bilirubin, LDH, alkaline phosphatase, Coombs' test monthly if patient is on long-term therapy
• Monitor electrolytes: potassium, sodium, chloride monthly if patient is on long-term therapy
• **Pseudomembranous colitis:** assess for diarrhea, abdominal pain, fever, fatigue, anorexia; possible anemia, elevated WBC and low serum albumin; stop product and usually give either vancomycin or **IV** metroNIDAZOLE
• Monitor for bleeding: ecchymosis, bleeding gums, hematuria, stool guaiac daily if on long-term therapy
• **Assess for overgrowth of infection:** perineal itching, fever, malaise, redness, pain, swelling, drainage, rash, diarrhea, change in cough, sputum

Nursing diagnoses
• Diarrhea (adverse reactions)
• Infection, risk for (uses)
• Injury, risk for (adverse reactions)
• Knowledge, deficient (teaching)
• Noncompliance (teaching)

Patient/family education
• Teach patient to report sore throat, bruising, bleeding, joint pain; may indicate **blood dyscrasias (rare)**
• Advise patient to contact prescriber if vaginal itching, loose foul-smelling stools, furry tongue occur; may indicate **superinfection**
• Advise patient to notify prescriber of diarrhea with blood or pus, which may indicate **pseudomembranous colitis**

Evaluation
Positive therapeutic outcome
• Absence of signs/symptoms of infection (WBC $<10,000/mm^3$, temp WNL, absence of red, draining wounds)
• Reported improvement in symptoms of infection

TREATMENT OF ANAPHYLAXIS: Withdraw product, maintain airway, administer EPINEPHrine, aminophylline, O_2, **IV** corticosteroids

---

piroxicam (Rx)
(peer-ox'i-kam)
Apo-Piroxicam ✚, Feldene, Gen-Piroxicam ✚
Func. class.: Nonsteroidal antiinflammatory
Chem. class.: Oxicam derivative
Pregnancy category C

ACTION: Inhibits COX-1, COX-2 by blocking arachidonate; antiinflammatory, antipyretic properties

Therapeutic outcome: Decreased pain, inflammation

USES: Mild to moderate pain, osteoarthritis, rheumatoid arthritis

CONTRAINDICATIONS:
Pregnancy **D** (3rd trimester); hypersensitivity to this product, NSAIDs, salicylates; asthma

BLACK BOX WARNING: Perioperative pain in CABG surgery

Precautions: Pregnancy **C,** avoid in late pregnancy, breastfeeding, children, bleeding disorders, GI/cardiac disorders, hypersensitivity to other antiinflammatory agents, CHF

BLACK BOX WARNING: GI bleeding, MI, stroke

Adverse effects: *italics* – common; **bold** = life-threatening

DOSAGE AND ROUTES
Adult: PO 20 mg/day or 10 mg bid

Available forms: Caps 10, 20 mg

Implementation
- Swallow caps whole; do not break, crush, or chew
- Give with food or milk to decrease gastric symptoms, water to enhance absorption
- Store at room temp in light-resistant container

ADVERSE EFFECTS
CNS: Dizziness, *drowsiness,* fatigue, tremors, confusion, insomnia, anxiety, depression, *headache*
CV: Tachycardia, peripheral edema, palpitations, **dysrhythmias,** hypertension, **MI, stroke,** CHF
EENT: Tinnitus, hearing loss, blurred vision
GI: *Nausea, anorexia, vomiting, diarrhea,* jaundice, **cholestatic hepatitis,** constipation, flatulence, cramps, dry mouth, peptic ulcer, **bleeding, ulceration, perforation,** dyspepsia
GU: Nephrotoxicity: dysuria, hematuria, oliguria, azotemia
HEMA: Blood dyscrasias
INTEG: Purpura, rash, pruritus, sweating, photosensitivity
MISC: Hyperkalemia, hypoglycemia
SYST: Anaphylaxis

Pharmacokinetics

Absorption	Well absorbed
Distribution	Unknown
Metabolism	Liver, extensively
Excretion	Kidneys, minimal; breast milk
Half-life	50 hr

Pharmacodynamics

Onset	1 hr
Peak	3-5 hr
Duration	48-72 hr

INTERACTIONS
Individual drugs
Alcohol, aspirin, cycloSPORINE, lithium, methotrexate: increased toxicity

Drug classifications
Anticoagulants (oral), corticosteroids: increased toxicity
Anticoagulants, antiplatelets, NSAIDs, SSRIs, SNRIs, thrombin inhibitors: increased bleeding risk
Antidiabetics (oral): hypoglycemia

Antihypertensives: decreased effect of antihypertensives
Diuretics: decreased effectiveness of diuretics

Drug/herb
Ginger, garlic, ginkgo: increased bleeding risk

Drug/lab
Increase: AST, ALT, LDH, BUN, creatinine
Decrease: Hgb/Hct, platelets, leukocytes

NURSING CONSIDERATIONS
Assessment
- Monitor blood counts during therapy; watch for decreasing platelets; if low, therapy may need to be discontinued, restarted after hematologic recovery; check for blood dyscrasia (thrombocytopenia): bruising, fatigue, bleeding, poor healing
- **Assess for pain:** location, duration, ROM, before, 1-2 hr after administration
- Assess for aspirin sensitivity, asthma, nasal polyps; these may develop into allergic reactions

Nursing diagnoses
- Injury, risk for (adverse reactions)
- Knowledge, deficient (teaching)
- Mobility, impaired physical (uses)
- Pain, chronic (uses)

Patient/family education
- Teach patient that product must be continued for prescribed time to be effective; to avoid aspirin, alcoholic beverages, and other OTC medications unless approved by prescriber
- Caution patient to report bleeding, bruising, fatigue, malaise, since blood dyscrasias do occur
- Instruct patient to use caution when driving; drowsiness, dizziness may occur
- Teach patient to take with a full glass of water to enhance absorption
- Instruct to inform all health care providers about product use

Evaluation
Positive therapeutic outcome
- Decreased pain
- Decreased inflammation
- Increased mobility

pitavastatin (Rx)

(pit′a-va-stat′in)
Livalo
Func. class.: Antilipidemic
Chem. class.: HMG-CoA reductase
inhibitor
Pregnancy category X

ACTION: Inhibits HMG-CoA reductase
enzyme, which reduces cholesterol synthesis,
high doses lead to plaque regression

Therapeutic outcome: Decreased cholesterol levels and LDLs, increased HDLs

USES: As an adjunct in primary hypercholesterolemia (types Ia, Ib), dysbetalipoproteinemia, elevated triglyceride levels; prevention of
cardiovascular disease by reduction of heart risk
in those with mildly elevated cholesterol

CONTRAINDICATIONS:

Pregnancy **X,** breastfeeding, hypersensitivity,
active liver disease, cholestasis

Precautions: Past liver disease, alcoholism,
severe acute infections, trauma, severe metabolic disorders, electrolyte imbalance, seizures,
surgery, organ transplant, endocrine disease,
females, hypotension, renal disease

DOSAGE AND ROUTES

Adult: PO 2 mg/day, usual range 1-4, max 4
mg/day

Renal dose

Adult: PO CCr 30-60 ml/min 1 mg qd, max
2 mg qd; CCr <30 ml/min on hemodialysis 1
mg qd, max 2 mg qd; CCr <30 ml/min not on
hemodialysis—not recommended

Available forms: Tabs 1, 2, 4 mg

Implementation

• Administer total daily dose at any time of day
• Store in cool environment in airtight, light-
resistant container

ADVERSE EFFECTS

CNS: Headache
GI: Constipation, diarrhea
INTEG: Rash, pruritus, alopecia
MS: Myalgia, **rhabdomyolysis,** arthralgia
RESP: Pharyngitis

Absorption	Unknown
Distribution	Concentrations are lower in healthy African-Americans
Metabolism	Liver
Excretion	Urine, feces
Half-life	12 hr

Pharmacodynamics

Unknown

INTERACTIONS

Individual drugs

Clofibrate, cycloSPORINE, erythromycin, gemfibrozil, niacin: increased risk of rhabdomyolysis
Colestipol: decreased action of atorvastatin
Erythromycin, red yeast rice: increased levels of
atorvastatin
Warfarin: increased action of warfarin

Drug classifications

Antifungals (azole): possible rhabdomyolysis

Drug/lab test

Increased: bilirubin, alkaline phosphatase, ALT,
AST
Interference: thyroid function tests

NURSING CONSIDERATIONS

Assessment

• Assess nutrition: fat, protein, carbohydrates;
nutritional analysis should be completed by
dietitian before treatment
• **Rhabdomyolysis:** assess for muscle pain,
tenderness; obtain CPK if these occur; product
may need to be discontinued
• Monitor bowel pattern daily; diarrhea may be
a problem
• Monitor triglycerides, cholesterol at baseline,
throughout treatment; LDL and VLDL should be
watched closely; if increased, product should be
discontinued
• Monitor liver function studies q1-2mo during
the first $1\frac{1}{2}$ yr of treatment; AST, ALT, liver function tests may be increased
• Monitor renal studies in patients with
compromised renal system: BUN, I&O ratio,
creatinine
• Assess eyes via ophthalmic exam 1 mo after
treatment begins, annually

Nursing diagnoses

• Diarrhea (adverse reactions)
• Knowledge, deficient (teaching)
• Noncompliance (teaching)

P

Adverse effects: *italics* – common; **bold** – life-threatening

Patient/family education

• Inform patient that compliance is needed for positive results to occur, not to double doses
• Teach patient that risk factors should be decreased: high-fat diet, smoking, alcohol consumption, absence of exercise
• Advise patient to notify prescriber if the GI symptoms of diarrhea, abdominal or epigastric pain, nausea, vomiting; chills, fever, sore throat; muscle pain, weakness occur
• Advise patient that treatment will take several years
• Advise patient that blood work will be necessary during treatment
• Advise patient not to take if pregnant, pregnancy **X**

Evaluation
Positive therapeutic outcome
• Decreased cholesterol levels, serum triglyceride
• Improved ratio of HDLs

---

plasma protein fraction (Rx)
Plasmanate
Func. class.: Hematological agent
Chem. class.: Plasma volume expander
Pregnancy category C

ACTION: Exerts similar oncotic pressure as human plasma, expands blood volume, shifts water from extravascular space to intravascular space

Therapeutic outcome: Shift of fluid from extravascular into intravascular space

USES: Hypovolemic shock, hypoproteinemia, ARDS, preoperative cardiopulmonary bypass, acute liver failure, nephrotic syndrome, cardiogenic shock

CONTRAINDICATIONS:
Hypersensitivity to this product or albumin, CHF, severe anemia, renal insufficiency, hyponatremia, cardiopulmonary bypass

Precautions: Pregnancy **C,** decreased salt intake, decreased cardiac reserve, lack of albumin deficiency, hepatic disease

DOSAGE AND ROUTES
Hypovolemia
Adult: **IV** INF 250-500 ml (12.5-25 g of protein), max 10 ml/min
Child: **IV** INF 10-30 ml/kg max 5-10 ml/min

Hypoproteinemia
Adult: **IV** INF 1000-1500 ml/day, max 8 ml/min

Available forms: Inj 5%

Implementation
• Give by **IV**; no dilution required; use inf pump, large-gauge needle ($\geq$20-G); discard unused portion; inf slowly to prevent hypotension; give within 4 hr of opening
• Provide adequate hydration before administration
• Do not use sol that has been frozen
• Adjust rate to changes in B/P
• Store at room temp, max 86° F

Additive compatibilities:
Carbohydrate and electrolyte sol, whole blood, packed RBCs, chloramphenicol, tetracycline

Additive incompatibilities:
Protein hydrolysate sol, amino acid sol, alcohol, norepinephrine

ADVERSE EFFECTS
CNS: Fever, chills, headache, paresthesias, flushing
CV: Fluid overload, hypotension, erratic pulse
GI: Nausea, vomiting, increased salivation
INTEG: Rash, urticaria, cyanosis
RESP: Altered respirations, dyspnea, **pulmonary edema**

Pharmacokinetics

Absorption	Completely absorbed
Distribution	Intravascular space
Metabolism	Unknown
Excretion	Unknown
Half-life	Unknown

Pharmacodynamics

Onset	15-30 min
Peak	Unknown
Duration	Unknown

INTERACTIONS
Drug/lab test
False increase: alkaline phosphatase

NURSING CONSIDERATIONS
Assessment
• Monitor blood studies: Hct, Hgb; electrolytes, serum protein; if serum protein declines, dyspnea, hypoxemia can result
• Monitor B/P (decreased), pulse (erratic), respiration during inf; CVP, jugular vein distention, PWP (increases if overload occurs); SOB,

---

anxiety, insomnia, expiratory crackles, frothy blood-tinged cough, cyanosis indicate pulmonary overload
• Monitor I&O ratio; urinary output may decrease
• Assess for allergy: fever, rash, itching, chills, flushing, urticaria, nausea, vomiting, or hypotension require discontinuation of inf; use new lot if therapy is reinstituted, premedicate with diphenhydrAMINE

Nursing diagnoses
• Cardiac output, decreased (uses)
• Fluid volume, deficient (uses)
• Fluid volume, excess (adverse reactions)

Patient/family education
• Explain reason for and expected result of medication

Evaluation
Positive therapeutic outcome
• Increased B/P
• Decreased edema
• Increased serum albumin

plerixafor (Rx)
(pler-ix′a-fore)
Mozobil
Func. class.: Biological modifier
Chem. class.: Colony-stimulating factor
Pregnancy category D

ACTION: Competitively inhibits the binding of stromal-derived factors, allowing hematopoietic stem cells to mobilize into peripheral blood

Therapeutic outcome: Successful collection of stem cells

USES: For peripheral blood stem cell (PBSC) mobilization for collection and autologous transplant in non-Hodgkin's lymphoma, multiple myeloma; used with a granulocyte colony stimulating factor (G-CSF)

CONTRAINDICATIONS:
Pregnancy **D**, hypersensitivity, breastfeeding

Precautions: Children, renal disease, thrombocytopenia

DOSAGE AND ROUTES
Adult: SUBCUT 0.24 mg/kg qd about 11 hr before initiating apheresis; give up to 4 consecutive days; give filgrastim 10 mcg/kg SUBCUT qd each AM beginning 4 days before the 1st evening dose of plerixafor and on each day of apheresis; give filgrastim before procedure

Available forms: Inj 300 mcg/ml, 480 mcg/1.6 ml, 480 mcg/0.8 ml, 3000 mcg/0.5 ml

Implementation
SUBCUT route
• Each single-use vial contains 24 mg of plerixafor (1.2 ml of 20 mg/ml sol); the volume is calculated by multiplying 0.012 by the actual body wt (kg)
• Give 11 hr before apheresis
• Max 40 mg/day, or 27 mg/day in renal disease
• Store at room temperature

ADVERSE EFFECTS
CNS: Syncope, dizziness, fatigue, headache, insomnia, malaise, paresthesias
GI: *Nausea,* vomiting, diarrhea, abdominal pain, constipation
HEMA: **Thrombocytopenia,** leukocytosis
INTEG: Rash, skin irritation, pruritus, inj site reaction, erythema, urticaria
MS: Musculoskeletal pain
RESP: Dyspnea, hypoxia

Pharmacokinetics
Absorption	Unknown
Distribution	Protein binding 58%
Metabolism	Unknown
Excretion	70% kidney as parent drug
Half-life	Terminal 3-5 hr

Pharmacodynamics
Onset	30-60 min
Peak	6-9 hr mobilization
Duration	Unknown

INTERACTIONS
Individual drugs
Lithium: increased adverse reactions, increased leukocytosis, do not use concomitantly

NURSING CONSIDERATIONS
Assessment
• Monitor blood studies: CBC/differential
• Monitor B/P, respirations, pulse before, during therapy
• Assess for bone pain; give mild analgesics

Nursing diagnoses
• Knowledge, deficient (teaching)

Patient/family education
• Explain reason for use and expected results

Evaluation
Positive therapeutic outcome
• Collection of stem cells

posaconazole (Rx)

(poe′sa-kon′a-zole)
Noxafil, Posanol ✤
Func. class.: Antifungal, systemic
Chem. class.: Triazole derivative
Pregnancy category C

ACTION: Inhibits a portion of cell wall synthesis; alters cell membranes and inhibits several fungal enzymes

Therapeutic outcome: Decreased fever, malaise, rash; negative C&S for infecting organism

USES: Prevention of aspergillus, candida infection, oropharyngeal candidiasis in the immunocompromised, chemotherapy-induced neutropenia, mucocutaneous candidiasis

CONTRAINDICATIONS:

Hypersensitivity to this product or other systemic antifungal or azoles, fungal meningitis, onchomycosis or dermatomycosis in cardiac dysfunction

Precautions: Pregnancy **C**, breastfeeding, children, hepatic/cardiac disease

DOSAGE AND ROUTES

Adult: PO 800 mg/day in 2-4 divided doses
Child: PO 100 mg tid

Available forms: Oral susp 200 mg/5 ml

Implementation
PO route
• **Oral susp:** give after shaking well; use calibrated measuring device; take only with a full meal or liquid nutritional supplements such as Ensure; rinse measuring device after each use
• Store in a tight container in refrigerator; do not freeze

ADVERSE EFFECTS

CNS: *Headache, dizziness,* insomnia, fever, rigors, weakness, anxiety
CV: Hypo/hypertension, tachycardia, anemia
GI: *Nausea, vomiting, anorexia, diarrhea,* cramps, abdominal pain, flatulence, **GI bleeding, hepatotoxicity**
GU: Gynecomastia, impotence, decreased libido
INTEG: *Pruritus,* fever, *rash,* **toxic epidermal necrolysis**
MISC: *Edema, fatigue,* malaise, hypokalemia, tinnitus, **rhabdomyolysis**

Pharmacokinetics

Absorption	Well absorbed, enhanced by food
Distribution	Protein binding 98%-99%
Metabolism	Liver
Excretion	Feces, 77% unchanged
Half-life	19-35 hr

Pharmacodynamics

Onset	Unknown
Peak	4-11 hr
Duration	Unknown

INTERACTIONS

Individual drugs
⚠ **BusPIRone, busulfan, clarithromycin, cycloSPORINE, diazepam, digoxin, felodipine, indinavir, isradipine, midazolam, niCARdipine, NIFEdipine, nimodipine, phenytoin, quiNIDine, ritonavir, saquinavir, tacrolimus, warfarin: increased levels, toxicity**
Haloperidol, chloroquine, droperidol, pentamidine; arsenic trioxide, levomethadyl: increased QT prolongation
Cimetidine, phenytoin: decreased posaconazole level
Didanosine, rifamycin: decreased posaconazole action
⚠ **Dofetilide, pimozide, quiNIDine, halofantrine: life-threatening reactions, increased QT prolongation**
Midazolam (oral), triazolam: increased sedation
Quinidine: increased tinnitus, hearing loss

Drug classifications
Antacids, H$_2$-receptor antagonists, rifamycins: decreased posaconazole action
Class IA/III antidysrhythmics, some phenothiazines, beta agonists, local anesthetics, tricyclics, CYP3A4 inhibitors (amiodarone, clarithromycin, erythromycin, telithromycin, troleandomycin), CYP3A4 substrates (methadone, pimozide, QUEtiapine, quiNIDine, risperidone, ziprasidone): increased QT prolongation
⚠ **Ergots: life-threatening reactions, increased QT prolongation**
Other hepatotoxic products: increased hepatotoxicity
Calcium channel blockers, HMG-CoA reductase inhibitors, vinca alkaloids: increased levels, toxicity
Oral contraceptives: decreased effect, use other contraceptives

⚠ Nurse Alert

Oral hypoglycemics: increased severe hypoglycemia

Drug/food
Food: increased absorption

NURSING CONSIDERATIONS
Assessment
• **Rhabdomyolysis:** assess for muscle pain, increased CPK, weakness, swelling of affected muscles; if these occur and if confirmed by CPK, product should be discontinued
• **QT prolongation:** monitor ECG for QT prolongation, ejection fraction; assess for chest pain, palpitations, dyspnea
• Assess for type of infection; may begin treatment before obtaining results
• Assess for infection: temp, WBC, sputum, baseline, periodically
• Monitor I&O ratio, potassium levels
• Monitor liver function tests (ALT, AST, bilirubin) if on long-term therapy
• Assess for allergic reaction: rash, photosensitivity, uricaria, dermatitis
⚠ Assess for hepatotoxicity: nausea, vomiting, jaundice, clay-colored stools, fatigue

Nursing diagnoses
• Infection, risk for (uses)
• Knowledge, deficient (teaching)

Patient/family education
• Teach patient that long-term therapy may be needed to clear infection (1 wk-6 mo depending on infection)
• Advise patient to avoid hazardous activities if dizziness occurs
• Advise patient to take 2 hr before administration of other products that increase gastric pH (antacids, H₂-blockers, omeprazole, sucralfate, anticholinergics); to notify health care provider of all medications taken
• Teach the patient the importance of compliance with product regimen; to use alternative method of contraception
• Teach patient to notify prescriber of GI symptoms, signs of hepatic dysfunction (fatigue, nausea, anorexia, vomiting, dark urine, pale stools)

Evaluation
Positive therapeutic outcome
• Decreased fever, malaise, rash, negative C&S for infecting organism

---

**potassium acetate/
potassium bicarbonate (Rx, OTC)**
K-Effervescent, Klor-Con EF, K-Vescent
**potassium bicarbonate/
potassium chloride (Rx, OTC)**
Neo-K ✦
**potassium bicarbonate/
potassium citrate (Rx, OTC)**
potassium chloride (Rx, OTC)
Epiklor, Klor-Con, K-Tab, Micro-K, Odan K-20 ✦
potassium gluconate (Rx, OTC)
Kaon, Kaylixir, K-G Elixir, Potassium-Rougier ✦
Func. class.: Electrolyte, mineral replacement
Chem. class.: Potassium
Pregnancy category C

ACTION: Needed for adequate transmission of nerve impulses and cardiac contraction, renal function, intracellular ion maintenance

Therapeutic outcome: Potassium level 3.0-5.0 mg/dl

USES: Prevention and treatment of hypokalemia

CONTRAINDICATIONS:
Renal disease (severe), severe hemolytic disease, Addison's disease, hyperkalemia, acute dehydration, extensive tissue breakdown

Precautions: Pregnancy C, cardiac disease, potassium-sparing diuretic therapy, systemic acidosis

DOSAGE AND ROUTES
Hypokalemia (prevention) (bicarbonate, chloride, gluconate)
Adult: PO 20 mEq/day in 1-2 divided doses
Child: PO 1-2 mEq/day in 1-2 divided doses

Hypokalemia, digoxin toxicity (acetate, chloride)
Adult: serum potassium conc > 2.5 mEq/L: IV max 10 mEq/l hr, with 24 hr dose max 200 mEq, initial dose of 20-40 mEq has been recom-

Adverse effects: *italics* = common; **bold** = life-threatening

mended; **PO** 40-100 mEq/day in 2-4 divided doses
Child: IV 0.25-0.5 mEq/g/dose, at 0.25-0.5 mEq/kg/hr; **PO** 2-5 mEq/day in divided doses

Available forms: Tabs for sol 6.5, 25 mEq; ext rel caps 8, 10 mEq; powder for sol 3.3, 5, 6.7, 10, 13.3 mEq/5 ml; tabs 2, 4, 5, 13.4 mEq; ext rel tabs 6.7, 8, 10 mEq; elix 6.7 mEq/5 ml; oral sol 2.375 mEq/5 ml; inj for prep of IV 1.5, 2, 2.4, 3, 3.2, 4.4, 4.7 mEq/ml

Implementation
PO route
• Do not break, crush, or chew ext rel tabs/ caps or enteric-coated products
• Give with meal or after meal; take cap with full glass of liquid; dissolve effervescent tab, powder in 8 oz of cold water or juice; do not give IM, SUBCUT
• Store at room temperature

IV route
• Give through large-bore needle to decrease vein inflammation; check for extravasation; administer in large vein, avoiding scalp vein in child
• After diluting in large volume of **IV** sol give as an **IV** inf slowly to prevent toxicity; never give **IV** bol or IM

Potassium acetate
Additive compatibilities: Metoclopramide
• **Potassium chloride** must be diluted, concentrated potassium injections are fatal

Continuous IV infusion route
• Conc max 80 mEq/L for peripheral line, 120 mEq/L central line
• Dehydrated patients should receive 1 L of potassium-free hydration sol; then infuse 10 mEq/hr; in severe hypokalemia rate may be 40 mEq/hr

Y-site compatibilities: Acyclovir, aldesleukin, allopurinol, amifostine, aminophylline, amiodarone, ampicillin, atropine, aztreonam, betamethasone, calcium gluconate, cefmetazole, cephalothin, cephapirin, chlordiazepoxide, chlorproMAZINE, ciprofloxacin, cladribine, cyanocobalamin, dexamethasone, digoxin, diltiazem, diphenhydrAMINE, DOBUTamine, DOPamine, droperidol, edrophonium, enalaprilat, EPINEPHrine, esmolol, estrogens, ethacrynate, famotidine, fentaNYL, filgrastim, fludarabine, fluorouracil, furosemide, gallium, granisetron, heparin, hydrALAZINE, IDArubicin, indomethacin, inamrinone, regular insulin, isoproterenol, kanamycin, labetalol, lidocaine, LORazepam,

magnesium sulfate, melphalan, meperidine, methicillin, methoxamine, methylergonovine, midazolam, minocycline, morphine, neostigmine, norepinephrine, ondansetron, oxacillin, oxytocin, paclitaxel, penicillin G potassium, pentazocine, phytonadione, piperacillin/ tazobactam, prednisoLONE, procainamide, prochlorperazine, propofol, propranolol, pyridostigmine, sargramostim, scopolamine, sodium bicarbonate, succinylcholine, tacrolimus, teniposide, theophylline, thiotepa, trimethaphan, trimethobenzamide, vinorelbine, zidovudine

Additive compatibilities: Aminophylline, amiodarone, atracurium, bretylium, calcium chloride, cefepime, cephalothin, cephapirin, chloramphenicol, cimetidine, ciprofloxacin, clindamycin, cloxacillin, corticotropin, cytarabine, dimenhyDRINATE, DOPamine, enalaprilat, erythromycin, floxacillin, fluconazole, furosemide, heparin, hydrocortisone, isoproterenol, lidocaine, metaraminol, methicillin, methyldopate, metoclopramide, mitoxantrone, nafcillin, netilmicin, norepinephrine, oxacillin, penicillin G potassium or sodium, phenylephrine, piperacillin, ranitidine, sodium bicarbonate, thiopental, vancomycin, verapamil, vit B/C

Potassium chloride
Y-site compatibilities: Aldesleukin, amifostine, granisetron, LORazepam, midazolam, thiotepa

ADVERSE EFFECTS
CNS: Confusion
CV: Bradycardia, *cardiac depression,* **dysrhythmias, arrest, peaking T waves, lowered R and depressed RST, prolonged P–R interval, widened QRS complex**
GI: *Nausea, vomiting, cramps,* pain, *diarrhea,* ulceration of small bowel
GU: Oliguria
INTEG: Cold extremities, rash

Pharmacokinetics

Absorption	Unknown
Distribution	Unknown
Metabolism	Unknown
Excretion	Kidneys, feces
Half-life	Unknown

Pharmacodynamics

	PO	IV
Onset	30 min	Immediate
Peak	Unknown	Unknown
Duration	Unknown	Unknown

⚠ Nurse Alert

INTERACTIONS
Drug classifications
Angiotensin-converting enzyme inhibitors, calcium, diuretics (potassium-sparing), magnesium, potassium phosphate, **IV,** other potassium products: increased hyperkalemia

NURSING CONSIDERATIONS
Assessment
• Assess ECG for peaking T-waves, lowered R, depressed RST, prolonged PR interval, widening QRS complex, hyperkalemia; product should be reduced or discontinued
• Monitor potassium level during treatment (3.5-5.0 mg/dl is normal level)
• Monitor hydration status, I&O ratio; watch for decreased urinary output; notify prescriber immediately; check urinary pH in patients receiving the product as a urinary acidifier
• Assess cardiac status: rate, rhythm, CVP, PWP, PAWP if being monitored directly

Nursing diagnoses
• Knowledge, deficient (teaching)
• Nutrition: less than body requirements, imbalanced (uses)

Patient/family education
• Teach patient to eat foods rich in potassium after medication is discontinued
• Advise patient to avoid OTC products: antacids, salt substitutes, analgesics, vit preparations, unless specifically directed by prescriber; avoid licorice in large amounts, may cause hypokalemia, sodium retention
• Advise patient to report hyperkalemia symptoms or continued hypokalemia symptoms
• Tell patient to take cap with full glass of liquid; to dissolve powder or tab completely in at least 120 ml of water or juice; not to crush, chew caps or tabs
• Emphasize importance of regular follow-up and periodic potassium levels

Evaluation
Positive therapeutic outcome
• Absence of fatigue, muscle weakness, and decreased thirst and urinary output, cardiac changes
• Potassium level normal

pramipexole (Rx)
(pra-mi-pex′ol)
Mirapex, Mirapex ER
Func. class.: Antiparkinsonian agent
Chem. class.: Dopamine receptor agonist, nonergot
Pregnancy category C

ACTION: Selective agonist for D_2 receptors (presynaptic/postsynaptic sites); binding at D_3 receptor contributes to antiparkinson effects

Therapeutic outcome: Decreased symptoms of Parkinson's disease (involuntary movements)

USES: Idiopathic Parkinson's disease, restless leg syndrome

CONTRAINDICATIONS: Hypersensitivity

Precautions: Pregnancy **C,** renal/cardiac disease, MI with dysrhythmias, affective disorders, psychosis, preexisting dyskinesias, history of falling asleep during daily activities

DOSAGE AND ROUTES
Initial treatment
Adult: PO from a starting dose of 0.375 mg/day given in 3 divided doses, increase gradually by 0.125 mg/dose at 5-7–day intervals until total daily dose of 4.5 mg is reached; ER 0.375 mg qd, may increase up to 0.75 mg/day, then increments of 0.75 mg/day ≤5-7 days, max 4.5 mg/day

Restless leg syndrome
Adult: PO 0.125 mg 2-3 hr before bedtime, increase gradually, max 0.5 mg/day

Renal dose
Adult: PO CCr 35-59 ml/min 0.125 mg bid, may increase q5-7day to 1.5 mg bid; CCr 15-34 ml/min 0.125 mg/day, may increase q5-7day to 1.5 mg/day

Available forms: Tabs 0.125, 0.25, 0.5, 1, 1.5 mg; cap ER 0.375, 0.75, 1.5, 3.0, 4.5 mg

Implementation
• Adjust dosage to patient's response
• Give with meals to decrease GI upset

ADVERSE EFFECTS
CNS: *Agitation, insomnia,* psychosis, hallucinations, depression, dizziness, headache, confusion, amnesia, dream disorder, asthenia,

dyskinesia, hypersomnolence, sudden sleep onset, impulse-control disorders
CV: *Orthostatic hypotension,* edema, syncope, tachycardia
EENT: Blurred vision
GI: *Nausea, anorexia,* constipation, dysphagia, dry mouth
GU: Impotence, urinary frequency
HEMA: Hemolytic anemia, leukopenia, agranulocytosis

Pharmacokinetics

Absorption	Well absorbed
Distribution	Widely distributed
Metabolism	Liver, minimally
Excretion	Kidneys, unchanged
Half-life	8 hr; 12 hr in geriatric

Pharmacodynamics

Onset	Unknown
Peak	2 hr
Duration	Unknown

INTERACTIONS

Individual drugs
Cimetidine, diltiazem, levodopa, quiNIDine, ranitidine, triamterine, verapamil: increased pramipexole levels
Metoclopramide: decreased pramipexole levels

Drug classifications
Butyrophenones, DOPamine agonists, phenothiazines: decreased pramipexole effect

NURSING CONSIDERATIONS

Assessment
• Monitor B/P, ECG, respiration during initial treatment; hypo/hypertension should be reported
• Assess mental status: affect, mood, behavioral changes, depression; complete suicide assessment
• Assess for involuntary movements in parkinsonism: akinesia, tremors, staggering gait, muscle rigidity, drooling; these symptoms should improve with therapy
⚠ **Assess for sleep attacks: may fall asleep during activities, without warning; may need to discontinue medication**

Nursing diagnoses
• Injury, risk for (uses)
• Knowledge, deficient (teaching)
• Mobility, impaired physical (uses)
• Noncompliance (teaching)

Patient/family education
• Advise patient that therapeutic effects may take several wk to a few mo
• Caution patient to change positions slowly to prevent orthostatic hypotension
• Instruct patient to use product exactly as prescribed; if product is discontinued abruptly, parkinsonian crisis may occur; if treatment is to be discontinued, taper over 1 wk; avoid alcohol, OTC sleeping products
• Advise patient to notify prescriber if pregnancy is planned or suspected

Evaluation
Positive therapeutic outcome
• Decreased akathisia, other involuntary movements
• Improved mood

pramlintide (Rx)
(pram′lin-tide)
Symlin
Func. class.: Antidiabetic
Chem. class.: Synthetic human amylin analog
Pregnancy category C

ACTION: Modulates and slows stomach emptying, prevents postprandial rise in plasma glucagon, decreases appetite, leads to decreased caloric intake and weight loss

Therapeutic outcome: Decreased polyuria, polydipsia, polyphagia; improved A1c

USES: As an adjunct to insulin therapy with uncontrolled type 1 or type 2 diabetes mellitus

CONTRAINDICATIONS:
Hypersensitivity to this product or cresol, gastroparesis

> **BLACK BOX WARNING:** Hypoglycemia

Precautions: Pregnancy **C,** breastfeeding

DOSAGE AND ROUTES

Type 1 diabetes
Adult: SUBCUT prior to each meal ($\geq$30 g CHO), titrate up from 15 mcg to target dose of 60 mcg/dose, each dose titration should occur after no nausea for 3 days

Type 2 diabetes
Adult: SUBCUT 60 mcg prior to each meal ($\geq$30 g CHO), titrate up to 120 mcg SUBCUT with each meal after no nausea for 3-7 days

Available forms: Inj 5-ml vials (0.6 mg/ml)

Implementation
• Pre-meal insulin should be decreased by 50% when starting and adjusted to therapeutic dose to prevent hypoglycemia

SUBCUT route
• Rotate inj sites, allow sol to warm to room temp before use
• Give immediately before mealtime or if 30 g of carbohydrates will be consumed
• Do not use if a meal is skipped
• Do not use if discolored; do not give in arm; absorption is variable
• Store at room temperature for up to 30 days; keep away from heat and sunlight; refrigerate all other supply

Syringe compatibilities: Do not mix with insulin, give separately

ADVERSE EFFECTS
CNS: *Headache,* fatigue, dizziness
GI: *Nausea, vomiting, anorexia,* abdominal pain
INTEG: Inj site reactions
META: Hypoglycemia
MS: Arthralgia
RESP: *Cough,* pharyngitis
SYST: *Systemic allergy*

Pharmacokinetics

Absorption	30%-40%
Distribution	Not bound to blood cells or albumin, 40% bound in plasma
Metabolism	Kidneys
Excretion	Unknown
Half-life	48 min

Pharmacodynamics

Onset	Unknown
Peak	20 min
Duration	3 hr

INTERACTIONS
Individual drugs
Acetaminophen: may increase effect of acetaminophen
Alcohol, disopyramide, insulin: increased hypoglycemia
Dextrothyroxine, niacin, triamterene: decreased hypoglycemia
Diphenoxylate, loperamide, octreotide: increased pramlintide action
Erythromycin, metoclopramide: do not use

Drug classifications
ACE inhibitors, anabolic steroids, androgens, corticosteroids, fibric acid derivatives: increased hypoglycemia
α-Glucosidase inhibitors, antimuscarinics, opiate agonist, tricyclics: increased pramlintide action
Estrogens, MAOIs, oral contraceptives, progestins, thiazide diuretics: decreased hypoglycemia
Phenothiazines: increased hyperglycemia

NURSING CONSIDERATIONS
Assessment
• Monitor fasting blood glucose, 2 hr postprandial (80-150 mg/dl, normal fasting level; 70-130 mg/dl, normal 2 hr level); A1c may also be drawn to identify treatment effectiveness; also monitor weight, appetite
• **Assess for hypoglycemic reaction** (sweating, weakness, dizziness, chills, confusion, headache, nausea, rapid weak pulse, fatigue, tachycardia, memory lapses, slurred speech, staggering gait, anxiety, tremors, hunger)
• **Assess for hyperglycemia:** acetone breath, polyuria, fatigue, polydipsia, flushed, dry skin, lethargy

Nursing diagnoses
• Injury, risk for (uses)
• Knowledge, deficient (teaching)
• Noncompliance (teaching)

Patient/family education
• Advise patient that product does not cure diabetes but controls symptoms
• Advise patient to carry emergency ID as diabetic
• Teach patient to recognize hypoglycemia reaction: headache, fatigue, weakness
• Teach patient the dosage, route, mixing instructions, if any diet restrictions, disease process
• Advise patient to carry a glucose source (candy or lump sugar) to treat hypoglycemia
• Teach patient symptoms of ketoacidosis: nausea, thirst, polyuria, dry mouth, decreased B/P, dry, flushed skin, acetone breath, drowsiness, Kussmaul respirations
• Advise patient that a plan is necessary for diet, exercise; all food on diet should be eaten; exercise routine should not vary
• Teach patient about blood glucose testing; make sure patient is able to determine glucose level
• Advise patient to avoid OTC products unless directed by prescriber, avoid alcohol

P

• Advise patient not to operate machinery or drive until effect is known

Evaluation
Positive therapeutic outcome
• Decrease in polyuria, polydipsia, polyphagia, clear sensorium; improved A1c, blood glucose; absence of dizziness; stable gait

TREATMENT OF OVERDOSE:
Glucose 25 g **IV**, via dextrose 50% sol, 50 ml or glucagon 1 mg SUBCUT

pramoxine topical
See Appendix B

prasugrel (Rx)
(pra′soo-grel)
Effient
Func. class.: Platelet aggregation inhibitor
Chem. class.: ADP receptor antagonist
Pregnancy category B

ACTION: Inhibits ADP-induced platelet aggregation

Therapeutic outcome: Absence of MI, stroke

USES: Reducing the risk of stroke, MI, vascular death, peripheral arterial disease in high-risk patients

CONTRAINDICATIONS:
Hypersensitivity, stroke, TIA

> **BLACK BOX WARNING:** Active bleeding

Precautions: Pregnancy **B**, breastfeeding, children, hepatic disease, increased bleeding risk, neutropenia, agranulocytosis, renal disease, surgery, trauma, thrombotic thrombocytopenia purpura, Asian patients, weight <60 kg, CABG, geriatric
Abrupt discontinuation

DOSAGE AND ROUTES
Adult/geriatric <75 yr and ≥60 kg: PO 60 mg loading dose, then 10 mg qd with aspirin (75-325 mg/day)
Adult/geriatric <75 yr and <60 kg: PO 60 mg loading dose, then 5 mg qd
Geriatric >75 yr: Not recommended

Available forms: Tabs 5, 10 mg

Implementation
• Give with food to decrease gastric symptoms
• Do not break tablets
• Do not discontinue therapy abruptly

ADVERSE EFFECTS
CNS: Headache, dizziness
CV: Edema, atrial fibrillation, bradycardia, chest pain, hyper/hypotension
GI: Nausea, vomiting, diarrhea
HEMA: Epistaxis, **leukopenia, thrombocytopenia, neutropenia, anaphylaxis, angioedema, anemia**
INTEG: Rash, hypercholesterolemia
MISC: Fatigue, **intracranial hemorrhage, secondary malignancy**
MS: Back pain

Pharmacokinetics

Absorption	Rapidly absorbed
Distribution	Unknown
Metabolism	Liver CYP3A4, CYP2B6
Excretion	Urine, feces
Half-life	7-8 hr

Pharmacodynamics

Onset	Unknown
Peak	30 min
Duration	Unknown

INTERACTIONS
Individual drugs
Abciximab, aspirin, eptifibatide, rifampin, tirofiban, ticlopidine, treprostinil: increased bleeding risk

Drug classifications
Anticoagulants, thrombolytics, NSAIDs, SSRIs: increased bleeding risk

NURSING CONSIDERATIONS
Assessment:
⚠ **Assess for thrombotic/thrombocytic purpura: fever, thrombocytopenia, neurolytic anemia**
• Monitor hepatic studies: AST, ALT, bilirubin, creatinine (long-term therapy)
• Monitor blood studies: CBC, differential, Hct, Hgb, PT, cholesterol (long-term therapy)

Nursing diagnoses
• Injury, risk for (uses)
• Knowledge, deficient (teaching)

Patient/family education
• Advise that blood work will be necessary during treatment

• Teach to report any unusual bruising, bleeding to prescriber; that it may take longer to stop bleeding
• Advise to take with food or just after eating to minimize GI discomfort
• Advise to report diarrhea, skin rashes, subcutaneous bleeding, chills, fever, sore throat
• Teach to tell all health care providers that prasugrel is used; may be withheld before surgery

Evaluation
Positive therapeutic outcome
• Absence of stroke, MI

---

pravastatin (Rx)
(pra'va-sta-tin)
Pravachol
Func. class.: Antilipidemic
Pregnancy category X

Do not confuse:
Pravachol/Prevacid

ACTION: Inhibits biosynthesis of VLDL, LDL, which are responsible for cholesterol development, by inhibiting the enzyme HMG-CoA reductase

Therapeutic outcome: Decreasing cholesterol levels and LDL, increased HDL

USES: As an adjunct in primary hypercholesterolemia types IIa, IIb, III, IV, artherosclerosis; to reduce the risk of recurrent MI, primary/secondary CV events; reduce stroke, TIAs

CONTRAINDICATIONS:
Pregnancy **X,** breastfeeding, hypersensitivity, active liver disease

Precautions: Past liver disease, alcoholism, severe acute infections, trauma, severe metabolic disorders, electrolyte imbalances

DOSAGE AND ROUTES
Adult: PO 40-80 mg/day at bedtime (range 20-80 mg/day), start at 10 mg/day if also on immunosuppressants
Adolescent 14-18 yr: PO 40 mg/day
Child 8-13 yr: PO 20 mg/day
Geriatric/renal/hepatic dose: PO 10 mg/day, initially

Renal dose
Adult: PO 10-20 mg daily at bedtime, increase at 4-wk intervals

Available forms: Tabs 10, 20, 40, 80 mg
Implementation
• Give at bedtime only; give 1 hr before or 2 hr after bile acid sequestrants
• Store in cool environment in airtight, light-resistant container

ADVERSE EFFECTS
CNS: Headache, dizziness, fatigue
CV: Chest pain
EENT: Lens opacities
GI: Nausea, constipation, diarrhea, flatus, abdominal pain, heartburn, **liver dysfunction, pancreatitis, hepatitis**
GU: Renal failure (myoglobinuria)
INTEG: Rash, pruritus
MS: Muscle cramps, myalgia, **myositis, rhabdomyolysis**
RESP: Common cold, rhinitis, cough

Pharmacokinetics
Absorption	Poorly absorbed, erratic
Distribution	Protein binding 80%
Metabolism	Liver, extensively
Excretion	Feces (70%-75%); kidneys, unchanged (20%); breast milk (minimal)
Half-life	2 hr

Pharmacodynamics
Onset	Unknown
Peak	1-1$^{1}/_2$ hr
Duration	Unknown

INTERACTIONS
Individual drugs
Clarithromycin, clofibrate, cycloSPORINE, erythromycin, gemfibrozil, itraconazole, niacin: increased risk for myopathy

Drug classifications
Bile acid sequestrants: decreased pravastatin bioavailability
Protease inhibitors: increased risk of myopathy

Drug/herb
St. John's wort: decreased effect
Red yeast rice: increased adverse reactions
Eucalyptus: increased hepatotoxicity

Drug/lab test
Increased: CPK, liver function tests
Altered: thyroid function tests

NURSING CONSIDERATIONS
Assessment
• Assess nutrition: fat, protein, carbohydrates; nutritional analysis should be completed by dietitian before treatment
• Monitor triglycerides, esterol, cholesterol at baseline, throughout treatment; LDL and HDL should be watched closely; if increased, product should be discontinued
⚠ **Rhabdomyolysis: assess for muscle tenderness, pain; obtain CPK; therapy should be discontinued**
• Monitor ophth status yearly

Nursing diagnoses
• Knowledge, deficient (teaching)
• Noncompliance (teaching)

Patient/family education
• Inform patient that compliance is needed for positive results to occur; not to double doses or skip doses
• Teach patient that risk factors should be decreased: high-fat diet, smoking, alcohol consumption, absence of exercise
• Advise patient to notify prescriber of weakness, tenderness, or limited mobility, blurred vision, severe GI symptoms, dizziness, headache, muscle pain, fever
⚠ **Explain to patient that contraception is necessary, since product produces teratogenic effects, pregnancy X, not to breastfeed**
• Advise patient to use sunscreen, protective clothing to prevent burns

Evaluation
Positive therapeutic outcome
• Decreased cholesterol, serum triglyceride levels and improved ratio with HDL

---

prazosin (Rx)
(pra′zoe-sin)
Minipress
Func. class.: Antihypertensive
Chem. class.: α_1-Adrenergic blocker, peripheral
Pregnancy category C

ACTION: Blocks α-mediated vasoconstriction of adrenergic receptors, inducing peripheral vasodilatation

Therapeutic outcome: Decreased B/P in hypertension; decreased cardiac preload, afterload

USES: Hypertension

Unlabeled uses: Benign prostatic hypertrophy to decrease urine outflow obstruction, posttraumatic stress disorder (PTSD)

CONTRAINDICATIONS:
Hypersensitivity

Precautions: Pregnancy **C**, breastfeeding, children, geriatric patients, renal/hepatic disease, prostate cancer, ocular surgery, orthostatic hypotension

DOSAGE AND ROUTES
Hypertension
Adult: PO 1 mg bid or tid, increasing to 20 mg/day in divided doses if required, usual range 6-15 mg/day; max 1 mg initially, max 20-40 mg/day
Child: PO 5 mcg/kg q6hr; max 400 mcg/kg/day or 15 mg/day

Benign prostatic hyperplasia (unlabeled)
Adult: PO 2 mg bid

Available forms: Caps 1, 2, 5 mg

Implementation
• Severe hypotension may occur after first dose of this medication; hypotension may be prevented by reducing or discontinuing diuretic therapy 3 days before beginning prazosin therapy
• Give same time each day
• Store in airtight container at 86° F (30° C) or less

ADVERSE EFFECTS
CNS: *Dizziness, headache, drowsiness,* anxiety, depression, vertigo, weakness, fatigue
CV: *Palpitations, orthostatic hypotension,* tachycardia, edema, rebound hypertension
EENT: Blurred vision, epistaxis, tinnitus, dry mouth, red sclera
GI: *Nausea,* vomiting, diarrhea, constipation, abdominal pain
GU: Urinary frequency, incontinence, impotence, priapism, water and sodium retention

Pharmacokinetics

Absorption	60%
Distribution	Widely distributed
Metabolism	Liver, extensively; protein binding 97%
Excretion	Kidneys, unchanged (10%); bile (90%)
Half-life	2-3 hr

Pharmacodynamics

Onset	2 hr
Peak	1-3 hr
Duration	6-12 hr

INTERACTIONS

Individual drugs
Alcohol, nitroglycerin: increased hypotension
CloNIDine: decreased antihypertensive effect

Drug classifications
Antihypertensives, β-adrenergic blockers, phosphodiesterase inhibitors (vardenafil, tadalafil, sildenafil), diuretics, MAOIs: increased hypotension
NSAIDs: decreased antihypertensive effect

Drug/herb
Hawthorn: increased antihypertensive effect

Drug/lab test
Increased: urinary norepinephrine, VMA

NURSING CONSIDERATIONS

Assessment
• **Hypertension/CHF:** Monitor B/P, orthostatic hypotension, syncope; check for edema in feet, legs daily; monitor I&O, weight daily; notify prescriber of changes
• Assess for allergic reactions: rash, fever, pruritus, urticaria; product should be discontinued if antihistamines fail to help
• Assess for orthostatic hypotension; tell patient to rise slowly from sitting or lying position

Nursing diagnoses
• Cardiac output, decreased (uses)
• Injury, risk for (adverse reactions)
• Knowledge, deficient (teaching)
• Noncompliance (teaching)

Patient/family education
• Instruct patient not to discontinue product abruptly; stress the importance of complying with dosage schedule, even if feeling better; if dose is missed, take as soon as remembered; take at same time each day
• Advise patient not to use OTC products (cough, cold, allergy) unless directed by prescriber; also to avoid large amounts of caffeine
• Emphasize the need to rise slowly to sitting or standing position to minimize orthostatic hypotension
• Teach patient to notify prescriber of mouth sores, sore throat, fever, swelling of hands or feet, irregular heartbeat, chest pain

• Caution patient to report excessive perspiration, dehydration, vomiting, diarrhea; may lead to fall in B/P
• Caution patient that product may cause dizziness, fainting, light-headedness; may occur during 1st few days of therapy; to avoid hazardous activities
• Teach patient how to take B/P and normal readings for age group; instruct to take B/P q7day

Evaluation
Positive therapeutic outcome
• Decreased B/P in hypertension

TREATMENT OF OVERDOSE:
Administer volume expanders or vasopressors, discontinue product, place patient in supine position

---

prednisoLONE (Rx)
(pred-niss'oh-lone)
Asmal Pred Plus, Millipred, Orapred, Orapred ODT, Prednoral, Prelone, Veripred
Func. class.: Corticosteroid, synthetic
Chem. class.: Intermediate-acting glucocorticoid
Pregnancy category C

Do not confuse:
prednisoLONE/predniSONE

ACTION: Decreases inflammation by suppressing migration of polymorphonuclear leukocytes, fibroblasts; reversal to increase capillary permeability and lysosomal stabilization

Therapeutic outcome: Decreased inflammation, decreased adrenal insufficiency

USES: Severe inflammation, immunosuppression, neoplasms

CONTRAINDICATIONS:
Child <2 yr, psychosis, hypersensitivity, idiopathic thrombocytopenia, acute glomerulonephritis, amebiasis, fungal infections, nonasthmatic bronchial disease, measles, varicella, Cushing's syndrome

Precautions: Pregnancy **C,** breastfeeding, children, diabetes mellitus, glaucoma, osteoporosis, seizure disorders, ulcerative colitis, CHF, myasthenia gravis

P

Adverse effects: *italics* = common; **bold** = life-threatening

DOSAGE AND ROUTES
Rheumatic disorders
Adult: PO 5-60 mg/day or in divided doses
Asthma/antiinflammatory
Adult: PO 40-80 mg/day in 1-2 divided doses
Child: PO 1 mg/kg/day in 2 divided doses

Available forms: Tabs 5 mg; syr 5 mg/5 ml, 15 mg/15 ml; oral liquid 5 mg/ml; tabs 1, 2.5, 5, 10, 20, 50 mg; oral sol 5 mg/ml, 5 mg/5 ml; syr 5 mg/5 ml; oral dissolving tab 10, 15, 30 mg

Implementation
• **Oral sol:** use calibrated measuring devices
• **Orally disintegrating tabs:** place on tongue, allow to dissolve, swallow; or swallow whole; do not cut, split

ADVERSE EFFECTS
CNS: *Depression,* flushing, sweating, headache, mood changes
CV: *Hypertension,* **circulatory collapse, thrombophlebitis, embolism,** tachycardia
EENT: Fungal infections, increased intraocular pressure, blurred vision
GI: *Diarrhea, nausea, abdominal distention,* **GI hemorrhage,** increased appetite, **pancreatitis**
HEMA: **Thrombocytopenia**
INTEG: Acne, poor wound healing, ecchymosis, petechiae
MS: Fractures, osteoporosis, weakness, arthralgia, myopathy, tendon rupture

Pharmacokinetics

Absorption	Well absorbed (PO, IM), completely absorbed (IV)
Distribution	Widely distributed, crosses placenta
Metabolism	Liver, extensively
Excretion	Kidney, breast milk
Half-life	2-4 hr

Pharmacodynamics

	PO	IM (phosphate)	IV	IA/IL
Onset	1 hr	Rapid	Rapid	Slow
Peak	2 hr	1 hr	Unknown	Unknown
Duration	1½ days	Unknown	Unknown	Up to 1 mo

INTERACTIONS
Individual drugs
Alcohol, amphotericin B, cycloSPORINE, digitalis, indomethacin: increased side effects
Ambenonium, isoniazid, neostigmine, somatrem: decreased effects of each specific product
Cholestyramine, colestipol, ePHEDrine, phenytoin, rifampin, theophylline: decreased action of prednisoLONE
Indomethacin, ketoconazole: increased action of prednisoLONE

Drug classifications
Antibiotics (macrolide), contraceptives (oral), estrogens, salicylates: increased action of prednisoLONE
Anticholinesterases, anticoagulants, anticonvulsants, antidiabetics, salicylates, toxoids, vaccines: decreased effects of each specific product
Barbiturates: decreased action of prednisoLONE
Diuretics, salicylates: increased side effects

Drug/lab test
Increased: cholesterol, sodium, blood glucose, uric acid, calcium, urine glucose
Decreased: calcium, potassium, T_4, T_3, thyroid ^{131}I uptake test, urine 17-OHCS, 17-KS, PBI
False negative: skin allergy tests

NURSING CONSIDERATIONS
Assessment
• Monitor potassium, blood glucose, urine glucose while patient is on long-term therapy; hypokalemia and hyperglycemia may occur
• Monitor weight daily; notify prescriber of weekly gain >5 lb; monitor I&O ratio; be alert for decreasing urinary output and increasing edema
• Monitor B/P q4hr, pulse; notify prescriber if chest pain occurs
• Monitor plasma cortisol levels during long-term therapy (normal level 138-635 nmol/L [SI units] when measured at 8 AM)
• Assess adrenal function periodically for hypothalamic-pituitary-adrenal axis suppression
• **Assess infection:** increased temp, WBC even after withdrawal of medication; product masks infection symptoms
• **Assess for potassium depletion:** paresthesias, fatigue, nausea, vomiting, depression, polyuria, dysrhythmias, weakness, edema, hypertension, cardiac symptoms
• **Adrenal insufficiency:** assess for nausea, vomiting, lethargy, restlessness, confusion

- Assess mental status: affect, mood, behavioral changes, aggression
- Monitor temp; if fever develops, product should be discontinued
- Assess for systemic absorption: increased temp, inflammation, irritation (topical)

Nursing diagnoses
- Infection, risk for (adverse reactions)
- Knowledge, deficient (teaching)
- Noncompliance (teaching)

Patient/family education
- Advise patient to carry/wear emergency ID as steroid user
- Advise patient to notify prescriber if therapeutic response decreases; dosage adjustment may be needed
- Caution patient not to discontinue abruptly; adrenal crisis can result; take exactly as prescribed
- Caution patient to avoid OTC products: salicylates, cough products with alcohol, cold preparations unless directed by prescriber
- Teach patient all aspects of product usage including cushingoid symptoms
- Teach patient symptoms of adrenal insufficiency: nausea, anorexia, fatigue, dizziness, dyspnea, weakness, joint pain
- Advise patient that long-term therapy may be needed to clear infection (1-2 mo depending on type of infection)

Evaluation
Positive therapeutic outcome
- Decreased inflammation

prednisoLONE ophthalmic
See Appendix B

predniSONE (Rx)
(pred'ni-sone)
Winpreo ✽
Func. class.: Corticosteroid
Chem. class.: Intermediate-acting glucocorticoid
Pregnancy category C

Do not confuse:
predniSONE/methylPREDNISolone/prednisoLONE/PriLOSEC

ACTION: Decreases inflammation by increasing capillary permeability and lysosomal stabilization, minimal mineralocorticoid activity

Therapeutic outcome: Decreased inflammation, decreased adrenal insufficiency

USES: Severe inflammation, immunosuppression, neoplasms, multiple sclerosis, collagen disorders, dermatologic disorders

CONTRAINDICATIONS:
Psychosis, hypersensitivity, idiopathic thrombocytopenia, acute glomerulonephritis, amebiasis, fungal infections, nonasthmatic bronchial disease, child <2 yr, AIDS, TB, measles

Precautions: Pregnancy C, diabetes mellitus, glaucoma, osteoporosis, seizure disorders, ulcerative colitis, CHF, myasthenia gravis, renal disease, esophagitis, peptic ulcer, cataracts, coagulopathy

DOSAGE AND ROUTES
Adult: PO 5-60 mg/day or divided bid-qid
Child: PO 0.05-2 mg/kg/day divided 1-4 ×/day

Nephrosis
Child: PO 2 mg/kg/day in divided doses, max 28 days, then 1-1.5 mg/kg/day every other day × 4 wk

Multiple sclerosis
Adult: PO 200 mg/day × 1 wk, then 80 mg every other day × 1 mo

Available forms: Tabs 1, 2.5, 5, 10, 20, 50 mg; oral sol 5 mg/5 ml; syr 5 mg/5 ml

Implementation
- Give with food or milk to decrease GI symptoms; use measuring device for liquid route
- For long-term use, alternative product therapy is recommended, to decrease adverse reactions

ADVERSE EFFECTS
CNS: Depression, flushing, sweating, headache, mood changes
CV: Hypertension, **circulatory collapse, thrombophlebitis, embolism,** tachycardia
EENT: Fungal infections, increased intraocular pressure, blurred vision
GI: Diarrhea, nausea, abdominal distention, **GI hemorrhage,** increased appetite, **pancreatitis**
HEMA: **Thrombocytopenia**
INTEG: Acne, poor wound healing, ecchymosis, petechiae
META: Hyperglycemia
MS: Fractures, osteoporosis, weakness

Pharmacokinetics

Pharmacokinetics

Absorption	Well absorbed
Distribution	Widely distributed, crosses placenta
Metabolism	Liver, extensively
Excretion	Kidney, breast milk
Half-life	3-4 hr

Pharmacodynamics

Onset	Unknown
Peak	1-2 hr
Duration	$1^1/_2$ days

INTERACTIONS

Individual drugs

Alcohol, amphotericin B, cycloSPORINE, digoxin: increased side effects

Ambenonium, isoniazid, neostigmine, sometrem: decreased effects of each specific product

Cholestyramine, colestipol, ePHEDrine, phenytoin, rifampin, theophylline: decreased action of predniSONE

Indomethacin: increased side effects, increased action of predniSONE

Ketoconazole: increased action of predniSONE

Drug classifications

Anticholinesterases, anticoagulants, anticonvulsants, antidiabetics, toxoids, vaccines: decreased effects of each specific product

Antiinfectives (macrolide), contraceptives (oral), estrogens: increased action of predniSONE

Barbiturates: decreased action of predniSONE

Diuretics: increased side effects

Salicylates: increased side effects, increased action of predniSONE, decreased effects of salicylates

Drug/herb

Ephedra (ma huang): decreased predniSONE effect

Drug/lab test

Increased: cholesterol, sodium, blood glucose, uric acid, calcium, urine glucose

Decreased: calcium, potassium, T_4, T_3, thyroid ^{131}I uptake test, urine 17-OHCS, 17-KS, PBI

False negative: skin allergy tests

NURSING CONSIDERATIONS

Assessment

• **Adrenal insufficiency:** assess for nausea, vomiting, anorexia, confusion, hypotension, weight loss before and during treatment; HPA suppression may be precipitated by abrupt withdrawal

• Monitor potassium, blood glucose, urine glucose while on long-term therapy; hypokalemia and hyperglycemia may occur

• Monitor weight daily; notify prescriber of weekly gain >5 lb; monitor I&O ratio; be alert for decreasing urinary output and increasing edema

• Monitor B/P q4hr, pulse; notify prescriber if chest pain occurs

• Monitor plasma cortisol levels during long-term therapy (normal level 138-635 nmol/L when measured at 8 AM)

• Assess adrenal function periodically for hypothalamic-pituitary-adrenal axis suppression

• **Assess infection:** increased temp, WBC even after withdrawal of medication; product masks infection symptoms

• **Assess for potassium depletion:** paresthesias, fatigue, nausea, vomiting, depression, polyuria, dysrhythmias, weakness, edema, hypertension, cardiac symptoms

• Assess mental status: affect, mood, behavioral changes, aggression

• Monitor temp; if fever develops, product should be discontinued

• Assess for systemic absorption: increased temp, inflammation, irritation (topical)

Nursing diagnoses

• Infection, risk for (adverse reactions)
• Knowledge, deficient (teaching)
• Noncompliance (teaching)

Patient/family education

• Advise patient that emergency ID as corticosteroid user should be carried or worn

• Advise patient to notify prescriber if therapeutic response decreases; dosage adjustment may be needed

⚠ **Caution patient not to discontinue abruptly; adrenal crisis can result**

• Caution patient to avoid OTC products: salicylates, cough products with alcohol, cold preparations unless directed by prescriber

• Teach patient all aspects of product use including cushingoid symptoms

• Teach patient symptoms of adrenal insufficiency: nausea, anorexia, fatigue, dizziness, dyspnea, weakness, joint pain

• Advise patient that long-term therapy may be needed to clear infection (1-2 mo depending on type of infection)

Evaluation

Positive therapeutic outcome

• Decreased inflammation

pregabalin (Rx)

(pre-gab'a-lin)
Lyrica
Func. class.: Anticonvulsant
Pregnancy category C
Controlled substance schedule V

ACTION: Binds to high-voltage–gated calcium channels in CNS tissues; this may lead to anticonvulsant action, similar to the inhibitory neurotransmitter GABA; anxiolytic, analgesic, and antiepileptic properties

Therapeutic outcome: Decreased seizure activity, decreased neuropathic pain

USES: Neuropathic pain associated with diabetic peripheral neuropathy, partial-onset seizures, postherpetic neuralgia, fibromyalgia

Unlabeled uses: Moderate pain, social anxiety disorder

CONTRAINDICATIONS:

Hypersensitivity, abrupt discontinuation

Precautions: Pregnancy **C**, breastfeeding, children <12 yr, geriatric, renal disease, PR interval prolongation, creatine kinase elevations, CHF (class III, IV), decreased platelets, drug abuse, dependence, glaucoma, myopathy, angioedema history, suicidal behavior

DOSAGE AND ROUTES

Diabetic peripheral neuropathic pain

Adult: PO 50 mg tid, may increase to 300 mg/day (max) within 1 wk, adjust in renal disease

Partial onset seizures

Adult: PO 75 mg bid or 50 mg tid; may increase to 600 mg/day (max)

Postherpetic neuralgia

Adult: 150 mg/day in 2-3 doses, may increase to 300 mg/day in 2-3 divided doses, if higher dose is needed in 2-4 wk, may increase to 600 mg/day in 2-3 divided doses

Fibromyalgia

Adult: PO 75 mg bid, may increase to 150 mg bid within 1 wk and 225 mg bid after 1 wk

Renal dose

PO CCr 30-60 ml/min 75-300 mg/day in 2-3 divided doses; CCr 15-30 ml/min 25-150 mg/day in 1-2 divided doses, CCr <15 ml/min 25-75 mg/day in a single dose

Available forms: Caps 25, 50, 75, 100, 150, 200, 225, 300 mg

Implementation

• Do not crush or chew caps; caps may be opened and contents put in applesauce or dissolved in juice
• Give without regard to meals
• Gradually withdraw over 7 days; abrupt withdrawal may precipitate seizures
• Store at room temperature away from heat and light
• Give hard candy, frequent rinsing of mouth, gum for dry mouth
• Provide assistance with ambulation during early part of treatment; dizziness occurs
• Provide seizure precautions: padded side rails; move objects that may harm patient
• Provide increased fluids, bulk in diet for constipation

ADVERSE EFFECTS

CNS: Dizziness, fatigue, confusion, euphoria, incoordination, nervousness, neuropathy, tremor, vertigo, somnolence, ataxia, amnesia, abnormal thinking
EENT: Dry mouth, blurred vision, nystagmus, amblyopia, sinusitis
GI: Constipation, flatulence, abdominal pain, weight gain
HEMA: Ecchymosis, **thrombocytopenia**
MS: Back pain, **rhabdomyolysis,** myopathy
MISC: Pruritus, orgasm/erectile dysfunction, peripheral edema, **angioedema, suicidal ideation**
RESP: Dyspnea

Pharmacokinetics

Absorption	Well absorbed, decreased by food
Distribution	Not bound to plasma proteins
Metabolism	Negligible
Excretion	90% unchanged, urine
Half-life	6 hr

Pharmacodynamics

Onset	Unknown
Peak	1.5 hr
Duration	Unknown

INTERACTIONS

Individual drugs

Alcohol: increased CNS depression

Drug classifications
Anxiolytics, barbiturates, general anesthetics, hypnotics, opiate agonists, phenothiazines, sedating H₁ blockers, sedatives, thiazolidinediones, tricyclics: increased CNS depression
Thiazolidinediones: increased weight gain/fluid retention; avoid use if possible

Drug/lab test
Increased: creatine kinase
Decreased: platelets

NURSING CONSIDERATIONS
Assessment
• Assess for seizures: aura, location, duration, activity at onset
• **Assess for pain:** location, duration, characteristics if using for diabetic neuropathy
• Monitor renal function tests: urinalysis, BUN, urine creatinine q3mo, creatine kinase; if markedly increased, discontinue
• Assess mental status: mood, sensorium, affect, behavioral changes, suicidal thoughts, behavior; if mental status changes, notify prescriber

Nursing diagnoses
• Knowledge, deficient (teaching)
• Pain, chronic (uses)

Patient/family education
• Advise patient to carry emergency ID stating patient's name, products taken, condition, prescriber's name and phone number
• Advise patient to avoid driving, other activities that require alertness: dizziness, drowsiness may occur
• Teach patient not to discontinue medication quickly after long-term use, taper over ≥1 wk; withdrawal-precipitated seizures may occur, not to double doses if dose is missed, take if 2 hr or more before next dose
• Teach patient to notify prescriber if pregnancy is planned or suspected; avoid breastfeeding
• Teach patient to report muscle pain, tenderness, weakness, when accompanied by fever, malaise
• Advise patient to avoid alcohol

Evaluation
Positive therapeutic outcome
• Decreased seizure activity; decrease in neuropathic pain

TREATMENT OF OVERDOSE:
Lavage, VS, hemodialysis

---

primidone (Rx)
(pri′mi-done)
Mysoline, Sertan ✤
Func. class.: Anticonvulsant
Chem. class.: Barbiturate derivative
Pregnancy category D

ACTION: Raises seizure threshold by conversion of product to phenobarbital; decreases neuron firing

Therapeutic outcome: Reduction in seizure activity

USES: Generalized tonic-clonic (grand mal), complex

CONTRAINDICATIONS:
Pregnancy **D**, hypersensitivity, porphyria, hepatic encephalopathy, breastfeeding

Precautions: COPD, renal/hepatic disease, hyperactive children, suicidal ideation/behavior

DOSAGE AND ROUTES
Adult and child >8 yr: PO 125-250 mg at bedtime, increase by 125-250 mg/day q3-7days, usual dose 750-1500 mg/day in 3-4 divided doses, max 2 g/day in divided doses
Child <8 yr: PO 50-125 mg at bedtime, increase by 50-125 mg/day q3-7day, usual dose 10-25 mg/kg/day in 3-4 divided doses

Neonate: PO 12-20 mg/kg/day in 2-4 divided doses, start at lower dose and titrate

Renal dose
Adult: CCr 10-15 ml/min: increase interval between doses to 8-12 hr; CCr <10 ml/min: increase interval to 12-24 hr

Available forms: Tabs 50, 250 mg; susp 250 mg/5 ml ✤; chew tabs 125 mg ✤

Implementation
• May give with food to decrease gastric irritation
• May crush tab and mix with food or fluid

ADVERSE EFFECTS
CNS: *Stimulation, drowsiness,* irritability, fatigue, emotional disturbances, mood changes, paranoia, psychosis, ataxia, *vertigo,* **suicidal ideation**
EENT: Diplopia, nystagmus, edema of eyelids
GI: *Nausea, vomiting, anorexia,* **hepatitis**
GU: Impotence
HEMA: **Thrombocytopenia, leukopenia, neutropenia, eosinophilia, megaloblastic**

---

anemia, decreased serum folate level, lymphadenopathy
INTEG: Rash, edema, alopecia, lupuslike syndrome

Pharmacokinetics

Absorption	60%-80%
Distribution	Widely distributed, crosses placenta
Metabolism	Liver, converted to phenobarbital + PEMA
Excretion	Kidneys, breast milk
Half-life	3-12 hr

Pharmacodynamics

Onset	Unknown
Peak	4 hr
Duration	Unknown

INTERACTIONS

Individual drugs

Acebutolol, lamotrigine, metoprolol, propranolol: decreased effectiveness

Acetazolamide, carBAMazepine: decreased primidone levels

Alcohol, heparin, isoniazid, nicotinamide, phenytoin: increased primidone levels

Drug classifications

Antidepressants (tricyclic), oral contraceptives, phenothiazines: decreased effectiveness

CNS depressants: increased primidone levels

CYP3A4 inducers (barbiturates, carBAMazepine, efavirenz, nevirapine), phenytoins: decreased primidone effect

CYP3A4 inhibitors (aprepitant, antiretroviral protease inhibitors, delavirdine, fluconazole, imatinib, voriconazole): increased toxicity

Succinimides: decreased primidone levels

Drug/herb

Ginkgo: increased effect

Ginseng, santonica: decreased effect

Kava, St. John's wort, valerian: avoid use

NURSING CONSIDERATIONS

Assessment

• Assess mental status: mood, sensorium, affect, memory (long, short), especially geriatric; suicidal thoughts/behavior

• Assess for blood dyscrasias: fever, sore throat, bruising, rash, jaundice, epistaxis (long-term treatment only)

• **Assess seizure activity** including type, location, duration, and character; provide seizure precaution

• Assess renal function tests: urinalysis, BUN, urine creatinine

• Monitor blood studies: RBC, Hct, Hgb, reticulocyte counts weekly for 4 wk then monthly

• Monitor liver function tests: ALT, AST, bilirubin, creatinine

• Monitor product levels during initial treatment: therapeutic level 5-15 mcg/ml; CBC, LFTs should be done q6mo

• Assess for signs of physical withdrawal if medication is suddenly discontinued

• Assess eye problems: need for ophth exam before, during, after treatment (slit lamp, funduscopy, tonometry)

• Assess allergic reaction: red raised rash; if this occurs, product should be discontinued

• Monitor for toxicity: bone marrow depression, nausea, vomiting, ataxia, diplopia, CV collapse

Nursing diagnoses

• Injury, risk for (side effects)
• Knowledge, deficient (teaching)

Patient/family education

• Teach patient to carry/wear emergency ID stating name, products taken, condition, prescriber's name, phone number

• Advise patient to avoid driving and other activities that require alertness

• Caution patient to avoid alcohol and CNS depressants; increased sedation may occur

• Teach patient not to discontinue medication quickly after long-term use; taper off over several wk

Evaluation
Positive therapeutic outcome
• Decreased seizure activity

---

procainamide (Rx)
(proe′kane-ah-mide)
Func. class.: Antidysrhythmic (class IA)
Chem. class.: Procaine HCl amide analog
Pregnancy category C

ACTION: Depresses excitability of cardiac muscle to electrical stimulation and slows conduction velocity in atrium, bundle of His, ventricle; increases refractory period

Therapeutic outcome: Prevention of dysrhythmias

USES: Life-threatening ventricular dysrhythmias

CONTRAINDICATIONS:
Hypersensitivity, severe heart block, torsades de pointes

> **BLACK BOX WARNING:** Lupus erythromatosis

Precautions: Pregnancy **C**, breastfeeding, children, renal/hepatic disease, CHF, respiratory depression, cytopenia, dysrhythmia associated with digoxin toxicity, myasthenia gravis, digoxin toxicity

> **BLACK BOX WARNING:** Bone marrow failure, cardiac arrhythmias

DOSAGE AND ROUTES
Ventricular tachycardia during CPR
Adult: IV loading dose 20 mg/min; either ventricular tachycardia resolves or patient becomes hypotensive; the QRS complex is widened by 50% of original width or total is 17 mg/kg (1.2 g for a 70 kg patient); may give up to 50 mg/min in urgent situations; maintenance 1-4 mg/min CONT IV INF; IM 50 mg/kg/day in divided doses q3-6hr
Child: IV PALS 15 mg/kg over 30-60 min

Renal dose
Adult: **IV** CCr 35-59 ml/min give 70% of maintenance dose; CCr 15-34 ml/min give 40%-60% maintenance dose; CCr <15 ml/min individualized

Available forms: inj 100, 500 mg/ml

Implementation
IM route
• IM inj in deltoid; aspirate to avoid intravascular administration, use only when unable to use IV

Direct IV route
• Dilute each 100 mg/10 ml of 0.9% NaCl, give at max 50 mg/min

Intermittent INF route
• Dilute 0.2-1 g/50-500 ml of D$_5$W (2-4 mg/ml) give over 30-60 min at max 25-50 mg/min, use inf pump

Y-site compatibilities: Alfentanil, amikacin, aminocaproic acid, aminophylline, amiodarone, amphotericin B lipid complex, amphotericin B liposome, anidulafungin, ascorbic acid, atenolol, atracurium, atropine, aztreonam, benztropine, bivalirudin, bleomycin, bumetanide, buprenorphine, butorphanol, calcium chloride/gluconate, caspofungin, ceFAZolin, cefmetazole, cefonicid, cefoperazone, cefotaxime, cefotetan, cefoxitin, ceftazidime, cefTRIAXone, cefuroxime, cephalothin, chlorproMAZINE, cimetidine, cisatracurium, CISplatin, clindamycin, cyanocobalamin, cyclophosphamide, cycloSPORINE, cytarabine, DACTINomycin, DAPTOmycin, dexamethasone, digoxin, diphenhydrAMINE, DOBUTamine, docetaxel, DOPamine, doxacurium, DOXOrubicin, doxycycline, enalaprilat, ePHEDrine, EPINEPHrine, epirubicin, epoetin alfa, eptifibatide, ertapenem, erythromycin, esmolol, etoposide, etoposide phosphate, famotidine, fenoldopam, fentaNYL, fluconazole, fludarabine, fluorouracil, folic acid, furosemide, gatifloxacin, gemcitabine, gentamicin, glycopyrrolate, granisetron, heparin, hydrocortisone, HYDROmorphone, IDArubicin, ifosfamide, indomethacin, insulin (regular), irinotecan, isoproterenol, ketorolac, labetalol, lidocaine, linezolid, LORazepam, magnesium sulfate, mannitol, mechlorethamine, meperidine, metaraminol, methicillin, methotrexate, methoxamine, methyldopate, methylPREDNISolone, metoclopramide, metoprolol, mezlocillin, miconazole, midazolam, mitoxantrone, morphine, moxalactam, multiple vitamins, mycophenolate, nafcillin, nalbuphine, naloxone, netilmicin, nitroglycerin, nitroprusside, norepinephrine, octreotide, ondansetron, oxacillin, oxaliplatin, oxytocin, paclitaxel, palonosetron, pamidronate, pancuronium, pantoprazole, papaverine, pemetrexed, penicillin G potassium/sodium, pentamidine, pentazocine, PENTobarbital, PHENobarbital, phenylephrine, phytonadione, piperacillin, piperacillin-tazobactam, polymyxin B, potassium chloride, prochlorperazine, promethazine, propranolol, protamine, pyridoxine, quiNIDine, quinupristin-dalfopristin, ranitidine, remifentanil, ritodrine, rocuronium, sodium bicarbonate, succinylcholine, SUFentanil, tacrolimus, teniposide, theophylline, thiamine, thiotepa, ticarcillin, ticarcillin-clavulanate, tigecycline, tirofiban, tobramycin, tolazoline, trimetaphan, urokinase, vancomycin, vasopressin, vecuronium, verapamil, vinCRIStine, vinorelbine, vitamin B complex/C, voriconazole, zoledronic acid

Y-site incompatibilities: Milrinone

ADVERSE EFFECTS
CNS: *Headache, dizziness,* confusion, psychosis, restlessness, irritability, weakness, depression
CV: *Hypotension,* **heart block, cardiovascular collapse, arrest, torsades de pointes**
GI: Nausea, vomiting, anorexia, diarrhea, hepatomegaly, pain, bitter taste

HEMA: Systemic lupus erythematosus syndrome, **agranulocytosis, thrombocytopenia, neutropenia, hemolytic anemia**
INTEG: Rash, urticaria, edema, swelling (rare), pruritus, flushing, **angioedema**
SYST: SLE

Pharmacokinetics

Absorption	Well absorbed
Distribution	Rapidly distributed, protein binding 15%
Metabolism	Liver
Excretion	Kidneys, unchanged (50%-70%)
Half-life	$2^{1}/_{2}$-$4^{1}/_{2}$ hr; increased in renal disease

Pharmacodynamics

	IV
Onset	Rapid
Peak	$^{1}/_{2}$-1 hr
Duration	3-4 hr

INTERACTIONS
Individual drugs
Cimetidine, quiNIDine, ranitidine, trimethoprim: increased procainamide effect
Thioridazine: increased toxicity

Drug classifications
Antidysrhythmics, quinolones: increased toxicity
β-Adrenergic blockers: increased procainamide effects
Neuromuscular blockers: increased neuromuscular blocking effect

Drug/lab test
Increased: ALT, AST, alkaline phosphatase, LDH, bilirubin

NURSING CONSIDERATIONS
Assessment
• Assess for oxygenation or perfusion deficit: decreased B/P, chest pain, dizziness, loss of consciousness
• Assess respiratory status: auscultate lung fields for bibasilar crackles in patients with advanced CHF
• Monitor I&O ratio; electrolytes: potassium, sodium, chloride; watch for decreasing urinary output, possible retention
• Monitor liver function tests: AST, ALT, bilirubin, alkaline phosphatase
⚠ **Monitor ECG continuously to determine product effectiveness; measure PR, QRS, QT intervals; check for PVCs, other dysrhyth-**mias; check B/P continuously for hypo/hypertension; for rebound hypertension after 1-2 hr; prolonged PR/QT intervals, QRS complex; if QT or QRS increases by 50% or more, withhold next dose, notify prescriber
• Monitor ANA titer; during long-term treatment, watch for lupuslike symptoms
• Monitor for dehydration or hypovolemia
⚠ **Monitor for CNS symptoms: confusion, seizures, psychosis, numbness, depression, involuntary movements; if these occur, product should be discontinued**
• Monitor blood levels (therapeutic level 3-10 mcg/ml), ANA titer or *N*-acetylprocainamide levels 10-20 mcg/ml; notify prescriber of abnormal results; assess for toxicity: confusion, drowsiness, nausea, vomiting, tachydysrhythmias, oliguria
• Assess cardiac rate, respiration: rate, rhythm, character, chest pain, ventricular tachycardia, supraventricular tachycardia or fibrillation

Nursing diagnoses
• Gas exchange, impaired (adverse reactions)
• Knowledge, deficient (teaching)

Patient/family education
• Advise patient to report side effects immediately to prescriber; to take exactly as prescribed; if dose is missed take when remembered if within 3-4 hr of next dose, do not double doses
• Caution patient that dark glasses may be needed for photophobia; to use sunscreen or stay out of sun to prevent burns; avoid temperature extremes; impairment of heat-regulating mechanism can occur
• Advise patient to complete follow-up appointment with prescriber, including pulmonary function tests, chest x-ray
• Instruct patient that dry mouth may be relieved by frequent sips of water, hard candy, sugarless gum
• Caution patient to make position changes from lying to standing slowly to prevent orthostatic hypotension
⚠ **Advise prescriber immediately if lupuslike symptoms (joint pain, butterfly rash, fever, chills, dyspnea), leukopenia symptoms (sore mouth, gums, throat), or thrombocytopenia symptoms (bleeding, bruising) occur**
• Teach patient how to take pulse and when to report to prescriber

Evaluation
Positive therapeutic outcome
• Decreased PVCs, ventricular tachycardia

TREATMENT OF OVERDOSE:
O_2, artificial ventilation, ECG, administer DOPamine for circulatory depression, diazepam or thiopental for seizures, isoproterenol

procarbazine (Rx)
(proe-kar'ba-zeen)
Matulane
Func. class.: Antineoplastic, alkylating agent
Chem. class.: Hydrazine derivative
Pregnancy category D

ACTION: Inhibits DNA, RNA, protein synthesis; has multiple sites of action; a nonvesicant

Therapeutic outcome: Prevention of rapidly growing malignant cells

USES: Lymphoma, Hodgkin's disease, cancers resistant to other therapy

Unlabeled uses: Brain, lung malignancies, other lymphomas, multiple myeloma, malignant melanoma, polycythemia vera

CONTRAINDICATIONS:
Pregnancy **D,** breastfeeding, hypersensitivity, thrombocytopenia

> **BLACK BOX WARNING:** Bone marrow depression

Precautions: Cardiac/renal/hepatic disease, radiation therapy, seizure disorder, anemia

DOSAGE AND ROUTES
Adult: PO 2-4 mg/kg/day for first wk; maintain dosage of 4-6 mg/kg/day until platelets and WBC fall; after recovery, 1-2 mg/kg/day
Child: PO 50 mg/m^2/day for 7 days, then 100 mg/m^2 until desired response, leukopenia, or thrombocytopenia occurs; 50 mg/m^2/day is maintenance after bone marrow recovery

Available forms: Caps 50 mg

Implementation
• Give with foods, fluids for GI upset; open cap and give with food/fluids for swallowing difficulty; administer as directed

ADVERSE EFFECTS
CNS: Headache, dizziness, **seizures,** insomnia, hallucinations, confusion, **coma,** pain, chills, fever, sweating, paresthesias, peripheral neuropathy

EENT: Retinal hemorrhage, nystagmus, photophobia, diplopia, dry eyes
GI: *Nausea, vomiting,* anorexia, diarrhea, constipation, dry mouth, stomatitis, elevated hepatic enzymes
GU: Azoospermia, cessation of menses
HEMA: Thrombocytopenia, anemia, leukopenia, myelosuppression, bleeding tendencies, purpura, petechiae, epistaxis, **hemolysis**
INTEG: *Rash,* pruritus, dermatitis, alopecia, herpes, hyperpigmentation
MS: Arthralgias, myalgias
RESP: Cough, pneumonitis
SYST: Secondary malignancy

Pharmacokinetics

Absorption	Well absorbed
Distribution	Widely distributed, crosses blood-brain barrier
Metabolism	Liver
Excretion	Kidneys
Half-life	1 hr

Pharmacodynamics
Unknown

INTERACTIONS
Individual drugs
Alcohol: increased CNS depression
Caffeine, guanethidine, levodopa, methyldopa, reserpine: increased hypertension
Meperidine: hypotension; do not use together

Drug classifications
Anticoagulants, NSAIDs, platelet inhibitors, thrombolytics: increased bleeding risk
Antidepressants (tricyclics), MAOIs, SSRIs, SNRIs: confusion, seizures, hypertension
Antihistamines, barbiturates, hypotensive agents, opiates, phenothiazines: increased CNS depression
Sympathomimetics: disulfiram-like reaction, life-threatening hypertensive crisis

Drug/food
Tyramine-containing foods: increased disulfiram-like reaction, hypertensive crisis

NURSING CONSIDERATIONS
Assessment
• **Bone marrow suppression:** monitor CBC, differential, platelet count weekly; withhold product if WBC is <4000/mm^3 or platelet count is <75,000/mm^3; notify prescriber of results if WBC <20,000/mm^3, platelets <150,000/mm^3

⚠ Nurse Alert

• Monitor pulmonary function tests, chest x-ray films before, during therapy; chest film should be obtained q2wk during treatment; check for dyspnea, crackles, unproductive cough, chest pain, tachypnea
• Monitor renal function tests: BUN, serum uric acid, urine CCr before, during therapy; I&O ratio; report fall in urine output of 30 ml/hr; check for decreased hyperuricemia
• Monitor hepatic studies before, during therapy: bilirubin, AST, ALT, ALK phos, LDH, PRN or qmo
• Monitor for cold, fever, sore throat (may indicate beginning of infection); identify edema in feet, joint and stomach pain, shaking; prescriber should be notified
• **Assess for bleeding:** hematuria, guaiac, bruising or petechiae, mucosa or orifices; no rectal temp
• Assess for tyramine-containing foods in the diet; hypertensive crisis can occur

Nursing diagnoses
• Body image, disturbed (adverse reactions)
• Infection, risk for (adverse reactions)
• Injury, risk for (adverse reactions)
• Knowledge, deficient (teaching)

Patient/family education
• Teach patient to avoid use of products containing aspirin or NSAIDs, razors, commercial mouthwash, since bleeding may occur; to report symptoms of bleeding (hematuria, tarry stools)
• Caution patient to report signs of anemia (fatigue, headache, irritability, faintness, shortness of breath); CNS changes, diarrhea
• Advise patient to report any changes in breathing or coughing even several mo after treatment; to avoid crowds and persons with respiratory tract or other infections
• Inform patient hair loss is common; discuss the use of wigs or hairpieces
• Caution patient not to have any vaccinations without the advice of the prescriber; serious reactions can occur
• Advise patient that contraception is needed during treatment and for several mo after the completion of therapy; may cause infertility; avoid breastfeeding
• Teach patient to avoid sunlight, UV exposure; wear sunscreen or protective clothing

Evaluation
Positive therapeutic outcome
• Absence of swelling at night
• Increased appetite, increased weight
• Decreasing malignancy

prochlorperazine (Rx)
(proe-klor-pair′a-zeen)
Compro
Func. class.: Antiemetic/antipsychotic
Chem. class.: Phenothiazine, piperazine derivative
Pregnancy category C

Do not confuse:
prochlorperazine/chlorproMAZINE

ACTION: Decreases DOPamine neurotransmission by increasing DOPamine turnover through blockade of the D_2 somatodendritic autoreceptor in the meso-limbic system

Therapeutic outcome: Decreased nausea, vomiting, decreased signs and symptoms of psychosis

USES: Nausea, vomiting, psychosis

CONTRAINDICATIONS:
Hypersensitivity to phenothiazines, coma, infants/neonates/child <2 yr, surgery

Precautions: Pregnancy **C**, breastfeeding, geriatric, seizure, encephalopathy, glaucoma, hepatic disease, Parkinson's disease, BPH

BLACK BOX WARNING: Dementia

P

DOSAGE AND ROUTES
Postoperative nausea/vomiting
Adult: IM 5-10 mg 1-2 hr before anesthesia; may repeat in 30 min; **IV** 5-10 mg 15-30 min before anesthesia; **IV** INF 20 mg/L D_5W or 0.9% NaCl 15-30 min before anesthesia, max 40 mg/day

Severe nausea/vomiting
Adult: PO 5-10 mg tid-qid; SUS REL 15 mg/day in AM or 10 mg q12hr; RECT 25 mg/bid; IM 5-10 mg; may repeat q3-4hr prn, max 40 mg/day
Child 18-39 kg: PO 2.5 mg tid or 5 mg bid; IM 0.132 mg/kg, q3-4hr prn, max 15 mg/day
Child 14-17 kg: PO/RECT 2.5 mg bid-tid; IM 0.132 mg/kg, q3-4hr prn, max 10 mg/day
Child 9-13 kg: PO/RECT 2.5 mg daily-bid; IM 0.132 mg/kg, q3-4hr prn, max 7.5 mg/day

Antipsychotic
Adult and child ≥12 yr: PO 5-10 mg tid-qid; may increase q2-3day, max 150 mg/day; IM 10-20 mg q2-4hr up to 4 doses, then 10-20 mg q4-6hr, max 200 mg/day; RECT 10 mg tid-qid, may increase by 5-10 mg q2-3day as needed

Child 2-12 yr: PO 2.5 mg bid-tid; IM 0.132 mg/kg

Antianxiety
Adult and child ≥12 yr: PO 5 mg tid-qid, max 20 mg/day or >12 wk; IM 5-10 mg q3-4hr, max 40 mg/day; **IV** 2.5-10 mg; max 40 mg/day
Child 2-12 yr: IM 0.132 mg/kg

Available forms: Syr 5 mg/ml; inj 5 mg/ml; tabs 5, 10, 25 mg; sus rel caps 10, 15 mg; supp 2.5, 5, 25 mg

Implementation
IM route
• Inject slowly in deep muscle mass; do not give SUBCUT; aspirate to avoid **IV** administration; do not administer sol with a precipitate; have patient lie down afterward for at least 30 min

Direct IV route
• Give by direct **IV** after diluting **IV** using 0.9% NaCl to 1 mg/1 ml; administer at 1 mg/min or less

Intermittent IV infusion route
• Administer after diluting 20 mg/L or less LR, Ringer's, dextrose, saline, or any combination

Syringe compatibilities: Atropine, butorphanol, chlorproMAZINE, cimetidine, diamorphine, diphenhydrAMINE, droperidol, fentanyl, glycopyrrolate, hydrOXYzine, meperidine, metoclopramide, nalbuphine, pentazocine, perphenazine, promazine, promethazine, ranitidine, scopolamine, SUFentanil

Syringe incompatibilities: Dimenhy-DRINATE, midazolam, PENTobarbital, thiopental

Y-site compatibilities: Amsacrine, calcium gluconate, CISplatin, cladribine, cyclophosphamide, cytarabine, DOXOrubicin, fluconazole, granisetron, heparin, hydrocortisone, melphalan, methotrexate, ondansetron, paclitaxel, potassium chloride, propofol, sargramostim, SUFentanil, teniposide, thiotepa, vinorelbine, vit B/C

Y-site incompatibilities: Foscarnet

ADVERSE EFFECTS
CNS: Tardive dyskinesia, *euphoria,* **depression, EPS,** restlessness, tremor, dizziness, **neuroleptic malignant syndrome,** drowsiness, headache
CV: Circulatory failure, tachycardia, hypotension, ECG changes
EENT: Blurred vision
GI: Nausea, vomiting, anorexia, dry mouth, diarrhea, constipation, weight loss, metallic taste, cramps

HEMA: Agranulocytosis
MISC: Impotence
RESP: Respiratory depression

Pharmacokinetics
Absorption	Variably absorbed (PO); well absorbed (IM)
Distribution	Widely distributed, high concentration in CNS, crosses placenta
Metabolism	Liver, extensively; GI mucosa
Excretion	Kidneys, breast milk
Half-life	Unknown

Pharmacodynamics
	PO	PO-SUS REL	RECT	IM	IV
Onset	½ hr	½ hr	1 hr	10-20 min	4-5 min
Peak	Unkn	Unkn	Unkn	Unkn	Unkn
Duration	3-4 hr	10-12 hr	3-4 hr	3-4 hr	3-4 hr

INTERACTIONS
Drug classifications
Antacids, barbiturates: decreased prochlorperazine effect
Anticholinergics, antidepressants, antiparkinson products: increased anticholinergic effects
SSRIs, SNRIs: increased serotonin syndrome, increased neuroleptic malignant syndrome
CNS depressants: increased CNS depression

Drug/herb
Betel palm, kava: increased EPS
Dong quai: avoid use

Drug/lab test
Increased: liver function tests, cardiac enzymes, cholesterol, blood glucose, prolactin, bilirubin, PBI, ^{131}I, alkaline phosphatase, leukocytes, granulocytes, platelets
Decreased: hormones (blood and urine)
False positive: pregnancy tests, urine bilirubin
False negative: urinary steroids, 17-OHCS, pregnancy tests

NURSING CONSIDERATIONS
Assessment
• Assess mental status: orientation, mood, behavior, presence and type of hallucinations before initial administration and monthly; this

product should significantly reduce psychotic behavior

• Check for swallowing of PO medication; check for hoarding or giving of medication to other patients

• Monitor I&O ratio; palpate bladder if low urinary output occurs, especially in geriatric; urinalysis recommended before, during prolonged therapy

⚠ Monitor bilirubin, CBC, liver function tests monthly; blood dyscrasias, hepatotoxicity may occur

• Assess affect, orientation, LOC, reflexes, gait, coordination, sleep pattern disturbances

• Monitor B/P with patient sitting, standing, and lying; take pulse and respirations q4hr during initial treatment; establish baseline before starting treatment; report drops of 30 mm Hg; obtain baseline ECG, Q-wave and T-wave changes

• Check for dizziness, faintness, palpitations, tachycardia on rising; severe orthostatic hypotension is common

⚠ Identify neuroleptic malignant syndrome: hyperpyrexia, muscle rigidity, increased CPK, altered mental status, seizures, fever, tachycardia, dyspnea, fatigue, loss of bladder control; notify prescriber immediately; product should be discontinued

• Assess for EPS including akathisia (inability to sit still, no pattern to movements), tardive dyskinesia (bizarre movements of the jaw, mouth, tongue, extremities), pseudoparkinsonism (ragged tremors, pill rolling, shuffling gait); an antiparkinsonism product should be prescribed

• Assess for constipation, urinary retention daily; if these occur, increase bulk, water in diet

Nursing diagnoses
• Coping, ineffective (uses)
• Knowledge, deficient (teaching)
• Noncompliance (teaching)

Patient/family education
• Teach patient to use good oral hygiene; frequent rinsing of mouth, sugarless gum for dry mouth since oral candidiasis may occur

• Caution patient to avoid hazardous activities until product response is determined; dizziness, blurred vision may occur

• Inform patient that orthostatic hypotension occurs often and to rise from sitting or lying position gradually; to remain lying down after IM inj for at least 30 min; tell patient to avoid hot tubs, hot showers, tub baths, since hypotension may occur; tell patient that in hot weather heat stroke may occur; take extra precautions to stay cool

• Advise patient to avoid abrupt withdrawal of this product, or EPS may result; product should be withdrawn slowly

• Teach patient to avoid OTC preparations (cough, hay fever, cold) unless approved by prescriber, since serious product interactions may occur; avoid use with alcohol, CNS depressants; increased drowsiness may occur; avoid activities requiring mental alertness

• Instruct patient to avoid sun or use sunscreen, sunglasses, and protective clothing to prevent burns

• Advise patient to take antacids 2 hr before or after taking this product

• Advise patient to report sore throat, malaise, fever, bleeding, mouth sores; if these occur, CBC should be done and product discontinued

• Teach patient not to double or skip doses

• Inform patient that urine may turn pink to reddish brown

• Instruct patient to report dark urine, clay-colored stools, bleeding, bruising, rash, blurred vision

• Advise patient that suppositories may contain coconut/palm oil

Evaluation
Positive therapeutic outcome
• Relief of nausea and vomiting
• Decrease in emotional excitement, hallucinations, delusions, paranoia
• Reorganization of patterns of thought, speech

TREATMENT OF OVERDOSE:
Lavage if orally ingested; provide airway; *do not induce vomiting or use EPINEPHrine*

progesterone (Rx)
(proe-jess′ter-one)
Crinone, Endometrin, First-Progesterone, Prochieve, Prometrium
Func. class.: Progestogen
Chem. class.: Progesterone derivative
Pregnancy category D

ACTION: Inhibits secretion of pituitary gonadotropins, which prevents follicular maturation, ovulation; stimulates growth of mammary tissue; antineoplastic action against endometrial cancer

Therapeutic outcome: Decreased abnormal uterine bleeding, absence of amenorrhea

USES: Contraception, amenorrhea, premenstrual syndrome, abnormal uterine bleeding, endometrial hyperplasia prevention, assisted reproductive technology (ART) gel

Unlabeled uses: Corpus luteum insufficiency

CONTRAINDICATIONS:
Pregnancy **D,** thromboembolic disorders, reproductive cancer, genital bleeding (abnormal, undiagnosed), cerebral hemorrhage, ectopic pregnancy, PID, STDs, hypersensitivity to this product or peanut oil

> **BLACK BOX WARNING:** Breast cancer

Precautions: Breastfeeding, hypertension, asthma, blood dyscrasias, gallbladder disease, CHF, diabetes mellitus, bone disease, depression, migraine headache, seizure disorders, renal/hepatic disease, family history of breast or reproductive tract cancer

> **BLACK BOX WARNING:** Cardiac disease, dementia

DOSAGE AND ROUTES
Infertility
Adult: Vag 90 mg/day (micronized gel); 100 mg 2-3 times/day, starting day after oocyte retrieval and up to 10 wk total

Amenorrhea/functional uterine bleeding
Adult: IM 5-10 mg/day × 6-8 doses

Endometrial hyperplasia prevention
Adult: PO 200 mg/day × 12 days

Assisted reproductive technology
Adult: GEL 90 mg (8%) vaginally daily, for supplementation; 90 mg (8%) vaginally bid for replacement; if pregnancy occurs, continue × 10-12 wk

Corpus luteum insufficiency (unlabeled)
Adult: VAG insert 100 mg bid-tid starting at oocyte retrieval and continuing up to 10-12 wk of gestation

Available forms: Caps 100, 200 mg; inj 50 mg/ml; powder micronized; vag gel 4%, 8%; vag insert 100 mg; supp 25, 100, 200, 500 mg, compounding kit 25, 50, 100, 200, 400 mg

Implementation
PO route
• Do not crush, break, chew caps, give one dose in AM

• With food or milk to decrease GI symptoms
• Start progesterone 14 days after estrogen dose, if given concomitantly
Vaginal route
• Wait at least 6 hr after any vaginal treatment before using vaginal gel
IM route
• Store in dark area
• Give titrated dose; use lowest effective dosage; give oil sol deep in large muscle mass; rotate sites; use after warming to dissolve crystals

ADVERSE EFFECTS
CNS: Dizziness, headache, migraines, depression, fatigue, mood swings, dementia, drowsiness
CV: Hypotension, **thrombophlebitis,** edema, **thromboembolism, stroke, pulmonary embolism, MI**
EENT: Diplopia, retinal thrombosis
GI: *Nausea,* vomiting, anorexia, cramps, increased weight, **cholestatic jaundice,** constipation
GU: Amenorrhea, cervical erosion, breakthrough bleeding, dysmenorrhea, vaginal candidiasis, breast changes, *gynecomastia, testicular atrophy, impotence,* endometriosis, **spontaneous abortion,** breast pain, ectopic pregnancy
INTEG: Rash, urticaria, acne, hirsutism, alopecia, oily skin, seborrhea, purpura, melasma
META: Hyperglycemia
SYST: Angioedema, anaphylaxis

Pharmacokinetics
Absorption	Unknown
Distribution	Unknown
Metabolism	Unknown
Excretion	Breast milk
Half-life	Unknown

Pharmacodynamics
	IM	RECT	VAG
Onset	Unknown	Unknown	Unknown
Peak	Unknown	Unknown	Unknown
Duration	24 hr	24 hr	24 hr

INTERACTIONS
Drug classifications
Barbiturates, phenytoins: decreased progesterone effect

CYP3A4 inhibitors (cimetidine, clarithromycin, danazol, diltiazem, erythromycin, fluconazole, itraconazole, ketoconazole, troleandomycin, verapamil, voriconazole): increased progesterone effect

Drug/lab test
Increased: alkaline phosphatase, nitrogen (urine), pregnanediol, amino acids, factors VII, VIII, IX, X
Decreased: GTT, HDL

NURSING CONSIDERATIONS

Assessment
• Monitor B/P at beginning of treatment and periodically; check weight daily; notify prescriber of weekly weight gain >5 lb
• Monitor I&O ratio: be alert for decreasing urinary output, increasing edema, hypertension
• Assess liver function tests: ALT, AST, bilirubin periodically during long-term therapy
• Assess edema, hypertension, cardiac symptoms, jaundice
• Assess mental status: affect, mood, behavioral changes, depression
• Assess for hypercalcemia
• Assess cervical cytology

Nursing diagnoses
• Injury, risk for (adverse reactions)
• Knowledge, deficient (teaching)
• Sexual dysfunction (uses)
• Tissue perfusion, ineffective (adverse reactions)

Patient/family education
• Teach patient to report breast lumps, vaginal bleeding, edema, jaundice, dark urine, clay-colored stools, dyspnea, headache, blurred vision, abdominal pain, numbness or stiffness in legs, chest pain
• Teach patient to report suspected pregnancy

Evaluation
Positive therapeutic outcome
• Decreased abnormal uterine bleeding
• Absence of amenorrhea
• Prevented pregnancy

promethazine (Rx)
(proe-meth′a-zeen)
Phenadoz, Phenergan, Promethagan
Func. class.: Antihistamine, H₁-receptor antagonist; antiemetic; sedative/hypnotic
Chem. class.: Phenothiazine derivative
Pregnancy category C

Do not confuse:
Phenergan/Theragran

ACTION: Acts on blood vessels, GI, respiratory system by competing with histamine for H₁-receptor site; decreases allergic response by blocking histamine

Therapeutic outcome: Absence of allergy symptoms and rhinitis, absence of nausea/vomiting, sedation

USES: Motion sickness, rhinitis, allergy symptoms, sedation, nausea, preoperative and postoperative sedation

CONTRAINDICATIONS:
Hypersensitivity to H₁-receptor antagonist, agranulocytosis, bone marrow suppression, breastfeeding, coma, jaundice, Reye's syndrome

> **BLACK BOX WARNING:** Infants, intraarterial/SUBCUT use, neonates, children, extravasation

Precautions: Pregnancy C, renal/cardiac/hepatic disease, asthma, seizure disorder, prostatic hypertrophy, bladder obstruction, glaucoma, COPD, GI obstruction, ileus, CNS depression, diabetes, sleep apnea, urinary retention

> **BLACK BOX WARNING:** IV use

DOSAGE AND ROUTES

Nausea/vomiting
Adult: PO/IM/IV/RECT 12.5-25 mg; q4-6hr prn
Child >2 yr: PO/IM/IV/RECT 0.25-0.5 mg/kg q4-6hr prn

Motion sickness
Adult: PO 25 mg bid; give 30-60 min before departure and q8-12hr prn
Child >2 yr: PO/IM/RECT 12.5-25 mg bid; give 30-60 min before departure and q8-12hr prn

Allergy/rhinitis (unlabeled)
Adult: PO 12.5 mg qid, or 25 mg at bedtime
Child ≥2 yr: PO 6.25-12.5 mg tid or 25 mg at bedtime

Sedation
Adult: PO/IM 25-50 mg at bedtime
Child ≥2 yr: PO/IM/RECT 12.5-25 mg at bedtime

Sedation (preoperative/postoperative)
Adult: PO/IM/IV 25-50 mg
Child ≥2 yr: PO/IM/IV 0.5-1.1 mg/kg

Available forms: Tabs 12.5, 25, 50 mg; supp 12.5, 25, 50 mg; inj 25, 50 mg/ml

Implementation
PO route
- With meals for GI symptoms; absorption may slightly decrease
- When used for motion sickness, 30 min-1 hr before travel

IM route
- IM inj in deep in large muscle; rotate site

Direct IV route

> **BLACK BOX WARNING:** Check for extravasation: burning, pain, swelling at **IV** site, can cause tissue necrosis

- Do not use if precipitate is present
- Rapid administration may cause transient decrease in B/P
- After diluting each 25-50 mg/9 ml of NaCl for inj; give 25 mg or less/2 min

Syringe compatibilities: Butorphanol, chlorproMAZINE, cimetidine, dihydroergotamine, diphenhydrAMINE, droperidol, fentaNYL, glycopyrrolate, HYDROmorphone, hydrOXYzine, meperidine, metoclopramide, midazolam, pentazocine, perphenazine, prochlorperazine, promazine, ranitidine, scopolamine

Y-site compatibilities: Alfentanil, amifostine, amikacin, aminocaproic acid, amsacrine, anidulafungin, ascorbic acid, atenolol, atracurium, atropine, aztreonam, benztropine, bivalirudin, bleomycin, bumetanide, buprenorphine, butorphanol, calcium chloride/gluconate, CARBOplatin, caspofungin, chlorproMAZINE, cimetidine, ciprofloxacin, cisatracurium, CISplatin, cladribine, codeine, cyanocobalamin, cyclophosphamide, cycloSPORINE, cytarabine, DACTINomycin, DAPTOmycin, dexmedetomidine, digoxin, diltiazem, diphenhydrAMINE, DOBUTamine, docetaxel, DOPamine, doxacurium, DOXOrubicin, doxycycline, enalaprilat, ePHEDrine, EPINEPHrine, epirubicin, epoetin, eptifibatide, erythromycin, esmolol, etoposide, famotidine, fenoldopam, fentaNYL, filgrastim, fluconazole, fludarabine, gemcitabine, gentamicin, glycopyrrolate, granisetron, HYDROmorphone, hydrOXYzine, IDArubicin, ifosfamide, insulin (regular), irinotecan, isoproterenol, labetalol, levofloxacin, lidocaine, linezolid, LORazepam, LR, magnesium sulfate, mannitol, mechlorethamine, melphalan, meperidine, metaraminol, methoxamine, methyldopa, metoclopramide, metoprolol, metroNIDAZOLE, miconazole, midazolam, milrinone, mitoxantrone, morphine, mycophenolate, nalbuphine, naloxone, netilmicin, nitroglycerin, norepinephrine, octreotide, ondansetron, oxaliplatin, oxytocin, paclitaxel, palonosetron, pamidronate, pancuronium, pemetrexed, pentamidine, pentazocine, phenylephrine, polymyxin B, procainamide, prochlorperazine, propranolol, protamine, pyridoxine, quiNIDine, quinupristin-dalfopristin, ranitidine, remifentanil, Ringer's, ritodrine, riTUXimab, rocuronium, sargramostim, sodium acetate, succinylcholine, SUFentanil, tacrolimus, teniposide, theophylline, thiamine, thiotepa, tigecycline, tirofiban, TNA, tobramycin, tolazoline, trastuzumab, trimetaphan, vancomycin, vasopressin, vecuronium, verapamil, vinCRIStine, vinorelbine, voriconazole

ADVERSE EFFECTS
CNS: *Dizziness, drowsiness,* poor coordination, fatigue, anxiety, euphoria, confusion, paresthesia, neuritis, EPS, **neuroleptic malignant syndrome**
CV: Hyper/hypotension, palpitations, tachycardia
EENT: Blurred vision, dilated pupils, tinnitus, nasal stuffiness, dry nose, throat, mouth, photosensitivity
GI: *Constipation,* dry mouth, nausea, vomiting, anorexia, diarrhea
GU: *Retention,* dysuria, frequency
HEMA: Thrombocytopenia, **agranulocytosis, hemolytic anemia**
INTEG: Rash, urticaria, photosensitivity
RESP: Increased thick secretions, wheezing, chest tightness, **apnea in pediatric patients**

Pharmacokinetics

Absorption	Well absorbed (PO, IM); erratically absorbed (RECT)
Distribution	Widely distributed; crosses the blood-brain barrier, placenta
Metabolism	Liver
Excretion	Kidneys, breast milk
Half-life	Unknown

Pharmacodynamics

	PO/IM/RECT	IV
Onset	20 min	3-5 min
Peak	Unknown	Unknown
Duration	4-12 hr	4-6 hr

INTERACTIONS
Individual drugs
Alcohol: increased CNS depression
Heparin: decreased oral anticoagulants effect

Drug classifications
Antidepressants (tricyclics), barbiturates, CNS
depressants, opiates, sedative/hypnotics:
increased CNS depression
MAOIs: increased promethazine effect

Drug/lab test
False negative: skin allergy tests (discontinue
antihistamines 3 days before testing)
False positive: urine pregnancy test
Interference: blood grouping (ABO), GTT

NURSING CONSIDERATIONS
Assessment
• **Neuroleptic malignant syndrome:** assess
for fever, confusion, diaphoresis, rigid muscles,
elevated CPK, encephalopathy, discontinue
product, notify prescriber
• Assess respiratory status: rate, rhythm, increase in bronchial secretions, wheezing, chest
tightness; provide fluids to 2 L/day to decrease
secretion thickness
• Monitor I&O ratio: be alert for urinary retention, frequency, dysuria, especially geriatric;
product should be discontinued if these occur
• Monitor CBC during long-term therapy; blood
dyscrasias may occur but are rare
• Monitor cardiac status: VS, palpitations,
increased pulse, hypo/hypertension

Nursing diagnoses
• Airway clearance, ineffective (uses)
• Injury, risk for (adverse reactions)
• Knowledge, deficient (teaching)
• Noncompliance (teaching, overuse)

Patient/family education
• Inform patient that a false-negative result may
occur with skin testing; these procedures should
not be scheduled until 3 days after discontinuing
use
• Advise patient to take 30 min before departure to prevent motion sickness
• Caution patient to avoid hazardous activities,
activities requiring alertness, since dizziness may
occur; instruct patient to request assistance with
ambulation
• Advise patient to avoid alcohol, other depressants; serious CNS depression may occur
• Teach patient all aspects of product use; to
notify prescriber if confusion, sedation, hypotension, jaundice, fever occur; to avoid driving and
other hazardous activity if drowsiness occurs
• Advise patient to take 1 hr before or 2 hr after
meals to facilitate absorption
• Caution patient not to exceed recommended
dosage; dysrhythmias may occur

• Inform patient hard candy, gum, frequent
rinsing of mouth may be used for dryness
• Advise that product may reduce sweating
(heat stroke)

Evaluation
Positive therapeutic outcome
• Absence of motion sickness
• Absence of nausea, vomiting

propafenone (Rx)
(pro-faff′e-nown)
Rythmol, Rythmol SR
Func. class.: Antidysrhythmic (Class IC)
Pregnancy category C

ACTION: Slows conduction velocity;
reduces membrane responsiveness; inhibits automaticity; increases ratio of effective refractory
period to action potential duration; β-blocking
activity

Therapeutic outcome: Absence of
arrhythmias

USES: Atrial fibrillation (single dose),
sustained ventricular tachycardia, paroxysmal
supraventricular tachycardia (PVST) prophylaxis, supraventricular dysrhythmias

CONTRAINDICATIONS:
2nd-, 3rd-degree AV block, right bundle branch
block, cardiogenic shock, hypersensitivity,
bradycardia, uncontrolled CHF, sick sinus
syndrome, marked hypotension, bronchospastic
disorders, electrolyte imbalance

Precautions: Pregnancy **C,** breastfeeding,
children, geriatric, CHF, hypo/hyperkalemia,
nonallergic bronchospasm, renal/hepatic
disease, hematologic disorders

BLACK BOX WARNING: Recent MI, cardiac
arrhythmias, QT prolongation, torsades de
pointes

DOSAGE AND ROUTES
Adult: PO 150 mg q8hr; allow a 3-4 day
interval before increasing dose, max 900 mg/day

Atrial fibrillation
Adult: PO 450 or 600 mg as a single dose; SR
225 mg q12hr, may increase to 325 mg q12hr,
max 425 mg q12hr

Available forms: Tabs 150, 225, 300 mg,
SR cap 225, 325, 425 mg

Implementation
- Begin treatment in hospital
- Remove other antiarrhythmics before starting propafenone
- Adjust dosage q3-4day, no sooner

ADVERSE EFFECTS
CNS: Headache, dizziness, abnormal dreams, syncope, confusion, **seizures,** insomnia, tremor, anxiety, fatigue
CV: Supraventricular dysrhythmia, ventricular dysrhythmia, bradycardia, prodysrhythmia, palpitations, AV block, intraventricular conduction delay, AV dissociation, hypotension, chest pain, asystole
EENT: Blurred vision, altered taste, tinnitus
GI: *Nausea, vomiting,* constipation, dyspepsia, cholestasis, abnormal hepatic studies, dry mouth, diarrhea, anorexia
HEMA: Leukopenia, agranulocytosis, granulocytopenia, thrombocytopenia, anemia, bruising
INTEG: Rash
RESP: Dyspnea

Pharmacokinetics

Absorption	Well absorbed
Distribution	Widely, crosses placenta
Metabolism	Rapid, liver, CYP1A2, CYP2D6, CYP3A4
Excretion	Kidneys
Half-life	2-32 hr

Pharmacodynamics (antiarrhythmic)

Onset	Hours to several days
Peak	4-5 days
Duration	Several hr

INTERACTIONS
Individual products
Arsenic trioxide, chloroquine, clarithromycin, droperidol, erythromycin, haloperidol, levomethadyl, methadone, pentamidine, chlorproMAZINE, mesoridazine, thioridazine: increased QT prolongation
Cimetidine, quiNIDine, rifampin: decreased propafenone effect
CycloSPORINE, digoxin: increased serum levels
Metropolol, propranolol: increased β-blocker effect
Warfarin: increased anticoagulation

Drug classifications
Local anesthetics: increased CNS effects
CYP1A2, CYP2D6, CYP3A4 inhibitors (protease inhibitors, quiNINE, PARoxetine, saquinavir, erythromycin, azole antifungals, sertraline, tricyclics): increased propafenone effects

Drug/lab test
Increased: CPK

NURSING CONSIDERATIONS
Assessment
- Monitor GI status: bowel pattern, number of stools
- ⚠ Assess cardiac status: rate, rhythm, quality; ECG or Holter monitor prior to, during therapy; watch for PR, QT prolongation
- Monitor chest x-ray film, pulmonary function test during treatment
- Monitor I&O ratio; check for decreasing output; daily weight
- Monitor B/P for fluctuations
- Assess lung fields; bilateral crackles, dyspnea, peripheral edema, weight gain, jugular venous distention may occur in CHF patient
- ⚠ Assess toxicity: fine tremors, dizziness, hypotension, drowsiness, abnormal heart rate

Nursing diagnoses
- Cardiac output, decreased (uses)
- Knowledge, deficient (teaching)

Patient/family education
- Advise patient to avoid hazardous activities until response is known
- Advise patient to report fever, chills, sore throat, bleeding, shortness of breath, chest pain, palpitations, blurred vision
- Advise patient to take medication with food
- Advise patient to carry emergency ID identifying medication and prescriber

Evaluation
Positive therapeutic outcome
- Absence of dysrhythmias

TREATMENT OF OVERDOSE:
O_2, artificial ventilation, defibrillation ECG; administer DOPamine for circulatory depression, diazepam or thiopental for seizures, isoproterenol

proparacaine ophthalmic
See Appendix B

⚠ Nurse Alert

🅰 HIGH ALERT

propofol (Rx)

(pro′poh-fole)

Diprivan, Fresenius, Propoven

Func. class.: General anesthetic

Pregnancy category B

ACTION: Produces dose-dependent CNS depression by activation of GABA receptor

Therapeutic outcome: Induction of anesthesia

USES: Induction or maintenance of anesthesia as part of balanced anesthetic technique; sedation in mechanically ventilated patients

CONTRAINDICATIONS:

Hypersensitivity to product or soybean oil, egg, benzyl alcohol (some products)

Precautions: Pregnancy **B**, breastfeeding, children, geriatric, respiratory depression, severe respiratory disorders, cardiac dysrhythmias, labor and delivery, renal disease, hyperlipidemia

DOSAGE AND ROUTES

Anesthesia

Adult <55 yr and ASA I/II IV (Diprivan or generic): IV 40 mg q10sec until induction onset; maintenance: 100-200 mcg/kg/min or **IV BOL** 20-50 mg prn, allow 3-5 min between adjustments; Fresenius Propoven 1% IV 20-40 q10sec until induction then 3-6 mg/kg/hr

Child ≥3 yr or ASA I or II: IV Induction: 2.5-3.5 mg/kg over 20-30 sec when not premedicated or lightly premedicated

Child 2 mo-16 yr maintenance: IV 125-300 mcg/kg/min, lower dose for ASA III or IV

ICU sedation

Adult: IV 5 mcg/kg/min over 5 min; may increase by 5-10 mcg/kg/min over 5-10 min until desired response (Diprivan or generic): 0.3-4 mg/kg/hr, max 4 mg/kg/hr (Fresenius Propoven)

Available forms: Inj 10 mg/ml in 20 ml ampule, 50 ml, 100 ml vials

Implementation

IV route

• Shake well before use; dilution is not necessary but if diluted, use only D₅W to ≥2 mg/ml; give over 3-5 min, titrate to needed level of sedation; use only glass containers when mixing, not stable in plastic; use aseptic technique when transferring from original container

• Fresenius Propoven 1%: Dilution is not necessary but if diluted use only D₅W or NS to ≥2 mg/ml (max dilution max 1 part Fresenius Propoven/4 parts D₅W or NS), do not admix, lidocaine can be used to reduce pain at site

• May be given by cont inf; give by inf pump

• Only with resuscitative equipment available, only by qualified persons trained in anesthesia

Y-site compatibilities: Acyclovir, alfentanil, aminophylline, ampicillin, aztreonam, bumetanide, buprenorphine, butorphanol, calcium gluconate, CARBOplatin, ceFAZolin, cefoperazone, cefotaxime, cefotetan, cefoxitin, ceftizoxime, cefTRIAXone, cefuroxime, chlorproMAZINE, cimetidine, CISplatin, clindamycin, cyclophosphamide, cycloSPORINE, cytarabine, dexamethasone, diphenhydrAMINE, DOBUTamine, DOPamine, doxycycline, droperidol, enalaprilat, ePHEDrine, EPINEPHrine, esmolol, famotidine, fentaNYL, fluconazole, fluorouracil, furosemide, ganciclovir, glycopyrrolate, granisetron, haloperidol, heparin, hydrocortisone, HYDROmorphone, hydrOXYzine, ifosfamide, imipenem/cilastatin, inamrinone, regular insulin, isoproterenol, ketamine, labetalol, levorphanol, lidocaine, LORazepam, magnesium sulfate, mannitol, meperidine, mezlocillin, miconazole, morphine, nafcillin, nalbuphine, naloxone, nitroglycerin, norepinephrine, ofloxacin, paclitaxel, PENTobarbital, PHENobarbital, piperacillin, potassium chloride, prochlorperazine, propranolol, ranitidine, scopolamine, sodium bicarbonate, sodium nitroprusside, succinylcholine, SUFentanil, thiopental, ticarcillin, ticarcillin/clavulanate, vecuronium, verapamil

Solution compatibilities: (If given together via Y-site) D₅W, D₅LR, LR, D₅/0.45% NaCl, D₅/0.2% NaCl

ADVERSE EFFECTS

CNS: Involuntary movement, headache, jerking, fever, dizziness, shivering, tremor, confusion, somnolence, paresthesia, agitation, abnormal dreams, euphoria, fatigue, **increased ICP, impaired cerebral flow, seizures**

CV: *Bradycardia, hypotension,* hypertension, PVC, PAC, tachycardia, abnormal ECG, ST segment depression, **asystole, bradydysrhythmias**

EENT: Blurred vision, tinnitus, eye pain, strange taste, diplopia

GI: *Nausea, vomiting, abdominal cramping,* dry mouth, swallowing, hypersalivation, **pancreatitis**

P

GU: Urine retention, green urine, cloudy urine, oliguria
INTEG: *Flushing, phlebitis, hives, burning/ stinging at inj site,* rash, pain of extremities
MS: Myalgia
RESP: Apnea, *cough, hiccups,* dyspnea, hypoventilation, sneezing, wheezing, tachypnea, hypoxia, respiratory acidosis
SYST: Propofol infusion syndrome

Pharmacokinetics

Absorption	Completely absorbed
Distribution	Rapid
Metabolism	Liver, conjugation to active metabolites; 95%-99% protein binding
Excretion	Urine
Half-life	3-12 hr

Pharmacodynamics

Onset	15-30 sec
Peak	Unknown
Duration	Unknown

INTERACTIONS

Individual drugs
Alcohol: increased CNS depression

Drug classifications
Antipsychotics, CNS depressants (sedative-hypnotics, opioid analgesics), inhalational anesthetics, skeletal muscle relaxants: increased CNS depression
MAOIs: do not use within 10 days

Drug/herb
St. John's wort: increased propofol effect

NURSING CONSIDERATIONS

Assessment
• Assess inj site: phlebitis, burning, stinging
• Monitor ECG for changes: PVC, PAC, ST segment changes; monitor VS
• Assess CNS changes: movement, jerking, tremors, dizziness, LOC, pupil reaction
• Assess allergic reactions: hives
⚠ **Assess respiratory dysfunction: respiratory depression, character, rate, rhythm; notify prescriber if respirations are <10/ min**
• **Propofol infusion syndrome:** assess for rhabdomyolysis, renal failure, hyperkalemia, metabolic acidosis, cardiac dysrhythmias, heart failure, usually between 35 and 93 hr after inf began, at >5 mg/kg/hr for >58 hr

Nursing diagnoses
• Breathing pattern, ineffective (adverse reactions)
• Injury, risk for (adverse reactions)
• Knowledge, deficient (teaching)

Patient/family education
• Teach patient that this medication will cause dizziness, drowsiness, sedation

Evaluation
Positive therapeutic outcome
• Induction of anesthesia

TREATMENT OF OVERDOSE:
Discontinue product; administer vasopressor agents or anticholinergics, artificial ventilation

---

propranolol (Rx)
(proe-pran'oh-lole)
Inderal, Inderal LA, InnoPran XL
Func. class.: Antihypertensive, antianginal, antidysrhythmic (class III)
Chem. class.: β-Adrenergic blocker
Pregnancy category C

Do not confuse:
Inderal/Toradol/Inderide/Adderall/Imuran
Propranolol/Pravachol

ACTION: Nonselective β-blocker with negative inotropic, chronotropic, dromotropic properties

Therapeutic outcome: Decreased B/P, heart rate

USES: Chronic stable angina pectoris, hypertension, supraventricular dysrhythmias, migraine prophylaxis, pheochromocytoma, cyanotic spells related to hypertrophic subaortic stenosis

Unlabeled uses: Parkinson's tremor, prevention of variceal bleeding caused by portal hypertension, akathisia induced by antipsychotics, lithium-induced tremor

CONTRAINDICATIONS:
Hypersensitivity to this product, cardiogenic shock, AV heart block, bronchospastic disease, sinus bradycardia, bronchospasm, asthma

Precautions: Pregnancy **C,** breastfeeding, children, diabetes mellitus, renal/hepatic disease, hyperthyroidism, COPD, myasthenia gravis, peripheral vascular disease, hypotension, cardiac failure, Raynaud's disease, sick sinus

---

⚠ Nurse Alert

syndrome, vasospastic angina, smoking, Wolff-Parkinson-White syndrome

> **BLACK BOX WARNING:** Abrupt discontinuation

DOSAGE AND ROUTES

Dysrhythmias
Adult: PO 10-30 mg tid-qid; **IV** BOL 1-3 mg given 1 mg/min; may repeat in 2 min; may repeat q4hr thereafter
Child: PO 1 mg/kg/day divided in 2 doses, **IV** 0.01-0.1 mg/kg over 5 min

Hypertension
Adult: PO 40 mg bid or 80 mg/day (EXT REL) initially; usual dosage 120-240 mg/day bid-tid or 120-160 mg/day (EXT REL)
Child: PO 0.5-1 mg/kg/day divided q6-12hr

Angina
Adult: PO 80-320 mg in divided doses bid-qid or 80 mg/day (EXT REL); usual dosage 160 mg/day (EXT REL)

MI prophylaxis
Adult: PO 180-240 mg/day tid-qid starting 5 days to 2 wk after MI

Pheochromocytoma
Adult: PO 60 mg/day × 3 days preoperatively in divided doses or 30 mg/day in divided doses (inoperable tumor)

Migraine
Adult: PO 80 mg/day (EXT REL) or in divided doses; may increase to 160-240 mg/day in divided doses
Child: PO 0.6-1.5 mg/kg/day divided q8hr

Essential tremor
Adult: PO 40 mg bid; usual dosage 120 mg/day

Available forms: Ext rel caps 60, 80, 120, 160 mg; tabs 10, 20, 40, 60, 80, 90 mg; inj 1 mg/ml; oral sol 4 mg, 8 mg/ml; conc oral sol 80 mg/ml

Implementation
PO route
• Do not break, crush, chew, or open ext rel cap
• Do not use ext rel cap for essential tremor, MI, cardiac dysrhythmias; do not use InnoPran XL in hypertropic subaortic stenosis, migraine, angina pectoris
• Ext rel caps should be taken daily; InnoPran XL should be taken at bedtime
• May mix oral sol with liquid or semisolid food; rinse container to get entire dose

• Give with 8 oz water with food; food enhances bioavailability
• Do not give with aluminum-containing antacid; may decrease GI absorption

Direct IV route
• IV undiluted or diluted 10 ml D_5W for inj; give 1 mg or less/min

Intermittent IV infusion route
• May be diluted in 50 ml NaCl and run 1 mg over 10-15 min

Y-site compatibilities: Acyclovir, alfentanil, alteplase, amikacin, aminocaproic acid, aminophylline, anidulafungin, ascorbic acid, atracurium, atropine, azaTHIOprine, aztreonam, benztropine, bivalirudin, bleomycin, bumetanide, buprenorphine, butorphanol, calcium chloride/gluconate, CARBOplatin, caspofungin, cefamandole, ceFAZolin, cefmetazole, cefonicid, cefoperazone, cefotaxime, cefotetan, cefoxitin, ceftazidime, ceftizoxime, cefTRIAXone, cefuroxime, cephalothin, cephapirin, chloramphenicol, chlorproMAZINE, cimetidine, CISplatin, clindamycin, cyanocobalamin, cyclophosphamide, cycloSPORINE, cytarabine, DACTINomycin, DAPTOmycin, dexamethasone, digoxin, diltiazem, diphenhydrAMINE, DOBUTamine, docetaxel, DOPamine, doxacurium, DOXOrubicin, doxycycline, enalaprilat, ePHEDrine, EPINEPHrine, epirubicin, epoetin alfa, eptifibatide, ertapenem, erythromycin, esmolol, etoposide, etoposide phosphate, famotidine, fenoldopam, fentaNYL, fluconazole, fludarabine, fluorouracil, folic acid, furosemide, ganciclovir, gatifloxacin, gemcitabine, gemtuzumab, gentamicin, glycopyrrolate, granisetron, heparin, hydrocortisone, HYDROmorphone, hydrOXYzine, IDArubicin, ifosfamide, imipenem-cilastatin, inamrinone, irinotecan, isoproterenol, ketorolac, labetalol, levofloxacin, lidocaine, linezolid, LORazepam, magnesium, mannitol, mechlorethamine, meperidine, metaraminol, methicillin, methotrexate, methoxamine, methyldopate, methylPREDNISolone, metoclopramide, metoprolol, metroNIDAZOLE, mezlocillin, miconazole, midazolam, milrinone, minocycline, mitoxantrone, morphine, moxalactam, multiple vitamins, mycophenolate, nafcillin, nalbuphine, naloxone, nesiritide, netilmicin, nitroglycerin, nitroprusside, norepinephrine, octreotide, ondansetron, oxacillin, oxaliplatin, oxytocin, palonosetron, pamidronate, pancuronium, papaverine, pemetrexed, penicillin G potassium/sodium, pentamidine, pentazocine, PENTobarbital, PHENobarbital, phenylephrine, phytonadione, piperacillin, polymyxin B, potassium chloride, procainamide, prochlorperazine, promethazine,

P

propofol, protamine, pyridoxine, quiNIDine, quinupristin-dalfopristin, ranitidine, ritodrine, rocuronium, sodium acetate/bicarbonate, succinylcholine, SUFentanil, tacrolimus, teniposide, theophylline, thiamine, thiotepa, ticarcillin, ticarcillin-clavulanate, tigecycline, tirofiban, tobramycin, tolazoline, trimetaphan, urokinase, vancomycin, vasopressin, vecuronium, verapamil, vinCRIStine, vinorelbine, vitamin B complcx/C, voriconazole, zoledronic acid

ADVERSE EFFECTS
CNS: Depression, hallucinations, dizziness, *fatigue*, lethargy, paresthesia, bizarre dreams, disorientation
CV: Bradycardia, *hypotension,* **CHF,** palpitations, AV block, peripheral vascular insufficiency, vasodilatation, **pulmonary edema, dysrhythmias,** cold extremities
EENT: Sore throat, **laryngospasm,** blurred vision, dry eyes
GI: Nausea, vomiting, diarrhea, colitis, constipation, cramps, dry mouth, hepatomegaly, gastric pain, acute pancreatitis
GU: Impotence, decreased libido, UTIs
HEMA: Agranulocytosis, thrombocytopenia
INTEG: Rash, pruritus, fever
META: Hyperglycemia, hypoglycemia
MISC: Facial swelling, weight change, Raynaud's phenomenon
MS: Joint pain, arthralgia, muscle cramps, pain
RESP: Dyspnea, respiratory dysfunction, **bronchospasm,** cough

Pharmacokinetics

Absorption	Well absorbed (PO); slowly absorbed (ext rel); completely absorbed (**IV**)
Distribution	Widely distributed, crosses blood-brain barrier, protein binding 90%
Metabolism	Liver, extensively
Excretion	Kidneys
Half-life	3-5 hr; ext rel 8-11 hr

Pharmacodynamics

	PO	PO-EXT REL	IV
Onset	$\frac{1}{2}$ hr	Unknown	Rapid
Peak	1-1$\frac{1}{2}$ hr	6 hr	1 min
Duration	6-12 hr	24 hr	4-6 hr

INTERACTIONS
Individual drugs
Cimetidine: increased β-blocking effect
Disopyramide: increased negative inotropic effects
Haloperidol, prazosin, quiNIDine: increased hypotension
Propafenone: increased propranolol levels
Smoking: decreased propranolol levels

Drug classifications
Barbiturates: decreased β-blocking effect
Calcium channel blockers, neuromuscular blockers: increased effects
Phenothiazines: increased toxicity

Drug/herb
Hawthorn: increased antihypertensive effect
Avoid use with feverfew, ma huang: decreased antihypertensive effect

Drug/lab test
Increased: serum potassium, serum uric acid, AST, ALT, alkaline phosphatase, LDH
Decreased: blood glucose
Interference: glaucoma testing

NURSING CONSIDERATIONS
Assessment
• Monitor B/P during beginning treatment, periodically thereafter; pulse q4hr; note rate, rhythm, quality; check apical/radial pulse before administration; notify prescriber of any significant changes (pulse <50 bpm or systolic B/P <90 mm Hg)
• Check for baselines in renal, liver function tests before therapy begins and periodically thereafter
• Assess for edema in feet, legs daily; monitor I&O, weight daily; check for jugular vein distention, crackles bilaterally; dyspnea (CHF)
• Monitor skin turgor, dryness of mucous membranes for hydration status, especially geriatric
• Assess for headache, light-headedness, decreased B/P; may indicate need for decreased dose; may aggravate symptoms of arterial insufficiency

Nursing diagnoses
• Cardiac output, decreased (uses)
• Injury, risk for (adverse reactions)
• Knowledge, deficient (teaching)
• Noncompliance (teaching)

Patient/family education
⚠ Teach patient not to discontinue product abruptly (life-threatening dysrhythmias, exacerbation of angina, MI); to take at same

⚠ Nurse Alert

time of day either with or without food consistently; taper over 2 wk
- Teach patient not to use OTC products containing α-adrenergic stimulants (such as nasal decongestants, cold preparations); to avoid alcohol, smoking and to limit sodium intake as prescribed
- Teach patient how to take pulse and B/P at home; advise when to notify prescriber
- Instruct patient to comply with weight control, dietary adjustments, modified exercise program
- Instruct patient to carry/wear emergency ID to identify product being taken, allergies; tell patient product controls symptoms but does not cure
- Caution patient to avoid hazardous activities if dizziness, drowsiness are present
- **Teach patient to report symptoms of CHF:** difficulty breathing, especially on exertion or when lying down, night cough, swelling of extremities or bradycardia, dizziness, confusion, depression, fever
- Advise patient that sensitivity to cold may occur
- Teach patient to monitor blood glucose; may mask symptoms of hypoglycemia
- Teach patient how to take pulse, B/P; withhold if <50 bpm or systolic B/P <90 mm Hg

Evaluation
Positive therapeutic outcome
- Decreased B/P in hypertension (after 1-2 wk)
- Decreased tremors
- Absence of dysrhythmias
- Decreased migraine headaches

TREATMENT OF OVERDOSE:
Lavage, **IV** atropine for bradycardia, **IV** theophylline for bronchospasm, digoxin, O_2, diuretic for cardiac failure, hemodialysis, **IV** glucose for hyperglycemia, **IV** diazepam (or phenytoin) for seizures

propylhexadrine nasal
See Appendix B

propylthiouracil (Rx)
(proe-pill-thye-oh-yoor′a-sill)
Propyl-Thyracil ♣
Func. class.: Thyroid hormone antagonist (antithyroid)
Chem. class.: Thioamide
Pregnancy category D

ACTION: Blocks synthesis peripherally of T_3, T_4, inhibits organification of iodine

Therapeutic outcome: Decreased T_3, T_4 levels, hyperthyroid symptoms

USES: Preparation for thyroidectomy, thyrotoxic crisis, hyperthyroidism, thyroid storm

CONTRAINDICATIONS:
Pregnancy **D**, breastfeeding, hypersensitivity, agranulocytosis, hepatitis, jaundice

Precautions: Infection, bone marrow depression, hepatic disease, fever

> **BLACK BOX WARNING:** Hepatic disease

DOSAGE AND ROUTES
Thyrotoxic crisis
Adult and child: PO 200-400 mg q4h for 1st 24 hr

Preparation for thyroidectomy
Adult: PO 600-1200 mg/day
Child: PO 10 mg/kg/day in divided doses

Hyperthyroidism
Adult: PO 100 mg tid increasing to 300 mg q8hr if condition is severe; continue to euthyroid state, then 100 mg daily-tid
Child >6 yr: PO 50 mg/day divided doses q8hr, titrate based on TSH/free T_4 levels
Neonate (unlabeled): PO 10 mg/kg/day in divided doses

Available forms: Tabs 50 mg

Implementation
- Give with meals to decrease GI upset
- Give at same time each day to maintain product level
- Give lowest dosage that relieves symptoms
- Store in light-resistant container
- Increase fluids to 3-4 L/day, unless contraindicated

ADVERSE EFFECTS
CNS: *Drowsiness, headache, vertigo, fever,* paresthesias, neuritis
GI: *Nausea, diarrhea, vomiting,* jaundice, **hepatitis,** loss of taste, **liver failure, death**
GU: Nephritis
HEMA: Agranulocytosis, leukopenia, thrombocytopenia, hypothrombinemia, lymphadenopathy, bleeding, vasculitis, periarteritis
INTEG: *Rash, urticaria, pruritus, alopecia, hyperpigmentation,* lupus-like syndrome
MS: Myalgia, arthralgia, nocturnal muscle cramps, osteoporosis

P

Adverse effects: *italics* = common; **bold** = life-threatening

Pharmacokinetics

Absorption	Rapidly absorbed
Distribution	Crosses placenta, concentration in thyroid gland
Metabolism	Liver
Excretion	Urine, bile, breast milk
Half-life	1-2 hr

Pharmacodynamics

Onset	30-40 min
Peak	Unknown
Duration	2-4 hr

INTERACTIONS

Individual drugs

Heparin: decreased anticoagulant effect
Lithium: increased antithyroid effect
Potassium/sodium iodide: increased effects
Radiation: increased bone marrow depression

Drug classifications

Anticoagulants (oral): decreased anticoagulant effect
Antineoplastics: increased bone marrow depression
Phenothiazines: increased agranulocytosis

Drug/lab test

Increased: pro-time, AST, ALT, alkaline phosphatase

NURSING CONSIDERATIONS

Assessment

• Monitor pulse, B/P, temp; I&O ratio; check for edema (puffy hands, feet, periorbits); indicates hypothyroidism
• Check weight daily with same clothing, scale, time of day
• Monitor T_3, T_4, which are increased; check serum TSH, which is decreased; assess free thyroxine index, which is increased if dosage is too low; discontinue product 3-4 wk before radioactive iodine uptake test
⚠ **Blood dyscrasias: Monitor CBC with differential; leukopenia, thrombocytopenia, agranulocytosis**
⚠ **Overdose: Assess for peripheral edema, heat intolerance, diaphoresis, palpitations, dysrhythmias, severe tachycardia, increased temp, delirium, CNS irritability**
⚠ **Hypersensitivity: Assess for rash, enlarged cervical lymph nodes; product may have to be discontinued**
• **Hypoprothrombinemia:** assess for bleeding, petechiae, ecchymosis

• **Bone marrow depression:** assess for sore throat, fever, fatigue
• **Hepatotoxicity:** monitor LFTs before and during treatment; jaundice, nausea, vomiting, abdominal pain, anorexia, diarrhea, fatigue
• Monitor clinical response: after 3 wk should include increased weight, decreased pulse, decreased T_4

Nursing diagnoses

• Knowledge, deficient (teaching)
• Noncompliance (teaching)

Patient/family education

• Advise patient to abstain from breastfeeding after delivery; product appears in breast milk
• Teach patient to take pulse daily and to keep graph of weight, pulse, mood
• Advise patient to report redness, swelling, sore throat, mouth lesions, which indicate blood dyscrasias
• Caution patient to avoid OTC products that contain iodine; that seafood, other iodine-containing foods may be restricted by prescriber
• Caution patient not to discontinue this medication abruptly; thyroid crisis may occur; stress patient compliance
• Teach patient that response may take several mo if thyroid is large
• Teach patient symptoms/signs of overdose: periorbital edema, cold intolerance, mental depression; notify prescriber at once
• Teach patient symptoms of inadequate dose: tachycardia, diarrhea, fever, irritability; prescriber should be notified to adjust dosage
• Teach patient to take medication exactly as prescribed, not to skip or double doses; missed doses should be taken when remembered up to 1 hr before next dose
• Instruct patient to carry/wear emergency identification indicating medication taken and condition being treated

Evaluation
Positive therapeutic outcome

• Weight gain
• Decreased pulse
• Decreased T_4
• Decreased B/P

⚠ Nurse Alert

protamine (Rx)
(proe'ta-meen)
Func. class.: Heparin antagonist
Chem. class.: Low-molecular-weight protein
Pregnancy category C

ACTION: Binds heparin, making it ineffective

Therapeutic outcome: Prevention of heparin overdose

USES: Heparin overdose; neutralizes heparin in procedures, hemorrhage

CONTRAINDICATION:
Hypersensitivity

Precautions: Pregnancy **C**, breastfeeding, fish allergy, diabetes, previous exposure to protamine, insulins, heparin rebound or bleeding

DOSAGE AND ROUTES
Heparin overdose
Adult and child: IV 1 mg of protamine/100 units of heparin given; administer slowly over 1-3 min; max 50 mg/10 min

Enoxaparin overdose
Adult: IV 1 mg of protamine/1 mg enoxaparin

Dalteparin/tinzaparin overdose
Adult: IV 1 mg of protamine/100 anti-Xa unit

Available forms: Inj 10 mg/ml

Implementation
Direct IV route
• After reconstituting 50 mg/5 ml sterile bacteriostatic water for inj, shake; give 20 mg or less over 1-3 min

Y-site compatibilities: Alfentanil, amikacin, aminophylline, ascorbic acid, atracurium, atropine, azaTHIOprine, aztreonam, benztropine, bumetanide, buprenorphine, butorphanol, calcium chloride/gluconate, ceftazidime, chlorproMAZINE, cimetidine, clindamycin, cyanocobalamin, cycloSPORINE, digoxin, diphenhydrAMINE, DOBUTamine, DOPamine, doxycycline, enalaprilat, ePHEDrine, EPINEPHrine, epoetin alfa, erythromycin, esmolol, famotidine, fentaNYL, fluconazole, ganciclovir, gentamicin, glycopyrrolate, hydrOXYzine, imipenem-cilastatin, inamrinone, iohexol, iopamidol, iothalamate, isoproterenol, labetalol, lidocaine, magnesium, mannitol, meperidine, metaraminol, methoxamine, methyldopate, metoclopramide, metoprolol, miconazole, midazolam, minocycline, morphine, multiple vitamins, nalbuphine, naloxone, netilmicin, nitroglycerin, nitroprusside, norepinephrine, ondansetron, oxytocin, papaverine, pentazocine, phenylephrine, polymyxin B, potassium chloride, procainamide, prochlorperazine, promethazine, propranolol, pyridoxine, quiNIDine, ranitidine, Ringer's, ritodrine, sodium bicarbonate, succinylcholine, SUFentanil, theophylline, thiamine, tobramycin, tolazoline, trimetaphan, urokinase, vancomycin, vasopressin, verapamil

ADVERSE EFFECTS
CNS: Lassitude, flushing
CV: Hypotension, bradycardia, **circulatory collapse**, capillary leak
GI: Nausea, vomiting, anorexia
HEMA: Bleeding
INTEG: *Rash*, dermatitis, urticaria
RESP: Dyspnea, **pulmonary edema, severe respiratory distress, bronchospasm**
SYST: **Anaphylaxis, angioedema**

Pharmacokinetics
Absorption	Completely absorbed
Distribution	Unknown
Metabolism	Unknown
Excretion	Unknown
Half-life	Unknown

Pharmacodynamics
Onset	5 min
Peak	Unknown
Duration	2 hr

NURSING CONSIDERATIONS
Assessment
• Monitor blood studies (Hct, platelets, occult blood stools) q3mo
• Monitor coagulation tests (aPTT, ACT) 15 min after dose, then in several hr
• Monitor VS, B/P, pulse q30min, plus 3 hr after dose
⚠ Assess for hypersensitivity: skin rash, urticaria, dermatitis, cough, wheezing, have emergency equipment nearby; men who have had a vasectomy may be more prone to hypersensitivity
⚠ Assess for allergy to salmon; use with caution in these patients

Nursing diagnoses
• Injury, risk for (uses)
• Knowledge, deficient (teaching)
• Tissue perfusion, ineffective (uses)

888   pseudoephedrine

Patient/family education
- Explain reason for medication and expected results; not to take if allergic to fish
- Caution patient to avoid contact activities that may result in bleeding

Evaluation
Positive therapeutic outcome
- Reversal of heparin overdose

---

pseudoephedrine (OTC)
(soo-doe-e-fed′rin)
Contac, Dimetapp Maximum Strength, Elix Sure Cold, Eltor ✚, Equaline Children's Nasal, Equaline Maximum Strength, Equate Suphedrine, Genaphed, Good Sense Nasal, Leader Pseuphedrine, Silfedrine, Sudafed, Sudafed 24 hour, Sudogest, Top Care Nasal, Wal-phed
Func. class.: Adrenergic
Chem. class.: Substituted phenylethyl-amine
Pregnancy category C

ACTION: Primary activity through α-adrenergic effects on respiratory mucosal membranes reducing congestion, hyperemia, edema; minimal bronchodilatation secondary to β-adrenergic effects

Therapeutic outcome: Decreased nasal congestion, swelling

USES: Nasal decongestant, otitis media adjunct, adjunct with antihistamines

CONTRAINDICATIONS:
Hypersensitivity to sympathomimetics, closed-angle glaucoma

Precautions: Pregnancy **C**, breastfeeding, cardiac disorders, hyperthyroidism, diabetes mellitus, prostatic hypertrophy, hypertension

DOSAGE AND ROUTES
Adult and child >12 yr: PO 60 mg q6hr; EXT REL 120 mg q12hr or 240 mg q24hr
Geriatric: PO 30-60 mg q6hr prn
Child 6-12 yr: PO 30 mg q6hr, max 120 mg/day
Child 2-6 yr: PO 15 mg q6hr, max 60 mg/day

Available forms: Ext rel caps 120, 240 mg; oral sol 15 mg, 30 mg/5 ml; drops 7.5 mg/0.8 ml; tabs 30, 60 mg; caps 60 mg; ext rel tabs 120, 240 mg

Implementation
- Swallow tab and ext rel cap whole; do not break, crush, or chew
- Give several hr before bedtime if insomnia occurs
- Store at room temperature

ADVERSE EFFECTS
CNS: *Tremors, anxiety,* stimulation, insomnia, headache, dizziness, hallucinations, **seizures** (geriatric)
CV: Palpitations, tachycardia, hypertension, chest pain, **dysrhythmias, CV collapse**
EENT: Dry nose, irritation of nose and throat
GI: *Anorexia, nausea, vomiting,* dry mouth
GU: Dysuria

Pharmacokinetics
Absorption	Well absorbed
Distribution	Enters CSF, crosses placenta
Metabolism	Liver, partially
Excretion	Kidneys, unchanged (75%); breast milk
Half-life	7 hr

Pharmacodynamics
	PO	PO-EXT REL
Onset	15-30 min	1 hr
Peak	Unknown	Unknown
Duration	4-6 hr	12 hr

INTERACTIONS
Drug classifications
Antidepressants (tricyclics), MAOIs: hypertensive crisis, do not use together
Urinary acidifiers: decreased effect of pseudoephedrine
Urinary alkalizers, adrenergics, β-blockers, phenothiazines, tricyclics: increased effect of pseudoephedrine

NURSING CONSIDERATIONS
Assessment
- Assess for CNS side effects in the geriatric: excitation, seizures, hallucinations
- Monitor for nasal congestion; auscultate lung sounds; check for tenacious bronchial secretions; children with otitis media should be assessed for eustachian tube congestion
- Monitor B/P and pulse throughout treatment

Nursing diagnoses
- Airway clearance, ineffective (uses)
- Knowledge, deficient (teaching)

Patient/family education
• Teach patient reason for product administration and expected results
• Instruct patient not to use continuously, or more than recommended dose; rebound congestion may occur
• Advise patient to check with prescriber before using other products, as product interactions may occur
• Advise patient to avoid taking near bedtime; stimulation can occur
• Caution patient not to use if stimulation, restlessness, tremors occur
• Notify parents of possible excessive agitation in children
⚠ Advise patient to notify prescriber of anxiety, slow or fast heart rate, dyspnea, seizures

Evaluation
Positive therapeutic outcome
• Decreased nasal congestion

pseudoephedrine nasal agent
See Appendix B

psyllium (OTC)
(sill'i-um)
Hydrocil, Leader Fiber Laxative, Metamucil, Natural Fiber, Natural Vegetable Fiber, Reguloid, Wal-Mucil
Func. class.: Laxative, bulk-forming
Chem. class.: Psyllium colloid
Pregnancy category C

ACTION: Bulk-forming laxative

Therapeutic outcome: Decreased constipation, decreased diarrhea in colitis

USES: Chronic constipation, ulcerative colitis, irritable bowel syndrome

CONTRAINDICATIONS:
Hypersensitivity, intestinal obstruction, abdominal pain, nausea/vomiting, fecal impaction

Precautions: Pregnancy **C**

DOSAGE AND ROUTES
Adult: PO 1-2 tsp in 8 oz of water bid or tid, then 8 oz of water; or 1 premeasured packet in 8 oz of water bid or tid, then 8 oz of water
Child >6 yr: 1 tsp in 4 oz of water at bedtime

Available forms: Chew pieces 1.7, 3.4 g/piece; powder effervescent 3.4, 3.7 g/packet; powder 3.3, 3.4, 3.5, 4.94 g/tsp; wafers 3.4 g/wafer

Implementation
• Give alone for better absorption; give after mixing with water immediately before use; administer with 8 oz of water or juice followed by another 8 oz of fluid
• Administer in AM or PM (oral dose)
• Shake susp well

ADVERSE EFFECTS
GI: *Nausea, vomiting, anorexia, diarrhea,* cramps, intestinal/esophageal blockage

Pharmacokinetics
Absorption	None
Distribution	None
Metabolism	Unknown
Excretion	Feces
Half-life	Unknown

Pharmacodynamics
Onset	12-24 hr
Peak	2-4 days
Duration	Unknown

INTERACTIONS
Drug classifications
Cardiac glycosides, oral anticoagulants, salicylates: decreased absorption of each specific product

Drug/herb
Flax, senna: increased laxative

NURSING CONSIDERATIONS
Assessment
• Monitor blood, urine electrolytes if used often by patient; check I&O ratio to identify fluid loss
• Assess for cramping, rectal bleeding, nausea, vomiting; if these symptoms occur, product should be discontinued; identify cause of constipation; identify whether fluids, bulk, or exercise is missing from lifestyle
• Assess stool for color, consistency, amount, presence of flatulence

Nursing diagnoses
• Constipation (uses)
• Knowledge, deficient (teaching)
• Noncompliance (teaching)

Patient/family education
• Discuss with patient that adequate fluid consumption is necessary
• Teach patient that normal bowel movements do not always occur daily

• Caution patient not to use in presence of abdominal pain, nausea, vomiting; tell patient to notify prescriber if constipation is unrelieved or if symptoms of electrolyte imbalance occur (muscle cramps, pain, weakness, dizziness, excessive thirst)
• Teach patient not to use laxatives for long-term therapy; bowel tone will be lost and will decrease
• Teach patient not to take at bedtime as a laxative; may interfere with sleep; also problems with lipid pneumonia
• Teach patient not to use with food or vitamin preparations; delays digestion and absorption of fat-soluble vitamins

Evaluation
Positive therapeutic outcome
• Decreased constipation in 12-24 hr

---

pyrazinamide (Rx)
(peer-a-zin'a-mide)
Tebrazid ✱
Func. class.: Antitubercular agent
Chem. class.: Pyrazinoic acid amine/ nicoturimide analog
Pregnancy category C

ACTION: Bactericidal interference with lipid; nucleic acid biosynthesis is possible

Therapeutic outcome: Bactericidal for *Mycobacterium* species

USES: Tuberculosis, as an adjunct when other products are not feasible

CONTRAINDICATIONS:
Hypersensitivity, severe hepatic damage, acute gout

Precautions: Pregnancy **C**, child <13 yr, renal failure, diabetes, porphyria, chronic gout

DOSAGE AND ROUTES
HIV negative
Adult/adolescent: PO 15-30 mg/kg/day max 30 mg/kg/day or 3 g/day; CDC max 50 mg/kg/ dose or 4 g max

Renal dose
Adult: PO CCr 10-50 ml/min, give dose q48-72hr; CCr <10 ml/min give dose q72hr

Available forms: Tabs 500 mg

Implementation
• Give with meals to decrease GI symptoms
• Give antiemetic if vomiting occurs

• May be given with other antitubercular products

ADVERSE EFFECTS
CNS: Headache
GI: Hepatotoxicity, abnormal liver function tests, peptic ulcer, nausea, vomiting, anorexia, cramps, diarrhea
GU: Urinary difficulty, increased uric acid
HEMA: Hemolytic anemia
INTEG: Photosensitivity, urticaria

Pharmacokinetics
Absorption	Well absorbed
Distribution	Widely distributed
Metabolism	Liver, extensively
Excretion	Kidneys, breast milk
Half-life	9-10 hr

Pharmacodynamics
Onset	Unknown
Peak	2 hr
Duration	$9^{1}/_{2}$ hr; metabolites 12 hr

INTERACTIONS
Drug/lab test
Increased: PBI
Decreased: 17-KS

NURSING CONSIDERATIONS
Assessment
• C&S studies should be done before treatment begins, periodically during treatment
• Monitor serum uric acid, which may be elevated and cause gout symptoms
• **Hepatotoxicity:** monitor liver function tests weekly: ALT, AST, bilirubin; hepatic status: decreased appetite, jaundice, dark urine, fatigue
• Monitor renal status before treatment, monthly thereafter: BUN, creatinine, output, specific gravity, urinalysis, uric acid
• Monitor mental status often: affect, mood, behavioral changes; psychosis may occur

Nursing diagnoses
• Diarrhea (adverse reactions)
• Infection, risk for (uses)
• Injury, risk for (adverse reactions)
• Knowledge, deficient (teaching)
• Noncompliance (teaching)

Patient/family education
• Instruct patient that compliance with dosage schedule, duration is necessary; that scheduled appointments must be kept or relapse may occur

---

⚠ Nurse Alert

- Advise diabetic patient to use blood glucose monitor to obtain correct result
- Advise patient to report weakness, fatigue, loss of appetite, nausea, vomiting, yellowing of skin or eyes, tingling/numbness of hands/feet

Evaluation
Positive therapeutic outcome
- Decreased symptoms of TB
- Sputum culture negative × 3

---

pyridostigmine (Rx)
(peer-id-oh-stig′meen)
Mestinon, Mestinon Timespan, Regonol
Func. class.: Cholinergic, anticholinesterase
Chem. class.: Tertiary amine carbamate
Pregnancy category C

ACTION: Inhibits destruction of acetylcholine, which increases concentration at sites where acetylcholine is released; this facilitates transmission of impulses across myoneural junction

Therapeutic outcome: Decreased action of nondepolarizing muscle relaxant; increased muscle strength in myasthenia gravis

USES: Nondepolarizing muscle relaxant antagonist, myasthenia gravis, pretreatment in nerve gas exposure (military only)

CONTRAINDICATIONS:
Bradycardia, hypotension, obstruction of intestine, renal system, bromide, benzyl alcohol sensitivity, cholinesterase inhibitor toxicity

Precautions: Pregnancy C, seizure disorders, bronchial asthma, coronary occlusion, hyperthyroidism, dysrhythmias, peptic ulcer, megacolon, poor GI motility

DOSAGE AND ROUTES
Myasthenia gravis
Adult: PO 600 mg/day in 5-6 divided doses, max 1.5 g/day; IM/IV 2 mg or 1/30 of PO dose; SUS REL 180-540 mg/day or bid at intervals of at least 6 hr
Child: PO 7 mg/kg/day in 5-6 divided doses; IM/IV 0.05-0.15 mg/kg/dose

Nondepolarizing neuromuscular blocker antagonist
Adult: 0.6-1.2 mg IV atropine, then 0.1-0.25 mg/kg/dose
Child: IV 0.1-0.25 mg/kg/dose

Nerve gas exposure prophylaxis (military)
Adult: PO 30 mg q8hr if threat of exposure to Soman gas is anticipated, start several hours before exposure and discontinue upon exposure; after this product is discontinued, give antidotes (atropine, pralidoxime)

Available forms: Tabs 60 mg; ext rel tabs 180 mg; syr 60 mg/5 ml; inj 5 mg/ml

Implementation
- Only with atropine sulfate available for cholinergic crisis
- Only after all other cholinergics have been discontinued
- Increased doses for tolerance, as ordered
- Larger doses after exercise or fatigue, as ordered
- Do not break, crush, or chew sus rel tabs

PO route
- On empty stomach for better absorption

IV route
- Undiluted (5 mg/ml), give through Y-tube or 3-way stopcock, give 0.5 mg or less/min (myasthenia gravis); 5 mg/min (reversal of nondepolarizing neuromuscular blockers)

Syringe compatibilities: Glycopyrrolate

Y-site compatibilities: Heparin, hydrocortisone, potassium chloride, vit B/C
- Storage at room temperature

ADVERSE EFFECTS
CNS: Dizziness, headache, sweating, weakness, **seizures,** uncoordination, paralysis, drowsiness, LOC
CV: Tachycardia, dysrhythmias, bradycardia, AV block, hypotension, ECG changes, **cardiac arrest,** syncope
EENT: Miosis, blurred vision, lacrimation, vision changes
GI: *Nausea, diarrhea, vomiting, cramps, increased salivary and gastric secretions, peristalsis*
GU: Frequency, incontinence, urgency
INTEG: Rash, urticaria, flushing
RESP: Respiratory depression, bronchospasm, constriction, laryngospasm, respiratory arrest
SYST: Cholinergic crisis

P

Pharmacokinetics

Absorption	Poorly absorbed (PO)
Distribution	Widely distributed, crosses placenta
Metabolism	Liver, plasma cholinesterase
Excretion	Kidneys
Half-life	2 hr (**IV**); 4 hr (PO)

Pharmacodynamics

	PO	PO-EXT REL	IM/IV
Onset	20-30 min	$^1/_2$-1 hr	2-15 min
Peak	Unknown	Unknown	Unknown
Duration	3-6 hr	3-6 hr	2-4 hr

INTERACTIONS

Individual drugs

Atropine, gallamine, metocurine, pancuronium, tubocurarine: decreased action

Succinylcholine: increased action of pyridostigmine

Magnesium, mecamylamine, polymyxin, procainamide, quiNIDine: decreased action of pyridostigmine

Drug classifications

Aminoglycosides, anesthetics, antidysrhythmics, corticosteroids, quinolones: decreased action of pyridostigmine

NURSING CONSIDERATIONS

Assessment

• **Myasthenia gravis:** assess for fatigue, ptosis, diplopia, difficulty swallowing, SOB, hand/gait before and after product, improvement should be seen after 1 hr

• Monitor I&O ratio; check for urinary retention or incontinence

• **Toxicity:** assess for bradycardia, hypotension, bronchospasm, headache, dizziness, seizures, respiratory depression; product should be discontinued if toxicity occurs

• Monitor VS, respiration; increased B/P during test and at baseline

• Monitor diabetic patient carefully, since this product lowers blood glucose

Nursing diagnoses

• Breathing pattern, ineffective (uses)
• Knowledge, deficient (teaching)

Patient/family education

• Advise patient to carry/wear emergency ID specifying myasthenia gravis, products taken

Evaluation

Positive therapeutic outcome

• Increased muscle strength, hand grasp, improved gait, absence of labored breathing (if severe); reversal of nondepolarizing neuromuscular blockers; prevention of nerve gas toxicity

TREATMENT OF OVERDOSE:

Discontinue product, atropine 1-4 mg **IV**

pyridoxine (vitamin B$_6$) (OTC, Rx)

(peer-i-dox'een)

Equaline Vitamin B$_6$, Neuro-K, Walgreens Finest B-6, Walgreens Gold Seal Vitamin B$_6$

Func. class.: Vitamin B$_6$, water soluble

Pregnancy category A

ACTION: Needed for fat, protein, carbohydrate metabolism; enhances glycogen release from liver and muscle tissue; needed as coenzyme for metabolic transformations of a variety of amino acids

Therapeutic outcome: Absence of vit B$_6$ deficiency

USES: Vitamin B$_6$ deficiency associated with the following: inborn errors of metabolism, seizures, isoniazid therapy, oral contraceptives, alcoholism, polyneuritis

Unlabeled uses: Palmar-plantar erythrodysesthesia syndrome

CONTRAINDICATION:

Hypersensitivity

Precautions: Pregnancy **A,** breastfeeding, children, Parkinson's disease, patients taking levodopa should avoid supplemental vitamins with >5 mg pyridoxine

DOSAGE AND ROUTES

RDA

Adult: PO (male) 1.7-2 mg; (female) 1.4-1.6 mg

Child 9-13 yr: PO 1 mg/day
Child 4-8 yr: PO 0.6 mg/day
Child 1-3 yr: PO 0.5 mg/day
Infant 7-12 mo: PO 0.3 mg/day

Vitamin B$_6$ deficiency

Adult: PO 5-25 mg/day × 3 wk
Child: PO 10 mg until desired response

Pyridoxine deficiency neuritis/seizure (not drug induced)
Adult: PO without neuritis 2.5-10 mg/day, after corrected 2-5 mg/day; with neuritis 100-200 mg/day × 3 wk, then 2-5 mg/day
Child: PO without neuritis 5-25 mg/day × 3 wk, then 1.5-2.5 mg/day in a multivitamin; with neuritis 10-50 mg/day × 3 wk, then 1-2 mg/day
Neonate with seizures: IM/IV 50-100 mg as a single dose

Deficiency caused by isoniazid, cycloSERINE, hydrALAZINE, penicillamine
Adult: PO 100-300 mg/day
Child: PO 10-50 mg/day

Prevention of deficiency caused by isoniazid, cycloSERINE, hydrALAZINE, penicillamine
Adult: PO 25-100 mg/day
Child: PO 1.2 mg/kg/day

Palmar-plantar erythrodysesthesia syndrome (unlabeled)
Adult: PO 50-150 mg/day

Available forms: Tabs 10, 25, 50, 100 mg; ext rel tabs 100 mg; inj 100 mg/ml; ext rel caps 150 mg

Implementation
PO route
• Swallow ext rel cap and ext rel tabs whole; do not break, crush, or chew
IM route
• Rotate sites to avoid pain; burning or stinging at site may occur; give by Z-track to minimize pain
• Store in airtight, light-resistant container
IV route
• Give IV undiluted or added to most IV sol; give 50 mg or less/1 min if undiluted

Syringe compatibilities: Doxapram

Additive incompatibilities: Erythromycin, iron salts, kanamycin, riboflavin, streptomycin

ADVERSE EFFECTS
CNS: Paresthesia, flushing, warmth, lethargy (rare with normal renal function)
INTEG: Pain at inj site

Absorption	Well absorbed (PO)
Distribution	Stored in liver, muscle, brain; crosses placenta
Metabolism	Unknown
Excretion	Kidneys, unchanged (not used)
Half-life	Unknown

Pharmacodynamics
Unknown

INTERACTIONS
Individual drugs
Chloramphenicol, cycloSERINE, hydrALAZINE, isoniazid, penicillamine: decreased effects of pyridoxine
Levodopa: decreased effects of levodopa

Drug classifications
Contraceptives (oral), immunosuppressants: decreased effects of pyridoxine

NURSING CONSIDERATIONS
Assessment
• Monitor pyridoxine levels throughout treatment
• Assess nutritional status: yeast, liver, legumes, bananas, green vegetables, whole grains
• Assess for pyridoxine (B$_6$) deficiency: nausea, vomiting, dermatitis, cheilosis, seizures, irritability, dermatitis before, during treatment
• Assess neurological status: paresthesia, lethargy
• Monitor blood tests: Hct, Hgb

Nursing diagnoses
• Knowledge, deficient (teaching)
• Noncompliance (teaching, overuse)
• Nutrition: less than body requirements, imbalanced (uses)

Patient/family education
• Teach patient to avoid other vitamin supplements unless directed by prescriber
• Advise patient to increase meat, bananas, potatoes, lima beans, whole grain cereals in diet which are high in vit B$_6$
• Caution patient not to increase dosage, since serious reactions may occur

Evaluation
Positive therapeutic outcome
• Absence of nausea, vomiting, anorexia, skin lesions, glossitis, stomatitis, edema, seizures, restlessness, paresthesia

pyrimethamine (Rx)

(peer-i-meth'a-meen)
Daraprim
Func. class.: Antimalarial, antiprotozoal
Chem. class.: Folic acid antagonist
Pregnancy category C

ACTION: Inhibits folic acid metabolism in parasite; prevents transmission by stopping growth of fertilized gametes

Therapeutic outcome: Prevention of malaria

USES: Malaria prophylaxis, antiprotozoal action against *Plasmodium vivax, Pneumocystis jiroveci*

CONTRAINDICATIONS:

Hypersensitivity, chloroquine-resistant malaria, megaloblastic anemia caused by folate deficiency

Precautions: Pregnancy **C,** breastfeeding, geriatric patients, blood dyscrasias, seizure disorder, glucose-6-phosphate dehydrogenase (G6PD) disease, renal/hepatic disease

DOSAGE AND ROUTES

Prophylaxis of malaria

• Begin 2 wk before entering endemic area and continue for 6-10 wk after return
Adult and child >10 yr: PO 25 mg qwk
Child 4-10 yr: PO 12.5 mg qwk
Child <4 yr: PO 6.25 mg qwk

Malaria treatment

Adult/adolescent/child >10 yr: PO 25 mg q day × 2 days with sulfonamide
Child 4-10 yr: 25 mg q day × 2 days

Toxoplasmosis

Adult: PO 50-75 mg, then reduce by about 50% for 4-5 wk, with 1-4 g sulfADIAZINE × 1-3 wk, then reduce by 50% for 4-5 wk
Child: PO 1 mg/kg/day in 2 divided doses or 2 mg/kg/day × 3 days, then 1 mg/kg/day or divided twice daily × 4 wk, max 25 mg/day

Toxoplasmosis in AIDS patients

Adult: PO 100-200 mg/day × 1-2 days, then 50-100 mg/day × 3-6 wk, then 25-50 mg/day for life (given with clindamycin or sulfADIAZINE)

Available forms: Tabs 25 mg; combo tabs 500 mg sulfadoxine/25 mg pyrimethamine

Implementation

PO route
• Give leucovorin IM 3-9 mg/day × 3 days if folic acid deficiency occurs
• Give before or after meals at same time each day to maintain product level, decrease GI symptoms
• **Extemporaneous susp:** tabs may be crushed and mixed with 25 ml distilled water, sucrose-containing sol (1 mg/ml), shake well, stable for 5-7 days at room temp if mixed with sucrose-containing sol
• Store in tight, light-resistant container

ADVERSE EFFECTS

CNS: Stimulation, irritability, **seizures,** tremors, ataxia, fatigue, fever
CV: Dysrhythmias
GI: *Nausea, vomiting, cramps, anorexia,* diarrhea, atrophic glossitis, gastritis
HEMA: Thrombocytopenia, leukopenia, pancytopenia, megaloblastic anemia, decreased folic acid, **agranulocytosis**
INTEG: Skin eruptions, photosensitivity, **Stevens-Johnson syndrome**
RESP: Respiratory failure

Pharmacokinetics

Absorption	Well absorbed
Distribution	Widely distributed; crosses placenta
Metabolism	Liver, extensively
Excretion	Kidneys, unchanged (30%); breast milk
Half-life	4 days

Pharmacodynamics

Onset	Unknown
Peak	2 hr
Duration	Unknown

INTERACTIONS

Individual drugs

Folic acid: increased synergistic action
Radiation: increased bone marrow suppression
Zidovudine: increased risk of megaloblastic anemia, agranulocytosis, thrombocytopenia

Drug classifications

Bone marrow depressants, folate antagonists: increased bone marrow suppression

NURSING CONSIDERATIONS

Assessment
- **Serious skin disorders:** assess for **Stevens-Johnson syndrome** (swelling of face, lips, throat, fever)
- Monitor folic acid level; megaloblastic anemia occurs
- ⚠ **Blood dyscrasias: assess blood studies, CBC, platelets; twice weekly if dosage is increased**
- ⚠ **Toxicity: assess for vomiting, anorexia, seizure, blood dyscrasia, glossitis; product should be discontinued immediately**

Nursing diagnoses
- Diarrhea (adverse reactions)
- Infection, risk for (uses)
- Injury, risk for (adverse reactions)
- Knowledge, deficient (teaching)
- Noncompliance (teaching)

Patient/family education
- Instruct patient that compliance with dosage schedule, duration is necessary; that scheduled appointments must be kept or relapse may occur
- Teach patient to report vision problems, fever, fatigue, bruising, bleeding, sore throat; may indicate **blood dyscrasias**
- Teach patient to report immediately skin rash; stop use

Evaluation
Positive therapeutic outcome
- Decreased symptoms of toxoplasmosis
- Decreased symptoms of *Pneumocystis jiroveci* pneumonia
- Decreased symptoms of malaria

TREATMENT OF OVERDOSE:
Gastric lavage, short-acting barbiturate, leucovorin, respiratory support if needed

---

QUEtiapine (Rx)
(kwe-tie′a-peen)
Seroquel, Seroquel XR
Func. class.: Antipsychotic
Chem. class.: Dibenzodiazepine
Pregnancy category C

ACTION: Functions as an antagonist at multiple neurotransmitter receptors in the brain including $5-HT_{1A}$, $5-HT_2$, DOPamine D_1, D_2, H_1, adrenergic α_1, α_2 receptors

Therapeutic outcome: Decreased hallucinations and disorganized thought

USES: Bipolar disorder, bipolar I disorder, depression, mania, schizophrenia

CONTRAINDICATIONS:
Hypersensitivity, breastfeeding

Precautions: Pregnancy **C**, geriatric, long-term use, seizures, hepatic disease, breast cancer, QT prolongation, CV disease, Parkinson's, brain tumor, hematological disease, torsades de pointes, cataracts, dehydration

> **BLACK BOX WARNING:** Children, suicide, dementia

DOSAGE AND ROUTES

Bipolar I disorder
Adult: PO (monotherapy or as adjunct to lithium or divalproex) 50 mg bid on day 1, 100 mg on day 2 in 2 divided doses as tolerated to 400 mg on day 4; range 400-800 mg/day

Psychotic disorders
Adult: PO 25 mg bid, titrate upward; XR: 300 mg/day in PM, range 400-800 mg/day

Depressive disorder (inadequate response to antidepressants alone)
Adult: PO EXT REL 50 mg/day in the PM on day 1, 2; on day 3 give 150 mg in the PM
Geriatric: PO EXT REL 50 mg; may increase by 50 mg/day based on response

Available forms: Tabs 25, 50, 100, 200, 300, 400 mg; ext rel tab 50, 150, 200, 300, 400 mg

Implementation
- Give reduced dosage in geriatric patients
- Give anticholinergic agent on order from prescriber to be used for EPS
- Avoid use of CNS depressants
- Give **immediate release** without regard to meals
- Give **extended release** without food or with light meal, swallow whole, do not split, crush, chew
- Supervise ambulation until patient is stabilized on medication; do not involve in strenuous exercise program because fainting is possible; patient should not stand still for a long time
- Sips of water, sugarless candy, gum for dry mouth
- Store in airtight, light-resistant container

ADVERSE EFFECTS
CNS: EPS, pseudoparkinsonism, akathisia, dystonia, tardive dyskinesia, drowsiness, in-

Adverse effects: *italics* = common; **bold** = life-threatening

896 QUEtiapine

somnia, agitation, anxiety, *headache,* **seizures, neuroleptic malignant syndrome,** dizziness, dystonia, restless legs syndrome
CV: Orthostatic hypotension, **tachycardia,** QT prolongation, CV disease, Parkinson's disease, cardiomyopathy, myocarditis
ENDO: SIADH, hyperglycemia
GI: Nausea, anorexia, constipation, abdominal pain, dry mouth
HEMA: Leukopenia, agranulocytosis
INTEG: Rash
META: Hyponatremia
MISC: Asthenia, back pain, fever, ear pain
MS: Rhabdomyolysis
RESP: Rhinitis
SYST: Stevens-Johnson syndrome, anaphylaxis

Pharmacokinetics

Absorption	Rapidly absorbed
Distribution	Widely distributed
Metabolism	Liver, extensively; inhibits P450 CYP3A4 enzyme system; 83% protein binding
Excretion	Urine, feces
Half-life	≥6 hr

Pharmacodynamics

Onset	Unknown
Peak	1.5 hr
Duration	Up to 12 hr

INTERACTIONS

Individual drugs
Alcohol: increased CNS depression
CarBAMazepine, phenytoin, rifampin, thioridazine: increased QUEtiapine clearance
Chloroquine, clarithromycin, droperidol, erythromycin, haloperidol, methadone, pentamidine: increased QT prolongation
Cimetidine: decreased QUEtiapine clearance
Erythromycin: increased effects of erythromycin
Fluconazole, itraconazole, ketoconazole: increased action of QUEtiapine
Levodopa: decreased effect of levodopa
LORazepam: decreased effect of LORazepam

Drug classifications
Analgesics (opioid), antihistamines, sedatives-hypnotics: increased CNS depression
Antihypertensives: increased hypotension
Barbiturates, glucocorticoids: increased clearance of quetiapine, decreased quetiapine effect

β-agonists, class IA/III antidysrhythmics, local anesthetics, phenothiazines (some), tricyclics: increased QT prolongation
DOPamine agonists: decreased effects of DOPamine agonists

NURSING CONSIDERATIONS
Assessment
• Assess CV status: QT prolongation, tachycardia, orthostatic B/P

> **BLACK BOX WARNING:** Mental status before initial administration, AIMS assessment; affect, orientation, LOC, reflexes, gait, coordination, sleep pattern disturbances; suicidal thoughts/behavior (child/young adult); dementia (geriatric patients)

• **Suicide:** restrict amount of product given, usually suicidal thoughts, behavior occur early in treatment and in children/adolescents/young adults
• Check that patient swallows all PO medication; check for hoarding or giving of medication to other patients
• Obtain baselines in blood glucose, liver function tests, neurologic status, ophthalmologic exam, cholesterol profile, weight
• Monitor B/P with patient in sitting, standing, and lying positions; take pulse and respirations q4hr during initial treatment; establish baseline before starting treatment; report drops of 30 mm Hg; obtain baseline ECG and monitor Q- and T-wave changes
• Check for dizziness, faintness, palpitations, tachycardia on rising; severe orthostatic hypotension is common
⚠ **Identify for neuroleptic malignant syndrome: hyperpyrexia, muscle rigidity, increased CPK, altered mental status, seizures, tachycardia, diaphoresis, hyper/hypotension, fatigue; product should be discontinued and prescriber notified immediately**
• **Assess for EPS** including akathisia (inability to sit still, no pattern to movements), tardive dyskinesia (bizarre movements of the jaw, mouth, tongue, extremities), pseudoparkinsonism (rigidity, tremors, pill rolling, shuffling gait); an antiparkinson product should be prescribed

Nursing diagnoses
• Coping, ineffective (uses)
• Knowledge, deficient (teaching)
• Noncompliance (teaching)

Patient/family education
• Teach patient to use good oral hygiene; frequent rinsing of mouth, sugarless gum for dry mouth
• Caution patient to avoid hazardous activities until product response is determined; dizziness, blurred vision may occur
• Inform patient that orthostatic hypotension occurs often; patient should rise from sitting or lying position gradually; avoid hot tubs, hot showers, and tub baths because hypotension may occur; inform patient that heat stroke may occur in hot weather, to take extra precautions to stay cool
• Advise patient to avoid abrupt withdrawal of this product or EPS may result; product should be withdrawn slowly
• Teach patient to avoid OTC preparations (cough, hayfever, cold) unless approved by prescriber; serious product interactions may occur; avoid use with alcohol, CNS depressants because increased drowsiness may occur
• Advise patient to take medication only as prescribed
• Advise patient that follow-up is necessary including LFTs, blood glucose, neurologic/oph-thalmic function, cholesterol profile, weight
• If drowsiness occurs, avoid hazardous activities such as driving
• Advise patient to notify prescriber if pregnancy is planned, suspected; do not breastfeed
• **Advise patient to notify prescriber immediately of fever, difficulty breathing, fatigue, sore throat, rash, bleeding**
• **Suicide: thoughts, behavior, primarily in children/adolescents/young adults**

Evaluation
Positive therapeutic outcome
• Decrease in emotional excitement, hallucinations, delusions, paranoia
• Reorganization of patterns of thought, speech

TREATMENT OF OVERDOSE:
Lavage, provide airway

quinapril (Rx)
(kwin'a-pril)
Accupril
Func. class.: Antihypertensive
Chem. class.: Angiotensin-converting enzyme (ACE) inhibitor
Pregnancy category D (2nd/3rd trimester
Pregnancy category C 1st trimester

ACTION: Selectively suppresses renin-angiotensin-aldosterone system; inhibits ACE, prevents conversion of angiotensin I to angiotensin II; results in dilatation of arterial, venous vessels

Therapeutic outcome: Decreased B/P in hypertension

USES: Hypertension, alone or in combination with thiazide diuretics, systolic CHF

CONTRAINDICATIONS:
Children, hypersensitivity to ACE inhibitors, angioedema

BLACK BOX WARNING: Pregnancy D (2nd/3rd trimester)

Precautions: Breastfeeding, geriatric, impaired renal/liver function, dialysis patients, hypovolemia, blood dyscrasias, COPD, asthma, bilateral renal stenosis, cough, pregnancy **C** 1st trimester, hyperkalemia

DOSAGE AND ROUTES
Hypertension
Adult: PO 10-20 mg/day initially, then 20-80 mg/day divided bid or daily (monotherapy), start at 2.5 mg/day (with diuretics)
Geriatric: PO 10 mg/day, titrate to desired response (monotherapy), start at 2.5 mg/day (with diuretics)

Congestive heart failure
Adult: PO 5 mg bid, may increase qwk until 20-40 mg/day in 2 divided doses

Renal dose
Adult: PO CCr 30-60 ml/min 5 mg/day initially; CCr <30 ml/min 2.5 mg/day initially

Available forms: Tabs 5, 10, 20, 40 mg

Implementation
• Tabs may be crushed if necessary, take 1-2 hr before food or antacids; avoid high-potassium foods

• Store in airtight container at 86° F (30° C) or less

• Severe hypotension may occur after 1st dose of this medication; may be prevented by reducing or discontinuing diuretic therapy 3 days before beginning quinapril therapy

ADVERSE EFFECTS

CNS: Headache, dizziness, fatigue, somnolence, depression, malaise, nervousness, vertigo
CV: Hypotension, postural hypotension, syncope, palpitations, angina pectoris, **MI, tachycardia,** vasodilatation, chest pain
GI: Nausea, diarrhea, constipation, vomiting, gastritis, **GI hemorrhage,** dry mouth
GU: Increased BUN, creatinine, decreased libido, impotence
INTEG: **Angioedema,** rash, sweating, photosensitivity, pruritus
META: Hyperkalemia
MISC: Back pain, amblyopia
MS: Myalgia
RESP: Cough, pharyngitis, dyspnea

Pharmacokinetics

Absorption	≥60%
Distribution	Protein binding 97%, crosses placenta
Metabolism	Liver (active metabolites quinaprilat)
Excretion	Metabolites urine (60%), feces (37%)
Half-life	2 hr

Pharmacodynamics

Onset	$^{1}/_{2}$-1 hr
Peak	1-2 hr
Duration	24 hr

INTERACTIONS

Individual drugs
Alcohol: increased hypotension (large amounts)
Lithium: increased toxicity
HydrALAZINE, prazosin: use caution
Tetracycline: decreased absorption of tetracycline

Drug classifications
Adrenergic blockers, antihypertensives, diuretics, ganglionic blockers, nitrates, phenothiazines: increased hypotension
Diuretics (potassium sparing), potassium supplements, sympathomimetics, ACE/angiotensin II receptor antagonists, vasodilators: use caution

NSAIDs: decreased hypotensive effect of quinapril

Drug/lab test
Increased: Potassium, creatinine, BUN, LFTs

NURSING CONSIDERATIONS

Assessment
• **Collagen vascular disease:** monitor blood studies: neutrophils, decreased platelets; WBC with differential baseline, periodically q3mo; if neutrophils <1000/mm³ discontinue treatment
• **Hypertension:** monitor B/P, check for orthostatic hypotension, syncope; if changes occur, dosage change may be required
• Monitor renal function tests (protein, BUN, creatinine) and periodically liver function tests, uric acid; glucose may be elevated; watch for increased levels that may indicate nephrotic syndrome and renal failure; monitor renal symptoms: polyuria, oliguria, frequency, dysuria
• Check potassium levels throughout treatment, although hyperkalemia rarely occurs
• **CHF:** check for edema in feet, legs daily, weight daily
• **Allergic reactions:** assess for allergic reactions: rash, fever, pruritus, urticaria; product should be discontinued if antihistamines fail to help

> **BLACK BOX WARNING:** Assess for pregnancy; pregnancy **D,** 2nd/3rd trimester; if pregnancy is suspected, discontinue product

Nursing diagnoses
• Cardiac output, decreased (uses)
• Injury, risk for (adverse reactions)
• Knowledge, deficient (teaching)
• Noncompliance (teaching)

Patient/family education
• Advise patient not to discontinue product abruptly; advise patient to tell all persons associated with care
• Teach patient not to use OTC products (cough, cold, allergy) unless directed by physician; serious side effects can occur; avoid high-fat meal at time of dose
• Inform patient that xanthines such as coffee, tea, chocolate, cola can prevent action of product
• Caution patient on the importance of complying with dosage schedule, even if feeling better; to continue with medical regimen to decrease B/P: exercise, cessation of smoking, decreasing stress, diet modifications

• Emphasize the need to rise slowly to sitting or standing position to minimize orthostatic hypotension; not to exercise in hot weather or increased hypotension can occur

• Teach patient to notify prescriber of mouth sores, sore throat, fever, swelling of hands or feet, irregular heartbeat, chest pain, coughing, shortness of breath

• Caution patient to report excessive perspiration, dehydration, vomiting, diarrhea; may lead to fall in B/P

• Caution patient that product may cause dizziness, fainting, light-headedness; may occur during 1st few days of therapy; to avoid activities that may be hazardous

• Teach patient how to take B/P, and normal readings for age group

• Teach patient product may cause skin rash or impaired taste perception

BLACK BOX WARNING: Pregnancy **D**, 2nd/3rd trimester, to report if pregnancy is planned or suspected, do not breastfeed

Evaluation
Positive therapeutic outcome
• Decreased B/P in hypertension

TREATMENT OF OVERDOSE:
0.9% NaCl **IV** inf, hemodialysis

quiNIDine gluconate (Rx)
(kwin'i dccn)
quiNIDine sulfate (Rx)
Func. class.: Antidysrhythmic (class IA)
Chem. class.: QuiNINE dextro isomer
Pregnancy category C

Do not confuse:
quiNIDine/quiNINE

ACTION: Prolongs action potential duration and effective refractory period, thus decreasing myocardial excitability; anticholinergic properties

Therapeutic outcome: Treatment of dysrhythmias

USES: Premature ventricular contractions (PVCs), atrial fibrillation, flutter; paroxysmal atrial tachycardia, ventricular tachycardia, malaria (**IV** quiNIDine gluconate)

CONTRAINDICATIONS:
Hypersensitivity or idiosyncratic response, digoxin toxicity, blood dyscrasias, myasthenia gravis

BLACK BOX WARNING: History of long QT syndrome, product-induced torsades de pointes, severe heart block

Precautions: Pregnancy C, breastfeeding, children, geriatric, renal/hepatic disease, potassium imbalance, CHF, respiratory depression, bradycardia, hypotension, syncope

BLACK BOX WARNING: Cardiac arrhythmias, MI

DOSAGE AND ROUTES
QuiNIDine sulfate
Atrial fibrillation/flutter
Adult: PO 200 mg q2-3hr × 5-8 doses; may increase daily until sinus rhythm is restored; max 4 g/day given only after digitalization; maintenance 200-300 mg tid-qid or 300-600 mg q8-12hr (EXT REL)

Paroxysmal supraventricular tachycardia
Adult: PO 400-600 mg q2-3hr, then 200-300 mg q6-8hr or 300-600 mg q8-12hr (EXT REL)

Premature atrial/ventricular contraction
Adult: PO 200-300 mg q6-8hr or 300-600 mg (EXT REL) q8-12hr, max 4 g/day
Child: PO 30 mg/kg/day or 900 mg/m^2/day in 5 divided doses

QuiNIDine gluconate
Adult: PO 324-648 mg q8-12hr (EXT REL); IM 600 mg, then 400 mg q2hr; **IV** give 16 mg/min

Available forms: Gluconate: ext rel tabs 324, 330 mg; inj gluconate 80 mg/ml; **sulfate:** tabs 200, 300 mg; ext rel tabs 300 mg

Implementation
• Give AV node blocker (digoxin) before starting quiNIDine to avoid increased ventricular rate
PO route
• Do not break, crush, or chew ext rel tab
• Give on an empty stomach with a full glass of water; may be given with meals if GI irritation occurs, absorption will be decreased
• Ext rel forms not interchangeable
• Tab may be crushed and mixed with fluid or foods for patients with swallowing difficulties
IM route
• Give IM injection in deltoid, aspirate to avoid intravascular administration

Q

Adverse effects: *italics* = common; **bold** = life-threatening

Intermittent IV infusion route
• Give after diluting 800 mg/50 ml or more D$_5$W (16 mg/ml); give max 0.25 mg/kg/min, quiNIDine is absorbed by PVC tubing, minimize length; use inf pump

Y-site compatibilities: Alfentanil, amikacin, anidulafungin, ascorbic acid, atenolol, atracurium, atropine, benztropine, bleomycin, bumetanide, buprenorphine, butorphanol, calcium gluconate, caspofungin, chlorproMAZINE, cimetidine, CISplatin, cyanocobalamin, cycloSPORINE, DACTINomycin, digoxin, diltiazem, diphenhydrAMINE, DOBUTamine, docetaxel, DOPamine, doxycycline, enalaprilat, ePHEDrine, EPINEPHrine, epoetin alfa, erythromycin, esmolol, etoposide, famotidine, fenoldopam, fentaNYL, fluconazole, fludarabine, gatifloxacin, gemcitabine, gentamicin, glycopyrrolate, granisetron, HYDROmorphone, IDArubicin, imipenem-cilastatin, irinotecan, isoproterenol, labetalol, lidocaine, linezolid, LORazepam, magnesium sulfate, mannitol, mechlorethamine, meperidine, metaraminol, methoxamine, methyldopa, metoclopramide, metoprolol, metroNIDAZOLE, miconazole, milrinone, mitoxantrone, morphine, multiple vitamins, mycophenolate, nalbuphine, naloxone, nesiritide, netilmicin, nitroglycerin, norepinephrine, octreotide, ondansetron, oxaliplatin, paclitaxel, palonosetron, pamidronate, pancuronium, papaverine, pentamidine, pentazocine, phenylephrine, phytonadione, polymyxin B, potassium chloride, procainamide, prochlorperazine, promethazine, propranolol, protamine, pyridoxine, ranitidine, ritodrine, succinylcholine, SUFentanil, tacrolimus, teniposide, theophylline, thiamine, thiotepa, tirofiban, tobramycin, tolazoline, trimetaphan, urokinase, vancomycin, vasopressin, verapamil, vinorelbine, voriconazole, zoledronic acid

ADVERSE EFFECTS

CNS: *Headache, dizziness,* involuntary movement, confusion, psychosis, restlessness, irritability, syncope, excitement, depression, ataxia
CV: **Hypotension**, *bradycardia, PVCs,* **heart block, cardiovascular collapse, arrest, torsades de pointes,** widening QRS complex, **ventricular tachycardia**

EENT: Cinchonism: tinnitus, blurred vision, hearing loss, mydriasis, disturbed color vision
GI: Nausea, vomiting, anorexia, *diarrhea,* **hepatotoxicity,** abdominal pain
HEMA: Thrombocytopenia, hemolytic anemia, agranulocytosis, hypoprothrombinemia
INTEG: Rash, urticaria, **angioedema,** swelling, photosensitivity, flushing with severe pruritus
RESP: Dyspnea, **respiratory depression**

Absorption	Well absorbed (PO, IM), slowly absorbed (sus rel)
Distribution	Widely distributed, crosses placenta, protein binding 80%-90%
Metabolism	Liver
Excretion	Kidney unchanged, 10%-50% breast milk
Half-life	6-7 hr

INTERACTIONS

Individual drugs

Amiodarone, cimetidine, NIFEdipine: increased quiNIDine level
Digoxin: increased digoxin level
NIFEdipine, sodium bicarbonate, verapamil: increased quiNIDine effect
Phenytoin, rifampin, sucralfate: decreased effects of quiNIDine
Propranolol: increased effect of propranolol
Reserpine: increased cardiac depression
Warfarin: increased levels of warfarin

Drug classifications

Antacids, carbonic anhydrase inhibitors, hydroxide suspensions: increased effects of quiNIDine
Anticholinergic blockers: increased vagolytic effects
Anticoagulants (oral): increased levels of anticoagulant
Antidepressants (tricyclics): increased effect of antidepressant
Antidysrhythmics: increased cardiac depression
Barbiturates, cholinergics: decreased effects of quiNIDine

	PO (SULFATE)	PO EXT REL	PO (GLUCONATE)	IM	IV
Onset	$1/2$ hr	Unknown	Unknown	$1/2$ hr	5 min
Peak	$1/2$-$1^1/_2$ hr	4 hr	4 hr	$1/2$-$1^1/_2$ hr	Unknown
Duration	6-8 hr	8-12 hr	6-8 hr	6-8 hr	6-8 hr

⚠ Nurse Alert

Neuromuscular blockers: increased neuromuscular blocking

Phenothiazines: increased cardiac depression

Drug/herb
Hawthorn: increased quiNIDine effect

Drug/food
Grapefruit juice: decreased absorption, decreased metabolism

Drug/lab test
Increased: CPK

Interference: triamterene therapy interferes with quiNIDine test levels

NURSING CONSIDERATIONS

Assessment
• Monitor ECG continuously to determine product effectiveness, measure PR, QRS, QT intervals, check for PVCs, other dysrhythmias; monitor B/P continuously for hypo/hypertension; for rebound hypertension after 1-2 hr; check for dehydration or hypovolemia

• Monitor blood levels (therapeutic level 2-7 mcg/ml)

• **Cinchonism:** assess for tinnitus, headache, nausea, dizziness, fever, vertigo, tremor, may lead to hearing loss

• Monitor I&O ratio, electrolytes (potassium, sodium, chloride); check weight daily; check for signs of CHF or pulmonary toxicity: dyspnea, fatigue, cough, fever, chest pain; if these occur, product should be discontinued

• Monitor liver function tests: AST, ALT, bilirubin, alkaline phosphatase

• Assess for CNS symptoms: confusion, psychosis, numbness, depression, involuntary movements; if these occur, product should be discontinued

• Monitor cardiac rate, respiration: rate, rhythm, character, chest pain; watch for ventricular tachycardia, supraventricular tachycardia, or fibrillation that indicates toxicity

Nursing diagnoses
• Cardiac output, decreased (uses)
• Gas exchange, impaired (adverse reactions)
• Knowledge, deficient (teaching)

Patient/family education
• Instruct patient to report adverse effects immediately to prescriber

• Caution patient that sunglasses may be needed for photophobia; to use sunscreen, protective clothing, or stay out of sun to prevent burns

• Instruct patient to complete follow-up appointments with health care provider including pulmonary function tests, chest x-ray, ophth and otoscopic exams

• Advise patients to report signs of cinchonism, diarrhea, anorexia, decreased B/P

• Avoid grapefruit

Evaluation
Positive therapeutic outcome
• Resolution of dysrhythmias

---

quiNINE (OTC, Rx)
(kwye′nine)

Apo-Quinine ✖, **Qualaquin**

Func. class.: Antimalarial

Chem. class.: Cinchona tree alkaloid

Pregnancy category C

ACTION: Inhibits parasite replications, transcription of DNA to RNA by forming complexes with DNA of parasite

Therapeutic outcome: Reduction/death of *Plasmodium falciparum*; decreased leg cramps

USES: *P. falciparum*, malaria

CONTRAINDICATIONS:
Hypersensitivity, G6PD deficiency, retinal field changes, myasthenia gravis

Precautions: Pregnancy **C**, blood dyscrasias, breastfeeding, severe GI/hepatic disease, neurologic disease, psoriasis, cardiac dysrhythmias, tinnitus, hypoglycemia

BLACK BOX WARNING: Nocturnal leg cramps

DOSAGE AND ROUTES

Malaria
Adult: PO 648 mg q8hr × 3 days or 7 days in SE Asia, given with tetracycline 250 mg q5hr × 7 days or clindamycin 900 mg q8hr × 7 days or doxycycline 100 mg q12hr × 7 days

Child: PO 25 mg/kg/day divided q8hr for 3-7 days in conjunction with another agent

Available forms: Tabs 324 mg

Implementation
• Give before or after meals at same time each day to maintain level

• Store in airtight, light-resistant container

ADVERSE EFFECTS
CNS: Headache, stimulation, fatigue, irritability, **seizures,** bad dreams, dizziness, fever, confusion, anxiety

Q

CV: Angina, dysrhythmias, tachycardia, hypotension, **acute circulatory failure**
EENT: *Blurred vision, corneal changes, retinal changes, difficulty focusing,* tinnitus, vertigo, deafness, photophobia, diplopia, night blindness
ENDO: Hypoglycemia
GI: *Nausea, vomiting, anorexia,* diarrhea, epigastric pain
GU: Renal tubular damage, **anuria**
HEMA: **Thrombocytopenia, purpura, hypothrombinemia, hemolysis**
INTEG: Pruritus, pigmentary changes, skin eruptions, lichen planus–like eruptions, flushing, facial edema, sweating
MISC: **Hemolytic uremic syndrome**
RESP: Dyspnea

Pharmacokinetics

Absorption	Rapidly absorbed, 80%
Distribution	Crosses placenta, excreted breast milk, protein binding 70%-90% in malaria
Metabolism	Liver, extensively 80%
Excretion	Urine, 20% unchanged
Half-life	8-12 hr, increases in malaria

Pharmacodynamics

Onset	Unknown
Peak	1-3 hr
Duration	8 hr

INTERACTIONS

Individual products
AcetaZOLAMIDE, sodium bicarbonate: increased toxicity
Digoxin, digitoxin: increased levels
QuiNIDine: increased QT prolongation
Rifampin: increased treatment failure

Drug classifications
CYP2D6 substrates (amoxapine, atomoxetine, carvedilol, metoprolol, propranolol, timolol, encainide, flecainide, mexiletine, clozapine, codeine, cyclobenzaprine, fenfluramine, darifenacin, dexfenfluramine, dextromethorphan, donepezil, FLUoxetine, galantamine, haloperidol, HYDROcodone, maprotiline, meperidine, methadone, methamphetamine, oxyCODONE, PARoxetine, risperidone, fluphenazine, perphenazine, thioridazine, traMADol, traZODone, venlafaxine, zolpidem): increased levels
Antacids (magnesium or aluminum salts): decreased absorption of quiNINE

Anticoagulants: increased levels of anticoagulants
CYP3A4 inhibitors (clarithromycin, cycloSPORINE, diltiazem, etravirine, azole antifungals, lapatinib, mifepristone, protease inhibitors): increased quiNINE levels
Neuromuscular blockers: increased effect of neuromuscular blockers
Tricyclics: increased levels of tricyclics

Drug/lab test
Increased: 17-ks
Interference: 17-ohcs

Drug/herb
St. John's wort: decreased quiNINE level

NURSING CONSIDERATIONS

Assessment
• Monitor B/P, pulse; watch for hypotension, tachycardia
• Assess liver studies qwk: ALT, AST, bilirubin
• Assess blood tests, CBC, since blood dyscrasias occur
• **Assess for cinchonism:** nausea, blurred vision, tinnitus, headache, difficulty focusing; quiNIDine levels >10 mcg/ml
• Assess for symptoms of malaria and improvement
• Assess frequency/duration of nocturnal leg cramps

Nursing diagnoses
• Infection, risk for (uses)
• Knowledge, deficient (teaching)
• Noncompliance (teaching)

Patient/family education
• Advise patient to avoid OTC preparations: cold preparations, tonic water
• Advise patient to take only as prescribed
• Teach patient visual changes may occur, to avoid driving or hazardous activities until response is known
• Teach patient to stop product and call prescriber if difficulty breathing, ringing in the ears, or allergic reaction occurs
• Teach patient to use insect repellant, protective clothing if in area with mosquitoes

Evaluation
Positive therapeutic outcome
• Decreased symptoms of malaria

rabeprazole (Rx)
(rab-ee-pray´zole)
Aciphex, Dariet ✣
Func. class.: Proton pump inhibitor
Chem. class.: Benzimidazole
Pregnancy category C

ACTION: Suppresses gastric secretion by inhibiting hydrogen/potassium ATPase enzyme system in the gastric parietal cell; characterized as a gastric acid pump inhibitor, since it blocks the final step of acid production

Therapeutic outcome: Absence of duodenal ulcers; decreased gastroesophageal reflux

USES: Gastroesophageal reflux disease (GERD), severe erosive esophagitis, poorly responsive systemic GERD, pathologic hypersecretory conditions (Zollinger-Ellison syndrome, systemic mastocytosis, multiple endocrine adenomas); treatment of duodenal ulcers with or without antiinfectives for *Helicobacter pylori;* daytime, nighttime heartburn

CONTRAINDICATIONS:
Hypersensitivity

Precautions: Pregnancy **C**, breastfeeding, children, Asian patients, diarrhea, geriatric patients, gastric cancer, hepatic/GI disease, IBS, osteoporosis, pseudomembranous colitis, ulcerative colitis, vit B_{12} deficiency

DOSAGE AND ROUTES
Healing of duodenal ulcers
Adult: PO 20 mg/day × ≤4 wk, to be taken after breakfast

Erosive esophagitis/GERD
Adult: PO 20 mg/day × 4-8 wk
Adolescent and child ≥12 yr: PO 20 mg/day up to 8 wk

Pathologic hypersecretory conditions
Adult: PO 60 mg/day; may increase to 120 mg in 2 divided doses

Available forms: Del rel tabs 20 mg

Implementation
PO route
• Do not break, crush, or chew del rel tab
• Give after breakfast daily with a full glass of water, without regard to food

ADVERSE EFFECTS
CNS: *Headache, dizziness, asthenia*
CV: Chest pain, angina, tachycardia, bradycardia, palpitations, peripheral edema
EENT: Tinnitus, taste perversion
GI: *Diarrhea, abdominal pain, vomiting, nausea, constipation, flatulence, acid regurgitation,* abdominal swelling, anorexia, irritable colon, esophageal candidiasis, dry mouth
GU: UTI, frequency, increased creatinine, **proteinuria, hematuria,** testicular pain, glycosuria
HEMA: Pancytopenia, thrombocytopenia, neutropenia, leukocytosis, anemia
INTEG: Rash, dry skin, urticaria, pruritus, alopecia
META: Hypoglycemia, increased hepatic enzymes, weight gain
MISC: *Back pain,* fever, fatigue, malaise, **Stevens-Johnson syndrome**
RESP: *Upper respiratory tract infections, cough,* epistaxis, **pneumonia**

Pharmacokinetics
Absorption	Unknown
Distribution	Protein binding 96.3%
Metabolism	Liver, extensively by CYP2C19
Excretion	Kidneys, feces, metabolites
Half-life	1-2 hr

Pharmacodynamics
Unknown

INTERACTIONS
Individual drugs
Digoxin, nelfinavir/omeprazole: increased levels
Ketoconazole, itraconazole, iron salts, atazanavir/ritonavir, ampicillin: decreased levels
Calcium carbonate, sucralfate, vitamin B_{12}: decreased rabeprazole levels
Clarithromycin, phenytoin: increased levels of rabeprazole
Warfarin, clopidogrel: increased bleeding risk

Drug classifications
Benzodiazepines, antacids, other proton pump inhibitors, H_2 blockers: increased levels of rabeprazole

Drug/herb
St. John's wort: decreased levels of rabeprazole

NURSING CONSIDERATIONS
Assessment
• Assess GI system: bowel sounds q8hr, abdomen for pain and swelling, anorexia

- Monitor hepatic enzymes: AST, ALT, increased alkaline phosphatase during treatment
- **Serious skin reactions:** assess for Stevens-Johnson syndrome
- **Blood dyscrasias (rare):** CBC with differential before and periodically during treatment

Nursing diagnoses
- Knowledge, deficient (teaching)
- Pain, chronic (uses)

Patient/family education
- Advise patient to report severe diarrhea; product may have to be discontinued
- Advise patient to notify prescriber if pregnancy is planned or suspected
- Teach patient to report diarrhea, black, tarry stools, product may need to be discontinued
- Inform diabetic patient that hypoglycemia can occur
- Caution patient to avoid driving and other hazardous activities until response to product is known
- Caution patient to avoid alcohol, salicylates, NSAIDs; may cause GI irritation
- Advise patient to wear sunscreen, protective clothing to prevent burns

Evaluation
Positive therapeutic outcome
- Absence of epigastric pain, swelling, fullness; decreased symptoms of GERD after 4-8 wk

---

raloxifene (Rx)
(ral-ox′ih-feen)
Evista
Func. class.: Bone resorption inhibitor
Chem. class.: Hormone modifier, selective estrogen receptor modulator (SERM)
Pregnancy category X

ACTION: Tissue-selective estrogen agonist/antagonist; agonist activity in bone and lipid metabolism, antagonistic activity on breast and uterus, reduces resorption of bone and decreases bone turnover

Therapeutic outcome: Absence or decrease of osteoporosis in postmenopausal women

USES: Prevention, treatment of osteoporosis in postmenopausal women, breast cancer prophylaxis in postmenopausal women with osteoporosis or in postmenopausal women at high risk for developing the disease

CONTRAINDICATIONS:
Pregnancy **X**, breastfeeding, hypersensitivity

> **BLACK BOX WARNING:** Women with active or history of venous thromboembolic events

Precautions: Hepatic/CV disease, cervical/uterine cancer, elevated triglycerides, pulmonary embolism

> **BLACK BOX WARNING:** Stroke

DOSAGE AND ROUTES
Hormone replacement
Adult: PO 60 mg/day, max 60 mg/day

Available forms: Tabs 60 mg

Implementation
- Administer without regard to meals
- Add calcium supplement, vit D if lacking

ADVERSE EFFECTS
CNS: Insomnia
CV: Hot flashes, peripheral edema, **thromboembolism, stroke**
EENT: Retinal vein occlusion (rare)
GI: *Nausea*, vomiting, diarrhea, dyspepsia
GU: Vaginitis, leukorrhea, *hot flashes*, cystitis, vaginal bleeding
INTEG: Rash, sweating
META: Weight gain, peripheral edema
MS: Arthralgia, myalgia, *leg cramps*, arthritis
RESP: Sinusitis, pharyngitis, increased cough, pneumonia, laryngitis, rhinitis, bronchitis, **pulmonary embolism**, flulike symptoms

Pharmacokinetics

Absorption	Unknown
Distribution	Highly protein bound
Metabolism	Unknown
Excretion	Feces, breast milk
Half-life	28-32 hr (elimination)

Pharmacodynamics
Unknown

INTERACTIONS
Individual drugs
Ampicillin, cholestyramine: decreased action of raloxifene
Desiccated thyroid, levothyroxine, liotrix: decreased action

Drug classifications
Anticoagulants: decreased action of anticoagulants

⚠ Nurse Alert

Highly protein-bound products, systemic estrogens: administer cautiously

Drug/food
Soy: decreased effect of raloxifene

Drug/lab test
Increased: apolipoprotein, corticosteroid-binding globulin, thyroxine-binding globulin (TBG)

Decreased: lipoprotein, LDL cholesterol, total cholesterol, calcium, total protein, albumin

NURSING CONSIDERATIONS
Assessment

BLACK BOX WARNING: For history of stroke, TIA, thrombosis, atrial fibrillation, hypertension, smoking; venous thrombosis may occur; avoid prolonged sitting, discontinue 3 days before surgery or other immobilization

• Obtain bone density test baseline, periodically throughout treatment; bone-specific alkaline phosphatase; osteocalcin, collagen breakdown
• Monitor B/P q4hr, watch for increase caused by H_2O and sodium retention

Nursing diagnoses
• Knowledge, deficient (teaching)
• Mobility, impaired physical (uses)

Patient/family education

BLACK BOX WARNING: Teach patients to discontinue product 72 hr before prolonged bedrest

• Advise patient to avoid maintaining one position for long periods
• Advise patient to take calcium supplements, vit D if intake is inadequate
• Advise patient to increase exercise using weights
• Advise patient to stop smoking and to decrease alcohol consumption
• Inform patient that this product does not help control hot flashes
• Instruct patient to report fever, acute migraine, insomnia, emotional distress, UTI, or vaginal itching

BLACK BOX WARNING: Teach patient to report swelling, warmth, or pain in calves

Evaluation
Positive therapeutic outcome
• Prevention, treatment of osteoporosis

raltegravir (Rx)
(ral-teg′ra-vir)
Isentress
Func. class.: Antiretroviral
Chem. class.: HIV integrase strand transfer inhibitor (ISTIs)
Pregnancy category C

ACTION: Inhibits catalytic activity of HIV integrase, which is an HIV-encoded enzyme needed for replication

Therapeutic outcome: Improvement in CD4, T-cell counts

USES: HIV in combination with other antiretrovirals

CONTRAINDICATIONS:
Hypersensitivity, breastfeeding

Precautions: Pregnancy C, children, geriatric, hepatic disease, immune reconstitution syndrome, hepatitis, antimicrobial resistance, lactase deficiency

DOSAGE AND ROUTES
Adult and adolescent ≥16 yr: PO 400 mg bid, if using with rifampin give 800 mg bid, max 800 mg/day with or without food

Available forms: Tabs 400 mg

Implementation
• Do not break, crush, or chew tabs
• May give without regard to meals, with 8 oz of water
• Store at room temperature

ADVERSE EFFECTS
CNS: *Fatigue,* fever, *dizziness, headache,* asthenia, **suicidal ideation**
CV: MI
GI: *Nausea,* vomiting, diarrhea, abdominal pain, gastritis, **hepatitis**
GU: Oliguria, proteinuria, hematuria, glomerulonephritis, **acute renal failure, renal tubular necrosis**
HEMA: Anemia, neutropenia
INTEG: Rash, urticaria, pruritus, pain or phlebitis at IV site, unusual sweating, alopecia
META: Hyperamylasia, hyperglycemia
MS: Myopathy, **rhabdomyolysis**

R

Absorption	Max 3 hr if taken on empty stomach
Distribution	Unknown
Metabolism	Liver by uridine diphosphate glucuronosyltransferase (UGT A1A enzyme system)
Excretion	51% feces, 32% urine
Half-life	Terminal 9 hr

Pharmacodynamics

Unknown

INTERACTIONS

Individual drugs
Rifampin, efavirenz, tenofovir, tipranavir/ritonavir: decreased raltegravir levels

Drug classifications
Fibric acid derivatives, HMG-CoA reductase inhibitors: increased rhabdomyolysis, myopathy, elevated CPK

H_2 blockers, protein pump inhibitors, UGT1A1 inhibitors (atazanavir): increased raltegravir effect

NURSING CONSIDERATIONS

Assessment
• **Rhabdomyolysis:** Assess for calf pain, increased CPK; product should be discontinued
• **HIV infection:** monitor CD4, T-cell count, plasma HIV RNA, viral load; resistance testing prior to therapy and at treatment failure
• **Suicidal thoughts, behavior: monitor for depression, more comon in those with mental illness**
• Assess skin eruptions: rash, urticaria, itching

Nursing diagnoses
• Infection, risk for (uses)
• Knowledge, deficient (teaching)
• Noncompliance (teaching)

Patient/family education
• Teach patient to take as prescribed; if dose is missed, take as soon as remembered up to 1 hr before next dose; do not double dose, do not share with others
• Teach patient that sexual partners need to be told that patient has HIV
• Advise patient that product does not cure infection, just controls symptoms, does not prevent infecting others
⚠ **Teach patient to report sore throat, fever, fatigue (may indicate superinfection)**

• Advise patient that product must be taken in equal intervals 2×/day to maintain blood levels for duration of therapy
• Advise patient to notify prescriber immediately of suicidal thoughts, behavior
• Advise patient to notify prescriber if pregnancy is planned or suspected, avoid breastfeeding

Evaluation
Positive therapeutic outcome
• Improvement in CD4, T-cell counts

---

ramelteon (Rx)
(rah-mel′tee-on)
Rozerem
Func. class.: Sedative-hypnotic, antianxiety
Chem. class.: Melatonin receptor agonist
Pregnancy category C

ACTION: Binds selectively to melatonin receptors (MT_1, MT_2); thought to be involved in circadian rhythm and the normal sleep-wake cycle

Therapeutic outcome: Ability to fall asleep easily and decrease early-morning awakenings

USES: Insomnia

CONTRAINDICATIONS:
Breastfeeding, infants, children, hypersensitivity, alcohol intoxication, hepatic encephalopathy

Precautions: Pregnancy **C,** hepatic disease, alcoholism, COPD, seizure disorder, sleep apnea, suicidal ideation, angioedema, depression, sleep-related behavior (sleepwalking), schizophrenia, bipolar disorder

DOSAGE AND ROUTES
Adult: PO 8 mg at bedtime

Hepatic dose
Do not use in severe hepatic disease; use with caution in mild to moderate hepatic disease

Available forms: Tabs 8 mg

Implementation
• Give within 30 min of bedtime for sleeplessness, give on empty stomach for fast onset
• Store in tight container in cool environment

ADVERSE EFFECTS
CNS: Dizziness, somnolence, fatigue, headache, insomnia, depression, complex sleep-

---

related reactions: sleep driving, sleep eating, **suicidal thoughts/behavior**
GI: Nausea, diarrhea, dysgeusia, vomiting
MISC: Myalgia, arthralgia, decreased blood cortisol, influenza, upper respiratory tract infection
SYST: Severe allergic reactions, angio-edema

Pharmacokinetics

Absorption	Rapidly absorbed
Distribution	Protein binding 82%
Metabolism	Rapid first-pass metabolism, liver
Excretion	84% urine, 4% feces
Half-life	2-5 hr

Pharmacodynamics

Onset	Unknown
Peak	0.75 hr
Duration	Unknown

INTERACTIONS

Individual drugs
Alcohol, ciprofloxacin, fluconazole, fluvoxamine, ketoconazole: increased ramelteon effect, toxicity
Rifampin: decreased effect of ramelteon

Drug classifications
Antiretroviral protease inhibitors: possible toxicity
Anxiolytics, azole antifungals, barbiturates, CYP1A2 inhibitors, hypnotics, sedatives: increased ramelteon effect, toxicity

Drug/food
High-fat/heavy meal: prolonged absorption, sleep onset reduced

NURSING CONSIDERATIONS

Assessment
• **Sleep characteristics:** assess type of sleep problem: falling asleep, staying asleep
• Assess mental status: mood, sensorium, affect, memory (long, short)

Nursing diagnoses
• Injury, risk for (adverse reactions)
• Knowledge, deficient (teaching)
• Sleep deprivation (uses)

Patient/family education
• Advise patient to avoid driving or other activities requiring alertness until product is stabilized

• Advise patient to avoid alcohol ingestion or CNS depressants
• Teach patient alternative measures to improve sleep: reading, exercise several hr before bedtime, warm bath, warm milk, TV, self-hypnosis, deep breathing
• Advise patient to take immediately before going to bed
• Advise patient not to ingest a high-fat/heavy meal before taking
• Teach patient to report cessation of menses, galactorrhea (women), decreased libido, infertility, worsening of insomnia, behavioral changes, suicidal thoughts/behavior

Evaluation
Positive therapeutic outcome
• Ability to sleep at night, decreased amount of early-morning awakening

---

ramipril (Rx)
(ra-mi′pril)
Altace
Func. class.: Antihypertensive
Chem. class.: Angiotensin-converting enzyme (ACE) inhibitor
Pregnancy category D

Do not confuse:
ramipril/enalapril, **Altace**/alteplase

ACTION: Selectively suppresses renin-angiotensin-aldosterone system; inhibits ACE; prevents conversion of angiotensin I to angiotensin II; results in dilatation of arterial, venous vessels

Therapeutic outcome: Decreased B/P in hypertension

USES: Hypertension, alone or in combination with thiazide diuretics; CHF (after MI), reduction in risk of MI, stroke, death from CV disorders

CONTRAINDICATIONS:
Breastfeeding, children, hypersensitivity to ACE inhibitors, history of ACE inhibitor–induced angioedema

BLACK BOX WARNING: Pregnancy **D** (2nd/3rd trimesters)

Precautions: Impaired renal/liver function, dialysis patients, hypovolemia, blood dyscrasias, COPD, CHF, asthma, geriatric, renal artery stenosis, cough

DOSAGE AND ROUTES

Hypertension
Adult: PO 2.5 mg/day initially, then 2.5-20 mg/day divided bid or daily

CHF/Post MI
Adult: PO 1.25-2.5 mg bid, may increase to 5 mg bid

Reduction in risk of MI, stroke, death
Adult: PO 2.5 mg/day × 7 days, then 5 mg/day × 21 days, then may increase to 10 mg/day

Renal impairment
Adult: PO CCr <40 ml/min; reduce by 50%, titrate upward to max 5 mg/day

Available forms: Caps 1.25, 2.5, 5, 10 mg

Implementation
• Caps may be opened and added to food
• Store in airtight container at 86° F (30° C) or less

ADVERSE EFFECTS

CNS: *Headache, dizziness,* anxiety, insomnia, paresthesia, fatigue, depression, malaise, vertigo
CV: *Hypotension,* chest pain, palpitations, angina, syncope, **dysrhythmia**
EENT: Hearing loss
GI: Nausea, constipation, vomiting, dyspepsia, dysphagia, anorexia, diarrhea, abdominal pain, **hepatitis, hepatic failure, pancreatitis, hepatic necrosis**
GU: **Proteinuria,** increased BUN, creatinine, impotence
HEMA: Decreased Hct, Hgb, **eosinophilia, leukopenia, pancytopenia, thrombocytopenia, agranulocytosis (rare)**
INTEG: Rash, sweating, photosensitivity, pruritus
META: *Hyperkalemia*
MISC: **Angioedema, toxic epidermal necrolysis, anaphylaxis, Stevens-Johnson syndrome**
MS: Arthralgia, arthritis, myalgia
RESP: Cough, dyspnea

Pharmacokinetics

Absorption	Well absorbed
Distribution	Not known, crosses placenta
Metabolism	Liver, extensively; protein binding 73%
Excretion	Urine
Half-life	Ramipril (5 hr), ramiprilat (24 hr)

Pharmacodynamics

Onset	$1/2$-1 hr
Peak	6-8 hr
Duration	24-72 hr

INTERACTIONS

Individual drugs
Alcohol: increased hypotension (large amounts)
Lithium: increased serum levels
HydrALAZINE, prazocin: increased toxicity
Indomethacin: decreased antihypertensive effect

Drug classifications
Adrenergic blockers, antihypertensives, diuretics, ganglionic blockers, nitrates: increased hypotension
Antacids: decreased absorption
Diuretics (potassium sparing), potassium supplements, sympathomimetics, vasodilators: increased toxicity
NSAIDs, salicylates: decreased antihypertensive effect

Drug/herb
Hawthorn: increased antihypertensive effect
Ephedra: decreased antihypertensive effect

Drug/lab test
False positive: urine acetone, ANA titer

NURSING CONSIDERATIONS

Assessment
• Monitor blood tests: neutrophils, decreased platelets; WBC with differential baseline, periodically q3mo; if neutrophils are <1000/mm³, discontinue treatment
• **Hypertension:** Monitor B/P, check for orthostatic hypotension, syncope; if changes occur, dosage may need to be changed
• **Renal disease:** Monitor renal function tests: protein, BUN, creatinine; watch for increased levels that may indicate nephrotic syndrome and renal failure; monitor renal symptoms: polyuria, oliguria, frequency, dysuria; establish baselines in renal, liver function tests before therapy begins and monitor periodically; liver function tests, uric acid, and glucose may be increased
• Check potassium levels throughout treatment, hyperkalemia occurs
• **CHF:** check for edema in feet, legs daily, weight daily
• **Allergic reactions:** angioedema, **Stevens-Johnson syndrome;** rash, fever, pruritus, urticaria; product should be discontinued if antihistamines fail to help

⚠ Nurse Alert

Nursing diagnoses
• Injury, risk for (side effects)
• Knowledge, deficient (teaching)
• Noncompliance (teaching)

Patient/family education
• Caution patient not to discontinue product abruptly; advise patient to tell all persons associated with care
• Teach patient not to use OTC products (cough, cold, allergy) unless directed by physician; serious side effects can occur; xanthines such as coffee, tea, chocolate, cola can prevent action of product
• Instruct patient on the importance of complying with dosage schedule, even if feeling better; to continue with medical regimen to decrease B/P: exercise, cessation of smoking, decreasing stress, diet modifications
• Emphasize the need to rise slowly to sitting or standing position to minimize orthostatic hypotension; not to exercise in hot weather because increased hypotension can occur
• Teach patient to notify prescriber of mouth sores, sore throat, fever, swelling of hands or feet, irregular heartbeat, chest pain, coughing, shortness of breath
• Caution patient to report excessive perspiration, dehydration, vomiting, diarrhea; may lead to fall in B/P
• Caution patient that product may cause dizziness, fainting, light-headedness; may occur during 1st few days of therapy; to avoid activities that may be hazardous
• Teach patient how to take B/P, and normal readings for age group

> **BLACK BOX WARNING:** Inform prescriber if pregnancy is planned or suspected, pregnancy **D,** do not breastfeed

Evaluation
Positive therapeutic outcome
• Decreased B/P in hypertension

TREATMENT OF OVERDOSE:
0.9% NaCl **IV** inf, hemodialysis

ranibizumab (Rx)
(ran-ih-biz′oo-mab)
Lucentis
Func. class.: Ophthalmic
Chem. class.: Selective vascular endothelial growth factor antagonist
Pregnancy category C

ACTION: Binds to receptor-binding site of active forms of vascular endothelial growth factor A (VEGF-A) that causes angiogenesis and cell proliferation

Therapeutic outcome: Prevention of increasing neovascular macular degeneration

USES: Macular degeneration (neovascular) (wet), macular edema after retinal vein occlusion (RVO)

CONTRAINDICATIONS:
Hypersensitivity, ocular infections

Precautions: Pregnancy **C,** breastfeeding, children, retinal detachment, increased intraocular pressure

DOSAGE AND ROUTES
Adult: Intravitreal 0.5 mg (0.05 ml) qmo

Available forms: Sol for inj 0.5 mg/0.05 ml

Implementation
• Given by ophthalmologist via intravitreal injection using adequate anesthesia; use 19-gauge filter
• Store in refrigerator; do not freeze
• Protect from light

ADVERSE EFFECTS
CNS: Dizziness, headache
EENT: Blepharitis, cataract, conjunctival hemorrhage/hyperemia, detachment of the retinal pigment epithelium, dryness/irritation/pain in the eye, visual impairment, vitreous floaters, ocular infection
GI: Constipation, nausea
MISC: Hypertension, UTI, **thromboembolism, non-ocular bleeding**
RESP: Bronchitis, cough, sinusitis, URI

Pharmacokinetics	
Absorption	Minimal
Distribution	None
Metabolism	None
Excretion	None
Half-life	Elimination 9 days

R

Adverse effects: *italics* = common; **bold** = life-threatening

Pharmacodynamics
Unknown

INTERACTIONS

Individual drugs
Verteporfin photodynamic therapy (PDT): increased severe inflammation

NURSING CONSIDERATIONS

Assessment
• Assess for eye changes: redness, sensitivity to light, vision change, intraocular pressure change; report to ophthalmologist immediately

Nursing diagnoses
• Knowledge, deficient (teaching)

Patient/family education
• Teach patient that if eye becomes red, sensitive to light, or painful or if there is a change in vision, seek immediate care from ophthalmologist
• Teach patient reason for treatment, expected results

Evaluation
Positive therapeutic outcome
• Prevention of increasing neovascular macular degeneration

---

ranitidine (Rx)
(ra-nit'i-deen)
Equaline Heartburn Relief, Nu-Ranit ✦, Top Care Heartburn Relief, Wal-Zan, Zantac, Zantac-C ✦, Zantac EFFER-dose
ranitidine bismuth citrate
Tritec
Func. class.: H₂ histamine receptor antagonist
Pregnancy category B

Do not confuse:
ranitidine/amantadine, **Zantac**/Xanax/Zofran

ACTION: Inhibits histamine at H₂ receptor site in the gastric parietal cells, which inhibits gastric acid secretion

Therapeutic outcome: Healing of duodenal ulcers or gastric ulcers; prevention of duodenal ulcers; decreased symptoms of gastroesophageal reflux disease (GERD), Zollinger-Ellison syndrome, or heartburn

USES: Short-term treatment of duodenal and gastric ulcers and maintenance; management of GERD, Zollinger-Ellison syndrome, active duodenal ulcers with *Helicobacter pylori* in combination with clarithromycin, hypersecretory conditions, stress ulcers, erosive esophagitis (maintenance), systemic mastocytosis, multiple endocrine adenoma syndrome, heartburn

Unlabeled uses: Prevention of aspiration pneumonitis, upper GI bleeding

CONTRAINDICATIONS:
Hypersensitivity

Precautions: Pregnancy **B**, breastfeeding, child <12 yr, renal/hepatic disease

DOSAGE AND ROUTES

Ranitidine

Erosive esophagitis
Adult: PO 150 mg qid for up to 12 wk
Child ≥1 mo: PO 5-10 mg/kg/day in 2-3 divided doses

Duodenal ulcer
Adult: PO 150 mg bid or 300 mg/day after PM meal or at bedtime, maintenance 150 mg at bedtime
Infant and child: PO 2-4 mg/kg bid, max 300 mg/day

Zollinger-Ellison syndrome
Adult: PO 150 mg bid, may increase if needed

Gastric ulcer
Adult: PO 150 mg bid × 6 wk, then 150 mg at bedtime
Infant/child: PO 2-4 mg/kg bid, max 300 mg/day

GERD
Adult: PO 150 mg bid

Renal dose
Adult: CCr <50 ml/min give 50% of dose or extend dosing interval

Ranitidine bismuth citrate
Adult: PO 400 mg bid × 4 wk with clarithromycin 500 mg tid × first 2 wk

Available forms: Ranitidine: tabs 75, 150, 300 mg; caps 150, 300 mg; syr 15 mg/ml; sol for inj 25 mg/ml; effervescent tabs 25 mg; ranitidine bismuth citrate: tabs 400 mg

---

Implementation

PO route
• May be given with or without meals; **EFFER-dose tab:** dissolves 25 mg/5 ml or more, give after dissolved; do not chew, swallow whole, or dissolve on tongue
• Give antacids 1 hr before or 1 hr after this product

IM route
• No dilution needed; inject in large muscle mass, aspirate

IV direct route
• Dilute to max 2.5 mg/ml (50 mg/20 ml) using 0.9% NaCl (nonpreserved) or D_5W, give dose over ≥5 min (max 4 mg/ml)

Intermittent IV INF route
• Dilute to max 0.5 mg/ml with D_5W, 0.9% NaCl, give over 15-20 min (5-7 ml/min); premixed ready-to-use bags as 1 mg/ml (50 mg/50 ml), inf over 15-20 min

Continuous 24 hr IV INF route
• **Adult:** dilute 150 mg/250 ml of D_5W or 0.9% NaCl, run over 24 hr (6.25 mg/hr or as directed); use inf device and use within 48 hr; *Zollinger-Ellison:* dilute in D_5W or 0.9% NaCl, max concentration 2.5 mg/ml, use inf device

Y-site compatibilities: Acyclovir, aldesleukin, alemtuzumab, alfentanil, allopurinol, amifostine, amikacin, aminophylline, amphotericin B liposome, amsacrine, anikinra, anidulafungin, ascorbic acid, atracurium, atropine, aztreonam, bivalirudin, bumetanide, buprenorphine, butorphanol, calcium chloride/gluconate, CARBOplatin, ccFAZolin, cefepime, cefonicid, cefoperazone, cefotaxime, cefotetan, cefoxitin, ceftazidime, ceftizoxime, cefTRIAXone, cefuroxime, chloramphenicol, chlorproMAZINE, cimetidine, ciprofloxacin, cisatracurium, CISplatin, clindamycin, cyanocobalamin, cyclophosphamide, cycloSPORINE, cytarabine, DACTINomycin, DAPTOmycin, dexamethasone, dexmedetomidine, digoxin, diltiazem, DOBUTamine, docetaxel, DOPamine, doripenem, doxacurium, doxapram, DOXOrubicin, DOXOrubicin liposome, doxycycline, enalaprilat, ePHEDrine, EPINEPHrine, epirubicin, epoetin alfa, ertapenem, erythromycin, esmolol, etoposide, etoposide phosphate, famotidine, fenoldopam, fentaNYL, filgrastim, fluconazole, fludarabine, fluorouracil, folic acid, foscarnet, furosemide, ganciclovir, gemcitabine, gentamicin, glycopyrrolate, granisetron, heparin, hydrocortisone, HYDROmorphone, IDArubicin, ifosfamide, imipenem/cilastatin, inamrinone, indomethacin, isoproterenol, ketorolac, labetalol, levofloxacin, lidocaine, linezolid, LORazepam, magnesium sulfate, mannitol, mechlorethamine, melphalan, meperidine, metaraminol, methotrexate, methoxamine, methyldopate, methylPREDNISolone, metoclopramide, metoprolol, metroNIDAZOLE, midazolam, milrinone, mitoxantrone, morphine, nalbuphine, naloxone, nesiritide, niCARdipine, nitroglycerin, nitroprusside, norepinephrine, octreotide, ondansetron, oxacillin, oxaliplatin, oxytocin, paclitaxel, palonosetron, pancuronium, papaverine, pemetrexed, penicillin G, pentamidine, pentazocine, PENTobarbital, PHENobarbital, phentolamine, phenylephrine, phytonadione, piperacillin/tazobactam, potassium chloride, procainamide, prochlorperazine, promethazine, propofol, propranolol, protamine, pyridoxine, remifentanil, riTUXimab, rocuronium, sargramostim, sodium acetate/bicarbonate, succinylcholine, SUFentanil, tacrolimus, teniposide, theophylline, thiamine, thiopental, thiotepa, ticarcillin/clavulanate, tigecycline, tirofiban, tobramycin, tolazoline, trastuzumab, trimetaphan, urokinase, vancomycin, vecuronium, vinCRIStine, vinorelbine, warfarin, zidovudine, zoledronic acid

Y-site incompatibilities: Amphotericin B cholesteryl, caspofungin, diazepam, diazoxide, insulin, pantoprazole, phenytoin, quinupristin/dalfopristin, trimethoprim/sulfamethoxazole

ADVERSE EFFECTS
CNS: Headache, sleeplessness, dizziness, confusion, agitation, depression; hallucinations (geriatric)
CV: Tachycardia, bradycardia, premature ventricular contractions
EENT: Blurred vision, increased ocular pressure
GI: Constipation, abdominal pain, diarrhea, nausea, vomiting, **hepatotoxicity**
GU: Impotence, **acute interstitial nephritis (rare)**
INTEG: Urticaria, rash, fever
RESP: Pneumonia
SYST: Anaphylaxis (rare)

Pharmacokinetics

Absorption	Well absorbed (PO, IM), completely absorbed (**IV**)
Distribution	Widely distributed, crosses placenta
Metabolism	Liver (30%)
Excretion	Kidneys unchanged (70%)
Half-life	2-3 hr, increased renal disease

R

Pharmacodynamics

	PO	IM/IV
Onset	Unknown	Unknown
Peak	2-3 hr	15 min
Duration	8-12 hr	8-12 hr

INTERACTIONS

Individual drugs
Adefovir, pramipexole, procainamide, trospium, triazolam, memantine, saquinavir: increased effect of each product

Diazepam, metoclopramide: decreased absorption of ranitidine

Ketoconazole: decreased effect of ketoconazole

NIFEdipine, ext rel products: increased GI obstruction risk

Procainamide: increased absorption, toxicity

Drug classifications
Anticholinergics, antacids: decreased ranitidine absorption

Anticoagulants, sulfonylureas: increased absorption, toxicity

Benzodiazepines, calcium channel blockers: increased effect of each product

Cephalosporins: decreased effects of cephalosporins

Iron salts: decreased effects of iron salts

Drug/lab test
Increased: alkaline phosphatase, AST, creatinine, LDH, ALT, bilirubin

False positive: urine protein

NURSING CONSIDERATIONS

Assessment
• **GI complaints:** assess patient with ulcers or suspected ulcers: epigastric or abdominal pain, hematemesis, occult blood in stools, blood in gastric aspirate before, throughout treatment

• Monitor I&O ratio, BUN, creatinine, CBC with differential monthly

• Assess mental status: confusion, dizziness, depression, anxiety, weakness, tremors, psychosis

Nursing diagnoses
• Knowledge, deficient (teaching)
• Pain, chronic (uses)

Patient/family education
• Caution patient that gynecomastia, impotence may occur and are reversible after treatment is discontinued

• Advise patient to avoid driving, other hazardous activities until stabilized on this medication; drowsiness or dizziness may occur

• Inform patient that smoking decreases the effectiveness of the product; that smoking cessation should be considered

• Instruct patient that product must be continued for prescribed time to be effective and taken exactly as prescribed; doses should not be doubled; a missed dose should be taken when remembered up to 1 hr before next dose

• Advise patient to report bruising, fatigue, malaise; blood dyscrasias may occur

• Inform patient to report diarrhea, black tarry stools, sore throat, rash, dizziness, confusion, or delirium to prescriber immediately

Evaluation
Positive therapeutic outcome
• Decreased pain in abdomen, heartburn
• Healing of ulcers
• Absence of gastroesophageal reflux

ranolazine (Rx)
(ruh-no′luh-zeen)
Ranexa
Func. class.: Antianginal
Pregnancy category C

ACTION: Antianginal, antiischemic; unknown, may work by inhibiting portal fatty-acid oxidation

Therapeutic outcome: Decreased anginal pain and number of episodes

USES: Chronic stable angina pectoris; use in those that have not responded to other treatment options; should be used in combination with other antianginals such as amlodipine, β-blockers, or nitrates

CONTRAINDICATIONS: Preexisting QT prolongation, hepatic disease (Child-Pugh class A, B, C), hypersensitivity, hypokalemia, renal failure, torsades de pointes, ventricular dysrhythmia, ventricular tachycardia, hepatic cirrhosis

Precautions: Pregnancy **C,** breastfeeding, children, geriatric, renal disease, hypotension

DOSAGE AND ROUTES
Adult: PO 500 mg bid and increased to 1000 mg bid based on response; max 1000 mg bid

Available forms: Ext rel tabs 500, 1000 mg

Implementation
• **Ext rel tabs:** Do not break, crush, or chew tabs; give products as prescribed; do not double or skip dose
• Give bid, without regard to meals

ADVERSE EFFECTS
CNS: *Headache, dizziness*
CV: Palpitations, **QT prolongation**
GI: Nausea, vomiting, constipation, dry mouth
MISC: Peripheral edema
RESP: Dyspnea

Pharmacokinetics

Absorption	Varied absorption
Distribution	Protein binding 62%
Metabolism	Liver, extensively by CYP3A, CYP2D6 (lesser)
Excretion	Urine 75%, feces 25%
Half-life	7 hr

Pharmacodynamics

Onset	Unknown
Peak	2-5 hr
Duration	Unknown

INTERACTIONS
Individual drugs
Haloperidol, chloroquine, droperidol, pentamidine, arsenic trioxide, levomethadyl; CYP3A4 substrates (methadone, pimozide, QUEtiapine, quiNIDine, risperidone, ziprasidone): increased QT prolongation
Digoxin, simvastatin: increased action of digoxin, simvastatin
Diltiazem, dofetilide, ketoconazole, PARoxetine, quiNIDine, sotalol, thioridazine, verapamil, ziprasidone: increased ranolazine action

Drug classifications
Anti-retroviral protease inhibitors: increased ranolazine absorption, toxicity
Class IA/III antidysrhythmics, some phenothiazines, β-agonists, local anesthetics, tricyclics; CYP3A4 inhibitors (amiodarone, clarithromycin, erythromycin, telithromycin, troleandomycin); CYP3A4 substrates (methadone, pimozide, QUEtiapine, quiNIDine, risperidone, ziprasidone): increased QT prolongation
Macrolide antibiotics, protease inhibitors: increased ranolazine action
Macrolides (clarithromycin, erythromycin, troleandomycin): increased QTc interval

Drug/food
Do not use with grapefruit or grapefruit juice

NURSING CONSIDERATIONS
Assessment
• Assess cardiac status: B/P, pulse, respiration, ECG; watch for prolongation of QT
• **QT prolongation:** ECG for QT prolongation, ejection fraction; assess for chest pain, palpitations, dyspnea
• **Angina:** characteristics of pain (intensity, location, duration, alleviating/precipitating factors)

Nursing diagnoses
• Knowledge, deficient (teaching)
• Pain, acute (uses)
• Tissue perfusion, ineffective (uses)

Patient/family education
• Teach patient to avoid hazardous activities until stabilized on product, dizziness is no longer a problem
• Advise patient to avoid OTC drugs, grapefruit juice, drugs prolonging QTc (quiNIDine, dofetilide, sotalol, erythromycin, thioridazine, ziprasidone or protease inhibitors, diltiazem, ketoconazole, macrolide antibiotics, verapamil) unless directed by prescriber
• Advise patient to comply in all areas of medical regimen
• Teach patient to notify prescriber of palpitations, fainting
• Teach patient to notify all health care providers of this product use

Evaluation
Positive therapeutic outcome
• Decreased anginal pain and number of episodes

R

---

rasagiline (Rx)
(ra-sa′-ji-leen)
Azilect
Func. class.: Antiparkinson agent
Chem. class.: MAOI, type B
Pregnancy category C

ACTION: Inhibits MAO type B at recommended doses; may increase DOPamine levels

Therapeutic outcome: Improved symptoms in those with Parkinson's disease

USES: Idiopathic Parkinson's disease monotherapy or with levodopa

CONTRAINDICATIONS:
Breastfeeding, hypersensitivity to this product or MAOIs, pheochromocytoma

---

Adverse effects: *italics* = common; **bold** = life-threatening

Precautions: Pregnancy C, children, psychiatric disorders, severe hepatic disorders

DOSAGE AND ROUTES

Monotherapy
Adult: PO 1 mg/day

Adjunctive therapy
Adult: PO 0.5 mg/day, may be increased to 1 mg/day; change of levodopa dose in adjunct therapy; reduced levodopa dose may be needed

Hepatic dose
Adult: PO 0.5 mg in mild hepatic disease

Concomitant ciprofloxacin, other CYP1A2 inhibitors
Adult: PO 0.5 mg; plasma concentrations of rasagiline may double

Available forms: Tabs 0.5, 1 mg

Implementation
• Give with meals to prevent nausea; continuing therapy usually reduces or eliminates nausea; do not give with foods/liquids containing large amounts of tyramine
• Give reduced dose of carbidopa/levodopa cautiously

ADVERSE EFFECTS
CNS: Drowsiness, hallucinations, depression, headache, malaise, paresthesia, vertigo, syncope
CV: Angina, **hypertensive crisis** (ingestion of tyramine products), orthostatic hypotension
GI: *Nausea*, diarrhea, dry mouth, dyspepsia
GU: Impotence, decreased libido
MISC: Conjunctivitis, fever, flu syndrome, neck pain, allergic reaction, alopecia
MS: Arthralgia, arthritis, dyskinesia, falls
RESP: Rhinitis

Pharmacokinetics

Absorption	Well absorbed
Distribution	Protein binding >88%-94%
Metabolism	Liver, CYP1A2
Excretion	Kidneys
Half-life	Unknown

Pharmacodynamics

Unknown

INTERACTIONS
Individual drugs
Ciprofloxacin: increased levels of rasagiline up to twofold

⚠ Meperidine: do not give; serious reaction including coma and death may occur

Drug classifications
⚠ Analgesics, sympathomimetics: do not give; serious reaction including coma and death may occur
⚠ Antidepressants (tricyclics, SSRIs, SNRIs, mirtazapine, cyclobenzaprine): increased severe CNS toxicity
CYP1A2 inhibitors (atazanavir, mexiletine, taurine): increased levels of rasagiline up to twofold
⚠ MAOIs: increased hypertensive crisis

Drug/herb
⚠ St. John's wort, yohimbe: do not give

Drug/food
Do not use with food/liquids that contain large amounts of tyramine

NURSING CONSIDERATIONS
Assessment
• **Assess for Parkinson's symptoms:** tremor, ataxia, muscle weakness and rigidity; baseline, periodically; assess for increased dyskinesia and postural hypotension if used in combination with levodopa
• Assess mental status: hallucinations, confusion, notify prescriber
• **Assess for hypertensive crisis:** severe headache, blurred vision, seizures, chest pain, difficulty thinking, nausea/vomiting, signs of stroke; any unexplained severe headache should be considered to be hypertensive crisis
• **Assess for melanomas** frequently, perform periodic skin exams by a dermatologist
• Monitor cardiac status: B/P, ECG; periodically during beginning treatment
• **Tyramine products:** assess for foods, other medications, may lead to hypertensive crisis (tachycardia, bradycardia, chest pain, nausea, vomiting, sweating, dilated pupils)

Nursing diagnoses
• Injury, risk for (uses, adverse reactions)
• Knowledge, deficient (teaching)
• Mobility, impaired physical (uses)

Patient/family education
• Advise patient to change position slowly to prevent orthostatic hypotension
• Instruct patient to avoid hazardous activities until stabilized; dizziness can occur
• Advise patient to rinse mouth frequently, use sugarless gum to alleviate dry mouth
• Teach patient to take as prescribed, not to miss dose or double doses; take missed dose

---

⚠ Nurse Alert

as soon as remembered if several hours before next dose
• Teach patient to prevent hypertensive crisis by avoiding tyramine foods >150 mg
• Teach patient to report signs of hypertensive crisis
• Teach patient to avoid CNS depressants, alcohol

Evaluation
Positive therapeutic outcome
• Improved symptoms in those with Parkinson's disease (decreasing tremors, ataxia, muscle weakness/rigidity)

rasburicase (Rx)
(rass-burr′i-case)
Elitek, Fasturtec ✤
Func. class.: Enzyme
Chem. class.: Recombinant urate-oxidase enzyme
Pregnancy category C

ACTION: Catalyzes enzymatic oxidation of uric acid into an inactive and a soluble metabolite (allantoin)

Therapeutic outcome: Decreased uric acid levels

USES: To reduce uric acid levels in children with leukemia, lymphoma, solid tumor malignancies who are receiving chemotherapy

CONTRAINDICATIONS:
Hypersensitivity

BLACK BOX WARNING: G6PD deficiency (Mediterranean, African descent), hemolytic reactions, or methemoglobinemia reactions to this product

Precautions: Pregnancy C, breastfeeding, children <2 yr, anemia

BLACK BOX WARNING: Acute bronchospasm, angina, angioedema, patients of African or Mediterranean ancestry, hypotension, urticaria

DOSAGE AND ROUTES
Adult/adolescent/child/infant: IV INF 0.2 mg/kg as a single daily dose given as **IV** INF over $^1/_2$ hr × 5 days

Available forms: Powder for inj 1.5, 7.5 mg/vial

Implementation
Intermittent IV INF route
• Reconstitute with diluent provided, add 1 ml of diluent/vial, swirl, withdraw amount needed and mix with 0.9% NaCl to final volume of 50 ml, use within 24 hr, give over 30 min, do not use filter, use different line, if not possible flush with ≥15 ml of NaCl before and after use
• Chemotherapy is started 4-24 hr after 1st dose

ADVERSE EFFECTS
CNS: *Headache,* fever
CV: Chest pain, hypotension
GI: *Nausea, vomiting, anorexia, diarrhea, abdominal pain, constipation, dyspepsia, mucositis*
HEMA: Neutropenia with fever, hemolysis, methemoglobinemia
INTEG: *Rash*
MISC: Edema
RESP: Bronchospasm, wheezing, dyspnea
SYST: Anaphylaxis, hemolysis, methemoglobinemia, sepsis

Pharmacokinetics
Absorption	Unknown
Distribution	Unknown
Metabolism	Unknown
Excretion	Unknown
Half-life	Elimination 16-21 hr

Pharmacodynamics
Unknown

INTERACTIONS
Individual drugs
Allopurinol: increased toxicity

NURSING CONSIDERATIONS
Assessment
• Monitor blood studies: BUN, serum uric acid, urine CCr, electrolytes, CBC with differential before, during therapy
• Monitor temp q4hr; fever may indicate beginning infection; no rectal temp
• **Assess for anaphylaxis** (dyspnea, urticaria, flushing, wheezing, swelling of lips, tongue, throat); have emergency equipment nearby
• **Assess for G6PD deficiency, hemolytic reactions, methemoglobinemia;** these patients should not be given this agent, screen patients who are higher risk for these disorders
• Assess GI symptoms: frequency of stools; cramping; if severe diarrhea occurs, fluid and electrolytes may need to be given

R

Nursing diagnoses
• Injury, risk for (adverse reactions, uses)
• Knowledge, deficient (teaching)

Patient/family education
• Advise of reason for therapy, expected results
• Advise to report trouble breathing, jaundice, chest pain

Evaluation
Positive therapeutic outcome
• Decreased uric acid levels in children when antineoplastics causing high uric acid levels are used

---

⚠ HIGH ALERT

remifentanil (Rx)
(re-me-fin′ta-nill)
Ultiva
Func. class.: Opiate agonist analgesic
Chem. class.: μ-Opioid agonist
Pregnancy category C
Controlled substance schedule II

ACTION: Inhibits ascending pain pathways in limbic system, thalamus, midbrain, hypothalamus

Therapeutic outcome: Maintenance of anesthesia

USES: In combination with other products in general anesthesia to provide analgesia

CONTRAINDICATIONS:
Hypersensitivity

Precautions: Pregnancy **C,** breastfeeding, geriatric, increased ICP, acute MI, severe heart disease, GI/renal/hepatic disease, asthma, respiratory conditions, seizure disorders, bradyarrhythmias, child <12 yr

DOSAGE AND ROUTES
Adult: Induction **IV** 0.5-1 mcg/kg/min with a hypnotic or volatile agent; maintenance with isoflurane (0.4-1.5 MAC) or propofol (100-200 mcg/kg/min); CONT INF 0.25-0.4 mcg/kg/min
Child 1-12 yr: CONT **IV** INF 0.25 mcg/kg/min with isoflurane
Full-term neonate and infant up to 2 mo:
CONT **IV** INF 0.4 mcg/kg/min with nitrous oxide

Available forms: Powder for inj, lyophilized 1, 2, 5 mg

Implementation
• Add 1 ml diluent/remifentanil
• Interruption of inf results in rapid reversal (no residual opioid effect within 5-10 min)
• Store in light-resistant area at room temperature

Direct IV route
• Use only during maintenance of general anesthesia; inject into tubing close to venous cannula, give in nonintubated patients over 30-60 sec

CONT IV INF route
• Use infusion device, max 16 hr, do not use same tubing as blood, do not admix

Y-site compatibilities: Acyclovir, alfentanil, amikacin, aminophylline, ampicillin, ampicillin/sulbactam, aztreonam, bretylium, bumetanide, buprenorphine, butorphanol, calcium gluconate, ceFAZolin, cefepime, cefotaxime, cefotetan, cefoxitin, ceftazidime, ceftizoxime, cefTRIAXone, cefuroxime, cimetidine, ciprofloxacin, cisatracurium, CISplatin, clindamycin, DACTINomycin, dexamethasone, digoxin, diltiazem, diphenhydrAMINE, DOBUTamine, docetaxel, DOPamine, doxacurium, doxycycline, droperidol, enalaprilat, EPINEPHrine, esmolol, etoposide, famotidine, fentaNYL, fluconazole, furosemide, ganciclovir, gatifloxicin, gemcitabine, gentamicin, granisetron, haloperidol, heparin, hetastarch, hydrocortisone sodium succinate, HYDROmorphone, hydrOXYzine, imipenem/cilastatin, inamrinone, isoproterenol, ketorolac, levofloxacin, lidocaine, LORazepam, magnesium sulfate, mannitol, meperidine, methylprednisoLONE sodium succinate, metoclopramide, metroNIDAZOLE, mezlocillin, midazolam, minocycline, morphine, nalbuphine, netilmicin, nitroglycerin, norepinephrine, ofloxacin, ondansetron, paclitaxel, palonsetron, phenylephrine, pipericillin, potassium chloride, procainamide, prochlorperazine, promethazine, ranitidine, sulfamethoxazole/trimethoprim, SUFentanil, teniposide, theophylline, thiopental, thiotepa, ticarcillin, ticarcillin/clavulate, tobramycin, vancomycin, voriconazole, zidovudine

Solution compatibilities: D_5, 0.45% NaCl, LR, D_5LR, 0.9% NaCl

ADVERSE EFFECTS
CNS: Drowsiness, *dizziness,* confusion, *headache,* sedation, euphoria, delirium, agitation, anxiety
CV: Palpitations, **bradycardia,** change in B/P; facial flushing, syncope, **asystole**
EENT: Tinnitus, blurred vision, miosis, diplopia

GI: *Nausea, vomiting,* anorexia, constipation, cramps, dry mouth
GU: Urinary retention, dysuria
INTEG: Rash, urticaria, bruising, flushing, diaphoresis, pruritus
MS: Rigidity
RESP: Respiratory depression, apnea

Pharmacokinetics

Absorption	Complete
Distribution	70% protein binding
Metabolism	Unknown
Excretion	Unknown
Half-life	Terminal 3-10 min

Pharmacodynamics

Onset	Immediate
Peak	Unknown
Duration	Unknown

INTERACTIONS

Individual drugs
Alcohol: increased respiratory depression, hypotension, profound sedation

Drug classifications
Antihistamines, CNS depressants, phenothiazines, sedative/hypnotics: increased respiratory depression, hypotension, profound sedation

Drug/herb
Kava: increased CNS depression

NURSING CONSIDERATIONS

Assessment
• Monitor I&O ratio, check for decreasing output; may indicate urinary retention, especially in geriatric
• Assess CNS changes: dizziness, drowsiness, hallucinations, euphoria, LOC pupil reaction
• Assess allergic reactions: rash, urticaria
• **Assess respiratory dysfunction:** respiratory depression, character, rate, rhythm; notify prescriber if respirations are <12/min; CV status, bradycardia, syncope
• Monitor GI status: nausea, vomiting, anorexia, constipation
• Use pain scoring to determine pain perception

Nursing diagnoses
• Knowledge, deficient (teaching)

Patient/family education
• Advise patient to call for assistance when ambulating or smoking; drowsiness, dizziness may occur

• Advise patient to make position changes slowly to prevent orthostatic hypotension

Evaluation
Positive therapeutic outcome
• Maintenance of anesthesia

repaglinide (Rx)
(re-pag'lih-nide)
Gluco Norm �, Prandin
Func. class.: Antidiabetic
Chem. class.: Meglitinides
Pregnancy category C

ACTION: Causes functioning β-cells in pancreas to release insulin, leading to drop in blood glucose levels; closes ATP-dependent potassium channels in the β-cell membrane; this leads to opening of calcium channels; increased calcium influx induces insulin secretion

Therapeutic outcome: Blood glucose controlled

USES: Type 2 diabetes mellitus

CONTRAINDICATIONS:
Hypersensitivity to meglitinides, diabetic ketoacidosis, type 1 diabetes

Precautions: Pregnancy C, breastfeeding, children, geriatric, cardiac disease, severe renal/hepatic disease, thyroid disease, severe hypoglycemic reactions

DOSAGE AND ROUTES
Adult: PO 1-2 mg with each meal, max 16 mg/day, adjust at weekly intervals; oral hypoglycemic-naïve patients or those with A1c <8% should start with 0.5 mg with each meal

Renal/hepatic dose
Adult: PO CCr 20-39 ml/min: 0.5 mg/day; titrate upward cautiously

Available forms: Tabs 0.5, 1, 2 mg

Implementation
• 15 min before meals: 2, 3, or 4 ×/day preprandially
• Skip dose if meal is skipped; add dose if meal is added
• Store in airtight container at room temperature

ADVERSE EFFECTS
CNS: *Headache, weakness,* paresthesia
ENDO: Hypoglycemia

GI: Nausea, vomiting, diarrhea, constipation, dyspepsia
INTEG: Rash, allergic reactions
MISC: Chest pain, UTI, allergy
MS: Back pains, arthralgia
RESP: URI, sinusitis, rhinitis, bronchitis

Pharmacokinetics

Absorption	Complete
Distribution	98% protein binding, crosses placenta
Metabolism	Liver
Excretion	Urine/feces
Half-life	1 hr

Pharmacodynamics

Onset	30 min
Peak	1 hr
Duration	<4 hr

INTERACTIONS

Individual drugs

CarBAMazepine, rifampin: increased repaglinide metabolism
Chloramphenicol, fenofibrate, gemfibrozil, probenecid, simvastatin: increased effect of repaglinide
Erythromycin, ketoconazole, miconazole: decreased repaglinide metabolism
Gemfibrozil: Do not use together
Isoniazid, phenobarbital, phenytoin, rifampin: decreased action of repaglinide
Levonorgestrel/ethinyl estradol: increase in both

Drug classifications

Antifungals, CYP450 inhibitors, macrolides: decreased repaglinide metabolism
Barbiturates, CYP450 inducers: increased repaglinide metabolism
β-Adrenergic blockers, coumarins, MAOIs, NSAIDs, salicylates, sulfonamides: increased repaglinide effect
Calcium channel blockers, contraceptives (oral), corticosteroids, diuretics (thiazide), estrogens, phenothiazines, sympathomimetics, thyroid preparations: decreased repaglinide effect

Drug/herb

Chromium, garlic, horse chestnut: increased antidiabetic effect

Drug/food

Decreased: repaglinide level; give before meals

NURSING CONSIDERATIONS

Assessment

• Assess for hypoglycemic or hyperglycemic reaction, which can occur soon after meals; dizziness, weakness, headache, tremor, anxiety, tachycardia, hunger, sweating, abdominal pain, monitor A1c, fasting, postprandial glucose during treatment

Nursing diagnoses

• Knowledge, deficient (teaching)
• Noncompliance (teaching)
• Nutrition: more than body requirements, imbalanced (uses)

Patient/family education

• Teach patient technique of blood glucose monitoring using blood glucose meter
• Teach patient the symptoms of hypoglycemia and hyperglycemia, what to do about each
• Teach patient that product must be continued on daily basis; explain consequence of discontinuing product abruptly
• Advise patient to avoid OTC medications unless ordered by prescriber
• Advise patient that diabetes is a lifelong illness; product will not cure disease
• Advise patient to eat all food included in diet plan to prevent hypoglycemia; to have glucagon emergency kit available; to take repaglinide 15-30 min before meals 2, 3, or 4×/day
• Instruct patient to carry/wear emergency ID for emergency purposes

Evaluation

Positive therapeutic outcome
• Decrease in polyuria, polydipsia, polyphagia; clear sensorium; absence of dizziness; stable gait; blood glucose, A1c improvement

retapamulin topical
See Appendix B

retinoic acid
See tretinoin

Rh₀ (D) immune globulin, standard dose IM
BayRho-D, HyperRHO SD, Rho Gam Ultra Filtered Plus
Rh₀ (D) immune globulin microdose IM
MICRhoGAM Ultra Filtered Plus
Rh₀ (D) immune globulin IV
Rhophylac, WinRho SDF
Func. class.: Immune globulins
Pregnancy category C

ACTION: Suppresses immune nonsensitized Rh₀ (D or Dᵘ)-negative patients who are exposed to Rh₀ (D or Dᵘ)-positive blood

Therapeutic outcome: Absence of Rh factor and transfusion error

USES: Prevention of isoimmunization in Rh-negative women exposed to Rh-positive blood given after abortions, miscarriages, amniocentesis, chronic idiopathic thrombocytopenic purpura (Rhophylac)

CONTRAINDICATIONS:
Previous immunization with this product, Rh₀ (D)-positive/Dᵘ-positive patient

Precautions: Pregnancy C

DOSAGE AND ROUTES

To reduce risk of Rh isoimmunization antepartum/suppression of Rh isoimmunization postpartum following delivery of full-term infant
Adult and adolescent ≥16 yr: IM (BayRho-D [HyperRHO SD] [full dose only]) 300 mcg (1500 international units) at 28 wk gestation, repeat within 72 hr of delivery of confirmed Rho(D)-positive infant; a dose is not needed after delivery, if delivery is within 3 wk of last dose and no fetal maternal hemorrhage of >15 ml of RBC; IM (RhoGam only) 300 mcg (1500 international units) at 26-28 wk gestation, repeat within 72 hr even if status of Rho is unknown or if 72 hr have passed; IM/IV (WinRho SDF only) 300 mcg (1500 international units) at 28 wk gestation; if given earlier in pregnancy, give at 12-wk intervals during pregnancy, a 120-mcg (600 international units) dose; IM/IV should be given as soon as possible and preferably within 72 hr of delivery of a confirmed Rho(D)-positive infant, and even if status is unknown give up to 28 days after delivery

Known or suspected massive feto-maternal hemorrhage (>15 ml of fetal RBC or >30 ml of fetal whole blood)
Adult and adolescent ≥16 yr: IM (BayRho-D [HyperRHO SD] [full dose only]) 300 mcg (1500 international units) per every 15 ml of fetal blood cells or 30 ml of whole blood, multiple syringes may be injected IM at the same time in different sites, give within 72 hr of exposure, repeat dose within 72 hr of delivery; IM (RhoGAM only) 300 mcg (1500 international units) for every 15 ml of fetal blood cells or 30 ml of whole blood, give total dose within 72 hr of exposure; IM/IV (WinRho SDF only) if large fetomaternal hemorrhage is suspected, give IV 9 mcg (45 international units) or IM 12 mcg (60 international units) for every ml of fetal whole blood, give IV 600 mcg (3000 international units) q8hr or IM 1200 mcg (6000 international units) q12hr until total dose is given, total dose should be given within 72 hr of exposure

Threatened abortion at any stage of pregnancy
Adult and adolescent ≥16 yr: IM (BayRho-D [HyperRHO SD] [full dose only]) 300 mcg (1500 international units) as soon as possible; if given 13-18 wk gestation, give another 300 mcg (1500 international units) at 26-28 wk gestation; repeat dose within 72 hr of delivery; IM (RhoGam only) 300 mcg (1500 international units) as soon as possible and within 72 hr; IM/IV (Rhophylac only) 300 mcg (1500 international units) as soon as possible and within 72 hr; IM/IV (WinRho SDF only) 300 mcg (1500 international units) as soon as possible and within 72 hr, repeat dose at 12-wk intervals during pregnancy and 120 mcg (600 international units) as soon as possible after delivery and within 72 hr

Following spontaneous abortion, induced termination of pregnancy, or ectopic pregnancy that occurs ≤12 wk gestation
Adult and adolescent ≥16 yr: IM (BayRho-D Minidose, HYperRHO Minidose, MICRORhoGAM only) 50 mcg (250 international units) as soon as possible, give within 3 hr of spontaneous or surgical removal, if possible within 72 hr

Following spontaneous abortion, induced termination of pregnancy, or ruptured tubal pregnancy that occurs ≥13 wk
Adult and adolescent ≥16 yr: IM(BayRho-D full dose [HyperRHO SD full dose] RhoGAM

R

only) 300 mcg (1500 international units) as soon as possible and within 72 hr of event

Following spontaneous abortion, induced termination of pregnancy, aminocentesis, chorionic villus sampling, abdominal trauma, ruptured tubal pregnancy, or percutaneous umbilical cord sampling up to 34 wk gestation

Adult and adolescent ≥16 wk: IM/IV (WinRho SDF only) 300 mcg (1500 international units) within 72 hr, repeat at 12-wk intervals during pregnancy, give 120 mcg (600 international units) as soon as possible and preferably within 72 hr of delivery

Available forms: BayRho-D sol for inj 300 mcg/ml (HyperRHO SD solution for injection); MICRhoGAM Ultra Filtered Plus Solution for inj 50 mcg/ml; RhoGam Ultra Filtered Plus Solution for inj 50 mcg; Rhophylac Pre-Filled Syringes Solution for inj 300 mcg/2 ml; WinRho SDF Liquid for inj; WinRho powder for inj

Implementation

• BayRho-D is being changed to HyperRHO SD
• BayRho-D (HyperRHO SD), MICRhoGAM, RhoGAM are given by IM only; do not give **IV**
• WinRho SDF and Rhophylac may be given IM or **IV**
• Inspect for particulate matter; do not use if particulate matter is present
• Reconstitution/dilution: no reconstitution or dilution is needed for BayRho-D (HyperRHO SD), Rhophylac, MICRoGAM, RhoGAM, or the liquid formulation of WinRho SDF
• WinRho SDF powder for **IV** use: if giving **IV**, reconstitute 600 international units or 1500 international units immediately before use with 2.5 ml of sterile diluent; reconstitute 5000 international units with 8.5 ml sterile diluent; add diluent to vial slowly down the wall of the vial; gently swirl until powder is dissolved; do not shake
• WinRho SDF powder for IM use: **IV** giving IM, reconstitute 600 international units or 1500 international units immediately before use with 1.25 ml of sterile diluent; 5000 international units with 8.5 ml of sterile diluent; add diluent to the vial slowly down the wall of the vial; gently swirl until powder is dissolved; do not shake
IM route
• Use aseptic technique, observe for 20 min after administration
• Bring Rhophylac to room temperature before using

• Inject into the deltoid muscle of upper arm or anterolateral portion of the upper thigh; do not inject into gluteal muscle
• If dose calculated will need multiple vials or syringes, use different sites at the same time

IV route
• Use aseptic technique
• WinRhoSDF: remove entire contents of vial to obtain calculated dose; if partial vial contents are required for dosage calculation, withdraw the entire vial contents to ensure correct calculation; inf correct calculated dose over 3-5 min; do not inf with other fluids or products
• Rhophylac: bring to room temperature; inf by slow **IV**; observe for 20 min

ADVERSE EFFECTS
CNS: Lethargy
CV: Hypo/hypertension
INTEG: Irritation at inj site, fever
MISC: Infection, **ARDS, anaphylaxis, pulmonary edema, DIC**
MS: Myalgia

Pharmacokinetics

Absorption	Well absorbed
Distribution	Unknown
Metabolism	Unknown
Excretion	Unknown
Half-life	Unknown

Pharmacodynamics

Onset	Rapid
Peak	Unknown
Duration	Unknown

INTERACTIONS
Drug classifications
Live virus vaccines (measles, mumps, rubella): decreased antibody response to vaccine

NURSING CONSIDERATIONS
Assessment
• Assess for allergies, reactions to immunizations; previous immunization with this product
• **Intravascular hemolysis:** assess for back pain, chills, hemoglobinuria, renal insufficiency
• Obtain type and cross-match of mother's blood and of neonate's cord blood; neonate must be Rh₀(D)-positive, mother must be Rh₀(D)-negative and (Dᵘ)-negative, medication should be given if there is a doubt

Nursing diagnoses
• Knowledge, deficient (teaching)

Patient/family education
• Teach patient how product works; that product must be given after subsequent deliveries if subsequent babies are Rh-positive
• **Intravascular hemolysis:** Teach patient to report immediately: shaking, fever, chills, dark urine, swelling of hand or feet, back pain, SOB

Evaluation
Positive therapeutic outcome
• Prevention of $Rh_o(D)$ sensitization in transfusion error
• Prevention of erythroblastosis fetalis in subsequent $Rh_o(D)$-positive neonates

---

ribavarin (Rx)
(rye-ba-vye′rin)
Virazole
Func. class.: Synthetic antiviral
Chem. class.: Tricyclic amine
Pregnancy category X

ACTION: Prevents replication of DNA and RNA synthesis

Therapeutic outcome: Resolution of severe lower respiratory tract infections

USES: Severe lower respiratory tract infections in infants and children

Unlabeled uses: Influenza A or B (early)

CONTRAINDICATIONS:
Pregnancy **X**, breastfeeding, children <1 yr, hypersensitivity

Precautions: Epilepsy, renal/hepatic disease

DOSAGE AND ROUTES
Infant and young child: INH 20 mg/ml × 12-18 hr/day × 3-7 days

Available forms: Powder for reconstitution for aerosol 6 g/vial

Implementation
• Give by the Viratek small particle aerosol generator (SPAG-2), do not use other inhalation equipment
• May be given by an oxygen hood for infants, or a face mask may be attached to the SPAG-2
• Reconstitute 6 g of sterile water for inj or inh, place sol in the Erlenmeyer flask and dilute further to 20 mg/ml

ADVERSE EFFECTS
CNS: Dizziness, faintness
CV: Hypotension, cardiac arrest
EENT: Eye irritation, conjunctivitis, blurred vision, photosensitivity
INTEG: Rash

Pharmacokinetics

Absorption	Inhalation (systemic)
Distribution	To respiratory tract
Metabolism	Liver
Excretion	Respiratory tract
Half-life	$9^{1}/_{2}$ hr

Pharmacodynamics

Onset	Unknown
Peak	Inhalation's end
Duration	Unknown

INTERACTIONS
Individual products
Zidovudine: decreased antiviral action, increased toxicity

Drug classification
Cardiac glycosides: increased toxicity

NURSING CONSIDERATIONS
Assessment
• Assess allergies before initiation of treatment, reaction of each medication; list allergies on chart in bright red letters
• Monitor respiratory status: rate, character, wheezing, tightness in chest
• Obtain C&S test results before starting treatment

Nursing diagnoses
• Gas exchange, impaired (uses)
• Infection, risk for (uses)
• Knowledge, deficient (teaching)

Patient/family education
• Teach patient and parents aspects of product therapy

Evaluation
Positive therapeutic outcome
• Absence of respiratory syncytial virus

R

riboflavin (vitamin B$_2$) (OTC)
(rye'boo-flay-vin)
Func. class.: Vitamin B$_2$, water soluble
Pregnancy category A

ACTION: Needed for respiratory reactions (catalyzes proteins) and for normal vision

Therapeutic outcome: Prevention or treatment of riboflavin deficiency

USES: Vitamin B$_2$ deficiency or polyneuritis; cheilosis adjunct with thiamine

Precautions: Pregnancy A

DOSAGE AND ROUTES
Deficiency
Adult: PO 5-30 mg/day
Child ≥12 yr: PO 3-10 mg/day, then 0.6 mg/1000 cal ingested

RDA
Adult: PO (Males) 1.3 mg; (females) 1.1 mg

Available forms: Tabs 5, 10, 25, 50, 100, 250 mg

Implementation
• Give with food for better absorption
• Store in airtight, light-resistant container

ADVERSE EFFECTS
GU: Yellow discoloration of urine (large doses)

Pharmacokinetics

Absorption	Well absorbed (by active transport)
Distribution	60% protein bound, widely distributed, crosses placenta
Metabolism	Unknown
Excretion	Kidneys (unchanged), excess amounts
Half-life	1-1^1/$_2$ hr

Pharmacodynamics
Unknown

INTERACTIONS

Individual drugs
Alcohol, probenecid: increased riboflavin need
Tetracycline: decreased action of tetracycline

Drug classifications
Antidepressants (tricyclics), phenothiazines: increased riboflavin need

Drug/lab test
False increase: urinary catecholamines

NURSING CONSIDERATIONS
Assessment
• Assess patient's nutritional status: liver, eggs, dairy products, yeast, whole grain, green vegetables
• Assess for vit B$_2$ deficiency: photophobia, cheilosis, stomatitis, ocular swelling

Nursing diagnoses
• Knowledge, deficient (teaching)
• Nutrition: less than body requirements, imbalanced (uses)

Patient/family education
• Inform patient that urine may turn bright yellow
• Instruct patient about needed addition of foods that are rich in riboflavin

Evaluation
Positive therapeutic outcome
• Absence of headache, GI problems, cheilosis, skin lesions, depression, burning itchy eyes, anemia

rifabutin (Rx)
(riff'a-byoo-tin)
Mycobutin
Func. class.: Antimycobacterial
Chem. class.: Rifamycin S derivative
Pregnancy category B

Do not confuse:
rifabutin/rifampin

ACTION: Inhibits DNA-dependent RNA polymerase in susceptible strains

Therapeutic outcome: Antimycobacterial death of *Escherichia coli, Bacillus subtilis;* mechanism of action against *Mycobacterium avium* unknown

USES: Prevention of *M. avium* complex (MAC) in patients with advanced HIV infection

Unlabeled uses: *Helicobacter pylori* that has not responded to other treatment

CONTRAINDICATIONS:
Hypersensitivity, active TB, WBC <1000/mm^3, platelets <50,000/mm^3

Precautions: Pregnancy **B**, breastfeeding, children, hepatic disease, blood dyscrasias

DOSAGE AND ROUTES
Adult: PO 300 mg/day (may take as 150 mg bid); max 600 mg/day

Renal dose
Adult: PO CCr <30 ml/min reduce dose by 50%

Available forms: Caps 150 mg

Implementation
• Give with meals to decrease GI symptoms; better to take on empty stomach 1 hr before or 2 hr after meals; high-fat food slows absorption, may take in 2 divided doses, may open capsule and mix with applesauce if unable to swallow whole
• Give antiemetic if vomiting occurs

ADVERSE EFFECTS
CNS: *Headache,* fatigue, anxiety, confusion, insomnia
GI: *Nausea, vomiting, anorexia, diarrhea,* heartburn, **hepatitis,** discolored saliva, **pseudomembranous colitis**
GU: Discolored urine
HEMA: Hemolytic anemia, eosinophilia, thrombocytopenia, leukopenia
INTEG: *Rash*
MISC: Flulike syndrome, shortness of breath, chest pressure
MS: Asthenia, arthralgia, myalgia

Pharmacokinetics

Absorption	Well absorbed
Distribution	Widely distributed
Metabolism	Liver
Excretion	Kidney
Half-life	45 hr

Pharmacodynamics

Onset	Unknown
Peak	2-3 hr
Duration	Unknown

INTERACTIONS
Individual drugs
Amprenavir, busPIRone, clofibrate, cycloSPORINE, dapsone, delavirdine, disopyramide, doxycycline, efavirenz, fluconazole, indinavir, ketoconazole, losartan, nelfinavir, nevirapine, phenytoin, quiNIDine, saquinavir, theophylline, zidovudine, zolpidem: decreased action of each specific product
Ritonavir: increased rifabutin level

Drug classifications
Anticoagulants, antidepressants (tricyclics), barbiturates, β-blockers, contraceptives (oral), corticosteroids, estrogens, sulfonylureas: decreased action of each specific product

Drug/food
High-fat foods: decreased absorption

Drug/lab test
Interference: folate level, vit B_{12}, BSP, gallbladder tests

NURSING CONSIDERATIONS
Assessment
• **Assess for active TB:** chest x-ray, sputum culture, blood culture, biopsy of lymph nodes, obtain PPD test; product should be given only for MAC and never for TB
• Monitor CBC for neutropenia, thrombocytopenia, eosinophilia
• **Pseudomembranous colitis:** assess for diarrhea, abdominal pain, fever, fatigue, anorexia; possible anemia, elevated WBC and low serum albumin; stop product and usually give either vancomycin or IV metroNIDAZOLE

Nursing diagnoses
• Diarrhea (adverse reaction)
• Infection, risk for (uses)
• Injury, risk for (adverse reaction)
• Knowledge, deficient (teaching)
• Noncompliance (teaching)

Patient/family education
• Caution patient that compliance with dosage schedule and duration is necessary
• Instruct patient that scheduled appointments must be kept or relapse may occur
• Instruct patient to notify prescriber if hepatitis, neutropenia, or thrombocytopenia occurs: sore throat, fever, bleeding, bruising, yellow sclera, anorexia, nausea, vomiting, fatigue, weakness; myositis: muscle or bone pain
• Advise patient that urine, feces, saliva, sputum, sweat, tears may be colored red-orange; soft contact lenses may become permanently stained
• Caution patients using oral contraceptives to use a nonhormonal method of birth control because rifabutin may decrease efficiency of oral contraceptives; to notify prescriber if pregnancy is planned or suspected

Evaluation
Positive therapeutic outcome
• Decreased symptoms of *M. avium* in patients with HIV

R

rifampin (Rx)

(rif'am-pin)
Rifadin, Rofact ✤
Func. class.: Antitubercular
Chem. class.: Rifamycin B derivative
Pregnancy category C

Do not confuse:
rifampin/rifabutin

ACTION: Inhibits DNA-dependent polymerase, decreases tubercle bacilli replication

Therapeutic outcome: Bactericidal against the following organisms: mycobacteria, *Staphylococcus aureus, Haemophilus influenzae, Neisseria meningitidis, Legionella pneumophila*

USES: Pulmonary TB, meningococcal carriers (prevention)

CONTRAINDICATIONS:
Hypersensitivity to this product or rifamycins, active *Neisseria meningitidis* infection

Precautions: Pregnancy **C**, breastfeeding, children <5 yr, hepatic disease, blood dyscrasias

DOSAGE AND ROUTES

Tuberculosis
Adult: PO/IV max 600 mg/day as single dose 1 hr before or 2 hr after meals, or 10 mg/kg/day 2-3 ×/wk
Child >5 yr: PO/IV 10-20 mg/kg/day as single dose 1 hr before or 2 hr after meals, max 600 mg/day, with other antitubercular products
6-mo regimen: 2-mo treatment of isoniazid, rifampin, pyrazinamide, and possibly streptomycin or ethambutol; then rifampin and isoniazid × 4 mo
9-mo regimen: Rifampin and isoniazid supplemented with pyrazinamide or streptomycin or ethambutol

Meningococcal carriers
Adult: PO/IV 600 mg bid × 2 days, max 600 mg/dose
Child >5 yr: PO/IV 10-20 mg/kg bid × 2 days, max 600 mg/dose
Infant 3 mo-1 yr: PO 5 mg/kg bid for 2 days

Available forms: Caps 150, 300 mg; powder for inj 600 mg/vial

Implementation
• Do not give IM or SUBCUT

PO route
• On empty stomach, 1 hr before or 2 hr after meals with a full glass of water
• Antiemetic if vomiting occurs
• Capsules may be opened and mixed with applesauce or gelatin

Intermittent IV INF route
• After diluting each 600 mg/10 ml of sterile water for inj (60 mg/ml), swirl, withdraw dose, and dilute in 100 ml or 500 ml of D$_5$W given as an inf over 3 hr, or if diluted in 100 ml, give over ¹/₂ hr; do not admix with other sol or medications

Y-site compatibilities: Amiodarone, bumetanide, midazolam, pantoprazole, vancomycin

ADVERSE EFFECTS

CNS: Headache, fatigue, anxiety, drowsiness, confusion
EENT: Visual disturbances
GI: *Nausea, vomiting, anorexia, diarrhea,* **pseudomembranous colitis,** *heartburn,* sore mouth and tongue, **pancreatitis,** elevated liver function tests
GU: **Hematuria, acute renal failure, hemoglobinuria**
HEMA: **Hemolytic anemia, eosinophilia, thrombocytopenia, leukopenia**
INTEG: Rash, pruritus, urticaria
MISC: Flulike syndrome, menstrual disturbances, edema, SOB, **Stevens-Johnson syndrome, toxic epidermal necrolysis, angioedema, anaphylaxis**
MS: Ataxia, weakness

Pharmacokinetics

Absorption	Well absorbed (PO), completely absorbed (**IV**)
Distribution	Widely distributed, crosses placenta
Metabolism	Liver—extensively
Excretion	Feces
Half-life	3 hr

Pharmacodynamics

	PO	IV
Onset	Rapid	Rapid
Peak	2-3 hr	Inf end
Duration	Unknown	Unknown

INTERACTIONS

Individual drugs
Acetaminophen, alcohol, chloramphenicol, clofibrate, cycloSPORINE, dapsone, digoxin,

⚠ Nurse Alert

diltiazem, doxycycline, haloperidol, NIFEdipine, phenytoin, theophylline, verapamil, zidovudine: decreased effect of specific product
Isoniazid: increased hepatotoxicity

Drug classifications

Anticoagulants, antidiabetics, barbiturates, benzodiazepines, β-blockers, contraceptives (oral), glucocorticoids, hormones, imidazole antifungals: decreased effect of each product
Protease inhibitors: do not use together

Drug/lab test

Interference: folate level, vit B_{12} gallbladder studies, dexamethasone suppression test
False positive: direct Coombs' test

NURSING CONSIDERATIONS

Assessment

• Monitor liver function tests qmo: ALT, AST, bilirubin
• Monitor renal status: before, qmo: BUN, creatinine, output, specific gravity, urinalysis
• **Pseudomembranous colitis:** assess for diarrhea, abdominal pain, fever, fatigue, anorexia; possible anemia, elevated WBC and low serum albumin; stop product and usually give either vancomycin or IV metroNIDAZOLE
• Monitor mental status often: affect, mood, behavioral changes; psychosis may occur
• Monitor hepatic status: decreased appetite, jaundice, dark urine, fatigue
• **Infection:** assess sputum culture, lung sounds
• C&S should be performed before beginning treatment, during, and after therapy is completed
• **Serious skin reactions:** assess for fever, sore throat, fatigue, ulcers, lesions in mouth, lips, rash; can be fatal

Nursing diagnoses

• Diarrhea (adverse reactions)
• Infection, risk for (uses)
• Injury, risk for (adverse reactions)
• Knowledge, deficient (teaching)
• Noncompliance (teaching)

Patient/family education

• Instruct patient that compliance with dosage schedule, duration is necessary
• Instruct patient that scheduled appointments must be kept or relapse may occur
• Instruct patient to notify prescriber if hepatitis, neutropenia, or thrombocytopenia occurs: sore throat, fever, bleeding, bruising, yellow sclera, anorexia, nausea, vomiting, fatigue, weakness, diarrhea with pus, mucus, blood

• Advise patient that urine, feces, saliva, sputum, sweat, tears may be colored red-orange; soft contact lenses may be permanently stained
• Caution patients using oral contraceptives to use a nonhormonal method of birth control because rifabutin may decrease the efficiency of oral contraceptives, to notify prescriber if pregnancy is planned or suspected
• Advise patient to avoid alcohol; hepatotoxicity may occur

Evaluation

Positive therapeutic outcome

• Decreased symptoms of TB

---

rifaximin (Rx)

(rif-ax'i-min)
Xifaxan
Func. class.: Misc. antiinfective
Chem. class.: Analog of rifampin
Pregnancy category C

R

Do not confuse:

rifaximin/rifampin

ACTION: Binds to bacterial DNA dependent RNA polymerase, thereby inhibiting bacterial RNA synthesis

Therapeutic outcome: Bacterial action against *E. coli*

USES: Traveler's diarrhea in those ≥12 yr old, caused by *E. coli,* hepatic encephalopathy

CONTRAINDICATIONS:

Hypersensitivity to this product or rifamycins, diarrhea with fever, blood in stool

Precautions: Pregnancy C, breastfeeding, children, geriatric patients

DOSAGE AND ROUTES

Traveler's diarrhea

Adult and child ≥12 yr: PO 200 mg tid × 3 days without regard to meals

Hepatic encephalopathy

Adult: PO 550 mg bid

Available forms: Tabs 200 mg

Implementation

• May be administered without regard to food

ADVERSE EFFECTS

CNS: Abnormal dreams, dizziness, insomnia
CV: Hypotension, chest pain, peripheral edema

GI: *Abdominal pain, constipation, defecation urgency, flatulence, nausea, rectal tenesmus,* vomiting, ascites, **pseudomembranous colitis**
MISC: *Headache, pyrexia,* motion sickness, tinnitus, rash, photosensitivity, **exfoliative dermatitis**
MS: Arthralgia
RESP: Dyspnea, cough, pharyngitis

Pharmacokinetics

Absorption	Unknown
Distribution	Unknown
Metabolism	Induces CYP3A4
Excretion	Feces
Half-life	6 hr

Pharmacodynamics
Unknown

NURSING CONSIDERATIONS

Assessment
• Assess for GI symptoms: amount and character of diarrhea, abdominal pain, nausea, vomiting
⚠ Assess for overgrowth of infection and pseudomembranous colitis

Nursing diagnoses
• Infection, risk for (uses)
• Knowledge, deficient (teaching)
• Noncompliance (teaching)

Patient/family education
• Instruct patient to discontinue rifaximin and notify prescriber if diarrhea persists for more than 24-48 hr, if diarrhea worsens, or if blood is in stools and fever is present
• Advise patient to avoid hazardous activities if dizziness occurs

Evaluation
Positive therapeutic outcome
• Absence of infection

---

rilpivirine
(ril-pi-vir′ine)
Edurant
Func. class.: Antiretroviral
Chem. class.: Non-nucleoside transcriptase inhibitors (NNTIs)

ACTION: Inhibits HIV-1 reverse transcriptase; unlike nucleoside reverse transcriptase inhibitors (NRTIs), it does not compete for binding nor does it require phosphorylation to be active. Binds directly to a site on reverse transcriptase; causing disruption of the enzyme's active site thereby blocking RNA-dependent and DNA-dependent DNA polymerase activities

USES: HIV in combination with other antiretrovirals

CONTRAINDICATIONS:
Hypersensitivity

Precautions: Pregnancy category **B**, breastfeeding, immune reconstitution syndrome, antimicrobial resistance, pancreatitis, depression, suicidal ideation, neonates, infants, children, adolescents <18 yr, QT prolongation, torsades de pointes, hyperlipidemia, hypertriglyceridemia, hypercholesterolemia

DOSAGE AND ROUTES
Treatment of antiretroviral treatment-naive adults with human immunodeficiency virus (HIV) in combination with other antiretroviral agents
Adult: PO 25 mg q day with a meal; give in combination with other antiretroviral agents. In antiretroviral-treatment–naive adults, rilpivirine is used as an alternative to efavirenz in NNRTI-based treatment regimens. Potential rilpivirine-based treatment regimens combine rilpivirine with either tenofovir plus emtricitabine or lamiVUDine, or abacavir plus emtricitabine or zidovudine plus emtricitabine or lamiVUDine

Available forms: Tab 25 mg

ADVERSE EFFECTS
CNS: Depressed mood, dizziness, drowsiness, dysphoria, fatigue, headache, major depression, mood alteration, negative thoughts, **suicide attempts**
GI: Abdominal pain, cholecystitis, cholelithiasis, decreased appetite, diarrhea, elevated hepatic enzymes, hyperbilirubinemia, hypercholesterolemia, nausea, vomiting
GU: Glomerulonephritis membranous/glomerulonephritis mesangioproliferative

Pharmacokinetics

Absorption	Increased effect 40% (food), decreased effect 50% (high protein drink)
Distribution	Protein binding (99.7%) to albumin
Metabolism	Via oxidation CYP3A system
Excretion	Feces 25% excreted unchanged (85%); urine (6.1%)
Half-life	Terminal elimination 50 hr

Pharmacodynamics

Onset	Unknown
Peak	4-5 hr
Duration	Unknown

INTERACTIONS
Individual drugs
Aminoglutethimide, bexarotene, bosentan, efavirenz, flutamide, griseofulvin, metyrapone, modafinil, nafcillin, nevirapine, pioglitazone, primidone, ritonavir, topiramate: Decreased rilpivirine effect, treatment failure

Abarelix, alfuzosin, amiodarone, amoxapine, apomorphine, artemether, asenapine, chloroquine, ciprofloxacin, citalopram, clozapine, cyclobenzaprine, dasatinib, dolasetron, dronedarone, droperidol, eribulin, flecainide, fluconazole, gatifloxacin, gemifloxacin, haloperidol, iloperidone, lapatinib, levofloxacin, lopinavir, lumefantrine, maprotiline, mefloquinem, moxifloxacin, nilotinib, norfloxacin, octreotide, ofloxacin, OLANZapine, ondansetron, paliperidone, palonosetron, pentamidine, posconazole, QUEtiapine, ranolazine, saquinavir: Increased QT prolongation

Fluconazole, voriconazole: Increased rilpivirine adverse reactions, fungal infections

Drug classifications
CYP3A4 inducers (phenytoin, fosphenytoin, barbiturates, OXcarbazepine, carBAMazepine, rifabutin, rifampin, rifapentine, dexamethasone), proton pump inhibitors (PPIs): Decreased rilpivirine effect, treatment failure

H_2 receptor antagonists (cimetidine, famotidine, nizatidine, ranitidine): Decreased rilpivirine effect, treatment failure; give 12 hr before or 4 hr after rilpivirine

Antacids: Decreased rilpivirine effect; use 2 hr or more before, or 4 hr after rilpivirine

CYP3A4 inhibitors (aldesleukin, amiodarone, aprepitant, atazanavir, basiliximab, boceprevir, bromocriptine, chloramphenicol, clarithromycin, conivaptan, dalopristin, danazol, darunavir, dasatinib, delavirdine, diltiazem, dronedarone, efavirenz, erythromycin, ethinyl estradiol, fluconazole, fluoxetine, fluvoxamine, fosamprenavir, fosaprepitant, IL-2, imatinib, indinavir, isoniazid, itraconazole, ketoconazole, lanreotide, lapatinib, miconazole, nefazodone, nelfinavir, niCARdipine, octreotide, posaconazole, quiNINE, ranolazine, rifaximin, tamoxifen, telaprevir, telithromycin, tipranavir, troleandomycin, verapamil, voriconazole, zafirlukast): Increased rilpivirine effect

Class IA/III antidysrhytmics, some phenothiazines, beta agonists, local anesthetics, tricyclics, CYP3A4 inhibitors (amiodarone, arsenic trioxide, clarithromycin, erythromycin, levomethadyl, telithromycin, troleandomycin); CYP3A4 substrates (methadone, pimozide, quetiapine, quiNIDine, risperidone, ziprasidone), halogenated anesthetics: Increased QT prolongation

Drug/food
Increased adverse reactions: grapefruit juice

NURSING CONSIDERATIONS
Nursing diagnoses
• Risk for infection (uses)
• Risk for injury (adverse reactions)

---

riluzole (Rx)
(ri-loo'zole)
Rilutek
Func. class.: Amyotropic lateral sclerosis (ALS) agent
Chem. class.: Benzathiazole
Pregnancy category C

ACTION: Unknown; may act by inhibiting glutamate, interfering with binding of amino acid receptors, inactivation of voltage-dependent sodium channels

Therapeutic outcome: Decreased symptoms of ALS

USES: ALS

CONTRAINDICATIONS: Hypersensitivity

Precautions: Pregnancy **C**, breastfeeding, children, geriatric, neutropenia, renal/hepatic disease, cigarette smoking, febrile illness, pneumonia

DOSAGE AND ROUTES
Adult: PO 50 mg q12hr; take 1 hr before or 2 hr after meals

Available forms: Tabs 50 mg

Implementation
• Give 1 hr before or 2 hr after meals; a high-fat meal decreases absorption

ADVERSE EFFECTS
CNS: Hypertonia, depression, dizziness, insomnia, somnolence, vertigo, paresthesia

CV: Hypertension, tachycardia, phlebitis, palpitation, postural hypertension
GI: Nausea, vomiting, dyspepsia, anorexia, diarrhea, flatulence, stomatitis, dry mouth, increased liver function tests, jaundice, abdominal pain
GU: UTI, dysuria
HEMA: Neutropenia
INTEG: Pruritus, eczema, alopecia, **exfoliative dermatitis**
MS: Arthralgia
RESP: Decreased lung function; rhinitis, increased cough, pneumonia

Pharmacokinetics

Absorption	Well
Distribution	Unknown
Metabolism	Liver, extensively
Excretion	Urine, feces
Half-life	Unknown

Pharmacodynamics

Unknown

INTERACTIONS
Individual drugs
Allopurinol, leflunomide, methotrexate, methyldopa, sulfasalazine, tacrine: increased hepatic injury
Amitriptyline, caffeine, theophylline: decreased elimination of riluzole
CarBAMazepine: increased liver function tests
Cigarette smoke, omeprazole, rifampin: increased elimination of riluzole

Drug classifications
Barbiturates: increased liver function tests
Quinolones: decreased elimination of riluzole

Drug/food
Charcoal-broiled foods: increased elimination of riluzole
High-fat meal: decreased absorption

NURSING CONSIDERATIONS
Assessment
• Assess for clinical improvement in neurologic function
• Monitor liver function tests: AST, ALT, bilirubin, GGT, baseline and qmo × 3 mo, then q3mo
• Assess for neutropenia (neutrophils <500/mm^3)

Nursing diagnoses
• Knowledge, deficient (teaching)
• Mobility, impaired physical (uses)

Patient/family education
• Advise to report febrile illness, may indicate neutropenia; cardiac/respiratory changes
• Teach reason for product and expected results

Evaluation
Positive therapeutic outcome
• Decreasing symptoms of ALS

rimantadine (Rx)
(ri-man'ti-deen)
Flumadine
Func. class.: Synthetic antiviral
Chem. class.: Tricyclic amine
Pregnancy category C

Do not confuse:
rimantadine/amantadine/ranitidine

ACTION: Prevents uncoating of nucleic acid in viral cell, preventing penetration of virus to host; causes release of DOPamine from neurons

Therapeutic outcome: Prevention of influenza type A

USES: Prophylaxis or treatment of influenza type A

CONTRAINDICATIONS:
Hypersensitivity to products of adamantine class (this product, amantadine)

Precautions: Pregnancy **C**, breastfeeding, children <1 yr, epilepsy, renal/hepatic disease

DOSAGE AND ROUTES
Influenza type A prophylaxis
Adult and child >10 yr: PO 100 mg bid
Child 1-10 yr: PO 5 mg/kg/day, max 150 mg

Treatment
Adult: PO 100 mg bid; start treatment at onset of symptoms, continue for at least 1 wk
Geriatric: PO 100 mg/day

Renal/hepatic dose
Adult: PO ≤10 ml/min 100 mg qd

Available forms: Tabs 100 mg; syr 50 mg/5 ml

Implementation
• Give before exposure to influenza; continue for 10 days after contact
• Give at least 4 hr before bedtime to prevent insomnia

⚠ Nurse Alert

• Administer after meals for better absorption, to decrease GI symptoms; cap may be opened and mixed with food for easy swallowing
• Give in divided doses to prevent CNS disturbances: headache, dizziness, fatigue, drowsiness
• Store in airtight, dry container

ADVERSE EFFECTS

CNS: *Headache, dizziness,* fatigue, depression, hallucinations, tremors, **seizures,** insomnia, poor concentration, asthenia, gait abnormalities, anxiety, confusion
CV: Pallor, palpitations, edema
EENT: Tinnitus, taste abnormality, eye pain
GI: *Nausea, vomiting,* constipation, *dry mouth, anorexia, abdominal pain, diarrhea,* dyspepsia
INTEG: Rash

Pharmacokinetics

Absorption	Minimally absorbed (PO)
Distribution	Widely distributed, crosses placenta, CSF concentration 50% plasma
Metabolism	Liver
Excretion	95% unchanged—kidneys
Half-life	13-65 hr, increased in renal disease

Pharmacodynamics

	PO
Onset	Unknown
Peak	$1^1/_2$-$2^1/_2$ hr
Duration	Unknown

INTERACTIONS

Individual drugs
Acetaminophen, aspirin, intranasal influenza vaccine: decreased peak concentration of rimantadine
Cimetidine: increased rimantadine concentration

NURSING CONSIDERATIONS

Assessment
• **Assess for seizures;** if seizures occur, product should be discontinued
• Monitor respiratory status: rate, character, wheezing, tightness in chest

Nursing diagnoses
• Infection, risk for (uses)
• Knowledge, deficient (teaching)

Patient/family education
• Instruct patient about aspects of product therapy: need to report dyspnea, dizziness, poor concentration, behavioral changes
• Advise patient to avoid hazardous activities if dizziness occurs
• Caution patient to consult prescriber before taking OTC medications, alcohol; serious product interactions may result

Evaluation
Positive therapeutic outcome
• Absence of fever, malaise, cough, dyspnea

---

risedronate (Rx)
(rih-sed'roh-nate)
Actonel, Atelvia
Func. class.: Bone resorption inhibitor
Chem. class.: Bisphosphonate
Pregnancy category C

ACTION: Inhibits bone resorption; absorbs calcium phosphate crystal in bone and may directly block dissolution of hydroxyapatite crystals of bone

Therapeutic outcome: Increased bone mass, activity without fractures

USES: Paget's disease; prevention, treatment of osteoporosis in postmenopausal women; glucocorticoid-induced osteoporosis; osteoporosis in men

CONTRAINDICATIONS:
Hypersensitivity to bisphosphonates, inability to stand or sit upright for ≥30 min, esophageal stricture, achalasia, hypocalcemia

Precautions: Pregnancy **C,** breastfeeding, children, renal disease, active upper GI disorders, dental disease, hyperparathyroidism, infection, vitamin D deficiency, coagulopathy, chemotherapy, asthma

DOSAGE AND ROUTES

Paget's disease
Adult: PO 30 mg/day × 2 mo; give calcium and vit D if dietary intake is lacking; if relapse occurs, retreatment is advised

Treatment/prevention of postmenopausal osteoporosis
Adult: PO 5 mg/day or 35 mg qwk or 75 mg/day × 2 consecutive days 2 × mo or 150 mg qmo

Glucocorticoid osteoporosis
Adult: PO 5 mg/day

Osteoporosis in men
Adult: PO 35 mg qwk

Renal dose
Adult: PO CCr <30 mg/min, avoid use

Available forms: Tabs 5, 30, 35, 75, 150 mg; tab gastro-resistant, weekly 35 mg; tab, weekly 35 mg

Implementation
• Give PO for 2 mo to be effective in Paget's disease
• Give with a full glass of water; patient should be in upright position
• Administer supplemental calcium and vit D in Paget's disease
• Give daily ≥30 min before meals
• Store in cool environment out of direct sunlight

ADVERSE EFFECTS
CNS: Dizziness, headache, depression
CV: Chest pain, hypertension, **atrial fibrillation**
GI: *Abdominal pain,* diarrhea, *nausea,* constipation, esophagitis
MS: *Severe muscle/joint/bone pain,* **osteonecrosis of the jaw**
MISC: Rash, UTI, pharyngitis, hypocalcemia, hypophosphatemia, increased PTH
SYST: Angioedema

Pharmacokinetics

Absorption	Unknown
Distribution	To bones (50%)
Metabolism	Unknown
Excretion	Kidneys
Half-life	Terminal 220 hr

Pharmacodynamics
Unknown

INTERACTIONS
Drug classifications
Aluminum, antacids, calcium, iron, magnesium salts: decreased absorption of risedronate
NSAIDs, salicylates: increased GI irritation

Drug/food
Food: decreased bioavailability; take ½ hr before food or drinks other than water

Drug/lab test
Increased: bone imaging agents

NURSING CONSIDERATIONS
Assessment
• **Paget's disease:** assess for headache, bone pain, increased head circumference
• **Osteoporosis:** in men or postmenopausal women; bone density study prior to and periodically during treatment
• **Hypocalcemia:** assess for paresthesia, twitching, laryngospasm, Chvostek's/Trousseau's signs
⚠ **Serious skin reactions: assess for angioedema**
⚠ **Assess for atrial fibrillation**
• Monitor phosphate, alkaline phosphatase, calcium; creatinine, BUN (renal disease)
• **Hypercalcemia:** assess for paresthesia, twitching, laryngospasm, Chvostek's/Trousseau's signs
⚠ **Assess dental health, cover with antiinfectives prior to dental extraction**

Nursing diagnoses
• Knowledge, deficient (teaching)
• Mobility, impaired physical (uses)
• Nutrition: less than body requirements, imbalanced (uses)

Patient/family education
• Advise patient to sit upright for ½ hr after dose to prevent irritation
• Instruct patient to comply with dietary restrictions, maintain good oral hygiene
• Advise patient to notify prescriber if pregnancy is planned or suspected

Evaluation
Positive therapeutic outcome
• Increased bone mass, absence of fractures

risperidone (Rx)
(res-pare′a-done)
Risperdal, Risperdal Consta, Risperdal M-TAB
Func. class.: Antipsychotic
Chem. class.: Benzisoxazole derivative
Pregnancy category C

Do not confuse:
Risperdal/reserpine

ACTION: Unknown; may be mediated through both DOPamine type 2 (D_2) and serotonin type 2 (5-HT_2) antagonism

Therapeutic outcome: Decreased hallucinations and disorganized thought

USES: Irritability associated with autism, bipolar disorder, mania, schizophrenia

CONTRAINDICATIONS:
Hypersensitivity, seizure

Precautions: Pregnancy C, children, geriatric, cardiac/renal/hepatic disease, breast cancer, Parkinson's disease, CNS depression, brain tumor, dehydration, diabetes, hematologic disease, seizure disorders, breastfeeding, abrupt discontinuation

> **BLACK BOX WARNING:** Dementia

DOSAGE AND ROUTES
Adult: PO 2 mg/day as a single dose or 2 divided doses, adjust dose at intervals of ≥24 hr and 1-2 mg/day as tolerated to 4-8 mg/day; IM establish dosing with PO prior to IM 25 mg q2wk, may increase to max 50 mg q2wk
Adolescent: PO 0.5 mg/q day in AM or PM, adjust dose at intervals of ≥24 hr and 0.5-1 mg/day as tolerated to 3 mg/day
Geriatric: PO 0.5 mg daily-bid, increase by 1 mg qwk; IM 25 mg q2wk

Hepatic dose/renal dose
Adult: PO 0.5 mg, increase by 0.5 mg bid, then increase to 1.5 mg bid

Available forms: Tabs 0.25, 0.5, 1, 2, 3, 4 mg; oral sol 1 mg/ml; orally disintegrating tabs 0.5, 1, 2, 3, 4 mg; long-acting inj kit (Risperdal Consta) 12.5, 25, 37.5, 50 mg

Implementation
PO route
• Reduced dosage in geriatric patients
• Anticholinergic agent on order from prescriber, to be used for EPS
• Avoid use with CNS depressants
• Conventional tabs: give without regard to meals
• *Oral disintegrating tab* (Risperdal M-Tab): do not open blister pack until ready to use; tear 1 of the 4 units apart at perforation; bend corner where indicated; peel back foil; do not push tab through foil; remove from pack and place on tongue; tab disintegrates in seconds and can be swallowed with or without liquids
• *Oral solution:* dilute 3-4 oz of a beverage, measure dose using calibrated pipette, not compatible with coffee, tea
IM route
• Only use diluent and needle provided; do not substitute, one needle is for deltoid use, one for gluteal, and are not interchangeable; allow to come to room temperature, reconstitute the powder using 2-ml prefilled syringe, shake vigorously, mixing is complete when suspension is uniform, thick, milky colored; do not combine different strengths in single administration; invert vial and withdraw dose, attach supplied label to syringe for ID purpose, unscrew the syringe from SmartSite Access Device and discard the vial and access device; attach Needle-Pro device as directed, inj deep IM into upper-outer quadrant of gluteal muscle or deltoid, use within 2 min of reconstitution
• Do not give IV
• When switching from oral to inj, give oral dose with first inj and continue for 3 wk, then discontinue

ADVERSE EFFECTS
CNS: *EPS (pseudoparkinsonism, akathisia, dystonia, tardive dyskinesia), drowsiness, insomnia, agitation, anxiety, headache,* **neuroleptic malignant syndrome,** dizziness, **seizures, suicidal ideation,** head titubation (shaking)
CV: Orthostatic hypotension, **tachycardia, heart failure, sudden death (geriatric),** AV block
EENT: Blurred vision, tinnitus
GI: *Nausea,* vomiting, *anorexia, constipation,* jaundice, weight gain
GU: Hyperprolactinemia, gynecomastia, dysuria
HEMA: **Neutropenia, granulocytopenia**
MS: **Rhabdomyolysis**
MISC: **Renal artery disease;** weight gain, hyperprolactinemia (child)
RESP: Rhinitis, sinusitis, upper respiratory infection, cough

Pharmacokinetics
Absorption	Unknown
Distribution	Unknown
Metabolism	Liver, extensively
Excretion	Urine 90%
Half-life	3-24 hr

Pharmacodynamics
Onset	Unknown
Peak	1-2 hr
Duration	Up to 12 hr

INTERACTIONS
Individual drugs
Alcohol: increased sedation

⚠ **Chloroquine, clarithromycin, droperidol, erythromycin, haloperidol, methadone, pentamidine: increased QT prolongation**

CarBAMazepine: increased risperidone excretion

⚠ **Furosemide: possible death in dementia-related psychosis**

Levodopa: decreased levodopa effect

Drug classifications
Antipsychotics: increased EPS

⚠ **β-agonists, class IA/III antidysrhythmics, local anesthetics, some phenothiazines, tricyclics: increased QT prolongation**

CNS depressants: increased sedation

CYP2D6 inducers (carBAMazepine, barbiturates, phenytoin, rifampin): decreased risperidone action

CYP2D6 inhibitors (selective serotonin reuptake inhibitors): serotonin syndrome, neuroleptic malignant syndrome

Drug/herb
Echinacea: decreased risperidone effect

Drug/lab test
Increased: prolactin levels

NURSING CONSIDERATIONS
Assessment
• **Suicidal thoughts, behaviors** often occur when depression is lessened; assess mental status: orientation, mood, behavior, presence and type of hallucinations before initial administration, monthly; this product should significantly reduce psychotic behavior

• Check that patient swallows all PO medication; check for hoarding or giving of medication to other patients

• Monitor I&O ratio; palpate bladder if low urinary output occurs, especially in geriatric; urinalysis recommended before, during prolonged therapy

• Monitor bilirubin, CBC, liver function tests monthly

• Assess affect, orientation, LOC, reflexes, gait, coordination, sleep pattern disturbances

• **QT prolongation:** Monitor B/P with patient in sitting, standing, and lying positions; take pulse and respirations q4hr during initial treatment; establish baseline before starting treatment; report drops of 30 mm Hg; obtain baseline ECG and monitor Q- and T-wave changes

• Check for dizziness, faintness, palpitations, tachycardia on rising; severe orthostatic hypotension is common

⚠ **Assess for neuroleptic malignant syndrome: hyperpyrexia, muscle rigidity, increased CPK, altered mental status; product should be discontinued**

• EPS: Assess for akathisia (inability to sit still, no pattern to movements), tardive dyskinesia (bizarre movements of the jaw, mouth, tongue, extremities), pseudoparkinsonism (rigidity, tremors, pill rolling, shuffling gait); an antiparkinsonian product should be prescribed

• Assess for constipation, urinary retention daily; if these occur, increase bulk, water in diet

Nursing diagnoses
• Coping, ineffective (uses)
• Knowledge, deficient (teaching)
• Noncompliance (teaching)

Patient/family education
• Teach patient to use good oral hygiene; frequent rinsing of mouth, sugarless gum for dry mouth

• Caution patient to avoid hazardous activities until product response is determined; dizziness, blurred vision may occur

• Inform patient that orthostatic hypotension occurs often; patient should rise from sitting or lying position gradually and remain lying down for at least 30 min after IM inj

• Instruct patient to avoid hot tubs, hot showers, tub baths; hypotension may occur

• Inform patient that heat stroke may occur in hot weather and to take extra precautions to stay cool

• Advise patient to avoid abrupt withdrawal of this product, or EPS may result; product should be withdrawn slowly

• Teach patient to avoid OTC preparations (cough, hay fever, cold) unless approved by prescriber; serious product interactions may occur; avoid use with alcohol, CNS depressants because increased drowsiness may occur

• Advise patient to use contraception, to inform prescriber if pregnancy is planned or suspected

Evaluation
Positive therapeutic outcome
• Decrease in emotional excitement, hallucinations, delusions, paranoia
• Reorganization of patterns of thought, speech

TREATMENT OF OVERDOSE:
Lavage, provide airway

⚠ Nurse Alert

ritonavir (Rx)

(ri-toe'na-veer)

Norvir

Func. class.: Antiretroviral

Chem. class.: Protease inhibitor

Pregnancy category B

Do not confuse:

ritonavir/retrovir

ACTION: Inhibits HIV-1 protease and prevents maturation of the infectious virus

Therapeutic outcome: Improvement of HIV-1 infection

USES: HIV-1 in combination with at least 2 other antiretrovirals

CONTRAINDICATIONS:

Hypersensitivity

> **BLACK BOX WARNING:** Coadministration with other drugs

Precautions: Pregnancy **B**, breastfeeding, children, liver disease, pancreatitis, diabetes, hemophilia, AV block, hypercholesterolemia, immune reconstitution syndrome, neonates, cardiomyopathy

DOSAGE AND ROUTES

Adult/adolescent >16 yr: PO 600 mg bid; if nausea occurs, begin dose at $^1/_2$ and gradually increase, max 1200 mg/day

Adolescent ≤16 yr/child/infant: PO 400 mg/m^2 bid up to 1200 mg/day; may start lower and escalate

Available forms: Caps 100 mg; oral sol 80 mg/ml, tab 100 mg

Implementation

• Oral sol: Shake oral sol well, use calibrated measuring device

• Store caps in refrigerator

• Mix liquid formulation with chocolate milk or liquid nutritional supplement to improve taste

• When switching from cap to tab, more GI symptoms may occur that will lessen over time

• Use dosage titration to minimize side effects

ADVERSE EFFECTS

CNS: *Paresthesia*, headache, **seizures**, dizziness, insomnia, fever, asthenia, **intracranial bleeding**

CV: QT, PR interval prolongation

GI: *Diarrhea*, buccal mucosa ulceration, *abdominal pain, nausea, taste perversion*, dry mouth, *vomiting, anorexia*

INTEG: Rash

MISC: Asthenia, **angioedema, anaphylaxis, Stevens-Johnson syndrome**, increased lipids, lipodystrophy

MS: Pain, **rhabdomyolysis**, myalgia

Pharmacokinetics

Absorption	Well
Distribution	Unknown
Metabolism	98% protein binding, liver
Excretion	Unknown
Half-life	3-5 hr

Pharmacodynamics

Onset	Unknown
Peak	2-4 hr
Duration	Unknown

INTERACTIONS

Individual drugs

Amiodarone, astemizole, buPROPion, cisapride, clozapine, desipramine, encainide, ergotamine, flecainide, meperidine, midazolam, pimozide, piroxicam, propafenone, propoxyphene, quiNIDine, ranolazine, saquinavir, terfenadine, triazolam, zolpidem: toxicity, do not use together

Atovaquone, divalproex, ethinyl estradiol, lamoTRIgine, phenytoin, sulfamethoxazole, theophylline, voriconazole, zidovudine: decreased levels of each drug

Bosentan: increased levels of bosentan

Clarithromycin: increased level of both products

ddI: increased levels of both products

Fluconazole: increased ritonavir level

Haloperidol, chloroquine, droperidol, pentamidine, arsenic trioxide, levomethadyl: increased QT prolongation

Nevirapine, phenytoin: decreased ritonavir levels

Drug classifications

Anticoagulants: decreased levels of anticoagulants

Azole antifungals, benzodiazepines, HMG-CoA reductase inhibitors, interleukins: toxicity, do not use together

Barbiturates, rifamycins: decreased ritonavir level

Class IA/III antidysrhythmics, some phenothiazines, β-agonists, local anesthetics, tricyclics, CYP3A4 inhibitors (amiodarone, clarithromycin, erythromycin, telithromycin, troleandomycin), CYP3A4 substrates (metha-

R

done, pimozide, QUEtiapine, quiNIDine, risperidone, ziprasidone): increased QT prolongation

Drug/herb
Red yeast rice: avoid use
St. John's wort: decreased ritonavir levels, avoid concurrent use

Drug/lab test
Increased: ALT, GGT, AST, CPK, cholesterol, triglycerides, uric acid
Decreased: Hct, RBC, Hgb, neutrophils, WBC

NURSING CONSIDERATIONS

Assessment
• **QT prolongation:** ECG for QT prolongation, ejection fraction; assess for chest pain, palpitations, dyspnea
• **Rhabdomyolysis:** muscle pain, increased CPK, weakness, swelling of affected muscles; if these occur and if confirmed by CPK, product should be discontinued
• Assess signs of infection, anemia
• Monitor viral load and CD4, blood glucose, plasma HIV RNA, serum cholesterol, lipid profile baseline, throughout therapy
• Resistance testing prior to starting therapy and after treatment failure
• Assess liver function tests: ALT, AST
• Monitor C&S before product therapy; product may be taken as soon as culture is done; repeat C&S after treatment; determine the presence of other STDs
• Assess bowel pattern before, during treatment; if severe abdominal pain with bleeding occurs, product should be discontinued; monitor hydration
• **Serious skin disorders: Stevens-Johnson syndrome,** angioedema; anaphylaxis

Nursing diagnoses
• Infection, risk for (uses)
• Knowledge, deficient (teaching)

Patient/family education
• Teach patient to take as prescribed; if dose is missed, take as soon as remembered up to 1 hr before next dose; do not double dose
• Teach patient that product must be taken in equal intervals around the clock to maintain blood levels for duration of therapy
• Teach patient that product is not a cure for HIV; opportunistic infections may continue to be acquired, and others may continue to contract HIV from the patient
• Advise patient not to use St. John's wort, that it decreases this product's effect

• Inform that redistribution of body fat or accumulation of body fat may occur

Evaluation
Positive therapeutic outcome
• Decreasing symptoms of HIV
• Improving viral load and CD4 cell counts

---

riTUXimab (Rx)
(rih-tuks'ih-mab)
Rituxan
Func. class.: Antineoplastic—miscellaneous; DMARD
Chem. class.: Murine/human monoclonal antibody
Pregnancy category C

ACTION: Directed against the CD20 antigen that is found on malignant B lymphocytes; CD20 regulates a portion of cell cycle initiation/differentiation

Therapeutic outcome: Decreased tumor size, prevention of spread of cancer

USES: Non-Hodgkin's lymphoma (CD20 positive, B-cell), bulky disease (tumors >10 cm), rheumatoid arthritis, Wegener's granulomatosis, microscopic polyangitis

CONTRAINDICATIONS:
Hypersensitivity, murine proteins

Precautions: Pregnancy C, breastfeeding, children, geriatric, cardiac/renal/pulmonary conditions

> **BLACK BOX WARNING:** Exfoliative dermatitis, infusion-related reactions, progressive multifocal leukoencephalopathy

DOSAGE AND ROUTES

Non-Hodgkin's Lymphoma (NHL), Chronic Lymphocytic Leukemia (CLL)
Adult: IV INF 375 mg/m^2 qwk × 4 doses; give at 50 mg/hr for 1st INF; if hypersensitivity does not occur, increase rate by 50 mg/hr q^1/$_2$hr, max 400 mg/hr; slow/interrupt INF if hypersensitivity occurs; other INF can be given at 100 mg/hr and increased by 100 mg/hr, max 400 mg/hr

Rheumatoid Arthritis
Adult: IV 100 mg on days 1, 15

Available forms: Inj 10 mg/ml

Implementation

Intermittent IV infusion route
- Hold antihypertensive 2 hr before administration
- Administer after diluting to a final conc of 1-4 mg/ml; use 0.9% NaCl, D₅W, gently invert bag to mix; do not mix with other products
- Increase fluid intake to 2-3 L/day to prevent dehydration, unless contraindicated

Y-site compatibilities: Acyclovir, amifostine, amikacin, aminophylline, ampicillin, ampicillin/sulbactam, aztreonam, bleomycin, bumetanide, buprenorphine, busulfan, butorphanol, calcium gluconate, CARBOplatin, carmustine, ceFAZolin, cefoperazone, cefotaxime, cefotetan, cefoxitin, ceftazidime, ceftizoxime, cefTRIAXone, cefuroxime, chlorproMAZINE, cimetidine, CISplatin, clindamycin, cyclophosphamide, cytarabine, DACTINomycin, DAUNOrubicin hydrochloride, dexamethasone, dexrazoxane, digoxin, diphenhydrAMINE, DOBUTamine, docetaxel, DOPamine, DOXOrubicin liposome, doxycycline, droperidol, enalaprilat, etoposide phosphate, famotidine, fentaNYL, filgrastim, floxuridine, fluconazole, fludarabine, fluorouracil, ganciclovir, gemcitabine, gentamicin, granisetron, haloperidol, heparin, hydrocortisone, HYDROmorphone, IDArubicin, ifosfamide, imipenem/cilastatin, irinotecan, leucovorin, levorphanol, LORazepam, magnesium sulfate, mannitol, meperidine, mesna, methotrexate, methylPREDNISolone, metoclopramide, metroNIDAZOLE, mitomycin, mitoxantrone, morphine, nalbuphine, netilmicin, paclitaxel, pentamidine, piperacillin/tazobactam, plicamycin, potassium chloride, prochlorperazine, promethazine, ranitidine, sargramostim, streptozocin, teniposide, theophylline, thiotepa, ticarcillin/clavulanate, tobramycin, trimethoprim/sulfamethoxazole, trimethobenzamide, vinBLAStine, vinCRIStine, vinorelbine, zidovudine

Y-site incompatibilities: Aldesleukin, amphotericin B colloidal, ciprofloxacin, cycloSPORINE, DAUNOrubicin liposome, DOXOrubicin hydrochloride, furosemide, levofloxacin, minocycline, ondansetron, quinupristin/dalfopristin, sodium bicarbonate, topotecan, vancomycin

Additive incompatibilities: Do not admix with other products
- Store vials at 36°-40° F, protect vials from direct sunlight, inf sol is stable at 36°-46° F × 24 hr and room temperature for another 12 hr

ADVERSE EFFECTS

CNS: Life-threatening brain infection (progressive multifocal leukoencephalopathy)
CV: Cardiac dysrhythmias, heart failure, MI, superventricular tachycardia, hypertension, angina
GI: *Nausea, vomiting, anorexia,* **GI obstruction/perforation**
GU: Renal failure
HEMA: Leukopenia, neutropenia, thrombocytopenia, anemia
INTEG: *Irritation at inj site, rash,* **fatal mucocutaneous infections (rare)**
MISC: *Fever,* chills, asthenia, *headache,* **angioedema,** hypotension, myalgia, bronchospasm, ARDs
SYST: Stevens-Johnson syndrome, exfoliative dermatitis, toxic epidermal necrolysis, tumor lysis syndrome

Pharmacokinetics

Absorption	Unknown
Distribution	Binds to CD20 sites on lymphoma cells
Metabolism	Unknown
Excretion	Unknown
Half-life	60-174 hr

Pharmacodynamics

Unknown

INTERACTIONS

Drug classifications
Anticoagulants, NSAIDs: increased bleeding risk

NURSING CONSIDERATIONS

Assessment
⚠ Assess for signs of fatal inf reaction: hypoxia, pulmonary infiltrates, ARDS, MI, ventricular fibrillation, cardiogenic shock; most fatal inf reactions occur with first inf, discontinue product
⚠ Assess for signs of severe mucocutaneous reactions: Stevens-Johnson syndrome, lichenoid dermatitis, toxic epidermal lysis; signs occur 1-13 wk after product was given
⚠ Assess for tumor lysis syndrome: acute renal failure requiring hemodialysis, hyperkalemia, hypocalcemia, hyperuricemia, hyperphosphatasemia
- **Multifocal leukoencephalopathy:** confusion, dizziness, lethargy, hemiparesis, monitor periodically

Adverse effects: *italics* = common; **bold** = life-threatening

• Monitor CBC, differential, platelet count weekly; withhold product if WBC is <3500/mm³ or platelet count <100,000/mm³; notify prescriber of these results; product should be discontinued
• Monitor ECG, serum creatinine/BUN, electrolytes, uric acid
• Assess GI symptoms: frequency of stools
• Assess signs of dehydration: rapid respirations, poor skin turgor, decreased urine output, dry skin, restlessness, weakness

Nursing diagnoses
• Injury, risk for (side effects)
• Knowledge, deficient (teaching)

Patient/family education
• Advise patient to report to prescriber possible infection (cough, fever, chills, sore throat), renal issues (painful urination, back/side pain), bleeding (gums, stools, bruising, urine, emesis, fatigue)
• Advise to avoid OTC products
• Teach to use contraception during and up to 12 mo after therapy
• Avoid use with vaccines, toxoids

Evaluation
Positive therapeutic outcome
• Prevention of increasing cancer progression

rivaroxaban
(ri-va-rox′a-ban)
Xarelto
Func. class.: Anticoagulant
Chem. class.: Factor Xa inhibitor
Pregnancy category C

ACTION: A novel, oral anticoagulant that selectively and potently inhibits coagulation factor Xa

Therapeutic outcome: Prevention of DVT, stroke, and systemic embolism

USES: For deep venous thrombosis (DVT) prophylaxis, which may lead to pulmonary embolism (PE), in patients undergoing knee or hip replacement surgery; for stroke prophylaxis and systemic embolism prophylaxis in patients with nonvalvular atrial fibrillation

CONTRAINDICATIONS: Severe hypersensitivity

Precautions: Moderate or severe hepatic disease (Child-Pugh Class B or C), hepatic disease associated with coagulopathy, creatinine clearance <30 ml/min for use as DVT prophylaxis and <15 ml/min for stroke and systemic embolism prophylaxis in nonvalvular atrial fibrillation, dental procedures, neonates, infants, children, adolescents, pregnancy category C, aneurysm, diabetes retinopathy, breastfeeding, diverticulitis, endocarditis, geriatrics, GI bleeding, hypertension, obstetric delivery, peptic ulcer disease, stroke, surgery

DOSAGE AND ROUTES

Deep venous thrombosis (DVT) prophylaxis, which may lead to pulmonary embolism (PE) (knee or hip replacement surgery):
Administer the initial dose at least 6–10 hr after surgery once hemostasis has been established
Adult: PO 10 mg daily for 12 days after knee replacement surgery or for 35 days after hip replacement

Stroke prophylaxis and systemic embolism prophylaxis (nonvalvular atrial fibrillation):
Adults: PO 20 mg daily with the evening meal (CrCl > 50 ml/min); **converting from warfarin to rivaroxaban:** discontinue warfarin and start rivaroxaban when INR is <3; **converting from another anticoagulant other than warfarin to rivaroxaban:** start rivaroxaban 0-2 hr before the next scheduled evening administration of anticoagulant (omit that dose of anticoagulant); for continuous infusion of unfractionated heparin, stop the infusion and initiate rivaroxaban simultaneously; **converting from rivaroxaban to another anticoagulant with rapid onset (not warfarin):** Discontinue rivaroxaban and give the first dose of the other anticoagulant (oral or parenteral) at the time that the next dose of rivaroxaban would have been administered

Available forms: Tab 10, 20, 50 mg

Implementation
• **For DVT prophylaxis**: give daily without regard to food, give initial dose ≥6-10 hr after surgery when hemostasis has been established
• For stroke/systemic embolism prophylaxis: give daily with evening meal
• If dose is not given at correct time, give as soon as possible on the same day
• Unless pathological bleeding occurs, do not discontinue rivaroxaban in the absence of alternative
• Store at room temperature

ADVERSE EFFECTS

GI: Cholestasis, **cytolytic hepatitis,** hyperbilirubinemia, increased hepatic enzymes, jaundice, nausea

HEMA: Adrenal bleeding, bleeding, cerebral hemorrhage, epidural hematoma, GI bleeding, hemiparesis, intracranial bleeding, retinal hemorrhage, retroperitoneal hemorrhage, subdural hematoma, thrombocytopenia

INTEG: Anaphylactic reaction, anaphylactic shock, blister, hypersensitivity, pruritus

SYST: Stevens-Johnson syndrome

> **BLACK BOX WARNING:** Active bleeding

> **BLACK BOX WARNING:** Abrupt discontinuation, epidermal/spinal anesthesia

Pharmacokinetics

Absorption	80%-100%
Distribution	Protein binding (92%-95%)
Metabolism	Oxidative degradation
Excretion	Urine (66%), feces (17%)
Half-life	5-9 hr; geriatric: 11-13 hr

Pharmacodynamics

Onset	Unknown
Peak	2-4 hrs
Duration	Unknown

INTERACTIONS

Individual drugs

Clarithromycin, conivaptan, erythromycin, itraconazole, ketoconazole, lopinavir/ritonavir, nicardipine: increased rivaroxaban effect, possible bleeding

CarBAMazepine, phenytoin, rifampin, ritonavir: decreased rivaroxaban effect

Amiodarone, azithromycin, darunavir, diltiazem, dronedarone, felodipineh, lapatinib, mifepristone, nelfinavir, pantoprazole, posaconazole, quiNIDine, ranolazine, saquinavir, tamoxifen, telithromycin, verapamil: increased rivaroxaban effect in renal impairment

Drug classifications

NSAIDs, other anticoagulants, platelet inhibitors, salicylates, thrombolytics: increased rivaroxaban effect, possible bleeding

Drug/herb

St. John's wort: decreased rivaroxaban effect

Drug/food

Grapefruit juice: increased rivaroxaban effect in renal disease

Food: decreased rivaroxaban effect

NURSING CONSIDERATIONS

Assessment

> **BLACK BOX WARNING: Bleeding:** Monitor for bleeding, including bleeding during dental procedures, easy bruising, blood in urine, stools, emesis, sputum, epistaxis; there is no specific antidote

> **BLACK BOX WARNING: Abrupt discontinuation:** Avoid the abrupt discontinuation unless an alternative anticoagulant is used in those with atrial fibrillation; discontinuing puts patients at increased risk for thrombotic events; if this product must be discontinued for reasons other than pathological bleeding, consider administering another anticoagulant

• **Pregnancy/breastfeeding:** pregnancy category C; identify if pregnancy is suspected or planned; pregnancy-related hemorrhage may occur, and anticoagulation cannot be monitored with standard laboratory testing; breastfeeding should be discontinued prior to use of this product

> **BLACK BOX WARNING: Epidural/spinal anesthesia:** Epidural or spinal hematomas that may result in long-term/permanent paralysis may occur in patients who have received anticoagulants and are receiving neuraxial anesthesia or undergoing spinal puncture. The epidural catheter should not be removed <18 hr after the last dose of rivaroxaban; do not administer the next rivaroxaban dose <6 hr after the catheter removal; delay rivaroxaban administration for 24 hr if traumatic puncture occurs. Monitor for neuro changes

• **Hepatic/Renal disease:** Increase in effect of this product in hepatic disease (Child-Pugh Class B or C), hepatic disease with coagulopathy; renal failure/severe renal impairment (creatinine clearance <30 ml/min in DVT prophylaxis and <15 ml/min for stroke/systemic embolism prophylaxis in nonvalvular atrial fibrillation); product should be discontinued in acute renal failure; reduce dose in those with atrial fibrillation and CrCl 15-50 ml/min; monitor renal function periodically (creatinine clearance, BUN)

R

Nursing diagnoses
• Risk for injury (Uses, adverse reactions)

Patient/family education
• Advise patient to report if pregnancy is planned or suspected, not to breastfeed
• Teach patient to report bleeding (bruising, blood in urine, stools, sputum, emesis, heavy menstrual flow) and to use soft toothbrush, electric shaver
• Advise patient to inform all health care providers of use
• Advise patient to avoid abrupt discontinuation without another blood thinner
• Instruct patients, especially those with dental disease, in proper oral hygiene, including caution in use of regular toothbrushes, dental floss, and toothpicks.

Evaluation
Positive therapeutic outcome
• Prevention of DVT, stroke and systemic embolism

rivastigmine (Rx)
(riv-as-tig′mine)
Exelon, Exelon Patch
Func. class.: Anti-Alzheimer's agent
Chem. class.: Cholinesterase inhibitor
Pregnancy category B

ACTION: Potent selective inhibitor of brain acetylcholinesterase (AChE) and butycholinerase (BChE)

Therapeutic outcome: Decreased signs and symptoms of Alzheimer's dementia

USES: Mild to moderate Alzheimer's dementia, mild to moderate Parkinson's disease dementia (PDD)

CONTRAINDICATIONS:
Hypersensitivity to this product, other carbamates

Precautions: Pregnancy **B**, breastfeeding, children, renal/hepatic/respiratory disease, seizure disorder, asthma, urinary obstruction, peptic ulcer, increased intracranial pressure, surgery, GI bleeding, jaundice

DOSAGE AND ROUTES
Adult: PO 1.5 mg bid with food for 4 wk or more, may increase to 3 mg bid after 4 wk or more; may increase to 4.5 mg bid and thereafter 6 mg bid, max 12 mg/day; transdermal apply 4.6 mg/24 hr after 4 wk or more, may increase to 9.5 mg/24 hr

Available forms: Caps 1.5, 3, 4.5, 6 mg; sol 2 mg/ml; transdermal patch 4.6, 9.5 mg/24 hr

Implementation
• Give with meals; take with AM and PM meal even though absorption may be decreased
• Provide assistance with ambulation during beginning therapy
• Discontinue treatment for several doses and restart at same or next lower dosage level if adverse reactions cause intolerance
• If treatment is interrupted for longer than several days treatment should be initiated with the lowest daily dose and titrated as indicated above

Transdermal route
• Apply to clean, hairless, dry skin; not in an area that clothing will rub; rotate sites daily; remove liner; apply firmly; may be used during water activities; avoid saunas, avoid excess sunlight or external heat, each 5 cm² patch contains 9 mg base, rate of 4.6 mg/24 hr, each 10 cm² patch is 18 mg base, rate of 9.5 mg/24 hr

ADVERSE EFFECTS
CNS: *Tremors, confusion, insomnia,* psychosis, hallucination, depression, dizziness, headache, anxiety, somnolence, fatigue, syncope, EPS, exacerbation of Parkinson's disease
CV: **QT prolongation, AV block, cardiac arrest, MI,** angina, palpitations
GI: *Nausea, vomiting, anorexia, abdominal distress, flatulence,* diarrhea, constipation, dyspepsia, colitis, eructation, fecal incontinence, **GI bleeding/obstruction,** GERD, gastritis, **pancreatitis**
MISC: UTI, asthenia, increased sweating, hypertension, flulike symptoms, weight change

Pharmacokinetics

Absorption	Rapidly, completely absorbed
Distribution	40% protein binding
Metabolism	To decarbamylated metabolite
Excretion	Kidney—metabolites, clearance lowered in geriatric, hepatic disease, increased nicotine use
Half-life	1½ hr

Pharmacodynamics
Unknown

⚠ Nurse Alert

INTERACTIONS

Individual drugs
Nicotine: increased metabolism, decreased blood level of rivastigmine

Drug classifications
Anticholinergics, phenothiazines, sedating H$_1$ blockers, tricyclics: decreased rivastigmine effect

Cholinergic agonists, other cholinesterase inhibitors: increased synergistic effect

NSAIDs: increased GI effects

NURSING CONSIDERATIONS

Assessment
• Monitor liver function tests: AST, ALT, alkaline phosphatase, LDH, bilirubin, CBC
• Assess for severe GI effects: nausea, vomiting, anorexia, weight loss
• Monitor B/P, respiration during initial treatment; hypo/hypertension should be reported
• **Cognitive/mental status:** affect, mood, behavioral changes, depression; complete suicide assessment

Nursing diagnoses
• Knowledge, deficient (teaching)

Patient/family education
• Teach patient procedure for giving oral sol; use instruction sheet provided; teach application of transdermal product, to fold in half and discard, not to get in eyes, to wash hands after application, to not use heating pad, sauna, tanning bed
• Teach patient to notify prescriber of severe GI effects
• Teach patient that product may cause dizziness, anorexia, weight loss

Evaluation
Positive therapeutic outcome
• Increased coherence, decreased symptoms of Alzheimer's disease, improved mood

rizatriptan (Rx)
(rye-zah-trip′tan)
Maxalt, Maxalt-MLT
Func. class.: Migraine agent
Chem. class.: 5-HT$_1$-like receptor agonist
Pregnancy category C

ACTION: Binds selectively to the vascular 5-HT$_{1B/1D}$ receptor subtype, exerts antimigraine effect; causes vasoconstriction in cranial arteries

Therapeutic outcome: After treatment, relief of migraine

USES: Acute treatment of migraine

CONTRAINDICATIONS:
Angina pectoris, history of MI, documented silent ischemia, Prinzmetal's angina, ischemic heart disease, concurrent ergotamine-containing preparations, uncontrolled hypertension, hypersensitivity, basilar or hemiplegic migraine

Precautions: Pregnancy C, breastfeeding, children, postmenopausal women, men >40 yr, geriatric, risk factors for CAD, hypercholesterolemia, obesity, diabetes, impaired renal/hepatic function

DOSAGE AND ROUTES
Adult: PO 5-10 mg single dose, redosing separate by 2 hr or more; max 30 mg/24 hr, use 5 mg in patient on propanolol; max 15 mg/24 hr

Available forms: Tabs (Maxalt) 5, 10 mg; orally disintegrating tabs (Maxalt-MLT) 5, 10 mg

Implementation
• Provide quiet, calm environment with decreased stimulation for noise, bright light, excessive talking
• Do not open blister pack until ready to use, put orally disintegrating tab on tongue to dissolve; swallow with saliva

ADVERSE EFFECTS
CNS: *Dizziness,* drowsiness, *headache, fatigue,* warm/cold sensation, flushing
CV: MI, ventricular fibrillation, ventricular tachycardia, coronary artery vasospasm
ENDO: Hot flashes, mild increase in growth hormone
GI: *Nausea,* dry mouth, diarrhea, abdominal pain
RESP: Chest tightness, pressure, dyspnea

Pharmacokinetics
Absorption	Unknown
Distribution	Unknown
Metabolism	Liver (metabolite)
Excretion	Urine/feces
Half-life	2-3 hr

Pharmacodynamics
Onset	10 min-2 hr
Peak	Unknown
Duration	Unknown

INTERACTIONS

Individual drugs

Cimetidine, isocarboxazide, pargyline, phenelzine, propranolol, trancyclomine: increased rizatriptan action

Ergot: increased vasospastic effects

Sibutramine: increased levels of sibutramine

Drug classifications

Contraceptives (oral), MAOIs, MAOIs (nonselective types A and B): increased rizatriptan action

Ergot derivatives, 5-HT$_1$ receptor agonists: increased vasospastic effects

Selective serotonin reuptake inhibitors: increased weakness, hyperreflexia, incoordination

Drug/herb

St. John's wort: serotonin syndrome

NURSING CONSIDERATIONS

Assessment

• Assess for stress level, activity, recreation, coping mechanisms

• Assess neurologic status: LOC, blurring vision, nausea, vomiting, tingling in extremities preceding headache

• **Ingestion of tyramine-containing foods:** Monitor for pickled products, beer, wine, aged cheese, food additives, preservatives, colorings, artificial sweeteners, chocolate, caffeine, which may precipitate these types of headaches

Nursing diagnoses

• Knowledge, deficient (teaching)

• Pain, acute (uses)

Patient/family education

• **Teach patient use of orally disintegrating tab:** instruct patient not to open blister until use, to peel blister open with dry hands, to place tab on tongue, where it will dissolve, and to swallow with saliva (contains phenylalanine)

• Advise patient to report any side effects to prescriber

• Advise patient to use alternative contraception while taking product if oral contraceptives are being used

• Teach patient that product does not prevent or reduce number of migraines, main action is abortive, if first dose does not relieve pain, do not use more, notify prescriber

Evaluation

Positive therapeutic outcome

• Decrease in frequency, severity of headache

roflumilast

(roe-flue'mi-last)

Daliresp

Func. class.: Respiratory anti-inflammatory agent

Chem. class.: Phosphodiesterase-4 (PDE4) inhibitor

Pregnancy category C

ACTION: Roflumilast and the active metabolite (roflumilast N-oxide), selectively inhibit phosphodiesterase-4 (PDE4); not a bronchodilator; instead, inhibition of the PDE4 enzyme blocks the hydrolyses and inactivation of cyclic adenosine monophosphate (cAMP), resulting in intracellular cAMP accumulation; decreases inflammatory activity, PDE4 inhibition may affect migration and actions of pro-inflammatory cells (neutrophils, other leukocytes, T-lymphocytes, monocytes, macrophages, fibroblasts)

Therapeutic outcome: Decreasing exacerbations in COPD

USES: For the prevention of COPD exacerbations in those with severe chronic obstructive pulmonary disease (COPD) associated with chronic bronchitis and a history of exacerbations

CONTRAINDICATIONS: Moderate to severe hepatic disease (Child-Pugh B or C)

Precautions: Pregnancy category C, breastfeeding, neonates, infants, children, and adolescents, acute bronchospasm, anxiety, insomnia, depression, and/or suicidal ideation or behavior

DOSAGE AND ROUTES

Adult: PO 500 mcg/day

Available forms: Tab 500 mcg

Implementation

PO route

• Give without regard to meals

• Store at room temperature

ADVERSE EFFECTS

CNS: Anxiety, depression, dizziness, headache, insomnia, suicidal ideation, tremor

EENT: Rhinitis, sinusitis

GI: Abdominal pain, anorexia, diarrhea, dyspepsia, gastritis, nausea, vomiting, weight loss

GU: Urinary tract infection

MS: Back pain, muscle cramps/spasm
SYST: Infections, influenza

Pharmacokinetics

Absorption	80%
Distribution	Protein binding 99%
Metabolism	Exclusively by CYP3A4, CYP1A2
Excretion	Unknown
Half-life	17 hr (parent); 30 hr (metabolite)

Pharmacodynamics

Onset	Unknown
Peak	1 hr (parent drug); 8 hrs (metabolite)
Duration	Unknown

INTERACTIONS

Drug classifications
CYP3A4 inducers (alcohol, barbiturates, bexarotene, bosentan, carBAMazepine, dexamethasone, erythromycin, etravirine, fluvoxamine, ketoconazole, metyrapone, modafinil, nevirapine, OXcarbazepine, PHENobarbital, phenytoin, rifabutin, rifampin, ritonavir: decreased roflumilast effect
CYP3A4/CYP1A2 inhibitors (cimetidine, dalfopristin, delavirdine, enoxacin, indinavir, isoniazid, itraconazole, quinupristin, tipranavir): increased roflumilast effect
Oral contraceptives (gestodene and ethinyl estradiol): increased roflumilast effect
Fosamprenavir: altered effect

Drug/herb
St. John's wort: decreased roflumilast effect

NURSING CONSIDERATIONS

Assessment
• Monitor lung sounds and respiratory function baseline and periodically thereafter
• Assess behavioral changes including mood, depression and suicidal thoughts/behaviors
• Monitor liver function tests baseline and periodically thereafter; if increases in liver function studies occur, product should be discontinued
• Monitor weight baseline and periodically, as weight loss is common

Nursing diagnoses
• Ineffective airway clearance (uses)
• Activity intolerance (uses)
• Knowledge deficit (teaching)

Patient/family education
• Advise patient to take product as directed, do not skip or double doses, take missed doses as soon as remembered unless almost time for next dose
• Teach patient not to use OTC or other products without prescriber approval; not to discontinue other respiratory products unless approved by prescriber
• Advise patient not to be used for acute bronchospasm, but may be continued during acute asthma attacks
• **Suicidal thoughts/behaviors: Instruct patient to notify prescriber of worsening depression or suicidal thoughts/behaviors**

Evaluation
Positive therapeutic outcome
• Decreasing exacerbations in COPD

---

romiplostim (Rx)
(roe-mi-ploe'stim)
Nplate
Func. class.: Thrombopoietin receptor agonist
Pregnancy category C

ACTION: A thrombopoietin-like fusion protein produced by DNA recombinant technology

Therapeutic outcome: Increase in platelet counts, absence of bleeding

USES: Chronic idiopathic thrombocytopenic purpura in patients who have had an insufficient response to corticosteroids, immunoglobulins, or splenectomy

CONTRAINDICATIONS:
Hypersensitivity to this product or mannitol

Precautions: Pregnancy C, breastfeeding, malignancies, bleeding, bone marrow suppression, children

DOSAGE AND ROUTES
Adult: SUBCUT 1 mcg/kg qwk, increase qwk by 1 mcg/kg until platelets ≥50,000/mm^3, max 10 mcg/kg/wk

Available forms: Inj vials 250, 500 mcg

Implementation
• Store vials in refrigerator, do not freeze; protect from light; diluted sol is stable refrigerated or at room temperature for 24 hrs

R

SUBCUT route
• Use 0.01 ml graduations syringe
• Discard any unused portion in vial; do not pool unused portions from vials
• Dilute 250 mcg/0.72 preservative-free sterile water for inj; 500 mcg/1.2 preservative-free sterile water for inj; final concentration 500 mcg/ml
• Gently swirl until dissolved; do not shake
• Do not use if discolored or if particulate matter is present
• Inj into outer aspect of upper arm or abdomen except for 2 inches around navel or front aspect of middle thigh; do not use areas that are bruised, scratched, or scarred
• Rotate inj sites

ADVERSE EFFECTS
CNS: *Dizziness, insomnia, headache,* fatigue
GI: Abdominal pain, dyspepsia, diarrhea
HEMA: Thromboembolism, thrombosis, bleeding, myelofibrosis, erythromelalgia
MS: Myalgia
SYST: Secondary malignancy, antibody formation

Pharmacokinetics

Absorption	Unknown
Distribution	Unknown
Metabolism	Unknown
Excretion	Unknown
Half-life	Terminal 1-34 days

Pharmacodynamics

Onset	Unknown
Peak	7-50 hr
Duration	Unknown

INTERACTIONS
Drug classifications
Anticoagulants, NSAIDs, platelet inhibitors, thrombolytics, salicylates: possible risk of bleeding

NURSING CONSIDERATIONS
Assessment
• Assess blood studies: CBC during treatment weekly and for 2 wks after discontinuing

Nursing diagnoses
• Injury, risk for (uses)
• Knowledge, deficient (teaching)

Patient/family education
• Instruct patient to report bleeding
• Inform the patient the reason for product and expected results

• Advise patient to report a missed dose to prescriber due to increased risk of bleeding

Evaluation
Positive therapeutic outcome
• Increase in platelet counts, absence of bleeding

ropinirole (Rx)
(roe-pin′e-role)
Requip, Requip XL
Func. class.: Antiparkinsonian agent
Chem. class.: Dopamine-receptor agonist, nonergot
Pregnancy category C

ACTION: Selective agonist for DOPamine D_2 receptors (presynaptic/postsynaptic sites); binding at D_3 receptor contributes to antiparkinson effects

Therapeutic outcome: Decreased symptoms of Parkinson's disease (involuntary movements)

USES: Parkinsonism, restless legs syndrome

CONTRAINDICATIONS:
Hypersensitivity

Precautions: Pregnancy **C**, cardiac/renal/hepatic disease, dysrhythmias, affective disorders, psychosis

DOSAGE AND ROUTES
Adult: PO 0.25 mg tid, titrate weekly to max of 24 mg/day; (XL) 2 mg/day × 1-2wk, may increase by 2 mg/day qwk

Restless leg syndrome
Adult: PO 0.25 mg 1-3 hr before bedtime, may increase until symptoms resolve

Available forms: Tabs 0.25, 0.5, 1, 2, 3, 4, 5 mg; ext rel tab 2, 4, 8, 12 mg

Implementation
• Give product until NPO before surgery
• Adjust dosage to patient's response
• Give with meals to decrease GI upset

ADVERSE EFFECTS
CNS: Dystonia, *agitation, insomnia,* dizziness, psychosis, hallucinations, depression, somnolence, **sleep attacks,** impulse-control disorders
CV: *Orthostatic hypotension,* hypotension, syncope, palpitations, **tachycardia,** hypertension

EENT: Blurred vision
GI: *Nausea, vomiting, anorexia, dry mouth,* constipation, dyspepsia, flatulence
GU: Impotence, urinary frequency
HEMA: Hemolytic anemia, leukopenia, agranulocytosis
INTEG: Rash, sweating
RESP: Pharyngitis, rhinitis, sinusitis, bronchitis, dyspnea

Pharmacokinetics

Absorption	Well absorbed
Distribution	Widely distributed
Metabolism	Liver, extensively by the liver by CYP450 CYP1A2 enzyme system
Excretion	Kidneys
Half-life	6 hr

Pharmacodynamics

Unknown

INTERACTIONS

Individual drugs
Cimetidine, ciprofloxacin, digoxin, diltiazem, enoxacin, erythromycin, fluvoxamine, levodopa, mexiletine, norfloxacin, tacrine, theophylline: increased effect of ropinirole
Metoclopramide: decreased ropinirole effect

Drug classifications
Butyrophenones, phenothiazines, thioxanthenes: decreased ropinirole effect

NURSING CONSIDERATIONS

Assessment
• Monitor B/P, respiration during initial treatment; hypotension or hypertension should be reported
• Assess mental status: affect, mood, behavioral changes, depression; complete suicide assessment
• **Parkinsonism:** assess for akinesia, tremors, staggering gait, muscle rigidity, drooling; these symptoms should improve with therapy
⚠ **Sleep attacks: assess for drowsiness, falling asleep without warning even during hazardous activities**

Nursing diagnoses
• Injury, risk for (uses)
• Knowledge, deficient (teaching)
• Mobility, impaired physical (uses)
• Noncompliance (teaching)

Patient/family education
• Advise patient that therapeutic effects may take several wk to a few mo
• Caution patient to change positions slowly to prevent orthostatic hypotension
• Instruct patient to use product exactly as prescribed; if product is discontinued abruptly, parkinsonian crisis may occur
• Teach patient that drowsiness, sleeping attacks may occur, to avoid driving or other hazardous activities until response is known
• Teach patient to avoid alcohol and CNS depressants (cough and cold products)
• Teach patient to notify prescriber of unusual urges

Evaluation
Positive therapeutic outcome
• Decreased akathisia, other involuntary movements
• Increased mood

---

ropivacaine (Rx)
(roe-pi′va-kane)
Naropin
Func. class.: Local anesthetic
Chem. class.: Amide
Pregnancy category B

ACTION: Competes with calcium for sites in nerve membrane that control sodium transport across cell membrane; decreases rise of depolarization phase of action potential

Therapeutic outcome: Maintenance of local anesthesia

USES: Peripheral nerve block, caudal anesthesia, central neural block, vaginal, epidural, spinal block

CONTRAINDICATIONS:
Children <12 yr, geriatric, hypersensitivity to amide local anesthetics, severe liver disease, severe hypotension, complete heart block

Precautions: Pregnancy **B,** severe product allergies, hyperthyroidism, CV, hepatic/neurologic disease

DOSAGE AND ROUTES

Lumbar epidural block for C-section
Adult: 20-30 ml of 0.5% SOL, or 15-20 ml of 0.75% SOL

R

Thoracic epidural
Adult: 5-15 ml of 0.5%-0.75% SOL

Major nerve block
Adult: 35-50 ml of 0.5% SOL or 10-40 ml of 0.75% SOL

Labor pain epidural
Adult: 10-20 ml of 0.2% SOL, then 6-14 ml/hr

Postoperative (lumbar/thoracic epidural)
Adult: 6-14 ml/hr of 0.2% SOL

Infiltration/minor nerve block
Adult: 1-100 ml of 0.2% SOL or 1-40 ml of 0.5% SOL

Available forms: Inj 2, 5, 7.5 mg/ml

Implementation
• Give only with resuscitative equipment nearby
• Give only products without preservatives for epidural or caudal anesthesia
• Use new sol; discard unused portions

ADVERSE EFFECTS

CNS: Anxiety, restlessness, **seizures, loss of consciousness,** drowsiness, disorientation, tremors, shivering, paresthesia
CV: **Myocardial depression, cardiac arrest, dysrhythmias,** bradycardia, *hypo*/hypertension, **fetal bradycardia**
EENT: Blurred vision, tinnitus, pupil constriction
ENDO: Hypokalemia
GI: Nausea, vomiting
GU: Urinary retention
INTEG: Rash, urticaria, allergic reactions, edema, burning, skin discoloration at injection site, tissue necrosis
RESP: **Status asthmaticus, respiratory arrest, anaphylaxis**

Pharmacokinetics

Absorption	Complete
Distribution	Unknown
Metabolism	Liver
Excretion	Kidneys
Half-life	Unknown

Pharmacodynamics

Onset	2-8 min
Peak	Unknown
Duration	3 hr, varies with inj site

INTERACTIONS

Individual drugs
Amiodarone, cimetidine, ciprofloxacin, fluvoxamine, imipramine, theophylline: increased effect
Chloroprocaine: decreased action of ropivacaine
Enflurane, EPINEPHrine, halothane: increased dysrhythmias

Drug classifications
Antidepressants (tricyclics), MAOIs, phenothiazines: increased hypertension
Azole antifungals: increased effect

NURSING CONSIDERATIONS

Assessment
• Assess B/P, pulse, respiration during treatment
• Assess fetal heart tones during labor
• Assess allergic reactions: rash, urticaria, itching
• Assess cardiac status: ECG for dysrhythmias, pulse, B/P during anesthesia

Nursing diagnoses
• Knowledge, deficient (teaching)

Evaluation
Positive therapeutic outcome
• Anesthesia necessary for procedure

TREATMENT OF OVERDOSE:
Airway, O_2, vasopressor, **IV** fluids, anticonvulsants for seizures

---

rosiglitazone (Rx)
(rose-i-glye′ta-zone)
Avandia
Func. class.: Antidiabetic, oral
Chem. class.: Thiazolidinedione
Pregnancy category C

ACTION: Improves insulin resistance by hepatic glucose metabolism, insulin receptor kinase activity, insulin receptor phosphorylation

Therapeutic outcome: Decreased symptoms of diabetes mellitus

USES: Stable type 2 diabetes mellitus alone or in combination with sulfonylureas, metformin, or insulin

Unlabeled uses: Increased ovulation frequency in those with polycystic ovary syndrome; reduced in-stent restenosis in those with diabetes

---

⚠ Nurse Alert

CONTRAINDICATIONS:
Breastfeeding, children, hypersensitivity to thia-zolidinediones, diabetic ketoacidosis, jaundice, type 1 diabetes

> **BLACK BOX WARNING:** NYHA III or IV acute heart failure, heart failure

Precautions: Pregnancy **C**, geriatric, thy-roid/renal/hepatic disease, heart failure, NYHA class I, II

> **BLACK BOX WARNING:** MI

DOSAGE AND ROUTES
Adult: PO 4 mg/day or in 2 divided doses, may increase to 8 mg/day or in 2 divided doses after 12 wk; may be added to metformin, sulfonyl-ureas at the adult dose

Available forms: Tabs 2, 4, 8 mg

Implementation
• Convert from other oral hypoglycemic agents if needed; change may be made without gradual dosage change; monitor blood glucose during conversion
• Give tabs crushed and mixed with meal or fluids for patients with difficulty swallowing
• Give once or in 2 divided doses without regard to food
• Store in airtight container in cool environment

ADVERSE EFFECTS
CNS: Fatigue, *headache*
CV: **CHF, MI, death (geriatric patients)**
ENDO: Hyper/hypoglycemia
GI: Weight gain, **hepatotoxicity**, increased total cholesterol, LDL, HDL, decreased free fatty acids
MISC: Accidental injury, upper respiratory tract infection, sinusitis, anemia, back pain, diarrhea, edema, bone fractures (female)
SYST: **Anaphylaxis, Stevens-Johnson syndrome, lactic acidosis**

Pharmacokinetics
Absorption	Unknown
Distribution	Protein binding 99.8%
Metabolism	Unknown
Excretion	Urine, feces, breast milk
Half-life	Elimination 3-4 hr

Pharmacodynamics
Onset	Unknown
Peak	6-12 wk
Duration	Unknown

INTERACTIONS
Individual drugs
Gemfibrozil: increased hypoglycemia
Insulin: avoid concurrent use

Drug classifications
CYP2C5 inducers/inhibitors: may increase/decrease effect
Nitrates: avoid concurrent use

Drug/herb
Horse chestnut: increased antidiabetic effect

NURSING CONSIDERATIONS
Assessment

> **BLACK BOX WARNING:** Use in NYHA III or IV acute heart failure is contraindicated; any deterioration in any cardiac status, discontinue product

• **CHF:** assess for dyspnea, edema, weight gain ≥5 lb, jugular vein distention; may need to change or discontinue
• **Lactic acidosis:** assess for dyspnea, abdominal pain, muscle pain; notify prescriber immediately
• Assess for hypoglycemic reactions (sweating, weakness, dizziness, anxiety, tremors, hunger), hyperglycemic reactions soon after meals
• **Assess for systemic reactions:** anaphy-laxis, Stevens-Johnson syndrome
• **Hepatotoxicity:** check liver function tests pe-riodically; AST, FBS, ALT (if ALT is >2.5 × ULN, do not use), HbA$_{2c}$, plasma lipids, lipoproteins, B/P, body weight during treatment

Nursing diagnoses
• Knowledge, deficient (teaching)
• Nutrition: more than body requirements, imbalanced (uses)

Patient/family education
• Teach patient to monitor capillary blood glucose test, that periodic liver function tests are mandatory; to report edema, weight gain
• Teach patient symptoms of hypo/hyperglyce-mia, what to do about each
• Advise patient that product must be continued on daily basis; explain consequence of discon-tinuing product abruptly

• Advise patient to avoid OTC medications, nitrates, insulin, or herbal preparations unless approved by prescriber
• Advise patient that diabetes is lifelong illness; that this product is not a cure, only controls symptoms
• Advise patient that all food included in diet plan must be eaten to prevent hypoglycemia
• Advise patient to carry/wear emergency ID and glucagon emergency kit for emergencies
• Instruct patient to notify prescriber if oral contraceptives are used
• Teach patient not to use if breastfeeding; may be secreted in breast milk
• **Hepatotoxicity:** advise patient to report nausea, vomiting, abdominal pain, fatigue, anorexia, dark urine, jaundice
• Teach patient that 2 wk is needed to see a reduction in blood glucose, 2-3 mo to see full effect

Evaluation
Positive therapeutic outcome
• Decrease in polyuria, polydipsia, polyphagia; clear sensorium; absence of dizziness; stable gait; blood glucose, A1c improvement

rosuvastatin (Rx)
(roe-soo′va-sta-tin)
Crestor
Func. class.: Antilipemic
Chem. class.: HMG-CoA reductase inhibitor
Pregnancy category X

ACTION: Inhibits HMG-CoA reductase, which reduces cholesterol synthesis

Therapeutic outcome: Decreasing cholesterol levels

USES: As an adjunct in primary hypercholesterolemia (types IIa, IIb), mixed dyslipidemia elevated serum triglycerides, homozygous/heterozygous familial hypercholesterolemia (FH), slowing of atherosclerosis, CV disease prophylaxis

CONTRAINDICATIONS:
Pregnancy **X**, breastfeeding, hypersensitivity, active liver disease

Precautions: Children, geriatric, past liver disease, alcoholism, severe acute infections, trauma, hypotension, uncontrolled seizure disorders, severe metabolic disorders, electrolyte imbalances, severe renal impairment, hypothyroidism, Asian patients

DOSAGE AND ROUTES
Patient should first be placed on a cholesterol-lowering diet

Hypercholesterolemia
Adult: PO 5-40 mg/day; initial dose 10 mg/day, reanalyze lipid levels at 2-4 wk and adjust dosage accordingly

Homozygous FH
Adult: PO 20 mg/day, max 40 mg

Dose in patients taking cycloSPORINE/gemfibrozil/lopinavir/ritonavir/atazanavir
Adult: 5 mg/day, max 10 mg/day

Heterozygous familial hypercholesterolemia
Females ≥1 yr post-menarche and ≥10 yr and males ≥10 yr: PO 5-20 mg q day individualized

Asian patients/predisposition for myopathy
Adult: PO 5 mg/day

Atherosclerosis slowing
Adult: PO 10 mg/day (for those not taking cycloSPORINE or gemfibrozil)

Renal/hepatic dose
Adult: PO CCr <30 ml/min 5 mg daily; max 10 mg daily; avoid use in hepatic disease

Available forms: Tabs 5, 10, 20, 40 mg

Implementation
• May be taken at any time of day, with or without food
• Store in cool environment in airtight, light-resistant container

ADVERSE EFFECTS
CNS: *Headache, dizziness,* insomnia, paresthesia
GI: *Nausea, constipation, abdominal pain, flatus, diarrhea, dyspepsia, heartburn,* **kidney failure, liver dysfunction,** vomiting
HEMA: Thrombocytopenia, hemolytic anemia, leukopenia
INTEG: *Rash, pruritus*
MS: *Asthenia, muscle cramps, arthritis, arthralgia, myalgia,* **myositis, rhabdomyolysis,** leg, shoulder, or localized pain
RESP: Rhinitis, sinusitis, *pharyngitis,* increased cough

Pharmacokinetics

Absorption	Unknown
Distribution	88% protein bound, crosses placenta
Metabolism	Minimal liver metabolism (about 10%)
Excretion	Primarily in feces (90%)
Half-life	19 hr

Pharmacodynamics

Onset	Unknown
Peak	3-5 hr
Duration	Unknown

INTERACTIONS

Individual drugs
Alcohol: increased hepatotoxicity
Clofibrate, cycloSPORINE, gemfibrozil, niacin: increased myalgia, myositis
Warfarin: increased bleeding

Drug classifications
Antifungals (azole), anti-retroviral protease inhibitors, fibric acid derivatives: increased myalgia, myositis
Bile acid sequestrants: increased effects

Drug/herb
St. John's wort: decreased rosuvastatin effect

Drug/lab test
Increased: CPK, liver function tests

NURSING CONSIDERATIONS

Assessment
• Assess diet: obtain diet history including fat, cholesterol in diet
• Monitor fasting cholesterol, LDL, HDL, triglycerides periodically during treatment
• Monitor liver function tests q1-2mo during the first $1\frac{1}{2}$ yr of treatment; AST, ALT, liver function tests may increase
• Monitor renal function in patients with compromised renal system: BUN, creatinine, I&O ratio
• Obtain ophthalmic exam before, 1 mo after treatment begins, annually; lens opacities may occur
⚠ Rhabdomyolysis: Assess for muscle pain, tenderness, obtain CPK; if these occur, product may need to be discontinued; for Asian ancestry: increased blood levels, rhabdomyolysis

Nursing diagnoses
• Knowledge, deficient (teaching)
• Noncompliance (teaching)

Patient/family education
• Advise to report suspected pregnancy, to use contraception while taking this product, pregnancy category **X**, not to breastfeed
• Advise that blood work and ophthalmic exam will be necessary during treatment
• Teach to report blurred vision, severe GI symptoms, dizziness, headache, muscle pain, weakness
• Teach that previously prescribed regimen will continue: low-cholesterol diet, exercise program, smoking cessation

Evaluation
Positive therapeutic outcome
• Cholesterol at desired level after 8 wk

---

rufinamide (Rx)
(roo-fin′a-mide)
Banzel
Func. class.: Anticonvulsant
Chem. class.: Triazole derivative
Pregnancy category C

ACTION: May act through action at sodium channels; exact action is unknown

Therapeutic outcome: Decrease in severity of seizures

USES: Lennox-Gastaut syndrome

CONTRAINDICATIONS: Hypersensitivity, familial short QT syndrome

Precautions: Pregnancy **C**, breastfeeding, renal/hepatic disease, geriatric patients, child <16 yr, depression, dialysis, hazardous activities, suicidal ideation

DOSAGE AND ROUTES
Adult: PO 400-800 mg/day divided bid, increase by 400-800 mg/day q2day to 3200 mg/day
Child ≥4 yr: PO 10 mg/kg/day divided equally bid; increase by 10 mg/kg/day every other day to 45 mg/kg/day or 3200 mg/day, whichever is less

Available forms: Tabs 200, 400 mg; oral susp 40 mg/ml

Implementation
• **PO tabs:** Give with food, may give whole, crushed, or halved

R

Adverse effects: *italics* = common; **bold** = life-threatening

• **Oral susp:** Shake well before use, use provided adapter and calibrated oral dosing syringe, insert adapter firmly in neck of bottle before use and keep in place for the duration of bottle use, insert dosing syringe into the adapter and withdraw dose from inverted bottle, replace cap after each use, use within 90 days of opening, give with food

ADVERSE EFFECTS

CNS: Dizziness, ataxia, drowsiness, fever, seizures, tremor, fatigue, headache, gait disturbance
EENT: Diplopia, blurred vision, nystagmus
GI: Nausea, hepatitis, vomiting
HEMA: Anemia, leukopenia, neutropenia, thrombocytopenia, lymphadenopathy
INTEG: Rash, urticaria
MISC: Edema, hematuria, influenzae, nephrolithiasis

Pharmacokinetics

Absorption	Unknown
Distribution	Unknown
Metabolism	Liver
Excretion	Kidneys
Half-life	Terminal 6-10 hr

Pharmacodynamics

Onset	Unknown
Peak	4-6 hr
Duration	Unknown

INTERACTIONS

Individual drugs
CarBAMazepine, PHENobarbital, phenytoin, primidone: decreased effect of rufinamide
Valproate: increased rufinamide effect

Drug classifications
Hormonal contraceptives: decreased effect

Drug/lab test
Increased: LFTs

NURSING CONSIDERATIONS

Assessment
• **Seizures:** Assess for duration, type, intensity precipitating factors
⚠ **Assess mental status: mood, sensorium, affect, memory (long, short), increased suicidal thoughts/actions**

Nursing diagnoses
• Injury, risk for (uses)
• Knowledge, deficient (teaching)

Patient/family education
• Caution patient not to discontinue product abruptly; seizures may occur
• Advise patient to avoid hazardous activities until stabilized on product
• Instruct patient to carry emergency ID stating product use
• Instruct patient to notify prescriber if pregnancy is planned or suspected, to use alternative form of contraception; hormonal contraceptives may be decreased
• Inform patient to take adequate fluids

Evaluation
Positive therapeutic outcome
• Decrease in severity of seizures

---

salicylic acid topical
See Appendix B

salmeterol (Rx)
(sal-met′er-ole)
Serevent, Serevent Diskus
Func. class.: Adrenergic β_2 agonist, bronchodilator
Pregnancy category C

ACTION: Causes bronchodilatation by action on β_2 (pulmonary) receptors by increasing levels of cyclic AMP, which relaxes smooth muscle; with very little effect on heart rate, maintains improvement in FEV from 3 to 12 hr; prevents nocturnal asthma symptoms

Therapeutic outcome: Ease of breathing

USES: Prevention of exercise-induced asthma, bronchospasm, COPD

CONTRAINDICATIONS:
Hypersensitivity to sympathomimetics, tachydysrhythmias, severe cardiac disease, monotherapy treatment of asthma

Precautions: Pregnancy **C,** breastfeeding, cardiac disorders, hyperthyroidism, diabetes mellitus, hypertension, prostatic hypertrophy, closed-angle glaucoma, seizures, acute asthma, as a substitute for corticosteroids, QT prolongation

> **BLACK BOX WARNING:** Asthma-related death

DOSAGE AND ROUTES
Adult/child ≥4 yr: INH 50 mcg (one inhalation as dry powder); exercise-induced bronchospasm: 50 mcg (2 INH) $^1/_2$-1 hr prior to exercise

Available forms: Inhalation powder 50 mcg/blister

Implementation
• Shake aerosol container, ask patient to exhale, then place mouthpiece in mouth, inhale slowly, hold breath, remove, exhale slowly; allow at least 1 min between inhalations
• Use this medication before other medications and allow at least 1 min between each
• Use spacing device for pediatric/geriatric patients
• Store in light-resistant container, do not expose to temperatures over 86° F (30° C)

ADVERSE EFFECTS
CNS: *Tremors, anxiety,* insomnia, headache, dizziness, fever
CV: Palpitations, **tachycardia,** angina, hypo/hypertension, **dysrhythmias**
EENT: Dry nose, irritation of nose and throat
GI: Heartburn, nausea, vomiting, abdominal pain
MS: Muscle cramps
RESP: **Bronchospasm,** cough

Pharmacokinetics	
Unknown	

Pharmacodynamics	
Onset	5-15 min
Peak	4 hr
Duration	12 hr

INTERACTIONS
Drug classifications
Antidepressants (tricyclics): increased salmeterol action
β-Adrenergic blockers: block therapeutic effect
Bronchodilators, aerosol: increased action of bronchodilator
CYP3A4 inhibitors (itraconazole, ketoconazole, nelfinavir, nefazodone, saquinavir): increased CV effects
MAOIs: increased action of salmeterol

Drug/herb
Betel palm, butterbur, coffee, cola nut, figwort, fumitory, guarana, hawthorn, lily of the valley, motherwort, plantain, tea (black, green), yerba maté: increased stimulation

NURSING CONSIDERATIONS
Assessment
• **Respiratory function:** assess vital capacity, FEV, ABGs, lung sounds, heart rate, rhythm (baseline)

• **Paradoxical bronchospasm:** monitor for dyspnea, wheezing, chest tightness

Nursing diagnoses
• Airway clearance, ineffective (uses)
• Gas exchange, impaired (uses)
• Knowledge, deficient (teaching)

Patient/family education
• Caution patient not to use OTC medications because extra stimulation may occur
• Instruct patient to use this medication before other medications and to allow at least 1 min between each, to prevent overstimulation
• Teach patient how to use inhaler; to avoid getting aerosol in eyes; blurring may result; to wash inhaler in warm water daily and dry; to avoid smoking, smoke-filled rooms, and persons with respiratory infections; review package insert with patient
• Instruct patient on administration of dose, not to use more than prescribed; serious side effects may occur
• Teach patient not to use for exercise-induced bronchospasm, never exhale into diskus, hold level, keep mouthpiece dry
• Teach patient not to use for treatment of acute exacerbation, a fast-acting β-blocker should be used instead
• Teach patient to report immediately dyspnea after use, if 1 canister or more is used in 2 mo time

Evaluation
Positive therapeutic outcome
• Absence of dyspnea, wheezing
• Improved airway exchange
• Improved ABGs

TREATMENT OF OVERDOSE:
Administer a β₂-adrenergic blocker

salsalate (Rx)
(sal-sa'late)
Func. class.: Nonopioid analgesic; nonsteroidal antiinflammatory agent
Chem. class.: Salicylate
Pregnancy category C

ACTION: Blocks formation of peripheral prostaglandins, which cause pain and inflammation; antipyretic action results from inhibition of hypothalamic heat-regulating center; does not inhibit platelet aggregation

Therapeutic outcome: Decreased pain, inflammation

USES: Mild to moderate pain or fever, including arthritis (osteoarthritis, rheumatoid arthritis)

CONTRAINDICATIONS:

Children <3 yr, hypersensitivity to salicylates, NSAIDs, GI bleeding, bleeding disorders, vit K deficiency

Precautions: Pregnancy **C** (1st trimester), breastfeeding, geriatric, anemia, renal/hepatic disease, Hodgkin's disease

DOSAGE AND ROUTES

Adult: PO 3 g/day in divided doses

Available forms: Caps 500 mg; tabs 500, 750 mg

Implementation

- Give with 8 oz of water and sit upright ½ hr after dose; with food or milk to decrease gastric symptoms
- Give antacids 1-2 hr after enteric products

ADVERSE EFFECTS

CNS: Stimulation, drowsiness, dizziness, confusion, **seizures,** headache, flushing, hallucinations, coma

CV: Rapid pulse, **pulmonary edema**

EENT: Tinnitus, hearing loss

ENDO: Hypoglycemia, hyponatremia, hypokalemia, alteration in acid-base balance

GI: *Nausea, vomiting, GI bleeding, diarrhea, heartburn,* anorexia, **hepatotoxicity**

HEMA: **Thrombocytopenia, agranulocytosis, leukopenia, neutropenia, hemolytic anemia,** increased pro-time

INTEG: *Rash,* urticaria, bruising, exfoliative dermatitis, **Stevens-Johnson syndrome,** toxic epidermal necrolysis, anaphylaxis, laryngeal edema

RESP: Wheezing, hyperpnea

Pharmacokinetics

Absorption	Absorbed in small intestine, full benefit 3-4 days
Distribution	Rapidly and widely distributed, crosses placenta
Metabolism	Not metabolized
Excretion	Unchanged—kidneys
Half-life	2-3 hr (low doses), 15-30 hr (high doses)

Pharmacodynamics

Onset	30 min
Peak	1-3 hr
Duration	3-6 hr

INTERACTIONS

Individual drugs

Alcohol, heparin, warfarin: increased bleeding

Insulin, methotrexate, phenytoin, probenecid: increased effects

Spironolactone, sulfinpyrazone: decreased effects

Drug classifications

Antacids, steroids, urinary alkalizers: decreased effects of salsalate

Anticoagulants, penicillins: increased effects

Salicylates: decreased blood glucose levels

Diuretics (loop), sulfonylamides: decreased effects

NSAIDs, platelet inhibitors, thrombolytics, SSRIs, SNRIs: increased bleeding risk

Drug/food

Foods causing acidic urine may increase level

Drug/lab test

Increased: coagulation studies, liver function tests, serum uric acid, amylase, CO_2, urinary protein

Decreased: serum potassium, cholesterol, blood glucose

Interference: urine catecholamines, pH, pregnancy test

NURSING CONSIDERATIONS

Assessment

- **Fever:** monitor temperature, sweating, chills
- **Pain:** assess location, duration, type, intensity, prior to dose and 1 hr after
- Monitor liver function tests: AST, ALT, bilirubin, creatinine if patient is on long-term therapy
- Monitor renal function tests: BUN, urine creatinine if patient is on long-term therapy
- Monitor blood tests: CBC, Hct, Hgb, Pro-time, stool guaiac, serum salicylate if patient is on long-term therapy
- Check I&O ratio; decreasing output may indicate renal failure if patient is on long-term therapy
- **Hepatotoxicity:** dark urine, clay-colored stools, yellowing of the skin and sclera, itching, abdominal pain, fever, diarrhea if patient is on long-term therapy
- **Serious skin reactions, allergic reactions:** rash, urticaria; if these occur, product may have to be discontinued; assess for asthma,

aspirin sensitivity, nasal polyps; may develop hypersensitivity, exfoliative dermatitis, Stevens-Johnson syndrome, toxic epidermal necrolysis, anaphylaxis
• **Ototoxicity:** assess for tinnitus, ringing, roaring in ears; audiometric testing needed before, after long-term therapy
• Assess for visual changes
• Check edema in feet, ankles, legs
• Identify prior product history; many product interactions are possible
• Monitor musculoskeletal status: ROM before dose
• Identify fever, length of time, and related symptoms

Nursing diagnoses
• Injury, risk for (side effects)
• Knowledge, deficient (teaching)
• Mobility, impaired physical (uses)
• Pain, chronic (uses)

Patient/family education
• Advise patient to report any symptoms of renal/hepatic toxicity, visual changes, ototoxicity, allergic reactions, bleeding (long-term therapy)
• Instruct patient to take with 8 oz of water and sit upright for $1/2$ hr after dose
• Caution patient not to exceed recommended dosage; acute poisoning may result
• Advise patient to read label on other OTC products; many contain aspirin
• Inform patient that the therapeutic response takes 2 wk (arthritis)
• Teach patient to report tinnitus, confusion, diarrhea, sweating, hyperventilation
• Caution patient to avoid alcohol ingestion; GI bleeding may occur
• Inform patient that patients who have allergies may develop allergic reactions

Evaluation
Positive therapeutic outcome
• Decreased pain
• Decreased inflammation

TREATMENT OF OVERDOSE:
Lavage, activated charcoal, monitor electrolytes, VS

saquinavir (Rx)
(sa-quen′a-ver)
Invirase
Func. class.: Antiretroviral
Chem. class.: Protease inhibitor
Pregnancy category B

ACTION: Inhibits HIV-1 protease

Therapeutic outcome: Prevents maturation of the infectious virus

USES: HIV-1 in combination with other antiretrovirals

CONTRAINDICATIONS:
Hypersensitivity

Precautions: Pregnancy **B**, breastfeeding, children, hepatic, diabetes, pancreatitis, immune reconstitution syndrome, hemophilia, hyperlipidemia

DOSAGE AND ROUTES
Adult: PO 1000 mg bid with 100 mg ritonavir

Available forms: Caps 200 mg; tab 500 mg

Implementation
• Give in equal intervals around the clock for duration of therapy

ADVERSE EFFECTS
CNS: *Paresthesia*, headache, **seizures**
CV: **QT/PR prolongation, 2nd/3rd degree AV block, torsades de pointes**
GI: *Diarrhea*, buccal mucosa ulceration, *abdominal pain, nausea,* vomiting
INTEG: *Rash*, **Stevens-Johnson syndrome**
MISC: Asthenia, *hyperglycemia*
MS: Pain

Pharmacokinetics

Absorption	Increased with food
Distribution	Protein binding 98%
Metabolism	Extensively
Excretion	Unknown
Half-life	Terminal 12 hr

Pharmacodynamics
Unknown

INTERACTIONS
Individual drugs
Clarithromycin, delavirdine, indinavir, ketoconazole, nelfinavir, ritonavir: increased saquinavir level

Adverse effects: *italics* = common; **bold** = life-threatening

CarBAMazepine, dexamethasone, nevirapine, phenobarbital, phenytoin, rifamycins: decreased saquinavir levels

Clindamycin, dapsone, quiNIDine: increased toxicity

Midazolam, triazolam: increased toxicity, increased CNS depression; do not use concurrently

Ritonavir with amiodarone, dofetilide, lovastatin, simvastatin: increased QT prolongation

Drug classifications

Calcium channel blockers: increased toxicity

Ergots: toxicity, increased vasoconstriction; do not use together

HMG-CoA reductase inhibitors: avoid use with saquinavir

Drug/herb

Garlic, St. John's wort: decreased saquinavir level, avoid concurrent use

Drug/food

Increased: bioavailability after high-fat meal

Grapefruit juice: increased saquinivir level

Drug/lab test

Interference: CPK, glucose (low)

NURSING CONSIDERATIONS

Assessment

• Assess signs of infection, anemia

• Monitor blood glucose, viral load, CD4+ T-cell count, plasma HIV RNA, serum cholesterol/lipid profile

• Obtain resistance testing at start of and at treatment failure

• Monitor liver function tests: ALT, AST

• Monitor C&S before product therapy; product may be taken as soon as culture is done; repeat C&S after treatment; determine the presence of other STDs

• **QT/PR prolongation, 2nd/3rd degree AV block, torsades de pointes:** monitor ECG for changes

• Assess bowel pattern before, during treatment; if severe abdominal pain with bleeding occurs, product should be discontinued; monitor hydration

• **Serious skin disorders: Stevens-Johnson syndrome;** assess skin eruptions, rash, urticaria, itching

Nursing diagnoses

• Infection, risk for (uses)

• Knowledge, deficient (teaching)

Patient/family education

• Advise patient to take as prescribed within 2 hr of a full meal; if dose is missed, take as soon as remembered up to 1 hr before next dose; do not double dose

• Advise patient that product must be taken in equal intervals around the clock to maintain blood levels for duration of therapy; that product is not a cure

• Advise to take precautions to prevent transmission

• Teach that there are significant drug interactions

Evaluation

Positive therapeutic outcome

• Decreasing symptoms of HIV

• Improving viral load and CD4 cell counts

sargramostim (Rx)

(sar-gram′oh-stim)

Leukine, rhu GM-CSF

Func. class.: Biological modifier: cytokine

Chem. class.: Granulocyte-macrophage colony-stimulating factor (GM-CSF)

Pregnancy category C

Do not confuse:

Leukine/leucovorin/Leukeran

ACTION: Stimulates proliferation and differentiation of hematopoietic progenitor cells (granulocyte, macrophage)

Therapeutic outcome: WBC and differential recovery

USES: Acceleration of myeloid recovery in patients with non-Hodgkin's lymphoma, acute lymphoblastic leukemia, acute myelogenous leukemia, autologous bone marrow transplantation in Hodgkin's disease; bone marrow transplantation failure or engraftment delay; mobilization and transplant of peripheral blood progenitor cells (PBPCs)

Unlabeled uses: Aplastic anemia, Crohn's disease, ganciclovir- or zidovudine-induced neutropenia

CONTRAINDICATIONS:

Hypersensitivity to GM-CSF, benzyl alcohol, yeast products; excessive leukemic myeloid blast in the bone marrow or peripheral blood, neonates

Precautions: Pregnancy C, breastfeeding, children, renal/hepatic/lung/cardiac disease, pleural/pericardial effusions, peripheral edema, leukocytosis, mannitol hypersensitivity, hepatic/renal disease

DOSAGE AND ROUTES

Myeloid reconstitution after autologous bone marrow transplantation

Adult: IV 250 mcg/m²/day × 3 wk; give over 2 hr, begin 2-4 hr after bone marrow INF, and not less than 24 hr after last dose of antineoplastics and 12 hr after last dose of radiotherapy, bone marrow transplantation failure, or engraftment delay

Acceleration of myeloid recovery

Adult: IV 250 mcg/m²/day × 14 days; give over 2 hr; may repeat in 7 days, may repeat 500 mcg/m²/day × 14 days after another 7 days if no improvement

Mobilization of PBPCs

Adult: IV/SUBCUT 250 mcg/m²/day during collection of PBPCs

After PBPC transplantation

Adult: IV/SUBCUT 250 mcg/m²/day until ANC >1500/mm³ × 3 days

Available forms: Powder for inj lyophilized 250 mcg

Implementation

SUBCUT route
• No further dilution of reconstituted sol is needed; take care not to inject intradermally

Intermittent IV infusion route
• After reconstituting with 1 ml sterile water for inj without preservative; do not reenter vial; discard unused portion; direct reconstitution sol at side of vial; rotate contents, do not shake
• Dilute in 0.9% NaCl to prepare IV inf; if final concentration is <10 mcg/ml, add human albumin to make a final concentration of 0.1% to NaCl before adding sargramostim to prevent adsorption; for a final concentration of 0.1% albumin, add 1 mg human albumin/1 ml 0.9% NaCl inj run over 2 hr **(bone marrow transplant or failure of graft); over 4 hr (chemotherapy for AML);** over 24 hr as cont inf **(PBPCs);** give within 6 hr after reconstitution

Y-site compatibilities: Amikacin, aminophylline, aztreonam, bleomycin, butorphanol, calcium gluconate, CARBOplatin, carmustine, ceFAZolin, cefepime, cefotaxime, cefotetan, ceftizoxime, cefTRIAXone, cefuroxime, cimetidine, CISplatin, clindamycin, cyclophosphamide, cycloSPORINE, cytarabine, dacarbazine, DACTINomycin, dexamethasone, diphenhydrAMINE, DOPamine, DOXOrubicin, doxycycline, droperidol, etoposide, famotidine, fentaNYL, floxuridine, fluconazole, fluorouracil, furosemide, gentamicin, granisetron, heparin, IDArubicin, ifosfamide, immune globulin, magnesium sulfate, mannitol, mechlorethamine, meperidine, mesna, methotrexate, metoclopramide, metroNIDAZOLE, minocycline, mitoxantrone, netilmicin, pentostatin, piperacillin/tazobactam, potassium chloride, prochlorperazine, promethazine, ranitidine, teniposide, ticarcillin, ticarcillin-clavulanate, trimethoprim-sulfamethoxazole, vinBLAStine, vinCRIStine, zidovudine

Y-site incompatibilities: Acyclovir, ampicillin, ampicillin/sulbactam, cefonicid, cefoperazine, ceftazidime, chlorproMAZINE, ganciclovir, haloperidol, hydrocortisone, HYDROmorphone, hydrOXYzine, IDArubicin, imipenem/cilastatin, LORazepam, methylPREDNISolone sodium succinate, mitomycin, morphine, nalbuphine, ondansetron, piperacillin, sodium bicarbonate, tobramycin

ADVERSE EFFECTS

CNS: Fever, malaise, CNS disorder, weakness, chills, dizziness, syncope, headache
CV: **Transient supraventricular tachycardia,** peripheral edema, **pericardial effusion,** hypotension, tachycardia
GI: Nausea, vomiting, diarrhea, anorexia, **GI hemorrhage,** stomatitis, **liver damage,** hyperbilirubinemia
GU: Urinary tract disorder, abnormal kidney function
HEMA: **Blood dyscrasias, hemorrhage**
INTEG: Alopecia, rash, peripheral edema
MS: Bone pain, myalgia
RESP: Dyspnea

Pharmacokinetics

Absorption	Completely absorbed
Distribution	Unknown
Metabolism	Unknown
Excretion	Unknown
Half-life	Elimination IV 60 min; SUBCUT 2-3 hr

Pharmacodynamics

Onset	Rapid
Peak	2 hr
Duration	Unknown

INTERACTIONS

Individual drugs
Lithium: increased myeloproliferation

S

Adverse effects: *italics* = common; **bold** = life-threatening

Drug classifications
Antineoplastics: do not use together
Corticosteroids: increased myeloproliferation

NURSING CONSIDERATIONS
Assessment
• Monitor blood studies: CBC, differential count before treatment and twice weekly; leukocytosis may occur (WBC >50,000 cells/mm³, ANC >20,000 cells/mm³), platelets; if ANC >20,000/mm³ or 10,000/mm³ after nadir has occurred or platelets >500,000/mm³, reduce dose by ¹/₂ or discontinue; if blast cells occur, discontinue
• Monitor renal/liver function tests before treatment: BUN, creatinine, urinalysis; AST, ALT, alkaline phosphatase; monitoring is needed twice a week in renal/hepatic disease
• Assess for **hypersensitivity reactions**/rashes and local inj site reactions; usually transient
• Assess for increased fluid retention in cardiac disease, body weight, hydration status, pulmonary function
• Assess for myalgia, arthralgia in legs, feet; use analgesics

Nursing diagnoses
• Infection, risk for (uses)
• Knowledge, deficient (teaching)

Patient/family education
• Teach patient reason for medication and expected results
• Advise patient to notify nurse or prescriber of dyspnea

Evaluation
Positive therapeutic outcome
• WBC and differential recovery
• Absence of infection

---

saxagliptin (Rx)
(sax-a-glip′tin)
Onglyza
Func. class.: Antidiabetic, oral
Chem. class.: Dipeptidyl-peptidase-4 (DPP-4) inhibitor
Pregnancy category C

ACTION: Slows the inactivation of incretin hormones, improves glucose homeostasis, improves glucose-dependent insulin synthesis, lowers glucagon secretions and slows gastric emptying time

Therapeutic outcome: Decrease in polyuria, polydipsia, polyphagia; clear sensorium; absence of dizziness; stable gait; blood glucose at normal level

USES: Type 2 diabetes mellitus as monotherapy or in combination with other antidiabetic agents

CONTRAINDICATIONS:
Hypersensitivity, diabetic ketoacidosis (DKA), type 1 diabetes mellitus

Precautions: Pregnancy **B**, geriatric, GI obstruction, thyroid disease, surgery, renal/hepatic disease, trauma

DOSAGE AND ROUTES
Adult: PO 2.5-5 mg; may use with other antidiabetic agents (metformin, pioglitazone, rosiglitazone)

Renal dose
Adult: PO CCr ≤50 ml/min 2.5 mg/day

Available forms: Tabs 2.5; 5 mg

Implementation
• May be taken with or without food
• Conversion from other antidiabetic agents; change may be made with gradual dosage change
• Store in tight container at room temperature

ADVERSE EFFECTS
CNS: *Headache*
ENDO: Hypoglycemia (renal impairment)
GI: *Nausea, vomiting,* abdominal pain
INTEG: Urticaria, **angioedema**
MISC: Lymphopenia, peripheral edema

Pharmacokinetics

Absorption	Rapidly
Distribution	Unknown
Metabolism	Unknown
Excretion	Kidneys 24% unchanged
Half-life	Terminal 2.5 hr, 3.1 hr metabolite

Pharmacodynamics

Onset	Unknown
Peak	1-4 hr
Duration	24 hr

INTERACTIONS
Individual drugs
Aripiprazole, clozapine, fosphenytoin, OLANZapine, phenytoin, QUEtiapine, risperidone, ziprasidone: decreased antidiabetic effect

---

⚠ Nurse Alert

Cimetidine, disopyramide: increased saxagliptin level

Cimetidine, FLUoxetine: increased hypoglycemia

Digoxin: increased levels of digoxin

Drug classifications

ACE inhibitors, estrogens, oral contraceptives, phenothiazines, progestins, protease inhibitors, sympathomimetics, thiazide diuretics: decreased antidiabetic effect

Androgens, β-blockers, corticosteroids, fibric acid derivatives, insulins, MAOIs, salicylates: increased hypoglycemia

Drug/herb

Garlic, horse chestnut: increased antidiabetic effect

NURSING CONSIDERATIONS

Assessment

• **Hypoglycemic reactions** (sweating, weakness, dizziness, anxiety, tremors, hunger); monitor blood glucose (BG) as needed

• Monitor CBC (baseline, q3mo) during treatment; check liver function tests periodically, AST, LDH, renal studies: BUN, creatinine during treatment; glycosylated hemoglobin HbA1c

Nursing diagnoses

• Knowledge, deficient (teaching)
• Noncompliance (teaching)
• Nutrition: more than body requirements, imbalanced (uses)

Patient/family education

• Teach patient to use regular self-monitoring of blood glucose using blood glucose meter

• Teach patient the symptoms of hypo/hyperglycemia; what to do about each

• Teach patient that product must be continued on daily basis; explain consequence of discontinuing product abruptly

• Advise patient to avoid OTC medications, alcohol, digoxin, exenatide, insulins, nateglinide, repaglinide, and other products that lower blood sugar, unless approved by prescriber

• Teach patient that diabetes is a lifelong illness; that this product is not a cure, only controls symptoms

• Teach patient that all food included in diet plan must be eaten to prevent hypo/hyperglycemia

• Teach patient to carry emergency ID

Evaluation

Positive therapeutic outcome

• Decrease in polyuria, polydipsia, polyphagia; clear sensorium; absence of dizziness; stable gait; blood glucose at normal level

---

scopolamine (Rx)

(skoe-pol′a-meen)

Maldemar, Scopace, Transderm-Scop

Func. class.: Cholinergic blocker

Chem. class.: Belladonna alkaloid

Pregnancy category C

ACTION: Inhibits acetylcholine at receptor sites in autonomic nervous system, which controls secretions, free acids in stomach; blocks central muscarinic receptors, which decreases involuntary movements

Therapeutic outcome: Absence of vomiting, secretions (preoperatively), involuntary movements

USES: Reduction of secretions before surgery, production of amnesia, prevention of motion sickness, Parkinson's symptoms

Unlabeled uses: Drooling (TD)

CONTRAINDICATIONS: Hypersensitivity, closed-angle glaucoma, myasthenia gravis, GI/GU obstruction, hypersensitivity to belladonna, barbiturates

Precautions: Pregnancy **C**, breastfeeding, children, geriatric, prostatic hypertrophy, CHF, hypertension, dysrhythmias, gastric ulcer, renal/hepatic disease, hiatal hernia, GERD, ulcerative colitis, hyperthyroidism

DOSAGE AND ROUTES

Prevention of motion sickness

Adult: Transdermal 1 patch placed behind ear 4 hr before travel, reapply q3day

Parkinson's symptoms

Adult: PO 0.4-0.8 mg q8hr

Preoperatively

Adult: IM/IV/SUBCUT 0.32-0.65 mg; TD apply 1 patch PM before surgery or 1 hr before C-section

Nausea and vomiting

Adult: SUBCUT 0.6-1 mg

Child: SUBCUT 0.006 mg/kg; max 0.3 mg/dose

Drooling (unlabeled)

Adult: Transdermal 1.5 mg patch q3day

Available forms: Patch 1.5 mg delivered in 72 hr; 0.4 mg/ml

S

Implementation

IM/SUBCUT/IV route
- Administer parenteral dose with patient recumbent to prevent postural hypotension

Transdermal route
- Instruct patient to wash, dry hands before and after applying to surface behind ear; to change patch q72hr; to apply at least 4 hr before traveling

Direct IV route
- Give by direct **IV** after diluting with sterile water; give slowly

Syringe compatibilities: Atropine, benzquinamide, butorphanol, chlorproMAZINE, cimetidine, dimenhyDRINATE, diphenhydrAMINE, droperidol, fentaNYL, glycopyrrolate, HYDROmorphone, hydrOXYzine, meperidine, metoclopramide, midazolam, morphine, nalbuphine, pentazocine, PENTobarbital, perphenazine, prochlorperazine, promazine, promethazine, ranitidine, SUFentanil, thiopental

Y-site compatibilities: Heparin, hydrocortisone, potassium chloride, propofol, SUFentanil, vit B/C

ADVERSE EFFECTS

CNS: Confusion, anxiety, restlessness, irritability, delusions, headache, fatigue, hallucinations, sedation, depression, incoherence, dizziness, excitement, delirium, flushing, weakness; transdermal: memory disturbances
CV: Palpitations, **tachycardia**, postural hypotension, paradoxical bradycardia
EENT: Transdermal: blurred vision, photophobia, dilated pupils, difficulty swallowing, mydriasis, cycloplegia
GI: *Dryness of mouth, constipation,* nausea, vomiting, abdominal distress, **paralytic ileus**
GU: Hesitancy, retention, difficult urination (patch)
INTEG: Urticaria, dry skin
MISC: Suppression of breastfeeding, nasal congestion, decreased sweating

Pharmacokinetics

Absorption	Well absorbed (IM, SUBCUT, TD)
Distribution	Crosses placenta, blood-brain barrier
Metabolism	Liver
Excretion	Unknown
Half-life	8 hr

Pharmacodynamics

	SUB-CUT/IM	IV	TRANS-DERMAL
Onset	30-45 min	10-15 min	4-5 hr
Peak	1 hr	1 hr	Unknown
Duration	6 hr	4 hr	72 hr

INTERACTIONS

Individual drugs
Alcohol: increased anticholinergic effect

Drug classifications
Antidepressants (tricyclics), antihistamines, opioids, phenothiazines: increased anticholinergic effect

NURSING CONSIDERATIONS

Assessment
- Monitor I&O ratio; retention commonly causes decreased urinary output
- **Parkinsonism, EPS:** assess for shuffling gait, muscle rigidity, involuntary movements; affect, mood, CNS depression, worsening of mental symptoms during early therapy
- Assess for urinary hesitancy, retention; palpate bladder if retention occurs
- Assess for constipation; increase fluids, bulk, exercise if this occurs
- Assess for tolerance over long-term therapy; dose may have to be increased or changed

Nursing diagnoses
- Fluid volume, deficient (uses)
- Knowledge, deficient (teaching)

Patient/family education
- Tell patient to avoid hazardous activities, activities requiring alertness; dizziness may occur
- Instruct patient to read labels of all OTC medications; if any scopolamine is found in product, avoid use
- Inform patient that blurred vision will decrease with repeated use of ophthalmic product
- Caution patient not to discontinue this product abruptly; to taper off over 1 wk

Transdermal route
- Apply with clean, dry hands; wash, dry hands before and after applying to surface behind ear, press patch firmly
- Teach patient to avoid hazardous activities, activities requiring alertness; dizziness may occur
- Teach patient to change patch q72hr
- Advise patient to discontinue use if blurred vision, severe dizziness, drowsiness occurs;

⚠ Nurse Alert

another type of antiemetic may be used or the patch rotated to the other ear
• Advise patient to keep medication out of children's reach
• Caution patient to report change in vision, blurring or loss of sight, trouble breathing, inhibition of sweating, flushing

Evaluation
Positive therapeutic outcome
• Decreased secretions
• Absence of motion sickness

scopolamine ophthalmic
See Appendix B

selegiline (Rx)
(se-le'ji-leen)
Apo-Selegiline ✸, Eldepryl, Emsam, Gen-Selegiline ✸, Zelapar
Func. class.: Antiparkinson agent
Chem. class.: MAOI, type B
Pregnancy category C

Do not confuse:
Eldepryl/enalapril

ACTION: Increased dopaminergic activity by inhibition of MAO type B activity; not fully understood

Therapeutic outcome: Decreased symptoms of Parkinson's disease

USES: Adjunct management of Parkinson's disease in patients being treated with levodopa/carbidopa who have responded poorly to therapy, depression (transdermal)

Unlabeled use: Alzheimer's disease, depression

CONTRAINDICATIONS:
Children/adolescents (suicide/hypertensive crisis), hypersensitivity, breastfeeding

Precautions: Pregnancy C

DOSAGE AND ROUTES
Adult: PO 10 mg/day in divided doses, 5 mg at breakfast and lunch with levodopa/carbidopa; after 2-3 days begin to reduce the dose of levodopa/carbidopa 10%-30%; **oral disintegrating tab** 1.25 mg (1 tab) initially, then 2.5 (2 tabs) dissolved on tongue daily before breakfast × 6 wk or more; max 2.5 mg/day; **transdermal** 6 mg/24 hr initially, increase by 3 mg/24 hr at ≥2 wk, up to 12 mg/24 hr if needed

Alzheimer's disease (unlabeled)
Adult: PO 5 mg bid AM, PM

Available forms: Tabs 5 mg, caps 5 mg; oral disintegrating tabs 1.25 mg; transdermal 6 mg/24 hr (20 mg/20 cm²), 9 mg/24 hr (30 mg/30 cm²), 12 mg/24 hr (40 mg/40 cm²)

Implementation
• Do not use in children due to risk for hypertensive crisis
• Adjust dosage to patient's response
• Give with meals; limit protein taken with product
• Give at doses <10 mg/day because of risks associated with nonselective inhibition of MAO
• **Oral disintegrating tab:** peel back foil, place tab on tongue, allow to dissolve, swallow with saliva
Transdermal route
• Apply to dry, intact skin on upper torso/thigh or outer surface of upper arm q12hr

ADVERSE EFFECTS
CNS: Increased tremors, chorea, restlessness, blepharospasm, increased bradykinesia, grimacing, tardive dyskinesia, dystonic symptoms, involuntary movements, increased apraxia, hallucinations, dizziness, mood changes, nightmares, delusions, lethargy, apathy, overstimulation, sleep disturbances, headache, migraine, numbness, muscle cramps, confusion, anxiety, tiredness, vertigo, personality change, back/leg pain, **suicide in children/adolescents, suicidal ideation in adults**
CV: Orthostatic hypotension, hypertension, **dysrhythmia,** palpitations; angina pectoris, hypotension, tachycardia, edema, sinus bradycardia, syncope, **hypertensive crisis (children)**
EENT: Diplopia, dry mouth, blurred vision, tinnitus
GI: *Nausea,* vomiting, constipation, weight loss, anorexia, diarrhea, heartburn, rectal bleeding, poor appetite, dysphagia, xerostomia
GU: Slow urination, nocturia, prostatic hypertrophy, hesitation, retention, frequency, sexual dysfunction
INTEG: Increased sweating, alopecia, hematoma, rash, photosensitivity, facial hair
RESP: Asthma, shortness of breath

S

Pharmacokinetics

Absorption	Well absorbed
Distribution	Widely distributed
Metabolism	Rapidly, liver
Excretion	Metabolites *N*-desmethyl-deprenyl, amphetamine, methamphetamine
Half-life	10 hr; oral disintegrating tab 1.3 hr

Pharmacodynamics

Onset	Unknown
Peak	$^1/_2$-2 hr
Duration	Unknown

INTERACTIONS

Individual drugs

Dextromethorphan: increased unusual behavior, psychosis

FLUoxetine, fluvoxamine, PARoxetine, sertraline: increased serotonin syndrome (confusion, seizures, fever, hypertension, agitation) discontinue 5 wk before selegiline

Levodopa/carbidopa: increased side effects

⚠ Meperidine: do not use, fatal reaction

Drug classifications

⚠ Antidepressants (tricyclics), opioids (especially meperidine): do not use, fatal reaction

Antihypertensives: increased hypotension

Drug/lab test

Decreased: VMA

False positive: urine ketones, urine glucose

False negative: urine glucose (glucose oxidase)

False increase: uric acid, urine protein

NURSING CONSIDERATIONS

Assessment

• Monitor cardiac status: tachycardia, bradycardia; B/P, respiration throughout treatment

• Assess mental status: affect, mood, behavioral changes, depression; perform suicide assessment

• **Parkinson's symptoms:** assess for rigidity, unsteady gait, weakness, tremors; these should decrease in severity

• Assess opioids; if patient has received, do not give selegiline; fatal reactions have occurred

Nursing diagnoses

• Knowledge, deficient (teaching)

• Mobility, impaired physical (uses)

Patient/family education

• Caution patient to change positions slowly to prevent orthostatic hypotension

• Advise patient to report side effects: twitching, eye spasms; may indicate overdose

• Caution patient to use product exactly as prescribed; if product is discontinued abruptly, parkinsonian crisis may occur

• Instruct patient to avoid foods high in tyramine: cheese, pickled products, wine, beer, large amounts of caffeine

• Instruct patient not to exceed recommended dose of 10 mg; might precipitate a hypertensive crisis; report severe headache or other unusual symptoms

Evaluation

Positive therapeutic outcome

• Decreased symptoms of Parkinson's disease

TREATMENT OF OVERDOSE:

IV fluids for hypertension, **IV** dilute pressure agent for B/P titration

selenium topical

See Appendix B

senna, sennosides (OTC)

(sin'na)

Black Draught, Equaline Senna, Ex-Lax, Fletcher's Laxative, Gentlax, Leader Laxative, Perdiem, Senexon, Senna-Gen, Senna-Lax, Senokot, Senokotxtra, Senolax, Seno Sol, Walgreens Senna

Func. class.: Laxative-stimulant

Chem. class.: Anthraquinone

Pregnancy category C

ACTION: Stimulates peristalsis by action on Auerbach's plexus; softens feces by increasing water and electrolytes in large intestine

Therapeutic outcome: Decreased constipation

USES: Acute constipation; bowel preparation for surgery or exam, prevention of constipation in those taking opiates long term

CONTRAINDICATIONS:

Breastfeeding, hypersensitivity, GI bleeding, intestinal obstruction, CHF, abdominal pain, nausea/vomiting, appendicitis, acute surgical abdomen

Precautions: Pregnancy **C**

⚠ Nurse Alert

DOSAGE AND ROUTES

Adult: PO (Senokot) 1-8 tabs/day or ¹/₂ to 4 tsp of granules (1 tsp = 4 ml) added to water or juice; RECT SUPP 1-2 at bedtime; SYR 1-4 tsp at bedtime (1 tsp = 4 ml), 7.5-15 ml; (Black Draught) ³/₄ oz dissolved in 2.5 oz of liquid given between 2-4 PM the day before procedure (X-Prep)

Child >27 kg: PO ¹/₂ adult dose; do not use Black Draught for children

Child 1 mo-1 yr: SYR 1.25-2.5 ml (Senokot) at bedtime

Available forms: Tabs 6, 8.6, 15, 25 mg; syr 8.8 mg/5 ml; liquid 33.3 mg/ml

Implementation
PO route
• Administer on empty stomach for more rapid results
• Give with a full glass of water in AM or PM (oral dose); evacuation occurs 6-12 hr later
• Dissolve granules in water or juice before administration
• Shake oral sol before giving

ADVERSE EFFECTS

GI: *Nausea, vomiting, anorexia, abdominal cramps,* diarrhea, flatulence
GU: Pink-red or brown-black discoloration of urine
META: Hypocalcemia, enteropathy, alkalosis, hypokalemia, **tetany**

Pharmacokinetics

Absorption	Minimally absorbed (PO)
Distribution	Unknown
Metabolism	Not metabolized
Excretion	Kidneys, feces
Half-life	Unknown

Pharmacodynamics

	PO	Rect
Onset	6-24 hr	Unknown
Peak	Unknown	Unknown
Duration	3-4 days	Unknown

INTERACTIONS

Individual drugs
Disulfiram: do not use together

Drug/herb
Flax, senna: increased laxative effect

NURSING CONSIDERATIONS

Assessment
• Stool: assess color, consistency, amount; cramping, rectal bleeding, nausea, vomiting; if these symptoms occur, product should be discontinued; identify cause of constipation; identify whether fluids, bulk, or exercise is missing from lifestyle

Nursing diagnoses
• Constipation (uses)
• Diarrhea (side effects)
• Knowledge, deficient (teaching)
• Noncompliance (teaching)

Patient/family education
• Discuss with patient that adequate fluid consumption is necessary
• Inform patient that normal bowel movements do not always occur daily
• Teach patient not to use in presence of abdominal pain, nausea, vomiting; tell patient to notify prescriber if constipation is unrelieved or if symptoms of electrolyte imbalance occur: muscle cramps, pain, weakness, dizziness, excessive thirst
• Teach patient to use other ways to decrease constipation: water, bulk in diet, exercise

Evaluation
Positive therapeutic outcome
• Decreased constipation in 8-10 hr

---

sertraline (Rx)
(ser'tra-leen)
Zoloft
Func. class.: Antidepressant
Chem. class.: Selective serotonin reuptake inhibitor (SSRI)
Pregnancy category C

S

Do not confuse:
Zoloft/Zocor

ACTION: Inhibits serotonin reuptake in CNS, thus increasing action of serotonin; does not affect DOPamine, norepinephrine

Therapeutic outcome: Relief of depression, obsessive-compulsive disorder (OCD), posttraumatic stress disorder (PTSD), panic disorder

USES: Major depression, OCD, PTSD, social anxiety disorder, panic disorder, premenstrual dysphoric disorder (PMDD)

Adverse effects: *italics* = common; **bold** = life-threatening

CONTRAINDICATIONS:
Hypersensitivity to this product or selective serotonin reuptake inhibitors

Precautions: Pregnancy **C,** breastfeeding, geriatric, renal/hepatic disease, epilepsy, recent MI, latex sensitivity (dropper of oral conc)

> **BLACK BOX WARNING:** Suicidal ideation, children

DOSAGE AND ROUTES
Adult/geriatric: PO 25-50 mg/day; may increase to a maximum of 200 mg/day, do not change dose at intervals of <1 wk; administer daily in AM or PM
Child 6-12 yr: PO 25 mg/day, max 200 mg/day

Premenstrual disorders
Adult: PO 50-150 mg nightly

Available forms: Tabs 25, 50, 100 mg; oral sol 20 mg/ml

Implementation
• Administer dosage at bedtime if oversedation occurs during day; may take entire dose at bedtime; may crush
• Give with food, milk for GI symptoms
• Give crushed if patient is unable to swallow medication whole
• Use sugarless gum, hard candy; frequent sips of water for dry mouth
• **Oral concentration:** dilute before use with 4 oz (½ cup) of water, orange juice, ginger ale, or lemon/lime soda; do not mix with other liquids
• Store at room temperature; do not freeze

ADVERSE EFFECTS
CNS: *Insomnia, agitation, somnolence, dizziness, headache, tremor, fatigue,* paresthesia, twitching, confusion, ataxia, gait abnormality (geriatric), **seizures, neuroleptic malignant syndrome–like reactions, serotonin syndrome, suicidal ideation**
CV: Palpitations, chest pain
EENT: Vision abnormalities, yawning
ENDO: Syndrome of inappropriate antidiuretic hormone (geriatric)
GI: *Diarrhea, nausea, constipation, anorexia, dry mouth,* dyspepsia, *vomiting, flatulence,* weight gain/loss
GU: *Male sexual dysfunction,* micturition disorder
INTEG: Increased sweating, rash, hot flashes
MISC: Hyponatremia

Pharmacokinetics
Absorption	Well absorbed
Distribution	Unknown, steady state 1 wk
Metabolism	Liver, extensively
Excretion	Feces (14%)
Half-life	26 hr

Pharmacodynamics
Onset	Unknown
Peak	4.5-8.4 hr
Duration	Unknown

INTERACTIONS
Individual drugs
Cimetidine, warfarin: increased sertraline effect
Clozapine: increased effects of clozapine
Diazepam: increased diazepam effect
Disulfiram: disulfiram reaction with oral conc due to alcohol content
Lithium: altered lithium levels
Phenytoin: increased effects of phenytoin
Pimozide: sertraline is contraindicated with pimozide, fatal reactions
Sibutramine, traZODone, busPIRone, linezolid, traMADol: increased serotonin syndrome, increased neuroleptic malignant syndrome
Sumatriptan: increased sumatriptan effects
TOLBUTamide: increased effect of TOLBUTamide
Warfarin: increased warfarin effect

Drug classifications
Anticoagulants, NSAIDs, thrombolytics, platelet inhibitors, salicylates: increased bleeding risk
Antidepressants (tricyclics), benzodiazepines: increased effect
Highly protein-bound products: increased sertraline levels
SSRIs, SNRIs, serotonin-receptor agonists, tricyclics: increased serotonin syndrome, increased neuroleptic malignant syndrome
⚠ MAOIs: fatal reactions

Drug/herb
Kava, valerian: increased CNS effect
SAM-e, St. John's wort, tryptophan: increased effect of SSRIs, serotonin syndrome; do not use together

Drug/lab test
Increased: AST, ALT

NURSING CONSIDERATIONS
Assessment

> **BLACK BOX WARNING:** Assess mental status: mood, sensorium, affect, suicidal tendencies (child/young adult); increase in psychiatric symptoms: depression, panic attacks, OCD, PTSD, social anxiety disorder

• Identify alcohol consumption; if alcohol is consumed, hold dose until AM

⚠ Serotonin syndrome: assess for hyperthermia, hypertension, rigidity, delirium, coma, myoclonus or neuroleptic malignant-like syndrome (muscle cramps, fever, unstable B/P, agitation, tremors, mental changes)

⚠ Bleeding (platelet serotonin depletion): assess for GI bleeding, ecchymoses, epistaxis, hematomas, petechiae, hemorrhage)

• LFTs baseline and periodically

• B/P (lying/standing), pulse q4hr; if systolic B/P drops 20 mm Hg, hold product, notify prescriber; VS q4hr in patients with CV disease

• Weight q wk; appetite may decrease with product

• Urinary retention, constipation, especially in geriatric patients

Nursing diagnoses
• Coping, ineffective (uses)
• Injury, risk for (adverse reactions)
• Knowledge, deficient (teaching)
• Noncompliance (teaching)

Patient/family education
• Teach patient that therapeutic effects may take 1 wk or longer

• Instruct patient to use caution in driving or other activities requiring alertness because of drowsiness, dizziness, blurred vision; to avoid rising quickly from sitting to standing, especially geriatric

• Advise patient to avoid alcohol ingestion, other CNS depressants

⚠ Teach patient not to discontinue medication quickly after long-term use: may cause nausea, headache, malaise

• Caution patient to wear sunscreen or large hat because photosensitivity can occur

• Teach patient to increase fluids, bulk in diet if constipation, urinary retention occur, especially geriatric

• Instruct patient to take gum, hard sugarless candy, or frequent sips of water for dry mouth

> **BLACK BOX WARNING:** Teach patient that suicidal thoughts/behavior may occur (children/adolescents)

Evaluation
Positive therapeutic outcome
• Decrease in depression, OCD
• Absence of suicidal thoughts

TREATMENT OF OVERDOSE:
ECG monitoring, induce emesis, lavage, activated charcoal, administer anticonvulsant

---

sildenafil (Rx)
(sil-den'a-fill)
Revatio, Viagra
Func. class.: Erectile agent; antihypertensive, peripheral vasodilator
Chem. class.: Selective inhibitor of cyclic GMP-PDE5
Pregnancy category B

ACTION: Enhances the effect of nitric oxide (NO) by inhibiting phosphodiesterase type 5 (PDE5), which is necessary for degrading cyclic GMP in the corpus cavernosum

Therapeutic outcome: Ability to achieve and maintain erection

USES: Treatment of erectile dysfunction, pulmonary hypertension; improvement in exercise ability

Unlabeled uses: Sexual dysfunction (women)

CONTRAINDICATIONS:
Hypersensitivity to this product or nitrates

Precautions: Pregnancy **B**, anatomical penile deformities, sickle cell anemia, leukemia, multiple myeloma, retinitis pigmentosa, bleeding disorders, active peptic ulceration, CV/renal/hepatic disease, multidrug antihypertensive regimens, geriatric patients

DOSAGE AND ROUTES

Erectile dysfunction (Viagra only)
Adult male <65 yr: PO 50 mg 1 hr before sexual activity; may be increased to 100 mg or decreased to 25 mg; max once/day
Adult ≥65 yr (male): PO 25 mg prn about 1 hr before sexual activity

Renal/hepatic dose
Adult: PO (Child-Pugh A, B) 25 mg, take 1 hr before sexual activity, do not use more than 1 ✕/day; CCr <30 ml/min 25 mg starting dose

Pulmonary hypertension (Revatio only)
Adult: PO 20 mg tid, take 4-6 hr apart; **IV** BOL 10 mg tid

Available forms: Tabs 20, 25, 50, 100 mg, sol for inj 10 mg/12.5 ml

Implementation
• **Erectile dysfunction:** give approximately 1 hr before sexual activity, do not use more than once a day, give on empty stomach for better absorption
• Tab may be split
• **Pulmonary hypertension:** Give 3✕/day, 4-6 hr apart

ADVERSE EFFECTS
CNS: *Headache, flushing, dizziness,* transient global amnesia, **seizures**
CV: MI, sudden death, CV collapse, TIAs, ventricular dysrhythmias, CV hemorrhage
MISC: *Dyspepsia, nasal congestion, UTI, abnormal vision, diarrhea, rash,* **NAION (nonarteritic ischemic optic neuropathy),** hearing loss, priapism, **sickle cell crisis**

Pharmacokinetics

Absorption	Rapidly, bioavailability (40%)
Distribution	Unknown
Metabolism	Liver (active metabolites)
Excretion	Feces, urine
Half-life	4 hr

Pharmacodynamics

Onset	Unknown
Peak	$^{1}/_{2}$-$1^{1}/_{2}$ hr
Duration	Unknown

INTERACTIONS
Individual drugs
Alcohol, amLODIPine: decreased B/P
Bosentan, rifampin, carBAMazepine, dexamethasone, phenytoin, nevirapine, rifabutin, troglitazone: decreased sildenafil levels
Cimetidine, erythromycin, itraconazole, ketoconazole, tacrolimus: increased sildenafil levels

Drug classifications
Antacids, barbiturates, CYP450 inducers: decreased sildenafil levels

Antiretroviral protease inhibitors: increased sildenafil levels
α-Blockers, angiotensin II receptor blockers: decreased B/P
⚠ **Nitrates: fatal fall in B/P; do not use together**

Drug/food
Grapefruit: increased product effect
High-fat meal: decreased absorption

NURSING CONSIDERATIONS
Assessment
⚠ **Identify organic nitrates that should not be used with this product**
⚠ **Assess for any severe loss of vision while taking this or any similar products; these products should not be used if vision loss has occurred**
• **Sickle cell crisis (vasoocclusive crisis):** when used for pulmonary hypertension, may require hospitalization

Nursing diagnoses
• Knowledge, deficient (teaching)
• Noncompliance (teaching)

Patient/family education
• Teach patient that product does not protect against STDs, including HIV
• Teach patient that product absorption is reduced with a high-fat meal
• Teach patient that product should not be used with nitrates in any form
• Teach patient that tab may be split
• Teach patient to notify prescriber immediately and stop taking product if vision loss occurs

Evaluation
Positive therapeutic outcome
• Ability to achieve and maintain an erection

silodosin (Rx)
(si-lo'do-seen)
Rapaflo
Func. class.: Selective α_1-adrenergic blocker
Chem. class.: Sulfamoylphenethylamine derivative
Pregnancy category B

ACTION: Binds preferentially to α_{1A}-adrenoceptor subtype located mainly in the prostate

Therapeutic outcome: Decreased symptoms of benign prostatic hyperplasia

⚠ Nurse Alert

USES: Symptoms of benign prostatic hyperplasia (BPH)

CONTRAINDICATIONS:
Hypersensitivity, renal failure, hepatic disease

Precautions: Pregnancy **B**, breastfeeding, children, renal/hepatic disease, females, hypotension, ocular surgery, orthostatic hypotension, prostate cancer, syncope, geriatric patients

DOSAGE AND ROUTES
Adult: PO 8 mg/day with a meal; max 8 mg/day

Renal dose
Adult: PO CCr 30-49 ml/min 4 mg/day; CCr <30 ml/min not recommended

Available forms: Tabs 8 mg

Implementation
• Give with meal at same time of day
• Store at room temperature; protect from light and moisture

ADVERSE EFFECTS
CNS: *Dizziness, headache,* asthenia, insomnia, syncope
CV: Orthostatic hypotension
EENT: Nasal congestion, rhinorrhea, sinusitis
GI: Diarrhea, abdominal pain, jaundice
GU: Abnormal ejaculation, priapism, urinary incontinence
HEMA: Purpura

Pharmacokinetics

Absorption	Decreased with high-fat/high-calorie meal
Distribution	Extensive protein binding 97%
Metabolism	Liver
Excretion	Urine
Half-life	24 hr (metabolite)

Pharmacodynamics

Unknown

INTERACTIONS

Drug classifications
CYP3A4 inhibitors (clarithromycin, itraconazole, ritonavir, anti-retroviral protease inhibitors, aprepitant, chloramphenicol, conivaptan, dalfopristin, danazol, delavirdine, efavirenz, fosaprepitant, fluconazole, fluvoxamine, imatinib, isoniazid, mifepristone, nefazodone, tamoxifen, telithromycin, troleandomycin, voriconazole, zileuton, zafirlukast): increased silodosin effect

Drug/food
Grapefruit juice: increased silodosin effect

Drug/lab test
Increased: LFTs

NURSING CONSIDERATIONS
Assessment
• **Prostatic hyperplasia:** assess for change in urinary patterns, baseline and throughout treatment
• Monitor CBC with diff and LFTs; B/P and heart rate
• Monitor BUN, uric acid, urodynamic studies (urinary flow rates, residual volume)
• Assess I&O ratios, weight daily, edema, report weight gain or edema

Nursing diagnoses
• Urinary elimination, impaired (uses)
• Knowledge, deficient (teaching)

Patient/family education
• Caution patient not to drive or operate machinery until effect is known
• Advise patient not to use with grapefruit juice

Evaluation
Positive therapeutic outcome
• Decreased symptoms of benign prostatic hyperplasia

---

silver nitrate 1% ophthalmic
See Appendix B

silver nitrate sulfacetamide sodium ophthalmic
See Appendix B

silver sulfADIAZINE topical
See Appendix B

simethicone (Rx, OTC)
(si-meth′i-kone)
Barriere ✦, Equaline Extra Strength Gas Relief, Gas Relief ✦, Gas-Relief, Gas-X, Good Sense Ultra Strength Gas Relief, Mylanta Gas, Mylanta Gas Relief, Mylicon, Ovol ✦, Phazyme, Top Care Gas Relief Extra Strength, Walgreens Gas Relief
Func. class.: Antiflatulent
Pregnancy category C

Do not confuse:
Mylicon/Mylanta Gas

Adverse effects: *italics* = common; **bold** = life-threatening

ACTION: Disperses, prevents gas pockets in GI system; lowers surface tension of gas bubbles

Therapeutic outcome: Belching or flatus

USES: Flatulence

Unlabeled uses: Dyspepsia

CONTRAINDICATIONS:
Hypersensitivity, GI obstruction/perforation

Precautions: Pregnancy **C,** abdominal pain, fistula, hiatal hernia

DOSAGE AND ROUTES
Adult and child >12 yr: PO 40-125 mg after meals and at bedtime prn, max 500 mg/day
Child 2-12 yr: PO 40 mg after meals and at bedtime prn, max 240 mg/day
Child <2 yr: PO 20 mg qid prn

Available forms: Chew tabs 40, 150, 166 mg; tabs 60, 80, 95, 125 mg; drops 20 mg/0.3 ml, 95 mg/1.425 ml; caps 95, 180 mg; caps, soft gel 125, 180 mg; oral dissolving film 62.5 mg

Implementation
• Give after meals and at bedtime
• Shake susp well before administering
• Chew tab should be chewed and not swallowed whole

ADVERSE EFFECTS
GI: Belching, rectal flatus, diarrhea

Pharmacokinetics

Absorption	None
Distribution	None
Metabolism	None
Excretion	None
Half-life	Unknown

Pharmacodynamics

Onset	Rapid
Peak	Unknown
Duration	3 hr

NURSING CONSIDERATIONS
Assessment
• Identify the reason for excess gas production: decreased bowel sounds, recent surgery, other GI conditions

Nursing diagnoses
• Knowledge, deficient (teaching)
• Pain, acute (uses)

Patient/family education
• Caution patient that tab must be chewed; to shake susp well before pouring

Evaluation
Positive therapeutic outcome
• Absence of flatulence

---

simvastatin (Rx)
(sim-va-stat′in)
Zocor
Func. class.: Antilipidemic
Chem. class.: HMG-CoA reductase inhibitor
Pregnancy category X

Do not confuse:
Zocor/Cozaar/Zoloft

ACTION: Inhibits HMG-CoA reductase enzyme, which reduces cholesterol synthesis; this enzyme is needed for cholesterol production

Therapeutic outcome: Decreasing cholesterol levels and LDLs, increased HDLs

USES: As an adjunct in primary hypercholesterolemia (types IIa, IIb), isolated hypertriglyceridemia (Frederickson type IV) and type III hyperlipoproteinemia, CAD, heterozygous familial hypercholesterolemia

CONTRAINDICATIONS:
Pregnancy **X,** breastfeeding, hypersensitivity, active liver disease

Precautions: Past liver disease, alcoholism, severe acute infections, trauma, severe metabolic disorders, electrolyte imbalances, Chinese patients

DOSAGE AND ROUTES
Adult: PO 20-40 mg/day in PM initially, usual range 5-40 mg/day daily in PM max, 40 mg/day for most patients; max 80 mg/day (for patients taking 80 mg/day chronically without myopathy); dosage adjustments may be made at 4-wk intervals or more; those taking verapamil and amiodarone max 20 mg/day, max <80 mg for Chinese patients taking lipid-modifying niacin doses

With diltiazem/verapamil
Adult: PO 5-10 mg q PM, max 10 mg/day with amiodarone/amLODIPine/ranolazine
Adult: PO 5-20 mg q PM, max 20 mg/day
Child and adolescents ≥10 yr including girls ≥1 yr postmenarche: PO 10 mg q PM, range 10-40 mg/day

---

Heterozygous familial hypercholesterolemia

Adolescent 10-17 yr: PO 10 mg daily, max 40 mg daily

Available forms: Tabs 5, 10, 20, 40, 80 mg

Implementation
• Give 30 min before AM and PM meals

ADVERSE EFFECTS

CNS: Headache
GI: Nausea, constipation, diarrhea, dyspepsia, flatus, abdominal pain, **liver dysfunction, pancreatitis**
INTEG: Rash, pruritus
MS: Muscle cramps, myalgia, **myositis, rhabdomyolysis,** myopathy
RESP: Upper respiratory tract infection

Pharmacokinetics

Absorption	85%
Distribution	Unknown
Metabolism	Liver—extensively
Excretion	70% feces, 20% kidneys
Half-life	3 hr

Pharmacodynamics

Unknown

INTERACTIONS

Individual drugs
Clarithromycin, clofibrate, cycloSPORINE, erythromycin, gemfibrozil, itraconazole, ketoconazole, niacin, danazol, delavirdine, nefazodone, verapamil, diltiazem, amiodarone, azole antifungals, telithromycin: increased myalgia, myositis, rhabdomyolysis
CycloSPORINE, gemfibrozil: do not use with simvastatin
Digoxin: increased digoxin levels
Warfarin: increased risk of bleeding

Drug classifications
Macrolide antiinfectives, protease inhibitors: increased myalgia, myositis, rhabdomyolysis

Drug/herb
St. John's wort: decreased effect

Drug/lab test
Increased: CPK, liver function tests

NURSING CONSIDERATIONS

Assessment
• Assess nutrition: fat, protein, carbohydrates; nutritional analysis should be completed by dietitian before treatment is initiated

⚠ **Rhabdomyolysis:** assess for muscle tenderness, increased CPK levels 10× ULN; therapy should be discontinued
• Monitor bowel pattern daily; diarrhea may be a problem
• Monitor triglycerides, cholesterol baseline, throughout treatment; LDL, HDL, triglycerides and cholesterol should be watched closely at 6-8 wk and q6mo; if increased, product should be discontinued

Nursing diagnoses
• Diarrhea (adverse reactions)
• Knowledge, deficient (teaching)
• Noncompliance (teaching)

Patient/family education
• Inform patient that compliance is needed for positive results to occur, not to double doses
• Advise patient to lower risk factors: high-fat diet, smoking, alcohol consumption, absence of exercise
• Advise patient to notify prescriber of planned or suspected pregnancy ✗

Evaluation
Positive therapeutic outcome
• Decreased cholesterol levels, serum triglycerides and improved ratio with HDLs

---

sipuleucel-T (Rx)
(si-pu-loo′sel tee)
Provenge
Func. class.: Antineoplastic-biologic response modifiers
Chem. class.: Active cellular immunotherapy

ACTION: Stimulates T-cell immunity against prostatic acid phosphatase (PAP), an antigen expressed in prostatic cancer tissue

Therapeutic outcome: Decreasing size of tumor, decreasing PSA

USES: Asymptomatic or minimally symptomatic metastatic, hormone-refractory prostate cancer

CONTRAINDICATIONS: Hypersensitivity

Precautions: Cardiac disease, chemotherapy, child/infant/neonate, immunosuppression, infusion reaction, pulmonary disease

DOSAGE AND ROUTES
Adult male: **IV** infusion: give entire contents of bag over 60 mins, q 2 wk × 3 doses; premedi-

cate with acetaminophen and diphenhydrAMINE 30 min before infusion to minimize acute infusion reactions

Available forms: Susp for injection

Implementation

Intermittent IV infusion route
• Premedicate with acetaminophen and antihistamine 30 min before infusion

Infusion route
• Visually inspect for particulate or discoloration prior to use; remove bag from container and check for leaks, do not use if leak, particulate, or discoloration is present, product is slightly cloudy cream to pink color, gently mix, check for clumps of clots; must begin infusion before expiration date and time indicated on cell product disposition form and product label
• Infuse entire volume over 60 min, do not use a cell filter; reactions may be treated with acetaminophen, H_1/H_2 blockers, low-dose meperidine, if acute reaction occurs, interrupt or slow infusion, do not resume if product has been at room temperature >3 hr
• Store in refrigerator of unopened bags, do not freeze

ADVERSE EFFECTS

CNS: Asthenia, dizziness, fatigue, fever, flushing, headache, insomnia, paresthesia, **stroke,** tremor, chills, hot flashes
CV: Hypertension, hypoxia, sinus tachycardia
GI: Anorexia, constipation, diarrhea, weight loss, nausea, vomiting
GU: Hematuria
HEMA: Anemia
MS: Arthralgia, back/bone pain, muscle cramps, myalgia
RESP: Bronchospasm

Pharmacokinetics

Absorption	Unknown
Distribution	T-cell stimulation at 8 wk was 8-fold higher than control
Metabolism	Unknown
Excretion	Unknown
Half-life	Unknown

Pharmacodynamics

Unknown

INTERACTIONS

Drug classifications
Antineoplastics, immunosuppressives: do not use together

NURSING CONSIDERATIONS

Assessment
• **Prostate cancer:** assess for more normal urinary patterns, hematuria, decreased tumor size
• **Bronchospasm, CV adverse reactions:** assess for ability to breathe easily, B/P, pulse, respirations, sinus tachycardia, hypertension

Nursing diagnoses
• Injury, risk for (uses, adverse reactions)

Patient/family education
• Instruct patient to notify health care provider of serious adverse reactions: inability to breathe, blood in urine, rapid heartbeat, allergic reactions
• Discuss reasons for product and expected results

Evaluation
Positive therapeutic outcome
• Decreasing size of tumor, decreasing PSA

sirolimus (Rx)
(seer-roe'-li-mus)
Rapamune
Func. class.: Immunosuppressant
Chem. class.: Macrolide
Pregnancy category C

ACTION: Produces immunosuppression by inhibiting T-lymphocyte activation and proliferation

Therapeutic outcome: Prevention of rejection in organ transplant

USES: Organ transplants: to prevent rejection, recommended use is with cycloSPORINE and corticosteroids

CONTRAINDICATIONS:
Breastfeeding, hypersensitivity to this product or to components of the product

Precautions: Pregnancy **C,** children <13 yr, severe cardiac/renal/hepatic disease, diabetes mellitus, hyperkalemia, hyperuricemia, hypertension, interstitial lung disease, hyperlipidemia

BLACK BOX WARNING: Lymphomas, infection, other malignancies

DOSAGE AND ROUTES
Adult/adolescent ≥40 kg: PO 2 mg daily with 6 mg loading dose

Child >13 yr <40 kg (88 lb): PO 1 mg/m²/day, 3 mg/m²/loading dose

Hepatic dose
Adult and child ≥13 yr <40 kg: PO reduce by 33% in maintenance dose (mild to moderate hepatic impairment); reduce by 50% in maintenance dose (severe hepatic impairment)

Available forms: Oral sol 1 mg/ml; tabs 1 mg, 2 mg

Implementation
• Administer prophylaxis for *Pneumocystis jiroveci* pneumonia for 1 yr after transplantation; prophylaxis for cytomegalovirus (CMV) is recommended for 90 days after transplantation in those at increased risk for CMV
• Use amber oral dose syringe and withdraw amount of oral sol needed from the bottle, empty correct dose into plastic/glass container holding 60 ml of water/orange juice, stir vigorously and have patient drink at once, refill container with additional 120 ml of water/orange juice, stir vigorously, and have patient drink at once; if using a pouch squeeze entire contents into container and follow preceding directions
• Give all medications PO if possible; avoid IM inj because bleeding may occur
• Give for 3 days before transplant surgery; patients should be placed in protective isolation, give at same time of day, give 4 hr after cycloSPORINE oral sol or caps, do not use with grapefruit juice
• Store protected from light; refrigerate; stable for 24 months

ADVERSE EFFECTS
CNS: *Tremors, headache, insomnia,* paresthesia, chills, fever
CV: Hypo/hypertension, **atrial fibrillation, CHF,** palpitations, **tachycardia,** peripheral edema, **thrombosis**
EENT: Blurred vision, photophobia
GI: Nausea, vomiting, diarrhea, constipation, **hepatotoxicity**
GU: UTI, **albuminuria, hematuria, proteinuria, renal failure,** nephrotic syndrome
HEMA: Anemia, **thrombocytopenia purpura, leukopenia**
INTEG: *Rash, acne,* photosensitivity
META: Increased creatinine, edema, hypercholesterolemia, *hyperlipemia,* hypophosphatemia, weight gain, hyperglycemia, hypo/hyperkalemia, hyperuricemia, hypomagnesemia
MS: Arthralgia
RESP: Pleural effusion, atelectasis, *dyspnea*
SYST: Lymphoma, exfoliative dermatitis

Pharmacokinetics
Absorption	Rapidly absorbed
Distribution	92% protein binding
Metabolism	Liver; extensively by CYP3A4 enzyme system
Excretion	Unknown
Half-life	Unknown

Pharmacodynamics
Onset	Unknown
Peak	1 hr single dose, 2 hr multiple dosing
Duration	Unknown

INTERACTIONS
Individual drugs
Bromocriptine, cimetidine, cycloSPORINE, danazol, erythromycin, metoclopramide: increased blood level
CarBAMazepine, PHENobarbital, phenytoin, rifamycin, rifapentine: decreased blood levels

Drug classifications
ACE inhibitors, angiotensin II receptor antagonists, cephalosporins, iodine-containing radiopaque contrast media, neuromuscular blockers, NSAIDs, penicillins, salicylates, thrombolytics: increased angioedema
Antifungal agents, calcium channel blockers, HIV protease inhibitors: increased blood levels
Live virus vaccines: decreased effect of vaccines

Drug/herb
St. John's wort: decreased sirolimus effect

Drug/food
Food: alters bioavailability, use consistently with or without food
Grapefruit juice: do not use with grapefruit juice

NURSING CONSIDERATIONS
Assessment
• **Bone marrow depression:** Hgb, WBC, platelets monthly during treatment; if leukocytes are <3000/mm³ or platelets <100,000/mm³, product should be discontinued or reduced; decreased Hgb level
• Monitor blood levels in those who may have altered metabolism, trough levels ≥15 ng/ml are associated with increased adverse reactions
• Monitor lipid profile: cholesterol, triglycerides; a lipid-lowering agent may be needed
• Assess for infection and development of lymphoma

S

• **Hepatotoxicity:** alk phos, AST, ALT, amylase, bilirubin: dark urine, jaundice, itching, light-colored stools; product should be discontinued

Nursing diagnoses
• Infection, risk for (uses)
• Knowledge, deficient (teaching)

Patient/family education
• Instruct patient to report fever, rash, severe diarrhea, chills, sore throat, fatigue because serious infections may occur; clay-colored stools, cramping may indicate hepatotoxicity
• Caution patient to avoid crowds or persons with known infections to reduce risk of infection
• Teach patient to use contraception before, during, and 12 wk after product has been discontinued, avoid breastfeeding
• Teach patient to use sunscreen, protective clothing to prevent burns
• Teach patient that lifelong use is required to prevent rejection
• Teach patient that continuing follow-up exams and blood work will be required

Evaluation
Positive therapeutic outcome
• Absence of graft rejection

sitagliptin (Rx)
(sit-a-glip′tin)
Januvia
Func. class.: Antidiabetic, oral
Chem. class.: Dipeptidyl-peptidase-4 inhibitor (DPP-4 inhibitor)
Pregnancy category B

ACTION: Slows the inactivation of incretin hormones; improves glucose homeostasis, improves glucose-dependent insulin secretion, lowers glucagon secretions and slows gastric emptying time

Therapeutic outcome: Decrease in polyuria, polydipsia, polyphagia; clear sensorium; absence of dizziness; stable gait; blood glucose at normal level

USES: Type 2 diabetes mellitus as monotherapy or in combination with other antidiabetic agents

CONTRAINDICATIONS:
Hypersensitivity, diabetic ketoacidosis (DKA)

Precautions: Pregnancy **B**, geriatric, hypersensitivity, GI obstruction, thyroid disease, surgery, renal/hepatic disease, trauma, breastfeeding, pancreatitis, hypercortisolism,

hyperglycemia, hyperthyroidism, hypoglycemia, ileus, pituitary insufficiency, surgery, type 1 diabetes mellitus

DOSAGE AND ROUTES
Adult: PO 100 mg/day; may use with other antidiabetic agents (metformin, pioglitazone, rosiglitazone) other than insulin

Renal dose
Adult: PO CCr 30-50 ml/min 50 mg qd; CCr <30 ml/min 25 mg qd

Available forms: Tabs 25, 50, 100 mg

Implementation
• May be taken with or without food
• Conversion from other antidiabetic agents; change may be made with gradual dosage change
• Store in tight container at room temperature

ADVERSE EFFECTS
CNS: *Headache*
ENDO: Hypoglycemia
GI: *Nausea, vomiting,* abdominal pain, diarrhea, **pancreatitis,** constipation
MISC: Peripheral edema
SYST: Anaphylaxis, Stevens-Johnson syndrome, angioedema

Pharmacokinetics
Absorption	Rapidly
Distribution	Unknown
Metabolism	Unknown
Excretion	Kidneys, 79% unchanged
Half-life	Terminal 12.4 hr

Pharmacodynamics
Onset	Unknown
Peak	1-4 hr
Duration	Unknown

INTERACTIONS
Individual drugs
Aripiprazole, clozapine, fosphenytoin, OLANZapine, phenytoin, QUEtiapine, risperidone, ziprasidone: decreased antidiabetic effect
Cimetidine, disopyramide: increased sitagliptin level
Cimetidine, FLUoxetine: increased hypoglycemia
Digoxin: increased levels of digoxin

Drug classifications
ACE inhibitors, estrogens, oral contraceptives, progestins, phenothiazines, protease inhibitors, sympathomimetics, thiazide diuretics: decreased antidiabetic effect

Androgens, β-blockers, corticosteroids, fibric acid derivatives, insulins, MAOIs, salicylates, sulfonylureas: increased hypoglycemia

Drug/herb
Garlic, green tea, horse chestnut: increased antidiabetic effect

NURSING CONSIDERATIONS
Assessment
• **Hypoglycemic reactions:** assess for sweating, weakness, dizziness, anxiety, tremors, hunger, hyperglycemic reactions soon after meals
• Monitor CBC (baseline, q3mo) during treatment; check liver function tests periodically, AST, LDH, renal studies: BUN, creatinine during treatment; Hgb A1c
• Monitor blood glucose (BG) as needed
• **Serious skin reactions:** assess for swelling of face, mouth, lips, dyspnea, wheezing
• **Pancreatitis:** assess for severe abdominal pain, nausea, vomiting; discontinue product
• **Renal studies:** monitor BUN, creatinine during treatment
• Monitor hemoglobin A1c; monitor blood glucose as needed

Nursing diagnoses
• Knowledge, deficient (teaching)
• Noncompliance (teaching)
• Nutrition: more than body requirements, imbalanced (uses)

Patient/family education
• Teach patient to use regular self-monitoring of blood glucose using blood glucose meter
• Teach patient the symptoms of hypo/hyperglycemia, what to do about each
• Teach patient that product must be continued on daily basis; explain consequence of discontinuing product abruptly
• Teach patient to notify prescriber if pregnancy is planned or suspected; to continue health regimen (diet, exercise)
• Advise patient to avoid OTC medications, alcohol, digoxin, exenatide, insulins, nateglinide, repaglinide, and other products that lower blood sugar, unless approved by prescriber
• Teach patient that diabetes is a lifelong illness; that this product is not a cure, only controls symptoms
• Teach patient that all food included in diet plan must be eaten to prevent hypo/hyperglycemia
• Teach patient to carry emergency ID
• Teach patient to notify prescriber immediately of hypersensitivity reactions (rash, swelling of face, trouble breathing)

Evaluation
Positive therapeutic outcome
• Decrease in polyuria, polydipsia, polyphagia; clear sensorium; absence of dizziness; stable gait, blood glucose, A1c improvement

---

sodium bicarbonate (Rx, OTC)
baking soda, Brosch-Neut, Citrocarbonate, Neut, Sellymin ❦
Func. class.: Alkalinizer; antacid
Chem. class.: $NaHCO_3$
Pregnancy category C

ACTION: Orally neutralizes gastric acid, which forms water, NaCl, CO_2; increases plasma bicarbonate, which buffers H^+ ion concentration; reverses acidosis **IV**

Therapeutic outcome: Correction of acidosis, gastric acid neutralization

USES: Acidosis (metabolic), cardiac arrest, alkalinization (systemic/urinary); antacid (PO); salicylate poisoning

CONTRAINDICATIONS:
Respiratory/metabolic alkalosis, hypochloremia, hypocalcemia

Precautions: Pregnancy **C**, CHF, cirrhosis, toxemia, renal disease, hypertension, hypokalemia, breastfeeding, hypernatremia, Bartter's syndrome, Cushing's syndrome, hyperaldosteronism, children

DOSAGE AND ROUTES
Acidosis, metabolic (not associated with cardiac arrest)
Adult and child: IV INF 2-5 mEq/kg over 4-8 hr depending on CO_2, pH

Cardiac arrest
Adult and child: IV BOL 1 mEq/kg of 7.5% or 8.4% SOL, then 0.5 mEq/kg q5-10min, then doses based on ABGs
Infant: IV 1 mEq/kg over several min (use only the 0.5 mEq/ml [4.2%] sol for inj)

Alkalinization of urine
Adult: PO 325 mg-2 g qid or 48 mEq/kg (4 g), then 12-24 mEq q4hr
Child: PO 84-840 mg/kg/day (1-10 mEq/kg), in divided doses q4-6hr

Antacid
Adult: PO 300 mg-2 g chewed, taken with water daily-qid

Available forms: Tabs 300, 325, 600, 650 mg; inj 4.2%, 5%, 7.5%, 8.4%

Implementation
PO route
- Antacid tab must be chewed and taken with 8 oz of water
- Dissolve effervescent tab in water
- May be used to neutralize gastric acid in peptic ulcer disease, given 1 and 3 hr after meals and at bedtime

Direct IV route
- Use in cardiac emergencies, use ampules or prefilled syringes only, give by rapid bolus dose, flush with 0.9% NaCl before and after use

Continuous IV infusion route
- Prepared sol or diluted in an equal amount of any dextrose/saline combination; administer 2-5 mEq/kg over 4-8 hr, max 50 mEq/hr; slower rate in children

Y-site compatibilities: Acyclovir, amifostine, asparaginase, aztreonam, bivalirudin, bumetanide, cefepime, cefmetazole, cefTRIAXone, chloramphenicol, cyclophosphamide, cytarabine, DAUNOrubicin, dexamethasone, DOXOrubicin, etoposide, famotidine, fentaNYL, filgrastim, fluconazole, fludarabine, furosemide, gallium nitrate, gemcitabine, gentamicin, granisetron, heparin, hydrocortisone sodium succinate, ifosfamide, indomethacin, insulin, ketorolac, labetalol, levofloxacin, lidocaine, linezolid, LORazepam, magnesium sulfate, melphalan, mesna, meperidine, methylPREDNISolone, metoclopramide, metoprolol, metroNIDAZOLE, milrinone, morphine, nafcillin, nitroglycerin, nitroprusside, paclitaxel, palonosetron, pantoprazole, pemetrexed, penicillin G potassium, phenylephrine, phytonadione, piperacillin/tazobactam, potassium chloride, procainamide, propofol, propranolol, protamine, ranitidine, remifentanil, tacrolimus, teniposide, thiotepa, ticarcillin/clavulanate, tirofiban, tobramycin, tolazoline, vasopressin, vitamin B complex with C, voriconazole

Y-site incompatibilities: Allopurinol, amiodarone, amphotericin B, amphotericin B cholesteryl sulfate complex, ampicillin, anidulafungin, calcium chloride, calicum gluconate, caspofungin, cefotaxime, cefoxitin, cefuroxime, diazepam, diphenhydrAMINE, DOBUTamine, DOXOrubicin liposome, doxycycline, EPINEPHrine, fenoldopam, ganciclovir, haloperidol, hydrOXYzine, IDArubicin, imipenem/cilastatin, inamrinone, isoproterenol, lansoprazole, leucovorin, midazolam, nalbuphine, norepinephrine, ondansetron, phenytoin, prochlorperazine, promethazine, quinupristin/dalfopristin, sargramostim, trimethoprim/sulfamethoxazole, verapamil, vinCRIStine, vinorelbine

ADVERSE EFFECTS
CNS: Irritability, headache, confusion, stimulation, tremors, *twitching, hyperreflexia,* **tetany,** weakness, **seizures** caused by alkalosis
CV: Irregular pulse, **cardiac arrest,** water retention, edema, weight gain
GI: Flatulence, *belching, distention*
GU: Calculi
META: *Alkalosis*
MS: Muscular twitching, tetany, irritability

Pharmacokinetics

Absorption	Unknown
Distribution	Widely distributed— extracellular fluids
Metabolism	Unknown
Excretion	Kidneys
Half-life	Unknown

Pharmacodynamics

	PO	IV
Onset	2 min	Rapid
Peak	$1/2$ hr	Rapid
Duration	1-3 hr	Unknown

INTERACTIONS
Individual drugs
Chlorpropamide, lithium: decreased effect of each specific product
Flecainide, mecamylamine, pseudoephedrine, quiNIDine, quiNINE: increased effects of each specific product

Drug classifications
Amphetamines, anorexiants, sympathomimetics: increased effects of each specific product
Barbiturates: decreased effects of barbiturates
Benzodiazepines: decreased effects of each specific product
Corticosteroids: increased sodium; decreased potassium, decreased effects of corticosteroids
Ketoconazoles: decreased effects of ketoconazoles
Salicylates: decreased effect of salicylates

Drug/herb
Oak bark: decreased action of sodium bicarbonate

⚠ Nurse Alert

Drug/lab test
Increased: sodium, lactate
Decreased: potassium

NURSING CONSIDERATIONS
Assessment
• Assess respiratory and pulse rate, rhythm, depth, lung sounds; notify prescriber of abnormalities
• Assess for CO_2 in GI tract; may lead to perforation if ulcer is severe
• **Fluid balance** (I&O ratio, weight daily, edema); notify prescriber of fluid overload, assess for edema, crackles, SOB
• Monitor electrolytes, blood pH, PO_2, HCO_3 during beginning treatment; ABGs frequently during emergencies
• Monitor extravasation with **IV** administration (tissue sloughing, ulceration, and necrosis)
• **Alkalosis:** irritability, confusion, twitching, hyperreflexia, stimulation, slow respirations, cyanosis, irregular pulse
• **Milk-alkali syndrome:** confusion, headache, nausea, vomiting, anorexia, urinary stones, hypercalcemia

Nursing diagnoses
• Fluid volume, excess (adverse reactions)
• Gas exchange, impaired (uses)
• Knowledge, deficient (teaching)

Patient/family education
• Instruct patient to chew antacid tab and drink 8 oz of water; not to take antacid with milk because milk-alkali syndrome may result; not to use antacid for more than 2 wk
• Advise patient to notify prescriber if indigestion is accompanied by chest pain; trouble breathing; diarrhea; dark, tarry stools; vomit that looks like coffee grounds; swelling of feet/ankles
• Teach patient about sodium-restricted diet; to avoid use of baking soda for indigestion

Evaluation
Positive therapeutic outcome
• ABGs, electrolytes, blood pH, HCO_3 normal levels
• Decreased gastric pain

sodium biphosphate/ sodium phosphate (OTC)
Fleet Enema, Phospho-soda
Func. class.: Laxative, saline
Pregnancy category C

ACTION: Increases water absorption in the small intestine by osmotic action; laxative effect occurs by increased peristalsis and water retention

Therapeutic outcome: Absence of constipation

USES: Constipation, bowel or rectal preparation for surgery, examination

CONTRAINDICATIONS:
Hypersensitivity, rectal fissures, abdominal pain, nausea/vomiting, appendicitis, acute surgical abdomen, ulcerated hemorrhoids, Na-restricted diets, renal failure, hyperphosphatemia, hypocalcemia, hypokalemia, hypernatremia, Addison's disease, CHF, ascites, bowel perforation, megacolon, imperforate anus

> **BLACK BOX WARNING:** GI obstruction, renal failure

Precautions: Pregnancy **C**

> **BLACK BOX WARNING:** Colitis, elderly, hypovolemia, renal disease

DOSAGE AND ROUTES
Adult: PO 20-30 ml (Phospho-soda)
Child: PO 5-15 ml (Phospho-soda)
Adult and child >12 yr: RECT enema (118 ml)
Child 2-12 yr: RECT $^1/_2$ enema (59 ml)

Available forms: Enema 7 g/phosphate and 19 g/biphosphate/118 ml; oral sol 18 g phosphate/48 g biphosphate/100 ml

Implementation
PO route
• Give on empty stomach
• Mix oral sol in cold water
• Take alone for better absorption; do not take within 1 hr of other products

ADVERSE EFFECTS
CV: Dysrhythmias, **cardiac arrest**, hypotension, widening QRS complex
GI: *Nausea, cramps,* diarrhea
META: Electrolyte, fluid imbalances

Pharmacokinetics

Absorption	Up to 20% (rec)
Distribution	Unknown
Metabolism	Unknown
Excretion	Kidneys
Half-life	Unknown

S

Pharmacodynamics

	PO	Rect
Onset	$1/2$-3 hr	5 min
Peak	Unknown	Unknown
Duration	Unknown	Unknown

NURSING CONSIDERATIONS

Assessment
• Assess stools: color, amount, consistency
• Assess for bowel pattern, bowel sounds (frequency, intensity), flatulence, distention, increased temp, dietary patterns (fluid, bulk), exercise
• Assess for cramping, rectal bleeding, nausea, vomiting; if these symptoms occur, product should be discontinued

Nursing diagnoses
• Constipation (uses)
• Knowledge, deficient (teaching)

Patient/family education
• Advise patient not to use laxatives or enema for long-term therapy; bowel tone will be lost
• Teach patient that normal bowel movements do not always occur daily
• Caution patient not to use in presence of abdominal pain, nausea, vomiting
• Caution patient to notify prescriber if constipation is unrelieved or if symptoms of electrolyte imbalance occur: muscle cramps, pain, weakness, dizziness, excessive thirst
• Instruct patient to maintain adequate fluid consumption to help prevent constipation

Evaluation
Positive therapeutic outcome
• Decrease in constipation

sodium polystyrene sulfonate (Rx)
(po-lee-stye′reen)
Kayexalate, Kionex, SPS
Func. class.: Potassium-removing resin
Chem. class.: Cation exchange resin
Pregnancy category C

ACTION: Removes potassium by exchanging sodium for potassium in body; occurs primarily in large intestine

Therapeutic outcome: Potassium levels within accepted range

USES: Hyperkalemia in conjunction with other measures

CONTRAINDICATIONS:
Hypersensitivity to saccharin or parabens that may be in some products; GI obstruction, neonate (reduced gut motility)

Precautions: Pregnancy C, geriatric, renal failure, CHF, severe edema, severe hypertension, sodium restriction, constipation, GI bleeding, hypocalcemia

DOSAGE AND ROUTES
Adult: PO 15 g daily-qid; RECT enema 30-50 q1-2hr initially prn, then q6hr prn
Child (unlabeled): PO 1 g/kg q6hr prn; RECT 1 g/kg q2-6hr prn

Available forms: Powder for susp 453.6 g, 454 g; oral susp 15 g/60 ml

Implementation
PO route
• Give oral dose as susp mixed with water or syr (20-100 ml)
• Give mild laxative as ordered to prevent constipation and fecal impaction
Rectal route
• Give by retention enema after mixing with warm water; introduce by gravity, continue stirring, flush with 100 ml of fluid, clamp, and leave in place for at least $1/2$-1 hr
• Complete irrigation of colon after enema with 1-2 qt of nonsodium sol, drain
• Store freshly prepared sol for 24 hr at room temperature

ADVERSE EFFECTS
GI: *Constipation,* anorexia, nausea, vomiting, diarrhea (sorbitol), *fecal impaction,* gastric irritation
META: Hypocalcemia, hypokalemia, hypomagnesemia, sodium retention

Pharmacokinetics

Absorption	None
Distribution	None
Metabolism	None
Excretion	Feces
Half-life	Unknown

Pharmacodynamics

	PO	Rect
Onset	2-12 hr	2-12 hr
Peak	Unknown	Unknown
Duration	6-24 hr	4-6 hr

INTERACTIONS
Individual drugs
Sorbitol: increased colonic necrosis, do not use concurrently

Lithium: decreased effect of lithium

Drug classifications
Diuretics (loop), cardiac glycosides: increased hypokalemia

Magnesium/calcium antacids: increased metabolic acidosis

Thyroid hormones: decreased effect of thyroid hormones

NURSING CONSIDERATIONS
Assessment
• Assess bowel function daily: amount of stool, color, characteristics
• Assess for hypotension: confusion, irritability, muscular pain, weakness
• Hyperkalemia: assess for confusion, dyspnea, weakness, dysrhythmias
• Monitor electrolytes: potassium, sodium, calcium, magnesium; I&O ratio, weight daily
• Monitor ECG for spiked T-waves, depressed ST segments, prolonged QT interval, and widening QRS complex
• Monitor I&O ratio, weight daily, crackles, dyspnea, jugular vein distention, edema
• Monitor for digoxin toxicity (nausea, vomiting, blurred vision, anorexia, dysrhythmia) in those receiving digoxin

Nursing diagnoses
• Constipation (adverse reactions)
• Diarrhea (adverse reactions)
• Knowledge, deficient (teaching)

Patient/family education
• Explain reason for medication and expected results
• Teach patient to avoid laxatives, antacids, electrolyte-based products unless approved by prescriber

Evaluation
Positive therapeutic outcome
• Potassium level 3.5-5 mg/dl

---

solifenacin (Rx)
(sol-i-fen′a-sin)
VESIcare
Func. class.: Urinary antispasmodic, anticholinergic
Chem. class.: Antimuscarinic receptor antagonist
Pregnancy category C

ACTION: Relaxes smooth muscles in urinary tract by inhibiting acetylcholine at postganglionic sites

Therapeutic outcome: Decreased dysuria, frequency, nocturia, incontinence

USES: Overactive bladder (urinary frequency, urgency, incontinence)

CONTRAINDICATIONS: Hypersensitivity, uncontrolled closed-angle glaucoma, urinary retention, gastric retention

Precautions: Pregnancy C, breastfeeding, children, geriatric patients, renal/hepatic disease, controlled closed-angle glaucoma, bladder outflow obstruction, GI obstruction, decreased GI motility, history of QT prolongation

DOSAGE AND ROUTES
Adult: PO 5 mg/day, max 10 mg/day

Renal/hepatic dose
Adult: PO CCr <30 ml/min 5 mg/day; Child-Pugh B max 5 mg/day

Available forms: Tabs 5, 10 mg

ADVERSE EFFECTS
CNS: Anxiety, paresthesia, fatigue, *dizziness,* headache, confusion
CV: Chest pain, hypertension, **QTc prolongation, peripheral edema**
EENT: *Vision abnormalities, xerophthalmia,* nasal dryness
GI: *Nausea, vomiting, anorexia,* abdominal pain, *constipation,* dry mouth, dyspepsia
GU: Dysuria, urinary retention, frequency, UTI
INTEG: Rash, pruritus, **angioedema**
MISC: Hyperthermia
RESP: Bronchitis, cough, pharyngitis, URI

Pharmacokinetics

Absorption	Rapid (90%)
Distribution	98% protein bound
Metabolism	Extensively metabolized by CYP3A4
Excretion	Excreted in urine (69%)/ feces (22%)
Half-life	Terminal half-life 45-68 hr

Pharmacodynamics

Unknown

INTERACTIONS

Drug classifications

Azoles, macrolides, fluoroquinolones, class I antidysrhythmics: increased QT prolongation

Benzodiazepines, hypnotics, opioids, sedatives: increased CNS depression

CYP3A4 inducers (carBAMazepine, nevirapine, phenobarbitol, phenytoin): decreased effects of solifenacin

CYP3A4 inhibitors (clarithromycin, diclofenac, doxycycline, erythromycin, isoniazid, ketoconazole, nefazodone, propofol, protease inhibitors, verapamil): increased action of solifenacin, max dose 5 mg

Drug/herb

St. John's wort: decreased effects

Drug/food

Grapefruit juice: increased effect

NURSING CONSIDERATIONS

Assessment

• **Urinary patterns:** assess for distention, nocturia, frequency, urgency, incontinence

• **Allergic reactions:** assess for rash; if this occurs, product should be discontinued

• **Cardiac patients:** monitor ECG for QT prolongation, avoid products that can increase QT prolongation

• **Angioedema:** assess for swelling of face, lips, tongue, larynx

Nursing diagnoses

• Knowledge, deficient (teaching)
• Urinary elimination, impaired (uses)

Patient/family education

• Caution patient to avoid hazardous activities; dizziness may occur

• Advise patient that constipation, blurred vision may occur

• Instruct patient to call prescriber if severe abdominal pain or constipation lasts for 3 or more days

• Advise patient that heat prostration may occur if used in a hot environment

Evaluation

Positive therapeutic outcome

• Urinary status: decreased dysuria, frequency, nocturia, incontinence

somatropin (Rx)

(soe-ma-troe′pin)

Genotropin, Humatrope, Norditropin, Norditropin Flexpro, Nutropin, Nutropin AQ, Omnitrope, Saizen, Serostim, Tev-Tropin, Zorbtive

Func. class.: Pituitary hormone
Chem. class.: Growth hormone

Pregnancy category C

Do not confuse:
Somatropin/SUMAtriptan

ACTION: Stimulates growth; similar to natural growth hormone—both preparations are developed by recombinant DNA technique

Therapeutic outcome: Increase in height as a result of skeletal growth in pituitary growth hormone deficiency

USES: Pituitary growth hormone deficiency (hypopituitary dwarfism), children with human growth hormone deficiency, AIDS wasting syndrome, cachexia, adults with somatropin deficiency syndrome (SDS), short stature in Noonan syndrome, SHOX deficiencies; Turner's syndrome, Prader-Willi syndrome

CONTRAINDICATIONS:
Hypersensitivity to benzyl alcohol, creosol, glycerin hypersensitivity (for medications that contain these products), closed epiphyses, acute respiratory failure, Prader-Willi syndrome with obesity, trauma

Precautions: Pregnancy C, breastfeeding, newborns, geriatric, diabetes mellitus, hypothyroidism, intracranial lesions, prolonged treatment in adults, scoliosis, sleep apnea, chemotherapy, respiratory disease

DOSAGE AND ROUTES

Genotropin

Child: SUBCUT 0.16-0.24 mg/kg/wk, divided into 6 or 7 daily inj, give in abdomen, thigh, buttocks

Adult: SUBCUT 0.4-0.8 mg/kg/wk divided in 6-7 daily doses

Humatrope
Child: SUBCUT/IM 0.006 mg/kg divided into equal doses either on 3 alternate days or 6 ×/wk, max 0.3 mg/kg/wk
Adult: IM 0.018 units/kg/day, max 0.0125 units/kg/day

Growth hormone deficiency

Nutropin/Nutropin AQ
Child: SUBCUT 0.3 mg/kg/wk

Serostim
Adult: SUBCUT at bedtime >55 kg 6 mg, 45-55 kg 5 mg, 35-45 kg 4 mg

Norditropin
Child: SUBCUT 0.024-0.034 mg/kg 6-7 ×/wk

Accretropin
Child: SUBCUT 0.18-0.3 mg/kg/wk divided into 6 or 7 equal daily inj

Replacement of GH in GH deficiency
Adult: SUBCUT (Saizen) 0.005 mg/kg/day; may increase after 4 wk to max 0.01 mg/kg/day

Available forms: Powder for inj (lyophilized) 1.5 mg (4 international units/ml), 4 mg (12 international units/vial), 5 mg (13 international units/vial), 5 mg (15 international units/vial), rDNA origin, 5.8 mg (15 international units/ml), 6 mg (18 international units/ml), 8 mg (24 international units/vial), 10 mg (26 international units/vial), inj 10 mg (30 international units/vial); 5, 10, 15 mg/1.5 ml

Implementation
• Store in refrigerator for <1 mo; if reconstituted, <1 wk; do not use discolored or cloudy sol

IM route
• **Accretropin:** Does not require reconstitution
• **Norditropin:** After reconstituting 4-8 mg/2 ml diluent
• **Humatrope:** 5 mg/1.5-5 ml dilute, do not shake
• **Nutropin/Nutropin AQ:** Reconstitute 5 mg/1-5 ml or 10 mg/1-10 ml of bacteriostatic water for inj (benzyl alcohol preserved)
• **Zorbtive:** Reconstitute 4, 5, 6 mg with 0.5-1 ml of sterile water for inj; reconstitute each 8.8 mg with 1-2 bacteriostatic water for inj

ADVERSE EFFECTS
CNS: Headache, growth of intracranial tumor, fever, aggressive behavior
ENDO: *Hyperglycemia, ketosis, hypothyroidism*
GI: Nausea, vomiting

GU: *Hypercalciuria*
INTEG: Rash, urticaria, pain, inflammation at inj site; hematoma
MS: Tissue swelling, joint and muscle pain
SYST: **Antibodies to growth hormone**

Pharmacokinetics

Absorption	Well absorbed (SUBCUT/IM)
Distribution	Unknown
Metabolism	Unknown
Excretion	Unknown
Half-life	15-60 min

Pharmacodynamics

	IM/SUBCUT (growth)
Onset	Unknown
Peak	Unknown
Duration	7 days

INTERACTIONS

Drug classifications
Androgens, thyroid hormones: increased epiphyseal closure
Glucocorticosteroids: decreased growth
Insulins, antidiabetics: decreased antidiabetic effect, adjust dosage

NURSING CONSIDERATIONS

Assessment
• Assess for signs/symptoms of diabetes
• Identify growth hormone antibodies if patient fails to respond to therapy
• Monitor thyroid function tests: T_3, T_4, T_7, TSH to identify hypothyroidism
• Assess for allergic reaction: rash, itching, fever, nausea, wheezing
• Assess for hypercalciuria: urinary stones; groin, flank pain; nausea, vomiting, frequency, hematuria, chills
• Monitor growth rate, bone age of child at intervals during treatment

Nursing diagnoses
• Body image, disturbed (uses)
• Knowledge, deficient (teaching)

Patient/family education
• Explain reason for medication and expected results; that treatment may continue for yr
• Advise patient that routine follow-up is needed to monitor growth rate
• Instruct parents on procedure for medication preparation and inj use; request demonstration, return demonstration; provide written instructions

S

Adverse effects: *italics* = common; **bold** = life-threatening

- Teach patient to maintain growth record, report knee, hip pain or limping
- Advise patient treatment is very expensive

Evaluation
Positive therapeutic outcome
- Growth in children until epiphyseal plates close

---

sorafenib (Rx)
(sore-ah-fen′ib)
Nexavar
Func. class.: Antineoplastic—miscellaneous
Chem. class.: Multikinase inhibitor, signal transduction inhibitor
Pregnancy category D

ACTION: Multikinase inhibitor that decreases tumor cell proliferation

Therapeutic outcome: Prevention of spread of malignancy

USES: Advanced/metastatic murine renal cell carcinoma, unresectable hematocellular cancer

CONTRAINDICATIONS:
Pregnancy **D,** hypersensitivity

Precautions: Breastfeeding, children, geriatric, cardiac/renal/hepatic disease, GI bleeding, infection, surgery, dental disease/work

DOSAGE AND ROUTES
Adult: PO 400 mg bid without food, continue until no longer benefiting or until unacceptable toxicity occurs

Available forms: Tabs 200 mg

Implementation
- Swallow tab whole; do not break, crush, or chew
- Give on empty stomach 1 hr before or 2 hr after meal
- Store at room temp, in dry place

ADVERSE EFFECTS
CNS: *Fatigue, weight loss, headache*
CV: Hypertension, cardiac ischemia, infarction, hypertensive crisis, cardiotoxicity, MI, thromboembolism
GI: *Nausea, diarrhea, vomiting,* anorexia, **pancreatitis,** mouth ulceration, *abdominal pain,* constipation, GI perforation

HEMA: Hemorrhage, leukopenia, lymphopenia, anemia, neutropenia, thrombocytopenia, pancytopenia
INTEG: *Rash,* pruritus, *dry skin,* erythema, *hand-foot syndrome,* exfoliative dermatitis, acne, flushing, *alopecia*
META: *Hypophosphatemia*
MS: *Arthralgia, myalgia*
RESP: *Hoarseness*

Pharmacokinetics
Absorption	38%-49%, high-fat meal decreases bioavailability
Distribution	Protein binding 99.5%
Metabolism	Liver, oxidative metabolism by CYP3A4, glucuronidation by UGT1A9
Excretion	77% feces
Half-life	Elimination 1-2 day

Pharmacodynamics
Onset	Unknown
Peak	3 hr
Duration	Unknown

INTERACTIONS
Individual drugs
CarBAMazepine, cimetidine, dexamethasone, PHENobarbital, phenytoin, ranitidine, rifampin, sodium bicarbonate: decreased sorafenib levels

Drug classifications
Anticoagulants, NSAIDs, platelet inhibitors, thrombolytics: increased bleeding risk
CYP3A4 inducers (barbiturates, bosentan, carBAMazepine, efavirenz, nevirapine, phenytoins, rifabutin, rifampin): may decrease sorafenib effect
UGT1A1 drugs (irinotecan, DOXOrubicin, morphine, naltrexone, estradiol, buprenorphine): increased effect of UGT1A1 substrates

Drug/lab test
Decreased: RBC, WBC, platelets
Increased: lipase, amylase, TSH, bilirubin, WBC, platelets

NURSING CONSIDERATIONS
Assessment
- Monitor CBC with differential LFTs
- Assess for **skin toxicities:** grade 1, continue therapy, topical treatment for relief; grade 2 (1st episode), continue therapy, if no improvement after 7 days, delay treatment until resolved to grade ≤1, resume dose by one dose level;

---

grade 2 (2nd or 3rd episode), delay treatment until resolved to grade ≤1, resume dose by one dose level; grade 2 (4th episode), discontinue therapy; grade 3 (1st or 2nd episode), delay treatment until resolved to grade ≤1, resume dose by one dose level; grade 3 (3rd episode), discontinue therapy
• **Cardiac events:** Monitor B/P weekly × 6 wk (hypertension); cardiac ischemia, bleeding, bruising
• Assess for **hand-foot reactions** during first 6 wk of therapy
• Monitor PT, INR (bleeding)

Nursing diagnoses
• Injury, risk for (uses, adverse reactions)

Patient/family education
⚠ **Teach patient to report adverse reactions immediately**
• Teach patient the reason for treatment, expected results
• Advise patient to use contraception during treatment, birth defects may occur (pregnancy **D**); avoid breastfeeding
• Advise patient not to double dose if missed
• Advise patient to avoid OTC products without approval of prescriber

Evaluation
Positive therapeutic outcome
• Decrease in renal cell carcinoma stabilization

sotalol (Rx)
(soe-ta'lole)
Betapace, Betapace AF, Sorine
Func. class.: Antidysrhythmic, group III
Chem. class.: Nonselective β-blocker
Pregnancy category B

ACTION: Blockade of β₁- and β₂-receptors leads to antidysrhythmic effect, prolongs action potential in myocardial fibers without affecting conduction, prolongs QT interval, no effect on QRS duration

Therapeutic outcome: Decreased B/P, heart rate, AV conduction

USES: Life-threatening ventricular dysrhythmias; Betapace AF: to maintain sinus rhythm in symptomatic atrial fibrillation/flutter

CONTRAINDICATIONS:
Hypersensitivity to β-blockers, cardiogenic shock, heart block (2nd or 3rd degree), sinus bradycardia, CHF, bronchial asthma, CCr <40 ml/min

> **BLACK BOX WARNING:** Congenital or acquired long QT syndrome, hypokalemia

Precautions: Pregnancy **B**, breastfeeding, major surgery, diabetes mellitus, renal/thyroid disease, COPD, well-compensated heart failure, CAD, nonallergic bronchospasm, electrolyte disturbances, bradycardia, peripheral vascular disease

> **BLACK BOX WARNING:** Cardiac dysrhythmias, torsades de pointes, ventricular dysrhythmias, ventricular fibrillation

DOSAGE AND ROUTES
Adult: PO initial 80 mg bid, may increase to total of 240-320 mg/day, each dosage increase is made after ≥3 days and QTc interval <550 msecs
Child >2 yr with normal renal function (unlabeled): PO 30 mg/m² tid, adjust dosage gradually after ≥36 hr to max 60 mg/m² tid

Renal dose
Adult: PO CCr 30-60 ml/min q24hr; CCr 10-29 ml/min q36-48hr; CCr <10 ml/min individualize dose

Life-threatening ventricular dysrhythmias
Adult: with CCr 40-60 ml/min **IV** 75 mg over 5 hr q day, monitor QTc at end of each infusion during initiation and titration; 80 mg PO = 75 mg **IV**; 120 mg PO = 112.5 mg **IV**; 160 mg PO = 150 mg **IV**

Betapace AF
Adult: PO initial 80 mg bid, titrate upward to 120 mg bid during initial hospitalization

Renal dose (Betapace AF)
Adult: CCr >60 ml/min q12hr; CCr 40-60 ml/min q24hr; CCr <40 ml/min do not use

Available forms: Tabs 80, 120, 160, 240 mg; (Betapace AF) 80, 120, 160 mg; inj 150 mg/10 ml (15 mg/ml)

Implementation
PO route
• Given before meals, at bedtime, tab may be crushed or swallowed whole; give with food to prevent GI upset; reduce dosage in renal dysfunction
• Betapace and Betapace AF are not interchangeable
• Store protected from light, moisture; place in cool environment

IV route

• Dilute to a volume of either 120 ml or 300 ml with D_5W, LR

• **75-mg dose:** withdraw 6 ml sotalol inj (90 mg), add 114 ml dilute to make 120 ml (0.75% mg/ml); or withdraw 6 ml sotalol inj (90 mg), add 294 ml, dilute to make 300 ml (0.3 mg/ml)

• **112.5-mg dose:** withdraw 9 ml sotalol inj, (135 ml), add 111 ml, dilute to 120 ml (1.125 mg/ml); or withdraw 9 ml sotalol (135 mg) and add 291 ml dilute to 300 ml (0.45 mg/ml)

• **150-mg dose:** withdraw 12 ml sotalol (180 mg), add 108 ml to 120 ml (1.5 mg/ml); or withdraw 12 ml of sotalol (180 mg), add 288 ml to 300 ml (0.6 mg/ml)

• Use inf pump and infuse 100 or 250 ml over 5 hr at a constant rate

ADVERSE EFFECTS

CNS: Dizziness, mental changes, drowsiness, fatigue, headache, catatonia, depression, anxiety, nightmares, paresthesia, lethargy, insomnia, decreased concentration

CV: Orthostatic hypotension, bradycardia, **CHF,** chest pain, **ventricular dysrhythmias, prolonged QT,** AV block, peripheral vascular insufficiency, palpitations, **prodysrhythmia, torsades de pointes; Betapace AF: life-threatening ventricular dysrhythmias**

EENT: Tinnitus, visual changes, sore throat, double vision, dry, burning eyes

GI: Nausea, vomiting, diarrhea, dry mouth, flatulence, constipation, anorexia, indigestion

GU: Impotence, dysuria, ejaculatory failure, urinary retention

HEMA: Agranulocytosis, thrombocytopenic purpura (rare), thrombocytopenia, leukopenia

INTEG: Rash, alopecia, urticaria, pruritus, fever, diaphoresis

MISC: Facial swelling, decreased exercise tolerance, weight change, Raynaud's disease

MS: Joint pain, arthralgia, muscle cramps, pain

RESP: Bronchospasm, dyspnea, wheezing, nasal stuffiness, pharyngitis

Pharmacokinetics

Absorption	Variable (30%)
Distribution	Crosses placenta, minimal penetration in CNS
Metabolism	Liver, protein binding 0%
Excretion	70% unchanged—kidneys
Half-life	10-24 hr, increased in renal disease

Pharmacodynamics

Onset	Several hr
Peak	Unknown
Duration	Unknown

INTERACTIONS

Individual drugs

Haloperidol, chloroquine, droperidol, pentamidine; arsenic trioxide, levomethadyl: increased QT prolongation

Insulin: increased hypoglycemia

Lidocaine: increased effects of lidocaine

Nitroglycerin: increased hypotension

Theophylline: decreased bronchodilating effects of theophylline

Drug classifications

Antihypertensives, diuretics: increased hypotension

β_2-Agonists: decreased bronchodilating effects

Class IA/III antidysrhythmics, some phenothiazines, β-agonists, local anesthetics, tricyclics, CYP3A4 inhibitors (amiodarone, clarithromycin, erythromycin, telithromycin, troleandomycin), CYP3A4 substrates (methadone, pimozide, QUEtiapine, quiNIDine, risperidone, ziprasidone): increased QT prolongation

Sulfonylureas: decreased hypoglycemic effects

Sympathomimetics: decreased β-blocker effects

Drug/lab test

False: increased urinary catecholamines

Interference: glucose, insulin tolerance tests

NURSING CONSIDERATIONS

Assessment

> **BLACK BOX WARNING: QT syndrome:**
> Monitor B/P during beginning treatment, periodically thereafter; pulse q4hr; note rate, rhythm, quality: apical/radial pulse before administration; notify prescriber of any significant changes (pulse <50 bpm); monitor ECG continuously (Betapace AF); use QT interval to determine patient eligibility; baseline QT must be ≤450 msec

• Check for baselines in renal function tests, before therapy begins

• Assess for edema in feet, legs daily, monitor I&O ratio, daily weight; check for jugular vein distention, crackles, bilaterally, dyspnea (CHF)

• Monitor skin turgor, dryness of mucous membranes for hydration status, especially in geriatric

Nursing diagnoses
• Cardiac output, decreased (uses)
• Injury, risk for (adverse reactions)
• Knowledge, deficient (teaching)
• Noncompliance (teaching)

Patient/family education
• Teach patient not to discontinue product abruptly, taper over 2 wk; may cause precipitate angina if stopped abruptly
• Teach patient not to use OTC products containing α-adrenergic stimulants (such as nasal decongestants, cold preparations); to avoid alcohol and smoking and to limit sodium intake as prescribed
• Teach patient how to take pulse and B/P at home, advise when to notify prescriber
• Instruct patient to comply with weight control, dietary adjustments, modified exercise program
• Caution patient to carry/wear emergency ID to identify product being taken, allergies
• Inform patient that product controls symptoms but does not cure
• Caution patient to avoid hazardous activities if dizziness, drowsiness are present
• Teach patient to report symptoms of **CHF:** difficulty breathing, especially on exertion or when lying down; night cough; swelling of extremities; bradycardia; dizziness; confusion; depression; fever
• Teach patient to take product as prescribed, not to double or skip doses; take any missed doses as soon as remembered if at least 4 hr until next dose

Evaluation
Positive therapeutic outcome
• Absence of dysrhythmias

TREATMENT OF OVERDOSE:
Lavage; **IV** atropine for bradycardia; **IV** theophylline for bronchospasm; digoxin, O_2, diuretic for cardiac failure; hemodialysis; **IV** glucose for hyperglycemia; **IV** diazepam (or phenytoin) for seizures

---

spironolactone (Rx)
(speer'on-oh-lak'tone)
Aldactone, Novo-Spiroton ✦
Func. class.: Potassium-sparing diuretic
Chem. class.: Aldosterone antagonist
Pregnancy category D

ACTION: Competes with aldosterone at receptor sites in the distal tubule in the renal system, resulting in excretion of sodium chloride, water, retention of potassium, phosphate

Therapeutic outcome: Diuretic and antihypertensive effect while retaining potassium; lowered aldosterone levels

USES: Edema of CHF, hypertension, diuretic-induced hypokalemia, primary hyperaldosteronism (diagnosis, short-term treatment, long-term treatment), edema of nephrotic syndrome, cirrhosis of the liver with ascites

Unlabeled uses: CHF, hirsutism in women

CONTRAINDICATIONS:
Pregnancy **D**, hypersensitivity, anuria, severe renal disease, hyperkalemia

Precautions: Breastfeeding, dehydration, renal/hepatic disease, electrolyte imbalances, metabolic acidosis, gynecomastia

> **BLACK BOX WARNING:** Secondary malignancy

DOSAGE AND ROUTES
Edema/hypertension
Adult: PO 25-200 mg/day in 1-2 divided doses

CHF
Adult: PO 12.5-25 mg/day, max 50 mg/day

Edema
Child: PO 1.5-3.3 mg/kg/day in single or divided doses

Hypertension
Child (unlabeled): PO 1.5-3.3 mg/kg in divided doses

Hypokalemia
Adult: PO 25-100 mg/day; if PO, potassium supplements must not be used

Primary hyperaldosteronism diagnosis
Adult: PO 400 mg/day × 4 days or 4 wk depending on the test, then 100-400 mg/day maintenance

Edema (nephrotic syndrome, CHF, hepatic disease)
Adult: PO 100 mg/day given as a single dose or in divided doses, titrate to response
Child: PO 1.5-3.3 mg/kg/day or 60 mg/m²/day given once daily or in 2-4 divided doses

Renal dose
Adult: PO CCr 10-50 ml/min; give dose q12-24hr; CCr <10 ml/min, avoid use

S

Polycystic ovary syndrome/ hirsutism in women (unlabeled)
Adult: PO 50-200 mg in 1-2 divided doses

Available forms: Tabs 25, 50, 100 mg

Implementation
• Give in AM to avoid interference with sleep
• Give with food if nausea occurs; absorption may be increased; take at same time each day

ADVERSE EFFECTS
CNS: Headache, confusion, drowsiness, lethargy, ataxia
ELECT: Hyperchloremic metabolic acidosis, **hyperkalemia,** hyponatremia
ENDO: Impotence, gynecomastia, irregular menses, amenorrhea, postmenopausal bleeding, hirsutism, deepening voice, breast pain
GI: Diarrhea, cramps, **bleeding,** gastritis, vomiting, anorexia, nausea, **hepatocellular toxicity**
HEMA: Agranulocytosis
INTEG: *Rash, pruritus,* urticaria

Pharmacokinetics

Absorption	GI tract; well absorbed
Distribution	Crosses placenta
Metabolism	Liver to canrenone (active metabolite)
Excretion	Renal; breast milk
Half-life	12-24 hr (canrenone)

Pharmacodynamics

Onset	24-48 hr
Peak	48-72 hr
Duration	Unknown

INTERACTIONS
Individual drugs
Aspirin: decreased action of spironolactone
Cholestyramine: increased hyperchloremic acidosis in cirrhosis
Digoxin: increased digoxin action
Lithium: increased action, toxicity

Drug classifications
ACE inhibitors, diuretics (potassium-sparing), potassium products, salt substitute: increased hyperkalemia
Anticoagulants: decreased effects of anticoagulants
Antihypertensives: increased action
NSAIDs: decreased effect of spironolactone

Drug/herb
St. John's wort: severe photosensitivity

Drug/lab test
Interference: 17-OHCS, 17-KS, radioimmunoassay, digoxin assay

NURSING CONSIDERATIONS
Assessment
• **Hypokalemia:** assess for polyuria, polydipsia, dysrhythmias including a U wave on ECG
• **Hyperkalemia:** assess for weakness, fatigue, dyspnea, dysrhythmias, confusion
• Assess fluid volume status: I&O ratios and record, count or weigh diapers as appropriate, weight, distended red veins, crackles in lung, color, quality, and specific gravity of urine, skin turgor, adequacy of pulses, moist mucous membranes, bilateral lung sounds, peripheral pitting edema; dehydration symptoms of decreasing output, thirst, hypotension, dry mouth and mucous membranes should be reported
• Monitor electrolytes: potassium, sodium, calcium, magnesium; also include BUN, ABGs, uric acid, CBC, blood glucose

Nursing diagnoses
• Fluid volume, deficient (adverse reactions)
• Fluid volume, excess (uses)
• Knowledge, deficient (teaching)
• Urinary elimination, impaired (adverse reactions)

Patient/family education
• Teach patient to take medication early in day to prevent nocturia
• Instruct patient to take with food or milk if GI symptoms of nausea and anorexia occur
• Teach patient to maintain a record of weight on a weekly basis and notify prescriber of weight loss of >5 lb
• Caution patient that this product causes an increase in potassium levels, that foods high in potassium should be avoided: oranges, bananas, salt substitutes, dried apricots, dates; avoid potassium salt substitutes; refer to dietitian for assistance planning
• Teach patient not to use alcohol or any OTC medications without prescriber's approval; serious product reactions may occur
• Emphasize the need to contact prescriber immediately if muscle cramps, weakness, nausea, dizziness, or numbness occur
• Teach patient to take own B/P and pulse and record
• Teach patient to notify prescriber of cramps, diarrhea, lethargy, thirst, headache, skin rash, menstrual abnormalities, deepening voice, breast enlargement

⚠ Nurse Alert

• Advise patient that dizziness and confusion may occur; avoid driving or other hazardous activities if alertness is decreased
• Teach patient to continue taking medication even if feeling better; this product controls symptoms but does not cure the condition
• Advise patient with hypertension to continue other treatment (exercise, weight loss, relaxation techniques, cessation of smoking)

Evaluation
Positive therapeutic outcome
• Prevention of hypokalemia (diuretic use)
• Decreased edema
• Decreased B/P
• Decreased aldosterone levels
• Increased diuresis

TREATMENT OF OVERDOSE:
• Lavage if taken orally, monitor electrolytes
• Administer sodium bicarbonate
• Monitor hydration, CV, renal status

---

stavudine d4t (Rx)
(sta′vu-deen)
Zerit
Func. class.: Antiretroviral
Chem. class.: Nucleoside reverse transcriptase inhibitor (NRTI)
Pregnancy category C

ACTION: Prevents replication of HIV-1 by inhibition of reverse transcriptase; causes DNA chain termination

Therapeutic outcome: Decreasing diarrhea, fatigue, night sweats; increased body weight

USES: Treatment of HIV-1; used in combination with other antiretrovirals

CONTRAINDICATIONS:
Hypersensitivity to this product or zidovudine, didanosine, zalcitabine; severe peripheral neuropathy

> **BLACK BOX WARNING:** Lactic acidosis

Precautions: Breastfeeding, advanced HIV infections, bone marrow suppression, renal, peripheral neuropathy, osteoporosis, obesity

> **BLACK BOX WARNING:** Pregnancy **C**, hepatic disease, pancreatitis

DOSAGE AND ROUTES
Adult >60 kg: PO 40 mg q12hr
Adult <60 kg: PO 30 mg q12hr
Child <30 kg: PO 1 mg/kg q12hr
Child ≥30 kg ≤60 kg: PO 30 mg q12hr
Child >60 kg: PO 40 mg q12hr

Renal dose
Adult >60 kg: CCr 26-50 ml/min 20 mg q12hr; CCr 10-25 ml/min 20 mg q24hr
Adult <60 kg: CCr 26-50 ml/min 15 mg q12hr; CCr 10-25 ml/min 15 mg q24hr

Available forms: Caps 15, 20, 30, 40 mg; oral powder for sol 1 mg/ml

Implementation
• Give with or without meals; absorption does not appear to be lowered when taken with food
• Give product q4hr around the clock, even during night
• Shake susp well before using

ADVERSE EFFECTS
CNS: *Peripheral neuropathy,* insomnia, anxiety, depression, dizziness, confusion, *headache,* chills/fever, malaise, neuropathy
CV: Chest pain, vasodilatation, hypertension
EENT: Conjunctivitis, abnormal vision
GI: **Hepatotoxicity,** *diarrhea, nausea, vomiting,* anorexia, dyspepsia, constipation, stomatitis, **pancreatitis**
HEMA: **Bone marrow suppression, leukopenia, macrocytosis**
INTEG: *Rash,* sweating, pruritus, benign neoplasms
MISC: **Lactic acidosis,** asthenia, lipodystrophy
MS: Myalgia, arthralgia
RESP: Dyspnea, pneumonia, asthma

Pharmacokinetics

Absorption	Rapidly absorbed, 82% bioavailability
Distribution	Cerebrospinal fluid
Metabolism	Unknown
Excretion	Kidneys, breast milk
Half-life	Elimination: 1-1.6 hr, intracellular: 3-3.5 hr

Pharmacodynamics

Onset	Unknown
Peak	1 hr
Duration	Unknown

S

Adverse effects: *italics* = common; **bold** = life-threatening

INTERACTIONS
Individual drugs
Chloramphenicol, dapsone, didanosine, ethambutol, hydrALAZINE, lithium, phenytoin, vinCRIStine, zalcitabine: increased peripheral neuropathy

Methadone, zidovudine: decreased stavudine effect

Probenecid: increased stavudine levels

Drug classifications
Myelosuppressants: increased myelosuppression

NURSING CONSIDERATIONS
Assessment
⚠ Assess for lactic acidosis and severe hepatomegaly with steatosis; death may result
- Monitor viral load and CD4 counts, plasma HIV RNA baseline, throughout treatment
- Monitor for peripheral neuropathy: tingling, pain in extremities; if these occur, discontinue product
- **Monitor for pancreatitis:** severe upper abdominal pain, nausea, vomiting throughout treatment; if these occur, discontinue product
- Monitor blood tests: WBC, differential, RBC, Hct, Hgb, platelets, serum amylase, lipase
- Monitor renal function tests: urinalysis, protein, blood, serum creatinine
- Obtain C&S before product therapy; product may be taken as soon as culture is performed; repeat C&S after therapy
- Monitor bowel pattern before, during treatment
- Monitor fluid overload; product requires large volume to stay in sol
- Assess for weakness, tremors, confusion, dizziness, psychosis; if these occur, product may have to be decreased or discontinued

Nursing diagnoses
- Infection, risk for (uses)
- Knowledge, deficient (teaching)

Patient/family education
- Teach patient signs of peripheral neuropathy: burning, weakness, pain, pricking feeling in the extremities
- Caution patient that this product should not be given with antineoplastics
- Inform patient that GI complaints and insomnia resolve after 3-4 wk of treatment
- Inform patient that product is not a cure for AIDS but controls symptoms
- Advise patient to call prescriber if sore throat, swollen lymph nodes, malaise, fever occur; may indicate presence of other infections
- Caution patient that even with product administration, virus is still infective and may be passed on to others
- Caution patient that follow-up visits must be continued because serious toxicity may occur; blood counts must be done q2wk
- Teach patient that product must be taken q4hr around the clock even during night
- Caution patient that serious product interactions with other medications may occur, check with prescriber first if taking chloramphenicol, dapsone, cisplatin, didanosine, ethambutol, lithium, antifungals
- Inform patient that other products may be necessary to prevent other infections
- Inform patient that product may cause fainting or dizziness

Evaluation
Positive therapeutic outcome
- Decreased symptoms of HIV infection

streptomycin (Rx)
(strep-toe-mye′sin)
Func. class.: Antiinfective, antituberculosis
Chem. class.: Aminoglycoside
Pregnancy category D

ACTION: Interferes with protein synthesis in bacterial cell by binding to ribosomal subunit, causing inaccurate peptide sequence to form in protein chain; bactericidal

Therapeutic outcome: Bactericidal effects for the following organisms: sensitive strains of *Mycobacterium tuberculosis,* nontuberculous infections caused by sensitive strains of *Yersinia pestis, Brucella, Haemophilus influenzae, Klebsiella pneumoniae, Escherichia coli, Enterobacter aerogenes, Streptococcus viridans, Francisella tularensis, Proteus*

USES: Active TB; used in combination for streptococcal and enterococcal infections; endocarditis, tularemia, plague

CONTRAINDICATIONS:
Hypersensitivity

BLACK BOX WARNING: Pregnancy D, severe renal disease

Precautions: Breastfeeding, geriatric, neonates, mild renal disease, myasthenia gravis, Parkinson's disease, hepatic disease

⚠ Nurse Alert

BLACK BOX WARNING: Hearing deficits, neuromuscular disease

DOSAGE AND ROUTES

General dosing
Adults: IM 1-2 g in divided doses q6-12hr
Child: IM 20-40 mg/kg/day in divided doses q6-12hr, max adult dose

Tuberculosis (HIV negative)
Adult: IM 15 mg/kg (max 1 g) daily × 2-3 mo, then 1 g 2-3 ×/wk given with other antitubercular products for up to 1 yr
Child: IM 20-40 mg/kg/day; max 1 g/day

Enterococcal endocarditis
Adult: IM, **IV** 15 mg/kg/day divided q12h
Child: IM/**IV** 20-30 mg/kg/day divided q12hr

Available forms: Inj 500 mg ✿, 1 g/ml

Implementation
• Give deeply in large muscle mass
• Reconstitute with 4.2-4.5 ml of sterile water for inj or 0.9% NaCl/1 g (200 mg/ml), 3.2-3.5 ml/1 g (250 mg/ml), 17 ml/5 g (250 mg/ml); give at 500 mg/ml or less

ADVERSE EFFECTS
CNS: Confusion, dizziness, depression, numbness, tremors, **seizures,** muscle twitching, **neurotoxicity,** dizziness, headache
CV: Hypotension, myocarditis, palpitations
EENT: *Ototoxicity,* tinnitus, deafness, visual disturbances
GI: *Nausea, vomiting, anorexia,* increased ALT, AST, bilirubin, hepatomegaly, **hepatic necrosis,** splenomegaly
GU: **Oliguria, hematuria, renal damage, azotemia, renal failure, nephrotoxicity**
HEMA: **Agranulocytosis, thrombocytopenia, leukopenia, eosinophilia, anemia**
INTEG: *Rash,* burning, urticaria, dermatitis, alopecia
MS: Arthralgia, weakness

Pharmacokinetics

Absorption	Well absorbed
Distribution	Widely distributed in extracellular fluids, poorly distributed in CSF; crosses placenta
Metabolism	Minimal—liver
Excretion	Mostly unchanged (>90%) kidneys
Half-life	2-2^1/$_2$ hr, increase in renal disease

Pharmacodynamics

Onset	Rapid
Peak	1-2 hr
Duration	Unknown

INTERACTIONS

Individual drugs
Amphotericin B, cidofovir, CISplatin, ethacrynic acid, furosemide, mannitol, methoxyflurane, polymyxin, tacrolimus, vancomycin: increased ototoxicity, neurotoxicity, nephrotoxicity
Succinylcholine, warfarin: increased effects of streptomycin

Drug classifications
Aminoglycosides, cephalosporins: increased ototoxicity, neurotoxicity, nephrotoxicity
Nondepolarizing neuromuscular blockers, NSAIDs: increased effects of streptomycin

NURSING CONSIDERATIONS

Assessment
• **Infection:** monitor urine, stool, sputum, wound characteristics, fever; monitor WBC for changes
• Assess patient for previous sensitivity reaction
• Complete C&S testing before, after product therapy to identify if correct treatment has been initiated
• **Assess for allergic reactions:** rash, urticaria, pruritus, chills, fever, joint pain; angioedema may occur a few days after therapy begins; EPINEPHrine, resuscitation equipment should be available for anaphylactic reaction
• **Severe renal disease:** identify urine output; if decreasing, notify prescriber (may indicate nephrotoxicity); also increased BUN, creatinine, urine CCr <80 ml/min
• Monitor blood tests: AST, ALT, CBC, Hct, bilirubin, LDH, alkaline phosphatase, Coombs' test monthly if patient is on long-term therapy
• Monitor electrolytes: potassium, sodium, chloride, magnesium monthly if patient is on long-term therapy
• Monitor for bleeding: ecchymosis, bleeding gums, hematuria, stool guaiac daily if on long-term therapy
• Assess for overgrowth of infection: perineal itching, fever, malaise, redness, pain, swelling, drainage, rash, diarrhea, change in cough, sputum
• Obtain weight before treatment; calculation of dosage is usually based on ideal body weight but may be calculated on actual body weight

S

• Monitor I&O ratio; urinalysis daily for proteinuria, cells, casts; report sudden change in urine output
• Obtain serum peak 30-60 min after IM inj, trough level drawn 30-60 min before next dose; therapeutic peak 15-40 mg/L, therapeutic trough <5 mg/L

> **BLACK BOX WARNING: Deafness:** assess by audiometric testing, ringing, roaring in ears, vertigo; assess hearing before, during, after treatment

• **Dehydration:** monitor for high specific gravity, decrease in skin turgor, dry mucous membranes, dark urine

Nursing diagnoses
• Diarrhea (adverse reactions)
• Infection, risk for (uses)
• Injury, risk for (adverse reactions)
• Knowledge, deficient (teaching)
• Noncompliance (teaching)

Patient/family education
• Teach patient to report sore throat, bruising, bleeding, joint pain, may indicate blood dyscrasias (rare); ringing, roaring in the ears
• Advise patient to contact prescriber if vaginal itching, loose foul-smelling stools, furry tongue occur; may indicate superinfection

Evaluation
Positive therapeutic outcome
• Absence of signs/symptoms of infection
• Reported improvement in symptoms of infection

TREATMENT OF OVERDOSE:
Withdraw product, hemodialysis, monitor serum levels of product, may give ticarcillin or carbenicillin

---

succimer (Rx)
(sux′i-mer)
Chemet
Func. class.: Heavy metal antagonist
Chem. class.: Chelating agent
Pregnancy category C

ACTION: Binds with ions of lead to form a water-soluble complex that is excreted by kidneys

Therapeutic outcome: Removal of lead from the body

USES: Lead poisoning in children with lead levels >45 mcg/dl; may be beneficial in mercury, arsenic poisoning

CONTRAINDICATIONS:
Hypersensitivity

Precautions: Pregnancy **C**, breastfeeding, children <1 yr, renal/hepatic disease

DOSAGE AND ROUTES
Adult: PO 10-30 mg/kg/day × 5 days
Child with lead level >45 mcg/dl: PO 10 mg/kg or 350 mg/m^2 q8hr × 5 days, then 10 mg/kg or 350 mg/m^2 q12hr × 2 wk; another course may be required depending on lead levels; allow 2 wk between courses

Available forms: Caps 100 mg

Implementation
• Give whole or cap contents mixed with food or fluid

ADVERSE EFFECTS
CNS: Drowsiness, dizziness, paresthesia, sensorimotor neuropathy
EENT: Otitis media, watery eyes, film in eyes, plugged ears
GI: *Nausea, vomiting, diarrhea, metallic taste, anorexia*
GU: Proteinuria, decreased urination, voiding difficulties
HEMA: Increased platelets, intermittent eosinophilia
INTEG: Rash, urticaria, pruritus
META: Increased AST, ALT, alkaline phosphatase, cholesterol
RESP: Sore throat, rhinorrhea, nasal congestion, cough
SYST: Back, stomach, head, rib, flank pain; abdominal cramps; chills; fever; flulike symptoms; head cold; headache

Pharmacokinetics

Absorption	Rapidly absorbed
Distribution	Unknown
Metabolism	Liver—extensively
Excretion	Kidneys—unchanged
Half-life	2 days

Pharmacodynamics

Onset	Up to 2 hr
Peak	2-4 hr
Duration	8-12 hr

INTERACTIONS
Drug classifications
Heavy metal antagonist, others: do not use together

NURSING CONSIDERATIONS
Assessment
• Assess VS, B/P, pulse, respirations, weigh daily
• Monitor I&O ratio, renal function tests, BUN, creatinine, CCr; watch for decreasing urine output
• Assess neurologic status: watch for paresthesias, beginning of seizures
• Monitor urine: pH, albumin, casts, blood, coproporphyrins, calcium
• Assess for febrile reactions that may occur 4-8 hr after product therapy
• Monitor for cardiac abnormalities: dysrhythmias, hypotension, tachycardia
• Assess for allergic reactions (rash, urticaria); if these occur, product should be discontinued

Nursing diagnoses
• Injury, risk for (uses, adverse reactions)
• Knowledge, deficient (teaching)
• Poisoning, risk for (uses)

Patient/family education
• Explain reason for medication and expected results
• Provide a referral to health department to assess lead levels in home or workplace
• Teach patient to increase fluid intake
• Advise patient that therapeutic effect may take 1-3 months
• Instruct patient to report rash; may occur every time product is used

Evaluation
Positive therapeutic outcome
• Decreased symptoms of lead intoxication
• Decreased lead level <50 mcg/dl

⚠ HIGH ALERT

succinylcholine (Rx)
(suk-sin-ill-koe'leen)
Anectine, Quelicin
Func. class.: Neuromuscular blocker (depolarizing—ultra short)
Pregnancy category C

ACTION: Inhibits transmission of nerve impulses by binding with cholinergic receptor sites, antagonizing action of acetylcholine; causes release of histamine

Therapeutic outcome: Paralysis of skeletal muscles

USES: Facilitation of endotracheal intubation, skeletal muscle relaxation during orthopedic manipulations

CONTRAINDICATIONS:
Hypersensitivity, malignant hyperthermia, trauma

Precautions: Pregnancy **C**, breastfeeding, geriatric or debilitated patients, severe burns, fractures (fasciculation may increase damage), electrolyte imbalances, dehydration, neuromuscular disease, respiratory disease, collagen diseases, glaucoma, eye surgery, renal/hepatic/cardiac disease

> **BLACK BOX WARNING:** Hyperkalemia, myopathy, rhabdomyolysis, children <2 yr

DOSAGE AND ROUTES
Adult: IV 0.3-1.1 mg/kg, max 150 mg, maintenance 0.04-0.07 mg/kg q5-10min as needed; CONT **IV** INF dilute to concentration of 1-2 mg/ml in D₅W or NS 10-100 mcg/kg/min
Child: **IV** initially 1-2 mg/kg; CONT **IV** INF not recommended

Available forms: Inj 20, 50, 100 mg/ml; powder for inj 100, 500 mg/vial, 1 g/vial

Implementation
IM route
• Give inj deep IM, preferably high in deltoid muscle
• Store in refrigerator; store powder at room temperature; close container tightly

IV route
• Use nerve stimulator by anesthesiologist to determine neuromuscular blockade
• Give anticholinesterase to reverse neuromuscular blockade
• Give by **IV** inf; dilute 1-2 mg/ml in D₅, isotonic saline sol, give 0.5-10 mg/min, titrate to patient response; may be given directly over 1 min

Syringe compatibilities: Heparin

Y-site compatibilities: Etomidate, heparin, potassium chloride, propofol, vit B/C

Additive compatibilities: Amikacin, cephapirin, isoproterenol, meperidine, methyldopate, morphine, norepinephrine, scopolamine

Additive incompatibilities: Barbiturates, nafcillin, sodium bicarbonate

---

Adverse effects: *italics* = common; **bold** = life-threatening

ADVERSE EFFECTS

CV: Bradycardia, tachycardia; increased, decreased B/P, **sinus arrest, dysrhythmias,** edema

EENT: Increased secretions, increased intra-ocular pressure

HEMA: Myoglobulinemia

INTEG: Rash, flushing, pruritus, urticaria

MS: Weakness, muscle pain, fasciculation, prolonged relaxation, myalgia, **rhabdomyolysis**

RESP: Prolonged apnea, bronchospasm, cyanosis, respiratory depression, wheezing, dyspnea

SYST: Anaphylaxis, angioedema

Pharmacokinetics

Absorption	Well absorbed (IM)
Distribution	Widely distributed, crosses placenta
Metabolism	Plasma (90%)
Excretion	Hydrolyzed in blood, excreted in urine (active/inactive metabolites)
Half-life	Unknown

Pharmacodynamics

	IM	IV
Onset	2-3 min	1 min
Peak	Unknown	2-3 min
Duration	10-30 min	6-10 min

INTERACTIONS

Individual products
Clindamycin, enflurane, isoflurane, lincomycin, lithium, oxytocin, procainamide, quiNIDine: increased neuromuscular blockade
Theophylline: dysrhythmias

Drug classifications
Aminoglycosides, anesthetics (local), antibiotics (polymyxin), β-adrenergic blockers, cardiac glycosides, magnesium salts, opioids, thiazides: increased neuromuscular blockade

Drug/herb
Melatonin: blocks succinylcholine

NURSING CONSIDERATIONS

Assessment
• Assess for electrolyte imbalances (potassium, magnesium); may lead to increased action of this product
• Monitor VS (B/P, pulse, respirations, airway) until fully recovered; rate, depth, pattern of respirations, strength of hand grip
• Monitor I&O ratio; check for urinary retention, frequency, hesitancy
• **Recovery:** assess for decreased paralysis of face, diaphragm, leg, arm, rest of body
• **Allergic reactions:** assess for rash, fever, respiratory distress, pruritus; product should be discontinued if these occur
• **Myopathy, rhabdomyolysis:** in pediatric patients (rare)

Nursing diagnoses
• Breathing pattern, ineffective (uses)
• Communication, impaired verbal (adverse reactions)

Patient/family education
• Explain reason for medication and expected results
• Provide reassurance if communication is difficult during recovery from neuromuscular blockade; postoperative stiffness is normal, soon subsides

Evaluation
Positive therapeutic outcome
• Paralysis of jaw, eyelid, head, neck, rest of body

TREATMENT OF OVERDOSE:
Edrophonium or neostigmine, atropine, monitor VS; may require mechanical ventilation

sucralfate (Rx)
(soo-kral′fate)
Carafate, Sulcrate ✴
Func. class.: Protectant; antiulcer
Chem. class.: Aluminum hydroxide/sulfated sucrose
Pregnancy category B

Do not confuse:
Carafate/Cafergot

ACTION: Forms a complex that adheres to ulcer site, adsorbs pepsin

Therapeutic outcome: Healing of ulcers

USES: Duodenal ulcer, oral mucositis, stomatitis after radiation of head and neck

Unlabeled uses: Gastric ulcers, gastro-esophageal reflux

CONTRAINDICATIONS:
Hypersensitivity

Precautions: Pregnancy **B**, breastfeeding, children, renal failure, hypoglycemia (diabetics)

DOSAGE AND ROUTES
Duodenal ulcers
Adult: PO 1 g qid 1 hr before meals and at bedtime
Child: PO 40-80 mg/kg/day divided

Available forms: Tabs 1 g; oral susp 1 g/10 ml

Implementation
• Do not break, crush, or chew tabs
• Give on empty stomach 1 hr before meals and at bedtime
• Avoid antacids $^{1}/_{2}$ hr before or 1 hr after taking this product
• Store at room temperature

ADVERSE EFFECTS
CNS: Drowsiness, dizziness
GI: *Dry mouth, constipation,* nausea, gastric pain, vomiting, bezoar (critically ill patients)
INTEG: Urticaria, rash, pruritus

Pharmacokinetics

Absorption	Minimally absorbed
Distribution	Unknown
Metabolism	Not metabolized
Excretion	Feces (90%)
Half-life	6-20 hr

Pharmacodynamics

Onset	$^{1}/_{2}$ hr
Peak	Unknown
Duration	6 hr

INTERACTIONS
Individual drugs
Cimetidine, ranitidine: decreased absorption of sucralfate
Digoxin, ketoconazole, phenytoin, tetracycline, theophylline: decreased action of each specific product

Drug classifications
Antacids: decreased absorption of sucralfate
Fat-soluble vitamins: decreased action of fat-soluble vitamins
Fluoroquinolones: decreased absorption

NURSING CONSIDERATIONS
Assessment
• **GI symptoms:** assess for abdominal pain, blood in stools
• **Hypoglycemia:** may occur in those with diabetes mellitus

Nursing diagnoses
• Constipation (adverse reactions)
• Knowledge, deficient (teaching)
• Pain, acute (uses)
• Pain, chronic (uses)

Patient/family education
• Instruct patient to take medication on empty stomach
• Caution patient to take full course of therapy, not to use >8 wk, to avoid smoking
• Caution patient to avoid antacids within $^{1}/_{2}$ hr of product or 1 hr after this product
• Advise patient to increase fluids, bulk, exercise to lessen constipation

Evaluation
Positive therapeutic outcome
• Absence of pain or GI complaints

---

sulfasalazine (Rx)
(sul-fa-sal'a-zeen)
Azulfidine, Azulfidine EN-tabs, Salazopyrin ✤
Func. class.: GI Antiinflammatory, antirheumatic (DMARD)
Chem. class.: GI Sulfonamide
Pregnancy category B

Do not confuse:
sulfasalazine/sulfiSOXAZOLE

ACTION: Proproduct to deliver sulfapyridine and 5-aminosalicylic acid to colon; antinflammatory in connective tissue

Therapeutic outcome: Treatment of ulcerative colitis, rheumatoid arthritis

USES: Ulcerative colitis, rheumatoid arthritis, juvenile rheumatoid arthritis (Azulfidine EN-tabs)

Unlabeled uses: Crohn's disease

CONTRAINDICATIONS:
Pregnancy at term, children <2 yr, hypersensitivity to sulfonamides or salicylates, intestinal, urinary obstruction, porphyria

Precautions: Pregnancy **B**, breastfeeding, impaired renal/hepatic function, severe allergy, bronchial asthma, megaloblastic anemia

DOSAGE AND ROUTES
Bowel disease
Adult: PO 3-4 g/day in divided doses; maintenance 2 g/day in divided doses q6hr

Child ≥6 yr: PO 40-60 mg/kg/day in 4-6 divided doses, then 30 mg/kg/day in 4 doses, max 2 g/day

Rheumatoid arthritis
Adult: PO 0.5-1 g/day, then increase daily dose by 500 mg qwk to 2 g/day in 2-3 divided doses

Juvenile rheumatoid arthritis
Child ≥6 yr: PO 30-50 mg/kg/24 hr, divided into 2 doses

Renal dose
Adult: PO CCr 10-30 ml/min give bid; CCr <10 ml/min give daily

Available forms: Tabs 500 mg; oral susp 250 mg/5 ml; del rel tabs 500 mg

Implementation
• Give with full glass of water to maintain adequate hydration; increase fluids to 2 L/day to decrease crystallization in kidneys; contact lenses, urine, skin may be yellow-orange
• Give total daily dose in evenly spaced doses and after meals to help minimize GI intolerance
• Give at bedtime
• Store in airtight, light-resistant container at room temperature

ADVERSE EFFECTS
CNS: Headache, confusion, insomnia, hallucinations, depression, vertigo, fatigue, anxiety, **seizures,** product fever, chills
CV: Allergic myocarditis
GI: *Nausea, vomiting, abdominal pain,* stomatitis, **hepatitis,** glossitis, **pancreatitis,** diarrhea
GU: Renal failure, toxic nephrosis, increased BUN, creatinine, crystalluria
HEMA: Leukopenia, neutropenia, thrombocytopenia, agranulocytosis, hemolytic anemia
INTEG: Rash, dermatitis, urticaria, Stevens-Johnson syndrome, erythema, photosensitivity
SYST: Anaphylaxis

Pharmacokinetics
Absorption	Partially absorbed
Distribution	Crosses placenta
Metabolism	Liver
Excretion	Kidneys, breast milk
Half-life	6 hr

Pharmacodynamics
Onset	1 hr
Peak	1¹/₂-6 hr
Duration	6-12 hr

INTERACTIONS
Individual drugs
AzaTHIOprine, mercaptopurine: increased leucopenia risk
CycloSPORINE: decreased effect of cycloSPORINE
Digoxin: decreased digoxin effect
Folic acid: decreased folic acid effect
Methotrexate: decreased renal excretion

Drug classifications
Anticoagulants (oral): increased anticoagulant effect
Hypoglycemics (oral): increased hypoglycemic response

Drug/food
Iron, folic acid will be poorly absorbed

Drug/lab test
False positive: urinary glucose test

NURSING CONSIDERATIONS
Assessment
• Monitor I&O ratio; note color, amount, character, pH of urine if product administered for UTIs; output should be 800 ml less than intake; if urine is highly acidic, alkalization may be needed
• Monitor kidney function tests: BUN, creatinine, urinalysis if on long-term therapy
⚠ **Blood dyscrasias: assess for rash, fever, sore throat, bruising, bleeding, fatigue, joint pain; monitor CBC before and q3mo**
⚠ **Allergic reaction: assess for rash, dermatitis, urticaria, pruritus, dyspnea, bronchospasm**
• **Ulcerative colitis, proctitis, other inflammatory bowel disease:** monitor character, amount, consistency of stools, abdominal pain, cramping, blood, mucus
• **Rheumatoid arthritis:** assess mobility, joint swelling, pain, activities of daily living

Nursing diagnoses
• Injury, risk for (uses)
• Knowledge, deficient (teaching)

Patient/family education
• Advise patient to take each oral dose with full glass of water to prevent crystalluria
• Teach patient to avoid sunlight or to use sunscreen to prevent burns
• Teach patient to avoid OTC medication (aspirin, vit C) unless directed by prescriber
• Advise patient to notify prescriber if skin rash, sore throat, fever, mouth sores, unusual bruising, bleeding occur

⚠ Nurse Alert

• Advise patient to use rectal susp at bedtime and retain all night

Evaluation
Positive therapeutic outcome
• Absence of fever, mucus in stools or pain in joints

---

sulindac (Rx)
(sul-in′dak)
Apo-Sulin ✤, **Clinoril**
Func. class.: Nonsteroidal antiinflammatory, antirheumatic
Chem. class.: Indeneacetic acid derivative
Pregnancy category C/D

Do not confuse:
Clinoril/Clozaril/Oruvail/Cleocin

ACTION: Metabolite inhibits COX-1, COX-2 by blocking arachidonate; analgesic, antiinflammatory, antipyretic

Therapeutic outcome: Decreased pain, inflammation

USES: Mild to moderate pain, osteoarthritis, rheumatoid, gouty arthritis, ankylosing spondylitis, bursitis, tendinitis

CONTRAINDICATIONS:
Hypersensitivity, asthma, severe renal/hepatic disease, active ulcers, pregnancy **D** 3rd trimester

> **BLACK BOX WARNING:** Perioperative pain, in CABG

Precautions: Pregnancy **C** (1st trimester), breastfeeding, children, bleeding disorders, GI/cardiac/renal disorders, hypersensitivity to other antiinflammatory agents, renal disease

> **BLACK BOX WARNING:** GI bleeding, MI stroke

DOSAGE AND ROUTES
Arthritis
Adult: PO 150 mg bid, may increase to 200 mg bid, max 400 mg/day
Child (unlabeled): PO 2-4 mg/kg/day in divided doses, max 6 mg/kg/day or 200 mg bid, whichever is less (safe/effective dose not established)

Bursitis/acute arthritis
Adult: PO 200 mg bid × 1-2 wk, then reduce dose

Available forms: Tabs 150, 200 mg

Implementation
• Do not break, crush, or chew tabs
• Give with full glass of water to enhance absorption
• Administer with food or milk to decrease gastric symptoms; food slows absorption slightly, does not decrease absorption

ADVERSE EFFECTS
CNS: Dizziness, drowsiness, fatigue, tremors, confusion, insomnia, anxiety, depression, *headache*
CV: Tachycardia, peripheral edema, palpitations, dysrhythmias, **MI, stroke, CHF**
EENT: Tinnitus, hearing loss, blurred vision
GI: *Nausea, anorexia, vomiting, diarrhea,* jaundice, **cholestatic hepatitis,** constipation, flatulence, cramps, dry mouth, peptic ulcer, **bleeding, ulceration, perforation;** dyspepsia
GU: **Nephrotoxicity: dysuria, hematuria, oliguria, azotemia**
HEMA: **Blood dyscrasias with prolonged use**
INTEG: Purpura, *rash, pruritus,* sweating, photosensitivity
SYST: **Anaphylaxis, Stevens-Johnson syndrome, toxic epidermal necrolysis**

Pharmacokinetics
Absorption	Well absorbed
Distribution	Not known
Metabolism	Converted to active product in liver
Excretion	Minimal unchanged kidneys, breast milk
Half-life	7.8 hr; 16.4 hr active metabolite

Pharmacodynamics
Onset	Unknown
Peak	2 hr
Duration	Unknown

INTERACTIONS
Individual drugs
Aspirin: increased GI reactions
Clopidogrel, eptifibatide, ticlopidine, tirofiban, valproic acid: increased bleeding risk
CycloSPORINE: increased nephrotoxicity
Methotrexate, probenecid: increased toxicity

Drug classifications
Antacids: decreased sulindac effect
Anticoagulants, SNRIs, SSRIs, thrombolytics: increased bleeding risk

---

Adverse effects: *italics* = common; **bold** = life-threatening

S

Antihypertensives: decreased antihypertensive effect

Glucocorticoids, NSAIDs: increased GI reactions

Quinolones (norfloxacin, floxacin, levofloxacin): increased CNS stimulation, seizures

Sulfonamides, sulfonylurea, aminoglycosides: increased toxicity

Drug/herb

Garlic, ginger: increased bleeding risk

Feverfew: decreased feverfew effect

NURSING CONSIDERATIONS

Assessment

> **BLACK BOX WARNING:** Do not use for perioperative pain in CABG

• Monitor blood counts during therapy; watch for decreasing platelets; if low, therapy may need to be discontinued, restarted after hematologic recovery; for blood dyscrasia (thrombocytopenia): bruising, fatigue, bleeding, poor healing

• Assess **pain:** frequency, intensity, characteristics, relief 1-2 hr after medication

• Assess for asthma, aspirin hypersensitivity, nasal polyps; hypersensitivity may develop, watch for rash

> **BLACK BOX WARNING: Cardiac status:** assess for CV thrombotic events, MI, stroke; may be fatal

> **BLACK BOX WARNING: GI status:** assess for ulceration, bleeding, perforation; may be fatal

Nursing diagnoses

• Injury, risk for (adverse reactions)
• Knowledge, deficient (teaching)
• Mobility, impaired physical (uses)
• Pain, chronic (uses)

Patient/family education

• Advise patient that product must be continued for prescribed time to be effective; to avoid aspirin, NSAIDs, alcoholic beverages

• Caution patient to report bleeding, bruising, fatigue, malaise because blood dyscrasias do occur

• Instruct patient to use caution when driving; drowsiness, dizziness may occur

• Teach patient to take with a full glass of water to enhance absorption

• Advise patient to inform all health care providers that product is used

Evaluation
Positive therapeutic outcome

• Decreased pain
• Decreased inflammation
• Increased mobility

SUMAtriptan (Rx)

(soo-ma-trip′tan)
ALSUMA Auto-injector, Imitrex, Sumavel Dose Pro
Func. class.: Antimigraine agent
Chem. class.: 5-HT$_1$ receptor agonist
Pregnancy category C

Do not confuse:
SUMAtriptan/somatropin

ACTION: Binds selectively to the vascular 5-HT$_1$ receptor subtype and exerts antimigraine effect; causes vasoconstriction in cranial arteries

Therapeutic outcome: Absence of migraines

USES: Acute treatment of migraine with or without aura and cluster headache

CONTRAINDICATIONS:

Angina pectoris, history of MI, documented silent ischemia, Prinzmetal's angina, ischemic heart disease, **IV** use, concurrent ergotamine-containing preparations, uncontrolled hypertension, hypersensitivity, basilar or hemiplegic migraine

Precautions: Pregnancy **C**, breastfeeding, children <18 yr, postmenopausal women, men >40 yr, geriatric, risk factors for CAD, hypercholesterolemia, obesity, diabetes, impaired renal/hepatic function

DOSAGE AND ROUTES

Adult: SUBCUT 6 mg or less, may repeat in 1 hr, max 12 mg/24 hr; PO 25 mg with fluids if no relief in 2 hr, give another dose, max 200 mg/day; NASAL 1 dose of 5, 10, or 20 mg in one nostril, may repeat in 2 hr, max 40 mg/24 hr, 1 puff each nostril q2hr

Hepatic dose

Adult: PO 25 mg, if no response after 2 hr, give up to 50 mg

Available forms: Inj 4, 6 mg/0.5 ml; tabs 25, 50, 100 mg; nasal spray 5 mg/100 mcl-units dose spray device 20 mg/100 mcl-units

---

Implementation
PO route
• Swallow tab whole; do not break, crush, or chew
• Take with fluids as soon as symptoms appear; may take a second dose >4 hr, max 200 mg/24 hr
SUBCUT route
• Give by SUBCUT route only, avoid IM or **IV** administration, use only for actual migraine attack
• Give 1st dose supervised by medical staff in those with CAD or those at risk for CAD
Nasal route
• Spray once in 1 nostril, may repeat if headache returns, do not repeat if pain continues after 1st dose

ADVERSE EFFECTS
CNS: *Tingling, hot sensation, burning, feeling of pressure, tightness, numbness, dizziness, sedation,* headache, anxiety, fatigue, cold sensation
CV: *Flushing,* **MI,** hypo/hypertension
EENT: Throat, mouth, nasal discomfort, vision changes
GI: Abdominal discomfort
INTEG: *Inj site reaction,* sweating
MS: *Weakness, neck stiffness,* myalgia
RESP: Chest tightness, pressure

Pharmacokinetics

Absorption	Well absorbed (SUBCUT)
Distribution	10%-20% plasma protein binding
Metabolism	Liver (metabolite)
Excretion	Urine, feces
Half-life	2 hr

Pharmacodynamics

	SUBCUT
Onset	10-20 min
Peak	10 min-2 hr
Duration	Up to 24 hr (pain relief)

INTERACTIONS
Individual drugs
Ergotamine: increased risk of vasospastic reaction

Drug classifications
Ergot derivatives: extended vasospastic effects
MAOIs, SSRIs, SNRIs, serotonin-receptor agonists: increased SUMAtriptan levels

Drug/herb
SAM-e, St. John's wort: serotonin syndrome

NURSING CONSIDERATIONS
Assessment
• **Serotonin syndrome:** assess for delirium, coma, agitation, diaphoresis, hypertension, fever, tremors, may resemble neuroleptic malignant syndrome (in patients taking SSRIs, SNRIs)
• Assess for tingling, hot sensation, burning, feeling of pressure, numbness, flushing, inj site reaction
• Assess B/P; signs/symptoms of coronary vasospasm
• Monitor stress level, activity, reaction, coping mechanisms of patient
• Assess neurologic status: LOC, blurring vision, nausea, vomiting, tingling in extremities preceding headache
• Assess for ingestion of tyramine-containing foods (pickled products, beer, wine, aged cheese), food additives, preservatives, colorings, artificial sweeteners, chocolate, caffeine, which may precipitate these types of headaches

Nursing diagnoses
• Knowledge, deficient (teaching)
• Pain, chronic (uses)

Patient/family education
• Caution patient not to take more than 2 doses/day or 12 mg/day; allow at least 1 hr between doses
• Caution patient to avoid driving or hazardous activities if dizziness or drowsiness occurs
• Teach patient to report chest tightness, heat, flushing, drowsiness, dizziness, fatigue, sudden severe abdominal pain or any allergic reactions that occur to prescriber immediately
• Inform patient to report any side effects to prescriber
• Caution patient to use contraception when taking product, to notify prescriber if pregnancy is suspected or planned
• **Nasal spray:** one spray in one nostril, may repeat if headache returns, do not repeat if pain continues after 1st dose

Evaluation
Positive therapeutic outcome
• Decrease in frequency, severity of headache

S

sunitinib (Rx)

(soo-nit'-in-ib)

Sutent

Func. class.: Antineoplastic—miscellaneous

Chem. class.: Protein-tyrosine kinase inhibitor

Pregnancy category D

ACTION: Inhibits multiple receptor tyrosine kinases (RTKs), some are responsible for tumor growth

Therapeutic outcome: Decrease in size of tumor

USES: Gastrointestinal stromal tumors (GIST) after disease progression or intolerance to imatinib; advanced renal carcinoma, pancreatic neuroendocrine tumors (pNET) in those with unresectable locally advanced/metastatic disease

CONTRAINDICATIONS:

Pregnancy **D**, breastfeeding, hypersensitivity

Precautions: Children, geriatric, active infections, QT prolongation, torsades de pointes, stroke, heart failure

DOSAGE AND ROUTES

Gastrointestinal stromal tumors (GIST)/renal cell cancer

Adult: PO 50 mg/day × 4 wk, then 2 wk off; may increase or decrease dose by 12.5 mg; if administered with CYP3A4 inducers, give 87.5 mg/day; if given with CYP3A4 inhibitors give 37.5 mg/day

Pancreatic neuroendocrine (pNET)

Adult: PO 37.5 mg q day continuously, increase or decrease by 12.5 mg based on tolerance, avoid potent CYP3A4 inhibitors/inducers, if used with CYP3A4 inhibitor decrease sunitinib dose to a minimum of 25 mg/day; if used with CYP3A4 inducer increase sunitinib to a max of 62.5 mg/day

Available forms: Caps 12.5, 25, 50 mg

Implementation

• Give with meal and large glass of water to decrease GI symptoms
• Give nutritious diet with iron, vitamin supplement, low fiber, few dairy products
• Store at 25°C (77°F)

ADVERSE EFFECTS

CNS: CNS hemorrhage, headache, dizziness, insomnia, seizures, fatigue

CV: Hypertension, left ventricular dysfunction; QT prolongation, cardiotoxicity, thrombotic microangiopathy, torsades de pointes

ENDO: Hyper/hypothyroidism

GI: *Nausea*, hepatotoxicity, vomiting, dyspepsia, *anorexia, abdominal pain,* altered taste, *constipation,* stomatitis, mucositis, pancreatitis, diarrhea, GI bleeding/perforation

GU: Nephrotic syndrome

HEMA: Neutropenia, thrombocytopenia, hemolytic anemia, leukopenia

INTEG: *Rash, yellow skin discoloration,* depigmentation of hair or skin, alopecia

MS: Pain, arthralgia, myalgia, myopathy, rhabdomyolysis

RESP: Cough, dyspnea, pulmonary embolism

SYST: Bleeding, electrolyte abnormalities, hand-foot syndrome, serious infection

Pharmacokinetics

Absorption	Unknown
Distribution	Protein binding 95%
Metabolism	By CYP3A4
Excretion	Feces, small amount in urine
Half-life	Terminal 40-60 hr (sunitinib); active metabolite 80-110 hr

Pharmacodynamics

Onset	Unknown
Peak	6-12 hr
Duration	Unknown

INTERACTIONS

Individual drugs

Acetaminophen: increased hepatotoxicity

Bevacizumab: microangiopathic hemolytic anemia; avoid concurrent use

Dexamethasone, carBAMazepine, PHENobarbital, phenytoin, rifampin: decreased sunitinib concentrations

Haloperidol, chloroquine, droperidol, pentamidine, arsenic trioxide, levomethadyl: increased QT prolongation

Simvastatin: increased plasma concentrations

Warfarin: increased plasma concentration; avoid use with warfarin, use low-molecular-weight anticoagulants instead

Drug classifications

Calcium channel blockers: increased plasma concentrations

Class IA/III antidysrhythmics, some phenothiazines, β-agonists, local anesthetics, tricyclics, CYP3A4 inhibitors (amiodarone, clarithromycin, erythromycin, telithromycin, troleandomycin), CYP3A4 substrates (methadone, pimozide, QUEtiapine, quiNIDine, risperidone, ziprasidone): increased QT prolongation

Drug/herb

St. John's wort: decreased sunitinib concentration

Drug/food

Grapefruit juice: increased plasma concentrations

NURSING CONSIDERATIONS

Assessment

• Monitor ANC and platelets; if ANC $<1 \times 10^9$/L and/or platelets $<50 \times 10^9$/L, stop until ANC $>1.5 \times 10^9$/L and platelets $>75 \times 10^9$/L; if ANC $<0.5 \times 10^9$/L and/or platelets $<10 \times 10^9$/L, reduce dose by 200 mg; if cytopenia continues, reduce dose by another 100 mg; if cytopenia continues for 4 wk, stop product until ANC $\geq 1 \times 10^9$/L

• Assess CV status: hypertension, QT prolongation can occur; monitor left ventricular ejection fraction (LVEF) (MUGA) baseline periodically, ECG, B/P

• Assess for **renal toxicity:** if bilirubin $>3 \times$ IULN, withhold sunitinib until bilirubin levels return to $<1.5 \times$ IULN; electrolytes

• **Hepatotoxicity:** monitor liver function tests, before treatment and qmo; if liver transaminases $>5 \times$ IULN, withhold sunitinib until transaminase levels return to $<2.5 \times$ IULN

• Assess for **CHF:** adrenal insufficiency in those experiencing trauma

• Assess for bleeding: epistaxis rectal, gingival, upper GI, genital, wound bleeding; tumor-related hemorrhage may occur rapidly

Nursing diagnoses

• Injury, risk for (uses, adverse reactions)
• Knowledge, deficient (teaching)

Patient/family education

• Advise patient to report adverse reactions immediately: shortness of breath, bleeding
• Teach patient reason for treatment, expected result
• Teach patient that many adverse reactions may occur: high B/P, bleeding, mouth swelling, taste change, skin discoloration, depigmentation of hair/skin
• Teach patient to avoid persons with known upper respiratory infections; immunosuppression is common
• Teach to avoid grapefruit juice
• Teach patient to report if pregnancy is planned or suspected, pregnancy **D**

Evaluation
Positive therapeutic outcome
• Decrease in size of tumor

suprofen ophthalmic
See Appendix B

tacrolimus (Rx) (PO, IV)
(tak-roe'li-mus)
Prograf
tacrolimus (topical) (Rx)
Protopic
Func. class.: Immunosuppressant
Chem. class.: Macrolide
Pregnancy category C

ACTION: Produces immunosuppression by inhibiting lymphocytes (T)

Therapeutic outcome: Prevention of rejection in organ transplant

USES: Organ transplants, to prevent rejection; **topical:** atopic dermatitis

Unlabeled uses: Severe recalcitrant psoriasis

CONTRAINDICATIONS:
Hypersensitivity to this product or to some kinds of castor oil, long-term use (topical), child <2 yr (topical)

Precautions: Pregnancy **C,** breastfeeding, children <12 yr, severe renal/hepatic disease, diabetes mellitus, hyperkalemia, hyperuricemia, lymphomas, hypertension

DOSAGE AND ROUTES

Kidney transplant rejection prophylaxis
Adult: IV 0.03-0.05 mg/kg/day as cont INF, give no sooner than 6 hr after transplantation

Liver transplant rejection prophylaxis
Adult: PO 0.10-0.15 mg/kg/day in 2 divided doses q12h, give no sooner than 6 hr after

T

transplantation; **IV** 0.03-0.05 mg/kg/day as a cont INF, give no sooner than 6 hr after transplantation

Heart transplant rejection prophylaxis
Adult: PO 0.075 mg/kg/day in 2 divided doses q12h, give no sooner than 6 hr after transplantation; **IV** 0.01 mg/kg/day as a cont INF, give no sooner than 6 hr after transplantation

Atopic dermatitis
Adult: TOP use 0.03% or 0.1% ointment, apply bid × 7 day after clearing of signs
Child 2-5 yr: TOP 0.03% ointment, apply bid × 7 day after clearing of signs

Available forms: Inj **IV** 5 mg/ml; caps 0.5, 1, 5 mg; ointment 0.03%, 0.1%

Implementation
PO route
- Give with meals to reduce GI upset; nausea is common
- Give for several days before transplant surgery; patients should be placed in protective isolation

Continuous IV infusion route
- Give after diluting in 0.9% NaCl or D₅W to a concentration of 0.004-0.02 mg/ml as a cont inf

Y-site compatibilities: Alemtuzumab, alfentanil, amifostine, amikacin, aminophylline, amiodarone, amphotericin B colloidal, amphotericin B liposome, anidulafungin, atracurium, aztreonam, benztropine, bivalirudin, bleomycin, bumetanide, buprenorphine, busulfan, butorphanol, calcium acetate/chloride/gluconate, CARBOplatin, carmustine, caspofungin, ceFAZolin, cefoperazone, cefotaxime, cefotetan, cefoxitin, ceftazidime, ceftizoxime, cefTRIAXone, cefuroxime, chloramphenicol, chlorproMAZINE, cimetidine, ciprofloxacin, cisatracurium, CISplatin, clindamycin, cyclophosphamide, cycloSPORINE, cytarabine, DACTINomycin, DAPTOmycin, dexamethasone, dexmedetomidine, dexrazoxane, digoxin, diltiazem, diphenhydrAMINE, DOBUTamine, docetaxel, dolasetron, DOPamine, doripenem, doxacurium, DOXOrubicin hydrochloride, doxycycline, droperidol, enalaprilat, ePHEDrine, EPINEPHrine, epirubicin, ertapenem, erythromycin, esmolol, etoposide, etoposide phosphate, famotidine, fenoldopam, fentaNYL, fluconazole, fludarabine, foscarnet, fosphenytoin, gemcitabine, gentamicin, glycopyrrolate, granisetron, haloperidol, heparin, hydrALAZINE, hydrocortisone, HYDROmorphone, IDArubicin, ifosfamide, imipenem/cilastatin, inamrinone, insulin, isoproterenol, ketorolac, labetalol, leucovorin, levofloxacin, levorphanol, lidocaine, linezolid, LORazepam, magnesium sulfate, mannitol, mechlorethamine, meperidine, meropenem, mesna, metaraminol, methotrexate, methyldopa, methylPREDNISolone, metoclopramide, metoprolol, metroNIDAZOLE, micafungin, midazolam, milrinone, mitomycin, mitoxantrone, mivacurium, morphine, multivitamins, nafcillin, nalbuphine, naloxone, nesiritide, niCARdipine, nitroglycerin, nitroprusside, norepinephrine, octreotide, ondansetron, oxacillin, oxaliplatin, oxytocin, paclitaxel, palonosetron, pancuronium, pemetrexed, penicillin G, pentamidine, pentazocine, perphenazine, phentolamine, phenylephrine, piperacillin/tazobactam, potassium chloride/phosphates, procainamide, prochlorperazine, promethazine, propranolol, quinupristin/dalfopristin, ranitidine, remifentanil, rocuronium, sodium acetate/bicarbonate/phosphates, streptozocin, succinylcholine, SUFentanil, teniposide, theophylline, thiotepa, ticarcillin/clavulanate, tigecycline, tirofiban, tobramycin, tolazoline, trimethobenzamide, vancomycin, vasopressin, vecuronium, verapamil, vinCRIStine, vinorelbine, voriconazole, zidovudine, zoledronic acid

Y-site incompatibilities: Acyclovir, allopurinol, azaTHIOprine, cefepime, dantrolene, diazepam, diazoxide, espmeprazole, folic acid, ganciclovir, iron sucrose, levothyroxine, omeprazole, phenytoin, thiopental

ADVERSE EFFECTS
CNS: *Tremors, headache,* insomnia, paresthesia, chills, fever, **seizures,** posterior reversible encephalopathy syndrome, BK-virus-associated nephropathy
CV: Hypertension, myocardial hypertrophy, **prolonged QTc**
EENT: Blurred vision, photophobia
GI: Nausea, vomiting, diarrhea, constipation, GI bleeding
GU: Urinary tract infections, **albuminuria, hematuria, proteinuria, renal failure**
HEMA: Anemia, **leukocytosis, thrombocytopenia, purpura**
INTEG: Rash, flushing, itching, alopecia
META: Hirsutism, hyperglycemia, hyperuricemia, hypo/hyperkalemia, hypomagnesemia
MS: Back pain, muscle spasms
RESP: Pleural effusion, atelectasis, dyspnea, **interstitial lung disease**
SYST: Anaphylaxis

Pharmacokinetics

Absorption	Erractically absorbed (PO), completely absorbed (**IV**)
Distribution	Crosses placenta, 75% protein binding
Metabolism	Liver to metabolite
Excretion	Kidney—minimal; breast milk, bile
Half-life	10 hr

Pharmacodynamics

	PO	IV
Onset	Unknown	Unknown
Peak	1-4 hr	Unknown
Duration	12 hr	12 hr

INTERACTIONS

Individual drugs

CarBAMazepine, PHENobarbital, phenytoin, rifamycin: decreased blood levels

Cimetidine, danazol, erythromycin, mycophenolate, mofetil: increased blood levels

CISplatin, cycloSPORINE: increased toxicity

Haloperidol, chloroquine, droperidol, pentamidine, arsenic trioxide, levomethadyl; CYP3A4 substrates (methadone, pimozide, QUEtiapine, quiNIDine, risperidone, ziprasidone): increased QT prolongation

Ibuprofen: increased oliguria

Drug classifications

Aminoglycosides: increased toxicity

Antifungals, calcium channel blockers: increased blood levels

Class IA/III antidysrhythmics, some phenothiazines, β-agonists, local anesthetics, tricyclics, CYP3A4 inhibitors (amiodarone, clarithromycin, erythromycin, telithromycin, troleandomycin), CYP3A4 substrates (methadone, pimozide, QUEtiapine, quiNIDine, risperidone, ziprasidone): increased QT prolongation

Vaccines: decreased effect

Drug/herb

Astragalus, echinacea, melatonin: decreased immunosuppression

Ginseng, St. John's wort: decreased effect

NURSING CONSIDERATIONS

Assessment

• Monitor blood studies: Hgb, WBC, platelets during treatment monthly; if WBC is <3000/mm³ or platelet count <100,000/mm³, product should be discontinued or reduced; decreased

Hgb level may indicate bone marrow suppression

• **QT prolongation:** ECG for QT prolongation, ejection fraction; assess for chest pain, palpitations, dyspnea

• Monitor liver function tests: alkaline phosphatase, AST, ALT, amylase, bilirubin, and for hepatotoxicity: dark urine, jaundice, itching, light-colored stools; product should be discontinued

• Monitor serum creatinine/BUN, serum electrolytes, lipid profile, serum tacrolimus concentration

⚠ **Assess for anaphylaxis: rash, pruritus, wheezing, laryngeal edema; stop inf, initiate emergency procedures**

Nursing diagnoses

• Infection, risk for (uses)
• Knowledge, deficient (teaching)

Patient/family education

> **BLACK BOX WARNING:** Advise patient to report if pregnancy is planned or suspected

> **BLACK BOX WARNING:** Advise patient to report symptoms of lymphoma

• Instruct patient to report fever, rash, severe diarrhea, chills, sore throat, fatigue because serious infections may occur; clay-colored stools, cramping may indicate hepatotoxicity, signs of diabetes mellitus

• Caution patient to avoid crowds or persons with known infections to reduce risk of infection, to avoid eating raw shellfish

Evaluation

Positive therapeutic outcome

• Absence of graft rejection
• Immunosuppression in autoimmune disorders

tadalafil (Rx)

(tah-dal′a-fil)

Adcirca, Cialis

Func. class.: Impotence agent

Chem. class.: Phosphodiesterase type 5 inhibitor

Pregnancy category B

ACTION: Inhibits phosphodiesterase type 5 (PDE5); enhances erectile function by increasing the amount of cyclic GMP, which causes smooth muscle relaxation and increased blood flow into the corpus cavernosum; improves erectile function for up to 36 hr

Therapeutic outcome: Erection

USES: Treatment of erectile dysfunction; pulmonary arterial hypertension (PAH) (Adcirca only)

CONTRAINDICATIONS:

Newborns, women, children, hypersensitivity, patients taking organic nitrates regularly or intermittently, patients taking any α-adrenergic antagonist other than 0.4 mg once-daily tamsulosin

Precautions: Pregnancy **B,** although not indicated for women, anatomic penile deformities, sickle cell anemia, leukemia, multiple myeloma, CV/renal/hepatic disease, bleeding disorders, active peptic ulcer, prolonged erection

DOSAGE AND ROUTES

Erectile dysfunction
Adult: PO CCr 51-80 ml/min erectile dysfunction no adjustment; 20 mg/day initially, pulmonary hypertension; 10 mg, taken prior to sexual activity, dose may be reduced to 5 mg or increased to a max of 20 mg; usual max dosing frequency is once per day; once-daily dosing 2.5 mg/day at same time each day

Renal dose
Adult: PO CCr 31-50 ml/min 5 mg/day, max 10 mg q48hr; CCr <30 ml/min, max 5 mg q72hr

Hepatic dose
Adult: PO Child-Pugh class A, B, max 10 mg/day or 20 mg/day (pulmonary hypertension) max 40 mg/day; Child-Pugh class C, not recommended

Concomitant medications
Ketoconazole, itraconazole, ritonavir, max 10 mg q72hr

Pulmonary hypertension
Adult: PO **(Adcirca only)** 40 mg qd; **Adult taking ritonavir:** PO 20 mg qd initially, then increase to 40 mg qd as tolerated

Available forms: Tabs 2.5, 5, 10, 20 mg; tab 20 mg (Adcirca)

Implementation
• **Sexual dysfunction:** give before sexual activity; do not use more than once a day
• **Pulmonary hypertension:** give Adcirca without regard to meals

ADVERSE EFFECTS
CNS: *Headache, flushing, dizziness,* seizures, transient global amnesia
CV: MI, hypotension, **QT prolongation**
INTEG: Stevens-Johnson syndrome, exfoliative dermatitis, urticaria
MISC: Back pain/myalgia, *dyspepsia, nasal congestion, UTI,* blurred vision, changes in color vision, *diarrhea,* pruritus, priapism, **nonarteritic ischemic optic neuropathy (NAION),** hearing loss

Pharmacokinetics

Absorption	Rapid; rate and extent of absorption of tadalafil are not influenced by food
Distribution	94% protein bound
Metabolism	Liver
Excretion	Excreted primarily as metabolites, feces, urine; plasma concentration 61% in feces, 36% in urine
Half-life	17.5 hr

Pharmacodynamics

Onset	Rapid
Peak	6 hr
Duration	Unknown

INTERACTIONS

Individual drugs
Alcohol, amlodipine, enalapril: decreased B/P
Bosentan: decreased effects of tadalafil
Itraconazole, ketoconazole, ritonavir: increased levels (although not studied, may also include other HIV protease inhibitors)

Drug classifications
⚠ Do not use with nitrates because of unsafe drop in B/P that could result in heart attack or stroke
α-blockers, angiotensin II receptor blockers: decreased B/P
Antacids: decreased effects of tadalafil

Drug/food
Grapefruit: increased tadalafil effect

NURSING CONSIDERATIONS
Assessment
• **Cialis:** assess for erectile dysfunction prior to treatment; organic nitrates that should not be used with this product; assess for severe loss of vision
• **Adcirca:** monitor hemodynamic parameters baseline and periodically

Nursing diagnoses
• Knowledge, deficient (teaching)
• Sexual dysfunction (uses)

Patient/family education
• Advise that product does not protect against STDs, including HIV
• Instruct to tell physician if patient has a bleeding problem
• Advise that product should not be used with nitrates in any form
• Advise that product has no effect in the absence of sexual stimulation
• Instruct to seek medical help if an erection lasts more than 4 hr
• Advise to tell physician of all medicines, vitamins, and herbs patient is taking, especially α-blockers, erythromycin, indinavir, itraconazole, ketoconozole, nitrates, ritonavir
• **Advise that tadalafil is contraindicated for use with α-blockers except 0.4 mg/daily tamsulosin**

Evaluation
Positive therapeutic outcome
• Sustainable erection
• Improvement in exercise ability (pulmonary hypertension)

tamoxifen (Rx)
(ta-mox′i-fen)
Apo-Tamox ✦, Nolvadex, Tamofen ✦
Func. class.: Antineoplastic
Chem. class.: Antiestrogen hormone
Pregnancy category D

ACTION: Inhibits cell division by binding to cytoplasmic estrogen receptors; resembles normal cell complex but inhibits DNA synthesis and estrogen response of target tissue

Therapeutic outcome: Prevention of rapidly growing malignant cells

USES: Advanced breast carcinoma that has not responded to other therapy in estrogen receptor–positive patients (usually postmenopausal), prevention of breast cancer, after breast surgery/radiation in ductal carcinoma in situ (DCIS)

Unlabeled uses: Mastalgia, pain/size of gynecomastia, ovulation stimulation, malignant carcinoid tumor, carcinoid syndrome, metaplastic melanoma, desmoid tumors, McCune-Albright syndrome (female pediatric patients)

CONTRAINDICATIONS:
Pregnancy **D**, breastfeeding, hypersensitivity

> **BLACK BOX WARNING:** Thromboembolic disease

Precautions: Leukopenia, thrombocytopenia, cataracts, women of childbearing age

> **BLACK BOX WARNING:** Endometrial cancer, stroke

DOSAGE AND ROUTES
Breast cancer
Adult: PO 20-40 mg/day × 5 yr, doses >20 mg/day divide AM/PM

High risk for breast cancer
Adult: PO 20 mg/day × 5 yr

Ductal carcinoma in situ
Adult: PO 20 mg/day × 5 yr

McCune-Albright syndrome (unlabeled)
Child 2-10 yr (girls): PO 20 mg/day for up to 1 yr

Available forms: Tabs 10, 20 mg

Implementation
• Do not break, crush, or chew tabs
• Give with food or fluids for GI upset; repeat dose may be needed if vomiting occurs
• Store in light-resistant container at room temperature

ADVERSE EFFECTS
CNS: *Hot flashes, headache, lightheadedness,* depression, mood changes
CV: Chest pain, stroke, fluid retention, flushing
EENT: Ocular lesions, cataracts, retinopathy, corneal opacity, blurred vision (high doses)
GI: *Nausea, vomiting,* altered taste (anorexia)
GU: Vaginal bleeding, pruritus vulvae, uterine malignancies, *altered menses, amenorrhea*
HEMA: Thrombocytopenia, leukopenia, deep vein thrombosis
INTEG: *Rash,* alopecia
META: Hypercalcemia
RESP: Pulmonary embolism

Pharmacokinetics
Absorption	Adequately absorbed
Distribution	Unknown
Metabolism	Liver—extensively
Excretion	Feces—slowly, small amounts (kidneys)
Half-life	1 wk

T

Adverse effects: *italics* = common; **bold** = life-threatening

Pharmacodynamics

Onset	Unknown
Peak	4-7 hr
Duration	Unknown

INTERACTIONS

Individual drugs

Aminoglutethimide, rifamycin: decreased tamoxifen levels

Bromocriptine: increased tamoxifen level

Letrozole: decreased levels of letrozole

PARoxetine: increased risk for death from breast cancer

Radiation: increased myelosuppression

Drug classifications

Anticoagulants: increased risk of bleeding

Cytotoxics: increased thromboembolic action

CYP2D6 inhibitors (antidepressants): decreased tamoxifen effect

CYP3A4 inducers (barbiturates, bosentan, carBAMazepine, efavirenz, phenytoin, nevirapine, rifabutin, rifampin): decreased tamoxifen effect

CYP3A4 inhibitors (aprepitant, antiretroviral protease inhibitors, clarithromycin, danazol, delavirdine, diltiazem, erythromycin, fluconazole, FLUoxetine, fluvoxamine, imatinib, ketoconazole, mibefradil, nefazodone, telithromycin, voriconazole): increased toxicity

Drug/herb

Black cohosh, dong quai, St. John's wort: avoid use

Drug/lab test

Increased: serum calcium, T_4, AST, ALT, cholesterol, triglycerides

NURSING CONSIDERATIONS

Assessment

• Monitor CBC, differential, platelet count weekly; withhold product if WBC is <4000/mm^3 or platelet count is <75,000/mm^3; notify prescriber of results; monitor calcium levels (hypercalcemia is common); breast exam, mammogram, pregnancy test, bone mineral density, LFTs, serum calcium, serum lipid profile

⚠ Assess for tumor flare: increase in bone, tumor pain during beginning treatment; give analgesics as ordered to decrease pain

• Assess for bleeding: hematuria, guaiac, bruising or petechiae, mucosa or orifices q8hr, no rectal temp

> **BLACK BOX WARNING: Assess for uterine malignancies:** symptoms of stroke, PE that may occur in women with DCIS and women at high risk for breast cancer

Nursing diagnoses

• Injury, risk for (adverse reactions)
• Knowledge, deficient (teaching)

Patient/family education

• Instruct patient to report any complaints, side effects to prescriber; if dose is missed, do not double next dose; that use may be 5 yr

• Advise patient that vaginal bleeding, pruritus, hot flashes can occur and are reversible after discontinuing treatment

• Instruct patient to report immediately decreased visual acuity, which may be irreversible; stress need for routine eye exams

• Inform patient about who should be told about tamoxifen therapy

• Advise patient to report vaginal bleeding immediately; that tumor flare (increase in size or tumor, increased bone pain) may occur and will subside rapidly; may take analgesics for pain; that premenopausal women must use mechanical birth control method because ovulation may be induced (teratogenic product)

• **Tumor flare:** Advise patient that increase in size of tumor, increased bone pain may occur and will subside rapidly; may take analgesics for pain

• Teach patient that hair loss may occur during treatment; a wig or hairpiece may make patient feel better; new hair may be different in color, texture

• Advise patient to increase fluids to 2 L/day unless contraindicated

Evaluation

Positive therapeutic outcome

• Decreased spread of malignant cells in breast cancer

---

tamsulosin (Rx)

(tam-sue-lo'sen)

Flomax

Func. class.: Selective α-adrenergic blocker, BPH agent

Chem. class.: Sulfamoyl phenethylamine derivative

Pregnancy category B

Do not confuse:
Flomax/Fosamax/Volmax

ACTION: Binds preferentially to α IA-adrenoceptor subtype located mainly in the prostate

Therapeutic outcome: Decreased symptoms of benign prostatic hyperplasia (BPH)

USES: Symptoms of BPH

CONTRAINDICATIONS:
Hypersensitivity

Precautions: Pregnancy **B**, breastfeeding, children, hepatic disease, CAD, severe renal disease, prostate cancer; cataract surgery (floppy iris syndrome)

DOSAGE AND ROUTES
Adult: PO 0.4 mg/day, increasing to 0.8 mg/day if required

Available forms: Caps 0.4 mg

Implementation
• Swallow caps whole; do not break, crush, or chew
• Store in airtight container at 86° F (30° C) or less
• May be given with food to prevent GI symptoms; ½ hr after same meal each day

ADVERSE EFFECTS
CNS: *Dizziness, headache,* asthenia, insomnia
CV: Chest pain, orthostatic hypotension
EENT: Amblyopia, floppy iris syndrome
GI: Nausea, diarrhea, dysgeusia
GU: Decreased libido, abnormal ejaculation, priapism
MS: Back pain
RESP: Rhinitis, pharyngitis, cough
SYST: **Angioedema**

Pharmacokinetics

Absorption	Well absorbed
Distribution	Not known; 98% plasma protein bound
Metabolism	Liver, extensively
Excretion	Kidneys
Half-life	9-15 hr

Pharmacodynamics
Unknown

INTERACTIONS
Individual drugs
Cimetidine: increased toxicity
Doxazosin, prazosin, terazosin, vardenafil: do not use together

Drug classifications
α-blockers: do not use together
Drug/food
Decreased: absorption with food

NURSING CONSIDERATIONS
Assessment
• Monitor CBC with differential and liver function tests; B/P and heart rate
• Monitor urodynamic studies/urinary flow rates, residual volume
• **Assess for BPH:** change in urinary patterns, baseline, throughout treatment; monitor I&O ratios, weight daily, edema, report weight gain or edema
• **Orthostatic hypotension:** monitor B/P standing, sitting

Nursing diagnoses
• Cardiac output, decreased (uses)
• Injury, risk for (side effects)
• Knowledge, deficient (teaching)
• Noncompliance (teaching)

Patient/family education
• Teach patient not to discontinue product abruptly; emphasize the importance of complying with dosage schedule, even if feeling better; if dose is missed take as soon as remembered; take at same time each day
• Teach patient not to use OTC products (cough, cold, allergy) unless directed by prescriber; also to avoid large amounts of caffeine
• Caution patient that product may cause dizziness, may occur during 1st few days of therapy; to avoid hazardous activities

Evaluation
Positive therapeutic outcome
• Decreased symptoms of BPH

tapentadol (Rx)
(ta-pen'ta-dol)
Nucynta
Func. class.: Analgesic, miscellaneous
Chem. class.: μ-Opioid receptor agonist
Controlled substance schedule II
Pregnancy category C

ACTION: Centrally acting synthetic analgesic; μ opioid agonist activity is thought to result in analgesia; inhibits norepinephrine uptake

Therapeutic outcome: Relief of pain

USES: Moderate to severe pain

CONTRAINDICATIONS:
Hypersensitivity, asthma, ileus, respiratory depression

Precautions: Pregnancy **C**, breastfeeding, children <18 yr, increased intracranial pressure, MI (acute), severe heart disease, respiratory depression, renal/hepatic disease, GI obstruction, ulcerative colitis, sleep apnea, seizure disorder

DOSAGE AND ROUTES
Adult: PO 50-100 mg q4-6hr; may give second dose 1 hr or more after 1st dose; max 700 mg on day 1, 600 mg/day thereafter

Available forms: Tab 50, 75, 100 mg

Implementation
• Give with antiemetic if nausea, vomiting occur
• Give when pain is beginning to return; determine dosing interval by response
• Store in light-resistant area at room temperature
• Provide assistance with ambulation
• Provide safety measures: night-light, call bell within easy reach

ADVERSE EFFECTS
CNS: *Drowsiness, dizziness, confusion, headache, euphoria,* hallucinations, restlessness, syncope, anxiety, flushing, psychological dependence, insomnia, lethargy, tremor, seizures
CV: Palpitations, bradycardia, hypo/hypertension, orthostatic hypotension, sinus tachycardia
GI: *Nausea, vomiting, anorexia, constipation, cramps,* gastritis, dyspepsia, biliary spasms
GU: Urinary retention/frequency
INTEG: *Rash,* urticaria, diaphoresis, pruritus
RESP: **Respiratory depression,** cough
SYST: **Anaphylaxis,** infection, serotonin syndrome

Pharmacokinetics
Absorption	32%
Distribution	Protein binding 20%
Metabolism	Liver, extensively
Excretion	Urine 99%
Half-life	Terminal 4 hr

Pharmacodynamics
Onset	Unknown
Peak	Unknown
Duration	Unknown

INTERACTIONS
Individual drugs
Alcohol: increased effects with other CNS depressants

Drug classifications
Antipsychotics, opioids, sedatives/hypnotics, skeletal muscle relaxants: increased effects with other CNS depressants
MAOIs: increased toxicity
Serotonin-receptor agonists, SSRIs, SNRIs, tricyclics: increased serotonin syndrome

Drug/herb
Kava, St. John's wort, valerian: increased sedative effect

NURSING CONSIDERATIONS
Assessment
• Monitor I&O ratio; check for decreasing output; may indicate urinary retention
• Assess CNS changes: dizziness, drowsiness, hallucinations, euphoria, LOC, pupil reaction
• Assess for allergic reactions: rash, urticaria, anaphylaxis
• **Serotonin syndrome:** Assess for increased heart rate, shivering, sweating, dilated pupils, tremors, high B/P, hyperthermia, headache, confusion; if these occur, stop product, administer a serotonin antagonist if needed
• **Assess for respiratory dysfunction:** respiratory depression, character, rate, rhythm; notify prescriber if respirations are <10/min; also B/P, pulse
• **Assess for pain:** intensity, location, type, characteristics; need for pain medication by pain/sedation scoring; physical dependence

Nursing diagnosis
• Pain, acute (uses)
• Knowledge, deficient (teaching)

Patient/family education
• Teach patient to report any symptoms of CNS changes, allergic reactions
• Advise that physical dependency may result from extended use
• Inform that withdrawal symptoms may occur: nausea, vomiting, cramps, fever, faintness, anorexia
• Teach to avoid CNS depressants, alcohol
• Advise to avoid driving, operating machinery if drowsiness occurs

Evaluation
Positive therapeutic outcome
• Decrease in pain

⚠ Nurse Alert

tazobactam
See piperacillin/tazobactam

telaprevir
(tel-a'pre-vir)
Incivek
Func. class.: Antiviral, antihepatitis agent
Chem. class.: NS3/4A protease inhibitor
Pregnancy category B (alone); X (combination therapy)

ACTION: Prevents hepatitis C viral (HCV) replication by blocking the proteolytic activity of HCV NS3/4A serine protease; hepatitis C virus NS3/4A serine protease is an enzyme responsible for the conversion of HCV-encoded polyproteins to mature/functioning viral proteins. These proteins (NS4A, NS4B, NS5A, NS5B), are needed for viral replication.

Therapeutic outcome: Decreasing hepatitis C viral infection

USES: Chronic hepatitis C

CONTRAINDICATIONS:
Pregnancy **X** in combination, male partners of women who are pregnant

Precautions: Breastfeeding, anemia, neutropenia, thrombocytopenia, HIV, hepatitis B, decompensated hepatic disease, in liver or other organ transplants, neonates, infants, children, adolescents <18 years of age, serious rashes

DOSAGE AND ROUTES
For the treatment of chronic hepatitis C infection (genotype 1) in adults with compensated liver disease

In patients without cirrhosis who are previously untreated or have relapsed after treatment with interferon and ribavirin therapy:
Adults: PO 750 mg tid (q7-9hr) with peginterferon alfa and ribavirin; duration is determined by the patient's IICV RNA level at treatment wk 4, 12. If the HCV RNA is undetectable at wk 4, 12, give the three-drug regimen for 12 wk, then give an additional 12 wk of only peginterferon alfa and ribavirin (24 wk total); if the HCV RNA is detectable but ≤1000 international units/ml at wk 4, or 12, give the three-drug regimen for 12 wk, then an additional 36 wk of only peginterferon alfa and ribavirin (48 wk total)

Those without cirrhosis who are previously partial or null responders to interferon and ribavirin therapy/or those with cirrhosis
Adults: PO 750 mg tid (q7-9hr) with peginterferon alfa and ribavirin; give the three drug regimen for 12 wk, then another 36 wk (48 wk total) of only peginterferon alfa and ribavirin

Available forms: Tab 375 mg

Implementation
• Only use in combination with peginterferon alfa and ribavirin; never give as monotherapy
• Discontinue in hepatitis C virus (HCV) RNA concentrations ≥1000 international units/ml at wk 4 or 12 or a confirmed detectable HCV RNA concentration at wk 24
• Any contraindication to peginterferon alfa or ribavirin also applies to this product. See ribavirin or peginterferon alfa monographs for additional information regarding contraindications and warnings associated with these products
• Give with food, not low-fat

ADVERSE EFFECTS
CNS: Fatigue
GI: Anorectal discomfort, diarrhea, dysgeusia, hemorrhoids, hyperbilirubinemia, nausea, pruritus ani, rectal burning, vomiting
HEMA: Anemia, decreased Hgb, leukopenia, lymphopenia, neutropenia, thrombocytopenia
INTEG: Drug reaction with eosinophilia and systemic symptoms (DRESS), pruritus, rash, Stevens-Johnson Syndrome (SJS); severe rashes (bullous rash, skin ulcerations, and vesicular rash)
META: Increased uric acid

Pharmacokinetics
Absorption	Unknown
Distribution	59%-76% protein binding
Metabolism	Liver
Excretion	82% (feces)
Half-life	9-11 hr

Pharmacodynamics
Onset	Unknown
Peak	4-5 hrs
Duration	Unknown

INTERACTIONS
Individual drugs
Acetaminophen, alfentanil, aliskiren, almotriptan, alosetron, ALPRAZolam, aminophylline, amiodarone, amitriptyline, amLODIPine,

T

aripiprazole, astemizole, atorvastatin, atorvastin, bepridil, boceprevir, bosentan, budesonide, bupivacaine, buprenorphine, busPIRone, carvedilol, cevimeline, chloroquine, cilostazol, cinacalcet, citalopram, clarithromycin, clomipramine, clonazePAM, clopidogrel, clozapine, colchicine, cyclobenzaprine, cycloSPORINE, dapsone, DAUNOrubicin, desipramine, desloratadine, dexamethasone, dexlansoprazole, dextromethorphan, diazepam, diclofenac, digoxin, diltiazem, disopyramide, disulfiram, docetaxel, dolasetron, donepezil, DOXOrubicin, droperidol, dutasteride, ebastine, eletriptan, eplerenone, erlotinib, erythromycin, estazolam, eszopiclone, ethosuximide, etoposide, exemestane, felodipine, fentaNYL, fexofenadine, finasteride, flecainide, flunitrazepam, flurazepam, galantamine, gefitinib, glyburide, granisetron, halofantrine, haloperidol, HYDROcodone, ifosfamide, imipramine, indiplon, isradipine, irinotecan, itraconazole, ivermectin, ixabepilone, ketoconazole, lansoprazole, lidocaine, loperamide, loratadine, losartan, maraviroc, mefloquine, meloxicam, mirtazapine, mitomycin, montelukast, morphine, nateglinide, niCARdipine, NIFEdipine, nisoldipine, nortriptyline, omeprazole, ondansetron, oxybutynin, oxyCODONE, paclitaxel, palonosetron, paricalcitol, plicamycin, posaconazole, prasugrel, praziquantel, propafenone, quazepam, QUEtiapine, quinacrine, quiNIDine, ramelteon, repaglinide, rifabutin, risperidone, ropivacaine, salmeterol, selegiline, sertraline, sibutramine, silodosin, sirolimus, sitaxsentan, solifenacin, SUFentanil, sunitinib, tacrolimus, telithromycin, teniposide, terfenadine, testosterone, theophylline, tiagabine, tinidazole, tolterodine, tolvaptan, traMADol, traZODone, vardenafil, venlafaxine, verapamil, vinBLAStine, vinCRIStine, voriconazole, warfarin, and others: use cautiously; may need to reduce dose: increased effect, adverse reactions of each product

Alfuzosin, cisapride, ezetimibe, lovastatin, niacin with simvastatin and boceprevir, pimozide, simvastatin; oral midazolam, triazolam; sildenafil, tadalafil (pulmonary arterial hypertension): do not use concurrently; increased, life-threatening reactions of each product

Atazanavir, efavirenz, lopinavir with ritonavir, ritonavir: possible treatment failure

Drosperinone: increased hyperkalemia

Ethinyl estradiol: Decreased estrogen levels

Methadone: decreased effect of methadone

Drug classifications

CYP3A4 inhibitors (carBAMazepine, PHENobarbital, phenytoin, rifampin): decreased telaprevir effect

Ergots (dihydroergotamine, ergotamine, ergonovine, methylergonovine): do not use concurrently; increased, life-threatening reactions of each product

Phosphodiesterase type 5 (PDE5) inhibitors (for erectile dysfunction), systemic corticosteroids: use cautiously; may need to reduce dose: increased effect, adverse reactions of each product

Drug/herb

Do not use with St. John's wort

NURSING CONSIDERATIONS

Assessment

• **Pregnancy:** Pregnancy (X) combination therapy; obtain a pregnancy test prior to, monthly during, and for 6 months after treatment is completed; those who are not willing to practice strict contraception should not receive treatment with these products; report any cases of prenatal ribavirin exposure to the Ribavirin Pregnancy registry at (800) 593-2214

• **Anemia:** Monitor hemoglobin prior to, at treatment wks 4, 8, and 12, and as needed. If Hgb is less than 10 g/dl, decrease ribavirin dosage; if Hgb is less than 8.5 g/dl, discontinuation of therapy is recommended; telaprevir dosage should not be altered based on adverse reactions; Anemia may be managed through ribavirin dose modifications; never alter the dose of telaprevir. If anemia persists despite a reduction in ribavirin dose, consider discontinuing telaprevir. If management of anemia requires permanent discontinuation of ribavirin, treatment with telaprevir must also be permanently discontinued. Once telaprevir has been discontinued, it must not be restarted; monitor CBC with differential at treatment wks 4, 8, 12, and at other treatment points as needed

• **Stevens-Johnson syndrome:** eosinophilia, fever, mucosal skin erosion, mucosal ulceration, target lesions; If serious skin reaction occurs, immediately discontinue all components of the three-drug regimen and refer the patient for urgent medical care. Thyroid function tests, LFTs, serum bilirubin/creatinine, BUN, bilirubin, serum electrolytes, serum uric acid, baseline and periodically during treatment

Nursing diagnoses

• Infection, risk for (Uses)

Patient/family education
• Instruct patient to use two forms of effective contraception (intrauterine devices and barrier methods) during treatment and for 6 months after treatment (pregnancy **X**), avoid breast feeding
• If a serious skin reaction occurs, patients should be instructed to seek urgent medical care and all components of the triple-drug regimen must be discontinued immediately

Evaluation
Positive therapeutic outcome
• Decreasing hepatitis C viral infection

telavancin (Rx)
(tel-a-van′sin)
Vibativ
Func. class.: Antiinfective—miscellaneous
Chem. class.: Lipoglycopeptide, a semi-synthetic derivative of vacomycin
Pregnancy category C

ACTION: Inhibits bacterial cell wall synthesis, blocks glycopeptides

Therapeutic outcome: Negative culture

USES: Skin/skin structure infections caused by *Enterococcus faecalis, E. faecium, Staphylococcus aureus* (MSRA), *S. aureus* (MSSA), *S. epidermidis, S. baemolyticus, Streptococcus agalactiae* (group B), *S. dysgalactiae, S. pyogenes* (group A beta tremolytic), *S. anginosus, S. intermedius, S. constellates*

Unlabeled uses: Nosocomial pneumonia caused by susceptible gram-positive bacteria

CONTRAINDICATIONS:
Hypersensitivity

Precautions: Breastfeeding, geriatric patients, renal disease, antimicrobial resistance, children, diabetes mellitus, diarrhea, GI disease, heart failure, hypertension, pseudomembranous colitis, QT prolongation, vancomycin hypersensitivity

> **BLACK BOX WARNING:** Pregnancy **C**, females

DOSAGE AND ROUTES
Adult: IV INF 10 mg/kg over 60 min q24hr × 7-14 days

Nosocomial pneumonia (unlabeled)
Adult: IV INF 10 mg/kg q24hr × 7-21 days

Available forms: Powder for inj 250, 750 mg

Implementation
• Use only for susceptible organisms to prevent drug-resistant bacteria
• Give antihistamine if red man syndrome occurs: decreased B/P, flushing of neck, face
• Store in refrigerator
• Have EPINEPHrine, suction, tracheostomy set, endotracheal intubation equipment on unit; anaphylaxis may occur
• Give adequate intake of fluids (2 L/day) to prevent nephrotoxicity

Intermittent IV infusion route
• Administer after reconstituting with 15 ml D_5W sterile water for inj; 0.9% NaCl (15 mg/ml) 250 mg vial; add 45 ml to 750 mg vial (15 mg/ml) for dose of 150-800 mg; further dilute with 100-250 ml of compatible sol; for dose <150 mg or 800 mg, further dilute to a conc of 0.6-8 mg/ml with compatible sol; give over 60 min

Solution compatibilities: D_5W, LR, 0.9% NaCl

ADVERSE EFFECTS
CNS: Anxiety, chills, flushing, headache, insomnia
CV: QT prolongation, irregular heartbeat
EENT: Hearing loss
GI: Nausea, vomiting, **pseudomembranous colitis,** abdominal pain, constipation, diarrhea, metallic taste
GU: Nephrotoxicity, *increased BUN, creatinine,* **renal failure,** foamy urine
HEMA: Leukopenia, eosinophilia, anemia, thrombocytopenia
INTEG: Chills, fever, rash, thrombophlebitis at inj site, urticaria, pruritus, necrosis (red man syndrome)
SYST: Anaphylaxis, superinfection

Pharmacokinetics
Absorption	Unknown
Distribution	Unknown
Metabolism	Unknown
Excretion	Urine 76%
Half-life	8-9 hr

Pharmacodynamics
Onset	Rapid
Peak	Unknown
Duration	Unknown

T

Adverse effects: *italics* = common; **bold** = life-threatening

INTERACTIONS
Individual drugs
Amphotericin B, bacitracin, cidofovir, CISplatin, colistin, polymyxin: increased toxicity, nephrotoxicity

Chloroquine, clarithromycin, dronedarone, droperidol, erythromycin, grepafloxacin, haloperidol, levomethadyl, methadone, pimozide, ziprasidone: increased QT prolongation

Drug classifications
Aminoglycosides, cephalosporins, nondepolarizing muscle relaxants: increased toxicity, nephrotoxicity

Class IA, III antidysrhythmics, some phenothiazines: increased QT prolongation

NURSING CONSIDERATIONS
Assessment
• Monitor I&O ratio; report hematuria, oliguria; nephrotoxicity may occur
• Monitor C&S throughout treatment
• Assess auditory function during, after treatment, hearing loss, ringing, roaring in ears; product should be discontinued
• Monitor B/P during administration; sudden drop may indicate red man syndrome
• Assess for skin eruptions
• Assess respiratory status: rate, character, wheezing, tightness in chest
• Assess allergies before treatment, reaction of each medication

Nursing diagnoses
• Infection, risk for (uses)
• Knowledge, deficient (teaching)

Patient/family education
• Teach all aspects of product therapy; culture may be taken after completed course of medication
• Advise to report sore throat, fever, fatigue; could indicate superinfection

Evaluation
Positive therapeutic outcome
• Negative culture

---

telbivudine (Rx)
(tel-bi′vyoo-deen)
Sebivo ✸, Tyzeka
Func. class.: Antiretroviral
Chem. class.: Nucleoside reverse transcriptase inhibitor (NRTI)
Pregnancy category B

ACTION: Inhibits replication of HBV DNA polymerase, which inhibits HBV replication

Therapeutic outcome: Decreased hepatitis B serology

USES: Treatment of chronic hepatitis B

CONTRAINDICATIONS:
Hypersensitivity, breastfeeding

Precautions: Pregnancy **B,** children, severe renal disease, anemia, organ transplant, dialysis, HIV, obesity, alcoholism; hispanic or African descent (safety not established)

> **BLACK BOX WARNING:** Impaired hepatic function, lactic acidosis

DOSAGE AND ROUTES
Adult and adolescent >16 yr: PO 600 mg/day; max 600 mg/day

Renal dose
Adult: PO CCr 30-49 ml/min 600 mg tab q48hr or 400 mg oral sol q day; CCr <30 ml/min (not requiring dialysis) 600 mg tab q72hr or 200 mg oral sol q day

Available forms: Tabs 600 mg

Implementation
• Give with or without food with a full glass of water
• Store at room temperature

ADVERSE EFFECTS
CNS: *Fever, headache, malaise,* weakness, *dizziness, insomnia*
EENT: Taste change, hearing loss, photophobia
GI: *Nausea, vomiting, diarrhea, anorexia,* abdominal pain, hepatomegaly
INTEG: *Rash*
MISC: Lactic acidosis
MS: Myalgia, arthralgia, muscle cramps
RESP: Cough

Pharmacokinetics

Absorption	Unknown
Distribution	Steady state 5-7 days, protein binding 3.3%
Metabolism	Unknown
Excretion	Kidneys, unchanged
Half-life	Terminal 40-49 hr

Pharmacodynamics
Unknown

⚠ Nurse Alert

INTERACTIONS
Individual drugs
CycloSPORINE, erythromycin, hydrochloro-
quine, niacin, penicillamine, zidovudine, ZDV:
increased myopathy risk

Drug classifications
Any agent altering renal function: altered telbivu-
dine levels

Azole antifungals, corticosteroids, fibric acid
derivatives, HMG-CoA reductase inhibitors:
increased myopathy risk

NURSING CONSIDERATIONS
Assessment

> **BLACK BOX WARNING:** Monitor liver function
> tests, hepatitis B serology, creatine kinase,
> periodically; monitor HBV DNA after 24 wk, if
> viral suppression is incomplete (≥300 copies/
> ml) start alternate therapy, monitor HBV DNA
> q6mo

Nursing diagnoses
• Infection, risk for (uses)
• Knowledge, deficient (teaching)

> **BLACK BOX WARNING: Lactic acidosis,
> severe hepatomegaly with steatosis:**
> obtain baseline LFTs, if elevated, discontinue
> treatment; discontinue even if LFTs are normal
> but lactic acidosis, hepatomegaly are present,
> may be fatal

Patient/family education
• Advise patient that GI complaints and insomnia may resolve after 3-4 wk of treatment
• Teach patient that product does not cure
hepatitis B and does not stop the spread to
others
• Teach patient that follow-up visits must be
continued
• Teach patient that serious product interactions may occur if OTC products are ingested;
check with prescriber before taking
• Advise patient that product may cause dizziness; avoid hazardous activities until response is
known
• Teach patient to report symptoms of cough,
difficulty sleeping or excessive headache, muscle
pain/weakness

Evaluation
Positive therapeutic outcome
• Decreased hepatitis B serology

telmisartan (Rx)
(tel-mih-sar'tan)
Micardis
Func. class.: Antihypertensive
Chem. class.: Angiotensin II receptor (type AT₁)

**Pregnancy category C (1st trimes-
ter) D (2nd/3rd trimesters)**

ACTION: Blocks the vasoconstrictor and
aldosterone-secreting effects of angiotensin II;
selectively blocks the binding of angiotensin II to
the AT₁ receptor found in tissues

Therapeutic outcome: Decreased B/P

USES: Hypertension, alone or in combination; stroke, MI prophylaxis (>55 yr) in those
unable to take ACE inhibitors

Unlabeled uses: Heart failure

CONTRAINDICATIONS:
Hypersensitivity

> **BLACK BOX WARNING:** Pregnancy **D** (2nd/3rd
> trimesters)

Precautions: Pregnancy **C** (1st trimester),
breastfeeding, children, geriatric, hypersensitivity to angiotensin-converting enzyme (ACE)
inhibitors, renal/hepatic disease, renal artery
stenosis, dialysis, CHF, hyperkalemia, hypotension, hypovolemia

DOSAGE AND ROUTES
Adult: PO 40 mg/day; range 20-80 mg/day

Stroke, MI prophylaxis
Adult >55 yr: PO 80 mg/day

Available forms: Tabs 20, 40, 80 mg

Implementation
• Give without regard to meals
• Give increased dose to African American,
hispanic patients, B/P response may be reduced

ADVERSE EFFECTS
CNS: Dizziness, insomnia, *anxiety,* headache,
fatigue
GI: *Diarrhea,* dyspepsia, *anorexia, vomiting*
MS: *Myalgia, pain*
RESP: Cough, *upper respiratory tract infec-
tion,* sinusitis, pharyngitis

Pharmacokinetics

Absorption	Unknown
Distribution	Highly protein bound
Metabolism	Liver, extensively
Excretion	Urine/feces
Half-life	Terminal 24 hr

Pharmacodynamics

Onset	3-hr
Peak	0.5-1 hr
Duration	Unknown

INTERACTIONS

Digoxin: increased digoxin peak, trough concentrations

Drug classifications

Antihypertensives, diuretics: increased antihypertensive action

NSAIDs, salicylates: decreased antihypertensive effect

Potassium-sparing diuretics, potassium salt substitutes: increased hyperkalemia

NURSING CONSIDERATIONS

Assessment

• Monitor B/P, pulse q4hr; note rate, rhythm, quality
• Monitor electrolytes: potassium, sodium, chloride
• Monitor baselines in renal, liver function tests before therapy begins
• Assess edema in feet, legs daily
• Assess skin turgor, dryness of mucous membranes for hydration status

Nursing diagnoses

• Knowledge, deficient (teaching)
• Noncompliance (teaching)

Patient/family education

• Instruct patient to comply with dosage schedule, even if feeling better
• Advise patient to notify prescriber of mouth sores, fever, swelling of hands or feet, irregular heartbeat, chest pain
• Teach patient that excessive perspiration, dehydration, vomiting, diarrhea may lead to fall in blood pressure; consult prescriber if these occur

> **BLACK BOX WARNING:** Teach patient that product may cause dizziness, fainting; light-headedness may occur

> **BLACK BOX WARNING:** Advise patient to use contraception while taking this product, pregnancy category **D**, 2nd/3rd trimester

• Teach patient to notify prescriber of all prescriptions, OTC preparations, and supplements taken

Evaluation

Positive therapeutic outcome
• Decreased B/P

---

temazepam (Rx)

(tem-az′a-pam)
Restoril
Func. class.: Sedative-hypnotic
Chem. class.: Benzodiazepine, short-intermediate acting
Pregnancy category X
Controlled substance schedule IV (USA), schedule F (Canada)

ACTION: Produces CNS depression at limbic, thalamic, hypothalamic levels of the CNS; may be mediated by neurotransmitter γ-aminobutyric acid (GABA); results are sedation, hypnosis, skeletal muscle relaxation, anticonvulsant activity, anxiolytic action

Therapeutic outcome: Decreased insomnia

USES: Insomnia

CONTRAINDICATIONS:
Pregnancy **X**, breastfeeding, hypersensitivity to benzodiazepines, intermittent porphyria

Precautions: Children <15 yr, geriatric, anemia, pulmonary/renal/hepatic disease, suicidal patients, product abuse, psychosis, acute closed-angle glaucoma, seizure disorders, angioedema, sleep-related behavior (sleep walking), pulmonary disease

DOSAGE AND ROUTES
Adult: PO 7.5-30 mg at bedtime
Geriatric: PO 7.5 mg at bedtime

Available forms: Caps 7.5, 15, 22.5, 30 mg

Implementation
• Give with food or milk to decrease GI symptoms; if patient is unable to swallow medication whole, tab may be crushed and mixed with foods or fluids

---

• Give sugarless gum, hard candy, frequent sips of water for dry mouth

ADVERSE EFFECTS
CNS: *Lethargy, drowsiness, daytime sedation,* dizziness, confusion, light-headedness, headache, anxiety, irritability, complex sleep-related reactions (sleep driving, sleep eating), fatigue
CV: Chest pain, pulse changes, hypotension
EENT: Blurred vision
GI: Nausea, vomiting, diarrhea, heartburn, abdominal pain, constipation, anorexia
SYST: Severe allergic reactions

Pharmacokinetics
Absorption	Well absorbed
Distribution	Widely distributed, crosses placenta, crosses blood-brain barrier
Metabolism	Liver
Excretion	Kidneys, breast milk
Half-life	10-20 hr

Pharmacodynamics
Onset	$^1/_2$ hr
Peak	2-3 hr
Duration	6-8 hr

INTERACTIONS
Individual drugs
Alcohol: increased actions of both products
Cimetidine, disulfiram: increased effect of each specific product
Rifampin: decreased action of rifampin
Theophylline: decreased effects of theophylline

Drug classifications
Antacids: decreased effect of antacids
Contraceptives (oral): increased effect
CNS depressants: increased action of both products

Drug/herb
Valerian: increased CNS depression

Drug/lab test
Increased: AST/ALT, serum bilirubin
Decreased: radioactive iodine uptake
False increase: 17-OHCS

NURSING CONSIDERATIONS
Assessment
• Assess mental status: mood, sensorium, anxiety, affect, sleeping pattern, drowsiness, dizziness, especially geriatric; physical dependency, withdrawal symptoms: anxiety, panic attacks, agitation, headache, nausea, vomiting, muscle pain, weakness; indications of increasing tolerance and abuse

Nursing diagnoses
• Anxiety (uses)
• Injury, risk for (adverse reactions)
• Knowledge, deficient (teaching)

Patient/family education
• Inform patient that product may be taken with food, and that tab may be crushed or swallowed whole
• Advise patient not to use for everyday stress or longer than 3 mo unless directed by prescriber; not to take more than prescribed amount; may be habit forming; not to double or skip doses
• Caution patient to avoid OTC preparations unless approved by prescriber; alcohol and CNS depressants will increase CNS depression
• Advise patient to avoid driving, activities that require alertness, drowsiness may occur; to avoid alcohol ingestion or other psychotropic medications; to rise slowly or fainting may occur, especially in geriatric; that drowsiness may worsen at beginning of treatment
• Caution patient not to discontinue medication abruptly after long-term use; withdrawal symptoms include vomiting, cramping, tremors, seizures
• Advise patient to use contraception while taking this product, to notify prescriber if pregnancy is planned or suspected, pregnancy **X**
• Advise patient that complex sleep-related behavior may occur (sleep driving/eating)
• Teach patient to limit to 7-10 days continuous use

Evaluation
Positive therapeutic outcome
• Decreased anxiety, restlessness, sleeplessness (short-term treatment only)

TREATMENT OF OVERDOSE:
Lavage, VS, supportive care

temozolomide (Rx)
(tem-oo-zole′oo-mide)
Temodar
Func. class.: Antineoplastic alkylating agents
Chem. class.: Imidazotetrazine derivative
Pregnancy category D

ACTION: A proproduct that undergoes conversion to 5-(3-methyl-1-triazeno) imidazole-4-carboxamide (MTIC); MTIC action prevents DNA transcription

Therapeutic outcome: Prevention of rapidly growing malignant cells

USES: Anaplastic astrocytoma with relapse, glioblastoma multiforme, malignant glioma

Unlabeled uses: Metastatic melanoma

CONTRAINDICATIONS:
Pregnancy **D**, breastfeeding, hypersensitivity to this product, carbazine, or gelatin

Precautions: Radiation therapy, renal/hepatic disease, bone marrow suppression, infection, geriatric, myelosuppression

DOSAGE AND ROUTES
Anaplastic astrocytoma
Adult: PO adjust dose based on nadir neutrophil and platelet counts 150 mg/m²/day × 5 days during 28-day cycle

Glioblastoma multiforme
Adult: PO/IV 75 mg/m²/day × 42 days with focal radiotherapy, then maintenance of 6 cycles

Malignant glioma
Adult: 150 mg/m²/day over 90 min day 1-5, q28day; may increase to 200 mg/m²/day on day 1-5, q28day if hematologic parameters permit

Available forms: Caps 5, 20, 100, 140, 180, 250 mg; powder for inj 100 mg

Implementation
PO route
• Give fluids **IV** or PO before chemotherapy to hydrate patient
• Give antiemetic 30-60 min before giving product to prevent vomiting, and prn; antibiotics for prophylaxis of infection
• Capsules should not be opened; if accidentally damaged, do not allow contact with skin, or inhale; take caps one at a time with 8 oz of water at the same time of day; use cytotic handling procedure
• Give on empty stomach at bedtime to prevent nausea/vomiting

IV route
• Bring vial to room temperature
• Inject 41 ml sterile water for inj into vial (2.5 mg/ml)
• Gently swirl, do not shake

Intermittent IV infusion route
• Withdraw up to 40 ml from each vial to make total dose and transfer to empty 250 ml PVC inf bag, flush before and after inf
• Run over 90 min
• Use reconstituted sol within 14 hr including inf time

ADVERSE EFFECTS
CNS: Seizures, *hemiparesis, dizziness, poor coordination, amnesia, insomnia, paresthesia, somnolence, paresis, ataxia, anxiety, dysphagia, depression, confusion*
GI: *Nausea, anorexia, vomiting,* abdominal pain, constipation
GU: *Urinary incontinence, UTI, frequency*
HEMA: Thrombocytopenia, leukopenia, anemia, myelosuppression, neutropenia
INTEG: *Rash, pruritus*
MISC: *Headache, fatigue, asthenia, fever, edema, back pain, weight increase, diplopia*
RESP: *Upper respiratory tract infection, pharyngitis, sinusitis, coughing*
SYST: Anaphylaxis, secondary malignancy

Pharmacokinetics
Absorption	Rapid, complete
Distribution	Crosses blood-brain barrier
Metabolism	To MTIC and metabolite
Excretion	Urine, feces
Half-life	1.8 hr

Pharmacodynamics
Onset	Unknown
Peak	1 hr
Duration	Unknown

INTERACTIONS
Individual drugs
Digoxin: decreased action of digoxin
Filgrastim, G-CSF, pegfilgrastim, sargramostim: do not use within 24 hr of these products
Radiation: increased toxicity, bone marrow suppression

Drug classifications
Anticoagulants, NSAIDs, platelet inhibitors, thrombolytics: increased bleeding risk
Antineoplastics: increased bone marrow suppression
Live virus vaccines, toxoids: increased adverse reactions, decreased antibody reaction

NURSING CONSIDERATIONS
Assessment
• Assess symptoms indicating severe allergic reaction: rash, pruritus, urticaria, purpuric skin lesions, itching, flushing; product should be discontinued
• Assess tumor response during treatment
• Obtain CBC on day 22 (21 days after 1st dose), CBC weekly until recovery if ANC is <1.5 × 10⁹/L and platelets <100 × 10⁹/L, do not

administer to patients that do not tolerate 100 mg/m²; myelosuppression usually occurs late in the treatment cycle
• Assess for seizures, mental status throughout treatment
• Monitor renal function studies: BUN, creatinine, urine CCr before, during therapy; I&O ratio; report fall in urine output to <30 ml/hr
• Monitor temp q4hr (may indicate beginning of infection)
• Monitor liver function tests before, during therapy (bilirubin, AST, ALT, LDH) as needed or monthly; note jaundice of skin or sclera, dark urine, clay-colored stools, itchy skin, abdominal pain, fever, diarrhea; hepatotoxicity can be serious and fatal
• Assess for bleeding: hematuria, stool guaiac, bruising or petechiae, mucosa or orifices; check for inflammation of mucosa, breaks in skin

Nursing diagnoses
• Body image, disturbed (adverse reactions)
• Infection, risk for (adverse reactions)
• Injury, risk for (adverse reactions)
• Knowledge, deficient (teaching)

Patient/family education
• Teach patient to avoid use of products containing aspirin or NSAIDs, razors, commercial mouthwash, since bleeding may occur; to report symptoms of bleeding (hematuria, tarry stools)
• Instruct patient to report signs of anemia (fatigue, headache, irritability, faintness, shortness of breath)
• Caution patient not to have any vaccinations without the advice of prescriber; serious reactions can occur
• Advise patient contraception is needed during treatment and for several months after completion of therapy; product has teratogenic properties, pregnancy **D**, not to breastfeed

Evaluation
Positive therapeutic outcome
• Prevention of rapid division of malignant cells

temsirolimus (Rx)
(tem-sir-oh′li-mus)
Torisel
Func. class.: Biological response modifier
Chem. class.: Kinase inhibitor, mTOR antagonist
Pregnancy category D

ACTION: Inhibits mammalian target of rapamycin (mTOR), a protein kinase

Therapeutic outcome: Decreased time of progression of renal cell carcinoma

USES: Renal cell carcinoma

CONTRAINDICATIONS:
Pregnancy **D**, breastfeeding, hypersensitivity to this product or to sirolimus, polysorbate 80

Precautions: Children <13 yr, females, severe pulmonary/renal/hepatic disease (bilirubin >1-1.5 × ULN or AST > ULN, but bilirubin ≤ULN), diabetes mellitus, hyperkalemia, hyperuricemia, hypertension, bone marrow suppression, hypertriglyceridemia/hyperlipidemia, surgery, brain tumor

DOSAGE AND ROUTES
Adult: IV 25 mg over 30-60 min qwk; treat until disease progression or severe toxicity occurs

Hepatic dose
Adult: IV (mild impairment) (bilirubin >1-1.5 × ULN or AST > ULN but bilirubin ≤ ULN)

Available forms: 25 mg/ml sol for inj kit

Implementation
• Premedicate with 25-50 mg diphenhydrAMINE **IV** 30 min before dose; if reaction occurs, stop for ¹/₂-1 hr; may resume at slower rate
• Use in-line filter ≤5 micrometers and inf pump; inf over 30-60 min; complete inf within 6 hr
• Dilute product with 1.8 ml of provided diluent; the result is 3 ml (10 mg/ml); invert to mix well; withdraw the required amount and inject rapidly into 250 ml of 0.9% NaCl; do not use PVC infusion bags/sets
• Protect from light during preparation; use only glass

ADVERSE EFFECTS
CNS: *Headache,* seizures
CV: Hypertension, **thrombophlebitis**
ENDO: Hypertriglyceridemia, hyperlipidemia, hyperglycemia
GI: Nausea, vomiting, diarrhea, constipation, **bowel perforation**
GU: UTIs, **albuminuria, hematuria, proteinuria, renal failure,** mucositis
HEMA: **Anemia, leukopenia, thrombocytopenia**
INTEG: *Rash,* pruritus
META: Metabolic acidosis, hyperglycemia, hyperlipidemia
RESP: **Interstitial lung disease**
SYST: **Lymphoma**

T

Adverse effects: *italics* = common; **bold** = life-threatening

Pharmacokinetics

Absorption	Rapidly absorbed
Distribution	Unknown
Metabolism	Extensively via liver by CYP3A4
Excretion	Eliminated via feces
Half-life	Unknown

Pharmacodynamics

Onset	Unknown
Peak	0.5-2 hr
Duration	Unknown

INTERACTIONS

Individual drugs

Bromocriptine, cimetidine, clarithromycin, cycloSPORINE, danazol, erythromycin, metoclopramide: increased blood levels

CarBAMazepine, dexamethasone, PHENobarbital, phenytoin, rifamycin, rifapentine: decreased blood levels

Sunitinib: increased toxicity

Drug classifications

Antifungals, benzodiazepines, calcium channel blockers, CYP3A4 inhibitors, HIV protease inhibitors, HMG-CoA reductase inhibitors: increased blood levels

CYP3A4 inducers: decreased blood levels

Vaccines: decreased effect of vaccines; avoid with vaccines

Drug/herb

Astragalus, echinacea, melatonin: decreased immunosuppression

Ginseng, maitake, mistletoe: increased effect

St. John's wort: may decrease the effect of sirolimus

Drug/food

Alters bioavailability; use consistently with or without food; do not use with grapefruit juice

NURSING CONSIDERATIONS

Assessment

• Assess cardiac status: B/P, heart rate
• Assess for interstitial lung disease
• Assess for hypersensitive reactions: anaphylaxis
• Monitor lipid profile: cholesterol, triglycerides, a lipid-lowering agent may be needed; blood glucose
⚠ **Assess for infection and development of lymphoma**
⚠ **Monitor blood tests: Hgb, WBC, platelets during treatment q mo**

• Monitor renal function tests: BUN, creatinine, phosphate potassium; proteinuria, hematuria, albuminemia may indicate renal failure
• **Hepatic disease:** monitor liver function test baseline and periodically

Nursing diagnoses

• Injury, risk for (uses, adverse reactions)
• Knowledge, deficient (teaching)

Patient/family education

• Advise patient to report fever, rash, severe diarrhea, chills, sore throat, fatigue; serious infections may occur; clay-colored stools, cramping (hepatotoxicity)
• Advise patient to avoid crowds, persons with known infections to reduce risk of infection
• Teach patient to use contraception before, during, and 12 wk after product has been discontinued; avoid breastfeeding; men should also use reliable contraception during and 12 wk after cessation of product, pregnancy **D**
• Advise to report excessive thirst, urinary frequency, new or worsening breathing problems, blood in stool, abdominal pain

Evaluation

Positive therapeutic outcome

• Decreased time of progression of renal cell carcinoma

⚠ HIGH ALERT

tenecteplase (TNK-tPA) (Rx)

(ten-ek′ta-place)

TNKase

Func. class.: Thrombolytic

Chem. class.: Tissue plasminogen activator

Pregnancy category C

ACTION: Activates conversion of plasminogen to plasmin (fibrinolysin): plasmin breaks down clots (fibrin), fibrinogen, factors V, VII; occlusion of venous access lines

Therapeutic outcome: Resolution of MI

USES: Acute MI, coronary artery thrombosis

CONTRAINDICATIONS:

Hypersensitivity, arteriovenous malformation, aneurysm, active bleeding, intracranial, intraspinal surgery or trauma within 2 mo, CNS neoplasms, severe hypertension, severe renal disease, hepatic disease, history of CVA, increased ICP, stroke

---

⚠ Nurse Alert

Precautions: Pregnancy **C**, breastfeeding, children, geriatric, arterial emboli from left side of heart, hypocoagulation, subacute bacterial endocarditis, rheumatic valvular disease, cerebral embolism/thrombosis/hemorrhage, intraarterial diagnostic procedure or surgery (10 days), recent major surgery, dysrhythmias, hypertension

DOSAGE AND ROUTES

Total dose, max 50 mg, based on patient's weight
Adult <60 kg: IV BOL 30 mg, give over 5 sec
Adult 60-70 kg: IV BOL 35 mg, give over 5 sec
Adult 70-80 kg: IV BOL 40 mg, give over 5 sec
Adult 80-90 kg: IV BOL 45 mg, give over 5 sec
Adult ≥90 kg: IV BOL 50 mg, give over 5 sec, max 50 mg total dose

Available forms: Powder for inj, lyophilized 50 mg

Implementation
Intermittent IV infusion route
• Give as soon as thrombi are identified; not useful for thrombi >1 wk old
• Administer cryoprecipitate or fresh frozen plasma if bleeding occurs
• Give heparin after fibrinogen level >100 mg/dl; heparin inf to increase PTT to 1.5-2 × baseline for 3-7 days; IV heparin with loading dose is recommended
• Aseptically withdraw 10 ml of sterile water for inj from diluent vial, use red cannula syringe-filling device, inject all contents of syringe into product vial, direct into powder, swirl, withdraw correct dose, discard any unused sol; stand the shield with dose vertically on flat surface and passively recap the red cannula; remove entire shield assembly by twisting counterclockwise; give by IV bol
• IV therapy: use upper extremity vessel that is accessible to manual compression
• Provide bed rest during entire course of treatment
• Avoid venous or arterial puncture, inj, rectal temp, any invasive treatment
• Treat fever with acetaminophen or aspirin
• Apply pressure for 30 sec to minor bleeding sites; inform prescriber if this does not attain hemostasis; apply pressure dressing

ADVERSE EFFECTS
CV: Dysrhythmias, hypotension, pulmonary edema, **PE, cardiogenic shock, cardiac arrest, heart failure, myocardial reinfarction,**

myocardial rupture, tamponade, pericarditis, pericardial effusion, thrombosis, CVA
HEMA: Decreased Hct, **bleeding**
INTEG: Rash, urticaria, phlebitis at **IV** inf site, itching, flushing
SYST: GI, GU, **intracranial, retroperitoneal bleeding, surface bleeding, anaphylaxis**

Pharmacokinetics
Absorption	Unknown
Distribution	Unknown
Metabolism	Liver
Excretion	Unknown
Half-life	20-24 min

Pharmacodynamics
Onset	Immediate
Peak	Unknown
Duration	Unknown

INTERACTIONS
Individual drugs
Aspirin, cefamandole, cefoperazone, cefotetan, clopidogrel, dipyridamole, indomethacin, phenylbutazone, ticlopidine: increased bleeding potential

Drug classifications
Anticoagulants, antithrombolytics, glycoprotein IIb, IIIa inhibitors, NSAIDs: increased bleeding potential

Drug/herb
Anise, basil, dong quai, fenugreek, feverfew, garlic, ginger, ginkgo, ginseng, green tea, horse chestnut: increased risk of bleeding

Drug/lab test
Increased: pro-time, aPTT, TT
Decreased: plasminogen, fibrinogen

NURSING CONSIDERATIONS
Assessment
• **Assess for allergy:** fever, rash, itching, chills; mild reaction may be treated with antihistamines
⚠ **Assess for bleeding during 1st hr of treatment; hematuria, hematemesis, bleeding from mucous membranes, epistaxis, ecchymosis; may require transfusion (rare), continue to assess for bleeding for 24 hr**
• Monitor blood tests (Hct, platelets, PTT, pro-time, TT, aPTT) before starting therapy; protime or aPTT must be less than 2 × control before starting therapy; PTT or pro-time q3-4hr during treatment

• Assess for hypersensitive reactions: fever, rash, dyspnea; product should be discontinued
• Monitor VS, B/P, pulse, respirations, neurologic signs, temp at least q4hr; temp >104° F (40° C) indicates internal bleeding; systolic pressure increase >25 mm Hg should be reported to prescriber
⚠ Assess for neurologic changes that may indicate intracranial bleeding
⚠ Assess for retroperitoneal bleeding: back pain, leg weakness, diminished pulses

Nursing diagnoses
• Cardiac output, decreased (uses)
• Knowledge, deficient (teaching)

Patient/family education
• Teach patient to notify prescriber immediately of severe headache
• Advise patient to notify prescriber of bleeding, hypersensitivity, fast, slow, or uneven heart rate, feeling of fainting, blood in urine/stools, nose bleeds

Evaluation
Positive therapeutic outcome
• Resolution of myocardial infarction

tenofovir (Rx)
(ten-oh-foh′veer)
Viread
Func. class.: Antiretroviral
Chem. class.: Nucleoside reverse transcriptase inhibitor (NRTI)
Pregnancy category B

ACTION: Inhibits replication of HIV-1 virus by competing with the natural substrate and then incorporating into cellular DNA by viral reverse transcriptase, thereby terminating cellular DNA chain

Therapeutic outcome: Improved symptoms of HIV-1 infection

USES: HIV-1 infection with at least 2 other antiretrovirals, hepatitis B

CONTRAINDICATIONS:
Hypersensitivity

> **BLACK BOX WARNING:** Lactic acidosis

Precautions: Pregnancy **B**, breastfeeding, children, geriatric, renal disease, hepatic insufficiency, CCr <60 ml/min, osteoporosis, immune reconstitution syndrome

> **BLACK BOX WARNING:** Hepatic disease, hepatitis

DOSAGE AND ROUTES
Adult: PO 300 mg with meal; if used with didanosine, give tenofovir 2 hr before or 1 hr after didanosine

Renal dose
Adult: PO CCr 30-49 ml/min 300 mg q48hr; CCr 10-29 ml/min 300 mg q72-96hr; CCr <10 ml/min not recommended

Available forms: Tabs 300 mg (300 mg of fumarate salt equivalent to 245 mg tenofovir disoproxil)

Implementation
• Administer PO without regard to meals
• Store at 25° C (77° F)
• Give product 2 hr before or 1 hr after taking didanosine (if used)

ADVERSE EFFECTS
CNS: *Headache,* asthenia
GI: *Nausea, vomiting, diarrhea,* anorexia, *flatulence, abdominal pain,* pancreatitis
GU: Renal failure, renal tubular acidosis/ necrosis, Fanconi syndrome
HEMA: Neutropenia, osteopenia
INTEG: *Rash,* angioedema
META: Lactic acidosis, hypokalemia, hypophosphatemia
MS: *Myopathy,* rhabdomyolysis
SYST: Lipodystrophy

Pharmacokinetics
Absorption	Rapidly absorbed
Distribution	Extravascular space; bound to serum plasma <0.7%, to serum proteins <7.2%
Metabolism	Unknown
Excretion	Urine, unchanged (70%-80%)
Half-life	Terminal 17 hr

Pharmacodynamics
Onset	Unknown
Peak	0.6-1.4 hr
Duration	Unknown

INTERACTIONS
Individual drugs
Acyclovir, cidofovir, ganciclovir, valacyclovir, valganciclovir: increased level of tenofovir
Didanosine: increased level of didanosine when coadministered with tenofovir

---

⚠ Nurse Alert

Drug classifications

Increased: levels of tenofovir with any product that decreases renal function

NURSING CONSIDERATIONS

Assessment

• Monitor viral load, CD4+ T cell count, plasma HIV RNA, serum creatinine/BUN/phosphate

• Resistance testing at start of therapy and at treatment failure

• Assess liver function tests: AST, ALT, bilirubin; amylase, lipase, triglycerides periodically during treatment

• Assess for bone, renal toxicity: if bone abnormalities are suspected, obtain tests: serum phosphorus, creatinine

• **Lactic acidosis, severe hepatomegaly with steatosis: Obtain baseline LFTs, if elevated discontinue treatment; discontinue even if LFTs are normal but lactic acidosis, hepatomegaly are present, may be fatal**

Nursing diagnoses

• Infection, risk for (uses)

• Injury, risk for (adverse reactions)

• Knowledge, deficient (teaching)

Patient/family education

• Instruct patient to take this product 2 hr before or 1 hr after taking didanosine (if used)

• Instruct patient to take product with meal

• Advise patients that GI complaints resolve after 3-4 wk of treatment

• Caution patient not to breastfeed while taking this product

• Inform patient that product must be taken daily even if patient feels better

• Advise patient to continue follow-up visits since serious toxicity may occur; blood counts must be done q2wk

• Inform patient that product controls symptoms but is not a cure for HIV; patient is still infectious, may pass HIV virus on to others

• Advise patient that other products may be necessary to prevent other infections

• Advise patient that changes in body fat distribution may occur

• **Lactic acidosis:** teach patient symptoms of lactic acidosis, to notify prescriber

Evaluation

Positive therapeutic outcome

• Decrease in signs/symptoms of HIV

---

terazosin (Rx)

(ter-ay′zoe-sin)
Func. class.: Antihypertensive
Chem. class.: α-Adrenergic blocker (peripherally acting)
Pregnancy category C

ACTION: Peripheral blood vessels are dilated, peripheral resistance is lowered; reduction in blood pressure results from α-adrenergic receptors being blocked

Therapeutic outcome: Decreased B/P in hypertension, decreased symptoms of benign prostatic hyperplasia (BPH)

USES: Hypertension, as a single agent or in combination with diuretics or β-blockers, BPH

CONTRAINDICATIONS:

Hypersensitivity

Precautions: Pregnancy **C**, breastfeeding, children, prostate cancer, renal disease, syncope

DOSAGE AND ROUTES

Hypertension

Adult: PO 1 mg at bedtime, may increase dosage slowly to desired response; max 20 mg/day

Benign prostatic hyperplasia

Adult: PO 1 mg at bedtime, gradually increase up to 5-10 mg, max 20 mg

Available forms: Caps 1, 2, 5, 10 mg

Implementation

• May be used in combination with other antihypertensives

• Give at same time each day

• May be given with food to prevent GI symptoms

• Store in airtight container at 86° F (30° C) or less

ADVERSE EFFECTS

CNS: *Dizziness, headache, drowsiness,* anxiety, depression, vertigo, weakness, fatigue
CV: Palpitations, orthostatic hypotension, tachycardia, edema, rebound hypertension
EENT: Blurred vision, epistaxis, tinnitus, dry mouth, red sclera, nasal congestion, sinusitis
GI: *Nausea,* vomiting, diarrhea, constipation, abdominal pain
GU: Urinary frequency, incontinence, impotence, priapism
RESP: Dyspnea, cough, pharyngitis

Pharmacokinetics

Absorption	Well absorbed
Distribution	Not known
Metabolism	Liver (50%)
Excretion	Kidneys unchanged (10%), feces unchanged (20%)
Half-life	9-12 hr

Pharmacodynamics

Onset	15 min
Peak	1 hr
Duration	24 hr

INTERACTIONS

Individual drugs

Alcohol, nitroglycerin, verapamil: increased hypotensive effects

Drug classifications

Antihypertensives (other): increased hypotension

β-Blockers: increased hypotensive effects

Estrogens, NSAIDs, salicylates, sympathomimetics: decreased antihypertensive effect

Drug/herb

Hawthorn: increased antihypertensive effect

Ephedra: decreased antihypertensive effect

NURSING CONSIDERATIONS

Assessment

• **Hypertension:** monitor B/P, orthostatic hypotension, syncope; check for edema in feet, legs daily; I&O ratio; weight daily; notify prescriber of changes

• **Benign prostatic hyperplasia (BPH):** assess urinary patterns (hesitancy, frequency, change in stream, dribbling, dysuria, urgency)

Nursing diagnoses

• Cardiac output, decreased (uses)

• Injury, risk for (adverse reactions)

• Knowledge, deficient (teaching)

• Noncompliance (teaching)

Patient/family education

• Caution patient not to discontinue product abruptly; the importance of complying with dosage schedule, even if feeling better; if dose is missed take as soon as remembered; take medication at same time each day

• Teach patient not to use OTC products (cough, cold, allergy) unless directed by prescriber; to avoid large amounts of caffeine

• Emphasize the need to rise slowly to sitting or standing position to minimize orthostatic hypotension

• Teach patient to notify prescriber of mouth sores, sore throat, fever, swelling of hands or feet, irregular heartbeat, chest pain

• Caution patient to report excessive perspiration, dehydration, vomiting, diarrhea; may lead to fall in B/P

• Caution patient that product may cause dizziness, fainting, light-headedness; may occur during 1st few days of therapy; to avoid hazardous activities

• **Hypertension:** teach patient how to take B/P and normal readings for age group; to take B/P q7day; to continue with regimen including diet and exercise

Evaluation

Positive therapeutic outcome

• Decreased B/P in hypertension

• Decreased symptoms of BPH

TREATMENT OF OVERDOSE:

Administer volume expanders or vasopressors; discontinue product; place patient in supine position

terbinafine (Rx)

(ter-bin′a-feen)

Lamisil

Func. class.: Antifungal, systemic

Chem. class.: Synthetic allylamine derivative

Pregnancy category B

Do not confuse:

LamISIL/lamoTRIgine

ACTION: Interferes with cell membrane permeability in fungi such as *Trichophyton rubrum, Trichophyton mentagrophytes, Trichophyton tonsurans, Epidermophyton floccosum, Microsporum canis, Microsporum audouinii, Microsporum gypseum, Candida,* broad-spectrum antifungal

Therapeutic outcome: Resolution of fungal infection

USES: Onychomycosis of the toenail or fingernail due to dermatophytes

Unlabeled uses: Cutaneous candidiasis, tinea versicolor

CONTRAINDICATIONS:

Hypersensitivity, chronic/active renal/hepatic disease GFR ≤50 mg/min

Precautions: Pregnancy **B**, breastfeeding, children, renal disease

DOSAGE AND ROUTES

Fingernail: PO 250 mg/day × 6 wk

Toenail: PO 250 mg/day × 12 wk

Available forms: Tabs 250 mg

Implementation
• **PO:** give without regard to food

ADVERSE EFFECTS

CNS: Depression
GI: *Diarrhea, dyspepsia, abdominal pain, nausea,* hepatitis
HEMA: Neutropenia
INTEG: Rash, pruritus, urticaria, **Stevens-Johnson syndrome**
MISC: Headache, hepatic enzyme changes, taste, visual/olfactory disturbance

Pharmacokinetics

Absorption	80%
Distribution	Extensive, most to hair, scalp, nails; excreted in breast milk; protein binding 99%
Metabolism	Liver, extensively
Excretion	Unknown
Half-life	22 days or longer

Pharmacodynamics

Onset	Up to 1 wk
Peak	Several days-weeks
Duration	Several weeks

INTERACTIONS

Individual drugs
Cimetidine: increased effect
CycloSPORINE: increased cycloSPORINE clearance
Dextromethorphan: increased levels
Rifampin: increased terbinafine clearance

Drug/herb
Cola nut, guarana, yerba maté, tea (black, green), coffee: side effects

NURSING CONSIDERATIONS

Assessment
• Assess hepatic studies (ALT, AST) before beginning treatment; do not use in presence of hepatic disease
• Monitor CBC in treatment >6 wk
• Assess for continuing infection

Nursing diagnoses
• Infection, risk for (uses)
• Knowledge, deficient (teaching)
• Noncompliance (teaching)

Patient/family education
• Teach patient to notify prescriber of nausea, vomiting, fatigue, jaundice, dark urine, clay-colored stool, RUQ pain, that may indicate hepatic dysfunction
• Teach patient to avoid using OTC medication unless approved by prescriber

Evaluation
Positive therapeutic outcome
• Decrease in size, number of lesions

terbinafine topical
See Appendix B

terbutaline (Rx)
(ter-byoo′te-leen)
Brethine, Bricanye ✦
Func. class.: Selective β$_2$-agonist; bronchodilator
Chem. class.: Catecholamine
Pregnancy category B

ACTION: Relaxes bronchial smooth muscle by direct action on β$_2$-adrenergic receptors through accumulation of cyclic AMP at β-adrenergic receptor sites; results are bronchodilatation, diuresis, and CNS and cardiac stimulation; relaxes uterine smooth muscle

Therapeutic outcome: Bronchodilatation with ease of breathing

USES: Bronchospasm

Unlabeled uses: Premature labor

CONTRAINDICATIONS:

Hypersensitivity to sympathomimetics; closed-angle glaucoma, tachydysrhythmias

Precautions: Pregnancy **B**, breastfeeding, geriatric, cardiac disorders, hyperthyroidism, diabetes mellitus, prostatic hypertension, hypertension, seizure disorder

BLACK BOX WARNING: Labor

DOSAGE AND ROUTES

Bronchospasm
Adult and child >12 yr: PO 2.5-5 mg q8hr; SUBCUT 0.25 mg q15-30min, max 0.5 mg in 4 hr

Adverse effects: *italics* = common; **bold** = life-threatening

Adolescent ≤15 yr and child ≥12 yr: PO 2.5 mg tid, max 7.5 mg/day

Renal dose
Adult: PO CCr 10-50 ml/min 50% of dose; CCr <10 ml/min avoid use

Severe renal failure
Adult: PO avoid if GFR <10 ml/min

Tocolytic (preterm labor) (unlabeled)
Adult: SUBCUT 0.25 mg q 20 min to 6 hr, hold if pulse >120 bpm

Available forms: Tabs 2.5, 5 mg; inj 1 mg/ml

Implementation
• Use this medication before other medications and allow 5 min between each to prevent overstimulation
PO route
• Give PO with meals to decrease gastric irritation; tab may be crushed and mixed with food or fluid
SUBCUT route
• May give by SUBCUT route; do not give by IM route
Aerosol route
• Give after shaking; ask patient to exhale, place mouthpiece in mouth, then inhale slowly; hold breath, remove, exhale slowly; allow at least 1 min between inhalations
• Store in light-resistant container, do not expose to temperatures over 86° F (30° C)

IV route
• Give at 5 mcg q10min until contractions are stopped; use inf pump for correct dose; after ¹/₂-1 hr with no contraction decrease dose by 5 mcg; switch to PO dose when possible

Y-site compatibilities: Regular insulin

ADVERSE EFFECTS
CNS: Tremors, anxiety, insomnia, headache, dizziness, stimulation
CV: Palpitations, tachycardia, hypertension, dysrhythmias, **cardiac arrest**
GI: Nausea, vomiting

Pharmacokinetics

Absorption	Well absorbed (SUBCUT), partially absorbed (PO)
Distribution	Unknown
Metabolism	Liver, partially
Excretion	Unknown
Half-life	Unknown

Pharmacodynamics

	PO	INH	SUB-CUT	IV
Onset	¹/₂ hr	5-15 min	10-15 min	Rapid
Peak	1-2 hr	1-2 hr	¹/₂-1 hr	Unknown
Duration	4-8 hr	4-6 hr	1¹/₂-4 hr	Unknown

INTERACTIONS
Individual drugs
Bleomycin: products are incompatible

Drug classifications
β-Adrenergic blockers: block therapeutic effect
MAOIs: increased chance of hypertensive crisis
Sympathomimetics: increased effects of both products

Drug/herb
Green tea (large amounts), guarana: increased effect

NURSING CONSIDERATIONS
Assessment
• Monitor respiratory function: vital capacity, FEV, ABGs, lung sounds, heart rate, rhythm (baseline)
• Determine that patient has not received theophylline therapy before giving dose; assess client's ability to self-medicate
• Monitor for evidence of allergic reactions; withhold dose and notify prescriber
• **Assess for paradoxical bronchospasm:** dyspnea, wheezing; keep emergency resuscitative equipment nearby

BLACK BOX WARNING: Assess for labor: maternal heart rate, B/P, contractions, fetal heart rate; can inhibit uterine contractions, labor; monitor for hypoglycemia

Nursing diagnoses
• Gas exchange, impaired (uses)
• Knowledge, deficient (teaching)
• Noncompliance (teaching)

Patient/family education
• Advise patient not to use OTC medications; extra stimulation may occur; to use this medication before other medications and allow at least 5 min between each to prevent overstimulation
• Teach patient how to use inhaler; to avoid getting aerosol in eyes because blurring may result; to wash inhaler in warm water daily and dry; to avoid smoking, smoke-filled rooms, persons

with respiratory infections; review package insert with patient
• Teach patient that paradoxical bronchospasm may occur; to stop product immediately and notify prescriber; to limit caffeine products such as chocolate, coffee, tea, and colas
• Instruct patient on administration of dose, not to use more than prescribed; serious side effects may occur; if taking PO regularly and dose is missed, take when remembered; space other doses on new time schedule

Evaluation
Positive therapeutic outcome
• Absence of dyspnea, wheezing after 1 hr
• Improved airway exchange
• Improved ABGs

TREATMENT OF OVERDOSE:
Administer a β_2-adrenergic blocker

terconazole vaginal antifungal
See Appendix B

teriparatide (Rx)
(tah-ree-par'ah-tide)
Forteo
Func. class.: Parathyroid hormone (rDNA)
Pregnancy category C

ACTION: Contains human recombinant parathyroid hormone, which stimulates new bone growth

Therapeutic outcome: Calcium levels at 9-10 mg/dl, decreased symptoms of hypocalcemia, hypoparathyroidism

USES: Postmenopausal women with osteoporosis, men with primary or hypogonadal osteoporosis who are at high risk for fracture, glucocorticoid-induced osteoporosis

CONTRAINDICATIONS:
Hypersensitivity, increased baseline risk of osteosarcoma (Paget's disease, open epiphyses, previous bone radiation), bone metastases, history of skeletal malignancies, other metabolic bone diseases, preexisting hypercalcemia

Precautions: Pregnancy **C**, breastfeeding, children, urolithiasis, hypotension, use >2 yr

BLACK BOX WARNING: Secondary malignancy

DOSAGE AND ROUTES
Adult: SUBCUT 20 mcg/day up to 2 yr (osteoporosis); use for years/lifetime is recommended (glucocorticoid-induced osteoporosis)

Available forms: Prefilled pen delivery device (delivers 20 mcg/day)

Implementation
• Store refrigerated; do not freeze
SUBCUT route
• Give by SUBCUT only, rotate inj sites

ADVERSE EFFECTS
CNS: Dizziness, headache, insomnia, depression, vertigo
CV: Hypertension, angina, syncope
GI: Nausea, diarrhea, dyspepsia, vomiting, constipation
INTEG: Rash, sweating
MISC: Pain, asthenia, hyperuricemia
MS: Arthralgia, leg cramps, back/leg pain, weakness, **osteosarcoma (rare)**
RESP: Rhinitis, cough, pharyngitis, pneumonia, dyspnea

Pharmacokinetics
Absorption	Extensively, rapidly
Distribution	Unknown
Metabolism	Liver
Excretion	Kidneys
Half-life	Unknown

Pharmacodynamics
Unknown

INTERACTIONS
Individual drug
Digoxin: increased digoxin toxicity

Drug/lab test
Calcium: increased levels

NURSING CONSIDERATIONS
Assessment
• **Secondary malignancy:** osteosarcoma depends on length of treatment, those at higher risk for osteosarcoma should not use this product
• Monitor uric acid, chloride, magnesium, electrolytes, urine pH, vit D, phosphate for normal serum levels; serum calcium may be transiently increased after dosing (max at 4-6 hr after dose)
• Assess for bone pain, headache, fatigue, changes in LOC, leg cramps

• Monitor for signs of persistent hypercalcemia: nausea, vomiting, constipation, lethargy, muscle weakness
• Assess nutritional status: diet for sources of vit D (milk, some seafood), calcium (dairy products, dark green vegetables), phosphates (dairy products)

Nursing diagnoses
• Injury, risk for (uses)
• Knowledge, deficient (teaching)
• Mobility, impaired physical (uses)

Patient/family education
• Advise patient of the symptoms of hypercalcemia
• Teach about foods rich in calcium
• Teach how to use delivery device, dispose of needles, not to share pen with others, use at same time of day
• Advise to sit or lie down if dizziness or fast heartbeat occurs after the first few doses

Evaluation
Positive therapeutic outcome
• Increased bone mineral density

tesamorelin
(tes-a-moe-rel′in)
Egrifta
Func. class.: Pituitary hormone, growth hormone modifiers
Pregnancy category X

ACTION: Binds to growth hormone releasing factor receptors on the pituitary somatotroph cells; binding stimulates the production, release of endogenous growth hormone (GH)

Therapeutic outcome: Decreasing lipodystrophy in HIV patients

USES: Treatment of excess abdominal fat in HIV-infected patients with lipodystrophy

CONTRAINDICATIONS:
Hypersensitivity to this product or mannitol, neoplastic disease, pregnancy **X**, disruption of the hypothalamic-pituitary axis (hypothalamic-pituitary-adrenal [HPA] suppression) resulting from hypophysectomy, hypopituitarism, pituitary tumor/surgery, radiation therapy of the head, head trauma, IV/IM administration

Precautions: Breastfeeding, CABG, diabetes, diabetic retinopathy, edema, geriatrics, children, infants, adolescents

DOSAGE AND ROUTES
Adult: SUBCUT 2 mg/day

Available forms: Powder for injection 1 mg

Implementation
SUBCUT route
• Visually inspect parenteral products for particulate matter and discoloration before use whenever solution and container permit
• To reconstitute, inject 2.1 ml sterile water for injection into the 2-mg vial; use the syringe with the needle already attached. To avoid foaming, push the plunger in slowly with the needle at a slight angle so the sterile water goes down the inside wall of the vial; with the needle and syringe attached to the vial, keep the vial upright and gently roll the vial for 30 sec until mixed; do not shake; withdraw 2.1 ml of the reconstituted solution
• Take the syringe out of the vial, place the needle cap on its side against a clean, flat surface; do not touch needle; hold syringe and slide the needle into cap; *push the cap all the way or until it snaps shut; do not touch cap until it covers the needle completely*
• Remove needle and insert a $1/2''$ 27-G safety injection needle onto the syringe; use immediately; throw away any unused product or used sterile water for injection
• Solution should be clear; do not use if discolored, cloudy, or has particles, but slight foaming is acceptable
• Inject subcut into abdomen; avoid scar tissues, bruises, or the navel; rotate injection sites in the abdomen; slowly push plunger down until all solution has been injected
• After removing the injection from the skin, flip back the needle shield until it snaps, covering the injection needle completely; keep pressing until you hear a click; that means the injection needle is protected
• Use a piece of sterile gauze to rub the injection site clean; if there is bleeding, apply pressure to the injection site with gauze for 30 seconds; if bleeding continues, apply a bandage to the site
• Properly dispose of used syringe, needles, vial, and sterile water for injection bottle in a sharps container

ADVERSE EFFECTS
CNS: Depression, flushing, headache, hypoesthesia, insomnia, night sweats, peripheral neuropathy paresthesias, spasms
CV: Chest pain, edema, hypertension, palpitations, peripheral edema

GI: Diarrhea, dyspepsia, nausea, upper abdominal pain, vomiting
INTEG: Flushing, injection site reactions, pruritus, rash, urticaria
MS: Arthralgia, carpal tunnel syndrome, joint swelling, myalgias, stiffness
RESP: *Upper respiratory tract infection*
SYST: Secondary malignancy

Pharmacokinetics

Absorption	Unknown
Distribution	Unknown
Metabolism	Unknown
Excretion	Unknown
Half-life	26 and 38 mins in healthy and HIV-infected patients, respectively, peak 0.15 hrs

Pharmacodynamics

Onset	Unknown
Peak	0.15 hrs
Duration	Unknown

INTERACTIONS
Individual drugs
Cortisone, predniSONE, simvastatin, ritonavir: decreased effect of each specific product

NURSING CONSIDERATIONS
Assessment
• Lipsodystrophy: Assess for sunken cheeks; thinning arms and legs; fat accumulation in the abdomen, jaws, and back of neck; after treatment these should lessen
• Monitor glycosylated hemoglobin A1c (HbA1c), serum IGF-1 concentrations, ophthalmologic exam

Nursing diagnoses
• Body image disturbance (uses)

Patient/family education
• Explain reason for product and expected result
• **Teach patient to use contraception (Pregnancy X)**

Evaluation
Positive therapeutic outcome
• Decreasing lipodystrophy in HIV patients

testosterone (Rx)
(tess-toss´te-rone)
testosterone enanthate (Rx)
Delatestryl
testosterone cypionate (Rx)
Depo-Testosterone
testosterone pellets (Rx)
Testopel
testosterone transdermal (Rx)
Androderm
testosterone gel (Rx)
AndroGel Fortesta, Testim
testosterone buccal (Rx)
Striant
testosterone topical solution (Rx)
Axiron
Func. class.: Androgenic anabolic steroid
Chem. class.: Halogenated testosterone derivative
Pregnancy category X
Controlled substance schedule III

ACTION: Increases weight by building body tissue; increases potassium, phosphorus, chloride, nitrogen levels; increases bone development; responsible for maintenance of secondary sex characteristics (male)

Therapeutic outcome: Increased hormone levels in eunuchoidism, decreased tumor growth in female breast cancer, onset of male puberty

USES: Female breast cancer, hypogonadism, eunuchoidism, male climacteric, oligospermia, impotence, osteoporosis, weight loss in AIDS patients, vulvar dystrophies, low testosterone levels, delayed male puberty (inj)

CONTRAINDICATIONS:
Pregnancy **X**, breastfeeding, severe renal/cardiac/hepatic disease, hypersensitivity, genital bleeding (rare), male breast/prostate cancer

Precautions: Diabetes mellitus, CV disease, MI, urinary tract disorders, prostate cancer, hypercalcemia

BLACK BOX WARNING: Children, accidental exposure

DOSAGE AND ROUTES

Replacement
Adult: IM 25-50 mg 2-3 ×/wk (base or propionate) or 50-400 mg q2-4wk (enanthate or cypionate); transdermal (Testoderm) 4-6 mg applied q24hr; (Androderm, AndroGel) 5 mg applied q24hr; once daily (gel); topical sol (Axiron) 60 mg (2 pump activations) each AM; BUCCAL 1 buccal system (30 mg) to the gum region q12hr before meals/PM
Adult (male) and child: SUBCUT (pellets) 150-450 mg (2-6 pellets) inserted q3-6mo

Breast cancer
Adult: IM 50-100 mg 3 ×/wk (propionate) or 200-400 mg q2-4wk (cypionate or enanthate)

Delayed male puberty
Child >12 yr: IM up to 100 mg/mo for up to 6 mo

Available forms: Enanthate: inj 200 mg/ml; **cypionate:** inj 100, 200 mg/ml; pellets 75 mg; **transdermal** 2.5, 4, 5, 6 mg/24 hr; gel 1% **buccal system** 30 mg; 1.62%, 10 mg/activation

Implementation
• Administer diet with increased calories, protein; decreased sodium if edema occurs
• Administer supportive product if anemia occurs
• Give titrated dose; use lowest effective dose
• Give IM inj deep into upper outer quadrant of gluteal muscle; route can be painful
Transdermal route
• Apply Testoderm to skin of scrotum, Androderm to skin of back, upper arms, thighs, abdomen; area must be clean and dry, free of hair
Gel route
• Products are not interchangeable, dosage and administration for AndroGel 1% differs from AndroGel 1.62%
• Apply daily to clean dry area on shoulders, upper arms, or abdomen; women, children should not touch gel or treated skin
Buccal system route
• Do not chew or swallow buccal system
• Rotate sites; place above incisor tooth on either side of mouth
• Open packet; place rounded side of surface against gum and hold firmly in place with finger over lip for 30 sec; if product falls off, replace with new system; discard in trash can away from children or pets

ADVERSE EFFECTS

CNS: Dizziness, headache, fatigue, tremors, paresthesias, flushing, sweating, anxiety, lability, insomnia, carpal tunnel syndrome

CV: Increased B/P
EENT: Conjunctival edema, nasal congestion
ENDO: Abnormal GTT
GI: Nausea, vomiting, constipation, weight gain, **cholestatic jaundice**
GU: Hematuria, amenorrhea, vaginitis, decreased libido, decreased breast size, clitoral hypertrophy, testicular atrophy, gynecomastia
HEMA: Polycythemia
INTEG: Rash, acneiform lesions, oily hair and skin, flushing, sweating, acne vulgaris, alopecia, hirsutism
MS: Cramps, spasms

Pharmacokinetics

Absorption	Well but slowly absorbed
Distribution	Crosses placenta
Metabolism	Liver
Excretion	Kidneys, breast milk
Half-life	8 days (cypionate)
	10-100 min (base)

Pharmacodynamics

	IM (base)	IM (cypionate)	IM (enanthate)	IM (propionate)
Onset	Unknown	Unknown	Unknown	Unknown
Peak	Unknown	Unknown	Unknown	Unknown
Duration	1-3 days	2-4 wk	2-4 wk	1-3 days

INTERACTIONS

Individual drugs
ACTH, buPROPion: increased edema
Insulin: decreased glucose levels may alter need for insulin
Oxyphenbutazone: increased effects of oxyphenbutazone

Drug classifications
Adrenal steroids: increased edema
Anticoagulants: increased pro-time
Antidiabetics, oral: decreased need for oral antidiabetics

Drug/lab test
Increased: serum cholesterol, blood glucose, urine glucose
Decreased: serum Ca, serum K, T_4, T_3, thyroid ^{131}I uptake test, urine 17-OHCS, 17-KS, PBI

NURSING CONSIDERATIONS

Assessment

• Monitor patient's weight daily; notify prescriber if weekly weight gain is >5 lb; assess I&O ratio; be alert for decreasing urinary output, increasing edema

• Monitor B/P q4hr, Hgb/Hct

• Assess growth rate, bone age in adolescent because growth rate may be uneven (linear/bone growth) if used for extended periods

• Monitor electrolytes: potassium, sodium, chloride, calcium; cholesterol

• Monitor liver function tests: ALT, AST, bilirubin

• Assess edema, hypertension, cardiac symptoms, jaundice

• Assess mental status: affect, mood, behavioral changes, aggression

• **Assess signs of masculinization** in female: increased libido, deepening of voice, decreased breast tissue, enlarged clitoris, menstrual irregularities; male: gynecomastia, impotence, testicular atrophy

• **Assess hypercalcemia:** lethargy, polyuria, polydipsia, nausea, vomiting, constipation; product may have to be decreased

• **Assess hypoglycemia** in diabetics because oral antidiabetic action is increased

Nursing diagnoses

• Infection, risk for (adverse reactions)
• Injury, risk for (adverse reactions)
• Knowledge, deficient (teaching)

Patient/family education

• Inform patient that product needs to be combined with complete health plan: diet, rest, exercise

• Caution patient to notify prescriber if therapeutic response decreases; not to discontinue this medication abruptly

• Inform women patients to report menstrual irregularities; about changes in sex characteristics

• Discuss that 1-3 mo course is necessary for response in breast cancer

• Inform patient about application of transdermal patches: Testoderm to skin of scrotum, Androderm to skin of back, upper arms, thighs, abdomen; area must be dry and free of hair; may be reapplied after bathing, swimming

• Teach about changes in sex characteristics: priapism, gynecomastia, increased libido

Evaluation

Positive therapeutic outcome

• Decrease size of tumor in breast cancer
• Increased androgen levels

tetracaine ophthalmic
See Appendix B

tetracaine topical
See Appendix B

tetracycline (Rx)
(tet-ra-sye′kleen)
Apo-Tetra ✤, Nu-Tetra ✤
Func. class.: Antiinfective—broad-spectrum
Chem. class.: Tetracycline
Pregnancy category D

ACTION: Inhibits protein synthesis and phosphorylation in microorganisms; bacteriostatic

Therapeutic outcome: Bactericidal action against susceptible organisms: gram-positive pathogens *Bacillus anthracis, Clostridium perfringens, Clostridium tetani, Listeria monocytogenes, Nocardia, Propionibacterium acnes, Actinomyces israelii;* gram-negative pathogens *Haemophilus influenzae, Legionella pneumophila, Yersinia enterocolitica, Yersinia pestis, Neisseria gonorrhoeae, Neisseria meningitidis*

USES: Syphilis, *Chlamydia trachomatis,* gonorrhea, lymphogranuloma venereum, uncommon gram-positive, gram-negative organisms, rickettsial infections

CONTRAINDICATIONS:
Pregnancy **D,** breastfeeding, children <8 yr, hypersensitivity to tetracyclines

Precautions: Renal/hepatic disease, UV exposure

DOSAGE AND ROUTES

Susceptible gram-positive/gram-negative infections
Adult: PO 250-500 mg q6hr
Child >8 yr: PO 25-50 mg/kg/day in divided doses q6hr

Chlamydia trachomatis
Adult: PO 500 mg qid × 7 days

Syphilis
Adult and adolescent: PO 500 mg qid × 2 wk; if syphilis duration >1 yr, must treat 30 days

---

Adverse effects: *italics* = common; **bold** = life-threatening

Brucellosis
Adult: PO 500 mg qid × 3 wk with 1 g of streptomycin IM 2 ×/day × 1 wk, and 1 ×/day the 2nd wk

Urethral, endocervical, rectal infections *(C. trachomatis)*
Adult: PO 500 mg qid × 7 days

Acne
Adult and adolescent: PO 250 mg q6hr, then 125-500 mg/day or every other day

Renal dose
Adult: PO CCr 51-90 ml/min give dose q8-12hr, CCr 10-50 ml/min give dose q12-24hr, CCr <10 ml/min give dose q24hr

Available forms: Caps 250, 500 mg

Implementation
PO route
• Give around the clock to maintain proper blood levels; give with food to increase absorption of product; do not give within 3 hr of other agents; product interactions may occur; take on an empty stomach
• Give with 8 oz of water
• Shake liquid preparation well before giving; use calibrated device for proper dosing

ADVERSE EFFECTS
CNS: Fever, headache, paresthesia
CV: Pericarditis
EENT: Dysphagia, glossitis, decreased calcification (permanent discoloration) of deciduous teeth, oral candidiasis, oral ulcers
GI: *Nausea,* abdominal pain, *vomiting, diarrhea,* anorexia, enterocolitis, **hepatotoxicity,** flatulence, abdominal cramps, epigastric burning, stomatitis, hepatitis, **pseudomembranous colitis**
GU: *Increased BUN,* **azotemia, acute renal failure**
HEMA: **Eosinophilia, neutropenia, thrombocytopenia, leukocytosis, hemolytic anemia**
INTEG: *Rash, urticaria, photosensitivity, increased pigmentation,* **exfoliative dermatitis,** pruritus, **angioedema, Stevens-Johnson syndrome**
MISC: Increased intracranial pressure, candidiasis

Pharmacokinetics
Absorption	60%-80% (PO), lower (IM)
Distribution	Widely distributed, some in CSF; crosses placenta
Metabolism	Not metabolized
Excretion	Unchanged—kidneys
Half-life	6-10 hr

Pharmacodynamics
Onset	1-2 hr
Peak	2-3 hr
Duration	Unknown

INTERACTIONS
Individual drugs
Cimetidine, NaHCO₃: decreased tetracycline effect
Digoxin: increased digoxin effect
Iron: forms chelates, decreased absorption
Methoxyflurane: fatal nephrotoxicity
Warfarin: increased warfarin effect

Drug classifications
Alkali products, antacids: decreased tetracycline effect
Contraceptives (oral): decreased oral contraceptive effect
Penicillins: decreased penicillin effect

Drug/herb
Dong quai: increased photosensitivity

Drug/food
Decreased: absorption with dairy products; forms insoluble chelate

Drug/lab test
False increase: urinary catecholamines

NURSING CONSIDERATIONS
Assessment
• **Serious skin reactions:** angioedema, Stevens-Johnson syndrome, exfoliative dermatitis, report immediately after stopping product
• Assess patient for previous sensitivity reaction
• Assess patient for signs and symptoms of infection including characteristics of wounds, sputum, urine, stool, WBC >10,000/mm³, temp; obtain baseline information before, during treatment
• Complete C&S testing before beginning product therapy to identify if correct treatment has been initiated
• **Assess for allergic reactions:** rash, urticaria, pruritus, chills, fever, joint pain; angioedema may occur a few days after therapy

begins; epinephrine, resuscitation equipment should be available for anaphylactic reaction
• Identify urine output; if decreasing, notify prescriber (may indicate nephrotoxicity); increased BUN, creatinine
• **Pseudomembranous colitis:** assess for diarrhea, abdominal pain, fever, fatigue, anorexia; possible anemia, elevated WBC and low serum albumin; stop product and usually give either vancomycin or IV metroNIDAZOLE
• Assess for overgrowth of infection: perineal itching, fever, malaise, redness, pain, swelling, drainage, rash, diarrhea, change in cough, sputum

Nursing diagnoses
• Diarrhea (adverse reactions)
• Infection, risk for (uses)
• Injury, risk for (adverse reactions)
• Knowledge, deficient (teaching)
• Noncompliance (teaching)

Patient/family education
• Teach patient to report sore throat, bruising, bleeding, joint pain; may indicate blood dyscrasias (rare)
• Advise patient to use sunscreen when outdoors to decrease photosensitivity reaction
• Advise patient to contact prescriber if vaginal itching, loose foul-smelling stools, furry tongue occur; may indicate superinfection; report itching, rash, pruritus, urticaria
• Instruct patient to take all medication prescribed for the length of time ordered; product must be taken around the clock to maintain blood levels; do not give medication to others
• Teach patient to notify prescriber immediately of diarrhea with pus, mucus, fever, abdominal pain
• Teach patient to notify prescriber if pregnancy is planned or suspected, pregnancy **D**

Evaluation
Positive therapeutic outcome
• Absence of signs/symptoms of infection (WBC <10,000/mm^3, temp WNL, absence of red, draining wounds)
• Reported improvement in symptoms of infection

---

tetrahydrozoline nasal agent
See Appendix B

tetrahydrozoline ophthalmic
See Appendix B

---

theophylline (Rx)
(thee-off'i-lin)
Elixophyllin, Theo-24, Theochron, Uniphyl
Func. class.: Spasmolytic, bronchodilator
Chem. class.: Xanthine, ethylenediamine
Pregnancy category C

ACTION: Relaxes smooth muscle of respiratory system by blocking phosphodiesterase, which increases cyclic AMP, exact action unknown

Therapeutic outcome: Ability to breathe without difficulty

USES: Bronchial asthma, bronchospasm of COPD, chronic bronchitis, emphysema

CONTRAINDICATIONS: Hypersensitivity to xanthines, tachydysrhythmias

Precautions: Pregnancy **C**, children, geriatric, CHF, cor pulmonale, hepatic disease, active peptic ulcer disease, diabetes mellitus, hyperthyroidism, hypertension, seizure disorder

DOSAGE AND ROUTES
Acute exacerbations of reversible airway obstructions
Adult: PO/IV 5 mg/kg loading dose over 20-30 min

COPD, chronic bronchitis
Adult: IV 0.4 mg/kg/hr in nonsmokers or 0.7 mg/kg/hr in smokers
Adult, child >45 kg: Maintenance PO (regular release) 10 mg/kg/day, in divided doses q1-8hr; after 3 days increase dosage to 400 mg in divided doses q6-8hr; after 3 more days increase to 600 mg in divided doses q6-8hr; max 800 mg/day

Apnea of prematurity
Neonate: IV 4 mg/kg over 20-30 min, then maintenance IV/PO neonate ≥24 days 1.5 mg/kg q12h

Available forms: Cap, ext rel 100, 200, 300, 400 mg; tab ext rel 100, 200, 400, 450, 600 mg; elixir 80 mg/15 ml; sol for inj 250 mg/10 ml, 500 mg/20 ml

Implementation
PO route
• Do not crush or chew time release products
• Contents of bead-filled cap may be sprinkled over food for children's use

T

• Give PO with 8 oz water; to decrease GI symptoms; avoid food, absorption may be affected

IV route
• Give loading dose over 20-30 min; max 20-25 mg/min; do not give by rapid **IV**; use only by cont inf

Y-site compatibilities: Acyclovir, ampicillin, aztreonam, ceFAZolin, cefotetan, ceftazidime, cefTRIAXone, cimetidine, clindamycin, dexamethasone, diltiazem, DOBUTamine, DOPamine, doxycycline, erythromycin, famotidine, fluconazole, gentamicin, haloperidol, heparin, hydrocortisone, lidocaine, methyldopate, methylPREDNISolone, metroNIDAZOLE, midazolam, nafcillin, nitroglycerin, nitroprusside, penicillin G potassium, piperacillin, potassium chloride, ranitidine, ticarcillin, ticarcillin/clavulanate, tobramycin, vancomycin

ADVERSE EFFECTS

CNS: *Anxiety, restlessness, insomnia, dizziness, seizures,* headache, light-headedness, muscle twitching, tremors
CV: *Palpitations, sinus tachycardia,* hypotension, **dysrhythmias,** fluid retention with tachycardia
ENDO: Hyperglycemia
GI: *Nausea, vomiting, anorexia,* diarrhea, bitter taste, dyspepsia, gastric distress
INTEG: Flushing, urticaria
MISC: SIADH, urinary frequency
RESP: Increased rate, tachypnea

Pharmacokinetics

Absorption	Well absorbed (PO), slowly absorbed (ext rel)
Distribution	Crosses placenta, widely distributed
Metabolism	Liver
Excretion	Kidneys, breast milk
Half-life	6.5-10.5 hr; increased in liver disease, CHF, geriatric

Pharmacodynamics

	PO	PO–TIME REL	IV
Onset	Rapid	Slow	Immediate
Peak	1 hr	4-8 hr	Inf end
Duration	6 hr	12-24 hr	6-8 hr

INTERACTIONS

Individual drugs
CarBAMazepine: decreased theophylline level
Cimetidine, disulfiram, erythromycin, fluvoxamine, influenza vaccine, mexiletine, propranolol: increased theophylline action

Lithium: decreased effect of lithium
PHENobarbital, phenytoin, rifampin: decreased theophylline

Drug classifications
Anticoagulants: increased anticoagulant level
β-Adrenergic blockers: cardiotoxicity
Contraceptives (oral), corticosteroids, fluoroquinolones, interferons: increased theophylline action
Smoking: decreased theophylline level

Drug/herb
Coffee, cola nut, guarana, ma huang (ephedra), tea (black, green), yerba maté: increased toxicity
St. John's wort: decreased theophylline level

NURSING CONSIDERATIONS

Assessment
• Monitor theophylline blood levels (therapeutic level is 5-15 mcg/ml); toxicity may occur with small increase above 15 mcg/ml
• Monitor I&O; diuresis occurs; dehydration may result in children or geriatric
• Assess for signs of toxicity: irritability, insomnia, restlessness, tremors, nausea, vomiting
• Monitor respiratory rate, rhythm, depth; auscultate lung fields bilaterally; notify prescriber of abnormalities
• Assess for allergic reactions: rash, urticaria; if these occur, product should be discontinued

Nursing diagnoses
• Knowledge, deficient (teaching)

Patient/family education
• Advise patient to check OTC medications, current prescription medications for ePHEDrine, which increases stimulation, and to avoid alcohol, caffeine
• Caution patient to avoid hazardous activities; dizziness may occur
• Inform patient that if GI upset occurs, to take product with 8 oz of water; avoid food; absorption may be decreased
• Advise patient to notify prescriber of toxicity: nausea, vomiting, anxiety, insomnia, seizures
• Advise patient to notify prescriber of change in smoking habit; dosage may have to be changed

Evaluation
Positive therapeutic outcome
• Ability to breathe more easily

thiamine (vitamin B₁) (PO, OTC; IV, IM, Rx)
Betaxin ✦, Betalin S, Biamine, Revitonus, Thiamilate
Func. class.: Vitamin B₁
Chem. class.: Water soluble
Pregnancy category A

Do not confuse:
thiamine/Tenormin

ACTION: Needed for pyruvate metabolism, carbohydrate metabolism

Therapeutic outcome: Prevention and treatment of thiamine deficiency

USES: Vit B₁ deficiency or polyneuritis, cheilosis adjunct with thiamine beriberi, Wernicke-Korsakoff syndrome, pellagra, metabolic disorders, alcoholism

CONTRAINDICATIONS:
Hypersensitivity

Precautions: Pregnancy A

DOSAGE AND ROUTES
RDA
Adult: PO (Male) 1.2-1.5 mg; (female) 1.1 mg; (pregnancy) 1.4 mg; (breastfeeding) 1.4 mg
Child 9-13 yr: PO 0.9 mg
Child 4-8 yr: PO 0.6 mg
Child 1-3 yr: PO 0.5 mg
Infant 6 mo-1 yr: PO 0.3 mg
Neonate and infant to 6 mo: PO 0.3 mg

Beriberi
Adult: PO 5-30 mg qd or given in 3 divided doses × 1 month; IM/IV 5-30 mg qd or in 3 doses, then convert to PO
Child/infant: PO 10-50 mg qd × 2 wk, then 5-10 mg qd × 1 mo; IV/IM 10-25 mg/day × 2 wk, then 5-10 mg qd × 1 mo

Available forms: Tabs 50, 100, 250, 500 mg; inj 100 mg/ml; enteric-coated tabs 20 mg

Implementation
IM route
• Give by IM inj; rotate sites if pain and inflammation occur; do not mix with alkaline sol; Z-track to minimize pain
• Application of cold compress may decrease pain
• Store in airtight, light-resistant container

Direct IV route
• IV undiluted given over 5 min
Continuous IV infusion route
• Dilute in compatible IV sol

Syringe compatibilities: Doxapram

Y-site compatibilities: Famotidine

ADVERSE EFFECTS
CNS: Weakness, restlessness
CV: Collapse, pulmonary edema, hypotension
EENT: Tightness of throat
GI: Hemorrhage, *nausea, diarrhea*
INTEG: Angioneurotic edema, cyanosis, sweating, warmth
SYST: Anaphylaxis

Pharmacokinetics

Absorption	Well absorbed (PO, IM), completely absorbed (**IV**)
Distribution	Widely distributed
Metabolism	Liver
Excretion	Kidneys (unchanged—excess amounts)
Half-life	Unknown

Pharmacodynamics
Unknown

NURSING CONSIDERATIONS
Assessment
• **Anaphylaxis (IV only):** assess for swelling of face, eyes, lips, throat, wheezing
• **Thiamine deficiency:** assess for anorexia, weakness, pain, depression, confusion, blurred vision, tachycardia
• Assess nutritional status: yeast, beef, liver, whole or enriched grains, legumes

Nursing diagnoses
• Knowledge, deficient (teaching)
• Nutrition: less than body requirements, imbalanced (uses)

Patient/family education
• Teach patient necessary foods to be included in diet: yeast, beef, liver, legumes, whole grains

Evaluation
Positive therapeutic outcome
• Absence of nausea, vomiting, anorexia, insomnia, tachycardia, paresthesias, depression, muscle weakness

T

Adverse effects: *italics* = common; **bold** = life-threatening

thioridazine (Rx)

(thye-or-rid′a-zeen)
Func. class.: Antipsychotic/neuroleptic
Chem. class.: Phenothiazine, piperidine
Pregnancy category C

Do not confuse:
Thioridazine/Thiothixene

ACTION: Depresses cerebral cortex, hypothalamus, limbic system, which control activity, aggression; blocks neurotransmission produced by dopamine at synapse; exhibits strong α-adrenergic, anticholinergic blocking action; mechanism for antipsychotic effects is unclear

Therapeutic outcome: Decreased signs and symptoms of psychosis

USES: Psychotic disorders, schizophrenia, behavioral problems in children, anxiety, major depressive disorders, organic brain syndrome

CONTRAINDICATIONS:

Children <2 yr, hypersensitivity, coma, CNS depression

> **BLACK BOX WARNING:** QT prolongation, cardiac dysrhythmias

Precautions: Pregnancy **C**, breastfeeding, seizure disorders, hypertension, hepatic/pulmonary disease, renal failure, BPH, glaucoma, phenothiazine hypersensitivity, suicidal ideation, smoking, Reye's syndrome, Parkinson's disease

> **BLACK BOX WARNING:** Cardiac disease, dementia, AV block, bundle branch block, torsades de pointes

DOSAGE AND ROUTES

Psychosis
Adult: PO 25-100 mg tid, max dose 800 mg/day; dose is gradually increased to desired response, then reduced to minimum maintenance

Depression/behavioral problems/organic brain syndrome
Adult: PO 25 tid, range from 10 mg bid-qid to 50 mg tid-qid; max 800 mg/day for short period
Geriatric: PO 10-25 mg daily-bid, increase 4-7 days by 10-25 mg to desired dose, max 300 mg/day for short period
Child 2-12 yr: PO 0.5-3 mg/kg/day in divided doses, max 3 mg/kg/day

Available forms: Tabs 10, 15, 25, 50, 100, 150, 200 mg

Implementation
• Decrease dosage in geriatric because metabolism is slowed
• Administer PO with full glass of water, milk; or give with food to decrease GI upset
• Give antacids 2 hr before or after this product
• Store in airtight, light-resistant container, oral sol in amber bottle

ADVERSE EFFECTS

CNS: *EPS (pseudoparkinsonism, akathisia, dystonia, tardive dyskinesia)*, **seizures,** *headache,* confusion, **neuroleptic malignant syndrome, dizziness,** drowsiness
CV: Orthostatic hypotension, **cardiac arrest,** ECG changes, **tachycardia, QT prolongation,** torsades de pointes
EENT: Blurred vision, glaucoma, dry eyes
GI: *Dry mouth, nausea, vomiting, anorexia, constipation,* diarrhea, jaundice, weight gain
GU: Urinary retention, urinary frequency, enuresis, impotence, amenorrhea, gynecomastia, ejaculation dysfunction, priapism
HEMA: Anemia, **leukopenia, leukocytosis, agranulocytosis**
INTEG: *Rash,* photosensitivity, dermatitis
RESP: **Laryngospasm,** dyspnea, **respiratory depression**

Pharmacokinetics
Absorption	Variably absorbed (tab)
Distribution	Widely distributed, high concentrations in CNS, crosses placenta, protein binding 91%-99%
Metabolism	Liver, extensively; GI mucosa
Excretion	Kidneys, breast milk
Half-life	26-36 hr

Pharmacodynamics
Onset	Erratic
Peak	2-4 hr
Duration	8-12 hr

INTERACTIONS

Individual drugs
Alcohol: oversedation
Aluminum hydroxide, magnesium hydroxide: decreased absorption

BLACK BOX WARNING: Haloperidol, chloroquine, droperidol, pentamidine, arsenic trioxide, levomethadyl: increased QT prolongation

Lithium: decreased thioridazine levels

Drug classifications
Anesthetics (barbiturate), CNS depressants: oversedation
Antacids: decreased absorption
Anticholinergics: increased anticholinergic effects
Antiparkinson agents: decreased effect of these agents
Barbiturates: decreased thioridazine effect
Centrally acting antihypertensives: decreased antihypertensive effect

BLACK BOX WARNING: Class IA/III antidysrhythmics, some phenothiazines, β-agonists, local anesthetics, tricyclics, CYP3A4 inhibitors (amiodarone, clarithromycin, erythromycin, telithromycin, troleandomycin); CYP3A4 substrates (methadone, pimozide, QUEtiapine, quiNIDine, risperidone, ziprasidone): increased QT prolongation

CYP2D6 inducers: decreased thioridazine levels
CYP2D6 inhibitors: increased thioridazine levels

Drug/lab test
Increased: liver function tests, cardiac enzymes, cholesterol, blood glucose, prolactin, bilirubin, cholinesterase, ^{131}I
Decreased: hormones (blood and urine)
False positive: pregnancy tests, PKU
False negative: urinary steroids, pregnancy test

NURSING CONSIDERATIONS
Assessment
• Assess mental status: orientation, mood, behavior, presence of hallucinations, and type before initial administration and monthly; this product should significantly reduce psychotic behavior
• Check for swallowing of PO medication; check for hoarding or giving of medication to other patients
• Monitor I&O ratio; palpate bladder if low urinary output occurs, especially in geriatric; urinalysis recommended before, during prolonged therapy
• Monitor bilirubin, CBC, liver function tests monthly
• Assess affect, orientation, LOC, reflexes, gait, coordination, sleep pattern disturbances
• Monitor B/P sitting, standing, and lying, take pulse and respirations q4hr during initial

treatment; establish baseline before starting treatment; report drops of 30 mm Hg; obtain baseline ECG, monitor Q- and T-wave changes
• Check for dizziness, faintness, palpitations, tachycardia on rising; severe orthostatic hypotension is common
• **QT prolongation:** monitor ECG for QT prolongation, ejection fraction; assess for chest pain, palpitations, dyspnea
⚠ Neuroleptic malignant syndrome: assess for hyperpyrexia, muscle rigidity, increased CPK, altered mental status, dyspnea, fatigue; product should be discontinued
• **EPS** including akathisia (inability to sit still, no pattern to movements), tardive dyskinesia (bizarre movements of the jaw, mouth, tongue, extremities), pseudoparkinsonism (ragged tremors, pill rolling, shuffling gate); an antiparkinsonian product should be prescribed
• Assess for constipation, urinary retention daily; if these occur, increase bulk, water in diet

Nursing diagnoses
• Coping, ineffective (uses)
• Knowledge, deficient (teaching)
• Noncompliance (teaching)

Patient/family education
• Teach patient to use good oral hygiene; frequent rinsing of mouth, sugarless gum for dry mouth
• Advise patient to avoid hazardous activities until product response is determined; dizziness, blurred vision are common
• Inform patient that orthostatic hypotension occurs often and to rise from sitting or lying position gradually; to avoid hot tubs, hot showers, tub baths because hypotension may occur
• Instruct patient that in hot weather, heat stroke may occur; take extra precautions to stay cool
• Caution patient to avoid abrupt withdrawal of this product, or EPS may result; product should be withdrawn slowly
• Teach patient to avoid OTC preparations (cough, hay fever, cold) unless approved by prescriber; serious product interactions may occur; avoid use with alcohol, CNS depressants; increased drowsiness may occur
• Advise patient to use sunglasses and sunscreen to prevent burns
• Teach patient about EPS and necessity for meticulous oral hygiene because oral candidiasis may occur
• Advise patient to take antacids 2 hr before or after this product
• Instruct patient to report sore throat, malaise, fever, bleeding, mouth sores; if these occur, CBC

T

should be performed and product discontinued; may cause vision impairment, report to prescriber
• Advise patient that urine may be discolored

Evaluation
Positive therapeutic outcome
• Decrease in emotional excitement, hallucinations, delusions, paranoia
• Reorganization of patterns of thought, speech

TREATMENT OF OVERDOSE:
Lavage if orally ingested; provide airway; *do not induce vomiting or use EPINEPHrine*, CV monitoring, continuous ECG

---

thyroid USP (desiccated) (Rx)
(thye′roid)
Armour Thyroid, Bio-Throid, Nature Thyroid, NP Thyroid
Func. class.: Thyroid hormone
Chem. class.: Active thyroid hormone in natural state and ratio
Pregnancy category A

Do not confuse:
Thyrar/Thyrolar

ACTION: Increases metabolic rate; increases cardiac output, O_2 consumption, body temp, blood volume, growth, development at cellular level

Therapeutic outcome: Correction of lack of thyroid hormone

USES: Hypothyroidism, cretinism (juvenile hypothyroidism), myxedema

CONTRAINDICATIONS:
Adrenal insufficiency, MI, thyrotoxicosis, porcine protein hypersensitivity

BLACK BOX WARNING: Obesity treatment

Precautions: Pregnancy A, breastfeeding, geriatric, angina pectoris, hypertension, ischemia, cardiac disease

DOSAGE AND ROUTES
Hypothyroidism
Adult: PO 60-65 mg/day, increased by 30 mg qmo until desired response; maintenance dose 65-120 mg/day

Geriatric: PO 7.5-15 mg/day, increase dose q6-8wk until desired response

Cretinism/juvenile hypothyroidism
Child: PO 15 mg/day, then 30 mg/day after 2 wk, then 60 mg/day after another 2 wk; maintenance dose 60-180 mg/day

Myxedema
Adult: PO 15 mg/day, double dose q2wk, maintenance 60-180 mg/day

Available forms: Tabs 16, 32, 60, 65, 98, 130, 195, 260, 325 mg; enteric-coated tabs 32, 65, 130 mg; sugar-coated tabs 32, 65, 130, 195 mg; caps 65, 130, 195, 325 mg

Implementation
• Give in AM if possible as a single dose to decrease sleeplessness; at same time each day to maintain product level
• Do not give with food because absorption will be decreased
• Give only for hormone imbalances; not to be used for obesity, male infertility, menstrual conditions, lethargy; give lowest dose that relieves symptoms; lower dosage in the geriatric and in cardiac diseases
• Store in airtight, light-resistant container
• Wean patient off medication 4 wk before RAIU test

ADVERSE EFFECTS
CNS: *Insomnia, tremors,* headache, **thyroid storm**
CV: *Tachycardia, palpitations, angina,* **dys-rhythmias,** hypertension, **cardiac arrest**
GI: Nausea, diarrhea, increased or decreased appetite, cramps
MISC: Menstrual irregularities, weight loss, sweating, heat intolerance, fever

Pharmacokinetics
Absorption	Well absorbed
Distribution	Widely distributed, does not cross placenta
Metabolism	Liver, tissues
Excretion	Feces via bile, breast milk
Half-life	T_3, 2 days; T_4, 1 wk

Pharmacodynamics
Onset	1 hr
Peak	12-48 hr
Duration	Unknown

INTERACTIONS
Individual drugs
Aluminum, calcium, magnesium: decreased thyroid absorption

Drug classifications

Anticoagulants, oral: increased effects of anticoagulants

Antidepressants (tricyclic): increased antidepressant (tricyclics) effect

Bile acid sequestrants: decreased thyroid absorption

Catecholamines: increased effects of catecholamines

Estrogens: decreased thyroid hormone effect

Sympathomimetics: increased effects of sympathomimetics

Drug/lab test

Increased: CPK, LDH, AST, PBI, blood glucose
Decreased: thyroid function tests

NURSING CONSIDERATIONS

Assessment

> **BLACK BOX WARNING: Obesity treatment:** use can lead to serious or life-threatening toxicity

- Identify if the patient is taking anticoagulants, antidiabetic agents; document on chart
- Take B/P, pulse before each dose; monitor I&O ratio and weight every day in same clothing, using same scale, at same time of day
- Monitor height, weight, psychomotor development, growth rate if given to a child
- Monitor T_3, T_4, FTIs, which are decreased; radioimmunoassay of TSH, which is increased; radioactive iodine uptake (RAIU), which is increased if patient's dose of medication is too low
- Monitor pro-time; patient may require decreased dosage of anticoagulant; check for bleeding, bruising
- **Hyperthyroidism:** assess for increased nervousness, excitability, irritability, which may indicate that dose of medication is too high, usually after 1-3 wk of treatment
- **Hypothyroidism:** lethargy, cold intolerance, weight gain, constipation, muscle cramps, may indicate dosage is too low
- Assess cardiac status: angina, palpitation, chest pain, change in VS; the geriatric patient may have undetected cardiac problems; baseline ECG should be completed before treatment

Nursing diagnoses

- Knowledge, deficient (teaching)
- Noncompliance (teaching)

Patient/family education

- Teach patient that product is not a cure but controls symptoms and that treatment is long-term, that strong odor is normal
- Instruct patient to report excitability, irritability, anxiety, sweating, heat intolerance, chest pain, palpitations, which indicate overdose
- Advise patient not to switch brands unless approved by prescriber; bioavailability may differ; do not take with food; absorption will be decreased
- Teach patient that product might be discontinued after giving birth; thyroid panel will be evaluated after 1-2 mo
- Teach patient that hyperthyroid child will show almost immediate behavior/personality change; that hair loss will occur in child and is temporary
- Caution patient that product is not to be taken to reduce weight
- Caution patient to avoid OTC preparations containing iodine; read labels; other medications should not be used unless approved by prescriber
- Teach patient to avoid iodine-containing food: iodized salt, soybeans, tofu, turnips, certain kinds of seafood and bread

Evaluation

Positive therapeutic outcome

- Absence of depression
- Weight loss, increased diuresis, pulse, appetite
- Absence of constipation, peripheral edema, cold intolerance, pale, cool dry skin, brittle nails, alopecia, coarse hair, menorrhagia, night blindness, paresthesias, syncope, stupor, coma, rosy cheeks
- Improved levels of T_3, T_4 by laboratory tests
- Child: Age-appropriate weight, height, and psychomotor development

TREATMENT OF OVERDOSE:

Withhold dose for up to 1 wk; acute overdose— gastric lavage or induce emesis, then activated charcoal; provide supportive treatment to control symptoms

tiagabine (Rx)

(tie-ah-ga′been)
Gabitril
Func. class.: Anticonvulsant
Pregnancy category C

ACTION: Inhibits reuptake and metabolism of GABA; may increase seizure threshold, structurally similar to GABA; tiagabine binding sites in neocortex, hippocampus

USES: Adjunct treatment of partial seizures in adults and children ≥12 yr

CONTRAINDICATIONS:
Hypersensitivity

Precautions: Pregnancy **C,** breastfeeding, child <12 yr, geriatric, renal/hepatic disease, suicidal ideation/behavior, status epilepticus, mania, bipolar disorder, abrupt discontinuation, depression

DOSAGE AND ROUTES
When not given with a CYP3A4 enzyme, effect of tiagabine is doubled; lower dosages are indicated
Adult: PO (those on an enzyme-inducing antiepileptic) 4 mg/day in divided doses, may increase by 4-8 mg qwk until desired response, max 56 mg/day
Child 12-18 yr: PO 4 mg/day, may increase by 4 mg at beginning of wk 2, may increase by 4-8 mg qwk until desired response, max 32 mg/day

Available forms: Tabs 2, 4, 12, 16 mg

Implementation
• Store at room temperature away from heat and light
• Provide assistance with ambulation during early part of treatment; dizziness occurs
• Provide seizure precautions: padded side rails; move objects that may harm patient

ADVERSE EFFECTS
CNS: *Dizziness, anxiety,* somnolence, ataxia, confusion, *asthenia,* unsteady gait, depression, **suicidal ideation**
CV: Vasodilatation
GI: Nausea, diarrhea, vomiting, increased appetite
INTEG: Pruritus, rash, **Stevens-Johnson syndrome**
RESP: Pharyngitis, coughing

Pharmacokinetics

Absorption	>95%
Distribution	Protein binding 96%
Metabolism	Liver
Excretion	Kidneys
Half-life	7-9 hr

Pharmacodynamics

Onset	Unknown
Peak	45 min
Duration	Unknown

INTERACTIONS

Individual drugs
CarBAMazepine, PHENobarbital, phenytoin, primidone: decreased effect of these products

Sevelamer: decreased tiagabine effect
Valproate: lower dose of tiagabine may be required

Drug classifications
CNS depressants: increased CNS depression

Drug/food
High-fat meal: decreased rate of absorption

NURSING CONSIDERATIONS

Assessment
• Monitor renal function tests: urinalysis, BUN, urine creatinine q3mo
• Monitor liver function tests: ALT, AST, bilirubin
• Assess description of seizures: location, duration, presence of aura
⚠ **Assess mental status: mood, sensorium, affect, behavioral changes, suicidal thoughts; if mental status changes, notify prescriber**

Nursing diagnoses
• Injury, risk for (uses, adverse reactions)
• Knowledge, deficient (teaching)
• Noncompliance (teaching)

Patient/family education
• Advise patient to carry/wear emergency ID stating patient's name, products taken, condition, prescriber's name and phone number
• Advise patient to avoid driving, other activities that require alertness
• Teach patient not to discontinue medication quickly after long-term use

Evaluation
Positive therapeutic outcome
• Decreased seizure activity; document on patient's chart

TREATMENT OF OVERDOSE:
Lavage, VS

ticagrelor
(tye-ka′gre-lor)
Brilinta
Func. class.: Platelet inhibitor
Chem. class.: ADP receptor antagonist
Pregnancy category C

ACTION: Reversibly binds to the platelet receptor, preventing platelet activation

Therapeutic outcome: Prevention of thromboembolism

USES: Arterial thromboembolism prophylaxis in acute coronary syndrome (ACS)

⚠ Nurse Alert

(unstable angina, acute MI), including in patients undergoing percutaneous coronary intervention (PCI)

CONTRAINDICATIONS:
Hypersensitivity, severe hepatic disease, bleeding

Precautions: Abrupt discontinuation, breastfeeding, children, infants, neonates, GI bleeding, hepatic disease, pregnancy C

DOSAGE AND ROUTES
Adult: PO Loading dose 180 mg with aspirin (usually 325 mg PO); then, give 90 mg bid with aspirin 75-100 mg/day, do not give maintenance doses of aspirin >100 mg/day

Available forms: Tab 90 mg

Implementation
• May be taken without regard to food
• Store at room temperature, in original container in dry place
• Discontinue 5-7 days before surgery

ADVERSE EFFECTS
CNS: Dizziness, fatigue, headache
CV: Atrial fibrillation, bradyarrhythmias, chest pain, hypertension, hypotension, syncope, ventricular pauses
GI: Diarrhea, nausea
HEMA: Fatal bleeding
MISC: Back pain, gynecomastia, hyperuricemia
RESP: Cough, dyspnea

> **BLACK BOX WARNING:** Bleeding, intracranial bleeding

> **BLACK BOX WARNING:** Coronary artery bypass graft (CABG) surgery

Pharmacokinetics

Absorption	36%
Distribution	Protein binding >99%
Metabolism	By CYP3A4
Excretion	26% (urine)
Half-life	7 hr; 9 hr metabolite

Pharmacodynamics

Onset	Unknown
Peak	1.5 hr (product), 2.5 hrs (metabolite)
Duration	≥8 hrs

INTERACTIONS
Individual drugs
Simvastatin, lovastatin: increased effect
Digoxin: change in effect

Drug classifications
Anticoagulants, NSAIDs, platelet inhibitors: increased bleeding risk
CYP3A4 inducers (carBAMazepine, dexamethasone, PHENobarbital, phenytoin, rifampin): decreased ticagrelor action
CYP3A4 inhibitors (atazanavir, clarithromycin, dalfopristin, delavirdine, indinavir, isoniazid, itraconazole, ketoconazole, lopinavir, nefazodone, nelfinavir, quinupristin, ritonavir, saquinavir, telithromycin, tipranavir, voriconazole): increased bleeding risk

Drug/lab
Serum creatinine: increased

NURSING CONSIDERATIONS
Assessment
• Thromboembolism: Monitor CBC differential with platelet count baseline and periodically during treatment

> **BLACK BOX WARNING:** Assess for bleeding that may occur when aspirin is combined with this product, some bleeding can be fatal

• Abrupt discontinuation: Do not discontinue abruptly, may increase risk for MI, stent thrombosis, death

Nursing diagnoses
• Risk for injury (uses)

Patient/family education
• Teach patient to take only as prescribed, do not skip or double doses, if a dose is missed, take next dose at scheduled time
• Advise patient to notify prescriber of chills, fever, bruising, bleeding
• Teach patient not to use any Rx, OTC products, herbs without approval of prescriber; products with aspirin, NSAIDs may cause bleeding
• Instruct patient to notify all health care providers of product use
• Advise patient that product can be taken without regard to meals
• Teach patient it may take longer for bleeding to stop

Evaluation
Positive therapeutic outcome
• Prevention of thromboembolism

T

Adverse effects: *italics* = common; **bold** = life-threatening

ticarcillin/clavulanate (Rx)
(tye-kar-sill'in)
Timentin
Func. class.: Extended-spectrum penicillin
Chem. class.: Antiinfective—broad-spectrum
Pregnancy category B

ACTION: Interferes with cell wall replication of susceptible organisms; osmotically unstable cell wall swells, bursts from osmotic pressure; clavulanate inhibits β-lactamase and protects against enzymatic degradation of ticarcillin

Therapeutic outcome: Resolution of infection

USES: Respiratory, soft tissue, urinary tract infections; bacterial septicemia; effective for gram-positive cocci *(Staphylococcus aureus, Streptococcus faecalis, Streptococcus pneumoniae)*, gram-negative cocci *(Neisseria gonorrhoeae)*, gram-positive bacilli *(Clostridium perfringens, Clostridium tetani)*, gram-negative bacilli *(Bacteroides, Fusobacterium nucleatum, Escherichia coli, Proteus mirabilis, Salmonella, Morganella morganii, Proteus rettgeri, Enterobacter, Pseudomonas aeruginosa, Serratia, Peptococcus, Peptostreptococcus, Eubacterium)*

CONTRAINDICATIONS: Hypersensitivity to penicillins; neonates

Precautions: Pregnancy **B,** hypersensitivity to cephalosporins, renal disease

DOSAGE AND ROUTES

Systemic/urinary tract infections, moderate/severe infections
Adult ≥60 kg: IV INF 3.1 g q4-6hr
Adult <60 kg: IV INF 200-300 mg/kg/day q4-6hr
Child >60 kg: IV INF 3.1 g q4hr
Child <60 kg: IV INF 300 mg/kg/day q4hr

Mild/moderate infections
Child ≥60 kg: IV INF 3.1 g q6hr
Child <60 kg: IV INF 200 mg/kg/day q6hr

Renal dose
Adult: IV INF loading dose 3.1 g; CCr 60 ml/min 3.1 g q4hr; CCr 30-60 ml/min 2 g q4hr; CCr 10-30 ml/min 2 g q8hr; CCr <10 ml/min 2 g q12hr; CCr <10 ml/min with hepatic dysfunction 2 g q24hr

Available forms: Inj IM, **IV** 3 g ticarcillin and 0.1 g clavulanate; **IV** inf 3 g ticarcillin and 0.1 g clavulanate; powder for inj 3 g ticarcillin, 0.1 g clavulanate

Implementation
• Give product after C&S has been completed
• Have adrenalin, suction, tracheostomy set, endotracheal intubation equipment available
• Obtain scratch test results to assess allergy after securing order from prescriber; usually done when penicillin is only product of choice
• Store at room temperature, reconstituted sol for 12-24 hr or 3-7 days refrigerated

Intermittent IV infusion route
• Give **IV** after diluting 3.1 g or less/13 ml of sterile water or 0.9% NaCl (200 mg/ml), shake; may further dilute in 50-100 ml or more 0.9% NaCl, D$_5$W, or LR and run over ½ hr

Y-site compatibilities: Allopurinol, amifostine, amikacin, anidulafungin, atropine, aztreonam, bivalirudin, bumetanide, ceFAZolin, cefepime, cefotaxime, cefoxitin, ceftazidime, ceftizoxime, cefTRIAXone, cefuroxime, chloramphenicol, cimetidine, clindamycin, cyclophosphamide, cycloSPORINE, dexamethasone, dexmedetomidine, digoxin, diltiazem, diphenhydrAMINE, docetaxel, DOPamine, DOXOrubicin liposome, doxycycline, enalaprilat, EPINEPHrine, esmolol, etoposide phosphate, famotidine, fenoldopam, filgrastim, fluconazole, furosemide, gemcitabine, gentamicin, granisetron, heparin, hydrocortisone, HYDROmorphone, imipenem/cilastatin, insulin, isoproterenol, labetalol, levofloxacin, lidocaine, linezolid, LORazepam, melphalan, meperidine, methylPREDNISolone, metoclopramide, metoprolol, metroNIDAZOLE, milrinone, morphine, nitroglycerin, nitroprusside, norepinephrine, ondansetron, palonosetron, pantoprazole, pemetrexed, penicillin G potassium, perphenazine, phenylephrine, procainamide, propofol, propranolol, ranitidine, remifentanil, sargramostim, sodium bicarbonate, tacrolimus, teniposide, theophylline, thiotepa, tirofiban, tobramycin, vasopressin, verapamil, vinorelbine, voriconazole

Y-site incompatibilities: Acyclovir, amphotericin B cholesteryl sulfate, azithromycin, caspofungin, diazepam, DOBUTamine, drotrecogin, erythromycin, ganciclovir, haloperidol, hydrOXYzine, lansoprazole, phenytoin, promethazine, protamine, quinupristin/dalfopristin, trimethoprim/sulfamethoxazole

ADVERSE EFFECTS

CNS: Lethargy, hallucinations, anxiety, depression, twitching, **coma, seizures,** confusion, drowsiness
GI: *Nausea, vomiting, diarrhea,* increased AST, ALT, abdominal pain, glossitis, colitis, **pseudomembranous colitis,** hepatotoxicity
GU: Oliguria, proteinuria, hematuria, *vaginitis, moniliasis,* **glomerulonephritis**
HEMA: Anemia, increased bleeding time, **bone marrow depression, granulocytopenia**
INTEG: Rash, urticaria, **toxic epidermal necrolysis**
META: Hypokalemia, hyperkalemia, alkalosis, hypernatremia
SYST: Anaphylaxis, Stevens-Johnson syndrome

Pharmacokinetics

Absorption	Completely absorbed (**IV**)
Distribution	Widely distributed, crosses blood-brain barrier
Metabolism	Liver
Excretion	Kidneys
Half-life	64-68 min

Pharmacodynamics

	IV
Onset	Unknown
Peak	30-45 min
Duration	4 hr

INTERACTIONS

Individual drugs

Chloramphenicol: decreased antimicrobial effect of ticarcillin
Heparin: increased effect of heparin
Methotrexate: increased methotrexate level
Probenecid, sulfinpyrazone: increased ticarcillin concentration

Drug classifications

Aminoglycosides (**IV**): decreased antimicrobial effect of ticarcillin
Anticoagulants: increased bleeding
Contraceptives (oral): decreased effect of oral contraceptives
Erythromycins: decreased absorption
Macrolides, sulfonamides, tetracyclines: decreased ticarcillin effect

Drug/lab test

False positive: urine glucose, urine protein, Coombs' test

NURSING CONSIDERATIONS

Assessment

• Monitor I&O ratio; report hematuria, oliguria because penicillin in high doses is nephrotoxic
• **Pseudomembranous colitis:** assess for diarrhea, abdominal pain, fever, fatigue, anorexia; possible anemia, elevated WBC, low serum albumin; stop product and usually give either vancomycin or IV metroNIDAZOLE
• Monitor liver function tests: AST, ALT
• Monitor blood tests: WBC, RBC, Hgb, Hct, bleeding time
• Monitor renal function tests: urinalysis, protein, blood
• Obtain C&S test results before initiating product therapy; product may be given as soon as culture is performed
• Assess bowel pattern before, during treatment
• Assess skin eruptions after administration of penicillin to 1 wk after discontinuing product
⚠ Assess for anaphylaxis: wheezing, rash, laryngeal edema; have emergency equipment nearby
• **Serious skin reactions:** Stevens-Johnson syndrome, toxic epidermal necrolysis

Nursing diagnoses

• Infection, risk for (uses)
• Knowledge, deficient (teaching)

Patient/family education

• Advise patient that C&S may be performed after completed course of medication
• Instruct patient to report sore throat, fever, fatigue (may indicate superinfection)
• Advise patient to carry/wear emergency ID if allergic to penicillins
• Advise patient to use alternative birth control methods instead of hormonal
• Advise patient to report persistent diarrhea with blood, pus, mucus, or fever

Evaluation
Positive therapeutic outcome
• Absence of fever, purulent drainage, redness, inflammation

TREATMENT OF OVERDOSE:

Withdraw product, maintain airway, administer EPINEPHrine, aminophylline, O_2, **IV** corticosteroids for anaphylaxis

Adverse effects: *italics* = common; **bold** = life-threatening

ticlopidine (Rx)

(tye-cloe'pi-deen)
Func. class.: Platelet aggregation inhibitor
Chem. class.: Thienopyridine compound
Pregnancy category B

ACTION: Irreversible inhibition of platelet aggregation through antagonism of ADP

Therapeutic outcome: Decreased stroke by decreasing platelet aggregation

USES: Reducing the risk of stroke in high-risk patients

Unlabeled uses: Intermittent claudication, chronic arterial occlusion, subarachnoid hemorrhage, uremic patients with AV shunts/fistulas, open heart surgery, coronary artery bypass grafts, primary glomerulonephritis, diabetic neuropathy

CONTRAINDICATIONS:

Hypersensitivity, severe liver disease, active bleeding, coagulopathy

> **BLACK BOX WARNING:** Agranulocytosis, neutropenia, thrombocytopenia, thrombotic thrombocytopenic purpura (TTP)

Precautions: Pregnancy **B,** breastfeeding, children, geriatric, past liver disease, renal disease, increased bleeding risk, peptic ulcer disease, surgery

> **BLACK BOX WARNING:** Anemia, hematological disease

DOSAGE AND ROUTES
Adult: PO 250 mg bid with food

Available forms: Tabs 250 mg

Implementation
• Give with food or after eating to decrease GI effects

ADVERSE EFFECTS
CNS: Dizziness
GI: Nausea, vomiting, diarrhea, GI discomfort, **cholestatic jaundice, hepatitis,** increased cholesterol LDL, VLDL, triglycerides
HEMA: Bleeding (epistaxis, hematuria, conjunctival hemorrhage, GI bleeding), agranulocytosis, neutropenia, thrombocytopenia, thrombotic thrombocytopenic purpura
INTEG: Rash, pruritus

Absorption	Well absorbed
Distribution	Unknown
Metabolism	Liver, extensively; 98% protein binding
Excretion	Kidneys, unchanged product
Half-life	Increased with repeat dosing; 4-5 days (multiple doses)

Onset	Unknown
Peak	1-3 hr
Duration	Unknown

INTERACTIONS
Individual drugs
Abciximab, aspirin, eptifibatide, tirofiban: increased bleeding tendencies
Ambrisentan, fosphenytoin, phenytoin, theophylline: increased levels of each specific drug
Cimetidine: increased effects of ticlopidine
CycloSPORINE: decreased plasma levels of cycloSPORINE
Digoxin: decreased plasma levels of digoxin

Drug classifications
Antacids: decreased plasma levels of ticlopidine
Anticoagulants, NSAIDs, salicylates, SSRIs, thrombin inhibitors, thrombolytics: increased bleeding risk
CYP2C19, CYP2DC substrates: increased levels of each specific drug

Drug/herb
Ginger, gingko, garlic, feverfew, horse chestnut, green tea: increased bleeding risk

NURSING CONSIDERATIONS
Assessment
• Monitor liver function tests: AST, ALT, bilirubin, creatinine if patient is on long-term therapy (4 mo or more)
• Monitor blood tests: CBC, Hct, Hgb, pro-time if patient is on long-term therapy; CBC q2wk × 3 mo therapy; thrombocytopenia, neutropenia may occur
• Monitor bleeding time baseline and throughout therapy, levels may be 2-5 × normal limit

Nursing diagnoses
• Injury, risk for (uses)
• Knowledge, deficient (teaching)

Patient/family education

• Advise patient that blood studies are necessary during treatment
• Advise patient to report any unusual bleeding to prescriber
• Instruct patient to take with food or just after eating to minimize GI discomfort, not to double missed dose
• Caution patient to report side effects such as diarrhea, skin rashes, subcutaneous bleeding, signs of cholestasis (yellow skin and sclera, dark urine, light-colored stools)
• Advise patient that product should be discontinued 10-14 days before surgery
• Advise there are many drug and herb interactions

Evaluation
Positive therapeutic outcome
• Absence of stroke

tigecycline (Rx)
(tye-ge-sye'kleen)
Tygacil
Func. class.: Broad-spectrum antiinfective
Chem. class.: Glycylcyclines
Pregnancy category D

ACTION: Inhibits protein synthesis and phosphorylation in microorganisms; bacteriostatic, structurally similar to the tetracyclines

Therapeutic outcome: Resolution of infection

USES: Complicated skin/skin structure infections: *Escherichia coli, Enterococcus faecalis* (vancomycin-susceptible only), *Staphylococcus aureus, Streptococcus agalactiae, S. anginosus* group, *S. pyogenes, Bacteroides fragilis;* complicated intraabdominal infections *(Citrobacter freundii), Enterobacter cloacae, Escherichia coli, Klebsiella oxytoca, K. pneumoniae, E. faecalis* (vancomycin-susceptible only), *S. aureus* (methicillin-susceptible only), *S. anginosus* group, *B. fragilis, Bacteroides thetaiotaomicron, B. uniformis, B. vulgatus, Clostridium perfringens, Peptostreptococcus micros,* community-acquired pneumonia

CONTRAINDICATIONS:
Pregnancy **D**, breastfeeding, children <18 yr, hypersensitivity to tigecycline

Precautions: Renal/hepatic disease, hypersensitivity to tetracyclines, ventricular-associated hospital-acquired pneumonias

DOSAGE AND ROUTES
Adult: **IV** 100 mg, then 50 mg q12hr, **IV INF** is given over 30 min to 60 min q12hr; given for 5-14 days depending on infection

Hepatic dose (Child-Pugh C)
Adult: **IV** 100 mg, then 25 mg q12hr

Available forms: Powder for inj, lyophilized 50 mg

Implementation
• Give after C&S obtained

Intermittent IV infusion route
• Reconstitute each vial with 5.3 ml of 0.9% NaCl, or D₅W (10 mg/ml); swirl to dissolve; immediately withdraw 5 ml of the reconstituted sol and add to a 100-ml **IV** bag for inf (1 mg/ml); may be yellow or orange, if not, sol should be discarded; do not give if particulate matter is present

Y-site compatibilities: Acyclovir, alfentanil, allopurinol, amifostine, amikacin, aminocaproic acid, aminophylline, amphotericin B liposome, ampicillin, ampicillin/sulbactam, argatroban, azithromycin, aztreonam, bivalirudin, bumetanide, buprenorphine, butorphanol, calcium chloride/gluconate, CARBOplatin, carmustine, caspofungin, ceFAZolin, cefepime, cefotaxime, cefotetan, cefoxitin, ceftazidime, ceftizoxime, cefTRIAXone, cefuroxime, cimetidine, ciprofloxacin, cisatracurium, CISplatin, clindamycin, cyclophosphamide, cycloSPORINE, cytarabine, dacarbazine, DACTINomycin, DAPTOmycin, DAUNOrubicin hydrochloride, dexamethasone, dexmedetomidine, dexrazoxane, digoxin, diltiazem, diphenhydrAMINE, DOBUTamine, docetaxel, dolasetron, DOPamine, doripenem, DOXOrubicin hydrochloride, DOXOrubicin liposome, droperidol, enalaprilat, EPINEPHrine, eptifibatide, ertapenem, erythromycin, esmolol, etoposide, etoposide phosphate, famotidine, fenoldopam, fentaNYL, fluconazole, fludarabine, fluorouracil, foscarnet, fosphenytoin, furosemide, ganciclovir, gemcitabine, gentamicin, glycopyrrolate, granisetron, haloperidol, heparin, hydrocortisone, HYDROmorphone, ifosfamide, imipenem/cilastatin, insulin, irinotecan, isoproterenol, ketorolac, labetalol, lansoprazole, lepirudin, leucovorin, levofloxacin, lidocaine, linezolid, LORazepam, magnesium sulfate, mannitol, mechlorethamine, melphalan, meperidine, meropenem, mesna, methohexital, methotrexate, methyldopa, metoclopramide, metoprolol, metroNIDAZOLE, midazolam, milrinone, mitomycin, mitoxantrone, morphine, moxifloxacin, mycophenolate, nafcillin, nalbuphine, naloxone, nesiritide, nitroglycerin, nitroprusside, norepinephrine, octreotide, ondansetron, oxaliplatin, oxytocin, paclitaxel, palonosetron, pamidronate, pancuronium, pantoprazole, pemetrexed, pentamidine, pentazocine, PENTobarbital, PHENobarbital, phenylephrine, piperacillin/tazobactam, potassium acetate/chloride/phosphate, procainamide, prochlorperazine, promethazine, propofol, propranolol, ranitidine, remifentanil, rocuronium, sodium acetate/bicarbonate/phosphate, streptozocin, succinylcholine, SUFentanil, tacrolimus, teniposide, theophylline, thiopental, thiotepa, ticarcillin/clavulanate, tirofiban, tobramycin, topotecan, trimethoprim/sulfamethoxazole, vancomycin, vasopressin, vecuronium, vinBLAStine, vinCRIStine, vinorelbine, zidovudine, zoledronic acid

Y-site incompatibilities: Amiodarone, amphotericin B colloidal, bleomycin, chloramphenicol, chlorpromazine, dantrolene, DAUNOrubicin liposome, diazepam, epirubicin, hydrALAZINE, IDArubicin, niCARdipine, phenytoin, quinapristin/dalfopristin, verapamil

• Store in tight, light-resistant container at room temperature

ADVERSE EFFECTS

CNS: Headache, dizziness, insomnia
CV: Hypo/hypertension, phlebitis
EENT: Tooth discoloration
GI: *Nausea, vomiting, diarrhea,* anorexia, constipation, dyspepsia, **hepatotoxicity, hepatic failure, pseudomembranous colitis**
HEMA: Anemia, leukocytosis, thrombocytopenia
INTEG: *Rash,* pruritus, sweating, photosensitivity
META: Increased ALT, AST, BUN, lactic acid, alkaline phosphatase, amylase, hyperglycemia, hypokalemia, hypoproteinemia, bilirubinemia
MISC: Back pain, fever, abnormal healing, abdominal pain, abscess, asthenia, infection, pain, peripheral edema, local reactions
RESP: Cough, dyspnea
SYST: Anaphylaxis

Pharmacokinetics

Absorption	Unknown
Distribution	Protein binding 71%-89%
Metabolism	Not extensively
Excretion	22% unchanged, urine; primarily biliarily excreted
Half-life	Terminal 42 hr

Pharmacodynamics

Unknown

INTERACTIONS

Individual drugs

Warfarin: increased effect of tigecycline

Drug classifications

Oral contraceptives: decreased effect of tigecycline

NURSING CONSIDERATIONS

Assessment

• **Pseudomembranous colitis:** assess for diarrhea, abdominal pain, fever, fatigue, anorexia; possible anemia, elevated WBC, low serum albumin; stop product and usually give either vancomycin or IV metroNIDAZOLE
• Assess for signs of anemia: Hct, Hgb, fatigue
• Monitor blood tests: PT, CBC, AST, ALT, BUN creatinine
• **Assess for allergic reactions:** rash, itching, pruritus, angioedema
• Assess for nausea, vomiting, diarrhea; administer antiemetic, antacids as ordered
• **Assess for overgrowth of infection:** fever, malaise, redness, pain, swelling, drainage, perineal itching, diarrhea, changes in cough or sputum

Nursing diagnoses

• Infection, risk for (use)
• Knowledge, deficient (teaching)

Patient/family education

• Teach patient to avoid sun exposure; sunscreen does not seem to decrease photosensitivity
• Teach patient to avoid pregnancy while taking this product; fetal harm may occur

Evaluation

Positive therapeutic outcome

• Decreased temp, absence of lesions, negative C&S

timolol (Rx)

(tye'moe-lole)
Apo-Timol ❋, Novo-Timol ❋
Func. class.: Antihypertensive; antiglaucoma
Chem. class.: Nonselective β-blocker
Pregnancy category C

ACTION: Competitively blocks stimulation of β-adrenergic receptor within vascular smooth muscle (decreases rate of SA node discharge, increases recovery time), slows conduction of AV node, decreases heart rate, which decreases O_2 consumption in myocardium; also decreases renin-aldosterone-angiotensin system; at high doses inhibits β_2 receptors in bronchial system

Therapeutic outcome: Decreased B/P, decreased arrhythmias, absence of death from MI, decreased aqueous humor in the eye, absence of migraine headaches

USES: Mild to moderate hypertension, migraine prophylaxis, to decrease mortality following MI

Unlabeled uses: Tremors, angina pectoris

CONTRAINDICATIONS:
Hypersensitivity to β-blockers, cardiogenic shock, heart block (2nd or 3rd degree), sinus bradycardia, CHF, cardiac failure, severe COPD, asthma

Precautions: Pregnancy **C**, breastfeeding, major surgery, diabetes mellitus, thyroid/renal/hepatic disease, COPD, well-compensated heart failure, CAD, nonallergic bronchospasm, peripheral vascular disease, diabetes mellitus

> **BLACK BOX WARNING:** Abrupt discontinuation

DOSAGE AND ROUTES
Hypertension
Adult: PO 10 mg bid, or 20 mg/day, may increase by 10 mg q7day, max 60 mg/day

Myocardial infarction
Adult: 10 mg bid beginning 1-4 wk after MI

Glaucoma
Adult: Ophth 1 gtt daily or bid
Child: Ophth 1 gtt daily or bid (0.25% SOL only)

Migraine headache prevention
Adult: PO 10 mg bid, or 20 mg/day; may increase to 30 mg/day, 20 mg in AM, 10 mg in PM; discontinue if not effective after 8 wk

Available forms: Tabs 5, 10, 20 mg

Implementation
• Given before meals, at bedtime; tab may be crushed or swallowed whole; give with food to prevent GI upset; reduce dosage in renal dysfunction
• Store protected from light, moisture; place in cool environment

ADVERSE EFFECTS
CNS: *Insomnia, dizziness,* hallucinations, anxiety, fatigue, depression, headache

CV: Hypotension, bradycardia, **CHF,** edema, chest pain, claudication, angina, AV block, ventricular dysrhythmias
EENT: *Vision changes,* sore throat, *double vision,* dry burning eyes
GI: *Nausea,* vomiting, **ischemic colitis,** diarrhea, *abdominal pain,* **mesenteric arterial thrombosis,** flatulence, constipation
GU: Impotence, urinary frequency
HEMA: Agranulocytosis, thrombocytopenia, purpura
INTEG: Rash, alopecia, pruritus, fever
META: Hypoglycemia
MUSC: *Joint pain, muscle pain*
RESP: Bronchospasm, dyspnea, cough, crackles, nasal stuffiness

Pharmacokinetics

Absorption	Well absorbed (PO), minimally absorbed (ophth)
Distribution	Protein binding <10%
Metabolism	Liver, extensively
Excretion	Breast milk
Half-life	3 hr

Pharmacodynamics

	PO
Onset	Unknown
Peak	2-4 hr
Duration	12-24 hr

INTERACTIONS
Individual drugs
Alcohol: increased hypotension, bradycardia (large amounts)
HydrALAZINE, methyldopa, prazosin, reserpine: increased hypotension, bradycardia
Insulin: decreased hypoglycemia
Thyroid hormones: decreased antihypertensive effect

Drug classifications
Anticholinergics, nitrates: increased hypotension, increased bradycardia
β_2-Adrenergic agonists: increased β-blocking effect
Calcium channel blockers: increased effects of calcium channel blockers
NSAIDs, salicylates, sympathomimetics: decreased antihypertensive effect
Sulfonylureas: decreased hypoglycemic effect
Theophyllines: decreased bronchodilatation

Drug/lab test
Increased: renal, liver function tests, uric acid
Interference: glucose, insulin tolerance test

T

Adverse effects: *italics* = common; **bold** = life-threatening

NURSING CONSIDERATIONS
Assessment

> **BLACK BOX WARNING: Abrupt discontinu-ation:** may result in myocardial ischemia, MI, severe hypotension, ventricular dysrhythmias in those with preexisting cardiovascular disease

• Assess for headaches: location, severity, dura-tion, frequency baseline, throughout treatment
• Monitor B/P during beginning treatment, periodically thereafter; pulse q4hr; note rate, rhythm, quality: apical/radial pulse before ad-ministration; notify prescriber of any significant changes (pulse <50 bpm)
• Check baselines in renal, liver function tests before therapy begins
• Assess for edema in feet, legs daily, monitor I&O ratio, daily weight; check for jugular vein distention, crackles bilaterally, dyspnea (CHF)
• Monitor skin turgor, dryness of mucous mem-branes for hydration status, especially geriatric

Nursing diagnoses
• Cardiac output, decreased (uses)
• Injury, risk for (side effects)
• Knowledge, deficient (teaching)
• Noncompliance (teaching)

Patient/family education

> **BLACK BOX WARNING:** Teach patient not to discontinue product abruptly; taper over 2 wk; may cause precipitate angina if stopped abruptly

• Advise patient not to use OTC products con-taining α-adrenergic stimulants (nasal decon-gestants, cold preparations); to avoid alcohol, smoking; to limit sodium intake as prescribed
• Teach patient how to take pulse and B/P at home; advise patient when to notify prescriber
• Instruct patient to comply with weight control, dietary adjustments, modified exercise program
• Advise patient to carry/wear emergency ID to identify product being taken, any allergies; tell patient product controls symptoms but does not cure
• Caution patient to avoid hazardous activities if dizziness, drowsiness are present
• Teach patient to report symptoms of CHF; dif-ficult breathing, especially on exertion or when lying down; night cough; swelling of extremities or bradycardia; dizziness; confusion; depres-sion; fever
• Teach patient to take product as prescribed, not to double dose, skip doses; take any missed doses as soon as remembered if at least 4 hr until next dose

Evaluation
Positive therapeutic outcome
• Decreased B/P in hypertension (after 1-2 wk)
• Absence of dysrhythmias

TREATMENT OF OVERDOSE:
Lavage, **IV** atropine for bradycardia, **IV** theoph-ylline for bronchospasm, digoxin, O_2, diuretic for cardiac failure, hemodialysis, **IV** glucose for hyperglycemia, **IV** diazepam (or phenytoin) for seizures

timolol ophthalmic
See Appendix B

tinidazole (Rx)
(tye-ni′da-zole)
Tindamax
Func. class.: Antiprotozoal
Chem. class.: Nitroimidazole derivative
Pregnancy category C

ACTION: Interferes with DNA/RNA synthe-sis in protozoa

Therapeutic outcome: Decrease in infection

USES: Amebiasis, giardiasis, trichomoniasis

CONTRAINDICATIONS:
Breastfeeding, hypersensitivity to this product or nitroimidazole derivative, pregnancy

Precautions: Pregnancy **C**, children, geriatric, hepatic disease, CNS depression, blood dyscrasias, candidiasis, seizures, viral infection, alcoholism

> **BLACK BOX WARNING:** Secondary malig-nancy

DOSAGE AND ROUTES
Amebic involvement (liver)
Adult: PO 2 g/day × 3-5 days
Child ≥3 yr: PO 50 mg/kg/day × 3-5 days, max 2 g

Giardiasis
Adult: PO 2 g as a single dose
Child ≥3 yr: PO 50 mg/kg as a single dose, max 2 g

Trichomoniasis
Adult: PO 2 g as a single dose

Bacterial vaginosis
Adult (not pregnant): PO 2 g/day × 2 days with food or 1 g/day × 5 days with food

Available forms: Tabs 250, 500 mg

Implementation
• Administer to those >3 yr old
• Give with food; tabs can be crushed and mixed with artificial cherry syrup

ADVERSE EFFECTS
CNS: *Dizziness, headache,* **seizures,** *peripheral neuropathy,* malaise, fatigue
GI: *Nausea, vomiting,* anorexia, increased AST and ALT, constipation, abdominal pain, indigestion, altered taste
HEMA: **Leukopenia,** neutropenia
INTEG: Pruritus, urticaria, *rash,* oral candidiasis
SYST: **Angioedema,** cramping

Pharmacokinetics

Absorption	Unknown
Distribution	Crosses blood-brain barrier
Metabolism	Extensively in the liver
Excretion	Unchanged (20%-25%) in urine, (12%) feces
Half-life	12-14 hr

Pharmacodynamics

Unknown

INTERACTIONS
Individual drugs
Do not use within 2 wk of taking disulfiram
Cholestyramine, oxytetracycline: decreased action of tinidazole
CycloSPORINE, fluorouracil, lithium, tacrolimus: increased action

Drug classifications
Anticoagulants, hydantoins: increased action
CYP3A4 inducers (phenobarbital, phenytoin, rifampin): decreased action of tinidazole
CYP3A4 inhibitors (cimetidine, ketoconazole): increased action of tinidazole

Drug/herb
St. John's wort: increased or decreased tinidazole level

Drug/lab test
Increase: triglycerides, LDH, AST/ALT, glucose
Decrease: WBCs

NURSING CONSIDERATIONS
Assessment
• **Assess for amebic liver abscess:** CBC, ESR, amebic gel diffusion test, ultrasound, total and differential leukocyte count
• Assess for signs of infection, anemia
• Assess bowel pattern before, during treatment

> **BLACK BOX WARNING: Secondary malignancy:** Avoid unnecessary use

Nursing diagnoses
• Infection, risk for (uses)
• Knowledge, deficient (teaching)

Patient/family education
• Instruct patient to take with food to increase plasma concentrations, minimize epigastric distress and other GI effects; not to use alcoholic beverages during or for 3 days afterward
• Advise patient that in cases of trichomoniasis, both partners should be treated at the same time

Evaluation
Positive therapeutic outcome
• Decrease in infection as evidenced by negative culture

⚠ HIGH ALERT

tinzaparin (Rx)
(tin-zay-par'in)
Innohep
Func. class.: Anticoagulant
Chem. class.: Unfractionated porcine heparin
Pregnancy category C

ACTION: Increases the inhibitory effect of antithrombin factor Xa, thrombin IIa

Therapeutic outcome: Resolution of DVT

USES: Treatment of DVT, pulmonary emboli after abdominal, knee, hip surgery or knee, hip replacement

Unlabeled uses: DVT prophylaxis

CONTRAINDICATIONS:
Hypersensitivity to this product, heparin, pork or benzyl alcohol, sulfites; hemophilia, leukemia with bleeding, peptic ulcer disease, thrombocytopenic purpura, heparin-induced thrombocytopenia

Precautions: Pregnancy **C,** breastfeeding, children, geriatric, alcoholism, severe renal/hepatic disease, blood dyscrasias, severe uncontrolled hypertension, subacute bacterial endocarditis, acute nephritis, elderly >70 yr (renal disease with DVT/PE)

> **BLACK BOX WARNING:** Spinal/epidural anesthesia, lumbar puncture

DOSAGE AND ROUTES

Treatment of deep vein thrombosis
Adult: SUBCUT 175 anti-Xa international units/kg daily ≥6 days and until adequate anticoagulation with warfarin (INR ≥2 for 2 consecutive days)

Prophylaxis of DVT/thromboembolism/PE (unlabeled)
Adult: 3500 anti-Xa units (50 anti-Xa units/kg) daily beginning 1-2 hr before surgery and continued for 5-10 days

Prophylaxis of deep vein thrombosis in orthopedic procedures (unlabeled)
Adult: 75 anti-Xa units/kg/day started 12-24 hr after surgery

Available forms: Inj 20,000 international units/ml

Implementation
• Give only after screening patient for bleeding disorders
• Give SUBCUT only; do not give IM
• Give for 6 days and until warfarin has been given to result in adequate coagulation
• Give SUBCUT to recumbent patient; rotate inj sites (left/right anterolateral, left/right posterolateral abdominal wall)
• Insert whole length of needle into skin fold held with thumb and forefinger
⚠ Use only this product when ordered; not interchangeable with heparin (unfractionated) or LMWHs
• Give at same time each day to maintain steady blood levels
• Do not massage area or aspirate when giving SUBCUT inj
• Alternate injection sites
• For excessive bruising at injection site, may use ice at site before subcut injection
• Do not mix with other products or inf fluids
• Store at 77° F (25° C); do not freeze

ADVERSE EFFECTS
CNS: Fever, confusion, dizziness, insomnia
CV: Angina, dysrhythmias, peripheral edema, tachycardia, hypo/hypertension
GI: Nausea, constipation, flatulence, dyspepsia, **hepatitis**
GU: UTI, hematuria, urinary retention, dysuria
HEMA: Hemorrhage, **anemia, thrombocytopenia,** bleeding
INTEG: Ecchymosis, inj site reaction
MISC: Headache, chest pain, hypersensitivity
SYST: Stevens-Johnson syndrome

Pharmacokinetics
Absorption	Unknown
Distribution	Unknown
Metabolism	Unknown
Excretion	Unknown
Half-life	4.5 hr

Pharmacodynamics
Onset	Unknown
Peak	3-5 hr (max antithrombin activity)
Duration	Unknown

INTERACTIONS
Individual drug
Clopidogrel, ticlopidine: increased tinzaparin action

Drug classifications
Anticoagulants (oral), NSAIDs, platelet inhibitors, salicylates, thrombolytics: increased tinzaparin action

NURSING CONSIDERATIONS
Assessment

> **BLACK BOX WARNING:** Spinal/epidermal anesthesia, lumbar puncture: monitor neurological impairment; if impairment occurs, urgent treatment is needed

• Monitor blood tests (Hct, platelets, occult blood in stools), anti-Xa; thrombocytopenia may occur
• **Assess for bleeding** gums, petechiae, ecchymosis, black tarry stools, hematuria

Nursing diagnoses
• Cardiac output, decreased (uses)
• Knowledge, deficient (teaching)

Patient/family education
• Instruct patient to report any signs of bleeding: gums, under skin, urine, stools

⚠ Nurse Alert

Evaluation
Positive therapeutic outcome
• Resolution of deep vein thrombosis

TREATMENT OF OVERDOSE:
Protamine 1 mg/100 anti-Xa international units of tinzaparin

---

tioconazole vaginal antifungal
See Appendix B

---

tiotropium (Rx)
(ty-oh'tro-pee-um)
Spiriva, HandiHaler
Func. class.: Anticholinergic, bronchodilator
Chem. class.: Synthetic quaternary ammonium compound
Pregnancy category C

ACTION: Inhibits interaction of acetylcholine at receptor sites on the bronchial smooth muscle, resulting in decreased cGMP and bronchodilatation

Therapeutic outcome: Improved breathing

USES: COPD, for long-term treatment, once daily maintenance of bronchospasm, associated with COPD including chronic bronchitis and emphysema

CONTRAINDICATIONS:
Hypersensitivity to this product, atropine, or its derivatives

Precautions: Pregnancy **C**, breastfeeding, children, geriatric, closed-angle glaucoma, prostatic hypertrophy, bladder neck obstruction, renal disease

DOSAGE AND ROUTES
Adult: INH content of 1 cap/day using Handi-Haler inhalation device

Available forms: Powder for inhalation 18 mcg in blister packs containing 6 caps with inhaler; 30 caps with inhaler

Implementation
Inhalation route
• Caps are for INH only; do not swallow
• Immediately before administration, peel back foil until cap is visible (until "stop" line); open dust cap of HandiHaler by pulling upward; then open mouthpiece
• Place cap in center chamber; firmly close mouthpiece until it clicks, leaving dust cap open
• Hold HandiHaler with mouthpiece upward; press button in once, completely, and release; this allows medication to be released
• Breathe out completely; do not breathe into mouthpiece at any time
• Raise device to mouth and close lips tightly around mouthpiece
• With head upright, breathe in slowly/deeply, but allowing the cap to vibrate; breathe until lungs fill; hold breath and remove mouthpiece; resume normal breathing
• Repeat
• Remove used capsule and discard; close the mouthpiece and dust cap; store

ADVERSE EFFECTS
CNS: Depression, paresthesia
CV: Chest pain, increased heart rate
EENT: Dry mouth, blurred vision, glaucoma
GI: *Vomiting*, abdominal pain, constipation, dyspepsia
INTEG: Rash, **angioedema**
MISC: Urinary difficulty, urinary retention
RESP: *Cough, worsening of symptoms,* sinusitis, URI, epistaxis, pharyngitis

Pharmacokinetics	
Absorption	Unknown
Distribution	Does not cross blood-brain barrier
Metabolism	Very little metabolized in the liver
Excretion	Excreted in urine
Half-life	5-6 days in animals

Pharmacodynamics
Unknown

INTERACTIONS
Drug classifications
Anticholinergics: avoid use with other anticholinergics

NURSING CONSIDERATIONS
Assessment
• For tolerance over long-term therapy; dose may have to be increased or changed
• **Respiratory status:** assess for dyspnea, rate, breath sounds before and during treatment; pulmonary function tests baseline and periodically; upper respiratory infection, cough, sinusitis

---

Nursing diagnoses
- Breathing pattern, ineffective (uses)
- Knowledge, deficient (teaching)

Patient/family education
- Teach patient how to use HandiHaler
- Teach patient signs of closed-angle glaucoma
- Advise patient that product is used for long-term maintenance, not for immediate relief of breathing problems
- Caution patient to avoid getting the powder in the eyes; may cause blurred vision and pupil dilatation

Evaluation
Positive therapeutic outcome
- Ability to breathe easier

tipranavir (Rx)
(ti-pran′a-veer)
Aptivus
Func. class.: Antiretroviral
Chem. class.: Protease inhibitor
Pregnancy category C

ACTION: Inhibits HIV protease; this prevents the maturation of virus

Therapeutic outcome: Prevention of worsening of HIV

USES: HIV in combination with other antiretrovirals

CONTRAINDICATIONS:
Hypersensitivity

> **BLACK BOX WARNING:** Hepatic disease (Child-Pugh B to C)

Precautions: Pregnancy C, breastfeeding, children, renal disease, history of renal stones, sulfa allergy, hemophilia, diabetes mellitus, pancreatitis, alcoholism, immune reconstitution syndrome, surgery, trauma, infection

> **BLACK BOX WARNING:** Intracranial bleeding, hepatitis

DOSAGE AND ROUTES
Reduce dosage in mild or moderate hepatic impairment and ketoconazole coadministration
Adult: PO 500 mg coadministered with ritonavir 200 mg bid with food
Adolescent and child ≥2 yr: PO 14 mg/kg given with ritonavir 6 mg/kg bid or 375 mg/m² given with ritonavir 150 mg/m² bid; max 500 mg with ritonavir 200 mg bid

Available forms: Caps 250 mg; oral sol 100 mg/ml

Implementation
- Swallow cap whole; do not break, crush, or chew
- Give after meals
- Give in equal intervals around the clock to maintain blood levels

ADVERSE EFFECTS
CNS: *Headache, insomnia,* dizziness, somnolence, fatigue, *fever,* **intracranial bleeding**
GI: *Diarrhea, abdominal pain, nausea, vomiting,* anorexia, dry mouth, **hepatitis B or C, fatalities when given with ritonavir, pancreatitis**
GU: Nephrolithiasis
INTEG: *Rash,* urticaria, lipodystrophy, serious rash
MS: Pain
OTHER: Asthenia, **insulin-resistant hyperglycemia,** *hyperlipidemia,* **ketoacidosis**

Pharmacokinetics
Absorption	Unknown
Distribution	Protein binding, 99.9%, steady state 7-10 days
Metabolism	CYP3A4
Excretion	80% feces
Half-life	Terminal 6 hr

Pharmacodynamics
Unknown

INTERACTIONS
Individual drugs
⚠ **Amiodarone, astemizole, cisapride, flecainide, midazolam, pimozide, propafenone, quiNIDine, rifabutin, rifampin, terfenadine, triazolam: life-threatening dysrhythmias**
Clarithromycin, zidovudine: increased levels of both products
Delavirdine, itraconazole, ketoconazole: increased tipranavir levels
Efavirenz, fluconazole, nevirapine: decreased tipranavir levels
Lovastatin, simvastatin: increased myopathy, rhabdomyolysis

Drug classifications
⚠ **Ergots: life-threatening dysrhythmias**
Oral contraceptives: increased levels of tipranavir
Rifamycins: decreased tipranavir levels

Drug/herb
St. John's wort: decreased tipranavir levels; avoid concurrent use

Drug/food
Grapefruit juice, high-fat, high-protein foods: decreased tipranavir absorption

Drug/lab test
Increased: AST, ALT

NURSING CONSIDERATIONS

Assessment
• Monitor for complaints of lower back, flank pain; indicates kidney stones
• Assess for signs of infection, anemia, the presence of other STDs

> **BLACK BOX WARNING:** Assess for hepatic studies: ALT, AST; total bilirubin, amylase, all may be elevated

• **HIV:** Monitor viral load, CD4, plasma HIV RNA, serum cholesterol/triglycerides during treatment
• Monitor bowel pattern before, during treatment; if severe abdominal pain with bleeding occurs, product should be discontinued; monitor hydration
• **Serious rash:** if a serious rash occurs, product should be discontinued
• Assess for allergies before treatment, reaction of each medication; place allergies on chart

Nursing Diagnoses
• Infection, risk for (use, adverse reactions)
• Knowledge, deficient (teaching)

Patient/family education
• Teach patient to take as prescribed; if dose is missed, take as soon as remembered up to 1 hr before next dose; do not double dose
• Teach patient that product must be taken in equal intervals around the clock to maintain blood levels for duration of therapy
⚠ Advise that hyperglycemia may occur; watch for increased thirst, weight loss, hunger, dry, itchy skin; notify prescriber
• Teach patient to increase fluids to prevent kidney stones; if stone formation occurs, treatment may need to be interrupted
• Advise patient that product does not cure AIDS, only controls symptoms; not to donate blood

Evaluation
Positive therapeutic outcome
• Prevention of viral replication

> **⚠ HIGH ALERT**

tirofiban (Rx)
(tie-roh-fee′ban)
Aggrastat
Func. class.: Antiplatelet
Chem. class.: Glycoprotein IIb/IIIa inhibitor
Pregnancy category B

ACTION: Antagonist of platelet glycoprotein (GP) IIb/IIIa receptor that leads to binding of fibrinogen and von Willebrand's factor, which inhibits platelet aggregation

Therapeutic outcome: Decreased platelet count

USES: Acute coronary syndrome in combination with heparin

CONTRAINDICATIONS:
Hypersensitivity, active internal bleeding, stroke, major surgery, severe trauma within 30 days, intracranial neoplasm, aneurysm, hemorrhage, acute pericarditis, platelets <100,000/mm³, history of thrombocytopenia, coagulopathy, systolic B/P >180 mm Hg or diastolic B/P >110 mm Hg

Precautions: Pregnancy **B,** breastfeeding, children, geriatric, renal disease, bleeding tendencies, hypertension, platelets <150,000/mm³

DOSAGE AND ROUTES
Adult: IV 0.4 mcg/kg/min × 30 min, then 0.1 mcg/kg/min for 12-24 hr after angioplasty or atherectomy

Renal dose
Adult: IV CCr <30 ml/min 0.2 mcg/kg/min × 30 min, then 0.05 mcg/kg/min, during angiography and for up to 24 hr after angioplasty

Available forms: Inj for sol 250 mcg/ml, inj 50 mcg/ml

Implementation
• Dilute inj: withdraw and discard 100 ml from a 500-ml bag of sterile 0.9% NaCl or D₅ and replace this vol with 100 ml of tirofiban inj from two vials
• Tirofiban inj for sol is premixed in containers of 500 ml 0.9% NaCl (50 mg/ml), give over 30 min
• Minimize other arterial/venous punctures, IM inj, catheter use, intubation to reduce bleeding risks

Y-site compatibilities: Acyclovir, alfentanil, allopurinol, amifostine, amikacin,

Adverse effects: *italics* = common; **bold** = life-threatening

aminocaproic acid, aminophylline, amiodarone, ampicillin, ampicillin/sulbactam, anidulafungin, argatroban, arsenic trioxide, atracurium, atropine, azithromycin, aztreonam, bivalirudin, bleomycin, bumetanide, buprenorphine, butorphanol, calcium chloride/gluconate, capreomycin, CARBOplatin, carmustine, caspofungin, ceFAZolin, cefepime, cefotaxime, cefotetan, cefoxitin, ceftazidime, ceftizoxime, cefTRIAXone, cefuroxime, chloramphenicol, chlorproMAZINE, cimetidine, ciprofloxacin, cisatracurium, CISplatin, clindamycin, cyclophosphamide, cycloSPORINE, cytarabine, DACTINomycin, DAPTOmycin, dexamethasone, dexmedetomidine, dexrazoxane, digoxin, diltiazem, diphenhydrAMINE, DOBUTamine, docetaxel, dolasetron, DOPamine, doxacurium, DOXOrubicin, DOXOrubicin liposome, doxycycline, droperidol, enalaprilat, ePHEDrine, EPINEPHrine, epirubicin, eptifibatide, ertapenem, erythromycin, esmolol, etoposide, etoposide phosphate, famotidine, fenoldopam, fentaNYL, fluconazole, fludarabine, fluorouracil, foscarnet, fosphenytoin, furosemide, ganciclovir, gemcitabine, gentamicin, glycopyrrolate, granisetron, haloperidol, heparin, hydrALAZINE, hydrocortisone, HYDROmorphone, IDArubicin, ifosfamide, imipenem/cilastatin, insulin, irinotecan, isoproterenol, ketorolac, labetalol, leucovorin, lidocaine, linezolid, LORazepam, magnesium sulfate, mannitol, mechlorethamine, melphalan, meperidine, meropenem, mesna, methylhexital, methotrexate, methyldopate, methylPREDNISolone, metoclopramide, metoprolol, metroNIDAZOLE, midazolam, milrinone, mitoxantrone, morphine, mycophenolate, nafcillin, nalbuphine, naloxone, nesiritide, niCARdipine, nitroglycerin, nitroprusside, norepinephrine, octreotide, ondansetron, oxaliplatin, oxytocin, paclitaxel, palonosetron, pamidronate, pancuronium, pantoprazole, pemetrexed, PENTobarbital, PHENobarbital, phentolamine, phenylephrine, piperacillin/tazobactam, potassium acetate/chloride/phosphates, procainamide, prochlorperazine, promethazine, propranolol, quinupristin/dalfopristin, ranitidine, remifentanil, rocuronium, sodium acetate/bicarbonate, streptozocin, succinylcholine, SUFentanil, tacrolimus, teniposide, theophylline, thiopental, thiotepa, ticarcillin/clavulanate, tigecycline, tobramycin, topotecan, vancomycin, vasopressin, vecuronium, verapamil, vinBLAStine, vinCRIStine, vinorelbine, voriconazole, zidovudine, zoledronic acid

Y-site incompatibilities: Amphotericin B colloidal, amphotericin B liposome, dantrolene, diazepam, phenytoin

ADVERSE EFFECTS
CNS: Dizziness, headache
CV: Bradycardia, hypotension
GI: Nausea, vomiting
HEMA: Bleeding, **thrombocytopenia**
INTEG: *Rash*
MISC: Dissection, edema, pain in legs/pelvis, sweating
SYST: Anaphylaxis

Pharmacokinetics

Absorption	Unknown
Distribution	Plasma clearance 20%-25%
Metabolism	Liver
Excretion	Urine/feces
Half-life	2 hr

Pharmacodynamics
Unknown

INTERACTIONS
Individual drugs
Abciximab, aspirin, cefamandole, cefoperazone, cefotetan, clopidogrel, dipyridamole, eptifibatide, heparin, ticlopidine, valproic acid: increased bleeding risk

Drug classifications
Heparins, NSAIDs, SNRIs, SSRIs, thrombin inhibitors: increased bleeding risk

NURSING CONSIDERATIONS
Assessment
• **Bleeding:** Monitor platelet counts, Hct, Hgb before treatment, within 6 hr of loading dose and at least daily thereafter; watch for bleeding from puncture sites, catheters, or in stools, urine
• **Multiple sclerosis, spinal cord injury:** assess muscle spasms, dizziness, drowsiness, difficulty moving, coordination, balance

Nursing diagnoses
• Injury, risk for (uses, adverse reactions)

Patient/family education
• Advise patient that it is necessary to quit smoking to prevent excessive vasoconstriction
• Teach signs/symptoms of bleeding, low platelets
• Advise that there are many drug and herb interactions

Evaluation
Positive therapeutic outcome
• Treatment of acute coronary syndrome

tizanidine (Rx)

(tye-za'na-deen)
Zanaflex
Func. class.: Skeletal muscle relaxant,
central acting
Chem. class.: Imidazole
Pregnancy category C

Do not confuse:
tizanidine/tiagabine

ACTION: Increases presynaptic inhibition
of motor neurons and reduces spasticity by
α_2-adrenergic agonism

Therapeutic outcome: Decreased pain/
spasticity in multiple sclerosis

USES: Acute/intermittent management of
increased muscle tone associated with spasticity,
symptoms of MS

CONTRAINDICATIONS:
Hypersensitivity

Precautions: Pregnancy **C**, breastfeeding, children, geriatric, renal/hepatic disease,
hypotension

DOSAGE AND ROUTES
Adult: PO 8 mg q6-8hr; max 36 mg/24 hr

Renal dose
Adult: PO CCr <25 ml/min, start with lower
dosage

Available forms: Tabs 2, 4 mg; caps 2,
4, 6 mg

Implementation
• Give with meals for GI symptoms
• Store in airtight container at room tempera-
ture
• Give consistently either with or without food;
food may affect absorption
• Titrate dose carefully

ADVERSE EFFECTS
CNS: *Dizziness,* somnolence, speech dis-
order, dyskinesia, nervousness, hallucination,
psychosis
CV: Hypotension, bradycardia
GI: *Constipation, vomiting, dry mouth,*
increased ALT, abnormal liver function tests
GU: Urinary frequency
OTHER: Blurred vision, pharyngitis, rhinitis,
tremor, rash, muscle weakness

Pharmacokinetics
Absorption	Completely absorbed
Distribution	Widely distributed
Metabolism	Liver, extensively
Excretion	Kidneys, feces
Half-life	$2^1/_2$ hr

Pharmacodynamics
Onset	Unknown
Peak	1-2 hr
Duration	3-6 hr

INTERACTIONS
Individual drugs
Acyclovir, alcohol, amiodarone, ciprofloxacin,
enoxacin, famotidine, fluvoxamine, norfloxacin,
propafenone, tacrine, verapamil, zileuton: increased tizanidine levels; avoid concurrent use
Rasagiline: increased effect of rasagiline

Drug classifications
Antihypertensive: increased hypotension
CNS depressants: increased CNS depression

Drug/herb
Kava, St. John's wort: increased CNS depression

Drug/lab test
Increased: AST, alkaline phosphatase, ALT,
serum glucose

NURSING CONSIDERATIONS
Assessment
• Assess for muscle spasticity baseline and
throughout treatment
• Monitor B/P, heart rate
• Perform neurologic exam in spasticity: deep
tendon reflexes, muscle tone, clonus, sensory
function
• Monitor renal/liver function tests, electrolytes,
CBC with differential during long-term treatment
• Assess for allergic reactions: rash, fever,
respiratory distress; severe weakness, numbness
in extremities
• Assess CNS depression: dizziness, drowsiness,
psychiatric symptoms
• Check dosage, because individual titration is
required

Nursing diagnoses
• Injury, risk for (adverse reactions)
• Knowledge, deficient (teaching)
• Mobility, impaired physical (uses)

Patient/family education
• Advise patient not to discontinue medication
quickly; spasticity will occur; product should be
tapered off over 1-2 wk

T

Adverse effects: *italics* = common; **bold** = life-threatening

• Advise patient not to take with alcohol, other CNS depressants; take as directed; if dose is missed, take as soon as remembered, unless it is almost time for next dose
• Caution patient to avoid altering activities while taking this product; to avoid hazardous activities if drowsiness or dizziness occurs; to rise from sitting or lying slowly to prevent fainting
• Teach patient to use gum, frequent sips of water for dry mouth
• Advise patient to avoid using OTC medications (cough preparations, antihistamines) unless directed by prescriber
• Notify prescriber if fainting, hallucinations, dark urine, stomach pain, yellowing of skin/eyes occurs
• Advise patient to rise slowly from lying or sitting to upright position to prevent orthostatic hypotension

Evaluation
Positive therapeutic outcome
• Decreased pain, spasticity

tobramycin (Rx)
(toe-bra-mye′sin)
TOBI
Func. class.: Antiinfective
Chem. class.: Aminoglycoside
Pregnancy category D

ACTION: Interferes with protein synthesis in bacterial cell by binding to ribosomal subunit, causing inaccurate peptide sequence to form in protein chain, causing bacterial death

Therapeutic outcome: Bactericidal effects for the following organisms: *Pseudomonas aeruginosa, Enterobacter, Escherichia coli, Providencia, Citrobacter, Staphylococcus, Proteus, Klebsiella, Serratia*

USES: Severe systemic infections of CNS, respiratory, GI, urinary tract, bone, skin, soft tissues, cystic fibrosis (nebulizer) for *P. aeruginosa*

CONTRAINDICATIONS:
Hypersensitivity to aminoglycosides

> **BLACK BOX WARNING:** Pregnancy **D,** severe renal disease

Precautions: Breastfeeding, geriatric, neonates, mild renal disease, myasthenia gravis, Parkinson's disease

> **BLACK BOX WARNING:** Hearing deficits, neuromuscular disease

DOSAGE AND ROUTES
Adult: IM/IV 3 mg/kg/day in divided doses q8hr; may give up to 6 mg/kg/day in divided doses q8-12hr; once-daily dosing (pulse dosing) (unlabeled) IV 5-7 mg/kg; dosing intervals are determined using a nomogram and are based on random levels drawn 8-12 hr after first dose
Child: IM/IV 6-7.5 mg/kg/day in 3-4 equal divided doses
Child ≥6 yr: NEB 300 mg bid in repeating cycles of 28 days on/28 days off; give inh over 10-15 min using a hand-held PARI LC PLUS reusable nebulizer with a DeVilbiss Pulmo-Aid compressor
Neonate <1 wk: IM/IV ≤4 mg/kg/day divided q12hr

Renal dose
Adult: IM/IV 1 mg/kg, then dose determined by blood levels, may be removed by dialysis

Available forms: Inj 10, 40 mg/ml; powder for inj 1.2 g; neb sol 300 mg/5 ml

Implementation
IM route
• Give inj deeply in large muscle mass
Nebulizer route
• Give as close to q12hr apart as possible; do not use <6 hr apart
• Do not mix with dornase alfa in the nebulizer
• Inhale sitting or standing; breathe normally through the mouthpiece; may use nose clips

Intermittent IV infusion route
• Give **IV** diluted in 50-100 ml of 0.9% NaCl, $D_{10}W$, D_5/0.9% NaCl, 0.9% NaCl, Ringer's, LR, D_5W (adult), inf over 30-60 min
• Flush after inf with D_5W, 0.9% NaCl
• Separate aminoglycosides and penicillins by ≥1 hr

Syringe compatibilities: Doxapram

Syringe incompatibilities: Cefamandole, clindamycin, heparin, sargramostim

Y-site compatibilities: Acyclovir, aldesleukin, alfentanil, alprostadil, amifostine, aminophylline, amiodarone, amsacrine, anidulafungin, ascorbic acid, atracurium, atropine, aztreonam, bivalirudin, bretylium, bumetanide, buprenorphine, butorphanol, calcium chloride/gluconate, CARBOplatin, caspofungin, chloramphenicol, cimetidine, ciprofloxacin, cisatracurium, CISplatin, clindamycin, cyanocobalamin, cyclophosphamide, cycloSPORINE, cytarabine, DACTINomycin, DAPTOmycin, dexmedetomidine, digoxin, diltiazem, diphenhydrAMINE, DOBUTamine, docetaxel, DOPamine, doripenem, doxacurium, DOXOrubicin hydrochloride, DOXOrubicin liposome, doxycycline, enalaprilat, ePHEDrine, EPINEPHrine, epirubicin, epoetin alfa, ertapenem, esmolol, etoposide, etoposide phosphate, famotidine, fenoldopam, fentaNYL, filgrastim, fluconazole, fludarabine, fluorouracil, foscarnet, furosemide, gemcitabine, gentamicin, glycopyrrolate, granisetron, HYDROmorphone, ifosfamide, imipenem/cilastatin, isoproterenol, ketorolac, labetalol, levofloxacin, lidocaine, linezolid, LORazepam, magnesium sulfate, mannitol, mechlorethamine, melphalan, meperidine, metaraminol, methicillin, methotrexate, methoxamine, methyldopate, methylPREDNISolone, metoclopramide, metoprolol, metroNIDAZOLE, miconazole, midazolam, milrinone, minocycline, mitoxantrone, morphine, moxalactam, multiple vitamins, nafcillin, nalbuphine, naloxone, niCARdipine, nitroglycerin, nitroprusside, norepinephrine, octreotide, ondansetron, oxaliplatin, oxytocin, paclitaxel, palonosetron, pantoprazole, papaverine, penicillin G, pentazocine, perphenazine, PHENobarbital, phentolamine, phenylephrine, phytonadione, potassium chloride, procainamide, prochlorperazine, promethazine, propranolol, protamine, pyridoxine, quinupristin/dalfopristin, ranitidine, remifentanil, riTUXimab, rocuronium, sodium acetate/bicarbonate, succinylcholine, SUFentanil, tacrolimus, teniposide, theophylline, thiamine, thiotepa, ticarcillin/clavulanate, tigecycline, tirofiban, tolazoline, trastuzumab, trimetaphan, urokinase, vancomycin, vasopressin, vecuronium, verapamil, vinCRIStine, vinorelbine, voriconazole, zidovudine

Y-site incompatibilities: Allopurinol, amphotericin B cholesteryl, amphotericin B colloidal, amphotericin B liposome, azaTHIOprine, azithromycin, ceFAZolin, cefoperazone, cefotetan, cefTRIAXone, dantrolene, dexamethasone, diazepam, diazoxide, drotrecogin, folic acid, ganciclovir, heparin, indomethacin, oxacillin, pemetrexed, pentamidine, PENTobarbital, phenytoin, piperacillin/tazobactam, propofol, sargramostim, trimethoprim/sulfamethoxazole

ADVERSE EFFECTS

CNS: Confusion, depression, numbness, tremors, **seizures,** muscle twitching, **neurotoxicity,** dizziness, vertigo
CV: Hypo/hypertension, palpitations

EENT: *Ototoxicity,* deafness, visual disturbances, tinnitus
GI: *Nausea, vomiting, anorexia,* increased ALT, AST, bilirubin, hepatomegaly, **hepatic necrosis,** splenomegaly
GU: Oliguria, hematuria, renal damage, azotemia, renal failure, nephrotoxicity
HEMA: Agranulocytosis, thrombocytopenia, leukopenia, eosinophilia, anemia
INTEG: *Rash,* burning, urticaria, dermatitis, alopecia

Pharmacokinetics

Absorption	Well absorbed (IM), completely absorbed (**IV**)
Distribution	Widely distributed in extracellular fluids
Metabolism	Minimal liver
Excretion	Mostly unchanged (>90%) kidneys
Half-life	2-3 hr, increased in renal disease, neonates

Pharmacodynamics

	IM	IV	OPHTH
Onset	Rapid	Rapid	Rapid
Peak	1 hr	Inf end	Unknown
Duration	Unknown	Unknown	Unknown

INTERACTIONS

Individual drugs
Acyclovir, amphotericin B, bacitracin, cidofovir, CISplatin, ethacrynic acid, furosemide, mannitol, methoxyflurane, polymyxin, vancomycin: increased ototoxicity, neurotoxicity, nephrotoxicity

Drug classifications
Aminoglycosides, cephalosporins, penicillins: increased ototoxicity, neurotoxicity, nephrotoxicity

NURSING CONSIDERATIONS

Assessment
• Assess patient for previous sensitivity reaction
Systemic route
• Assess patient for signs and symptoms of infection including characteristics of wounds, sputum, urine, stool, WBC >10,000/mm^3, temp baseline, during treatment
• Complete C&S testing before beginning product therapy to identify if correct treatment has been initiated

---

• Assess for allergic reactions: rash, urticaria, pruritus, chills, fever, joint pain

> **BLACK BOX WARNING: Renal disease:**
> Identify urine output; if decreasing, notify prescriber (may indicate nephrotoxicity); also, obtain BUN, creatinine, urine CCr (<80 ml/min) values; urinalysis daily for proteinuria, cells, casts; report sudden change in urine output

• Monitor blood studies: AST, ALT, CBC, Hct, bilirubin, LDH, alkaline phosphatase, Coombs' test monthly if patient is on long-term therapy
• Monitor electrolytes: potassium, sodium, chloride, magnesium monthly if patient is on long-term therapy
• Monitor for bleeding: ecchymosis, bleeding gums, hematuria, stool guaiac daily if patient is on long-term therapy
• **Assess for overgrowth of infection:** perineal itching, fever, malaise, redness, pain, swelling, drainage, rash, diarrhea, change in cough, sputum
• Obtain weight before treatment; calculation of dosage is usually based on ideal body weight but may be calculated on actual body weight
• Monitor VS during inf, watch for hypotension, change in pulse
• Assess **IV** site for thrombophlebitis including pain, redness, swelling q30min; change site if needed; apply warm compresses to discontinued site
• Obtain serum peak, drawn at 30-60 min after **IV** inf or 60 min after IM inj, trough level drawn just before next dose; peak 4-12 mcg/ml, trough 1-2 mcg/ml

> **BLACK BOX WARNING:** Monitor for deafness by audiometric testing, ringing, roaring in ears, vertigo; assess hearing before, during, after treatment

Nursing diagnoses
• Diarrhea (adverse reactions)
• Infection, risk for (uses)
• Injury, risk for (adverse reactions)
• Knowledge, deficient (teaching)
• Noncompliance (teaching)

Patient/family education
• Teach patient to report sore throat, bruising, bleeding, joint pain; may indicate blood dyscrasias (rare)
• Advise patient to contact prescriber if vaginal itching, loose foul-smelling stools, furry tongue occur; may indicate superinfection

> **BLACK BOX WARNING:** Advise patient to notify prescriber if pregnancy is planned or suspected, pregnancy **D**

• Advise patient to notify prescriber of diarrhea with blood or pus; may indicate pseudomembranous colitis

Nebulizer route
• Advise patient to use multiple therapies first, then tobramycin

Evaluation
Positive therapeutic outcome
• Absence of signs/symptoms of infection (WBC <10,000/mm^3, temp WNL, absence of red, draining wounds)
• Reported improvement in symptoms of infection

TREATMENT OF OVERDOSE:
Withdraw product, hemodialysis, exchange transfusion in the newborn, monitor serum levels of product, may give ticarcillin or carbenicillin

tobramycin ophthalmic
See Appendix B

tocilizumab (Rx)
(toe'si-liz'oo-mab)
Actemra
Func. class.: DMARDs (Disease modifying anti-rheumatoid drugs)/tumor necrosis factor (TNF) modifier
Pregnancy category C

ACTION: Interleukin- 6 (IL-6) receptor inhibiting monoclonal antibody

Therapeutic outcome: Ability to move more easily with less pain

USES: Rheumatoid arthritis, active systemic juvenile idiopathic arthritis

CONTRAINDICATIONS:
Serious infections, risk for GI perforation, active hepatic disease, severe neutropenia/thrombocytopenia, demyelinating disorders

Precautions: Breastfeeding, pregnancy **C**

DOSAGE AND ROUTES
Adult: IV 4 mg/kg over 1 hr q4wk, may increase to 8 mg/kg q4wk based on clinical response, max dose 800 mg/inf; do not initiate if ANC is >2000 and platelets are <100,000.

Juvenile idiopathic arthritis
Child ≥2 yr/adolescent ≥30 kg: IV 8 mg/kg over 1 hr q2wk
Child ≥2 yr/adolescent <30 kg: IV 12 mg/kg over 1 hr

Available forms: Sol for inj 80 mg/4 ml, 200 mg/10 ml, 400 mg/20 ml

Implementation
Intermittent IV route
• Visually inspect for particulate matter and discoloration before administration whenever solution and container permit, colorless to pale yellow liquid
• From a 100-ml infusion bag or bottle, withdraw a volume of 0.9% NaCl for inj equal to the volume of the tocilizumab solution required for the patient's dose
• Slowly add tocilizumab from each vial into the infusion bag or bottle. Gently invert the bag to avoid foaming. Fully diluted solutions are compatible with polypropylene, polyethylene, and polyvinyl chloride infusion bags and polypropylene, polyethylene, and glass infusion bottles
• The fully diluted sol for inf may be stored refrigerated or at room temp for up to 24 hours and should be protected from light. Do not use unused product remaining in vials; no preservatives
• Allow the fully diluted solution to reach room temp before infusing
• Give over 60 min with an infusion set. Do not administer as an IV push or bolus
• Do not infuse concomitantly in the same intravenous line with other drugs

ADVERSE EFFECTS
CNS: Headache, dizziness
CV: Hypertension
GI: Perforation, abdominal pain, gastritis, mouth ulcerations
HEMA: Neutropenia, thrombocytopenia
INTEG: Rash, infusion reactions
RESP: Upper respiratory infections, nasopharyngitis, bronchitis
SYST: Serious infections, anaphylaxis, infusion-related reactions, anti-tocilizumab antibody formation

Pharmacokinetics
Absorption	Unknown
Distribution	Unknown
Metabolism	Unknown
Excretion	Unknown
Half-life	~6 days with a single dose and ~11 days with multiple (steady state) doses

Pharmacodynamics
Unknown

INTERACTIONS
Drug classifications
Live virus vaccines: Do not use together
TNF modifiers, DMARDs, immunosuppressives: avoid use due to increased risk of infection

NURSING CONSIDERATIONS
Assessment
• **Rheumatoid arthritis:** assess ROM, pain, stiffness baseline and periodically
• Monitor blood studies: CBC with differential, LFTs, platelet count, serum lipid profile, baseline and periodically
• Assess for infection before and periodically, obtain TB screening before beginning treatment

Nursing diagnoses
• Activity intolerance (uses)
• Injury, risk for (adverse reactions)

Patient/family education
• Teach patient that this treatment must continue unless safety or effectiveness is an issue; reason for use and expected result
• Advise patient to avoid use of live vaccines
• Instruct patient to report signs/symptoms of infection (including TB and Hepatitis B)

Evaluation
Positive therapeutic outcome
• Ability to move more easily with less pain

tolcapone (Rx)
(toll'cah-pone)
Tasmar
Func. class.: Antiparkinson agent
Chem. class.: Catecholamine inhibitor (COMT)
Pregnancy category C

ACTION: Selective, reversible inhibitor of catecholamine; used as adjunct to levodopa/carbidopa therapy

Therapeutic outcome: Increased ability to move and speak

USES: Parkinsonism

CONTRAINDICATIONS:
Hypersensitivity

Precautions: Pregnancy **C,** breastfeeding, cardiac/renal disease, hypertension, asthma, history of rhabdomyolysis

BLACK BOX WARNING: Hepatic disease

DOSAGE AND ROUTES
Adult: PO 100-200 mg tid, with levodopa/carbidopa therapy; max 600 mg/day; discontinue if no benefit in 3 wk

Available forms: Tabs 100, 200 mg

Implementation
• Administer tid with levodopa/carbidopa therapy
• Food taken within 1 hr before or 2 hr after meals increases action of product by 20%
• Provide assistance with ambulation during beginning therapy

ADVERSE EFFECTS
CNS: Dystonia, dyskinesia, dreaming, *fatigue, headache, confusion,* psychosis, hallucination, dizziness, sleep disorders
CV: *Orthostatic hypotension,* chest pain, hypotension
EENT: Cataract, eye inflammation
GI: *Nausea, vomiting, abdominal distress,* diarrhea, constipation, **fatal liver failure,** elevated liver function tests
GU: UTI, urine discoloration, uterine tumor, micturition disorder, hematuria
HEMA: Hemolytic anemia, leukopenia, agranulocytosis
INTEG: Sweating, alopecia
MS: Rhabdomyolysis

Pharmacokinetics

Absorption	Rapidly absorbed
Distribution	Protein binding 99%
Metabolism	Liver, extensively
Excretion	Urine (60%), feces (40%)
Half-life	2-3 hr

Pharmacodynamics

Onset	Unknown
Peak	2 hr
Duration	Unknown

INTERACTIONS
Individual drugs
Apomorphine, DOBUTamine, isoproterenol, α-methyldopa: may influence pharmacokinetics

Drug classifications
MAOIs: decreased normal catecholamine metabolism; MAO-B inhibitor may be used

NURSING CONSIDERATIONS
Assessment
• **Hepatic disease:** monitor liver function tests: AST, ALT, alkaline phosphatase, LDH, bilirubin, CBC
• Assess involuntary movements in parkinsonism: akinesia, tremors, staggering gait, muscle rigidity, drooling
• Monitor B/P, respiration during initial treatment; hypo/hypertension should be reported
• Monitor mental status: affect, mood, behavioral changes

Nursing diagnoses
• Injury, risk for (uses)
• Knowledge, deficient (teaching)
• Mobility, impaired physical (uses)

Patient/family education
• Advise patient to change positions slowly to prevent orthostatic hypotension
• Advise patient that urine, sweat may change color

BLACK BOX WARNING: Advise patient to report signs of hepatic injury: clay-colored stools, jaundice, fatigue, appetite loss, lethargy

• Teach patient to report nausea, vomiting, anorexia

Evaluation
Positive therapeutic outcome
• Decrease in akathisia, improved mood

tolnaftate topical
See Appendix B

tolterodine (Rx)
(tol-tehr'oh-deen)
Detrol, Detrol LA
Func. class.: Overactive bladder product
Chem. class.: Muscarinic receptor antagonist
Pregnancy category C

ACTION: Relaxes smooth muscles in urinary tract by inhibiting acetylcholine at postganglionic sites

Therapeutic outcome: Decreased symptoms of overactive bladder

USES: Overactive bladder (frequency, urgency), urinary incontinence

CONTRAINDICATIONS:
Hypersensitivity, uncontrolled closed-angle glaucoma, urinary retention, gastric retention

Precautions: Pregnancy **C**, breastfeeding, children, renal/hepatic disease, controlled closed-angle glaucoma, bladder obstruction, QT prolongation, decreased GI motility

DOSAGE AND ROUTES
Adult and geriatric: PO 2 mg bid, may decrease to 1 mg bid; EXT REL 4 mg/day, may decrease to 2 mg if needed, max 4 mg/day

Hepatic disease
Adult: PO 1 mg bid (50% dose) or EXT REL 2 mg/day

Renal dose
Adult: PO CCr ≤30 ml/min reduce by 50%

Available forms: Tabs 1, 2 mg; ext rel caps 2, 4 mg

Implementation
• Swallow whole; give with liquids

ADVERSE EFFECTS
CNS: *Anxiety,* paresthesia, fatigue, *dizziness,* headache, increasing dementia, memory impairment
CV: Chest pain, hypertension, **QT prolongation**
EENT: Vision abnormalities, xerophthalmia
GI: *Nausea, vomiting, anorexia,* abdominal pain, constipation, dry mouth, dyspepsia
GU: Dysuria, retention, frequency, UTI
INTEG: Rash, pruritus
RESP: Bronchitis, cough, pharyngitis, upper respiratory tract infection
SYST: **Angioedema, Stevens-Johnson syndrome**

Pharmacokinetics	
Absorption	Rapidly absorbed
Distribution	Highly protein bound
Metabolism	Liver, extensively by CYP2D6, a portion of the population may be poor metabolizers
Excretion	Urine/feces
Half-life	Unknown

Pharmacodynamics	
Unknown	

INTERACTIONS
Individual drugs
Chloroquine, clarithromycin, droperidol, erythromycin, grepafloxacin, halofantrine, haloperidol, methadone, pentamidine: increased QT prolongation

Drug classifications
Antibiotics (macrolide), antifungal agents, antiretroviral protease inhibitors: increased action of tolterodine
Antimuscarinics: increased anticholinergic effect
β-agonists, class IA/III antidysrhythmics, local anesthetics, some phenothiazines, tricyclics: increased QT prolongation
Diuretics: increased urinary frequency

Drug/food
Increased: bioavailability of tolterodine

NURSING CONSIDERATIONS
Assessment
• **Assess urinary patterns:** distention, nocturia, frequency, urgency, incontinence
• **Serious skin disorders:** assess for angioedema, Stevens-Johnson syndrome; assess allergic reactions: rash; if this occurs, product should be discontinued
• **QT prolongation:** ECG for QT prolongation, ejection fraction; assess for chest pain, palpitations, dyspnea

Nursing diagnoses
• Activity intolerance (uses)
• Knowledge, deficient (teaching)
• Urinary elimination, impaired (uses)

Patient/family education
• Advise patient to avoid hazardous activities; dizziness may occur
• Advise patient not to drink liquids before bedtime
• Teach patient importance of bladder maintenance
• Teach patient to take with liquids; swallow whole

Evaluation
Positive therapeutic outcome
• Decreased urinary frequency, urgency

tolvaptan (Rx)
(tole-vap′tan)
Samsca
Func. class.: Vasopressin receptor antagonist, V2
Pregnancy category C

ACTION: Arginine vasopressin (AVP) antagonist with affinity for V₂ receptors; level of circulating AVP in circulating blood is critical for regulation of water, electrolyte balance and is usually elevated in euvolemic/hypervolemic hyponatremia

---

Adverse effects: *italics* = common; **bold** = life-threatening

Therapeutic outcome: Normal serum sodium level

USES: Hypervolemic/euvolemic hyponatremia in heart failure, cirrhosis, SIADH

CONTRAINDICATIONS:
Hypersensitivity, hypovolemia, anuria

Precautions: Pregnancy **C**, breastfeeding, children, dehydration, geriatric patients, hepatic disease, hyperkalemia

> **BLACK BOX WARNING:** Alcoholism, malnutrition

DOSAGE AND ROUTES
Adult: PO 15 mg qd; after 24 hr, may increase to 30 mg qd; max 60 mg/day

Available forms: Tab 15, 30 mg

Implementation
- Give PO with or without food
- Avoid fluid restriction the first 24 hr
- Initiate in hospital setting

ADVERSE EFFECTS
CNS: Fever
CV: Ventricular fibrillation, DIC, stroke, thrombosis
GI: Nausea, vomiting, constipation, colitis
GU: Polyuria
HEMA: Bleeding
META: Dehydration, hyperglycemia, hyperkalemia, hypernatremia
MS: Rhabdomyolysis
RESP: Respiratory depression, pulmonary embolism

Pharmacokinetics

Absorption	Unknown
Distribution	Protein binding 99%
Metabolism	CYP3A4
Excretion	Unknown
Half-life	Terminal 12 hr

Pharmacodynamics

Onset	Unknown
Peak	2-4 hr
Duration	Unknown

INTERACTIONS

Drug classifications
CYP3A4 inducers (carBAMazepine, dexamethasone, etravirine, flutamide, griseofulvin, metyrapsone, modafinil, nafacillin, nevirapine, OXcarbazepine, phenytoin, rifampin, rifabutin, rifapendine, topiramate): decreased plasma concentrations of tolvaptan
CYP3A4 inhibitors (efavirenz, fosamprenavir, quiNINE), P-gp inhibitors (azithromycin, cycloSPORINE, mefloquine, palperidone, propafenone, quiNIDine, testosterone): increased plasma concentrations of tolvaptan

Drug/herb
St. John's wort: decreased tolvaptan effect

NURSING CONSIDERATIONS

Assessment
- Assess renal, hepatic function
- Monitor frequent sodium volume status; overly rapid correction of sodium concentration ($>$12 mEq/L per 24 hr) may result in osmotic demyelination syndrome
- Assess CV status: ventricular fibrillation, hypertension, monitor B/P, pulse
- Monitor electrolytes (sodium, potassium)

Nursing diagnoses
- Injury, risk for (uses)
- Knowledge, deficient (teaching)

Patient/family education
- Teach patient to avoid pregnancy, breastfeeding while taking this product
- Advise of administration procedure and expected result

Evaluation
Positive therapeutic outcome
- Correction of serum sodium levels

---

topiramate (Rx)
(to-pi-ra'mate)
Topamax, Topamax Sprinkle, Topiragen
Func. class.: Anticonvulsant— miscellaneous
Chem. class.: Monosaccharide derivative
Pregnancy category D

ACTION: Increased GABA activity; may prevent seizure spread as opposed to an elevation of seizure threshold

Therapeutic outcome: Absence of seizures

USES: Partial seizures in adults and children 2-16 yr old; tonic-clonic seizures; seizures in Lennox-Gastaut syndrome, migraine prophylaxis

Unlabeled uses: Infantile spasms

⚠ Nurse Alert

CONTRAINDICATIONS:
Hypersensitivity, metabolic acidosis, pregnancy **D**

Precautions: Breastfeeding, children, renal/hepatic disease, acute myopia, secondary closed-angle glaucoma, behavioral disorders, COPD, dialysis, encephalopathy, status asthmaticus, status epilepticus, surgery, paresthesias, maculopathy

DOSAGE AND ROUTES
Adjunctive therapy
Adult/adolescent/child ≥ 10 yr: PO 25-50 mg/day initially, titrate by 25-50 mg/wk, up to 200-400 mg/day in 2 divided doses
Child 2-9 yr: PO week 1 25 mg q PM, then 25 mg bid if tolerated (week 2), then increase by 25-50 mg/day each week as tolerated over 5-7 wk titration period, maintenance given in 2 divided doses; <11 kg minimum 150 mg/day, max 250 mg/day; 12-22 kg minimum 200 mg/day, max 300 mg/day; 23-31 kg minimum 200 mg, max 350 mg/day, 32-38 kg minimum 250 mg/kg, max 350 mg/day; >38 kg minimum 250 mg/day, max 400 mg/day

Migraine prophylaxis
Adult: PO 25 mg/day initially, increase by 25 mg/day qwk up to 100 mg/day in 2 divided doses

Renal dose
Adult: PO CCr <70 ml/min ½ dose

Available forms: Tabs 25, 50, 100, 200 mg; sprinkle caps 15, 25 mg

Implementation
• Do not break, crush, or chew tabs; very bitter
• May take without regard to meals
• Sprinkle cap can be given whole or opened and sprinkled on soft food; do not chew

ADVERSE EFFECTS
CNS: Dizziness, fatigue, cognitive disorder, *insomnia,* anxiety, depression, paresthesia, motor retardation, **suicidal ideation,** memory loss, tremor
EENT: Diplopia, vision abnormality
GI: *Diarrhea, anorexia,* nausea, dyspepsia, abdominal pain, constipation, dry mouth, **pancreatitis**
GU: Breast pain, dysmenorrhea, menstrual disorder
INTEG: Rash
MISC: Weight loss, **leukopenia,** metabolic acidosis, increased body temperature, **unexplained death (epilepsy)**

RESP: Upper respiratory tract infection, pharyngitis, sinusitis

Pharmacokinetics
Absorption	Well absorbed
Distribution	Crosses placenta, plasma protein binding (9%-17%), steady state 4 days
Metabolism	Unknown
Excretion	Kidneys unchanged 55%-97%
Half-life	19-25 hr

Pharmacodynamics
Onset	Unknown
Peak	2-4 hr
Duration	Unknown

INTERACTIONS
Individual drugs
Alcohol: increased CNS depression
Amitriptyline: increased effect of amitriptyline
CarBAMazepine, phenytoin, probenecid: decreased levels of topiramate
Digoxin: decreased levels of digoxin
Estrogen: decreased levels of estrogen
Hydrochlorothiazide, lamoTRIgine, metformin: increased topiramate levels
Lithium: decreased levels of lithium
Risperidone: decreased levels of risperidone
Valproic acid: decreased levels of both products

Drug classifications
Carbonic anhydrase inhibitors: increased kidney stone formation
CNS depressants: increased CNS depression
Oral contraceptives: decreased level of oral contraceptives

NURSING CONSIDERATIONS
Assessment
• **Bipolar disorder:** assess mood, behavior
⚠ **Assess mental status: mood, sensorium, affect, memory (long, short), especially in geriatric; suicidal thoughts/behavior**
• Assess for blood dyscrasias: fever, sore throat, bruising, rash, jaundice, epistaxis (long-term treatment only)
• **Assess seizure activity** including type, location, duration, and character; provide seizure precaution
• Monitor CBC during long-term therapy; serum bicarbonate
• Assess body weight and evidence of cognitive disorder

Adverse effects: *italics* = common; **bold** = life-threatening

Nursing diagnoses
- Injury, risk for (side effects)
- Knowledge, deficient (teaching)

Patient/family education
- Teach patient to carry/wear emergency ID stating name, products taken, condition, prescriber's name and phone number
- Advise patient to avoid driving, other activities that require alertness
- Teach patient not to discontinue medication abruptly after long-term use
- Advise patient to use nonhormonal contraceptive; effect of oral contraceptives is decreased, pregnancy **D**

Evaluation
Positive therapeutic outcome
- Decreased seizure activity

TREATMENT OF OVERDOSE:
Lavage, VS

⚠ HIGH ALERT

topotecan (Rx)
(to-poe′ti-kan)
Hycamtin
Func. class: Antineoplastic natural; topoisomerase inhibitor
Chem. class.: Camptothecin analog
Pregnancy category D

ACTION: Antitumor product with topoisomerase I–inhibitory activity; topoisomerase I relieves torsional strain in DNA by causing single-strand breaks; causes double-strand DNA damage

Therapeutic outcome: Decreased tumor size

USES: Metastatic ovarian cancer after failure of traditional chemotherapy, relapsed small cell lung cancer, cervical cancer

CONTRAINDICATIONS:
Pregnancy **D**, breastfeeding, hypersensitivity, severe bone marrow depression

BLACK BOX WARNING: Neutropenia

Precautions: Children, renal disease

DOSAGE AND ROUTES
Adult: IV INF 1.5 mg/m^2 over 30 min/day × 5 days starting on day 1 of a 21-day course × 4 courses; may be reduced to 0.25 mg/m^2 for subsequent courses if severe neutropenia occurs; PO 2.3 mg/m^2/day on days 1-5 of a 21-day course (relapsed small cell lung cancer in those with prior response)

Renal dose
Adult: IV CCr 20-39 ml/min 0.75 mg/m^2/day × 5 days on day 1 of a 21-day course

Available forms: Lyophilized powder for inj 4 mg; cap 0.25, 1 mg

Implementation
- Provide increased fluid intake to 2-3 L/day to prevent dehydration, unless contraindicated
- Change **IV** site q48hr

ADVERSE EFFECTS
CNS: Arthralgia, *asthenia, headache,* myalgia, *pain,* weakness
GI: *Abdominal pain, constipation,* diarrhea, obstruction, *nausea,* stomatitis, *vomiting,* increased ALT, AST, anorexia
HEMA: Neutropenia, leukopenia, thrombocytopenia, anemia, sepsis
INTEG: *Total alopecia*
RESP: Dyspnea, cough, **interstitial lung disease**

Pharmacokinetics

Absorption	Rapidly, completely absorbed
Distribution	7%-35% protein binding
Metabolism	Liver
Excretion	Urine, feces to metabolites
Half-life	2.8 hr

Pharmacodynamics

Unknown

INTERACTIONS

Individual drugs
CISplatin: increased myelosuppression
Itraconazole, mefloquine, niCARdipine, quiNIDine, RU-486, tamoxifen, testosterone, verapamil: avoid giving together

Drug classifications
Anticoagulants, NSAIDs, platelet inhibitors, thrombolytics: increased bleeding risk
P-glycoprotein, breast cancer resistance protein inhibitors (amiodarone, clarithromycin, diltiazem, erythromycin, indinavir vaccines, toxoids: avoid using together

Drug/food
Grapefruit juice: avoid use

NURSING CONSIDERATIONS

Assessment

• Monitor liver function tests: AST, ALT, alkaline phosphatase, which may be elevated; creatinine, BUN

> **BLACK BOX WARNING:** Monitor CBC, differential, platelet count weekly; withhold product if WBC is <3500/mm³ or platelet count is <100,000/mm³; notify prescriber of these results; product should be discontinued

• Assess buccal cavity for dryness, sores or ulceration, white patches, oral pain, bleeding, dysphagia
• Assess GI symptoms: frequency of stools, cramping
• Assess signs of dehydration: rapid respiration, poor skin turgor, decreased urine output, dry skin, restlessness, weakness

Nursing diagnoses

• Infection, risk for (adverse reactions)
• Knowledge, deficient (teaching)

Patient/family education

• Advise patient to avoid foods with citric acid or hot flavor or rough texture if stomatitis is present; to drink adequate fluids
• Provide patient with nutritious diet of iron, vit K supplements, low fiber, few dairy products
• Advise patient that total alopecia may occur; hair grows back but may be different in color and texture
• Advise patient to report stomatitis; any bleeding, white spots, ulcerations in mouth; tell patient to examine mouth daily; report symptoms
• Teach patient to report signs of anemia; fatigue, headache, faintness, shortness of breath, irritability
• Teach patient to rinse mouth tid-qid with water, club soda; brush teeth bid-tid with soft brush or cotton-tipped applicator for stomatitis; use unwaxed dental floss
• Teach patient to use effective contraception during treatment and up to 6 mo after, avoid breastfeeding
• Advise patient to avoid OTC products without approval of prescriber
• Advise to avoid driving or other activities requiring alertness
• Advise to avoid vaccines, toxoids

Evaluation

Positive therapeutic outcome

• Decreased tumor size, spread of malignancy

toremifene (Rx)

(tore′me-feen)
Fareston
Func. class.: Antineoplastic
Chem. class.: Antiestrogen hormone
Pregnancy category D

ACTION: Inhibits cell division by binding to cytoplasmic estrogen receptors; resembles normal cell complex but inhibits DNA synthesis and estrogen response of target tissue

Therapeutic outcome: Prevention of rapidly growing malignant cells

USES: Advanced breast carcinoma that has not responded to other therapy in estrogen-receptor-positive patients (usually postmenopausal)

CONTRAINDICATIONS:
Pregnancy **D,** hypersensitivity, history of thromboembolism

> **BLACK BOX WARNING:** QT prolongation

Precautions: Breastfeeding, children, cataracts, leukopenia, thrombocytopenia, hypercalcemia, hepatic disease, endometrial hyperplasia

DOSAGE AND ROUTES

Adult: PO 60 mg/day

Available forms: Tabs 60 mg

Implementation

• Do not break, crush, or chew tabs
• Give with food or fluids to decrease GI upset; repeat dose may be needed if vomiting occurs
• Store in light-resistant container at room temperature

ADVERSE EFFECTS

CNS: *Hot flashes, headache, lightheadedness,* depression
CV: Chest pain, **CHF, MI, PE,** chest pain, angina
EENT: Ocular lesions, retinopathy, corneal opacity, blurred vision (high doses)
GI: *Nausea, vomiting,* altered taste (anorexia)
GU: Vaginal bleeding, pruritus vulvae
HEMA: Thrombocytopenia, leukopenia, thrombosis
INTEG: *Rash,* alopecia, sweating
META: Hypercalcemia
RESP: Pulmonary embolism

Pharmacokinetics

Absorption	Adequately absorbed
Distribution	99% protein binding
Metabolism	Liver, extensively
Excretion	Feces, slowly, small amounts (kidneys)
Half-life	Terminal 5-6 days

Pharmacodynamics

Onset	Unknown
Peak	3 hr
Duration	Unknown

INTERACTIONS

Individual drugs
Warfarin: increased warfarin effect

> **BLACK BOX WARNING:** Haloperidol, chloroquine, droperidol, pentamidine, arsenic trioxide, levomethadyl: increased QT prolongation

Drug classifications

> **BLACK BOX WARNING:** Class IA/III antidysrhythmics, some phenothiazines, β-agonists, local anesthetics, tricyclics, pentamidine; CYP3A4 inhibitors (amiodarone, clarithromycin, erythromycin, telithromycin, troleandomycin); CYP3A4 substrates (methadone, pimozide, QUEtiapine, quiNIDine, risperidone, ziprasidone): increased QT prolongation

CYP3A4 inducers (barbiturates, bosentan, carBAMazepine, efavirenz, phenytoins, nevirapine, rifabutin, rifampin): decreased toremifene effect

CYP3A4 inhibitors (aprepitant, antiretroviral protease inhibitors, clarithromycin, danazol, delivirdine, diltiazem, erythromycin, fluconazole, FLUoxetine, fluvoxamine, imatinib, ketoconazole, mibefradil, nefazodone, telithromycin, voriconazole): increased toxicity

Drug/herb
St. John's wort: avoid use

Drug/lab test
Increased: serum Ca

NURSING CONSIDERATIONS

Assessment
• Monitor CBC, differential, platelet count weekly; withhold product if WBC is <4000/mm³ or platelet count is <75,000/mm³; notify prescriber of results; monitor calcium levels (hypercalcemia is common), LFTs, serum calcium

• **Assess for tumor flare:** increase in bone, tumor pain during beginning treatment; give analgesics as ordered to decrease pain

• Assess for bleeding: hematuria, guaiac, bruising or petechiae, mucosa or orifices q8hr, no rectal temp

• **QT prolongation:** ECG for QT prolongation, ejection fraction; assess for chest pain, palpitations, dyspnea

> **BLACK BOX WARNING: Allergic reactions:** assess for rash, pruritus, urticaria, purpuric skin lesions, itching, flushing

Nursing diagnoses
• Injury, risk for (adverse reactions)
• Knowledge, deficient (teaching)

Patient/family education
• Instruct patient to report any complaints, side effects to prescriber; if dose is missed, do not double next dose

• Advise patient that vaginal bleeding, pruritus, hot flashes can occur and are reversible after discontinuing treatment

• Instruct patient to report immediately decreased visual acuity, which may be irreversible; stress need for routine eye exams

• Inform patient about who should be told about toremifene therapy

• Advise patient to report vaginal bleeding immediately; that tumor flare (increase in size of tumor, increased bone pain) may occur and will subside rapidly; may take analgesics for pain; that premenopausal women must use mechanical birth control method because ovulation may be induced (teratogenic product)

• Caution patient to use sunscreen and protective clothing to prevent burns because photosensitivity is common

• Teach patient that hair loss may occur during treatment; a wig or hairpiece may make patient feel better; new hair may be different in color, texture

• Inform patient rash or lesions are temporary and may become large during beginning therapy

Evaluation
Positive therapeutic outcome
• Decreased spread of malignant cells in breast cancer

trace elements (chromium, copper, iodide, manganese, selenium, zinc) (Rx)
Concentrated Multiple Trace Elements, ConTE-PAK-4, M.T.E.-4, M.T.E.-4 Concentrated, M.T.E.-5, M.T.E.-5 Concentrated, M.T.E.-6, M.T.E.-6 Concentrated, M.T.E.-7, MulTE-PAK-4, MulTE-PAK-5, Multiple Trace Element, Multiple Trace Element Neonatal, Multiple Trace Element Pediatric, Neotrace 4, Ped TE-PAK-4, Pedtrice-4, P.T.E.-4, P.T.E.-5
Func. class.: Mineral supplement
Pregnancy category C

ACTION: Needed for adequate absorption and synthesis of amino acids

Therapeutic outcome: Replacement for mineral deficiencies

USES: Prevention of trace element deficiency, a component of TPN

Precautions: Pregnancy **C**, breastfeeding, liver, biliary disease, vomiting or diarrhea

DOSAGE AND ROUTES
Usual dosage may be given in TPN SOL

Chromium
Adult: **IV** 10-15 mcg/day
Child: **IV** 0.14-0.20 mcg/ kg/day

Copper
Adult: **IV** 0.5-1.5 mg/day
Child: **IV** 0.05-0.2 mg/kg/day

Iodide
Adult: **IV** 1 mcg/kg/day

Manganese
Adult: **IV** 0.15-0.8 mg/day

Selenium
Adult: **IV** 20-40 mcg/day
Child: **IV** 3 mcg/kg/day

Zinc
Adult: **IV** 2-4 mg/day
Child: **IV** 0.05 mg/kg/day

Available forms: Many forms available; see particular elements

Implementation
• Give by **IV** inf, often mixed with TPN sol
• Discard unused portions

• Give by continuous inf diluted in 1 L or more **IV** sol; give at prescribed rate

ADVERSE EFFECTS
CHROMIUM: Seizures, coma, nausea, vomiting, ulcers, **renal/hepatic toxicity**
COPPER: Personality changes, diarrhea, weakness, photophobia, muscle weakness
IODINE: Headache, edema of eyelids, acne, metallic taste, sore mouth, runny nose
MANGANESE: Incoordination, headache, irritability, lability, slurred speech, impotence
SELENIUM: Alopecia, depression, vomiting, GI cramping, nervousness, garlic smell
ZINC: Vomiting, oliguria, **hypothermia**, vision changes, **tachycardia**, jaundice, **coma**

Pharmacokinetics
Absorption	Completely absorbed
Distribution	Widely distributed
Metabolism	Unknown
Excretion	Depends on element
Half-life	Unknown

Pharmacodynamics
Unknown

NURSING CONSIDERATIONS
Assessment
• Assess trace element levels; notify prescriber if low; copper 0.07-0.15 mg/ml, zinc 0.05-0.15 mg/100 ml, manganese 4-20 mcg/100 ml, selenium 0.1-0.19 mcg/ml
• Assess trace element deficiency if patient is receiving TPN for extended period
• Obtain calorie count to identify nutritional deficiencies
• Assess for toxicity of individual element (see Adverse Effects)

Nursing diagnoses
• Knowledge, deficient (teaching)
• Nutrition: less than body requirements, imbalanced (uses)

Patient/family education
• Explain to patient reason for and expected results of medication

Evaluation
Positive therapeutic outcome
• Absence of element deficiency

T

traMADol (Rx)

(trah'mah-dol)

Rybix, Ryzolt, Ultram, Ultram ER, Zytram ❦

Func. class.: Analgesic, miscellaneous

Pregnancy category C

Do not confuse:
traMADol/Toradol

ACTION: Binds to μ-opioid receptors and inhibits reuptake of norepinephrine, serotonin

Therapeutic outcome: Relief of pain

USES: Management of moderate to severe pain, chronic pain

CONTRAINDICATIONS:

Hypersensitivity, acute intoxication with any CNS depressant, alcohol, asthma, respiratory depression

Precautions: Pregnancy **C**, breastfeeding, children, geriatric, seizure disorder, renal/hepatic disease, respiratory depression, head trauma, increased ICP, acute abdominal condition, product abuse, depression, suicidal ideation

DOSAGE AND ROUTES

Mild to moderate pain

Adult: PO 50-100 mg prn q4-6hr, max 400 mg/day; orally disintegrating tab 50 mg/day, titrate by 50 mg q3days, separate doses to 200 mg/day (50 mg qid)

Geriatric >75 yr: PO <300 mg/day in divided dose

Hepatic dose

Adult: PO 50 mg q12hr

Renal dose

Adult (Child-Pugh C): PO CCr <30 ml/min q12hr, max 200 mg/day; do not use ext rel tabs

Moderate to severe chronic pain

Adult: PO-ER (Ultram ER) 100 mg, titrate upward q5day by 100 mg, max 300 mg/day; (Ryzolt) 100 mg, titrate upward q2-3day in 100-mg increments; max 300 mg/day; products are not interchangeable

Available forms: Tabs 50 mg; ext rel tab 100, 200, 300 mg; orally disintegrating tab 50 mg

Implementation

• Do not break, crush, or chew ext rel product
• Give with antiemetic for nausea, vomiting
• Administer when pain is beginning to return; determine dosage interval by patient response
• Ext rel products (Ryzolt/Ultram ER) are not interchangeable
• Store in cool environment, protect from sunlight

ADVERSE EFFECTS

CNS: Dizziness, CNS stimulation, somnolence, headache, anxiety, confusion, euphoria, **seizures,** hallucinations, sedation, **neuroleptic malignant syndrome–like reactions**

CV: Vasodilatation, orthostatic hypotension, tachycardia, hypertension, abnormal ECG

EENT: Visual disturbances

GI: Nausea, constipation, vomiting, dry mouth, diarrhea, abdominal pain, anorexia, flatulence, GI bleeding

GU: Urinary retention/frequency, menopausal symptoms, dysuria, menstrual disorder

INTEG: Pruritus, rash, urticaria, vesicles, flushing

SYST: Anaphylaxis, Stevens-Johnson syndrome, toxic epidermal necrolysis, serotonin syndrome

Pharmacokinetics

Absorption	Rapidly, almost completely absorbed
Distribution	Steady state 2 days
Metabolism	Extensively in liver, may cross blood-brain barrier
Excretion	Unchanged product 30% in urine
Half-life	Unknown

Pharmacodynamics

Unknown

INTERACTIONS

Individual drugs

Alcohol: increased CNS depression
CarBAMazepine: decreased tramadol level

Drug classifications

CYP3A4 inducers (barbiturates, bosentan, carBAMazepine, efavirenz, nevirapine, phenytoin, rifabutin, rifampin): decreased tramadol effect

CYP3A4 inhibitors (aprepitant, antiretroviral protease inhibitors, clarithromycin, danazol, delavirdine, diltiazem, erythromycin, fluconazole, FLUoxetine, fluvoxamine, imatinib, ketoconazole, mibefradil, nefazodone, telithromycin, voriconazole): increased tramadol levels

⚠ Nurse Alert

MAOIs: inhibition of norepinephrine and serotonin reuptake; use together with caution

Opiates, sedative/hypnotics: increased CNS depression

SSRIs, SNRIs, serotonin-receptor agonists: increased serotonin syndrome

Drug/herb

Chamomile, hops, kava, skullcap, valerian: increased CNS depression

St. John's wort: avoid use

Drug/lab test

Increased: creatinine, liver enzymes

Decreased: Hgb

NURSING CONSIDERATIONS

Assessment

• **Pain:** assess location, type, character; give before pain becomes extreme

• Assess for increased side effects in renal/hepatic disease

• Monitor I&O ratio: check for decreasing output; may indicate urinary retention

• Assess need for product

• Assess for constipation and bowel pattern; increase fluids, bulk in diet

• Monitor CNS changes: dizziness, drowsiness, hallucinations, euphoria, LOC, pupil reaction

• Determine allergic reactions: rash, urticaria

• **Serotonin syndrome, neuroleptic malignant syndrome:** assess for increased heart rate, shivering, sweating, dilated pupils, tremors, high B/P, hyperthermia, headache, confusion; if these occur, stop product, administer a serotonin antagonist if needed

Nursing diagnoses

• Injury, risk for (adverse reactions)

• Knowledge, deficient (teaching)

• Pain, acute (uses)

• Pain, chronic (uses)

Patient/family education

• Teach patient to report any symptoms of CNS changes, allergic reactions

• Teach patient that drowsiness, dizziness, and confusion may occur; to call for assistance

• Instruct patient to make position changes slowly; orthostatic hypotension may occur

• Tell patient to avoid OTC medication and alcohol unless approved by prescriber

Evaluation

Positive therapeutic outcome

• Decreased pain

---

trandolapril (Rx)

(tran-doe'la-prill)

Mavik

Func. class.: Antihypertensive

Chem. class.: Angiotensin-converting enzyme (ACE) inhibitor

Pregnancy category D (2nd/3rd trimester), pregnancy C (1st trimester)

ACTION: Selectively suppresses renin-angiotensin-aldosterone system; inhibits ACE; prevents conversion of angiotensin I to angiotensin II, resulting in dilatation of arterial and venous vessels and lowered B/P

Therapeutic outcome: Decreased B/P in hypertension

USES: Hypertension alone or in combination, heart failure, after MI, LV dysfunction after MI

CONTRAINDICATIONS:

Breastfeeding, hypersensitivity, history of angioedema

> **BLACK BOX WARNING:** Pregnancy **D** (2nd/3rd trimester), pregnancy **C** (1st trimester)

Precautions: Geriatric, hyperkalemia, hepatic disease, bilateral renal stenosis, after kidney transplant, aortal/mitral valve stenosis, cirrhosis, severe renal disease, untreated CHF, autoimmune diseases, cough

DOSAGE AND ROUTES

Hypertension

Adult: PO 1 mg/day, 2 mg/day in African Americans, make dosage adjustment ≥1 wk; up to 8 mg/day

Heart failure (after MI/left ventricular dysfunction)

Adult: PO 1 mg/day, titrate upward to 4 mg/day if tolerated

Renal dose/hepatic dose

Adult: PO CCr <30 ml/min or hepatic disease 0.5 mg/day

Available forms: Tabs 1, 2, 4 mg

Implementation

• Store in airtight container at ≤77° F (≤25° C) or less

ADVERSE EFFECTS

CNS: *Dizziness,* paresthesias, headache, *syncope,* fatigue, drowsiness, depression, sleep disturbances, anxiety

CV: *Hypotension,* **MI,** palpitations, angina, TIAs, **stroke,** bradycardia, dysrhythmias

GI: Nausea, vomiting, cramps, diarrhea, constipation, **pancreatitis,** *dyspepsia*

GU: Proteinuria, renal failure

HEMA: Agranulocytosis, neutropenia, leukopenia, anemia

INTEG: Rash, purpura, pruritus

MISC: Hyperkalemia, hyponatremia, impotence, *myalgia,* **angioedema,** muscle cramps, asthenia, hypocalcemia, gout

RESP: Dyspnea, cough

Pharmacokinetics

Absorption	40%-60%
Distribution	Unknown
Metabolism	Liver
Excretion	Kidneys, feces
Half-life	0.6-1.1 hr, 16-24 hr

Pharmacodynamics

Onset	$1/2$ hr
Peak	4-10 hr
Duration	>8 days

INTERACTIONS

Individual drugs

Levodopa, lithium, reserpine: increased effect of each specific product

Drug classifications

Antacids, NSAIDs, salicylates: decreased effect of trandolapril

Antihypertensives, diuretics: increased severe hypotension

Barbiturates, ergots, hypoglycemics, neuromuscular blocking agents: increased effects of each specific product

Diuretics (potassium-sparing): increased potassium levels

Phenothiazines: increased antihypertensive effects

Potassium supplements: increased potassium levels

Salt substitutes: increased potassium levels

NURSING CONSIDERATIONS

Assessment

• Monitor blood tests: neutrophils, decreased platelets

• Monitor B/P, orthostatic hypotension, syncope; if changes occur dosage change may be required

• Monitor renal studies: protein, BUN, creatinine; increased levels may indicate nephrotic syndrome and renal failure

• Monitor renal symptoms: polyuria, oliguria, frequency, dysuria

• Establish baselines in renal, liver function tests before therapy begins

• Check potassium levels throughout treatment, although hyperkalemia rarely occurs

• Check for edema in feet, legs daily

• Assess for allergic reactions: rash, fever, pruritus, urticaria; product should be discontinued if antihistamines fail to help

Nursing diagnoses

• Cardiac output, decreased (uses)
• Injury, risk for (adverse reactions)
• Knowledge, deficient (teaching)
• Noncompliance (teaching)

Patient/family education

• Advise patient not to discontinue product abruptly; advise patient to tell all persons associated with health care

• Teach patient not to use OTC products (cough, cold, allergy) unless directed by physician; serious side effects can occur; xanthines, such as coffee, tea, chocolate, cola, can prevent action of product

• Instruct patient on the importance of complying with dosage schedule, even if feeling better; to continue with medical regimen to decrease B/P: exercise, cessation of smoking, decreasing stress, diet modifications

• Emphasize the need to rise slowly to sitting or standing position to minimize orthostatic hypotension; not to exercise in hot weather, which can cause increased hypotension

• Advise patient to notify prescriber of mouth sores, sore throat, fever, swelling of hands or feet, irregular heartbeat, chest pain, coughing, shortness of breath

• Caution patient to report excessive perspiration, dehydration, vomiting, diarrhea; may lead to fall in B/P

• Caution patient that product may cause dizziness, fainting, light-headedness; may occur during 1st few days of therapy; to avoid activities that may be hazardous

• Teach patient how to take B/P and normal readings for age group

BLACK BOX WARNING: Teach patient to notify prescriber if pregnancy is suspected or planned, pregnancy **D**

Evaluation
Positive therapeutic outcome
• Decreased B/P in hypertension

TREATMENT OF OVERDOSE:
Lavage, **IV** atropine for bradycardia, **IV** theophylline for bronchospasm, digoxin, O₂, diuretic for cardiac failure, hemodialysis

---

⚠ HIGH ALERT

trastuzumab (Rx)
(tras-tuz′uh-mab)
Herceptin
Func. class.: Antineoplastic—miscellaneous
Chem. class.: Humanized monoclonal antibody
Pregnancy category D

ACTION: DNA-derived monoclonal antibody selectively binds to extracellular portion of human epidermal growth factor receptor 2 (HER2); it inhibits proliferation of cancer cells

Therapeutic outcome: Decreasing symptoms of breast cancer

USES: Breast cancer; metastatic with overexpression of HER2, early breast cancer (adjuvant, neoadjuvant), gastric cancer

CONTRAINDICATIONS:
Pregnancy **D**, hypersensitivity to this product, Chinese hamster ovary cell protein

Precautions: Breastfeeding, children, geriatric, pulmonary disease, anemia, leukopenia

> **BLACK BOX WARNING:** Cardiac disease, respiratory distress syndrome, respiratory insufficiency, infusion-related reactions

DOSAGE AND ROUTES
Breast cancer
Several regimens may be used
Adult: **IV** 4 mg/kg given over 90 min, then maintenance 2 mg/kg given over 30 min; do not give as **IV** PUSH or BOL; may be given in combination with other antineoplastics

Gastric cancer
Adult: **IV** 8 mg/kg over 90 min on day 1, then 6 mg/kg over 30-90 min q21days from day 22, give with CISplatin 80 mg/m² on day 1 plus 5-fluorouracil 800 mg/m² CONT INF on days 1-5

or capecitabine 1000 mg/m² bid on days 1-14, repeat cycle q3wk

Available forms: Lyophilized powder 440 mg

Implementation
• Give acetaminophen as ordered to alleviate fever and headache
• Increase fluid intake to 2-3 L/day

Intermittent IV infusion route
• Administer after reconstituting vial with 20 ml of bacteriostatic water for inj, 1.1% benzyl alcohol preserved (supplied) to yield 21 mg/ml, mark date on vial 28 days from reconstitution date; if patient is allergic to benzyl alcohol, reconstitute with sterile water for inj; use immediately; inf over 90 min; q3wk give 8 mg/kg loading dose over 90 min; subsequent doses 6 mg/kg may be given over 30-60 min
• Do not mix or dilute with other products or dextrose sol

ADVERSE EFFECTS
CNS: *Dizziness, numbness, paresthesias,* depression, *insomnia,* neuropathy, peripheral neuritis
CV: **Tachycardia, CHF**
GI: Nausea, vomiting, *anorexia, diarrhea,* abdominal pain, **hepatotoxicity**
HEMA: *Anemia,* leukopenia
INTEG: *Rash,* acne, herpes simplex
META: Edema, peripheral edema
MISC: *Flulike symptoms; fever, headache, chills*
MS: Arthralgia, *bone pain*
RESP: *Cough, dyspnea, pharyngitis, rhinitis,* sinusitis, **pneumonia, pulmonary edema/fibrosis**
SYST: Anaphylaxis, angioedema

Pharmacokinetics

Absorption	Unknown
Distribution	Unknown
Metabolism	Unknown
Excretion	Unknown
Half-life	1-32 days

Pharmacodynamics
Unknown

INTERACTIONS
Individual drugs
Cyclophosphamide: increased cardiomyopathy risk; avoid use
Warfarin: increased bleeding risk

Adverse effects: *italics* = common; **bold** = life-threatening

Drug classifications
Anthracyclines: increased cardiomyopathy risk
Vaccines/toxoids: decreased immune response

NURSING CONSIDERATIONS

Assessment
• Monitor CBC, HER2 overexpression
• Assess for symptoms of infection; may be masked by product
• Assess CNS reaction: LOC, mental status, dizziness, confusion

> **BLACK BOX WARNING: CHF** and other cardiac symptoms: assess for dyspnea, coughing, gallop; obtain a full cardiac workup including ECG, echocardiogram, multigated angiogram

• Hypersensitivity reactions, anaphylaxis

> **BLACK BOX WARNING: Potentially fatal infusion reactions:** assess for fever, chills, nausea, vomiting, pain, headache, dizziness, hypotension; discontinue product

Nursing diagnoses
• Infection, risk for (side effects)
• Knowledge, deficient (teaching)
• Nutrition: less than body requirements, imbalanced (side effects)

Patient/family education
• Advise patient to take acetaminophen for fever
• Teach patient to avoid hazardous tasks, since confusion, dizziness may occur
• Teach patient to report signs of infection: sore throat, fever, diarrhea, vomiting
• Inform patient that emotional lability is common; instruct patient to notify prescriber if severe or incapacitating
• Advise patient to use contraception while taking this product, pregnancy **D**; avoid breastfeeding

Evaluation
Positive therapeutic outcome
• Decrease in size of tumors

travoprost ophthalmic
See Appendix B

traZODone (Rx)
(tray′zoe-done)
Oletpro
Func. class.: Antidepressant—miscellaneous
Chem. class.: Triazolopyridine
Pregnancy category C

ACTION: Selectively inhibits serotonin, norepinephrine uptake by brain, potentiates behavioral changes

Therapeutic outcome: Decreased symptoms of depression after 2-3 wk

USES: Depression

CONTRAINDICATIONS:
Hypersensitivity to tricyclics, recovery phase of MI, seizure disorders, prostatic hypertrophy

Precautions: Pregnancy **C**, suicidal patients, severe depression, increased intraocular pressure, closed-angle glaucoma, urinary retention, cardiac/hepatic disease, hyperthyroidism, electroshock therapy, elective surgery, bleeding, abrupt discontinuation, bipolar disorder, breastfeeding, dehydration, hyponatremia, hypovolemia

> **BLACK BOX WARNING:** Suicidal ideation in children/adolescents

DOSAGE AND ROUTES:
Adult: PO 150 mg/day in divided doses; may increase by 50 mg/day q3-4day, max 400 mg/day (outpatient), 600 mg/day (inpatient); EXT REL 150 mg q day in the evening, may increase gradually by 75 mg/day at 3 day intervals, max 375 mg/day
Geriatric: PO 25-50 at bedtime, increase by 25-50 mg q3-7day to desired dose, usual 75-150 mg/day
Child 6-18 yr (unlabeled): PO 1.5-2 mg/kg/day in divided doses, may increase q3-4day up to 6 mg/kg/day or 400 mg/day in divided doses, whichever is less

Available forms: Tabs 50, 100, 150, 300 mg; ext rel tabs 150, 300 mg

Implementation
• Give with food or milk for GI symptoms; crush if patient is unable to swallow medication whole
• Give dose at bedtime if oversedation occurs during day; may take entire dose at bedtime; geriatric may not tolerate once/day dosing
• Store at room temperature; do not freeze

ADVERSE EFFECTS

CNS: *Dizziness, drowsiness,* confusion, headache, anxiety, tremors, stimulation, weakness, insomnia, nightmares, EPS (geriatric), increase in psychiatric symptoms, **suicide in children/adolescents**

CV: *Orthostatic hypotension, ECG changes, tachycardia,* **hypertension,** palpitations

EENT: *Blurred vision,* tinnitus, mydriasis

GI: *Diarrhea, dry mouth,* nausea, vomiting, **paralytic ileus,** increased appetite, cramps, epigastric distress, jaundice, **hepatitis,** stomatitis, constipation

GU: *Retention,* **acute renal failure, priapism**

HEMA: Agranulocytosis, thrombocytopenia, eosinophilia, leukopenia

INTEG: Rash, urticaria, sweating, pruritus, photosensitivity

Pharmacokinetics

Absorption	Well absorbed
Distribution	Widely distributed
Metabolism	Liver, extensively
Excretion	Kidneys, minimally unchanged
Half-life	$4^{1}/_{2}$-$7^{1}/_{2}$ hr

Pharmacodynamics

Onset	Unknown
Peak	1 hr without food, 2 hr with food
Duration	Unknown

INTERACTIONS

Individual drugs

Alcohol, carBAMazepine, digoxin, phenytoin: increased effect of each product

FLUoxetine, nefazodone: increased levels, increased toxicity, serotonin syndrome

Guanethidine, cloNIDine: decreased effects of each product

Warfarin: increased or decreased effects of warfarin

Drug classifications

Barbiturates, benzodiazepines, CNS depressants: increased effects

CYP3A4, 2D6 inhibitors (phenothiazenes, protease inhibitors, azole antifungals): increased effects of trazodone

MAOIs: increased hyperpyretic crisis, seizures, hypertensive episode, do not use within 14 days

SNRIs, SSRIs: increased toxicity, serotonin syndrome

Sympathomimetics (direct-acting): increased sympathomimetic effects

Sympathomimetics (indirect-acting): decreased effects

Drug/herb

Hops, kava, lavender, valerian: increased CNS depression

SAM-e, St. John's wort: increased serotonin syndrome

Drug/lab test

Increased: serum bilirubin, blood glucose, alkaline phosphatase

Decreased: VMA, 5-HIAA

False increase: urinary catecholamines

NURSING CONSIDERATIONS

Assessment

• **Pain:** assess for location, duration, intensity before, 1-2 hr after medication

• Monitor B/P (lying, standing), pulse q4hr; if systolic B/P drops 20 mm Hg hold product, notify prescriber; take vital signs q4hr in patients with CV disease

• Monitor blood tests: CBC, leukocytes, differential, cardiac enzymes if patient is receiving long-term therapy

• Monitor liver function tests: AST, ALT, bilirubin

• Check weight qwk; appetite may increase with product

• Assess ECG for flattening of T wave, bundle branch block, AV block, dysrhythmias in cardiac patients

• Assess for EPS primarily in geriatric: rigidity, dystonia, akathisia

> **BLACK BOX WARNING:** Assess mental status: mood, sensorium, affect, suicidal tendencies in children/adolescents; increase in psychiatric symptoms: depression, panic

• Monitor urinary retention, constipation; constipation is more likely to occur in children or geriatric

• **Withdrawal symptoms:** assess for headache, nausea, vomiting, muscle pain, weakness; do not usually occur unless product was discontinued abruptly

• Identify alcohol consumption; if alcohol is consumed, hold dose until AM

• **Serotonin syndrome, neuroleptic malignant syndrome:** assess for increased heart rate, shivering, sweating, dilated pupils, tremors, high B/P, hyperthermia, headache, confusion; if these occur, stop product, administer a serotonin antagonist if needed

T

Nursing diagnoses
• Coping, ineffective (uses)
• Injury, risk for (adverse reactions)
• Knowledge, deficient (teaching)
• Noncompliance (teaching)

Patient/family education
• Teach patient that therapeutic effects may take 2-3 wk
• Teach patient to use caution in driving or other activities requiring alertness because of drowsiness, dizziness, blurred vision; to avoid rising quickly from sitting to standing, especially geriatric
• Caution patient to avoid alcohol ingestion, other CNS depressants
• Teach patient not to discontinue medication quickly after long-term use: may cause nausea, headache, malaise
• Advise patient to wear sunscreen or large hat because photosensitivity occurs
• Teach patient to increase fluids, bulk in diet if constipation, urinary retention occur, especially geriatric
• Advise patient to take gum, hard sugarless candy, or frequent sips of water for dry mouth

BLACK BOX WARNING: Teach family to watch for suicidal ideation or tendencies, usually in children/adolescents

Evaluation
Positive therapeutic outcome
• Decrease in depression
• Absence of suicidal thoughts

TREATMENT OF OVERDOSE:
ECG monitoring, induce emesis, lavage, activated charcoal, administer anticonvulsant

treprostinil (Rx)
(treh-prah'stin-ill)
Remodulin, Tyvaso
Func. class.: Antiplatelet agent
Chem. class.: Tricyclic benzidine prostacyclin analog
Pregnancy category B

ACTION: Direct vasodilatation of pulmonary, systemic arterial vascular beds, inhibition of platelet aggregation

Therapeutic outcome: Decreased pulmonary arterial hypertension (PAH)

USES: PAH, NYHA class II through IV

CONTRAINDICATIONS:
Hypersensitivity to this product or other prostacyclin analogs

Precautions: Pregnancy **B**, breastfeeding, children, geriatric, past hepatic disease, renal/thromboembolic disease, abrupt discontinuation, **IV** administration

DOSAGE AND ROUTES
Adult: SUBCUT INF 1.25 ng/kg/min by cont INF, may reduce to 0.625 ng if not tolerated; may increase by 1.25 ng/kg/min qwk for first 4 wk, then 2.5 ng/kg/min qwk for remainder of INF; oral INH 3 breaths via Tyvaso INH system qid

Hepatic dose
Adult: SUBCUT INF 0.625 ng/kg ideal body weight/min and increase cautiously

Available forms: Inj 1, 2.5, 5, 10 mg/ml; neb sol 1.74 mg/2.9 ml

Implementation
SUBCUT INF route
• By continuous subcut infusion
• No dilution required

CONT IV INF route
• By surgically placed CV catheter using an ambulatory inf pump
• The IV pump, product, and patient education can be obtained from Priority Healthcare in the United States
• Must be diluted with sterile water for inj or 0.9% NaCl
• Calculate the concentration using this formula: diluted conc = [dose (ng/kg/min) × weight (kg) × 0.00006]/inf rate (ml/hr)
• Sudden decreased doses or abrupt withdrawal may worsen pulmonary atrial hypertension symptoms

Oral inhalation route
• Avoid skin or eyes, do not take orally; use Tyvaso Inhalation System only
• Patient should have a backup Optineb-ir device to avoid interruptions
• Follow instructions for use and cleaning
• Do not mix with other medications in Optineb-ir device
• Twist off cap and squeeze total contents into medicine cup, volume is sufficient for 4 treatments

ADVERSE EFFECTS
CNS: Dizziness, headache
CV: Vasodilatation, hypotension, edema
GI: Nausea, *diarrhea*
INTEG: *Rash,* pruritus

⚠ Nurse Alert

OTHER: Jaw pain
SYST: Infusion site reactions, inf site pain, increased risk of infection

Pharmacokinetics

Absorption	Unknown
Distribution	Unknown
Metabolism	Liver, 90% protein binding
Excretion	Urine, feces
Half-life	2-4 hr, terminal

Pharmacodynamics

Unknown

INTERACTIONS

Individual drug
Aspirin: increased risk of bleeding

Drug classifications
Anticoagulants, NSAIDs, SSRIs, thrombin inhibitors: increased risk of bleeding
Antihypertensives, β-blockers, calcium channel blockers, diuretics, MAOIs, vasodilators: increased hypotension

NURSING CONSIDERATIONS

Assessment
• Monitor liver function tests: AST, ALT, bilirubin, creatinine (long-term therapy)
⚠ Monitor blood tests: CBC; CBC q2wk × 3 mo, Hct, Hgb, pro-time (long-term therapy)
⚠ Monitor bleed time baseline and throughout; levels may be 2-5 × normal limit

Nursing diagnoses
• Knowledge, deficient (teaching)
Patient/family education
• Teach patient that blood work will be necessary during treatment
• Teach patient to report side effects such as diarrhea, skin rashes
• Teach patient that therapy will be needed for prolonged periods of time, sometimes years
• Advise patient that aseptic technique must be used in preparing and administering to prevent infection
• Teach that there are many drug and herb interactions
• Teach signs/symptoms of bleeding: blood in urine, stools

Evaluation
Positive therapeutic outcome
• Decreased pulmonary arterial hypertension

tretinoin (vitamin A acid, retinoic acid) (Rx)

(tret′i-noyn)
Avita, Renova, Retin-A, Retin-A Micro, Stieva-A ✽
Func. class.: Vitamin A acid/acne product, antineoplastic—miscellaneous
Chem. class.: Tretinoin derivative
Pregnancy category C (TOPICAL), D (PO)

ACTION: (Topical) Decreases cohesiveness of follicular epithelium, decreases microcomedone formation; (PO) induces maturation of acute promyelocytic leukemia, exact action is unknown

Therapeutic outcome: Decreased signs/symptoms of leukemia

USES: (Topical) Acne vulgaris (grades 1-3); (PO) acute promyolocytic leukemia, facial wrinkles, photoaging

Unlabeled uses: Acne rosacea, actinic keratosis, ichthyosis, Kaposi's sarcoma, keloids, keratosis follicularis, melasma

CONTRAINDICATIONS:
Hypersensitivity to retinoids or sensitivity to parabens

BLACK BOX WARNING: Pregnancy **D** (PO)

Precautions: Pregnancy **C** (topical), breastfeeding, eczema, sunburn, sun exposure

BLACK BOX WARNING: Rapid-evolving leukocytosis, respiratory compromise, acute promyelocytic leukemia differentiation syndrome

DOSAGE AND ROUTES
Adult and child: TOP cleanse area, apply 0.025%-0.1% cream or 0.05% liquid at bedtime; cover lightly

Promyelocytic leukemia
Adult: PO 45 mg/m²/day given as 2 evenly divided doses until remission; discontinue treatment 30 days after remission or after 90 days of treatment, whichever is first

Available forms: Topical cream 0.01%, 0.02%, 0.025%, 0.05%, 0.1%; topical gel 0.025%, 0.04%, 0.05%, 0.1%; topical liquid 0.05%; caps 10 mg

T

Adverse effects: *italics* = common; **bold** = life-threatening

Implementation
Topical route
• Apply using gloves or cotton, once daily before bedtime; cover area lightly using gauze
• Store at room temperature
• Wash hands after application
• Apply only to affected areas

ADVERSE EFFECTS

PO route
CNS: Headache, fever, sweating, fatigue
CV: Cardiac dysrhythmias, pericardial effusion
GI: Nausea, vomiting, **hemorrhage,** abdominal pain, diarrhea, constipation, dyspepsia, distention, **hepatitis**
META: Hypercholesterolemia, hypertriglyceridemia
RESP: Pneumonia, upper respiratory tract disease

Topical route
INTEG: Rash, stinging, warmth, redness, erythema, blistering, crusting, peeling, contact dermatitis, hypo/hyperpigmentation, dry skin, pruritus, scaly skin, retinoic acid syndrome (RAS)

Pharmacokinetics	
Absorption	Small amounts
Distribution	Unknown
Metabolism	Unknown
Excretion	Kidneys
Half-life	Unknown

Pharmacodynamics
Unknown

INTERACTIONS

Individual drugs
Aminocaproic acid, aprotinin, tranexamic acid: increased thrombotic complications
Benzoyl peroxide, resorcinol, salicylic acid (topical), sulfur: increased peeling
Ketoconazole: increased plasma concentrations of tretinoin (oral)

Drug classifications
Alcohol, astringents, cleansers with drying effect, medicated, abrasive soaps: use with caution (topical)
Diuretics (thiazide), phenothiazines, quinolones, retinoids, sulfonamides, sulfonylureas: increased photosensitivity
Tetracyclines: increased ICP, risk of pseudotumor cerebri; do not use together

Drug/lab test
Increased: AST, ALT

NURSING CONSIDERATIONS

Assessment
Topical route
• Assess part of body involved, including time involved, what helps or aggravates condition, cysts, dryness, itching; lesions may become worse at beginning of treatment
PO route
• Monitor hepatic function, coagulation, hematologic parameters, also cholesterol, triglycerides

Nursing diagnoses
• Body image, disturbed (uses)
• Knowledge, deficient (teaching)
• Skin integrity, impaired (uses)

Patient/family education
Topical route
• Instruct patient to avoid application on normal skin, to avoid getting cream in eyes, nose, other mucous membranes
• Advise patient to avoid sunlight, sunlamps or to use protective clothing or sunscreen to prevent burns
• Advise patient that treatment may cause warmth, stinging; dryness, peeling will occur
• Inform patient that cosmetics may be used over product; not to use shaving lotions
• Inform patient that rash may occur during first 1-3 wk of therapy
• Caution patient that product does not cure condition, only relieves symptoms; that therapeutic results may be seen in 2-3 wk but may not be optimal until after 6 wk
PO route

> **BLACK BOX WARNING:** Advise patient to report to prescriber if pregnancy is planned or suspected, pregnancy **D** (PO)

Evaluation
Positive therapeutic outcome
• Decrease in size and number of lesions

tretinoin topical
See Appendix B

⚠ Nurse Alert

triamcinolone (Rx)

(trye-am-sin'oh-lone)
**Aristospan, Kenalog-10, Kenalog-40,
Tac-3, Tac-40, Triesence**
Func. class.: Corticosteroid, synthetic;
antiinflammatory
Chem. class.: Glucocorticoid, intermedi-
ate-acting
Pregnancy category C

ACTION: Decreases inflammation by
suppressing migration of polymorphonuclear
leukocytes, fibroblasts, reversal of increased
capillary permeability and lysosomal stabilization

Therapeutic outcome: Decreased
inflammation, normal immune response

USES: Severe inflammation, immunosuppression, neoplasms, asthma (steroid
dependent), collagen, respiratory, dermatologic
disorders, rheumatic disorders

CONTRAINDICATIONS:

Children <2 yr, psychosis, hypersensitivity,
idiopathic thrombocytopenia, acute glomerulonephritis, amebiasis, fungal infections, nonasthmatic bronchial disease, AIDS, TB, adrenal
insufficiency, acute bronchospasm, neonatal
prematurity, epidural/intrathecal administration
(triamcinolone acetonide injections [Kenalog])

Precautions: Pregnancy **C**, breastfeeding,
diabetes mellitus, glaucoma, osteoporosis,
seizure disorders, ulcerative colitis, CHF,
myasthenia gravis, renal disease, esophagitis,
peptic ulcer, acne, cataracts, coagulopathy, head
trauma

DOSAGE AND ROUTES

Adult: PO 4-12 mg/day in divided doses
daily-qid; IM 40 mg qwk (acetonide, diacetate),
5-48 mg into neoplasms (diacetate, acetonide),
2-40 mg into joint or soft tissue (hexacetonide), 0.5 mg/sq in of affected intralesional skin
(hexacetonide), 2-20 mg into joint or soft tissue
(hexacetonide)
Child: PO 117 mcg/kg/day in divided doses

Asthma
Adult: INH 2 tid-qid, max 16 INH/day
Child 6-12 yr: INH 1-2 tid-qid, max 12 INH/day

Severe/incapacitating allergic conditions such as asthma
Adult: IM (Trivaris) 60 mg, titrate; usual range
40-80 mg

Child: IM (Trivaris) 0.11-1.6 mg/kg/day (3.2-
48 mg/m²/day) given in 3-4 divided doses

Available forms: Inj 25, 40 mg/ml diacetate; inj 3, 10, 40 mg/ml acetonide; inj 5, 20
mg/ml hexacetonide; inh 100 mcg/spray

Implementation
PO route
• Give with food or milk to decrease GI symptoms; tablet may be crushed
IM route
• Give IM inj deeply in large muscle mass;
rotate sites; avoid deltoid; use 21-G needle
• Give in one dose in AM to prevent adrenal
suppression; avoid SUBCUT administration, may
damage tissue
Inhalation route
• Use spacer device for geriatric
• Give inh with water to decrease possibility of
fungal infections; titrated dose, use lowest effective dose
• Give after cleaning aerosol top daily with
warm water, dry thoroughly
• Store in cool environment; do not puncture or
incinerate container
Topical route
• Apply only to affected areas; do not get in eyes
• Apply medication, then cover with occlusive
dressing (only if prescribed), seal to normal
skin, change q12hr; systemic absorption may
occur
• Apply only to dermatoses; do not use on
weeping, denuded, or infected areas
• Cleanse skin before applying product
• Continue treatment for a few days after area
has cleared
• Store at room temperature
Nasal route
• Have patient clear nasal passages before
administration; use decongestant if needed;
shake inhaler, invert, tilt head backward, insert
nozzle into nostril, away from septum; hold
other nostril closed and depress activator, inhale
through nose, exhale through mouth

ADVERSE EFFECTS

CNS: *Depression, flushing, sweating,* headache, mood changes
CV: *Hypertension,* **circulatory collapse,
thrombophlebitis, embolism,** tachycardia,
edema
EENT: Fungal infections, increased intraocular
pressure, blurred vision
GI: *Diarrhea, nausea, abdominal distention,* **GI hemorrhage,** *increased appetite,*
pancreatitis
HEMA: Thrombocytopenia

T

INTEG: Acne, poor wound healing, ecchymosis, petechiae

MS: Fractures, osteoporosis, weakness

Pharmacokinetics

Absorption	Well absorbed (PO, IM)
Distribution	Crosses placenta, widely distributed
Metabolism	Liver, extensively
Excretion	Kidney, breast milk
Half-life	2-5 hr, adrenal suppression 3-4 days

INTERACTIONS

Individual drugs

Alcohol, amphotericin B, cycloSPORINE, digoxin, indomethacin: increased side effects

Ambenonium, isoniazid, neostigmine, somatrem: decreased effects of each specific product

Cholestyramine, colestipol, ePHEDrine, phenytoin, rifampin, theophylline: decreased action of triamcinolone

Indomethacin, ketoconazole: increased action of triamcinolone

Drug classifications

Anticholinesterases, anticoagulants, anticonvulsants, antidiabetics, salicylates: decreased effects of each specific product

Antidiabetic agents: increased need for antidiabetic agents

Antiinfectives (macrolide), contraceptives (oral), estrogens, salicylates: increased action of triamcinolone

Barbiturates: decreased action of triamcinolone

Diuretics, salicylates: increased side effects

Toxoids, vaccines: decreased effects of toxoids, vaccines

Drug/herb

Aloe, cascara sagrada, senna: increased hypokalemia

Drug/lab test

Increased: cholesterol, sodium, blood glucose, uric acid, calcium, urine glucose

Decreased: calcium, potassium, T_4, T_3, thyroid ^{131}I uptake test, urine 17-OHCS, 17-KS

False negative: skin allergy tests

NURSING CONSIDERATIONS

Assessment

• Monitor potassium, blood glucose, urine glucose while on long-term therapy; hypokalemia and hyperglycemia

• Monitor weight daily; notify prescriber of weekly gain >5 lb; I&O ratio; be alert for decreasing urinary output and increasing edema

• Monitor B/P q4hr, pulse; notify prescriber if chest pain occurs

• Monitor plasma cortisol levels during long-term therapy (normal level 138-635 nmol/L [SI units] when measured at 8 AM); adrenal function periodically for hypothalamic-pituitary-adrenal axis suppression

• Assess for infection: increased temp, WBC even after withdrawal of medication; product masks infection symptoms

• Assess for potassium depletion: paresthesias, fatigue, nausea, vomiting, depression, polyuria, dysrhythmias, weakness

• Assess mental status: affect, mood, behavioral changes, aggression

• Assess nasal passages during long-term treatment for changes in mucus (nasal)

• Monitor temp; if fever develops, product should be discontinued

• Assess for systemic absorption: increased temp, inflammation, irritation (topical)

Nursing diagnoses

• Infection, risk for (adverse reactions)
• Knowledge, deficient (teaching)
• Noncompliance (teaching)

Patient/family education

• Advise patient that emergency ID as corticosteroid user should be carried/worn

• Instruct patient to notify prescriber if therapeutic response decreases; dosage adjustment may be needed; not to discontinue abruptly; adrenal crisis can result

• Caution patient to avoid OTC products: salicylates, alcohol in cough products, cold preparations unless directed by prescriber

• Advise patient on all aspects of product use including cushingoid symptoms

• Teach patient symptoms of adrenal insufficiency: nausea, anorexia, fatigue, dizziness, dyspnea, weakness, joint pain

Pharmacodynamics

	PO	IM	TOPICAL	INH	INTRANASAL
Onset	Unknown	Unknown	Min to hr	1-2 wk	Unknown
Peak	1-2 hr	1-2 hr	Hr to days	Unknown	2-3 wk
Duration	3 days	Unknown	Hr to days	Unknown	Unknown

⚠ Nurse Alert

• Teach patient that long-term therapy may be needed to clear infection (1-2 mo depending on type of infection)
Inhalation route
• Teach patient proper administration technique; to wash inhaler with warm water and dry after each use
• Teach patient all aspects of product use including cushingoid symptoms
Topical route
• Instruct patient to avoid sunlight on affected area; burns may occur
Nasal route
• Instruct patient to clear nasal passages if sneezing attack occurs, repeat dose
• Advise patient to continue using product even if mild nasal bleeding occurs; is usually transient
• Teach patient method of instillation after providing written instruction from manufacturer

Evaluation
Positive therapeutic outcome
• Decrease in runny nose (nasal)
• Decreased dyspnea, wheezing, dry crackles on auscultation (inh)
• Ease of respirations, decreased inflammation
• Absence of severe itching, patches on skin, flaking (topical)

triamcinolone nasal agent
See Appendix B

triamcinolone ophthalmic
See Appendix B

triamcinolone topical
See Appendix B

triazolam (Rx)
(trye-az'oh-lam)
Apo-Triazo ✤, Gen-Triazolam ✤, Halcion
Func. class.: Sedative-hypnotic, antianxiety
Chem. class.: Benzodiazepine, short acting
Pregnancy category X
Controlled substance schedule IV (USA), targeted (CDSA IV) (Canada)

ACTION: Produces CNS depression at limbic, thalamic, hypothalamic levels of CNS; may be mediated by neurotransmitter; γ-aminobutyric acid (GABA); results are sedation, hypnosis, skeletal muscle relaxation, anticonvulsant activity, anxiolytic action

Therapeutic outcome: Decreased anxiety, insomnia

USES: Insomnia (short-term), sedative/hypnotic

CONTRAINDICATIONS:
Pregnancy **X,** breastfeeding, hypersensitivity to benzodiazepines, intermittent porphyria

Precautions: Children <15 yr, geriatric, anemia, renal/hepatic disease, suicidal individuals, product abuse, psychosis, acute closed-angle glaucoma, seizure disorders, angioedema, respiratory disease, depression, sleep-related behaviors (sleep walking)

DOSAGE AND ROUTES
Adult: PO 0.125-0.5 mg at bedtime, max 0.5 mg/day
Geriatric: PO 0.0625-0.125 mg at bedtime, max 0.25 mg/day

Available forms: Tabs 0.125, 0.25 mg
Implementation
• Give with food or milk to decrease GI symptoms; if patient is unable to swallow medication whole, tab may be crushed and mixed with food or fluid
• Give sugarless gum, hard candy, frequent sips of water for dry mouth

ADVERSE EFFECTS
CNS: *Headache, lethargy, drowsiness, daytime sedation,* dizziness, confusion, lightheadedness, anxiety, irritability, amnesia, poor coordination, complex sleep-related reactions (sleep driving, sleep eating)
CV: Chest pain, pulse changes
GI: Nausea, vomiting, diarrhea, heartburn, abdominal pain, constipation, **hepatic injury**
HEMA: Leukopenia, granulocytopenia (rare)
SYST: Severe allergic reactions

Pharmacokinetics	
Absorption	Well absorbed
Distribution	Widely distributed, crosses placenta, crosses blood-brain barrier
Metabolism	Liver
Excretion	Kidneys, breast milk
Half-life	2-3 hr

Pharmacodynamics

Onset	$^{1}/_{2}$ hr
Peak	Unknown
Duration	6-8 hr

INTERACTIONS

Individual drugs

Alcohol: increased action of both products

Cimetidine, clarithromycin, disulfiram, erythromycin, isoniazid, probenecid: increased effects; do not use concurrently

Rifampin: decreased action of rifampin

Theophylline: decreased effects of theophylline

Drug classifications

Antacids: decreased effects of antacids

Antiinfectives (clarithromycin): increased effects

CNS depressants: increased effects of both products

Contraceptives (oral): increased effects; do not use concurrently

CYP3A4 inhibitors, protease inhibitors: increased triazolam levels

Smoking: decreased hypnotic effects

Drug/herb

Chamomile, hops, kava, lavender, valerian: increased CNS depression

Drug/lab test

Increased: AST, ALT, serum bilirubin

Decreased: radioactive iodine uptake

False increase: 17-OHCS

NURSING CONSIDERATIONS

Assessment

• Assess patient's mental status: mood, sensorium, anxiety, affect, sleeping pattern, drowsiness, dizziness, especially geriatric; physical dependency, withdrawal symptoms: anxiety, panic attacks, agitation, seizures, headache, nausea, vomiting, muscle pain, weakness; suicidal tendencies; for indications of increasing tolerance and abuse

• Monitor patient's B/P (lying, standing), pulse; if systolic B/P drops 20 mm Hg, hold product, notify prescriber

• Monitor blood tests: CBC during long-term therapy; blood dyscrasias have occurred rarely; decreased hematocrit, neutropenia may occur

• Monitor liver function tests: AST, ALT, bilirubin, creatinine LDH, alkaline phosphatase

• Monitor I&O ratio; indicate renal dysfunction

Nursing diagnoses

• Anxiety (uses)

• Injury, risk for (adverse reactions)

• Knowledge, deficient (teaching)

Patient/family education

• Advise patient that product may be taken with food or fluids, and tab may be crushed or swallowed whole

• Caution patient not to use for everyday stress or longer than 3 mo unless directed by prescriber; not to take more than prescribed amount; may be habit forming; not to double doses or skip doses

• Instruct patient to avoid OTC preparations unless approved by prescriber; alcohol and CNS depressants will increase CNS depression

• Caution patient to avoid driving, activities that require alertness because drowsiness may occur; to avoid alcohol ingestion or other psychotropic medications; to rise slowly or fainting may occur, especially geriatric; that drowsiness may worsen at beginning of treatment

• Teach patient to use reliable contraception, pregnancy **X**

• Teach patient that complex sleep-related behaviors (sleep eating/driving) may occur

• Advise patient not to discontinue medication abruptly after long-term use; withdrawal symptoms include vomiting, cramping, tremors, seizures; decrease dosage by 50% q2nights until 0.125 mg for 2 nights, then stop

Evaluation
Positive therapeutic outcome

• Decreased anxiety, restlessness, sleeplessness (short-term treatment only)

TREATMENT OF OVERDOSE:
Lavage, VS, supportive care

---

trifluridine ophthalmic
See Appendix B

trimethobenzamide (Rx)
(trye-meth-oh-ben′za-mide)
Tigan
Func. class.: Antiemetic, anticholinergic
Chem. class.: Ethanolamine derivative
Pregnancy category C

ACTION: Acts centrally by blocking chemoreceptor trigger zone, which in turn acts on vomiting center

Therapeutic outcome: Absence of nausea and vomiting

USES: Nausea, vomiting, prevention of postoperative vomiting

CONTRAINDICATIONS:

Children (parenterally), hypersensitivity to opioids, shock

Precautions: Pregnancy **C**, children, geriatric, cardiac dysrhythmias, acute febrile illness, encephalitis, gastroenteritis, dehydration, electrolyte imbalances, Reye's syndrome

DOSAGE AND ROUTES

Postoperative vomiting
Adult: IM 200 mg followed by a second dose 1 hr later

Nausea/vomiting
Adult: PO 300 mg tid-qid; IM 200 mg tid-qid

Renal dose
Adult: IM CCr 15-30 ml/min give 50% of dose

Available forms: Caps 300 mg; inj 100 mg/ml

Implementation
PO route
• Cap may be swallowed whole or opened and mixed with food or fluids
IM route
• Administer IM inj in large muscle mass; aspirate to avoid **IV** administration
• Patient should remain lying down for 30 min after IM inj

Syringe compatibilities: Glycopyrrolate, HYDROmorphone, midazolam, nalbuphine

ADVERSE EFFECTS

CNS: *Drowsiness,* headache, dizziness, confusion, *vertigo,* EPS, disorientation, **coma, seizures,** depression
CV: Hyper/hypotension, palpitations, **cardiac dysrhythmias**
EENT: Dry mouth, blurred vision, photosensitivity
GI: Nausea, diarrhea, vomiting, difficulty swallowing
INTEG: Rash, urticaria, fever, chills, flushing, hyperpyrexia

Pharmacokinetics

Absorption	Unknown
Distribution	Unknown
Metabolism	Liver, extensively
Excretion	Kidneys
Half-life	Unknown

Pharmacodynamics

	PO	IM	RECT
Onset	20-40 min	15 min	10-40 min
Peak	Unknown	Unknown	Unknown
Duration	3-4 hr	2-3 hr	3-4 hr

INTERACTIONS

Individual drugs
Alcohol: increased effect

Drug classifications
CNS depressants: increased effect

NURSING CONSIDERATIONS

Assessment
• Monitor VS, B/P; check patients with cardiac disease more often
• Assess for signs of toxicity of other products or masking of symptoms of disease: brain tumor, intestinal obstructions
• Observe for drowsiness, dizziness
• Assess for nausea, vomiting before and after treatment

Nursing diagnoses
• Knowledge, deficient (teaching)

Patient/family education
• Teach patient to use good oral hygiene; frequent rinsing of mouth, sugarless gum for dry mouth
• Caution patient to avoid hazardous activities until product response is determined; drowsiness may occur
• Inform patient that orthostatic hypotension occurs often and to rise from sitting or lying position gradually; avoid hot tubs, hot showers, and tub baths because hypotension may occur
• Advise patient to remain lying down after IM inj for at least 30 min
• Inform patient that in hot weather, heat stroke may occur; take extra precautions to stay cool
• Teach patient to avoid OTC preparations (cough, hay fever, cold) unless approved by prescriber, serious product interactions may occur; avoid use with alcohol, CNS depressants, increased drowsiness may occur
• Teach patient about EPS
• Instruct patient to report sore throat, malaise, fever, bleeding, mouth sores; if these occur, CBC should be performed and product discontinued

Evaluation
Positive therapeutic outcome
• Decreased nausea, vomiting

trimethoprim/ sulfamethoxazole (cotrimoxazole) (Rx)

(trye-meth'oh-prim/sul-fa-meth-ox'a-zole [ko-trye-mox'a-zole])

Bacter-Aid DS, Bactrim DS, Novo-Trimel ✦, Nu-Cotrimox ✦, Septra, Septra DS, SMZ/TMP, Sultrex

Func. class.: Antiinfective
Chem. class.: Sulfonamide—miscellaneous

Pregnancy category C

ACTION: Sulfamethoxazole (SMZ) interferes with bacterial biosynthesis of proteins by competitive antagonism of PABA when adequate levels are maintained; trimethoprim (TMP) blocks synthesis of tetrahydrofolic acid; combination blocks two consecutive steps in bacterial synthesis of essential nucleic acids, protein

Therapeutic outcome: Absence of infection, based on C&S

USES: UTI, otitis media, acute and chronic prostatitis, shigellosis, *Pneumocystis jiroveci* pneumonitis, chronic bronchitis, chancroid, traveler's diarrhea

CONTRAINDICATIONS:
Pregnancy at term, breastfeeding, infants <2 mo, hypersensitivity to trimethoprim or sulfonamides, megaloblastic anemia, CCr <15 ml/min, porphyria, hyperkalemia

Precautions: Pregnancy C, infants, geriatric, renal disease, G6PD deficiency, impaired renal/hepatic function, possible folate deficiency, severe allergy, bronchial asthma, UV exposure

DOSAGE AND ROUTES
Based on TMP content

UTI
Adult: PO 160 mg TMP q12hr × 10-14 days
Child: PO 8 mg/kg TMP daily in 2 divided doses q12hr

Otitis media
Child: PO 8 mg/kg TMP daily in 2 divided doses q12hr × 10 days

Chronic bronchitis
Adult: PO 160 mg TMP q12hr × 10-14 days

***Pneumocystis jiroveci* pneumonitis**
Adult and child: PO 15-20 mg/kg TMP daily in 4 divided doses q6hr × 14 days; IV 15-20 mg/ kg/day (based on TMP) in 3-4 divided doses for up to 14 days

Renal dose
Dosage reduction necessary in moderate to severe renal impairment (CCr <30 ml/min)

Available forms: Tabs 80 mg TMP/400 mg SMZ, 160 mg TMP/800 mg SMZ; susp 40 mg/200 mg/5 ml; IV 16 mg/80 mg/ml

Implementation
• Give with full glass of water to maintain adequate hydration; increase fluids to 2 L/day to decrease crystallization in kidneys
• Give medication after C&S; repeat C&S after full course of medication
• Store in airtight, light-resistant container at room temp

Intermittent IV infusion route
• Dilute 5 ml ampule/100-125 ml of D₅W, stable for 6 hr, give over ¹/₂ hr, do not refrigerate

Y-site compatibilities: Acyclovir, aldesleukin, allopurinol, amifostine, atracurium, aztreonam, cefepime, cyclophosphamide, diltiazem, enalaprilat, esmolol, filgrastim, fludarabine, gallium, granisetron, hydromorphone, labetalol, LORazepam, magnesium sulfate, melphalan, meperidine, morphine, pancuronium, perphenazine, piperacillin/tazobactam, sargramostim, tacrolimus, teniposide, thiotepa, vecuronium, zidovudine

Y-site incompatibilities: Alfentanil, amikacin, aminophylline, amphotericin B colloidal, ampicillin, ampicillin/sulbactam, ascorbic acid, atropine, azaTHIOprine, benztropine, bumetanide, buprenorphine, butorphanol, calcium chloride/gluconate, caspofungin, ceFAZolin, cefotaxime, cefoxitin, ceftazidime, cefTRIAXone, chloramphenicol, chlorproMAZINE, cimetidine, clindamycin, codeine, cyanocobalamin, cycloSPORINE, dantrolene, dexamethasone, diazepam, diazoxide, digoxin, diphenhydrAMINE, DOBUTamine, DOPamine, DOXOrubicin, doxycycline, ePHEDrine, EPINEPHrine, epirubicin, epoetin alfa, erythromycin, famotidine, fentaNYL, fluconazole, folic acid, furosemide, ganciclovir, gentamicin, glycopyrrolate, haloperidol, heparin, hydrALAZINE, hydrocortisone, hydrOXYzine, IDArubicin, imipenem/cilastatin, inamrinone, indomethacin, insulin, isoproterenol, ketorolac, lidocaine, mannitol, mechlorethamine, metaraminol, methoxamine, methyldopa, methylPREDNISolone, metoclopramide, metoprolol, metroNIDAZOLE, midazolam, multi-vitamins, nafcillin, nalbuphine, naloxone, nitroglycerin, nitroprusside, norepinephrine, ondansetron, oxacillin, oxytocin, papaverine, penicillin G, pentamidine, pentazocine, PENTobarbital, PHENobarbital, phentolamine, phenylephrine, phenytoin, phytonadione, potassium chloride, procainamide, prochlorperazine, promethazine, propranolol, protamine, quinupristin/dalfo-pristin, ranitidine, sodium bicarbonate, suc-cinylcholine, SUFentanil, thiamine, ticarcillin/clavulanate, tobramycin, tolazoline, trimetaphan, urokinase, vancomycin, verapamil, vinorelbine

ADVERSE EFFECTS

CNS: Headache, insomnia, hallucinations, depression, vertigo, fatigue, anxiety, seizures, product fever, chills, **aseptic meningitis**
CV: Allergic myocarditis
EENT: Tinnitus
GI: *Nausea, vomiting, abdominal pain,* stomatitis, **hepatitis,** glossitis, pancreatitis, diarrhea, **enterocolitis,** anorexia, **pseudomembranous colitis**
GU: Renal failure, toxic nephrosis; increased BUN, creatinine; crystalluria
HEMA: Leukopenia, neutropenia, thrombocytopenia, agranulocytosis, hemolytic anemia, hypoprothrombinemia, Henoch-Schölein purpura, methemoglobinemia, eosinophilia I
INTEG: Rash, dermatitis, urticaria, erythema, photosensitivity, pain, inflammation at injection site, **toxic epidermal necrolysis, erythema multiforme**
RESP: Cough, shortness of breath
SYST: Anaphylaxis, systemic lupus erythematosus, Stevens-Johnson syndrome

Pharmacokinetics

Absorption	Rapid
Distribution	Breast milk, crosses placenta, 68% protein bound
Metabolism	Liver
Excretion	Kidneys
Half-life	8-13 hr

Pharmacodynamics

Onset	Unknown
Peak	1-4 hr
Duration	Unknown

INTERACTIONS

Individual drugs

CycloSPORINE: decreased response
Dofetilide: increased levels of dofetilide
Methenamine: increased crystalluria
Methotrexate: increased bone marrow depression

Phenytoin: decreased hepatic clearance of phenytoin

Drug classifications

Anticoagulants (oral): increased anticoagulant effect
CYP2C9, CYP3A4 inducers: decreased hepatic clearance
Diuretics (potassium-sparing), potassium supplements: increased potassium levels
Diuretics (thiazide): increased thrombocytopenia
Sulfonylureas: increased hypoglycemic response

Drug/lab test

Increased: alkaline phosphatase, creatinine, bilirubin, AST, ALT

NURSING CONSIDERATIONS

Assessment

• Monitor I&O ratio; note color, character, pH of urine if product administered for UTI; output should be 800 ml less than intake; if urine is highly acidic, alkalization may be needed
• Monitor renal function tests: BUN, creatinine, urinalysis (long-term therapy)
• Assess type of infection; obtain C&S before starting therapy
• Assess blood dyscrasias, skin rash, fever, sore throat, bruising, bleeding, fatigue, joint pain
• Assess allergic reaction: rash, dermatitis, urticaria, pruritus, dyspnea, bronchospasm, AIDS patients are more susceptible

Nursing diagnoses

• Infection, risk for (uses)
• Knowledge, deficient (teaching)
• Noncompliance (teaching)

Patient family education

• Teach patient to take each oral dose with full glass of water to prevent crystalluria; drink 8-10 glasses of water/day
• Teach patient to complete full course of treatment to prevent superinfection
• Teach patient to avoid sunlight or use sunscreen to prevent burns
• Teach patient to avoid OTC medications (aspirin, vit C) unless directed by prescriber
• If diabetic, teach patient to use Clinistix or Tes-Tape
• Teach patient to use alternative contraceptive measures; decreased effectiveness of oral contraceptives may result
• Teach patient to notify prescriber if skin rash, sore throat, fever, mouth sores, unusual bruising, bleeding occur

T

Evaluation
Positive therapeutic outcome
• Absence of pain, fever, C&S negative

triptorelin (Rx)
(trip-toe'rel-in)
Trelstar, Trelstar Depot, Trelstar LA
Func. class.: Gonadotropin-releasing hormone antagonist
Chem. class.: Synthetic decapeptide analog of LHRH
Pregnancy category X

ACTION: Inhibitor of pituitary gonadotropin secretion; initially increases LH and FSH, with increases in testosterone, reduction in sex steroid levels

Therapeutic outcome: Decreased signs/symptoms of advanced prostate cancer

USES: Advanced prostate cancer

CONTRAINDICATIONS:
Pregnancy **X**, breastfeeding, hypersensitivity to this product or other LHRH agonists or LHRH

Precautions: Metastatic vertebral lesions, urinary tract obstruction, spinal cord compression, renal disease

DOSAGE AND ROUTES
Adult: IM 3.75 mg q4wk; 11.25 mg q12wk, 22.5 mg q24wk

Available forms: Microgranules, depot inj 3.75 mg, 11.25 mg

Implementation
• Give IM using implant, inserted by qualified person
• Use syringe with 20-G needle, withdraw 2 ml of sterile water for inj, inject into vial, shake well, withdraw vial contents, inject immediately

ADVERSE EFFECTS
CNS: Headache, insomnia, dizziness, lability, fatigue
CV: *Hypertension,* peripheral edema
ENDO: Gynecomastia, breast tenderness, hot flashes
GI: Nausea, vomiting, diarrhea
GU: Impotence, urinary retention, UTI
INTEG: Rash, pain on injection, pruritus, hypersensitivity
MISC: Anaphylaxis, angioedema
MS: Osteoneuralgia

Pharmacokinetics

Absorption	Unknown
Distribution	Unknown
Metabolism	CYP450
Excretion	Liver, kidneys
Half-life	3 hr

Pharmacodynamics

Unknown

INTERACTIONS
Drug/lab test
Increased: alk phos, estradiol, FSH, LH, testosterone levels
Decreased: testosterone levels, progesterone

NURSING CONSIDERATIONS
Assessment
• **Assess for severe hypersensitivity:** discontinue product and give antihistamines, have emergency equipment nearby
• Monitor I&O ratios; palpate bladder for distention in urinary obstruction
• Monitor for relief of bone pain (back pain)
• Assess levels of testosterone and PSA

Nursing diagnoses
• Diarrhea (adverse reactions)
• Knowledge, deficient (teaching)

Patient/family education
• Teach patient that gynecomastia may occur but will decrease after treatment is discontinued
• Advise patient to report allergic reaction immediately
• Teach patient that disease flare may occur at beginning of therapy

Evaluation
Positive therapeutic outcome
• More normal levels of PSA, acid phosphatase, alkaline phosphatase, testosterone level of <25 ng/dl, tumor response

tropicamide ophthalmic
See Appendix B

trospium (Rx)

(trose'pee-um)

Sanctura, Sanctura XR

Func. class.: Anticholinergic, overactive bladder product

Chem. class.: Muscarinic receptor antagonist

Pregnancy category C

ACTION: Relaxes smooth muscles in bladder by inhibiting acetylcholine effect on muscarinic receptors

Therapeutic outcome: Absence of bladder distention, nocturia, frequency, urgency, incontinence

USES: Overactive bladder (urinary frequency, urgency)

CONTRAINDICATIONS:

Hypersensitivity, uncontrolled closed-angle glaucoma, urinary retention, gastric retention, myasthenia gravis

Precautions: Pregnancy **C**, breastfeeding, children, renal/hepatic disease, controlled closed-angle glaucoma, ulcerative colitis, intestinal atony, bladder outflow obstruction

DOSAGE AND ROUTES

Adult: PO 20 mg bid, give 5 ml ≥1 hr prior to meals or on empty stomach ER 60 mg qAM

Renal dose

Adult: PO CCr < 30 ml/min 20 mg/day at bedtime

Geriatric ≥75 yr: PO titrate down to 20 mg/day based on response and tolerance

Available forms: Tabs 20 mg caps ER 60 mg

Implementation

• Take 1 hr before meals or on empty stomach

ADVERSE EFFECTS

CNS: Fatigue, dizziness, headache

CV: Tachycardia

EENT: Dry eyes, vision abnormalities

GI: Flatulence, abdominal pain, *constipation,* *dry mouth,* dyspepsia

GU: Urinary retention, UTI

INTEG: Dry skin, **angioedema**

MISC: **Heat stroke,** fever

Pharmacokinetics

Absorption	Rapidly absorbed (10%)
Distribution	Protein bound (50%-85%)
Metabolism	Not fully understood in humans; extensively metabolized
Excretion	Urine (6%), feces (85%); excreted in urine by active tubular secretion
Half-life	Unknown

Pharmacodynamics

Unknown

INTERACTIONS

Individual drugs

Alcohol: increased drowsiness

Metformin, procainamide, quiNIDine, ranitidine, tenofovir, triamterene, vancomycin: increased or decreased action of trospium

Drug classifications

CNS depressants: increased drowsiness

Products excreted by active renal secretion (aMILoride, digoxin, morphine): increased or decreased action of trospium

Drug/food

High-fat meal: decreased absorption

NURSING CONSIDERATIONS

Assessment

• **Assess urinary patterns:** distention, nocturia, frequency, urgency, incontinence

Nursing diagnoses

• Knowledge, deficient (teaching)
• Urinary elimination, impaired (uses)

Patient/family education

• Advise patient to avoid hazardous activities; dizziness may occur
• Caution patient that alcohol may increase drowsiness
• Inform patient about anticholinergic effects that may occur

Evaluation

Positive therapeutic outcome

• Correction of urinary status: absence of dysuria, frequency, nocturia, incontinence

T

ulipristal (Rx)
(ue'li-pris'tal)
Ella
Func. class.: Progesterone agonist/antagonist-abortifacient
Pregnancy category X

ACTION: Binds to the progesterone receptor and prevents progesterone from occupying the receptor, postpones follicular rupture when taken immediately prior to ovulation

Therapeutic outcome: Absence of pregnancy

USES: Emergency contraception

CONTRAINDICATIONS:
Pregnancy **X,** children/infants/neonates, postmenopausal females

Precautions: History of ectopic pregnancy, HIV

DOSAGE AND ROUTES
Adult/adolescent females: PO 30 mg (1 tab) as soon as possible within 120 hr (5 days) of unprotected intercourse or a known or suspected contraceptive failure

Available forms: Tab 30 mg

Implementation
• Administer without regard to food
• Store at room temperature, protect from light

ADVERSE EFFECTS
CNS: Dizziness, headache, fatigue
GI: Nausea, vomiting, abdominal pain
GU: Dysmenorrhea, breakthrough bleeding
INTEG: Acne vulgaris

Pharmacokinetics

Absorption	Unknown
Distribution	Protein binding >94%
Metabolism	Metabolized by CYP3A4
Excretion	Unknown
Half-life	Terminal half-life 27-38 hrs

Pharmacodynamics

Onset	Unknown
Peak	1 hr
Duration	Unknown

INTERACTIONS
Individual drugs
Bosentan, carBAMazepine, felbamate, griseofulvin, OXcarbazepine, phenytoin, rifampin, St. John's wort, topiramate, bexarotene, dexamethasone, etravirine, flutamide, metyrapone, modafinil, nafcillin, nevirapine, pioglitazone, rifabutin, itraconazole, ketoconazole: decreased effect of ulipristal

Aldesleukin, IL-2, amiodarone, atazanavir, basiliximab, chloramphenicol, cimetidine, clarithromycin, dalfopristin, danazol, darunavir, delavirdine, diltiazem, dronedarone, erythromycin, fluconazole, FLUoxetine, fluvoxamine, imatinib, isoniazid, lapatinib, nefazodone, nelfinavir, niCARdipine, octreotide, pantoprazole, quinupristin, ranolazine, saquinavir, tamoxifen, telithromycin, tipranavir, verapamil, voriconazole, zafirlukast: increased ulipristal effect and adverse reactions

Aprepitant, fosaprepitant, efavirenz, fosamprenavir, quiNINE, ritonavir: increased or decreased ulipristal effect

Drug classifications
Regular hormonal contraceptive methods: decreased contraceptive action
CYP3A4 inducers, barbiturates: decreased effect of ulipristal
CYP3A4 inhibitors: increased ulipristal effect and adverse reactions

Drug/herb
St. John's wort: decreased effect of ulipristal

NURSING CONSIDERATIONS
Assessment
• **Assess need for emergency contraception,** pregnancy planned or suspected, obtain pregnancy test before use (pregnancy **X**)
• Assess medications taken, many drug interactions may occur

Nursing diagnoses
• Noncompliance (teaching)

Patient/family education
• Instruct patient that if vomiting occurs within 3 hours of taking the tablet, consider repeating the dose
• Advise patient to report to provider any side effects
• Explain reason for medication and expected results
• Advise patient to avoid use in breastfeeding

Evaluation
Positive therapeutic outcome
• Absence of pregnancy

undecylenic acid topical
See Appendix B

unoprostone ophthalmic
See Appendix B

⚠ HIGH ALERT

urokinase (Rx)
(yoor-oh-kin'ase)
Kinlytic
Func. class.: Thrombolytic
Chem. class.: β-Hemolytic *Streptococcus* filtrate (purified)
Pregnancy category B

ACTION: Promotes thrombolysis by directly converting plasminogen to plasmin

Therapeutic outcome: Lysis of emboli, or thrombosis in various parts of the body

USES: Pulmonary embolism

CONTRAINDICATIONS:
Hypersensitivity to this product or other thrombolytic enzymes, internal active bleeding, intraspinal surgery, neoplasms of CNS, ulcerative colitis/enteritis, severe uncontrolled hypertension, renal/ hepatic disease, hypocoagulation, COPD, subacute bacterial endocarditis, rheumatic valvular disease, cerebral embolism/ thrombosis/hemorrhage, intraarterial diagnostic procedure or surgery (10 days), recent major surgery/trauma, aneurysm, AV malformation

Precautions: Pregnancy **B,** arterial emboli from left side of heart, hepatic disease

DOSAGE AND ROUTES
Lysis of pulmonary emboli
Adult: IV 4400 international units/kg/hr over 10 min (90 ml/hr); CONT IV INF 4400 international units/kg/hr × 12 hr (15 ml/hr); flush line at end of INF

Acute MI
Adult: Intracoronary administration instill 6000 international units/min into occluded artery for 1-2 hr after giving **IV** BOL of heparin 2500-10,000 units; may also give as **IV** INF of 2-3 million units over 45-90 min

Venous catheter occlusion (unlabeled)
Adult and child: Instill 5000 international units into line, wait 5 min, then aspirate; repeat aspiration attempts q5min × $1/2$ hr; if occlusion has not been removed, then cap line and wait $1/2$-1 hr, then aspirate; may need 2nd dose if still occluded

Available forms: Powder for inj, lyophilized: 250,000 international units/vial; powder for catheter clearance

Implementation
Intermittent IV route
• Use programmable inf pump, terminal filter (0.45 μm or smaller)
• Reconstitute only with 5 ml sterile water for inj (not bacteriostatic water)/ 250,000 international units urokinase (Kinlytic), and roll (not shake) to enhance reconstitution; further dilute with 190 ml; give as intermittent inf or give to clear cannula by using 1 ml of diluted product; inject into cannula slowly, clamp 5 min, aspirate clot; avoid excessive pressure when urokinase is injected into catheter; force could rupture catheter or expel clot into circulation
• Give as soon as thrombi identified; not useful for thrombi >1 wk old
• Cryoprecipitate or fresh frozen plasma if bleeding occurs
• Loading dose at beginning of therapy; may require increased loading doses
• Heparin therapy after thrombolyic therapy is discontinued, TT or aPTT <2× control (-3-4 hr)

Y-site compatibilities: Alfentanil, amikacin, aminophylline, ascorbic acid, atracurium, atropine, aztreonam, benztropine, bumetanide, buprenorphine, butorphanol, calcium chloride/ gluconate, ceFAZolin, cefoperazone, cefotaxime, cefotetan, cefoxitin, ceftazidime, cefuroxime, chloramphenicol, cimetidine, clindamycin, cyanocobalamin, cycloSPORINE, dexamethasone, digoxin, diphenhydrAMINE, DOBUTamine, DOPamine, doxycycline, enalaprilat, ePHEDrine, EPINEPHrine, epoetin, erythromycin, esmolol, famotidine, fentaNYL, fluconazole, folic acid, furosemide, gentamicin, glycopyrrolate, heparin, hydrocortisone, imipenem/cilastatin, insulin, isoproterenol, ketorolac, labetalol, lidocaine, magnesium sulfate, mannitol, meperidine, metaraminol, methoxamine, methyldopate, metoclopramide, metoprolol, midazolam, morphine, multivitamins, nafcillin, nalbuphine, naloxone, nitroglycerin, nitroprusside, norepinephrine, ondansetron, oxytocin, papaverine, penicillin

U

Adverse effects: *italics* = common; **bold** = life-threatening

G, pentamidine, pentazocine, PENTobarbital, PHENobarbital, phenylephrine, phytonadione, potassium chloride, procainamide, propranolol, protamine, pyridoxime, ranitidine, sodium bicarbonate, streptokinase, succinylcholine, SUFentanil, theophylline, thiamine, ticarcillin/clavulanate, tobramycin, tolazoline, trimetaphan, vasopressin, verapamil

Y-site incompatibilities: Amphotericin B colloidal, dantrolene, diazepam, diazoxide, hydralazine, inamrinone, phenytoin, prochlorperazine, promethazine, trimethoprim/sulfamethoxazole, vasopressin

ADVERSE EFFECTS
CNS: *Headache,* fever
CV: Hypotension, dysrhythmias
GI: *Nausea,* vomiting
HEMA: *Decreased Hct,* **bleeding**
INTEG: *Rash, urticaria,* phlebitis at **IV** inf site, itching, flushing
MS: Low back pain
RESP: Altered respirations, cyanosis, shortness of breath, **bronchospasm**
SYST: **GI, GU, intracranial, retroperitoneal bleeding;** surface bleeding; **anaphylaxis** (rare)

Pharmacokinetics
Absorption	Completely
Distribution	Unknown
Metabolism	Liver
Excretion	Kidneys
Half-life	10-20 min

Pharmacodynamics
Onset	Rapid
Peak	Rapid
Duration	12 hr

INTERACTIONS
Individual drugs
Abciximab, aspirin, clopidogrel, dipyridamole, eptifibatide, heparin, indomethacin, phenylbutazone, plicamycin, ticlopidine, tirofiban, valproic acid: increased bleeding potential

Drug classifications
Anticoagulants (oral), cephalosporins (some), NSAIDs: increased bleeding potential
Glycoprotein IIb, IIIa inhibitors: increased bleeding risk

Drug/lab test
Increased: pro-time, APTT, TT

NURSING CONSIDERATIONS
Assessment
• Monitor VS, B/P, pulse, respirations (including peripheral), neurologic signs, temp at least q4hr; temp >104° F (40° C) indicates internal bleeding; monitor rhythm closely; ventricular dysrhythmias may occur with hyperfusion; monitor heart, breath sounds, neurologic status, peripheral pulses
• **Assess for bleeding** during 1st hr of treatment: hematuria, hematemesis, bleeding from mucous membranes, epistaxis, ecchymosis; guaiac, all body fluids, stools; blood studies (Hct, platelets, PTT, pro-time, TT, aPTT) before starting therapy (pro-time or aPTT must be less than 2 × control); TT or pro-time q3-4hr during treatment
• **Assess hypersensitivity:** fever, rash, itching, chills, facial swelling, dyspnea; mild reaction may be treated with antihistamines; notify prescriber of severe reactions, stop product, keep resuscitative equipment nearby
• Monitor ECG on monitor, watch for segment changes, changes in rhythm; sinus bradycardia, ventricular tachycardia, accelerated idioventricular rhythm may occur because of reperfusion

Nursing diagnoses
• Gas exchange, impaired (uses)
• Injury, risk for (adverse reactions)
Patient/family education
• Teach patient reason for medication, signs and symptoms of bleeding, allergic reactions, when to notify health care prescriber

Evaluation
Positive therapeutic outcome
• Lysis of thrombi or emboli

---

valacyclovir (Rx)
(val-a-sye′kloh-vir)
Valtrex
Func. class.: Antiviral
Chem. class.: Acyclic purine nucleoside analog
Pregnancy category B

Do not confuse:
valacyclovir/valganciclovir, **Valtrex**/Valcyte

ACTION: Interferes with DNA synthesis by conversion to acyclovir, causing decreased viral replication, time of lesional healing

---

Therapeutic outcome: Absence of itching, painful lesions; crusting and healing of lesions

USES: Treatment or suppression of herpes zoster (shingles), recurrent genital herpes, herpes labialis (cold sores), varicella, varicella-zoster

Unlabeled uses: Prevention of CMV infection in advanced HIV, posttransplant patients, Bell's palsy, herpes simplex virus prophylaxis

CONTRAINDICATIONS:
Hypersensitivity to this product, acyclovir, valganciclovir

Precautions: Pregnancy **B**, breastfeeding, geriatric, renal/hepatic disease, electrolyte imbalance, dehydration, hypersensitivity to penciclovir, famciclovir, ganciclovir, varicella

DOSAGE AND ROUTES
Genital herpes (suppressive initial)
Adult: PO 1 g bid × 10 days initially

Genital herpes (recurrent episodes)
Adult: PO 500 mg bid × 3 days

Genital herpes (suppressive therapy)
Adult: PO 1 g/day with normal immune function; 500 mg/day for those with ≤9 recurrences/yr; 500 mg bid in HIV-infected patients with CD4 ≥100

Reduction of transmission
Adult: PO 500 mg/day for source partner

Herpes zoster
Adult: PO 1 g tid × 1 wk

Herpes labialis
Adult: PO 2 g bid × 1 day at first sign of lesions

Varicella (chickenpox) in immunocompetent patients
Adolescent and child ≥2 yr: PO 20 mg/kg/dose tid × 5 days, max 3 g/day; start at first sign, preferably within 24 hr of rash

Renal dose
Adult: PO CCr 30-49 ml/min 1g q12hr (herpes zoster); 1 g q12hr × 1 day (herpes labialis); CCr 10-29 ml/min 1 g q24hr (genital herpes/herpes zoster); 500 mg q24hr (recurrent genital herpes); CCr <10 ml/min 500 mg q24hr (genital herpes/herpes zoster), 500 mg q24hr (recurrent genital herpes)

Available forms: Tabs 500, 1000 mg

Implementation
• Give within 72 hr of outbreak (herpes zoster); as soon as possible (herpes labialis, genital herpes)
• Give orally before infection occurs

ADVERSE EFFECTS
CNS: Tremors, lethargy, *dizziness, headache, weakness,* depression
ENDO: *Dysmenorrhea*
GI: *Nausea, vomiting, diarrhea, abdominal pain, constipation,* increased AST
HEMA: Thrombocytopenic purpura, hemolytic uremic syndrome
INTEG: *Rash*

Pharmacokinetics

Absorption	Unknown
Distribution	Crosses placenta, enters breast milk, protein binding 13.5%-17.9%
Metabolism	Converts to acyclovir
Excretion	Urine, as acyclovir
Half-life	2½-3½ hr

Pharmacodynamics
Unknown

INTERACTIONS
Individual drugs
Cimetidine, probenecid: increased blood levels of valacyclovir (only if renal disease is significant)

NURSING CONSIDERATIONS
Assessment
• **Assess for signs of infection;** characteristics of lesions; therapy should be started at first sign of herpes and is most effective within 72 hr of outbreak
• Assess C&S before product therapy; product may be given as soon as culture is performed; repeat C&S after treatment; determine the presence of other STDs
• Assess bowel pattern before, during treatment
• Assess for skin eruptions: rash
• Assess allergies before treatment, reaction of each medication
⚠ Assess for thrombocytopenic purpura, hemolytic uremic syndrome, may be fatal

Nursing diagnoses
• Infection, risk for (uses)

V

Patient/family education

- Advise patient to take as prescribed; if dose is missed, take as soon as remembered up to 2 hr before next dose; do not double dose
- Instruct patient to take product orally before infection occurs; product should be taken when itching or pain occurs, usually before eruptions
- Inform patient that partners need to be told that patient has herpes; they can become infected; condoms must be worn to prevent reinfections
- Tell patient that product does not cure infection, just controls symptoms and does not prevent infection to others

Evaluation
Positive therapeutic outcome

- Absence of itching, painful lesions; crusting and healed lesions

valganciclovir (Rx)
(val-gan-sy'kloh-veer)
Valcyte
Func. class.: Antiviral
Chem. class.: Synthetic nucleoside
Pregnancy category C

Do not confuse:
valganciclovir/valacyclovir, Valcyte/Valtrex

ACTION: Valganciclovir is metabolized to ganciclovir; inhibits replication of human CMV in vivo and in vitro by selectively inhibiting viral DNA synthesis

Therapeutic outcome: Decreased proliferation of virus responsible for CMV retinitis

USES: Cytomegalovirus (CMV) retinitis in immunocompromised persons, including those with AIDS, after indirect ophthalmoscopy confirms diagnosis; prevention of CMV in transplantation; prevention of CMV in patients at risk going through transplant (kidney, heart, pancreas)

CONTRAINDICATIONS:
Breastfeeding, hypersensitivity to ganciclovir or valacyclovir, absolute neutrophil count <500/mm³, platelet count <25,000/mm³, hemodialysis, liver transplant

Precautions: Pregnancy C, children, geriatric, renal function impairment, hypersensitivity to acyclovir, penciclovir, famciclovir

> **BLACK BOX WARNING:** Preexisting cytopenias, secondary malignancy, infertility, anemia

DOSAGE AND ROUTES
Treatment of CMV
Adult: PO induction 900 mg bid × 21 days with food; maintenance 900 mg/day with food

Transplant (CMV prophylaxis)
Adult/adolescent >16 yr: PO 900 mg/day with food starting within 10 days before transplantation until 100 days after transplantation
Infant ≥4 mo/child/adolescent ≤16 yr: PO give within 10 days of heart/kidney transplant; calculate dose as 7 × BSA × CCr and give a single daily dose

Renal dose
CCr ≥60 ml/min same dosage as above; CCr 40-59 ml/min 450 mg bid × 21 days, then 450 mg/day; CCr 25-39 ml/min 450 mg/day × 21 days, then 450 mg q2day; CCr 10-24 ml/min 450 mg q2day, then 450 mg 2 ×/week

Available forms: Tabs 450 mg; powder for oral sol 50 mg/ml

Implementation
PO tab
- Give with food for better absorption, avoid getting on skin, do not break tab
Oral SOL
- Measure 9 ml of purified water in graduated cylinder, shake bottle to loosen powder, add ½ liquid, shake well, add remaining water, shake, remove child-resistant cap and push bottle adapter into neck of bottle, close with cap, give using the dispenser provided

ADVERSE EFFECTS
CNS: *Fever,* chills, **coma**, *confusion,* abnormal thoughts, dizziness, bizarre dreams, *headache,* psychosis, tremors, somnolence, *paresthesia, weakness,* seizures, insomnia
EENT: Retinal detachment in CMV retinitis
GI: *Abnormal liver function tests, nausea, vomiting, anorexia, diarrhea, abdominal pain,* hemorrhage
GU: Hematuria, increased creatinine, BUN
HEMA: Granulocytopenia, thrombocytopenia, irreversible neutropenia, anemia, eosinophilia
INTEG: *Rash,* alopecia, *pruritus,* urticaria, pain at inj site, phlebitis, **Stevens-Johnson syndrome**
MISC: Local and systemic infections and sepsis

Pharmacokinetics

Absorption	Well absorbed from GI tract
Distribution	Plasma protein binding unknown; crosses blood-brain barrier, CSF
Metabolism	Rapidly metabolized in intestinal wall and liver to ganciclovir
Excretion	Kidneys (ganciclovir)
Half-life	$3-4^1/_2$ hr

Pharmacodynamics

Onset	Unknown
Peak	1-3 hr
Duration	Unknown

INTERACTIONS

Individual drugs

Adriamycin, amphotericin B, cycloSPORINE, dapsone, DOXOrubicin, flucytosine, pentamidine, trimethoprim/sulfamethoxazole, vinBLAStine, vinCRIStine: increased toxicity

Didanosine: increased effect

Imipenem/cilastatin: increased seizures

Probenecid: decreased renal clearance of valganciclovir

Radiation, zidovudine: severe granulocytopenia; do not coadminister

Drug classifications

Antineoplastics: severe granulocytopenia; do not coadminister

Nucleoside analogs, other: increased toxicity

Drug/food

Absorption: increased with high-fat meal

NURSING CONSIDERATIONS

Assessment

> **BLACK BOX WARNING:** Assess for leukopenia/neutropenia/thrombocytopenia: WBCs, platelets q2day during 2 ×/day dosing and then qwk

• Assess serum creatinine or CCr ≥ q2wk
• Assess for CMV retinitis by ophthalmoscopy before beginning treatment and q2wk
• Obtain culture for CMV
• **Assess for infection:** sore throat, cough, fever, chills, back pain; notify prescriber

Nursing diagnoses

• Infection, risk for (uses)
• Injury, risk for (uses, adverse reactions)
• Knowledge, deficient (teaching)

Patient/family education

• Inform patient that product does not cure condition, that regular ophthalmologic and blood tests are necessary
• Caution patient that major toxicities may necessitate discontinuing product
• Caution patient to use contraception during treatment and that infertility may occur; men should use barrier contraception for 90 days after treatment
• Instruct patient to take with food
A Instruct patient to report infection: fever, chills, sore throat; blood dyscrasias: bruising, bleeding, petechiae
• Advise patient to avoid crowds, persons with respiratory infections
• Caution patient to use sunscreen to prevent burns

Evaluation
Positive therapeutic outcome
• Decreased symptoms of CMV

TREATMENT OF OVERDOSE:

Maintain adequate hydration; dialysis may help reduce serum concentrations; consider use of hematopoietic growth factors

---

valproate (Rx)
(val-proh'ate)
Depacon
valproic acid (Rx)
Depakene, Stavzor
divalproex sodium (Rx)
Depakote, Depakote ER, Epival ✦
Func. class.: Anticonvulsant, vascular headache suppressant
Chem. class.: Carboxylic acid derivative
Pregnancy category D

ACTION: Increases levels of γ-aminobutyric acid (GABA) in the brain, which decreases seizure activity

Therapeutic outcome: Decreased symptoms of epilepsy, bipolar disorder

USES: Simple (petit mal), complex (petit mal), absence, mixed seizures, manic episode associated with bipolar disorder, prophylaxis of migraine, adjunct in schizophrenia, tardive dyskinesia, aggression in children with ADHD, organic brain syndrome, tonic-clonic (grand mal)/myoclonic seizures

Unlabeled uses: Rectal for seizures (valproic acid)

V

Adverse effects: *italics* = common; **bold** = life-threatening

CONTRAINDICATIONS:
Hypersensitivity, urea cycle disorders

> **BLACK BOX WARNING:** Pregnancy **D**, hepatic disease, pancreatitis

Precautions: Breastfeeding, geriatric

> **BLACK BOX WARNING:** Children <2 yr

DOSAGE AND ROUTES
Epilepsy
Adult and child: PO 10-15 mg/kg/day divided in 2-3 doses, may increase by 5-10 mg/kg/day qwk, max 60 mg/kg/day in 2-3 divided doses; **IV** ≤20 mg/min over 1 hr

Mania (divalproex sodium)
Adult: PO 750 mg/day in divided doses, max 60 mg/kg/day or 3000 mg/day

Mania (valproic acid: Stavzor)
Adult: DEL REL cap 750 mg/day in divided doses

Migraine (divalproex sodium)
Adult: PO 250 mg bid, may increase to 1000 mg/day; or 500 mg (Depakote ER) daily × 7 days, then 1000 mg/day

Available forms: Valproic acid: caps 250 mg; syr 250 mg/5 ml del rel cap (Stavzor) 125 mg; divalproex: del rel tabs 125, 250, 500 mg; ext rel tabs 250, 500 mg; sprinkle caps 125 mg; valproate: inj 100 mg/ml

Implementation
• Swallow tabs and caps whole; do not break, crush, or chew
• Sprinkle cap contents on food
• Give elixir alone; do not dilute with carbonated beverage; do not give syrup to patients on sodium restriction
• Give with food or milk to decrease GI symptoms

ADVERSE EFFECTS
CNS: *Sedation, drowsiness,* dizziness, headache, incoordination, depression, hallucinations, behavioral changes, tremors, aggression, weakness, **coma, suicidal ideation**
EENT: Visual disturbances, taste perversion
GI: *Nausea, vomiting, constipation, diarrhea,* dyspepsia, anorexia, cramps, **hepatic failure, pancreatitis, toxic hepatitis,** stomatitis, weight gain
GU: Enuresis, irregular menses

HEMA: Thrombocytopenia, leukopenia, lymphocytosis, increased pro-time, bruising, epistaxis
INTEG: *Rash,* alopecia, photosensitivity, dry skin

Pharmacokinetics
Absorption	Unknown
Distribution	Breast milk, crosses placenta, widely distributed, protein binding 90%
Metabolism	Liver
Excretion	Kidneys
Half-life	6-16 hr

Pharmacodynamics
Onset	15-30 min
Peak	1-4 hr
Duration	4-6 hr

INTERACTIONS
Individual drugs
Abciximab, cefoperazone, cefotetan, eptifibatide, heparin, tirofiban: increased bleeding risk
Alcohol: increased CNS depression
CarBAMazepine, ethosuximide, lamoTRIgine, LORazepam, rufinamide, zidovudine: increased action and toxicity of these products
CarBAMazepine, lamoTRIgine, rifampin: decreased valproic acid level
Cimetidine: decreased metabolism of valproic acid
Chlorpromazine, erythromycin, felbamate: increased valproic acid level
Phenytoin: increased action of phenytoin

Drug classifications
Antidepressants (tricyclics), barbiturates: increased action
Antihistamines, barbiturates, MAOIs, opioids, sedative/hypnotics: increased CNS depression
Antiplatelets, NSAIDs, thrombolytics: increased bleeding risk
Salicylates: increased toxicity of valproic acid

Drug/lab test
False positive: ketones, urine
Interference: thyroid function tests

NURSING CONSIDERATIONS
Assessment
• Monitor blood tests: Hct, Hgb, RBC, serum folate, ammonia, platelets, pro-time, PTT, vit D if on long-term therapy
• Monitor liver function tests: AST, ALT, bilirubin, creatinine, failure

⚠ Nurse Alert

• Monitor blood levels: therapeutic level 50-100 mcg/ml
• Assess seizure disorder; location, aura, activity, duration; seizure precautions should be in place
⚠ **Assess bipolar disorder: mood, activity, sleeping, eating, behavior; suicidal thoughts/behaviors**
• **Assess migraines:** frequency, intensity
• **Assess respiratory dysfunction:** respiratory depression, character, rate, rhythm; hold product if respirations are <12/min or if pupils are dilated

> **BLACK BOX WARNING:** Assess for pancreatitis, may be fatal

Nursing diagnoses
• Injury, risk for (uses, adverse reactions)
• Knowledge, deficient

Patient/family education
• Teach patient that physical dependency may result from extended use
• Instruct patient to avoid driving, other activities that require alertness
• Advise patient not to discontinue medication quickly after long-term use; seizures may result
• Advise patient to report visual disturbances, rash, diarrhea, light-colored stools, jaundice, protracted vomiting to prescriber
• Advise patient to use contraception while taking this product, pregnancy **D**

Evaluation
Positive therapeutic outcome
• Decreased seizures

---

valsartan (Rx)
(val-zar′tan)
Diovan
Func. class.: Antihypertensive
Chem. class.: Angiotensin II receptor antagonist (type AT₁)
Pregnancy category D

ACTION: Blocks the vasoconstrictor and aldosterone-secreting effects of angiotensin II; selectively blocks the binding of angiotensin II to the AT₁ receptor found in tissues

Therapeutic outcome: Decreased B/P

USES: Hypertension, alone or in combination, in patients >6 yr; CHF, after MI with left ventricular dysfunction/failure in stable patients

CONTRAINDICATIONS:
Hypersensitivity, severe hepatic disease, bilateral renal artery stenosis

> **BLACK BOX WARNING:** Pregnancy **D** 2nd/3rd trimester

Precautions: Breastfeeding, children, geriatric, CHF, hypertrophic cardiomyopathy, aortic/mitral valve stenosis, CAD, angioedema, renal/hepatic disease, hypersensitivity to ACE inhibitors, hyperkalemia, hypovolemia

DOSAGE AND ROUTES
Adult: PO 80 or 160 mg/day alone or in combination with other antihypertensives, may increase to 320 mg CHF
Child/adolescent 6-16 yr: PO 1.3 mg/kg/day, max 40 mg/day

CHF
Adult: PO 40 mg bid, up to 60 mg bid

Post MI
Adult: PO 20 mg bid as early as 12 hr after MI, may be titrated within 7 days to 40 mg bid, then titrate to maintenance of 160 mg bid

Available forms: Tabs 80, 160, 320 mg

Implementation
• Administer without regard to meals

ADVERSE EFFECTS
CNS: *Dizziness, insomnia,* drowsiness, vertigo, headache, fatigue
CV: Angina pectoris, 2nd-degree AV block, **cerebrovascular accident,** hypotension, **MI, dysrhythmias**
EENT: Conjunctivitis
GI: *Diarrhea,* abdominal pain, nausea, **hepatotoxicity**
GU: Impotence, **nephrotoxicity**
HEMA: *Anemia,* neutropenia
META: Hyperkalemia
MISC: Vasculitis
MS: Cramps, myalgia, pain, stiffness
RESP: *Cough*

Pharmacokinetics
Absorption	Well absorbed
Distribution	Bound to plasma proteins
Metabolism	Extensive
Excretion	Feces, urine, breast milk
Half-life	9 hr

Adverse effects: *italics* = common; **bold** =

Pharmacodynamics

Onset	Up to 2 hr
Peak	4-6 hr
Duration	24 hr

INTERACTIONS

Individual drugs
Lithium: increased effects of lithium

Drug classifications
Diuretics (potassium-sparing, potassium supplements, ACE inhibitors): increased hyperkalemia

NSAIDs, salicylates: decreased antihypertensive effects

NURSING CONSIDERATIONS

Assessment
• Assess B/P (lying, sitting, standing), pulse q4hr; note rate, rhythm, quality periodically
• Monitor electrolytes: potassium, sodium, chloride; total CO_2
• Assess for angioedema: facial swelling, shortness of breath
• Obtain baselines in renal, liver function tests before therapy begins
• Assess blood tests: BUN, creatinine, before treatment
• Monitor for edema in feet, legs daily
• Assess for skin turgor, dryness of mucous membranes for hydration status; correct volume depletion before initiating therapy

Nursing diagnoses
• Fluid volume, deficient (side effects)
• Knowledge, deficient (teaching)
• Noncompliance (teaching)

Patient/family education
• Teach patient not to take this product if breastfeeding or pregnant, or have had an allergic reaction to this product
• If a dose is missed, instruct patient to take as soon as possible, unless it is within an hour before next dose
• Advise patient to comply with dosage schedule, even if feeling better
• Teach patient to notify prescriber of fever, swelling of hands or feet, irregular heartbeat, chest pain, persistent cough
Advise patient excessive perspiration, hydration, diarrhea may lead to fall in blood pressure; consult prescriber if these occur
Inform patient that product may cause dizziness, fainting; light-headedness may occur

• Caution patient to rise slowly to sitting or standing position to minimize orthostatic hypotension; how to take B/P

> **BLACK BOX WARNING:** Teach patient not to take this medication if pregnant (D) or breastfeeding

Evaluation
Positive therapeutic outcome
• Decreased B/P

vancomycin
(van-koe-mye'sin)
Vancocin
Func. class.: Antiinfective—miscellaneous
Chem. class.: Tricyclic glycopeptide
Pregnancy category B

ACTION: Inhibits bacterial cell wall synthesis, blocks glycopeptides

Therapeutic outcome: Bactericidal for the following organisms: staphylococci, streptococci, *Corynebacterium, Clostridium*

USES: Resistant staphylococcal infections, pseudomembranous colitis, staphylococcal enterocolitis, group A β-hemolytic streptococci, endocarditis prophylaxis for dental procedures, diphtheroid endocarditis

CONTRAINDICATIONS: Hypersensitivity, previous hearing loss

Precautions: Pregnancy **B**, breastfeeding, neonates, geriatric, renal disease

DOSAGE AND ROUTES

Serious staphylococcal infections
Adult: IV 500 mg (7.5 mg/kg) q6-8hr or 1 g (15 mg/kg) q12hr
Child: IV 40-60 mg/kg/day divided q6-8hr
Neonate: IV 15 mg/kg initially followed by 10 mg/kg q8-24hr

Pseudomembranous/ staphylococcal enterocolitis
Adult: PO 125 mg qid × 10-14 days
Child: PO 40 mg/kg/day divided q6hr × 7-10 days, max 2 g/day

Endocarditis prophylaxis for dental procedure
Adult: IV 1 g over 1 hr; 1 hr before dental procedure

Child: IV 20 mg/kg over 1 hr; 1 hr before procedure

Renal dose
Adult: IV CCr >70 ml/min no dosage adjustment; CCr 50-70 ml/min loading dose of 15 mg/kg, reduce dose to 750 mg-1 g q18-24hr; CCr <49 ml/min initial loading dose of 15 mg/kg, with subsequent dosing based on concentration, may be q24-72hr or longer

Available forms: Pulvules 125, 250 mg; powder for inj IV 500 mg; vials 1, 5, 10 g

Implementation
• Give antihistamine if red man syndrome occurs: decreased B/P, flushing of neck, face
• Give dose based on serum conc
• Give in equal intervals around the clock to maintain blood levels
• Store at room temp for up to 2 wk after reconstitution
• Have adrenaline, suction, tracheostomy set, endotracheal intubation equipment on unit; anaphylaxis may occur
• Provide adequate intake of fluids (2 L) to prevent nephrotoxicity
• Retention enema: Dilute 500 mg/1000 ml NS, q6hr

IT route
• Use preservative-free 0.9% NaCl (2-5 mg/ml final conc), instill into ventricular cerebrospinal fluid

Intermittent IV INF route
• Give after reconstitution with 10 ml of sterile water for inj (500 mg/10 ml); further dilution is needed for IV, 500 mg/100 ml of 0.9% NaCl, D₅W given as intermittent inf over 1 hr; decrease rate of inf if red man syndrome occurs

Continuous IV INF route
• Reconstitute, then may inf 1-2 g in volume to give over 24 hr if intermittent IV route cannot be used

Y-site compatibilities: Acyclovir, allopurinol, amiodarone, amsacrine, atracurium, cyclophosphamide, diltiazem, enalaprilat, esmolol, filgrastim, fluconazole, fludarabine, gallium, granisetron, hydromorphone, insulin (regular), labetalol, LORazepam, magnesium sulfate, melphalan, meperidine, meropenem, midazolam, morphine, ondansetron, paclitaxel, pancuronium, perphenazine, propofol, sodium bicarbonate, tacrolimus, teniposide, theophylline, thiotepa, tolazoline, vecuronium, vinorelbine, warfarin, zidovudine

Additive compatibilities: Amikacin, atracurium, calcium gluconate, cefepime, cimetidine, corticotropin, dimenhyDRINATE, hydrocortisone, meropenem, ofloxacin, potassium chloride, ranitidine, verapamil, vit B/C

ADVERSE EFFECTS
CV: Cardiac arrest, vascular collapse **(rare)**, hypotension
EENT: *Ototoxicity, permanent deafness,* tinnitus, nystagmus
GI: Nausea, pseudomembranous colitis
GU: Nephrotoxicity: increased BUN, creatinine, albumin, fatal uremia
HEMA: Leukopenia, eosinophilia, neutropenia
INTEG: Chills, fever, rash, thrombophlebitis at inj site, urticaria, pruritus, necrosis (red man syndrome), skin/subcutaneous tissue disorders
RESP: Wheezing, dyspnea
SYST: Anaphylaxis, superinfection

Pharmacokinetics

Absorption	Poorly absorbed (PO), completely absorbed (**IV**)
Distribution	Widely distributed, crosses placenta
Metabolism	Liver
Excretion	PO, feces; **IV**, kidneys
Half-life	4-8 hr

Pharmacodynamics

	IV
Onset	Immediate
Peak	Inf end
Duration	Unknown

INTERACTIONS
Individual drugs
Amphotericin B, bacitracin, cidofovir, CISplatin, colistin, polymyxin B: increased ototoxicity or nephrotoxicity

Drug classifications
Aminoglycosides, cephalosporins, nondepolarizing muscle relaxants: increased ototoxicity or nephrotoxicity

NURSING CONSIDERATIONS
Assessment
• **Assess for infection:** WBC, urine, stools, sputum, wound characteristics, throughout treatment
• Monitor I&O ratio; report hematuria, oliguria because nephrotoxicity may occur

Adverse effects: *italics* = common; **bold** = life-threa[...]

V

- Monitor blood tests: WBC; serum levels; peak 1 hr after 1-hr inf 25-40 mg/L; trough before next dose 5-10 mg/L
- Obtain C&S before product therapy; product may be given as soon as culture is performed
- Assess auditory function during, after treatment; hearing loss, ringing, roaring in ears; product should be discontinued
- Monitor B/P during administration; sudden drop may indicate red man syndrome
- Assess for signs of infection
- Assess respiratory status: rate, character, wheezing, tightness in chest
- Identify allergies before treatment, reaction of each medication

Nursing diagnoses
- Infection, risk for (uses)
- Knowledge, deficient (teaching)

Patient/family education
- Teach patient aspects of product therapy: need to complete entire course of medication to ensure organism death (7-10 days); culture may be performed after completed course of medication
- Advise patient to report sore throat, fever, fatigue; could indicate superinfection
- Instruct patient that product must be taken in equal intervals around the clock to maintain blood levels

Evaluation
Positive therapeutic outcome
- Absence of fever, sore throat
- Negative culture after treatment

vardenafil (Rx)
(var-den'a-fil)
Levitra, Staxyn
Func. class.: Impotence agent
Chem. class.: Phosphodiesterase type 5 inhibitor
Pregnancy category B

ACTION: Inhibits phosphodiesterase type 5 (PDE5); enhances erectile function by increasing the amount of cyclic GMP, which causes smooth muscle relaxation and increased blood flow into the corpus cavernosum

Therapeutic outcome: Erection

USES: Treatment of erectile dysfunction

CONTRAINDICATIONS:
Hypersensitivity, coadministration of α-blockers or nitrates, renal failure, congenital or acquired QT prolongation

Precautions: Pregnancy **B**; not indicated for women, children, or newborns; hepatic impairment; retinitis pigmentosa; cardiovascular disease; anatomic penile deformities; sickle cell anemia; leukemia; multiple myeloma; bleeding disorders; active peptic ulceration; renal disease

DOSAGE AND ROUTES
Adult: PO 10 mg, taken 1 hr before sexual activity, dose may be reduced to 5 mg or increased to a max of 20 mg; max dosing frequency is once/day; orally disintegrating tab 10 mg 60 min before sexual activity; do not use with potent CYP3A4 inhibitors
Geriatric >65 yr: PO 5 mg initially, titrate as needed/tolerated

Hepatic dose (Child-Pugh B)
Adult: PO 5 mg, max 10 mg

Concomitant medications
Ritonavir, max 2.5 mg q72hr; for indinavir, ketoconazole 400 mg/day and itraconazole 400 mg/day, max 2.5 mg/day; for ketoconazole 200 mg/day, itraconazole 200 mg/day and erythromycin, max 5 mg/day

Available forms: Tabs 2.5, 5, 10, 20 mg; orally disintegrating tab 10 mg

Implementation
- Take approximately 1 hr before sexual activity; do not use more than once a day
- Orally disintegrating tabs are not interchangeable with film-coated tabs

ADVERSE EFFECTS
CNS: *Headache, flushing, dizziness, insomnia,* **seizures,** transient global amnesia
CV: Hypertension, **MI, CV collapse,** chest pain
EENT: Conjunctivitis, tinnitus, photophobia, diminished vision, glaucoma, hearing loss
GU: Abnormal ejaculation, priapism
MISC: Rash, GERD, GGTP increased, **NAION (nonarteritic ischemic optic neuropathy),** dyspepsia
MS: Myalgia, arthralgia, neck pain
RESP: Rhinitis, sinusitis, dyspnea, pharyngitis, epistaxis

Pharmacokinetics

Absorption	Rapid; reduced absorption with high-fat meal
Distribution	Bioavailability 15%; protein binding 95%
Metabolism	Liver
Excretion	Primarily in feces (91%-95%)
Half-life	4-5 hr

Pharmacodynamics

Onset	20 min
Peak	$\frac{1}{2}$-$1\frac{1}{2}$ hr
Duration	<5 hr

INTERACTIONS

Individual drugs
Alcohol, amLODIPine, metoprolol, NIFEdipine: increased hypotension, do not use concurrently

Cimetidine, erythromycin, itraconazole, ketoconazole: increased levels

Clarithromycin, droperidol, procainamide, quiNIDine: serious dysrhythmias; do not use concurrently

Drug classifications
⚠ **Do not use with nitrates because of unsafe decrease in B/P that could result in heart attack or stroke**

α-Blockers, protease inhibitors: increased hypotension; do not use concurrently

Angiotensin II receptor blockers: increased hypotension; do not use concurrently

Antidysrhythmics class Ia, III, quinolones: serious dysrhythmias; do not use together

Antiretroviral protease inhibitors: increased vardenafil levels

Drug/food
High-fat meal: decreased absorption

Drug/lab test
Increase: CK

NURSING CONSIDERATIONS

Assessment
• Assess for use of organic nitrates that should not be used with this product
• Assess for severe loss of vision while taking this or any similar products; these products should not be used if vision loss has occurred

Nursing diagnoses
• Knowledge, deficient (teaching)
• Sexual dysfunction (uses)

Patient/family education
• Advise that product does not protect against STDs, including HIV
• Teach that product absorption is reduced with a high-fat meal
• Instruct that product should not be used with nitrates in any form
• Inform that product has no effect in the absence of sexual stimulation
• Teach that patient should seek immediate medical attention if erection lasts for more than 4 hr
• Advise to inform physician of all medications being taken
• Teach patient to notify prescriber immediately and stop taking product if vision loss occurs

Evaluation
Positive therapeutic outcome
• Sustainable erection

varenicline (Rx)
(var-e-ni'kleen)
Champix ✹, **Chantix**
Func. class.: Smoking cessation agent
Pregnancy category C

ACTION: Partial agonist for nicotine receptors; partially activates receptors to help curb cravings; occupies receptors to prevent nicotine binding

Therapeutic outcome: Smoking cessation

USES: Smoking deterrent

CONTRAINDICATIONS:
Hypersensitivity, eating disorders

Precautions: Pregnancy C, breastfeeding, children <18 yr, geriatric, renal disease, recent MI, angioedema

BLACK BOX WARNING: Bipolar disorder, depression, schizophrenia, suicidal ideation

DOSAGE AND ROUTES
Adult: PO therapy should begin 1 week prior to smoking stop date (i.e., take product plus tobacco for 7 days); titrate for 1 wk, days 1 through 3, 0.5 mg/day; days 4 through 7, 0.5 mg bid; day 8 through end of treatment 1 mg bid; treatment is 12 wk and may repeat for another 12 wk

Renal dose

Adult: PO CCr ≤50 ml/min, titrate to max 0.5 mg bid

Available forms: Tabs 0.5, 1 mg, Chantix continuing month PAK; Chantix starting month PAK

Implementation

• Do not break, crush, or chew tabs
• Give increased fluids, bulk in diet if constipation occurs
• Give with a full glass of water after eating
• Give sugarless gum, hard candy, or frequent sips of water for dry mouth

ADVERSE EFFECTS

CNS: Headache, agitation, dizziness, insomnia, abnormal dreams, fatigue, malaise, behavior changes, depression, **suicidal ideation, suicide,** amnesia, hallucinations, hostility, mania, psychosis, tremor
CV: **Dysrhythmias,** hypertension, palpitations, **tachycardia,** angina, hypotension, **MI**
EENT: *Blurred vision,* tinnitus
GI: *Nausea, vomiting,* anorexia, *dry mouth,* increased/decreased appetite, *constipation,* flatulence, GERD
GU: Erectile dysfunction, urinary frequency, menstrual irregularities
INTEG: Rash, pruritus, **angioedema, Stevens-Johnson syndrome**
MISC: Weight loss or gain
RESP: Dyspnea, rhinorrhea

Pharmacokinetics

Absorption	Unknown
Distribution	Steady state 4 days
Metabolism	Minimal
Excretion	Urine 92%, unchanged
Half-life	Elimination 24 hr

Pharmacodynamics

Unknown

NURSING CONSIDERATIONS

Assessment

• Assess for renal function in geriatric
• Assess for smoking cessation after 12 wk; if progress has not been made, product may be used for an additional 12 wk
• Assess mental status: mood, sensorium, affect

Nursing diagnoses

• Coping, ineffective (uses)
• Knowledge, deficient (teaching)

Patient/family education

• Teach patient that treatment for smoking cessation lasts 12 wk and another 12 wk may be required
• Teach patient to use caution in driving, other activities requiring alertness; blurred vision may occur
• Advise patient to set a date to quit smoking and initiate treatment 1 wk prior to that date
• Teach patient how to titrate product
• Advise patient not to use with nicotine patches unless directed by prescriber; may increase B/P
• Advise patient to notify prescriber if pregnancy is suspected or planned
• Teach patient common side effects to be expected

Evaluation
Positive therapeutic outcome

• Smoking cessation

---

vasopressin (Rx)
(vay-soe-press'in)
Pitressin, Pressyn ✦
Func. class.: Pituitary hormone
Chem. class.: Lysine vasopressin
Pregnancy category C

ACTION: Promotes reabsorption of water by action on renal tubular epithelium; causes vasoconstriction on muscles in the GI system

Therapeutic outcome: Increased osmolality, decreased urine output in diabetes insipidus

USES: Diabetes insipidus (nonnephrogenic/nonpsychogenic), abdominal distention postoperatively, bleeding esophageal varices

CONTRAINDICATIONS: Hypersensitivity, chronic nephritis

Precautions: Pregnancy **C,** breastfeeding, CAD, asthma, renal/vascular disease, migraines, seizures

DOSAGE AND ROUTES

Diabetes insipidus

Adult: IM/SUBCUT 5-10 units bid-qid prn; CONT **IV** INF 0.0005 units/kg/hr, (0.05 milliunit/kg/hr), double dose q30min as needed
Child: IM/SUBCUT 2.5-10 units bid-qid prn; IM/SUBCUT 1.25-2.5 units q2-3day (Pitressin Tannate) for chronic therapy

Abdominal distention
Adult: IM 5 units, then q3-4hr, increasing to 10 units if needed (aqueous)

Available forms: Inj 20, 5 units/ml (tannate)

Implementation
IM/SUBCUT route
• May be given IM/SUBCUT for diagnosis of diabetes insipidus
• Give patient 16 oz water at administration to prevent nausea, vomiting, cramping

ADVERSE EFFECTS
CNS: Drowsiness, headache, lethargy, flushing, vertigo
CV: Increased B/P, dysrhythmias, chest pain, **cardiac arrest, shock, MI**
EENT: Nasal irritation, congestion, rhinitis
GI: Nausea, heartburn, cramps, vomiting, flatus
GU: Vulval pain, uterine cramping
MISC: Tremor, sweating, vertigo, urticaria, bronchial constriction

Pharmacokinetics
Absorption	Erratically absorbed (IM)
Distribution	Widely distributed extracellular fluid
Metabolism	Liver, rapidly
Excretion	Kidneys, unchanged
Half-life	10-20 min

Pharmacodynamics
	IM	IV
Onset	1 hr	Unknown
Peak	Unknown	Unknown
Duration	3-8 hr	3-8 hr

INTERACTIONS
Individual drugs
CarBAMazepine, chloropromide, clofibrate, fludrocortisone, urea: decreased antidiuretic effect
Demeclocycline, lithium: increased antidiuretic effect

Drug classifications
Tricyclics: increased antidiuretic effect

NURSING CONSIDERATIONS
Assessment
• Assess intranasal use: nausea, congestion, cramps, headache; usually decreased with decreased dose

• Monitor pulse, B/P when giving product **IV** or SUBCUT
• Monitor I&O ratio, weight daily, fluid/electrolyte balance; check for edema in extremities; if water retention is severe, diuretic may be prescribed; **check for water intoxication: lethargy, behavioral changes, disorientation, neuromuscular excitability**
• Small doses may precipitate coronary adverse effects; keep emergency equipment nearby

Nursing diagnoses
• Fluid volume, deficient (uses)
• Fluid volume, excess (side effects)
• Knowledge, deficient (teaching)

Patient/family education
• Teach patient technique for nasal instillation: to insert tube into nasal cavity to instill product
• Caution patient to avoid OTC products for cough, hay fever because these preparations may contain epinephrine, decrease product response; do not use with alcohol
• Advise patient to carry/wear emergency ID specifying therapy, disease process (diabetes insipidus)
• Teach patient to measure/record I&O
• Teach patient to avoid alcohol, all OTC medications unless approved by prescriber

Evaluation
Positive therapeutic outcome
• Absence of severe thirst
• Decreased urine output, osmolality

⚠ HIGH ALERT

vecuronium (Rx)
(ve-kure-oh'nee-yum)
Func. class.: Neuromuscular blocker—nondepolarizing
Chem. class.: Synthetic curariform
Pregnancy category C

ACTION: Inhibits transmission of nerve impulses by binding with cholinergic receptor sites, antagonizing action of acetylcholine

Therapeutic outcome: Skeletal muscle paralysis during anesthesia

USES: Facilitation of endotracheal intubation; skeletal muscle relaxation during mechanical ventilation, surgery, or general anesthesia

CONTRAINDICATIONS: Hypersensitivity

Precautions: Pregnancy C, breastfeeding, children <2 yr, electrolyte imbalances, dehydration, neuromuscular/cardiac/hepatic disease

> **BLACK BOX WARNING:** Respiratory disease

DOSAGE AND ROUTES
Adult and child >1 yr: IV initially 0.08-0.1 mg/kg or 0.04-0.06 mg/kg if given with succinylcholine, maintenance 0.01-0.015 mg/kg 25-40 min after initial dose, then 0.01-0.015 mg/kg q12-15min

Infant 1 yr->7 wk: IV 0.08-0.1 mg/kg, maintenance 0.05-0.1 mg/kg q60min as needed

Neonate: IV 0.1 mg/kg/dose, maintenance 0.03-0.15 mg/kg/dose q1-2hr as needed

Available forms: 10 mg/5 ml vial

Implementation
• Use peripheral nerve stimulator by anesthesiologist to determine neuromuscular blockade; deep tendon reflexes should be monitored during extended periods
• Give by direct **IV** after reconstituting with bacteriostatic water, over 5 min, D₅W, 0.9% NaCl or LR
• Give by direct **IV** after reconstituting dose in 5-10 ml of provided diluent; give by titrating to patient response
• Give by continuous inf after diluting to 10-20 mg/100 ml and by titrating to patient response (only by qualified person, usually an anesthesiologist); do not administer IM
• Store in light-resistant area

Syringe incompatibilities: Barbiturates

Y-site compatibilities: Aminophylline, ceFAZolin, cefuroxime, cimetidine, diltiazem, DOBUTamine, DOPamine, EPINEPHrine, esmolol, fentaNYL, fluconazole, gentamicin, heparin, hydrocortisone, HYDROmorphone, isoproterenol, labetalol, LORazepam, midazolam, milrinone, morphine, niCARdipine, nitroglycerin, nitroprusside, norepinephrine, propofol, ranitidine, trimethoprim/sulfamethoxazole, vancomycin

Y-site incompatibilities: Barbiturates

ADVERSE EFFECTS
CNS: Skeletal muscle weakness or paralysis (rarely), flushing
INTEG: Urticaria
MISC: Myopathy, hypotension

RESP: Prolonged apnea, possible respiratory paralysis, bronchospasm, tachycardia, flushing, wheezing, dyspnea
SYST: Anaphylaxis

Pharmacokinetics

Absorption	Completely absorbed
Distribution	Rapid, to extracellular fluids
Metabolism	Liver (20%)
Excretion	Kidneys, unchanged (35%)
Half-life	1½ hr, increased in hepatic disease

Pharmacodynamics

Onset	1 min
Peak	3-5 min
Duration	15-25 min (recovery index)

INTERACTIONS
Individual products
Amphotericin B, clindamycin, enflurane, isoflurane, lincomycin, lithium, phenytoin, piperacillin, polymyxin B, quiNIDine, succinylcholine, verapamil: increased neuromuscular blockade
Theophylline: dysrhythmias

Drug classifications
Aminoglycosides, analgesics (opioid), local anesthetics, polymyxin antibiotics, thiazides: increased neuromuscular blockade

NURSING CONSIDERATIONS
Assessment
• Monitor for electrolyte imbalances (potassium, magnesium) before product is used; electrolyte imbalances may lead to increased action of this product

> **BLACK BOX WARNING:** Monitor patient's vital signs (B/P, pulse, respirations, airway) until fully recovered; rate, depth, pattern of respirations, strength of hand grip; patient should be intubated before use

• Monitor patient's recovery: decreased paralysis of face, diaphragm, leg, arm, rest of body; residual weakness and respiratory problems may occur during recovery period
• Monitor allergic reactions: rash, fever, respiratory distress, pruritus; product should be discontinued

Nursing diagnoses
• Breathing pattern, ineffective (uses)
• Knowledge, deficient (teaching)

Patient/family education
• Provide patient reassurance if communication is difficult during recovery from neuromuscular blockade
• Provide explanation to patients regarding all procedures or treatments; patient will remain conscious if anesthesia is not given also

Evaluation
Positive therapeutic outcome
• Paralysis of jaw, eyelid, head, neck, rest of body as evaluated by peripheral nerve stimulator

TREATMENT OF OVERDOSE:
Edrophonium or neostigmine, atropine, monitor VS; may require mechanical ventilation

vemurafenib
(vem-ue-raf'e-nib)
Zelboraf
Func. class.: Biologic response modifiers; signal transduction inhibitors (STIs)
Pregnancy category D

ACTION: Inhibitor of some mutated forms of BRAF serine threonine kinase, thereby blocking cellular proliferation in melanoma cells with the mutation. It also inhibits other kinases including CRAF, ARAF, wild-type BRAF, SRMA, ACK1, MAP4H5, and FGR. It is a potent adenosine triphosphate-competitive inhibitor of RAFs with a modest preference for mutant BRAF and CRAF as compared with wild-type BRAF.

Therapeutic outcome: Decreased spread of malignancy

USES: Unresectable or metastatic malignant melanoma with V600E mutation of the BRAF gene

CONTRAINDICATIONS:
Hypersensitivity

Precautions: Pregnancy D, breastfeeding, children, infants, neonates, hepatic disease, QT prolongation, secondary malignancy, torsades de pointes, hypokalemia, hypomagnesium, sunlight exposure

DOSAGE AND ROUTES
Adult: PO 960 mg (4 tabs) bid about q12h

Dose adjustments for toxicity due to symptomatic adverse reactions or QTc prolongation for Grade 1 or tolerable Grade 2 adverse events:
No dosage change

For Intolerable Grade 2 or Grade 3 adverse events (1st episode):
Interrupt treatment until toxicity resolves to grade ≤1; when resuming, reduce dosage to 720 mg (3 tabs) bid

For Intolerable Grade 2 or Grade 3 adverse events (2nd episode):
Interrupt treatment until toxicity resolves to grade ≤1; when resuming, reduce dose to 480 mg (2 tabs) bid

For Intolerable Grade 2 or Grade 3 adverse events (3rd episode)
Discontinue treatment permanently

For Grade 4 adverse events (1st episode):
Discontinue permanently or interrupt until toxicity resolves to grade ≤1; when resuming, reduce dose to 480 mg (2 tablets) bid

For Grade 4 adverse events (2nd episode):
Discontinue permanently

Available forms: Tab 240 mg

Implementation
• Continue until disease progresses or unacceptable toxicity occurs
• Missed doses can be taken up to 4 hr before the next dose is due; take about 12 hr apart; take without regard to meals
• Swallow whole with a full glass of water; do not crush or chew
• Store at room temperature in original container

ADVERSE EFFECTS
CNS: Asthenia, fatigue, fever, dizziness, headache, muscle paralysis, peripheral neuropathy
CV: Atrial fibrillation, hypotension, peripheral edema, QT prolongation
EENT: Blurred vision, iritis, photophobia, uveitis
GI: Constipation, decreased appetite, diarrhea, dysgeusia, nausea, vomiting, weight loss
INTEG: Actinic keratosis, alopecia, hyperkeratosis, maculopapular rash, palmar-plantar erythrodysesthesia (hand and foot syndrome), papular rash, photosensitivity, pruritus, xerosis/dry skin

V

MS: Arthralgia, arthritis, back pain, extremity
pain, musculoskeletal pain, myalgias
RESP: Cough
SYST: Anaphylaxis, secondary malignancy

Pharmacokinetics

Absorption	Unknown
Distribution	Protein binding 99%
Metabolism	Unknown
Excretion	94% feces
Half-life	30-120 hr

Pharmacodynamics

Onset	Unknown
Peak	Unknown
Duration	Unknown

INTERACTIONS

Individual drugs

Abarelix, alfuzosin, amoxapine, apomorphine,
arsenic trioxide, asenapine, chloroquine,
ciprofloxacin, citalopram, clarithromycin,
clozapine, cyclobenzaprine, dasatinib,
dolasetron, dronedarone, droperidol,
eribulin, erythromycin, ezogabine, flecainide,
fluconazole, gatifloxacin, gemifloxacin,
grepafloxacin, halofantrine, haloperidol, iloperidone, indacaterol, lapatinib, levofloxacin,
levomethadyl, lopinavir/ritonavir, magnesium
sulfate, maprotiline, mefloquine, methadone,
moxifloxacin, nilotinib, norfloxacin, octreotide, ofloxacin, OLANZapine, ondansetron,
paliperidone, palonosetron, pentamidine,
pimozide, posaconazole, potassium sulfate,
probucol, propafenone, QUEtiapine, quiNI-
Dine, ranolazine, rilpivirine, risperidone,
saquinavir, sodium, sparfloxacin, sunitinib,
tacrolimus, telavancin, telithromycin,
tetrabenazine, troleandomycin, vardenafil,
vemurafenib, venlafaxine, vorinostat, ziprasidone: increased QT prolongation, torsades
de pointes

Drug classifications

Beta-agonists, Class IA antiarrhythmics (disopyramide, procainamide, quiNIDine), Class
III antiarrhythmics (amiodarone, dofetilide,
ibutilide, sotalol), halogenated anesthetics,
local anesthetics, certain phenothiazines
(chlorproMAZINE, fluphenazine, mesoridazine, perphenazine, prochlorperazine,
thioridazine and trifluoperazine), tricyclic
antidepressants: increased QT prolongation,
torsades de pointes

CYP3A4 inducers (alcohol, barbiturates,
bexarotene, carBAMazepine, erythromycin,
etravirine, fluvoxamine, ketoconazole, metyrapone, modafinil, nevirapine, OXcarbazepine,
phenytoin, rifabutin, rifampin, ritonavir):
decreased vemurafenib effect
CYP3A4/CYP1A2 inhibitors (cimetidine, dalfopristin, delavirdine, enoxacin, indinavir, isoniazid, itraconazole, quinupristin, tipranavir):
increased vemurafenib effect

Drug/lab test

Alkaline phosphatase, bilirubin, LFTs, serum
creatinine: increase

NURSING CONSIDERATIONS

Assessment

• **Hepatic disease:** Liver function test (LFT)
abnormalities, altered bilirubin levels, may
occur during treatment; monitor LFTs and
bilirubin levels prior to treatment, then monthly;
more frequent testing is needed in those
presenting with grade 2 or greater toxicities;
Laboratory alterations should be managed
with dose reduction, treatment interruption, or
discontinuation
• **QT prolongation:** has been reported with
the use of crizotinib; therefore, crizotinib should
be avoided in patients with QT prolongation;
Monitor ECG and electrolytes in those with
congestive heart failure, bradycardia, electrolyte
imbalance (hypokalemia, hypomagnesemia),
or in those who are taking concomitant medications known to prolong the QT interval; treatment interruption, dosage adjustment, treatment
discontinuation may be needed in those who
develop QT prolongation
• **Pregnancy/breastfeeding:** Identify if
pregnancy is planned or suspected, pregnancy
category D, avoid breastfeeding
• Serum electrolytes

Nursing diagnoses

• Risk for injury (uses)

Patient/family education

• Decreased spread of malignancy

---

venlafaxine (Rx)
(ven-la-fax′een)
Effexor, Effexor XR
Func. class.: Second-generation SNRI
antidepressant—miscellaneous
Pregnancy category C

ACTION: Potent inhibitor of neuronal
serotonin and norepinephrine uptake, weak

inhibitor of dopamine; no muscarinic, histaminergic, or α-adrenergic receptors in vitro

Therapeutic outcome: Relief of depression

USES: Prevention/treatment of major depression, to treat depression at end of life; long-term treatment of generalized anxiety disorder, panic disorder, social anxiety disorder (Effexor XR only)

CONTRAINDICATIONS:
Hypersensitivity, bipolar disorder, interstitial lung disease

Precautions: Pregnancy **C**, breastfeeding, geriatric, mania, recent MI, cardiac/renal/hepatic disease, seizure disorder, hypertension, eosinophilic pneumonia, desvenlafaxine hypersensitivity

> **BLACK BOX WARNING:** Children, suicidal ideation

DOSAGE AND ROUTES
Depression
Adult: PO 75 mg/day in 2 or 3 divided doses; taken with food, may be increased to 150 mg/day; if needed may be further increased to 225 mg/day; increments of 75 mg/day should be made at intervals of no less than 4 days; some hospitalized patients may require up to 375 mg/day in 3 divided doses; EXT REL 37.5-75 mg PO daily, max 225 mg/day; give Effexor XR daily

Anxiety disorders
Adult: PO 75 mg/day or 37.5 mg/day × 4-7 days initially, max 225 mg/day

Hepatic dose
Adult: PO moderate impairment 50% of dose

Renal dose
Adult: PO CCr 10-70 ml/min reduce dose by 25%-50%; CCr <10 ml/min reduce by 50%

Hot flashes (unlabeled)
Adult (male, prostate cancer): PO 12.5 mg bid × 4 wk
Adult female: PO 37.5-75 mg/day

Available forms: Tabs scored (Effexor) 25, 37.5, 50, 75, 100 mg; ext rel caps (Effexor XR) 37.5, 75, 150, 225 mg

Implementation
• Give with food or milk for GI symptoms
• Crush if patient is unable to swallow medication whole
• Store at room temperature; do not freeze

ADVERSE EFFECTS
CNS: *Emotional lability, vertigo, dizziness, weakness,* apathy, ataxia, CNS stimulation, euphoria, hallucinations, hostility, increased libido, hypertonia, hypotonia, psychosis, insomnia, anxiety, **suicidal ideation in children/adolescents, seizures,** neuroleptic malignant syndrome–like reaction
CV: *Migraine,* angina pectoris, extrasystoles, postural hypotension, syncope, thrombophlebitis, hypertension, sustained hypertension, change in QTc interval, increased pulse, increased cholesterol
EENT: *Abnormal vision,* taste, *ear pain,* cataract, conjunctivitis, corneal lesions, dry eyes, otitis media, photophobia
GI: *Dysphagia, eructation,* colitis, gastritis, gingivitis, **rectal hemorrhage,** stomatitis, stomach and mouth ulceration, nausea, anorexia, dry mouth
GU: *Anorgasmia,* abnormal ejaculation, *dysuria, hematuria, metrorrhagia, vaginitis, impaired urination,* albuminuria, amenorrhea, kidney calculus, cystitis, nocturia, breast and bladder pain, polyuria, *uterine hemorrhage, vaginal hemorrhage,* moniliasis
HEMA: **Agranulocytosis, aplastic anemia, neutropenia, pancytopenia, abnormal bleeding**
INTEG: Ecchymosis, acne, alopecia, brittle nails, dry skin, photosensitivity, sweating, **angioedema (ext rel)**
META: *Peripheral edema, weight loss or gain,* diabetes mellitus, edema, glycosuria, hyperlipemia, hypokalemia
MS: Arthritis, bone pain, bursitis, myasthenia, tenosynovitis, arthralgia
RESP: *Bronchitis, dyspnea,* asthma, chest congestion, epistaxis, hyperventilation, laryngitis
SYST: *Malaise, neck pain,* enlarged abdomen, cyst, facial edema, hangover effect, hernia

Pharmacokinetics
Absorption	Well absorbed
Distribution	Widely distributed, 27% protein binding
Metabolism	Liver, extensively
Excretion	Kidneys, 87%
Half-life	5 hr, 11 hr (active metabolite)

Pharmacodynamics
Unknown

INTERACTIONS

Individual drugs
Alcohol: increased CNS depression
Cimetidine: increased venlafaxine effect
Clozapine, desipramine, haloperidol, warfarin: increased levels of these products
Cyproheptadine: decreased venlafaxine effect
Indinavir: decreased effect of indinavir
Sibutramine, sumatriptan, traMADol, traZODone: increased serotonin syndrome

Drug classifications
Antihistamines, opioids, sedative-hypnotics: increased CNS depression
MAOIs: hyperthermia, rigidity, rapid fluctuations of vital signs, mental status changes, neuroleptic malignant syndrome
Salicylates, NSAIDs, platelet inhibitors, anticoagulants: increased bleeding risk
SSRIs, SNRIs, serotonin-receptor agonists: increased serotonin syndrome

Drug/herb
Kava, valerian: increased CNS depression
St. John's wort: serotonin syndrome

Drug/lab test
Increased: alkaline phosphatase, bilirubin, AST, ALT, BUN, creatinine, serum cholesterol, CPK, LDH

NURSING CONSIDERATIONS

Assessment
• Monitor B/P (lying, standing), pulse q4hr; if systolic B/P drops 20 mm Hg hold product, notify prescriber; take vital signs q4hr in patients with CV disease
• Monitor blood tests: CBC, leukocytes, differential, cardiac enzymes if patient is receiving long-term therapy
• Monitor liver function tests: AST, ALT, bilirubin
• Check weight qwk; weight loss or gain; appetite may increase, peripheral edema may occur

> **BLACK BOX WARNING:** Assess mental status: mood, sensorium, affect; increase in psychiatric symptoms: depression, panic; for suicidal ideation in children/adolescents

• Monitor urinary retention, constipation; constipation is more likely to occur in children or geriatric
• **Assess for withdrawal symptoms:** headache, nausea, vomiting, muscle pain, weakness; do not usually occur unless product was discontinued abruptly
• Identify alcohol consumption; if alcohol is consumed, hold dose

• **Serotonin syndrome, neuroleptic malignant syndrome:** assess for increased heart rate, shivering, sweating, dilated pupils, tremors, high B/P, hyperthermia, headache, confusion; if these occur, stop product, administer a serotonin antagonist if needed

Nursing diagnoses
• Coping, ineffective (uses)
• Injury, risk for (side effects)
• Knowledge, deficient (teaching)
• Noncompliance (teaching)

Patient/family education
• Advise patient to notify prescriber of rash, hives, or allergic reactions
• Teach patient that therapeutic effects may take 2-3 wk
• Teach patient to use caution in driving or other activities requiring alertness because of drowsiness, dizziness, blurred vision; to avoid rising quickly from sitting to standing, especially geriatric
• Teach patient to avoid alcohol ingestion, other CNS depressants
• Advise patient to avoid pregnancy, breastfeeding while taking this product
• **Teach patient that worsening of symptoms, suicidal thoughts/behavior may occur in children, young adults**

Evaluation
Positive therapeutic outcome
• Decreased depression, anxiety; sense of well-being
• Absence of suicidal thoughts

TREATMENT OF OVERDOSE:
ECG monitoring, induce emesis, lavage, activated charcoal, administer anticonvulsant

> **verapamil (Rx)**
> (ver-ap′a-mil)
> **Apo-Verap, Calan, Calan SR, Covera-HS, Isoptin, Isoptin SR, Nu-Verap ✦, Verelan, Verelan PM**
> *Func. class.:* Calcium-channel blocker; antihypertensive; antianginal, antidysrhythmic (Class IV)
> *Chem. class.:* Diphenylalkylamine
> **Pregnancy category C**

ACTION: Inhibits calcium ion influx across cell membrane during cardiac depolarization; produces relaxation of coronary vascular smooth muscle, peripheral vascular smooth muscle; dilates coronary vascular arteries; decreases SA/AV node conduction; dilates peripheral arteries

Therapeutic outcome: Decreased angina pectoris, dysrhythmias, B/P

USES: Chronic stable vasospastic, unstable angina; dysrhythmias, hypertension, supraventricular tachycardia, atrial flutter or fibrillation

Unlabeled uses: Prevention of migraine headaches, claudication, mania

CONTRAINDICATIONS:
Sick sinus syndrome, 2nd- or 3rd-degree heart block, hypotension <90 mm Hg systolic, cardiogenic shock, severe CHF

Precautions: Pregnancy **C**, breastfeeding, children, geriatric, CHF, hypotension, hepatic injury, renal disease, concomitant β-blocker therapy

DOSAGE AND ROUTES
Angina
Adult: PO 80-120 mg tid, increase qwk, max 480 mg/day

Dysrhythmias
Adult: PO 240-320 mg/day in 3-4 divided doses in digitalized patients
Adult: IV BOL 5-10 mg (0.075-0.15 mg/kg) over 2 min, may repeat 10 mg (0.15 mg/kg) ¹/₂ hr after first dose
Child 1-15 yr: IV BOL 0.1-0.3 mg/kg over >2 min, repeat in 30 min, max 5 mg in a single dose
Child 0-1 yr: IV BOL 0.1-0.2 mg/kg over ≥2 min, may repeat after 30 min

Hypertension
Adult: PO 80 mg tid, may titrate upward; EXT REL 120-240 mg/day as a single dose, may increase to 240-480 mg/day

Hepatic dose/geriatric/compromised ventricular function
Adult: PO 40 mg tid initially, increase as tolerated

Available forms: Tabs 40, 80, 120 mg; ext rel tabs 120, 180, 240 mg; inj 2.5 mg/ml in ampules, syringes, vials; ext rel caps 100, 200, 240, 300 mg

Implementation
PO route
• Do not crush or chew ext rel products
• Cap may be opened and contents sprinkled on food; do not dissolve, chew cap
• Give once a day before meals at bedtime; sus rel give with food to decrease GI symptoms

Direct IV route
• Give by direct **IV** undiluted (Y-site, 3-way stopcock) over at least 2 min, or 3 min geriatric; discard unused sol; to prevent serious hypotension, patient should be recumbent for 1 hr or more

Y-site compatibilities: Alfentanil, amikacin, argatroban, ascorbic acid, atracurium, atropine, aztreonam, bivalirudin, bumetanide, buprenorphine, butorphanol, calcium chloride/gluconate, CARBOplatin, caspofungin, ceFAZolin, cefonicid, cefotaxime, cefotetan, cefoxitin, ceftizoxime, cefTRIAXone, cefuroxime, chlorproMAZINE, cimetidine, ciprofloxacin, clindamycin, cyanocobalamin, cyclophosphamide, cycloSPORINE, cytarabine, DACTINomycin, DAPTOmycin, dexamethasone, dexmedetomidine, digoxin, diltiazem, diphenhydrAMINE, DOBUTamine, docetaxel, DOPamine, doxacurium, DOXOrubicin hydrochloride, doxycycline, enalaprilat, ePHEDrine, EPINEPHrine, epirubicin, epoetin alfa, eptifibatide, erythromycin, esmolol, etoposide, etoposide phosphate, famotidine, fenoldopam, fentaNYL, fluconazole, fludarabine, gemcitabine, gentamicin, glycopyrrolate, granisetron, heparin, hydrALAZINE, hydrocortisone, HYDROmorphone, ifosfamide, imipenem/cilastatin, inamrinone, insulin, isoproterenol, ketorolac, labetalol, levofloxacin, lidocaine, linezolid, LORazepam, magnesium sulfate, mannitol, mechlorethamine, meperidine, metaraminol, methotrexate, methoxamine, methyldopa, methylPREDNISolone, metoclopramide, metoprolol, metroNIDAZOLE, miconazole, midazolam, milrinone, mitoxantrone, morphine, multivitamins, nalbuphine, naloxone, nesiritide, nitroglycerin, nitroprusside, norepinephrine, octreotide, ondansetron, oxaliplatin, oxytocin, paclitaxel, palonosetron, papaverine, pemetrexed, penicillin G, pentamidine, pentazocine, phentolamine, phenylephrine, phytonadione, piperacillin/tazobactam, potassium chloride, procainamide, prochlorperazine, promethazine, propranolol, protamine, pyridoxime, quinupristin/dalfopristin, ranitidine, rocuronium, sodium acetate, succinylcholine, SUFentanil, tacrolimus, teniposide, theophylline, thiamine, ticarcillin/clavulanate, tirofiban, tobramycin, tolazoline, trimethaphan, urokinase, vancomycin, vasopres-

V

sin, vecuronium, vinCRIStine, vinorelbine, voriconazole

Y-site incompatibilities: Acyclovir, albumin, aminophylline, amphotericin B cholesteryl, amphotericin B colloidal, amphotericin B liposome, ampicillin, ampicillin/sulbactam, azaTHIOprine, cefoperazone, ceftazidime, chloramphenicol, dantrolene, diazepam, diazoxide, ertapenem, fluorouracil, folic acid, furosemide, ganciclovir, indomethacin, pantoprazole, PENTobarbital, PHENobarbital, phenytoin, piperacillin/tazobactam, propofol, sodium bicarbonate, thiotepa, tigecycline, trimethoprim/sulfamethoxazole

ADVERSE EFFECTS

CNS: *Headache, drowsiness,* dizziness, anxiety, depression, weakness, asthenia, fatigue, insomnia, confusion, light-headedness
CV: *Edema,* **CHF,** bradycardia, hypotension, palpitations, AV block, **dysrhythmias**
GI: *Nausea,* diarrhea, gastric upset, *constipation,* elevated liver function tests
GU: Impotence, nocturia, polyuria, gynecomastia
HEMA: Bruising, petechiae, bleeding
INTEG: Rash, bruising
MISC: Gingival hyperplasia
SYST: **Stevens-Johnson syndrome**

Pharmacokinetics

Absorption	Well absorbed (PO)
Distribution	Not known
Metabolism	Liver, extensively
Excretion	Kidneys (70%)
Half-life	Biphasic 4 min, 3-7 hr

Pharmacodynamics

	PO	PO-EXT REL	IV
Onset	1-2 hr	Unknown	1-5 min
Peak	$\frac{1}{2}$-$1\frac{1}{2}$ hr	5-7 hr	3-5 min
Duration	3-7 hr	24 hr	2 hr

INTERACTIONS

Individual drugs

CarBAMazepine, cycloSPORINE, digoxin, theophylline: increased levels of each specific product
Cimetidine, telithromycin: increased effect of verapamil
FentaNYL, prazosin, quiNIDine: increased hypotension
Lithium: decreased lithium levels

Drug classifications

Antihypertensive, β-adrenergic blockers, nitrates: increased effects of verapamil
Nondepolarizing muscle relaxants: increased effect
NSAIDs: decreased antihypertensive effect

Drug/food

Grapefruit juice: increased hypotension

Drug/lab test

Increased: alkaline phosphatase, AST, ALT, BUN, creatinine, serum cholesterol

NURSING CONSIDERATIONS

Assessment

• **CHF:** Assess fluid volume status: I&O ratio and record; weight; distended red veins; crackles in lung; color; quality, specific gravity of urine; skin turgor; adequacy of pulses; moist mucous membranes; bilateral lung sounds; peripheral pitting edema; dehydration symptoms of decreasing output, thirst, hypotension, dry mouth, and mucous membranes should be reported
• Monitor B/P and pulse, pulmonary capillary wedge pressure (PCWP), central venous pressure, index, often during inf; notify prescriber if <50 bpm, systolic B/P <90 mm Hg
• Monitor ALT, AST, bilirubin daily; if these are elevated, hepatotoxicity is suspected
• Monitor platelets; if <150,000/mm³, product is usually discontinued and another product started
• Assess for extravasation; change site q48hr
• **Monitor cardiac status:** B/P, pulse, respiration, ECG
• Monitor renal/hepatic function tests during long-term treatment, serum potassium, periodically

Nursing diagnoses

• Cardiac output, decreased (uses)
• Knowledge, deficient (teaching)

Patient/family education

• Advise patient to increase fluids/fiber to counteract constipation
• Caution patient to avoid hazardous activities until stabilized on product and dizziness is no longer a problem
• Teach patient how to take pulse, B/P before taking product; to keep record or graph
• Instruct patient to limit caffeine consumption; to avoid alcohol, grapefruit, and OTC products unless directed by prescriber
• Advise patient to comply with medical regimen: diet, exercise, stress reduction,

product therapy; to notify prescriber of irregular heartbeat, shortness of breath, swelling of feet and hands, pronounced dizziness, constipation, nausea, hypotension, **IV** calcium
• Teach patient to use as directed even if feeling better; may be taken with other CV products (nitrates, β-blockers)
• Caution patient not to discontinue abruptly; chest pain may occur
• Advise to report chest pain, palpitations, irregular heart beats, swelling of extremities, skin irritation, rash, tremors, weakness

Evaluation
Positive therapeutic outcome
• Decreased anginal pain
• Decreased dysrhythmias
• Decreased B/P

TREATMENT OF OVERDOSE:
Defibrillation, atropine for AV block, vasopressor for hypotension, **IV** calcium

vidarabine ophthalmic
See Appendix B

vigabatrin (Rx)
(vye-ga'ba-trin)
Sabril
Func. class.: Anticonvulsant
Chem. class.: GABA transaminase inhibitor
Pregnancy category C

ACTION: May inhibit reuptake and metabolism of GABA, may increase seizure threshold; structurally similar to GABA

Therapeutic outcome: Prevention of seizure activity

USES: Adjunct treatment of partial seizures in adults and children ≥12 yr, infantile spasm

CONTRAINDICATIONS:
Hypersensitivity to this product

Precautions: Pregnancy **C**, breastfeeding, children <2 yr, geriatric patients, renal/hepatic disease, suicidal ideation/behavior, abrupt discontinuation

BLACK BOX WARNING: Visual disturbance

DOSAGE AND ROUTES
Partial seizures
Adult: PO 500 mg bid, titrate in 500-mg increments at weekly intervals, up to 1.5 g bid

Infantile spasm
Infant >1 mo, child ≤2 yr: PO 50 mg/kg/day in 2 divided doses titrate in 25-50 mg/kg/day increments q3days, max 150 mg/kg/day

Renal dose
Adult: PO CCr 50-80 ml/min, reduce dosage by 25%; PO CCr 30-50 ml/min, reduce dosage by 50%; PO CCr 10-30 ml/min, reduce dosage by 75%

Available forms: powder for solution; tablet 500 mg

Implementation
PO route (tab)
• Give without regard to meals
PO route (oral solution)
• Reconstitute immediately before using
• Empty contents into a clean cup
• For each packet, dissolve 10 ml of water, conc. 50 mg/ml; do not use other liquids
• Stir until dissolved; solution should be clear
• Use calibrated oral syringe to measure correct dosage
• Discard any unused solution

ADVERSE EFFECTS
CNS: *Dizziness,* irritability, lethargy, **malignant hyperthermia**, insomnia
CV: Edema
EENT: Vision impairment
GI: Nausea, vomiting, diarrhea, increased appetite, abdominal pain, GI bleeding, hemorrhoids, weight gain, constipation
HEMA: Anemia
INTEG: Pruritus, rash
RESP: Coughing, **respiratory depression, pulmonary embolism**

Pharmacokinetics	
Absorption	>95%
Distribution	Widely; no protein binding
Metabolism	Not metabolized
Excretion	Urine 80% parent drug, slowed in renal disease
Half-life	7.5 hr

Pharmacodynamics	
Onset	Unknown
Peak	2 hr
Duration	Unknown

V

INTERACTIONS
Individual drugs
AzaTHIOprine, chloroquine, deferoxamine, ethambutol, hydroxychloroquine, interferons, loxapine, mecasermin, rh-IGF-1, pentostatin, tamoxifen, thiothixene: Serious ophthalmic effects (glaucoma, retinopathy); avoid concurrent use

Drug classifications
CNS depressants: increased CNS depression
Corticosteroids, phenothiazines, phosphodiesterase inhibitors: Serious ophthalmic effects (glaucoma, retinopathy)

NURSING CONSIDERATIONS
Assessment
• Monitor renal studies: urinalysis, BUN, urine creatinine q3mo
• Monitor hepatic studies: ALT, AST, bilirubin
• Assess description of seizures: location, duration, presence of aura
• Assess mental status: mood, sensorium, affect, behavioral changes; if mental status changes, notify prescriber

Nursing diagnoses
• Injury, risk for (uses)
• Noncompliance (teaching)
• Knowledge deficit (teaching)

Perform/provide
• Store at room temperature
• Provide assistance with ambulation during early part of treatment; dizziness occurs
• Provide seizure precautions: padded side rails; move objects that may harm patient

Patient/family education
• Teach patient to carry emergency ID stating patient's name, products taken, condition, prescriber's name and phone number
• Advise patient to avoid driving, other activities that require alertness
• Inform patient not to discontinue medication quickly after long-term use

Evaluation:
• Therapeutic response: decreased seizure activity; document on patient's chart

vilazodone (Rx)
(vil-az′oh-done)
Viibryd
Func. class.: Antidepressant, miscellaneous
Pregnancy category C

ACTION: A novel antidepressant unrelated to other antidepressants, enhances serotoninergic action by a dual mechanism

Therapeutic outcome: Remission of depressive symptoms

USES: Major depression

CONTRAINDICATIONS:
Concomitant use of MAOIs or within 14 days after discontinuing an MAOI or within 14 days after discontinuing vilazodone

Precautions: Abrupt discontinuation, bipolar disorder, bleeding, operating machinery, ECT, geriatrics, hepatic disease, hyponatremia, hypovolemia, infants, labor, pregnancy **C**, substance abuse, history of seizures, serotonin syndrome, neuroleptic malignant syndrome, use with serotonin precursors (e.g., tryptophan) or serotonergic drugs, suicidal ideation and worsening depression or behavior

> **BLACK BOX WARNING:** Child, suicidal ideation

DOSAGE AND ROUTES
Adult: PO 10 mg ×7 days, then 20 mg ×7 days, then 40 mg/day; if taking a potent CYP3A4 inhibitor, the max is 20 mg/day

Available forms: Tabs 10, 20, 40 mg

Implementation
• Administer with food to increase absorption
• Store at room temperature, away from moisture, heat

ADVERSE EFFECTS
CNS: Restlessness, dizziness, drowsiness, fatigue, mania, insomnia, migraine, **neuroleptic malignant-like syndrome,** paresthesias, **seizures, suicidal ideation,** tremor, night sweats, dream disorders
EENT: Cataracts, blurred vision
GI: Nausea, vomiting, flatulence, diarrhea, xerostomia, altered taste, gastroenteritis
GU: Decreased libido, ejaculation disorder, increased frequency of urination, sexual dysfunction

HEMA: Bleeding, decreased platelets
MS: Arthralgia
SYST: Neonatal abstinence syndrome, withdrawal, **serotonin syndrome**

Pharmacokinetics

Absorption	Unknown
Distribution	Protein binding 96-99%
Metabolism	Metabolized by the liver by CYP 3A4 (major) and CYP2C19 and CYP2D (minor) and non-CYP pathways
Excretion	Unknown
Half-life	25 hr

Pharmacodynamics

Onset	Unknown
Peak	4-5 hr
Duration	Unknown

INTERACTIONS

Individual drugs
Selegline, busPIRone, dextromethorphan, fenfluramine, dexfluramine, lithium, meperidine, fentaNYL, methylphenidate, dexmethylphenidate, metoclopramide, mirtazapine, nefazodone, pentazocine, phenothiazines, haloperidol, loxapine, thiothixene, molidone: increased serotonin syndrome

Drug classifications
MAO inhibitors: do not use together
SSRIs, SNRIs, serotonin receptor agonists, ergots, amphetamines: increased serotonin syndrome
Anticoagulants, thrombolytics, platelet inhibitors, salicylates: increased bleeding
CYP3A4 inhibitors: increased vilazodone levels

Drug/herb
St. John's wort: increased serotonin syndrome

Drug/food
Grapefruit juice: avoid use

NURSING CONSIDERATIONS

Assessment
• Assess mental status: orientation, mood behavior initially and periodically.

> **BLACK BOX WARNING:** Initiate suicide precautions if indicated

• Assess for history of seizures, mania
• Monitor renal, hepatic status: hyponatremia

Nursing diagnoses
• Ineffective coping (uses)
• Risk for injury (adverse reactions)
• Sexual dysfunction (adverse reactions)

Patient/family education
• Teach patient to take as directed, do not double doses
• Advise patient to avoid abrupt discontinuation unless approved by prescriber
• Instruct patient not to drive or operate machinery until effects are known
• Instruct patient not to use other products unless approved by prescriber
• Advise patient to contact prescriber if allergic reactions, personality changes (aggression, anxiety, anger, hostility), extreme sleepiness or drowsiness, confusion, nervousness, restlessness, clumsiness, numbness, tingling or burning pain in hands, arms, legs or feet, tremors, or having unusual behavior or thoughts about self-harm

Evaluation
Positive therapeutic outcome
• Remission of depressive symptoms

⚠ HIGH ALERT

vinBLAStine (VLB) (Rx)
(vin-blast'een)
Velbe ✦
Func. class.: Antineoplastic
Chem. class.: Vinca rosea alkaloid
Pregnancy category D

Do not confuse:
vinBLAStine/vinCRIStine

ACTION: Inhibits mitotic activity, arrests cell cycle at metaphase; inhibits RNA synthesis, blocks cellular use of glutamic acid needed for purine synthesis; a vesicant

Therapeutic outcome: Prevention of rapid growth of malignant cells; immunosuppression

USES: Breast, testicular cancer; lymphomas; neuroblastoma; Hodgkin's, non-Hodgkin's lymphomas; mycosis fungoides; histiocytosis; Kaposi's sarcoma, Langerhan's cell histiocytosis

CONTRAINDICATIONS:
Pregnancy **D**, breastfeeding, infants, hypersensitivity, leukopenia, granulocytopenia, bone marrow suppression, infection

BLACK BOX WARNING: Intrathecal use

Precautions: Renal/hepatic disease, tumor lysis syndrome

BLACK BOX WARNING: Extravasation

DOSAGE AND ROUTES
Breast cancer
Adult: **IV** 4.5 mg/m^2 on day 1 of every 21 days in combination with DOXOrubicin and thiotepa

Hodgkin's disease
Adult: **IV** 6 mg/m^2 on days 1 and 15 q28 days with DOXOrubicin (ABVD)
Child: **IV** 2.5-6 mg/m^2/day once q 1-2 wk × 3-6 wks; max weekly dose 12.5 mg/m^2

Available forms: Inj powder 10 mg for 10 ml **IV** inj; sol for inj 1 mg/ml

Implementation
IV inj route
• Administer **IV** after diluting 10 mg/10 ml NaCl; give through Y-tube or 3-way stopcock or directly over 1 min

Intermittent IV INF route
• Further dilute in 50-100 ml of NS, inf over 15-30 min
• Give by intermittent inf
• Sol should be prepared by qualified personnel only under controlled conditions
• Use Luer-Lok tubing to prevent leakage; do not let sol come in contact with skin; if contact occurs, wash well with soap and water

BLACK BOX WARNING: Give hyaluronidase 150 units/ml in 1 ml of NaCl, warm compress for extravasation for vesicant activity treatment

BLACK BOX WARNING: Do not administer intrathecally: fatal

Syringe compatibilities: Bleomycin, CISplatin, cyclophosphamide, droperidol, fluorouracil, leucovorin, methotrexate, metoclopramide, mitomycin, vinCRIStine

Y-site compatibilities: Allopurinol, amifostine, aztreonam, bleomycin, CISplatin, cyclophosphamide, DOXOrubicin, droperidol, filgrastim, fludarabine, fluorouracil, granisetron, heparin, leucovorin, melphalan, methotrexate, metoclopramide, mitomycin, ondansetron, pa-

clitaxel, piperacillin/tazobactam, sargramostim, teniposide, thiotepa, vinCRIStine, vinorelbine

Y-site incompatibilities: Furosemide

Additive compatibilities: Bleomycin

ADVERSE EFFECTS
CNS: Paresthesias, peripheral neuropathy, depression, headache, **seizures,** malaise
CV: Tachycardia, orthostatic hypotension, hypertension
GI: *Nausea, vomiting,* ileus, *anorexia, stomatitis, constipation,* abdominal pain, GI and rectal bleeding, **hepatotoxicity,** pharyngitis
GU: Urinary retention, **renal failure,** hyperuricemia
HEMA: **Thrombocytopenia, leukopenia, myelosuppression,** agranulocytosis, granulocytosis, aplastic anemia, neutropenia, pancytopenia
INTEG: *Rash, alopecia,* photosensitivity, **extravasation, tissue necrosis**
META: SIADH
SYST: **Tumor lysis syndrome (TLS)**
RESP: **Fibrosis, pulmonary infiltrate, bronchospasm**

Pharmacokinetics
Absorption	Complete bioavailability
Distribution	Crosses blood-brain barrier slightly
Metabolism	Liver—active antineoplastic
Excretion	Biliary, kidneys
Half-life	Triphasic <5 min, 50-155 min, 23-85 hr

Pharmacodynamics
Unknown

INTERACTIONS
Individual drugs
Bleomycin: increased synergism
Methotrexate: increased methotrexate action
Mitomycin: increased bronchospasm
Phenytoin: decreased phenytoin level
Radiation: increased toxicity, bone marrow suppression; do not use together

Drug classifications
Anticoagulants, NSAIDs: increased bleeding risk
Antineoplastics: increased toxicity, bone marrow suppression
CYP3A4 inducers (barbiturates, bosentan, carBAMazepine, efavirenz, phenytoin, nevirapine, rifabutin, rifampin): decreased vinBLAStine effect

CYP3A4 inhibitors (aprepitant, antiretroviral protease inhibitors, clarithromycin, danazol, delavirdine, diltiazem, erythromycin, fluconazole, fluoxetine, fluvoxamine, imatinib, ketoconazole, mebefradil, nefazodone, telithromycin, voriconazole): increased toxicity

Live virus vaccines: increased adverse reactions

Drug/herb
St. John's wort: avoid use

NURSING CONSIDERATIONS

Assessment
• Monitor B/P (baseline and q15min) during administration
• Monitor CBC, differential, platelet count weekly; withhold product if WBC is <2000/mm³ or platelet count is <75,000/mm³; notify prescriber of results; recovery will take 3 wk; RBC, Hct, Hgb may be decreased
• Assess for dyspnea, crackles, unproductive cough, chest pain, tachypnea
• Monitor renal function tests: BUN, serum uric acid, urine CCr before, during therapy; I&O ratio; report fall in urine output of 30 ml/hr; for decreased hyperuricemia
• Monitor for cold, fever, sore throat (may indicate beginning of infection); notify prescriber if these occur
• Assess for bleeding: hematuria, guaiac, bruising or petechiae, mucosa or orifices q8hr, no rectal temp; avoid IM inj; use pressure to venipuncture sites
• Identify nutritional status: an antiemetic may need to be prescribed
• Assess for gout, joint pain, swelling, increased uric acid; allopurinol or other treatment may be used
• Assess for symptoms indicating severe allergic reactions: rash, pruritus, urticaria, itching, flushing, bronchospasm, hypotension; epinephrine and resuscitative equipment should be nearby

Nursing diagnoses
• Body image, disturbed (adverse reactions)
• Infection, risk for (adverse reactions)
• Injury, risk for (adverse reactions)
• Knowledge, deficient (teaching)

Patient/family education
• Teach patient to avoid use of products containing aspirin or NSAIDs, razors, commercial mouthwash because bleeding may occur; to report symptoms of bleeding (hematuria, tarry stools)

• Instruct patient to report signs of anemia, (fatigue, headache, irritability, faintness, shortness of breath)
• Caution patient to report any changes in breathing or coughing even several mo after treatment; avoid breastfeeding; may cause male infertility
• Advise patient that contraception will be necessary during treatment; teratogenesis may occur
• Advise patient to use sunscreen, wear protective clothing and sunglasses
• Inform patient that hair may be lost during treatment; a wig or hairpiece may make patient feel better; new hair will be different in color, texture
• Advise patient to avoid vaccinations during treatment; serious reactions may occur
• Teach patient to report signs/symptoms of infection: fever, chills, sore throat; patient should avoid crowds and persons with known infections
• Teach patient to use effective contraception, pregnancy **D**, avoid breastfeeding, may cause male infertility

Evaluation
Positive therapeutic outcome
• Decreased spread of malignant cells

⚠ HIGH ALERT

vinCRIStine (VCR) (Rx)
(vin-kris'teen)
Vincasar PFS
Func. class.: Antineoplastic—miscellaneous
Chem. class.: Vinca alkaloid
Pregnancy category D

Do not confuse:
vinCRIStine/vinBLAStine

ACTION: Inhibits mitotic activity, arrests cell cycle at metaphase; inhibits RNA synthesis, blocks cellular use of glutamic acid needed for purine synthesis; a vesicant

Therapeutic outcome: Prevention of rapid growth of malignant cells, immunosuppression

USES: Lymphomas, neuroblastomas, Hodgkin's disease, acute lymphoblastic and other leukemias, rhabdomyosarcoma, Wilms' tumor, non-Hodgkin's lymphoma, malignant glioma, soft-tissue sarcoma

V

Adverse effects: *italics* = common; **bold** = life-threatening

CONTRAINDICATIONS:
Pregnancy **D**, breastfeeding, infants, hypersensitivity, radiation therapy

> **BLACK BOX WARNING:** Intrathecal use

Precautions: Renal/hepatic disease, hypertension, neuromuscular disease

> **BLACK BOX WARNING:** Extravasation

DOSAGE AND ROUTES
Adult: IV 0.4-1.4 mg/m²/wk, max 2 mg
Child >10 kg: IV 1-2 mg/m²/wk, max 2 mg

Available forms: Inj 1 mg/ml; powder for inj 5 mg/vial

Implementation

> **BLACK BOX WARNING:** Do not give intrathecally: fatal

• Administer **IV** after diluting with diluent provided or 1 mg/10 ml of sterile water or 0.9% NaCl; give through Y-tube or 3-way stopcock or directly over 1 min

> **BLACK BOX WARNING:** Hyaluronidase 150 units/ml in 1 ml of NaCl; apply warm compress for extravasation

Syringe compatibilities: Bleomycin, CISplatin, cyclophosphamide, doxapram, DOXOrubicin, droperidol, fluorouracil, heparin, leucovorin, methotrexate, metoclopramide, mitomycin, ondansetron, vinCRIStine

Syringe incompatibilities: Furosemide

Y-site compatibilities: Allopurinol, amifostine, aztreonam, bleomycin, CISplatin, cladribine, cyclophosphamide, DOXOrubicin, droperidol, filgrastim, fludarabine, fluorouracil, granisetron, heparin, leucovorin, methotrexate, metoclopramide, mitomycin, ondansetron, paclitaxel, sargramostim, teniposide, thiotepa, vinCRIStine, vinorelbine

Y-site incompatibilities: Furosemide

ADVERSE EFFECTS
CNS: *Decreased reflexes, numbness, weakness, motor difficulties,* CNS depression, cranial nerve paralysis, **seizures,** peripheral neuropathy
CV: Orthostatic hypotension
EENT: *Diplopia*

GI: *Nausea, vomiting, anorexia, stomatitis, constipation,* **paralytic ileus, abdominal pain, hepatotoxicity**
GU: Renal tubular obstruction
HEMA: Thrombocytopenia, leukopenia, myelosuppression, anemia
INTEG: *Alopecia,* extravasation
SYST: Tumor lysis syndrome (TLS)

Pharmacokinetics
Absorption	Complete bioavailability
Distribution	Rapidly, widely distributed; crosses blood-brain barrier
Metabolism	Liver
Excretion	Biliary, in feces, crosses placenta
Half-life	Triphasic <5 min, 50-155 min, 23-85 hr

Pharmacodynamics
Onset	Unknown
Peak	Unknown
Duration	1 wk

INTERACTIONS
Individual drugs
Digoxin: decreased digoxin level
Mitomycin-C: increased acute pulmonary reactions
Radiation: increased toxicity, bone marrow suppression; do not use together

Drug classifications
CYP3A4 inducers (barbiturates, bosentan, carBAMazepine, efavirenz, phenytoins, nevirapine, rifabutin, rifampin): decreased vinCRIStine effect
CYP3A4 inhibitors (aprepitant, antiretroviral protease inhibitors, clarithromycin, danazol, delavirdine, diltiazem, erythromycin, fluconazole, FLUoxetine, fluvoxamine, imatinib, ketoconazole, mibefradil, nefazodone, telithromycin, voriconazole): increased toxicity
Peripheral nervous system products: neurotoxicity
Vaccines/toxoids: decreased immune response

Drug/herb
St. John's wort: avoid use

NURSING CONSIDERATIONS
Assessment
• Monitor CBC, differential, platelet count weekly; withhold product if WBC is <4000/

mm^3 or platelet count is <75,000/mm^3; notify prescriber of results; platelets may increase or decrease
• Assess neurologic status: paresthesia, weakness, cranial nerve palsies, orthostatic hypotension, lethargy, agitation, psychosis; notify prescriber
• Monitor renal function tests: BUN, serum uric acid, urine CCr before, during therapy; I&O ratio; report fall in urine output of 30 ml/hr; for decreased hyperuricemia, hyponatremia, and increased fluid retention (SIADH)
• Monitor for cold, fever, sore throat (may indicate beginning of infection)
• Identify for increased uric acid levels, joint pain in extremities; increase fluid intake to 2-3 L/day unless contraindicated

Nursing diagnoses
• Body image, disturbed (adverse reactions)
• Infection, risk for (adverse reactions)
• Injury, risk for (adverse reactions)
• Knowledge, deficient (teaching)

Patient/family education
• Teach patient to avoid use of products containing aspirin or NSAIDs, razors, commercial mouthwash because bleeding may occur; to report symptoms of bleeding (hematuria, tarry stools)
• Instruct patient to report signs of anemia (fatigue, headache, irritability, faintness, shortness of breath)
• Caution patient to report any changes in breathing or coughing, even several mo after treatment
• Advise patient that contraception will be necessary during and 2 mo after treatment; may be teratogenic, pregnancy **D,** avoid breastfeeding
• Inform patient that hair may be lost during treatment; a wig or hairpiece may make patient feel better; new hair will be different in color, texture
• Advise patient to avoid vaccinations during treatment; serious reactions may occur
• Teach patient to report signs/symptoms of infection: fever, chills, sore throat; patient should avoid crowds or persons with known infections
• Advise patient to increase fluids, bulk in diet, exercise to prevent constipation

Evaluation
Positive therapeutic outcome
• Decreased spread of malignancies

⚠ HIGH ALERT

vinorelbine (Rx)
(vi-nor′el-bine)
Navelbine
Func. class.: Antineoplastic—miscellaneous
Chem. class.: Semisynthetic vinca alkaloid
Pregnancy category D

ACTION: Inhibits mitotic spindle activity, arrests cell cycle at metaphase; inhibits RNA synthesis, blocks cellular use of glutamic acid needed for purine synthesis; a vesicant

Therapeutic outcome: Decreased spread of malignancy

USES: Unresectable, advanced non–small-cell lung cancer (NSCLC) stage IV; may be used alone or in combination with cisplatin for stage III or IV NSCLC

CONTRAINDICATIONS:
Pregnancy **D,** breastfeeding, hypersensitivity, infants, granulocyte count <1000 cells/mm^3 pretreatment

BLACK BOX WARNING: Severe neutropenia, intrathecal use

Precautions: Children, geriatric, hepatic/pulmonary/neurologic/renal disease, bone marrow suppression

BLACK BOX WARNING: Extravasation

DOSAGE AND ROUTES
Adult: IV 30 mg/m^2 qwk

ANC: 1000-1499, give 50% dose; <1000 hold dose; <1000 × 3 wk, discontinue

Hepatic dose
Adult: IV total bilirubin 2.1-3 mg/dl 15 mg/m^2 qwk; total bilirubin ≥3 mg/dl 7.5 mg/m^2/day

Available forms: Inj 10 mg/ml

Implementation

BLACK BOX WARNING: Do not give intrathecally: fatal

BLACK BOX WARNING: Hyaluronidase 150 units/ml in 1 ml of 0.9% NaCl, warm compress for extravasation for vesicant activity treatment

---

• Antacid before oral agent; give product after evening meal before bedtime
• Antiemetic 30-60 min before giving product and prn to prevent vomiting

Intermittent IV infusion route
• Dilute to 0.5-2 mg/ml with 0.9% NaCl, 0.45% NaCl, D₅W, D₅/0.45% NaCl, LR, Ringer's; give over 6-10 min into Y-site or central line; flush line

Continuous IV infusion route
• Give 40 mg/m² q3wk after **IV** bol of 8 mg/m²; may be given in combination with DOXOrubicin, fluorouracil, cisplatin

Y-site compatibilities: Amikacin, aztreonam, bleomycin, buprenorphine, butorphanol, calcium gluconate, CARBOplatin, cefotaxime, CISplatin, cimetidine, clindamycin, dexamethasone, enalaprilat, etoposide, famotidine, filgrastim, fluconazole, fludarabine, gentamicin, hydrocortisone, LORazepam, meperidine, morphine, netilmicin, ondansetron, plicamycin, streptozocin, teniposide, ticarcillin, tobramycin, vancomycin, vinBLAStine, vinCRIStine, zidovudine

ADVERSE EFFECTS

CNS: Paresthesias, peripheral neuropathy, depression, headache, **seizures**, weakness, jaw pain, asthenia
CV: Chest pain
GI: *Nausea, vomiting,* ileus, *anorexia, stomatitis,* constipation, abdominal pain, *diarrhea,* **hepatotoxicity, GI obstruction/ perforation**
HEMA: **Neutropenia, anemia, thrombocytopenia, granulocytopenia**
INTEG: *Rash, alopecia,* photosensitivity, inj site reaction, necrosis
META: Syndrome of inappropriate diuretic hormone
MS: Myalgia
RESP: Shortness of breath

Pharmacokinetics

Absorption	Poor bioavailability (<50%)
Distribution	Highly bound to platelets, lymphocytes
Metabolism	Liver, to metabolite
Excretion	Bile
Half-life	43 hr

Pharmacodynamics

Onset	Unknown
Peak	1-2 hr
Duration	Unknown

INTERACTIONS
Drug classifications
NSAIDs, anticoagulants: increased bleeding risk
CYP3A4 inhibitors (antiretroviral protease inhibitors, aprepitant, clarithromycin, danazol, delavirdine, diltiazem, erythromycin, fluconazole, FLUoxetine, fluvoxamine, imatinib, ketoconazole, mibefradil, nefazodone, telithromycin, voriconazole): increased toxicity
CYP3A4 inducers (barbiturates, bosentan, carBAMazepine, efavirenz, phenytoins, nevirapine, rifabutin, rifampin): decreased vinorelbine effect

Drug/herb
• St. John's wort: avoid use

NURSING CONSIDERATIONS
Assessment
• Monitor B/P (baseline and q15min) during administration

> **BLACK BOX WARNING:** Monitor CBC, differential, platelet count before each dose; withhold product if WBC is <4000/mm³ or platelet count is <75,000/mm³; notify prescriber of results; recovery will take 3 wk; liver function tests: AST, ALT, bilirubin, LDH

• Assess for dyspnea, crackles, unproductive cough, chest pain, tachypnea
• Monitor renal function tests: BUN, serum uric acid, urine CCr before, during therapy, I&O ratio; report fall in urine output of 30 ml/hr; for decreased hyperuricemia
• Monitor for cold, fever, sore throat (may indicate beginning **infection**); notify prescriber if these occur; effects of alopecia on body image
• **Assess for bleeding:** hematuria, guaiac, bruising or petechiae, mucosa or orifices q8hr: no rectal temp; avoid IM inj; use pressure on venipuncture sites
• Identify nutritional status: an antiemetic may need to be prescribed
• **Assess for symptoms indicating severe allergic reactions:** rash, pruritus, urticaria, itching, flushing, bronchospasm, hypotension; epinephrine and resuscitative equipment should be nearby

• Assess neurologic status: numbness, pain, tingling, loss of Achilles reflex, weakness, palsies
• **Assess for gout:** pain, swelling, increased uric acid levels

Nursing diagnoses
• Body image, disturbed (adverse reactions)
• Infection, risk for (adverse reactions)
• Injury, risk for (adverse reactions)
• Knowledge, deficient (teaching)

Patient/family education
• Teach patient to use liquid diet: cola, gelatin; dry toast or crackers may be added if patient is not nauseated or vomiting
• Advise patient to rinse mouth 3-4 ×/day with water and brush teeth 2-3 ×/day with soft brush or cotton-tipped applicators for stomatitis; use unwaxed dental floss
• Advise patient to avoid crowds, people with infections, vaccinations
• Advise patient to use effective contraception during and for ≥2 mo after product is discontinued; pregnancy **D,** avoid breastfeeding
• Teach patient hair may be lost but will grow back; new hair may be different texture, color

Evaluation
Positive therapeutic outcome
• Decreased spread of malignant cells

vitamin A (PO, OTC; IM, Rx)
Aquasol A, Del-Vi-A, Vitamin A
Func. class.: Vitamin, fat-soluble
Chem. class.: Retinol
Pregnancy category C (PO); X (parenteral)

ACTION: Needed for normal bone and tooth development, visual dark adaptation, skin disease, mucosa tissue repair; assists in production of adrenal steroids, cholesterol, RNA

Therapeutic outcome: Prevention, absence of vit A deficiency

USES: Vit A deficiency

CONTRAINDICATIONS:
Pregnancy **X** (parenteral), hypersensitivity to vit A, malabsorption syndrome (PO), hypervitaminosis A, parenteral, **IV** administration

Precautions: Pregnancy **C** (PO), breastfeeding, impaired renal function, children, hepatic disease, infants, alcoholism, hepatitis

DOSAGE AND ROUTES
Adult and child >8 yr: PO 100,000-500,000 international units/day × 3 days, then 50,000 international units/day × 2 wk; dose based on severity of deficiency; maintenance 10,000-20,000 international units for 2 mo
Child 1-8 yr: IM 5000-15,000 international units/day × 10 days
Infant <1 yr: IM 5000-15,000 international units × 10 days

Maintenance
Child 4-8 yr: IM 15,000 international units/day × 2 mo
Child <4 yr: IM 10,000 international units/day × 2 mo

Available forms: Caps 10,000, 25,000, 50,000 international units; drops 5000 international units; inj 50,000 international units/ml; tabs 10,000, 25,000, 50,000 international units

Implementation
PO route
• Give with food (PO) for better absorption; do not give **IV** because anaphylaxis may occur, IM only
• Oral preparations are not indicated for vit A deficiency in those with malabsorption syndrome
• Store in airtight, light-resistant container
IM route
• Give deep in large muscle mass; do not use deltoid muscle for administration of >1 ml

ADVERSE EFFECTS
CNS: Headache, increased ICP, intracranial hypertension, lethargy, malaise
EENT: Gingivitis, papilledema, exophthalmos, inflammation of tongue and lips
GI: Nausea, vomiting, anorexia, abdominal pain, *jaundice*
INTEG: Drying of skin, pruritus, increased pigmentation, night sweats, alopecia
META: Hypomenorrhea, hypercalcemia
MS: Arthralgia, retarded growth, hard areas on bone

Pharmacokinetics

Absorption	Rapidly absorbed
Distribution	Stored in liver, kidneys, lungs
Metabolism	Liver
Excretion	Breast milk
Half-life	Unknown

V

Adverse effects: *italics* = common; **bold** = life-threatening

Pharmacodynamics

Unknown

INTERACTIONS

Individual drugs

Cholestyramine, colestipol, mineral oil: decreased absorption of vit A

Drug classifications

Contraceptives (oral), corticosteroids: increased levels of vit A

Drug/lab test

False increase: bilirubin, serum cholesterol

NURSING CONSIDERATIONS

Assessment

• Assess nutritional status: increase intake of yellow and dark green vegetables, yellow/orange fruits, vit A–fortified foods, liver, egg yolks
• Assess vit A deficiency: decreased growth; night blindness; dry, brittle nails; hair loss; urinary stones; increased infection; hyperkeratosis of skin; drying of cornea
• Identify vit A deficiency by plasma vit A, carotene level
• Assess for chronic vit A toxicity: increased calcium, BUN, glucose, cholesterol, triglyceride level

Nursing diagnoses

• Knowledge, deficient (teaching)
• Nutrition, less than body requirements, imbalanced (uses)

Patient/family education

• Instruct patient that if dose is missed, it should be omitted
• Inform patient that ophth exams may be required periodically throughout therapy
• Instruct patient not to use mineral oil while taking this product because absorption will be decreased
• Advise patient to notify prescriber of nausea, vomiting, lip cracking, loss of hair, headache
• Caution patient not to take more than the prescribed amount

Evaluation
Positive therapeutic outcome

• Increase in growth rate, weight
• Absence of dry skin and mucous membranes, night blindness

TREATMENT OF OVERDOSE:

Discontinue product

vitamin A acid
See tretinoin

vitamin B₁
See thiamine

(vitamin B₁₂) cyanocobalamin (PO, OTC; IM/SUBCUT, Rx)
(sye-an-oh-koe-bal′a-min)
Alphamin ✦, Anacobin ✦, Bedoz ✦, Cobex, Cobolin-M Crystamine, Crysti-1000, Cyanabin ✦, Cyanoject, Cyomin, Ener-B, Hydrobexan, Hydro Cobex, Hydro-Crysti-12
Func. class.: Vitamin B₁₂, water-soluble vitamin

(vitamin B₁₂a) hydroxocobalamin (vit B₁₂) (Rx)
(hye-drox′-o-ko-bal′-a-min)
Hydro Cobex, Hydroxycobal, LA-12, Nascobal, Neuroforter, Rubesol-1000, Rubramin PC, Shovite, Vibral LA, Vibral, Vitamin B₁₂
Pregnancy category A

ACTION: Needed for adequate nerve functioning, protein and carbohydrate metabolism, normal growth, RBC development and cell reproduction

Therapeutic outcome: Prevention, correction of vit B₁₂ deficiency

USES: Vit B₁₂ deficiency; pernicious anemia; vit B₁₂ malabsorption syndrome; Schilling test; increased requirements with pregnancy, thyrotoxicosis, hemolytic anemia, hemorrhage, renal and hepatic disease

CONTRAINDICATIONS:

Hypersensitivity, optic nerve atrophy

Precautions: Pregnancy **A,** breastfeeding, children

DOSAGE AND ROUTES

Cyanocobalamin
Adult: PO up to 1000 mcg/day; SUBCUT/IM 30-100 mcg/day × 1 wk, then 100-200 mcg/mo

Shilling test
Adult and child: IM 1000 mcg in 1 dose

⚠ Nurse Alert

Child: PO up to 1000 mcg/day; SUBCUT/IM 30-50 mcg/day × 2 wk, then 100 mcg/mo; NASAL 500 mcg qwk

Hydroxocobalamin
Adult: SUBCUT/IM 30-50 mcg/day × 5-10 days, then 100-200 mcg/mo
Child: SUBCUT/IM 30-50 mcg/day × 5-10 days, then 30-50 mcg/mo

Available forms: Cyanocobalamin: tabs 25, 50, 100, 250, 500, 1000, 5000 mcg; ext rel tabs 100, 200, 500, 1000 mcg; lozenges: 100, 250, 500 mcg; nasal gel 500 mcg/spray; inj 100, 1000 mcg/ml; hydroxocobalamin: inj 1000 mcg/ml

Implementation
PO route
• Give with fruit juice to disguise taste; administer immediately after mixing
• Give with meals if possible for better absorption; large doses should not be used because most is excreted
IM route
• Give by IM inj for pernicious anemia for life unless contraindicated
IV route
• May be mixed with TPN sol, but **IV** route is not recommended

Y-site compatibilities: Heparin, hydrocortisone sodium succinate, potassium chloride

Solution compatibilities: Dextrose/Ringer's or LR's combinations, dextrose/saline combinations, D₅W, D₁₀W, 0.45% NaCl, Ringer's or LR's sol, ascorbic acid

ADVERSE EFFECTS
CNS: Flushing, optic nerve atrophy
CV: **CHF,** peripheral vascular thrombosis, **pulmonary edema**
GI: *Diarrhea*
INTEG: Itching, rash, pain at inj site
META: Hypokalemia
SYST: **Anaphylactic shock**

Pharmacokinetics

Absorption	Well absorbed (IM, SUBCUT)
Distribution	Crosses placenta
Metabolism	Stored in liver, kidney, stomach
Excretion	50%-90% (urine), breast milk
Half-life	Unknown

Pharmacodynamics
Unknown

INTERACTIONS
Individual drugs
Aminosalicylic acid, chloramphenicol, cimetidine, colchicine: decreased absorption
PredniSONE: increased absorption

Drug classifications
Aminoglycosides, anticonvulsants, potassium products: decreased absorption

Drug/herb
Goldenseal: decreased vit B₁₂ absorption

Drug/lab test
False positive: intrinsic factor

NURSING CONSIDERATIONS
Assessment
• Assess for deficiency: anorexia, dyspepsia on exertion, palpitations, paresthesias, psychosis, visual disturbances, pallor, red inflamed tongue, neuropathy, edema of legs
• Monitor potassium levels during beginning treatment in patients with megaloblastic anemia
• Monitor CBC for increase in reticulocyte count during 1st wk of therapy, then increase in RBC and hemoglobin; folic acid levels, vit B₁₂ levels
• Assess nutritional status: egg yolks, fish, organ meats, dairy products, clams, oysters, which are good sources of vit B₁₂
• Monitor for pulmonary edema or worsening of CHF in cardiac patients

Nursing diagnoses
• Knowledge, deficient (teaching)
• Noncompliance (teaching) (overuse)
• Nutrition, less than body requirements, imbalanced (uses)

Patient/family education
• Instruct patient that treatment must continue for life if diagnosed as having pernicious anemia
• Advise patient to eat well-balanced diet from the food pyramid and comply with dietary recommendation
• Caution patient not to exceed the RDA of vit B₁₂ because adverse reactions may occur

Evaluation
Positive therapeutic outcome
• Decreased anorexia, dyspnea on exertion, palpitations, paresthesias, psychosis, visual disturbances, edema of legs
• Prevention or correction of vit B₁₂ deficiency

V

TREATMENT OF OVERDOSE:
Discontinue products

---

vitamin D (cholecalciferol, vitamin D₃ or ergocalciferol, vitamin D₂) (Rx, OTC)
Calciferol, Delta-D, Drisdol, Radiostol ✹, Radiostol Forte ✹, vitamin D, vitamin D₃
Func. class.: Vitamin D
Chem. class.: Fat-soluble vitamin
Pregnancy category C

Do not confuse:
Calciferol/calcitriol

ACTION: Needed for regulation of calcium, phosphate levels; normal bone development; parathyroid activity; neuromuscular functioning

Therapeutic outcome: Prevention of rickets, osteomalacia, normal calcium/phosphate levels

USES: Vit D deficiency, rickets, renal osteodystrophy, hypoparathyroidism, hypophosphatemia, psoriasis, rheumatoid arthritis

CONTRAINDICATIONS:
Hypersensitivity, hypercalcemia, renal dysfunction, hyperphosphatemia

Precautions: Pregnancy C, CV disease, renal calculi

DOSAGE AND ROUTES
Deficiency
Adult: PO/IM 12,000 international units/day, then increased to 500,000 international units/day
Child: PO/IM 1500-5000 international units/day × 2-4 wk, may repeat after 2 wk or 600,000 international units as single dose

Hypoparathyroidism
Adult and child: PO/IM 200,000 international units given with 4 g calcium tab

Available forms: Tabs 400, 1000, 50,000 international units; caps 25,000, 50,000 international units; oral sol 8000 international units/ml; inj 500,000 international units/ml, 500,000 international units/5 ml

Implementation
PO route
• PO may be increased q4wk depending on blood level

• Store in airtight, light-resistant container at room temperature
IM route
• Give inj deeply in large muscle mass, administer slowly, aspirate to avoid **IV** administration, rotate inj site

ADVERSE EFFECTS
CNS: Fatigue, weakness, drowsiness, **seizures,** headache, psychosis
CV: Hypertension, dysrhythmias
GI: Nausea, vomiting, anorexia, cramps, diarrhea, constipation, metallic taste, dry mouth
GU: Polyuria, nocturia, **hematuria, albuminuria, renal failure,** decreased libido
INTEG: Pruritus, photophobia
MS: Decreased bone growth, early joint pain, early muscle pain

Pharmacokinetics

Absorption	Well absorbed
Distribution	Stored in liver
Metabolism	Liver, sun
Excretion	Bile, kidney
Half-life	12-22 hr

Pharmacodynamics

	PO	IM
Onset	Unknown	Unknown
Peak	4 hr	Unknown
Duration	15-20 days	Unknown

INTERACTIONS
Individual drugs
Cholestyramine, colestipol, PHENobarbital, phenytoin: decreased effects of vit D
Verapamil: increased toxicity

Drug classifications
Antacids, diuretics (thiazide): increased toxicity

NURSING CONSIDERATIONS
Assessment
• Monitor BUN, urinary calcium, AST, ALT, cholesterol, creatinine, uric acid, chloride, magnesium, electrolytes, urine pH, phosphate—may increase; calcium should be kept at 9-10 mg/dl; vit D at 50-135 international units/dl, phosphate at 70 mg/dl; alkaline phosphatase may be decreased
• Monitor for increased blood level; toxic reactions may occur rapidly
• Assess for dry mouth, metallic taste, polyuria, bone pain, muscle weakness, headache, fatigue, tinnitus, change in LOC, irregular pulse, dysrhythmias, increased respirations, anorexia,

⚠ Nurse Alert

nausea, vomiting, cramps, diarrhea, constipation; may indicate hypercalcemia

• Assess renal status: decreased urinary output (oliguria, anuria), edema in extremities, weight gain ≥5 lb, periorbital edema

• Assess nutritional status, diet for sources of vit D (milk, cod, halibut, salmon, sardines, egg yolk), calcium (dairy products, dark green vegetables), phosphates (dairy products)

Nursing diagnoses
• Knowledge, deficient (teaching)
• Nutrition, less than body requirements, imbalanced (uses)

Patient/family education
• Advise patient to omit dose if missed; to avoid vitamin supplements unless directed by prescriber
• Inform patient of necessary foods to be included in diet
• Advise patient to keep appointments for evaluation because therapeutic and toxic levels are narrow
• Instruct patient to report weakness, lethargy, headache, anorexia, loss of weight; to report nausea, vomiting, abdominal cramps, diarrhea, constipation, excessive thirst, polyuria, muscle and bone pain
• Caution patient to decrease intake of antacids and laxatives containing magnesium

Evaluation
Positive therapeutic outcome
• Calcium levels 9-10 ml/dl
• Decreasing symptoms of bone disease

---

vitamin E (OTC)
Amino-Opti-E, Aquasol E, Daltose ✦, E-Complex-600, E-Ferol, E-Vitamin Succinate, E-200 I.U. Softgels, Gordo-Vite E, Tocopherol, Vita-Plus E Softgels, Vitec
Func. class.: Vitamin E
Chem. class.: Fat-soluble vitamin
Pregnancy category A

ACTION: Needed for digestion and metabolism of polyunsaturated fats, decreases platelet aggregation, decreases blood clot formation, promotes normal growth and development of muscle tissue, prostaglandin synthesis

Therapeutic outcome: Prevention and treatment of vit E deficiency

USES: Vit E deficiency, impaired fat absorption, hemolytic anemia in premature neonates,

prevention of retrolental fibroplasia, sickle cell anemia, supplement in malabsorption syndrome

CONTRAINDICATIONS:
IV use in infants

Precautions: Pregnancy **A,** anemia, breastfeeding, hypothrombinemia

DOSAGE AND ROUTES
Deficiency
Adult: PO 60-75 international units/day
Child: PO 1 international unit/kg (malabsorption)

Prevention of deficiency
Adult: PO 30 international units/day
Infant: PO 5 international units/day

Topical route
Adult and child: TOP apply to affected areas as needed

Available forms: Caps 100, 200, 400, 500, 600, 1000 international units; tabs 100, 200, 400 international units; drops 50 mg/ml; chew tabs 400 units; ointment, cream, lotion, oil

Implementation
PO route
• Chew chewable tabs well
• Sol may be dropped in mouth or mixed with food
• Store in airtight, light-resistant container
Topical route
• Apply topical to moisturize dry skin

ADVERSE EFFECTS
CNS: Headache, fatigue
CV: Increased risk of thrombophlebitis
EENT: Blurred vision
GI: Nausea, cramps, diarrhea
GU: Gonadal dysfunction
INTEG: Sterile abscess, contact dermatitis
META: Altered metabolism of hormones (thyroid, pituitary, adrenal), altered immunity
MS: Weakness

Pharmacokinetics

Absorption	20%-80% (PO)
Distribution	Widely distributed, stored in fat
Metabolism	Liver
Excretion	Bile
Half-life	Unknown

Adverse effects: *italics* = common; **bold** = life-threatening

Pharmacodynamics
Unknown

INTERACTIONS

Individual drugs
Cholestyramine, colestipol, mineral oil, sucralfate: decreased absorption

Drug classification
Anticoagulants (oral): increased action of anticoagulants

NURSING CONSIDERATIONS

Assessment
• Assess nutritional status: intake of wheat germ, dark green leafy vegetables, nuts, eggs, liver, vegetable oils, dairy products, cereals
• Assess for vit E deficiency (usually in neonates): irritability, restlessness, hemolytic anemia

Nursing diagnoses
• Knowledge, deficient (teaching)
• Nutrition, less than body requirements, imbalanced (uses)

Patient/family education
• Inform patient necessary foods to be included in diet high in vit E
• Instruct patient to omit if dose is missed
• Instruct patient to avoid vit supplements unless directed by prescriber because overdose may occur

Evaluation
Positive therapeutic outcome
• Absence of hemolytic anemia
• Adequate vit E levels
• Improvement in skin lesions
• Decrease in edema

---

voriconazole (Rx)
(vohr-i-kahn'a-zol)
Vfend
Func. class.: Antifungal
Pregnancy category D

ACTION: Inhibits fungal CYP 450-mediation demethylation, needed for biosynthesis, causing leakage from cell membrane

Therapeutic outcome: Decreasing signs, symptoms of infection

USES: Invasive aspergillosis, serious fungal infections (*Candida* sp., *Scedosporium apiospermum, Fusarium* sp.), *Monosportum, Apiospermum*

CONTRAINDICATIONS:
Pregnancy **D**, breastfeeding, children, hypersensitivity, severe bone marrow depression, severe hepatic disease

Precautions: Renal disease (**IV**); Asian/African descent, cardiomyopathy, cholestasis, chemotherapy, lactase deficiency, visual disturbances, renal failure, pancreatitis, QT prolongation, hypokalemia, ventricular dysrhythmias, torsades de pointes

DOSAGE AND ROUTES
Adult/geriatric/child ≥12 yr: PO give 1 hr before or after meals; ≥40 kg, loading dose 400 mg q12hr on day 1, then 200 mg q12hr; <40 kg, loading dose 200 mg q12hr on day 1, then 100 mg q12hr
Adult/geriatric/child ≥12 yr: IV loading dose 6 mg/kg q12hr × 2 dose, then 4 mg/kg q12hr; may switch to oral dosing

Renal dose
Adult: PO CCr <50 ml/min, use only orally

Hepatic dose
Adult: PO 6 mg/kg q12hr × 2 doses, then 2 mg/kg q12hr or 100 mg q12hr if ≥40 kg; 50 mg q12hr if <40 kg

Available forms: Tabs 50, 200 mg; powder for inj, lyophilized 200 mg voriconazole, powder for oral susp 45 g (40 mg/ml after reconstitution)

Implementation
• Give 1 hr before or after meals
• Store at room temperature (powder, tabs)

Intermittent IV infusion route
• Give product only after C&S confirms organism, product needed to treat condition; make sure product is used in life-threatening infections
• Reconstitute powder with 19 ml water for inj to 10 mg/ml, shake until dissolved; infuse over 1-2 hr at a conc of 5 mg/ml or less; do not admix with other products, 4.2% sodium bicarbonate inf

Y-site compatibilities: Acyclovir, alfentanil, allopurinol, amifostine, amikacin, aminocaproic acid, aminophylline, amiodarone, amphotericin B liposome, ampicillin, ampicillin/sulbactam, anidulafungin, azithromycin, aztreonam, bivalirudin, bleomycin, bumetanide, buprenorphine, butorphanol, calcium acetate/chloride/gluconate, CARBOplatin, carmustine, caspofungin, ceFAZolin, cefotaxime, cefotetan, cefoxitin, ceftazidime, ceftizoxime, cefTRIAXone, chloramphenicol, chlorproMAZINE,

⚠ Nurse Alert

cimetidine, ciprofloxacin, cisatracurium, CISplatin, clindamycin, cyclophosphamide, cytarabine, dacarbazine, DACTINomycin, DAPTOmycin, DAUNOrubicin, dexamethasone, dexmedetomidine, dexrazoxane, digoxin, diltiazem, diphenhydrAMINE, DOBUTamine, docetaxel, dolasetron, DOPamine, doripenem, doxacurium, doxycycline, droperidol, enalaprilat, ePHEDrine, EPINEPHrine, epirubicin, ertapenem, erythromycin, esmolol, etoposide, etoposide phosphate, famotidine, fenoldopam, fentaNYL, fluconazole, fludarabine, fluorouracil, foscarnet, fosphenytoin, furosemide, ganciclovir, gemcitabine, gentamicin, glycopyrrolate, granisetron, haloperidol, heparin, hydrALAZINE, hydrocortisone, ifosfamide, imipenem/cilastatin, inamrinone, insulin, irinotecan, isoproterenol, ketorolac, labetalol, leucovorin, levofloxacin, lidocaine, linezolid, LORazepam, magnesium sulfate, mannitol, mechlorethamine, melphalan, meperidine, meropenem, mesna, metaraminol, methohexital, methotrexate, methyldopa, methylPREDNISolone, metoclopramide, metoprolol, metroNIDAZOLE, midazolam, milrinone, mitomycin, morphine, nafcillin, nalbuphine, naloxone, niCARdipine, nitroglycerin, norepinephrine, octreotide, ondansetron, oxaliplatin, oxytocin, paclitaxel, palonosetron, pancuronium, pentamidine, pentazocine, PENTobarbital, PHENobarbital, phentolamine, phenylephrine, piperacillin/tazobactam, potassium chloride/ phosphates, procainamide, promethazine, propranolol, quinupristin/dalfopristin, remifentanil, rocuronium, sodium acetate/bicarbonate/ phosphates, streptozocin, succinylcholine, SUFentanil, tacrolimus, teniposide, theophylline, thiotepa, ticarcillin/clavulanate, tirofiban, tobramycin, topotecan, trimethobenzamide, trimethoprim/sulfamethoxazole, vancomycin, vasopressin, vecuronium, verapamil, vinBLAStine, vinCRIStine, vinorelbine, zidovudine

Y-site incompatibilities: Amphotericin B colloidal, busulfan, cefepime, cyclopSPORINE, dantrolene, diazepam, DOXOrubicin, IDArubicin, mitoxantrone, nitroprusside, pantoprazole, phenytoin, thiopental

ADVERSE EFFECTS

CNS: *Headache,* paresthesias, peripheral neuropathy, hallucinations, psychosis, EPS, depression, Guillain-Barré syndrome, insomnia, **suicidal ideation,** dizziness
CV: **Tachycardia,** hyper/hypotension, vasodilatation, **atrial dysrhythmias, atrial fibrillation, AV block, bradycardia, CHF, MI, QT prolongation, torsades de pointes**

EENT: Blurred vision, eye hemorrhage
INTEG: *Burning, irritation,* pain, necrosis at inj site with extravasation, dermatitis, rash, photosensitivity
GI: *Nausea, vomiting, anorexia,* diarrhea, cramps, **hemorrhagic gastroenteritis, acute liver failure, hepatitis, intestinal perforation, pancreatitis**
GU: *Hypokalemia,* azotemia, **renal tubular necrosis, permanent renal impairment, anuria, oliguria**
HEMA: Anemia, **eosinophilia,** hypomagnesemia, **thrombocytopenia, leukopenia, pancytopenia**
MISC: Respiratory disorder
SYST: **Stevens-Johnson syndrome, toxic epidermal necrolysis, sepsis, melanoma (photosensitivity reaction)**

Pharmacokinetics

Absorption	Unknown
Distribution	Protein binding 58%
Metabolism	CYP3A4/CYP2C9
Excretion	Via hepatic metabolism
Half-life	Elimination 6 hr (dose dependent)

Pharmacodynamics

Onset	Unknown
Peak	1-2 hr
Duration	Unknown

INTERACTIONS

Individual drugs

CISplatin, cycloSPORINE, polymyxin B, vancomycin: increased nephrotoxicity
CycloSPORINE, phenytoin, pimozide, prednisoLONE, quiNIDine, rifabutin, sirolimus, tacrolimus, warfarin: increased effects of each specific product
Digoxin: increased hypokalemia
Haloperidol, chloroquine, droperidol, pentamidine; arsenic trioxide, levomethadyl: increased QT prolongation

Drug classifications

Aminoglycosides: increased nephrotoxicity
Benzodiazepines, calcium channel blockers, ergots, HMG-CoA reductase inhibitors, nonnucleoside reverse transcriptase inhibitors, protease inhibitors, proton pump inhibitors, sulfonylureas, vinca alkaloids: increased effects of each specific product
Class IA/III antidysrhythmics, some phenothiazines, beta agonists, local anesthetics, tricyclics, CYP3A4 inhibitors (amiodarone,

V

clarithromycin, erythromycin, telithromycin, troleandomycin); CYP3A4 substrates (methadone, pimozide, QUEtiapine, quiNIDine, risperidone, ziprasidone): increased QT prolongation

Corticosteroids, diuretics (thiazide), skeletal muscle relaxants: increased hypokalemia

Drug/herb

St. John's wort: do not use together

Drug/food

High-fat foods: avoid use with high-fat meals, take 1 hr before or after a meal

NURSING CONSIDERATIONS

Assessment

• Monitor VS q15-30min during first inf; note changes in pulse, B/P

• Monitor I&O ratio; watch for decreasing urinary output, change in specific gravity; discontinue product to prevent permanent damage to renal tubules

• Monitor blood tests: CBC, K, Na, Ca, Mg q2wk; BUN, creatinine weekly

• Monitor weight weekly; if weight increases >2 lb/wk, edema is present; renal damage should be considered

⚠ Assess for renal toxicity: increasing BUN, serum creatinine; if BUN is >40 mg/dl or if serum creatinine >3 mg/dl, product may be discontinued or dosage reduced

⚠ Assess for hepatotoxicity: increasing AST, ALT, alkaline phosphatase, bilirubin

• Assess for allergic reaction: dermatitis, rash; product should be discontinued, antihistamines (mild reaction) or epinephrine (severe reaction) administered

• Assess for hypokalemia: anorexia, drowsiness, weakness, decreased reflexes, dizziness, increased urinary output, increased thirst, paresthesias

• Assess for ototoxicity: tinnitus (ringing, roaring in ears), vertigo, loss of hearing (rare)

• QT prolongation: ECG for QT prolongation, ejection fraction; assess for chest pain, palpitations, dyspnea

Nursing diagnoses

• Infection, risk for (uses)
• Injury, risk for (uses, adverse reactions)
• Knowledge, deficient (teaching)

Patient/family education

• Teach that long-term therapy may be needed to clear infection (2 wk-3 mo depending on type of infection)

• Advise patient to notify prescriber of bleeding, bruising, or soft tissue swelling

• Teach to take 1 hr before or after meal
• Advise patient not to drive at night because of vision changes
• Advise to avoid strong, direct sunlight
• Advise women of childbearing age to use effective contraceptive

Evaluation

Positive therapeutic outcome

• Decreased fever, malaise, rash, negative C&S for infecting organism

---

⚠ HIGH ALERT

warfarin (Rx)

(war'far-in)

Coumadin, Jantoven

Func. class.: Anticoagulant

Pregnancy category X

Do not confuse:
Coumadin/Cardura/Compazine

ACTION: Interferes with blood clotting by indirect means; depresses hepatic synthesis of vit K–dependent coagulation factors (II, VII, IX, X)

Therapeutic outcome: Prevention of clotting

USES: Antiphospholipid antibody syndrome, arterial thromboembolism prophylaxis, deep vein thrombosis, MI prophylaxis, post MI, stroke prophylaxis, thrombosis prophylaxis

CONTRAINDICATIONS:

Pregnancy **X,** breastfeeding, hypersensitivity, hemophilia, leukemia with bleeding, peptic ulcer disease, thrombocytopenic purpura, hepatic disease (severe), malignant hypertension, subacute bacterial endocarditis, acute nephritis, blood dyscrasias, preeclampsia, eclampsia, hemorrhagic tendencies, surgery of CNS, eye, traumatic surgery with large open surface, bleeding tendencies of GI/GU/respiratory, stroke, aneurysms, pericardial effusion, spinal puncture, major regional/lumbar block anesthesia

BLACK BOX WARNING: Bleeding

Precautions: Alcoholism, geriatric, CHF, debilitated patients, trauma, indwelling catheters, severe hypertension, active infections, protein C deficiency, polycythemia vera, vasculitis, severe diabetes, Asian patients (CYP2C9, VKORC1)

⚠ Nurse Alert

DOSAGE AND ROUTES
Adult: PO/IV 2.5-10 mg/day × 3 days, then titrated to INR/pro-time
Adolescent/child/infant: PO/IV 0.2 mg/kg/day titrated to INR

Available forms: Tabs 1, 2, 2.5, 3, 4, 5, 6, 7.5, 10 mg; 5.4 mg powder for inj

Implementation
PO route
• Warfarin is usually given with **IV** heparin for 3 or more days, warfarin blood level may take several days

Direct IV route
• Reconstitute with 2.7 ml of sterile water for inj; do not use solution that is discolored or has particulates
• Give over 1-2 min into peripheral vein

Y-site compatibilities: CeFAZolin, cefTRIAXone, DOPamine, heparin, lidocaine, morphine, nitroglycerin, potassium chloride, ranitidine

ADVERSE EFFECTS
CNS: *Fever,* dizziness, fatigue, headache, lethargy
CV: Angina, chest pain, edema, hypotension, syncope
GI: *Diarrhea,* nausea, vomiting, anorexia, stomatitis, cramps, **hepatitis,** cholestatic jaundice
GU: **Hematuria**
HEMA: **Hemorrhage, agranulocytosis, leukopenia, eosinophilia,** ecchymosis, anemia, petechiae
INTEG: *Rash,* dermatitis, urticaria, alopecia, pruritus
MISC: Epistaxis, hemoptysis, mouth ulcers, taste disturbances, priapism, dyspnea
MS: Bone fractures
SYST: **Anaphylaxis,** coma, cholesterol, microembolisms, **exfoliative dermatitis, purple toe syndrome**

Pharmacokinetics
Absorption	Well absorbed (PO), completely absorbed
Distribution	Crosses placenta, 99% plasma protein binding
Metabolism	Liver
Excretion	Kidney, feces (active, inactive metabolites)
Half-life	Effective $^1/_2$-2$^1/_2$ days

Pharmacodynamics
	PO
Onset	12-24 hr
Peak	$^1/_2$-4 days
Duration	3-5 days

INTERACTIONS
Individual drugs
Allopurinol, amiodarone, chloral hydrate, chloramphenicol, cimetidine, clofibrate, clotrimoxazole, dextrothyroxine, diflunisal, disulfiram, erythromycin, furosemide, glucagon, heparin, indomethacin, isoniazid, mefenamic acid, metroNIDAZOLE, mifepristone, phenylbutazone, quiNIDine, RU-486, sulfinpyrazone, sulindac, thyroid: increased warfarin action
Aprepitant, azoTHIOprine, bosentan, carBAMazepine, dicloxacillin, ethchlorvynol, factor IX/VIIa, griseofulvin, nafcillin, phenytoin, rifampin, sucralfate, sulfasalazine, thyroid, vitamin K: decreased warfarin action
Phenytoin: increased toxicity

Drug classifications
Antidepressants (tricyclic), ethacrynic acids, HMG-CoA reductase inhibitors, NSAIDs, oxyphenbutazones, COX-2 selective inhibitors, penicillins, quinolones, salicylates, selective serotonin reuptake inhibitors, steroids, sulfonamides, thrombolytics: increased warfarin action
Barbiturates, bile acid sequestrants, contraceptives (oral), estrogens: decreased warfarin action
Sulfonylureas (oral): increased toxicity

Drug/herb
Angelica, anise, basil, chamomile, chondroitin, dong quai, evening primrose, feverfew, garlic, ginger, ginkgo, ginseng, horse chestnut, kava, licorice, melatonin, red yeast rice, saw palmetto: increased risk of bleeding
Coenzyme Q10, St. John's wort: decreased anticoagulant effect

Drug/food
Vit K foods: decreased warfarin action

Drug/lab test
Increased: T_3 uptake, liver function tests
Decreased: uric acid

W

Adverse effects: *italics* = common; **bold** = life-threatening

NURSING CONSIDERATIONS
Assessment

> **BLACK BOX WARNING:** Monitor blood studies (Hct, PT, platelets, occult blood in stools) q3mo; INR: in hospital daily after 2nd or 3rd dose; once in therapeutic range for 2 consecutive days, monitor 2-3× wk for 1-2 wk, then less frequently depending on stability of INR results; *Outpatient:* monitor every few days until stable dose, then periodically thereafter depending on stability of INR results

> **BLACK BOX WARNING:** Assess for bleeding gums, petechiae, ecchymosis, black tarry stools, hematuria; fatal hemorrhage can occur

• Monitor B/P, watch for increasing signs of hypertension
• Assess for fever, skin rash, urticaria
• Assess for needed dosage change q1-2wk

Nursing diagnoses
• Injury, risk for (uses, adverse reactions)
• Knowledge, deficient (teaching)
• Tissue perfusion, ineffective (uses)

Patient/family education
• Caution patient to avoid OTC preparations unless directed by prescriber; may cause serious product interactions
• Advise patient that product may be withheld during active bleeding (menstruation), depending on condition
• Advise patient to use soft-bristle toothbrush to avoid bleeding gums, avoid contact sports, use electric razor, avoid IM inj
• Instruct patient to carry/wear emergency ID identifying product taken
• Advise patient to report any signs of bleeding: gums, under skin, urine, stools
• Teach patient to read food labels; limited intake of vit K foods (green leafy vegetables) is necessary to maintain consistent prothrombin levels

Evaluation
Positive therapeutic outcome
• Decrease of deep vein thrombosis
• Pro-time (1.3-2.0 × control)

xylometazoline nasal agent
See Appendix B

zafirlukast (Rx)
(za-feer'loo-cast)
Accolate
Func. class.: Bronchodilator
Chem. class.: Leukotriene receptor antagonist
Pregnancy category B

ACTION: Antagonizes the contractile action of leukotrienes (LTC_4, LTD_4, LTE_4) in airway smooth muscle; inhibits bronchoconstriction caused by antigens

Therapeutic outcome: Ability to breathe more easily

USES: Prophylaxis and chronic treatment of asthma in adults/children >5 yr

CONTRAINDICATIONS: Hypersensitivity, hepatic disease, hepatic encephalopathy

Precautions: Pregnancy **B,** breastfeeding, children, geriatric, hepatic disease, Churg-Strauss syndrome, acute bronchospasm

DOSAGE AND ROUTES
Adult and child ≥12 yr: PO 20 mg bid, take 1 hr before or 2 hr after meals
Child 5-11 yr: PO 10 mg bid

Available forms: Tabs 10, 20 mg

Implementation
• Give PO 1 hr before or 2 hr after meals; absorption may be decreased if given with food
• Give with 8 oz of water if GI upset occurs

ADVERSE EFFECTS
CNS: Headache, dizziness, **suicidal ideation,** fever, insomnia
GI: Nausea, diarrhea, abdominal pain, vomiting, dyspepsia, **hepatic failure, hepatitis**
HEMA: **Agranulocytosis**
MISC: Infections, pain, asthenia, myalgia, fever, increased ALT, urticaria, rash, **angioedema**

Pharmacokinetics

Absorption	Rapidly absorbed
Distribution	Unknown
Metabolism	Extensively by CYP2C9, CYP3A4 enzyme systems, protein binding (99%)
Excretion	Feces
Half-life	10 hr

Pharmacodynamics

Onset	Unknown
Peak	3 hr
Duration	Unknown

INTERACTIONS

Individual drugs
Aspirin: increased plasma levels of zafirlukast
Erythromycin, theophylline: decreased plasma levels of zafirlukast
Warfarin: increased pro-time

Drug classifications
CYP3A4 metabolizers (alfentanil, aripiprazole, busPIRone, buprenorphine, carBAMazepine, many corticosteroids, cyclobenzaprine, cycloSPORINE, darifenacin, disopyramide, calcium channel blockers, eplerenone, ergots, fentaNYL, galantamine, halofantrine, levomethadyl, systemic lidocaine, lovastatin, oxybutynin, paricalcitol, quiNIDine, simvastatin, solifenacin, tadalafil, tolterodine, zonisamide): dosage reduction may be needed; avoid use
CYP2C9 metabolizers (some COX-2 inhibitors, chlorpropamide, diclofenac, dronabinol, THC, flurbiprofen, fluvastatin, glimepiride, glipiZIDE, glyBURIDE, ibuprofen, indomethacin, irbesartan, losartan, meloxicam, naproxen, nateglinide, phenytoin, piroxicam, rosiglitazone, TOLBUTamide, valsartan): dosage reduction may be needed; avoid use

Drug/herb
Green tea (large amounts), guarana: increased effect

Drug/food
Decreased: bioavailability of zafirlukast

NURSING CONSIDERATIONS

Assessment
• Assess respiratory rate, rhythm, depth; auscultate lung fields bilaterally; notify prescriber of abnormalities
• **Churg-Strauss syndrome (rare):** assess adults carefully (eosinophilia, vasculitic rash, worsening pulmonary symptoms, cardiac complications, neuropathy)
• **Hepatic disease:** Monitor liver function tests

Nursing diagnoses
• Breathing pattern, ineffective (uses)
• Knowledge, deficient (teaching)
• Noncompliance (teaching)

Patient/family education
• Advise patient to check OTC medications, current prescription medications that may increase stimulation
• Advise patient to avoid hazardous activities; dizziness may occur
• Advise patient that if GI upset occurs, to take product with 8 oz of water; avoid food if possible; absorption may be decreased
• Advise to take even if symptom-free
• Advise patient to notify prescriber of nausea, vomiting, diarrhea, abdominal pain, fatigue, jaundice, anorexia, flulike symptoms (hepatic dysfunction)
• Advise patient not to use for acute asthma episodes, or to use while breastfeeding

Evaluation
Positive therapeutic outcome
• Ability to breathe more easily

---

zaleplon (Rx)
(zale′plon)
Sonata
Func. class.: Sedative-hypnotic, non-barbiturate
Chem. class.: Pyrazolopyrimidine
Pregnancy category C
Controlled substance schedule IV

ACTION: Binds selectively to ω-1 receptor of the γ-aminobutyric acid type A (GABA$_A$) receptor complex; results are sedation, hypnosis, skeletal muscle relaxation, anticonvulsant activity, anxiolytic action

Therapeutic outcome: Ability to sleep

USES: Insomnia

CONTRAINDICATIONS:
Hypersensitivity, severe hepatic disease

Precautions: Pregnancy **C**, breastfeeding, children <15 yr, geriatric, renal/hepatic disease, psychosis, angioedema, respiratory disease, depression, sleep-related behavior (sleep walking)

DOSAGE AND ROUTES
Adult: PO 10 mg at bedtime; may increase dosage to 20 mg at bedtime if needed; 5 mg may be used in low-weight persons
Geriatric: PO 5 mg at bedtime; may increase if needed

Z

Adverse effects: *italics* = common; **bold** = life-threatening

Available forms: Caps 5, 10 mg

Implementation
• Give ¹/₂-1 hr before bedtime for sleeplessness; give on empty stomach

ADVERSE EFFECTS
CNS: *Drowsiness,* amnesia, depersonalization, hallucinations, hyperesthesia, paresthesia, somnolence, tremor, vertigo, dizziness, anxiety, *lethargy, daytime sedation,* confusion, complex sleep-related reactions (sleep driving, sleep eating)
EENT: Vision changes, ear/eye pain, hyperacusis, parosmia
GI: Nausea, anorexia, colitis, dyspepsia, dry mouth, constipation, abdominal pain
MISC: Asthenia, fever, headache, myalgia, dysmenorrhea
SYST: Severe allergic reactions

Pharmacokinetics

Absorption	Rapidly absorbed
Distribution	Extravascular tissues, crosses blood-brain barrier; crosses placenta
Metabolism	Extensively, liver to inactive metabolites
Excretion	Kidneys
Half-life	1 hr

Pharmacodynamics

Onset	Rapid
Peak	1 hr
Duration	Unknown

INTERACTIONS

Individual drugs
Cimetidine: increased action of zaleplon
Rifampin: decreased zaleplon levels

Drug classifications
CYP3A4 inhibitors/inducers: increased or decreased zaleplon levels

Drug/herb
Chamomile, hops, kava, valerian: increased CNS depression

Drug/food
High-fat/heavy meal: prolonged absorption, sleep onset reduced

NURSING CONSIDERATIONS

Assessment
• **Sleep disorders:** assess for type of sleep problem, falling asleep, staying asleep

• Assess for previous product dependence or tolerance; if product dependent or tolerant, amount of medication should be restricted
• Monitor patient's mental status: mood, sensorium, affect, sleeping patterns, drowsiness, dizziness, suicidal tendencies, excessive sedation, impaired coordination

Nursing diagnoses
• Knowledge, deficient (teaching)
• Noncompliance (teaching)
• Sleep deprivation (uses)

Patient/family education
• Inform patient that product is for short-term use only
• Teach patient to take immediately before going to bed
• Advise patient that product may cause memory problems, dependence (if used for longer periods of time), changes in behavior/thinking, complex sleep-related behavior (sleep eating/driving)
• Advise patient not to ingest a high-fat/heavy meal before taking
• Advise patient to avoid OTC preparations unless approved by a physician, to avoid alcohol ingestion or other psychotropic medications unless prescribed by a health care provider, that 1-2 wk of therapy may be required before therapeutic effects occur
• Caution patient to avoid driving, activities requiring alertness; drowsiness may occur; until medication response is known, tell patient that drowsiness may worsen at beginning of treatment
• Instruct patient not to discontinue medication abruptly after long-term use

Evaluation
Positive therapeutic outcome
• Decreased sleeplessness

---

zanamivir (Rx)
(zan-a-mee′veer)
Relenza
Func. class.: Antiviral
Chem. class.: Neuramidase inhibitor
Pregnancy category C

ACTION: Inhibits neuramidase enzyme needed for influenza virus replication

Therapeutic outcome: Decreased symptoms of influenza types A and B for those who have been symptomatic for no more than 2 days

USES: Treatment of influenza types A and B for those who have been symptomatic for no more than 2 days

Unlabeled uses: Prophylaxis against influenza A and B infections; swine flu (H1N1)

CONTRAINDICATIONS:
Hypersensitivity

Precautions: Pregnancy **C**, breastfeeding, children <7 yr, geriatric, respiratory disease, angioedema, milk protein hypersensitivity, Reye's syndrome

DOSAGE AND ROUTES
Adult and child >7 yr: INH 2 inh (two 5-mg blisters) q12hr × 5 days, on the 1st day 2 doses should be taken with at least 2 hr between doses

H1N1 (swine flu) (unlabeled)
Adult/adolescent/child ≥7 yr: INH 2 inh bid × 5 days

Available forms: Blisters of powder for inhalation 5 mg

Implementation
• Give before exposure to influenza; continue for 5 days after contact
• Store in airtight, dry container

ADVERSE EFFECTS
CNS: *Headache, dizziness,* fatigue, **seizures,** self-injury, delirium (child)
EENT: Ear, nose, throat infections
GI: *Nausea, vomiting, diarrhea*
RESP: Nasal symptoms, cough, sinusitis, bronchitis, **bronchospasm**
SYST: Angioedema

Pharmacokinetics

Absorption	4%-17% absorbed
Distribution	<10% protein binding
Metabolism	Not metabolized
Excretion	Kidneys unchanged
Half-life	2½-5 hr

Pharmacodynamics

Unknown

INTERACTIONS
Individual drugs
Intranasal influenza vaccine: decreased effect; separate by ≥48 hr, do not restart antiviral drugs for ≥2 wk

NURSING CONSIDERATIONS
Assessment
• Assess for symptoms of influenza A: increased temp, malaise, aches and pains
• Assess for skin eruptions, photosensitivity after administration of product
• Monitor respiratory status: rate, character, wheezing, tightness in chest
• Assess for allergies before initiation of treatment, reaction of each medication

Nursing diagnoses
• Infection, risk for (uses)
• Knowledge, deficient (teaching)

Patient/family education
• Give patient "Patient's instructions for use" and review all points before using delivery system
• Teach patient to avoid hazardous activities if dizziness occurs
• Teach patient to take product exactly as prescribed; to use for the entire 5 days
• Inform patient that this product does not reduce transmission risk of influenza to others
• Advise patients with asthma or COPD to carry a fast-acting inhaled bronchodilator since bronchospasm may occur; to use scheduled inhaled bronchodilators before using this product

Evaluation
Positive therapeutic outcome
• Absence of fever, malaise, cough, dyspnea in influenza A

zidovudine (Rx)
(zye-doe′vue-deen)
Apo-Zidovudine ✦, Novo-AZT ✦, Retrovir
Func. class.: Antiretroviral
Chem. class.: Nucleoside reverse transcriptase inhibitor (NRTI)
Pregnancy category C

ACTION: Inhibits replication of HIV-1 by incorporating into cellular DNA by viral reverse transcriptase, thereby terminating the cellular DNA chain

Therapeutic outcome: Decreased symptoms of HIV-1 infection

USES: Used in combination with at least 2 other antiretrovirals for HIV-1 infection

CONTRAINDICATIONS:
Hypersensitivity

Precautions: Pregnancy **C**, breastfeeding, children, granulocyte count <1000/mm³ or Hgb <9.5 g/dl, severe renal disease, obesity

> **BLACK BOX WARNING:** Impaired hepatic function, anemia, lactic acidosis, myopathy, neutropenia

DOSAGE AND ROUTES
Adult: PO 600 mg/day in divided doses, either 200 mg tid or 300 mg bid in combination with other antiretrovirals; **IV** 1-mg/kg q4hr, initiate PO as soon as possible, up to 1000 mg
Child 6 wk-12 yr: PO 160 mg/m² q8hr (480 mg/m²/day, max 200 mg q8hr) in combination with other antiretrovirals; **IV** same as adult

Neonate: PO 2-3 mg/kg/dose q6hr; **IV** 1.5 mg/kg INF over 30 min q6hr

Treatment of HIV in combination with other antiretrovirals
Adult/adolescent/child ≥30 kg: PO 300 mg bid or 200 mg tid
Child ≥4 wk and weight 4-<9 kg/infant: PO total daily dose 24 mg/kg/day given 12 mg/kg bid or 8 mg/kg tid

Perinatal transmission prophylaxis
Full-term neonate: PO 2 mg/kg or **IV** 1.5 mg/kg q6hr starting 12 hr after birth; continue up to 6 wk of age

Preterm neonate: PO 2 mg/kg or **IV** 1.5 mg/kg q12hr; if >30 wk gestation at birth, advance to q8hr at 2 wk of age; if <30 wk gestation at birth, advance to q8hr at 4 wk of age

Prevention of maternal-fetal HIV transmission
Neonatal: PO 2 mg/kg/dose q6hr × 6 wk beginning 8-12 hr after birth; **IV** 1.5 mg/kg/dose over 30 min q6hr until able to take PO

Maternal (>14 wk gestation): PO 100 mg 5 ×/day until start of labor, then during labor/delivery **IV** 2 mg/kg over 1 hr followed by **IV** INF 1 mg/kg/hr until umbilical cord is clamped

Symptomatic HIV infection
Child 3 mo-12 yr: PO 90-180 mg/m² q6hr (max 200 mg q6hr); **IV** 1-2 mg/kg over 1 hr q4hr
Adult: PO 100 mg q4hr; **IV** 1-2 mg/kg over 1 hr q4hr

Prevention of HIV after needlestick
Adult: PO 200 mg tid plus lamiVUDine 150 mg bid, plus a protease inhibitor for high-risk exposure; begin within 2 hr of exposure

Available forms: Caps 100 mg; tabs 300 mg; inj 200 mg/20 ml; oral syr 50 mg/5 ml

Implementation
PO route
- Give on empty stomach, bid or tid
- Do not take dapsone at same time as didanosine

Intermittent IV infusion route
- Give after diluting with D₅W; give over 1 hr (<4 mg/ml), do not give by direct **IV**

Y-site compatibilities: Acyclovir, allopurinol, amikacin, amphotericin B, aztreonam, ceftazidime, cefTRIAXone, cimetidine, clindamycin, dexamethasone, DOBUTamine, DOPamine, erythromycin, fluconazole, fludarabine, gentamicin, heparin, imipenem/cilastatin, lorazepam, metoclopramide, morphine, nafcillin, ondansetron, oxacillin, pentamidine, phenylephrine, piperacillin, potassium chloride, ranitidine, sargramostim, tobramycin, trimethoprim/sulfamethoxazole, vancomycin

Additive incompatibilities: Blood products or protein solutions

ADVERSE EFFECTS
CNS: *Fever, headache, malaise,* diaphoresis, *dizziness, insomnia,* paresthesia, somnolence, chills, tremor, twitching, anxiety, confusion, depression, lability, vertigo, loss of mental acuity, **seizures,** malaise
EENT: Taste change, hearing loss, photophobia
GI: *Nausea, vomiting, diarrhea,* anorexia, cramps, *dyspepsia, constipation,* dysphagia, *flatulence,* rectal bleeding, mouth ulcer, abdominal pain, hepatomegaly
GU: Dysuria, polyuria, frequency, hesitancy
HEMA: Granulocytopenia, anemia
INTEG: *Rash,* acne, pruritus, urticaria
MS: Myalgia, arthralgia, muscle spasm
RESP: Dyspnea
SYST: Lactic acidosis

Pharmacokinetics

Absorption	Well absorbed (PO), completely absorbed (**IV**)
Distribution	Widely distributed—crosses placenta, CSF, protein binding 38%
Metabolism	Liver, mostly
Excretion	Kidneys
Half-life	Terminal $\frac{1}{2}$-3 hr

Pharmacodynamics

	PO	IV
Onset	Unknown	Rapid
Peak	$\frac{1}{2}$-$1\frac{1}{2}$ hr	Inf end
Duration	Unknown	Unknown

INTERACTIONS

Individual drugs
Fluconazole, probenecid: increased toxicity
Ganciclovir, radiation, SMZ/TMP, valganciclovir: increased bone marrow suppression
Methadone: increased zidovudine level

Drug classifications
Antineoplastics: increased bone marrow suppression

NURSING CONSIDERATIONS

Assessment
• **Assess for peripheral neuropathy:** tingling or pain in hands and feet, distal numbness; if these occur, product may be decreased or discontinued
• **Assess for pancreatitis:** abdominal pain, nausea, vomiting, elevated liver enzymes; product should be discontinued because condition can be fatal
• Assess children by dilated retinal examination q6mo to rule out retinal depigmentation

> **BLACK BOX WARNING:** Monitor CBC, differential, platelet count qmo; withhold product if WBC is <4000/mm³ or platelet count is <75,000/mm³; notify prescriber of results; monitor viral load, CD4 counts, LFTs, plasma HIV RNA, serum creatinine/BUN baseline, throughout treatment

• **Lactic acidosis, severe hepatomegaly with steatosis:** obtain baseline LFTs; if elevated, discontinue treatment; discontinue even if LFTs are normal but lactic acidosis, hepatomegaly are present: may be fatal

Nursing diagnoses
• Infection, risk for (uses)
• Injury, risk for (adverse reactions)
• Knowledge, deficient (teaching)

Patient/family education
• Caution patient to take on empty stomach; to use exactly as prescribed
• Advise patient to report signs of infection: increased temp, sore throat, flulike symptoms; to avoid crowds and those with known infections
• Instruct patient to report signs of anemia: fatigue, headache, faintness, shortness of breath, irritability
• Advise patient to report bleeding; avoid use of razors or commercial mouthwash
• Inform patient that hair may be lost during therapy (rare); a wig or hairpiece may make patient feel better
• Caution patient to avoid OTC products or other medications without approval of prescriber
• Caution patient not to have any sexual contact without use of a condom; needles should not be shared; blood from infected individual should not come in contact with another's mucous membranes

Evaluation
Positive therapeutic outcome
• Decreased infection; decreased symptoms of HIV infection

---

zinc (PO, OTC; IV, Rx)
(zink sul'fate)
Orazinc, PMS Egozinc ✤, Verazinc, Zinca-Pak, Zincate, Zinc 15, Zinc-220
Func. class.: Trace element; nutritional supplement
Pregnancy category C, parenteral

ACTION: Needed for adequate healing, bone and joint development, (23% zinc)

Therapeutic outcome: Replacement of zinc

USES: Prevention of zinc deficiency, adjunct to vit A therapy

Unlabeled uses: Wound healing

Precautions: Pregnancy C (parenteral), breastfeeding, hypocupremia, neonatal prematurity, neonates, renal disease

Adverse effects: *italics* = common; **bold** = life-threatening

DOSAGE AND ROUTES

Dietary supplement (elemental zinc)
Adult/adolescent pregnant females: PO 11-13 mg/day

Nutritional supplement (IV)
Adult: IV 2.5-4 mg/day, may increase by 2 mg/day if needed
Child 1-5 yr: IV 50 mcg/kg/day
Adult and lactating female: PO 12-14 mg/day × 12 mo
Adult and adolescent male ≥14 yr: PO 11 mg/day
Adult female ≥19 yr: PO 8 mg/day
Adolescent female ≥14 yr: PO 9 mg/day
Child 9-13 yr: PO 8 mg/day
Child 4-8 yr: PO 5 mg/day
Child 1-3 yr: PO 3 mg/day
Infant 7-12 mo: PO 3 mg/day
Infant birth to 6 mo: PO 2 mg/day (adequate intake)

Wound healing
Adult: PO 50 mg tid until healed (elemental iron)

Available forms: Tabs 66, 110 mg; caps 220 mg; inj 1, 5 mg/ml

Implementation
PO route
• Give with meals to decrease gastric upset; restrict dairy products, caffeine, which decrease absorption

IV route
• Part of TPN

ADVERSE EFFECTS
GI: Nausea, vomiting, cramps, heartburn, ulcer formation
OVERDOSE: Diarrhea, rash, dehydration, restlessness

Pharmacokinetics

Absorption	Poorly absorbed (PO), completely absorbed (IV)
Distribution	Widely distributed
Metabolism	Liver
Excretion	90% (feces), 10% (kidneys)
Half-life	Unknown

Pharmacodynamics
Unknown

INTERACTIONS
Drug classifications
Fluoroquinolones, tetracyclines: decreased absorption

NURSING CONSIDERATIONS
Assessment
• Monitor zinc levels during treatment

Nursing diagnoses
• Knowledge, deficient (teaching)
• Nutrition, less than body requirements, imbalanced (uses)

Patient/family education
• Inform patient that element must be taken for 3 mo to be effective
• Advise patient to report immediately nausea, diarrhea, rash, severe vomiting, restlessness, abdominal pain, tarry stools

Evaluation
Positive therapeutic outcome
• Absence of zinc deficiency
• Improved wound healing

ziprasidone (Rx)
(zi-praz′ih-dohn)
Geodon, Zeldox ✲
Func. class.: Antipsychotic/neuroleptic
Chem. class.: Benzisoxazole derivative
Pregnancy category C

ACTION: Unknown; may be mediated through both dopamine type 2 (D_2) and serotonin type 2 (5-HT_2) antagonism

Therapeutic outcome: Decreased signs/symptoms of psychosis

USES: Schizophrenia, acute agitation, acute psychosis, bipolar disorder, mania, psychotic depression

CONTRAINDICATIONS:
Hypersensitivity, breastfeeding

Precautions: Pregnancy C, children, geriatric, renal/cardiac/hepatic disease, breast cancer, diabetes, AV block, CNS depression, seizure disorders

> **BLACK BOX WARNING:** Dementia

DOSAGE AND ROUTES

Schizophrenia
Adult: PO 20 mg bid with food, adjust dosage every 2 days upward to max of 80 mg bid; IM 10-20 mg; may give 10 mg q2hr, doses of 20 mg may be given q4hr, max 40 mg/day

Bipolar disorder
Adult: PO 40 mg bid with food, on day 2 increase to 60 or 80 mg bid, then adjust to response; maintenance as adjunct to lithium/valproate 40-80 mg bid

Available forms: Tabs 20, 40, 60, 80 mg; inj 20 mg/ml

Implementation
- Give reduced dosage in geriatric
- Give antiparkinsonian agent on order from prescriber, to be used for EPS
- Provide decreased stimulus by dimming lights, avoiding loud noises
- Provide supervised ambulation until patient is stabilized on medication; do not involve in strenuous exercise program because fainting is possible; patient should not stand still for a long time

PO route
- Food increases absorption
- Store in airtight, light-resistant container

IM route
- Add 1.2 ml sterile water for inj to vial, shake vigorously until product is dissolved, do not admix

ADVERSE EFFECTS

CNS: *EPS (pseudoparkinsonism, akathisia, dystonia, tardive dyskinesia), drowsiness, insomnia, agitation, anxiety, headache,* **seizures, neuroleptic malignant syndrome,** dizziness, tremor, facial droop
CV: Orthostatic hypotension, **tachycardia, prolonged QT/QTc, sudden death, heart failure (geriatric), torsades de pointes**
EENT: Blurred vision, diplopia
ENDO: Metabolic changes
GI: *Nausea,* vomiting, *anorexia, constipation,* jaundice, weight gain, diarrhea, dry mouth, abdominal pain
GU: Enuresis, urinary incontinence, gynecomastia, impotence, priapism
RESP: Rhinitis, dyspnea, infection, cough

Pharmacokinetics

Absorption	Unknown
Distribution	Protein binding 90%
Metabolism	Liver, extensively to metabolite
Excretion	Unknown
Half-life	Terminal 7 hr

Pharmacodynamics

Onset	Unknown
Peak	6-8 hr
Duration	Unknown

INTERACTIONS

Individual drugs
Alcohol: increased sedation
Chloroquine, clarithromycin, droperidol, erythromycin, grepafloxacin, haloperidol, methadone, moxifloxacin, pentamidine: increased QT prolongation
CarBAMazepine: increased excretion of ziprasidone
Ketoconazole: increased ziprasidone level
Lithium: increased EPS

Drug classifications
Antihypertensives: increased hypotension
Antipsychotics: increased EPS
β-agonists, class IA/III antidysrhythmics, local anesthetics, phenothiazines (some), tricyclics: increased QT prolongation
CNS depressants: increased sedation
SSRIs, SNRIs: increased serotonin syndrome, increased neuroleptic malignant syndrome

Drug/herb
Chamomile, hops, kava, skullcap, valerian: increased CNS depression

NURSING CONSIDERATIONS

Assessment

> **BLACK BOX WARNING:** Assess geriatric with dementia closely; heart failure, sudden death have occurred

- Assess mental status before initial administration
- Check swallowing of PO medication; check for hoarding or giving of medication to other patients
- Monitor I&O ratio; palpate bladder if urinary output is low
- Monitor bilirubin, CBC, liver function tests, fasting blood glucose qmo

Z

Adverse effects: *italics* = common; **bold** = life-threatening

- Monitor urinalysis before, during prolonged therapy
- Assess affect, orientation, LOC, reflexes, gait, coordination, sleep pattern disturbances
- Monitor B/P standing and lying; also pulse, respirations; take these q4hr during initial treatment; establish baseline before starting treatment; report drops of 30 mm Hg; watch for ECG changes
- Assess dizziness, faintness, palpitations, tachycardia on rising
- **Assess EPS,** including akathisia (inability to sit still, no pattern to movements), tardive dyskinesia (bizarre movements of the jaw, mouth, tongue, extremities), pseudoparkinsonism (rigidity, tremors, pill rolling, shuffling gait)
- **⚠ Assess for neuroleptic malignant syndrome: hyperthermia, increased CPK, altered mental status, muscle rigidity**
- Assess constipation, urinary retention daily; if these occur, increase bulk and water in diet

Nursing diagnoses
- Coping, ineffective (uses)
- Knowledge, deficient (teaching)
- Noncompliance (teaching)

Patient/family education
- Advise patient that orthostatic hypotension may occur and to rise from sitting or lying position gradually; avoid hot tubs, hot showers, tub baths because hypotension may occur
- Advise patient to avoid abrupt withdrawal of this product; EPS may result; product should be withdrawn slowly
- Advise patient to avoid OTC preparations (cough, hay fever, cold) unless approved by prescriber, since serious product interactions may occur; avoid use with alcohol, CNS depressants; increased drowsiness may occur
- Teach patient to avoid hazardous activities if drowsy or dizzy
- Advise patient to increase fluids to prevent constipation
- Teach patient to use sips of water, candy, gum for dry mouth
- Teach patient compliance with product regimen
- Teach patient to report impaired vision, tremors, muscle twitching
- Teach patient that in hot weather, heat stroke may occur; take extra precautions to stay cool

Evaluation
Positive therapeutic outcome
- Decrease in emotional excitement, hallucinations, delusions, paranoia; reorganization of patterns of thought, speech

TREATMENT OF OVERDOSE:
Lavage if orally ingested; provide airway; *do not induce vomiting*

zoledronic acid (Rx)
(zoh'leh-drah'nick ass'id)
Reclast, Zometa
Func. class.: Bone-resorption inhibitor
Chem. class.: Bisphosphonate
Pregnancy category D

ACTION: Inhibits normal and abnormal bone resorption; potent inhibitor of osteoclastic bone resorption; inhibits osteoclastic activity, reduces bone resorption and inhibits skeletal calcium release caused by stimulating factors released by tumors; reduction of abnormal bone resorption is responsible for therapeutic effect in hypercalcemia; may directly block dissolution of hydroxyapatite bone crystals

Therapeutic outcome: Serum calcium at normal level

USES: Moderate to severe hypercalcemia associated with malignancy; multiple myeloma; bone metastases from solid tumors (used with antineoplastics), active Paget's disease, osteoporosis, glucocorticoid-induced osteoporosis, osteoporosis prophylaxis in postmenopausal women

CONTRAINDICATIONS:
Pregnancy **D**, breastfeeding, hypocalcemia, hypersensitivity to this product or bisphosphonates

Precautions: Children, geriatric, renal dysfunction, aspirin-sensitive asthma, asthmatic patients, asthma, acute bronchospasm, anemia, chemotherapy, coagulopathy, dehydration, dental disease, diabetes mellitus, renal disease, electrolyte imbalance, hypertension, hypomagnesemia, hypophosphatemia, hypovolemia, phosphate hypersensitivity, infection, multiple myeloma

DOSAGE AND ROUTES
Hypercalcemia of malignancy
Adult: IV INF 4 mg, given as a single INF over ≥15 min, may re-treat with 4 mg if serum calcium does not return to normal within 1 wk

Multiple myeloma/metastatic bone lesions
Adult: IV INF 4 mg, given over 15 min q3-4wk

Osteoporosis
Adult: IV 5 mg over 15 min or more q12mo

Active Paget's disease
Adult: **IV** INF 5 mg over ≥15 min

Osteoporosis prophylaxis (Reclast), postmenopausal women
Adult: **IV** INF 5 mg every other yr

Osteoporosis prophylaxis (Reclast) taking systemic glucocorticoids
Adult: **IV** 5 mg qyr

Available forms: Sol for inj 4 mg/5 ml (Zometa); inj 5 mg/100 ml (Reclast)

Implementation
• Give acetaminophen before and for 72 hr after to decrease pain
• Sol reconstituted with sterile water may be stored under refrigeration for up to 24 hr **IV**
• Administer in separate **IV** line from all other products

Zometa
• Administer after reconstituting by adding 5 ml of sterile water for inj to each vial, then add up to ≥100 ml of sterile 0.9% NaCl, D₅W, run over ≥15 min

Reclast
• No further dilution required; inf over ≥15 min at constant rate; max 5 mg

ADVERSE EFFECTS
CNS: Dizziness, headache, anxiety, confusion, insomnia, agitation
CV: Hypotension, leg edema, **atrial fibrillation,** chest pain
GI: Abdominal pain, anorexia, constipation, nausea, diarrhea, vomiting, taste change
GU: UTI, possible reduced renal function, **renal damage**
META: Anemia, hypokalemia, hypomagnesemia, hypophosphatemia, hypocalcemia, increased serum creatinine
MISC: *Fever, chills, flulike symptoms*
MS: Severe bone pain, *arthralgias, myalgias,* osteonecrosis of the jaw

Pharmacokinetics

Absorption	Rapidly cleared from circulation
Distribution	Taken up mainly by bones; plasma protein binding ~22%
Metabolism	Not metabolized
Excretion	Kidneys (~50% eliminated in urine within 24 hr)
Half-life	Terminal 167 hr

Pharmacodynamics

Onset	Unknown
Peak	15 min
Duration	Max effect 7 days

INTERACTIONS
Individual drugs
Calcium, vitamin D: decreased zoledronic acid effect
Digoxin: hypomagnesemia, hypokalemia
Infusion solutions (calcium-containing): do not mix with calcium-containing inf sol such as lactated Ringer's sol

Drug classifications
Aminoglycosides, NSAIDs, radiopaque contrast agents: increased neurotoxicity
Aminoglycosides, loop diuretics: decreased serum calcium

NURSING CONSIDERATIONS
Assessment
• Assess renal function tests and calcium, phosphate, magnesium, potassium, creatinine; if creatinine is elevated hold treatment
• **Assess for hypocalcemia:** paresthesia, twitching, laryngospasm; Chvostek's/Trousseau's signs
• Assess dental status; cover with antiinfectives for dental extraction
• Assess for atrial fibrillation

Nursing diagnoses
• Fluid volume, excess (side effects)
• Injury, risk for (uses, adverse reactions)
• Knowledge, deficient (teaching)

Patient/family education
• Instruct patient to report hypercalcemic relapse: nausea, vomiting, bone pain, thirst
• Advise patient to continue with dietary recommendations including calcium and vit D; take a multiple vitamin daily, 500 mg of calcium, 400 international units vit D in multiple myeloma
• Teach patient if nausea/vomiting occur, eat small meals, use lozenges or chewing gum
• Advise patient if bone pain occurs, notify prescriber to obtain analgesic
• Advise patient to avoid pregnancy
• Instruct patient to continue good oral hygiene

Evaluation
Positive therapeutic outcome
• Calcium levels decreased to normal

Z

TREATMENT OF OVERDOSE:
Correct clinically relevant reductions in serum calcium by administering **IV** calcium gluconate; in serum phosphorus, with potassium or sodium phosphate; in serum magnesium, with magnesium sulfate

zolmitriptan (Rx)

(zole-mih-trip′tan)
Zomig, Zomig-ZMT
Func. class.: Migraine agent, abortive
Chem. class.: 5HT$_{1B}$/5HT$_{1D}$ receptor agonist (triptan)
Pregnancy category C

ACTION: Binds selectively to the vascular serotonin type 1 (5HT$_{1B}$/5HT$_{1D}$) receptor subtype, exerts antimigraine effect; causes vasoconstriction in cranial arteries

Therapeutic outcome: Decreased severity, frequency of headache

USES: Acute treatment of migraine with or without aura

CONTRAINDICATIONS:
Angina pectoris, history of MI, documented silent ischemia, ischemic heart disease, uncontrolled hypertension, hypersensitivity, basilar or hemiplegic migraine, risk of CV events

Precautions: Pregnancy **C**, breastfeeding, children, postmenopausal women, men >40 yr, geriatric, risk factors for CAD, hypercholesterolemia, obesity, diabetes, impaired renal/hepatic function

DOSAGE AND ROUTES:
Adult: PO start at 2.5 mg or lower (tab may be broken), may repeat after 2 hr, max 10 mg/24 hr; NASAL 1 spray in 1 nostril at onset of migraine, repeat in 2 hr if no relief

Available forms: Tabs 2.5, 5 mg; orally disintegrating tabs 2.5, 5 mg; nasal spray 5 mg

Implementation
• Give with fluids as soon as symptoms of migraine occur
• Provide quiet, calm environment with decreased stimulation for noise, bright light, excessive talking

ADVERSE EFFECTS
CNS: *Tingling, hot sensation, burning, feeling of pressure, tightness, numbness, dizziness, sedation*

CV: Palpitations, chest pain
GI: Abdominal discomfort, nausea, dry mouth, dyspepsia, dysphagia
MISC: Odd taste (spray)
MS: *Weakness, neck stiffness,* myalgia
RESP: Chest tightness, pressure

Pharmacokinetics

Absorption	Unknown
Distribution	25% plasma protein binding
Metabolism	Liver
Excretion	Urine, feces
Half-life	3-3½ hr

Pharmacodynamics

Onset	Unknown
Peak	Unknown
Duration	2-3½ hr

INTERACTIONS
Individual drugs
Cimetidine: increased half-life of zolmitriptan
Ergot: increased vasospastic effects
FLUoxetine, fluvoxamine, PARoxetine, sertraline: increased weakness, hyperreflexia, incoordination
Sibutramine: increased zolmitriptan levels

Drug classifications
Contraceptives (oral): increased half-life of zolmitriptan
Ergot derivatives: increased vasospastic effects
MAOIs: do not use within 2 wk
Selective serotonin reuptake inhibitors: increased weakness, hyperreflexia, incoordination

Drug/herb
SAM-e, St. John's wort: serotonin syndrome

NURSING CONSIDERATIONS
Assessment
• Assess for tingling, hot sensation, burning, feeling of pressure, numbness, flushing
• Assess for stress level, activity, recreation, coping mechanisms
• Assess neurologic status: LOC, blurring vision, nausea, vomiting, tingling in extremities preceding headache
• Monitor ingestion of tyramine foods (pickled products, beer, wine, aged cheese), food additives, preservatives, colorings, artifical sweeteners, chocolate, caffeine, which may precipitate these types of headaches

⚠ Nurse Alert

• **Assess for serotonin syndrome** if also taking an SSRI

Nursing diagnoses
• Knowledge, deficient (teaching)
• Noncompliance (teaching)
• Pain, acute (uses)

Patient/family education
• Teach patient to report any side effects to prescriber
• Advise patient to use contraception while taking product

Evaluation
Positive therapeutic outcome
• Decrease in frequency, severity of headache

---

zolpidem (Rx)
(zole-pi′dem)
Ambien, Ambien CR, Edluar, Zolpimist
Func. class.: Sedative-hypnotic
Chem. class.: Nonbenzodiazepine of imidazopyridine class
Pregnancy category C
Controlled substance schedule IV

ACTION: Produces CNS depression at limbic, thalamic, hypothalamic levels of CNS; may be mediated by neurotransmitter γ-aminobutyric acid (GABA); results are sedation, hypnosis, skeletal muscle relaxation, anticonvulsant activity, anxiolytic action

Therapeutic outcome: Ability to sleep, sedation

USES: Insomnia, short-term treatment; insomnia with difficulty of sleep onset/maintenance (ext rel)

CONTRAINDICATIONS:
Hypersensitivity to benzodiazepines

Precautions: Pregnancy **C**, breastfeeding, children <18 yr, geriatric, anemia, renal/hepatic disease, suicidal individuals, product abuse, psychosis, seizure disorders, angioedema, depression, respiratory disease, sleep apnea, sleep-related behavior (sleep walking), myasthenia gravis

DOSAGE AND ROUTES
Adult: PO 10 mg at bedtime × 7-10 days only; total dose max 10 mg; EXT REL 12.5 mg immediately before bedtime, may be useful for up to 24 wk in people 18-64 yr with primary insomnia; oral spray (Zolpimist) 10 mg (2 sprays) immediately before bedtime, max 10 mg/day; SL (Edluar) 10 mg just before bedtime
Geriatric: PO 5 mg at bedtime; EXT REL 6.25 mg

Available forms: Tabs 5, 10 mg; ext rel tabs 6.25, 12.5 mg; SL 5, 10 mg; oral spray 5 mg/spray

Implementation
PO route
• Do not break, crush, or chew ext rel product or orally disintegrating tab
• Give $1/2$-1 hr before bedtime for sleeplessness; give several hr before patient is to rise (to avoid hangover)
• Give with food or fluids; tab may be crushed or swallowed whole
• Do not use spray with or after a meal
• Store in airtight container in cool environment

ADVERSE EFFECTS
CNS: Headache, lethargy, drowsiness, daytime sedation, dizziness, confusion, light-headedness, anxiety, irritability, amnesia, poor coordination, complex sleep-related reactions (sleep driving, sleep eating), depression, somnolence, **suicidal ideation,** abnormal thinking/behavioral changes
CV: Chest pain, palpitation
GI: Nausea, vomiting, diarrhea, heartburn, abdominal pain, constipation
HEMA: Leukopenia, granulocytopenia (rare)
MISC: Myalgia
SYST: Severe allergic reactions

Pharmacokinetics
Absorption	Rapidly absorbed
Distribution	Unknown
Metabolism	Liver—inactive metabolite
Excretion	Kidneys, breast milk
Half-life	$2^{1}/_{2}$ hr, increased in geriatric

Pharmacodynamics
Onset	PO up to 1.5 mg

INTERACTIONS
Individual drugs
Alcohol: increased action of both products

Drug classifications
CNS depressants: increased action of both products

Adverse effects: *italics* = common; **bold** = life-threatening

Z

CYP3A4 inhibitors/inducers: increased or decreased zolpidem levels

NURSING CONSIDERATIONS

Assessment

• Assess mental status: mood, sensorium, anxiety, affect, sleeping pattern, drowsiness, dizziness, especially geriatric; physical dependency, withdrawal symptoms: anxiety, panic attacks, agitation, seizures, headache, nausea, vomiting, muscle pain, weakness; suicidal tendencies; for indications of increasing tolerance and abuse
• Monitor B/P (lying, standing), pulse; if systolic B/P drops 20 mm Hg, hold product, notify prescriber
• Monitor I&O ratio for renal dysfunction

Nursing diagnoses

• Anxiety (uses)
• Injury, risk for (adverse reactions)
• Knowledge, deficient (teaching)

Patient/family education

• Advise patient that complex sleep-related behavior may occur (sleep driving/eating)
• Instruct patient that product may be taken with food or fluids
• Caution patient not to use for everyday stress or longer than 3 mo unless directed by prescriber; not to take more than prescribed amount; may be habit forming; not to double or skip doses
• Caution patient to avoid OTC preparations unless approved by prescriber; alcohol and CNS depressants will increase CNS depression
• Advise patient to avoid driving, activities that require alertness, because drowsiness may occur; to avoid alcohol ingestion or other psychotropic medications; to rise slowly or fainting may occur, especially geriatric; that drowsiness may worsen at beginning of treatment
• Instruct patient not to discontinue medication abruptly after long-term use; withdrawal symptoms include vomiting, cramping, tremors, seizures
• Teach patient use of orally disintegrating tabs: place on tongue, allow to dissolve before swallowing

Evaluation

Positive therapeutic outcome
• Ability to sleep at night
• Decreased amount of early-morning awakening if taking product for insomnia

TREATMENT OF OVERDOSE:

Lavage, VS, supportive care

---

zonisamide (Rx)

(zone-is'a-mide)
Zonegran
Func. class.: Anticonvulsant
Chem. class.: Sulfonamides
Pregnancy category C

ACTION: May act through sodium and calcium channels, but exact action is unknown; serotoninergic action

Therapeutic outcome: Decreased seizures

USES: Epilepsy, adjunctive therapy of partial seizures

CONTRAINDICATIONS:

Hypersensitivity to this product or sulfonamides, psychiatric condition, hepatic failure

Precautions: Pregnancy **C**, breastfeeding, children <16 yr, geriatric, allergies, renal/hepatic disease

DOSAGE AND ROUTES

Adults and child >16 yr: PO 100 mg/day, may increase after 2 wk to 200 mg/day, may increase q2wk, max dose 600 mg/day

Available forms: Caps 25, 50, 100 mg

ADVERSE EFFECTS

CNS: Dizziness, insomnia, paresthesias, depression, fatigue, headache, confusion, somnolence, agitation, irritability, speech disturbance, **suicidal ideation**
EENT: Diplopia, verbal difficulty, speech abnormalities, taste perversion
GI: Nausea, constipation, anorexia, weight loss, diarrhea, dyspepsia
HEMA: Aplastic anemia, granulocytopenia (rare)
INTEG: Rash
SYST: Stevens-Johnson syndrome, metabolic acidosis

Pharmacokinetics

Absorption	Unknown
Distribution	Protein binding 40%
Metabolism	Liver
Excretion	Kidneys
Half-life	In RBCs 105 hr

Pharmacodynamics

Onset	Unknown
Peak	2-6 hr
Duration	Unknown

INTERACTIONS

Individual drugs
Alcohol: increased CNS depression

Drug classifications
CarBAMazepine, PHENobarbital, phenytoin: decreased half-life of zonisamide

CYP3A4 inducers, inhibitors: altered product levels

Drug/herb
St. John's wort: increased effect of zonisamide

Drug/food
Grapefruit: do not use together

NURSING CONSIDERATIONS

Assessment
• Assess for seizures: duration, type, intensity, precipitating factors

• Renal function: albumin conc, BUN, creatinine; serum bicarbonate baseline, periodically

⚠ Assess mental status: mood, sensorium, affect, memory (long, short); suicidal thoughts/behavior

• Assess for rash, hypersensitivity reaction

Nursing diagnoses
• Injury, risk for (uses, adverse reactions)
• Knowledge, deficient (teaching)
• Noncompliance (teaching)

Patient/family education
• Advise patient not to discontinue product abruptly; seizures may occur

• Advise patient to avoid hazardous activities until stabilized on product

• Advise patient to carry/wear emergency ID stating product use

• Teach patient to take adequate fluids; not to use grapefruit juice

Evaluation
Positive therapeutic outcome
• Decrease in severity of seizures

Alpha-adrenergic Blockers

ACTION: α-Adrenergic blockers bind to α-adrenergic receptors, causing dilatation of peripheral blood vessels and lower peripheral resistance resulting in decreased blood pressure.

USES: α-Adrenergic blockers are used for benign prostatic hyperplasia, pheochromocytoma, prevention of tissue necrosis, and sloughing associated with extravasation of IV vasopressors.

CONTRAINDICATIONS:

Hypersensitive reactions may occur, and allergies should be identified before these products are given. Patients with myocardial infarction, coronary insufficiency, angina, or other evidence of coronary artery disease should not use these products.

IMPLEMENTATION
PO route
• Start with low dose, gradually increasing to prevent side effects
• Give with food or milk for GI symptoms

ADVERSE EFFECTS: The most common side effects are hypotension, tachycardia, nasal stuffiness, nausea, vomiting, and diarrhea.

PHARMACOKINETICS: Onset, peak, and duration vary among products.

INTERACTIONS: Vasoconstrictive and hypertensive effects of epinephrine are antagonized by α-adrenergic blockers.

NURSING CONSIDERATIONS
Assessment
• Monitor electrolytes: potassium, sodium chloride, carbon dioxide
• Monitor weight daily, I&O
• Monitor B/P with patient lying, standing before starting treatment, q4hr thereafter
• Assess for nausea, vomiting, diarrhea
• Assess for skin turgor, dryness of mucous membranes for hydration status

Nursing diagnoses
• Injury, risk for (adverse reactions)
• Sleep deprivation (adverse reactions)
• Tissue perfusion, ineffective (uses)

Patient/family education
• Caution patient to avoid alcoholic beverages
• Advise patient to report dizziness, palpitations, fainting

• Instruct patient to change position slowly or fainting may occur
• Teach patient to take product exactly as prescribed; to avoid all OTC products (cough, cold, allergy) unless directed by prescriber

Evaluation
Positive therapeutic outcome
• Decreased B/P
• Increased peripheral pulses

Generic Names

α 1 blockers:
silodosin

Anesthetics—general/local

ACTION: Anesthetics (general) act on the CNS to produce tranquilization and sleep before invasive procedures. Anesthetics (local) inhibit conduction of nerve impulses from sensory nerves.

USES: General anesthetics are used to premedicate for surgery, and for induction and maintenance in general anesthesia. For local anesthetics, refer to individual product listing for indications.

CONTRAINDICATIONS:

Persons with CVA, increased ICP, severe hypertension, and cardiac decompensation should not use these products since severe adverse reactions can occur.

Precautions: Anesthetics (general) should be used with caution in the geriatric, children <2 yr, and those with cardiovascular disease (hypotension, bradydysrhythmias), renal/hepatic disease, and Parkinson's disease. The precaution for anesthetics (local) is pregnancy.

IMPLEMENTATION
• Give anticholinergic preoperatively to decrease secretions
• Administer only with resuscitative equipment nearby
• Provide quiet environment for recovery to decrease psychotic symptoms

ADVERSE EFFECTS: The most common side effects are dystonia, akathisia, flexion of arms, fine tremors, drowsiness, restlessness, and hypotension. Also common are chills, respiratory depression, and laryngospasm.

Adverse effects: *italics* = common; **bold** = life-threatening

PHARMACOKINETICS: Onset, peak, and duration vary widely among products. Most products are metabolized in the liver and excreted in urine.

INTERACTIONS: AOIs, tricyclics, and phenothiazines may cause severe hypo/hypertension when used with local anesthetics. CNS depressants will potentiate general and local anesthetics.

NURSING CONSIDERATIONS
Assessment
• Monitor VS q10min during **IV** administration, q30min after IM dose

Nursing diagnoses
General
• Injury, risk for (adverse reactions)
• Knowledge, deficient (teaching)
Local
• Pain, acute (uses)
• Knowledge, deficient (teaching)

Evaluation
Positive therapeutic outcome
• Maintenance of anesthesia
• Decreased pain

Generic Names

General anesthetics:
droperidol (high alert), **fentaNYL** (high alert), fentaNYL/droperidol, fentaNYL transdermal, fospropofol, midazolam, **propofol** (high alert)

Local anesthetics:
lidocaine, parenteral (high alert), penicillin G procaine, ropivacaine

Antacids

ACTION: Antacids are basic compounds that neutralize gastric acidity and decrease the rate of gastric emptying. Products are divided into those containing aluminum, magnesium, calcium, or a combination of these.

USES: Antacids decrease hyperacidity in conditions such as peptic ulcer disease, reflux esophagitis, gastritis, or hiatal hernia.

CONTRAINDICATIONS:
Sensitivity to aluminum or magnesium products may cause hypersensitive reactions. Aluminum products should not be used by persons sensitive to aluminum. Magnesium products should not be used by persons sensitive to magnesium. Check for sensitivity before administering.

Precautions: Magnesium products should be given cautiously to patients with renal insufficiency, and during pregnancy and breastfeeding. Sodium content of antacids may be significant. Use with caution for patients with hypertension, or CHF or those on a low-sodium diet.

IMPLEMENTATION
• Advise patient not to take other products within 1-2 hr of antacid administration, since antacids may impair absorption of other products
• Give all products with an 8-oz glass of water to ensure absorption in the stomach
• Give another antacid if constipation occurs with aluminum products

ADVERSE EFFECTS: The most common side effect caused by aluminum-containing antacids is constipation, which may lead to fecal impaction and bowel obstruction. Diarrhea occurs often when magnesium products are given. Alkalosis may occur when systemic products are used. Constipation occurs more frequently than laxation with calcium carbonate. The release of CO_2 from carbonate-containing antacids causes belching, abdominal distention, and flatulence. Sodium bicarbonate may act as a systemic antacid and produce systemic electrolyte disturbances and alkalosis. Calcium carbonate and sodium bicarbonate may cause rebound hyperacidity and milk-alkali syndrome. Alkaluria may occur when products are used on a long-term basis, particularly in persons with abnormal renal function.

PHARMACOKINETICS: Duration is 20-40 min. If ingested 1 hr after meals, acidity is reduced for at least 3hr.

INTERACTIONS: Products whose effects may be increased by some antacids include quinidine, amphetamines, pseudoephedrine, levodopa, valproic acid, and dicumarol. Products whose effects may be decreased by some antacids include cimetidine, corticosteroids, ranitidine, iron salts, phenothiazines, phenytoin, digoxin, tetracyclines, ketoconazole, salicylates, and isoniazid.

NURSING CONSIDERATIONS
Assessment
• Assess for aggravating and alleviating factors of epigastric pain or hyperacidity; identify the

location, duration, and characteristics of epigastric pain
• Assess GI symptoms, including constipation, diarrhea, abdominal pain; if severe abdominal pain with fever occurs, these products should not be given
• Assess renal symptoms, including increasing urinary pH, electrolytes

Nursing diagnoses
• Constipation (adverse reactions)
• Diarrhea (adverse reactions)
• Pain, chronic (uses)

Evaluation
Positive therapeutic outcome
• Absence of epigastric pain
• Decreased acidity

Generic Names
aluminum hydroxide, bismuth subsalicylate, calcium carbonate, magaldrate, magnesium oxide, sodium bicarbonate

Anti-Alzheimer Agents

ACTION: Anti-Alzheimer agents improve cognitive functioning by increasing acetylcholine and inhibiting cholinesterase in the CNS. They do not cure the condition, but improve symptoms.

USES: Anti-Alzheimer agents are used for the treatment of Alzheimer's symptoms.

CONTRAINDICATIONS: Persons with hypersensitivity reactions should not use these products.

Precautions: Anti-Alzheimer agents should be used cautiously in pregnancy **(C)**, breastfeeding, sick sinus syndrome, GI bleeding, bladder obstruction, and seizures.

IMPLEMENTATION
• Give lowest possible dose for therapeutic result; adjust dose to response
• Provide assistance with ambulation during beginning therapy if dizziness, ataxia occur

ADVERSE EFFECTS: The most common side effects are nausea, vomiting, diarrhea, dry mouth, insomnia, dizziness, urinary frequency, incontinence, and rash. The most serious side effects are seizures and dysrhythmias.

PHARMACOKINETICS: Onset, peak, and duration vary widely among products. Most products are metabolized in the liver and excreted by the kidneys.

INTERACTIONS: Increased synergistic reactions may occur with succinylcholine, cholinesterase inhibitors, and cholinergic agonists. There may be a decrease in the action of anticholinergics, and there may be additive effects when used with cholinergic agents.

NURSING CONSIDERATIONS
Assessment
• B/P, hypo/hypertension
• Mental status: affect, mood, behavioral changes, depression, confusion
• GI status: nausea, vomiting, anorexia, diarrhea
• GU status: urinary frequency, incontinence

Nursing diagnoses
• Knowledge, deficient (teaching)
• Noncompliance (teaching)
• Thought processes, disturbed (uses)

Patient/family education
• Instruct patient to report side effects, adverse reactions to healthcare provider
• Advise patient to use exactly as prescribed, at regular intervals
• Caution patient not to increase or abruptly decrease dose; serious consequences may result
• Inform patient that product is not a cure, but relieves symptoms

Evaluation
Positive therapeutic outcome
• Decrease in confusion
• Improved mood

Generic Names
donepezil, memantine, rivastigmine

Antianginals

ACTION: Antianginals are divided into the nitrates, calcium channel blockers, and β-adrenergic blockers. The nitrates dilate coronary arteries, causing decreased preload, and dilate systemic arteries, causing decreased afterload. Calcium channel blockers dilate coronary arteries and decrease SA/AV node conduction. β-Adrenergic blockers decrease heart rate so that myocardial O_2 use is decreased. Dipyridamole selectively dilates coronary arteries to increase coronary blood flow.

USES: Antianginals are used in chronic stable angina pectoris, unstable angina, and vasospastic angina. Some (i.e., calcium channel blockers and β-blockers) may be used as dysrhythmics and in hypertension.

CONTRAINDICATIONS:
Persons with known hypersensitivity, increased ICP, or cerebral hemorrhage should not use some of these products.

Precautions: Antianginals should be used with caution in pregnancy, breastfeeding, children, postural hypotension, renal disease, and hepatic injury.

IMPLEMENTATION
• Store protected from light, moisture; place in cool environment

ADVERSE EFFECTS:
The most common side effects are postural hypotension, headache, flushing, dizziness, nausea, edema, and drowsiness. Also common are rash, dysrhythmias, and fatigue.

PHARMACOKINETICS:
Onset, peak, and duration vary widely among coronary products. Most products are metabolized in the liver and excreted in urine.

INTERACTIONS:
Interactions vary widely among products. Check individual monographs for specific information.

NURSING CONSIDERATIONS
Assessment
• Monitor orthostatic B/P, pulse
• Assess for pain: duration, time started, activity being performed, character
• Assess for tolerance if taken over long period
• Assess for headache, light-headedness, decreased B/P; may indicate a need for decreased dosage

Nursing diagnoses
• Cardiac output, decreased (adverse reactions)
• Injury, risk for (uses)
• Knowledge, deficient (teaching)
• Pain, acute (uses)
• Tissue perfusion, ineffective (uses)

Patient/family education
• Instruct patient to keep tabs in original container
• Instruct patient not to use OTC products unless directed by prescriber

• Advise patient to report bradycardia, dizziness, confusion, depression, fever
• Teach patient to take pulse at home; advise when to notify prescriber
• Advise patient to avoid alcohol, smoking, sodium intake
• Advise patient to comply with weight control, dietary adjustments, modified exercise program
• Teach patient to carry/wear emergency ID to identify product being taken, allergies
• Caution patient to make position changes slowly to prevent fainting

Evaluation
Positive therapeutic outcome
• Decrease, prevention of anginal pain

Generic Names

Nitrates:
isosorbide, nitroglycerin

β-Adrenergic blockers:
atenolol, dipyridamole, metoprolol, nadolol, propranolol

Calcium channel blockers:
amLODIPine, diltiazem (high alert), niCARdipine, NIFEdipine, verapamil

Miscellaneous:
ranolazine

Antianxiety Agents

ACTION: Benzodiazepines potentiate the action of GABA, including any other inhibitory transmitters in the CNS, resulting in decreased anxiety. Most agents cause a decrease in CNS excitability.

USES: Anxiety is relieved in conditions such as generalized anxiety disorder and phobic disorders. Benzodiazepines are also used for acute alcohol withdrawal to prevent delirium tremens, and some products are used for relaxation before surgery.

CONTRAINDICATIONS:
These products are contraindicated in hypersensitivity, acute closed-angle glaucoma, breastfeeding (diazepam), children <6 mo, and hepatic disease (clonazepam).

Precautions: Antianxiety agents should be used cautiously in geriatric or debilitated patients. Usually smaller doses are needed since metabolism is slowed. Persons with renal/hepatic disease may show delayed excretion.

Clonazepam may increase the incidence of seizures.

IMPLEMENTATION
• Give with food or milk for GI symptoms; may give crushed if patient is unable to swallow whole (tabs only, no controlled or sustained-release products)

ADVERSE EFFECTS: The most
common side effects are dizziness, drowsiness, blurred vision, and orthostatic hypotension. Most adverse reactions are mediated through the CNS. There is potential for abuse and physical dependence with some products.

PHARMACOKINETICS: Most of
these agents are metabolized by the liver and excreted via the kidneys.

INTERACTIONS: Increased CNS
depression may occur when given with other CNS depressants. These products should be used together cautiously. Alcohol should not be used, as fatal reactions have occurred. The serum concentration and toxicity may be increased when used with benzodiazepines.

NURSING CONSIDERATIONS

Assessment
• Assess B/P (lying and standing), pulse; if systolic B/P drops 20 mm Hg, hold product and notify prescriber; orthostatic hypotension can be severe
• Monitor renal/hepatic function tests: AST, ALT, bilirubin, creatinine, LDH, alkaline phosphatase
• Monitor physical dependency and withdrawal with some products, including headache, nausea, vomiting, muscle pain, and weakness after long-term use

Nursing diagnoses
• Anxiety (uses)
• Injury, risk for, physical (adverse reactions)
• Knowledge, deficient (teaching)

Patient/family education
• Inform patient that product should not be used for everyday stress or long-term use; not to take more than prescribed amount since product is habit forming
• Caution patient to avoid driving and activities that require alertness since drowsiness and dizziness may occur
• Instruct patient to abstain from alcohol, other psychotropic medications unless directed by prescriber

• Caution patient not to discontinue abruptly; after extended periods, withdrawal symptoms may occur

Evaluation
Positive therapeutic outcome
• Decreased anxiety
• Increased relaxation

Generic Names

Benzodiazepines:
ALPRAZolam, chlordiazePOXIDE, clonazePAM, diazepam, LORazepam, midazolam, triazolam

Miscellaneous:
busPIRone, doxepin, hydrOXYzine, PARoxetine, venlafaxine

Antiasthmatics

ACTION: Bronchodilators are divided
into anticholinergics, α/β-adrenergic agonists, β-adrenergic agonists, and phosphodiesterase inhibitors. Also included in antiasthmatic agents are corticosteroids, leukotriene antagonists, mast cell stabilizers, and monoclonal antibodies. Anticholinergics act by inhibiting interaction of acetylcholine at receptor sites on bronchial smooth muscle. α/β-Adrenergic agonists act by relaxing bronchial smooth muscle and increasing diameter of nasal passages. β-Adrenergic agonists act by action on β_2-receptors, which relaxes bronchial smooth muscle. Phosphodiesterase inhibitors act by blocking phosphodiesterase and increasing cAMP, which mediates smooth muscle relaxation in the respiratory system. Corticosteroids act by decreasing inflammation in the bronchial system. Leukotriene receptor antagonists decrease leukotrienes, and mast cell stabilizers decrease histamine; both act to decrease bronchospasm.

USES: Antiasthmatics are used for bronchial
asthma; bronchospasm associated with bronchitis, emphysema, or other obstructive pulmonary diseases; Cheyne-Stokes respirations; and prevention of exercise-induced asthma. Some products are used for rhinitis and other allergic reactions.

CONTRAINDICATIONS:
Persons with hypersensitivity, closed-angle glaucoma, tachydysrhythmias, and severe cardiac disease should not use some of these products.

Precautions: Antiasthmatics should be used with caution in pregnancy, breastfeeding, hyperthyroidism, hypertension, prostatic hypertrophy, and seizure disorders.

IMPLEMENTATION

• Give inhaled product after shaking; exhale, place mouthpiece in mouth, inhale slowly, hold breath, remove, exhale slowly
• Give PO product with meals to decrease gastric irritation
• Store inhaled product in light-resistant container; do not expose to temperatures >86° F (30° C)
• Give gum, small sips of water for dry mouth

ADVERSE EFFECTS: The most common side effects are tremors, anxiety, nausea, vomiting and irritation in the throat. The most serious adverse reactions are bronchospasm and dyspnea.

PHARMACOKINETICS: Onset, peak, and duration vary widely among products. Most products are metabolized by the liver and excreted in urine.

INTERACTIONS: Interactions vary widely among products. Check individual monographs for specific information.

NURSING CONSIDERATIONS

Assessment
• Monitor respiratory function: vital capacity, forced expiratory volume, ABGs, lung sounds, heart rate and rhythm, aggravating and alleviating factors

Nursing diagnoses
• Activity intolerance (uses)
• Airway clearance, ineffective (uses)
• Injury, risk for, physical (adverse reactions)
• Knowledge, deficient (teaching)
• Noncompliance (teaching)

Patient/family education
• Caution patient to avoid hazardous activities; drowsiness or dizziness may occur with some products
• Instruct patient to obtain bloodwork as required; some products require blood levels to be drawn
• Advise patient to avoid all OTC medications unless approved by provider
• Instruct patient to report side effects, including insomnia, heart palpitations, light-headedness; these side effects may occur with some products

Evaluation
Positive therapeutic outcome
• Decreased severity and number of asthma attacks
• Absence of dyspnea, wheezing

Generic Names

Bronchodilators:
albuterol, arformoterol, **atropine** (high alert), formoterol, ipratropium, levalbuterol, terbutaline, theophylline, tiotropium

Adrenergics:
EPINEPHrine (high alert)

Corticosteroids:
beclomethasone, betamethasone, budesonide, cortisone, dexamethasone, flunisolide, fluticasone, hydrocortisone, methylPREDNISolone, predniSONE, triamcinolone

Leukotriene antagonists:
zafirlukast

Monoclonal antibodies:
omalizumab

Anticholinergics

ACTION: Anticholinergics inhibit the muscarinic actions of acetylcholine at receptor sites in the autonomic nervous system. Anticholinergics are also known as antimuscarinic products.

USES: Anticholinergics are used for a variety of conditions: decreasing involuntary movements in parkinsonism (benztropine, trihexyphenidyl); bradydysrhythmias (atropine); nausea and vomiting (scopolamine); and as cycloplegic mydriatics (atropine, hematropine, scopalamine, cyclopentolate, tropicamide). Gastrointestinal anticholinergics are used to decrease motility (smooth muscle tone) in the GI, biliary, and urinary tracts and for their ability to decrease gastric secretions (propantheline, glycopyrrolate).

CONTRAINDICATIONS:
Persons with closed-angle glaucoma, myasthenia gravis, or GI/GU obstruction should not use some of these products.

Precautions: Anticholinergics should be used with caution in pregnant,breastfeeding, or geriatric patients, or in those with prostatic hypertrophy, CHF, or hypertension. Use with caution in the presence of high environmental temperature.

IMPLEMENTATION
PO route
• Give with or after meals to prevent GI upset; may give with fluids other than water
• Store at room temperature
• Give hard candy, frequent drinks, sugarless gum to relieve dry mouth

IM/IV route
• Give parenteral dose with patient recumbent to prevent postural hypotension
• Give parenteral dose slowly; keep in bed for at least 1 hr after dose; monitor VS
• Give after checking dose carefully; even slight overdose could lead to toxicity

ADVERSE EFFECTS: The most common side effects are dry mouth, constipation, urinary retention, urinary hesitancy, headache, and dizziness. Also common is paralytic ileus.

PHARMACOKINETICS: Onset, peak, and duration vary widely among products. Most products are metabolized in the liver and excreted in urine.

INTERACTIONS: Increased anticholinergic effects may occur when used with MAOIs, tricyclics, and amantadine. Anticholinergics may cause a decreased effect of phenothiazines and levodopa.

NURSING CONSIDERATIONS
Assessment
• Assess I&O ratio; retention commonly causes decreased urinary output
• Assess for urinary hesitancy, retention; palpate bladder if retention occurs
• Assess for constipation; increase fluids, bulk, exercise if this occurs
• Identify tolerance over long-term therapy; dosage may need to be increased or changed
• Assess mental status: affect, mood, CNS depression, worsening of mental symptoms during early therapy

Nursing diagnoses
• Cardiac output, decreased (uses)
• Constipation (adverse reactions)
• Knowledge, deficient (teaching)

Patient/family education
• Caution patient to avoid driving and other hazardous activities; drowsiness may occur
• Advise patient to avoid OTC medication: cough, cold preparations with alcohol, antihistamines unless directed by prescriber

Evaluation
Positive therapeutic outcome
• Decreased secretions
• Absence of nausea and vomiting

Generic Names
atropine (high alert), benztropine, glycopyrrolate, hyoscyamine, scopolamine (transdermal), solifenacin

Anticoagulants

ACTION: Anticoagulants interfere with blood clotting by preventing clot formation.

USES: Anticoagulants are used for DVT, pulmonary emboli, myocardial infarction, open heart surgery, disseminated intravascular clotting syndrome, atrial fibrillation with embolization, and in transfusion and dialysis.

CONTRAINDICATIONS:
Persons with hemophilia and related disorders, leukemia with bleeding, peptic ulcer disease, thrombocytopenic purpura, blood dyscrasias, acute nephritis, and subacute bacterial endocarditis should not use these products.

Precautions: Anticoagulants should be used with caution in pregnancy, geriatric, and alcoholism.

IMPLEMENTATION
• Store in tight container (PO dose)
SUBCUT route
• Give at same time each day to maintain steady blood levels
• Do not massage area or aspirate when giving SUBCUT inj; give in abdomen between pelvic bones; rotate sites; do not pull back on plunger, leave in for 10 sec; apply gentle pressure for 1 min
• Do not change needles
• Avoid all IM inj that may cause bleeding

ADVERSE EFFECTS: The most serious adverse reactions are hemorrhage, agranulocytosis, leukopenia, eosinophilia, and thrombocytopenia, depending on the specific product. The most common side effects are diarrhea, rash, and fever.

PHARMACOKINETICS: Onset, peak, and duration vary widely among products. Most products are metabolized in the liver and excreted in urine.

Adverse effects: *italics* = common; **bold** = life-threatening

INTERACTIONS: Salicylates, steroids, and nonsteroidal antiinflammatories will potentiate the action of anticoagulants. Anticoagulants may cause serious effects. Check individual monographs for specific information.

NURSING CONSIDERATIONS

Assessment

• Monitor blood tests (Hct, platelets, occult blood in stools) q3mo
• Monitor PTT, which should be $1^{1}/_{2}$-2 × control, PPT; daily, APTT, ACT, INR
• Monitor B/P; watch for increasing signs of hypertension
• Monitor for bleeding gums, petechiae, ecchymosis, black tarry stools, hematuria
• Monitor for fever, skin rash, urticaria
• Monitor for needed dosage change q1-2wk

Nursing diagnoses

• Injury, risk for (side effects)
• Knowledge, deficient (teaching)
• Tissue perfusion, ineffective (uses)

Patient/family education

• Advise patient to avoid OTC preparations that may cause serious product interactions unless directed by prescriber
• Inform patient that product may be held during active bleeding (menstruation), depending on condition
• Caution patient to use soft-bristle toothbrush to prevent bleeding gums; avoid contact sports; use electric razor
• Instruct patient to carry/wear emergency ID identifying product taken
• Instruct patient to report any signs of bleeding: gums, under skin, urine, stools

Evaluation
Positive therapeutic outcome
• Decrease of DVT

Generic Names
argatroban, dabigatran, **dalteparin** (high alert), **enoxaparin** (high alert), fondaparinux, **heparin** (high alert), **lepirudin** (high alert), **tinzaparin** (high alert), **warfarin** (high alert)

Anticonvulsants

ACTION: Anticonvulsants are divided into the barbiturates, benzodiazepines, hydantoins, succinimides, and miscellaneous products. Barbiturates and benzodiazepines are discussed in separate sections. Hydantoins act by inhibiting the spread of seizure activity in the motor cortex. Succinimides act by inhibiting spike and wave formation; they also decrease amplitude, frequency, duration, and spread of discharge in seizures.

USES: Hydantoins are used in generalized tonic-clonic seizures, status epilepticus, and psychomotor seizures. Succinimides are used for absence (or petit mal) seizures. Barbiturates are used in generalized tonic-clonic and cortical focal seizures.

CONTRAINDICATIONS:
Hypersensitive reactions may occur, and allergies should be identified before these products are given.

Precautions: Persons with renal/hepatic disease should be watched closely.

IMPLEMENTATION
PO route
• Give with food, milk to decrease GI symptoms
• Provide good oral hygiene as it is important for patients taking hydantoins

ADVERSE EFFECTS: Bone marrow depression is the most life-threatening adverse reaction associated with hydantoins or succinimides. The most common side effects are GI symptoms. Other common side effects for hydantoins are gingival hyperplasia and CNS effects such as nystagmus, ataxia, slurred speech, and confusion.

PHARMACOKINETICS: Onset, peak, and duration vary widely among products. Most products are metabolized in the liver and excreted in urine, bile, and feces.

INTERACTIONS: Hydantoins cause decreased effects of estrogens, and oral contraceptives.

NURSING CONSIDERATIONS
Assessment
• Monitor renal function tests, including BUN, creatinine, serum uric acid, urine CCr before, during therapy
• Monitor blood tests: RBC, Hct, Hgb, reticulocyte counts weekly for 4 wk then monthly
• Monitor hepatic function tests: AST, ALT, bilirubin, creatinine
• Assess mental status, including mood, sensorium, affect, behavioral changes; if mental status changes, notify prescriber

---

- Assess for eye problems, including need for ophth examinations before, during, and after treatment (slit lamp, fundoscopy, tonometry)
- Assess for allergic reaction, including red, raised rash; if this occurs, product should be discontinued
- Assess for blood dyscrasias, including fever, sore throat, bruising, rash, jaundice
- Monitor toxicity, including bone marrow depression, nausea, vomiting, ataxia, diplopia, cardiovascular collapse, Stevens-Johnson syndrome

Nursing diagnoses
- Injury, risk for (uses)
- Noncompliance (teaching)
- Sleep deprivation (adverse reactions)

Patient/family education
- Advise patient to carry/wear emergency ID stating products taken, condition, prescriber's name, phone number
- Advise patient to avoid driving, other activities that require alertness

Evaluation
Positive therapeutic outcome
- Decreased seizure activity; document on patient's chart

Generic Names

Succinimides:
ethosuximide

Hydantoins:
fosphenytoin, phenytoin

Miscellaneous:
acetaZOLAMIDE, carBAMazepine, clonazePAM, diazepam, ezogabine, gabapentin, lacosamide, lamoTRIgine, **magnesium sulfate** (high alert), rufinamide, tiagabine, topiramate, valproate/valproic acid/divalproex sodium, vigabatrin, zonisamide

Barbiturates:
PHENobarbital (high alert), primidone, **thiopental** (high alert)

Antidepressants

ACTION: Antidepressants are divided into the tricyclics, MAOIs, and miscellaneous antidepressants (SSRIs). The tricyclics work by blocking reuptake of norepinephrine and serotonin into nerve endings and increasing action of norepinephrine and serotonin in nerve cells. MAOIs act by increasing concentrations of endogenous epinephrine, norepinephrine, serotonin, and dopamine in storage sites in the CNS by inhibition of MAO; increased concentration reduces depression.

USES: Antidepressants are used for depression and, in some cases, enuresis in children.

CONTRAINDICATIONS:
The contraindications for antidepressants are seizure disorders, prostatic hypertrophy, and severe renal/hepatic/cardiac disease depending on the type of medication.

Precautions: Antidepressants should be used cautiously in pregnant, geriatric, and suicidal patients; severe depression; schizophrenia; hyperactivity; and diabetes mellitus.

IMPLEMENTATION
PO route
- Give increased fluids, bulk in diet if constipation, urinary retention occur
- Give with food or milk for GI symptoms
- Give gum, hard candy, or frequent sips of water for dry mouth
- Store in airtight container at room temperature; do not refreeze
- Provide assistance with ambulation during beginning therapy since drowsiness/dizziness occurs

ADVERSE EFFECTS: The most serious adverse reactions are paralytic ileus, acute renal failure, hypertension, and hypertensive crisis, depending on the specific product. Common side effects are dizziness, drowsiness, diarrhea, dry mouth, urinary retention, and orthostatic hypotension.

PHARMACOKINETICS: Onset, peak, and duration vary widely among products. Most products are metabolized in the liver and excreted in urine.

INTERACTIONS: Interactions vary widely among products. Check individual monographs for specific information.

NURSING CONSIDERATIONS
Assessment
- Monitor B/P (lying, standing), pulse q4hr; if systolic B/P drops 20 mm Hg, hold product, notify prescriber; take VS q4hr in patients with CV disease
- Monitor blood tests: CBC, leukocytes, differential, cardiac enzymes if patient is receiving long-term therapy

• Monitor hepatic function tests: AST, ALT, bilirubin, creatinine
• Monitor weight weekly; appetite may increase with product
• Monitor for EPS primarily in geriatric: rigidity, dystonia, akathisia
• Assess mental status: mood, sensorium, affect, suicidal tendencies, increase in psychiatric symptoms (depression, panic)
• Check for urinary retention, constipation; constipation is more likely to occur in children, geriatric patients
• Assess for withdrawal symptoms: headache, nausea, vomiting, muscle pain, weakness; do not usually occur unless product was discontinued abruptly
• Identify alcohol consumption; if alcohol is consumed, hold dose until AM

Nursing diagnoses
• Coping, ineffective (uses)
• Injury, risk for (uses/adverse reactions)
• Knowledge, deficient (teaching)

Patient/family education
• Teach patient that therapeutic effects may take 2-3 wk
• Advise patient to use caution in driving or other activities requiring alertness because of drowsiness, dizziness, blurred vision
• Caution patient to avoid alcohol ingestion, other CNS depressants
• Instruct patient not to discontinue medication quickly after long-term use; may cause nausea, headache, malaise
• Instruct patient to wear sunscreen or large hat, since photosensitivity may occur

Evaluation
Positive therapeutic outcome
• Decreased depression

Generic Names

Tetracyclics:
mirtazapine

Tricyclics:
amitriptyline, clomiPRAMINE, desipramine, doxepin, imipramine, nortriptyline

Miscellaneous:
buPROPion, DULoxetine, traZODone, venlafaxine

SSRIs:
citalopram, escitalopram, FLUoxetine, PARoxetine, sertraline

Antidiabetics

ACTION: Antidiabetics are divided into the insulins that decrease blood glucose, phosphate, and potassium and increase blood pyruvate and lactate and oral antidiabetics that cause functioning β-cells in the pancreas to release insulin and improve the effect of endogenous and exogenous insulin.

USES: Insulins are used for ketoacidosis and diabetes mellitus types 1 and 2; oral antidiabetics are used for diabetes mellitus type 2.

CONTRAINDICATIONS:
Hypersensitive reactions may occur, and allergies should be identified before these products are given. Oral antidiabetics should not be used in juvenile or brittle diabetes, diabetic ketoacidosis, or severe renal/hepatic disease.

Precautions: Oral antidiabetics should be used with caution in pregnancy, breastfeeding, geriatric, cardiac disease, and in the presence of alcohol.

IMPLEMENTATION
PO route
• Give oral antidiabetic 30 min before meals
SUBCUT route
• Give insulin after warming to room temperature by rotating in palms to prevent lipodystrophy from injecting cold insulin
• Give human insulin to those allergic to beef or pork
• Rotate inj sites when giving insulin; use abdomen, upper back, thighs, upper arm, buttocks; keep a record of sites

ADVERSE EFFECTS: The most common side effect of insulin and oral antidiabetics is hypoglycemia. Other adverse reactions for oral antidiabetics include blood dyscrasias, hepatotoxicity, and, rarely, cholestatic jaundice. Adverse reactions for insulin products include allergic responses and, more rarely, anaphylaxis.

PHARMACOKINETICS: Onset, peak, and duration vary widely among products. Oral antidiabetics are metabolized in the liver, with metabolites excreted in urine, bile, and feces.

INTERACTIONS: Interactions vary widely among products. Check individual monographs for specific information.

⚠ Nurse Alert

NURSING CONSIDERATIONS

Assessment

• Monitor blood, urine glucose levels during treatment to determine diabetes control (oral products)
• Monitor fasting blood glucose, 2 hr PP (60-100 mg/dl normal fasting level) (70-130 mg/dl—normal 2-hr level)
• Assess for hypoglycemic reaction that can occur during peak time

Nursing diagnoses

• Nutrition: more than body requirements, imbalanced (uses)

Patient/family education

• Advise patient to avoid alcohol and salicylates except on advice of prescriber
• Teach patient symptoms of ketoacidosis: nausea, thirst, polyuria, dry mouth, decreased B/P, dry, flushed skin, acetone breath, drowsiness, Kussmaul respirations
• Teach patient symptoms of hypoglycemia: headache, tremors, fatigue, weakness; that candy or sugar should be carried to treat hypoglycemia
• Advise patient to test urine for glucose/ketones tid if this product is replacing insulin
• Advise patient to continue weight control, dietary restrictions, exercise, hygiene

Evaluation

Positive therapeutic outcome

• Decrease in polyuria, polydipsia, polyphagia
• Clear sensorium
• Absence of dizziness
• Stable gait

Generic Names

glipiZIDE, glyBURIDE, **insulin aspart** (high alert), **insulin detemir** (high alert), **insulin glargine** (high alert), **insulin glulisine** (high alert), **insulin lispro** (high alert), **insulin, regular** (high alert), **insulin, regular concentrated** (high alert), insulin, zinc suspension (Lente), insulin, zinc suspension extended (Ultralente), liraglutide, linagliptin, metformin, miglitol, pioglitazone, repaglinide, rosiglitazone, saxagliptin, sitagliptin

Antidiarrheals

ACTION: Antidiarrheals work by various actions including direct action on intestinal muscles to decrease GI peristalsis or by inhibiting prostaglandin synthesis responsible for GI hypermotility, acting on mucosal receptors responsible for peristalsis, or decreasing water content of stools.

USES: Antidiarrheals are used for diarrhea of undetermined causes.

CONTRAINDICATIONS:

The contraindications are persons with severe ulcerative colitis, and pseudomembranous colitis with some products.

Precautions: Antidiarrheals should be used with caution in pregnancy, breastfeeding, children, geriatric patients, dehydration.

IMPLEMENTATION

PO route

• Give for 48 hr only

ADVERSE EFFECTS: The most serious adverse reactions of some products are paralytic ileus, toxic megacolon, and angioneurotic edema. The most common side effects are constipation, nausea, dry mouth, and abdominal pain.

PHARMACOKINETICS: Onset, peak, and duration vary widely among products. Most products are metabolized in the liver and excreted in urine.

INTERACTIONS: Interactions vary widely among products. Check individual monographs for specific information.

NURSING CONSIDERATIONS

Assessment

• Monitor electrolytes (potassium, sodium, chloride) if on long-term therapy
• Monitor bowel pattern before; for rebound constipation after termination of medication
• Assess response after 48 hr; if no response, product should be discontinued
• Identify dehydration in children

Nursing diagnoses

• Constipation (adverse reactions)
• Diarrhea (uses)
• Fluid volume, risk for deficient (adverse reactions)
• Knowledge, deficient (teaching)

Patient/family education

• Advise patient to avoid OTC products
• Caution patient not to exceed recommended dose

Adverse effects: *italics* = common; **bold** = life-threatening

Evaluation
Positive therapeutic outcome
• Decreased diarrhea

Generic Names
bismuth subsalicylate, kaolin/pectin, loperamide

Antidysrhythmics

ACTION: Antidysrhythmics are divided into four classes and miscellaneous antidysrhythmics:
• Class I increases the duration of action potential and the effective refractory period and reduces disparity in the refractory period between a normal and infarcted myocardium; further subclasses include Ia, Ib, Ic
• Class II decreases the rate of SA node discharge, increases recovery time, slows conduction through the AV node, and decreases heart rate, which decreases O_2 consumption in the myocardium
• Class III increases the duration of action potential and the effective refractory period
• Class IV inhibits calcium ion influx across the cell membrane during cardiac depolarization; decreases SA node discharge, decreases conduction velocity through the AV node
• Miscellaneous antidysrhythmics include those such as adenosine, which slows conduction through the AV node, and digoxin, which decreases conduction velocity and prolongs the effective refractory period in the AV node

USES: Antidysrhythmics are used for PVCs, tachycardia, hypertension, atrial fibrillation, and angina pectoris.

CONTRAINDICATIONS:
Contraindications vary widely among products.

Precautions: Precautions vary widely among products.

ADVERSE EFFECTS: Side effects and adverse reactions vary widely among products.

PHARMACOKINETICS: Onset, peak, and duration vary widely among products.

INTERACTIONS: Interactions vary widely among products. Check individual monographs for specific information.

NURSING CONSIDERATIONS

Assessment
• Monitor ECG continuously to determine product effectiveness, PVCs, or other dysrhythmias
• Assess for dehydration or hypovolemia
• Monitor B/P continuously for hypo/hypertension
• Monitor I&O ratio
• Monitor serum potassium
• Assess for edema in feet and legs daily

Nursing diagnoses
• Cardiac output, decreased (uses)
• Diarrhea (adverse reactions)
• Gas exchange, impaired (adverse reactions)
• Tissue perfusion, ineffective (uses)

Patient/family education
• Advise patient to comply with dosage schedule, even if patient is feeling better
• Instruct patient to report bradycardia, dizziness, confusion, depression, fever

Evaluation
Positive therapeutic outcome
• Decrease in B/P in hypertension
• Decreased B/P, edema, moist crackles in CHF

Generic Names
Class Ia:
disopyramide, procainamide, quiNIDine

Class Ib:
lidocaine, parenteral (high alert), phenytoin

Class Ic:
flecainide, propafenone

Class II:
acebutolol, esmolol, propranolol, sotalol

Class III:
amiodarone (high alert), **dronedarone** (high alert), **ibutilide** (high alert)

Class IV:
verapamil

Miscellaneous:
adenosine (high alert), **atropine** (high alert), **digoxin** (high alert)

Antiemetics

ACTION: The antiemetics are divided into the 5-HT$_3$ receptor antagonists, the phenothiazines, and the miscellaneous products. The 5-HT$_3$ receptor antagonists work by blocking serotonin peripherally, centrally, and in the small intestine. The phenothiazines act by blocking the chemoreceptor trigger zone in the brain. The miscellaneous products work by either decreasing motion sickness or delaying gastric emptying.

USES: Antiemetics are used to prevent nausea and vomiting due to cancer chemotherapy, radiotherapy, and surgery (5-HT$_3$ receptor antagonists); some of the miscellaneous products (antihistamines) work by decreasing motion sickness. Most other products are used for many types of nausea and vomiting.

CONTRAINDICATIONS:
Persons developing hypersensitive reactions should not use these products.

Precautions: Antiemetics should be used cautiously in pregnancy, breastfeeding, hepatic disease, and some GI disorders.

IMPLEMENTATION
• Give prophylactically, before nausea and vomiting occur, in cancer chemotherapy
• Store at room temperature vial/ampules, oral products

ADVERSE EFFECTS: The most common side effects are headache, dizziness, fatigue, and diarrhea.

PHARMACOKINETICS: Onset, peak, and duration vary widely among products. Most products are metabolized by the liver and excreted by the kidneys.

INTERACTIONS: Interactions vary widely among products. Check individual monographs for specific information. Other CNS depressants increase CNS depression.

NURSING CONSIDERATIONS
Assessment
• Assess reason for nausea, vomiting; absence of nausea and vomiting after giving product
• Monitor hypersensitivity reactions: rash, bronchospasm with some products

Nursing diagnoses
• Fluid volume, risk for deficient (uses)
• Injury, risk for, physical (uses, adverse reactions)
• Knowledge, deficient (teaching)
• Nutrition: less than body requirements, imbalanced (uses)

Patient/family education
• Caution patient to avoid hazardous activities if dizziness occurs; ask for assistance if hospitalized
• Instruct patient to rise slowly to prevent orthostatic hypotension
• Teach patient all aspects of product usage
• Teach patient conservative methods to control nausea and vomiting such as sips of water or other fluids and dry crackers

Evaluation
Positive therapeutic outcome
• Absence or decreasing nausea and vomiting after use

Generic Names
5-HT$_3$ antagonists:
dolasetron, granisetron, ondansetron, palonosetron

Phenothiazines:
chlorproMAZINE, prochlorperazine, promethazine

Miscellaneous:
aprepitant, meclizine, metoclopramide, scopolamine, trimethobenzamide

Antifungals (systemic)

ACTION: Antifungals act by increasing cell membrane permeability in susceptible organisms by binding sterols and decreasing potassium, sodium, and nutrients in the cell.

USES: Antifungals are used for infections of histoplasmosis, blastomycosis, coccidioidomycosis, cryptococcosis, aspergillosis, phycomycosis, candidiasis, sporotrichosis causing severe meningitis, septicemia, and skin infections.

CONTRAINDICATIONS:
Persons with severe bone marrow depression or hypersensitivity should not use these products.

Precautions: Antifungals should be used with caution in renal/hepatic disease and pregnancy.

IMPLEMENTATION
IV route
• Give by **IV** using in-line filter (mean pore diameter >1 μm) using distal veins; check for extravasation, necrosis q8hr
• Give product only after C&S confirms organism, make sure product is used in life-threatening infections

• Provide protection from light during infusion; cover with foil
• Give symptomatic treatment as ordered for adverse reactions: aspirin, antihistamines, antiemetics, antispasmodics
• Store protected from moisture and light; diluted sol is stable for 24 hr

ADVERSE EFFECTS: The most serious adverse reactions include renal tubular acidosis, permanent renal impairment, anuria, oliguria, hemorrhagic gastroenteritis, acute liver failure, and blood dyscrasias. Some common side effects include hypokalemia, nausea, vomiting, anorexia, headache, fever, and chills.

PHARMACOKINETICS: Onset, peak, and duration vary widely among products. Most products are metabolized in the liver and excreted in urine.

INTERACTIONS: Interactions vary widely among products. Check individual monographs for specific information.

NURSING CONSIDERATIONS

Assessment
• Monitor VS q15-30min during first infusion; note changes in pulse,B/P
• Monitor I&O ratio; watch for decreasing urinary output, change in specific gravity; discontinue product to prevent permanent damage to renal tubules
• Monitor blood tests; CBC, potassium, sodium, calcium, magnesium q2wk
• Monitor weight weekly; if weight increases over 2 lb/wk, edema is present; renal damage should be considered
• Assess for renal toxicity: increasing BUN, if >40 mg/dl or if serum creatinine >3 mg/dl; product may be discontinued or dosage reduced
• Assess for hepatotoxicity: increasing AST, ALT, alkaline phosphatase, bilirubin
• Assess for allergic reaction: dermatitis, rash; product should be discontinued; antihistamines (mild reaction) or epINEPHrine (severe reaction) administered
• Assess for hypokalemia: anorexia, drowsiness, weakness, decreased reflexes, dizziness, increased urinary output, increased thirst, paresthesias
• Assess for ototoxicity: tinnitus (ringing, roaring in ears), vertigo, loss of hearing (rare)

Nursing diagnoses
• Infection, risk for (uses)
• Injury, risk for (adverse reactions)
• Knowledge, deficient (teaching)

⚠ Nurse Alert

Patient/family education
• Teach patient that long-term therapy may be needed to clear infection (2 wk-3 mo depending on type of infection)

Evaluation
Positive therapeutic outcome
• Decreased fever, malaise, rash
• Negative C&S for infecting organism

Generic Names
amphotericin B, anidulafungin, fluconazole, itraconazole, ketoconazole, micafungin, nystatin, posaconazole, voriconazole

Antihistamines

ACTION: Antihistamines compete with histamines for H_1 receptor sites. They antagonize in varying degrees most of the pharmacologic effects of histamines.

USES: Antihistamines are used to control the symptoms of allergies, rhinitis, and pruritus.

CONTRAINDICATIONS: Hypersensitivity to H_1-receptor antagonists occurs rarely. Patients with acute asthma and lower respiratory tract disease should not use these products since thick secretions may result. Other contraindications include closed-angle glaucoma, bladder neck obstruction, stenosing peptic ulcer, symptomatic prostatic hypertrophy, breastfeeding, and in the newborn.

Precautions: Antihistamines must be used cautiously in conjunction with intraocular pressure since they increase intraocular pressure. Caution should also be used in pregnancy, breastfeeding, and geriatric patients and patients with renal/cardiac disease, hypertension, and seizure disorders.

ADVERSE EFFECTS: Most products cause drowsiness; however, loratadine and fexofenadine produce little, if any, drowsiness. Other common side effects are headache and thickening of bronchial secretions. Serious blood dyscrasias may occur, but are rare. Urinary retention, GI effects occur with many of these products.

PHARMACOKINETICS: Onset varies from 20-60 min, with duration lasting 4-24 hr. In general, pharmacokinetics vary widely among products.

INTERACTIONS: Barbiturates, opioids, hypnotics, tricyclics, and alcohol can increase CNS depression when taken with antihistamines.

NURSING CONSIDERATIONS

Assessment
• Check I&O ratio; be alert for urinary retention, frequency, dysuria; product should be discontinued if these occur
• Assess for blood dyscrasias: thrombocytopenia, agranulocytosis (rare)
• Assess for respiratory status, including rate, rhythm, increase in bronchial secretions, wheezing, chest tightness
• Assess for cardiac status, including palpitations, increased pulse, hypotension
• Assess CBC during long-term therapy, since hemolytic anemia, although rare, may occur
• Administer with food or milk to decrease GI symptoms; absorption may be decreased slightly
• Administer whole (sus rel tab)
• Provide hard candy, gum, frequent rinsing of mouth for dryness

Nursing diagnoses
• Airway clearance, ineffective (uses)

Patient/family education
• Advise patient to notify prescriber if confusion, sedation, hypotension occur
• Caution patient to avoid driving and other hazardous activity if drowsiness occurs
• Instruct patient to avoid concurrent use of alcohol and other CNS depressants
• Inform patient to discontinue a few days before skin testing

Evaluation
Positive therapeutic outcome
• Absence of allergy symptoms, itching

Generic Names
brompheniramine, budesonide, cetirizine, chlorpheniramine, cyproheptadine, desloratadine, diphenhydrAMINE, fexofenadine, levocetirizine, loratadine, promethazine

Antihypertensives

ACTION: Antihypertensives are divided into angiotensin converting enzyme (ACE) inhibitors, β-adrenergic blockers, calcium channel blockers, centrally acting adrenergics, diuretics, peripherally acting antiadrenergics, and vasodilators. β-Blockers, calcium channel blockers, and diuretics are discussed in separate sections. ACE inhibitors selectively suppress conversion of renin-angiotensin I to angiotensin II; dilatation of arterial and venous vessels occurs. Centrally acting adrenergics act by inhibiting the sympathetic vasomotor center in the CNS, which reduces impulses in the sympathetic nervous system; blood pressure, pulse rate, and cardiac output decrease. Peripherally acting antiadrenergics inhibit sympathetic vasoconstriction by inhibiting release of norepinephrine and/or depleting norepinephrine stores in adrenergic nerve endings. Vasodilators act on arteriolar smooth muscle by producing direct relaxation or vasodilatation; a reduction in blood pressure, with concomitant increases in heart rate and cardiac output, occurs.

USES: Antihypertensives are used for hypertension and for heart failure not responsive to conventional therapy. Some products are used in hypertensive crisis, angina, and for some cardiac dysrhythmias.

CONTRAINDICATIONS:
Hypersensitive reactions may occur, and allergies should be identified before these products are given. Antihypertensives should not be used in children or in patients with heart block.

Precautions: Antihypertensives should be used with caution in geriatric and dialysis patients, and in the presence of hypovolemia, leukemia, and electrolyte imbalances.

IMPLEMENTATION
• Place patient in supine or Trendelenburg position for severe hypotension

ADVERSE EFFECTS: The most common side effects are marked hypotension, bradycardia, tachycardia, headache, nausea, and vomiting. Side effects and adverse reactions may vary widely between classes and specific products.

PHARMACOKINETICS: Onset, peak, and duration vary widely among products. Most products are metabolized in the liver, with metabolites excreted in urine, bile, and feces.

INTERACTIONS: Interactions vary widely among products. Check individual monographs for specific information.

NURSING CONSIDERATIONS
Assessment
• Monitor blood tests: neutrophil; decreased platelets occur with many of the products

• Monitor renal function tests: protein, BUN, creatinine; watch for increased levels, which may indicate nephrotic syndrome; obtain baselines in renal/hepatic function tests before beginning treatment
• Assess for edema in feet and legs daily
• Identify allergic reaction, including rash, fever, pruritus, urticaria: product should be discontinued if antihistamines fail to help
• Identify symptoms of CHF: edema, dyspnea, wet crackles, B/P
• Assess for renal symptoms: polyuria, oliguria, frequency

Nursing diagnoses
• Cardiac output, decreased (uses)
• Diarrhea (adverse reactions)
• Gas exchange, impaired (adverse reactions)
• Tissue perfusion, ineffective (uses)

Patient/family education
• Instruct patient to comply with dosage schedule, even if feeling better
• Advise patient to rise slowly to sitting or standing position to minimize orthostatic hypotension

Evaluation
Positive therapeutic outcome
• Decrease in B/P in hypertension
• Decreased B/P, edema, moist crackles in CHF

Generic Names

Angiotensin-converting enzyme inhibitors:
benazepril, enalapril, fosinopril, lisinopril, quinapril, ramipril, trandolapril

Angiotensin II receptor blockers:
azilsartan, candesartan, eprosartan, irbesartan, losartan, olmesartan, telmisartan, valsartan

Centrally acting adrenergics:
cloNIDine, guanfacine, methyldopa

Peripherally acting antiadrenergics:
doxazosin, prazosin, reserpine

Vasodilators:
ambrisentan, fenoldopam, hydrALAZINE, minoxidil, **nitroprusside** (high alert)

Antiadrenergic: Combined α/β-blocker:
labetalol

Direct renin inhibitors:
aliskiren

Antiinfectives

ACTION: Antiinfectives are divided into several groups, which include but are not limited to penicillins, cephalosporins, aminoglyco-

sides, sulfonamides, tetracyclines, monobactam, erythromycins, and quinolones. These products inhibit the growth and replication of susceptible bacterial organisms.

USES: Antiinfectives are used for infections of susceptible organisms. These products are effective against bacterial, rickettsial, and spirochete infections.

CONTRAINDICATIONS:
Hypersensitive reactions may occur, and allergies should be identified before these products are given. Cross-sensitivity can occur between products of different classes (penicillins or cephalosporins). Often persons allergic to penicillins are also allergic to cephalosporins.

Precautions: Antiinfectives should be used with caution in persons with renal/hepatic disease.

IMPLEMENTATION
• Give for 10-14 days to ensure organism death, prevention of superinfection
• Give after C&S completed; product may be taken as soon as culture is obtained

ADVERSE EFFECTS: The most
common side effects are nausea, vomiting, and diarrhea. Adverse reactions include bone marrow depression and anaphylaxis.

PHARMACOKINETICS: Onset,
peak, and duration vary widely among products. Most products are metabolized in the liver. Metabolites are excreted in urine, bile, and feces.

INTERACTIONS: Interactions vary
widely among products. Check individual monographs for specific information.

NURSING CONSIDERATIONS
Assessment
• Assess for nephrotoxicity: increased BUN, creatinine
• Monitor blood tests: AST, ALT, CBC, Hct, bilirubin; test monthly if patient is on long-term therapy
• Monitor bowel pattern daily; if severe diarrhea occurs, product should be discontinued
• Monitor urine output; if decreasing, notify prescriber; may indicate nephrotoxicity
• Assess for allergic reaction: rash, fever, pruritus, urticaria; product should be discontinued
• Assess for bleeding: ecchymosis, bleeding gums, hematuria, stool guaiac daily

• Assess for overgrowth of infection: perineal itching, fever, malaise, redness, pain, swelling, drainage, rash, diarrhea, change in cough, sputum

Nursing diagnoses
• Diarrhea (adverse reactions)
• Infection, risk for (uses)

Patient/family education
• Teach patient to comply with dosage schedule, even if feeling better
• Advise patient to report sore throat, bruising, bleeding, joint pain; may indicate blood dyscrasias (rare)

Evaluation
Positive therapeutic outcome
• Absence of fever, fatigue, malaise, draining wounds

Generic Names

Aminoglycosides:
amikacin, azithromycin, clarithromycin, gentamicin, neomycin, streptomycin, tobramycin

Cephalosporins:
cefaclor, cefadroxil, ceFAZolin, cefdinir, cefditoren, cefepime, cefixime, cefotaxime, cefprozil, ceftibuten, cefuroxime, cephalexin, cephradine

Fluoroquinolones:
ciprofloxacin, gemifloxacin, levofloxacin, norfloxacin, ofloxacin

Ketolides:
telithromycin

Miscellaneous:
adefovir, daptomycin, doripenem, ertapenem, fidaxomicin, meropenem, peginterferon alfa-2a, telavancin, vancomycin

Penicillins:
amoxicillin/clavulanate, ampicillin/sulbactam, imipenem/cilastatin, nafcillin, penicillin G benzathine, penicillin G, penicillin G procaine, penicillin V, piperacillin/tazobactam, ticarcillin, ticarcillin/clavulanate

Sulfonamides:
sulfasalazine

Tetracyclines:
doxycycline, minocycline, tetracycline

Antilipidemics

ACTION: Antilipidemics are divided into three categories or subclassifications; HMG-CoA reductase inhibitors (statins), bile acid sequestrants, and miscellaneous products. The HMG-CoA reductase inhibitors work by reduction of an enzyme that is responsible for the beginning step in cholesterol production. Bile acid sequestrants work by binding cholesterol in the GI system. The miscellaneous products work by various actions.

USES: Primary hypercholesterolemia in individuals as an adjunct with other lifestyle changes.

CONTRAINDICATIONS:
Persons breastfeeding (some products) or those with hypersensitivity to any product or severe hepatic disease should not take these products. Antilipidemics are identified as pregnancy category **X** on some products.

Precautions: Some products are identified as pregnancy category **C**.

IMPLEMENTATION
• Give as directed by health care provider; times will vary with medication used
• Provide protection from sunlight and heat

ADVERSE EFFECTS: The most common side effects are headache, dizziness, fatigue, insomnia, peripheral edema, dysrhythmias, sinusitis, pharyngitis, abdominal pain, diarrhea, constipation, flatulence, and back pain.

PHARMACOKINETICS: Pharmacokinetics and pharmacodynamics vary with each product.

INTERACTIONS: Interactions vary widely among products. Check individual monographs for specific information.

NURSING CONSIDERATIONS
Assessment
• Obtain a diet and lifestyle history, including exercise, smoking, alcohol, and stress-related activities

Nursing diagnoses
• Constipation (adverse reactions)
• Diarrhea (adverse reactions)
• Knowledge, deficient (teaching)
• Noncompliance (teaching)

Patient/family education
• Teach patient all aspects of medication use
• Instruct patient to combine medication with lifestyle changes, including low-cholesterol diet,

---

decreasing LDL in diet; avoid smoking, alcohol, and sedentary daily routine

Evaluation
Positive therapeutic outcome
• Decrease in triglycerides and LDL cholesterol levels

Generic Names

HMG-CoA reductase inhibitors:
atorvastatin, fluvastatin, lovastatin, pitavastatin, pravastatin, simvastatin

Bile acid sequestrants:
cholestyramine, colesevelam

Miscellaneous:
ezetimibe, fenofibrate, fenofibric acid, gemfibrozil, niacin, niacinamide

Antineoplastics

ACTION: Antineoplastics are divided into alkylating agents, antimetabolites, antibiotic agents, hormonal agents, and miscellaneous agents. Alkylating agents act by cross-linking strands of DNA. Antimetabolites act by inhibiting DNA synthesis. Antibiotic agents act by inhibiting RNA synthesis and by delaying or inhibiting mitosis. Hormones alter the effect of androgens, luteinizing hormone, follicle-stimulating hormone, or estrogen by changing the hormonal environment.

USES: Antineoplastics vary widely among products and classes of products. They are used to treat leukemia, Hodgkin's disease, lymphomas, and other tumors throughout the body.

CONTRAINDICATIONS:
Hypersensitive reactions may occur, and allergies should be identified before these products are given. Also, persons with severe renal/hepatic disease should not use these products unless the benefits outweigh the risks.

Precautions: Persons with bleeding, severe bone marrow depression, or renal/hepatic disease should be watched closely.

IMPLEMENTATION
• Check **IV** site for irritation; phlebitis
• Have epINEPHrine available for hypersensitivity reaction
• Give antibiotics for prophylaxis of infection
• Provide strict medical asepsis, protective isolation if WBC levels are low

• Provide comprehensive oral hygiene, using careful technique and soft-bristle brush

ADVERSE EFFECTS: Most products cause thrombocytopenia, leukopenia, and anemia. If these reactions occur, the product may need to be stopped until the problem is corrected. Other side effects include nausea, vomiting, glossitis, and hair loss. Some products also cause hepatotoxicity, nephrotoxicity, and cardiotoxicity.

PHARMACOKINETICS: Onset, peak, and duration vary widely among products. Most products cross the placenta and are excreted in breast milk and in urine.

INTERACTIONS: Toxicity may occur when used with other antineoplastics or radiation.

NURSING CONSIDERATIONS

Assessment
• Monitor CBC, differential, platelet count weekly; withhold product if WBC is <4000 or platelet count is <75,000; notify prescriber of results
• Monitor renal function tests: BUN, creatinine, serum uric acid, and urine creatinine clearance before, during therapy
• Monitor I&O ratio; report fall in urine output of 30 ml/hr
• Monitor temp q4hr (may indicate beginning infection)
• Monitor hepatic function tests before, during therapy (bilirubin, AST, ALT, LDH) monthly or as needed
• Assess for bleeding, including hematuria, guaiac, bruising or petechiae, mucosa, or orifices q8hr; obtain prescription for viscous lidocaine (Xylocaine)
• Identify jaundice of skin, sclera, dark urine, clay-colored stools, itchy skin, abdominal pain, fever, diarrhea
• Assess for edema in feet, joint pain, stomach pain, shaking
• Assess for inflammation of mucosa, breaks in skin

Nursing diagnoses
• Infection, risk for (adverse reactions)
• Nutrition: less than body requirements, imbalanced (adverse reactions)
• Oral mucous membrane, impaired (adverse reactions)

⚠ Nurse Alert

Patient/family education
• Advise patient to report signs of infection, including increased temp, sore throat, malaise
• Instruct patient to report signs of anemia, including fatigue, headache, faintness, shortness of breath, irritability
• Instruct patient to report bleeding and to avoid use of razors and commercial mouthwash

Evaluation
Positive therapeutic outcome
• Decreased tumor size

Generic Names

Alkylating agents:
bendamustine, **busulfan** (high alert), **CAR-BOplatin** (high alert), **carmustine** (high alert), chlorambucil, **CISplatin** (high alert), **cyclophosphamide** (high alert), **dacarbazine** (high alert), **melphalan** (high alert), oxaliplatin

Antimetabolites:
capecitabine, **cytarabine** (high alert), decitabine, **etoposide** (high alert), **fluorouracil** (high alert), mercaptopurine, **methotrexate** (high alert), pemetrexed

Antibiotic agents:
bleomycin (high alert), **DACTINomycin** (high alert), **DAUNOrubicin** (high alert), **DOXOrubicin** (high alert), **mitomycin** (high alert), **mitoxantrone** (high alert)

Hormonal agents:
flutamide, fulvestrant, goserelin, **irinotecan** (high alert), **leuprolide** (high alert), megestrol, tamoxifen, **topotecan** (high alert)

Miscellaneous agents:
alemtuzumab, anastrozole, azacitidine, bortezomib, brentuximab, cabazitaxel, cetuximab, crizotinib, dasatinib, eribulin, erlotinib, gemcitabine, ibritumomab, imatinib, interferon alfa-2a, interferon alfa-2b, ipilimumab, irinotecan, ixabepilone, lapatinib, nilotinib, panitumumab, procarbazine, ranibizumab, riTUXimab, sipuleucel-T, vemurafenib, **vinBLAStine** (high alert), **vinCRIStine** (high alert), **vinorelbine** (high alert)

Antiparkinsonian Agents

ACTION: Antiparkinsonian agents are divided into cholinergics, dopamine agonists, and monoamine oxidase type B inhibitors. Cholinergics work by blocking or competing at central acetylcholine receptors. Dopamine agonists work by decarboxylation to dopamine or by activation of dopamine receptors. Monoamine oxidase type B inhibitors increase dopamine activity by inhibiting MAO type B activity.

USES: Antiparkinson agents are used alone or in combination for patients with Parkinson's disease.

CONTRAINDICATIONS:
Persons with hypersensitivity, closed-angle glaucoma, and undiagnosed skin lesions should not use these products.

Precautions: Antiparkinsonian agents should be used with caution in pregnancy, breastfeeding, children, renal/cardiac/hepatic disease, and affective disorder.

IMPLEMENTATION
• Give product up until NPO before surgery
• Adjust dosage depending on patient response
• Give with meals; limit protein taken with product
• Give only after MAOIs have been discontinued for 2 wk
• Assist with ambulation during beginning therapy if needed
• Test for diabetes mellitus and acromegaly if on long-term therapy

ADVERSE EFFECTS: Side effects and adverse reactions vary widely among products. The most common side effects include involuntary movements, headache, numbness, insomnia, nightmares, nausea, vomiting, dry mouth, and orthostatic hypotension.

PHARMACOKINETICS: Onset, peak, and duration vary widely among products. Most products are metabolized in the liver and excreted in urine.

INTERACTIONS: Interactions vary widely among products. Check individual monographs for specific information.

NURSING CONSIDERATIONS
Assessment
• Monitor B/P, respiration
• Assess mental status: affect, behavioral changes, depression, complete suicide assessment

Nursing diagnoses
• Injury, risk for (uses)
• Knowledge, deficient (teaching)
• Mobility, impaired physical (uses)

Patient/family education
• Advise patient to change positions slowly to prevent orthostatic hypotension
• Instruct patient to report side effects: twitching, eye spasm; indicate overdose
• Advise patient to use product exactly as prescribed; if product is discontinued abruptly, parkinsonian crisis may occur

Evaluation
Positive therapeutic outcome
• Decrease in akathisia
• Improvement in mood

Generic Names
amantadine, benztropine, bromocriptine, carbidopa-levodopa, pramipexole, rasagiline, selegiline, tolcapone

Antiplatelets

ACTION: The antiplatelets are divided into the platelet aggregation inhibitors, platelet adhesion inhibitors, and the glycoprotein IIb, IIIa inhibitors. The platelet aggregation inhibitors work by action on thrombin; the platelet adhesion inhibitors work by inhibition of phosphodiesterase; and the glycoprotein IIb, IIIa inhibitors work by preventing fibrin from binding to glycoprotein IIb, IIIa receptors.

USES: Antiplatelets are used to prevent myocardial infarction and stroke; other products are used for coronary syndromes.

CONTRAINDICATIONS:
Persons developing hypersensitive reactions should not use these products.

Precautions: Antiplatelets should be used cautiously in pregnancy, breastfeeding, and bleeding disorders.

IMPLEMENTATION
• Give with heparin or other aspirin (some products)
• Store at room temperature vial/ampules, oral products

ADVERSE EFFECTS: The most common side effects are headache, dizziness, bleeding, and diarrhea.

PHARMACOKINETICS: Onset, peak, and duration vary widely among products. Most products are metabolized by the liver and excreted by the kidneys.

INTERACTIONS: Interactions vary widely among products. Check individual monographs for specific information.

NURSING CONSIDERATIONS
Assessment
• Assess reason for use of these products
• Monitor hypersensitivity reactions with some products
• Monitor bleeding from orifices, stool urine
• Monitor blood tests: platelets, Hgb, Hct, PT/APTT, and INR

Nursing diagnoses
• Injury, risk for, physical (uses, adverse reactions)
• Knowledge, deficient (teaching)

Patient/family education
• Caution patient to avoid hazardous activities if drowsiness, dizziness occurs; ask for assistance if hospitalized
• Teach patient all aspects of product usage

Evaluation
Positive therapeutic outcome
• Absence of MI, stroke, or other coronary syndromes

Generic Names

Platelet aggregation inhibitors:
cilostazol, clopidogrel, ticagrelol, ticlopidine

Platelet adhesion inhibitors:
dipyridamole

Glycoprotein IIb, IIIa inhibitors:
eptifibatide (high alert), **tirofiban** (high alert)

Antipsychotics

ACTION: Antipsychotics/neuroleptics are divided into several subgroups: phenothiazines, thioxanthenes, butyrophenones, dibenzoxazepines, dibenzodiazepines, and indolones and other heterocyclic compounds. Although chemically different, these subgroups share many pharmacologic and clinical properties. All antipsychotics work to block postsynaptic dopamine receptors in the brain that are responsible for psychotic behavior, including hallucinations, delusions, and paranoia.

USES: Antipsychotic behavior is decreased in conditions such as schizophrenia, paranoia, and mania. These agents are also effective for severe anxiety, intractable hiccups, nausea, vomiting, behavioral problems in children, and for relaxation before surgery.

CONTRAINDICATIONS:
Persons with liver damage, severe hypertension or coronary disease, cerebral arteriosclerosis, blood dyscrasias, bone marrow depression, parkinsonism, severe depression, or closed-angle glaucoma; children <12 yr; persons withdrawing from alcohol or barbiturates should not use antipsychotics until these conditions are corrected.

Precautions: Caution must be used when antipsychotics are given to geriatric patients, since metabolism is slowed and adverse reactions can occur rapidly. Renal/hepatic disease may cause poor metabolism and excretion of the product. Seizure threshold is decreased with these products; increases in the dose of anticonvulsants may be required. Persons with diabetes mellitus, prostatic hypertrophy, chronic respiratory disease, and peptic ulcer disease should be monitored closely.

IMPLEMENTATION
• Give antiparkinsonian agent if extrapyramidal symptoms occur
• Administer liquid conc mixed in glass of juice or cola since taste is unpleasant; avoid contact with skin when preparing liquid conc or parenteral medications
• Supervise ambulation until stabilized on medication; do not involve in strenuous exercise program, since fainting is possible; patient should not stand still for long periods
• Increase fluids to prevent constipation
• Give sips of water, candy, gum for dry mouth
• Patient should remain lying down for at least 30 min after IM inj

ADVERSE EFFECTS:
The most common side effects include extrapyramidal symptoms such as pseudoparkinsonism, akathisia, dystonia, and tardive dyskinesia, which may be controlled by use of antiparkinsonian agents. Serious adverse reactions such as hypotension, agranulocytosis, cardiac arrest, and laryngospasm have occurred. Other common side effects include dry mouth and photosensitivity.

PHARMACOKINETICS:
Onset, peak, and duration vary widely with different products and routes. Products are metabolized by the liver, are excreted in urine as metabolites, are highly bound to plasma proteins, cross the placenta, and enter breast milk. Half-life can be extended over 3 days.

INTERACTIONS:
Because other CNS depressants can cause oversedation, these combinations should be used carefully. Anticholinergics may decrease the therapeutic actions of phenothiazines and also cause increased anticholinergic effects.

NURSING CONSIDERATIONS

Assessment
• Monitor bilirubin, CBC, hepatic function tests monthly, since these products are metabolized in the liver and excreted in urine
• Monitor I&O ratio: palpate bladder if low urinary output occurs, since urinary retention occurs with many of these products
• Assess affect, orientation, LOC, reflexes, gait, coordination, sleep pattern disturbances
• Assess dizziness, faintness, palpitations, tachycardia on rising
• Check B/P with patient lying and standing; wide fluctuations between lying and standing B/P may require dosage or product change, since orthostatic hypotension is occurring
• Assess for EPS, including akathisia, tardive dyskinesia, pseudoparkinsonism

Nursing diagnoses
• Sensory perception, disturbed (uses)
• Thought processes, disturbed (uses)

Patient/family education
• Advise patient to rise from sitting or lying position gradually, since fainting may occur
• Caution patient to avoid hot tubs, hot showers, or tub baths, since hypotension may occur
• Advise patient to wear sunscreen or protective clothing to prevent burns
• Advise patient to take extra precautions during hot weather to stay cool; heat stroke can occur
• Caution patient to avoid driving and other activities requiring alertness until response to medication is known
• Inform patient that drowsiness or impaired mental/motor activity is evident the first 2 wk, but tends to decrease over time

Evaluation
Positive therapeutic outcome
• Decrease in excitement, hallucinations, delusions, paranoia
• Reorganization of thought patterns, speech

Generic Names

Phenothiazines:
chlorproMAZINE, fluphenazine

Butyrophenone:
haloperidol

Miscellaneous:
aripiprazole, asenapine, iloperidone, loxapine, OLANZapine, paliperidone, QUEtiapine, risperidone, ziprasidone

Antipyretics

ACTION: The antipyretics act on the CNS to control fever and also inhibit prostaglandin production.

USES: Antipyretics are used to decrease fever.

CONTRAINDICATIONS:
Persons developing hypersensitive reactions should not use these products.

Precautions: Antipyretics should be used cautiously in pregnancy, breastfeeding, geriatric patients, hepatic disease, and those with certain GI disorders.

IMPLEMENTATION
* Give around the clock to keep fever reduced
* Store at room temperature

ADVERSE EFFECTS: The most common side effects are nausea, vomiting, and rash.

PHARMACOKINETICS: Onset, peak, and duration vary widely among products. Most products are metabolized by the liver and excreted by the kidneys.

INTERACTIONS: Interactions vary widely among products. Check individual monographs for specific information.

NURSING CONSIDERATIONS
Assessment
* Monitor temp frequently
* Assess reason for use and expected outcome
* Monitor hypersensitivity reactions: rash, bronchospasm with some products

Nursing diagnoses
* Injury, risk for, physical (uses, adverse reactions)
* Knowledge, deficient (teaching)

Patient/family education
* Teach patient all aspects of product usage

Evaluation
Positive therapeutic outcome
* Absence or decreasing fever after use

Generic Names
acetaminophen, aspirin, choline/magnesium salicylates, ibuprofen, ketoprofen, magnesium salicylate, naproxen, salsalate

Antiretrovirals

ACTION: Antiretrovirals act by blocking DNA synthesis.

USES: Antiretrovirals are used in HIV infections, chronic hepatitis C to slow the progression of the disease.

CONTRAINDICATIONS:
Persons with hypersensitivity should not use these products.

Precautions: Antiretrovirals should be used cautiously in pregnancy, breastfeeding, and renal/hepatic disease. Protease inhibitors should be used cautiously in diabetes.

IMPLEMENTATION
* Give in equal intervals around the clock
* Store at room temperature

ADVERSE EFFECTS: The most common side effects are nausea, vomiting, anorexia, headache, and diarrhea. The most serious adverse reactions are nephrotoxicity and blood dyscrasias.

PHARMACOKINETICS: Onset, peak, and duration vary widely among products. Most products are metabolized by the liver and excreted by the kidneys.

INTERACTIONS: Interactions vary widely among products. Check individual monographs for specific information.

NURSING CONSIDERATIONS
Assessment
* Monitor for signs of HIV infection: increased CD4 counts, decreased viral load; signs of chronic hepatitis C
* Monitor patients with compromised renal system; since product is excreted slowly in poor renal system function, toxicity may occur rapidly

Nursing diagnoses
- Infection, risk for (uses)
- Injury, risk for (adverse reactions)
- Knowledge, deficient (teaching)
- Noncompliance (teaching)

Patient/family education
- Instruct patient to report sore throat, fever, fatigue; may indicate superinfection
- Caution patient that product does not cure condition or prevent infecting others, but controls symptoms
- Instruct patient that product must be taken around the clock, in equal intervals to maintain blood levels for duration of therapy
- Instruct patient to notify prescriber of side effects such as bruising, bleeding, fatigue, malaise; may indicate blood dyscrasias

Evaluation
Positive therapeutic outcome
- Decreased viral load
- Increased CD4 count
- Improvement in the symptoms of HIV/AIDS

Generic Names

Nonnucleoside reverse transcriptase inhibitors:
delavirdine, efavirenz, etravirine, nevirapine, rilpivirine

Nucleoside reverse transcriptase inhibitors:
abacavir, didanosine, emtricitabine, lamiVUDine, stavudine d4t, tenofovir, zidovudine

Protease inhibitors:
atazanavir, boceprevir, fosamprenavir, indinavir, nelfinavir, ritonavir, saquinavir, telaprevir, tipranavir

Fusion inhibitors:
enfuvirtide

Miscellaneous:
raltegravir

Antituberculars

ACTION: Antituberculars act by inhibiting RNA or DNA, or interfering with lipid and protein synthesis, thereby decreasing tubercle bacilli replication.

USES: Antituberculars are used for pulmonary tuberculosis.

CONTRAINDICATIONS:
Persons with severe renal disease or hypersensitivity should not use these products.

Precautions: Antituberculars should be used with caution in pregnancy, breastfeeding, and hepatic disease.

IMPLEMENTATION
- Give some of these agents on empty stomach, 1 hr before meals (only for isoniazid and rifampin) or 2hr after meals
- Give antiemetic if vomiting occurs
- Give after C&S is completed; monthly to detect resistance

ADVERSE EFFECTS: Adverse effects vary widely among products. Most products can cause nausea, vomiting, anorexia, and rash. Serious adverse reactions include renal failure, nephrotoxicity, ototoxicity, and hepatic necrosis.

PHARMACOKINETICS: Onset, peak, and duration vary widely among products. Most products are metabolized in the liver and excreted in urine.

INTERACTIONS: Interactions vary widely among products. Check individual monographs for specific information.

NURSING CONSIDERATIONS
Assessment
- Assess for signs of anemia: Hct, Hgb, fatigue
- Monitor hepatic function tests weekly: ALT, AST, bilirubin
- Monitor renal status before treatment and monthly thereafter: BUN, creatinine, output, specific gravity, urinalysis
- Monitor hepatic status: decreased appetite, jaundice, dark urine, fatigue

Nursing diagnoses
- Infection, risk for (uses)
- Injury, risk for (adverse reactions)
- Knowledge, deficient (teaching)
- Noncompliance (teaching)

Patient/family education
- Teach patient that compliance with dosage schedule, duration is necessary
- Teach patient that scheduled appointments must be kept; relapse may occur
- Advise patient to avoid alcohol while taking product
- Advise patient to report flulike symptoms: excessive fatigue, anorexia, vomiting, sore throat; unusual bleeding, yellowish discoloration of skin/eyes

Evaluation
Positive therapeutic outcome
- Decreased symptoms of TB
- Negative culture

Generic Names
ethambutol, isoniazid, pyrazinamide, rifabutin, rifampin, streptomycin

Antitussives/Expectorants

ACTION: Antitussives suppress the cough reflex by direct action on the cough center in the medulla. Expectorants act by liquefying and reducing the viscosity of thick, tenacious secretions.

USES: Antitussives/expectorants are used to treat cough occurring in pneumonia, bronchitis, TB, cystic fibrosis, and emphysema; as an adjunct in atelectasis (expectorants); and for nonproductive cough (antitussives).

CONTRAINDICATIONS:
Some products are contraindicated in pregnancy, breastfeeding, and hypothyroidism

Precautions: Some products should be used cautiously with asthma and in geriatric and debilitated patients.

IMPLEMENTATION
- Give decreased dosage to geriatric patients; their metabolism may be slowed
- Increase fluids to liquefy secretions
- Humidify patient's room

ADVERSE EFFECTS: The most common side effects are drowsiness, dizziness, and nausea.

PHARMACOKINETICS: Onset, peak, and duration vary widely among products. Some products are metabolized in the liver and excreted in urine.

INTERACTIONS: Interactions vary widely among products. Check individual monographs for specific information.

NURSING CONSIDERATIONS

Assessment
- Assess cough: type, frequency, character including sputum

Nursing diagnoses
- Airway clearance, ineffective (uses)
- Breathing pattern, ineffective (uses)
- Knowledge, deficient (teaching)

Patient/family education
- Advise patient to avoid driving and other hazardous activities until stabilized on this medication
- Caution patient to avoid smoking, smoke-filled rooms, perfumes, dust, environmental pollutants, cleaners that increase cough

Evaluation
Positive therapeutic outcome
- Absence of cough

Generic Names
acetylcysteine, codeine, dextromethorphan, diphenhydrAMINE, guaiFENesin, HYDROcodone

Antivirals

ACTION: Antivirals act by interfering with DNA synthesis that is needed for viral replication.

USES: Antivirals are used for mucocutaneous herpes simplex virus, herpes genitalis (HSV-1, HSV-2), varicella infections, herpes zoster, and herpes simplex encephalitis.

CONTRAINDICATIONS:
Persons with hypersensitivity or immunosuppressed individuals should not use these products.

Precautions: Antivirals should be used cautiously in pregnancy, breastfeeding, and renal/hepatic disease.

IMPLEMENTATION
- Give increased fluids to 3 L/day to decrease crystalluria when given **IV**
- Store at room temperature for up to 12 hr after reconstitution

ADVERSE EFFECTS: The most common side effects are nausea, vomiting, anorexia, headache, and diarrhea. The most serious adverse reactions are nephrotoxicity and blood dyscrasias.

PHARMACOKINETICS: Onset, peak, and duration vary widely among products. Most products are metabolized by the liver and excreted by the kidneys.

INTERACTIONS: Interactions vary widely among products. Check individual monographs for specific information.

NURSING CONSIDERATIONS
Assessment
• Monitor for signs of infection, anemia
• Monitor patients with a compromised renal system; since product is excreted slowly in poor renal system function, toxicity may occur rapidly
• Monitor renal function tests: urinalysis, BUN, serum creatinine or decreased CCr may indicate nephrotoxicity; I&O ratio; report hematuria, oliguria, fatigue, weakness; check for protein in the urine during treatment
• Assess C&S before treatment; agent may be given as soon as culture is taken; repeat C&S after treatment
• Monitor bowel pattern before, during treatment; if severe abdominal pain with bleeding occurs, agent should be discontinued
• Monitor skin reactions: rash, urticaria, itching
• Monitor hepatic function tests: AST, ALT
• Monitor blood tests: WBC, RBC, Hct, Hgb, bleeding time; blood dyscrasias

Nursing diagnoses
• Infection, risk for (uses)
• Injury, risk for (adverse reactions)
• Knowledge, deficient (teaching)

Patient/family education
• Instruct patient to report sore throat, fever, fatigue; may indicate superinfection
• Caution patient that product does not prevent infecting others or cure condition but controls symptoms
• Instruct patient that product must be taken around the clock in equal intervals to maintain blood levels for duration of therapy
• Instruct patient to notify prescriber of side effects such as bruising, bleeding, fatigue, malaise; may indicate blood dyscrasias

Evaluation
Positive therapeutic outcome
• Absence or control of infection

Generic Names
acyclovir, amantadine, cidofovir, docosanol, entecavir, famciclovir, foscarnet, ganciclovir, lamiVUDine, maraviroc, oseltamivir, penciclovir, ribavirin, valacyclovir, valganciclovir, zanamivir

β-Adrenergic Blockers

ACTION: β-Blockers are divided into selective and nonselective blockers. Selective β-blockers competitively block stimulation of $β_1$-receptors in cardiac smooth muscle; these products produce chronotropic and inotropic effects. Nonselective blockers produce a fall in blood pressure without reflex tachycardia or reduction in heart rate through a mixture of β-blocking effects; elevated plasma renins are reduced.

USES: β-Blockers are used for hypertension, ventricular dysrhythmias, and prophylaxis of angina pectoris.

CONTRAINDICATIONS: Hypersensitive reactions may occur, and allergies should be identified before these products are given. β-Adrenergic blockers should not be used in heart block, CHF, or cardiogenic shock.

Precautions: β-Blockers should be used with caution in pregnant and geriatric patients or in renal/thyroid disease, COPD, CAD, diabetes mellitus, and asthma.

IMPLEMENTATION
• Give PO before meals and at bedtime; tab may be crushed or swallowed whole
• Give reduced dosage in renal dysfunction

ADVERSE EFFECTS: The most common side effects are orthostatic hypotension, bradycardia, diarrhea, nausea, and vomiting. Serious adverse reactions include blood dyscrasias, bronchospasm, and CHF.

PHARMACOKINETICS: Onset, peak, and duration vary widely among products. Most products are metabolized in the liver, with metabolites excreted in urine, bile, and feces.

INTERACTIONS: Interactions vary widely among products. Check individual monographs for specific information.

NURSING CONSIDERATIONS
Assessment
• Monitor renal function tests: protein, BUN, creatinine; watch for increased levels that may indicate nephrotic syndrome; obtain baselines in renal/hepatic function tests before beginning treatment
• Monitor I&O ratio, weight daily

• Monitor B/P during beginning of treatment and periodically thereafter, pulse q4hr; note rate, rhythm, quality
• Monitor apical/radial pulse before administration; notify prescriber of significant changes
• Check for edema in feet and legs daily

Nursing diagnoses
• Cardiac output, decreased (uses)
• Diarrhea (adverse reactions)
• Gas exchange, impaired (adverse reactions)
• Tissue perfusion, ineffective (uses)

Patient/family education
• Instruct patient to comply with dosage schedule, even if feeling better
• Caution patient to rise slowly to sitting or standing position to minimize orthostatic hypotension
• Advise patient to report bradycardia, dizziness, confusion, depression, fever
• Teach patient to take pulse at home; advise when to notify prescriber
• Instruct patient to comply with weight control, dietary adjustment, modified exercise program
• Advise patient to wear support hose to minimize effects of orthostatic hypotension
• Advise patient not to discontinue product abruptly; taper over 2 wk; may precipitate angina

Evaluation
Positive therapeutic outcome
• Decrease in B/P in hypertension
• Decreased B/P, edema, moist crackles in CHF

Generic Names

Selective β₁-receptor blockers:
acebutolol, atenolol, esmolol, metoprolol, nebibolol

β₂-receptor blocker:
indacaterol

Nonselective β₁ and β₂-blockers:
carteolol, nadolol, propranolol, timolol

Combined α₁, β₁, and β₂-receptor blocker:
labetalol

Bone Resorption Inhibitors

ACTION: Bone resorption inhibitors are divided into the biphosphonates and the selective estrogen receptor modulators. The biphosphonates act by absorbing calcium phosphate crystals in bone and may directly block dissolution of hydroxyapatite crystals of bone, inhibiting normal and abnormal bone resorption and mineralization. Selective estrogen receptor modulators act by reducing resorption of bone and decreasing bone turnover, mediated through estrogen receptor binding.

USES: Bone resorption inhibitors are used for prevention and treatment of osteoporosis in postmenopausal women, treatment of Paget's disease, and treatment of osteoporosis in men.

CONTRAINDICATIONS:
Persons developing hypersensitive reactions or those with hypocalcemia should not use these products.

Precautions: Bone resorption inhibitors should be used cautiously in pregnancy, breastfeeding, the geriatric patient, renal/hepatic disease, and some GI disorders.

IMPLEMENTATION
• Give for 6 months or more in Paget's disease
• Store at room temperature

ADVERSE EFFECTS: The most common side effects are nausea, vomiting, headache, bone pain, and rash.

PHARMACOKINETICS: Onset, peak, and duration vary widely among products. Most products are taken up by the bones and excreted by the kidneys.

INTERACTIONS: Interactions vary widely among products. Check individual monographs for specific information.

NURSING CONSIDERATIONS
Assessment
• Assess reason for use and expected outcome
• Monitor bone density test; hormonal status (women) before starting treatment and thereafter
• Monitor hypercalcemia: paresthesia, twitching, laryngospasm; Chvostek's, Trousseau's signs

Nursing diagnoses
• Injury, risk for, physical (uses, adverse reactions)
• Knowledge, deficient (teaching)

Patient/family education
• Instruct patient to remain upright for at least 30 min after taking to prevent esophageal irritation
• Teach patient all aspects of product usage
• Instruct patient to use weight-bearing exercise to increase bone density

Evaluation
Positive therapeutic outcome
• Increase in bone mass
• Absence of fractures

Generic Names

Bisphosphonates:
alendronate, etidronate, ibandronate, pamidronate, risedronate

Selective estrogen receptor modulator:
raloxifene

Monoclonal antibody:
denosumab

Calcium Channel Blockers

ACTION: Calcium channel blockers inhibit calcium ion influx across the cell membrane in cardiac and vascular smooth muscle. This action produces relaxation of coronary vascular smooth muscle, dilates coronary arteries, slows SA/AV node conduction, and dilates peripheral arteries.

USES: Calcium channel blockers are used for chronic stable angina pectoris, vasospastic angina, dysrhythmias, hypertension, and unstable angina.

CONTRAINDICATIONS:
Persons with 2nd- or 3rd-degree heart block, sick sinus syndrome, hypotension of <90 mm Hg systolic, Wolff-Parkinson-White syndrome, or cardiogenic shock should not use these products, since worsening of those conditions may occur.

Precautions: CHF may worsen since edema may be increased. Hypotension may worsen, since B/P is decreased. Patients with renal/hepatic disease should use these products cautiously since they are metabolized in the liver and excreted by the kidneys.

IMPLEMENTATION
• Give PO before meals and at bedtime

ADVERSE EFFECTS: The most common side effects are dysrhythmias and edema. Also common are headache, fatigue, drowsiness, and flushing.

PHARMACOKINETICS: Onset, peak, and duration vary widely with route of administration. Products are metabolized by the liver and excreted in the urine primarily as metabolites.

INTERACTIONS: Increased levels of digoxin and theophylline may occur when used with these products. Increased effects of β-blockers and antihypertensives may occur with calcium channel blockers.

NURSING CONSIDERATIONS
Assessment
• Monitor cardiac system: B/P, pulse, respirations, ECG intervals (PR, QRS, QT)

Nursing diagnoses
• Cardiac output, decreased (adverse reactions)
• Tissue perfusion, ineffective (uses)

Patient/family education
• Teach patient how to take pulse before taking product; patient should record or graph pulses to identify changes
• Advise patient to avoid hazardous activities until stabilized on this product since dizziness occurs frequently
• Inform patient of the need for compliance to all areas of medical regimen, including diet, exercise, stress reduction, and product therapy

Evaluation
Positive therapeutic outcome
• Decreased anginal pain
• Decreased B/P, dysrhythmias

Generic Names
amLODIPine, clevidipine, **diltiazem** (high alert), felodipine, isradipine, niCARdipine, NIFEdipine, verapamil

Cardiac Glycosides

ACTION: Cardiac glycosides act by inhibiting sodium and potassium ATPase and then making more calcium available to activate contracted proteins. Cardiac contractility and cardiac output are increased.

USES: Cardiac glycosides are used for CHF, atrial fibrillation, atrial flutter, atrial tachycardia, and rapid digitalization in these disorders.

CONTRAINDICATIONS:
Hypersensitive reactions may occur, and allergies should be identified before these products are given. Also, persons with ventricular tachycardia, ventricular fibrillation, and carotid sinus syndrome should not use these products.

Precautions: Persons with acute MI and those who have or may develop serum potassium, calcium, or magnesium imbalances should use these products cautiously. Also, geriatric patients and those with AV block, severe respiratory disease, hypothyroidism, or renal/hepatic disease should exercise caution when these products are prescribed.

IMPLEMENTATION
• Give potassium supplements if ordered for potassium levels <3

ADVERSE EFFECTS:
The most common side effects are cardiac disturbances, headache, hypotension, and GI symptoms. Also common are blurred vision and yellow-green halos.

PHARMACOKINETICS:
Onset, peak, and duration vary widely with the route of administration. Digitoxin is inactivated by the liver, and inactive metabolites are excreted in urine. Digoxin is excreted in urine mainly as the parent product and metabolites.

INTERACTIONS:
Toxicity may occur when used with diuretics, succinylcholine, quinidine, and thioamines. Increased blood levels may occur with propantheline bromide, spironolactone, quinidine, verapamil, aminoglycosides (PO), amiodarone, anticholinergics, and quinine. Diuretics may increase toxicity.

NURSING CONSIDERATIONS
Assessment
• Montior cardiac system: B/P, pulse, respirations, and increased urine output
• Monitor apical pulse for 1 min before giving product; if pulse <60, take again in 1 hr; if <60 notify prescriber
• Monitor electrolytes: potassium, sodium, chloride, calcium, magnesium; renal function tests, including BUN and creatinine; and blood tests, including AST, ALT, bilirubin
• Monitor I&O ratio, daily weights
• Monitor therapeutic product levels

Nursing diagnoses
• Cardiac output, decreased (adverse reactions)
• Tissue perfusion, ineffective (uses)

Patient/family education
• Teach patient how to take pulse before taking product; patient should record or graph pulse to identify changes

• Advise patient to avoid hazardous activities until stabilized on this product since dizziness occurs frequently
• Inform patient of the need for compliance to all areas of medical regimen, including diet, exercise, stress reduction, product therapy

Evaluation
Positive therapeutic outcome
• Decreased weight, edema, pulse, respiration
• Increased urine output

Generic Names
digoxin (high alert)

Cholinergics

ACTION:
Cholinergics act by preventing destruction of acetylcholine, which increases concentration at sites where acetylcholine is released. This exaggerates the effects of acetylcholine and facilitates transmission of impulses across the myoneural junction. Cholinergics may also act by stimulating receptors for acetylcholine.

USES:
Cholinergics are used for myasthenia gravis, as antagonists of nondepolarizing neuromuscular blockade, postoperative bladder distention and urinary distention, postoperative ileus.

CONTRAINDICATIONS:
Persons with obstruction of the intestine or renal system should not use these products.

Precautions: Caution should be used in patients with bradycardia, hypotension, seizure disorders, bronchial asthma, coronary occlusion, and hyperthyroidism, and in breastfeeding and children.

IMPLEMENTATION
• Give only with atropine sulfate available for cholinergic crisis
• Give only after all other cholinergics have been discontinued
• Give increased dosages if tolerance occurs
• Give larger doses after exercise or fatigue
• Give on empty stomach for better absorption
• Store at room temperature

ADVERSE EFFECTS:
The most serious adverse reactions are respiratory depression, bronchospasm, constriction, laryngospasm, respiratory arrest, convulsions, and

paralysis. The most common side effects are nausea, diarrhea, and vomiting.

PHARMACOKINETICS: Onset, peak, and duration vary widely among products. Most products are metabolized in the liver and excreted in urine.

INTERACTIONS: Interactions vary widely among products. Check individual monographs for specific information.

NURSING CONSIDERATIONS

Assessment
• Monitor VS, respiration q8hr
• Monitor I&O ratio; check for urinary retention or incontinence
• Assess for bradycardia, hypotension, bronchospasm, headache, dizziness, seizures, respiratory depression; product should be discontinued if toxicity occurs

Nursing diagnoses
• Breathing pattern, ineffective (uses)
• Knowledge, deficient (teaching)
• Noncompliance (teaching)
• Urinary elimination, impaired (uses)

Patient/family education
• Inform patient that product is not a cure; it only relieves symptoms (myasthenia gravis)
• Advise patient to carry/wear emergency ID specifying myasthenia gravis, products taken

Evaluation
Positive therapeutic outcome
• Increased muscle strength, hand grasp
• Improved muscle gait
• Absence of labored breathing (if severe)

Generic Names
bethanechol, physostigmine, pyridostigmine

Cholinergic Blockers

ACTION: Cholinergic blockers inhibit or block acetylcholine at receptor sites in the autonomic nervous system.

USES: Many cholinergic blockers are used to decrease secretions before surgery, to reverse neuromuscular blockade, and to decrease motility of the GI, biliary, and urinary tracts. Other products are used for parkinsonian symptoms, including dystonia associated with neuroleptic products.

CONTRAINDICATIONS: Hypersensitivity can occur, and allergies should be identified before administering these products. Persons with GI and GU obstruction should not use these products, since constipation and urinary retention may occur. They are also contraindicated in closed-angle glaucoma and myasthenia gravis.

Precautions: Caution must be used when these products are given to the geriatric patient, since metabolism is slowed. Also, persons with tachycardia or prostatic hypertrophy should use these products with caution.

IMPLEMENTATION
• Give with food or milk to decrease GI symptoms
• Give parenteral dose with patient recumbent to prevent postural hypotension; give dose slowly, monitoring VS
• Give hard candy, gum, frequent rinsing of mouth for dryness

ADVERSE EFFECTS: The most common side effects are dryness of the mouth and constipation, which can be prevented by frequent rinsing of the mouth and increasing water and bulk in the diet.

PHARMACOKINETICS: Onset, peak, and duration vary with route.

INTERACTIONS: Increase in anticholinergic effect occurs when used with opioids, barbiturates, antihistamines, MAOIs, phenothiazines, amantadine.

NURSING CONSIDERATIONS

Assessment
• Assess I&O ratio; be alert for urinary retention, frequency, dysuria; product should be discontinued if these occur
• Assess urinary hesitancy, retention; palpate bladder if retention occurs
• Assess constipation; increase fluids, bulk, exercise
• Assess for tolerance over long-term therapy; dosage may need to be changed
• Assess mental status: affect, mood, CNS depression, worsening of mental symptoms during early therapy

Nursing diagnoses
• Mobility, impaired physical (uses)
• Pain, chronic (uses)

Patient/family education
• Caution patient to avoid driving and other hazardous activities if drowsiness occurs
• Advise patient to avoid concurrent use of cough, cold preparations with alcohol, antihistamines unless directed by prescriber
• Caution patient to use with caution in hot weather, since medication may increase susceptibility to heat stroke

Evaluation
Positive therapeutic outcome
• Absence of cramps
• Absence of EPS

Generic Names
atropine (high alert), benztropine, glycopyrrolate, scopolamine

Corticosteroids

ACTION: Corticosteroids are divided into glucocorticoids and mineralocorticoids. Glucocorticoids decrease inflammation by the suppression of migration of polymorphonuclear leukocytes, fibroblasts, increased capillary permeability, and lysosomal stabilization. They also have varied metabolic effects and modify the body's immune responses to many different stimuli. Mineralocorticoids act by increasing resorption of sodium by increasing hydrogen and potassium excretion in the distal tubule.

USES: Glucocorticoids are used to decrease inflammation and for immunosuppression. In addition, some products may be given for allergy, adrenal insufficiency, or cerebral edema. Mineralocorticoids are given for adrenal insufficiency or adrenogenital syndrome.

CONTRAINDICATIONS:
Hypersensitivity may occur and should be identified before administering. Since these products mask infection, they should not be used in systemic fungal infections or amebiasis. Mothers taking pharmacologic doses of corticosteroids should not breastfeed.

Precautions: Caution must be used when these products are prescribed for diabetic patients since hyperglycemia may occur. Also, patients with glaucoma, seizure disorders, peptic ulcer, impaired renal function, CHF, hypertension, ulcerative colitis, or myasthenia gravis should be monitored closely if corticosteroids are given. Use with caution during pregnancy, in children, and in the geriatric patient.

IMPLEMENTATION
• Give with food or milk to decrease GI symptoms
• Give single daily or alternate-day doses in the morning before 9 AM (for replacement therapy)

ADVERSE EFFECTS: The most common side effects include change in behavior, including insomnia and euphoria; GI irritation, including peptic ulcer; metabolic reactions, including hypokalemia, hyperglycemia, and carbohydrate intolerance; and sodium and fluid retention. Most adverse reactions are dose dependent.

PHARMACOKINETICS: For oral preparations the onset of action occurs between 1-2 hr, and duration can be up to 2 days, with a half-life of 2-4 days. Pharmacokinetics vary widely among products. These products cross the placenta and appear in breast milk.

INTERACTIONS: Decreased corticosteroid effect may occur with barbiturates, rifampin, and phenytoin; corticosteroid dosage may need to be increased. There is a possibility of GI bleeding when used with salicylates and indomethacin. Steroids may reduce salicylate levels. When using with digoxin, glycosides, potassium-depleting diuretics, and amphotericin, serum potassium levels should be monitored.

NURSING CONSIDERATIONS
Assessment
• Monitor potassium, blood glucose, urine glucose while on long-term therapy; hypokalemia and hyperglycemia are common
• Monitor weight daily; notify prescriber if weekly gain of >5 lb since these products alter fluid and electrolyte balance
• Assess for potassium depletion: paresthesias, fatigue, nausea, vomiting, depression, polyuria, dysrhythmias, weakness
• Assess for mental status: affect, mood, behavioral changes, aggression; if severe personality changes occur, including depression, product may need to be tapered and then discontinued
• Monitor I&O ratio; be alert for decreasing urinary output and increasing edema
• Monitor plasma cortisol levels during long-term therapy (normal level is 138-635 nmol/L when drawn at 8 AM)
• Assess for infection: increased temp, WBC, even after withdrawal of medication; product masks symptoms of infection
• Assess for adrenal insufficiency: nausea,

anorexia, fatigue, dizziness, dyspnea, weakness, joint pain

Nursing diagnoses

- Body image, disturbed (adverse reactions)
- Infection, risk for (adverse reactions)
- Suicide, risk for (adverse reactions)

Patient/family education

- Advise patient that emergency ID as steroid user should be carried/worn
- Advise patient not to discontinue this medication abruptly; adrenal crisis can result
- Teach patient all aspects of product use, including cushingoid symptoms
- Instruct patient to take with meals or a snack
- Teach patient to avoid exposure to chickenpox or measles if taking immunosuppressives

Evaluation

Positive therapeutic outcome

- Decreased inflammation

Generic Names

Glucocorticoids:
beclomethasone, betamethasone, cortisone, dexamethasone, hydrocortisone, hydrocortisone sodium succinate, methylPREDNISolone, predniSOLONE, predniSONE, triamcinolone

Diuretics

ACTION: Diuretics are divided into subgroups: thiazides and thiazide-like diuretics, loop diuretics, carbonic anhydrase inhibitors, osmotic diuretics, and potassium-sparing diuretics. Each one of these subgroups differs in its mechanism of action. Thiazides and thiazide-like diuretics increase excretion of water and sodium by inhibiting resorption in the early distal tubule. Loop diuretics inhibit resorption of sodium and chloride in the thick ascending limb of the loop of Henle. Carbonic anhydrase inhibitors increase sodium excretion by decreasing sodium-hydrogen ion exchange throughout the renal tubule. Carbonic anhydrase inhibitors also decrease secretion of aqueous humor in the eye and thus decrease intraocular pressure. Osmotic diuretics increase the osmotic pressure of glomerular filtrate, thus decreasing net absorption of sodium. The potassium-sparing diuretics interfere with sodium resorption at the distal tubule, thus decreasing potassium excretion.

USES: Blood pressure is reduced in hypertension; edema is reduced in CHF; intraocular pressure is decreased in glaucoma.

CONTRAINDICATIONS: Persons with electrolyte imbalances (sodium, chloride, potassium), dehydration, or anuria should not be given these products until the problem is corrected.

Precautions: Caution must be used when diuretics are given to the geriatric patient, since electrolyte disturbances and dehydration can occur rapidly. Renal/hepatic disorders may cause poor metabolism and excretion of the product.

IMPLEMENTATION

- Give in AM to avoid interference with sleep if using product as a diuretic
- Give potassium replacement if potassium is less than 3 mg/dl

ADVERSE EFFECTS: Hypokalemia, hyperuricemia, and hyperglycemia occur most frequently with thiazide diuretics. Aplastic anemia, blood dyscrasias, volume depletion, and dehydration may occur when thiazide-like diuretics, loop diuretics, or carbonic anhydrase inhibitors are given. Side effects and adverse reactions vary widely for the miscellaneous products.

PHARMACOKINETICS: Onset, peak, and duration vary widely among the different subgroups of these products.

INTERACTIONS: Cholestyramine and colestipol decrease the absorption of thiazide diuretics. Concurrent use of thiazides with diazoxide may increase hyperuricemia, hyperglycemia, and antihypertensive effects of thiazides. Ototoxicity may occur when loop diuretics are used with aminoglycosides. Thiazide and loop diuretics may increase therapeutic and toxic effects of lithium.

NURSING CONSIDERATIONS

Assessment

- Monitor weight, I&O ratio daily to determine fluid loss; check skin turgor for dehydration
- Monitor electrolytes: potassium, sodium, chloride; include BUN, blood glucose, CBC, serum creatinine, blood pH, ABGs, uric acid, calcium; electrolyte imbalances may occur quickly
- Monitor B/P with patient lying, standing; postural hypotension may occur since fluid loss occurs from intravascular spaces first
- Assess for signs of metabolic alkalosis, including drowsiness and restlessness

• Assess for signs of hypokalemia with some products: postural hypotension, malaise, fatigue, tachycardia, leg cramps, weakness

Nursing diagnoses
• Cardiac output, decreased (adverse reactions)
• Fluid volume, excess (uses)

Patient/family education
• Teach patient to take product early in the day (diuretic) to prevent nocturia

Evaluation
Positive therapeutic outcome
• Improvement in edema of feet, legs, sacral area daily if medication is being used in CHF
• Improvement in B/P if medication is being used as a diuretic
• Improvement in intraocular pressure if medication is being used to decrease aqueous humor in the eye

---

Generic Names

Thiazides:
chlorothiazide, hydrochlorothiazide

Thiazide-like:
chlorthalidone, indapamide, metolazone

Loop:
bumetanide, furosemide

Carbonic anhydrase inhibitors:
acetaZOLAMIDE

Potassium-sparing:
amiloride, spironolactone

Osmotic:
mannitol, urea

Histamine H₂ Antagonists

ACTION: Histamine H₂ antagonists act by inhibiting histamine at H₂ receptor site in parietal cells, which inhibits gastric acid secretion.

USES: Histamine H₂ antagonists are used for short-term treatment of duodenal and gastric ulcers and maintenance therapy for duodenal ulcer and for gastroesophageal reflux disease.

CONTRAINDICATIONS:
Persons with hypersensitivity should not use these products.

Precautions: Caution should be used in pregnancy, breastfeeding, children <16 yr, organic brain syndrome, and renal/hepatic disease.

IMPLEMENTATION
• Give with meals for prolonged product effect
• Give antacids 1 hr before or 1 hr after cimetidine
• Give **IV** slowly; bradycardia may occur; give over 30 min
• Store diluted sol at room temperature for up to 48 hr

ADVERSE EFFECTS:
The most serious adverse reactions are agranulocytosis, thrombocytopenia, neutropenia, aplastic anemia, and exfoliative dermatitis. The most common side effects are confusion (not with rantidine), headache, and diarrhea.

PHARMACOKINETICS:
Onset, peak, and duration vary widely among products. Most products are metabolized in the liver and excreted in urine.

INTERACTIONS:
Antacids interfere with absorption of histamine H₂ antagonists. Check individual monographs for specific information.

NURSING CONSIDERATIONS
Assessment
• Monitor gastric pH (>5 should be maintained)
• Monitor I&O ratio, BUN, creatinine

Nursing diagnoses
• Injury, risk for (bleeding)
• Knowledge, deficient (teaching)
• Pain, chronic (uses)

Patient/family education
• Advise patient that gynecomastia, impotence may occur but is reversible
• Caution patient to avoid driving and other hazardous activities until patient is stabilized on this medication
• Caution patient to avoid black pepper, caffeine, alcohol, harsh spices, extremes in temperature of food
• Caution patient to avoid OTC preparations: aspirin, cough, cold preparations
• Inform patient that product must be continued for prescribed time to be effective
• Advise patient to report bruising, fatigue, malaise; blood dyscrasias may occur

Evaluation
Positive therapeutic outcome
• Decreased pain in abdomen

⚠ Nurse Alert

Generic Names
cimetidine, famotidine, ranitidine

Immunosuppressants

ACTION: Immunosuppressants produce immunosuppression by inhibiting T lymphocytes.

USES: Most immunosuppressants are used for organ transplants to prevent rejection.

CONTRAINDICATIONS: Products are contraindicated in hypersensitivity.

Precautions: Caution should be used in pregnancy and severe renal/hepatic disease.

IMPLEMENTATION
• Give for several days before transplant surgery
• Give with meals for GI upset or place product in chocolate milk
• Give with oral antifungal for *Candida* infections

ADVERSE EFFECTS: The most serious adverse reactions are albuminuria, hematuria, proteinuria, renal failure, and hepatotoxicity. The most common side effects are oral *Candida* infection, gum hyperplasia, tremors, and headache. The most serious adverse reactions for azathioprine are hematologic (leukopenia and thrombocytopenia) and GI (nausea and vomiting). There is a risk of secondary infection.

PHARMACOKINETICS: Onset, peak, and duration vary widely among products. Most products are metabolized in the liver and excreted in urine.

INTERACTIONS: Interactions vary widely among products. Check individual monographs for specific information.

NURSING CONSIDERATIONS
Assessment
• Monitor renal function tests: BUN, creatinine at least monthly during treatment, 3 mo after treatment
• Monitor hepatic function tests: alkaline phosphatase, AST, ALT, bilirubin
• Monitor product blood levels during treatment

• Assess for hepatotoxicity: dark urine, jaundice, itching, light-colored stools; product should be discontinued

Nursing diagnoses
• Infection, risk for (adverse reactions)
• Injury, risk for (uses)
• Knowledge, deficient (teaching)

Patient/family education
• Advise patient to report fever, chills, sore throat, fatigue since serious infections may occur
• Caution patient to use contraceptive measures during treatment and for 12 wk after ending therapy

Evaluation
Positive therapeutic outcome
• Absence of rejection

Generic Names
azaTHIOprine, **basiliximab** (high alert), cycloSPORINE, everolimus, muromonab-CD3, sirolimus, tacrolimus

Laxatives

ACTION: Laxatives are divided into bulk products, lubricants, osmotics, saline laxative stimulants, and stool softeners. Bulks work by absorbing water and expanding to increase moisture content and bulk in the stool. Lubricants increase water retention in the stool, causing reabsorption of water in the bowel. Saline draws water into the intestinal lumen. Osmotics increase distention and promote peristalsis. Stimulants act by increasing peristalsis by direct effect on the intestine. Stool softeners reduce surface tension of liquid in the bowel.

USES: Laxatives are used as a preparation for bowel or rectal examination, for constipation, or as stool softeners.

CONTRAINDICATIONS: Persons with GI obstruction, perforation, gastric retention, toxic colitis, megacolon, abdominal pain, nausea, vomiting, and fecal impaction should not use these products.

Precautions: Caution should be used in rectal bleeding, large hemorrhoids, and anal excoriation.

IMPLEMENTATION
• Give alone only with water for better absorption; do not take within 1 hr of antacids, milk, or cimetidine

• Swallow tab whole; do not break, crush, or chew

ADVERSE EFFECTS: The most common side effects are nausea, abdominal cramps, and diarrhea.

PHARMACOKINETICS: Onset, peak, and duration vary among products.

INTERACTIONS: Interactions vary widely among products. Check individual monographs for specific information.

NURSING CONSIDERATIONS

Assessment
• Monitor blood, urine electrolytes if product is used often by patient
• Monitor I&O ratio to identify fluid loss
• Determine cause of constipation; identify whether fluids, bulk, or exercise is missing from lifestyle
• Assess for cramping, rectal bleeding, nausea, vomiting; if these symptoms occur, product should be discontinued

Nursing diagnoses
• Constipation (uses)
• Diarrhea (adverse reactions)
• Knowledge, deficient (teaching)

Patient/family education
• Caution patient not to use laxatives for long-term therapy; bowel tone will be lost; that normal bowel movements do not always occur daily
• Caution patient not to use in presence of abdominal pain, nausea, vomiting
• Advise patient to notify prescriber of abdominal pain, nausea, vomiting
• Advise patient to notify prescriber if constipation is unrelieved or if symptoms of electrolyte imbalance occur: muscle cramps, pain, weakness, dizziness

Evaluation
Positive therapeutic outcome
• Decrease in constipation

Generic Names

Bulk laxative:
psyllium

Osmotic agent:
lactulose

Saline laxatives:
magnesium salts, sodium biphosphate/sodium phosphate

Stimulants:
bisacodyl, senna

Stool softener:
docusate

Neuromuscular Blocking Agents

ACTION: Neuromuscular blocking agents are divided into depolarizing and nondepolarizing blockers. They act by inhibiting transmission of nerve impulses by binding with cholinergic receptor sites.

USES: Neuromuscular blocking agents are used to facilitate endotracheal intubation and skeletal muscle relaxation during mechanical ventilation, surgery, or general anesthesia.

CONTRAINDICATIONS:
Persons who are hypersensitive should not be given this product.

Precautions: Caution should be used in pregnancy, breastfeeding, children <2 yr, thyroid disease, collagen disease, cardiac disease, electrolyte imbalances, dehydration, neuromuscular disease (myasthenia gravis), and respiratory disease.

IMPLEMENTATION
• Administer using nerve stimulator by anesthesiologist to determine neuromuscular blockade
• Administer anticholinesterase to reverse neuromuscular blockade
• Give **IV** undiluted over 1-2 min (only by qualified person, usually an anesthesiologist)
• Store in light-resistant, cool area
• Reassure patient if communication is difficult during recovery from neuromuscular blockade

ADVERSE EFFECTS: The most serious adverse reactions are prolonged apnea, bronchospasm, cyanosis, respiratory depression, and malignant hyperthermia. The most common side effects are bradycardia and decreased motility.

PHARMACOKINETICS: Onset, peak, and duration vary widely among products. Most products are metabolized in the liver and excreted in urine.

INTERACTIONS: Aminoglycosides potentiate neuromuscular blockade. Check individual monographs for specific information.

NURSING CONSIDERATIONS

Assessment
• Monitor for electrolyte imbalances (potassium, magnesium); may lead to increased action of this product
• Monitor VS (B/P, pulse, respirations, airway) q15min until fully recovered; rate, depth, pattern of respirations, strength of hand grip
• Monitor I&O ratio; check for urinary retention, frequency, hesitancy
• Assess for recovery: decreased paralysis of face, diaphragm, leg, arm, rest of body
• Assess for allergic reactions: rash, fever, respiratory distress, pruritus; product should be discontinued

Nursing diagnoses
• Breathing pattern, ineffective (uses)
• Injury, risk for (adverse reactions)
• Knowledge, deficient (teaching)

Evaluation
Positive therapeutic outcome
• Paralysis of jaw, eyelid, head, neck, rest of body

Generic Names
pancuronium (high alert), **succinylcholine** (high alert), **vecuronium** (high alert)

Nonsteroidal Antiinflammatories

ACTION: Nonsteroidal antiinflammatories decrease prostaglandin synthesis by inhibiting an enzyme needed for biosynthesis.

USES: Nonsteroidal antiinflammatories are used to treat mild to moderate pain, osteoarthritis, rheumatoid arthritis, and dysmenorrhea.

CONTRAINDICATIONS:
Persons with hypersensitivity, asthma, or severe renal/hepatic disease should not use these products.

Precautions: Caution should be used in pregnancy, breastfeeding, children, geriatric patients, bleeding/GI/cardiac disorders, and hypersensitivity to other antiinflammatory agents.

IMPLEMENTATION
• Give with food to decrease GI symptoms; however, best to take on empty stomach to facilitate absorption
• Store at room temperature

ADVERSE EFFECTS: The most serious adverse reactions are nephrotoxicity (dysuria, hematuria, oliguria, azotemia), blood dyscrasias, and cholestatic hepatitis. The most common side effects are nausea, abdominal pain, anorexia, dizziness, and drowsiness.

PHARMACOKINETICS: Onset, peak, and duration vary widely among products. Most products are metabolized in the liver and excreted in urine.

INTERACTIONS: Interactions vary widely among products. Check individual monographs for specific information.

NURSING CONSIDERATIONS

Assessment
• Monitor renal, hepatic, blood tests: BUN, creatinine, AST, ALT, Hgb, before treatment, periodically thereafter
• Monitor audiometric, ophth examination before, during, and after treatment.
• Check for eye, ear problems: blurred vision, tinnitus; may indicate toxicity

Nursing diagnoses
• Knowledge, deficient (teaching)
• Mobility, impaired physical (uses)
• Noncompliance (teaching)
• Pain, chronic (uses)

Patient/family education
• Advise patient to report blurred vision, ringing, roaring in ears; may indicate toxicity
• Caution patient to avoid driving, other hazardous activities if dizziness, drowsiness occurs, especially in geriatric patients
• Advise patient to report change in urine pattern, increased weight, edema, increased pain in joints, fever, blood in urine; indicate nephrotoxicity
• Inform patient that therapeutic effects may take up to 1 mo to occur

Evaluation
Positive therapeutic outcome
• Decreased pain, stiffness in joints
• Decreased swelling in joints
• Ability to move more easily

Generic Names

celecoxib, diclofenac, etodolac, ibuprofen, indomethacin, ketoprofen, ketorolac, nabumetone, naproxen, piroxicam, sulindac

Opioid Analgesics

ACTION: These agents depress pain impulse transmission at the spinal cord level by interacting with opioid receptors. Products are divided into opiates and nonopiates.

USES: Most opioid analgesics are used to control moderate to severe pain and are used before and after surgery.

CONTRAINDICATIONS:

Hypersensitive reactions occur frequently. Check for sensitivity before administering. These products should not be used if opioid addiction is suspected.

Precautions: Caution must be used when these products are given to persons with an addictive personality, since the possibility of addiction is so great. Also, persons with increased ICP may experience an even greater increase in ICP. Persons with severe heart disease, renal/hepatic disease, respiratory conditions, and seizure disorders should be monitored closely for worsening condition.

IMPLEMENTATION

• Give with antiemetic if nausea or vomiting occurs
• Give when pain is beginning to return; determine dosage interval by patient response
• Provide assistance with ambulation; patient should not be ambulating during product peak

ADVERSE EFFECTS: GI symptoms, including nausea, vomiting, anorexia, constipation, and cramps are the most common side effects. Other common side effects include lightheadedness, dizziness, and sedation. Serious adverse reactions such as respiratory depression, respiratory arrest, circulatory depression, and increased ICP may result but are less common and usually dose dependent.

PHARMACOKINETICS: Onset of action is immediate by IV route and rapid by IM and PO routes. Peak occurs from 1-2 hr, depending on route, with a duration of 2-8 hr. These agents cross the placenta and appear in breast milk.

INTERACTIONS: Barbiturates, other opioids, hypnotics, antipsychotics, or alcohol can increase CNS depression when taken with opioids.

NURSING CONSIDERATIONS

Assessment

• Monitor I&O ratio; be alert for urinary retention, frequency, dysuria; product should be discontinued if these occur
• Assess for respiratory dysfunction: respiratory depression, rate, rhythm, character; notify prescriber if respirations are <12/min
• Assess for CNS changes: dizziness, drowsiness, hallucinations, euphoria, LOC, pupil reaction
• Assess for allergic reactions: rash, urticaria
• Assess for need for pain medication, use pain scoring

Nursing diagnoses

• Gas exchange, impaired (adverse reactions)
• Pain, acute (uses)

Patient/family education

• Advise patient to report any symptoms of CNS changes, allergic reactions, or shortness of breath
• Caution patient that physical dependency may result when used for extended periods
• Teach patient that withdrawal symptoms may occur, including nausea, vomiting, cramps, fever, faintness, anorexia
• Advise patient to avoid alcohol and other CNS depressants

Evaluation

Positive therapeutic outcome
• Decrease in pain

Generic Names

buprenorphine, butorphanol, codeine, fentaNYL (high alert), fentaNYL transdermal, **HYDROmorphone** (high alert), **meperidine** (high alert), **methadone** (high alert), **morphine** (high alert), nalbuphine, **oxyCODONE** (high alert), **oxymorphone** (high alert), **pentazocine** (high alert), **remifentanil** (high alert)

Salicylates

ACTION: Salicylates have analgesic, antipyretic, and antiinflammatory effects. The analgesic and antiinflammatory activities may be mediated through the inhibition of prostaglandin synthesis. Antipyretic action results from inhibition of the hypothalamic heat-regulating center.

⚠ Nurse Alert

USES: The primary uses of salicylates are relief of mild to moderate pain and fever and ininflammatory conditions such as arthritis, thromboembolic disorders, and rheumatic fever.

CONTRAINDICATIONS:
Hypersensitivity to salicylates is common. Check for sensitivity before administering. Persons with bleeding disorders, GI bleeding, and vit K deficiency should not use these products since salicylates increase pro-time. Children should not use these products since salicylates have been associated with Reye's syndrome.

Precautions: Caution is needed when salicylates are given to patients with anemia, renal/hepatic disease, and Hodgkin's disease. Caution should also be exercised in pregnancy and breastfeeding.

IMPLEMENTATION
• Give with food or milk to decrease gastric irritation; give 30 min before or 1 hr after meals with a full glass of water

ADVERSE EFFECTS:
The most common side effects are GI symptoms and rash. Serious blood dyscrasias and hepatotoxicity may result when used for long periods at high doses. Tinnitus or impaired hearing may indicate that blood salicylate levels are reaching or exceeding the upper limit of the therapeutic range.

PHARMACOKINETICS:
Onset of action occurs in 15-30 min, with a peak of 1-2 hr and a duration up to 6 hr. These products are metabolized by the liver and excreted by the kidneys.

INTERACTIONS:
Increased effects of anticoagulants, insulin, methotrexate, heparin, valproic acid, and oral sulfonylureas may occur when used with salicylates. Aspirin may decrease serum concentrations of nonsteroidal antiinflammatory agents.

NURSING CONSIDERATIONS
Assessment
• Monitor renal/hepatic function tests: AST, ALT, bilirubin, creatinine, LDH, alkaline phosphatase, BUN if patient is on long-term therapy since these products are metabolized and excreted by the liver and kidney
• Monitor blood tests: CBC, Hct, Hgb, and pro-time if patient is on long-term therapy, since these products increase the possibility of bleeding and blood dyscrasias

• Assess for hepatotoxicity: dark urine, clay-colored stools, jaundiced skin and sclera, itching, abdominal pain, fever, diarrhea, which may occur with long-term use
• Assess for ototoxicity: tinnitus, ringing, roaring in ears; audiometric testing is needed before and after long-term therapy

Nursing diagnoses
• Activity intolerance (uses)
• Mobility, impaired physical (uses)
• Pain, acute (uses)
• Pain, chronic (uses)
• Sensory perception, disturbed (adverse reactions)
• Thermoregulation, ineffective (uses)

Patient/family education
• Advise patient that blood sugar levels should be monitored closely if patient is diabetic
• Caution patient not to exceed recommended dosage; acute poisoning may result
• Inform patient that therapeutic response takes 2 wk in arthritis
• Caution patient to avoid use of alcohol since GI bleeding may result
• Advise patient to notify prescriber if ringing in the ears or persistent GI pain occurs
• Advise patient to take with full glass of water to reduce risk of lodging in esophagus

Evaluation
Positive therapeutic outcome
• Decreased pain, fever

Generic Names
aspirin, magnesium salicylate, salsalate

Sedatives/Hypnotics

ACTION: The sedatives/hypnotics depress the CNS; some products at the cerebral cortex, others inhibit transmitters in the CNS.

USES: Sedatives/hypnotics are used for the treatment of sleep disorders, seizures, muscle spasms, and alcohol withdrawal.

CONTRAINDICATIONS:
Persons with hypersensitivity reactions should not use these products.

Precautions: Sedatives/hypnotics should be used cautiously in pregnancy (**C**) and breastfeeding.

IMPLEMENTATION
• Give lowest possible dose for therapeutic result; adjust dose to response
• Provide assistance with ambulation during beginning therapy if dizziness, ataxia occur

ADVERSE EFFECTS:
The most common side effects are nausea and drowsiness. The most serious side effects are Stevens-Johnson syndrome, blood dyscrasias, and risk of dependency.

PHARMACOKINETICS:
Onset, peak, and duration vary widely among products. Most products are metabolized in the liver and excreted by the kidneys.

INTERACTIONS:
Increased CNS depression may occur with other CNS depressants such as alcohol, opiates, antipsychotics, and antidepressants.

NURSING CONSIDERATIONS
Assessment
• Monitor mental status: affect, mood, behavioral changes, depression, confusion; seizure activity

Nursing diagnoses
• Knowledge, deficient (teaching)
• Noncompliance (teaching)
• Sleep deprivation (uses)

Patient/family education
• Inform patient that these products should only be used for short-term insomnia
• Caution patient not to drive or engage in other hazardous activities while taking these products
• Instruct patient to avoid breastfeeding while taking these products
• Instruct patient to avoid alcohol or other CNS depressants as drowsiness will increase
• Teach patient that some of the products take two nights to be effective
• Advise patient to report side effects, adverse reactions to health care provider
• Instruct patient to use exactly as prescribed, at regular intervals

Evaluation
Positive therapeutic outcome
• Ability to sleep throughout the night
• Absence or decreasing seizure activity

Generic Names

Barbiturates:
PHENobarbital (high alert)

Benzodiazepines:
chlordiazePOXIDE, clorazepate, diazepam, flurazepam, LORazepam, midazolam, oxazepam, temazepam, triazolam

Miscellaneous products:
chloral hydrate, dexmedetomidine, **droperidol** (high alert), eszopiclone, hydrOXYzine, promethazine, ramelteon, zaleplon, zolpidem

Skeletal Muscle Relaxants

ACTION:
Most skeletal muscle relaxants inhibit synaptic responses in the CNS by stimulating receptors and decreasing neurotransmission, decreasing pain and spasticity.

USES:
Skeletal muscle relaxants are used for musculoskeletal disorders with pain or spasticity related to spinal cord injuries.

CONTRAINDICATIONS:
Persons with hypersensitivity should not use these products.

Precautions: Skeletal muscle relaxants should be used cautiously in pregnancy (**C**), breastfeeding, the geriatric patient, peptic ulcer, renal/hepatic disease, stroke, seizure disorder, and diabetes.

IMPLEMENTATION
• Give when pain is beginning to return, not after pain is severe
• Store in dry area, away from heat and sunlight

ADVERSE EFFECTS:
The most common side effects are dizziness, weakness, fatigue, drowsiness, and headache. Some products can cause seizures, cardiovascular collapse, and severe CNS depression.

PHARMACOKINETICS:
Pharmacokinetics vary widely among products. Check individual monographs for specific information.

INTERACTIONS:
CNS depressants used with skeletal muscle relaxants may lead to increased CNS depression.

NURSING CONSIDERATIONS
Assessment
• Monitor pain: character, location, duration, alleviating/aggravating factors

Nursing diagnoses
- Injury, risk for (adverse reactions)
- Knowledge, deficient (teaching)
- Mobility, impaired physical (uses)
- Pain, acute (uses)
- Pain, chronic (uses)

Patient/family education
- Advise patient not to use with other CNS depressant unless prescriber approved
- Inform patient that many products require 1-2 mo of treatment for full effect
- Caution patient to avoid hazardous activities until response to medication is known
- Caution patient that most products should not be discontinued quickly, but tapered over 1-2 wk

Evaluation
Positive therapeutic outcome
- Decrease in pain or spasticity

Generic Names

Centrally acting:
baclofen, carisoprodol, cyclobenzaprine, diazepam, methocarbamol

Direct-acting:
dantrolene

Thrombolytics

ACTION: Thrombolytics activate conversion of plasminogen to plasmin (fibrinolysin). Plasmin is able to break down clots (fibrin).

USES: Thrombolytics are used to treat DVT, PE, arterial thrombosis, arterial embolism, arteriovenous cannula occlusion, lysis of coronary artery thrombi after MI, and acute evolving transmural MI.

CONTRAINDICATIONS:
Persons with hypersensitivity, active bleeding, intraspinal surgery, neoplasms of the CNS, ulcerative colitis/enteritis, severe hypertension, renal/hepatic disease, hypocoagulation, COPD, subacute bacterial endocarditis, rheumatic valvular disease, cerebral embolism/thrombosis/hemorrhage, intra-arterial diagnostic procedure or surgery (10 days), and recent major surgery should not use these products.

Precautions: Caution should be used in arterial emboli from left side of heart and pregnancy.

IMPLEMENTATION
- Administer as soon as thrombi identified; not useful for thrombi over 1wk old
- Administer cryoprecipitate or fresh, frozen plasma if bleeding occurs
- Give loading dose at beginning of therapy; may require increased loading doses
- Give heparin after fibrinogen level is over 100 mg/dl; heparin INF to increase PTT to 1.5-2 × baseline for 3-7 days
- About 10% of patients have high streptococcal antibody titers requiring increased loading doses
- Give **IV** therapy using 0.8-μm filter
- Store reconstituted sol in refrigerator; discard after 24 hr
- Provide bed rest during entire course of treatment

ADVERSE EFFECTS: Serious adverse reactions include GI, GU, intracranial, and retroperitoneal bleeding and anaphylaxis. The most common side effects are decreased Hct, urticaria, headache, and nausea.

PHARMACOKINETICS: Onset, peak, and duration vary widely among products. Most products are metabolized in the liver and excreted in urine.

INTERACTIONS: Interactions vary widely among products. Check individual monographs for specific information.

NURSING CONSIDERATIONS
Assessment
- Monitor VS, B/P, pulse, respirations, neurologic signs, temp at least q4hr (increased temp is an indicator of internal bleeding), cardiac rhythm following intracoronary administration; systolic pressure increase of >25 mm Hg should be reported to prescriber
- Assess for neurologic changes that may indicate intracranial bleeding
- Assess retroperitoneal bleeding: back pain, leg weakness, diminished pulses
- Assess for allergy: fever, rash, itching, chills; mild reaction may be treated with antihistamines
- Assess for bleeding during 1st hr of treatment: hematuria, hematemesis, bleeding from mucous membranes, epistaxis, ecchymosis
- Monitor blood tests (Hct, platelets, PTT, PT, TT, APTT) before starting therapy; PT or APTT must be less than 2 times control before starting therapy; TT or PT q3-4hr during treatment

Nursing diagnoses
• Injury, risk for (uses)

Patient/family education
• Teach patient to avoid venous or arterial puncture, injection, rectal temp
• Teach patient to treat fever with acetaminophen or aspirin
• Teach patient to apply pressure for 30 sec to minor bleeding sites; inform prescriber if this does not attain hemostasis; apply pressure dressing

Evaluation
Positive therapeutic outcome
• Resolution of thrombosis, embolism

Generic Names
alteplase (high alert), drotrecogin alfa, **tenecteplase** (high alert), **urokinase** (high alert)

Thyroid Hormones

ACTION: Thyroid hormones increase metabolic rates, resulting in increased cardiac output, O_2 consumption, body temp, blood volume, growth, development at cellular level, respiratory rate, and enzyme system activity.

USES: Thyroid hormones are used for thyroid replacement.

CONTRAINDICATIONS:
Persons with adrenal insufficiency, myocardial infarction, or thyrotoxicosis should not use these products.

Precautions: Caution should be used in pregnancy (A) and breastfeeding. Geriatric patients and those with angina pectoris, hypertension, ischemia, cardiac disease, or diabetes mellitus or insipidus should be watched closely when using these products.

IMPLEMENTATION
• Give at same time each day to maintain product level
• Give only for hormone imbalances; not to be used for obesity, male infertility, menstrual conditions, lethargy
• Remove medication 4 wk before RAIU test

ADVERSE EFFECTS: The most
common side effects include insomnia, tremors, tachycardia, palpitations, angina, dysrhythmias, weight loss, and changes in appetite. Serious adverse reactions include thyroid storm.

PHARMACOKINETICS: Pharmacokinetics vary widely among products. Check individual monographs for specific information.

INTERACTIONS
• Impaired absorption of thyroid products may occur when administered with cholestyramine, iron products (separate by 4-5 hr).
• Increased effects of anticoagulants, sympathomimetics, tricyclics, catecholamines may occur.
• Decreased effects of digoxin, glycosides, insulin, hypoglycemics may occur.
• Decreased effects of thyroid products may occur with estrogens.

NURSING CONSIDERATIONS
Assessment
• Monitor B/P, pulse before each dose
• Monitor I&O ratio
• Monitor weight daily in same clothing, using same scale, at same time of day
• Monitor height, growth rate if given to a child
• Monitor T_3, T_4, which are decreased; radioimmunoassay of TSH, which is increased; ratio uptake, which is decreased if patient is on too low a dosage of medication
• Assess for increased nervousness, excitability, irritability; may indicate too high a dosage of medication, usually after 1-3 wk of treatment
• Assess for cardiac status: angina, palpitation, chest pain, change in VS

Nursing diagnoses
• Body image, disturbed (adverse reactions)
• Knowledge, deficient (teaching)
• Noncompliance (teaching)

Patient/family education
• Advise patient/family that hair loss will occur in children and is temporary
• Advise patient to report excitability, irritability, anxiety; indicates overdose
• Caution patient not to switch brands unless directed by prescriber
• Caution family that hypothyroid children will show almost immediate behavior/personality change
• Advise patient that treatment product is not to be taken to reduce weight
• Advise patient to avoid OTC preparations with iodine; read labels; to avoid iodine-containing foods: iodized salt, soybeans, tofu, turnips, some seafood, some bread

Evaluation
Positive therapeutic outcome
• Absence of depression
• Increased weight loss, diuresis, pulse, appetite

• Absence of constipation, peripheral edema, cold intolerance, pale, cool, dry skin, brittle nails, alopecia, coarse hair, menorrhagia, night blindness, paresthesias, syncope, stupor, coma, rosy cheeks

Generic Names
levothyroxine, liothyronine (T₃), liotrix, thyroid USP

Vasodilators

ACTION: Vasodilators act in various ways. Check individual monographs for specific action.

USES: Vasodilators are used to treat intermittent claudication, arteriosclerosis obliterans, vasospasm and muscular ischemia, ischemic cerebral vascular disease, hypertension, and angina.

CONTRAINDICATIONS: Some products are contraindicated in acute MI, paroxysmal tachycardia, and thyrotoxicosis.

Precautions: Caution should be used in uncompensated heart disease or peptic ulcer disease.

IMPLEMENTATION
• Give with meals to reduce GI symptoms
• Store in tight container at room temperature

ADVERSE EFFECTS: The most common side effects are headache, nausea, hypotension, hypertension, and ECG changes.

PHARMACOKINETICS: Onset, peak, and duration vary widely among products. Most products are metabolized in the liver and excreted in urine.

INTERACTIONS: Interactions vary widely among products. Check individual monographs for specific information.

NURSING CONSIDERATIONS
Assessment
• Assess bleeding time in individuals with bleeding disorders
• Assess cardiac status: B/P, pulse, rate, rhythm, character; watch for increasing pulse

Nursing diagnoses
• Cardiac output, decreased (uses)
• Knowledge, deficient (teaching)
• Tissue perfusion, ineffective (uses)

Patient/family education
• Inform patient that medication is not cure, may need to be taken continuously
• Advise patient that it is necessary to quit smoking to prevent excessive vasoconstriction
• Advise patient that improvement may be sudden, but usually occurs gradually over several weeks
• Instruct patient to report headache, weakness, increased pulse, since product may need to be decreased or discontinued
• Instruct patient to avoid hazardous activities until stabilized on medication; dizziness may occur

Evaluation
Positive therapeutic outcome
• Ability to walk without pain
• Increased temp in extremities
• Increased pulse volume

Generic Names
amyl nitrite, bosentan, dipyridamole, hydrALAZINE, minoxidil, nesiritide

Vitamins

ACTION: The action of vitamins varies widely among products and classes. Check individual monographs for specific action.

USES: Vitamins are used to correct and prevent vitamin deficiencies.

CONTRAINDICATIONS: Hypersensitive reactions may occur, and allergies should be identified before these products are given.

IMPLEMENTATION
• Give PO with food for better absorption
• Store in tight, light-resistant container

ADVERSE EFFECTS: There is an absence of side effects or adverse reactions with the water-soluble vitamins (C, B). However, fat-soluble vitamins (A, D, E, K) may accumulate in the body and cause adverse reactions (refer to individual monographs).

PHARMACOKINETICS: Onset, peak, and duration vary widely among products. Check individual monographs for specific information.

NURSING CONSIDERATIONS

Nursing diagnoses
• Nutrition: less than body requirements, imbalanced (uses)

Patient/family education
• Advise patient not to take more than prescribed amount

Evaluation
Positive therapeutic outcome
• Absence of vitamin deficiency

Generic Names

Fat-soluble:
phytonadione (vitamin K_1), vitamin A, vitamin D, vitamin E

Water-soluble:
ascorbic acid (C), cyanocobalamin (B_{12}), pyridoxine (B_6), riboflavin (B_2), thiamine (B_1)

Miscellaneous:
multivitamins

Appendix A

Selected New Drugs

abiraterone
(a-bir-a'ter-one)
Zytiga
See p. 4

aflibercept
(a-fli-ber'cept)
EYLEA
Func. class.: Biologic response modifier; signal transduction inhibitor (STIs) (Ophthalmic)
Pregnancy category C

ACTION: A recombinant fusion protein consisting of portions of human VEGF receptors 1 and 2 extracellular domains fused to human IgG1; acts as a soluble decoy receptor that binds vascular endothelial growth factor-A (VEGF-A) and placental growth factor (PIGF); can act as mitogenic, chemotactic, vascular permeability factors for endothelial cells; VEGF-A interacts with VEGFR-1 and VEGFR-2 on the surface of endothelial cells; results in neovascularization and vascular permeability; binding of aflibercept to VEGF-A and PIGF prevents activation of these receptors

Therapeutic outcome: Prevention of further vision loss

USES: Neovascular (wet) age-related macular degeneration (AMD)

CONTRAINDICATIONS:
Hypersensitivity, ocular/periocular infection, active intraocular inflammation

Precautions: Neonates, infants, children, adolescents, pregnancy (C), breastfeeding; history of glaucoma, ocular surgery; driving or operating machinery

DOSAGE AND ROUTES
Adult: Intravitreal INJ 2 mg (0.05 ml) into affected eye(s) q4wk × 12 wk, then 2 mg (0.05 ml) q8wk

Available forms: Solution for injection 2 mg/0.05 ml

Implementation
Intravitreal route
• Visually inspect for particulate matter, discoloration before use; do not use if particulates, cloudiness, discoloration are visible; only for use by physicians trained in administration
• Use controlled aseptic conditions (sterile gloves, sterile drape, sterile eyelid speculum); adequate anesthesia, topical broad-spectrum antiinfective should be given before use
• Use each vial for treatment of single eye only; if other eye is being treated, use new vial and change the sterile field, syringe, gloves, drapes, eyelid speculum, filter, injection needles before administering to the other eye
• Use aseptic technique, withdraw all of vial contents through a 5-micron 19-G filter needle attached to 1-ml syringe supplied by manufacturer; after vial contents are withdrawn, discard filter needle and replace with sterile 30-G × ½ inch needle for intravitreal injection; expel any air bubbles and contents of syringe until plunger tip is aligned with line that marks 0.05 ml
• Immediately after the intravitreal injection, monitor patient for elevation in intraocular pressure (IOP); appropriate monitoring may consist of a check for perfusion of optic nerve head or tonometry; sterile paracentesis needle should be available if required
• Storage: do not freeze, protect from light, refrigerate, store in original package until time of use

ADVERSE EFFECTS
CV: Thromboembolism, nonfatal stroke, nonfatal myocardial infarction, vascular death
EENT: *Ocular hemorrhage, ocular pain, cataracts, vitreous detachment, vitreous floaters,* conjunctival hyperemia, corneal erosion, detachment of retinal pigment epithelium, injection site pain, foreign body sensation, increased lacrimation, blurred vision, retinal pigment epithelium tear, injection site hemorrhage, blepharedema, corneal edema
SYST: Hypersensitivity

Pharmacokinetics

Absorption	Complete
Distribution	Systemic circulation
Metabolism	Unknown
Excretion	Unknown
Half-life	Terminal 5-6 days

Pharmacodynamics

Onset	Unknown
Peak	Unknown
Duration	Unknown

NURSING CONSIDERATIONS

Assessment
• Assess for infection: monitor for infection during week after injection to permit early treatment of any ocular infection that may develop; proper aseptic injection technique should be used to minimize infection
• Assess for increased intraocular pressure: monitor for acute increases in intraocular pressure within 60 min of injection; sustained increases in intraocular pressure have been reported after repeated intravitreal dosing; monitor intraocular pressure and optic nerve head perfusion, a sterile paracentesis needle should be available
• Assess for further vision loss

Patient/family education
• Advise patient to seek immediate care if symptoms of endophthalmitis or retinal detachment develop (ocular pain, hyperemia of the conjunctiva, photophobia, blurry vision)

Evaluation
Positive therapeutic outcome
• Prevention of further vision loss

---

aminophylline (theophylline ethylenediamine) (Rx)
(am-in-off′i-lin)
Hepsera
Added here due to extensive dosing revisions

DOSAGE AND ROUTES

For treatment of reversible airways obstruction (bronchospasm prophylaxis) associated with asthma or chronic obstructive pulmonary disease (COPD, emphysema, chronic bronchitis)
Calculate initial mg/kg dose based on ideal body weight as theophylline distributes poorly into body fat

For adjunct treatment of acute exacerbations of the symptoms and reversible airflow obstruction associated with asthma and other chronic lung diseases (COPD) along with inhaled beta-2 selective agonists and systemic corticosteroids
Adult <60 yr and adolescent ≥16 yr: IV CONT INF expressed in theophylline; Initially, 0.4 mg/kg/hr; up to max 900 mg/day (otherwise healthy nonsmokers); patients who smoke may require an increased dose; Give 0.2 mg/kg/hr (up to 400 mg/day) in CHF, cor pulmonale, liver dysfunction, sepsis with multiorgan failure, shock; reduced doses may be needed in patients receiving other drugs that decrease theophylline clearance; adjust dosage based on serum concentrations
Adult ≥60 yr: IV CONT INF: Initially, 0.3 mg/kg/hr; give 0.2 mg/kg/hr in CHF, cor pulmonale, liver dysfunction, sepsis with multiorgan failure, shock; reduced doses may be needed in patients receiving other drugs that decrease theophylline clearance; adjust dosage-based serum concentrations; max 400 mg/day unless serum concentration and patient condition require a higher dose
Child ≥12 yr and adolescent ≤15 yr: IV CONT INF: Initially, 0.5 mg/kg/hr in healthy nonsmokers (up to 900 mg/day); 0.7 mg/kg/hr in smokers; 0.2 mg/kg/hr (up to 400 mg/day) in cardiac decompensation, cor pulmonale, liver dysfunction, sepsis with multiorgan failure, or shock; adjust dosage based on serum concentrations
Child 9 to 11 yr: IV CONT INF: Initially, 0.7 mg/kg/hr; reduced doses may be needed in patients receiving other drugs that decrease theophylline clearance; give 0.2 mg/kg/hr (up to 400 mg/day) in cardiac decompensation, cor pulmonale, liver dysfunction, sepsis with multiorgan failure, or shock; adjust dosage based on serum concentrations
Child 1 to 8 yr: IV CONT INF: Initially, 0.8 mg/kg/hr; reduced doses may be needed in patients receiving other drugs that decrease theophylline clearance; 0.2 mg/kg/hr (up to 400 mg/day) in cardiac decompensation, cor pulmonale, liver dysfunction, sepsis with multiorgan failure, or shock; adjust dosage based on serum concentrations
Infant 6 to 52 wk: IV CONT INF: Calculate initial dosage using the following equation: $(0.008 \times$ age in wk$) + 0.21 =$ theophylline dosage in mg/kg/hr; reduced doses may be needed in patients with risk factors for reduced

theophylline clearance (cimetidine therapy, cardiac or liver dysfunction, renal impairment in infant <3 mo); adjust dosage based on serum concentrations

For maintenance therapy of asthma or COPD

Adult, adolescent, and child >45 kg: PO (expressed in theophylline and reg release products): Initially, 300 mg/day in divided doses q6-8hr; after 3 days, if tolerated, increase dose to 400 mg/day in divided doses q6-8hr; after 3 more days, if tolerated, increase dose to 600 mg/day PO in divided doses q6-8hr; adjust dose to maintain therapeutic range; doses of 400-1600 mg/day may be needed, max 400 mg/day in patients with risk factors for decreased theophylline clearance (elderly >60; NIH recommends initial dose for asthma of 10 mg/kg/day (max: 300 mg/day) titrated to serum concentration of 5-15 mcg/ml (usual max: 800 mg/day in children ≥12 yr and 16 mg/kg/day in children 1-11 yr)

Child and adolescent ≤15 yr and ≤45 kg: PO: Initially, 12-14 mg/kg (max 300 mg) per day in divided doses q4-6 hr; after 3 days, if tolerated, may increase to 16 mg/kg (max: 400 mg) per day in divided doses q4-6hr; after 3 more days, if tolerated and if needed, increase dose to 20 mg/kg (max 600 mg) per day in divided doses q4-6hr; adjust dose to maintain therapeutic range (doses of 10-36 mg/kg/day in child 1-9 yr may be needed); max 16 mg/kg (400 mg) per day in patients with risk factors for decreased theophylline clearance or who cannot receive recommended serum concentration monitoring; NIH recommends initial dose for asthma of 10 mg/kg/day (max 300 mg/day) titrated to serum concentration of 5-15 mcg/ml (usual max 800 mg/day in patients ≥12 yr and 16 mg/kg/day in children 1-11 yr)

Neonates and infants up to 52 wk: PO: Calculate initial dose using the following equation: $[(0.2 \times \text{age in wk}) + 5] \times (\text{kg body weight})$ = theophylline dosage in mg/day; In infants up to 26 wk old, divide dose and administer q8hr and in infant >26 wk , divide dose and give q6hr; adjust dose to maintain a steady-state serum concentration of 5-10 mcg/ml in neonates and 10-15 mcg/ml in infants; NIH recommends initial dose for asthma of 10 mg/kg/day titrated to theophylline serum concentration of 5-15 mcg/ml, max in mg/kg/day = $\lfloor (0.2 \times \text{age in weeks}) + 5 \rfloor$

Extended-release products are to be used only for chronic disease management; do not use in treatment of acute symptoms of asthma and reversible bronchospasm

Adults, adolescents, and children ≥12 yr and >45 kg (Theo-24 Cap): PO: Initially, 300-400 mg/day q24hr; evening dosing is not recommended; after 3 days, if tolerated, increase to 400-600 mg/day q24hr; adjust dose to maintain therapeutic range; doses of 400-1600 mg/day may be needed; max 400 mg/day in with decreased theophylline clearance, (elderly >60 yr), and in those who cannot receive recommended serum concentration monitoring

Child >12 yr and adolescent <16 yr and <45 kg (Theo-24 Cap): Initially, 12-14 mg/kg (max 300 mg) per day q24hr; evening dosing is not recommended; after 3 days, if tolerated, may increase to 16 mg/kg (max 400 mg) per day; after 3 more days, if tolerated and if needed, increase to 20 mg/kg (max 600 mg) per day; adjust dose to maintain therapeutic range; max 16 mg/kg/day up to 400 mg/day in those with decreased theophylline clearance

Treatment of methotrexate toxicity (unlabeled)

Adults, adolescents, and children ≥3 yr: IV 2.5 mg/kg over 45-60 min

asparaginase *Erwinia chrysanthemi*
Erwinaze
Func. class.: Antineoplastic, natural and semisynthetic
Pregnancy category C

ACTION: Contains an asparaginase specific enzyme L-asparaginase derived from *Erwinia chrysanthemi*, which catalyzes asparagine to aspartic acid and ammonia and causes reduced circulating concentrations of asparagine; efficacy of asparaginase *Erwinia chrysanthemi* may be leukemic cell cytotoxicity from asparagine deficiency

Therapeutic outcome: Decreased spread of malignancy

USES: Treatment of acute lymphocytic leukemia (ALL) in combination with other chemotherapeutic agents in patients who have developed hypersensitivity to *E. coli*-derived asparaginase

CONTRAINDICATIONS:
Hypersensitivity, breastfeeding, history of serious pancreatitis, bleeding, or serious thrombosis with prior L-asparaginase therapy

Precautions: Pregnancy (C), children <2 yr, hepatic disease, diabetes mellitus

DOSAGE AND ROUTES
Adult, adolescent, child ≥2 yr (substitute for pegaspargase): IM 25,000 IU/m² 3 ×/ wk (Monday/Wednesday/Friday) × 6 doses for each planned dose of pegaspargase within a treatment
Adult (substitute for L-asparaginase *E. coli*): IM 25,000 IU/m² for each scheduled dose of native *E. coli* asparaginase within a treatment

Available forms: Powder for inj 10,000 Units

Implementation
• Slowly inject 1 or 2 ml of preservative-free sterile sodium chloride (0.9%) inj against inner vial wall; do not forcefully inject sol directly onto or into powder; if 1 ml of NS is used, conc is 10,000 IU/ml; if 2 ml of NS is used, conc is 5000 IU/ ml; dissolve contents by gentle mixing or swirling; do not shake or invert vial
• Reconstituted sol should be clear and color-less; discard if any visible particles or protein aggregates are present
• Calculate the volume needed to obtain dose; withdraw volume containing calculated dose from vial into polypropylene syringe within 15 min of reconstitution
• Do not freeze or refrigerate the reconstituted solution; discard any unused portions
IM route
• Administer dose by IM inj within 4 hr of reconstitution; limit volume to 2 ml per inj site; multiple inj sites may be needed

ADVERSE EFFECTS
ENDO: Hyperglycemia
GI: Pancreatitis
HEMA: Bleeding, serious thrombosis
INTEG: Local inj site reaction
MISC: Hyperammonemia (seizure, headache), neurotoxicity, elevated hepatic enzymes, hyperbilirubinemia
SYST: Anaphylaxis

Pharmacokinetics

Absorption	Unknown
Distribution	Unknown
Metabolism	Unknown
Excretion	Unknown
Half-life	Unknown

Pharmacodynamics

Onset	Unknown
Peak	Unknown
Duration	Unknown

INTERACTIONS
Individual drugs
Cytarabine: increased pancreatitis risk
Methotrexate: Synergistic or antagonistic effect, depending on administration schedule
VinCRIStine: increased neurotoxicity

Drug classifications
Anticoagulants, NSAIDs, platelet inhibitors, salicylates, thrombolytics: increased bleeding risk

Drug/lab test
Increased: liver function tests, ammonia
Decreased: fibrinogen, protein C activity, protein S activity, anti-thrombin III

NURSING CONSIDERATIONS
Assessment
• Assess for anaphylaxis: give only with resuscitation equipment and other agents necessary to treat anaphylaxis; if a serious hypersensitivity reaction occurs, discontinue product
• Assess for bleeding: identify if NSAIDs, salicylates, thrombolytics, platelet inhibitors, anticoagulants have been used; grade 1 or 2 bleeding or coagulation abnormalities may occur (serious thrombosis, sagittal sinus thrombosis); discontinue for a thrombotic or hemorrhagic event until symptoms resolve; after resolution, treatment may be resumed; coagulation proteins were decreased in most patients after a 2-wk course: fibrinogen, protein C activity, protein S activity, antithrombin III
• Assess for pancreatitis: discontinue for severe or hemorrhagic pancreatitis (abdominal pain >72 hr and amylase elevation ≥2 × upper limit of normal); mild pancreatitis, hold until the signs, symptoms subside and amylase concentrations return to normal, then resume
• Assess for hyperglycemia: glucose intolerance that is irreversible in some cases; monitor baseline and periodic glucose concentration; administer insulin therapy as needed
• Assess for hyperammonemia/neurotoxicity: seizures, headache; asparagine rescue may be used to treat acute CNS toxicity; doses of asparagine used were 1-2 mmol/kg/day continuous IV infusion × 5 days
• Monitor liver function tests and assess for hyperbilirubinemia

• Assess for local injection site reaction: no more than 2 ml of the reconstituted product is to be administered at a single injection site

Patient/family education
• Advise patient to get immediate medical advice if they experience abdominal pain, nausea, vomiting, diarrhea; pancreatitis may occur
• Advise patient to get immediate medical advice if experiencing anaphylactic reactions
• Advise patient to contact provider if patient experiences excessive thirst or any increase in volume or frequency of urination; hyperglycemia may occur

Evaluation
Positive therapeutic outcome
• Decreased spread of malignancy

axitinib
Inlyta
Func. class.: Antineoplastic, biologic response modifier, signal transduction inhibitor (STI)
Chem. class.: Tyrosine kinase inhibitor
Pregnancy category D

ACTION: Inhibits receptor tyrosine kinases including vascular endothelial growth factor receptors (VEGFR)-1, VEGFR-2, and VEGFR-3; inhibits tumor growth and phosphorylation of VEGFR-2 and VEGF-mediated endothelial cell proliferation

Therapeutic outcome: Decreased spread of malignancy

USES: Treatment of advanced renal cell cancer after failure of one prior systemic therapy

CONTRAINDICATIONS:
Pregnancy (D), breastfeeding

Precautions: Risk for or history of thromboembolic disease, recent bleeding, untreated brain metastasis, recent GI bleeding, GI perforation, fistula, surgery, moderate hepatic disease, uncontrolled hypertension, hyper/hypothyroidism, proteinuria, infertility, end-stage renal disease (CrCl <15 ml/min); not intended for use in adolescents, children, infants, neonates

DOSAGE AND ROUTES
Adult: **PO** 5 mg bid (at 12 hr intervals), may increase to 7 mg bid and then to 10 mg bid in those not receiving antihypertensives who toler-

ate the lower dosage for at least 2 consecutive wk with no more than grade 2 adverse reactions. Reduce to 3 mg bid if a dose reduction is needed; if further reduction is necessary, reduce to 2 mg bid
Adult receiving a strong CYP 3A4/5 inhibitor: Reduce dose by 1/2, adjust as needed

Available forms: Tab 1, 5 mg

Implementation
• Give with or without food; swallow tablet whole with a glass of water
• If patient vomits or misses a dose, an additional dose should not be taken; the next dose should be taken at the usual time
• Store at room temperature

ADVERSE EFFECTS
CNS: Dizziness, headache, reversible posterior leukoencephalopathy syndrome (RPLS), fatigue
CV: Hypertension, arterial thromboembolic events (ATE), venous thromboembolic events (VTE)
ENDO: Hypothyroidism, hyperthyroidism
GI: Lower GI bleeding/perforation/fistula. abdominal pain, constipation, diarrhea, dysgeusia, dyspepsia, dysphonia, hemorrhoids, nausea, mucosal inflammation, stomatitis, vomiting, increased ALT/AST
GU: Proteinuria
HEMA: Bleeding intracranial bleeding, anemia, polycythemia, decreased/increased hemoglobin, lymphopenia thrombocytopenia, neutropenia
INTEG: Palmar-plantar erythrodysesthesia (hand and foot syndrome) rash, dry skin, pruritus, alopecia, erythema
MISC: Weight loss dehydration metabolic and electrolyte laboratory abnormalities included
MS: Asthenia, arthralgia, musculoskeletal pain, myalgia
RESP: Cough, dyspnea

Pharmacokinetics
Absorption	Unknown
Distribution	Protein binding >99%
Metabolism	Liver
Excretion	Unknown
Half-life	2.5-6.1 hr

Pharmacodynamics
Onset	Unknown
Peak	Unknown
Duration	Unknown

INTERACTIONS
Individual drugs
CYP3A4/5 inhibitor, strong, moderate (ketoconazole, boceprevir, chloramphenicol, conivaptan, delavirdine, fosamprenavir, imatinib, indinavir, isoniazid, itraconazole, dalfopristin; quinupristin, posaconazole, ritonavir, telithromycin, tipranavir [boosted with ritonavir], darunavir [boosted with ritonavir], aldesleukin, IL-2, amiodarone, aprepitant, fosaprepitant atazanavir, bromocriptine, clarithromycin, crizotinib, danazol, diltiazem, dronedarone, erythromycin, fluvoxamine, lanreotide, lapatinib, miconazole, mifepristone, nefazodone, nelfinavir, niCARdipine, octreotide, pantoprazole, saquinavir, tamoxifen, verapamil, voriconazole, grapefruit juice): increased axitinib effect

CYP3A4/5 inducers, strong/moderate (rifampin, carBAMazepine, dexamethasone, phenytoin, PHENobarbital, rifabutin, rifapentine, St. John's wort, ethanol, bexarotene, bosentan, efavirenz, etravirine, griseofulvin, metyrapone, modafinil, nafcillin, nevirapine, OXcarbazepine, vemurafenib, pioglitazone, topiramate): decreased effect of axitinib

CYP3A4/5 inhibitor and inducers (quiNINE): increased or decreased axitinib effect

Drug/lab test
Increase: creatinine, lipase, amylase, sodium, potassium, glucose
Decrease: bicarbonate, calcium, albumin, glucose, phosphate, sodium
Increase or decrease: sodium, glucose

Drug/herb
St. John's wort: decreased effect of axitinib

NURSING CONSIDERATIONS
Assessment
• Bleeding: monitor for GI bleeding or perforation; temporarily discontinue therapy if a patient develops any bleeding that requires treatment
• Surgery: discontinue ≥24 hr before surgery, may be resumed after adequate wound healing
• Hepatic/renal disease: dosage should be reduced in patients with moderate (Child-Pugh Class B) hepatic disease, monitor liver function tests (ALT, AST, bilirubin) before and periodically during therapy; monitor CCr before and during treatment
• Hypertension: B/P should be well controlled before starting treatment; monitor patients for hypertension and administer antihypertensive therapy as needed before and during therapy; dose should be reduced for persistent hypertension; therapy should be discontinued if B/P remains elevated after a dosage reduction or if there is evidence of hypertensive crisis; after discontinuation monitor B/P for hypotension in those receiving antihypertensives
• Hyper/hypothyroidism: monitor thyroid function tests before and periodically during therapy; thyroid disease should be treated with thyroid medications
• Monitor for proteinuria before and periodically during therapy; product may need to be decreased or discontinued if moderate to severe proteinuria occurs
• Pregnancy/breastfeeding: pregnancy category D; determine if the patient is pregnant or breastfeeding before using this product; may also cause infertility

Patient/family education:
• Instruct patient to use contraception during treatment (pregnancy category D) or to avoid use of this product; to notify prescriber if pregnancy is planned or suspected, not to breastfeed
• Instruct patient to notify prescriber of bleeding that is severe or that requires treatment
• Teach patient that product will be discontinued ≥24 hr before surgery; may be resumed after adequate wound healing
• Teach patient that laboratory testing will be required before and periodically during product use
• Teach patient how to monitor B/P and that B/P products should be continued as directed by prescriber

Evaluation
Positive therapeutic outcome
• Decreased spread of malignancy

azilsartan
Edarbi
See p. 100

belatacept
Nulojix
See p. 108

belimumab
Benlysta
See p. 110

boceprevir
Victrelis
See p. 130

brentuximab
Adcetris
See p. 135

crizotinib
XALKORI
See p. 265

desvenlafaxine
Pristiq
See p. 306

ezogabine
Potiga
See p. 425

fidaxomicin
Dificid
See p. 448

glucarpidase
(gloo-kar'pi-dayz)
Voraxaze
Func. class.: Recombinant bacterial enzyme
Pregnancy category C

ACTION: A recombinant bacterial enzyme that hydrolyzes glutamate residue from methotrexate and provides an alternate nonrenal pathway for methotrexate elimination in patients with renal dysfunction during high-dose methotrexate treatment. As a result of its enzymatic action, glucarpidase converts methotrexate to its inactive metabolites

Therapeutic outcome: Resolution of methotrexate toxicity

USES: The treatment of methotrexate toxicity (methotrexate plasma concentration >1 micromole/liter) in those with delayed methotrexate clearance due to impaired renal function

Precautions: Pregnancy (C), breastfeeding

DOSAGE AND ROUTES
Adult/adolescent/child: IV 50 Units/kg over 5 min; continue to give leucovorin, IV hydration, urinary alkalinization as needed

Available forms: Sol for IV

Implementation
IV direct route
• Visually inspect parenteral products for particulate matter and discoloration prior to administration
• Reconstitution: Add 1 ml of sterile saline for injection to vial, roll and tilt the vial gently to mix; do not shake; flush the IV line then inject as a bolus inj over 5 min; flush the IV line again
• Do not administer to patients who exhibit the expected clearance of methotrexate (plasma methotrexate concentrations within 2 standard deviations of the mean methotrexate excretion curve specific for the dose of methotrexate administered)
• Do not administer to patients with normal or mildly impaired renal function because of the potential risk of subtherapeutic exposure to methotrexate
• Continue to administer leucovorin after glucarpidase, but do not administer leucovorin within 2 hr before or after glucarpidase. For the first 48 hr after glucarpidase administration, administer the same leucovorin dose as given before glucarpidase. After 48 hr after glucarpidase, administer leucovorin based on the measured methotrexate concentration. Do not discontinue therapy with leucovorin based on the determination of a single methotrexate concentration below the leucovorin treatment threshold. Continue leucovorin until the methotrexate concentration has been maintained below the leucovorin treatment threshold for a minimum of 3 days; use of a chromatographic method to determine methotrexate concentrations is needed for the first 48 hr after glucarpidase receipt
• Continue hydration and alkalinization of the urine as needed
• Store reconstituted solution refrigerated ≤4 hr, discard any unused product; no preservative is present

ADVERSE EFFECTS
CNS: Paresthesia, headache
CV: Hypo/hypertension
EENT: Throat irritation or tightness
GI: Nausea, vomiting
INTEG: Flushing, hot, burning sensation; rash, hypersensitivity, serious allergic reactions
SYST: Antibody formation

Pharmacokinetics

Absorption	Unknown
Distribution	Unknown
Metabolism	Unknown
Excretion	Unknown
Half-life	Unknown

Pharmacodynamics

Onset	Unknown
Peak	Unknown
Duration	Unknown

INTERACTIONS

Individual drugs

Pemetrexed, pralatrexate: decreased glucarpidase level—avoid concurrent use

NURSING CONSIDERATIONS

Assessment

• Continue monitoring of methotrexate blood levels, renal status (creatinine/BUN) after glucarpidase is given. Methotrexate concentrations within 48 hr of glucarpidase are the only reliable measure by a chromatographic method. Leucovorin receipt is needed until the methotrexate level has been maintained below the leucovorin treatment threshold for a minimum of 3 days

Patient/family education

• Instruct patient to immediately report any infusion-related reactions: fever, chills, flushing, feeling hot, rash, hives, itching, throat tightness or breathing problems, tingling, numbness, or headache

Evaluation

Positive therapeutic outcome

• Resolution of methotrexate toxicity

indacaterol

Arcapta Neohaler

See p. 557

ipilimumab

Yervoy

See p. 574

linagliptin

Tradjenta

See p. 626

norepinephrine

Levophed

See p. 774

rilpivirine

Edurant

See p. 926

rivaroxaban

Xarelto

See p. 936

roflumilast

Daliresp

See p. 940

telaprevir

Incivek

See p. 1001

tesamorelin

Egrifta

See p. 1018

ticagrelor

Brilinta

See p. 1030

vemurafenib

Zelboraf

See p. 1091

Appendix B

Ophthalmic, Nasal, Topical, and Otic Products

OPHTHALMIC PRODUCTS

α-ADRENERGIC BLOCKER
dapiprazole (Rx)
(da-pip'ra-zole)
Rev-Eyes

ANESTHETICS
lidocaine (Rx)
(lye'doe-kane)
Akten

proparacaine (Rx)
(proe-par'a-kane)
Alcaine, Diocaine ❀, Ophthaine, Ophthetic

tetracaine (Rx)
(tet'ra-kane)
Minims Tetracaine ❀, Pontocaine, Tetracaine

ANTIHISTAMINES
alcaftadine
(al-caf'tah-deen)
Lastacalf

azelastine (Rx)
(ay-zell'ah-steen)
Optivar

emedastine (Rx)
(ee-med'-a-steen)
Emadine

epinastine (Rx)
(ep-een-as'teen)
Elestat

ketotifen (Rx, OTC)
(kee-toh-tif'en)
Zaditor

levocabastine (Rx)
(lee-voh-cab'ah-steen)
Livostin

olopatadine (Rx)
(oh-loh-pat'ah-deen)
Patanol

ANTIINFECTIVES
azithromycin (Rx)
(ay-zi-thro-my'sin)
AzaSite

besifloxacin (Rx)
(be'si-flox'a-sin)
Besivance

chloramphenicol (Rx)
(klor-am-fen'i-kole)
AK-Chlor, Chloramphenicol, Chloromycetin Ophthalmic, Chloroptic, Chloroptic S.O.P., Fenicol ❀, Isopto Fenical ❀, Pentamycin ❀

ciprofloxacin (Rx)
(sip-ro-floks'a-sin)
Ciloxan

erythromycin (Rx)
(er-ith-roe-mye'sin)
Erythromycin, Ilotycin

ganciclovir (Rx)
(gan-sye'kloe-vir)
Virgan

gatifloxacin (Rx)
(gat-ih-floks'ah-sin)
Zymar, Zymaxid

gentamicin (Rx)
(jen-ta-mye'sin)
Garamycin Ophthalmic, Genoptic Ophthalmic, Genoptic S.O.P., Gentacidin, Gentamicin Ophthalmic, Gentak

levofloxacin (Rx)
(lee-voh-flock'sah-sin)
Quixin

moxifloxacin (Rx)
(mox-i-flox'a-sin)
Vigamox

natamycin (Rx)
(nat-a-mye'sin)
Natacyn

norfloxacin (Rx)
(nor-floks'a-sin)
Chibroxin
ofloxacin (Rx)
(oh-floks'a-sin)
Ocuflox
silver nitrate 1% (Rx)
silver nitrate
sulfacetamide sodium (Rx)
(sul-fa-seet'a-mide)
**AK-Sulf, Bleph-10, Bleph-10
S.O.P., Cetamide, Isopto Cetamide,
Ocusulf-10, Sodium Sulamyd, Sodium
Sulfacetamide, Storzsulf, Sulf-10,
Sulster**
tobramycin (Rx)
(toe-bra-mye'sin)
AKTob, Defy, Tobrex
trifluridine (Rx)
(trye-floor'i-deen)
Viroptic
vidarabine (Rx)
(vye-dare'a-been)
Vira-A

β-ADRENERGIC BLOCKERS
betaxolol (Rx)
(beh-tax'oh-lole)
Betoptic, Betoptic S
carteolol (Rx)
(kar-tee'oh-lole)
Carteolol HCl, Ocupress
levobetaxolol (Rx)
(lee-voh-beh-tax'oh-lohl)
Betaxon
levobunolol (Rx)
(lee-voe-byoo'no-lole)
AK Beta, Betagen
metipranolol (Rx)
(met-ee-pran'oh-lole)
OptiPranolol
timolol (Rx)
(tym'-moe-lole)
**Apo-Timop ❋, Betimol, Timoptic,
Timoptic-XE**

**CARBONIC ANHYDRASE
INHIBITORS**
brinzolamide (Rx)
(brin-zoh'la-mide)
Azopt
dorzolamide (Rx)
(dor-zol'a-mide)
Trusopt

**CHOLINERGICS
(Direct-acting)**
acetylcholine (Rx)
(ah-see-til-koe'leen)
Miochol-E
carbachol (Rx)
(kar'ba-kole)
**Carbastat, Carboptic, Isopto
Carbachol, Miostat**
pilocarpine (Rx)
(pye-loe-kar'peen)
**Adsorbocarpine, Akarpine, Isopto
Carpine, Ocu-Carpine, Ocusert Pilo-
20, Ocusert Pilo-40, Pilagan, Pilocar,
pilocarpine, Pilopine HS, Piloptic-$\frac{1}{2}$,
Piloptic-1, Piloptic-2, Piloptic-3,
Piloptic-4, Piloptic-6, Pilostat,
Pilopto-Carpine**

**CHOLINESTERASE
INHIBITORS**
demecarium (Rx)
(dem-e-kare'ee-um)
Humorsol
ecothiophate (Rx)
(ek-oh-thye'oh-fate)
Phospholine Iodide
isoflurophate (Rx)
(i-se'flur-e'fate)
Floropryl
physostigmine (Rx)
(fi-zoe-stig'meen)
Eserine Salicylate, Isopto Eserine

CORTICOSTEROIDS
dexamethasone (Rx)
(dex-a-meth'a-sone)
**AK-Dex, Decadron Phosphate,
Dexamethasone Ophthalmic
Suspension, Maxidex, Ozurdex**

fluocinolone (Rx)
(floo-oh-sin'oh-lone)
Retisert
fluorometholone (Rx)
(flure-oh-meth'oh-lone)
Flarex, Fluor-Op, FML, FML Forte, FML S.O.P.
loteprednol (Rx)
(loe-tee-pred-nole)
Alrex, Lotemax
medrysone (Rx)
(me'dri-sone)
HMS
prednisoLONE (Rx)
(pred-niss'oh-lone)
Econopred, Econopred Plus, AK-Pred, Inflamase Forte, Inflamase Mild, Pred-Forte
rimexolone (Rx)
(ri-mex'a-lone)
Vexol
triamcinolone (Rx)
(trye-am-sin'oh-lone)
Triesence

MYDRIATICS
atropine (Rx)
(a'troe-peen)
Atropine-1, Atropine Care, Atropine Sulfate Ophthalmic, Atropisol, Isopto Atropine
cyclopentolate (Rx)
(sye-kloe-pen'toe-late)
AK-Pentolate, Cyclogyl, Cyclopentolate HCl
homatropine (Rx)
(home-a'troe-peen)
Homatropine HBr, Isopto Homatropine, Minims Homatropine ✤
phenylephrine (OTC)
(fen-ill-ef'rin)
AK-Dilate, AK-Nefrin, Isopto Frin, Neo-Synephrine 2.5%, Neo-Synephrine 10%, phenylephrine HCl, 2.5% Mydfrin, Phenoptic Relief, Prefrin
scopolamine (Rx)
(skoe-pol'a-meen)
Isopto Hyoscine

tropicamide (Rx)
(troe-pik'a-mide)
Mydriacyl, Opticyl, Tropicacyl, Tropicamide

NONSTEROIDAL ANTIINFLAMMATORIES
bromfenac (Rx)
(brome'fen-ak)
Xibrom
diclofenac (Rx)
(dye-kloe'fen-ak)
Voltaren
flurbiprofen (Rx)
(flure-bi'pro-fen)
Ocufen
ketorolac (Rx)
(kee-toe'role-ak)
Acular, Acuvail
nepafenac (Rx)
(ne-pa-fen'ak)
Nevanac
suprofen (Rx)
(soo-proe'fen)
Profenal

SYMPATHOMIMETICS
apraclonidine (Rx)
(a-pra-klon'i-deen)
Iopidine
brimonidine (Rx)
(brem-on'i-dine)
Alphagan, Alphagan P
dipivefrin (Rx)
(dye-pi'vef-rin)
Propine, AKPro
epINEPHrine/epinephryl borate (Rx)
(ep-i-nef'rin)
Epifrin, Glaucon/Epinal, Eppy ✤

OPHTHALMIC DECONGESTANTS/ VASOCONSTRICTORS
Iodoxamide
(loe-dox'ah-mide)
Alomide

naphazoline (Rx, OTC)
(naf-az'oh-leen)
20/20 Eye Drops, AK-Con, Albalon, Allerest Eye Drops, Allergy Drops, Clear Eyes, Clear Eyes ACR, Comfort Eye Drops, Degest 2, Maximum Strength Allergy Drops, Nafazair, naphazoline HCl, Naphcon, Naphcon Forte, Opcon, Vasoclear, Vasocon Regular

oxymetazoline (Rx)
(ox-i-met-ah-zoh'leen)
OcuClear, Visine L.R.

tetrahydrozoline (OTC)
(tet-ra-hye-dro'zoe-leen)
Collyrium Fresh, Eyesine, Geneye, Geneye Extra, Mallazine Eye Drops, Murine Plus, Optigene 3, tetrahydrozoline HCl, Tetrasine, Tetrasine Extra, Visine Moisturizing

MISCELLANEOUS OPHTHALMICS

bimatoprost (Rx)
(bih-mat'o-prost)
Latisse, Lumigan

latanoprost (Rx)
(la-tan'oh-prost)
Xalatan

travoprost (Rx)
(tra'voe-prost)
Travatan

unoprostone (Rx)
(yoo-noe-pros'tone)
Rescula

β-Adrenergic blockers
ACTION: Reduces production of aqueous humor by unknown mechanism

USES: Ocular hypertension, chronic open angle glaucoma

Anesthetics
ACTION: Decreases ion permeability by stabilizing neuronal membrane

USES: Cataract extraction, tonometry, gonioscopy, removal of foreign objects, corneal suture removal, glaucoma surgery (ophthalmic); pruritus, sunburn, toothache, sore throat, cold sores, oral pain, rectal pain and irritation, control of gagging (topical)

Antiinfectives
ACTION: Inhibits folic acid synthesis by preventing PABA use, which is necessary for bacterial growth

USES: Conjunctivitis, superficial eye infections, corneal ulcers, prophylaxis against infection after removal of foreign matter from the eye

Antiinflammatories
ACTION: Decreases inflammation, resulting in decreased pain, photophobia, hyperemia, cellular infiltration

USES: Inflammation of eye, eyelids, conjunctiva, cornea; uveitis, iridocyclitis, allergic conditions, burns, foreign bodies, postoperatively in cataract

Carbonic anhydrase inhibitor
ACTION: Converted to epINEPHrine, which decreases aqueous production and increases outflow

USES: Open angle glaucoma, ocular hypertension

Direct-acting miotic
ACTION: Acts directly on cholinergic receptor sites; induces miosis, spasm of accommodation, fall in intraocular pressure, caused by stimulation of ciliary, pupillary sphincter muscles, which leads to pulling away of iris from filtration angle, resulting in increased outflow of aqueous humor

USES: Primary glaucoma, early stages of wide angle glaucoma (less useful in advanced stages), chronic open angle glaucoma, acute closed angle glaucoma before emergency surgery; also neutralizes mydriatics used during eye exam; may be used alternately with mydriatics to break adhesions between iris and lens

CONTRAINDICATIONS: Hypersensitivity

Precautions: Pregnancy, breastfeeding, children, aphakia, hypersensitivity to carbonic anhydrase inhibitors, sulfonamides, thiazide diuretics, ocular inhibitors, renal/hepatic insufficiency

Implementation
• Storage at room temperature away from light

ADVERSE EFFECTS
CNS: Headache
CV: Hypertension, tachycardia, dysrhythmias
EENT: Burning, stinging
GI: Bitter taste

NURSING CONSIDERATIONS

Assessment
• Monitor ophthalmic exams and intraocular pressure readings
• Monitor blood counts; renal/hepatic function tests and serum electrolytes during long-term treatment

Nursing diagnoses
• Knowledge, deficient (teaching)
• Sensory perception, disturbed: visual (uses)

Patient/family education
• Teach how to instill drops
• Advise patient that product may cause burning, itching, blurring, dryness of eye area

Evaluation
Positive therapeutic outcome
• Absence of increased intraocular pressure

NASAL AGENTS

NASAL ANTIHISTAMINES
olopatadine (Rx)
(oh-low-pat'uh-deen)
Patanase

NASAL DECONGESTANTS
azelastine (Rx)
(ay-zell'ah-steen)
Astelin, Astepro
desoxyephedrine (OTC)
(des-oxy-e-fed'rin)
Vicks Vapor Inhaler
ePHEDrine (OTC)
(e-fed'rin)
Pretz-D
EPINEPHrine (OTC)
(ep-i-neff'rin)
Adrenalin
naphazoline (OTC)
(naff-a-zoe'leen)
Privine

oxymetazoline (OTC)
(ox-i-met-az'oh-leen)
12 Hour Nasal, Afrin 12 Hour Original, Afrin 12-Hour Original Pump Mist, Afrin Severe Congestion with Menthol, Afrin Sinus with Vapornase, Afrin No-Drip 12-Hour, Afrin No-Drip 12-Hour Extra Moisturizing, Dristan, Duramist Plus, Duration, Genasal, Nafrine ❋, Neo-Synephrine 12 Hour, Nostrilla, oxymetazoline HCl, Nasal Relief, Nasal Decongestant Maximum Strength, Vicks Sinex 12 Hour Long-Acting, Vicks Sinex 12-Hour Ultra Fine Mist for Sinus Relief
phenylephrine (OTC)
(fen-ill-eff'rin)
Alconefrin 12, Children's Nostril, Neo-Synephrine, Sinex
propylhexadrine (OTC)
(proe-pil-hex'a-dreen)
Benzedrex Inhaler
pseudoephedrine (Rx, OTC)
(soo-doe-e-fed'rin)
Cenafed, Decofed, Dimetapp, Genaphed, Sudafed, Triaminic
tetrahydrozoline (OTC)
(tet-ra-hye-dro'zoe-leen)
Tyzine, Tyzine Pediatric
xylometazoline (OTC)
(zye-loh-meh-tazz'oh-leen)
Natru-vent, Otrivin, Otrivin Pediatric Nasal

NASAL STEROIDS
beclomethasone (Rx)
(be-kloe-meth'a-sone)
Beconase AQ Nasal, Beconase Inhalation, Vancenase AQ Nasal, Vancenase Pocket Inhaler
budesonide (Rx)
(byoo-des'oh-nide)
Rhinocort, Rhinocort Aqua
flunisolide (Rx)
(floo-niss'oh-lide)
Nasalide, Nasarel
fluticasone (Rx)
(floo-tic'a-son)
Flonase, Veramyst

triamcinolone (Rx)
(trye-am-sin'oh-lone)
Nasacort AQ

NONSTEROIDAL ANTIINFLAMMATORY

ketorolac (Rx)
(kee'toe-role-ak)
Sprix

ACTION: Produces vasoconstriction (rapid, long acting) of arterioles, thereby decreasing fluid exudation, mucosal engorgement by stimulation of α-adrenergic receptors in vascular smooth muscle

Therapeutic outcome: Absence of nasal congestion

USES: Nasal congestion

CONTRAINDICATIONS:
Hypersensitivity to sympathomimetic amines

Precautions: Pregnancy **C**, children <6 yr, geriatric, diabetes, CV disease, hypertension, hyperthyroidism, increased ICP, prostatic hypertrophy, glaucoma

DOSAGE AND ROUTES

Desoxyephedrine
Adult and child >6 yr: 1-2 INH in each nostril q2hr or less

EPHEDrine
Adult: Fill dropper to the level marked, then use in each nostril q4hr or less

EPINEPHrine
Adult and child >6 yr: Apply with swab, drops, spray prn

Naphazoline
Adult and child >6 yr: 1-2 drops/spray q6hr or less

Oxymetazoline
Adult and child >6 yr: INSTILL 2-3 gtt or sprays to each nostril bid
Child 2-6 yr: INSTILL 2-3 gtt or sprays 0.025 SOL bid, max 3 days

Phenylephrine
Adult and child >12 yr: 2-3 drops/spray (0.25-0.5) in each nostril q3-4hr or less; or 2-3 drops/spray (1%) in each nostril q4hr or less
Child 6-12 yr: 2-3 drops/spray (0.25%) in each nostril q3-4hr

Infant >6 mo: 1-2 drops (0.16%) in each nostril q3hr

Propylhexadrine
Adult and child >6 yr: 1-2 INH in each nostril q2hr or less

Tetrahydrozoline
Adult and child >6 yr: 2-4 drops (0.1%) q3-4hr prn or 3-4 sprays in each nostril q4hr prn
Child 2-6 yr: 2-3 drops (0.05%) in each nostril q4-6hr prn

Xylometazoline
Adult and child >12 yr: 2-3 drops/spray (0.1%) in each nostril q8-10hr
Child 2-12 yr: 2-3 drops (0.05%) in each nostril q8-10hr

Available forms: Nasal sol 0.025%, 0.05%

Implementation
• Have patient tilt head back, squeeze bulb to create a vacuum, and draw correct amount of sol into dropper; insert 2 gtt of sol into nostril; repeat in other nostril
• Store in light-resistant container; do not expose to high temperature or let sol come into contact with aluminum
• Give for <4 consecutive days
• Provide environmental humidification to decrease nasal congestion, dryness

ADVERSE EFFECTS
CNS: Anxiety, restlessness, tremors, weakness, insomnia, dizziness, fever, headache
EENT: Irritation, burning, sneezing, stinging, dryness, rebound congestion
GI: Nausea, vomiting, anorexia
INTEG: Contact dermatitis

NURSING CONSIDERATIONS

Assessment
• Assess for redness, swelling, pain in nasal passages before, during treatment
• Assess for systemic absorption; hypertension, tachycardia; notify prescriber; systemic absorption occurs at high doses or after prolonged use

Nursing diagnoses
• Airway clearance, ineffective (uses)
• Knowledge, deficient (teaching)
• Noncompliance (teaching)

Patient/family education
• Advise patient that stinging may occur for several applications; drying of mucosa may be decreased by environmental humidification

• Caution patient to notify prescriber if irregular pulse, insomnia, dizziness, or tremors occur
• Teach patient proper administration to avoid systemic absorption
• Advise patient to rinse dropper with very hot water to prevent contamination

Evaluation
Positive therapeutic outcome
• Decreased nasal congestion

TOPICAL GLUCOCORTICOIDS

betamethasone (Rx)
(bay-ta-meth'a-sone)
Alphatrex, Beben ✤,
Betacort ✤, Betatrex, Beta-Val,
Betnovate ✤, Celestoderm ✤,
Diprosone, Ectosone ✤, Luxiq,
Maxivate, Metaderm ✤, Psorion,
Valisone

betamethasone (augmented) (Rx)
(bay-ta-meth'a-sone)
Diprolene, Diprolene AF

clobetasol (Rx)
(kloe-bay'ta-sol)
Clobex, Cormax, Dermovate ✤,
Embeline E 0.05%, Temovate

desonide (Rx)
(dess'oh-nide)
Verdeso Foam

desoximetasone (Rx)
(dess-ox-i-met'a-sone)
Topicort, Topicort LP

dexamethasone (Rx)
(dex-a-meth'a-sone)
Aeroseb-Dex, Decaspray

fluocinolone (Rx)
(floo-oh-sin'oh-lone)
Derma-Smoothe/FS oil, Fluocin,
Licon, Lidemol ✤, Lidex, Lyderm ✤,
Topsyn ✤, Vasoderm

flurandrenolide (Rx)
(flure-an-dren'oh-lide)
Cordran, Cordran SP, Drenison 1/4 ✤,
Drenison Tape ✤

fluticasone (Rx)
(floo-tik'a-sone)
Cutivate

halcinonide (Rx)
(hal-sin'oh-nide)
Halog, Halog-E

hydrocortisone (Rx)
(hye-droe-kor'ti-sone)
Actiocort, Aeroseb-HC, Ala-Cort,
Allercort, Alphaderm, Anusol HC,
Bactine, Barriere-HC ✤, CaldeCORT
Anti-Itch, Carmol HC, Cetacort,
Cortacet ✤, Cortaid, Cortalo,
Cortate ✤, Cort-Dome, Cortef ✤,
Corticaine, Corticreme ✤, Cortifair,
Cortizone, Cortoderm ✤, Cortril,
Delcort, Dermacort, DemiCort,
Dermtex HC, Emo-Cort, Epifoam,
FoilleCort, Gly-Cort, Gynecort, Hi-
Cor, Hycort, Hyderm ✤, Hydro-Tex,
Hytone, Lacti-Care-HC, Lanacort,
Lemoderm, Locoid, Locoid Lotion, My
Cort, Novoehydrocort ✤, Nutracort
Pharm, Pharmacort, Pentacort,
Rederm, Rhulicort S-T Cort, Synacort,
Sarna HC ✤, Texa-Cort,
Unicort ✤, Westcort

triamcinolone (Rx)
(trye-am-sin'oh-lone)
Aristocort, Delta-Tritex, Flutex,
Kenac, Kenalog, Kenonel, Triaderm,
Trianide ✤, Triderm, Trymex

ACTION: Antipruritic, antiinflammatory

Therapeutic outcome: Decreased itching, inflammation

USES: Psoriasis, eczema, contact dermatitis, pruritus; usually reserved for severe dermatoses that have not responded to less potent formulation

CONTRAINDICATIONS:
Hypersensitivity, viral infections, fungal infections

Precautions: Pregnancy **C**

DOSAGE AND ROUTES
Adult and child: Apply to affected area

Implementation
• Apply only to affected areas; do not get in eyes
• Apply and leave site uncovered or lightly covered; occlusive dressing is not recommended—systemic absorption may occur

- Use only on dermatoses; do not use on weeping, denuded, or infected area
- Cleanse area before application of product
- Continue treatment for a few days after area has cleared
- Store at room temperature

ADVERSE EFFECTS
INTEG: *Acne, atrophy, epidermal thinning, purpura, striae*

NURSING CONSIDERATIONS
Assessment
- Monitor temp; if fever develops, product should be discontinued
- Monitor for systemic absorption, increased temp, inflammation, irritation

Nursing diagnoses
- Knowledge, deficient (teaching)
- Pain, chronic (uses)
- Skin integrity, impaired (uses)

Patient/family education
- Teach patient to avoid sunlight on affected area; burns may occur
- Teach patient to limit treatment to 14 days

Evaluation
Positive therapeutic outcome
- Absence of severe itching, patches on skin, flaking

TOPICAL ANTIFUNGALS

clotrimazole (OTC)
(kloe-trye'ma-zole)
Canestew ✿, Clotrimaderm ✿, Clotrimazole, Cruex, Desenex, Lotrimin AF, Myclo ✿, Neozol ✿
econazole (OTC)
(ee-kon'a-zole)
Spectazole
ketoconazole (OTC)
(kee-toe-kon'a-zole)
Nizoral, Xolegel
miconazole (OTC)
(mye-kon'a-zole)
Absorbine Antifungal Foot Powder, Breeze Mist Antifungal, Fungoid Tincture, Lotrimin AF, Maximum Strength Desenex Antifungal, Micatin, Monistat-Derm, Ony-Clear, Tetterine, ZeaSob-AF
nystatin (OTC)
(nye-stat'in)
Mycostatin, Nodostine ✿, Nilstat, Nyoderm ✿, Nystex
selenium (OTC)
(see-leen'ee-um)
Exsel, Head and Shoulders Intensive Treatment, Selenium Sulfide, Selsun, Selsun Blue
terbinafine (OTC)
(ter-bin'a-feen)
Lamisil
tolnaftate (OTC)
(tole-naf'tate)
Absorbine Athlete's Foot Cream, Aftate for Athlete's Foot, Aftate for Jock Itch, Genaspor, Quinsana Plus, Tinactin, Ting, tolnaftate
undecylenic acid (OTC)
(un-deh-sih-len'ik)
Blis-To-Sol, Breeze Mist, Caldesene, Cruex, Decylenes, Desenex, Desenex Maximum Strength, Pedi-Pro, Phicon F, Protectol

ACTION: Interferes with fungal cell membrane permeability

Therapeutic outcome: Absence of itching and white patches of the skin

USES: Tinea cruris, tinea pedis, diaper rash, minor skin irritations; amphotericin B is used for *Candida* infections

CONTRAINDICATIONS:
Hypersensitivity

Precautions: Pregnancy **B**, breastfeeding, children

DOSAGE AND ROUTES
Massage into affected area, surrounding area daily or bid, continue for 7-14 days, max 4 wk

Implementation
- Apply to affected area, surrounding area; do not cover with occlusive dressings
- Store below 30° C (86° F)

ADVERSE EFFECTS
INTEG: Burning, stinging, dryness, itching, local irritation

NURSING CONSIDERATIONS

Assessment
• Assess skin for fungal infections: peeling, dryness, itching before, throughout treatment
• Assess for continuing infection; increased size, number of lesions

Nursing diagnoses
• Infection, risk for (uses)
• Knowledge, deficient (teaching)
• Skin integrity, impaired (uses)

Patient/family education
• Instruct to apply with glove to prevent further infection; not to cover with occlusive dressings
• Teach patient that long-term therapy may be needed to clear infection (2 wk-6 mo depending on organism); compliance is needed even after feeling better
• Teach patient proper hygiene: hand-washing technique, nail care, use of concomitant top agents if prescribed
• Caution patient to avoid use of OTC creams, ointments, lotions unless directed by prescriber
• Instruct patient to use medical asepsis (hand washing) before, after each application; to change socks and shoes once a day during treatment of tinea pedis
• Advise patient to report to health care prescriber if infection persists or recurs; if blisters, burning, oozing, swelling occur
• Caution patient to avoid alcohol because nausea, vomiting, hypertension may occur
• Caution patient to use sunscreen or avoid direct sunlight to prevent photosensitivity
• Advise patient to notify prescriber of sore throat, fever, skin rash, which may indicate overgrowth of organisms

Evaluation
Positive therapeutic outcome
• Decrease in size, number of lesions

TOPICAL ANTIINFECTIVES

azelaic acid (Rx)
(a-zuh-lay'ic)
Azelex, Finacea
bacitracin (OTC)
(bass-i-tray'sin)
Bacitin ✤, Bacitracin
clindamycin (Rx)
(klin-da-my'sin)
Cleocin T, Clindets, Clindagel, ClindaMax

---

erythromycin (Rx, OTC)
(er-ith-roe-mye'sin)
A/T/S, Akne-Mycin, Eryderm, Erygel, Erythromycin, Staticin, T-Stat
gentamicin (Rx)
(jen-ta-mye'sin)
Gentamicin
mafenide (Rx)
(ma'fe-nide)
Sulfamylon
metronidazole (Rx)
(met-roh-nye'da-zole)
MetroGel, MetroCream, MetroLotion, Noritate
mupirocin (Rx)
(myoo-peer'oh-sin)
Bactroban
neomycin (OTC)
(nee-oh-mye'sin)
Neomycin Sulfate
nitrofurazone (Rx)
(nye-troe-fyoor'a-zone)
Furacin, Nitrofurazone
retapamulin (Rx)
(re-tap'a-mue'lin)
Altabax
salicylic acid (Rx)
(sal'i-sil'ik)
Salitop
silver sulfADIAZINE (Rx)
(sul-fa-dye'a-zeen)
Flamazine ✤, Silvadene, SSD, SSD AF, Thermazene
tretinoin (Rx)
(treh'tih-noyn)
Atralin

ACTION: Interferes with bacterial protein synthesis

Therapeutic outcome: Resolution of infection

USES: Skin infections, minor burns, wounds, skin grafts, primary pyodermas, otitis externa

CONTRAINDICATIONS: Hypersensitivity, large areas, burns, ulcerations

Precautions: Pregnancy **C**, breastfeeding, impaired renal function, external ear or perforated eardrum

Implementation
• Apply enough medication to cover lesions completely
• Apply after cleansing with soap, water before each application; dry well
• Apply to less than 20% of body surface area when patient has impaired renal function
• Store at room temperature in dry place

ADVERSE EFFECTS
INTEG: Rash, urticaria, scaling, redness

NURSING CONSIDERATIONS
Assessment
• Assess for allergic reaction: burning, stinging, swelling, redness
• Assess for signs of nephrotoxicity or ototoxicity

Nursing diagnoses
• Infection, risk for (uses)
• Knowledge, deficient (teaching)
• Skin integrity, impaired (uses)

Evaluation
Positive therapeutic outcome
• Decrease in size, number of lesions

TOPICAL ANTIVIRALS

---

acyclovir (Rx)
(ay-sye′kloe-ver)
Zovirax
penciclovir (Rx)
(pen-sye′kloe-ver)
Denavir

ACTION: Interferes with viral DNA replication

Therapeutic outcome: Resolution of infection

USES: Simple mucocutaneous herpes simplex, in immunocompromised clients with initial herpes genitalis

CONTRAINDICATIONS:
Hypersensitivity

Precautions: Pregnancy **C**, breastfeeding

Implementation
• Apply with finger cot or rubber glove to prevent further infection
• Apply enough medication to cover lesions completely
• Apply after cleansing with soap, water before each application; dry well
• Store at room temperature in dry place

ADVERSE EFFECTS
INTEG: Rash, urticaria, stinging, burning, pruritus, vulvitis

NURSING CONSIDERATIONS
Assessment
• Assess for allergic reaction: burning, stinging, swelling, redness, rash, vulvitis, pruritus
• Assess for signs of nephrotoxicity or ototoxicity

Nursing diagnoses
• Infection, risk for (uses)
• Knowledge, deficient (teaching)
• Skin integrity, impaired (uses)

Patient/family education
• Teach patient not to use in eyes or when there is no evidence of infection
• Advise patient to apply with glove to prevent further infection
• Advise patient to avoid use of OTC creams, ointments, lotions unless directed by prescriber
• Advise patient to use medical asepsis (hand washing) before, after each application and avoid contact with eyes
• Advise patient to adhere strictly to prescribed regimen to maximize successful treatment outcome
• Advise patient to begin taking product when symptoms arise

Evaluation
Positive therapeutic outcome
• Decrease in size, number of lesions

TOPICAL ANESTHETICS

benzocaine (OTC)
(ben'zoe-kane)
**Americaine Anesthetic, Anbesol
Maximum Strength, Baby Anbesol,
Biozene, Boil-Ease, Children's
Chloraseptic, Dermoplast, Foille,
Foille Plus, Hurricaine, Lanacane,
Medamint, Orabase, Oracin, Ora-Jel**

dibucaine (OTC)
(dye'byoo-kane)
Dibucaine, Nupercainal

lidocaine (Rx, OTC)
(lye'doe-kane)
**Anestacon, Burn-O-Jel, Dentipatch,
Derma Flex, ELA-Max, Lidoderm,
Numby Staff, Solarcaine Aloe Extra
Burn Relief, Xylocaine, Xylocaine
10% Oral, Xylocaine Viscous,
Zilactin-L**

pramoxine (OTC)
(pra-mox'een)
Itch-X, PrameGel, Prax, Tronothane

tetracaine (OTC, Rx)
(tet'ra-cane)
Pontocaine, Viractin

ACTION: Inhibits conduction of nerve impulses from sensory nerves

Therapeutic outcome: Decreasing inflammation, itching, pain

USES: Oral irritation, sore throat, toothache, cold sore, canker sore, sunburn, minor cuts, insect bites, pain, itching

CONTRAINDICATIONS:
Hypersensitivity, infants <1 yr, application to large areas

Precautions: Pregnancy **C**, children <6 yr, sepsis, denuded skin

DOSAGE AND ROUTES
Adult and child: TOP apply qid as needed; RECT insert tid and after each BM

Implementation
• Store in tight, light-resistant container; do not freeze, puncture, or incinerate aerosol container

ADVERSE EFFECTS
INTEG: Rash, irritation, sensitization

NURSING CONSIDERATIONS
Assessment
• Assess pain: location, duration, characteristics before, after administration
• Assess for infection: redness, drainage, inflammation; this product should not be used until infection is treated

Nursing diagnoses
• Knowledge, deficient (teaching)
• Pain, acute (uses)

Patient/family education
• Teach patient to avoid contact with eyes
• Teach patient not to use for prolonged periods: use for <1 wk; if condition remains, prescriber should be contacted

Evaluation
Positive therapeutic outcome
• Decreased redness, swelling, pain

TOPICAL MISCELLANEOUS

docosanol (OTC)
(doh-koh'sah-nohl)
Abreva

pimecrolimus (Rx)
(pim-eh-kroh-ly'mus)
Elidel

ACTION: Docosanol unknown; pimecrolimus may bind with macrophilin and inhibit calcium-dependent phosphatase

Therapeutic outcome: Decreased redness, swelling, pain

USES: Docosanol applied to fever blisters to promote more rapid healing; pimecrolimus used to treat mild to moderate atopic dermatitis in nonimmunocompromised patients ≥2 yr who are unresponsive to other treatment

CONTRAINDICATIONS:
Hypersensitivity

Precautions: Pregnancy **C**, breastfeeding, dermal infections

DOSAGE AND ROUTES

Docosanol
Adult: TOP rub into blisters 5 ×/day until healing occurs

Pimecrolimus
Adult and child ≥2 yr: TOP apply thin layer 2 ×/day and rub in; use as long as needed

Implementation
• Apply to skin, rub in gently

ADVERSE EFFECTS

Docosanol
NONE known

Pimecrolimus
INTEG: Burning

NURSING CONSIDERATIONS

Assessment
• Assess skin condition (color, pain, inflammation) before, after administration
• Assess for signs and symptoms of skin infections (redness, draining lesions); if present, avoid use of product (pimecrolimus)

Nursing diagnoses
• Skin integrity, impaired (uses)
• Infection, risk for (uses)
• Knowledge, deficient (teaching)

Patient/family education
• Advise patient to avoid contact between medication and eyes
• Instruct patient to discontinue use of product when condition clears

Evaluation
Positive therapeutic outcome
• Decreased inflammation, redness

VAGINAL ANTIFUNGALS

butoconazole (OTC)
(byoo-toh-kone′ah-zole)
Femstat-3, Gynazol-1, Mycelex-3

clotrimazole (OTC)
(kloe-trye′ma-zole)
Canesten ✦, Clotriamazole, Gyne-Lotrimin 3, Gyne-Lotrimin 7, Mycelex 7, Myclo ✦

miconazole (OTC)
(mye-kon′a-zole)
Femizole-M, Monistat, Monistat 3, Monistat 7, Monistat Dual Pak, M-Zole 7 Dual Pack

nystatin (OTC)
(nye-stat′in)
Nystatin

terconazole (OTC)
(ter-kone′ah-zole)
Terazol 7, Tetrazol 3

tioconazole (OTC)
(tye-oh-kone′ah-zole)
Gyne-Trosyd ✦, Monistat 1, Vagistat-1

ACTION: Interferes with fungal DNA replication; binds sterols in fungal cell membranes, which increases permeability, leaking of nutrients

Therapeutic outcome: Fungistatic/fungicidal against susceptible organisms: *Candida* only

USES: Vaginal, vulval, vulvovaginal candidiasis (moniliasis)

CONTRAINDICATIONS: Hypersensitivity

Precautions: Pregnancy, breastfeeding, children <2 yr

DOSAGE AND ROUTES

Butoconazole
Adult: VAG 5 g (1 applicator) at bedtime × 3-6 days

Clotrimazole
Adult: 100 mg (1 vag tab, 100 mg) at bedtime × 1 wk, or 200 mg (2 vag tab, 100 mg) at

bedtime × 3 nights, or 500 mg (1 vag tab, 500 mg), or 5 g (1 applicator) at bedtime × 1-2 wk

Miconazole
Adult: 200 mg SUPP at bedtime × 3 days or 100 mg SUPP × 1 wk

Nystatin
Adult: 100,000 units/day × 2 wk

Terconazole
Adult: VAG 5 g (1 applicator) at bedtime × 7 days

Tioconazole
Adult: 1 applicator at bedtime × 1 wk

Implementation
Topical route
• Administer one full applicator every night high into the vagina
• Store at room temperature in dry place

ADVERSE EFFECTS
GU: Vulvovaginal burning, itching, pelvic cramps
INTEG: Rash, urticaria, stinging, burning
MISC: *Headache,* body pain

NURSING CONSIDERATIONS

Assessment
• Assess for allergic reaction: burning, stinging, itching, discharge, soreness

Nursing diagnoses
• Infection, risk for (uses)
• Knowledge, deficient (teaching)
• Skin integrity, impaired (uses)

Patient/family education
• Instruct patient in asepsis (hand washing) before, after each application
• Teach patient to apply with applicator only; to avoid use of any other vaginal product unless directed by prescriber; sanitary napkin may prevent soiling of undergarments
• Instruct patient to abstain from sexual intercourse until treatment is completed; reinfection and irritation may occur
• Advise patient to notify prescriber if symptoms persist

Evaluation
Positive therapeutic outcome
• Decrease in itching or white discharge (vaginal)

OTIC ANTIINFECTIVES

boric acid (OTC)
(bor′ik as′id)
Auro-Dri, Dri/Ear, Ear Dry
chloramphenicol (Rx)
(klor-am-fen′i-kole)
Chloromycetin Otic
ciprofloxacin (Rx)
(sip′roe-flox′a-sin)
Cetraxel

ACTION: Inhibits protein synthesis in susceptible microorganisms

USES: Ear infection (external), short-term use

CONTRAINDICATIONS:
Hypersensitivity, perforated eardrum

Precautions: Pregnancy C

Implementation
• After removing impacted cerumen by irrigation
• After cleaning stopper with alcohol
• After restraining child if necessary
• After warming sol to body temp

ADVERSE EFFECTS
EENT: Itching, irritation in ear
INTEG: Rash, urticaria

NURSING CONSIDERATIONS

Assessment
• Assess for redness, swelling, fever, pain in ear, which indicates superinfection

Nursing diagnoses
• Infection, risk for (uses)
• Knowledge, deficient (teaching)

Patient/family education
• Teach patient correct method of instillation using aseptic technique, including not touching dropper to ear
• Inform patient that dizziness may occur after instillation

Evaluation
Positive therapeutic outcome
• Decreased ear pain

Appendix C Vaccines and toxoids

GENERIC NAME	TRADE NAME	USES	DOSAGE AND ROUTES	CONTRAINDICATIONS
adenovirus vaccine		Prevention of adenovirus types 4/7	Adult ≤50 yr/adolescent ≥17 yr in the military PO 1 tab of each 4/7 as a single dose	Pregnancy
avian influenza A (H5N1) virus vaccine		Prophylaxis	Adult: IM 1 ml (90 mcg) 2 doses, 28 days apart	IV
anthrax vaccine	BioThrax	Pre-/postexposure prophylaxis	**Preexposure** Adult: SUBCUT 0.5 ml at 0, 2, 4 wk, then 0.5 ml at 6, 12, 18 mo **Postexposure** Adult: SUBCUT 0.5 ml 0, 2, 4 wk, with antibiotics	Hypersensitivity
BCG vaccine	TICE BCG	TB exposure	Adult and child >1 mo: 0.2–0.3 ml Child <1 mo: Reduce dose by 50% using 2 ml of sterile water after reconstituting	Hypersensitivity, hypogamma-globulinemia, positive TB test, burns
cholera vaccine	No trade name	Immunization for cholera outside the United States	Adult and child >10 yr: IM/SUBCUT 2× of 0.5 ml, 7–30 days before traveling to cholera areas Booster is used q6mo 0.5 ml prn	Hypersensitivity, acute febrile illness
diphtheria and tetanus toxoids, adsorbed	No trade name	Induces antitoxins to provide immunity to diphtheria and tetanus	Adult and child ≥7 yr: IM (adult strength) 0.5 ml q4-8wk × 2 doses, then 3rd dose 6-12 mo after 2nd dose, booster IM 0.5 ml q10yr Child 1-6 yr: IM (pediatric strength) 0.5 ml q4wk × 2 doses, booster 6-12 mo after 2nd dose Infant 6 wk-1 yr: IM (pediatric strength) 0.5 ml q4wk × 3 doses, booster 6-12 mo after 3rd dose	Hypersensitivity to mercury; thimerosal; immunocompromised patients; radiation; corticosteroids; acute illness
diphtheria and tetanus toxoids and whole-cell pertussis vaccine (DPT, DTP)	DTwP, Tri-Immunol	Prevention of diphtheria, tetanus, pertussis	Doses vary Check product information	Hypersensitivity, active infection, poliomyelitis outbreak, immunosuppression, febrile illness
diphtheria and tetanus toxoids and acellular pertussis vaccine	Adacel, Boostrix, Daptacel, Infanrix, Tripedia			
diphtheria, tetanus, pertussis, haemophilus, polio IPV	Pentacel	Immunity to diphtheria, tetanus, pertussis, haemophilus, polio IPV	Infant >6 wk and child ≤5 yr: IM 0.5 ml at 2, 4, 6, and 15-18 mo	Hypersensitivity, polio outbreak, acute infection, immunosuppression
diphtheria, tetanus, pertussis, polio vaccine IPV	Kinrix	Immunity to diphtheria, tetanus, pertussis, polio vaccine IPV	Child: IM 0.5 ml	Hypersensitivity, polio outbreak, acute infection, immunosuppression

H1N1 influenza A (swine flu) virus vaccine	Influenza A (H1N1)	Immunity to H1N1	Adult <50 yr, adolescent, child ≥2 yr: Intranasal 1 dose (roughly 0.1 ml) into each nostril; child 2-9 repeat dose ≥4 wk later Adult, adolescent, child ≥3 yr: IM 0.5 ml as a single dose; child 3-9 yr repeat dose ≥4 wk later (Sanofi) (CSL); child 4-9 yr repeat dose ≥4 wk later (Novartis); infants ≥6 mo, child <36 mo: IM 0.25 ml, repeat in 4 wk (Sanofi) Adult: IM 0.5 ml as a single dose (GSK)	Hypersensitivity, febrile illness active infection
haemophilus b conjugate vaccine, diphtheria CRM₁₉₇ protein conjugate (HbOC)	HibTITER	Polysaccharide immunization of children 2-6 yr against *H. influenzae* b, conjugate	**HibTITER (IM only)** Child: IM 0.5 ml Child 2-6 mo: 0.5 ml q2mo × 3 inj	
haemophilus b conjugate vaccine, meningococcal protein conjugate (PRP-OMP)	PedvaxHIB	Immunization of child 2, 4, 6 mo	Child 7-11 mo: Previously unvaccinated 0.5 ml q2mo inj Child 12-14 mo: Previously unvaccinated 0.5 ml × 1 inj **PedvaxHIB (IM only)** Child 2-14 mo: 0.5 ml × 2 inj at 2, 4 mo of age (6 mo dose not needed), then booster at 12-18 mo against invasive disease Child ≥15 mo: Previously unvaccinated 0.5 ml inj	
hepatitis A vaccine, inactivated	Havrix, VAQTA	Active immunization against hepatitis A virus	Adult: IM 1440 EL units (Havrix) or 50 units (VAQTA) as a single dose; booster dose is the same given at 6, 12 mo Child 2-18 yr: IM 720 EL units (Havrix) or 25 units (VAQTA) as a single dose, booster dose is the same given at 6, 12 mo	Hypersensitivity
hepatitis B vaccine, recombinant	Engerix-B, Recombivax HB	Immunization against all subtypes of hepatitis B virus	Varies widely	Hypersensitivity to this vaccine or yeast
herpes zoster virus vaccine	Zostavax	Prevention of herpes zoster	Adult ≥60 yr: SUBCUT 0.65 ml	<60 yr, child, infant, AIDS, IM/IV, leukemia, lymphoma, pregnancy
human papillomavirus recombinant vaccine, quadrivalent	Gardasil	Prevention of HPV types 6, 11, 15, 18, cervical cancer, genital warts, precancerous dysplasic lesions, anal cancer/anal intraepithelial neoplasia	Adult up to 26 yr and child >9 yr to 26 yr: IM give as 3 separate doses; 1st dose as elected; 2nd dose 2 mo after 1st dose; 3rd dose 6 mo after 1st dose	Child <9 yr, pregnancy, breastfeeding, geriatric, active disease, hypersensitivity

Continued

Appendix C Vaccines and toxoids—cont'd

GENERIC NAME	TRADE NAME	USES	DOSAGE AND ROUTES	CONTRAINDICATIONS
influenza virus vaccine	Afluria, FluMist, Fluogen, Flu-Shield, Fluviral*, Fluvirin, Fluzone, influenza virus vaccine, trivalent	Prevention of Russian, Chilean, Philippine influenza	Adult and child >12 yr: IM 0.5 ml in 1 dose Adult 18-64 yr: ID 0.1 ml as a single dose Child 3-12 yr: IM 0.5 ml, repeat in 1 mo (split) unless 1978-1985 vaccine was given; also given nasal Child 6 mo to 3 yr: IM 0.25 ml, repeat in 1 mo (split) unless 1978-1985 vaccine was given; also given nasal child ≤2 yr	Hypersensitivity, active infection, chicken egg allergy, Guillain-Barré syndrome, active neurologic disorders
Japanese encephalitis virus vaccine, inactivated	JE-VAX	Active immunity against Japanese encephalitis (JE)	Adult and child ≥3 yr: SUBCUT 1 ml, days 0, 7, 30; booster SUBCUT 1 ml 2 yr after last dose Child 1-3 yr: SUBCUT 0.5 ml, days 0, 7, 30; booster SUBCUT 0.5 ml 2 yr after last dose	Hypersensitivity to murine, thimerosal; allergic reactions to previous dose
Lyme disease vaccine (recombinant OspA)	LYMErix	Immunization against Lyme disease	Adult and adolescent 15-70 yr: IM 30 mcg in deltoid, repeat at 1, 12 mo after first dose	Hypersensitivity, antibiotic refractory Lyme arthritis
measles and rubella virus vaccine, live attenuated	M-R-Vax II	Immunity to measles and rubella by antibody production	Adult and child ≥15 mo: SUBCUT 0.5 ml (1000 units)	Hypersensitivity; immunocompromised patients, active untreated TB, cancer, blood dyscrasias, radiation, corticosteroids, pregnancy; allergic reactions to neomycin, eggs
measles, mumps, and rubella vaccine, live	M-M-R-II	Prevention of measles, mumps, rubella	Adult: SUBCUT 1 vial; 2 vials separated by 1 mo, in person born after 1957 Child >15 mo and adult: SUBCUT 0.5 ml	Hypersensitivity, blood dyscrasias, anemia, active infection, immunosuppression; egg, chicken allergy; pregnancy, febrile illness, neomycin allergy; neoplasms
measles, mumps, rubella, varicella	ProQuad	Immunity to measles, mumps, rubella, varicella	Child: SUBCUT 0.5 ml	Hypersensitivity to eggs, neomycin, cancer, radiation, corticosteroids, blood dyscrasias, active untreated TB
measles virus vaccine, live attenuated	Attenuvax	Immunity to measles by antibody production	Adult and child ≥15 mo: SUBCUT 0.5 ml (1000 units), 1 dose 15 mo, 2nd dose age 4-6 or 11-12	Hypersensitivity to eggs, neomycin; cancer, radiation, corticosteroids, pregnancy, immunocompromised patients, blood dyscrasias, active untreated TB
meningococcal diphtheria toxoid conjugate vaccine	Menomune, Menactra, Menveo	Prophylaxis to meningococcal meningitis/diphtheria	All doses are different; check product information	Latex hypersensitivity
meningococcal polysaccharide vaccine	Menomune-A/C/Y/W-135, Menactra	Prophylaxis to meningococcal meningitis	Adult and child >2 yr: SUBCUT 0.5 ml	Hypersensitivity to thimerosal, pregnancy, acute illness

mumps virus vaccine, live	Mumpsvax	Active immunity to mumps	Adult and child ≥1 yr: SUBCUT 0.5 ml (20,000 units)	Hypersensitivity to eggs, neomycin; cancer; radiation, corticosteroids, pregnancy, immunocompromised patients, blood dyscrasias, active untreated TB
plague vaccine	No trade name	Active immunity to *Yersinia pestis* plague	Adult: IM 1 ml, then 0.2 ml in 4-12 wk, then 0.2 ml 5-6 mo after 2nd dose; booster 0.1-0.2 ml q6mo when in plague area	Hypersensitivity to phenol, sulfites, formaldehyde, beef, soy, casein; pregnancy, coagulation disorders
pneumococcal 7-valent conjugate vaccine	Prevnar	Immunity against *Streptococcus pneumoniae*	Child: IM 0.5 ml ×3 doses (7-11 mo); ×2 doses (12-23 mo); ×1 dose >2-9 yr	Hypersensitivity to diphtheria toxoid or this product
pneumococcal vaccine, polyvalent	Pneumovax 23, Pnu-Imune 23	Pneumococcal immunization	Adult and child >2 yr: IM/SUBCUT 0.5 ml	Hypersensitivity, Hodgkin's disease, ARDS
poliovirus vaccine, live, oral, trivalent (TOPV) poliovirus vaccine (IPV)	Orimune, IPOL	Prevention of polio	Adult and child >2 yr: PO 0.5 ml, given q8wk ×2 doses, then 0.5 ml 1/2-1 yr after dose 2 Infant: PO 0.5 ml at 2, 4, 18 mo; booster at 4-6 yr; may also be given: IPV at 2, 4 mo, then TOPV at 12-18 mo, booster at 4-6 yr	Hypersensitivity, active infection, allergy to neomycin/streptomycin, immunosuppression, vomiting, diarrhea
rabies vaccine, adsorbed	No trade name	Active immunity to rabies	**Preexposure** Adult and child: IM 1 ml day 0, 7, 21, or 28 days (total 3 doses); booster IM 1 ml prn q2-5yr **Postexposure** Adult and child not vaccinated: IM 20 international units/kg of human rabies immune globulin (HRIG), give 5 total doses of 1-ml inj of rabies vaccine on days 0, 3, 7, 14, 28	Severe hypersensitivity to previous inj of vaccine, thimerosol
rabies vaccine, human diploid cell (HDCV)	Imovax Rabies, Imovax Rabies I.D.	Active immunity to rabies	**Preexposure** Adult and child: IM 1 ml day 0, 7, 21, or 28 (total 4 doses) **Postexposure** Adult and child: IM 1 ml on day 0, 3, 7, 14, 28 (total 5 doses)	No contraindications
rotavirus	RotaTeq, Rotarix	Prevents rotavirus	Infant: PO 3 doses given between 6 and 32 wk of age; 1st dose between 6-12 wk of age; 2nd and 3rd doses q4-10wk	Hypersensitivity to this product or latex, immunocompromised, blood products given within 6 wk, lymphatic disorders

*Canada only.

Continued

Appendix C Vaccines and toxoids—cont'd

GENERIC NAME	TRADE NAME	USES	DOSAGE AND ROUTES	CONTRAINDICATIONS
rubella and mumps virus vaccine, live	Biavax II	Immunity to rubella and mumps by antibody production	Adult and child ≥1 yr: SUBCUT 0.5 ml	Hypersensitivity to eggs, neomycin; cancer, radiation, corticosteroids, pregnancy; immunocompromised patients, blood dyscrasias, active untreated TB
rubella virus vaccine, live attenuated (RA 27/3)	Meruvax II	Immunity to rubella by antibody production	Adult and child ≥1 yr: SUBCUT 0.5 ml (1000 units)	Hypersensitivity to eggs, neomycin; cancer, radiation, corticosteroids
smallpox vaccine	ACAM 2000, Dry Vax	Prevention of smallpox	See package insert	No contraindications
tetanus toxoid, adsorbed/tetanus toxoid	No trade name	Tetanus toxoid: Used for prophylactic treatment of wounds	Adult and child: IM 0.5 ml q4-6wk × 2 doses, then 0.5 ml 1 yr after dose 2 (adsorbed); SUBCUT/IM 0.5 ml q4-8wk × 3 doses, then 0.5 ml ½-1 yr after dose 3, booster dose 0.5 ml q10yr	Hypersensitivity, active infection, poliomyelitis outbreak, immunosuppression
typhoid vaccine, parenteral typhoid vaccine, oral	No trade name Vivotif Berna Vaccine	Active immunity to typhoid fever	Adult: PO 1 cap 1 hr before meals × 4 doses, booster q5yr Adult and child >10 yr: SUBCUT 0.5 ml, repeat in 4 wk, booster q3yr Child 6 mo-10 yr: SUBCUT 0.25 ml, repeat in 4 wk, booster q3yr	Parenteral: Systemic or allergic reaction, acute respiratory or other acute infection, intensive physical exercise in high temperatures Oral: Hypersensitivity, acute febrile illness, suppressive or antibiotic products
typhoid Vi polysaccharide vaccine	Typhim Vi	Active immunity to typhoid fever	Adult and child ≥2 yr: IM 0.5 ml as a single dose, reimmunize q2yr 0.5 ml IM, if needed	Hypersensitivity, chronic typhoid carriers
varicella virus vaccine	Varivax	Prevention of varicella-zoster (chickenpox)	Adult and child ≥13 yr: SUBCUT 0.5 ml, 2nd dose SUBCUT 0.5 ml 4-8 wk later	Hypersensitivity to neomycin; blood dyscrasias, immunosuppression, active untreated TB, acute illness, pregnancy, diseases of lymphatic system
yellow fever vaccine	YF-Vax	Active immunity to yellow fever	Adult and child ≥9 mo: SUBCUT 0.5 ml deeply, booster q10yr Child 6-9 mo: same as above if exposed	Hypersensitivity to egg or chicken embryo protein, pregnancy, child <6 mo, immunodeficiency
zoster vaccine, live	Zostavax	Herpes zoster prevention	Reconstitute immediately after removing from freezer; give SUBCUT as a single dose; inject total amount of single-dose vial	Immunosuppression; neomycin, gelatin allergy; children, TB, pregnancy (C)

Appendix D

Abbreviations and Pregnancy Categories

abd	abdomen	GPC	giant papillary conjunctivitis
ABG	arterial blood gas	gr	grain
ac	before meals	GTT	glucose tolerance test
ACE	angiotensin-converting enzyme	gtt	drops
ACT	activated clotting time	GU	genitourinary
ADA	American Diabetes Association	GVHD	graft-versus-host disease
ADH	antidiuretic hormone	H_2	histamine$_2$
ALT	alanine aminotransferase	hCG	human chorionic gonadotropin
ANA	antinuclear antibody	Hct	hematocrit
AP	anteroposterior	HDCV	human diploid cell rabies vaccine
APLA	antiphospholipid antibody syndrome	Hgb	hemoglobin
APTT	activated partial thromboplastin time	H&H	hematocrit and hemoglobin
ASA	acetylsalicylic acid, aspirin	5-HIAA	5-hydroxyindoleacetic acid
ASHD	arteriosclerotic heart disease	HIV	human immunodeficiency virus (AIDS)
AST	aspartate aminotransferase (SGOT)	H_2O	water
AV	atrioventricular	HOB	head of bed
bid	twice a day	HR	heart rate
BM	bowel movement	hr	hour
BMR	basal metabolic rate	IBD	inflammatory bowel disease
B/P	blood pressure	IC	intracardiac
BPH	benign prostatic hypertrophy	ICP	intracranial pressure
BPM	beats per minute	ID	intradermal
BS	blood sugar	IgG	immunoglobulin G
BUN	blood urea nitrogen	IM	intramuscular
C	Celsius (centigrade)	inf	infusion
CAD	coronary artery disease	INH	inhalation
cap	capsule	inj	injection
Cath	catheterization or catheterize	I&O	intake and output
CBC	complete blood cell count	IPPB	intermittent positive-pressure breathing
CHF	congestive heart failure	IT	intrathecal
CHo	carbohydrates	ITP	idiopathic thrombocytopenic purpura
cm	centimeter	IUD	intrauterine device
CNS	central nervous system	IV	intravenous
CO_2	carbon dioxide	IVP	intravenous pyelogram
cont	continuous	K	potassium
COPD	chronic obstructive pulmonary disease	kg	kilogram
CPAP	continuous positive airway pressure	L	liter
CPK	creatinine phosphokinase	lb	pound
CPR	cardiopulmonary resuscitation	LDH	lactic dehydrogenase
CCr	creatinine clearance	LE	lupus erythematosus
C&S	culture and sensitivity	LH	luteinizing hormone
C sect	cesarean section	LLQ	left lower quadrant
CSF	cerebrospinal fluid	LMP	last menstrual period
CTCL	cutaneous T-cell lymphoma	LOC	level of consciousness
CV	cardiovascular	LR	lactated Ringer's solution
CVA	cerebrovascular accident	LUQ	left upper quadrant
CVP	central venous pressure	M	meter
D&C	dilatation and curettage	m	minim
dir inf	direct infusion	m^2	square meter
dr	dram	MAOI	monoamine oxidase inhibitor
D_5W	5% glucose in distilled water	mcg	microgram
DVT	deep vein thrombosis	mEq	milliequivalent
ECG	electrocardiogram (EKG)	mg	milligram
EDTA	ethylenediamine tetraacetic acid	MI	myocardial infarction
EEG	electroencephalogram	min	minute
EENT	ear, eye, nose, and throat	ml	milliliter
EPS	extrapyramidal symptoms	mm	millimeter
ESR	erythrocyte sedimentation rate	mo	month
ext rel	extended release	Na	sodium
FBS	fasting blood sugar	neg	negative
FHT	fetal heart tones	NGU	nongonococcal urethritis
FSH	follicle-stimulating hormone	NHL	non-Hodgkin's lymphoma
g	gram	NPO	nothing by mouth (Lat. *nulla per os*)
GABA	γ-aminobutyric acid	NS	normal saline
GI	gastrointestinal	O_2	oxygen

OBS	organic brain syndrome		RUQ	right upper quadrant
OD	right eye		Rx	prescription
OR	operating room		SARS	severe acute respiratory syndrome
OS	left eye		SCr	serum creatinine
OTC	over-the-counter		SIMV	synchronous intermittent mandatory ventilation
OU	each eye		SL	sublingual
oz	ounce		SLE	systemic lupus erythematosus
p̄	after		SOB	shortness of breath
P56	Plasma-Lyte 56		sol	solution
PaCO₂	arterial carbon dioxide tension (pressure)		sp gr	specific gravity
PaO₂	arterial oxygen tension (pressure)		ss	one half
PAT	paroxysmal atrial tachycardia		STD	sexually transmitted disease
PBI	protein-bound iodine		SUBCUT	subcutaneous
pc	after meals		supp	suppository
PCI	percutaneous coronary intervention		sus rel	sustained release
PCWP	pulmonary capillary wedge pressure		syr	syrup
PEEP	positive end-expiratory pressure		T&A	tonsillectomy and adenoidectomy
PERRLA	pupils equal, round, react to light and accommodation		tab	tablet
			tbsp	tablespoon
pH	hydrogen ion concentration		TD	transdermal
PO	by mouth		temp	temperature
postop	postoperative		tid	three times daily
PP	postprandial		tinc	tincture
PPHN	persistent pulmonary hypertension of the newborn		TPN	total parenteral nutrition
preop	preoperative		TOP	topical
prn	as required		TSH	thyroid-stimulating hormone
PT	prothrombin time		tsp	teaspoon
PTT	partial thromboplastin time		TT	thrombin time
PVC	premature ventricular contraction		UA	urinalysis
q	every		UTI	urinary tract infection
q<small>AM</small>	every morning		UV	ultraviolet
qhr	every hour		vag	vaginal
q2hr	every 2 hours		VMA	vanillylmandelic acid
q3hr	every 3 hours		vol	volume
q4hr	every 4 hours		VS	vital sign
q6hr	every 6 hours		WBC	white blood cell count
q12hr	every 12 hours		wk	week
qid	four times daily		wt	weight
qmo	every month		yr	year
q<small>PM</small>	every night		>	greater than
qs	sufficient quantity		<	less than
qt	quart		=	equal
qwk	every week		°	degree
R	right		%	percent
RAIU	radioactive iodine uptake		α	alpha
RBC	red blood count or cell		γ	gamma
RLQ	right lower quadrant		β	beta
ROM	range of motion			

- For a list of the Institute for Safe Medicine Practices (ISMP) error-prone abbreviations, symbols, and dose designations, please see http://www.ismp.org/tools/errorproneabbreviations.pdf.
- For frequently asked questions regarding the 2010 National Patient Safety Goals, please visit The Joint Commission website at http://www.jointcommission.org/PatientSafety/NationalPatientSafetyGoals.

FDA Pregnancy Categories

A No risk demonstrated to the fetus in any trimester

B No adverse effects in animals, no human studies available

C Only given after risks to the fetus are considered; animal studies have shown adverse reactions, no human studies available

D Definite fetal risks, may be given despite risks if needed in life-threatening conditions

X Absolute fetal abnormalities; not to be used any time during pregnancy

Note: **UK** = Unknown fetal risk (used in this text but not an official FDA pregnancy category).

Immunization Schedules

Recommended Childhood and Adolescent Immunization Schedule—United States, 2010
Immunization Schedule for Persons Aged 0-6 Years

Vaccine ▼ Age ▶	Birth	1 month	2 months	4 months	6 months	12 months	15 months	18 months	19-23 months	2-3 years	4-6 years
Hepatitis B[*]	HepB	HepB			HepB						
Rotavirus[*]			Rota	Rota	Rota						
Diphtheria, Tetanus, Pertussis[*]			DTaP	DTaP	DTaP		DTaP				DTaP
Haemophilus Influenzae Type b[*]			Hib	Hib	Hib[*]	Hib					
Pneumococcal[*]			PCV	PCV	PCV	PCV				PPSV	
Inactivated Poliovirus[*]			IPV	IPV		IPV					IPV
Influenza[*]						Influenza (Yearly)					
Measles, Mumps, Rubella[*]						MMR					MMR
Varicella[*]						Varicella					Varicella
Hepatitis A[*]						HepA (2 doses)				HepA Series	
Meningococcal[*]										MCV	

Range of recommended ages

Certain high-risk groups

This schedule indicates the recommended ages for routine administration of currently licensed childhood vaccines, as of December 15, 2009, for children aged 0-6 years. Any dose not administered at the recommended age should be administered at any subsequent visit, when indicated and feasible. Additional vaccines may be licensed and recommended during the year. Licensed combination vaccines may be used whenever any components of the combination are indicated and other components of the vaccine are not contraindicated and if approved by the Food and Drug Administration for that dose of the series. **Providers should consult the respective Advisory Committee on Immunization Practices statement for detailed recommendations, including for high-risk conditions: http://www.cdc.gov/vaccines/pubs/ACIP-list.htm.** Clinically significant adverse events that follow immunization should be reported to the Vaccine Adverse Event Reporting System (VAERS). Guidance about how to obtain and complete a VAERS form is available at http://www.vaers.hhs.gov or by telephone, 800-822-7967.

[*]For complete information go to http://www.cdc.gov/vaccines/schedules/index

Immunization Schedule for Persons Aged 7-18 Years

Vaccine ▼ Age ▶	7-10 years	11-12 years	13-18 years
Tetanus, Diphtheria, Pertussis*		Tdap	Tdap
Human Papillomavirus*	*	HPV (3 doses)	HPV Series
Meningococcal*	MCV	MCV	MCV
Influenza*		Influenza (Yearly)	
Pneumococcal*		PPSV	
Hepatitis A*		HepA Series	
Hepatitis B*		HepB Series	
Inactivated Poliovirus*		IPV Series	
Measles, Mumps, Rubella*		MMR Series	
Varicella*		Varicella Series	

Legend:
- Range of recommended ages
- Catch-up immunization
- Certain high-risk groups

This schedule indicates the recommended ages for routine administration of currently licensed childhood vaccines, as of December 15, 2009, for children aged 7-18 years. Any dose not administered at the recommended age should be administered at any subsequent visit, when indicated and feasible. Additional vaccines may be licensed and recommended during the year. Licensed combination vaccines may be used whenever any components of the combination are indicated and other components of the vaccine are not contraindicated and if approved by the Food and Drug Administration for that dose of the series. **Providers should consult the respective Advisory Committee on Immunization Practices statement for detailed recommendations, including for high-risk conditions: http://www.cdc.gov/vaccines/pubs/ACIP-list.htm.** Clinically significant adverse events that follow immunization should be reported to the Vaccine Adverse Event Reporting System (VAERS). Guidance about how to obtain and complete a VAERS form is available at http://www.vaers.hhs.gov or by telephone, 800-822-7967.

*For complete information go to http://www.cdc.gov/nip/recs/child-schedule.htm#printable.

Appendix F

Standard Precautions

The following precautions are used in the care of all patients regardless of their diagnosis or disease. They are also applied when handling or cleaning equipment or supplies that are potentially contaminated.

1. Wear gloves any time that you may contact blood, any moist body fluid (except sweat), secretions, excretions, nonintact skin, or mucous membranes.
2. Remove your gloves, wash your hands, and reapply clean gloves if your gloves become soiled with infective material.
3. Even if you are wearing gloves, remove them, wash your hands, and apply clean gloves *immediately before* contact with mucous membranes or nonintact skin.
4. Wear a protective cover gown of waterproof material if your clothing is likely to have substantial contact with infective material or if splashing of body fluids is likely.
5. Wear a face shield or goggles to protect your eyes if splashing of secretions is likely.
6. Any time a face shield or goggles are worn, wear a surgical mask to protect the mucous membranes of your nose and mouth. A surgical mask may be worn during certain sterile procedures without protective eyewear. However, protective eyewear is *never* worn without a surgical mask.
7. Handle needles, razors, broken glass, and other sharp objects with care. Needles should never be recapped. All sharps should be disposed of in a puncture-resistant sharps container.
8. Wash your hands before and after each patient contact.
9. Wash your hands before you apply and after you remove gloves. Do not assume that hand washing is unnecessary because gloves were worn. Do not wash your hands with gloves on them.
10. Gloves are used for the care of one patient only, then discarded.
11. Follow your facility policy for disposal of gloves and other contaminated items. These items are generally not disposed of in open trash containers. Facilities have designated disposal sites for these biohazardous waste materials.
12. Use resuscitation barrier devices as an alternative to mouth-to-mouth resuscitation.
13. Linen should be handled in a manner that prevents contamination of the outside of the container. Linen from isolation rooms was previously double bagged. Double bagging is no longer recommended since all linen is handled as potentially infectious. Double bag linen only if the outside of the bag becomes contaminated during the bagging process.

Appendix G
Illustrated Mechanisms and Sites of Action

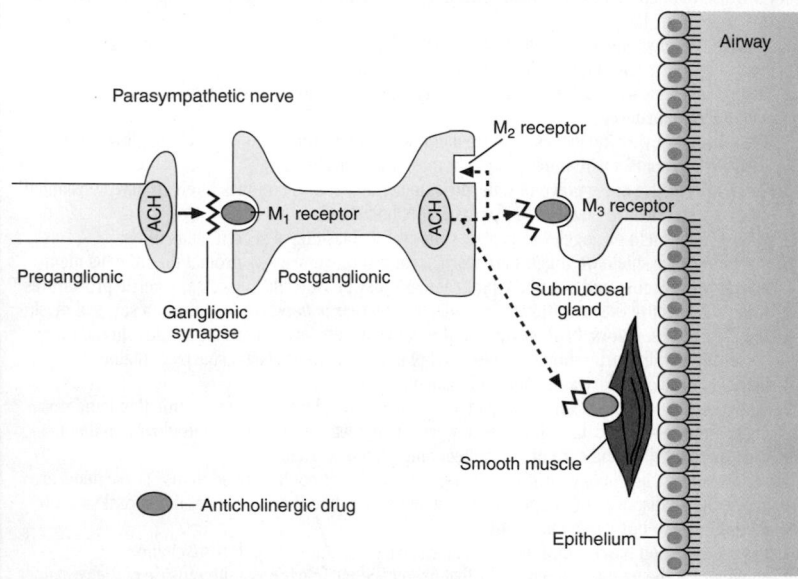

Fig. G-1 Sites and Mechanisms of Action: Anticholinergic Bronchodilators: Anticholinergic bronchodilators, such as ipratropium, work by blocking muscarinic-1 (M_1) receptors on postganglionic parasympathetic nerve endings and muscarinic-3 (M_3) receptors on the cell membranes of bronchial smooth muscles and submucosal glands. Normally, stimulation of the M_1 and M_3 receptors by acetylcholine (ACH) causes bronchoconstriction and mucus secretion from submucosal glands. Anticholinergic bronchodilators block these specific muscarinic receptors from the effects of acetylcholine, causing bronchial smooth muscle relaxation, bronchodilatation, and decreased mucus production. (From Gardenhire OS: *Rau's Respiratory Care Pharmacology,* ed 7, St. Louis, 2008, Mosby.)

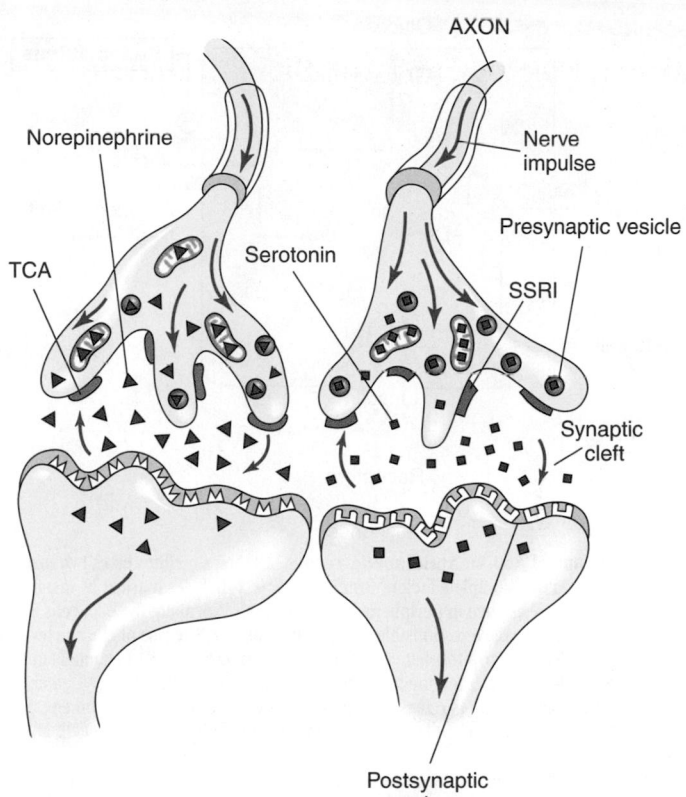

Fig. G-2 Mechanisms of Action: Antidepressants. Depression is thought to occur when levels of neurotransmitters, such as norepinephrine and serotonin, are reduced at postsynaptic receptor sites. These neurotransmitters affect a wide array of functions, including mood, obsessions, appetite, and anxiety. Antidepressants work by increasing the availability of these neurotransmitters at postsynaptic membranes and by enhancing and prolonging their effects. As a result, these agents improve mood, reduce anxiety, and minimize obsessions.

Antidepressants typically are classified as tricyclic antidepressants (TCAs), monoamine oxidase inhibitors (not shown), selective serotonin reuptake inhibitors (SSRIs), and atypical antidepressants (not shown). TCAs, such as amitriptyline and desipramine, primarily block norepinephrine reuptake at presynaptic membranes, thereby increasing the norepinephrine concentration at synapses and making more available at postsynaptic receptors.

SSRIs, such as fluoxetine and paroxetine, selectively inhibit serotonin uptake at presynaptic membranes. This action leads to increased serotonin availability at postsynaptic receptors. (From Gutierrez K: *Pharmacotherapeutics: Clinical Decision Making in Nursing,* ed 2, Philadelphia, 2008, Saunders.)

Fig. G-3 Mechanisms of Action: Antidiabetic Agents. Diabetes mellitus takes two forms: type 1 diabetes characterized by a complete lack of insulin and type 2 diabetes marked by insufficient insulin secretion, insulin resistance in peripheral tissues, or both. Normally, the beta cells in the pancreatic islets of Langerhans are responsible for secreting insulin. The rise of glucose levels in the beta cell triggers adenosine triphosphate (ATP)-dependent potassium (K^+) channels in the membranes of beta cells to close. Then the beta cells depolarize and calcium (Ca^{++}) enters the cell through Ca^{++} channel, and insulin is released from the cell. When circulating insulin engages with insulin receptors on cell membranes, it facilitates the movement of glucose into the cell, among other actions.

Type 1 diabetes is treated with the use of exogenous insulin, which mimics natural insulin in the body. Insulin takes many forms with varying degrees of onset, peak, and duration, including rapid, regular, intermediate, and long acting.

Type 2 diabetes is usually treated with oral agents. Sulfonylureas, such as glyburide, block ATP-dependent K^+ channels in the cell membranes of beta cells, ultimately resulting in the release of insulin. (From Taylor: *Mosby's Crash Course Pharmacology,* St. Louis, 1998, Mosby.)

Fig. G-4 Sites and Mechanisms of Action: Antifungal Agents. Antifungal agents primarily affect fungi at one of two sites: the cell membrane or the cell nucleus. Most of these agents, such as polyene, imidazole, and allylamine antifungals, act on the fungal cell membrane. Polyene antifungals, such as amphotericin B, bind to ergosterol and increase cell membrane permeability. Imidazole antifungals, such as fluconazole and ketoconazole, interfere with ergosterol synthesis by inhibiting the cytochrome P_{450} enzyme system, altering the cell membrane, and inhibiting fungal growth. Allylamine antifungals, such as terbinafine, inhibit the enzyme squaline epoxidase, which disrupts ergosterol production—and cell membrane integrity. When cell membrane permeability increases, cellular components, including potassium (K^+) and magnesium (Mg^{++}), leak out. Loss of these cellular components leads to cell death.

Another antifungal agent, griseofulvin, directly affects the fungal nucleus, interfering with mitosis. By binding to structures in the mitotic spindle, it prevents cells from dividing, which eventually leads to their death. (From Gutierrez K: *Pharmacotherapeutics: Clinical Decision Making in Nursing,* ed 2, Philadelphia, 2008, Saunders.)

Fig. G-5 Sites and Mechanisms of Action: Antiinfective Agents. The goal of antiinfective therapy is to kill or inhibit the growth of microorganisms such as bacteria, viruses, and fungi. To achieve this goal, antiinfective agents must reach their targets, which usually occurs through absorption and distribution by the circulatory system. When the target is reached, a drug can kill or suppress microorganisms by:

• Inhibiting cell wall synthesis or activating enzymes that disrupt the cell wall, which leads to cellular weakening, lysis, and death. Penicillins (ampicillin), cephalosporins (cefazolin), carbapenems (imipenem), monobactams (aztreonam), and tricyclic glycopeptides (vancomycin) act in this way.

• Altering cell membrane permeability through direct action on the cell wall, which allows intracellular substances to leak out and destabilizes the cell. Polyene antifungals (amphotericin) work by this mechanism.

• Altering protein synthesis by binding to bacterial ribosomes (50/30) or affecting ribosomal function, which leads to cell death or slowed growth respectively. Aminoglycosides (gentamicin), macrolides (erythromycin), tetracyclines (doxycycline), lincosamides (clindamycin), and the miscellaneous antiinfective chloramphenicol use this action.

• Inhibiting DNA or RNA, including messenger RNA (mRNA), synthesis by binding to nucleic acids or interacting with enzymes required for their synthesis. Antitubercular agents (rifampin), nitroimidazoles (metronidazole), antiviral agents (acyclovir), antiretroviral agents (stavudine), and quinolones (ciprofloxacin) act like this.

• Inhibiting the metabolism of folic acid and folinic acid or other cellular components that are essential for bacterial cell growth. The miscellaneous antiinfective trimethoprim employs this mechanism of action. (From Page C et al: *Integrated Pharmacology,* ed 3, St. Louis, 2006, Mosby.)

Fig. G-6 Mechanisms and Sites of Action: Antiretroviral Agents. When viruses reproduce, the infectious viral particle, or virion **(A)**, enters the host cell. The virion attaches to the cell's surface and then inserts itself into the host cell **(B)**. Once inside, the virion uncoats, and the enzyme reverse transcriptase makes two copies of the viral RNA: one copy is identical; the other is a mirror image. These two copies form double-stranded viral DNA that enters the host cell's nucleus, where it inserts itself into the host cell's DNA with the help of the enzyme integrase. Then viral DNA reprograms the host cell to produce additional viral RNA, which begins the process of forming new viruses. Specifically, messenger RNA (mRNA) instructs ribosomal RNA (rRNA) to produce a new chain of proteins and enzymes that are used to form new viruses. Protease cuts the chains, creating individual proteins. These combine with new RNA to create new virions, which bud and are released from the host cell **(C)**.

Antiretroviral agents target specific enzymes during viral reproduction. Nucleoside reverse transcriptase inhibitors, such as stavudine, interfere with the action of reverse transcriptase by mimicking naturally occurring nucleosides. Nucleotide reverse transcriptase inhibitors, such as tenofovir, block reverse transcriptase by competing with the natural substrate deoxyadenosine triphosphate and by causing DNA chain termination. Nonnucleoside reverse transcriptase inhibitors, such as delavirdine, work by directly binding to reverse transcriptase. As a result, no viral DNA is available to insert itself into the host cell's DNA. Protease inhibitors, such as indinavir, bind to and interfere with the action of protease; thus, the new chain of proteins formed by rRNA cannot be cut into individual proteins to make new viruses. (From Gutierrez K: *Pharmacotherapeutics: Clinical Decision Making in Nursing,* ed 2, Philadelphia, 2008, Saunders.)

Fig. G-7 Mechanisms of Action: Benzodiazepines. Benzodiazepines reduce anxiety by stimulating the action of the inhibitory neurotransmitter, gamma-aminobutyric acid (GABA), in the limbic system. The limbic system plays an important role in the regulation of human behavior. Dysfunction of GABA neurotransmission in the limbic system may be linked to the development of certain anxiety disorders.

The limbic system contains a highly dense area of benzodiazepine receptors that may be linked to the antianxiety effects of benzodiazepines. These benzodiazepine receptors are located on the surface of neuronal cell membranes and are adjacent to GABA receptors. The binding of a benzodiazepine to its receptor enhances the affinity of a GABA receptor for GABA. In the absence of a benzodiazepine, the binding of GABA to its receptor causes the chloride channel in the cell membrane to open, which increases the influx of chloride into the cell. This influx of chloride results in hyperpolarization of the neuronal cell membrane and reduces the neuron's ability to fire, which is why GABA is considered an inhibitory neurotransmitter.

A benzodiazepine acts only in the presence of GABA. When it binds to a benzodiazepine receptor, it prolongs the time that the chloride channel remains open. This results in greater depression of neuronal function and a reduction in anxiety. (From Gutierrez K: *Pharmacotherapeutics: Clinical Decision Making in Nursing,* ed 2, Philadelphia, 2008, Saunders.)

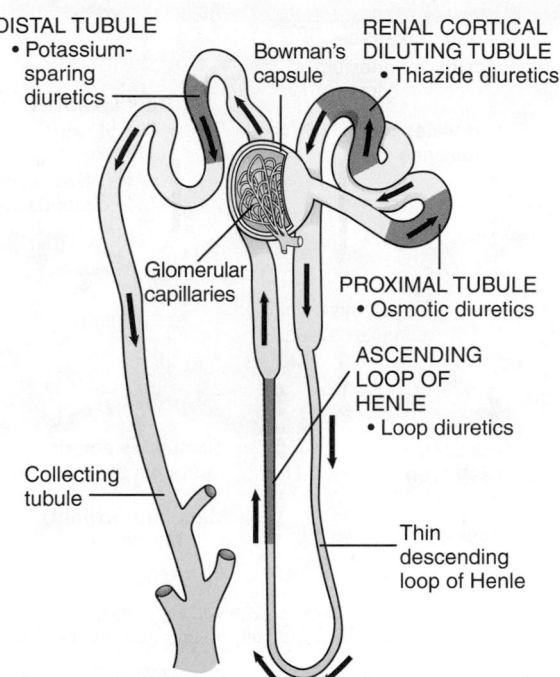

Fig. G-8 Sites of Action: Diuretics. Diuretics act primarily to increase water and sodium excretion by the kidneys, thereby increasing urine output. In the process, chloride, potassium, and other electrolytes may also be excreted. Most diuretics act by blocking sodium, water, and chloride reabsorption by peritubular capillaries in the nephrons. As a result, water and electrolytes remain in the convoluted tubules to be excreted as urine. The increased water and electrolyte excretion reduces blood volume—and ultimately blood pressure.

Diuretics belong to four major subclasses:

1. Thiazide diuretics, such as hydrochlorothiazide, act in the early portion of the distal convoluted tubule, called the cortical diluting segment. These drugs block sodium, chloride, and water reabsorption and promote their excretion along with potassium.

2. Loop diuretics, such as furosemide, act primarily in the thick ascending limb of the loop of Henle, blocking sodium, water, and chloride reabsorption. Then these substances are excreted along with potassium.

3. Potassium-sparing diuretics, such as spironolactone, act in the late portion of the distal convoluted tubule and collecting tubule. Here, they inhibit the action of aldosterone, leading to sodium excretion and potassium retention. Although triamterene and amiloride, two other potassium-sparing diuretics, act at the same site, they do not affect aldosterone. Instead, these drugs directly block the exchange of sodium and potassium, leading to decreased sodium reabsorption and decreased potassium excretion.

4. Osmotic diuretics, such as mannitol, work in the proximal convoluted tubule. As their name implies, these diuretics increase the osmotic pressure of the glomerular filtrate, inhibiting the passive reabsorption of water, sodium, and chloride. (From Gutierrez K: *Pharmacotherapeutics: Clinical Decision Making in Nursing,* ed 2, Philadelphia, 2008, Saunders.)

Fig. G-9 Mechanisms of Action: Laxatives. Laxatives ease or stimulate defecation. Typically, they are classified by their mechanism of action as bulk-forming, osmotic, stimulant, or surfactant laxatives.

Bulk-forming laxatives, such as psyllium, act in the small and large bowel. Because ingredients in these laxatives are undigestible, they remain within the stool and increase the fecal mass by drawing in water. These agents also enhance bacterial growth in the colon, further adding to the fecal mass.

Osmotic laxatives, such as lactulose, draw water into the intestinal lumen, causing the fecal mass to soften and swell. This osmotic action may be enhanced by the metabolism of colonic bacteria to lactate and other organic acids. These acids decrease colonic pH and increase colonic motility.

Stimulant (or irritant) laxatives, such as senna, act on the intestinal wall to increase water and electrolytes in the intestinal lumen. In addition, they directly irritate the colon, increasing motility.

Surfactant laxatives (or fecal softeners), such as docusate, reduce the surface tension of the stool, allowing water to enter it. These laxatives may also help to increase water and electrolyte excretion into the intestinal lumen, softening and increasing the fecal mass. (From Page C et al: *Integrated Pharmacology,* ed 3, St. Louis, 2006, Mosby.)

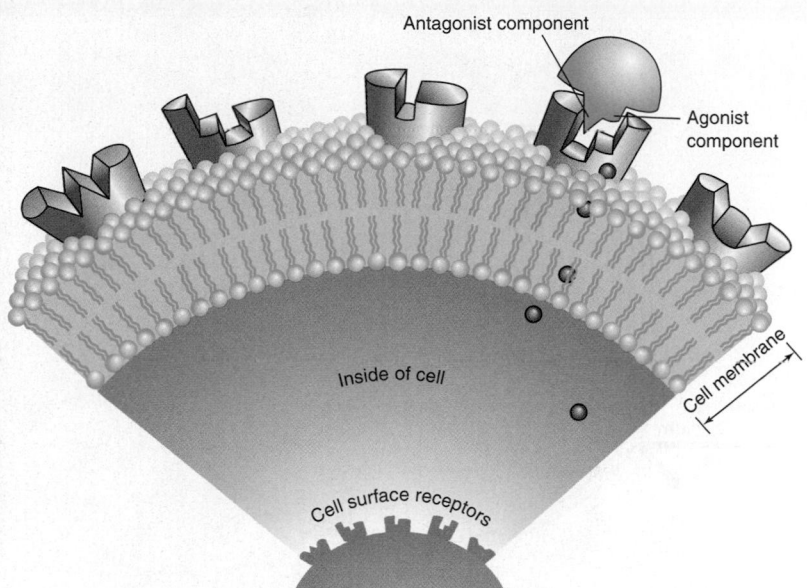

Fig. G-10 Mechanisms of Action: Narcotic Agonist-Antagonist Analgesics. Cell membranes have different types of opioid receptors, such as mu, kappa, and delta receptors. Opioid agonist-antagonists work by stimulating one type of receptor, while simultaneously blocking another type. As agonists, they work primarily by activating kappa receptors to produce analgesia and such other effects as CNS and respiratory depression, decreased GI motility, and euphoria. As antagonists, they compete with opioids at mu receptors, helping to reverse or block some of the other effects of agonists. (From Gutierrez K: *Pharmacotherapeutics: Clinical Decision Making in Nursing,* ed 2, Philadelphia, 2008, Saunders.)

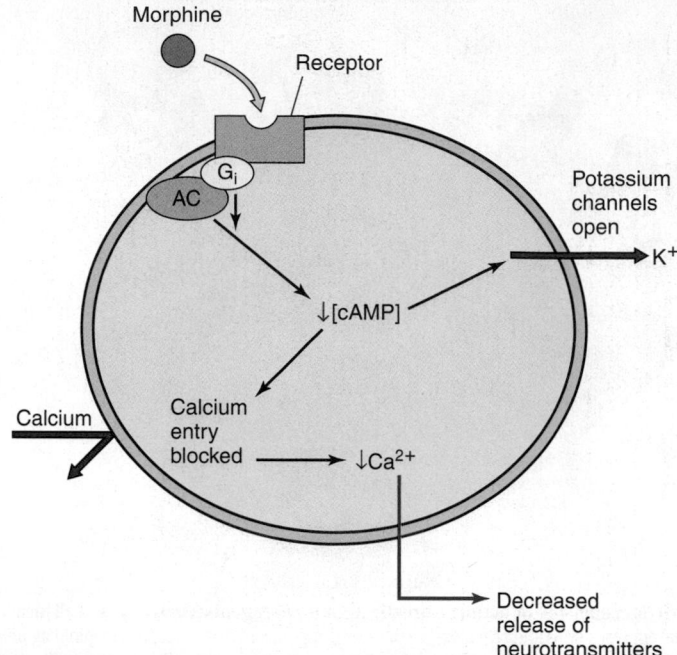

Fig. G-11 Mechanisms of Action: Narcotic Analgesics. Narcotic analgesics bind to three types of opioid receptors: mu, kappa, and delta receptors. They produce analgesia primarily by activating mu receptors. However, they also engage with and activate kappa and delta receptors, producing other effects, such as sedation and vasomotor stimulation.

When morphine or another narcotic analgesic binds to opioid receptors, activation occurs. The receptors send signals to the enzyme adenyl cyclase (AC) to slow activity by way of G proteins (G_i). Decreased adenyl cyclase activity causes reduced production of cyclic adenosine monophosphate (cAMP). A secondary messenger substance, cAMP is important for regulating cell membrane channels. A reduced cAMP level allows fewer potassium ions to leave the cell and blocks calcium ions from entering the cell. This ion imbalance—especially the reduced intracellular calcium level—ultimately decreases the release of neurotransmitters from the cell, thereby blocking or reducing pain impulse transmission. (From Minneman KP, Wecker L: *Brody's Human Pharmacology: Molecular to Clinical*, ed 4, St. Louis, 2005, Mosby.)

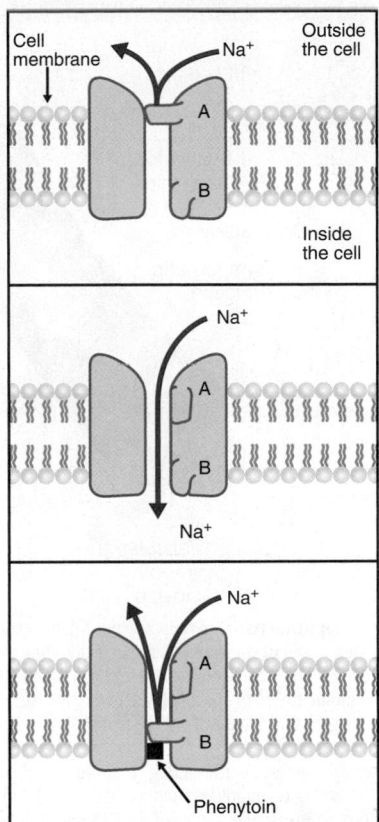

Fig. G-12 Mechanisms of Action: Phenytoin. Phenytoin, which is used to treat tonic-clonic seizures, acts in the motor cortex and brain stem, where the tonic phase of tonic-clonic seizures originates. By altering sodium transport across neuronal cell membranes, phenytoin stabilizes the cell membrane, reduces repetitive firing of the neurons, and halts or limits the spread of seizures. The first illustration shows a neuronal cell membrane in its resting state. The activation gate **(A)** of the sodium channel in the cell membrane is closed and blocks sodium (Na$^+$) from entering the cell. In the second illustration, a nerve impulse has caused depolarization and opening of the activation gate, allowing Na$^+$ to move into the cell. In the third illustration, depolarization continues and an inactivation gate **(B)** moves into the channel. This prevents Na$^+$ from moving into the cell. Phenytoin prolongs the inactivated state of the sodium channel by preventing reopening of the inactivation gate. By further preventing Na$^+$ from entering the cell, phenytoin slows impulse transmission, and thus slows the rate at which neurons fire. (From Minneman KP, Wecker L: *Brody's Human Pharmacology: Molecular to Clinical,* ed 4, St. Louis, 2005, Mosby.)

Fig. G-13 Sites of Action: Sympatholytics. Sympatholytics inhibit sympathetic nervous system (SNS) activity, which plays a major role in regulating B/P. Normally when the SNS is stimulated, nerve impulses travel from the cardiovascular center of the CNS to the sympathetic ganglia. From there, the impulses travel along postganglionic fibers to specific effector organs, such as the heart and blood vessels. SNS stimulation also triggers the release of norepinephrine, which acts primarily at alpha-adrenergic receptors.

Sympatholytics fall into two subclasses: central-acting α_2 agonists and peripheral-acting α_1-adrenergic antagonists. Central-acting α_2 agonists, such as methyldopa and clonidine, stimulate α_2-adrenergic receptors in the cardiovascular center of the CNS and reduce activity in the vasomotor center of the brain, interfering with sympathetic stimulation of the heart and blood vessels. This causes blood vessel dilatation and decreased cardiac output, which leads to reduced B/P.

Peripheral-acting α_1-adrenergic antagonists, such as prazosin, inhibit the stimulation of α_1-adrenergic receptors by norepinephrine in vascular smooth muscle, interfering with SNS-induced vasoconstriction. As a result, the blood vessels dilate, reducing peripheral vascular resistance and venous return to the heart. These effects, in turn, lead to decreased B/P. (From Prosser S, Worster B, Dewar K: *Applied Pharmacology for Nurses and Other Health Care Professionals,* St. Louis, 2000, Mosby.)

Appendix H

Photo Atlas of Drug Administration

Fig. H-2 Intradermal Injection. For an intradermal injection, note formation of small bleb approximately 6 mm ($^1/_4$ in) in diameter at injection site. (From Potter PA, Perry AG: *Fundamentals of Nursing,* ed 7, St. Louis, 2009, Mosby.)

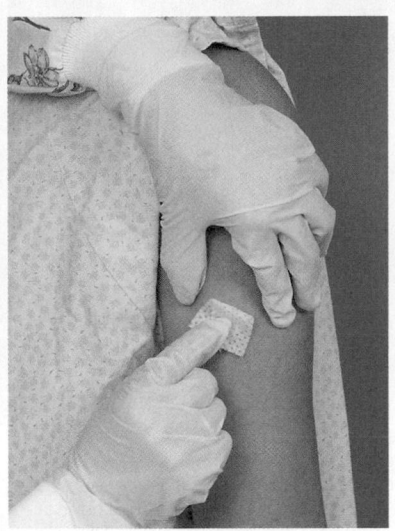

Fig. H-1 Administering an Injection. Cleanse site with antiseptic swab. Apply swab at center of site and rotate outward in circular direction for about 5 cm (2 in). (From Potter PA, Perry AG: *Fundamentals of Nursing,* ed 7, St. Louis, 2009, Mosby.)

Fig. H-3 Subcutaneous Injection. A, For a subcutaneous injection, hold the syringe between the thumb and forefinger of the dominant hand as a dart, with the palm down. **B,** After injecting the needle at a 45- to 90-degree angle, grasp lower end of syringe barrel with nondominant hand to end of plunger. Avoid moving syringe while slowly pulling back on plunger to aspirate drug. If blood appears in syringe, remove needle, discard medication and syringe, and repeat procedure. *Exception:* Do not aspirate when giving heparin. (From Potter PA, Perry AG: *Fundamentals of Nursing,* ed 7, St. Louis, 2009, Mosby.)

Fig. H-4 Subcutaneous Injection. A, Sites recommended for subcutaneous injections. **B,** Giving subcutaneous injection in the abdomen. (From Potter PA, Perry AG: *Fundamentals of Nursing,* ed 6, St.Louis, 2005, Mosby.)

Fig. H-5 Deltoid Intradermal Injection. A, Landmarks for IM injection into the deltoid muscle. **B,** Giving IM injection in deltoid muscle. (From Potter PA, Perry AG: *Fundamentals of Nursing,* ed 7, St. Louis, 2009, Mosby.)

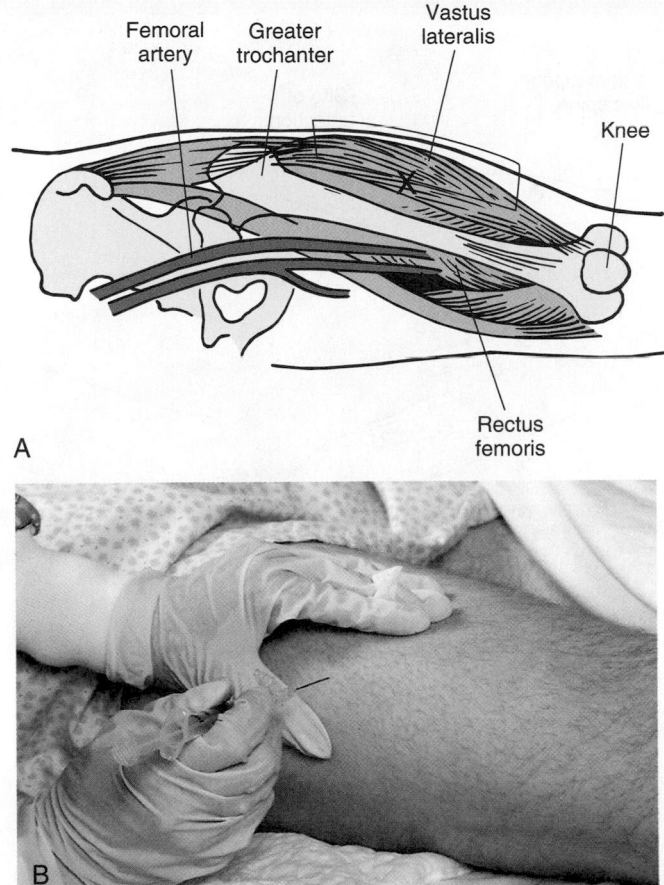

Fig. H-6 Vastus Lateralis Intramuscular Injection. A, Landmarks for IM injection in vastus lateralis. **B,** Giving IM injection in vastus lateralis site. (From Potter PA, Perry AG: *Fundamentals of Nursing,* ed 7, St. Louis, 2009, Mosby.)

Fig. H-7 Ventrogluteal Intramuscular Injection. A, Anatomical view of ventrogluteal site. **B,** Giving IM injection into ventrogluteal muscle to avoid major nerves and blood vessels. (From Potter PA, Perry AG: *Fundamentals of Nursing,* ed 7, St. Louis, 2009, Mosby.)

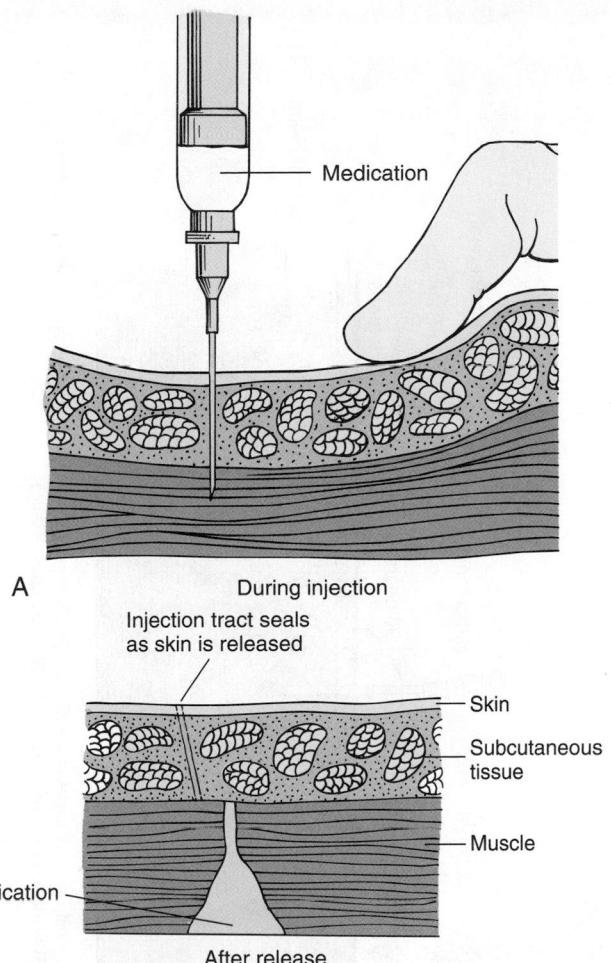

Fig. H-8 Z-Track Method of Injection. A, Pulling on overlying skin during IM injection moves tissues to prevent later tracking. **B,** The Z-track left after injection prevents the deposit of medication through sensitive tissue. (From Potter PA, Perry AG: *Fundamentals of Nursing,* ed 7, St. Louis, 2009, Mosby.)

Fig. H-9 Comparison of Needle Angles. Comparison of angles of insertion for IM (90 degrees), SUBCUT (45 degrees and 90 degrees), and ID (15 degrees) injections. (From Potter PA, Perry AG: *Fundamentals of Nursing*, ed 7, St. Louis, 2009, Mosby.)

Fig. H-10 Administering Medication by IV Bolus (push). A, Needle system: Insert small-gauge needle of syringe containing prepared drug through center of injection port. **B,**Needleless system: Remove cap of needleless injection port. Connect tip of syringe directly. (From Potter PA, Perry AG: *Fundamentals of Nursing,* ed 6, St. Louis, 2005, Mosby.)

Continued

Fig. H-10, cont'd C, Occlude **IV** line by pinching tubing just above injection port. Pull back gently on syringe's plunger to aspirate blood return. **D,** After noting blood return, continue to occlude tubing and inject medication slowly over several minutes (read directions on drug package). Use watch to time administration. **E, IV** lock: Insert needle of syringe containing prepared drug through center of diaphragm. (From Potter PA, Perry AG: *Fundamentals of Nursing,* ed 6, St. Louis, 2005, Mosby.)

Fig. H-11 Administering IV Medication by Piggyback, Volume Administration Sets of Miniinfusors (Syringe Pump). Use needle-lock device to secure needle of secondary piggyback line through injection port of main line. (From Potter PA, Perry AG: *Fundamentals of Nursing,* ed 6, St. Louis, 2005, Mosby.)

Index

Entries can be identified as follows: generic name, Trade Name, DRUG CATEGORY

Entries can be identified as follows: generic name, Trade Name, DRUG CATEGORY

Entries can be identified as follows: generic name, Trade Name, DRUG CATEGORY

Entries can be identified as follows: generic name, Trade Name, DRUG CATEGORY

Entries can be identified as follows: generic name, Trade Name, DRUG CATEGORY

Entries can be identified as follows: generic name, Trade Name, DRUG CATEGORY

Entries can be identified as follows: generic name, Trade Name, DRUG CATEGORY

- Does the patient have any allergies?
- Is the patient NPO?
- Is the patient taking any other medication and/or herbal supplements that may interact with this drug?
- Are there any vital signs that I need to check before administering the drug?
- Do I need to check any lab values (i.e., glucose)?
- Are there any other assessments that I need to make before giving this drug?

The 5 rights of medication administration

Always adhere to the 5 rights of medication administration when transcribing, preparing, administering, and documenting medications:

1. **Right patient:** Compare the patient's armband with the medication administration record. Compare the patient's name on the medication administration record (MAR) with that on the medication drawer or computerized equipment.
2. **Right drug:** Verify the correct medication by comparing the name on the label on the drug container with that written on the MAR.
3. **Right route:** Check the ordered route by reading the medication order, and verify the appropriateness of the route based on knowledge of the patient's condition.
4. **Right dose:** Always independently double-check dosages of medications with the pharmacy's calculations or with a second nurse. The nurse must also be aware of therapeutic dosages for each medication and question an order that is not within that range.
5. **Right time:** All medications should be administered within 30 minutes of the scheduled time. The medications must also be prepared to correlate appropriately with meal times and to avoid drug interactions.

Following appropriate drug administration, assess the patient for the expected therapeutic outcome and/or potential side effects.

Nomogram for Calculation of Body Surface Area

Place a straight edge from the patient's height in the left column to his or her weight in the right column. The point of intersection on the body surface area column indicates the body surface area (BSA). (Reproduced in Behrman RE, Kliegman RM, Jenson HB: *Nelson Textbook of Pediatrics*, ed 18, Philadelphia, 2007, WB Saunders; nomogram modified from data of E. Boyd by CD West.)

Alternative (Mosteller's formula):

Surface area (m²) $= \sqrt{\dfrac{\text{Height (cm)} \times \text{Weight (kg)}}{3600}}$

Surface area rule:

Child dose $= \dfrac{\text{Surface area (m}^2) \times \text{Adult dose}}{1.73 \text{ m}^2}$

BMI formula:

BMI $= \dfrac{\text{Weight (kg)}}{\text{Height (m}^2)}$

Syringe Compatibility

	Atropine	Buprenorphine	Butorphanol	ChlorproMAZINE	Codeine	Diazepam	DimenhyDRINATE	DiphenhydrAMINE	Droperidol	Fentanyl	Glycopyrrolate	Heparin
Atropine			C	C		I	C	C	C	C	C	
Buprenorphine												
Butorphanol	C			C		I	I	C	C	C		
ChlorproMAZINE	C		C			I	I	C	C	C	C	C
Codeine						I						
Diazepam	I		I	I	I		I	I	I	I	I	
DimenhyDRINATE	C		I	I		I		C	C	C	I	
DiphenhydrAMINE	C		C	C		I	C		C	C	C	
Droperidol	C		C	C		I	C	C		C	C	I
Fentanyl	C		C	C		I	C	C	C		C	
Glycopyrrolate	C			C		I	I	C	C	C		
Heparin			I	C	I				I			
HydrOXYzine	C		C	C		I	I	C	C	C	C	
Meperidine	C		C	C		I	C	C	C	C	C	I
Metoclopramide	C		C	C		I	C	C	C	C		
Midazolam	C		C	C		I	C	C	C	C		
Morphine	C		C	C		I	C	C	C	C	C	I
Nalbuphine	C					I			C			
Pentazocine	C		C	C		I	C	C	C	C	I	I
Pentobarbital	C		I	I	I	I	I	I	I	I	I	
Perphenazine	C		C	C		I	C	C	C	C		
Prochlorperazine	C		C	C		I	I	C	C	C	C	
Promazine	C			C		I	I	C	C	C	C	
Promethazine	C		C	C		I	I	C	C	C	C	
Ranitidine	C			C			C	C		C	C	
Scopolamine Hbr	C		C	C		I	C	C	C	C	C	
Secobarbital	I		I	I	I	I	I	I	I	I	I	
Thiethylperazine			C			I						

Developed by Providence Memorial Hospital, El Paso, Texas.
NOTE: Give within 15 minutes of mixing.
C = compatible; I = incompatible; □ = no documented information.
* = compatibility depends on manufacturer, Wyeth and DuPont forms are incompatible.